GREEN'S
OPERATIVE
HAND
SURGERY

FIFTH EDITION

VOLUME TWO

GREEN'S OPERATIVE HAND SURGERY

FIFTH EDITION

VOLUME TWO

David P. Green, MD
Clinical Professor
Department of Orthopaedics
The University of Texas Health Science
  Center at San Antonio
Founding President
The Hand Center of San Antonio
San Antonio, Texas

Robert N. Hotchkiss, MD
Associate Attending Orthopedic
  Surgeon
Hospital for Special Surgery
Director
Alberto Vilar Center for Research of the
  Hand and Upper Extremity
New York, New York

William C. Pederson, MD
Clinical Associate Professor of Surgery
  and Orthopaedic Surgery
The University of Texas Health Science
  Center at San Antonio
Director of Fellowship Training
The Hand Center of San Antonio
San Antonio, Texas

Scott W. Wolfe, MD
Professor of Orthopedic Surgery
Weill Medical College of Cornell
  University
Chief, Hand and Upper Extremity
  Surgery
Attending Orthopedic Surgeon
Hospital for Special Surgery
New York, New York

Illustrator:
Elizabeth Roselius, MS, FAMI

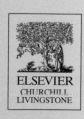

ELSEVIER
CHURCHILL
LIVINGSTONE

ELSEVIER
CHURCHILL
LIVINGSTONE

The Curtis Center
170 S Independence Mall W 300E
Philadelphia, Pennsylvania 19106

GREEN'S OPERATIVE HAND SURGERY   ISBN 0-443-06626-4
Copyright © 2005, 1999, 1993, 1988, 1982 by Elsevier Inc.

VOL 1: P/N 996002403
VOL 2: P/N 996002462

NOTICE

Orthopaedic surgery is an ever-changing field. Standard safety precautions must be followed, but as new research and clinical experience broaden our knowledge, changes in treatment and drug therapy may become necessary or appropriate. Readers are advised to check the most current product information provided by the manufacturer of each drug to be administered to verify the recommended dose, the method and duration of administration, and contraindications. It is the responsibility of the licensed prescriber, relying on experience and knowledge of the patient, to determine dosages and the best treatment for each individual patient. Neither the publisher nor the author assumes any liability for any injury and/or damage to persons or property arising from this publication.

International Standard Book Number 0-443-06626-4

Acquisitions Editor: Daniel Pepper
Developmental Editor: Arlene Chappelle
Publishing Services Manager: Tina Rebane
Design Manager: Gene Harris

Printed in the United States of America.

Last digit is the print number: 9   8   7   6   5   4   3   2   1

CONTRIBUTORS

Brian D. Adams, MD
Professor, Orthopaedic Surgery and Biomedical Engineering, University of Iowa, Iowa City, Iowa
Distal Radioulnar Joint Instability

David W. Altchek, MD
Associate Professor of Clinical Surgery, Weill Medical College of Cornell University; Associate Attending Orthopedic Surgeon, Hospital for Special Surgery, New York, New York
Arthroscopy and the Thrower's Elbow

Peter C. Amadio, MD
Professor of Orthopedics, Mayo Clinic College of Medicine; Consultant, Department of Orthopedic Surgery and Surgery of the Hand, Mayo Clinic, Rochester, Minnesota
Stiff Finger Joints; Fractures of the Carpal Bones

Dimitri J. Anastakis, MD, MEd, FRCS, FACS
Associate Professor, Divisions of Plastic and Orthopaedic Surgery, Department of Surgery, University of Toronto; Associate Director, Surgical Services, University Health Network, Toronto Western Hospital, Toronto, Ontario, Canada
Free Functioning Muscle Transfers

Douglas M. Anderson, MD
Department of Veterans Affairs, Audie L. Murphy Memorial Veterans Hospital Division, San Antonio, Texas
Anesthesia

George A. Anderson, MBBS, MS Orth, D Orth, MNAMS Orth, MCh Orth (Liverpool), FAMS-PNS (Vienna), FACS Orth
Professor of Orthopaedic Surgery, Head of Dr. Paul Brand Department of Hand Surgery and Leprosy Reconstructive Surgery, and Course Director, Hand Therapy and Leprosy Physiotherapy, Christian Medical College Hospital, Vellore, Tamil Nadu, India
Ulnar Nerve Palsy

Edward A. Athanasian, MD
Associate Professor of Clinical Orthopedic Surgery, Weill Medical College of Cornell University; Associate Attending Orthopedic Surgeon, Hospital for Special Surgery, and Assistant Attending Surgeon, Memorial Sloan-Kettering Cancer Center, New York, New York
Bone and Soft Tissue Tumors

Mark E. Baratz, MD
Vice Chairman, Research and Educational Program, and Director, Division of Hand and Upper Extremities, Department of Orthopaedic Surgery, Allegheny General Hospital; Allegheny Orthopaedic Associates, Pittsburgh, Pennsylvania
Extensor Tendon Injuries

David P. Barei, MD, FRCS(C)
Assistant Professor of Orthopaedics and Sports Medicine, University of Washington School of Medicine, Harborview Medical Center, Seattle, Washington
Fractures of the Distal Humerus

O. Alton Barron, MD
Assistant Clinical Professor of Orthopaedic Surgery, Columbia College of Physicians and Surgeons; Senior Attending Hand Surgeon, C. V. Starr Hand Surgery Center, St. Luke's–Roosevelt Hospital Center, New York, New York
Dislocations and Ligament Injuries in the Digits

Michael S. Bednar, MD
Associate Professor, Department of Orthopaedic Surgery and Rehabilitation, Loyola University Health System, Maywood, Illinois
Congenital Deformities of the Wrist and Forearm

Rolfe Birch, MChir, FRCS
Professor in Neurological Orthopaedic Surgery, University College London; Visiting Professor, Department of Academic Neurology, Imperial College, London; Honorary Consultant Surgeon, Hospital for Sick Children, London, National Hospital for Neurology and Neurosurgery, London, Raigmore Hospital, Inverness, and Birmingham Children's Hospital; Honorary Surgeon to the Royal Navy; Peripheral Nerve Injury Unit, Royal National Orthopaedic Hospital, Middlesex, United Kingdom
Nerve Repair

Allen T. Bishop, MD
Professor of Orthopedic Surgery, Mayo Clinic College of Medicine; Consultant, Department of Orthopedic Surgery, and Chair, Division of Hand Surgery, Mayo Clinic, Rochester, Minnesota
Vascularized Bone Grafting

Martin I. Boyer, MD, MSc, FRCS(C)
Associate Professor, Department of Orthopaedic
Surgery, Chief, Orthopaedic Hand Surgery Service, and
Coordinator, Third and Fourth Year Orthopaedic
Surgery Rotations, Washington University School of
Medicine at Barnes-Jewish Hospital, St. Louis, Missouri
Flexor Tendon Injury (Acute Injuries)

Richard E. Brown, MD, FACS
Clinical Professor, Division of Plastic Surgery, Southern
Illinois University; The Center for Plastic Surgery,
Springfield Clinic, Springfield, Illinois
The Perionychium

Earl Z. Browne, Jr., MD
Section Head, Microsurgery, Department of Plastic
Surgery, The Cleveland Clinic, Cleveland, Ohio
Skin Grafts and Skin Flaps (Skin Grafting)

Michelle Gerwin Carlson, MD
Assistant Professor of Surgery (Orthopedics), Weill
Medical College of Cornell University; Assistant
Attending Orthopedic Surgeon, Hospital for Special
Surgery, New York, New York
Cerebral Palsy

Louis W. Catalano III, MD
Clinical Instructor, Department of Orthopaedic Surgery,
Columbia College of Physicians and Surgeons;
Attending Hand Surgeon, C. V. Starr Hand Surgery
Center, St. Luke's–Roosevelt Hospital Center,
New York, New York
Dislocations and Ligament Injuries in the Digits

Kevin C. Chung, MD, MS, FACS
Associate Professor of Surgery, Section of Plastic
Surgery, Department of Surgery, The University of
Michigan Hand Center, Ann Arbor, Michigan
Skin Tumors

Mark S. Cohen, MD
Professor, Director, Hand and Elbow Section, and
Director, Orthopaedic Education, Department of
Orthopaedic Surgery, Rush University Medical Center,
Chicago, Illinois
Total Elbow Arthroplasty

Struan H. Coleman, MD, PhD
Instructor in Orthopedics, Weill Medical College of
Cornell University; Sports Medicine and Shoulder
Service, Hospital for Special Surgery, New York,
New York
Arthroscopy and the Thrower's Elbow

Randall W. Culp, MD
Associate Professor of Orthopedic, Hand and
Microsurgery, Thomas Jefferson University,
Philadelphia; The Philadelphia Hand Center, P.C.,
King of Prussia, Pennsylvania
Wrist Arthroscopy: Operative Procedures

Timothy R. C. Davis, FRCS, ChM
Special Professor in Trauma and Orthopaedic Surgery,
Nottingham University; Consultant Hand Surgeon,
Queens Medical Centre, Nottingham, United Kingdom
Median Nerve Palsy

Kazuteru Doi, MD, PhD
Clinical Professor, Department of Orthopedic Surgery,
Yamaguchi University School of Medicine, Ube,
Yamaguchi; President, Ogori Daiichi General Hospital,
and Director, Department of Orthopedic Surgery, Ogori
Daiichi General Hospital, Ogori, Yamaguchi, Japan
Traumatic Brachial Plexus Injury

Marybeth Ezaki, MD
Associate Professor of Orthopaedic Surgery, University
of Texas Southwestern Medical Center; Director, Hand
and Upper Extremity Service, Texas Scottish Rite
Hospital for Children, Dallas, Texas
Congenital Contracture

Paul Feldon, MD
Associate Clinical Professor of Orthopaedic Surgery,
Tufts University School of Medicine; Hand Surgical
Associates, Boston, Massachusetts
*Rheumatoid Arthritis and Other Connective Tissue
Diseases*

Diego L. Fernandez, MD
Professor of Orthopaedic Surgery, University of Bern;
Department of Orthopaedic Surgery, Lindenhof
Hospital, Bern, Switzerland
Distal Radius Fractures

Guy Foucher, MD
Professor, Trauma Department, University of Las
Palmas, Gran Canaria, Spain
Vascularized Joint Transfers

Marc Garcia-Elias, MD, PhD
Consultant, Hand Surgery, Institut Kaplan, Barcelona,
Spain
Carpal Instability

William B. Geissler, MD
Professor, Division of Hand and Upper Extremity
Surgery; Chief, Arthroscopic Surgery and Sports
Medicine; Director, Hand and Upper Extremity
Fellowship; Team Consultant, Ole Miss, Department of
Orthopaedic Surgery and Rehabilitation, University of
Mississippi Medical Center, Jackson, Mississippi
Carpal Instability

Günter Germann, MD, PhD
Chairman, Department of Hand, Plastic, and
Reconstructive Surgery, BG-Trauma
Center–Ludwigshafen; Plastic and Hand Surgery,
The University of Heidelberg, Ludwigshafen, Germany
The Burned Hand

Steven Z. Glickel, MD
Associate Clinical Professor of Orthopaedic Surgery,
Columbia College of Physicians and Surgeons;
Director, C. V. Starr Hand Surgery Center, St.
Luke's–Roosevelt Hospital Center, New York,
New York
Dislocations and Ligament Injuries in the Digits

Richard D. Goldner, MD
Associate Professor, Department of Orthopaedic
Surgery, Duke University Medical Center, Durham,
North Carolina
Replantation

David P. Green, MD
Clinical Professor, Department of Orthopaedics,
University of Texas Health Science Center at San
Antonio; Founding President, The Hand Center of San
Antonio, San Antonio, Texas
General Principles; Radial Nerve Palsy

John R. Griffin, MD
Division of Plastic Surgery, Surgery of the Hand,
Children's Hospital of Oakland, Oakland, California
Congenital Contracture

Ayan Gulgonen, MD
Istanbul, Turkey
Compartment Syndrome

Douglas P. Hanel, MD
Professor of Orthopaedics and Adjunct Professor of
Plastic Surgery, University of Washington; Department
of Orthopaedics and Sports Medicine, Harborview
Medical Center, Seattle, Washington
*Fractures of the Distal Humerus; The Mangled Upper
Extremity*

Hill Hastings II, MD
Clinical Professor of Orthopaedic Surgery, Indiana
University Medical Center; Hand and Upper Extremity
Surgeon, The Indiana Hand Center, Indianapolis,
Indiana
Wrist Arthrodesis (Partial and Complete)

Vincent R. Hentz, MD
Professor of Surgery, Robert A. Chase Center for Hand
and Upper Limb Surgery, Stanford University School of
Medicine, Palo Alto, California
Traumatic Brachial Plexus Injury

Robert N. Hotchkiss, MD
Associate Attending Orthopedic Surgeon, Hospital for
Special Surgery; Director, Alberto Vilar Center for
Research of the Hand and Upper Extremity, New York,
New York
*Complex Traumatic Elbow Dislocation; Treatment of the
Stiff Elbow*

Thomas B. Hughes, MD
Drexel University College of Medicine, Department of
Orthopaedic Surgery, Allegheny General Hospital,
Pittsburgh, Pennsylvania
Extensor Tendon Injuries

Michelle A. James, MD
Assistant Chief of Orthopaedic Surgery, Shriners
Hospital for Children, Northern California,
Sacramento, California
Congenital Deformities of the Wrist and Forearm

Peter J. L. Jebson, MD
Associate Professor and Chief, Division of Elbow, Hand
and Microsurgery, Department of Orthopaedic Surgery,
University of Michigan Health System, Ann Arbor,
Michigan
Amputations

Karen Johnston Jones, MD
Associate Clinical Professor, Department of
Orthopaedic Surgery, The University of Texas Health
Science Center at San Antonio; Hand Surgeon, The
Hand Center of San Antonio, San Antonio, Texas
Thoracic Outlet Compression Syndrome

Neil F. Jones, MD, FRCS
Professor, Department of Orthopedic Surgery, Division
of Plastic and Reconstructive Surgery, University of
California, Los Angeles, School of Medicine; Chief of
Hand Surgery, UCLA Medical Center, Los Angeles,
California
Free Skin and Composite Flaps

Jesse B. Jupiter, MD
The Hansjorg Wyss/AO Professor of Orthopaedic
Surgery, Harvard Medical School; Chief, Hand and
Upper Extremity Service, Department of Orthopaedic
Surgery, Massachusetts General Hospital, Boston,
Massachusetts
Fractures of the Proximal Ulna

Morton L. Kasdan, MD, FACS
Clinical Professor of Plastic Surgery, University of
Louisville, Louisville, Kentucky
Factitious Disorders

Leonid I. Katolik, MD
Assistant Professor, Department of Orthopaedics and
Sports Medicine, University of Washington School of
Medicine; Section of Hand, Upper Extremity, and
Microvascular Surgery, Harborview Medical Center,
Seattle, Washington
Total Elbow Arthroplasty

Robert A. Kaufmann, MD
Assistant Professor, Hand and Upper Extremity Surgery,
University of Pittsburgh School of Medicine, Pittsburgh,
Pennsylvania
*Flexor Tendon Injury (Flexor Tendon Reconstruction);
Wrist Arthroscopy: Operative Procedures*

Simon P. Kay, FRCS
Professor of Hand Surgery, University of Leeds;
Consultant, Plastic and Hand Surgery, Department of
Plastic Surgery, St. James's University Hospital, Leeds,
United Kingdom
*Congenital Deformities of the Hand and Fingers;
Congenital Contracture*

Mary Ann E. Keenan, MD
Professor of Orthopaedic Surgery, University of
Pennsylvania School of Medicine; Chief, Neuro-
Orthopaedics Service, Hospital of the University of
Pennsylvania, Philadelphia, Pennsylvania
Upper Extremity Dysfunction After Stroke or Brain Injury

Graham J. W. King, MD, MSc, FRCS(C)
Professor, Division of Orthopaedic Surgery, University
of Western Ontario; Hand and Upper Limb Centre,
St. Joseph's Health Centre, London, Ontario, Canada
Fractures of the Head of the Radius

John King, MD
Lakelands Orthopaedic Clinic, Greenwood, South Carolina
Thumb Basal Joint Arthritis

L. Andrew Koman, MD
Vice Chair and Professor, Department of Orthopaedic
Surgery, and Professor, Department of Pediatrics, Wake
Forest University School of Medicine, Wake Forest
University Baptist Medical Center, Winston-Salem,
North Carolina
Complex Regional Pain Syndrome; Vascular Disorders

Scott H. Kozin, MD
Assistant Professor, Department of Orthopaedic
Surgery, Temple University School of Medicine;
Director of Hand Surgery, Shriners Hospital for
Children, Philadelphia, Pennsylvania
*Editor of the Congenital Section; Embryology; Deformities
of the Hand and Fingers; Deformities of the Thumb;
Congenital Contracture*

W. P. Andrew Lee, MD
Professor of Surgery and Chief, Division of Plastic
Surgery, University of Pittsburgh School of Medicine,
Pittsburgh, Pennsylvania
Thumb Reconstruction

Michel Leit, MD, MS
Fellow, Department of Orthopaedics, University of
Rochester Medical Center, Rochester, New York
Thumb Basal Joint Arthritis

Graham D. Lister, MB, ChB
Formerly Professor, Department of Surgery, University
of Utah School of Medicine; Formerly Chief, Division
of Plastic and Reconstructive Surgery, University of
Utah Medical Center, Salt Lake City, Utah
*Skin Grafts and Skin Flaps (Skin Flaps); Free Skin and
Composite Flaps*

Dean S. Louis, MD
Active Professor Emeritus, Department of Orthopaedic
Surgery, University of Michigan Health System,
Ann Arbor, Michigan
Amputations; Factitious Disorders

Susan E. Mackinnon, MD, FRCS(C), FACS
Shoenberg Professor of Surgery, and Chief, Division of
Plastic and Reconstructive Surgery, Washington
University School of Medicine, St. Louis, Missouri
Compression Neuropathies

Govind Narain Malaviya, MB, MS, MSc, FICS, DHRM
Deputy Director and Head, Plastic and Reconstructive
Surgery Unit, Central JALMA Institute for Leprosy,
Taj Ganj, Agra, India
Chronic Infections

Ralph T. Manktelow, MD, FRCS(C)
Professor, Division of Plastic Surgery, Department of
Surgery, University of Toronto, Toronto General
Hospital, Toronto, Ontario, Canada
Free Functioning Muscle Transfers

David McCombe, MB, BS, FRACS
Department of Surgery, University of Melbourne;
Department of Orthopaedic Surgery, St. Vincent's
Hospital, Melbourne, Australia
Congenital Deformities of the Hand and Fingers

Duncan Angus McGrouther, MBChB, FRCS, MSc, MD
Professor, Plastic and Reconstructive Surgery Research,
The University of Manchester, Manchester, United
Kingdom
Dupuytren's Contracture

Lewis H. Millender, MD*
Formerly Clinic Professor, Department of Orthopedic
Surgery, Tufts University School of Medicine;
Formerly Assistant Chief, Hand Surgery Service,
New England Baptist Hospital, Boston,
Massachusetts
*Rheumatoid Arthritis and Other Connective Tissue
Diseases*

Steven L. Moran, MD
Assistant Professor of Plastic Surgery, Mayo Clinic
College of Medicine, Rochester, Minnesota
Fractures of the Carpal Bones

Edward A. Nalebuff, MD
Clinical Professor of Orthopaedics, Tufts University
School of Medicine; Chief, Hand Surgery Service,
New England Baptist Hospital, Boston,
Massachusetts
*Rheumatoid Arthritis and Other Connective Tissue
Diseases*

Christine B. Novak, PT, MS
Research Associate Professor, Division of Plastic and
Reconstructive Surgery, Washington University School
of Medicine, St. Louis, Missouri
Compression Neuropathies

Shawn W. O'Driscoll, MD, PhD, FRCS(C)
Professor of Orthopedics, Mayo Clinic College of
Medicine; Consultant, Department of Orthopedics,
Mayo Clinic, Rochester, Minnesota
Recurrent Instability of the Elbow

---

*Deceased

A. Lee Osterman, MD
Professor of Orthopedic and Hand Surgery, Jefferson Medical College of Thomas Jefferson University, Philadelphia; Director, The Philadelphia Hand Center, P.C., King of Prussia, Pennsylvania
Wrist Arthroscopy: Operative Procedures

Mukund R. Patel, MD, FACS
Clinical Associate Professor of Orthopedic Surgery, Downstate Medical Center, State University of New York, Brooklyn; Chief of Hand Surgery, Victory Memorial Hospital, Brooklyn; Senior Attending Hand Surgeon, Maimonides Medical Center, Brooklyn; Staten Island University Hospital, St. Vincent's Catholic Medical Center, Staten Island, New York
Chronic Infections

William C. Pederson, MD
Clinical Associate Professor of Surgery and Orthopaedic Surgery, The University of Texas Health Science Center at San Antonio; Director of Fellowship Training, The Hand Center of San Antonio, San Antonio, Texas
Principles of Microvascular Surgery; Skin Grafts and Skin Flaps (Skin Grafting; Skin Flaps; Coverage of the Elbow); The Management of Snake (Pit Viper) Bites

Katrin Philipp, MD
Resident, Department of Hand, Plastic, and Reconstructive Surgery, Burn Center, BG-Trauma Center, Plastic and Hand Surgery, University of Heidelberg, Ludwigshafen, Germany
The Burned Hand

Gary G. Poehling, MD
Professor and Chair, Department of Orthopaedic Surgery, Wake Forest University School of Medicine, Winston-Salem, North Carolina
Wrist Arthroscopy: Anatomy and Diagnosis; Complex Regional Pain Syndrome

Somayaji Ramamurthy, MD
Professor, Department of Anesthesiology, University of Texas Health Science Center at San Antonio, San Antonio, Texas
Anesthesia

David Ring, MD
Instructor, Orthopaedic Surgery, Harvard Medical School; Hand and Upper Extremity Service, Department of Orthopaedic Surgery, Massachusetts General Hospital, Boston, Massachusetts
Fractures of the Proximal Ulna

Spencer A. Rowland, MD, MS
Clinical Professor, Department of Orthopaedics, The University of Texas Health Science Center at San Antonio, San Antonio, Texas
The Management of Snake (Pit Viper) Bites

David S. Ruch, MD
Professor, Department of Orthopaedic Surgery, Wake Forest University School of Medicine, Winston-Salem, North Carolina
Wrist Arthroscopy: Anatomy and Diagnosis; Vascular Disorders

A. Neil Salyapongse, MD
Plastic and Hand Surgery Associates, Belleville, Illinois
Thumb Reconstruction

Christopher C. Schmidt, MD
Drexel University College of Medicine, and Director, Microsurgical Reconstruction of the Upper Limb, Department of Orthopacdic Surgery, Allegheny General Hospital, Pittsburgh, Pennsylvania
Extensor Tendon Injuries

William H. Seitz, Jr., MD
Director, Hand and Upper Extremity Center, Cleveland Orthopaedic and Spine Hospital at Lutheran, Cleveland, Ohio
Distraction Lengthening in the Hand and Upper Extremity

Frances E. Sharpe, MD
Orthopedic Surgeon, Kaiser Permanente, Fontana Medical Center, Fontana, California
Acute Infections in the Hand; Skin Grafts and Skin Flaps (Coverage of the Elbow)

Alexander Y. Shin, MD
Consultant and Associate Professor of Orthopedic Surgery, Mayo Clinic College of Medicine; Division of Hand Surgery, Department of Orthopedic Surgery, Mayo Clinic, Rochester, Minnesota
Stiff Finger Joints

Beth Paterson Smith, PhD
Associate Professor, and Director, Orthopaedic Research Laboratory, Department of Orthopaedic Surgery, Wake Forest University School of Medicine, Winston-Salem, North Carolina
Complex Regional Pain Syndrome; Vascular Disorders

Thomas L. Smith, PhD
Associate Professor, Department of Orthopaedic Surgery, Wake Forest University School of Medicine, Winston-Salem, North Carolina
Complex Regional Pain Syndrome; Vascular Disorders

Nicole Z. Sommer, MD
Assistant Professor, The Plastic Surgery Institute, Southern Illinois University School of Medicine, Springfield, Illinois
The Perionychium

Dean G. Sotereanos, MD
Professor Orthopaedic Surgery, Drexel University School of Medicine; Vice Chairman, Department of Orthopaedic Surgery, Allegheny General Hospital, Pittsburgh, Pennsylvania
Complex Traumatic Elbow Dislocation

Peter J. Stern, MD
Norman S. and Elizabeth C. A. Hill Professor and Chairman, Department of Orthopaedic Surgery, University of Cincinnati College of Medicine, Cincinnati, Ohio
Fractures of the Metacarpals and Phalanges

Milan V. Stevanovic, MD, PhD

Professor of Orthopaedics and Surgery, Hand and Microsurgery, and Director, Joseph H. Boyes Microsurgery Laboratory, Keck School of Medicine, Department of Orthopaedic Surgery, University of Southern California, Los Angeles, California

Acute Infections in the Hand; Skin Grafts and Skin Flaps (Coverage of the Elbow)

Alan M. Sugar, MD

Professor of Medicine, Boston University School of Medicine, Boston; Medical Director, HIV/AIDS and Hepatitis Viruses Infection Programs and Infectious Disease Clinical Services, Cape Cod Hospital; Chief, Infection Control Program, Cape Cod Healthcare, Hyannis, Massachusetts

Chronic Infections

John S. Taras, MD

Associate Professor of Orthopedic Surgery, Thomas Jefferson University School of Medicine; Associate Professor of Orthopedic Surgery, and Chief, Hand Surgery, Drexel University School of Medicine; The Philadelphia Hand Center, P.C., Philadelphia, Pennsylvania

Flexor Tendon Injury (Flexor Tendon Reconstruction)

Andrew L. Terrono, MD

Associate Clinical Professor of Orthopaedic Surgery, Tufts University School of Medicine; New England Baptist Hospital; Hand Surgical Associates, Boston, Massachusetts

Rheumatoid Arthritis and Other Connective Tissue Diseases

Matthew M. Tomaino, MD, MBA

Professor of Orthopaedics, and Chief, Division of Hand, Shoulder and Elbow Surgery, University of Rochester Medical Center, Rochester, New York

Thumb Basal Joint Arthritis

James R. Urbaniak, MD

Virginia Flowers Baker Professor and Vice Chairman, Department of Surgery, Duke University Medical Center, Durham, North Carolina

Replantation

Ann E. Van Heest, MD

Associate Professor, Department of Orthopedic Surgery, University of Minnesota; Shriners Hospital–Twin Cities Unit; Pediatric Hand and Upper Extremity Service, Gillette Children's Hospital, Minneapolis, Minnesota

Tetraplegia

Nicholas B. Vedder, MD, FACS

Professor of Surgery and Orthopaedics, and Chief, Division of Plastic Surgery, University of Washington, Seattle, Washington

The Mangled Upper Extremity

Peter M. Waters, MD

Associate Professor of Orthopaedic Surgery, Harvard Medical School; Director, Brachial Plexus and Hand/Upper Extremity Programs, Department of Orthopaedic Surgery, Children's Hospital, Boston, Massachusetts

Pediatric Brachial Plexus Palsy

Fu-Chan Wei, MD, FACS

Professor, Department of Plastic Surgery, Chang-Gung Memorial Hospital; Dean, Medical College, Chang-Gung University, Taipei, Taiwan, Republic of China

Toe-to-Hand Transplantation

Scott W. Wolfe, MD

Professor of Orthopedic Surgery, Weill Medical College of Cornell University; Chief, Hand and Upper Extremity Surgery, and Attending Orthopedic Surgeon, Hospital for Special Surgery, New York, New York

Distal Radius Fractures; Tenosynovitis

PREFACE

The positive acceptance and widespread use of *Operative Hand Surgery* in its previous editions has been most gratifying, but there is always room for improvement and we have tried to make the fifth edition even better. The most noticeable changes for the reader include the following:

1 **Organization.** The entire format and location of chapters have been radically altered. New chapters have been created, deleting relatively obsolete material, introducing new concepts and techniques, and in some instances merging parts of several old chapters into new composites.

2 **Authors.** The major strength of this book has always been the quality of the contributors. Many of the authors who wrote chapters for the first three or four editions are at or near retirement age, but the hand surgery world is blessed with a tremendous pool of exceptional new talent. We have very carefully selected some of these best and brightest to revise old chapters or write new ones, in most instances liberally retaining the core elements of old chapters.

3 **References.** From its conception in 1982, one of the objectives of *Operative Hand Surgery* has been to provide the reader with a comprehensive reference list of virtually everything about a topic that has been written in the English language. Continued adherence to this principle has resulted in an inordinate number of pages being devoted to exhaustive lists of references, which in turn squeezes the amount of space available for text and illustrations. Computer technology has provided a satisfactory compromise: the fifth edition will continue to have comprehensive reference lists for each chapter, but they will reside on a companion CD-ROM. At the end of each chapter, however, the reader will find a list of annotated references compiled by each author, with his or her comments on those articles deemed to be the most important to that subject.

4 **Internet Access.** Another advantage of computer technology makes it possible to have the entire text and all illustrations accessible via the Internet. Not only does this give the reader freer access to the content of the book, but this **e-dition** creates a mechanism to provide more frequent updates than is possible with only the printed version.

5 **Operative Techniques.** Although the emphasis of this book has always been on *operative* treatment, an effort has been made in the fifth edition to incorporate even more specific details of surgical technique. At the same time, attention has not been lessened on the important indications for and alternative methods of specific treatments, and even more has been added regarding expected outcomes.

Perhaps less obvious to the reader, but critical to the ongoing improvement of this book, is the expanded editorial staff. The first two editions of *Operative Hand Surgery* had a single editor; for this fifth edition there have been four, bringing broader expertise and enhanced quality of ideas to the table.

DAVID P. GREEN, MD
ROBERT N. HOTCHKISS, MD
WILLIAM C. PEDERSON, MD
SCOTT W. WOLFE, MD

ACKNOWLEDGMENTS

Over the two-decade life span of *Operative Hand Surgery,* massive changes have taken place in the medical publishing world. Globalization, business mergers, personnel changes, and different priorities have radically altered what goes on behind the scenes in bringing a book to publication. Although some contacts at Elsevier have come and gone, we have been fortunate to have had the steady hand of Developmental Editor Arlene Chappelle guiding, cajoling, and sometimes goading us to complete our assigned tasks in this fifth edition. She has kept us focused on what needed to be done, and we are grateful to her for her clear direction and guidance. Dan Pepper, Acquisitions Editor, inherited this project in mid stream and has been of tremendous help. Tina Rebane, Publishing Services Manager, has done a superb job arranging and overseeing the actual production of this book.

One aspect of medical publishing has not changed—the commitment of very busy surgeons to devote enormous chunks of their time and energy to writing chapters for *Operative Hand Surgery.* We, the editors—on behalf of readers of this book and students of hand surgery throughout the world—again express our appreciation to these men and women for their unselfish efforts.

One of our contributors deserves special mention. Scott Kozin took on the unenviable task of section editor for the chapters on congenital abnormalities. From the inception of this book in 1982, that group of chapters has posed the most daunting editorial challenge, probably because the subject virtually defies a clear and precise organizational format. When Dr. Kozin agreed to take on this assignment, he probably did not appreciate its complexity, but despite the predictable difficulty, he stayed the course and saw the job to its completion.

Elizabeth Roselius is one of the major reasons that this book has been successful. She is a world-class medical illustrator whose talents have enhanced numerous books and whose efforts have been widely acknowledged; the first edition of *Operative Hand Surgery* received the Illustrated Medical Book Award, Clinical Text, from the Association of Medical Illustrators. She has added a substantial number of new illustrations for this fifth edition.

Above all, I wish to thank my good friends Bob Hotchkiss, Chris Pederson, and Scott Wolfe. I am grateful to them not only for bringing to the book new insights, but also for assuming an increasingly heavier share of the editorial load.

DAVID P. GREEN, MD

CONTENTS

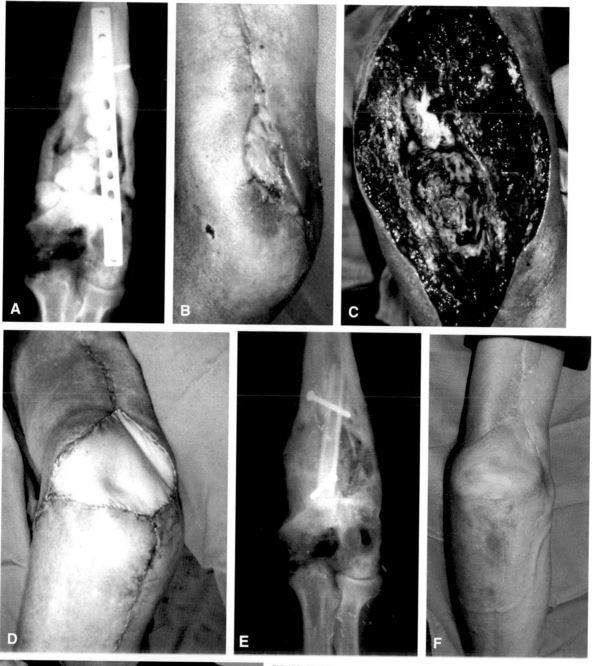

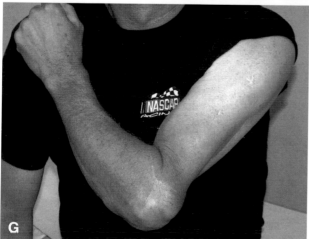

FIGURE 47-75. A 36-year-old truck driver involved in a roll-over motor vehicle accident sustained a severely crushed supracondylar left humerus fracture. Open reduction and internal fixation was performed. The fracture did not heal and deep infection ensued. A total of seven procedures had been performed before presentation to our department. The patient underwent a staged reconstruction. After removal of hardware and control of infection, soft tissue coverage was achieved using a rotational radial forearm flap. After 6 weeks of intravenous antibiotic therapy, the patient was returned to the operating room for bone reconstruction using a vascularized free fibula graft. **A,** Initial presentation radiographs of the distal humerus. Partial hardware removal and placement of tobramycin antibiotic beads had been done before presentation. **B,** Skin appearance at the posterior distal humerus. Wound dehiscence and soft tissue loss resulted from chronic infection. **C,** Soft tissue defect after débridement. **D,** Soft tissue defect covered with a radial forearm rotational flap. **E,** Radiographic appearance 6 months after vascularized free fibula grafting of bony defect of the distal humerus. **F,** Soft tissue appearance 6 months after vascularized free fibula grafting. Patient lacked 15 degrees of extension. **G,** Elbow flexion at 6 months after vascularized free fibula grafting. Flexion was to 105 degrees.

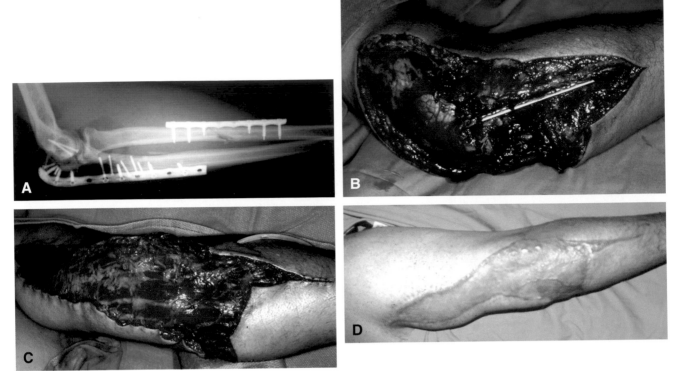

FIGURE 47-79. A 40-year-old man sustained a severe open fracture-dislocation of the elbow. A large soft tissue defect was present, leaving exposed bone and joint. After irrigation and débridement, open reduction and internal fixation was performed of the radius, ulna, and capitellum. The following day, the patient underwent repeat débridement, primary bone grafting, and soft tissue coverage with a latissimus dorsi rotational flap. At 3-month follow-up, his range of motion was from 15 to 105 degrees. **A,** Radiographic appearance immediately after fixation. **B,** Soft tissue defect after second débridement. **C,** Soft tissue defect covered with rotational latissimus dorsi muscle flap. **D,** Soft tissue appearance at 3-month follow-up.

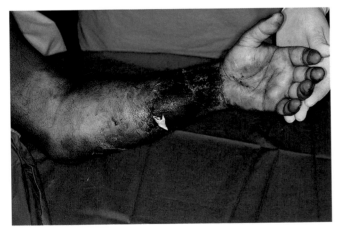

FIGURE 56-4. An earthquake victim whose forearm was exposed to prolonged direct pressure up to 10 hours under a collapsed wall developed an acute compartment syndrome.

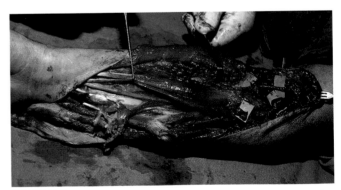

FIGURE 56-9. Repair of the brachial artery at the elbow 12 hours after injury. Below the arterial repair, the separated ends of the ulnar nerve are seen that will be repaired at this stage. The already necrotic parts of the muscles are to be excised meticulously.

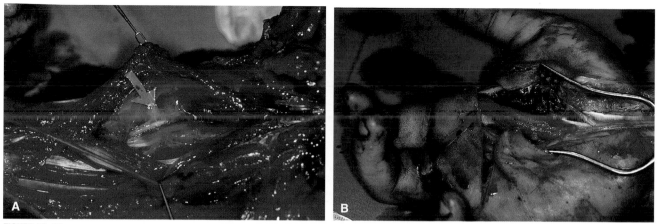

FIGURE 56-13. **A,** Dirty pale color of part of the deep flexor and pronator muscles around the median nerve immediately after the release of tourniquet in reactive hyperemic phase indicates irreversible necrosis. **B,** Lumbrical of the index finger with its pale color and insensitivity to stimulation is an indication that it will become necrotic and fibrotic and therefore is to be resected at this stage.

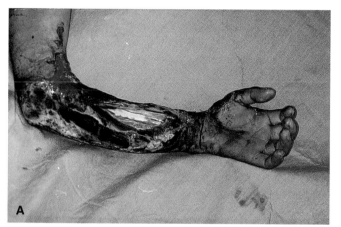

FIGURE 56-17. **A,** Severe necrosis of the soft tissues and muscles from a crushing injury.

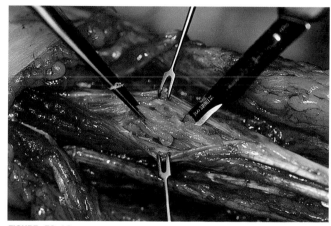

FIGURE 56-18. Resection of the yellow friable necrotic tissue after epimysiotomies of the individual muscle fascia.

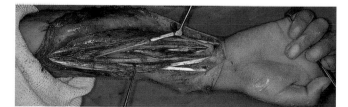

FIGURE 56-22. Ischemic necrosis of the distal bellies of superficial flexors in a Holden II, mild type after tight casting.

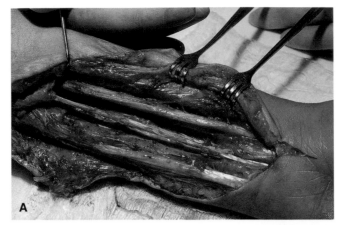

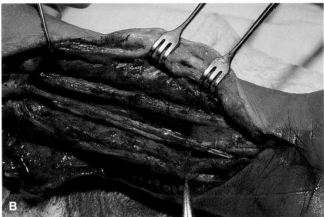

FIGURE 56-31. A, The external neurolysis of the median nerve after resection of the ischemic muscles. The tourniquet is still up. **B,** Return of circulation immediately after tourniquet release. Petechial bleedings and homogeneous circulation along the epineurium can be seen; there the procedure is sufficient.

CHAPTER 33

Ulnar Nerve Palsy

George A. Anderson

ETIOLOGY

The common causes of ulnar nerve palsy are (1) lacerations to the fascicles in the medial cord of the brachial plexus, (2) injury to the ulnar nerve itself, as far distally as its terminal deep motor branch in the hand, and (3) primary involvement of the ulnar nerve in leprosy.[14,19,50,55,69] Less common causes are the residual paralysis of a part or whole of the ulnar nerve due to primary neurologic disease, including poliomyelitis,[6,123] syringomyelia, or Charcot-Marie-Tooth disease,[123] and the neglected cubitus valgus deformity that progresses to tardy ulnar nerve palsy. Anatomic causes include pressure on the ulnar nerve at the cubital tunnel due to osteoarthritis, an enlarging synovial cyst in a patient with rheumatoid arthritis, or anomalous accessory muscles, fibrous bands, or ligaments in the cubital tunnel or Guyon's canal.

Characteristics

In lacerations or other forms of injuries to the ulnar nerve, there is a predictable pattern of sensory and motor deficit in the hand depending on the location of the injury[73,82,111,131] In leprosy (Hansen's disease), sensory changes frequently precede motor paralysis and, after a variable period of time, the total picture of proximal or distal sensorimotor dysfunction emerges.[14,16,19] In poliomyelitis, there is lower motor neuron type of flaccid paralysis without sensory loss. In cases of poliomyelitis, the exact extent of paralysis cannot be initially determined but there is a fairly rapid improvement of muscle power between the first to fourth months and 93% of possible recovery occurs by the end of the first year.[129] In Charcot-Marie-Tooth disease and syringomyelia there is often more extensive weakness, with characteristic dissociated sensory loss in the latter.

Patterns of Motor Paralysis

In proximal ulnar nerve palsy all the extrinsic and intrinsic muscles supplied by the ulnar nerve are affected. In distal ulnar nerve palsy the extrinsic muscles are spared and the intrinsic muscles are involved. Paralysis affecting the deep branch of the ulnar nerve in the palm spares the hypothenar muscle function while the rest of the intrinsic muscles are affected.

Patterns of Sensory Loss

In proximal ulnar nerve lesions, sensory loss is on the palmar and dorsal aspects of the medial third of the hand together with sensory loss on the palmar and dorsal aspects of the whole of the little finger and the ulnar half of the ring finger. In medial cord palsy, there may be additional sensory loss in the medial antebrachial and medial brachial cutaneous nerve distributions. In distal ulnar nerve lesions the sensory loss is only on the palmar aspect of the medial third of the palm, the whole of the palmar aspect of the little finger and the ulnar half of the ring finger, and the dorsal aspects of the little finger and ulnar side of the ring finger distal to the proximal interphalangeal (PIP) joints. This difference in sensory loss in distal ulnar nerve lesions is due to the sparing of the dorsal cutaneous branch of the ulnar nerve usually given off from the ulnar nerve trunk at 6 to 8 cm proximal to the wrist crease, to supply the dorsum of the medial third of the hand as far as the PIP joint of the dorsum of the little finger and the ulnar aspect of the dorsum of the ring finger. There is no sensory loss if the deep branch of the ulnar nerve is injured or compressed in the palm. Because of a distinct lack of an overt "physical" sign of sensory loss in the vital ulnar nerve distribution of the hand in the early stages of a proximal or distal ulnar nerve lesion, the pattern of sensory loss has to be examined and recorded after taking a clinical history.

In previous editions of this chapter, **George Omer** gave a detailed account of the deficits in ulnar nerve palsy with descriptions of the approach and management as applied to ulnar nerve palsy due to injury. I gratefully acknowledge the wealth of information that he has imparted to the chapter, and I used part of his format and many of his illustrations and references. My additions included some features that characterize other causes of ulnar palsy, a regrouping of clinical tests, a discussion of the pertinent mechanics of clawing in the fingers, and explanations for other deformities. I have added my thoughts on preoperative evaluation, classifications of specific deformities facilitating surgical management, some new concepts in surgical techniques, and my approach to optimize the care of the diverse problems that ulnar nerve palsy produces in the hand.

Ulnar Nerve Palsy in Leprosy

In 1948, Dr. Paul Brand pioneered reconstructive surgery on patients afflicted with leprosy and performed the first correction of claw hand at the Christian Medical College Hospital, Vellore, India. He evolved a system of detailed clinical evaluation and introduced modalities of preoperative approach for correction of deformity and new procedures for claw hands.[14] Some of these have remained the "workhorse" for surgeons treating leprosy and are used as *the* standard by which all other procedures are evaluated.[3,114,143] Since 1948, more than 9600 patients with claw hands and related deformities have undergone surgical reconstruction by Dr. Brand, his colleagues, and different surgical teams. I have observed through the years how leprosy, the world's most common cause of ulnar nerve palsy, has unwittingly served as a surgical model for the correction of all deformities due to ulnar nerve paralysis.

In leprosy there is a profound loss of sensation along the ulnar nerve distribution. Patients may present with blisters or ulceration in the little and ring fingers, which in some instances may be the actual reason for them to seek medical attention rather than for nerve pain, weakness, or hypopigmented patches on the skin.[19] This is primarily due to the insidious nature of the clinical manifestations of leprosy while the patient unknowingly delays seeking medical attention.[14,19,50,69] The delay may be compounded by the routine need for clinicians to confirm the diagnosis by skin smears, biopsy of the skin itself, or, in some situations, a biopsy of a cutaneous nerve to aid in the classification of the disease.[119] Treatment of the manifestations of ulnar nerve involvement must await appropriate and adequate chemotherapy to obtain bacterial clearance. When this is done the patient is referred for treatment of persistent nerve pain or enlargement of the nerve or of a deformity in the hand along with the former problems. Absorption of parts of the distal segments of the little or the ring finger is in keeping with paralysis of long duration.

In patients with ulnar nerve palsy of traumatic etiology or due to entrapment there is only a "local" component to their problem, and an early decision can be made as to whether surgical intervention is necessary at the time of first consultation.

CLINICAL FEATURES OF ULNAR NERVE PARALYSIS

The physical signs of ulnar nerve palsy are among the earliest to be recorded in the medical literature for peripheral nerve injuries. The appearance of the hand at rest, the deformity patterns that unravel as the hand is tested, and the weakness of specific muscle groups during physical examination constitute the overall clinical picture and denote structural alterations and substitution patterns that patients acquire.

Clinical examination should preferably begin with observing the outstretched hand. The obvious characteristic is a "claw" deformity, also referred to as the "benediction hand" because of conspicuous flexion deformities in the little and ring fingers with a lesser degree of involvement of the middle and index fingers. The palmar aspect of the hand is next viewed by placing it palm up on the table to note the flattened palm and wasting of the hypothenar region as well as a shallow midpalmar receptacle distal to the thenar and hypothenar eminences. Supple and delicate hands show longitudinal palmar furrows between prominent long flexors beneath the palmar skin that indicate wasting of the lumbricals. The dorsum of the hand shows pronounced wasting, with shallow concavities between the intermetacarpal space of the interosseous muscles and particularly of the thumb web. The hand proper takes on the shape of an isosceles triangle with its base distally, rather than the normal rectangular contour. This change of configuration is mainly due to the absence of the hypothenar muscle bulge medial to the fifth metacarpal and the combined adductor pollicis/first dorsal interosseous muscle fullness of the thumb web space. Manual workers or those engaged in heavy hands-on rural farming demonstrate the dorsal wasting and contour changes in the ulnar palsied hand remarkably well.

MECHANICS OF PARALYTIC CLAW HAND

Claw fingers are the most obvious of all the deformities in ulnar nerve palsy, and patients find it difficult to hide them. The mechanical and electrophysiologic aspects of claw hand have attracted anatomists, kinesiologists, and surgeons alike, and an understanding of the nuances of the deformity has led to a better appreciation of the problem and to surgical strategies that benefit the patient.

The lumbrical muscles bring about flexion of the metacarpophalangeal (MP) joint[8,34,45,51,85,86,132,134,140] and extension of the PIP joint.[8,34,45,51,132,134,140] Interossei also bring about MP joint flexion and interphalangeal (IP) joint extension,[51,85,86,132,134,140,150] in addition to the adduction and abduction. The claw finger represents a defective mechanical system brought about by the altered equilibrium in the small joints resulting from paralysis of these intrinsic muscles. The reader is referred to the detailed description of the biarticular model of digital mechanics by Landsmeer[75,96] and to the findings of others[8,85,86,132,134,157] regarding the production and clinical manifestation of this deformity to fully appreciate the rationale for corrective surgery for claw hand. The approach to the correction of the abnormal posture of claw deformity due to intrinsic paralysis has a well-founded scientific basis that should be utilized by the surgeon.

In short, according to Landsmeer,[75] the movements of the MP joints and the IP joints in the finger are normally independent but the movements of the two IP joints are limited or, rather, coordinated because flexion of the distal interphalangeal (DIP) joint brings about flexion of the PIP joint. This is because (1) the flexion of the distal phalanx draws the dorsal expansion distally by loosening the tension on the central tendon; (2) flexion of the DIP joint tenses the oblique retinacular ligament (the volar reins of the extensor assembly)[75] causing this ligament to slide volarward and impart a flexion force to the PIP joint, and (3) as the PIP joint flexes, the lateral tendons at the PIP joint also slide volarward and their extension moment is reduced.

Therefore, Landsmeer considered this to be a biarticular system comprising the MP and PIP joints, with the proximal phalanx forming the intercalated bone. This biarticular system will be stable in any given posture if the ratios of the moment arm (flexor vs. extensor) of the opposing tendons at the two joints are equal. He has shown that in the finger the extensor to flexor moment arm ratio at the MP joint is greater than that of the PIP joint. In the absence of a functioning intrinsic system the biarticular system will not be stable in a straight position because it will be controlled only by the long flexor and extensor tendons. In the normal situation while the patient attempts to extend his or her finger, with the MP joints in neutral, the tension placed on the extensor tendon is transmitted distally to extend the IP joints. In the paralytic finger, long extensor function is "blocked" at the MP joint by the diversion of this tension to the sagittal band,[96] producing hyperextension and effectively blocking the extensor's ability to extend the PIP joint.[96,157] Without intrinsic function, the middle and distal phalanges collapse into flexion. The normal cascade of digital extension is disrupted, in that during any attempt to actively open the finger, the MP joint extends first and will extend more than the PIP joint, and even after the MP joint reaches maximum extension the PIP joint will never attain neutral extension. The normal sequence of digital closure is also reversed, in that the IP joint flexion precedes the MP joint flexion. The independence of MP and IP joint motion is lost.

Therefore, in a finger deprived of functioning intrinsic muscles, clawing is the principal longitudinal axial deformity and the loss of independence of movement at the MP and PIP joints is the principal disability. To improve this clinical situation a third muscle-tendon unit needs to run volar to the center of curvature of the metacarpal (MP joint) and dorsal to the center of curvature of the head of the proximal phalanx (PIP joint) to counterbalance the system and provide the equilibrium and independence of the normally functioning intrinsic muscles. Alternatively, the MP joint needs to be statically prevented from hyperextension to allow the long extensors to extend the IP joints. Improved function through restoration of the mechanical balance reduces substitution patterns that patients with paralytic hands habitually adopt.

The surgeon may choose to release soft tissue or other periarticular structures in correcting claw-like deformity due to nonparalytic origin.

The "Claw" Thumb

The thumb has a complex array of movements in its three articulations, the carpometacarpal (CMC) joint, MP joint, and IP joint. To study one of its principal axes of movements that take place in the flexion-extension plane, and the resulting instability that arises due to ulnar nerve palsy, again we need to appreciate the extensor to flexor moment arm ratio of the forces that move these joints. The basal CMC joint has the largest extensor to flexor moment, followed by the MP joint and then the IP joint.[24] The basal joint in ulnar nerve palsy is affected in part by the paralysis of the adductor pollicis, the flexor pollicis brevis (FPB), and the first dorsal interosseous. Normally the first dorsal interosseous prevents the tendency for the CMC joint to sublux posteriorly,[24] but in the presence of the functioning abductor pollicis brevis (APB), opponens pollicis, and the extrinsic muscle units, the basal joint remains a fairly stable articulation. Therefore, for the purpose of studying the behavior of the distal two joints, Landsmeer's biarticular chain model can be applied.

With the paralysis of the adductor pollicis and a part or whole of the FPB, the MP and IP joints of the thumb are totally under the control of the extrinsic flexors and extensors, with the proximal phalanx behaving like an intercalated bone. The MP joint will go into hyperextension and the IP joint into flexion because of the greater extensor moment at the MP joint and the lesser extensor moment at the IP joint, respectively. The system collapses into a "Z"-thumb deformity. In this unstable equilibrium, reconstruction has often been approached by providing a primary adductor that also is expected to restore short flexor function. Reconstructive procedures have attained satisfactory results by the transfer of one extrinsic tendon to one of three known sites (adductor tubercle, APB insertion, or proximal phalanx).

EVALUATION FOR SURGICAL RECONSTRUCTION

Specific Signs and Tests of Motor Dysfunction (Table 33-1)

The Finger Intrinsic Muscles

1. The ring and little fingers and, to a lesser extent, the middle and index fingers adopt an attitude of hyperextension of the proximal phalanges and flexion of the middle and distal phalanges (Duchenne's sign, 1867).[45,88] The claw deformity is also referred to as the "intrinsic minus" deformity or "intrinsic zero" disability and is due to the paralysis of the interosseous and the ulnar two lumbricals. If the extrinsic flexor muscle function is near normal, the claw deformity will be more pronounced.

2. Application of dorsal pressure over the proximal phalanx to passively flex the MP joint results in straightening of the distal joints and temporary correction of claw deformity (Bouvier's maneuver, 1851).[157] The extensor digitorum tendon can extend the middle and distal phalanges when the proximal phalanx is stabilized. A positive sign is pathognomonic of claw finger caused by intrinsic muscle paralysis.

3. An increase of the claw deformity is brought about by an unconscious effort on the part of the patient to further extend the fingers by palmar flexing the wrist (Andre-Thomas sign, 1917).[88] This is due to the tenodesis effect of the long extensor tendons and exaggeration of the hyperextension deformity at the MP joints.

4. An inability to cross the long finger dorsally over the index finger and vice versa with the palm placed flat on the table tests the first volar interosseous and second dorsal interosseous muscles.[46,109]

5. An inability to actively move the long finger in radial and ulnar deviation with the palm placed flat on the table (Pitres-Testut sign, 1925) demonstrates the paralysis of the second and third dorsal interosseous muscles.[46,88]

6. Loss of integration of MP and IP flexion occurs because of paralysis of the lumbrical muscles to the ring and little fingers.[52] Normal finger flexion is initiated at the MP joint followed by IP joint flexion. In intrinsic paralysis, the MP joint does not flex until IP joint flexion is completed. The fingers curl or roll into the palm, and objects are pushed away instead of grasped.

7. Flattened metacarpal arch (palmar arch) and loss of hypothenar elevation (Masse's sign, 1916)[46] is caused by

Table 33-1

SIGNS, TESTS, AND MANEUVERS USED TO IDENTIFY ULNAR NERVE PARALYSIS

Claw deformity of fingers: hyperextension at MP joint and flexion at IP joints	1867: Duchenne sign[45,88]
Active extension of middle and distal phalanges (by the extensor digitorum) on dorsal passive restraint of the proximal segment (i.e., preventing the proximal phalanx from going into hyperextension)	1851: Bouvier's maneuver[157]
Increase in claw deformity when patient makes an effort to extend the fingers by flexing the wrist (i.e., attempting to tenodese the extensor tendons)	1917: Andre-Thomas sign[88]
Inability to abduct the extended middle finger to the radial and ulnar side when the hand is placed on a flat surface (a test for second and third dorsal interosseous muscles)	1925: Pitres-Testut sign[46,88]
Inability to cross the middle finger dorsally over the index finger, or the index over the middle finger, the "cross your fingers" test (a test of the first volar interosseous and second dorsal interosseous muscles)	1980: Earle, Valstou[46]
Loss of integration of MP and IP flexion: MP joint does not flex until IP joint flexion has been completed (due to paralysis of the lumbrical muscles to the ring and little fingers)	1961: Flatt[52]
The fingers curl or roll into the palm and objects are pushed away instead of grasped.	1961: Brand[18]
Hyperextension of the MP joint of thumb during key pinch or gross grip (due to paralysis of the adductor pollicis muscle, which acts as a first metacarpal adductor, a flexor of the thumb MP joint, and an extensor of the thumb IP joint)	1915: Jeanne's sign[30,126]
Flattened palmar (metacarpal) arch (due to paralysis of the opponens digiti quinti and decreased range of flexion of the little finger MP joint)	1916: Masse's sign[46]
Thumb IP joint flexion (80 to 90 degrees) (due to paralysis of first volar and second dorsal interosseous and adductor pollicis muscles with the flexor pollicis longus substituting their function)	1915: Froment's sign[30,126]
Combined hyperextension at MP joint and hyperflexion of IP joint (noticed when patient makes a pulp to pulp pinch with thumb and index finger)	1956: Bunnell's O sign[12,34,88]
Loss of active lateral mobility with the fingers in extension (due to paralysis of the interosseous and hypothenar muscles)	1974: Smith[132,133]
Inability to bring tips of the extended fingers together into a cone (due to paralysis of the adductor pollicis muscle)	1925: Pitres-Testut sign[88]
Inability to adduct the extended little finger to the extended ring finger (due to the continued activity of the extensor digiti minimi, unopposed by the third palmar interosseous, which is paralyzed)	1930: Wartenberg's sign[73,88,154]
Loss of extrinsic power with inability to flex the distal joint of the ring and little fingers (due to weakness of the FDPR and FDPL innervated by the ulnar nerve)	1919: Pollock's sign[46]
Partial loss of wrist flexion with inability to perform power grip with a neutral wrist (due to paralysis of the flexor carpi ulnaris)	1961: Bowden and Napier[12]

paralysis of the opponens digiti quinti and decreased range of flexion of the MP joint of the little finger.[86,144]

8. Loss of active mediolateral mobility (adduction and abduction) with the fingers in extension is due to paralysis of the interossei and hypothenar muscles (Pitres-Testut sign).[132,133] Because there is also paralysis of the adductor pollicis muscle, the tips of the extended digits cannot be brought together into a cone.[88] The resulting effect is impairment of precision grip.

9. An inability to adduct the extended little finger to the extended ring finger is Wartenberg's sign.[73,88,154] This sign is characteristic of isolated deep motor branch involvement, in which the functioning abductor digiti minimi is unopposed by the paralyzed third palmar interosseous.

The Thumb

1. In hyperextension of the MP joint of the thumb by 10 to 15 degrees during key pinch or gross grip (Jeanne's sign, 1915)[30,126] there is loss of lateral or key pinch of the thumb because of paralysis of the adductor pollicis muscle, which normally acts as a first metacarpal adductor, a flexor of the thumb MP joint, and an extensor of the thumb IP joint. The residual strength for palmar adduction of the thumb (key pinch) may be diminished as much as 77% to 80% in ulnar nerve palsy.[88]

2. Hyperflexion of the IP joint of the thumb may occur while attempting to perform a lateral pinch (Froment's sign, 1915).[30,126] The IP joint flexion of the thumb may hyperextend as much as 80 to 90 degrees owing to the substitution of the action of the flexor pollicis longus (FPL) to hold an object.

3. A combined hyperextension at the MP joint and hyperflexion of the IP joint of the thumb makes the interval between the index finger and thumb more circular, rather than the normal spindle configuration on attempting to hold an object (Bunnell's O sign, 1956).[12,34,88]

The Extrinsic Muscles

1. Loss of extrinsic power to the ulnar-innervated portion of the flexor digitorum profundus (FDP) leads to weakness or an inability to flex the distal phalanges of the ring and little fingers (Pollock's sign, 1919).[46] I observe the clenched fist from the medial side and note whether the DIP joint of the little finger remains extended. Normally, the little and ring fingers are tucked up well into the palm on closing the fist to give an X configuration to the folded creases of the little finger. Loss of DIP flexion converts the X configuration to a Y.
2. Partial loss of wrist flexion may occur because of paralysis of the flexor carpi ulnaris (FCU). The wrist is held in the neutral position during power grip and is dorsiflexed until the thumb lies in line with the radius during precision grip.[12] The impairment in power grip is greater than the loss of power for precise grasp.[12]

Anomalous Innervation Patterns

Anomalous innervation patterns of muscles controlling the hand unit are not uncommon and need to be recognized to avoid errors in diagnosis and management. Careful voluntary muscle testing, precise evaluation of sensibility and sudomotor activity, anesthetic blocks of intact nerves, and electrodiagnostic studies that include conduction times across selected segments of the ulnar nerve need to be performed.[78,105,108,153]

The ulnar nerve normally contains axons from the anterior divisions of C8 and T1, but it may contain axons from the anterior division of the C7 or T2 roots as well. In 5% to 10% of upper extremities, the motor axons to the FCU arise from the C7 root rather than from the C8 and T1 roots[73]; therefore, in cases with complete C8 and T1 root lesions that normally demonstrate intrinsic and extrinsic muscle paralysis in the hand, the FCU will still be functioning.

Innervation of the FDP may vary from all ulnar to all median to a completely dual nerve supply.

Motor neural connections that take place between the median and ulnar nerves in the forearm are termed Martin (1763)-Gruber (1870) anomalous connections.[73,76,88,131] This occurs adjacent to the ulnar artery in the proximal forearm and is between the median nerve (or its anterior interosseous branch) and the ulnar nerve. There is a 17% overall occurrence of this anomaly,[76,153] and four types of Martin-Gruber connections have been described: 60% are type I, in which motor branches from the median nerve travel with the ulnar nerve to innervate "median" muscles; 35% are type II, in which motor branches from the median nerve innervate the "ulnar" muscles; 3% are type III, in which motor fibers from the ulnar nerve travel with the median nerve and innervate "median" muscles; and 1% are type IV, in which motor fibers from the ulnar nerve travel with the median nerve to innervate "ulnar" muscles.[76]

Within the hand the Riche (1897)-Cannieu (1897) anomalous connection occurs between the motor branch of the ulnar nerve and the recurrent branch of the median nerve.[73]

These anomalies gain clinical importance when a patient presents without detectable intrinsic deformity despite a complete ulnar nerve injury in zone V and complete sensory loss in the autonomous zone.[41] This exemplifies median nerve innervation of all of the lumbricals. Alternatively, there may be continued function of the median nerve–innervated muscles in spite of severance of the median nerve and anesthesia in a median nerve distribution.[41] The third lumbrical has dual innervation in 50% of upper extremities,[73] and in such a hand a complete distal ulnar nerve palsy would result in clawing deformity in only the little finger. The first dorsal interosseous is innervated completely or partially by the median nerve in 10% of hands and by the radial nerve in 1% of hands.[73]

The dorsal cutaneous sensory branch of the ulnar nerve perforates the fascia 6 to 8 cm proximal to the wrist and supplies the dorsoulnar surface of the hand and the little finger. However, this area can be supplied by the superficial branch of the radial nerve, which may lead to confusion concerning the level of an ulnar nerve lesion.

INDICATIONS FOR SURGERY

Ulnar Nerve Laceration

Nerve repair is the basic approach to nerve laceration.[10,78,94,147] Successful repairs of divided nerves in the upper extremity have been shown to occur if the repair has been carried out within 3 months.[107,109] In proximal ulnar nerve repair the potential for recovery of sensibility is reported to be better than the potential for functional motor recovery in the hand.[104] In situations in which the patient is referred late for definitive care the critical limit of delay beyond which motor recovery is unlikely to return is considered as 6 to 9 months for lesions at the elbow and 12 to 15 months for lesions at the wrist level[71] and is age dependent. The critical limit of delay beyond which sensation is unlikely to return is as much as 2 years. After primary ulnar nerve repair, there may be a discrepancy between the return of sensory function and intrinsic motor function, the latter often being minimal or clinically nonexistent.[78] After nerve repair, if the electrodiagnostic tests show no signs of reinnervation within 6 to 9 months, then the surgeon has to consider the option of reconstructive surgery. In a child or an adolescent, and depending on the circumstances of the primary repair, some consideration can be given to exploration of the repair and/or microneurolysis or nerve grafting. As a corollary to early tendon transfer to improve muscle coordination and sensory re-education, the author does nerve repair or nerve grafting even if the patient seeks treatment late (i.e., beyond the critical limit of delay for motor recovery) to provide an opportunity for gradual return of some protective sensation to the vital tactile areas.

Homeostasis of the involved extremity must be established before reconstructive surgery.[102,112] The vascularity of the extremity should be adequate, there should be stable skeletal alignment, and the joints should have full painless passive range of motion. Preoperative joint contractures, unless corrected, tend to worsen after tendon transfer. The power and amplitude of muscles to be transferred must be adequate. Soft tissues should be free of scar contracture, and chronic wounds should be fully settled for 3 months before surgery is performed for elective tendon transfers. While waiting, the planned supervised rehabilitation program can be coordinated with the surgical team.[6]

The appropriate use of splints, fabricated for each patient and altered or changed whenever indicated,[91,98] can help to manage claw deformity. Maintenance of the distal transverse palmar arch and the thumb-index web space with adequate lumbrical and thenar stops to obtain the functional position can be difficult.[91] Splints interfere with the rehabilitation of sensibility and are generally used intermittently. Preoperative counseling is important to help the patient understand the discipline and duration of the postoperative rehabilitation protocol. It is important to ascertain whether the patient desires increased functional performance or cosmetic improvement. Tendon transfers, tenodesis, or arthrodesis can be used in isolation or in combination,[21,23,112,137] and making judicious use of these diverse methods may strike a balance. Staged reconstruction ensures a better outcome after each surgery, especially when the surgical requirements in a patient appear elaborate. It stands to reason that the removal of functional motors, even if done in stages, will lead to residual weakness at the donor sites. Therefore, the surgeon should ensure that the patient understands that reconstructive surgery is a planned equitable redistribution of available assets. Briefing patients on the expected pattern of deformity correction and anticipated return of power will make their expectations realistic.

Ulnar Palsy Due to Leprosy

It is the propensity for nerve damage in leprosy that results in disability.[14,19,70,119] The ulnar nerve is the most common nerve to be paralyzed.[14,19,55,70] Currently, a multi-drug therapy regimen is used to arrest most forms of the disease. However, the long-term function of the nerve in leprosy is actually determined by the duration and level of nerve impairment at the commencement of definitive therapy.[50,68] Delays in diagnosis can result in permanent loss of ulnar nerve function. Recent implementation of a short, fixed-duration course of multi-drug therapy has resulted in a dramatic fall in the prevalence of leprosy; however, the incidence of new cases has yet to fall significantly and the pool of patients with potential nerve damage remains large.[138] When the bacillus infiltrates the ulnar nerve, resultant intraneural edema causes local compression within the normal anatomic boundaries of the cubital tunnel and Guyon's canal and is compounded by secondary local ischemia due to compression of perineural blood vessels. Schwann cells and axons are destroyed by a CD4$^+$ T-cell–mediated granulomatous process,[69,70,119] and postinflammatory fibrosis leads to irreversible nerve damage.[69] Historically, nerve decompression was advocated to prevent progression of nerve paralysis. Recently, this approach has been challenged by a randomized controlled trial that demonstrated that decompression of the ulnar nerve combined with medical therapy showed no additional benefit over medical therapy alone, at a follow-up after 1 or 2 years.[47] Therefore, decompression surgery for ulnar nerve involvement is now reserved for the rare situation of intraneural abscess[6] or intractable pain despite vigorous immunosuppressive therapy.

Prerequisites for reconstructive surgery on patients with ulnar nerve palsy due to leprosy include an understanding of the stage and activity of the disease, the presence of intact, healthy skin, and patient motivation.[50,55] Reconstructive surgery for leprosy is recommended when a patient's medical treatment is optimized, skin smears for the bacillus are negative, the bacteriological index is negative on two successive tests, the disease activity is quiescent for at least a year before the date of intended surgery, and the paralysis is established. Ideally, the patient should be free of corticosteroid treatment for several months before surgery. The surgeon should work in collaboration with a dermatologist/leprologist before the contemplated surgery to optimize preparation for surgery. If the patient's disease is still active and there are features of acute neuritis, the stress of surgery poses a threat for additional nerve progression in the same limb or at other sites.

In the past, afflicted individuals lacked interest in reconstructive surgery, in large part owing to inadequate or incomplete medical treatment and delayed presentation with permanent impairment.[14,19,50] Patients developed fixed compensatory substitution patterns that made it difficult to re-educate newly transferred muscles.[2,3,50] These obstacles have been considerably overcome now with educational programs, and patients wish to have earlier surgical correction for their deformity. Preoperative corrective splinting has been advised together with home physical therapy to gradually minimize severe contractures and strengthen the functioning muscles.[2,3] Periodic review to evaluate progress prepares the patient and the surgical team for the eventual surgical correction.

In ulnar nerve palsy due to leprosy, the objective of surgical reconstruction is to apply standard surgical procedures with the aim of enabling the patient to be gainfully employed and integrated into society. The paralyzed hand should be functional, and its appearance should not attract undue attention. Health education for ongoing care of the insensate hand should accompany surgical reconstruction. Early signs of infection to the fingertips and pulp must be managed urgently to prevent tissue loss.

Ulnar Nerve Palsy Due to Poliomyelitis

In paralysis secondary to poliomyelitis, the ulnar innervated lumbricals can be paralyzed, sparing a part of or the whole of the interosseous muscles or vice versa. The severity of a deformity will depend on the extent to which either of these muscle groups is paralyzed. The paralysis is typically nonprogressive and with no loss of sensation. Children are most frequently affected, and their joints are often hypermobile.[6] Surgery should be delayed until the child is at least 5 years of age, so that the child will be able to cooperate with the postoperative re-education program.

PREOPERATIVE ANGLE MEASUREMENTS

Measurements of the specific angle at the PIP joints reveal the status of the claw hand and facilitate the identification of deficiencies as well as hidden secondary problems. Five sets of angles are measured at the PIP joint of each finger and the IP joint of the thumb using a goniometer placed on the dorsal aspect of the joint.

1. *Unassisted angle.*[55,74,146] The patient is asked to maintain a "lumbrical-plus" position of MP flexion and IP exten-

sion, and the examiner measures the extension deficit at the PIP joint. This tests the ability of the intrinsic mechanism to bring about active IP extension. Patients with a greater PIP extension deficit have less likelihood of complete correction after surgery.[55]

2. *Assisted angle.*[55,74,146] The examiner supports the proximal segment of the finger to maintain flexion at the MP joint and instructs the patient to extend the IP joints (viz., Bouvier's maneuver). In the absence of a contracture of the IP joints, this angle should become 0 degrees in a paralytic claw hand. The extent to which a patient can fully extend the IP joints can be used as a prognostic indicator for tendon transfer. A finger with incomplete extension is not ideal for claw correction because the long extensors will not extend the IP joints even after the MP joint is prevented from fully extending by the procedure.

3. *Contracture angle.*[55,74,146] Incomplete passive extension should be noted as a fixed flexion contracture; and, depending on the chronicity, there may be contracture with deficiency of volar skin and contracture of the volar plate and/or the capsule of the PIP joint.

4. *Adaptive shortening angle of extrinsic flexors.*[3,6] Habitual posturing of the wrist in flexion to minimize the claw deformity can lead over time to adaptive shortening of the extrinsic flexors, characterized by an increased angulation at the PIP joint as the wrist is passively moved into extension.[2,3,6]

5. *Hypermobile angle.*[3,6] Patients with ligamentous laxity, as characterized by hypermobile joints[18,55] with passive hyperextension of the PIP joints more than 20 degrees,[3,5] should be approached with care regarding tension adjustment of transferred tendons because of the likelihood of producing an intrinsic-plus deformity in the finger.[3,18,55]

ASSOCIATED ADVERSE CONDITIONS IN CLAW HANDS

Additional adverse affects can be observed in some claw hands, and these must be identified and documented at the preoperative assessment. The management of these problems is done as an adjuvant procedure during claw correction or even at an early stage before the definitive claw correction.

1. *"Guttering" of the long extensor tendons.*[17-19,55] This refers to ulnar subluxation of the extensor tendons at the MP joints when the digits are flexed. This indicates laxity of the sagittal bands at MP joints and can be compounded by contracture of the long extensors in neglected deformities.

2. *Radioulnar deviation at the MP joint.* With digital extension, radial or ulnar deviation of the digits can occur without volar subluxation of the MP joint and can measure as much as 30 degrees. This problem has been noted also after claw hand correction by dynamic transfers.[114]

3. *Integrity of the extensor apparatus over the PIP joint.* Long-standing deformities can attenuate the central slip over the PIP joint and compromise the ability of the extensor mechanism to extend the middle phalanx. With

the MP joints passively stabilized in flexion, the PIP joint exhibits an extension lag, with a compensatory hyperextension deformity of the DIP joint via the oblique retinacular ligament. I have noted this rare combination in the dominant hands of young patients with ulnar nerve palsy who were not referred early for surgical management. In chronic cases the lateral bands subluxate volarward and impart a persistent flexion moment at the PIP joint that eventually leads to a boutonnière deformity.[17,19,55,74,146] Claw corrective surgery by tendon transfer will be unsuccessful in the presence of this deformity.[56]

4. *Reversal of the distal transverse metacarpal arch*[55,114, 117,118] (viz., Masse's sign).[46] In ulnar nerve palsy there is a relative flattening of the normal distal transverse metacarpal arch. This is best observed when the hand is viewed end on by noting the movement of the MP joints as the patient clenches the fist. I measure this arch by using a small goniometer placed with its center at the dorsum of the third MP joint level. The normal slope toward the ulnar side is approximately 20 degrees in a fully clenched fist.

CLASSIFICATION OF PARALYTIC CLAW HANDS

Based on the physiologic characteristics of hypermobility and other features[18,55] and on the chronicity and etiology of the deformity, I developed a simple classification of claw hand. By understanding the type of claw hand, the selection of the appropriate corrective procedure is more straightforward.[3]

Type I: Supple claw hands with no hypermobile joints and no contractures at the IP joints
Type II: Hypermobile joints as demonstrated by 20 degrees or more of painless passive hyperextension, measured at the PIP joints
Type III: Mobile joints in association with adaptive shortening of the long flexors, usually the superficialis tendons (myostatic contractures), with no IP joint contracture
Type IV: Contracted claw hands demonstrating PIP joint flexion contracture of 15 degrees or more, related either to the volar skin, joint capsule, or volar plate contracture and with or without adaptive shortening of long flexors
Type V: Claw hands with attrition of the dorsal extensor apparatus at the PIP joint with "hooding deformity," fibrous or bony ankylosis of the PIP joint, and MP joint extension contracture

RECONSTRUCTIVE SURGERY FOR ULNAR PALSY

The list of deformities or deficiencies in the hand that can be addressed surgically are presented in Table 33-2.

The choice of surgical procedures depends on the level of ulnar nerve injury. Each of the deficiencies can be corrected in staged surgery for proximal ulnar palsy and can be modified based on a patient's particular requirements. Attention to the first seven in the list is necessary for hands with distal ulnar nerve palsy. For paralysis of the deep branch of the ulnar nerve, selective procedures can be done excluding the

Table 33-2
DEFORMITIES AND DEFICIENCIES CORRECTABLE BY SURGERY

Claw finger

Unstable thumb (claw thumb, Z thumb)

Flattened or reversed distal transverse metacarpal arch

Loss of strong adduction of the first metacarpal

Loss of abduction of the index finger

Abnormal abduction of the little finger

Loss of sensibility in the autonomous area of the little finger

Weakness of the FDP of the ring and little fingers

Weakness of flexion in ulnar deviation of the wrist (i.e., the action of FCU)

Hollow defects/wasting of the intermetacarpal spaces (web spaces)

need for restoring the transverse metacarpal arch, providing sensibility, or improving power to the flexor digitorum profundus of the little finger (FDPL) and flexor digitorum profundus of the ring finger (FDPR).

ROLE OF PREOPERATIVE HAND THERAPY

If dynamic procedures have been planned for claw hand correction, the preoperative assisted angle should be 0 degrees. If the hand has "hooding" deformity,[17,19,55,74,146] in any of the digits with flexion angles between 30 and 60 degrees, preoperative correction of the angle can be attempted with physical therapy. Wax bath, oil massage, exercises, and various modalities of splinting are used.[16,17,19,55,74,146] For boutonnière deformity, a dynamic splint and home exercise program can be used for 6 to 8 weeks to reduce the assisted angle in preparation for tendon transfer.[2,3] For PIP joint contractures of 45 degrees or more, supervised therapy with serial static plaster splinting is indicated. If correction has reached a plateau, further efforts may be counterproductive and consideration should be given to surgical release of skin and volar plate contracture, with or without skin graft. Reconstructive surgery may be done at the time of release or in a staged fashion. Similarly, when planning dynamic tendon transfers for other deformities such as "Z" thumb and hyperabduction of the little finger, normal range of passive motion of the joints should be demonstrable and there should be no defect due to injury or stretch at the proposed site of insertion of the motor tendon.

METHODS OF CLAW HAND RECONSTRUCTION

Claw hand correction is broadly grouped into *static* and *dynamic* procedures. Static procedures are performed to maintain the MP joint in some degree of flexion or to limit MP joint hyperextension; in either case the claw posture is reversed by the functioning long extensors. Flexion of the MP joint is unrestricted in static procedures. Dynamic correction involves the transfer of a normally functioning

but dispensable motor to a predetermined location in the digit to bring about correction of deformity while introducing additional motor power to carry out specific functions that had been lost.

Proximal Phalangeal Flexion

Static Techniques

Flexor Pulley Advancement. Bunnell[33,34] performed flexor pulley advancement (partial release) as an isolated procedure to correct claw deformity. Each side of the proximal pulley system was split 1.5 to 2.5 cm up to the middle of the proximal phalanx. The flexor tendons then "bow string," to bring about flexion at the MP joint. Mechanically there is gross increase in the extrinsic flexor moment at the MP joint with corresponding increase in power of the long flexors across this joint. The procedure is not effective if there is damage to the extrinsic extensors or the dorsal apparatus of the finger.

Fasciodermadesis. Zancolli[157] described excision of 2 cm of the palmar skin (dermadesis) at the MP joint level combined with shortening of the pretendinous band of the palmar aponeurosis (fasciodermadesis) to correct claw hands with weak extensor muscles. He found the procedure insufficient to prevent recurrence of MP joint hyperextension if the extensors were normal. The disadvantages are the loss of palmar skin and a transverse scar that can stretch out and lead to recurrence of deformity.

Volar Capsulodesis. Zancolli's innovative volar MP joint capsulodesis consists of an A1 pulley release with MP joint volar plate advancement.[156] The procedure may be modified depending on the strength of the extensors and may be performed in children.

A transverse incision is made over the distal palmar crease. The A1 pulley is divided in the center along its entire length to expose the volar plate, and the flexor tendons are retracted to one side. As the retraction on the flexor tendon is continued, the volar plate is identified and incised along the longitudinal midline to create two capsular flaps, and these are next detached from the metacarpal origin. The joint is better visualized and exposed by hyperextending the proximal phalanx fully. A small transverse bone tunnel is created in the metacarpal neck with a finely pointed awl or Kirschner wire, and a monofilament wire is passed through the tunnel and both flaps of the volar plate to maintain the MP joint in 5 degrees of flexion. The limbs of the wire are twisted firmly and cut to lie flat on the bone. The position of the MP joint is tested to ascertain the adequacy of fixation. The capsuloplasty is performed sequentially from the index MP joint to the small MP joint. The retraction on the long flexors is released, and skin closure is completed. Soft gauze dressings are placed in the interdigital intervals, and the palm and soft-roll gauze is applied all around. A cast or splint is applied to maintain the wrist in neutral position, the MP joints are in 20 degrees flexion, and the IP joints are left free. Postoperatively, the cast is retained for 5 weeks and then re-education is commenced.

For complicated claw hands that had MP joint contracture Zancolli incorporated collateral ligament release on both sides of the MP joint with the volar capsuloplasty. In this combined procedure the MP joints were maintained in 20 degrees of flexion during the capsuloplasty and the postoperative immobilization of the MP joints was in 45 degrees of flexion.

Omer advanced the volar plate by cutting away a triangular portion of the deep transverse metacarpal ligament (DTML) on each side of the volar plate flap[99] (Fig. 33-1). A 1.5-cm-wide ellipse of palmar skin was excised to prevent stretching of the volar plate,[29] and postoperative immobilization was maintained for 6 weeks. [77]

This procedure spares available motors for the restoration of other important dynamic functions.

There is some restriction of the lateral mobility of the fingers, and grip strength is not augmented as it is in dynamic transfers.[156] Flexion contracture can result if the volar plate is advanced too far proximally on the metacarpal or the pulley release is continued beyond the A1 pulley. Long-term follow-up studies have demonstrated recurrence of clawing in some patients.[29]

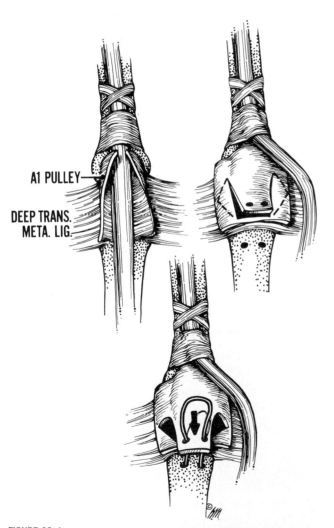

FIGURE 33-1. Capsulodesis of the MP joint in static correction of claw finger deformity. Excision of triangular segments of the deep transverse metacarpal ligament on either side allows the flap of volar plate to be proximally advanced in a straight line. The volar plate is anchored into the metacarpal neck.

 # Author's Preferred Method of Treatment

I release the volar plate in a parallel fashion as suggested by Omer[99] but avoid excising a triangular portion of the DTML. I position the MP joint in 10 to 15 degrees of flexion and score the volar aspect of the neck of the metacarpal before anchoring the volar plate through the bone with a nonabsorbable suture. The MP joints are positioned in 30 to 45 degrees of flexion in a well-padded circumferential cast for 4 weeks. The patient is allowed to move his or her IP joints as comfort permits from the second or third postoperative day. After the plaster is removed at 4 weeks the patient is provided with a knuckle bender splint to be used for an additional 4 to 6 weeks.

I have found this procedure useful in patients who do not have sufficient strength of the usual transferable motors (MRC grade V) and in patients with postpolio residual paralysis of the intrinsic muscles who lack strong extrinsic muscle power (Fig. 33-2). I have not found this procedure beneficial in patients with leprosy whose insensate hands do not stand up to the strain of the continuous stretch that they place on their digits. Recurrence within a year is often seen with flattening of the transverse metacarpal arch. These and other static procedures are not ideal for those engaged in heavy manual labor in the factory, farm, or fields.

Dorsal Methods (Howard[34]; Mikhail[90]). There are two methods under this group designed to provide a bony block to proximal phalangeal extension. This enables the long extensors to extend the IP joints and correct the deformity.

Mikhail inserted a bone block on the dorsum of the metacarpal head and reported on six patients monitored for up to 4 years.[90] Howard suggested an elevation of a bone wedge as a block from the dorsal aspect of the metacarpal head itself.[34]

I do the metacarpal head dorsal bone block procedure for a long established paralytic hand with absent intrinsic muscle function and weak extrinsic muscles. Because the patients also have associated MP joint extension contracture, a dorsal MP joint capsulotomy and unilateral collateral ligament release is done before the dorsal bone block procedure. This helps the patient to overcome the claw deformity while leaving the existing long flexor/extensor muscle balance undisturbed.

Static Tenodesis Techniques (Parkes[115]; Riordan[120-122])

Riordan Static Tenodesis (Dorsal Side)—Without Additional Tendon Grafts. One half of the normally functioning extensor carpi radialis longus (ECRL) and extensor carpi ulnaris (ECU) tendons are made use of as "grafts" to prevent hyperextension of the MP joint while the remaining half continue to actively extend the wrist. The ECRL and ECU tendons are split in the middle through their length, and one half is divided transversely at the junction of the middle and distal thirds of the forearm. The divided halves are turned distally, leaving their insertions at the dorsal base of the metacarpals undisturbed. These two halves are further split longitudinally to yield a total of four slips. The lateral bands of the dorsal extensor apparatus are exposed on the

CRITICAL POINTS: MODIFIED MP JOINT VOLAR CAPSULODESIS

INDICATION

- Intrinsic paralysis in residual poliomyelitis
- Probably for late post-traumatic ulnar palsy without contractures at the PIP joint

PEARLS

- Ensure there is no lag or contracture at the PIP joint
- Reasonably strong long flexor and extensor extrinsic muscles

TECHNICAL POINTS

- Release only the A1 pulley.
- Make two parallel incisions on the volar plate and capsule 6 to 8 mm apart.
- Raise a distally based flap of volar plate and capsule.
- Create a transverse bone tunnel at the neck of the metacarpal.

- Advance the volar plate/capsular flap sufficiently to flex the MP joint 10 to 15 degrees.
- Anchor the flap through the bone tunnel with a nonabsorbable suture.
- Immobilize with the MP joints in 40 to 45 degrees of flexion.
- Allow movement of IP joints from the second to third postoperative day.
- Remove cast after 4 weeks.
- Provide a knuckle bender splint for a minimum of 6 weeks thereafter.

PITFALL

- Ensure that the thick portion of the volar plate/capsule combination is anchored to the neck of the metacarpal.

LATE POSTOPERATIVE PRECAUTION

- Avoid passive stretching of the MP joint.

---

radial side of the proximal base of each finger through separate skin incisions. Each slip is passed into the lumbrical canal remaining volar to the DTML to emerge radial to the respective metacarpals and go on to the radial lateral band of the corresponding finger. The tenodesis is sutured with the wrist in 30 degrees of dorsiflexion and the MP joints in 80 degrees of flexion. The ECU can be used in isolation if only the ring and little fingers are involved.

Parkes Static Tenodesis (Volar Side)—With Free Tendon Grafts (Fig. 33-3A). Two free tendon grafts, from the plantaris tendon, the palmaris tendon, or toe extensors, are required for four fingers to be corrected. In the proximal segments of each finger the radial side of the dorsal extensor expansion (DEE) is exposed through midlateral incisions that are curved slightly dorsally at the level of the PIP joint. Parkes advised scarifying the superficial surfaces of the DEE at the site of attachment. A palmar incision is made in the shape of a "7" with its transverse limb located at the distal palmar crease. The palmar skin and aponeurosis are reflected together to expose the lumbrical muscles. The lumbrical sheaths are opened, and segments of grafts are tunneled distally to the corresponding finger incision. The distal step of the operation is completed first by suturing the grafts to the

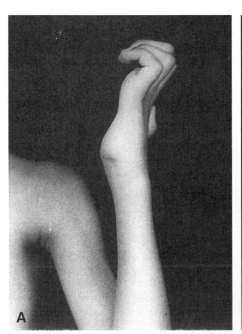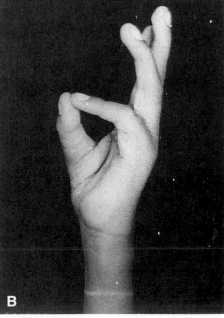

FIGURE 33-2. **A,** Claw hand due to residual poliomyelitis in a 14-year old with hypermobile joints and decreased strength of the extrinsic flexors and extensors. **B,** Volar capsulodesis with good correction of claw hand deformity at a 3-year follow-up.

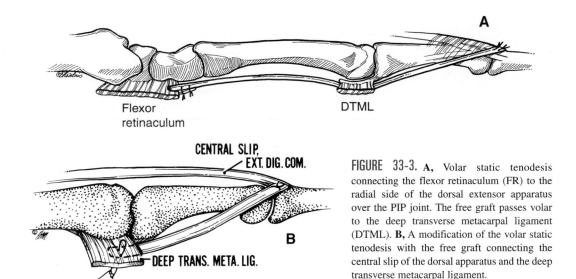

FIGURE 33-3. A, Volar static tenodesis connecting the flexor retinaculum (FR) to the radial side of the dorsal extensor apparatus over the PIP joint. The free graft passes volar to the deep transverse metacarpal ligament (DTML). **B,** A modification of the volar static tenodesis with the free graft connecting the central slip of the dorsal apparatus and the deep transverse metacarpal ligament.

lateral bands in each finger with a nonabsorbable suture followed by skin closure. Next the proximal part of the palmar incision is retracted to expose the flexor retinaculum and the proximal end of each graft is passed through the retinaculum. With the IP joints in full extension, the tension on the grafts is adjusted by maintaining the MP joints in gently increasing degrees of flexion (index: 30 degrees; little: 45 degrees). Hemostasis is secured, and the hand is immobilized in the "intrinsic-plus" position.

This is a predictable static tenodesis procedure that corrects the claw deformity, allowing the grafts to function independently on each finger with their tensions unaffected by movements of the wrist. As in all tenodesis procedures, some degree of flexion at the IP joints will take place before active flexion of the MP joints during grip, as a residual claw hand pattern of closure.

Omer modified Parkes' procedure to obtain equivalent tension between adjacent fingers and minimize the length of tendon graft. In this modification, the tendon graft is first attached to the ulnar dorsal band of the ring finger and then passed around the DTML before suturing it to the radial dorsal band of the little finger (see Fig. 33-3B). A similar tenodesis is done with the index and long fingers. I have no experience with this latter modification.

The disadvantages of all static procedures are that they will restore normal finger coordination and sequence and do not provide an additional motor to restore MP flexion. Recurrence is the rule unless there is a radical change in the patient's work style and the paralyzed hand is more protected than used. Metacarpal arch reversal can in due course become troublesome.

Integration of Finger Flexion

Wrist Tenodesis Technique (Fowler[53,120])
In 1946, Fowler reported a simple dynamic tenodesis to control claw hand deformity that preceded the other static procedures. The procedure incorporates active wrist motion to tension static tendon grafts. Free tendon grafts are sutured to the extensor retinaculum of the wrist and passed in a

dorsal to palmar direction through the intermetacarpal spaces, volar to the DTML, through the lumbrical canals, and onto the lateral bands of the dorsal extensor expansion of the four fingers (Fig. 33-4). The grafts were tensioned with the wrist in 30 degrees of dorsiflexion, the MP joints in 80 degrees of flexion, and the IP joints in full extension.

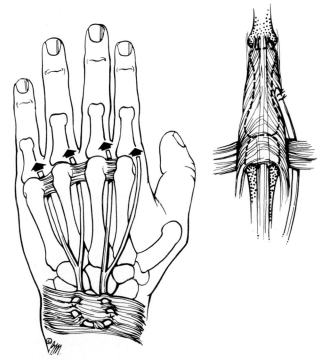

FIGURE 33-4. Dynamic dorsal tenodesis to control claw finger deformity. The free tendon graft is attached to the central part of the extensor retinaculum, and four individual strips are passed in a dorsal to palmar direction through the intermetacarpal spaces to remain volar to the deep transverse metacarpal ligament and through the lumbrical canal to be inserted into the lateral bands of the dorsal extensor expansion of the fingers.

This wrist-powered tenodesis was effective only when the patient flexed the wrist to tighten the graft and produce active MP flexion with IP joint extension.

A modification of Fowler's tenodesis has been described for the proximal attachment of the graft to the distal radius through drill holes.[148]

Disadvantages. As the tenodesis tension loosens with time, the deformity may begin to recur. To achieve simultaneous MP flexion and IP joint extension, increasing amounts of wrist flexion are required, and this may lead to adaptive shortening or myostatic contracture of the extrinsic flexors of the fingers.

Dynamic Tendon Transfers

The transfer of normally functioning muscle tendon units for ulnar palsy was first reported by Sir Harold Stiles and Forrester-Brown in 1922.[141] By passing the tendon graft slips volar to the deep transverse metacarpal ligament and into the lateral band of the dorsal extensor apparatus, the procedure was designed to improve synchronous motion of the finger joints and duplicate lumbrical muscle action.[14,33,53,82,120,133,137]

The procedure was subsequently modified with the description of different insertions, including the proximal phalanx,[23,26] the pulley system,[3,28,123,157] and the interosseous tendons.[3,114,158] Other variations focused on correcting the abduction posture of the index and middle fingers[158] and the reversed transverse metacarpal arch,[3,114] preventing swan neck deformity,[3,4,18,55,98,114] and improving coordination of finger closure.[3,114]

Zancolli[157] studied the flexion moment arm of structures coursing volar to the MP joint and showed that a tendon slip that was attached to or passed via the flexor pulley system would exert a greater flexion force than a tendon graft that passed nearer to the center of the MP joint through the lumbrical canal. The flexor moment was the least for interosseous tendons.

Transfer of Extrinsic Finger Flexors

Superficialis Tendon Transfer Techniques and Modifications (Stiles[141]; Bunnell[17,33]; Littler[82])

Sir Harold Stiles and Forrester-Brown (1922) reported the first clinical application of tendon transfer for correction of intrinsic paralysis in two patients, by transferring one slip of each superficialis tendon into the corresponding extensor digitorum tendon over the proximal phalanx.

Bunnell (1942) popularized the Stiles' superficialis tendon transfer by rerouting both slips of all superficialis tendons through the lumbrical canals and anchored them to both sides of the lateral band of the dorsal extensor expansion (*Stiles-Bunnell procedure*). The complex transfer involved passage of:

- The split superficialis of index finger (FDSI) for the radial side of the lateral bands of the index and middle fingers
- The split superficialis of the middle finger (FDSM) for the ulnar side lateral band of the index, middle, and ring fingers
- The split superficialis of the ring finger (FDSR) to the radial side of ring and little fingers

- The split superficialis of the little finger (FDSL) to the ulnar side of the little finger

Bunnell's aim was twofold: to bring about claw correction as well as the much needed abduction and adduction of the paralyzed fingers. The latter ingenious idea had not previously been addressed by a tendon transfer procedure. The Stiles-Bunnell operation, however, was beset with problems resulting from the complexity and adhesion potential of crisscrossing tendon grafts, as well as the loss of a powerful motor from the digits and the potential for excessive force and intrinsic plus deformities of the fingers.[17,155]

Littler, in 1949,[82] proposed an important modification of the Stiles-Bunnell procedure by using only the long finger superficialis tendon (FDSM). This became the standard technique and was referred to as the modified Stiles-Bunnell procedure. The FDSM is detached through an incision on the lateral side of the middle finger at the PIP joint level. The distal end of the tendon is retrieved through a palmar incision and split lengthwise into four equal slips for use in the four fingers. The routing and distal attachment (reinsertion) of the tendon slips remained the same, that is, through the lumbrical canal of each finger volar to the deep transverse metacarpal ligament and into the radial lateral band of the dorsal apparatus (Fig. 33-5A). Each slip was sutured with the wrist in 30 degrees of palmar flexion, the MP joints in 80 to 90 degrees of flexion, and the IP joints in full extension (0 degrees). The use of the ring finger superficialis tendon for this procedure is contraindicated in proximal ulnar nerve palsy or when the profundus of the ring finger is weak.

Disadvantages. PIP flexion contractures and DIP extension lag have been documented in the donor finger,[17,26,38,118] most frequently when the superficialis was removed through a conventional midlateral approach.[17,26,118] The midlateral approach exposed the distal part of the lateral band to injury and contributed to DIP extension lag.[4] Brand's long-term follow-up studies[17] has shown a high incidence of swan neck deformity in one or more of the operated fingers owing to excessive tension on the transferred tendon slip. The complication was particularly troublesome in hands with ligamentous laxity and hypermobile joints.[17,55] A "superficialis-minus" deformity has also been reported to occur after removal of the superficialis from a finger.[143] Loss of PIP joint flexion has been attributed to adhesions between the profundus and superficialis tendon remnant[17,26,55] and is more pronounced in fingers with a weak profundus tendon.

To prevent these complications, North and Littler recommend removal of the superficialis through a volar incision between the A1 and A2 pulleys.[98] The removal of the FDS through a volar skin incision and sectioning between A2 and C1 pulleys has reduced the DIP joint extension lag and PIP joint flexion contracture.[4] Tendon transfers using the superficialis transfers do not result in increased gross grip strength.[64,65] The procedure will have a better long-term result in deformity correction when the tendon slips are sutured under correct tension, that is, with the wrist in neutral flexion-extension, MP joints in 45 to 55 degrees of flexion, and the IP joints in neutral position. In contracted claw hands that had preoperative physiotherapy, this

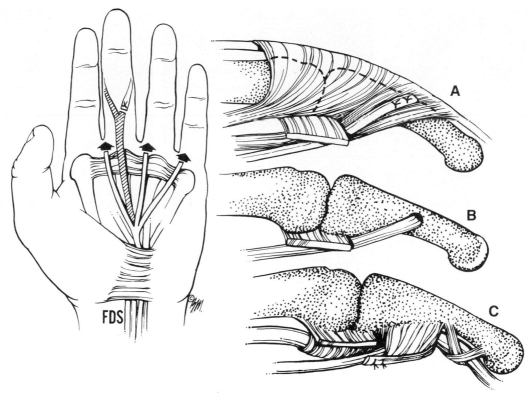

FIGURE 33-5. Transfer of flexor digitorum superficialis to correct claw deformity. Half of the distal tendon of the donor tendon is tenodesed across the PIP joint to prevent hyperextension. The FDS is split into four tails, passed volar to the deep transverse metacarpal ligament and anchored either to (**A**) the lateral band of the dorsal apparatus or (**B**) the proximal phalanx or (**C**) the A2 pulley or the extended A1 and A2a pulley insertion.

procedure enables the superficialis slips to exert a continued corrective force and prevent recurrence.[2,3]

Brand[18,20] believes that ulnar nerve palsy results in claw deformities in all four fingers, although this may be apparent in the index and middle fingers only during power pinch. Weakness is not limited only to the fingers with obvious clawing.[38,64] Therefore, the recommendation is that surgery be done in all fingers of a claw hand.[19,20,38,64]

Studies on the single superficialis transfer to the lateral band insertion on 20 contracted claw hands (type IV) in treated leprosy patients with ulnar nerve palsy revealed excellent and good results of claw correction in 95% of the fingers at an average follow-up of 2 years[3] (Fig. 33-6). The outcome of this procedure with removal of the tendon through the lateral route for transfer to the lateral band studied on 200 hands selected by systematic sampling showed satisfactory results in 95% of claw hands.[143]

Modifications in Insertion of the Superficialis Transfer (Burkhalter[35,39]; Zancolli[99,157])

Based on the premise that the FDS transfers can provide adequate integration of MP and IP motion, the concept of varying its insertion to enhance these functions and to keep the secondary effects to a minimum came about. The four primary insertion sites are classified as:

A. Lateral band insertion—intrinsic replacement (Stiles and Forrester-Brown [1922], Bunnell [1942], Littler [1949], Brand [1952], Riordan [1953], Lennox-Fritschi [1971])
B. Phalangeal insertion (Burkhalter [1974])

C. Pulley insertion (Riordan [1969], Zancolli [1979], Brooks and Jones [1975], Anderson [1988])
D. Interosseous insertion (Zancolli [1979], Palande [1983], Anderson [1988])

Phalangeal Insertion (Burkhalter[35,39]). Burkhalter recommended insertion of the superficialis tendon slips directly to the proximal phalanx in patients with ulnar nerve palsy due to trauma (see Fig. 33-5B). The aim was to avoid the risk of PIP joint hyperextension noted with transfers to the lateral band of the dorsal apparatus.

Pulley Insertions (Zancolli's "Lasso"[99,157]). Riordan (1969)[123] was probably the first to suggest that the tendon slip be inserted into the annular pulley of the flexor tendon sheath if the patient has a normally hyperextensible IP joint.

However, Zancolli preferred to loop the tendon slip beneath the entire A1 pulley and termed the procedure the *lasso technique.* He delineated the A1 pulleys through a transverse skin incision at the level of the distal palmar crease. The flexor superficialis tendon is sectioned in the finger and divided into two slips. Each tendon slip is retained volar to the deep transverse metacarpal ligament and looped through the A1 proximal pulley and sutured to itself.

Interosseous Insertions (Zancolli[158]; Palande[114]; Anderson[3]). The interosseous tendons were used as insertion sites with different motors: a superficialis tendon,[3,154] ECRL,[114] or palmaris longus.[3,114] Zancolli[158] described the

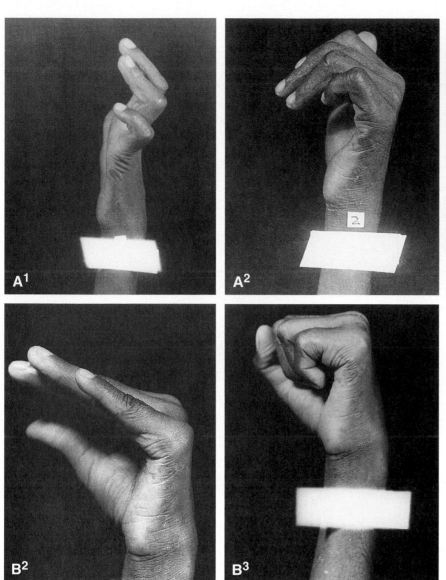

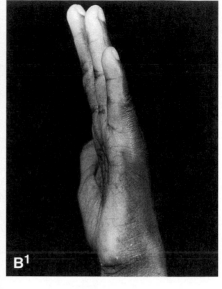

FIGURE 33-6. Type IV claw hand in proximal ulnar palsy seen at 2 years. **A1** and **A2,** Clawing of all four fingers with contractures and excessive unassisted angles at the PIP joints of all fingers. Preoperative physiotherapy was followed by transfer of a single superficialis tendon split into four tails to the lateral bands of extensor apparatus (modified Stiles-Bunnell procedure). **B1 to B3,** Results of claw correction in the outstretched hand, lumbrical position, and full closure as seen at a 4-year follow-up.

use of the first and second dorsal interosseous as insertion sites to attach slips of a superficialis tendon with the goal of obtaining proximal phalangeal flexion and restore digital abduction. He termed this procedure *direct interosseous activation.* Palande[114] extended this principle to correct intrinsic-minus hands associated with reversal of the transverse metacarpal arch.

Modification of the Pulley Insertion Using FDS. Omer preferred the use of the A2 pulley as the insertion site instead of the A1 pulley (see Fig. 33-5C) to improve the mechanics of MP flexion. The tendon is tensioned with the forearm supinated and wrist kept flat on the table with MP joints in 45 degrees of flexion. Transfers for the little finger are intentionally tightened in excess of that required for the ring finger because failure to correct claw deformity was seen to occur most often in the little finger.[44] Good deformity correction was reported in a small number of hands when used for ring and little finger claw correction.[128]

Anderson[3] performs an extended pulley insertion (EPI) by looping a slip of the superficialis tendon around both the A1 and proximal A2 pulleys (Fig. 33-7) in each finger.

The EPI technique provides a better hold for primary flexor function of the proximal phalanx. It demonstrates less tendency for attenuation and avoids the possibility of exaggerating the flexor moment when the whole length of A2 pulley alone is used.[89]

Description of the EPI Procedure (Anderson, 1988). The middle finger superficialis is sectioned between C1 and A2 pulleys through an oblique incision in the finger.[3] A small transverse incision is made in the mid palm, and the tendon is retrieved and split lengthwise into four tails. A transverse palmar incision is made between the distal palmar crease and the palmar-digital crease across the palm. The pulley system is identified from the A1 proximal edge to the A2 distal edge on each digit. With a curved hemostat the ends of the slips of the FDSM are routed sequentially beneath the bridge of intervening palmar skin and volar to the DTML through the lumbrical canals of each finger. A custom right-angled mosquito hemostat or baby Mixter clamp is used to pass each slip beneath the A1 and A2 pulleys until a "palpable" dent is felt just beyond the A2a distal margin. Each tendon end is inserted through the flexor sheath and

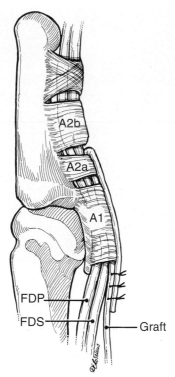

FIGURE 33-7. Technique of extended pulley insertion using A1 and A2a pulleys. A slip of the flexor superficialis tendon is passed under A1 as far as the distal end of the A2a pulley; the slip is folded back and sutured to itself.

retrieved with a straight clamp. The wrist is positioned in neutral and the MP joints in 60 degrees of flexion, and the tendon slips are folded back and sutured to themselves. The hand and wrist are immobilized to the level of the PIP joint, with the wrist in 10 degrees of flexion and the MP joints in full flexion. The patient is encouraged to mobilize the IP joints as comfort permits. The cast is removed after 3 weeks and muscle re-education is begun. After the initial 4 weeks of therapy the patient is allowed to use the hand with a knuckle bender splint for 6 to 8 weeks and advanced to routine activities and vocation thereafter.

In 20 hands with features of adaptive shortening of the long flexors (type IV claw hands), the procedure gave excellent and good results of claw correction in 92% of the fingers (Fig. 33-8). Patients averaged a 10-degree MP joint flexion contracture but had no impairment of vocational activities.[3] Because of the strong flexion moment, the procedure may not be ideally suited for patients with hypermobile joints (i.e., type II claw hands), nor is it ideal for contracted hands (type IV), unless the contractures have been completely corrected by hand physiotherapy. The theoretical possibility of a trigger finger developing in a digit because of addition to the contents of the flexor sheath has not occurred.

Finger Level Extensor Motor

Extensor Indicis Proprius and Extensor Digiti Minimi Transfer and Modification (Fowler[53,122]; Riordan[120,121,136,137])

Fowler originally described the technique[53,122] of using the extensor indicis proprius (EIP) and the extensor digiti minimi (EDM) tendons as transfers to the lateral bands of the dorsal apparatus. Longitudinal or small curved incisions are made on the dorsal aspect of the second and fifth MP joints and the EIP and EDM are sectioned at the joint level. A transverse incision is made just distal to the wrist, and the two tendons are retrieved through the incision and split lengthwise into two. The four slips are tunneled subcutaneously to the dorsal apparatus of the radial side of the fingers and sutured at this site.

This procedure may produce excessive tension in the extensor apparatus and lead to intrinsic-plus deformities. It may also cause reversal of the normal metacarpal arch and, occasionally, extensor weakness in the little finger; thus, the procedure has been abandoned by some surgeons.[53]

Modification I. Riordan[89,90,102,103] modified the procedure by splitting the EIP into two slips and transferring them through the intermetacarpal space between the ring and little digits. The tendon slips were routed palmar to the transverse metacarpal ligament and onto the radial lateral bands of the ring and little fingers. If there was a combined median nerve

---

CRITICAL POINTS: EXTENDED PULLEY INSERTION PROCEDURE FOR CLAW CORRECTION

INDICATIONS

- Type III claw hand
- Type IV claw hand with release of contractures and preoperative corrective splinting

PEARLS

- "Palpable" dent in the A2 pulley system just at the distal end of the A2a pulley

TECHNICAL POINTS

- Section the FDSM tendon proximal to C1 pulley in the long finger.
- Make a transverse palmar incision distal to the distal palmar crease.

- Retrieve the FDSM through midpalmar incision and split into four tails.
- Reroute the tails through lumbrical canal volar to the DTML.
- Pass one slip at a time into the pulley system with a fine right-angled mosquito hemostat.
- Pass each tendon slip through palpable "dent" distal to A2a pulley.
- Suture the tendon slip to itself with MP joints in 60 degrees of flexion.
- Immobilize the wrist in 10 degrees of flexion, with MP joints fully flexed and IP joints free.
- Begin transfer training at 3 to 4 weeks; use knuckle bender splint for 6 to 8 weeks.

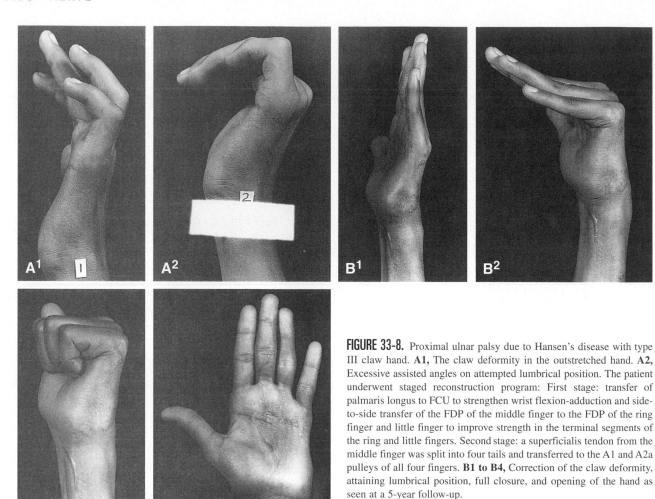

FIGURE 33-8. Proximal ulnar palsy due to Hansen's disease with type III claw hand. **A1,** The claw deformity in the outstretched hand. **A2,** Excessive assisted angles on attempted lumbrical position. The patient underwent staged reconstruction program: First stage: transfer of palmaris longus to FCU to strengthen wrist flexion-adduction and side-to-side transfer of the FDP of the middle finger to the FDP of the ring finger and little finger to improve strength in the terminal segments of the ring and little fingers. Second stage: a superficialis tendon from the middle finger was split into four tails and transferred to the A1 and A2a pulleys of all four fingers. **B1 to B4,** Correction of the claw deformity, attaining lumbrical position, full closure, and opening of the hand as seen at a 5-year follow-up.

palsy, he attached a free tendon graft onto this common motor and directed the tendon slips to the radial lateral band of the long and index fingers as well.

Author's Modification. I harvest additional length of both the EIP and the EDM by incising an additional length of about 1 cm of the extensor apparatus at the MP joint in line with the tendons but not beyond the capsule of the joint. The extensor apparatus is tightly closed with a running monofilament suture. This technique solves the relative deficiency in length of these tendons that occurs when they are transferred from the dorsal to the volar side. Incisions are made on the dorsoradial aspects of the little to middle fingers and the dorsoulnar aspect of the index finger to expose the lateral bands of the dorsal extensor apparatus. A tendon passer can be used to sequentially deliver the tendon slips from the dorsal incisions into the lumbrical canal and volar to the DTML. With the wrist in 45 degrees of extension, the MP joint in 60 degrees of flexion, and the IP joints straight, each tendon slip is sutured to the lateral bands of the dorsal extensor apparatus.

The modified Fowler procedure has a limited role in the management of claw deformities, particularly when there is extensive scarring on the flexor side of the distal forearm or palm. The metacarpal arch is not improved with this operation, and this transfer does not add appreciable grip strength.

Wrist-Level Motors for Proximal Phalanx Power and Integration of Finger Flexion (Brand[15,18]; Burkhalter[35,39]; Brooks[28]; Fowler[49,91]; Riordan[49,120-124])

To simultaneously correct the claw deformity and gain grip strength, it is necessary to add an additional muscle-tendon unit to the power train for flexion of the proximal phalanx. This is best achieved by transferring a wrist motor or the brachioradialis to flex the proximal phalanges.

All wrist motors require free grafts to provide sufficient length to reach the insertion site. Available donor grafts include the plantaris, palmaris, fascia lata, or toe extensors. The incidence of absence of the palmaris longus tendon is in the range of 11% to 14% of individuals, and the plantaris is absent in 8% to 19%.[63] Ultrasound has a sensitivity of 95% for detecting a plantaris tendon suitable for grafting.[130]

Dorsal Route Transfer of ECRB (Brand[15]) (Fig. 33-9). Brand described a technique to transfer a wrist extensor through a dorsal route to the lateral band of the extensor expansion (EE4T procedure: extensor tendon, extensor route, four-tailed graft).[15] The extensor carpi radialis brevis or longus (ECRL or ECRB) was lengthened by a plantaris

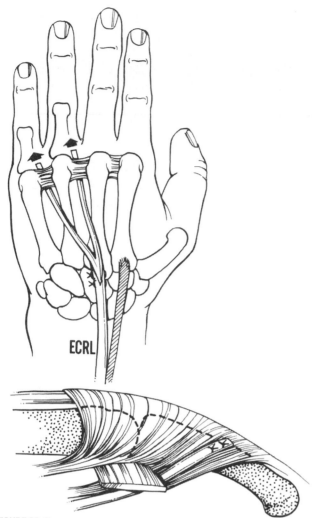

FIGURE 33-9. Increased strength of proximal phalangeal flexion is obtained by transfer of the ECRL or lengthened brachioradialis with a free graft. The slips are taken through the dorsal route and passed volar to the deep transverse metacarpal ligament and through the lumbrical canals to be inserted to the lateral bands of the dorsal extensor expansion.

tendon that was split into four tails. The tendon slips were passed through the intermetacarpal spaces, into the lumbrical canal and palmar to the DTML, to be attached to the radial lateral bands of the long, ring, and little fingers and the ulnar lateral band of the index finger. This method shared the disadvantages of the EIP transfer in that it did not improve the flattened transverse metacarpal arch or the weakness of grip. This procedure was superseded by the extensor to flexor route transfer (see later).

Riordan's Flexor Carpi Radialis Transfer. Riordan[120,121] elongated the flexor carpi radialis (FCR) with a brachioradialis, plantaris, or palmaris longus free graft and passed it from the flexor to the extensor side of the forearm. The slips were routed in a similar fashion to the radial lateral bands of the involved fingers. The transfer was intended to simultaneously correct the wrist flexion deformity that is seen among patients who habitually use a wrist tenodesis maneuver to attempt to extend their clawed fingers. The operation, however, removes the only wrist flexor in a proximal ulnar

palsy, and this may be detrimental to wrist stability and positioning.

Flexor Route Transfer of ECRL (Brand[18]) (Fig. 33-10). Brand introduced another modification of the procedure by recommending passage of a dorsal tendon graft to the flexor side through the carpal tunnel (EF4T procedure: extensor tendon, flexor route, four-tailed graft).[18] The ECRL tendon was preferred over the ECRB as the motor. A transverse incision is made over the second metacarpal base, and the insertion of the ECRL is divided (Fig 33-10A). A second transverse incision is made on the dorsoradial aspect of the forearm 8 to 10 cm proximal to the radial styloid, and the ECRL is retrieved into the wound. The tendon is lengthened by a suitable tendon graft using a weaving technique to invaginate the cut edges (Fig. 33-10B).

CRITICAL POINTS: BRAND'S WRAPAROUND TECHNIQUE FOR LENGTHENING ECRL TENDON WITH FREE GRAFT

FREE GRAFT

- Palmaris longus tendon
- Plantaris tendon
- Fascia lata
- One tendon slip of extensor digitorum of the foot

TECHNICAL POINTS (See Fig. 33-10)

- Make a longitudinal incision on the ECRL tendon 2 cm proximal to its end for up to half its thickness.
- Hold the incised edges with two fine hemostats and gently pull them apart to create a spindle-shaped segment on the ECRL tendon.
- Incise the center of this spindle-shaped portion with a No. 15 scalpel blade.
- Pull one end of the free graft proximally through the ECRL and anchor it to the "floor" of the spread using three sutures with fine monofilament material.
- Invaginate cut edges of ECRL over free graft with a running stitch using the same suture material.
- Repeat the above steps by next spreading the free graft at the level of the distal end of ECRL.
- Suture the ECRL to the "floor" of the free graft and invaginate the free graft over ECRL tendon.
- The ends of the ECRL and the free graft will now be completely covered.
- Gentle pull on the ECRL–free graft combination can ascertain the strength and adequacy of the anastomosis.

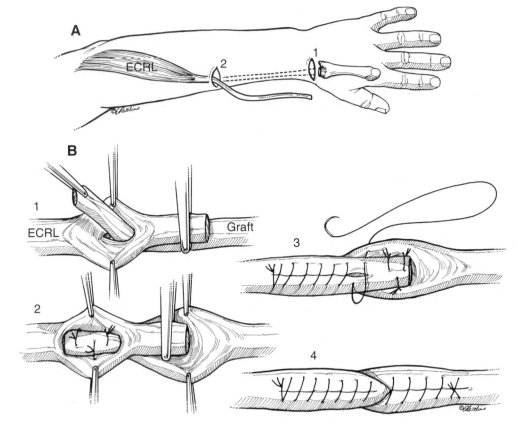

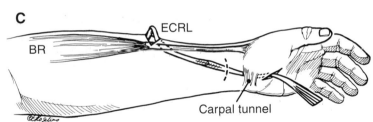

C

BR

ECRL

Carpal tunnel

FIGURE 33-10. Transfer of ECRL tendon for claw hand correction. **A,** Sectioning of the ECRL at its insertion to the base of the second metacarpal (1) and another incision (2) for retrieval of the tendon proximally in the forearm. **B,** The wraparound anastomosis of the ECRL with free graft (see text for steps of this technique). **C,** A tendon passer is passed from a midpalmar incision, through the carpal tunnel and into the forearm incision under the brachioradialis to retrieve the lengthened ECRL tendon and complete the transfer to the lateral bands.

Next an incision is made in the midpalmar region along the thenar crease, and the palmar fascia is separated to expose the superficial palmar arch. A long tendon retriever is passed dorsal to the palmar arch and through the carpal tunnel toward the dorsoradial incision in the forearm (Fig. 33-10C). The distal end of the lengthened ECRL is retrieved into the midpalmar incision. Here the graft is split into four tails, and each tail is passed in a similar fashion along the lumbrical canal and into separate incisions at the base of the index through small digits. The wounds on the wrist, forearm, and palm are closed before tensioning the graft. With the wrist positioned in 30 degrees of flexion, the MP joints in 60 degrees of flexion, and the IP joints straight[3,6,55] the graft slips are then sutured to the lateral band of the dorsal extensor expansion, taking care that the four tails have equal tension.

The tourniquet is released and hemostasis is secured before skin closure. The skin incisions are closed with a continuous monofilament suture, so that they may be retained for the entire 3-week immobilization period. The hand is placed in a well-padded plaster cast with the wrist in neutral position, the MP joints in 80 degrees of flexion, and the IP joints straight.

CRITICAL POINTS: TENSIONING THE FOUR TAILS OF A WRIST-LEVEL MOTOR

1. First tension the index finger to take up the slack and suture to the lateral band.
2. Next tension the small finger tendon slip to take up the slack, and advance an additional 6 mm before suturing.
3. Lastly, suture the ring and middle slips with no additional tension.
4. Maintain IP joints in full extension during tensioning.

 ## Author's Preferred Method of Treatment

Approximately 2 cm of the distal end of the ECRL is excised so that the junction of tendon and free graft stays well proximal to the carpal tunnel. I make an additional transverse incision just proximal to the wrist crease to pilot the tendon passer deep to all the flexors as advised by Brand to avoid injury to vital structures. With the hand and wrist in proper position, I grasp the most proximal edge of the lateral band with a mosquito clamp (Fig. 33-11) and gently apply traction to remove the slack from the extensor expansion and maintain the IP joints in full extension. An assistant holds this position while the graft slips are sutured to the lateral bands.[6]

While several methods of tension adjustment have been described,[18,55,114,145] no method can perfectly compensate for the altered viscoelastic properties of the donor muscle-tendon units under anesthesia, and each is aided by the donor muscle's ability to compensate for moderate changes in its length-tension relationship. In one study it was suggested that passive tension to guide intraoperative decision may result in overstretch of the muscle-tendon unit and lead to low active force generation.[54] Therefore, there has been an effort to provide the surgeon with a reliable method for predicting the functional effect of tendon transfer by measuring the intraoperative sarcomere length combined with the information on the biomechanical modeling generated from normative values of the muscle architecture, tendon compliance, and joint moment.[80] This may well be the future direction if the last factor is standardized for all extrinsic muscles used as transfers. I favor the tried and tested method of Brand[18] and Fritschi[55] with simple tension adjustment technique on a positioning frame and the manual removal of slack at the dorsal apparatus.[6]

A study of the EF4T procedure done on 32 type I hands (no preoperative contractures) showed fair to good correction in both appearance and adequacy of attaining lumbrical position in 92% of the hands at a 2-year follow-up.[114] In a longer follow-up study of 10 years, in two cohorts of 20 type II (hypermobile) and type IV (contracted) hands, 79% maintained excellent or good correction.[3] In type III hands (adaptive shortening of the long flexors), the procedure resulted in good-to-excellent correction in 86% of the fingers at a 10-year follow-up study[3] (Fig. 33-12).

Disadvantages. The need for a free tendon or fascia lata graft to lengthen the wrist extensor motor unit can result in adhesions, and meticulous technique is required to pass the graft dorsal to contents of the carpal canal to avoid injury.[18,25] The multiple steps of the EF4T procedure require increased operative time. A postoperative physiotherapy program is a necessity, because re-education of extensor motors for claw correction is more difficult than that for flexor motors.[18] No increased incidence of median nerve compromise was noted in a long-term study comparing tendon grafts passed within and outside of the carpal tunnel in cured leprosy patients.[25]

Modifications in the Volar Route Transfer

ECRL Volar Transfer With Proximal Phalanx Insertion (Burkhalter and Strait[39]). Burkhalter and Strait modified the Brand extensor route (EE4T) transfer (1954)[15] by correcting only the ring and small digits and by inserting the tendon slips into transosseous tunnels at the base of the respective proximal phalanges. The ECRL is lengthened with a split tendon graft and passed through the third and fourth intermetacarpal spaces. It is important to remove enough intermetacarpal fascia to minimize adhesions of the tendons. At the finger, each tendon slip is passed through a transverse drill hole in the respective phalanx and held with a pull-out suture technique. Postoperative immobilization is continued for 4 weeks, with the wrist maintained in 45 degrees of dorsiflexion with the MP joints in 60 degrees of flexion. Postoperative re-education is by contracting the ECRL to obtain finger flexion. IP joint extension is not dynamically augmented by this transfer but is improved through a tenodesis effect. This is a reliable procedure that

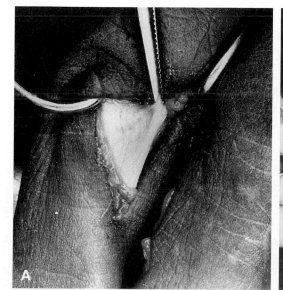
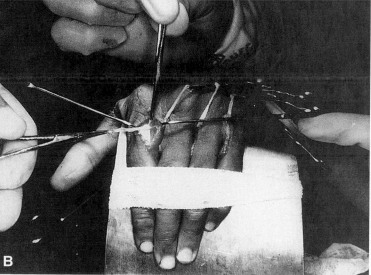

FIGURE 33-11. Lateral band insertion technique. **A,** Exposure of the lateral band on the dorsal extensor apparatus on the finger with a fine hemostat holding the edge of the lateral band to exert a proximal traction to remove the slack on the apparatus. **B,** The hand and wrist are positioned while the assistant gently holds the lateral bands as the tension is adjusted on the tendon slips before they are sutured to the ulnar lateral band of the index finger and to the radial lateral bands of the little, ring, and middle fingers sequentially.

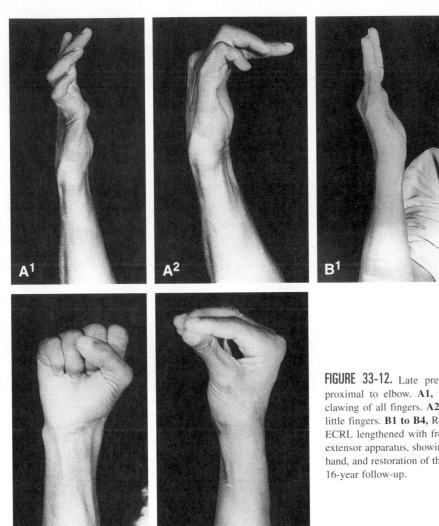

FIGURE 33-12. Late presentation of high ulnar nerve injury proximal to elbow. **A1,** Preoperative wasting of the hand with clawing of all fingers. **A2,** High unassisted angles in the ring and little fingers. **B1 to B4,** Result of reconstruction by transfer of the ECRL lengthened with free graft to the lateral band of the dorsal extensor apparatus, showing correction of deformity, closure of the hand, and restoration of the transverse metacarpal arch as seen at a 16-year follow-up.

gives good results of claw correction in patients with post-traumatic ulnar nerve palsy.[39] The ECRB or the brachio-radialis can also serve as the motor for this procedure.

Brooks and Jones Volar Route Transfer to A2 Pulley Insertion Site.[27,28] Brooks and Jones modified the EF4T procedure (Brand, 1961)[18] by using either the FCR or the ECRL donor, lengthened with toe extensor tendon grafts, and passed through the carpal tunnel to the A2 pulleys of the respective digits. Each slip of the graft is sutured back on itself, with the wrist held in maximum flexion and the MP joints in neutral position. Smith[136,137] mentioned the risk of median nerve compression in post-traumatic ulnar nerve palsy, when four tendon grafts are added to the contents of the carpal canal. Median nerve compromise can be avoided by using thin grafts with a donor-graft junction that is situated well proximal to the carpal tunnel.

Palmaris Four-Tail (PL4T) Transfer
(Lennox-Fritschi, 1971)

Fritschi[55] described and popularized an operation that he attributed to his colleague Lennox, who first performed it during the 1960s. The palmaris longus is used as a motor when it is present. The tendon is divided at its insertion into the palmar fascia, withdrawn proximally in the forearm about 4 to 6 cm from the wrist crease, lengthened with a tendon graft, and tunneled subcutaneously into a midpalmar incision. The rest of the procedure is as described for the Brand's EF4T procedure. Though a relatively weak donor, this procedure is most successful in younger patients with supple hands who demonstrate a strong palmaris longus (Fig. 33-13).

ECRL Volar Route Transfer to an Interosseous Tendon Insertion

The interosseous tendons have been used as insertion sites with different motors: a superficialis tendon,[3,158] ECRL,[114] or palmaris longus.[3,114]

Zancolli[158] described the use of the first and second dorsal interosseous as insertion sites to attach slips of a superficialis tendon with the goal of obtaining proximal phalangeal flexion and restore digital abduction. He termed this procedure *direct interosseous activation.* Palande[114] extended this principle to correct intrinsic-minus hands associated with reversal of the transverse metacarpal arch. The motor was either a lengthened ECRL or a lengthened

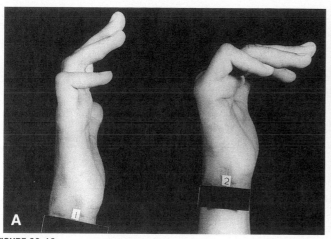

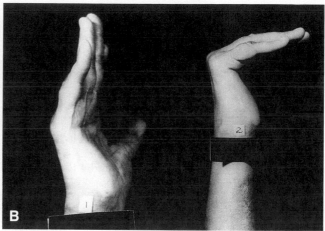

FIGURE 33-13. Proximal ulnar nerve palsy in a patient with tuberculoid type Hansen's disease. **A,** Mobile claw hands are demonstrated in the outstretched hand and lumbrical positions. As a first stage, tendon transfer with lengthened palmaris longus was done into the lateral bands of the dorsal apparatus. **B,** A 19-year follow-up view shows the good correction maintained in all fingers.

palmaris longus tunneled through the carpal tunnel. The graft was split into five slips and distributed in sequence: the first slip around the hypothenar muscle tendon mass, the next three around the adjacent interossei between the fingers, and the last around the first dorsal interossei muscle tendon. The slips were routed volar to the DTML and passed through the interosseous muscle tendon unit and folded back on itself. The fingers are positioned with the MP joints in 55 degrees of flexion and the IP joints straight. An effect of the procedure was to restore the metacarpal arch during the contraction of the motor by convergence of the extreme medial and lateral tendon graft slips. The proximal migration of the transferred tendon slips in the immediate postoperative period was prevented by passage of the graft volar to the DTML before its dorsal insertion on the interossei tendons.

Author's Technique of the "Interosseous Insertion" Procedure. Because the interosseous tendons have the smallest flexor moment at the MP joint, an interosseous tendon transfer is capable of delivering only a limited force distally. The palmar interossei behave like the lumbricals[86] and serve as useful sites in correcting supple and hypermobile claw hands (type I and II claw hands). The procedure can be used to minimize secondary deformities seen in claw correction.

I prefer the palmaris longus as the motor for transfer or, in its absence, one of the FDS tendons (Fig. 33-14A). The palmaris longus is divided through a small transverse incision on the flexor crease of the wrist, and its end is retrieved 4 cm proximally through a small transverse incision in the forearm. It is lengthened with the plantaris tendon or a strip of fascia lata by Brand's wraparound method (see

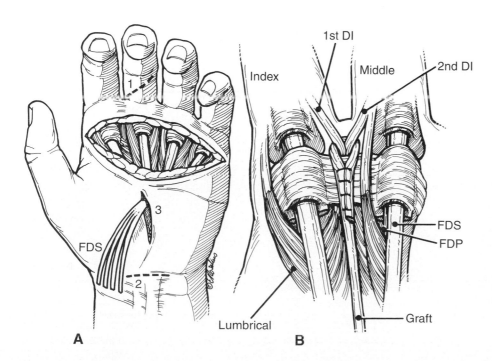

A **B**

FIGURE 33-14. Interosseous insertion technique for claw hand correction for all four fingers with supple or hypermobile joints. **A,** (1) Incision for sectioning FDS between A2 and C1 pulleys, (2) incision for sectioning the palmaris longus tendon, (3) midpalmar incision to retrieve the motor and divide it into four slips. A transpalmar incision is used to identify the wing tendons of the adjacent interossei distal to the deep transverse metacarpal ligament. **B,** The graft is taken volar to the deep transverse metacarpal ligament and looped around the wing tendons of the adjacent first palmar interossei of the index finger and second dorsal interossei of the middle finger and the graft is sutured to itself. The lumbricals are not part of the insertion site.

Fig 33-10B). A midpalmar incision is made, the lengthened palmaris longus is passed through the carpal tunnel using a tendon retriever, and the graft is divided into four slips. A transpalmar incision is then made at the distal palmar crease, and wide flaps are raised proximally and distally. The graft slips are passed sequentially into the distal palmar incision from the midpalmar incision along the lumbrical canals using a tendon passer. The slips are kept moist in saline gauze. Next the lumbrical muscles are identified and used as guides to the DTML and the wing tendons of the interossei in the interdigital spaces. The fascia that lies over the interossei tendons on either side of the interdigital spaces is incised, and the tendons are cleanly exposed. A fine right-angled clamp is initially passed dorsally around the dorsal interosseous tendon of the index and the adjacent palmar and dorsal interossei tendons of each web space to prepare these spaces to receive a graft slip and a suture. Now a 3-0 nonabsorbable suture is placed in the end of each tendon slip, and one slip is passed around the first dorsal interosseous muscle tendon area, the next around the adjacent "wing" interosseous tendons between the index and middle fingers, and then around the adjacent interossei between the middle and ring fingers and lastly between the ring and little fingers. (It is optional to place a fifth slip around the hypothenar muscle mass proximal to their insertion in the little finger, when the preoperative transverse metacarpal arch is reversed by 10 to 15 degrees in supple hands.) With the hand placed supine on the table, the MP joints are flexed to 60 degrees and the IP joints are held straight. Slack is removed with gentle traction and the sutures tied, beginning with the index finger, followed by the slip between the ring and little fingers and then the two intermediate slips. The hand is now lifted off the table to verify claw correction in all fingers and to ensure that no finger is out of step with its neighbor. A simple passive way to confirm this is to utilize the wrist flexion and extension tenodesis maneuver to verify correct tension. If there is doubt about the laxity of a slip then that slip is adjusted with

a gentle proximal pull as it is folded back and sutured finally to itself (see Fig. 33-14B). After hemostasis and closure, the hand is immobilized in the lumbrical-plus position with the wrist in neutral position, MP joints in 80 degrees of flexion, and IP joints straight for 3 weeks. The dorsal portion of the splint over the PIP joints can be removed after 2 to 3 days to allow gentle side-to-side motion of the digits.

Although transfer training is easier with flexor motors than the extensor motors (Brand, 1961), it is advisable to begin a staged regimen of hand therapy.

Author's Staged Regimen of Postoperative Hand Therapy for Claw Correction. In the first week the patient is supervised to attain and maintain the lumbrical-plus position and uses a thermoplastic splint between exercises. Over the next 7 to 10 days active IP joint flexion is begun while the MP joints remain in flexion. At no point during the first and second stages is the patient allowed to extend the MP joints. During the third stage the patient is encouraged to maintain the IP joint in absolute neutral extension and then extend the MP joints. The exercises at this stage are combined with supervised light functional activities that encourage the lumbrical posture. Patients with insensate hands are particularly at risk of loosening tendon transfers, and it is critical that the reconstruction team remind the patient of their vulnerability to injury during the postoperative period.

Results. In one series, the interosseous insertion led to good-excellent claw finger correction in 85% of hands and satisfactory restoration of the arch when the ECRL was used as the motor.[114] Notably, postoperative hyperextension of the PIP joint of the finger was significantly less than that seen after more distal attachments. At 2-year follow-up of a group of patients with type II (hypermobile) hands, good-to-excellent results were obtained in 96% for the interosseous insertion procedure using either the palmaris longus (Fig. 33-15) or the FDS as motor.[3] When the interosseous insertion was compared with the distal insertion of the EF4T

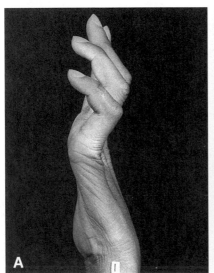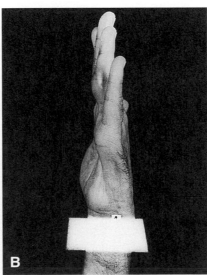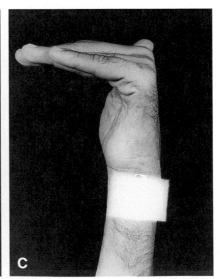

FIGURE 33-15. Hypermobile claw hand (type II claw hand) owing to proximal ulnar nerve injury. The outstretched hand demonstrates claw deformity in all fingers, more prominent on the ulnar side. Each PIP joint had passive hyperextension above 20 degrees. Reconstructive surgery by transfer of a lengthened palmaris longus tendon divided into four slips for insertion serially into the first dorsal interossei on the radial side of the index and the wing tendons of the interossei lying between the three adjacent sides of the fingers was done. **B** and **C,** A 9-year follow-up demonstrates maintenance of excellent correction.

CRITICAL POINTS: INTEROSSEOUS INSERTION PROCEDURE FOR CLAW CORRECTION

INDICATION

- Type I and type II claw hands

PEARLS

- Dissect structures beyond the DTML with care to identify the adjacent palmar and dorsal interossei "wing" tendons

TECHNICAL POINTS

- It is the most technically demanding claw reconstructive procedure.
- Retract the neurovascular structures toward the ulnar side proximal to the DTML.
- Follow the lumbrical muscle as a guide to the wing tendons of the interossei.
- Remove fascia in the region of the interossei to expose the wing tendons.
- Use a fine-tipped right-angled hemostat to prepare the space to swing the graft slip through.
- Gentle abduction and rotation of the adjacent finger helps in better visualization of the wing tendons.

- Remove slack from all tendons starting with the radial side of the index finger.
- Position the hand with MP joints in 60 degrees of flexion and IP joints in extension.
- Tie the suture around the slip and the adjacent interossei.
- Verify claw correction by passive tenodesis of the wrist to detect smooth arrangement of fingers without MP joint hyperextension. Then suture the folded back slip to itself.

POSTOPERATIVE CARE

- Immobilize the hand in the lumbrical-plus position.
- Remove dorsal plaster distal to the PIP joints after 2 days.
- Perform a supervised staged tendon transfer rehabilitation.
- Discourage strong activities with the operated hand for a 3-month period.

---

for similar type of claw hands, the intrinsic-plus deformity was seen in 6.25% of the fingers in the former and 13.75% of fingers in the latter.[3]

The main advantage of this procedure is the small flexor moment of the interossei serving as the insertion sites and the decreased chance of overcorrection. Insertion into wing tendons allows the force to be spread over a broader area than when it is concentrated at the lateral band of the dorsal extensor expansion. The goal is to diminish the chances of an undesirable intrinsic-plus deformity, and the ideal candidate is one with a type I (supple) or type II (hypermobile) claw hand.

Special Note on Chronic Claw Hand Deformities in Hansen's Disease

Based on the successful outcome of surgery on the hands of leprosy patients who presented early after medical treatment for surgical reconstruction, the same procedures were performed on the hands of patients who presented with chronic or fixed deformities of 5 years or greater. A recurrence rate of the claw deformity was seen in 45% of 136 claw hands that were treated by various operative procedures.[2] The causes for this were multifactorial and included the presence of severe PIP flexion contractures, the development of strong habitual substitution patterns of hand function, the difficulty to consciously control the transferred muscles in the postoperative period, and the occasional injudicious choice of operative procedures. Better results followed the use of flexor motors as donors. Suggested measures to improve the results of reconstruction for chronic deformity included the introduction of activities of

daily living and occupational orientation using corrective splinting 3 months before surgery, careful choice of the surgical procedure and technique, and a renewed campaign for early surgery for inactive disease.[2]

RESTORATION OF THUMB-INDEX KEY PINCH AND TIP PINCH

Loss of adductor pollicis action and FPB action results in the collapse of the biarticular system with a "Z" deformity, functionally translated as poor key and tip pinches in the thumb and loss of power grip of the whole hand when the thumb has to work in consonance with other digits. The EPL and the FPL muscles are the remaining extrinsic motors that contribute to adduction,[135,136] and their function in the absence of ulnar intrinsic muscles contributes to the collapse in the anteroposterior plane.

In the normal hand the adduction force is achieved by the adductor pollicis, and the first dorsal interosseous prevents distraction and dorsal subluxation of the CMC joint.[24] Biomechanical studies have demonstrated a 75% to 80% loss of power pinch in patients with ulnar nerve palsy.[59,88] This is explained by the combined tension capability of the adductor pollicis and FPB of 4.3%, nearly double that of the FPL (2.7%).[24] These two powerful intrinsic muscles of the thumb achieve their effectiveness because of their large moment at the CMC joint.[24]

In the ulnar palsied thumb with a "Z"-collapse deformity, CMC joint hyperextension and hyperabduction is initially prevented by a strong dermal-fascial cradle around the basal joint.[24] Restoration of strong adduction of the first metacarpal, active flexion of the hyperextended MP joint, and active extension of the hyperflexed IP joint can help the patient regain function in this vital pillar for power and precision. It is important to know that the range of movement at the MP joint of the thumb does not compare with the ranges at other MP joints but the IP joint of the thumb has greater range of motion than any other distal joint of the hand. The combination of a stable MP joint and a highly mobile IP joint makes it possible to hold an array of objects with different shapes and sizes.

Thumb Adduction Techniques (Bunnell[34]; Boyes[13]; Goldner[58,59]; Littler[30,48,52,53,82,83]; Smith[135-137]; Robinson et al[125])

Most tendon transfers for adduction of the thumb provide power pinch only in the range of 25% to 50% of normal strength.[29,59,88,135] Potential donors include a wrist motor, the brachioradialis, or one of the digital tendons.

ECRB as Motor (Smith[136])

This is one of the most reliable procedures for adduction for the thumb. The ECRB is detached and retrieved into a proximal incision in the mid forearm, where it is lengthened with a free tendon graft. The lengthened unit is routed dorsal to the extensor retinaculum to retain some potential for dorsiflexion of the wrist. It is tunneled from this site through the third intermetacarpal space. With a curved hemostat, further tunneling of the graft is done superficial to the muscle belly of the adductor pollicis and deep to the flexor tendons toward its insertion on the ulnar base of the proximal phalanx of the thumb. A counter-incision is made in the ulnar midaxial line of the thumb over the MP joint. The graft is adjusted and sutured to the adductor pollicis insertion site with sufficient tension to allow the thumb to rest just palmar to the long axis of the index finger when the wrist is in 0 degrees of extension. When the wrist is in palmar flexion, the thumb falls into abduction; with the wrist actively extended, the thumb is drawn firmly against the palm (Fig. 33-16). The average key pinch is doubled by the operation.[64,135]

Omer[101] favored suturing the ECRB to the strong fascia over the abductor tubercle of the first metacarpal. The use of the abductor tubercle as the insertion site adds pronation for improved pinch.[48]

Brachioradialis as Motor (Boyes[13])

Boyes advocated the use of the brachioradialis and recommended that the direction of pull parallel the fibers of the transverse head of the adductor pollicis so that the donor exerts maximal power as it pulls at a right angle to the axis of the thumb. This procedure is done in a reverse order, that is, by first attaching one end of a tendon graft to the adductor tubercle of the proximal phalanx with a pull-out wire suture. The free end is then routed along the volar surface of the paralyzed adductor to the third intermetacarpal space and brought out through a dorsal incision. From there the graft is passed deep to the extensor tendons to emerge in a subcuticular plane on the radial side of the forearm. The brachioradialis is detached through a separate incision and attached to the distal graft. An adequately mobilized brachio-

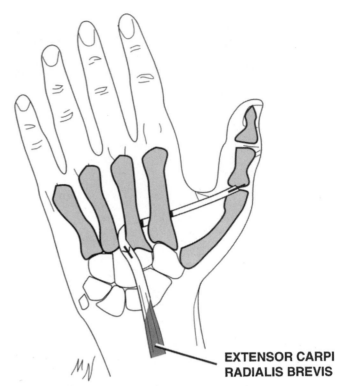

FIGURE 33-16. Transfer of the ECRB extended with a free tendon graft, through the interspace between the third and fourth metacarpals across the palm volar to the adductor pollicis muscle and dorsal to the finger flexor tendons and neurovascular structures, to insert into the fascia over the abductor tubercle of the first metacarpal. (The brachioradialis also may be used as the motor for the transfer.) This transfer will add power to key pinch and will continue to align and provide the power for wrist extension. It is preferable to a "volar" transfer (see Figure 33-17).

radialis has a sufficient amplitude of motion to allow thumb action whether the wrist is flexed or extended. Other motors used for thumb adduction are the ECU[13] and the ECRL.[139]

FDS as Motor, Transferred to the Adductor Pollicis Insertion (Littler[82,83]; Brown[30])

The long finger FDS or the ring FDS is used as a donor in patients with hyperextension deformity of the MP joint of the thumb.[82,83] The FDS tendon is detached in the finger between the A1 and A2 pulley by cutting the tendon at its decussation and leaving one limb long enough to prevent a recurvatum at the PIP joint.[30,98] The tendon is withdrawn into the palm and tunneled across the volar surface of the adductor pollicis and sutured to the adductor tubercle insertion. Hamlin and Littler[62] reported a return of pinch power to 70% of the uninvolved hand with this procedure.

FDS as Motor, Transferred to Abductor Tubercle (Edgerton and Brand[48])

This modification of the procedure of the FDS into the abductor tubercle was described to improve key pinch. The vertical septum of the palmar fascia attached to the third metacarpal is used as the pulley.[48,100] This step is necessary for flexor tendon motors because otherwise the tendon will gradually migrate radialward and make the procedure ineffective (Fig. 33-17).

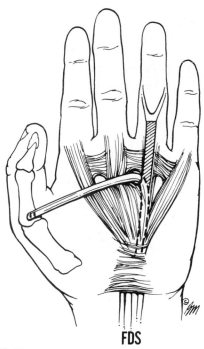

FIGURE 33-17. Transfer of the FDS through a palmar fascia pulley to the abductor tubercle of the thumb. This transfer will add power to key pinch but will further weaken power grip.

FDSM as Motor With Dual Insertion to the Thumb (Goldner[58,59])

The FDSM is used for the transfer, with one slip sutured to the ulnar aspect of the proximal phalanx and the other slip sutured to the adductor tendon insertion. The released FDSM is withdrawn at the ulnar side of the pronator quadratus muscle in the distal forearm. From here the tendon is then passed to the dorsum of the wrist, taken around the ECU (which serves as a pulley), and finally passed deep to the dorsal structures of the hand to two insertion sites on the thumb. Each of these transfers is reinforced by action of the FPL and EPL acting as secondary adductors.

Extensor Indicis as Motor (Brown[30])

Bunnell had preferred the use of the extensor digitorum of the index finger because he considered it to be a stronger donor. Brown[30] preferred this tendon because of its functional independence and passed it through the fourth intermetacarpal space, across the transverse muscle belly of the adductor pollicis, and sutured it to the adductor pollicis insertion. Proper tension is achieved by holding the wrist in neutral, and moderate tension is exerted on the tendon before sutures are placed. Brand[24] emphasized the requirements of strength and stability in restoring thumb adduction in ulnar nerve palsy and considered the EDC (index) as too weak to adduct the thumb.

Combination of EI and ED (Little) Tendon Transfers for Pinch (Robinson et al[125])

To improve pinch and abduction of the index finger, the ulnar slip of the EDC (little) is transferred across the dorsum of the hand to the adductor tubercle of the thumb and the

EIP is divided at the dorsal hood of the MP joint and passed around the thumb extensor tendons, looped around the first dorsal interosseous and attached to the radial base of the index proximal phalanx. This changes the vector of pull and makes the EIP an abductor of the index finger. In six patients who had this combination procedure, pinch improved by up to 45% and index abduction to 30% to 40% of normal after 40 months.[125]

Index Abduction Techniques (Bunnell[13,34]; Bruner[32]; Graham and Riordan[61]; Hirayama et al[66]; Neviaser et al[97]; Omer[92,113])

The thumb is more important in pinch,[42] but the index finger also needs to be stabilized to provide effective pinch. For tip pinch the index finger should be in abduction and slight radial rotation.

Accessory Slip of APL Transfer (Neviaser et al.[97])

Neviaser and coworkers recommended transferring one accessory slip of the APL elongated with a palmaris longus or plantaris free graft to the tendon of the first dorsal interosseous (Fig. 33-18). The APL is exposed distal to the first dorsal compartment, and the insertion of one of its slips is detached, lengthened, and routed to the first dorsal

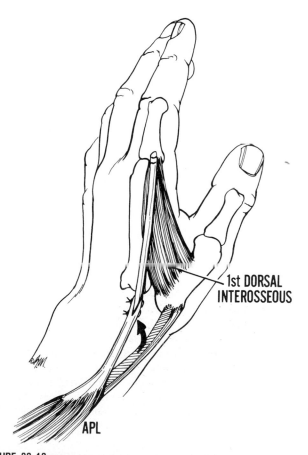

FIGURE 33-18. Extension of an accessory slip of the APL with a free tendon graft into the tendon insertion of the first dorsal interosseous to improve index abduction. The brachioradialis may be used as an alternative motor.

interosseous. This transfer does not appreciably increase the force of tip pinch, but it stabilizes the index finger.[136,137]

EIP Transfer to First Dorsal Interosseous

Bunnell reported transfer of the EIP to the first dorsal interosseous muscle. The tendon is divided from the index dorsal hood and withdrawn at the wrist through a short transverse incision, passed distally around the radial border of the second metacarpal, and inserted into the first dorsal interosseous tendon volar to the axis of motion of the MP joint. The dorsal apparatus should be carefully closed to prevent extension lag of the index finger.[31,95,137] The transfer is sutured under considerable tension for adequate performance.[30] Modifications in the use of EIP transfer for index abduction include improving the force vector by rerouting the tendon at the wrist to pass around the extensor tendons[139] or by splitting the EIP into two slips and inserting one slip into the first dorsal interosseous and the other into the adductor pollicis.

Disadvantages. Clippinger and Goldner[28,40] believe that this transfer is not a satisfactory procedure, perhaps because of a short moment arm and a narrow angle of approach. Smith[136] noted that some patients develop an undesirable radial-deviated posture of the index finger after this procedure.

Palmaris Longus to the First Dorsal Interosseous

Hirayama[66] lengthened the palmaris longus muscle-tendon unit with a strip of palmar fascia and transferred this unit subcutaneously to the dorsum of the hand and distally to the insertion of the first dorsal interosseous. The course of the transposed tendon aligns with the course of the first dorsal interosseous.[21-23] The wrist is immobilized for 3 weeks in 10 degrees of dorsiflexion with 30 degrees of flexion and 20 degrees of abduction of the MP joint of the index finger.

Extensor Pollicis Brevis (EPB) Transfer

Bruner[32] transferred the EPB to the tendon of the first dorsal interosseous (Fig. 33-19). Graham and Riordan[61] stated that the EPB lacked the strength to carry out adequate abduction. DeAbreu[43] combined the transfer of two relatively weak muscles, the EPB tendon to the tendinous insertion of the first dorsal interosseous and the EI tendon to the insertion of the adductor pollicis muscle.

FDSR Transfer (Graham and Riordan[61])

Graham and Riordan transferred the FDSR to the first dorsal interosseous to produce strong abduction of the index finger. The superficialis is withdrawn to the wrist level and redirected subcutaneously over the anatomic snuffbox to the radial aspect of the index finger. The tendon can be inserted into the proximal phalanx or the first dorsal interosseous tendon insertion. Postoperative immobilization includes holding the index finger in abduction and extension with the wrist slightly flexed. Active motion is permitted at the end of 3 weeks.

Goldner[59] believed that all these transfers provide improved stability, a moderate degree of tenodesis, and definite improvement in pinch, but only in the range of 10% to 15%. The technique should not be used in high ulnar nerve palsies.

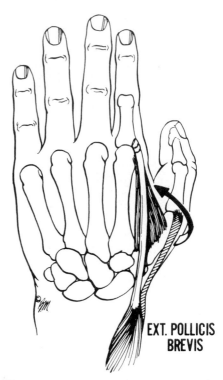

FIGURE 33-19. Transfer of the EPB to the insertion of the first dorsal interosseous to improve index abduction.

Stabilization of the Thumb MP and IP Joints to Restore Pinch

Split FPL to EPL Transfer-Tenodesis (Tsuge and Hashizume[149]; House and Walsh[67])

To make pulp pinch possible with the thumb, it is necessary to correct the problem of IP joint hyperflexion in addition to MP joint stabilization. A split transfer of the FPL effectively neutralizes the IP joint without weakening pinch power.[149] The radial half of the FPL is detached at its insertion and reattached to the volar aspect of the proximal phalanx of the thumb by a pull-out wire technique or alternatively sewn to the EPL tendon at the DIP joint. The split FPL transfer was also recommended in the two-stage reconstruction of tetraplegic hands[67,93] when hyperflexion of the IP joint developed after tendon transfer to restore FPL function. The transfer distributes FPL flexion force to the dorsal and palmar bases of the distal phalanx, effectively stabilizing the joint against hyperflexion while maintaining strong and accurate pinch power.[67] Key pinch was restored effectively in 47 tetraplegic hands without postoperative complications and was preferred over IP joint fusion using Kirschner wires or screws.[93]

Author's Method of Split-FPL Tendon Transfer

I reserve the split-FPL to EPL transfer for patients with supple hands and persistent IP joint hyperflexion with only mild (10 degree) MP joint hyperextension collapse deformity. I do not recommend it on thumbs with IP joint flexion contracture, MP joint contracture, instability, or pain in either of these joints. In splitting the FPL, the ulnar half should be left undisturbed so that the delicate arterial supply of the vincula is preserved.[7]

A zigzag incision is made on the volar aspect of the thumb angled at the IP joint crease (Fig. 33-20). The FPL flexor sheath is exposed, and a small longitudinal incision is made in the middle of the FPL tendon at its insertion and extended proximally while preserving the A2 pulley. The radial half of the FPL tendon is detached at its insertion, and a blunt hook is used to retrieve it proximal to the oblique pulley. Next, an oblique or longitudinal incision is made over the dorsum of the proximal phalanx to expose the EPL as far as the IP joint. A fine curved hemostat is used to create a tunnel that passes deep to the neurovascular structures along the radial side of the proximal phalanx and dorsal to the EPL. The end of the radial half of the FPL is passed dorsally and sutured into the EPL proximal to the IP joint with nonabsorbable sutures. Tension is adjusted by pulling on the transferred FPL slip to set the MP joint flexion at 15 degrees while maintaining the IP joint in neutral extension and the thumb base extended (i.e., lying naturally anterior to the plane of the palm). A Kirschner wire is used to transfix the IP joint in this position. The hand is immobilized with the wrist in neutral flexion, the thumb in full palmar abduction, and the MP joint flexed 20 degrees. After 4 weeks of immobilization the cast and the Kirschner wire are removed. Light activities are begun, and forceful flexion of the IP joint is discouraged. An IP extension splint is used between exercises for 6 to 8 weeks (Fig. 33-21).

Arthrodesis of Thumb Joints (Brand[21]; Brown[30]; Omer[100,108]; Tubiana[151,152])

Brown[30] noted that splinting of an ulnar-palsied thumb increased pinch strength by 1 to 2 kg. Arthrodesis of the thumb has also been reported to stabilize key pinch and improve tip pinch.[108] Arthrodesis would seem a logical

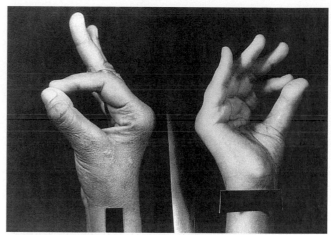

FIGURE 33-21. The patient had mild MP joint hyperextension and gradually developed increasing IP joint flexion while attempting power pinch in this dominant hand. There was no instability of these joints, but the patient found it difficult to work. The radial half of the FPL tendon was transferred dorsally to the EPL, providing good correction of the deformity at the MP and IP joints as seen at an 8-year follow-up of this second stage. (Same patient as in Figure 33-13.)

compromise because of the inability to simultaneously restore the complex flexor-pronator function of the FPB and the adductor-supinator function of the adductor pollicis with tendon transfers. Mechanically, arthrodesis of one of the joints in the thumb would abolish the biarticular system and enable the extrinsic flexor and extensors to better stabilize the remaining joint. Fixed deformity of the remaining joint is a contraindication for arthrodesis of either one.

Arthrodesis of the MP joint to allow the terminal joint to be controlled by the long extrinsic muscles is the most widely used method and is indicated when there is severe hyperextension contracture or excessive Jeanne's sign with pain and instability.[82,99] It is also indicated when a positive Jeanne sign develops after an FDS transfer.[64]

Arthrodesis of the MP joint

Omer[99,104] recommended arthrodesis of the MP joint to correct instability in the longitudinal arch of the thumb and also to improve the distal stability for tip pinch.[82] A dorsal longitudinal incision was used and the extensor apparatus split. A saw was used to produce a chevron-shaped mortise, with the point of the chevron directed proximally. The joint was held in 10 to 15 degrees of flexion and stabilized with two crossed Kirschner wires. Slight pronation is important to improve pulp-to-pulp pinch. A thumb spica cast is worn for 6 weeks, followed by light unresisted use of the thumb until radiographic healing is evident. The chevron technique is technically straightforward and offers a large surface area of cancellous bone to expedite fusion.[116]

Brand places the MP joint in 15 degrees of flexion, 5 degrees of abduction, and 15 degrees of pronation. Barden[9] reported normal motion of the IP joint after arthrodesis of the MP joint of the thumb, with correction of Froment's sign.

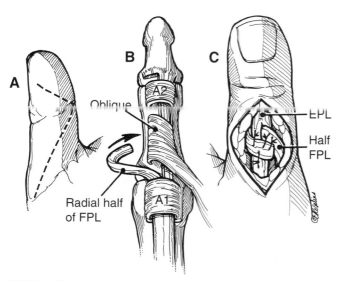

FIGURE 33-20. Half of FPL tendon transfer to the EPL tendon for restoring stability to the MP joint and IP joint of thumb to improve pinch. Zigzag incision on the volar aspect of the thumb to expose the FPL. **A,** Radial half of FPL is sectioned distal to A2 pulley, and it is slit farther proximally to the distal end of A1 pulley. **B,** It is transferred dorsally and sutured to the EPL tendon just proximal to the IP joint.

Author's Preferred Method of Treatment

If the patient manifests a "Z" deformity only while holding an object against resistance this would indicate that there is sufficient median-innervated FPB power to provide an acceptable though weak pinch. For dominant hands, or if there is marked reduction of key and tip pinch strengths in comparison with the unaffected hand, the patient is given the option of tendon transfer. If the patient experiences fatigue or pain with the use of the thumb, I prefer MP joint arthrodesis and an adductorplasty with brachioradialis or the APL as the motor. For this transfer, I prefer motors that leave little or no donor deficit. If there is obvious hyperextension deformity at the MP joint in the resting hand, I prefer to do an MP joint arthrodesis as the first stage. The option of a second stage adductorplasty is offered for power pinch if the remaining extrinsic muscles are not satisfactory to provide adduction power.

In a patient with poor bone stock, I use a slight modification of the Lister technique of intraosseous wiring.[81] Flush opposing surfaces of the MP joint are prepared by removing a 15- to 20-degree closing wedge with a power saw. The joint is stabilized by an oblique radial-to-ulnar Kirschner wire and reinforced with an interosseous loop of stainless steel in the coronal plane, exiting approximately 1 cm from the cut surface.

In a patient with good bone stock, I prefer Segmüller's tension band cerclage arthrodesis technique.[127] Functional use of the thumb compresses the site and encourages early fusion. The initial preparation of the joint for arthrodesis is the same for both techniques.

In either method, a hand-based thumb spica cast is applied that includes the IP joint. The cast is retained for 4 weeks with the interosseous wire technique and for 3 weeks with the tension band technique. Light activities are introduced and restricted activity continued for 2 to 3 months. These two techniques are simple, and I have had uniformly successful fusion at this joint by both the methods.

Notes on the Hypermobile Hands with "Z" Thumbs

Tendon transfers in hypermobile hands test the surgeon's experience and skill. Delicate balance of these joints is required to provide stability and enhance power.[5] For these hands, I favor the adductor tubercle as the insertion site for a lengthened brachioradialis or APL transfer, routed through the third intermetacarpal space. Patients with CMC laxity may present with wide thumb abduction, such that the tip of the fully flexed index finger is still unable to reach the thumb pulp.[24] Arthrodesis of the MP joint is my first choice to provide a stable thumb in this cohort.

Arthrodesis of the IP Joint

Tubiana prefers IP joint arthrodesis to fusion of the MP joint.[151,152] Brown reserved this procedure for patients in whom the IP joint is noticeably unstable.[17] The position for fusion of the IP joint of the thumb is 20 to 30 degrees of flexion.[75] The reported disadvantage is the loss of motion that some patients consider an even greater problem than the loss of pinch.[64,108]

I prefer to arthrodese the IP joint only when there is a fixed flexion deformity in excess of 30 degrees or when there is instability or arthritic changes. I prefer a Kirschner wire/interosseous wire combination technique as described earlier.[81] I augment this with an adductorplasty using a lengthened brachioradialis or a slip of the APL to the adductor tubercle if the preoperative functional assessment demonstrates a loss of over 50% power when compared with the unaffected hand.

RESTORATION OF TRANSVERSE METACARPAL ARCH

Tubiana and Valentin,[150] Stack,[140] and Backhouse and Catton[8] have all drawn attention to the importance of the intrinsic muscles in adduction, abduction, and flexion at the MP joints—motions that can combine to produce digital rotation during precision grip. This is observed in the functions of the normal transverse metacarpal arch for precision grip, tool handling, and the cupping of the hand that facilitates the grasping of large objects. The interossei are essential to produce rotation of the digits that enable the hands to be competent and elegant in performing specific tasks of prehension. In ulnar nerve palsy, the normal stability of the distal transverse metacarpal arch is lost owing to the paralysis of the interossei, and the hypothenar muscles and the metacarpals remain together as though held by a transverse sling, the strong deep transverse metacarpal ligaments, while the fingers are in a collapsed state. This abolishes the ability of a palsied hand to contour itself around an object placed within its domain. The simple act of opening the lid of a jar or turning a valve becomes clumsy and the palm is unable to be "cupped" to hold fluid, gather grain, or mold dough. Even a claw hand that has been corrected by a lumbrical replacement procedure is likely to recur if the transverse metacarpal arch remains unstable or flat.[118]

Bunnell,[13,34] Littler,[82,83] and Ranney[117,118] have described procedures that partly improve this complex situation.

Bunnell's "Tendon T" Operation

An FDS is detached from the finger, retrieved proximally, and attached to the middle of a free tendon graft. This graft is passed dorsal to the flexor tendons with one of its two ends inserted to the base of the proximal phalanx of the thumb on the radial side and the other to the neck of the metacarpal of the little finger on the ulnar side to form a "T." On voluntary contraction of the superficialis, there is adduction/flexion of the thumb and the little finger and the "T" is converted into a "Y" to restore the metacarpal arch.

Littler's Split Superficialis Tendon Procedure

Littler modified Bunnell's procedure by avoiding the use of the free tendon graft and altering the insertion sites. An FDS tendon is detached, and one division is taken and sutured to the adductor tubercle of the thumb and the other to the ulnar base of the proximal phalanx of the little finger.

Ranney's EDM Transfer

Ranney concentrated only on the ulnar side by stressing the importance of depressing the metacarpal arch with a volar transfer of an extensor tendon to the neck of the fifth metacarpal. The extensor digiti minimi (EDM) is removed by a step-cut at its normal insertion, leaving the remaining strip sutured to the ED (little). The EDM tendon is withdrawn to the wrist and passed to the palmar forearm between the APL and the FCR. From here the EDM tendon is passed subcutaneously in a diagonal course to be anchored to the periosteum of the neck of the fifth metacarpal.

Omer, in 1995, mentioned that Ahern, in 1969, had produced an effect similar to that of Ranney's procedure by looping the FDS of the little finger around the DTML between the fourth and fifth metacarpals. I have done this as a concomitant procedure during claw hand correction for leprosy patients by inserting the FDSL to the tendinous insertion of the hypothenar muscles at the ulnar aspect of the fifth MP joint with satisfactory correction.

Omer[100,104,110,113] modified Bunnell's "tendon T" operation to provide combined restoration of the metacarpal arch and claw correction of the fourth and fifth digits. He divided the FDSR or FDSM into two slips and transferred the radial slip to the abductor tubercle of the thumb and the ulnar slip to the little and ring fingers. He used the lateral bands of the dorsal apparatus as the insertion point if there was an assisted angle in the clawed ring and little fingers or the A2 pulley if there was no assisted angle in the clawed fingers (Fig. 33-22). When activated, the "Y" transfer glided proximally over the distal edge of the vertical fascial septum of the third metacarpal as a pulley, to provide key pinch for the thumb and claw correction for the ring and little fingers, with the added benefit of an improved metacarpal arch.

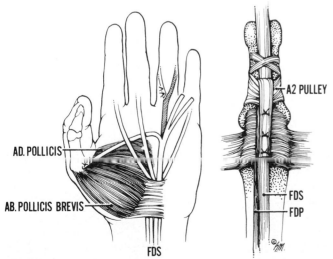

FIGURE 33-22. Transfer off the FDS as an internal splint for low distal ulnar palsy. The tendon is detached at the PIP joint level with tenodesis of the radial half across the joint. The tendon is further split, and the radial half of the tendon passes volar to the adductor pollicis muscle and dorsal to the FDP tendons into the insertion of the APB. The ulnar half of the tendon is again split into two slips that are directed distally and volar to the deep transverse metacarpal ligament and looped through the A2 annular pulley of the flexor sheath for the ring and little fingers. The result is improved key pinch, and active flexion returns to the MP joint of the ring and little fingers.

Advantages. The objectives of this transfer are to improve the integration of MP and IP joint flexion, provide key pinch for the thumb, and correct the flattened metacarpal arch, in distal ulnar nerve palsy. It can also be used as an internal splint while awaiting nerve regeneration after repair.[108]

Disadvantages. The split tendon distal to the vertical septum of the palmar fascia may lead to adhesions and limit its effective excursion. Either of the two slips may take the entire force of FDS contraction to provide function in one direction while the other slip slackens gradually. Omer cautioned that this transfer decreases grip strength because the superficialis tendon is dissipated into several insertions. When performing the "Y" transfer, Omer recommends an MP joint arthrodesis to improve thumb adduction and key pinch. However, this transfer does not add appreciable strength for proximal phalanx flexion or power grip, which is a major problem in ulnar nerve palsy.[64,106]

Author's Preferred Method of Treatment

I prefer a separate transfer for restoration of the metacarpal arch. I do the Ranney procedure and tunnel the EDM only under the APL and not under the FCR and then route the tendon across the palm. It is important to avoid injury to the palmar cutaneous branch of the median nerve during tunneling. I insert the tendon to the hypothenar tendon insertion at the ulnar aspect of the fifth MP joint. With the wrist positioned in 10 degrees of flexion and the pulps of the little finger and thumb passively opposed, the slack from the tendon is removed and then the suturing is completed. Postoperative immobilization for 3 weeks in a light cast is followed by exercises that simulate the cupping action of the palm. A circular broad rubber band or garter rubber is used around the fingers and thumb to bunch the pulps together so that the tips appear as a rosette. The patient is encouraged to purposefully attempt to fan out the digits held with this rubber. The program is continued at home for 6 to 12 weeks. I gauge the success of the procedure by a patient's ability to flex the fourth and fifth metacarpals volarward by 15 degrees on clenching the fist (Fig. 33-23). Most patients continue to have difficulty with holding circular objects even after this surgery but gradually accommodate, in part by the acquisition of substitution patterns, for these prehensile functions.

LITTLE FINGER ABDUCTION (Blacker et al[11]; Goldner[59]; Voche and Merle[154])

Blacker and colleagues demonstrated that the EDM has the potential to abduct the little finger through its indirect insertion into the abductor tubercle on the proximal phalanx. The third palmar interosseous counters this effect in normal hands. In ulnar nerve palsy the intrinsic paralysis leaves the EDM unopposed (Wartenberg's sign).

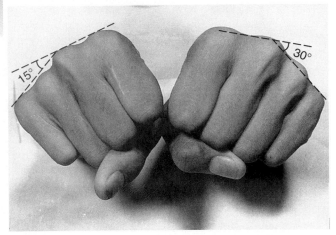

FIGURE 33-23. Correction of the reversed transverse metacarpal arch. This was done as a second stage after good result of claw correction by the palmaris longus transfer to the lateral bands in a mobile claw hand. The transverse metacarpal arch was satisfactorily restored by transfer of the EDM to the hypothenar tendon insertion at the ulnar base of the little finger.

Split-EDM Transfer

Half of the EDM tendon is detached from the extensor hood at the MP joint and retrieved through an incision just distal to the extensor retinaculum. A palmar incision that extends obliquely from the distal palmar crease to the proximal digital crease is made to expose the deep transverse metacarpal ligament and the flexor sheath of the little finger. A tunneller is passed through the fourth intermetacarpal space to emerge in the dorsal incision, and the end of the half EDM slip is retrieved into the palm. If the little finger is clawed as well as abducted, the tendon slip is inserted into a radially based flap of the flexor tendon sheath just distal to the A1 pulley (Brooks' insertion).[27,28] If the little finger is not clawed, the tendon slip is passed dorsal to the deep transverse metacarpal ligament and sutured into the radial collateral ligament attachment on the proximal phalanx of the little finger (Fig. 33-24). For tensioning, the wrist is held in neutral and the MP joint is in 20 degrees of flexion. The ring and little fingers are splinted for 4 weeks with the wrist extended, and the MP joint is flexed. The IP joints are left free, and motion is encouraged to prevent adhesions of the flexor tendons.

Complete EDM Transfer

Goldner[59] used the *entire* EDM by detaching it at the MP joint and withdrawing the tendon just distal to the extensor retinaculum. He directed it beneath the ECRL to create a pulley and then to the dorsal surface of the base of the little finger. The tendon was inserted into the oblique fibers of the dorsal apparatus or directly into bone.

Junctura Tendinum and Medial ED Slip of Ring Finger Transfer

Voche and Merle[154] described the correction of Wartenberg's sign by using a central or an ulnar slip from the ED of the ring finger and extended it by detaching the junctura tendinum from the neighboring little finger ED tendon. The

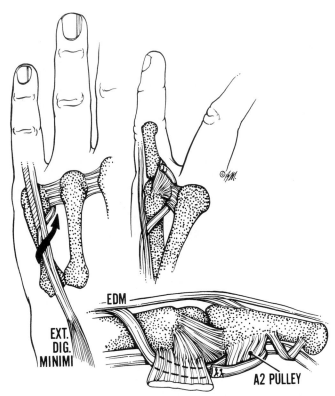

FIGURE 33-24. Transfer of the ulnar half of the EDM to correct persistent abduction of the little finger. The ulnar half of the tendon is directed volar to the deep transverse metacarpal ligament and sutured to the phalangeal attachment of the radial collateral ligament of the MP joint of the little finger. If the little finger is clawed as well as abducted, the other half tendon is inserted through the A2 pulley of the flexor sheath.

junctura tendinum attachment to the little finger is first dissected and surgically extended distally over the MP joint of the little finger and the gap in the extensor hood closed. The distal tip of this extended junctura tendinum is gently pulled proximally and freed up to its origin on the ED of the ring finger. The tendon slip is passed volar to the deep transverse metacarpal ligament and sutured either to the radial collateral ligament on the proximal phalanx of the little finger or to the radial aspect of the extensor hood. The adequacy in length of this slip largely depends on the actual length of the junctura tendinum bridging the ED of the little and ring fingers, and the surgeon must harvest sufficient length from the dorsal hood of the little finger. A short slip will invariably slacken the extensor mechanism of the ring finger and tighten the dorsal apparatus over the MP joint of the little finger.

Author's Preferred Method of Treatment

Corrections of this sometimes vexing problem are fortunately few in my clinical practice. Tendon transfers that use the radial lateral band of the dorsal extensor expansion to correct claw hand deformity often simultaneously address the problem. If preoperative evaluation defines ulnar sub-luxation of the sagittal band of the extensor apparatus over the MP joint, reefing the sagittal band on the radial side and a releasing incision on the ulnar sagittal band can be followed by the lateral band insertion of a dynamic transfer. In the uncommon situation in which the little finger abducts even after claw finger correction I use one entire slip of the EDM or an accessory ED tendon to the ring finger and dissect them as far distally as possible. Careful closure of the gap in the extensor apparatus on the donor finger is necessary. I use a pull-out wire technique to insert the tendon into the proximal phalanx of the little finger because of limitations in working space.

RESTORING FINGER AND WRIST FLEXION WEAKNESS

Physical examination of a hand with marked weakness of the ring and little fingers is characterized by the patient's inability to tuck the tips of these fingers into the palm at the level of the distal palmar crease, with the DIP joint remaining extended. Manual muscle testing and assessment of grip with a Jamar dynamometer confirm subjective weakness.

FDPL and FDPR Transfer to FDPM (Omer[99,103,110]; Omer and Pirela-Cruz[113])

Omer attaches the profundus tendons of the ring and little fingers to the profundus tendon of the long finger in the forearm. The index profundus is left free (Fig. 33-25). Simple DIP tenodesis using the respective flexor digitorum profundus of the ring and little fingers has also been suggested,[95,99] in addition to transfers for proximal phalanx flexion and integration of finger flexion and restoration of the metacarpal arch.

For restoring strong flexion and ulnar deviation at the wrist, Omer proposed the transfer of the FCR to the FCU in patients with proximal ulnar nerve palsy.

Bunnell[34] believed it inadvisable to join the ring and little profundus to the profundus of the long finger because functional extrinsic digital flexors actually accentuate the claw hand deformity. Brand[23] did not consider loss of the FCU and the ulnar half of the FDP to be a functional problem and recommended against tendon transfers unless there was concomitant median or radial nerve loss.

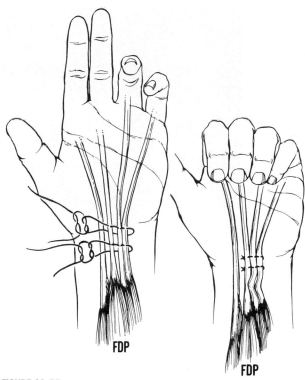

FIGURE 33-25. Tenodesis of the ulnar-innervated profundus tendons of the ring and little fingers to the active median-innervated FDP of the long finger to increase power for gross grip. Double line of sutures is important to prevent "whipsawing" of the tendons during power grip.

side transfer of the FDPM to the FDPR and FDPL just proximal to flexor zone V in the distal forearm. However, it is essential that the patient understand that this operation will most likely exaggerate the claw deformity. After 3 weeks of immobilization, muscle strengthening exercises are supervised for the next 4 weeks. A knuckle bender splint is worn, and instructions are given regarding prevention of contractures at the IP joints during this interim period before the next stage of reconstruction is done.

For weak wrist flexion and ulnar deviation in proximal ulnar nerve lesions, I have transferred the palmaris longus to the FCU if the tendon appears stout on physical examination and is not necessary for correction of intrinsic paralysis. Alternatively and in the absence of the palmaris longus, I have sectioned the ulnar half of the FCR just proximal to the wrist crease and split it proximally for 10 to 12 cm before transferring this to the FCU.

RESTORATION OF SENSIBILITY

Loss of sensibility in the ulnar border of the hand and loss of proprioception in the little finger are significant functional limitations. Repeated ulceration at the tips of the digits can lead to absorption and shortening despite the success of tendon transfers in correcting the claw deformity (Fig. 33-26). In patients who have leprosy, successful medical treatment does not restore sensation and their insensate digits remain a liability for life. Health education is reinforced in many different ways so that individuals can care for their hands. Brand's approach through the "New Life

Author's Preferred Method of Treatment

For a patient with proximal ulnar nerve palsy, it is inadvisable to correct the intrinsic muscle paralysis before restoration of adequate extrinsic flexion power, because the patient will find it difficult to close the hand fully and continue to have a weak grip despite the claw correction. The sequence of corrective surgery is important: there is a need to first restore extrinsic power before providing prehension with intrinsic muscle functional transfers. I perform a side-to-

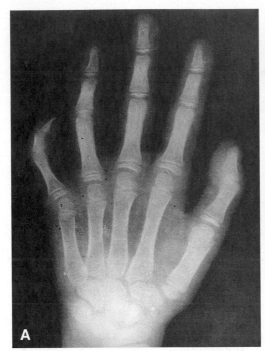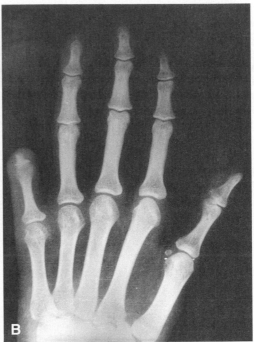

FIGURE 33-26. Radiologic appearance of the progressive absorption of the little finger due to persisting sensory loss in Hansen's disease after successful corrective surgery of claw hand and "Z" thumb. **A,** The anteroposterior view of claw hand due to proximal ulnar palsy in a 13-year-old patient with inactive Hansen's disease shows minimal absorption of the terminal phalanx. Surgery consisted of an EF4T procedure and a transfer of the FDSM to the abductor tubercle of the thumb. **B,** Radiograph of the hand taken at a review 9 years later shows maintenance of sustained correction of the claw fingers and thumb but marked absorption of the little finger up to the base of the middle phalanx in the little finger.

Centers" in this country has helped preserve many hands by enabling a change of vocation to carpentry, weaving, knitting, lathe machine work, and the like, vocations in which there is the need for the individual to regularly observe his or her hands as he or she completes the task.

Digital Nerve Transfer (Lewis et al[79]; Stocks et al[142])

Lewis,[79,142] transferred a functioning median-supplied digital nerve to a nonfunctioning ulnar digital nerve of the little finger to restore sensation. These authors reported that 85% of their patients obtained sensibility levels of S3+ or S4 after surgery. Patients who returned to work after surgery rated their sensibility significantly better than those who did not work. This procedure has obvious advantages in late-presenting ulnar nerve injuries and in cases in which the patients already show tell-tale signs of trophic changes. Frank tissue loss precludes attempts at reinnervation.

I have transferred a neurovascular cutaneous island flap from the ulnar side of the pulp of the middle finger to the pulp of the little finger in selected patients with a history of chronic ulnar nerve injury due to trauma or burns. This is technically straightforward, and the patient notices an early appreciation of sensation.

WASTED INTERMETACARPAL SPACES

Severe intermetacarpal atrophy can be quite disfiguring and disturbing to patients, despite successful functional restoration for ulnar nerve palsy. This is particularly true for patients treated for leprosy and may represent a barrier to integration

with family and colleagues at work. Surgical insertion of a dermal graft can mask interosseous wasting and is most successful between the thumb and index metacarpals.[72] Suitable candidates are those who have had the motor component of the deformities corrected 2 to 3 months previously with appreciable functional restoration. The patient must be informed that this "cosmetic" procedure may only be 50% successful in long-term correction of the deformity. As the transplanted fascia becomes atrophic and the remnant of subcutaneous fat gets absorbed, the fullness of the intermetacarpal space will recede to a level just beneath the metacarpal edges in a "successful" procedure. Wasting of all intermetacarpal spaces can be treated at the same sitting.

Description of Dermal Graft Procedure (Johnson[72])

A transverse incision is made along the entire width of the web margin of the first intermetacarpal space (Fig. 33-27). Gentle blunt dissection is carried out in the subcutaneous space above the atrophic muscle, taking care not to make the pocket any larger than required. The aim is to get a snug fit of the graft and leave no space for a seroma to form. The pocket is packed with a sponge soaked in 1:200,000 adrenaline solution while the dermal graft is being obtained. The dermal graft is taken from the lateral aspect of the buttocks where it is thick, by first folding back a split-thickness skin graft overlying the proposed site. The dermal graft is harvested by incising and removing an ellipse or a rectangle of dermal tissue depending on the size required for the number of spaces to be filled. If only a single graft is harvested, the split-skin graft can usually be discarded and

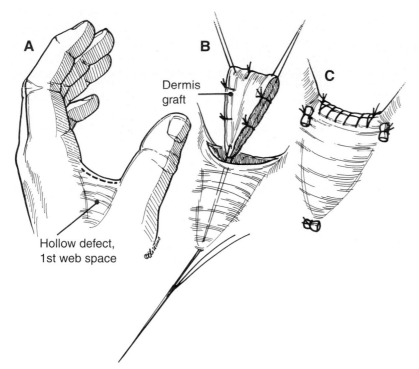

FIGURE 33-27. Free dermal graft transfer for atrophy of the first web space. **A,** Incision along thumb web margin (*hatched area* represents wasting). **B,** Dermal graft from the ipsilateral thigh folded and piloted into the defect with a straight needle and brought out dorsally at the angle of the web. **C,** Dermal graft held in place with tie over sutures on small rubber tubing. The web is closed. This is repeated as required for other intermetacarpal spaces.

a primary closure performed after undermining the edges of the defect. When all the intermetacarpal spaces are being treated, the split-skin graft is turned back to cover the underlying fat and anchored with interrupted sutures. A tie-down bolus dressing is applied. Next the harvested dermal graft is folded on itself to form two layers and shaped to conform to the triangular web spaces to be filled. A few interrupted sutures are placed on the three sides. Each doubled graft is tacked in three corners using absorbable sutures, by leaving the suture at the advancing corner long and threaded onto a straight needle. After obtaining complete hemostasis in the pocket using bipolar cautery, the straight needles are used to guide the graft to fill the entire pocket. The sutures at the three angles are tied over a cotton pledge or button. The web incisions are closed with a continuous monofilament nylon suture. The hand is dressed in a bulky conforming dressing with the thumb web fully abducted and lightly padded plaster. Postoperative elevation is advised for 48 hours, and the thumb web is maintained in abduction splinting for 3 weeks. Complications include hematoma and persistent edema. The former may have to be drained if not resolved by elevation and hand therapy.

The avascular dermal transplants should be made using as little fat as possible because most of the fat is resorbed. I have filled all four intermetacarpal spaces in younger patients whose ulnar palsy affected their dominant hand. As expected, a large part of the grafts were absorbed but the ultimate appearance was quite satisfying to the few who had the procedure.

Early Tendon Transfers (Internal Splints) for Nerve Injuries

Burkhalter[35] introduced the concept of early tendon transfers after nerve repair to allow early function of the hand while awaiting nerve regeneration. The performance of certain basic functions during this period allowed the hand to remain conditioned and gradually attain maximal function. Early tendon transfers can prevent deformities that lead to contractures, improve the coordination of residual muscle-tendon units, and stimulate sensory re-education during nerve recovery.[35,37] The transfers function as internal splints for the paralyzed muscles and in the event of a failure of nerve recovery will remain and function as a permanent solution.[35,37,103]

Unlike external splinting, which can be cumbersome and where compliance can be a problem, internal splinting has a distinct advantage. The surgeon can use as few transfers as required to maintain dynamic positions for functional coordination and sensory re-education. Tendon transfers as internal splints for distal ulnar nerve palsy are listed in Table 33-3. Early tendon transfers have been shown to improve function more in the dominant than in the nondominant hand.[40]

Author's Preferred Method of Treatment

Ulnar nerve palsy results in a hand with so many functional problems that there is no "standard" accepted program that is suitable for reconstruction in all patients. Available tendon assets must be invested wisely. For example, the ubiquitous FDS has been overused for proximal phalanx flexion, as a substitute for the lumbricals, as a thumb adductor, for restoration of the metacarpal arch, and as an index abductor, yet it provides the only flexor power in the ring and little fingers in high (proximal) ulnar nerve palsy!

Table 33-3

INTERNAL SPLINTS (TENDON TRANSFERS) ONLY FOR POST-TRAUMATIC DISTAL ULNAR PALSY

Needed Function	Transfer*
Proximal phalanx flexion for ring and little fingers	Ulnar half of FDSR with split insertion to ring and little fingers to lateral band of DEE[79,84] or A1, A2, or A1 + A2a pulleys[26,30,103]
Restoration of transverse metacarpal arch and adduction of little finger	FDSR Y insertion[4,15,21,49,50,67]
Thumb adduction for key pinch	FDSR radial half to abductor tubercle[21,33,67,75] FDSL to hypothenar insertion, near fifth MP joint

*Note only the FDS from two fingers can at the most be used. The author suggests the FDSR and FDSL.

The prognosis for reinnervation after early repair of a distal ulnar nerve laceration has improved in recent times.[10,57,87,92,94] In these patients, selected tendon transfers may be performed as internal splints to support partial function, decrease cortical exclusion, and prevent deformity while awaiting potential nerve recovery. A complete motor reconstruction program should be performed in patients with severe extremity injuries, a long nerve graft, or a high (proximal) ulnar nerve lesion. The author's preferred methods are listed in Table 33-4. The surgeon needs to carefully choose what is most suited to the patient's needs and do them in stages if necessary. It is important to remember that in patients with proximal ulnar nerve injury, the potential for return of functional motor function with tendon transfers is better than the potential for recovery of sensibility.

I do not recommend the use of one tendon to fulfill different functions at opposite ends of the hand; such transfers are likely not to be effective, owing to differential tension requirements on the two slips. Placement of multiple graft slips to similar insertion sites in the fingers in claw correction is an exception, because the movements to be restored are in the same plane and the digits work in tandem. Given an adequate number and power of potential donors, tendon transfer within the hand should attempt to satisfactorily replace one function and be durable.

The reconstructive methods to restore balance and improve function on each patient is a decision that the surgeon needs to consider carefully, by adopting staged management and by avoiding ambitious combinations of surgery. Treatment of ulnar nerve palsy for different causes differs only slightly. Table 33-5 lists my preference in children with ulnar nerve palsy, and Table 33-6 is the surgical program for the few individuals with intrinsic paralysis due to residual paralysis of poliomyelitis.

Table 33-4

AUTHOR'S PREFERENCE FOR RECONSTRUCTIVE PROCEDURE IN ULNAR PALSY*

Required Functions	Preferred Options
MP and IP joint integration: claw finger correction	*Type I claw hand:* EF4T[18,55,114]; PL4T[55] int. insertion with PL[3,114]; FDSR[3] *Type II claw hand:* int. insertion with PL4T[3,114] or FDSR[3]; EF4T[3,18,55]; PL4T[3,55] *Type III claw hand:* FDSM to A1 + A2a[3] pulley; EF4T[55] *Type IV claw hand:* FDSM to lateral band[3,18,55]; EF4T to lateral band[3,55] *Type V claw hand:* repair/relocate lateral band, then modified Stiles-Bunnell transfer to central tendon of dorsal apparatus[3,55]
Thumb adduction	BR to add. tubercle[13] ECRB to prox. phalanx[136]
Index abduction	E1 to first DI[30]
Thumb MP joint hyperextension	Half FPL to EPL
Thumb MP joint instability	MP joint fusion[77,102,127]
Thumb IP joint fixed contracture	IP joint fusion[77]
Metacarpal arch reversal	EDM to hypothenar insertion base little finger[11] FDSL to hypothenar insertion base little finger
Profundus weakness FDPL and R	FDPL and R tenodesis to FDPM[99,103,113]
Wrist flexion-adduction weakness	PL to FCU[99] Half FCR to FCU (yoke transfer)
Ring and little finger sensibility	Proximal digital nerve from medial side of middle finger transfer to common digital nerve between ring and little fingers[79,142]
Sensation to the pulp of little finger	Neurovascular island from medial side of middle finger translocated to little finger pulp
Gross wasting intermetacarpal space	Dermofascial flap from thigh to fill spaces[72]

*Selection to be based on location of lesion: i.e., proximal, distal, or distal motor branch paralysis.

Table 33-5

AUTHOR'S PREFERENCE OF RECONSTRUCTIVE SURGERY IN CHILDREN WITH ULNAR NERVE PALSY*

Required Function	Preferred Options
Claw hand	PL4T, EF4T, interosseous insertion of PL
"Z" thumb	BR to adductor tubercle
Hypermobile "Z" thumb	MP joint arthrodesis after the 14th year
Arch reversal	FDSL to hypothenar insertion base little finger

*Additional reconstruction can be done for any other deficiencies that appear marked. Adopting a staged reconstructive surgical program is ideal.

Table 33-6

AUTHOR'S PREFERENCE OF RECONSTRUCTIVE SURGERY FOR POST-POLIO RESIDUAL PARALYTIC HANDS WITH INTRINSIC WEAKNESS*

Specific Deficits	Preferred Surgery
Claw fingers	MP volar capsulodesis
"Z" thumb	MP joint arthrodesis

*Additional deformities must be carefully evaluated for correction based on the available assets. The remarkable adaptation and substitution in these sensate hands should *not* be disturbed by an ambitious program of corrective procedures that can restrict mobility.

ANNOTATED REFERENCES

8. Backhouse KM, Catton WI: An experimental study of the functions of the lumbrical muscles in the human hand. J Anat 88:133-141, 1954.

   This study of the lumbrical muscles by electromyography and electrical stimulation provided a valuable insight into the true functions of the lumbricals by clearly showing that they are primarily extensors of the IP joint. Their function as an MP joint flexor was found to be weak and only in IP joint extension. It prompted even more detailed study by anatomists and kinesiologists.

18. Brand PW: Tendon grafting: Illustrated by a new operation for intrinsic paralysis of the fingers. J Bone Joint Surg Br 43:444-453, 1961.

   Following on the author's earlier report with the Stiles-Bunnell and modified Stiles-Bunnell procedures using the superficialis tendon for claw hands due to leprosy done for large numbers of patients since 1948, this was a comprehensive work revolving around a "phasic" transfer of the author's for claw hands of the same etiology. Valuable information on his method of lengthening the wrist motors and introduction of the flexor route for transfer through the carpal tunnel besides the detailed documentation of the outcome of claw correction and the complications can be found. This continues to serve as a reference for comparing the outcome of different dynamic claw correction procedures.

33. Bunnell S: Surgery of the intrinsic muscles of the hand other than those producing opposition of the thumb. J Bone Joint Surg 24:1-3, 1942.

   This is the earliest report on the deformities resulting from intrinsic muscle paralysis of the hand that bears the hallmark of the father of modern hand surgery. Bunnell's craftsmanship and scientific basis for transfers has no parallel as he lays the foundations of surgical mechanics, tendon dynamics, the routes, and the importance of "pulleys" in tendon transfers for intrinsic muscle paralysis. The making of a reconstructive surgeon for paralytic conditions in the hand begins with the assimilation of this report.

35. Burkhalter WE: Early tendon transfers in upper extremity peripheral nerve injury. Clin Orthop 104:68-79, 1974.

   A vital and much needed break from tradition is reported about the functional restoration by early tendon transfers in the hand. It is the antecedent report for the innovative internal splinting methods to improve muscle-tendon coordination and to stimulate sensory re-education. The author's extensive experience as a leading surgeon for the war wounded provided an impetus for this philosophy of management that is the recommended norm.

75. Landsmeer JMF: The coordination of finger-joint motions. J Bone Joint Surg Am 45:1652-1662, 1963.

   Johann Landsmeer's article summarizes major aspects of his life's work in the field of biomechanics of the complex deformities in the digits. His monumental work on the digital articulations explained by the biarticular model with the intercalated segment represents an area that has not much caught the attention of hand surgeons. In understanding this report, it is likely that the reader will be prompted to access Landsmeer's complete works and to pursue the technical aspects of reconstructive surgery through an appreciation of the mechanics of causation of deformity.

82. Littler JW: Tendon transfers and arthrodesis in combined median and ulnar nerve palsies. J Bone Joint Surg Am 31:225-234, 1949.

   This is one of the early reports to carry much information on the methods of reconstructive procedures for the multiple problems met with in the paralytic hand. Some of the proposals, modifications, and contributions in the areas of claw correction, restoration of thumb adduction, and correction of the reversed metacarpal arch are very informative and stand to this day as useful options.

86. Long C: Intrinsic-extrinsic muscle control of the fingers: Electromyographic studies. J Bone Joint Surg Am 50:973-984, 1968.

   Evaluation of the actual functioning of the intrinsic and extrinsic muscles that control the hand in motion is presented through EMG analysis. In Dr. Charles Long's studies of the combination of motions with respect to MP and IP joints, the lumbricals and interossei were shown as being separate kinesiologic entities but that the palmar interossei behaved like the lumbricals in extending the IP joints during any position of the MP joints. This further strengthens the decision to make use of the interossei as an insertion site.

115. Parkes A: Paralytic claw fingers—a graft tenodesis operation. Hand 5:192-199, 1973.

   An impressive presentation of an effective graft tenodesis operation follows the analysis of the dynamic procedures and their limitations. Coming 15 years after the description of the MP joint volar capsulodesis, this static procedure came to be realized as predictable to preserve the individuality of the finger after claw correction. Strange although it may sound, this is the only procedure that can be safely "undone," and this feature has not been put to good use for the program of internal splinting while awaiting ulnar nerve recovery.

118. Ranney DA: The mechanism of arch reversal in the surgically corrected claw hand. Hand 6:266-272, 1974.

A transverse deformity of the hand like the reversed metacarpal arch is as disabling as the axial deformity of the hand is disfiguring. The author provides some valuable insights into the mechanism of causation of this deformity. It draws the attention of reconstructive surgeons to the surgical procedures that aggravate the problem and how this could be partly overcome.

156. Zancolli EA: Claw-hand caused by paralysis of the intrinsic muscles. A simple surgical procedure for its correction. J Bone Joint Surg Am 39:1076-1080, 1957.

A successful answer to claw correction without the need for tendon transfer came about after the description of the volar stabilization of the MP joint in flexion through capsulodesis. This detailed report also covers an elaborate aspect of the mechanism of claw deformity, and it is of historical importance to review this paper because of the need for any surgical team to find recourse to this method of correction.

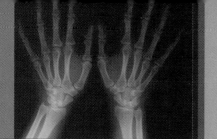

CHAPTER 34

Cerebral Palsy

Michelle Gerwin Carlson

Cerebral palsy is a musculoskeletal deformity caused by an irreversible, static, perinatal brain injury. The extent of involvement of motor function, sensibility, and intelligence is variable.[85,100] Cerebral palsy is usually classified by the number of limbs involved: monoplegia (one extremity), hemiplegia (one arm, one leg), diplegia (two legs), tetraplegia (two legs, one arm), and quadriplegia (all four extremities). Motor involvement can take the form of spasticity or flaccidity,[115] and in athetosis it can vary between the two. Spastic involvement of a muscle is often coupled with flaccid involvement of its antagonist, potentiating the deformity. Spastic deformities in the upper extremity most often result in shoulder internal rotation, elbow flexion, forearm pronation, wrist flexion, finger flexion, intrinsic spasticity, and thumb-in-palm deformity.

Identification of upper limb dysfunction is usually noted by 1 year of age, as the normal infant develops a refined pinch with opposition of the thumb to the index finger. Infants with cerebral palsy do not reach this milestone, although they may develop a more primitive key pinch (thumb to side of index finger).

PREOPERATIVE EVALUATION

Evaluation of the patient with cerebral palsy should involve a team approach, including the pediatrician, occupational therapist, physical therapist, and social worker. Often multiple visits to the treating orthopedist are required until a full evaluation is completed. It is imperative to eliminate other treatable diagnoses as potential causes for cerebral dysfunction. The team should ensure that the child is getting adequate therapy and accommodation in school. Treatment should be aimed at improving function of the upper extremity, but it can rarely yield restoration of a normal limb. Surgery of the upper extremity in cerebral palsy is reparative, not curative.[13,63]

Historically, 50% of operations on the upper extremity are performed to achieve functional improvement. In the remaining operations, cosmesis and hygiene are the major factors influencing treatment.[9,10,38] In identifying surgical candidates, it is equally important to properly identify those patients who have little voluntary control of the extremity and thus will not benefit from surgical intervention. A careful examination of the patient, including motor, sensory, and intellectual function, is critical in determining the most successful treatment.

Physical Examination

Physical examination of the spastic upper extremity is difficult. Despite their best efforts, patients often have difficulty cooperating during the examination. Asking patients to perform activities with both extremities simultaneously can ensure that the patient comprehends instructions. Evaluation for voluntary activity and for differentiation of muscle spasticity from muscle contracture and joint contracture is important.[115] Muscle spasticity, with relaxation, allows full range of motion of the joint, whereas muscle contracture does not. Muscle contracture and joint contracture often coexist in the adult; joint contractures are less common in the child. Observation of the patient performing routine activities assists in determining true functional deficits and patterns of hand function. Often the patient (or the parent) can verbalize what activities he or she is unable to perform as a result of the spastic extremity, and treatment can be tailored accordingly. Multiple visits are paramount to a thorough evaluation; videotaping of the child during functional activities and ambulation is very helpful.

The examination must accomplish several tasks. First, notation should be made of the position of rest of the extremity. Passive as well as active range of motion of all joints should be measured. The strength of all potential donor muscles for transfer should be measured. Patterned hand function should be identified. Flexor tendon spasticity and tightness should be identified. Muscle spasticity can be overcome by the application of gentle sustained resistance to the spastic force. Inspection should be made of potential hygiene problems in the axilla, antecubital fossa, volar wrist flexion crease, palm, and interdigital spaces.

Shoulder. If the position of rest is in internal rotation, spasticity and possible contracture exist (Fig. 34-1A). A determination should be made as to whether this interferes with the patient's ability to use the extremity. Patients who are wheelchair bound may have no loss of use of the extremity with an internal rotation contracture, because the entire use of that extremity is in front of them on a work board.

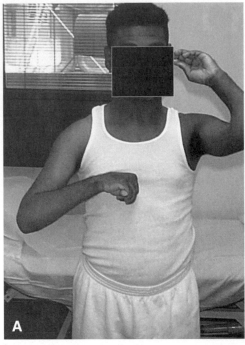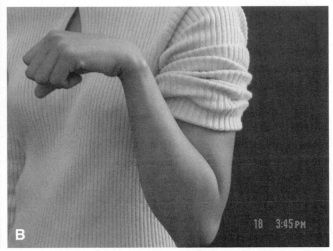

FIGURE 34-1. Spastic posturing in the upper extremity in cerebral palsy. **A,** Shoulder internal rotation. **B,** Elbow flexion, forearm pronation, and wrist flexion. (**A** and **B,** © Michelle Gerwin Carlson.)

Elbow. The biceps and brachioradialis are palpated in terminal extension for spasticity. The position of rest of the elbow when the patient is walking, running, and performing other activities should be observed. Wheelchair-bound patients rarely need more than 45 degrees of terminal extension of the elbow, because most of their use is at tabletop level, whereas ambulatory patients with assistive devices will have difficulty with elbow spasticity.

Forearm. Palpation of the pronator teres during passive supination of the forearm can identify spasticity. Evaluation for active supination and pronation should also be determined, as well as the position of the forearm at rest.

Wrist and Digits. Observation of the wrist during flexion and extension often demonstrates causes of spasticity. If the wrist ulnarly deviates with flexion (see Fig. 34-1B), spasticity of the flexor carpi ulnaris (FCU) tendon is suspected. If ulnar deviation of the wrist occurs in extension, the extensor carpi ulnaris (ECU) tendon is the cause. Incomplete passive extension is usually secondary to contracture of the FCU. In addition to evaluating for active wrist extension, active flexion should be tested while palpating the flexor carpi radialis (FCR) tendon. It is critical that the FCR be functional if the FCU is to be considered as a potential transfer.

Flexor Tightness. Digital flexor tendon tightness can be assessed using Volkmann's angle (Fig. 34-2). With the wrist flexed and the digits held completely extended, the wrist is then passively brought into maximal extension.[98] In the absence of flexor tendon tightness, full wrist extension and finger extension can be simultaneously achieved. With digital flexor contracture, the wrist cannot be extended to neutral. It is possible to assess whether the spasticity is in the flexor digitorum superficialis (FDS) or profundus (FDP) by holding the wrist in extension while passively extending the digits. When passive proximal interphalangeal (PIP) joint extension is limited, FDS spasticity should be suspected (FDP spasticity may also be present). If the PIP joints have full passive extension but the distal interphalangeal (DIP) joints do not, then FDP spasticity is suspected.

Grasp and Release. Evaluation for grasp and release should be performed with the wrist flexed and extended. Poor grasp is secondary to weak or absent *wrist* extension, because a flexed wrist slackens the digital flexor muscles and minimizes potential for force production. Inability to extend the wrist may be caused by weak or absent wrist extensors or by spastic wrist flexors. The strength of grasp can be improved with a transfer to increase wrist extensor power.

Poor release is the result of weak or absent *digital* extensors. Patients with impaired release are unable to actively extend the digits or are able to extend the digits only when the wrist is flexed; when the wrist is passively held extended, active digital extension is not possible. It is important to rule out flexor tendon spasticity as a cause, because a transfer to improve wrist extension may leave this patient unable to extend the digits. This patient would benefit from a transfer to augment digital extension, not wrist extension.

Intrinsic Tightness. Intrinsic muscle tightness can be identified by a resting position of metacarpophalangeal (MCP) joint flexion and interphalangeal (IP) joint extension.

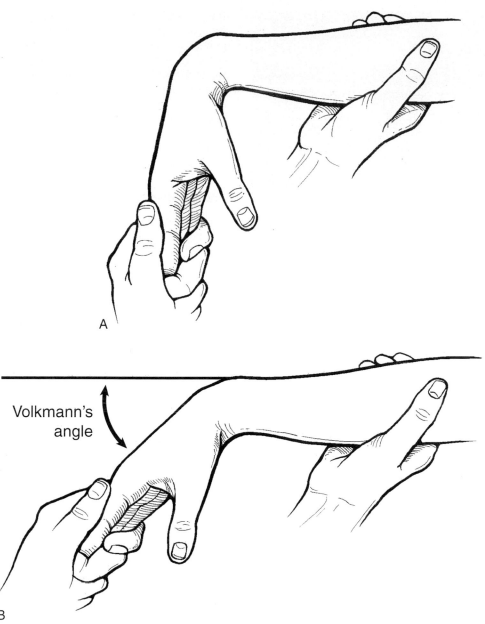

FIGURE 34-2. Volkmann's test for digital flexor tendon tightness. **A,** The digits are held extended with the wrist flexed. **B,** The wrist is extended with the digits extended. With no flexor tendon tightness, full extension of the wrist should be possible. Wrist extension to less than neutral (Volkmann's angle) indicates the need for surgical intervention.

If a patient is a candidate for digital flexor tendon lengthening, the intrinsics must be carefully examined. If the intrinsics are spastic, release of the digital flexors without release of the intrinsics will result in a hand with flexed MCP joints and extended PIP joints.

Intrinsic tightness is best evaluated by the Bunnell test, performed by passive flexion of the PIP joints while the MCP joints are held first in full extension and subsequently in flexion. When fixed intrinsic tightness is present, passive motion of the PIP joint is greater with the MCP joints flexed than when extended. (See Chapter 33 for more detailed description and illustrations of the intrinsic tightness test.) If swan neck deformities of the PIP joints are present, they should be evaluated for flexibility. Local anesthetic block of the ulnar nerve at the wrist can be very effective in demonstrating the effect of intrinsic muscle release for the surgeon, as well as the patient. Ulnar nerve block can also help to differentiate intrinsic spasticity from fixed intrinsic or PIP contractures.

Thumb. Correction of the thumb-in-palm deformity is a careful balancing act between multiple muscles, tendons, and joints. Correction of the thumb-in-palm deformity is often performed concurrently with wrist extension augmentation, so testing of the deformity should be done in both wrist flexion and extension. Thumb extension occurs in a radial direction in the plane of the hand, and thumb abduction occurs in the plane perpendicular to the palmar

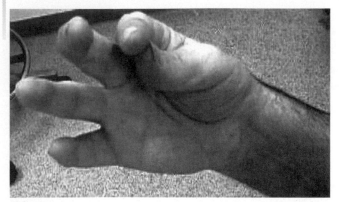

FIGURE 34-3. Thumb-in-palm deformity. Undesired flexion of the thumb into the palm interferes with grasp, and the inability to abduct the thumb prevents manipulation of large objects. (© Michelle Gerwin Carlson.)

surface (Fig. 34-3). Examination of the deformity should include evaluation of four key points:

1. Web space contracture with measurement of the passive and active web space angle
2. Spasticity or contracture of the adductor pollicis brevis (APB), flexor pollicis brevis (FPB), and first dorsal interosseous, and spasticity of the flexor pollicis longus (FPL) with the wrist flexed and extended
3. Strength of the abductor pollicis longus (APL) and extensor pollicis brevis (EPB) with the wrist flexed and extended, and strength of the extensor pollicis longus (EPL) with the wrist flexed and extended
4. Hyperextension of the thumb MCP joint

Dynamic Electromyography

Dynamic electromyography (EMG) is helpful to identify spastic and flaccid muscles and to determine phasic activity. EMGs have been advocated in the decision process for surgery,[38-43,45,48,66,85] although some believe that the information gained is not more valuable than that obtained from serial physical examinations.[55] Dynamic EMGs often require a combination of surface electrodes and fine-needle examination of the muscles of the elbow, forearm, and hand. Volitional activity as well as patterned activity should be evaluated to identify muscles that are firing normally in phase versus those that are firing out of phase, firing continuously, or not firing at all (Fig. 34-4).

In the elbow, the biceps, brachialis, and brachioradialis can be evaluated for spasticity and possible surgical release, as can the adductor pollicis in the hand. Weak or absent wrist extension (grasp) or digital extension (release) can be identified by the EMG response of the wrist extensors and digital flexor muscles, respectively. Dynamic EMGs can help to identify inappropriate muscle firing, as well as those muscles that would be best for transfer. Out-of-phase or continuous firing of the flexor carpi ulnaris and digital flexors is frequently seen, as is absent firing of the digital and radial wrist extensors. Extensor carpi ulnaris function is more variable.

Muscles firing during digital release are good candidates for transfers to improve digital extension, and those firing in grasp are good choices for wrist extension transfers.[38] The

flexor carpi ulnaris, flexor carpi radialis, brachioradialis, pronator teres, extensor carpi ulnaris, and extensor carpi radialis longus all should be studied to determine which are active in grasp and which in release, and therefore best for transfer.[38,40] Continuous activity in a muscle is not an *absolute* contraindication for use as a transfer, because there are some data to suggest that phasic activity can develop after transfer.[66,85]

Unfortunately, specially trained personnel are required to perform dynamic EMGs, and many laboratories do not have the technical support to perform these tests.

Preoperative Therapy and Other Modalities

Preoperative therapy should be aimed at maintaining function and preventing contracture. Range-of-motion exercises can help prevent joint contractures. Splinting and serial casting can stretch tight flexor muscles, but the results are usually temporary.[47,102] Splints are a useful adjunct in planning surgical intervention. A patient with a chronically flexed wrist can "test" the functional effect of the wrist in a neutral position by using a wrist splint. Similarly, potential thumb-in-palm correction can be evaluated with a thumb abduction splint, and potential swan neck deformity correction can be evaluated with an extension block splint. These splints are usually too cumbersome to be practical or effective in providing long-term functional improvement. Contraction of the stretched flexor muscles tends to lead to "flexing out" of the splint (Fig. 34-5). Adaptive devices, however, can be very useful to enable patients to independently perform activities of daily living.

Electrical stimulation has been advocated in the upper extremity for patients with cerebral palsy, but large studies with long-term follow-up have not been performed and improvement in fine motor control has not been documented.[8,86,111,112] In stroke patients it has been shown that electrical stimulation does not improve digital extensor function or decrease finger flexor tightness.[37] Systemic medications have been advocated to decrease spasticity.[67] Botulinum A toxin, which denervates the muscle by blocking presynaptic acetylcholine release, has gained some interest. Some have found it useful in the lower extremity, but its effects are temporary.[50] Injection of botulinum A toxin[2,14,20,50,106,113] is still experimental, and long-term results have not been demonstrated. Constraint-induced therapy has been used to inhibit the uninvolved arm so as to encourage the involved arm to perform more tasks. Studies have shown improvement in hand function and quality of use in the short term,[155,272] but long-term benefits have yet to be demonstrated.

Grading of Hand Function

Many classifications have been proposed to grade hand function. All are used to assess operative results and not to identify patients for surgery. Classifications vary from four subgroups to nine subgroups, identifying functional use of the hand. The rating system of Green and Banks,[34] modified by Samilson and Morris,[85] contains four subgroups:

Poor: Use of the hand only as a paperweight, poor or absent grasp and release, and poor control

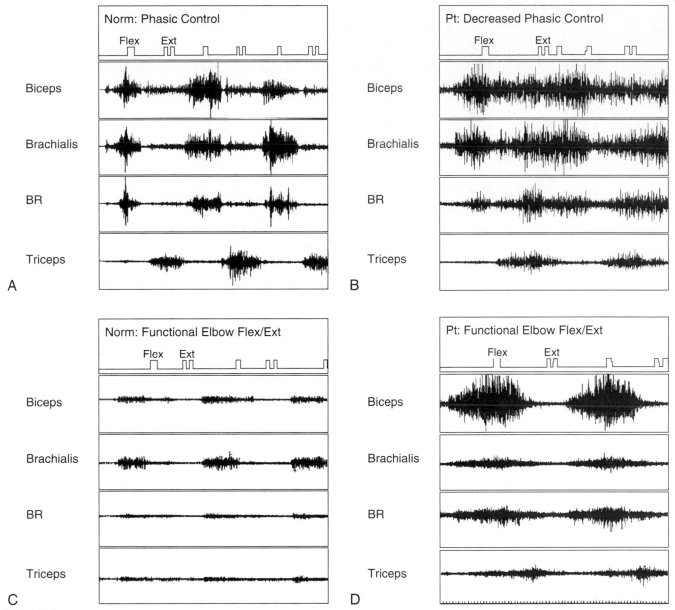

FIGURE 34-4. Dynamic electromyograms of the elbow. **A,** Normal phasic control in maximal contraction. Note the alternation in firing between flexion and extension. **B,** In this patient there is loss of phasic control and the elbow flexors fire in flexion and extension. **C,** Normal functional use. A patient is asked to lift a light object and the amount of contraction decreases from maximal effort (compare with **A**). **D,** In this patient there is loss of functional grading, because even with lifting a light object there is still significant functional contraction.

Fair: Use of the hand as a helping hand but no effectual use of the hand in dressing, moderate grasp and release, and fair control

Good: Use of the hand as a help in dressing and eating and general activities, effectual grasp and release, excellent control

Excellent: Good use of the hand in dressing and eating, effectual grasp and release, and good control

House and colleagues[44] described a classification system containing nine subgroups, making identification of small improvement in function possible (Table 34-1). Other classification systems have also been described to evaluate function of the upper extremity in cerebral palsy.[96,103]

TYPES OF OPERATIONS

Guidelines for Surgical Intervention

Several guidelines for selection of surgical candidates have appeared throughout the literature, and include voluntary use and sensibility of the hand, age and intelligence of the patient, and the presence of athetosis. All of these are relative indications or contraindications and need to be considered in light of the entire patient and expected goals.[16,38,55,68,104,107]

Voluntary Hand Use. Quantification of voluntary hand use is difficult. Hoffer[38] described the ability to place the hand from the head to the knee in an alternating fashion

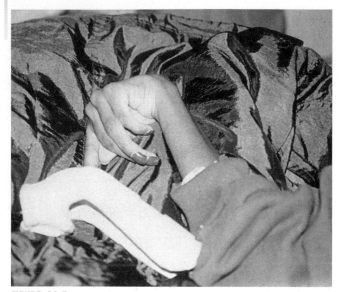

FIGURE 34-5. Splinting of the severely flexed wrist is difficult. Volar splinting of the wrist stimulates the palm, increasing the pathologic flexion response, which tends to make the patient "flex out" of the splint. Dorsal splinting lacks the mechanical advantage necessary to be effective. (© Michelle Gerwin Carlson.)

every 5 seconds as a way of estimating voluntary hand use. Hand placement is dependent on good shoulder and elbow control without contracture. Good hand placement is not possible with significant ataxia, athetosis, or dyskinesia.

It is important to examine the hand and wrist for voluntary flexion and extension. The digits should be examined with the wrist flexed and extended. Flexion of the wrist may allow active digital extension that is not possible with the wrist extended. Similarly, extension of the wrist may allow active digital flexion that is not possible with the wrist flexed.

Patients who do not have voluntary use of the hand will not have functional improvement with reconstructive surgery.[53] Limbs that have at least helper function preoperatively are much more likely to benefit functionally from surgery than those that have no useful function.[44] However, surgery may still be of benefit to improve the appearance of the extremity or to prevent hygiene problems.

Sensibility. Impairment of two-point discrimination, stereognosis, and proprioception is found in 50% to 90% of patients.[4,17,32,100,105,114] Sensibility is best tested by texture discrimination in the child younger than age 3 years, object identification in the 4- to 5-year old, graphesthesia in the 6- to 9-year old, and two-point discrimination in the older child.[4,38,39] Improved functional results after upper extremity surgery are more likely in patients with less than 10 mm of two-point discrimination, three of five object discrimination, or number discrimination in the palm (graphesthesia).[30,64,100] Sensory impairment, however, should not preclude reconstructive surgery.[29] Decreased stereognostic ability may in fact be more related to motor impairment and inability to manipulate objects than to actual sensory impairment. Impaired sensibility can be compensated for by hand-eye visual control.[44,100]

Intelligence Quotient (IQ). For reconstructive surgery, many believe that surgery should not be undertaken if the patient has an IQ less than 70.[28,34] However, it has been demonstrated that IQ tests may not be accurate in patients with cerebral palsy.[83,85] Moreover, IQ is not applicable in muscle release procedures and is unimportant if the planned procedure is not dependent on motor or sensory re-education.[55,63]

Athetosis. Fluctuations in tone make reconstructive procedures difficult.[38] Observation for the predominant direction of spasticity may be helpful,[55] but overcorrection is easy. Often fusions produce more reliable results in athetoid patients.[44]

Table 34-1
CLASSIFICATION OF HAND FUNCTION

Class	Designation	Activity Level
0	Does not use	Does not use
1	Poor passive assist	Uses as stabilizing weight only
2	Fair passive assist	Can hold onto object placed in hand
3	Good passive assist	Can hold object and stabilize for use by other hand
4	Poor active assist	Can actively grasp object and hold it weakly
5	Fair active assist	Can actively grasp object and stabilize it well
6	Good active assist	Can actively grasp object, stabilize it well, and manipulate it against other hand
7	Spontaneous use, partial	Can perform bimanual activities easily; occasionally uses hand spontaneously
8	Spontaneous use, complete	Uses hand completely independently without reference to the other hand

From House JH, Gwathmey FW, Fidler MO: A dynamic approach to the thumb-in-palm deformity in cerebral palsy: Evaluation and results in fifty-six patients. J Bone Joint Surg Am 63:216-225, 1981.

Summary of Guidelines. Hygiene should be the primary goal in patients with IQ less than 50, hand placement greater than 5 seconds, and poor sensibility.[38] Patients with IQ greater than 50 but poor placement and sensibility should also be considered for procedures to improve the contracted appearance of the limb. Patients with IQ greater than 50, hand placement less than 5 seconds, and good sensibility are ideal candidates for functional improvement of the extremity.

Goals of Surgical Procedures

The goals for surgery are threefold: (1) to rebalance the muscles in the limb to improve function, (2) to decrease hygiene problems, and (3) to improve cosmesis. Muscular rebalancing involves release of spastic muscles and/or augmentation of antagonist muscles. Because a spastic muscle is, by definition, already firing out of phase, it is often a good choice for transfer to its antagonist. In severe cases of spasticity in which a tendon has sustained firing in phase and out of phase, transfer of that tendon can serve to tether the joint in the opposite direction of the deformity and thus can still be of use in correction of the deformity.[50] Return of phasic activity has occasionally been seen after transfer.[66,85] Results of tendon transfers in properly selected patients have been good, with improvement of function in many hands.[78]

Muscular release can take several forms: release of the origin of the muscle, release of the insertion of the muscle, and lengthening of the muscle by either fractional lengthening through the musculotendinous junction or "Z"-lengthening through the tendon. Motor neurectomy and skeletal shortening can also be used to decrease muscle spasticity or contracture. Any release or lengthening procedure necessarily weakens the muscle. Fractional lengthening is effective when smaller amounts of lengthening are required and can be easily fine tuned at the time of surgery by application of passive stretch to the lengthened muscle. "Z"-lengthening allows for more extensive lengthening, approaching almost twice the length of the tendon. Fine-tuning of this lengthening procedure is more difficult; overlengthening and rupture of the reapproximated tendon can occur.

Release of the origin of the muscle will maintain more function than will tenotomy or release of the tendon insertion. After release, the origin slides distally and will reattach to local soft tissues and still maintain function, although with less strength. Complete release of the muscle insertion allows separation of the muscle from the joint upon which it is acting, causing permanent loss of function.

Joint capsular releases are required if fixed deformities are present and are more commonly necessary in the older child or adult. Arthrodeses may be required for longstanding contractures or when motors are weak or absent. Wrist motion is important to preserve when possible, because it is necessary to initiate a tenodesis effect on the digital flexors and extensors, thus enabling opening and closing of the hand. Wrist fusion will eliminate this tenodesis effect and decrease the patient's voluntary finger motion and thus should be used cautiously.

It is important to address the entire extremity when planning surgical correction. When possible, correction of elbow and wrist flexion deformity should be performed concurrently. Correction of the elbow deformity without correction of the wrist deformity can decrease overall functional ability (Fig. 34-6). Similarly, correction of the wrist deformity without correction of the elbow deformity may improve finger function but does not increase the functional range of the hand in space.

Timing of Surgical Procedures

The effects of cerebral palsy are often recognized soon after birth. Most believe that surgery should be delayed until a clear evaluation of functional use of the hand is possible (between 6 and 12 years of age),[23,54,55,90,109] although some have advocated early surgical correction of the hand at 18 months to 5 years.[11] Reliance on strict age criteria should probably be avoided, and correction should be undertaken when predominant hand use patterns become apparent. Often, because of referral patterns, the child is not referred until the teenage years. This should not be a contraindication to surgery.[55] Even adult patients can benefit from reconstructive surgery, although functional improvement will probably be less.[3] Reconstruction in adults should not be undertaken lightly, however, because they often have learned to compensate for their disabilities. They may be reticent to change, and function may be worsened by attempts at upper limb "improvement."

SHOULDER

Condition

Typical posturing of the shoulder is in internal rotation and adduction. The deformity is caused by spasm or contracture of the subscapularis and pectoralis major muscles and can usually be treated with stretching.[21] Much less frequently, external rotation and abduction posturing of the shoulder may be seen (Fig. 34-7).

Operative Procedures

Lengthening or release of the subscapularis and pectoralis major muscles is usually sufficient to release the internal rotation and adduction contracture. A proximal humeral external rotation osteotomy is occasionally necessary for severe contractures.[90] External rotation spasticity is relieved by release of the supraspinatus, infraspinatus, and teres minor. In athetoid patients, recurrent dislocation of the glenohumeral joint should be treated with glenohumeral arthrodesis.[41]

Release of Shoulder Internal Rotation Deformity

Indication. Release of the shoulder internal rotators is indicated for problems of hygiene within the axilla.

Contraindication. Release of the internal rotators should not be performed in patients with subluxation or dislocation of the shoulder because this may exacerbate the instability.[49] These patients are better candidates for shoulder fusion.

Technique
An axillary incision is made in the axillary fold. The tendon of the pectoralis major is identified anteriorly on the greater

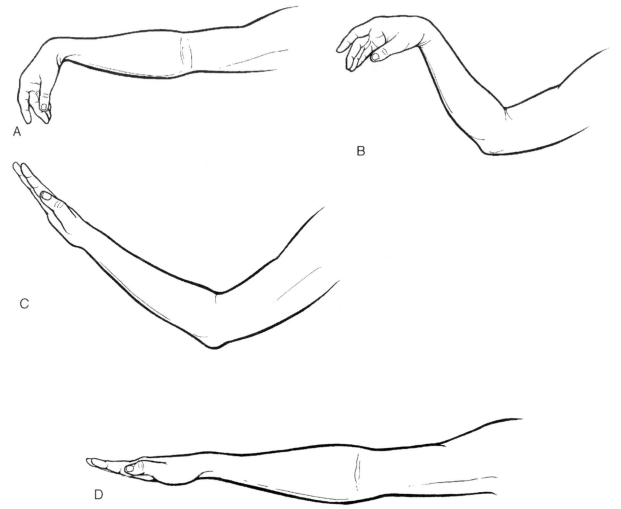

FIGURE 34-6. Concurrent correction of elbow and wrist flexion deformities is important to improve function of the limb. **A,** Wrist and elbow flexion deformity. **B,** Correction of the elbow alone leaves the hand palmarly oriented. **C,** Correction of the wrist alone does not improve the patient's ability to position the hand in space. **D,** Correction of the wrist and elbow places the hand in a neutral position with maximal reach.

tuberosity of the humerus and divided or "Z"-lengthened. The subscapularis tendon insertion is identified on the lesser tuberosity and divided or "Z"-lengthened. "Z"-lengthening should always be attempted, because it will preserve some of the function of the tendon and help prevent anterior dislocation of the shoulder. With severe internal rotation

contracture, "Z"-lengthening will not produce enough length to allow external rotation of the shoulder, and division of the tendon is necessary. The capsule of the shoulder joint is not divided.

An external rotation abduction splint is worn for 3 weeks, followed by progressive range-of-motion exercises.

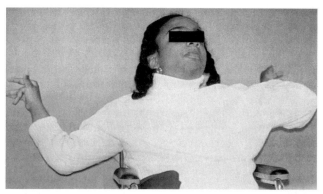

FIGURE 34-7. External rotation and abduction posturing of the shoulder. (© Michelle Gerwin Carlson.)

Author's Preferred Method of Treatment

In the nonfunctional shoulder with severe internal rotation contracture, I lengthen the subscapularis and pectoralis major to address hygiene problems. I rarely address external rotation spasticity because it tends to be episodic, and it usually occurs in a functional shoulder in which overcorrection would cause loss of shoulder function.

ELBOW

Condition

In cerebral palsy, the predominant elbow deformity is a flexion contracture. The initial cause of the deformity is the spastic contracture of any or all of the muscles on the anterior surface of the elbow (biceps, brachialis, brachioradialis), but long-standing deformities can result additionally in soft tissue and joint contractures that also may need to be addressed operatively. The severity of the flexion deformity can range from none to severe chronic hyperflexion of the elbow, causing skin breakdown in the antecubital fossa. Within this spectrum are patients whose elbows remain flexed at 90 degrees throughout use but can be passively extended and patients whose elbows rest at full extension but involuntarily contract with walking or use of the hand. The decision on operative intervention depends on the extent of deformity.

Traditionally, an elbow flexion contracture was considered mostly a cosmetic or hygienic problem.[38] Severe flexion deformity leads to skin breakdown in the antecubital fossa as well as difficulty with dressing. Appearance is an important factor, especially for hemiplegic patients, and cosmetic correction is a commonly expressed desire for the upper extremity. However, the functional limitations of the elbow flexion deformity should not be overlooked. In severe hyperflexion deformities, release of the contracture can allow a patient to assist in wheelchair transfers with the forearms, touch a pictureboard to communicate, reach the tray top of a wheelchair, or touch a wider sphere of objects in his or her environment. In less severe flexion deformities, release of the contracture can allow for use of crutches and walkers, facilitate two-handed manipulation of objects away from the body and, importantly, enable use of a keyboard.

Operative Procedures

Release of the elbow flexion contracture can be addressed in two ways: release of the muscles crossing the anterior elbow or denervation of these muscles. Release of the muscles crossing the elbow includes either individual releases of the biceps, brachialis, and brachioradialis or a flexor-pronator slide. In long-standing contractures, the anterior elbow capsule may also need to be addressed. Dynamic EMGs may be helpful preoperatively in assessing which muscles are spastic, those that are firing out of phase, and those that need to be addressed surgically.

Musculocutaneous Neurectomy[38,41,75]

Indication. Musculocutaneous neurectomy is effective for spastic deformity of less than 30 degrees. Full passive range of motion of the joint is mandatory, because this procedure will not correct soft tissue contractures about the joint. Lidocaine block of the musculocutaneous nerve along the proximal medial aspect of the biceps may assist in differentiating abnormal muscle tone from fixed contracture and will help delineate the degree of potential passive elbow extension possible after neurectomy. The test will also identify the amount of elbow flexion possible through the intact brachioradialis.

Contraindication. Musculocutaneous neurectomy is contraindicated in patients with functional elbows that depend on biceps and brachialis flexion. This procedure is an "all or none" treatment, and no fine-tuning of tension in the muscles or independent biceps or brachialis release is possible. It only addresses muscular spasticity and is contraindicated when muscular contracture exists. Additionally, it will leave a sensory deficit in the lateral arm in the distribution of the lateral antebrachial cutaneous nerve.

Technique
The musculocutaneous nerve is exposed through an axillary approach after visualization of the lateral cord of the brachial plexus and the biceps tendon.[38] It is identified as it penetrates the biceps muscle and can be stimulated at this point to confirm identification. The nerve is then transected at this level.

No postoperative immobilization is necessary.

Elbow Flexor Lengthening[21,27,38,49,53,55,62,63,90]

Indication. Lengthening of the biceps, brachialis, and brachioradialis is the most direct way to approach the flexion contracture of the elbow. It can be expected to achieve an increase in elbow extension of 40 degrees,[62,63] with minimal loss of flexion or functional flexion power.[62]

Technique
It is important to use preoperative dynamic EMGs and serial clinical examinations to properly identify the tendons that require lengthening. An "S"-shaped antecubital incision is used. The lacertus fibrosus is identified and transected. The lateral antebrachial cutaneous nerve, emerging from the interval between the biceps and brachialis lateral to the biceps tendon, is identified and retracted laterally. The median nerve and brachial artery are identified medial to the biceps tendon. If the decision has been made to lengthen the biceps tendon, it is done at this point. For mild contractures, a fractional lengthening of the tendon can be performed at the musculotendinous junction. Two transverse and slightly oblique cuts, 1 to 2 cm apart, are made through the entire tendinous portion of the musculotendinous junction, with care taken to leave the muscle fibers intact. Passive extension of the elbow will allow for separation of these tenotomy sites, keeping the muscle in continuity. In more severe contractures, "Z"-lengthening of the biceps is necessary. "Z"-lengthening of the tendon should be performed over as much length of the tendon as possible, because this will facilitate reattachment. After lengthening of the biceps, the brachialis muscle is identified. Fractional lengthening can be performed though the aponeurotic fibers, although for more severe contractures, myotomy of the muscle is necessary. At this point, assessment of the spasticity of the brachioradialis muscle can be made. If preoperative EMGs have demonstrated significant spasticity, or intraoperatively it prevents extension of the elbow, then release of its origin from the distal humerus can be performed. Care should be taken to identify and protect the radial nerve along the medial aspect of the brachioradialis. In adults, anterior capsular contracture may further limit extension and should be released through this incision after elevation or division of the brachialis. In severe deformities, extension of the elbow

may ultimately be limited by the shortened neurovascular bundle.

Before skin closure, the "Z"-lengthened biceps is reattached. This should be done with the elbow in 30 degrees of flexion, with maximal tension on the proximal and distal ends of the tendon. A Pulvertaft weave of the tendon ends yields a strong repair.

The elbow is immobilized in a long-arm cast in 30 to 45 degrees of extension for 1 month after surgery. Extension splinting should be continued for another month, with removal of the splint several times a day for active and passive range-of-motion exercises. After 2 months, daytime splinting is discontinued. Night-time splinting should be continued if there is a tendency for recurrence of the deformity, especially during growth spurts.

Flexor-Pronator Muscle Slide

Indication. The flexor pronator muscle mass crosses the elbow and can contribute to elbow flexion contracture. However, a flexor-pronator muscle slide alone does not provide enough functional benefit at the elbow to be considered an effective treatment of elbow flexion deformity and is often performed in conjunction with brachialis fractional lengthening.[45] It does release the pronator muscle as well as addressing the wrist and digital flexors and is discussed in the section on the forearm.

 ## Author's Preferred Method of Treatment

The decision for surgical intervention in the elbow depends on the extent of deformity. I separate the elbow deformities into two groups: those with fixed contractures greater than 40 degrees, and those with fixed contractures less than 40 degrees but with an additional dynamic component. Dynamic elbow deformities are best treated with fractional lengthening of the elbow flexor muscles. Flexion contractures greater than 40 degrees will require more extensive release.

Fractional Elbow Muscle Lengthening (Fig. 34-8)

Indication. Fractional lengthening of the elbow flexors is indicated when the fixed elbow flexion contracture is less than 40 degrees and dynamic deformity occurs causing unwanted elbow flexion during activities and ambulation.

Contraindication. Patients must have strong elbow flexion or lengthening of the flexors will weaken their elbow.

Technique

A transverse incision is made over the antecubital fossa and carried down through subcutaneous tissue with sharp and blunt dissection. The lacertus fibrosis is identified and transected. The neurovascular bundle is identified and retracted medially. The lateral antebrachial cutaneous nerve is iden-

tified and protected as it exits between the biceps and brachialis. A fractional lengthening of the brachialis is performed through two incisions 1 cm apart in the tendinous portion of the musculotendinous junction. These are begun medially and then extended laterally, after the radial nerve has been identified and protected in the interval between the brachialis and brachioradialis. The proximal incision should be performed first; if not, the proximal portion of the musculotendinous junction slides proximally after the distal division and is hard to reach within the wound. Next, the anterior half of the brachioradialis is taken down from its

---

CRITICAL POINTS: FRACTIONAL ELBOW MUSCLE LENGTHENING

INDICATIONS

- Dynamic elbow flexion contracture greater than 40 degrees
- Static flexion contracture less than 40 degrees

PREOPERATIVE EVALUATION

- Dynamic EMGs may be helpful in identifying involved muscles.

PEARLS

- Use electrocautery to perform the fractional lengthening of the brachialis.
- Perform the proximal cut first in the fractional lengthening of the brachialis.

TECHNICAL POINTS

- Make a transverse antecubital incision.
- Identify the lateral antebrachial cutaneous nerve.
- Transect the lacertus fibrosus.
- Elevate the neurovascular bundle from the anterior surface of the brachialis.
- Fractionally lengthen the brachialis.
- Identify the radial nerve in the interval between the brachialis and brachioradialis.
- Release the proximal anterior origin of the brachioradialis.
- Lengthen the biceps, proximal laterally, distal medially. Secure with horizontal mattress sutures.

PITFALL

- Perform biceps lengthening last so as not to rupture the musculotendinous junction.

POSTOPERATIVE CARE

- No immobilization is required
- Immediately begin active and passive range-of-motion exercises.

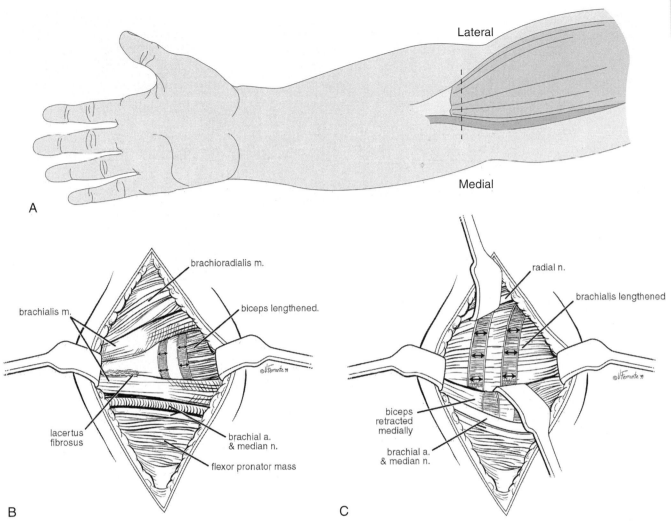

FIGURE 34-8. Fractional lengthening of the elbow flexors. **A,** Through a transverse incision in the antecubital fossa, the lacertus fibrosus is transected and the neurovascular bundle and lateral antebrachial cutaneous nerves are identified and protected. **B,** Fractional lengthening of the biceps tendon through the musculotendinous junction. **C,** Fractional lengthening of the brachialis through the musculotendinous junction and subperiosteal release of the proximal brachioradialis from the distal humerus through the same incision.

origin on the humerus with a combination of electrocautery and blunt dissection with careful retraction of the radial nerve. Lastly, the biceps tendon is isolated and lengthened by dividing the medial half distally and the lateral half proximally. Full passive extension of the elbow is then performed, allowing the biceps tendon fibers to slide on themselves. Two nonabsorbable 3-0 horizontal mattress sutures are placed in the tendon to secure the lengthening.

No postoperative immobilization is necessary. Patients are allowed full active and passive range of motion of their elbows. If a concurrent pronator rerouting is performed, then the patient is placed in a sugar tong splint postoperatively and unrestricted range of motion is delayed for 4 weeks postoperatively.

Patients are told to expect a 45-degree improvement in the carrying angle of the extremity and a decrease in spastic flexion, as well as a 10-degree improvement in flexion contracture. They should have no observable loss in elbow flexion power.

Full Elbow Release (Fig. 34-9)

Indication. In the functional upper extremity, flexion contractures of more than 40 degrees should be addressed. In the nonfunctional upper extremity, a flexion contracture of 40 degrees can be addressed for cosmetic purposes. If appearance is not a concern, then the deformity is only addressed if it causes a problem with hygiene and nursing care. With contractures of 100 degrees or more, skin maceration or breakdown may become a problem. In the wheelchair-bound patient, flexion deformities of more than 100 degrees make assistance during transfers difficult and manipulation of objects on a tabletop or use of a pictureboard impossible. Release of elbow flexion contracture can often have surprising improvement of function for those individuals.

Contraindication. Patients with weak elbow flexion may have a functional loss of elbow flexion after full elbow

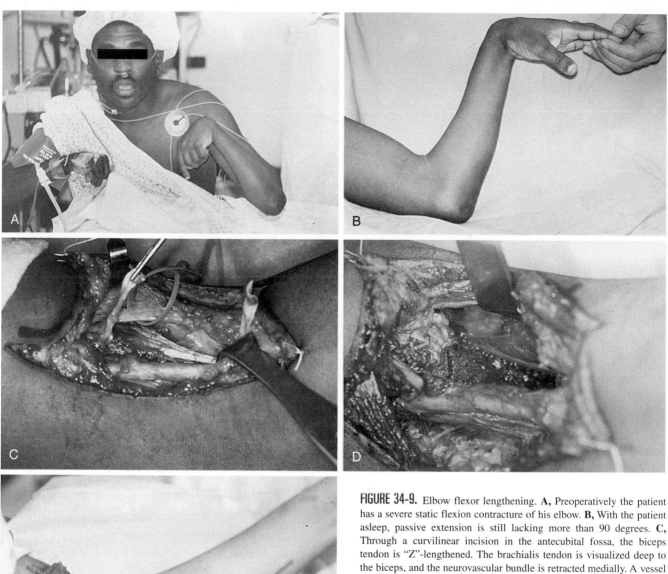

FIGURE 34-9. Elbow flexor lengthening. **A,** Preoperatively the patient has a severe static flexion contracture of his elbow. **B,** With the patient asleep, passive extension is still lacking more than 90 degrees. **C,** Through a curvilinear incision in the antecubital fossa, the biceps tendon is "Z"-lengthened. The brachialis tendon is visualized deep to the biceps, and the neurovascular bundle is retracted medially. A vessel loop has been placed around the lateral antebrachial cutaneous nerve, which is protected. **D,** The brachialis muscle has been transected, and the brachioradialis has been subperiosteally dissected off the humerus. Note that the radial nerve branches to the brachioradialis are preserved. **E,** After complete release of the anterior capsule, the neurovascular bundle is the only tight structure preventing complete extension of the elbow and can be seen anteriorly, bowstringing across the antecubital fossa.   *Continued*

release. The risks and benefits of loss of elbow flexion compared with improvement of hygienic care of the extremity must be weighed. The effects of surgery can be simulated with a trial of botulinum toxin.

Technique

A transverse antecubital incision can usually be used to approach the elbow. In cases of flexion contracture greater than 90 degrees, an "S"-shaped incision will probably be necessary to allow for exposure of the anterior elbow and closure of the wound. The lacertus fibrosus is identified and transected. The neurovascular bundle is identified and retracted medially. The lateral antebrachial cutaneous nerve is identified and protected as it exits between the biceps

and brachialis. The biceps tendon is identified, and a "Z"-lengthening of the biceps tendon is performed. A fractional lengthening of the brachialis is performed through two incisions 1 cm apart in the tendinous portion of the musculotendinous junction, and an additional myotomy of the anterior half of the brachialis is performed. The lengthenings are begun medially and then extended laterally, after the radial nerve has been identified and protected in the interval between the brachialis and brachioradialis. Next attention is directed to the brachioradialis, which is taken down completely from its origin on the humerus with a combination of electrocautery and blunt dissection with careful retraction of the radial nerve. If the elbow does not come out to full extension at this point, the brachialis is

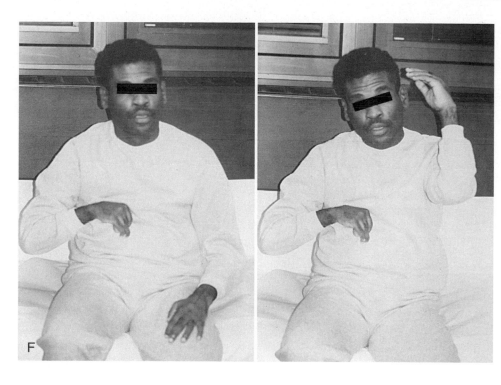

FIGURE 34-9—cont'd. F, Postoperatively, the patient has improved extension and retained flexion of the left elbow. (**A-F,** © Michelle Gerwin Carlson.)

elevated and electrocautery is used to release the anterior elbow capsule. The biceps tendon lengthening is then woven together with the elbow in 30 degrees of flexion and maximum traction on the tendon ends. Three 2-0 horizontal nonabsorbable sutures are used to repair the reapproximated tendon ends.

Patients are placed in a long-arm extension splint for 1 month. One month postoperatively the dressing is removed and an orthoplast extension splint is worn at night. Active and passive range of motion of the elbow is addressed in therapy for 3 months.

An improvement of 45 degrees in the flexion contracture of the extremity is usually obtained. Many patients are able to accomplish tasks that were difficult before. For wheelchair-bound patients, the procedure improves their ability to work at table top and assist in transfers. Ambulatory patients can

CRITICAL POINTS: FULL ELBOW RELEASE

INDICATIONS

- Elbow flexion contracture greater than 40 degrees in functional extremity
- Elbow flexion contracture greater than 100 degrees in nonfunctional extremity

PREOPERATIVE EVALUATION

- Assess functional needs of nonambulatory patients.

PEARLS

- Use electrocautery to myotomize the brachialis to decrease bleeding.
- Use electrocautery to incise the anterior joint capsule.

TECHNICAL POINTS

- Make a transverse or "S"-shaped antecubital incision.
- Identify the lateral antebrachial cutaneous nerve.

- Transect the lacertus fibrosus and "Z"-lengthen the biceps.
- Myotomize the anterior half of the brachialis.
- Identify the radial nerve on the medial brachioradialis.
- Elevate the origin of the brachioradialis.
- Retract the brachialis and incise the anterior capsule.
- Repair the biceps with maximum tension at 30 degrees of elbow flexion.

PITFALLS

- Tension needs to be reset carefully in the repaired biceps or elbow flexion weakness will result.

POSTOPERATIVE CARE

- Apply long-arm plaster extension splint for 4 weeks.
- Use Orthoplast night extension splint for 3 months.
- Begin active and passive range-of-motion exercises at 4 weeks postoperatively.

expect an improvement in the use of their arm in two-handed activities and in the reach of the extremity.

FOREARM

Condition

Pronation deformity of the forearm is caused by spasticity of the pronator teres and pronator quadratus. It interferes with the use of the extremity in two-handed manipulation of objects. With a pronation contracture, the palms cannot face each other and manipulation of small objects between the hands is difficult. With large objects, the spastic hand cannot be used as an assistive hand to carry objects and patients often use the radial aspect of the hand to support an object instead of the palm and fingers. With severe spasticity, patients are forced to use a reverse grasp posture, using the ulnar aspect of the hand to grasp objects because they are unable to present the radial aspect of the hand.[55] Internal rotation contracture of the shoulder aggravates the problem. Rarely, radial head dislocation (in 2% of patients)[73] or distal radioulnar joint dislocation may occur and limit the passive range of motion of the forearm.

Operative Procedures

Several operative procedures have been described to decrease the deforming pronation force. It is important to consider the entire operative plan for an extremity because other operative procedures to improve wrist extension can also improve supination. FCU to extensor carpi radialis brevis (ECRB) transfer for wrist extension may increase supination by an average of 22 degrees.[3]

Release of the pronator can be performed at its origin by flexor-pronator muscle slide or at its insertion by pronator tenotomy or rerouting. The flexor-pronator muscle slide is effective in relieving a pronation contracture, but overcorrection and a supination deformity can result.[6] Results of some studies of pronator rerouting have demonstrated an increase in active supination of 46 to 78 degrees[3,56,81,94] compared with 54 degrees for pronator tenotomy.[94] However, the arc of motion is unchanged after pronator rerouting, suggesting that it may serve more to reposition the forearm than to function as an active supinator.[78,81] It is important

that the pronator quadratus not be released in conjunction with the pronator teres release or rerouting because this may result in loss of pronation.[81]

Gschwind and Tonkin[35] have described four types of pronation deformities and recommended surgical correction for each (Table 34-2).

Flexor-Pronator Muscle Slide[18,21,45,70,109]

Indication. The flexor-pronator muscle slide releases the pronator teres as well as the wrist and digital flexors. In addition to releasing the pronation contracture of the forearm, it is helpful when releasing contractures about the elbow as well as the long flexors of the wrist and digits.

Contraindication. The flexor-pronator muscle slide is an extensive procedure in which fine-tuning of the relative release of the involved muscle groups is not possible. It may cause excessive weakness of the finger flexors and overcorrection of pronation deformity.[38] It should be reserved for the treatment of less functional extremities.

Technique

The skin incision is made from 5 cm proximal to the medial epicondyle to the ulnar aspect of the midportion of the forearm. The ulnar nerve and its branches to the flexor carpi ulnaris are identified and protected. The lacertus fibrosus is divided, and the median nerve and brachial artery are identified and protected. The flexor-pronator muscle mass is then dissected from the periosteum beginning at the medial epicondyle and coronoid process of the ulna. It is dissected en masse, with release of the origins of the flexor carpi ulnaris and flexor digitorum profundus from the ulna and interosseous membrane. Care is taken to protect the medial collateral ligament. The flexor pollicis longus origin is released from the radius. The elbow, wrist, and digits are passively extended to complete the release. The ulnar nerve may be transposed anteriorly before closure.

The arm is immobilized in a splint for 4 weeks with the elbow extended to 45 degrees, the forearm supinated, the wrist in 30 degrees of extension, and the fingers in a resting posture. A removable splint is continued for 4 weeks, allowing for removal for range of motion and therapy. After 2 months, splinting is discontinued unless there is a tendency for recurrence of deformity.

Table 34-2

TYPES OF PRONATION DEFORMITIES AND RECOMMENDED TREATMENT

Type	Function	Treatment
I	Active supination beyond neutral	No surgery
II	Active supination to less than neutral	Pronator quadratus release and flexor aponeurotic release
III	No active supination, free passive supination	Pronator teres transfer
IV	No active supination, tight passive supination	Pronator quadratus release and flexor aponeurotic release

Release of Pronator Insertion[6,21,27,34,35,44,74,85,93,94,115]

Indication. Release of the pronator insertion will release the deforming force of the pronator teres muscle. Release alone is indicated in two populations: patients who have no voluntary control of pronation, and patients who have good active supination. In patients who do not have active supination, a tendon transfer may be necessary to augment supination after release of the pronator.

Contraindication. Isolated pronator release in patients who have no active supination will not improve the deformity.

Pronator Teres Rerouting[35,53,56,63,78,81,94]

Indication. Rerouting of the pronator converts this muscle to a supinator. Results have demonstrated a 50% increase in supination and correction of the reverse grasp position.[56,94] It is indicated in patients who have active control of the pronator and who are lacking active supination. The tendon can be released and rerouted through the interosseous space, or, alternatively, the pronator can be "Z"-lengthened and the distal portion brought around the radius and through the interosseous membrane from dorsal to volar, where it is woven into the proximal tendon.[35]

Contraindication. Pronator teres rerouting is contraindicated in patients who have no active pronation control.

Author's Preferred Method of Treatment

Pronation contracture of the forearm is best treated by release or rerouting of the distal pronator teres insertion (Fig. 34-10). In patients who have active supination, I prefer a pronator tenotomy. If the patient has active pronation

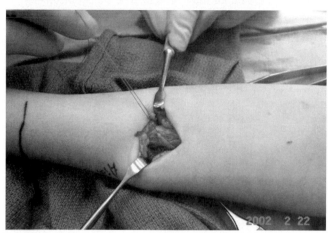

FIGURE 34-10. Pronator rerouting. Through a longitudinal incision in the middle aspect of the forearm the pronator is taken down from its insertion on the radius, routed through the interosseous septum (from volar to dorsal), and reattached to a drill hole in the dorsoradial radius. The wrist is to the left and the elbow to the right in this photograph. (© Michelle Gerwin Carlson.)

CRITICAL POINTS: PRONATOR TENOTOMY OR REROUTING

INDICATIONS
- Pronator tenotomy: active supination short of neutral
- Pronator rerouting: weak to no active supination

CONTRAINDICATION
- No active pronation control.

PREOPERATIVE EVALUATION
- Test for active supination and pronation.

PEARLS
- Release of proximal attachments of the pronator to the radius ensures good pull-through.

TECHNICAL POINTS
- Make a longitudinal incision on the radial aspect of the mid forearm.
- Protect the medial antebrachial cutaneous nerve and superficial radial nerve.
- Develop the interval between the brachioradialis and wrist extensors.

- Subperiosteally elevate the insertion of the pronator with a periosteal tail.
- Extraperiosteally strip the radius at the level of the insertion.
- Incise the interosseous membrane at this level over a 2-cm distance.
- Pass the pronator from volar to dorsal through the interosseous membrane with a right angled clamp.
- Suture the pronator to a drill hole in the radial aspect of the radius.

PITFALL
- When performing a rerouting, do not use the periosteal tail if it is thin.

POSTOPERATIVE CARE
- Wear a "sugar tong" postoperative splint for 1 month.
- Remove dressing at 1 month and apply an Orthoplast "sugar tong" splint for another month.
- During the second month the Orthoplast splint is removed only for therapy.
- Discontinue the splint at 2 months after surgery.

but no active supination, then rerouting of the pronator is advisable. If there is neither active pronation nor supination but the forearm is positioned in pronation, then rerouting of the pronator can create a tenodesis of the forearm in a more neutral position.

Technique

A longitudinal incision is made over the insertion of the pronator in the radial mid forearm. The subcutaneous tissue is dissected and the medial antebrachial cutaneous nerve and superficial radial nerve are identified and protected. The interval between the brachioradialis and wrist extensors is developed and the insertion of the pronator is identified. If a tenotomy is to be performed, this can be done sharply at this point. If a rerouting is to be performed, then the insertion of the pronator is elevated subperiosteally from the radius with a distal slip of periosteum. Care should be taken to ensure that any proximal attachments of the pronator to the radius are released. The radius is stripped extraperiosteally at the level of the pronator insertion, and the interosseous membrane is incised over a 2-cm distance. A right-angled clamp is then introduced from the dorsal aspect of the radius through the interosseous membrane emerging volarly. The pronator is then delivered to this clamp and passed dorsally through the interosseous membrane. A drill hole is made in the radial aspect of the radius beginning dorsally and exiting volarly. One of the tails of the sutures tagging the pronator is passed through this drill hole and then tied to the other tail, allowing the pronator to snug up against the drill hole. The securing of this suture should be done after all other procedures on the arm are performed so as not to loosen the fixation during manipulation of the forearm.

A sugar tong splint is used for 1 month, after which the operative dressing is removed and an Orthoplast splint is applied and removed only for therapy for active and passive range of motion. At 2 months postoperatively the splint is discontinued.

Patients with active pronation preoperatively are told to expect an improvement in active supination that may range from 45 to 90 degrees. It is important that patients understand that they may have mild losses of supination. In patients without active pronation preoperatively, the goal is to tenodese the forearm in neutral position, but results are less reliable.

WRIST AND DIGITAL EXTENSION

Condition

In cerebral palsy, the wrist often assumes a flexed posture. An absence of active wrist extension can have several causes: weak wrist extensors, tight or spastic wrist flexors, and volar wrist capsular contracture. The flexed attitude of the wrist causes two functional problems: it decreases the mechanical advantage of the digital flexors, which weakens grip, and it places the hand in a position in which the fingers are obstructed from visual feedback.

There are multiple procedures to augment wrist extension, but the degree of contracture or spasticity of the wrist and digital flexors must be taken into consideration when evaluating the wrist for surgical intervention. If difficult to

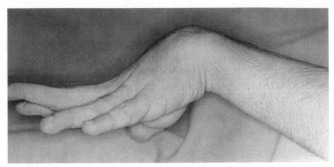

FIGURE 34-11. A patient with good active digital extension but absent wrist extension. (© Michelle Gerwin Carlson.)

assess, median and ulnar nerve blocks at the elbow can temporarily eliminate the flexor spasticity and allow a better evaluation of wrist extension.[55] Ulnar deviation of the wrist may compound a flexion deformity and may be caused by a spastic or contracted FCU. Often the muscle causing the deformity can be used in transfer to augment its antagonist. Care must be taken before transferring the FCU tendon to be certain that the FCR tendon is functioning, or a wrist extension deformity may be created.

It is imperative to evaluate digital extension when evaluating wrist extension (Fig. 34-11). Grasp and release must be evaluated to ensure that improvements in wrist extension will not decrease digital extension. In addition, the patient may rely on ulnar deviation of the wrist to increase thumb abduction through a tenodesis maneuver. If wrist ulnar deviation is altered, it may be necessary to concurrently perform a procedure to augment thumb abduction.

Operative Procedures

There are several operative procedures to augment wrist extension and improve function. Appropriate donors to transfer to the ECRB include the ECU,[21,49,53,55,79] FCU,* pronator teres,[12,21,34,71] and brachioradialis.[44,61,71] When transferring the FCU, an alternate route through the interosseous membrane has been described to decrease the ulnar-deviating force on the wrist,[78] but this also decreases the supination effect of the transfer.

In patients with severe fixed wrist capsular contracture, a proximal row carpectomy may be necessary to allow extension of the wrist to neutral, before tendon transfers can be performed.[54] Wrist arthrodesis can be used to improve hygiene or cosmesis[1,36,77] at the wrist but may cause loss of function because of the loss of the tenodesis effect on the digital motors.[84,98] In the child, an epiphyseal arthrodesis (wrist fusion that preserves the physeal plate) can be performed so as to allow continued growth.[27] Alternatively, a tendon transfer can be done in the child to create a tenodesis of the wrist that can later be converted to a wrist arthrodesis if necessary.[27,55]

FCU to extensor digitorum communis (EDC) transfer† will improve digital extension while also improving wrist

---

*See references 10, 21, 27, 24, 33-35, 40, 43, 44, 47, 53, 79, 84, 85, 99, 101, 103, and 110.

†See references 21, 24, 38, 40, 43, 47, 53, 84, 85, and 99.

Table 34-3
FINGER EXTENSION DEFORMITIES AND THEIR TREATMENT

Type	Deformity	Treatment
I	Active digital extension possible with wrist extended less than 20 degrees from neutral	No treatment or minimal digital fractional lengthening
II	Active digital extension possible with wrist flexed more than 20 degrees from neutral	Fractional lengthening of the digital flexors in addition to augmentation of wrist extension and/or flexor carpi ulnaris tenotomy
III	No active digital extension	Augmentation of digital extension with flexor carpi ulnaris transfer to extensor digitorum communis

extension. It is useful in patients who are unable to actively extend the fingers when the wrist is passively extended. Weak digital extension is less common than weak wrist extension.[55] Zancolli and Zancolli defined three types of finger extension deformities and suggested a treatment algorithm (Table 34-3).[116]

It is infrequent that patients have both poor wrist and digital extension.[55] In this situation, FCU to EDC and either ECU or pronator teres to ECRB is usually an effective approach.

Results of wrist extension transfers have demonstrated improved function in approximately 80% of patients.[3,34] FCU to ECRB transfer has shown good results, with an average improvement of resting wrist posture from 41 degrees of flexion to 11 degrees and an improvement in the location of the arc of motion, with increased wrist extension and a compensatory loss of flexion. The total range of motion is unchanged after this procedure, although wrist extension has been shown to improve by 35 to 45 degrees.[3,78,101,103,108] The greatest improvement in function of the hand is seen in patients without flexion contractures who use a wrist flexion tenodesis maneuver when attempting digital extension.[34]

FCU to ECRB Transfer

Indication. FCU to ECRB transfer is indicated in patients who have a tight FCU and absent or weak wrist extension (less than neutral).

Contraindication. Absence of a functioning FCR will result in loss of active wrist flexion and a wrist extension deformity.

Technique (Fig. 34-12)
The FCU can be harvested through two transverse incisions. The first incision is made over the FCU insertion on the pisiform at the wrist flexion crease. Tension on the tendon then allows the proximal aspect of the tendon to be palpated. The second transverse incision is made at the most proximal palpable point on the tendon. Transverse incisions are more aesthetic, but care must be taken to protect the ulnar neurovascular bundle during harvest. The FCU is transected at its insertion on the pisiform, and its attachments to the subcutaneous tissue are freed. It is then withdrawn through the proximal incision and dissected as far proximally as

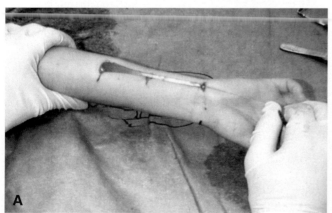
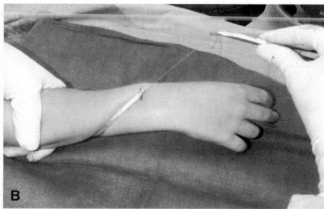

FIGURE 34-12. FCU to ECRB transfer. **A,** The FCU tendon is harvested through two volar incisions, one distal at the pisiform and the other over the mid-forearm. The FCU can be harvested using a tendon stripper inserted distally. **B,** The tendon is wrapped over the forearm to mark the site of attachment to the ECRB tendon. A small transverse incision can then be made at this spot and the tendon tunneled subcutaneously. The length gained from the subcutaneous tunnel will allow for easy weaving in a Pulvertaft fashion. (**A** and **B,** © Michelle Gerwin Carlson.)

CRITICAL POINTS: FCU TO ECRB TRANSFER

INDICATIONS

- Inability to actively extend wrist to neutral with functioning FCU and FCR
- Occasionally possible in patients with static wrist flexion contractures, although more likely to need arthrodesis

CONTRAINDICATION

- No active control of flexor carpi radialis (FCR)

PEARLS

- After tendon transfer, the wrist should passively rest in 20 degrees of flexion.

PITFALLS

- If weak digital extension is not addressed concurrently, wrist extensor transfer will worsen digital extension.
- Overtightening of the transfer will weaken digital extension.

TECHNICAL POINTS

- Harvest FCU through transverse incision just proximal to pisiform.
- Use tendon stripper to strip tendon to mid-forearm region.
- Make counterincision in volar, ulnar mid forearm over the FCU.
- Deliver FCU into this wound.
- Drape FCU over skin from volar wound to dorsal forearm over the ECRB and locate level of tendon weave.
- Make a transverse incision over the ECRB tendon.
- Perform a Pulvertaft weave of the FCU into the ECRB with maximum tension and the wrist in neutral.

POSTOPERATIVE CARE

- Apply postoperative dressing with wrist splinted in 30 degrees of extension.
- At 1 month after surgery, apply removable Orthoplast wrist extension splint and begin range-of-motion exercises.
- At 2 months, discontinue splinting.

transverse or longitudinal incision is made over the ECRB at this point. A subcutaneous tunnel is created from the dorsal wound to the volar ulnar wound. The tunnel should be deep to the subcutaneous adipose tissue but superficial to all tendons. Care should be taken to ensure that this tunnel is as direct as possible; otherwise, as the transfer is used, it will ultimately find the most direct route and this may result in effective lengthening of the transfer. The FCU is then passed through this tunnel to the ECRB. A Pulvertaft weave is performed between the two tendons, with each weave secured with two 3-0 nonabsorbable sutures. The weave should be done with maximal tension on the tendon ends while the wrist is held in neutral. Interval checks should be made while the tendon weave is performed to be sure that the wrist assumes a position of 20 degrees of flexion when allowed to rest against gravity. If passive flexion of the wrist

CRITICAL POINTS: ECU TO ECRB TRANSFER

INDICATIONS

- Weak extension of the wrist with absent FCU or FCR, and ulnar deviation with extension
- Weak extension of the wrist and FCU used for FCU to EDC transfer

PEARLS

- Always perform lengthening of the FCU concurrently.
- After transfer, the wrist should passively rest in 20 degrees of flexion.

PITFALLS

- If weak digital extension is not addressed concurrently, wrist extensor transfer will worsen digital extension.
- Overtightening of the transfer will weaken digital extension.

TECHNICAL POINTS

- Make a transverse incision over the dorsal forearm extending from ECRB to ECU, approximately 2 cm proximal to Lister's tubercle.
- Transect the ECU as distally as possible.
- Identify the ECRB and perform Pulvertaft weave of ECU into ECRB with maximal tension with the wrist in neutral.

POSTOPERATIVE CARE

- Apply postoperative dressing with wrist splinted in 30 degrees of extension.
- At 1 month, apply removable Orthoplast wrist extension splint and begin range-of-motion exercises.
- At 2 months, discontinue splinting.

possible to allow a direct line of pull to the transfer. To ensure adequate length, the tendon is passed around the ulnar aspect of the forearm, over the skin, to the point where it intersects with the ECRB. This maneuver will ensure enough distal length on the tendon to allow for a Pulvertaft weave after the tendon is tunneled subcutaneously. A

to 20 degrees is not possible, the tendon repair is too tight and should be loosened.[85] Care should be taken to ensure that the weave will not encroach on the intersection with the APL and EPB with wrist extension or with the extensor retinaculum with wrist flexion. If this does occur, the retinaculum can be divided.

The wrist is immobilized in 30 degrees of extension for 4 weeks. A removable splint is then worn for 4 weeks, followed by range-of-motion exercises. After 8 weeks, splinting is discontinued unless there is a tendency for the deformity to recur, in which case a volar wrist extension splint is worn at night.

ECU to ECRB Transfer

Indications. This transfer is performed in patients whose radial wrist extensors are weak, resulting in an ulnar deviation deformity with wrist extension. It is also indicated when the FCU has been used as a transfer to the digital extensors.

Contraindication. This procedure is contraindicated in patients without active extension of the wrist.

Technique

The incision may be either a single longitudinal midline incision or a transverse incision extending from the ECU to the ECRB. The ECU tendon is transected distally at its insertion at the base of the fifth metacarpal and dissected to its musculotendinous junction to ensure a direct line of pull. Repair of the ECU to the ECRB is performed external to the extensor retinaculum using a Pulvertaft weave as described previously. This transfer should always be done in conjunction with fractional lengthening of the FCU.

Immobilization is as described for the FCU to ECRB transfer.

FCU to EDC Transfer

Indication. The FCU to EDC transfer is indicated in patients with weak or absent active digital extension.

Contraindication. This transfer is contraindicated in patients with good digital extension and weak wrist extension. The FCR must be functional or a loss of active wrist flexion will result.

Technique

The FCU is harvested as previously described. The point of attachment to the EDC is identified, with the FCU tendon draped across the skin. A transverse or longitudinal incision is made over the EDC, and the tendons to the index through little finger are identified. A subcutaneous tunnel is created between the dorsal and ulnar incisions, and the FCU is passed through this tunnel and out the dorsal wound over the EDC. Tension is applied to the EDC tendons to position the MCP joints in full extension with the wrist in neutral. The four EDC tendons are sutured together distally to allow for a normal cascade to the fingers before transfer. The FCU is then passed through the EDC tendons in an ulnar to radial direction, beginning at the fifth EDC tendon and progressing through to the index tendon. Each weave is sewn into place with 3-0 nonabsorbable sutures. The FCU is then passed back in a radial to ulnar direction through the EDC tendons and sutured in place. Length permitting, it may be passed a third time and sutured; and the excess tendon is excised.

The extremity is immobilized for 4 weeks in a splint with the wrist in 30 degrees of extension and the digits fully extended. A removable Orthoplast forearm-based splint for digital extension is applied for 4 additional weeks and removed for therapy and range-of-motion exercises. Night splinting is continued as necessary to avoid recurrence of the deformity.

CRITICAL POINTS: FCU TO EDC TRANSFER

INDICATIONS

- Weak or absent active digital extension, with full passive digital extension
- Functioning FCU and FCR

PEARLS

- If digital flexors are tight, test for active digital extension with the wrist flexed.

PITFALL

- FCR must be strong or wrist extension deformity may result.

TECHNICAL POINTS

- Harvest FCU tendon as in FCU to ECRB transfer.
- Identify location of transfer as in FCU to ECRB protocol.
- Make a transverse incision in the dorsal forearm over EDC junction.
- Identify EDC tendons to index, long, ring, and little fingers and suture together distally while applying tension proximally.
- Make subcutaneous tunnel from volar wound to dorsal wound and pass FCU tendon.
- Perform Pulvertaft weave of FCU into EDC with wrist in neutral and maximal tension on EDC.

POSTOPERATIVE CARE

- Apply dressing with forearm-based digital extension splint for 4 weeks.
- Apply removable Orthoplast splint for 4 weeks and begin range-of-motion exercises.
- Discontinue splinting at 8 weeks after surgery.

Pronator Teres to ECRB Transfer

Indication. This procedure is an option in patients without a functioning FCR, in whom harvest of the FCU is contraindicated. Fractional lengthening of the FCU should be done in conjunction with pronator transfer. In cases where the FCU is transferred for digital extension, and if the ECU is not available, the pronator teres is a good candidate to augment wrist extension.

Contraindications. This procedure limits the arc of motion of the wrist as a result of the short excursion of the pronator and should be used with caution in patients with pronator spasticity. Patients who are dependent on wrist flexion for digital extension may have more difficulty opening their hand. It may also cause an increase in the elbow flexion deformity.

Technique

A longitudinal incision is made over the insertion of the pronator in the radial mid forearm. The subcutaneous tissue is dissected, and the medial antebrachial cutaneous nerve and superficial radial nerve, as it emerges from under the brachioradialis, are identified and protected. The interval between the brachioradialis and wrist extensors is developed and the insertion of the pronator is identified. The ECRB tendon is separated from the extensor carpi radialis longus (ECRL) tendon. A Pulvertaft weave can then be performed into the ECRB with the pronator teres, extended by its periosteal sleeve. Tension is set with maximum tension on each tendon and the wrist at neutral. It is important that the resting posture of the wrist be in 20 degrees of flexion.

Immobilization is as described for the FCU to ECRB transfer.

Brachioradialis to ECRB Transfer

Indication. The brachioradialis can be an effective transfer when other motors are not available. Freeing of the muscle proximally can increase the excursion from 1.5 to 3 cm and gain approximately 25 degrees of extension, with obligatory loss in active and passive wrist flexion.[61]

Technique

The brachioradialis can be approached either through one longitudinal dorsoradial incision or through multiple transverse incisions. The brachioradialis insertion on the distal radius is identified and transected, while protecting the radial artery and nerve. The brachioradialis is mobilized proximally and freed from the ECRL and the FCR. It is then ready for transfer to the ECRB as previously described. The transfer is tensioned with the elbow flexed and the wrist at neutral, maintaining maximum tension of the brachioradialis during the weave.

The arm is immobilized for 4 weeks with the elbow flexed 90 degrees and supinated and the wrist extended 30 degrees. A removable splint is worn for 4 more weeks while range-of-motion exercises and therapy are begun. Night splinting is continued after 8 weeks if there is a tendency for recurrence of the deformity.

Epiphyseal Wrist Arthrodesis

Indication. Arthrodesis of the wrist is performed for hygiene or cosmesis in a hand with little or no function and capsular contracture. Epiphyseal arthrodesis allows continued growth at the wrist.

Contraindication. This procedure should be used cautiously in patients with weak digital extension, because arthrodesis of the wrist will decrease the tenodesis effect on the digital extensors.

Technique

The wrist is exposed through a longitudinal incision. The extensor retinaculum is divided longitudinally and the extensor tendons retracted. The capsule is divided longitudinally, and the scaphoid and lunate are exposed. The articular surfaces of the scaphoid and lunate are removed with a knife and/or bur down to cancellous bone. Similarly, the articular cartilage of the distal radius is removed down to the epiphyseal bone, with care taken not to disturb the physis. The radiocarpal joint is held reduced in neutral and is secured with two crossed Kirschner wires in the small child and smooth Steinmann pins in the older child. These are cut off just below the skin. Bone graft may be added but is usually not necessary.

The wrist is immobilized in a short-arm cast until fusion is identified by serial monthly radiographs. The Kirschner wires or Steinmann pins are removed at this point.

Wedge Resection Wrist Arthrodesis

Indications. When release of all the wrist flexors in a skeletally mature patient still does not allow the wrist to be passively extended to a neutral position, wedge resection arthrodesis of the wrist is necessary. It also allows the wrist to be placed in a neutral position without tightening the flexor tendons. Arthrodesis of the wrist is also indicated when there are no available donors for wrist extension.

Contraindication. This procedure may weaken digital extension, owing to the effective lengthening of the extensor tendons and the loss of tenodesis effect due to the loss of wrist flexion. It should be performed only in the skeletally mature patient.

Technique

Through a dorsal longitudinal incision, the extensor retinaculum is transected over the third dorsal compartment, and subperiosteal dissection of the distal radius and carpus is performed. The angle of maximum passive extension of the wrist, when the digits are held fully extended (Volkmann's angle), is measured. An oscillating saw is used to remove the articular cartilage of the radius. A second cut is made through the carpus to resect a wedge of bone equivalent to Volkmann's angle. The carpus between the two saw cuts is then subperiosteally dissected and removed. Closure of the osteotomy site will then result in repositioning of the wrist in neutral without increased tension on the flexor tendons. The arthrodesis is completed by decortication of the remaining carpal articular surfaces (including the second and third carpometacarpal [CMC] joints). Internal fixation is accomplished with a 3.5-mm straight wrist fusion plate extending from the distal radius to the third metacarpal. The cancellous bone of the resected carpal bones provides an excellent source of bone graft; iliac crest bone graft is usually not required.

The wrist is immobilized in a short-arm cast until the fusion is healed radiographically.

Author's Preferred Method of Treatment

In the functional hand, the decision for transfer to the wrist or digital extensors is based on a series of tests of active and passive wrist and digital extension. First, testing of active digital extension is performed with the wrist held in a neutral position (Fig. 34-13). If full active extension is possible, then no transfer is necessary for the digital extensors. If full active digital extension is not possible, but the digits can be extended passively, a transfer to motor the digital extensors is necessary. I prefer an FCU to EDC transfer for this deformity. Patients with this deficiency are

considered to have *weak release*. A transfer to the *wrist* extensors in this situation will only worsen this patient's hand because the patient will be unable to open the fingers with the wrist extended.

If passive extension of the digits is limited when the wrist is held in full extension, then a fractional lengthening of the

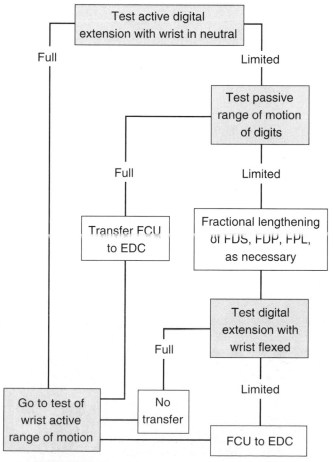

FIGURE 34-13. Algorithm for evaluation of digital extension.

CRITICAL POINTS: WEDGE RESECTION WRIST ARTHRODESIS

INDICATIONS
- Patients with no active wrist flexion or extension
- For patients with active wrist extension, inability to passively extend the wrist intraoperatively after release of the FCU and palmaris longus and lengthening of the FCR
- Allows wrist to be placed in a neutral position without increasing the tightness of the digital flexors

CONTRAINDICATION
- Skeletally immature patient

PEARLS
- Check active digital extension preoperatively because a transfer may be necessary.

PITFALL
- May weaken digital extension if patient does not have good preoperative digital extension with the wrist held in neutral

TECHNICAL POINTS
- Perform subperiosteal dissection of distal radius and carpus.
- Measure Volkmann's angle (maximal wrist extension with digits extended).
- Use oscillating saw to remove articular surface of radius.
- Excise carpal bone wedge to match Volkmann's angle.
- Make sure cuts meet at volar cortex of carpus.
- Close osteotomy site and decorticate remaining articular surfaces including the second and third CMC joints.
- Use straight wrist fusion plate from the distal radius to third metacarpal.
- Resected carpal bones may be used for bone graft.

POSTOPERATIVE CARE
- Immobilize wrist in a short-arm splint or cast until radiographic fusion is evident (usually 6 to 8 weeks).

digital flexors will be necessary. Active digital extension is then tested with the wrist flexed. Good digital extension indicates that a transfer will probably not be necessary after release of the tight digital flexors. Limited active digital extension with the wrist flexed, however, indicates that a transfer will be necessary to augment extension in addition to lengthening of the digital flexors. Usually the FCU to EDC transfer is a good option.

After testing digital extension, wrist extension should be tested next. It is helpful to think of wrist flexion deformity in three groups: functional, dynamic, and static.

Functional Deformities. Patients with functional deformities of the wrist may have good active range of motion of the wrist but on performing activities the wrist drops into flexion. Treatment involves fractional lengthening of the spastic flexors (usually the FCU). No transfer for wrist extension is needed.

Dynamic Deformities. Dynamic deformities of the wrist have no static contracture. Patients may or may not have some active extension but cannot extend their wrist to neutral. Passive extension of the wrist and digits should be evaluated. If there is full passive extension of the wrist and digits, a transfer to augment wrist extension is indicated. I prefer an FCU to ECRB transfer, assuming the FCR is adequate. For patients without a functioning FCR, the FCU is lengthened and the ECU to ECRB transfer should be performed. If the FCU is nonfunctional or being used as a transfer to the digital extensors, then an ECU to ECRB transfer can be used. This will provide adequate wrist extension, because the FCU to EDC transfer also aids in extending the wrist.

Static Deformities. Static wrist deformities have a static flexion contracture of greater than 45 degrees. This usually occurs in the older patient and often necessitates wrist fusion to correct the deformity. Occasionally tendon transfer is possible and the decision can be made intraoperatively. After release of the FCU from the pisiform, an assessment is made of the tightness of the FCR and palmaris longus. The FCR can be fractionally lengthened or "Z"-lengthened as necessary. A tenotomy of the palmaris longus should be performed. If passive extension of the wrist is not possible after release of these tendons, a wrist arthrodesis should be done. If passive extension to neutral is possible, then an

FCU to ECRB transfer may be performed. In the wrist with no active flexion or extension preoperatively, I perform a wrist arthrodesis. Tenotomy of the FCR, FCU, and palmaris longus may be necessary. If the digital flexors or wrist capsule is tight as the wrist is brought into neutral, then a wedge resection (or proximal row carpectomy) and arthrodesis are appropriate.

WRIST AND DIGITAL FLEXOR TENDON TIGHTNESS

Condition

Wrist flexion deformity is caused primarily by spasticity or contracture of the FCU tendon, although the FCR and the palmaris longus can contribute. Digital flexor tightness can also contribute to the wrist flexion deformity and is measured by Volkmann's angle (see Fig. 34-2). In extreme digital flexor tendon tightness, no extension of the wrist is possible when the digits are held extended. Extension of the wrist to less than neutral identifies flexor tendon tightness that will need to be addressed surgically (Fig. 34-14).

Operative Procedures

There are several procedures to lengthen the flexor tendons, including flexor-pronator slide,[45,70,103,109] fractional lengthening,[21,24,25,28,53,57,59,60,103] "Z"-lengthening,[24,25,28] superficialis to profundus transfer,[5,6] and, less commonly, bony shortening (proximal row carpectomy[47,69,88,103] or wedge resection arthrodesis[55]). Wrist flexor tendons may be lengthened by fractional lengthening or "Z"-lengthening. If both the FCR and FCU are involved, at least one should be kept in continuity to enable active wrist flexion, although it may be lengthened.

All flexor tendon lengthenings weaken the power of the muscle, but this is compensated for by an increase in grip strength owing to improved extension of the wrist. Weakening of the flexors is minimized by fractional lengthening and is most pronounced with superficialis to profundus transfer. Superficialis to profundus transfer is used when hygiene is the primary goal and limited function of the hand is expected.[6] The effect of "Z"-lengthening falls in between these two.

Bony procedures are reserved for the skeletally mature patient and often have the unwanted effect of weakening

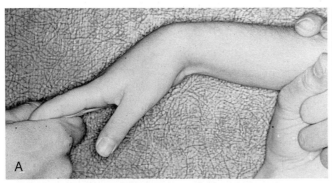
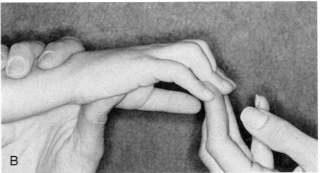

FIGURE 34-14. Flexor tendon tightness. **A,** Tight digital flexors allow wrist extension to only −45 degrees with the digits held extended. **B,** With the wrist held extended, the digits cannot be passively fully extended. (**A** and **B,** © Michelle Gerwin Carlson.)

the extensors. Maintenance of wrist mobility and tendon transfers is more desirable when possible.

Flexor-Pronator Muscle Slide

Indication. This procedure is indicated when significant function of the digits is not expected. Selective lengthening of the digital and wrist flexors is not possible.

Technique
See Forearm section.

Fractional Tendon Lengthening

Indication. This procedure is indicated in the functional hand. It is the optimal way of lengthening the flexor tendons, with the least risk of excessive lengthening of the tendons and weakened grip.

Contraindication. If the digits cannot be fully extended with the wrist flexed, then fractional tendon lengthening is not likely to produce enough length. "Z"-lengthening or superficialis to profundus transfer should be considered in these cases.

Technique
The musculotendinous junctions of the digital flexor tendons can be palpated on the mid aspect of the volar forearm. Exposure is gained through a 4-cm longitudinal incision centered over the musculotendinous junction. Enough of the musculotendinous junction must be exposed to allow for two tenotomies in this region. Two oblique tenotomies are made at least 1 cm apart in the musculotendinous junction of each tendon to be lengthened (Fig. 34-15). The distal tenotomy should be at least 2 cm proximal to the distal aspect of the musculotendinous junction. The muscular portion of the musculotendinous junction *must be kept*

CRITICAL POINTS: FRACTIONAL TENDON LENGTHENING

INDICATION

- For patients unable to fully passively extend their fingers with the wrist in neutral

PEARLS

- Patients must be able to fully passively extend their fingers with their wrists flexed or this procedure will not produce enough lengthening of the tendons.

PITFALL

- Resist the temptation to passively extend the digits fully intraoperatively because this may lead to overlengthening.

TECHNICAL POINTS

- Make a 4-cm longitudinal incision centered over the musculotendinous junction of the digital flexors in the forearm.
- Make two oblique tenotomies in the musculotendinous junction of each tendon spaced 1 cm apart.
- Make tenotomies at least 2 cm proximal to the most distal aspect of the musculotendinous junction.

POSTOPERATIVE CARE

- Immobilize the wrist in neutral for 4 weeks with the digits not included.
- Immediately begin digital active and passive range-of-motion exercises.
- If the patient has difficulty extending the digits, add a volar digital extension splint.

CRITICAL POINTS: TENDON "Z"-LENGTHENING

INDICATIONS

- For tight wrist flexors or FPL tendon lengthening
- Produces more tendon lengthening than fractional lengthening

PEARLS

- Always make the arms of the "Z" as long as possible.
- Effective lengthening will be two times the length of the split minus the length of the repair.

PITFALLS

- If the arms of the "Z" are too short, sufficient lengthening of the tendon will not occur.

TECHNICAL POINTS

- Make a longitudinal split in the tendon.
- Divide the hemi-tendon slip on opposite sides of the tendon proximally and distally.
- Overlap the proximal and distal ends of the tendon in a side-to-side fashion with the desired tension, and suture with three horizontal mattress sutures.

POSTOPERATIVE CARE

- Immobilize the wrist and thumb (for FPL) lengthening in neutral for 4 weeks.
- Begin active and passive range-of-motion exercises at 4 weeks.
- Wear removable splint for 4 weeks.

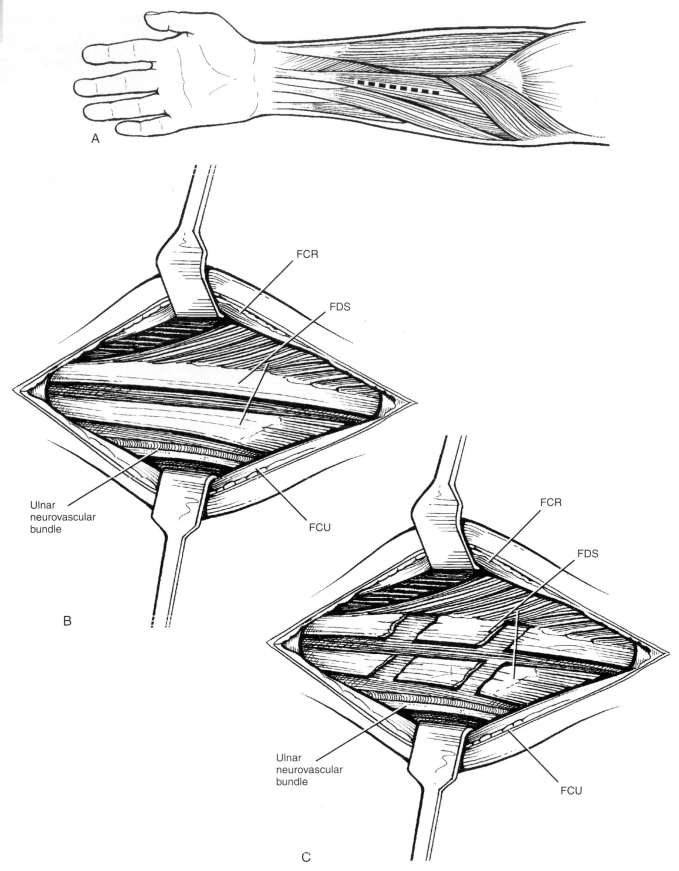

FIGURE 34-15. Fractional lengthening of the digital flexors. **A,** The incision is planned over the musculotendinous junction of the digital flexors. **B,** The ulnar neurovascular bundle and flexor carpi radialis (FCR) are retracted, and the superficial flexors (FDS) are exposed. **C,** Two oblique incisions are made in the tendinous portion of each musculotendinous junction (see text for precise locations). The bridging muscle fibers are preserved. The FDS can then be retracted and the FDP addressed in a similar fashion.

intact. The wrist is held in neutral, and gentle passive extension of the digits short of the desired length is performed. The digits should not be fully extended. Overcorrection of the digits intraoperatively will result in overweakening of the flexor tendons and possible swan neck deformities of the fingers.

The arm is immobilized in a plaster splint with the wrist in neutral for 4 weeks. Unrestricted finger motion is allowed immediately postoperatively, and the patient is given instruction on digital extension exercises. Postoperatively, if the patient has difficulty in extending the digits, a volar extension splint may be added. The plaster splint is removed at 4 weeks, and a removable wrist splint is applied to allow for wrist range of motion and therapy. At 8 weeks, splinting is discontinued unless recurrence of deformity requires night splinting.

Tendon "Z"-Lengthening

Indication. "Z"-lengthening produces a greater amount of tendon lengthening than fractional lengthening. It is frequently used for lengthening of the FPL tendon when it cannot be fully extended even with the wrist fully flexed. In this situation, it is unlikely that fractional lengthening will be sufficient. For the FPL, the amount of lengthening performed should be 0.5 mm for every degree of desired correction (e.g., 2.5 cm for a 50-degree contracture).[31]

Contraindication. "Z"-lengthening is not used for the digital flexors, because superficialis to profundus transfer is equally effective and less tedious.

Technique

A longitudinal incision is made in the volar forearm over the tendon to be lengthened. As much of the tendon as possible is exposed. A longitudinal split is made in the tendon in a proximal to distal fashion as long as possible. The effective lengthening of the tendon will be twice the length of this longitudinal split minus the length needed for the repair. The hemi-tendon is divided radially at one end and ulnarly at the other to complete the transection of the tendon. The ends are woven with a Pulvertaft or side-to-side technique at the desired tension. For the wrist flexors, the tension should be set with the wrist in a neutral position. For the thumb, the tension should be set with the wrist at neutral and thumb MCP and IP joints slightly flexed. With extension of the wrist, the thumb should cross the index finger. With flexion of the wrist, the thumb should be able to be fully extended out of the palm.

After wrist flexor tendon lengthening, the wrist is immobilized in slight flexion for 4 weeks. For the FPL, the wrist is immobilized in slight flexion and the thumb in neutral position for 4 weeks. After 4 weeks, a removable splint is applied and therapy and range-of-motion exercises are begun. Splinting is discontinued at 8 weeks.

Superficialis to Profundus Transfer ("STP" Procedure)

Indication. The STP transfer is indicated when significant contracture of the digital flexors is present and the fingers cannot be passively extended even with the wrist fully flexed. If the FPL is contracted, it is usually treated with "Z"-lengthening.

CRITICAL POINTS: STP TRANSFER

INDICATIONS

- Significant contracture of the digital flexors
- No ability to passively extend fingers even with wrist flexed
- Difficulties with hygiene

PEARLS

- In patients with severe involvement this can be done under local anesthesia.
- If the FPL is contracted it will require "Z"-lengthening.

PITFALL

- Overlengthening of the transfer will significantly weaken digits.

TECHNICAL POINTS

- Make a longitudinal incision over the volar forearm centered over the musculotendinous junction.
- Transect the superficialis tendons distally and the profundus tendons proximally.
- Suture tendons individually if there is function of the digits and together if there is little function.
- If tendons are to be sutured as a group, suture the profundus together distally and the superficialis tendons proximally before transection to maintain the normal cascade.
- Tension the repair with the wrist in neutral and the digits flexed 45 degrees at the MCP and PIP joints.
- With wrist extension the fingers should touch the palm, and with wrist flexion the fingers should be able to be fully extended.
- Repair the tendon ends in a side-to-side fashion.

POSTOPERATIVE CARE

- Immobilize the wrist in neutral with the MCP joints flexed 90 degrees and the PIP joints in extension for 4 weeks.
- Use a removable splint for 4 weeks and begin active and passive range-of-motion exercises.

Contraindication. This procedure should be used with caution in patients with functional use of their hand, because it may result in significant weakening of the grip.

Technique

Through a longitudinal incision in the distal forearm, the superficialis and profundus tendons are identified. With the fingers in a normal cascade, the profundus tendons are sutured together distally and the superficialis tendons proximally before transection. The superficialis tendons are then transected distally, and the profundus tendons are transected proximally. Tension during repair is set with the wrist at neutral and the digits flexed 45 degrees at the MCP and PIP joints[55] (or alternatively, with the wrist flexed 20 degrees and the MCP and PIP joints flexed 20 degrees).[6] With the wrist extended 45 degrees, the digits should touch the palm; and with wrist flexion, the digits should be able to be extended completely. The repair is performed in a side-to-side fashion.

The arm is immobilized for 4 weeks with the wrist in neutral, the MCP joints flexed 90 degrees, and the PIP joints in extension. A removable splint is then used for 4 weeks, and range-of-motion exercises and therapy are begun. At 8 weeks, splinting is discontinued.

Author's Preferred Method of Treatment

If the wrist cannot be extended at all from the fully flexed position, then "Z"-lengthening of the wrist flexor tendons (FCR, FCU) is usually necessary. If partial extension is possible, then fractional lengthening is usually sufficient.

If the fingers can be fully passively extended with the wrist flexed, I perform fractional lengthening to give sufficient length to allow for extension of the digits with the wrist extended. Fractional lengthening has the added benefit of minute adjustments in tension and the ability of the patient in the immediate postoperative period to increase the lengthening with active digital extension. If the digits cannot be fully extended with the wrist flexed, then "Z"-lengthening or superficialis to profundus transfer is necessary. "Z"-lengthening of the digital flexors is tedious, because nine "Z"-lengthenings are usually required (four FDS, four FDP, FPL), and I prefer STP transfer with "Z"-lengthening of the FPL. In a nonfunctional hand with tight wrist and digital flexors, I perform wedge resection arthrodesis.

THUMB-IN-PALM DEFORMITY

Condition

Flexion of the thumb into the palm of the hand is one of the greatest deterrents to good hand function in the patient with cerebral palsy. The etiology of thumb-in-palm deformity is multifactorial. When evaluating the child with this deformity, four key elements must be considered: (1) spastic flexors and adductors, (2) flaccid extensors and abductors, (3) hypermobile MCP joint, and (4) web space skin contrac-

ture. The spastic flexors and adductors are the FPL, the adductor pollicis, the first dorsal interosseous, and the FPB. Spasticity of the short flexor, adductor, and first dorsal interosseous can be identified by examining the extremity during use and by passively abducting the thumb while palpating the tendons. During use, the thumb metacarpal assumes an adducted position when the adductor and first dorsal interosseous are spastic. Similarly the MCP joint flexes if the FPB is spastic. FPL spasticity is examined with the wrist held in both flexion and extension, to demonstrate flexion of the thumb MCP and IP joints. If the thumb IP joint is fixed in full flexion when the wrist is positioned at neutral and the thumb metacarpal gently abducted, the FPL needs to be lengthened.[71]

Extensor and abductor function of the thumb are performed by the EPB, the EPL, and APL. Function of these muscles should be tested with the wrist flexed and extended. Often the EPL functions well, despite an adduction deformity of the thumb, and when a patient reaches for an object the IP joint extends despite the flexion and adduction of the thumb metacarpal.[54]

MCP joint hypermobility is a concern when considering tendon transfers to augment abduction and extension. If the MCP joint can be passively extended beyond neutral, these transfers may produce undesirable hyperextension of the MCP joint instead of abduction and extension of the thumb ray. A soft tissue contracture of the skin of the web space can exacerbate the deformity and may need to be addressed at the time of surgery.

Several classification systems of thumb-in-palm deformity have been created to describe the deformity seen.[44,63,80,82] House and colleagues[44] and Sakellarides and coworkers[82] both described four-part classifications (Table 34-4).

Operative Procedures

Operative procedures are directed at each of the four elements of the deformity: (1) release of the spastic flexor and adductor muscles, (2) augmentation of weak extensor and abductor muscles, (3) stabilization of the thumb MCP joint, and (4) release of skin web space contracture.

Spasticity of the thumb intrinsics is present in almost all thumb-in-palm deformities. Attention should be addressed to the adductor pollicis, FPB, and first dorsal interosseous muscles. If flexion of the thumb MCP joint is not a significant component of the deformity, then the FPB is probably not involved. Release of the adductor can be performed at its origin* or insertion.† Hoffer and colleagues recommended that if selective control of the adductor can be demonstrated by dynamic EMG, then release of its origin to preserve function should be performed. If there is no voluntary control of the adductor, then release of the muscle from its insertion should be performed.[42] The FPL should be lengthened if it is spastic.[29,44,57,71,85,98]

Augmentation of thumb extension and abduction with a variety of tendon transfers has been described, including brachioradialis,[29,61,78,89] palmaris longus,[29,44] FCR and

---

*See references 21, 22, 31, 42, 44, 46, 49, 53, 57, 58, 71, 89, 90, 95-97, 101, and 115.

†See references 11, 23, 29, 31, 42, 44, 47, 57, 61, and 99.

Table 34-4

CLASSIFICATIONS OF THUMB-IN-PALM DEFORMITY

Type (House, et al.[44])	Description	Involved Elements
I	Simple metacarpal adduction contracture	Spastic adductor and first dorsal interosseous
II	Metacarpal adduction contracture with MCP flexion deformity	Spastic adductor, first dorsal interosseous, flexor pollicis brevis
III	Metacarpal adduction contracture with MCP hyperextension/instability	Spastic adductor, first dorsal interosseous, extensor pollicis brevis
IV	Metacarpal adduction contracture, MCP and IP flexion deformities	Spastic adductor, first dorsal interosseous, flexor pollicis longus

Type (Sakellarides, et al.[82])	Elements	Treatment
I	Weak extensor pollicis longus	Palmaris or FCR to EPL transfer
II	Spastic or contracted thumb intrinsics	Release of thenar muscles, first dorsal interosseous, contracted thumb release, web space release as needed
III	Weak abductor pollicis longus	Rerouting of abductor pollicis longus around flexor carpi radialis
IV	Spastic or contracted FPL	"Z"-lengthening of FPL

FCU,[22,29,44,46,47,85,89,98] ECRL and ECRB,[57,58,89] and FDS.[9,21,24,29,71,85] Results of brachioradialis to APL transfer have not demonstrated significant improvement in active abduction,[78,89] but transfer to the EPB may be more successful.

Other procedures to improve extension include rerouting of the EPL and FPL abductorplasty.[6a,24,26,27,53,55,76,80,84] Imbrication of the APL and EPB has also been described[21,24,57,58,65,99] and is effective when EPL function is weak.

Augmentations to thumb extension and abduction will cause undesirable MCP joint hyperextension and be less effective for thumb ray abduction if the MCP joint can hyperextend passively more than 20 degrees. Arthrodesis of the MCP joint prevents hyperextension,* and the resulting limitation of flexion is an advantage in the correction of the thumb-in-palm deformity. MCP joint capsulodesis has been described but may be less reliable.[11,51,87] Metacarpal bone block with fusion of the thumb CMC joint has been described[9,10,22,74,84,85,93] but is rarely performed now because it significantly decreases pinch and makes the hand difficult to get into small places.

Finally, in hands with no functional motors available for transfer to abduct the thumb, transfer of the abductor end-to-side into the substance of the FCR tendon can provide a passive tenodesis.[44] Soft tissue contracture of the skin of the first web space should be addressed in these patients with a four-flap "Z"-plasty.[21,41,44,46,71,90]

Release of the Origin of Spastic Thumb Intrinsics

Indication. Release of the origin of the thumb intrinsics is indicated when there is selective control of the muscles.

Contraindication. If there is no selective control of the adductor pollicis, release of the muscle from its origin is less

likely to be effective, and release of its insertion should be performed.

Technique[55-58]

A curved incision is made in the thenar crease extending from the volar carpal ligament to the base of the index finger. The adductor pollicis is exposed in the interval between the common digital nerve of the index and long fingers and the flexor tendons of the long finger. The origin of the muscle from the third metacarpal is dissected free in a distal to proximal direction. The deep palmar arch and motor branch of the ulnar nerve are identified and protected as the proximal aspect of the muscle is dissected. Complete detachment of the muscle origin is necessary to provide release of the contracture. The proximal extent of the deep exposure is limited by the superficial vascular arch. The FPB can be identified in the proximal part of the incision and detached from the volar carpal ligament if an MCP flexion deformity is present. The origin of the first dorsal interosseous can be released through this incision or through a separate longitudinal incision over the dorsal aspect of the thumb metacarpal. The muscle's origin is dissected off the metacarpal, with care taken to protect the princeps pollicis vessels at the base of the metacarpal.

The wrist is immobilized for 4 weeks in neutral position with the thumb abducted. A removable thumb spica splint is worn for 4 more weeks while therapy and range-of-motion exercises are begun. Splinting is discontinued at 8 weeks, unless a tendency for recurrence of deformity requires night splinting.

Release of the Insertion of the Spastic Thumb Intrinsics

Indications. If there is no voluntary control of the adductor pollicis and FPB, then tenotomy at their insertion is effective. If selective control of the muscles is present,

---
*See references 19, 21, 27, 44-46, 84, 96, 98, and 99.

then release of the myotendinous junction can be performed, leaving some of the muscle fibers in continuity. Alternatively, the muscle insertion can be reattached to the middle aspect of the metacarpal, effectively lengthening the muscle.

Technique

The adductor pollicis, FPB, and first dorsal interosseous are approached through a double opposing "Z"-plasty of the thumb web space (Fig. 34-16). The oblique and transverse heads of the adductor tendon are identified and can be completely detached from the metacarpal and sesamoid or fractionally lengthened. To fractionally lengthen the adductor, an oblique incision of the tendon is made near the myotendinous junction and the thumb is gently abducted to allow sliding of the muscle fibers. The first dorsal interosseous

CRITICAL POINTS: RELEASE OF THE INSERTION OF THE SPASTIC THUMB INTRINSICS

INDICATION

- For adduction deformity of the thumb without voluntary control of the adductor and flexor brevis. If selective control of the adductor muscle is present, then reattachment of the tendon to the middle aspect of the metacarpal should be performed.

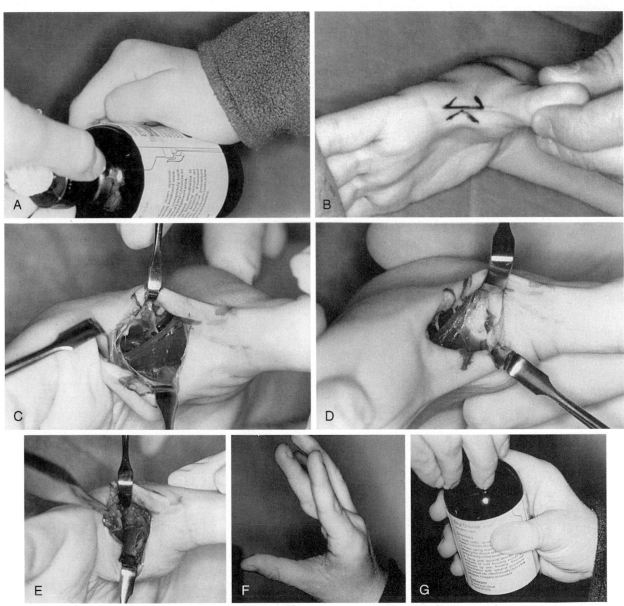

FIGURE 34-16. Correction of thumb-in-palm deformity. **A,** Thumb-in-palm prevents this patient from being able to grasp a bottle. **B,** A double opposing "Z"-plasty for release of the adductor pollicis and the first dorsal interosseous. **C,** The adductor is visualized volarly and the first dorsal interosseous dorsally. **D,** Release of the tendinous portion of the adductor with muscular attachment left intact. **E,** Complete release of the adductor and the first dorsal interosseous muscle. **F,** Postoperative appearance of the hand. **G,** The patient is now able to grip a bottle. (A-G, © Michelle Gerwin Carlson.)

CRITICAL POINTS: RELEASE OF THE INSERTION OF THE SPASTIC THUMB INTRINSICS—cont'd

PREOPERATIVE EVALUATION

- The thumb should be examined in wrist flexion and extension to note contribution of FPL spasticity.
- Active and passive thumb web spaces should be measured to differentiate spasticity from contracture.
- Patients should be evaluated during functional activities because thumb adduction spasticity may increase with use.

PEARLS

- If spasticity of the FPL is evidenced by flexion of the IP joint when the wrist is held in neutral, then this tendon will need to be addressed.
- A fractional lengthening of the FPL will be sufficient if the FPL is not tight in wrist flexion.
- If the FPL is tight in wrist flexion, then a "Z"-lengthening of the tendon will be necessary.

PITFALL

- Be sure to augment thumb abduction/extension if it is weak.

TECHNICAL POINTS

- Make a double opposing "Z"-plasty of the first web space.
- Detach the adductor tendon from the metacarpal and sesamoid.
- Elevate the origin of the first dorsal interosseous muscle from the thumb metacarpal.
- Protect the princeps pollicis artery on the ulnar periosteum of the metacarpal.
- Reattach the adductor to the periosteum on the middle aspect of the thumb metacarpal.
- If necessary, perform MCP joint capsulodesis by incising the volar capsule and suturing periosteum of the ulnar sesamoid to the metacarpal periosteum, producing 10 degrees of flexion of the MCP joint.
- Fix CMC joint in maximum extension with a 0.45-inch Kirschner wire.
- Stabilize the MCP joint in 10 degrees of flexion if a capsulodesis has been performed with a 0.35-inch Kirschner wire.

POSTOPERATIVE CARE

- Apply a short-arm/thumb spica splint for 4 weeks.

CRITICAL POINTS: RELEASE OF THE INSERTION OF THE SPASTIC THUMB INTRINSICS—cont'd

POSTOPERATIVE CARE—cont'd

- Remove pins at 4 weeks and begin active and passive range-of-motion exercises.
- Use an Orthoplast thumb spica splint for 4 more weeks.
- Discontinue splinting at 8 weeks.

origin from the first metacarpal can be visualized in the depths of the wound dorsal to the adductor and can be subperiosteally dissected off of the metacarpal, with care taken to preserve the princeps pollicis artery. The adductor tendon can be reattached to the periosteum in the mid aspect of the metacarpal with 4-0 nonabsorbable suture. If the MCP joint is unstable, then a capsulodesis can be performed through this incision. The capsule is incised just proximal to the ulnar sesamoid and two nonabsorbable sutures are placed between the sesamoid and the periosteum of the metacarpal, tightening the capsule and bringing the MCP joint into slight flexion. A 0.45-inch Kirschner wire is used to stabilize the CMC joint in maximal extension and abduction, and another 0.35-inch Kirschner wire is placed across the MCP joint in 10 degrees of flexion.

The wrist is immobilized for 4 weeks in neutral position with the thumb abducted. At 4 weeks the Kirschner wires are removed and a removable thumb spica splint is worn for 4 more weeks while therapy and range-of-motion exercises are begun. Splinting is discontinued at 8 weeks, unless a tendency for recurrence of deformity requires night splinting.

EPL Redirection

Indication. This procedure is indicated in patients who have a functioning EPL and is performed in conjunction with release of the thumb intrinsics.

Contraindication. Absence of a functioning EPL is a contraindication to this procedure.

Technique[54,55]

The EPL is exposed through a longitudinal incision radial to Lister's tubercle, just proximal to the extensor retinaculum. A second incision is made over the dorsal aspect of the MCP joint to expose the EPL and extensor aponeurosis. The EPL is transected at this level with a 10×4-mm strip of extensor aponeurosis dissected out from its midportion. A running 4-0 monofilament suture is used to close the extensor aponeurosis. The tendon is withdrawn through the proximal incision. A hemostat or small tendon passer is passed from the thumb incision, through the first dorsal compartment, and out the dorsal wrist incision. An incision may need to be made over the first dorsal compartment to accomplish this. The instrument is then used to draw the EPL through the first dorsal compartment and out the thumb wound. The EPL is passed along the radial side of the APL before being passed through an incision in the MCP joint capsule and sutured into place. If the MCP joint passively hyperextends, the repair should be done into the proximal metacarpal side of the capsule to decrease its effect on the proximal phalanx. The repair should be done with enough tension to hold the thumb metacarpal extended.

The hand is placed in a short-arm/thumb spica cast for 1 month with the thumb metacarpal maximally extended and abducted, the MCP joint slightly flexed, and the wrist extended 30 degrees. A removable splint is applied for an additional 4 weeks, and range-of-motion exercises and therapy are begun. The splint is discontinued at 2 months and night splinting instituted only for a tendency for recurrence of the deformity.

FPL Abductorplasty

Indication. This procedure is indicated when the FPL is spastic and needs to be released or when the EPL is not functioning and cannot be used for transfer.

Contraindications. It is contraindicated in patients who already have a weak pinch. It is also contraindicated in patients who have an MCP fusion, because IP fusion is required after this procedure.

Technique[26]
The FPL tendon is identified through a radial midlateral incision from the middle of the distal phalanx to the neck of the thumb metacarpal. The FPL is transected midways over the proximal phalanx. The distal stump can be used as a tenodesis of the IP joint. A second longitudinal incision is made over the volar wrist radial to the tendon of the FCR and proximal to the wrist flexion crease. The FPL is identified deep in this wound and withdrawn. A subcutaneous tunnel is then created from the proximal wound to the distal wound through which the FPL is passed. It is sutured to the MCP joint capsule as described for EPL redirection.

The arm is immobilized in a short-arm cast for 4 weeks with the wrist in 30 degrees of flexion and the thumb metacarpal fully extended and abducted. A removable splint is worn for an additional 4 weeks while range-of-motion exercises and therapy are started. After 8 weeks, night splinting is used as needed if there is a tendency for recurrence of the deformity.

Imbrication of APL and EPB

Indication. Imbrication of APL and EPB tendons can augment thumb abduction and extension in patients with weak EPL function who are not candidates for EPL rerouting.

Technique
A skin incision is made over the first dorsal compartment, and the retinaculum is incised along its dorsal aspect. The tendons of the APL and EPB are plicated with a hemostat and sewn together with 3-0 nonabsorbable suture.

Alternatively, the tendons can be plicated distally, through a small incision at the APL's insertion on the metacarpal base, so as to avoid release of the first dorsal retinacular pulley and attendant loss of abduction moment. The tendons can also be joined proximally in the forearm if another procedure necessitates a proximal forearm incision.

The wrist is immobilized for 4 weeks in 30 degrees of extension with the thumb metacarpal in full abduction and extension. A removable splint is then used for 4 weeks to allow for therapy and range of motion. Splinting is discontinued at 8 weeks, and night splinting is used only for recurrence of deformity.

Thumb MCP Joint Epiphyseal Arthrodesis

Indication. MCP joint epiphyseal arthrodesis is indicated for the hyperextensible MCP joint in the growing child, when tendon transfers to augment extension or abduction are planned.

Contraindication. Arthrodesis is contraindicated when an IP arthrodesis is contemplated.

Technique[31]
The MCP joint is approached through a dorsal incision. The interval between the EPL and EPB is split, and subperiosteal dissection of the articular surface of the proximal phalanx and metacarpal head is performed. Care should be taken not to extend the dissection proximally on the metacarpal or distally on the proximal phalanx to expose the physes. The articular surface is removed first with a knife to expose the ossification center, then the subchondral bone can be removed with an oscillating saw. The osteotomies should be performed to position the joint in 10 degrees of flexion. The MCP joint is fixed with two 0.035-inch Kirschner wires.

Immobilization of the wrist and MCP joint is accomplished with a thumb spica cast until bony union is observed.

Author's Preferred Method of Treatment

I find that the easiest way to address the thumb-in-palm problem is to identify and address the four key issues in the deformity: spastic or contracted flexors and adductors, weak or absent extensors and abductors, MCP hypermobility, and skin web space contracture. I correct the spastic flexors and adductors, MCP hypermobility, and skin web space contracture simultaneously through a single incision, using a double opposing "Z"-plasty of the web space. I release the insertion of the adductor and reattach it to the middle aspect of the thumb metacarpal, release the first dorsal interosseous origin off the thumb metacarpal, and transect the FPB insertion. An MCP joint capsulodesis is performed for MCP joint hyperextension. If spasticity of the FPL is evidenced by flexion of the IP joint when the wrist is held in neutral, then a fractional lengthening will be sufficient. If the FPL is tight when the wrist is held in flexion, a "Z"-lengthening of the tendon is necessary.

For weak abduction and extension, I reroute the EPL if there is good EPL function. Rerouting of the EPL allows the tendon to become a thumb *ray* abductor instead of an IP extensor and thumb ray adductor. I have found that release of the adductors alone improves the abduction/extension arc approximately 20 degrees, but with EPL rerouting the arc improves approximately 40 degrees.[6a] When EPL function is not good, I perform brachioradialis to EPB transfer. This transfer will need some re-education postoperatively, because patients need to initially reinforce thumb extension with elbow flexion against resistance. I have been less satisfied with simple plication of the APL and EPB because they tend to stretch.

If the digital flexors and extensors have no function, then I may not perform transfers to augment thumb extension. The only use the patient may have of the hand may be the adducted thumb against the palm. Correction of the thumb-in-palm deformity may eliminate function of the extremity because of inability to flex the digits to an abducted thumb.

EPL Rerouting (Fig. 34-17)

Indication. Patients lacking thumb abduction and extension with active EPL function. To determine optimum candidates, the patient is asked to actively extend the IP joint while the wrist is held in the neutral position. This procedure should be performed concurrently with a release of the insertion of the thumb intrinsics.

Contraindication. Absence of active EPL function is a contraindication to this procedure.

Technique

Through a transverse incision just proximal to Lister's tubercle, the retinaculum over the third dorsal compartment is incised. The EPL is removed from its tunnel and allowed to migrate in a radial direction, by releasing any subcutaneous septa that might prevent its translocation. Through a second transverse incision just distal to the first dorsal compartment, a proximally based slip of APL is harvested. The EPL tendon is identified in the distal incision, and the slip of abductor is looped about the EPL and sewn to the most volar aspect of the retinaculum of the first dorsal compartment or the volar radial periosteum. The EPL is freed from surrounding attachments to ensure a direct line of pull for the tendon. The adequacy of the radial pulley is checked intraoperatively by traction on the EPL at the wrist, producing thumb ray extension and abduction instead of adduction and IP joint extension. The CMC joint is pinned temporarily in maximal extension with a 0.045-inch Kirschner wire.

Patients are placed in a short-arm thumb spica splint for 4 weeks, at which time the Kirschner wires are removed and a removable Orthoplast splint is applied. Hand therapy is recommended for approximately 12 weeks. Initially, therapy seeks to enable the patient to inhibit thumb adduction during the performance of exercises. After this is achieved, active EPL/EPB firing is attempted, usually at 2 weeks. Therapy then progresses to include light cylindrical grasp and lateral or opposed pinch of small objects with use of balanced

---

CRITICAL POINTS: EPL REROUTING

INDICATIONS

- Poor thumb abduction/extension
- Release of the thumb intrinsics performed concurrently

PREOPERATIVE EVALUATION

- Patients must have good active EPL function with the wrist held in neutral.

PEARLS

- The adequacy of the radial pulley is checked intraoperatively by traction on the EPL at the wrist: this should produce thumb metacarpal extension instead of adduction and IP extension.

TECHNICAL POINTS

- Make a transverse incision proximal to Lister's tubercle.

- Open the retinaculum of the third dorsal compartment.
- Translocate the EPL tendon radially.
- Through a second transverse incision distal to the first dorsal compartment create a proximally based slip of APL.
- Free the EPL up through this incision proximally and distally.
- Wrap the slip of APL around the EPL and suture to the volar periosteum of the radius or the volar first dorsal compartment.
- Pin the CMC joint in maximal thumb abduction and extension.

POSTOPERATIVE CARE

- Manage as in thumb intrinsic release protocol.
- Remove Kirschner wire at 4 weeks postoperatively.
- Attempt active EPL/EPB firing at 6 weeks postoperatively.

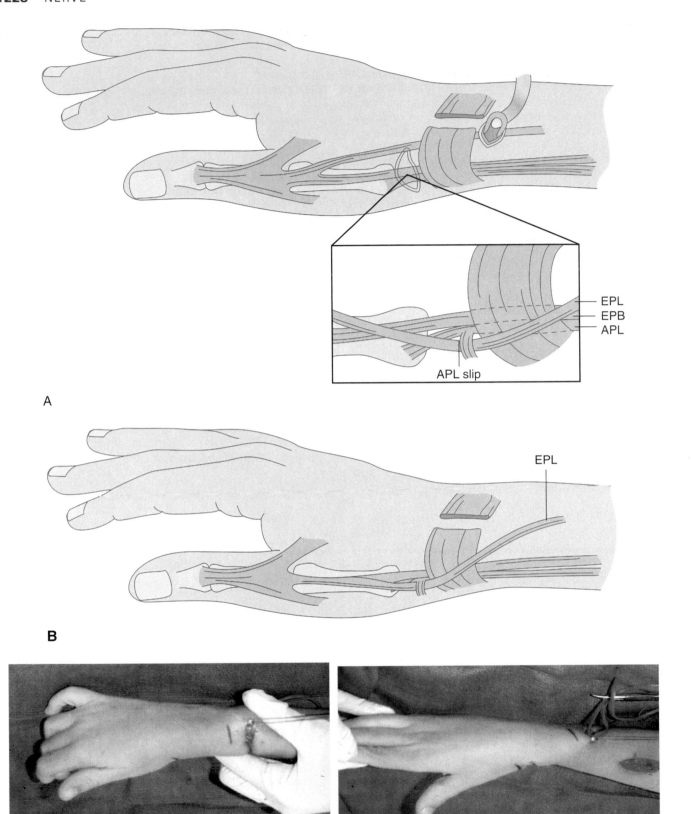

FIGURE 34-17. EPL rerouting. **A,** After release of the EPL from the third dorsal compartment, the EPL is identified through a radial incision distal to the styloid. A proximally based slip of APB is harvested and sutured to the radial periosteum, creating a radial pulley for the EPL. **B,** After rerouting, the EPL has an abduction/extension line of pull. **C,** Intraoperative photograph demonstrating the pull of the untreated EPL causing adduction of the thumb ray and IP extension. **D,** After rerouting the EPL, its pull causes thumb abduction. (**C** and **D,** © Michelle Gerwin Carlson.)

abduction and extension. After 4 weeks the splint is removed and activities of daily living are encouraged.

Brachioradialis to EPB Transfer

Indication. Patients lack thumb extension and abduction with poor EPL function.

Contraindication. This procedure is contraindicated in patients who do not have voluntary control of the brachioradialis with elbow flexion.

Technique (Fig. 34-18)

A 2-cm transverse incision is made 3 cm proximal to the tip of the radial styloid. The subcutaneous tissues are spread bluntly, with care taken to avoid injury to the superficial branches of the radial nerve. The brachioradialis tendon is identified and released from its insertion on the distal radius as distal as possible. The first dorsal compartment is inspected, and the EPB identity is confirmed using a traction maneuver. The APL will have no effect on the MCP joint, while the EPB tendon will extend the MCP joint. If the EPB is not present or is too small, a rerouted EPL can be used instead. The EPB is transected as proximally as possible at the musculotendinous junction and woven into the brachioradialis tendon in a Pulvertaft fashion. Maximum tension is placed on the two tendon ends with the wrist in neutral and the elbow flexed during the weave. It is important for this transfer to be tight.

The postoperative regimen is the same as for EPL rerouting, with occasional re-education necessary to reinforce thumb extension with elbow flexion against resistance.

INTRINSIC MUSCLE SPASTICITY AND DIGITAL SWAN NECK DEFORMITY

Condition

Intrinsic spasticity in the hand causes flexion at the MCP joints and extension at the PIP joints. Over time, swan neck deformities of the digits result, although some evidence exists that the digital extensors may also contribute to this deformity.[98] Swan neck deformity is rarely a functional problem unless the PIP joints tend to "stick" in hyperextension and the patient has difficulty initiating flexion. More commonly, the deformity is a cosmetic concern. The functional and cosmetic benefit of correcting PIP hyperextension can be demonstrated to the patient preoperatively with the use of figure-of-eight extension block splints.

Similarly, the MCP flexion component causes difficulty only if severe, because it is usually overpowered by the

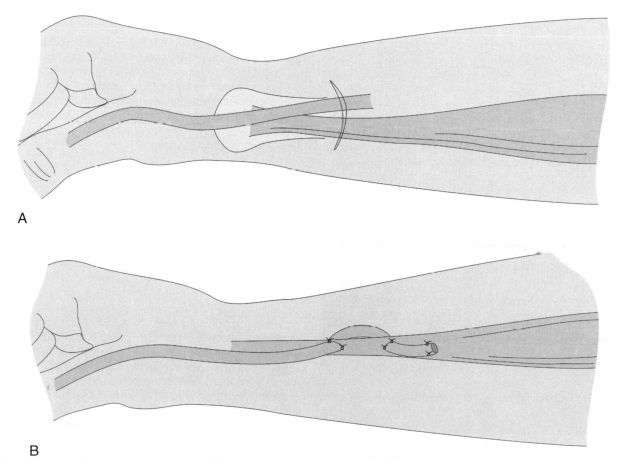

A

B

FIGURE 34-18. Brachioradialis to EPB transfer. **A** and **B**, Through a transverse incision, the brachioradialis is harvested distally and the EPB proximally. The EPB is then woven into the brachioradialis, or, alternatively, a surgeon's knot may be performed between the two tendons.

CRITICAL POINTS: BRACHIORADIALIS TO EPB TRANSFER

INDICATION

■ Patients lacking thumb abduction and extension with poor EPL function

PREOPERATIVE EVALUATION

■ Patients should have voluntary control of the brachioradialis with elbow flexion.

PEARLS

■ EPB tendon is identified as the most ulnar tendon in the first dorsal compartment.
■ If the EPB is too small, the rerouted EPL can be used instead.

PITFALL

■ This transfer must be tight; if it is too loose, adequate thumb abduction will not be accomplished.

TECHNICAL POINTS

■ Make a 2-cm transverse incision 3 cm proximal to the tip of the radial styloid.
■ Dissect deep tissues protecting the branches of the radial nerve.
■ Release the brachioradialis at its insertion into the radius.
■ Transect the EPB tendon as proximally as possible at the musculotendinous junction.
■ Weave the EPB into the brachioradialis in a Pulvertaft fashion with maximal tension on the two tendons with the wrist in neutral and the elbow in flexion.

POSTOPERATIVE CARE

■ Manage as described for EPL rerouting.
■ Re-education is occasionally necessary to reinforce thumb extension with elbow flexion against resistance.

EDC. However, the deformity may become more pronounced after correction of a wrist flexion deformity because of the effective weakening of the EDC tendons. Lengthening procedures for the digital flexors may unmask intrinsic spasticity (Fig. 34-19).

Operative Procedures

Intrinsic spasticity can be treated by two methods: intrinsic muscle origin slide and ulnar motor neurectomy. Intrinsic muscle origin slide will correct the spasticity of the muscle, decrease the contracture, and retain some function. Ulnar

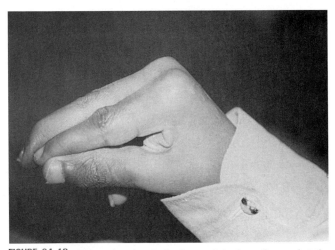

FIGURE 34-19. This patient has had release of the long flexors, but the intrinsic muscles were not addressed. The severe MCP flexion and PIP extension of the fingers significantly limit function, and he still has an interdigital hygiene problem. (© Michelle Gerwin Carlson.)

motor neurectomy will eliminate the spasticity of the intrinsics[89] at the expense of *all* intrinsic function but will not reduce any component of myostatic contracture. The effectiveness of an ulnar motor neurectomy can be tested with an ulnar nerve block at the wrist.

PIP hyperextension can also be corrected with superficialis tenodesis or central slip tenotomy. The end of the superficialis tendon can be repaired either to bone[21,84,90,95-99] or to the fibro-osseous pulley.[21,55]

Interosseous Muscle Slide

Indication. This procedure should be performed when significant MCP flexion is decreasing hand function and/or causing a problem with interdigital hygiene. Some intrinsic function is retained, and the contracture across the MCP joint is decreased.

Contraindication. This procedure should not be performed for cosmesis.

Technique

A transverse incision is made on the dorsum of the hand at the mid-metacarpal level, or two longitudinal incisions are made in the index-long and ring-little interspaces. The interosseous muscles are identified with retraction of the extensor tendons. Subperiosteal dissection is performed to release both the dorsal and volar interosseous muscles. The MCP joints are brought into full passive extension with the PIP joints flexed. If MCP joint extension is still tight, a Kirschner wire can be used for 4 weeks to hold the MCP joints extended.

The MCP joints are immobilized in full extension for 4 weeks. A removable splint is then applied for 4 weeks, and therapy and range-of-motion exercises are begun. Splinting is discontinued at 8 weeks and night splinting instituted only if there is a tendency for recurrence of the deformity.

Ulnar Motor Neurectomy

Indication. Ulnar motor neurectomy is a straightforward approach to decreasing intrinsic muscle spasticity but results in complete loss of intrinsic function. It should be used when good digital function is not anticipated and hygiene is the primary goal.

Contraindication. This is contraindicated when good digital function is expected. It may result in a clawhand deformity.

Technique (Fig. 34-20)

A 3- to 4-cm incision is made over the ulnar nerve and artery in Guyon's canal. The ulnar neurovascular bundle is identified proximally and traced distally by releasing the volar carpal ligament. The ulnar nerve divides into a superficial sensory branch and a deep motor branch within Guyon's canal. The deep motor branch is isolated as it courses around the hook of the hamate, and a section of the motor branch is excised. A nerve stimulator can be used to confirm the identity of the motor branch before transection.

No postoperative immobilization is necessary.

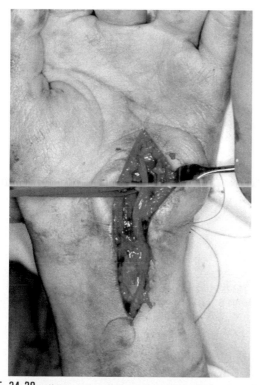

FIGURE 34-20. Ulnar motor neurectomy. The ulnar nerve has been dissected out from above the wrist. The vessel loop is around the motor branch, which is transected. (© Michelle Gerwin Carlson.)

Superficialis PIP Tenodesis

Indication. This procedure is indicated for PIP hyperextension that is hindering active flexion of the digit.

Contraindication. This procedure is contraindicated if the FDP is nonfunctional in the involved finger.

Technique

A midaxial incision is made over the radial side of the middle phalanx, and the flexor sheath is identified and incised. The radial slip of the FDS tendon is identified. A second incision is made over the A1 pulley in the palm, and the A1 pulley is incised. The radial slip of the FDS tendon is positively identified beneath the A1 pulley using a traction maneuver and transected proximally. It is then withdrawn through the distal incision. This involves division of the chiasm, which can be done through the proximal and distal incisions. A third midaxial incision is made over the ulnar aspect of the proximal phalanx. The radial slip of the FDS tendon is passed from the radial incision to the ulnar incision by passing it deep to both neurovascular bundles and the remaining flexor tendons. A transverse drill hole, large enough to pass the tendon, is made through the middle to distal third of the proximal phalanx in an ulnar to radial direction. A tagging suture is placed on the distal end of the tendon, and the tendon is delivered into the drill hole by passing two Keith needles through the drill hole and out the radial side of the digit. The tendon should be long enough to just enter the drill hole but not emerge from the radial side. The sutures are tied over a button on the skin on the radial aspect of the digit, with enough tension to produce a 20-degree flexion contracture of the PIP joint. The PIP joint is then held in this position with a Kirschner wire. Alternatively, the superficialis tendon can be fixed with a suture anchor into the proximal phalanx, or it can be sutured to the fibro-osseous flexor sheath. (See Chapter 9 for another technique of superficialis PIP tenodesis.)

The Kirschner wire is removed at 2 weeks, and range of motion is begun with active and passive flexion and an extension block splint that limits extension to 20 degrees. Full range of motion is allowed after 8 weeks.

 ## Author's Preferred Method of Treatment

I find severe MCP flexion deformity from intrinsic spasticity a very difficult problem to correct. Ulnar motor block identifies the correction possible with ulnar motor neurectomy, and I prefer this procedure to interosseous muscle slide in patients with poorly functioning hands. Often ulnar block incompletely corrects the deformity because of fixed capsular contractures of the MCP joints, and in these patients I have found MCP arthrodesis to successfully improve the position of the fingers and retain some function of the hand. Additionally, shortening can be accomplished through the arthrodesis, helping to relatively lengthen the

CRITICAL POINTS: MCP JOINT ARTHRODESIS

INDICATION

- Patients with MCP flexion deformity not improved with an ulnar nerve block

PREOPERATIVE EVALUATION

- Ulnar nerve block will identify flexible deformities.
- The function of the long digital flexors should be assessed.

PEARLS

- If there is significant spasticity of the flexors or extensors, intraoperative botulinum toxin may allow for a smoother postoperative course.

TECHNICAL POINTS

- Make a longitudinal incision over each MCP joint to be arthrodesed.
- Incise the extensor hood ulnar to the EDC tendon.
- Incise the capsule longitudinally, and release the collateral ligaments.

- Remove the articular surface of the metacarpal and phalanx with an oscillating saw.
- Produce a cascade of flexion of 20 degrees in index finger to 40 degrees in little finger.
- Fix MCP fusion with a 2.0-mm plate, two to three screws on each side
- Close capsule and extensor hood.

PITFALL

- Arthrodesis in too much MCP flexion, especially of the fifth finger, will make it difficult to clear the digits in grasp

POSTOPERATIVE CARE

- Apply forearm-based extension splint for 4 weeks.
- Use palm-based thermoplastic splint across MCP joints with PIP joints free until union.

---

tight extrinsic flexors. It is important to ensure that the intrinsics are not the only functioning muscles in the hand and that the patient has good extrinsic flexor function, or hand function will be adversely affected.

MCP Joint Arthrodesis

Indication. Patients with MCP flexion deformity may not improve with ulnar nerve block.

Contraindication. Patients must have functioning long digital flexors or MCP fusion will remove any functional flexion of the digit.

Technique

A longitudinal incision is made over each MCP joint to be arthrodesed. The extensor hood is incised ulnar to the extensor tendon, and the capsule is incised longitudinally. The collateral ligaments are released from the metacarpal head, and the articular surface of the metacarpal head and base of the proximal phalanx are removed with an oscillating saw. The metacarpal osteotomy should be performed to create a cascade of flexion through the arthrodesis from 20 degrees for the index finger to 40 degrees for the little finger. Care must be taken not to produce a radial or ulnar angular deformity through the fusion site. A 2.0-mm plate is contoured and used to fix the metacarpal to the proximal phalanx with two to three screws proximally and distally. The capsule is closed when possible with nonabsorbable suture, and the extensor hood is repaired with interrupted nonabsorbable suture.

The hand is immobilized for 4 weeks in a forearm-based extension splint with the wrist in neutral and the digits extended. At 4 weeks, a thermoplastic palm-based splint across the MCP joints with the PIP joints free is worn until union is demonstrated on radiographs. I tell patients to expect improved use of the hand because of the ability to place objects in the palm with the MCP joints extended. As long as patients have digital flexion, the improved position of the MCP joints outweighs the loss of MCP motion.

Central Slip Tenotomy

For swan neck deformity of the PIP joints, I have found central slip tenotomy to be a very effective treatment. It is important to verify that patients have active digital flexion when the digits are held passively in the corrected position, or recurrence of the deformity is likely. PIP tenodesis is effective to treat the deformity but is a difficult procedure to set appropriate tension and often requires significant rehabilitation postoperatively.

Indication. This procedure is indicated in patients with active swan neck deformity of the PIP joints greater than 20 degrees.

Contraindication. Patients who cannot actively flex their PIP joints when the digit is held in the corrected position are likely to have a recurrence of deformity.

Technique (Fig. 34-21)[7a]

A transverse incision is made dorsally, approximately 1 cm proximal to the PIP joint, and the extensor mechanism is identified. A forceps is used to grasp the center of the tendon, and gentle traction facilitates identification of the separation between central slip and lateral bands. The central slip is transected transversely, and the lateral bands are

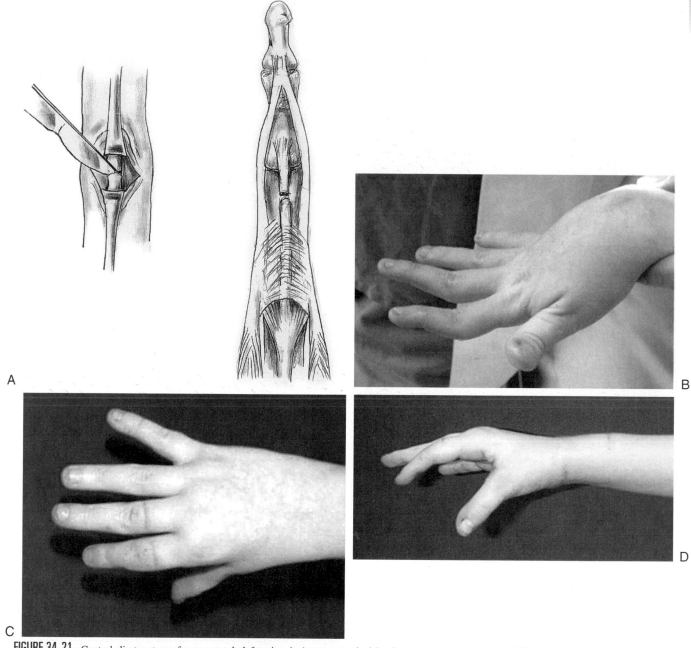

FIGURE 34-21. Central slip tenotomy for swan neck deformity. **A,** A transverse incision is made just proximal to the PIP joint and a tenotomy of the central slip is performed leaving the lateral bands intact. **B,** Preoperative swan neck deformity. **C,** The healed incision is visible proximal to the PIP joint. **D,** Postoperative correction of the swan neck deformity. (**B-D,** © Michelle Gerwin Carlson.)

left intact. As the central slip is transected the demarcation between it and the lateral bands becomes more apparent. The skin is reapproximated with absorbable sutures, and the PIP joint is fixed with a 0.35-inch Kirschner wire in 10 degrees of flexion.

The digits are splinted in extension for 4 weeks, at which point the splint and Kirschner wires are removed. Molded oval figure-of-eight splints are applied to the PIP joints and active flexion is begun. Active extension should be limited to −10 degrees by the oval figure-of-eight splint. At 8 weeks postoperatively the splints are discarded and full range of motion is allowed. Patients are told to expect correction of the deformity to within 10 degrees of neutral.

DIRECTIONS FOR THE FUTURE

The most important advancement for the future will be restoration of function to hands that lack voluntary control. The key dysfunctional component of cerebral palsy is not the muscle or its peripheral nerve but the damaged central nervous system pathways. If a normal impulse pathway can be redirected to the dysfunctional muscle and its nerve, it may be possible to restore normal function. Work with computerized neurostimulation generated by brain electroencephalographic waves may eventually solve this problem.

CRITICAL POINTS: CENTRAL SLIP TENOTOMY

INDICATION

■ Patients with active swan neck deformity greater than 20 degrees

PREOPERATIVE EVALUATION

■ Check for active digital flexion when the PIP is held in neutral.

PEARLS

■ Grasping the extensor mechanism and lifting with a forceps facilitates identification of the demarcation between central slip and lateral bands.

TECHNICAL POINTS

■ Make a transverse incision 1 cm proximal to the PIP joint.

■ Transect the central slip, leaving the lateral bands intact.

■ Transfix the PIP joint in 10 degrees of flexion with a 0.035-inch Kirschner wire.

PITFALL

■ Be sure to transect the entire central slip but not the lateral bands.

POSTOPERATIVE CARE

■ Splint digit in extension for 4 weeks.

■ Remove pin at 4 weeks and apply oval figure-of-eight splint.

■ Splint limits extension to −10 degrees.

■ At 8 weeks, allow full range of motion and discontinue splint.

ANNOTATED REFERENCES

33. Green WT: Tendon transplantation of the flexor carpi ulnaris for pronation-flexion deformity of the wrist. Surg Gynecol Obstet 75:337-342, 1942.

34. Green WT, Banks HH: Flexor carpi ulnaris transplant and its use in cerebral palsy. J Bone Joint Surg Am 44:1343-1352, 1962.

These two articles describe the classic FCU to ECRB transfer as described by Dr. William Green in the treatment of spastic, obstetrical, and infantile paralysis. Although almost all patients improved in function, no data are given in either paper on the range of motion achieved with the transfer, and some of the photographs may demonstrate a wrist extension contracture in a few patients. This is a gold standard procedure, but care must be taken to use it for the correct indications.

35. Gschwind C, Tonkin M: Surgery for cerebral palsy: Part I. Classification and operative procedures for pronation deformity. J Hand Surg [Br] 17:391-395, 1992.

The authors divide pronation deformity into four distinct groups and simplify the approach to the treatment of this deformity, with indications for each procedure.

40. Hoffer MM, Lehman M, Mitani M: Long-term follow-up on tendon transfers to the extensors of the wrist and fingers in patients with cerebral palsy. J Hand Surg [Am] 11:836-840, 1986.

Hoffer and colleagues in this article first describe the concept of grasp versus release. They advocate transfer to the finger extensors for poor release and to the wrist extensors for poor grasp. Before this distinction, most transfers were done to the wrist extensors with occasional weakening of digital extension and thus detrimental effect on hand function.

44. House JH, Gwathmey FW, Fidler MO: A dynamic approach to the thumb-in-palm deformity in cerebral palsy: Evaluation and results in fifty-six patients. J Bone Joint Surg Am 63:216-225, 1981.

The authors give an organized and concise description of different types of thumb-in-palm deformities and how to address treatment.

49. Koman LA, Gelberman RH, Toby EB, Poehling GG: Cerebral palsy: Management of the upper extremity. Clin Orthop 253:62-74, 1990.

104. Van Heest AE, House JH, Cariello C: Upper extremity surgical treatment of cerebral palsy. J Hand Surg [Am] 24:323-330, 1999.

107. Waters PM, Van Heest AE: Spastic hemiplegia of the upper extremity in children. Hand Clin 14:119-134, 1998.

These are three excellent articles on the treatment of the entire upper extremity in cerebral palsy.

50. Koman LA, Mooney JF III, Smith B, et al: Management of cerebral palsy with botulinum A toxin: Preliminary investigation. J Pediatr Orthop 13:489-495, 1993.

This is the landmark article in the use of Botox to treat spasticity in cerebral palsy. It has since been used frequently in the treatment and evaluation of patients with spasticity.

54. Manske PR: Redirection of extensor pollicis longus in the treatment of spastic thumb-in-palm deformity. J Hand Surg [Am] 10:553-560, 1985.

Manske first describes redirecting the EPL tendon to make it more effective in abduction-extension. Many modifications of this technique have since been described.

62. Mital MA: Lengthening of the elbow flexors in cerebral palsy. J Bone Joint Surg Am 61:515-522, 1979.

This article was one of the pivotal articles in the treatment of spasticity of the elbow. Instead of addressing the flexor pronator mass, it addressed the actual elbow flexors individually with excellent results.

81. Sakellarides HT, Mital MA, Lenzi WD: Treatment of pronation contractures of the forearm in cerebral palsy by changing the insertion of the pronator radii teres. J Bone Joint Surg Am 63:645-652, 1981.

This is the original article first describing the use of pronator rerouting in the treatment of pronation deformity. Most patients gained significant active supination, but the specific indications for this procedure are not discussed.

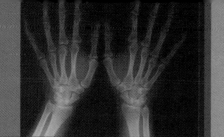

CHAPTER 35

Upper Extremity Dysfunction After Stroke or Brain Injury

Mary Ann E. Keenan

CHARACTERISTICS OF NEUROLOGIC IMPAIRMENTS

Cerebrovascular accident and traumatic brain injury are distinct diagnoses but both result in upper motor neuron syndrome and share many features.[7,58,80,109] Upper motor neuron syndrome is characterized by impairment of motor control, spasticity, muscle weakness, stereotypical patterns of movement (synergy), and the stimulation of distant movement by noxious stimuli (synkinesia).

Impairment of movement after head injury and stroke should be considered both phenomenologically and functionally. Syndromes of restricted limb motion are the most common type of movement impairment. Syndromes of excessive motion are less frequent (Table 35-1). Diffuse axonal injury, multifocal vascular pathology, and diffuse hypoxic encephalopathy lead to a large variety of post-traumatic motor phenomena, which are functionally significant. Cognitive, memory, and sensory deficits are also commonly seen in these patients.

Lesions of the central nervous system, the peripheral nervous system, and the musculoskeletal system and lesions causing pain may lead directly or indirectly to syndromes of restricted or excessive motion of the limbs. A distinction between restricted versus excessive motion is made because the functional implications of each type of motion disorder and the treatment approaches for the problems they generate are very different.

Syndromes of restricted limb motion are manifested by impaired access of the limb to targets in the environment during voluntary movement. Limbs are unable or are poorly able to move toward objects or places because motion across joints is restricted by central or peripheral pathology. An example is a patient with spastic finger flexors who attempts to open the hand to grasp an object. Accessing the object is impaired because spastic finger flexors restrict the voluntary amplitude and speed of finger extension. Another example seen after head injury is heterotopic bone formation about the elbow, which restricts joint motion and impairs use of the upper extremity even in the presence of voluntary muscle action. Limbs with restricted motion lose their operating range and are unable to be positioned adequately for

<table>
<tr><td colspan="2">Table 35-1</td></tr>
<tr><td colspan="2">CLINICAL PHENOMENA ASSOCIATED WITH IMPAIRED MOVEMENT THAT FUNCTIONALLY LEADS TO RESTRICTED OR EXCESSIVE MOTION AFTER TRAUMATIC BRAIN INJURY OR CEREBROVASCULAR ACCIDENT</td></tr>
<tr><td>Limbs With Restricted Motion</td><td>Limbs With Excessive Motion</td></tr>
<tr><td>Spasticity, stiffness and contracture</td><td>Cerebellar ataxia</td></tr>
<tr><td>Upper motoneuron patterns of dysfunction</td><td>Brain stem syndrome</td></tr>
<tr><td>Heterotopic ossification</td><td>Clonus</td></tr>
<tr><td>Bony malalignment/fracture malunion</td><td>Ballismus</td></tr>
<tr><td>Pain syndromes</td><td>Chorea</td></tr>
<tr><td>Pseudobulbar athetoid syndrome</td><td>Tremors</td></tr>
<tr><td>Brain stem syndrome</td><td>Myoclonus</td></tr>
<tr><td>Rigidity and bradykinesia</td><td>Tics</td></tr>
<tr><td>Dystonia, torticollis, bruxism, locked jaws</td><td>Ligamentous and capsular instabilities</td></tr>
<tr><td>Decorticate and decerebrate rigidity</td><td>Sensory disturbance</td></tr>
</table>

function. The general treatment strategy for limbs with restricted motion is to identify and reduce sources of limb restriction.

Syndromes of excessive limb motion are manifested by impaired tolerances in the production of voluntary movement parameters such as movement amplitude, accuracy, timing, and force. Clinical conditions resulting from head injury and associated with excessive motion include movement disorders such as hemiballismus, athetosis, tremor, and cerebellar ataxia. Biomechanical laxity in the musculoskeletal system may also be associated with excessive motion. For example, subluxation or frank dislocation of the shoulder joint may lead to excessive motion in the shoulder girdle.

Because of the similarities between stroke and traumatic brain injury, there is a great deal of overlap in the surgical and nonsurgical management of the upper extremity dysfunction caused by these conditions.[11]

RECONSTRUCTIVE SURGERY AS A REHABILITATION TOOL

The effects of injury to the brain extend beyond its cognitive function, and the musculoskeletal system is profoundly affected. Hypertonicity, the unmasking of primitive reflexes, and impaired motor control all contribute to the abnormal limb positions, contractures, and impaired mobility that are frequently encountered in persons with brain injury.

The converse is also true. The brain is strongly affected by dysfunction of the musculoskeletal system. Just as the shoulder and elbow position the hand for grasping and manipulating objects, the musculoskeletal system gives mobility to the brain and positions it to interact with the world. Independent mobility is a key element of human life and is of fundamental importance to our well-being.

Professionals working in the field of brain injury and stroke rehabilitation are knowledgeable about the cognitive and behavioral deficits that accompany brain injury. It has been my colleagues' and my experience that less importance has been given to the musculoskeletal impairment that results from brain trauma or stroke. The penalties of musculoskeletal limitations for the individual can be devastating. Improvement in an individual's physical mobility is therapeutic and often leads to increases in the person's cognitive, behavioral, and emotional capacities.

Wellness promotion has become an objective of medical care in recent years. This cannot mean the complete prevention of disease, injury, and disability. In the physically disabled population, wellness promotion means maximizing function and mobility to avoid the complications of chronic incapacity. Potential complications of physical immobility include decubiti, infection, pain, social isolation, and physical and emotional dependence. The societal costs can be measured in terms of loss of productivity for the patient and his or her family.

EXPECTATIONS AND TIMING OF RECONSTRUCTIVE SURGERY

When evaluating patients with central nervous system dysfunction, questions commonly arise regarding the indications for surgery, the cost, the expected outcomes, and the practicality of a surgical approach. These issues should be considered on an individual basis for each patient. General principles have been delineated that can serve as guidelines for decision making.

Operate early—before deformities are severe and fixed. Surgery is a powerful rehabilitation tool. It is often the only treatment that will correct a limb deformity or improve function. Surgery should not be considered a treatment of last resort when "conservative" measures have failed. Physical and occupational therapy cannot effect a permanent change in motor control. Systemic drug therapy for increased muscle tone has generalized effects and cannot be targeted to specific offending muscles. Phenol blocks and botulinum toxin injections provide only temporary modulation of muscle tone. When a permanent treatment is needed to decrease muscle tone or redirect a muscle force, surgery should be considered. The results of surgical intervention are improved when deformities are corrected early. Less muscle lengthening is needed when deformities are mild and there is little or no fixed contracture to overcome. Early surgery preserves maximum muscle strength, joint capsule and ligament flexibility, and articular cartilage integrity. In general, the patient will also be in better physiologic condition to undergo surgery if there has not been a prolonged period of immobility.

Better underlying motor control means better function for the extremity. Surgery cannot impart control to a muscle. Lengthening a spastic muscle can improve its function by diminishing the overactive stretch response and uncovering any control that was present. Successful surgery depends on a careful preoperative evaluation to determine the amount of volitional control present in each muscle in the affected limb.

Motor performance can be considered on a continuous scale, with the disabled patient at the lower end and the elite athlete at the upper end. Infinitesimal improvements in the performance of elite athletes distinguish between the winner and the runner-up. Incremental changes in limb function also result in performance improvements for the disabled individual. Surgery should not be reserved for patients with severe impairment and deformity. Individuals with milder degrees of impairment can benefit greatly from relatively simple procedures such as lengthening of the extrinsic finger flexors to improve intricate hand function. The amount of improvement correlates best with the degree of residual motor control and not with the severity of the deformity.

Distinguish between the function of the extremity and the function of the individual. We commonly speak of "functional" and "nonfunctional" surgical procedures. These terms refer to the expected outcomes for a limb but do not indicate the outcome for the person. Surgical releases of a contracted arm in a hemiplegic patient can allow the individual to become independent in dressing even though the arm itself remains nonfunctional.

Consider the cost of not correcting limb deformities. The cost of motor control evaluation using dynamic electromyography (EMG) is relatively modest when compared with its potential benefits. Dynamic EMG is a one-time expense. The cost of performing an incorrect surgical procedure that fails to correct or worsens a limb deformity is much greater. The cost of performing a surgical procedure is likewise limited when compared with a lifetime of attendant care, spasticity medications, repeated blocks, orthotics, complications of skin ulceration and infection, and lost productivity for the patient and caretakers.

STROKE

A cerebrovascular accident remains one of the most serious medical problems in the United States. Stroke is responsible for 200,000 deaths per year and is the leading cause of hemiplegia in the adult.[14,15,47] Management of stroke has become a major priority for physicians treating the elderly.

The overall incidence of cerebrovascular accident is 1 per 1000 annually, with 250,000 survivors per year. There are over 2 million people with permanent neurologic deficits secondary to cerebrovascular accidents in the United States. The average patient who survives beyond the first few months has a life expectancy of greater than 6 years.[48] The survival and longevity of these patients justifies an aggressive approach to rehabilitation.[14,15]

Pathophysiology

Cerebral function depends on a continuous supply of oxygen. Any significant interruption of oxygenation by thrombosis, emboli, or hemorrhage will result in neuron death and subsequent deficits in cognitive, sensory, and motor functions. Thrombosis is the most common cause of infarction and accounts for nearly three fourths of all cerebrovascular accidents.[47,48] Arteriosclerosis is the most significant predisposing factor. The pathogenesis is multifactorial and related to platelet interaction with endothelial cells, serum lipid concentration and vessel deposition, and smooth muscle cell proliferation in the arterial wall.

Cranial hemorrhage accounts for approximately one sixth of all cerebrovascular accidents and includes spontaneous intracerebral hemorrhage and subarachnoid hemorrhage. Hypertension is common among these patients. Embolic events account for less than 10% of cerebrovascular accidents and are related to extracranial vascular pathology, such as carotid atherosclerosis, cardiac valve pathology, or cardiac arrhythmia.

Predisposing factors to cerebrovascular accidents include atherosclerosis, increasing age, genetic predisposition, hypertension, hyperlipidemia, hypercholesterolemia, obesity, cardiac anomalies (e.g., arrhythmias, myocardial infarction, hypotension, mural thrombosis), diabetes mellitus, collagen vascular disease (e.g., vasculitis, polyarteritis), hyperviscosity states (e.g., polycythemia, sickle cell anemia), oral contraceptive use, tobacco use, migraine headaches, and septic vasculitis (e.g., tuberculosis, syphilis, and mucormycosis).

Neurologic Impairment After Stroke

Distinct clinical syndromes arise from insults to specific areas of the cerebral cortex.[7,24,103,105] The middle cerebral artery supplies the largest area of the cerebral cortex. This area controls sensory and motor function of the trunk, upper extremity, and face, as well as the functions of speech. Cerebrovascular accidents involving the middle cerebral artery are the most common and produce the typical hemiplegic picture of greater impairment in the upper extremity, face, and speech, compared with lower extremity involvement.

The anterior cerebral artery supplies the mid cortex in the sagittal plane. This area of cerebral cortex controls sensory and motor function predominantly in the lower extremity. Cerebrovascular accidents involving the anterior cerebral artery result in a hemiplegic picture of sensory and motor deficits chiefly involving the lower extremity.

The posterior cerebral artery supplies the visual cortex in the occipital region. Involvement of this artery typically results in visual impairment. Bilateral cortical involvement may lead to severe mental impairment, frontal release signs, loss of short-term memory, and inability to learn.

Cerebrovascular accidents in the vertebral basilar system are rare. Deficits in balance and coordination arise from interruption of afferent and efferent pathways between the brain and spinal cord. Balance and reactions are also dependent on limb control and proprioception.

Cognitive Impairment

Cognitive deficits can follow cerebrovascular accidents, and patients must be carefully evaluated to assess rehabilitation potential. Impairment of mentation, decreased learning ability, and loss of short-term memory may occur. These deficits may be severe in patients with extensive frontal lobe deficits. These patients show clinical features similar to senility, with lack of attention span and little motivation for recovery. Their prognosis for rehabilitation is poor.

Aphasia is defined as a loss of ability to communicate. It may be expressive or receptive, although it usually involves both components. Aphasia occurs with lesions of the left hemisphere, usually without regard to hand dominance. A receptive aphasia hinders rehabilitation most strongly because the patient cannot understand instructions. Persistent receptive loss has a poor prognosis.

An expressive aphasia, on the other hand, may be compatible with rehabilitation because affected patients retain the ability to comprehend and follow instructions. Occasionally, patient frustration may inhibit progress, but improvement in communication takes place over a long period. Expressive aphasia may substantially resolve with time.

Apraxia, or impairment of execution, is characterized by a loss of ability to perform a previously learned action, such as tying shoelaces or waving good-bye. It occurs more commonly with right hemispheric involvement. Apraxia is not a result of motor or sensory loss. The impairment occurs on the nonhemiplegic side of the body as well. The prognosis with severe apraxia is usually poor, although minor involvement may result only in slight clumsiness. Some improvement with practice and repetition may occur, but if impairment persists after 3 months, further improvement is unlikely.

Sensory Impairment

A wide span of sensory loss, from minimal to severe, may occur after cerebrovascular accident. Sensory perception occurs in the cerebral cortex and is most often affected by lesions of the middle cerebral artery. Sensory loss may be manifest by impairment of touch; pinprick; two-point discrimination; proprioception; discrimination of size, shape, texture, or point localization; or the presence of astereognosis. Impairment of these functions in the upper extremity is a poor prognostic sign, even though motor function may be intact or only minimally impaired.[68,70,71,81]

Lesions of the parietal lobe of the nondominant hemisphere may result in a lack of awareness of the involved side of the body. A failure to recognize and use the involved side may occur despite minimal motor involvement.

Disturbances of vision may occur. Manifestations include hemianopia (blindness in one eye), disturbance of perception, poor perceptual organization, loss of geometric sense, inability to copy figures, and failure to perform tasks involving spatial analysis. Hemianopia is likely to be permanent, yet it may have little impact on rehabilitation potential. Disturbances in visual perception are more significant and may result in failures of activities of daily living.[139]

Motor Impairment

Motor impairment is the most obvious sequela of stroke. Recovery follows a fairly typical pattern. A period of flaccid paralysis occurs and lasts from 24 hours to several weeks. This is followed by a period of increasing muscle tone. In general, the longer that flaccidity persists, the poorer is the prognosis for functional recovery. If the arm is not supported during this time, inferior subluxation of the shoulder may result. With time, the shoulder adductor and internal rotator muscles become tight and the elbow, wrist, and finger flexors develop increased tone. These changes usually become evident within 48 hours after the stroke. Any paralysis remaining after 3 months will usually persist, although some slight improvement may occur over 6 months.[139] Functional improvement may continue as a result of further sensorimotor re-education. Increasing muscle tone usually leads to muscle spasticity. Hyperactive deep tendon reflexes and clonus may appear.

Voluntary movement returns first in the most proximal muscle groups of the limbs and follows in a proximal-to-distal direction of recovery. Voluntary shoulder function should be sought during the early recovery phase when flaccidity is present.

Motor control is graded using a clinical scale (Table 35-2). The extremity may be hypotonic or flaccid and without any volitional movement (grade 1). A spastic extremity may also be postured rigidly without volitional or reflexive movement (grade 2). Patterned or synergistic motor control is defined as a mass flexion or extension response involving the entire extremity (grade 3). A mass flexion pattern in the upper extremity consists of shoulder abduction, forearm pronation, and flexion of the elbow, wrist, and fingers. This mass patterned movement may be reflexive in response to a stimulus and without volitional control. Other patients can volitionally initiate a mass movement (grade 4). Selective motor control with pattern overlay is defined as the ability to move a single joint or digit with minimal movement in the adjacent joints and is usually best controlled when performing an activity slowly. Rapid movements or physiologic stress make the mass pattern more pronounced (grade 5). Selective motor control is the ability to volitionally move a

single joint or digit independently of the adjacent joints (grade 6). Spasticity can mask underlying motor control.

Even when patterned movement can be initiated volitionally it is a neurologically primitive form of motor control and of no functional use in the upper extremity. The lower extremity can more successfully use synergistic motions for functional activities, such as transfers or walking. The patient can be taught to use the flexion movement to advance the limb and the extension pattern to provide limb stability during stance. The upper extremity requires a measure of selective control (grade 5 or 6) for functional use.

The final processes in sensory perception occur in the cerebral cortex, where basic sensory information is integrated to complex sensory phenomena such as proprioception, spatial relationships, shape, sight, and texture. Patients with severe parietal dysfunction and sensory loss may lack sufficient perception of space and awareness of the involved segment of their body to ambulate. Patients with severe perceptual loss may lack balance to sit, stand, or walk.

The Role of the Surgeon in the Management of Stroke

The Period of Acute Injury. The reconstructive surgeon is rarely involved in the acute care of the stroke patient. Efforts at this time are directed toward the medical stabilization of the patient. In some cases the surgeon or therapist may be asked to assist with splinting extremities to prevent limb deformities.

The Period of Physiologic Recovery. Spontaneous neurologic recovery occurs primarily during the first 6 months after a stroke. During the subacute phase, limb flaccidity is changing to spasticity. The patient is commonly in a rehabilitation facility for a portion of this time. Muscle weakness can result in joint subluxation if the limb is not protected with a sling to support the shoulder or a splint to support the wrist. When spasticity becomes pronounced, intervention is needed to prevent contracture formation until spontaneous neurologic recovery has ceased.

The Period of Functional Adaptation to Residual Deficits. After 6 months the patient is usually neurologically stable. Definitive decisions can then be made regarding bracing or

Table 35-2
CLINICAL SCALE OF MOTOR CONTROL

	Motor Control	Description
Grade 1	Flaccid	Hypotonic, no active motion
Grade 2	Rigid	Hypertonic, no active motion
Grade 3	Reflexive mass pattern (synergy)	Mass flexion or extension in response to stimulation
Grade 4	Volitional mass pattern	Patient-initiated mass flexion or extension movement
Grade 5	Selective with pattern overlay	Slow volitional movement of specific joints Physiologic stress results in mass action
Grade 6	Selective	Volitional control of individual joints

surgery to correct limb deformities and rebalance muscle forces. This is the time of greatest contribution by the reconstructive surgeon.

TRAUMATIC BRAIN INJURY

Injury to the brain is a leading cause of disability and death in the United States.[11,51,56,105,133a,141] An epidemiologic study of physician documented cases of traumatic brain injuries occurring in San Diego County, California, in 1981 determined an annual incidence of 180 per 100,000 population.[84] Applying this rate to the U.S. population provides an estimate of 410,000 new cases of traumatic brain injury cases each year. Eleven percent of these patients will die shortly after the injury. Approximately 80% of the survivors will have a good or moderate neurologic recovery. Most traumatic brain injuries occur in individuals who are younger than 45 years old, and those who survive have a normal life span.[51]

Prognosis

Prognosis after traumatic brain injury has traditionally been predicted relative to the Glasgow Coma Scale (GCS) (Table 35-3).[61,63-67,143,144] The GCS evaluates three areas of a patient's reactions: eye opening, motor responses, and verbal responses. The Glasgow Outcome Scale (GOS) is frequently used to determine outcome after brain injury (Table 35-4). Using the GCS score obtained within 24 hours

Table 35-3
GLASGOW COMA SCALE

Eye Opening:	
Spontaneous	4
Speech	3
Pain	2
None	1
Motor Response:	
Obeys	6
Localizes	5
Withdrawal	4
Abnormal flexion	3
Extension	2
None	1
Verbal Response:	
Oriented	5
Confused	4
Inappropriate	3
Incomprehensible	2
None	1

The Glasgow Coma Score is the total of the eye opening, motor response and verbal scores.

From Teasdale G, Jennett B: Assessment of coma and impaired consciousness: A practical scale. Lancet 2:81-84, 1974.

Table 35-4
GLASGOW OUTCOME SCALE

Dead
Persistent vegetative state
Severely disabled
Moderately disabled
Good recovery

The Glasgow Outcome Scale is used to grade the long-term recovery after traumatic brain Injury.

From Jennett B, Teasdale G, Braakman R, et al: Prognosis of patients with severe head injury. Neurosurgery 4:283, 1979.

of the patient's admission to the hospital, a coma score of 11 or greater is associated with an 82% probability of moderate or good neurologic recovery. A coma score of 8 to 10 results in a 68% of a moderate or good recovery. Coma scores of 5 to 7 indicate severe injuries and result in only a 34% incidence of moderate or good neurologic recovery. Lower scores have a significantly higher incidence of severe sequelae.

Age is an important determinant of neurologic outcome after brain injury, regardless of the severity of injury. It has been demonstrated that patients younger than the age of 20 at the time of brain injury have a 62% expectation of moderate to good neurologic recovery. Patients between the ages of 20 and 30 can expect a 46% chance of moderate or good neurologic recovery. In a series of pediatric patients with brain injury, 90% achieved a moderate or good neurologic recovery and only 8% died or remained in a persistent vegetative state.[63] Young children with a GCS score of 5 or better have a good prognosis for recovery.

The duration of coma is another prognostic indicator. If emersion from coma occurs within the first 2 weeks of brain injury, 70% of patients can be expected to achieve a good recovery. If the coma persists beyond 4 weeks, the chance of good recovery lessens considerably. Brain stem involvement, as indicated by the presence of decerebrate or decorticate posturing, has a poor prognosis for outcome. If decerebrate posturing occurs and resolves within the first week after injury, 40% of patients will achieve a good neurologic recovery. If decerebrate posturing persists beyond the first week, only 9% of patients will achieve a good neurologic recovery. In a similar manner, the duration of post-traumatic confusion can also be an indicator of prognosis. If the period of post-traumatic confusion persists for more than 4 weeks, then one third of these patients will have a poor neurologic outcome. It should be remembered, however, that prognosis is a probability statement; although various factors can be used as guidelines, none is an absolute indicator in the individual patient.

Management of Brain Injury

The Period of Acute Injury

Management of brain injury can be divided into three distinct time periods.[43] The initial phase of management occurs immediately after the injury in the acute care hospital. The majority of traumatic brain injuries are the result of a motor vehicle accident, and multiple skeletal and visceral injuries are common. Because of the multitrauma nature of the injury, an orthopedic consultant plays a pivotal role in patient management. Aggressive treatment of orthopedic injuries at this stage can dramatically affect functional outcome.

The first rule of orthopedic care is to make an early and accurate diagnosis of skeletal injury. In the turmoil of a multiple trauma situation with potential life-threatening injuries and ongoing resuscitation efforts, missed fractures or major peripheral nerve injuries are not uncommon.[29, 39,68,139] In a study performed at Rancho Los Amigos Medical Center, Garland reported an 11% incidence of delayed diagnosis of fractures, with an average time to diagnosis of 57 days.[39] Upper extremity injuries were the most frequently missed. In the comatose patient, screening radiographs of all major joints, spine, and pelvis should be obtained on a routine basis. It is also important to look for peripheral as well as central causes for neurologic deficits. Stone and Keenan reported that 34% of brain-injured patients have missed peripheral nerve injuries.[139] Especially in the presence of a limb fracture, a peripheral nerve injury should be suspected.[39,78,101,116]

Pain in patients with traumatic brain injury is often caused by complex regional pain syndrome, deep vein thrombophlebitis, spasticity, occult fracture, or heterotopic ossification.[49,50,140] If pain is treated promptly (and this depends on accurate and early diagnosis), prolonged restriction of motion may be preempted. Heterotopic ossification, fracture, and fracture malunion may restrict motion on the basis of lost structural integrity. Peripheral nerve injury produces weakness and pain, and both are potential causes of restricted motion.

Brachial plexus injuries can be particularly problematic. Plexopathies have been reported in up to 10% of patients with traumatic brain injury. They are particularly prevalent after motorcycle accidents and ejections from a motor vehicle. Fifty percent are associated with upper extremity skeletal trauma, including fractures of the clavicle, humerus, and scapula or shoulder dislocation. Ten to 20 percent involve vascular injury to the subclavian or brachial arteries. Humeral fractures in patients with concurrent complete plexopathies have an increased incidence of delayed union.[21]

The second rule of orthopedic care is to assume that the patient will make a good neurologic recovery. Therefore, all orthopedic injuries should be treated appropriately. Internal fixation is best, when possible. Cast or splint treatment of a fracture in the presence of rigidity, spasticity, and diminished sensibility can be problematic. Spasticity develops rapidly after traumatic brain injuries, and casting a spastic joint in a flexed position may result in a joint contracture or an unsatisfactory reduction. Fracture healing is accelerated, presumably by the same humoral factors that contribute to heterotopic bone formation. Fracture malunion is a common and potentially avoidable complication (Fig. 35-1).

The third rule of orthopedic care is to expect a lack of patient cooperation. As patients emerge from coma, they may be anticipated to go through a period of agitation and confusion. Fracture care should be made as foolproof as possible since patient cooperation cannot be expected. Anticipating a possible period of agitation, traction and external fixators for treatment of extremity fractures should be avoided when possible.

The Period of Physiologic Recovery

After traumatic brain injury, spontaneous neurologic recovery can proceed for a prolonged period of time. Overall neurologic improvement can be made for up to 18 months. In general, the majority of improvement in motor control occurs within the first 6 months after injury. After this period the patient can be assumed to have achieved maximum spontaneous improvement in motor control. Cognitive changes are made most rapidly in the early phases after brain injury but can continue for years (Table 35-5).

During the subacute or recovery phase the patient is generally in a rehabilitation facility. Serious head injury is usually complicated by upper motor neuron syndrome. Upper motor neuron syndrome is a complex of neurologic phenomena characterized by various impairments of motor control, increased muscle tone in the form of spasticity and rigidity, and stereotypical patterns of movement (synergy).

Spasticity is often severe and prevents adequate joint range of motion. Spasticity also interferes with the maintenance of limb position despite the most conscientious and aggressive treatment attempts by family members, nursing staff, and therapists. Even in those situations in which joint motion can be maintained by a knowledgeable therapist, the degree of force required can be painful and potentially harmful for the patient. Lesser degrees of spasticity can be functionally disabling or can require the use of positioning devices that may interfere with the use of an extremity.

Multiple complications can occur in the presence of spasticity (Table 35-6). Contractures are common. Limited positioning and myostatic contractures in patients with diminished nutritional status can result in pressure sores or hygiene problems. Malunion of unstabilized fractures can occur due to uncontrolled muscle tone. Joint subluxation can occur from prolonged spasticity or the attempts to range a joint in the presence of severe spasticity. If a ligamentous injury occurred at the time of injury, frank dislocation of a joint can be caused by hypertonicity. Spasticity also appears to be one of several etiologic factors underlying heterotopic ossification in periarticular locations (Figs. 35-2 and 35-3). Another common complication of spasticity is acquired peripheral neuropathy. The most common peripheral neuropathies acquired with severe spasticity and contracture formation are ulnar neuropathy at the elbow and median neuropathy at the wrist (Fig. 35-4).

During the subacute period, the temporary control of spasticity is the major focus of treatment. Prevention of additional complications such as disuse muscle atrophy, joint contracture, heterotopic ossification, and peripheral neuropathy is critical to a good functional outcome. Early joint contractures are best corrected during the subacute period, first by a reduction of spasticity and subsequently by splinting, casting, and range-of-motion therapy. When tone and contractures are controlled, functional training can progress.

The Period of Functional Adaptation to Residual Deficits

When neurologic recovery has ceased to occur, the brain-injured patient is left with residual limb deformities from spasticity, contracture, and muscle imbalance. It is at this time that definitive surgical procedures are performed to rebalance the muscle forces and correct the residual deformities.

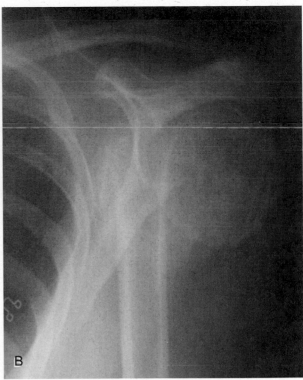

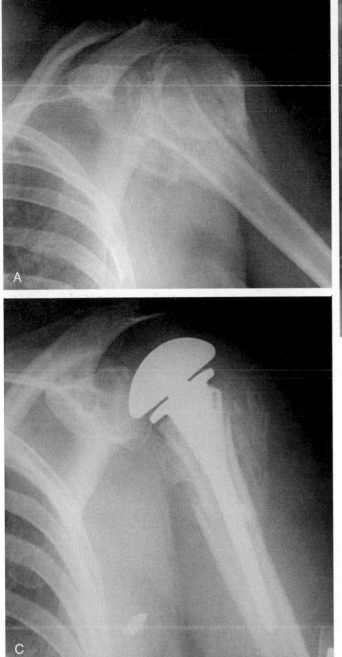

FIGURE 35-1. This 55-year-old woman had sustained traumatic brain injury and proximal humerus fracture (**A** and **B**) among other injuries. The fracture remained untreated because it was presumed that she would not survive. When she regained cognitive function and motor control, the resultant malunion necessitated hemiarthroplasty (**C**), with good functional result.

Timing of intervention is variable, and the surgeon must consider factors such as the rate of improvement in volitional motor control when deciding to intervene surgically. If waiting for additional improvement in motor control will be overridden by potential complications of contracture formation, osteopenia, peripheral nerve compression, and muscle atrophy, then early surgical intervention is appropriate.

Heterotopic Ossification

Heterotopic ossification presents clinically as an intense inflammatory periarticular reaction, characterized by redness, warmth, severe pain, and rapidly decreasing range of motion.[40] Heterotopic ossification is usually demonstrated on radiographs as spotty periarticular calcification within 2 months after traumatic brain injury.[37,137] The incidence of periarticular heterotopic ossification after traumatic brain injury is 11%, with hips most commonly involved, followed by shoulders and elbows.[40] An increased incidence of up to 85% is seen in patients who have concomitant musculoskeletal injuries,[40,59,84] and consideration should be given to prophylaxis. Several modalities have been used with varying success. High-dose diphosphonates (Didronel) and nonsteroidal anti-inflammatory drugs (indomethacin) have been used in the early postinjury period. Radiation (800 cGy via limited fields) has been used within several days after injury.

Table 35-5
RANCHO LOS AMIGOS LEVELS OF COGNITIVE FUNCTIONING

I	No response
II	Generalized response
III	Localized response
IV	Confused-agitated
V	Confused-inappropriate, nonagitated
VI	Confused-appropriate
VII	Automatic-appropriate
VIII	Purposeful-appropriate

From Hagen C, Malkmus D, Durham P, et al: Levels of cognitive functioning. *In* Rehabilitation of the Brain Injured Adult: Comprehensive Physical Management. Downey, CA, Professional Staff Association of Rancho Los Amigos Hospital, 1979, pp. 87-89.

Table 35-6
COMPLICATIONS OF SPASTICITY

Contractures

Decubitus ulcers

Hygiene difficulties

Fracture malunion

Joint subluxation or dislocation

Heterotopic ossification

Peripheral neuropathy

From Keenan MA, Waters RL: Surgical treatment of the upper extremity after stroke or brain injury. *In* Chapman M (ed): Operative Orthopaedics. Philadelphia, JB Lippincott, 1993, pp 1529-1544.

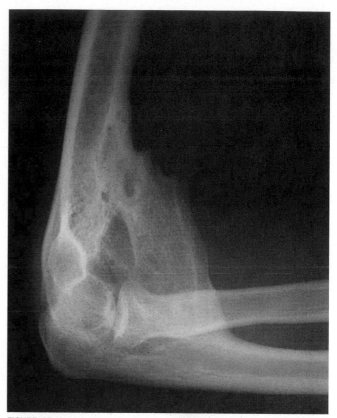

FIGURE 35-2. Preoperative radiograph of the elbow of a patient with a traumatic brain injury and joint ankylosis secondary to anterior heterotopic ossification.

The formation of heterotopic ossification can be followed with radiographs. Bone scans and alkaline phosphatase levels are of limited value. The heterotopic ossification is mature when the radiographs show a well-defined, corticated bone mass. Surgical excision has been demonstrated among spinal cord–injured patients to carry a higher risk of recurrence if attempted before maturation, although this has not been shown to apply to patients with traumatic brain injury. Early excision should be considered in cases in which the heterotopic ossification is causing progressive nerve or vascular compromise or is threatening ankylosis.

Complex Regional Pain Syndrome

Complex regional pain syndrome (previously referred to as causalgia or reflex sympathetic dystrophy [see Chapter 57]) is characterized by "constant, spontaneous, severe, burning pain and is usually associated with hypoesthesia and hyperesthesia, hyperpathia, and allodynia, along with vasomotor and sudomotor disturbances that, if persistent, result in trophic changes."[50] It commonly develops after cerebrovascular accident (posthemiplegic dystrophy), traumatic brain injury, and surgery. It may be associated with concurrent musculoskeletal trauma, although the severity of the initial injury is unrelated to the severity of the pain syndrome.[49,50]

Onset after trauma is usually within the first several weeks, but with stroke and brain injury the onset may be delayed and atypical. Because of this, complex regional pain syndrome may remain undiagnosed in the stroke or brain injury population until it becomes irreversible. Complex regional pain syndrome has three phases: acute, dystrophic, and atrophic.[50]

The acute phase is characterized by constant burning pain, usually localized to a recently injured area. The pain is aggravated by motion or repetitive stimuli. There may be local edema and muscle spasm. During the dystrophic phase, the edema spreads, nearby joints become stiff, and muscle wasting begins. Pain remains the chief complaint, and non-noxious stimuli become progressively more irritating. Nails become ridged and brittle, hair becomes coarse, and skin becomes cyanotic, moist, and cool. Muscular atrophy becomes more pronounced. In the atrophic phase the trophic changes become irreversible. There is further smoothing and tightening of the skin. Involved joints become progressively stiff and may eventually ankylose.

Radiographs that show patchy periarticular demineralization (Sudeck's atrophy) during the first phase may help confirm the diagnosis. Subperiosteal resorption, tunneling of the cortex, and striation may be evident on good quality

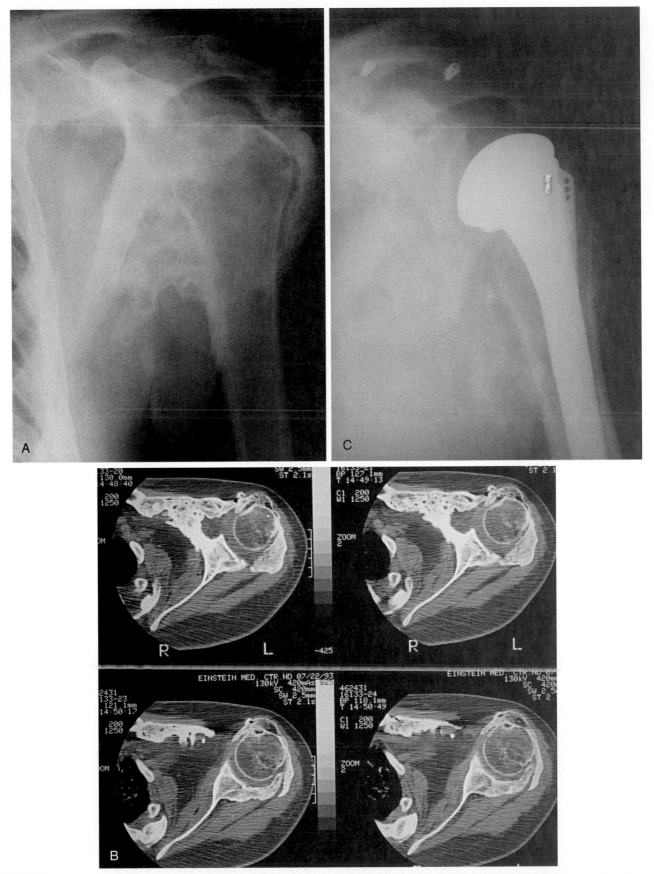

FIGURE 35-3. Preoperative and postoperative radiograph (**A**) and computed tomogram (**B**) of an individual with post-traumatic heterotopic ossification causing shoulder ankylosis. The patient required hemi-arthroplasty (**C**), which resulted in greatly improved function.

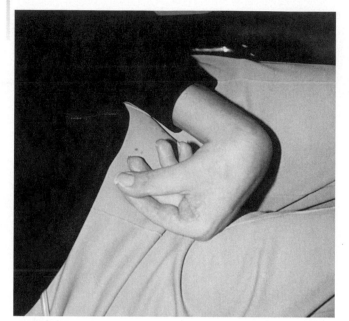

FIGURE 35-4. Severe wrist flexion deformity in this patient resulted in carpal tunnel syndrome.

films. Unfortunately, none of these changes is specific for complex regional pain syndrome, and triple-phase bone scan, although studied extensively, is not considered a highly accurate diagnostic modality. In treating complex regional pain syndrome in the brain-injured patient, I use a regimen of amitriptyline, physical therapy, and sympathetic blockade. For a more detailed discussion of diagnosis and treatment, the reader is referred to Chapter 57.

General Considerations for Treatment Decision Making

Prognosis for Recovery

A major consideration in the treatment of spasticity is whether the neurologic condition is stable. If significant changes in the neurologic status can be anticipated within a relatively short time frame, treatments that are reversible or temporary should be chosen. Tendon lengthening or transfer procedures result in permanent changes and are best done when the neurologic condition has stabilized.

Timing of Neurologic Recovery

Spontaneous neurologic recovery occurs for up to 18 months after a traumatic brain injury. The period of neurologic recovery after stroke is generally 12 months. In both cases, however, the time of meaningful recovery of motor function is approximately 6 months. When possible, definitive surgical procedures are delayed until the patient shows no further improvement in motor control. The prolonged period of recovery combined with the intense level of spasticity, the common additional problem of rigidity (resistance to slow stretch), and the strong muscles found in young patients with brain injury make the temporary control of spasticity much more difficult. Phenol nerve blocks, botulinum toxin injections, and casting techniques are used commonly in these situations.

Pattern of Neurologic Recovery

The majority of stroke patients have hemiplegic involvement with a nonfunctional upper extremity and less involvement of the lower extremity. The surgical procedures designed for deformities of the upper extremity are more likely to be for the correction of contractures than for improvement in function. Even when functional procedures are employed, the gains from these procedures are more moderate than in the brain-injured patient.

The young brain-injured patient is more likely to have quadriplegic involvement, concomitant peripheral nerve injuries, residual deformities from fractures, and heterotopic ossification but good return of motor control. Functional surgical procedures are more common in these patients. Because patient compliance is diminished in brain-injured patients because of cognitive deficits, more durable casting is needed postoperatively to protect tendon transfers.

Degree of Spasticity

The majority of stroke patients have a period of limb flaccidity before the gradual onset of increasing muscle tone or spasticity. Because these patients are typically older than brain-injured patients, their muscles are also comparably weaker. This weakness, combined with a shorter period of spontaneous neurologic recovery, makes the temporary control of spasticity an easier task in stroke patients. The use of temporary blocks is therefore less common in the stroke patient.

Active and Passive Function

Extremity use can be classified as either active or passive. Active function of an extremity requires the volitional inauguration and control of the muscles by the nervous system. Passive function implies that the limb cannot be moved volitionally by the patient. Good passive function means that the limb is flexible, is pain free, and does not cause difficulties with positioning, skin care, or activities of daily living. A contracted arm can cause pain and problems with dressing, sitting, lying in bed, or skin care. An arm with uncontrolled athetotic movements can similarly cause problems and be painful. Impaired passive function of an extremity directly impacts on the overall function of the patient.

Components of Deformity

Limitations of limb mobility are most often the result of a combination of both neurogenic and mechanical factors. The mechanical problems include fracture malunions, joint subluxation, capsular contracture, heterotopic ossification, and soft tissue contractures. Together these are considered to be the static component of the deformity. The dynamic component of the deformity or dysfunction is the result of neurogenic factors such as weakness, spasticity, rigidity, impaired motor control, and spastic reactions triggered by stimulation. It is important to distinguish the contribution of these factors to the limb deformity because treatment options will vary considerably.

Temporary Control of Spasticity

The treatment of spasticity depends on the time since injury and the prognosis for further recovery. In the period of neurologic recovery, temporizing interventions are used because permanent changes may result in chronic imbalance of forces across joints. Prevention of additional complications such as disuse muscle atrophy, joint contractures, heterotopic ossification, and peripheral neuropathies is critical to a good functional outcome. Several choices are available for treatment.

Oral Drug Therapy

Oral antispastic agents may be used during this period. Antispastic agents that have sedating properties such as baclofen (Lioresal), diazepam (Valium), and clonidine may further impair patients with attention deficits and/or memory disorders. Baclofen inhibits both polysynaptic and monosynaptic reflexes at the spinal cord level. It does, however, have general central nervous system depressant actions. The drug tizanidine (Zanaflex) has been reported to affect the central nervous system less than other agents and may be useful.

Dantrolene (Dantrium) is another drug that can be used to control spasticity. Dantrolene is the drug of choice for treating clonus. Dantrolene produces relaxation by directly affecting the contractile response of skeletal muscle at a site beyond the myoneural junction. It causes dissociation of the excitation-contraction coupling mechanism by interfering with the release of calcium from the sarcoplasmic reticulum. Although it does not affect the central nervous system directly, it does cause drowsiness, dizziness, and generalized weakness, which may interfere with the patient's overall function. Use of dantrolene for the control of spasticity is indicated in upper motor neuron diseases, such as spinal cord injury, cerebral palsy, stroke, or multiple sclerosis. The most serious problem encountered with the use of dantrolene is hepatotoxicity. The risk appears greatest in females, those older than 35 years of age, and in patients taking other medications. When using dantrolene, the lowest effective dose should be used and liver enzyme functions should be monitored closely. If no beneficial effect is noted after 45 days of use, the drug should be stopped.

Casts and Splints

A combination of anesthetic peripheral nerve blocks and casting/splinting techniques can be used to give temporary relief of spasticity. Casting maintains muscle fiber length and diminishes muscle tone by decreasing sensory input. Local anesthetic nerve blocks are very helpful when done before cast application, to relieve spasticity and improve limb positioning. Serial casts are used to correct joint contractures by changing casts on a weekly basis. Serial casting is most successful for contractures when present for less than 6 months. Although some carryover effect on spasticity can be seen, this is generally not a practical treatment modality.

Dynamic splinting has a very limited role in treating spastic contractures and may trigger increased muscle tone if not used carefully. Both dynamic splints and serial casting may be very helpful after surgical release to correct the residual static contracture.

Intrathecal Baclofen

Baclofen pump technology has an advantage over oral drug therapy because it directly applies small concentrations of medication to the intrathecal space. The smaller doses

control spasticity effectively while minimizing central side effects. The pump is placed in a subfascial pocket in the abdominal wall. A catheter is routed subcutaneously from the intrathecal space to the pump. The pump can be refilled by injection into the reservoir chamber. The dosage and rate of administration can be easily adjusted by using a laptop computer that sends radio signals to the pump. Continuous infusion of intrathecal baclofen has been reported to be useful in managing spasticity secondary to spinal cord injury with diminished cognitive impairment.[97]

Chemodenervation and Neurolytic Blocks

Focal injection with neurolytic or chemodenervating agents is the most suitable approach for treating focally restricted motion secondary to spasticity. Neurolytic agents such as phenol or alcohol and chemodenervation agents such as botulinum toxin A are used during the period of neurologic recovery, because their effects last only 3 to 5 months. When these agents "wear off," clinical re-evaluation of motor function is performed to assess whether additional recovery has taken place and whether further injections are necessary. To be maximally effective, it is critical that the functional problems of the patient can be accurately ascribed to specific spastic muscles. This can be assessed using multi-channel dynamic EMG. If many muscles are found to contribute, multiple targeted injections can be performed and thus minimize central nervous system side effects. For patients with athetosis, focal injections are less effective, and other modalities, such as environmental modification, weights, bracing, and oral medications should be considered during the period of physiologic recovery.

Phenol Blocks

Phenol, a derivative of benzene, denatures the protein membrane of peripheral nerves when used in aqueous concentrations of 5% or more. When phenol is injected in or near a nerve, it reduces neural traffic along the nerve and hence it is useful as a temporary treatment of spasticity. The onset of the destructive process may begin to show effects several days after injection, but phenol also has a local anesthetic feature that allows a clinician and the patient to see "partial results" shortly after the phenol block is performed.[6] The denaturing process induced by phenol continues for several weeks, but eventually regeneration occurs within 3 to 5 months.

Histologically it has been shown that phenol destroys axons of all sizes in a patchy distribution, but the effect is more pronounced on the outer aspect of the nerve bundle, onto which phenol is dripped. When phenol is percutaneously injected, it is likely that the nerve block will be incomplete. This effect is particularly beneficial in situations in which a spastic muscle has retained volitional capacity, because under these circumstances it is desirable to reduce spasticity while still preserving volitional capacity of a given muscle or muscle group.

The technique of phenol injection is based on electrical stimulation. Nerve branches are injected as close as possible to the motor points of the involved muscle. A surface stimulator is briefly used to approximate the percutaneous stimulation site in advance. A 25-gauge Teflon-coated hypodermic is advanced toward the motor nerve. Electrical stimulation is adjusted by noting whether muscle contraction of the index muscle takes place. As one gets closer to the motor nerve, less current intensity is required to produce a contractile response. The motor nerve is injected when minimal current produces a visible or palpable contraction of the muscle. Generally, 4 to 7 mL of 5% to 7% aqueous phenol is injected at each site. As with any injection, care needs to be taken to avoid injection into a blood vessel, and this is done by aspirating the syringe before the injection.[107]

Botulinum Toxin Blocks

The use of botulinum toxin also exemplifies a localized approach toward functional problems associated with spasticity. Ordinarily, an action potential propagating down a motor nerve to the neuromuscular junction triggers the release of acetylcholine from presynaptic storage sites in the nerve terminal into the synaptic space. The released quanta of acetylcholine, after traversing the synapse and attaching onto receptors located on the postsynaptic muscle membrane, cause its depolarization. This activates a biochemical sequence that ultimately leads to forceful muscle contraction. Botulinum toxin type A is a protein produced by *Clostridium botulinum* that inhibits this calcium-mediated release of acetylcholine at the neuromuscular junction. Botulinum toxin A attaches to the presynaptic nerve terminal, and a component of the toxin crosses the nerve cell membrane. This component interferes with "fusion proteins" affiliated with vesicles of acetylcholine and thereby prevents the release of acetylcholine from their storage vesicles.

Botulinum toxin injection has been used to treat a variety of dystonias and is currently approved by the U.S. Food and Drug Administration for the treatment of blepharospasm, facial spasm, and strabismus. A number of studies have reported its use in treating spasticity in individuals with cerebral palsy, stroke, head trauma, and multiple sclerosis. Clinical benefit lasts 3 to 5 months but may be more variable. Botulinum toxin is injected directly into an offending muscle and, depending on the size of the muscle being injected, dosing has ranged between 10 and 200 units, depending on the size of the muscle. Current practice is to wait at least 12 weeks before re-injection and not to administer a total of more than 400 units in a single treatment session. Because this upper limit of 400 units may be reached rather quickly when injecting a few large proximal muscles or many smaller-sized distal muscles, a different strategy is needed for the limb requiring many proximal and distal injections. In this circumstance, botulinum toxin A and phenol may be combined, the former being injected into smaller distal muscles and the latter aimed at larger proximal ones. A 3- to 7-day delay between injections of botulinum toxin A and the onset of its clinical effect is typical.

The technique of injection varies. Some physicians prefer to inject through a syringe attached to a hypodermic needle that doubles as a monopolar EMG recording electrode. Patients may be asked to make an effort to contract the targeted muscle, or the muscle may be contracting involuntarily. After inserting the needle electrode, injection is made when EMG activity is recorded. For deep or small spastic muscles (e.g., tibialis posterior, long toe flexors, or finger flexors), electrical stimulation is preferred as a means of localizing the muscle before injection.

Block Techniques for Common Deformities

Shoulder Adduction Spasticity. Shoulder adduction and internal rotation spasticity are common problems in both stroke and brain-injured patients. This deformity interferes with hygiene and dressing. Botulinum toxin and phenol motor point blocks of the pectoralis major, latissimus dorsi, and teres major muscles are effective in reducing tone and improving shoulder abduction during the physiologic recovery phase. Phenol block of the thoracodorsal nerve can also be performed.

The onset of muscle relaxation with phenol occurs gradually over the first 24 hours. The onset of botulinum toxin occurs over a 2-week period. Physical therapy is then instituted using both active and passive techniques to increase shoulder range of motion. Blocks can be repeated as needed during the period of time in which neurologic recovery can be expected to continue.

Elbow Flexor Spasticity. During the physiologic recovery phase, control of elbow flexor spasticity is helpful to upper extremity function. The brachioradialis muscle has been shown by dynamic EMG studies to be the most spastic of the elbow flexor muscles.[77] The biceps and brachialis muscles are also significant contributors to the deformity.

Botulinum toxin or phenol motor point blocks are done as described earlier to provide temporary relief. Active and passive range of motion of the elbow is performed after the block. Every attempt is made to incorporate functional activities of the upper extremity into the therapy program. When an elbow contracture is present, serial casting or dynamic splints can be used to correct the deformity.

Wrist and Finger Flexor Spasticity. Spastic forearm flexor muscles causing wrist and finger flexion deformities are treated during the physiologic recovery phase by phenol motor point blocks or by chemodenervation using botulinum toxin.

Because of the large sensory components of both the median ulnar nerves, direct injection of the nerves with phenol is undesirable. Surgical dissection to expose the motor branches would be extensive and would cause excessive scarring for only temporary relief of spasticity. For these reasons an attempt is made to localize the point of entry of the motor branches into the muscles using surface electrical stimulation and targeted motor point injection as described earlier. No more than five points should be injected in a forearm in 1 day to avoid excessive swelling and inflammation.

In recent years, botulinum toxin has become the preferred method of temporary control of spasticity in the arm. The technique is less demanding than phenol injections because the motor points of the muscles do not need to be located as accurately, and permanent scarring of the nerve is avoided. EMG is helpful to localize the individual muscles to be injected.

Residual spasticity and mild contracture are commonly present despite motor point blocks. The blocks can be supplemented with functional electrical stimulation of the wrist and finger extensor muscles and by casting or splinting techniques. Gentle passive range of motion of the wrist and fingers is performed. When motor control is present, a program of active exercise and functional training is also employed.

Intrinsic Spasticity in the Hand. Spasticity involving the intrinsic muscles of the hand is common but may be masked by spastic deformities in the extrinsic finger flexors. An adducted thumb, limited extension of the metacarpophalangeal (MCP) joints, or swan neck positioning of the fingers should alert the physician to the possibility of underlying intrinsic spasticity. In the past, phenol block of the motor branch of the ulnar nerve in Guyon's canal was done after surgical exposure (Fig. 35-5).[82] The close proximity of the sensory branch of the nerve made percutaneous injection undesirable because loss of sensation in the hand or painful dysesthesia could develop from phenol injection of the sensory nerve. The preferred technique now is to inject botulinum toxin into the offending muscles and thus prevent a permanent deformity.

Thumb-in-Palm Deformity. The thumb-in-palm deformity is heterogeneous in appearance and etiology and may be secondary to spasticity of multiple muscles. If flexion of the interphalangeal (IP) joint of the thumb is present, then an injection of the flexor pollicis longus with botulinum toxin is performed. When the thumb metacarpal is severely adducted, chemodenervation of the thenar muscles and adductor pollicis is done.

Casting or splinting may be needed after the block if a contracture is present. Active and passive range-of-motion exercises are performed. Functional training is performed when any motor control is present in the upper extremity.

Evaluation of Residual Limb Deformities

Assessment of Cognition and Communication

At the conclusion of the period of physiologic recovery, the patient is evaluated for surgical procedures that have the potential to rebalance muscle function and correct deformity. Upper extremity function requires complex and highly sophisticated mechanisms working together in unison. Improving upper extremity function requires careful systematic evaluation before surgery. The goals of surgery must be practical and clearly understood by the patient and the family. Assessment includes an evaluation of cognition and communication skills.[70,139] The patient must be capable of following simple commands and should also be able to cooperate with a postoperative therapy program. In addition, the patient should have sufficient cognition to incorporate the improved motor function into their use of the extremity. Adequate memory is needed to retain what is taught during the postoperative therapy.

Sensory Evaluation

Intact sensation is essential to functional use of the hand.[70,71,139] The basic modalities of pain, light touch, and temperature must be present. Two-point discrimination is a valuable predictive test. A patient will rarely use the hand for functional activities if the discrimination is greater than 10 mm. Proprioception and kinesthetic awareness of the limb in space are important. Kinesthetic awareness is tested in a hemiplegic individual by placing the spastic limb in a position and asking the patient to duplicate this position with the sound limb while keeping the eyes closed. Stereognosis is not a practical test in spastic patients.

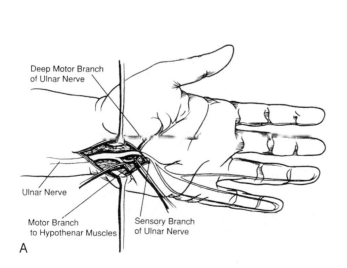

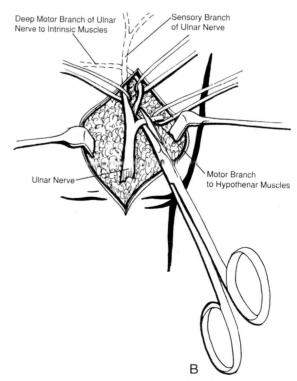

FIGURE 35-5. A and **B,** Isolation of the motor branches of the ulnar nerve distal to Guyon's canal. (From Keenan MA, Kozin SH, Berlet AC: Manual of Orthopaedic Surgery for Spasticity. New York, Raven Press, 1993.)

Affected patients lack the fine motor control necessary to manipulate an object in the hand.

It is helpful to observe the patient's spontaneous use of the hand. A patient with impaired sensation will often use a hand on request, by relying on visual feedback. The patient, however, may not use the extremity in activities of daily living even as a functional assist. Visual perceptual deficits add increased problems involving motion of the limb and even awareness of the limb itself.

Evaluation of Limb Deformity and Potential Functional Capability

Diffuse axonal injury, multifocal vascular pathology, and diffuse hypoxic encephalopathy lead to a wide variety of motor dysfunction. Lesions affecting the corticospinal system, the cerebellum, and the extrapyramidal system are common in head-injured patients. In a study of residual motor system involvement 10 years after head injury, Evans found hemiparesis to be the most common residual, but many patients had a brain stem syndrome consisting of ipsilateral ataxia and contralateral spastic hemiparesis. A small percentage had a pseudobulbar athetoid type of picture.[33] The literature also identifies patients with residuals of bilateral hemiparesis, patients with relatively "pure" ataxia involving both sides of the body, as well as patients with severe dystonic forms such as decerebrate posturing or rigidity. Many patients, especially during the early recovery stage from head injury, have mixed signs such as spasticity combined with tremor and ataxia. Hemiballismus has been reported after head injury, although frank parkinsonism is said to be rare. Concurrent peripheral neuropathy is not uncommon after head injury, and focal dystonia, although unusual, is also seen. Because so many different aspects of the motor control system may be affected by head injury, I have compiled a way of organizing the somewhat unwieldy array of clinical signs and symptoms that emerge from a damaged nervous system. The perspective taken is a functional one, taking into account the impact of restricted or excessive movement disorders on the patient's ability to function.

Treatment of spasticity is most effective when functional problems are formulated and described in focal rather than diffuse terms. Treatment of focal problems lends itself well to surgical intervention to target particular muscles. Surgical lengthening or release and tendon transfer of targeted muscles can provide very effective solutions to problems of function that are clearly identified from the outset. Identifying the specific offending muscles is critically important to localized strategies of intervention. For example, if the clinical problem is an adducted shoulder that hinders access to the axilla for purposes of bathing and deodorant application, blocking the pectoralis major or surgically releasing it will not solve the problem if teres major and latissimus dorsi are responsible for the problem.

In a neurologically impaired patient it may be difficult to distinguish between the many potential causes of limited joint motion. The possibilities include increase muscle tone, a myostatic contracture, the presence of periarticular heterotopic ossification, an undetected fracture or dislocation, joint subluxation, pain, or diminished cognition and cooperation on the part of the patient.

Clinical Evaluation of Motor Control

In broad terms, evaluation of spasticity focuses on identification of three factors: (1) the clinical pattern of motor dysfunction, (2) the patient's ability to control muscles involved in the clinical pattern, and (3) the role of muscle stiffness and contracture in relation to the functional problem. For purposes of convenience, 13 clinical patterns of motor dysfunction are most commonly seen, organized by joint or limb segment, and typically found in patients with traumatic brain injury and upper motor neuron lesions.[108] Six of these apply to the upper extremity (Table 35-7). Other variations of motor dysfunction occur but are less common. Various muscles may contribute to motor dysfunction across joints and limb segments in these clinical patterns. The evaluation focuses on the following characteristics: (1) voluntary or selective control, (2) spastic reactivity, (3) rheologic stiffness, and (4) contracture. Does the patient have voluntary control over a given muscle? Is the muscle spastic to passive stretch? Is the muscle, as an antagonist, activated during active movement generated by an agonist? Does the muscle have increased stiffness when stretched? Does the muscle have fixed shortening (contracture)? When many muscles cross a joint, the characteristics of each muscle may vary. Because each muscle may contribute to movement of the joint, information about each muscle's contribution is useful to the assessment as a whole.[107]

Spasticity often masks underlying motor control. In the upper extremity the most common pattern of spasticity is one of flexion. Passive range of motion of each joint should be established first. This is tested by slow extension of the joint to avoid the velocity-sensitive response of the muscle spindle. When spasticity is significant and passive motion is incomplete, it is necessary and advisable to perform a nerve block to assess whether a concomitant myostatic contracture is present.[44,70] Blocks can be easily performed without the use of special devices. By temporarily eliminating pain and muscle tone, patient cooperation is gained and the amount of myostatic contracture can be determined. Using local anesthetic blocks the strength and motor control of the antagonistic muscle group can also be evaluated (Fig. 35-6). To evaluate passive motion in the entire upper extremity, a brachial plexus block using a local anesthetic can be performed.

Table 35-7

COMMON CLINICAL PATTERNS OF MOTOR DYSFUNCTION IN THE UPPER EXTREMITY

Adducted/internally rotated shoulder
Flexed elbow
Pronated forearm
Flexed wrist
Clenched fist
Thumb-in-palm

From Mayer NH, Esquenazi A, Keenan MAE: Analysis and management of spasticity, contracture, and impaired motor control. *In* Horn LK, Zasler ND (eds): Rehabilitation of Traumatic Brain Injury, 3rd ed. Philadelphia, Hanley & Belfus, 1996, pp 411-458.

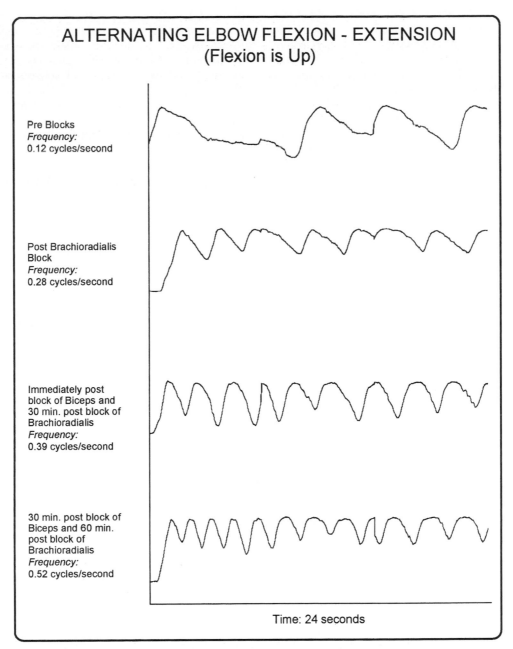

FIGURE 35-6. This series of tracings records the maximum frequency of flexion-extension movement in a patient with upper motor neuron lesions secondary to traumatic brain injury. The first tracing is maximal effort before placement of a block. The second tracing shows improvement after motor point block of the brachioradialis. Further improvement is noted immediately after bupivacaine (Marcaine) block of the biceps and 30 minutes after block of the brachioradialis. After the biceps block has been allowed to set up, further improvement is noted. This is an example of spasticity of antagonist muscles masking underlying motor control.

Unmasking of primitive patterning reflexes further contributes to the motor impairment. Spasticity (hyperactive response to quick stretch), rigidity (resistance to slow movement), or movement dystonias may be present. The degree of spasticity within selected muscles can be graded clinically in response to a quick stretch as mild, moderate, or severe. There is surprising consistency between observers using this simple grading system.[16] Another method of quantifying muscle tone is to measure the amount of intramuscular pressure generated by a passive quick stretch or during functional use of the limb. Intramuscular pressure can be measured using a wick or slit catheter technique. The pressure generated within the muscle is proportional to the force of contraction.[4]

As reviewed earlier, the degree of volitional motor control should be graded in the extremity using a clinical scale (see Table 35-2). Only patients with grades 5 or 6 are considered to have functional volitional motor control.

Laboratory Assessment of Motor Control

Given the degree of clinical effort, patient morbidity and procedural costs involved in treating complicated movement dysfunction in patients with cardiovascular accident and traumatic brain injury, clinical examination alone is not sufficient to answer questions of selective voluntary control and synergy with a high degree of confidence. Laboratory assessments may include formal gait and motion analysis and dynamic EMG studies. Dynamic multi-channel EMG can be acquired with simultaneous measurements of joint motion (kinematics) in the upper and lower extremities and with ground reaction forces (kinetics) obtained from force plate measurements in the lower extremities. Kinetic, kinematic, and dynamic EMG data can assist the clinician in interpreting whether voluntary function (effort-related initiation, modulation, and termination of activity) is present in a given muscle and whether that muscle's behavior is also dyssynergic (sometimes referred to as "out of phase" behavior). Combined with clinical information, laboratory measurements of muscle function often provide the degree of detail and confidence necessary for making surgical treatment decisions.

My colleagues and I reviewed the findings in several previous studies of spastic patients from our institution and devised the following classification of EMG activity to standardize terminology for either the upper or lower extremity (Table 35-8).[77] Class I constitutes a normal phasic pattern with appropriate on and off EMG activity. Class II consists of EMG activity that, although phasic, begins prematurely and continues for a short period beyond the normal duration of activity for that muscle. This is more commonly seen in the lower extremity. Class III consists of phasic activity with prolongation beyond the normal timing of the muscle. Class III activity can be further subdivided into three patterns depending on the degree of prolongation. Class IIIA consists of phasic activity with a short period of low-intensity EMG activity extending into the next phase of the flexion-extension cycle and is secondary to mild spasticity. Class IIIB consists of phasic activity with prolongation extending for at least half of the next phase of motion. This is indicative of a moderate amount of spasticity. Class IIIC consists of phasic activity with severe prolongation in which EMG activity is continued throughout the next phase of motion at a high intensity but the underlying phasic nature of the muscle activity is still distinguishable. This is representative of severe spasticity. Class IV consists of

continuous EMG activity without phasic variations. Class V consists of EMG activity seen only in response to a quick stretch by the antagonist muscles. There is no volitional activation of the muscle. This pattern is commonly seen in the finger extensors.[81] Class VI consists of absent EMG activity.

The next section illustrates how to apply strategies of focal evaluation and localized treatment, using a joint-by-joint approach in spastic patients with familiar patterns of upper motor neuron dysfunction.

Management of Common Upper Extremity Deformities

General Considerations

The patterns of limb spasticity seen after stroke and traumatic brain injury are very similar. Therefore, the same procedures can be used in both patient populations and are described together. However, these procedures are not applied equally to both patient groups. The degree of spasticity, the timing of neurologic recovery, and the pattern of spontaneous neurologic recovery are different between stroke and brain-injured patients. These differences account for the variation in the need for specific treatments between the two groups.

Patients who have had traumatic brain injury or stroke present unique challenges to the surgical team. The patients may have behavioral deficits or cognitive limitations that would make them difficult to manage with regional anesthesia and sedation. Therefore, general anesthesia is preferred. Brain-injured patients have often previously had a tracheostomy; therefore an anesthesia team familiar with airway difficulties is important. Great care must be taken when positioning these patients for long procedures because joint contractures may increase the risk of pressure ulcer formation.

Multiple contractures often exist on one or both upper extremities. To avoid exposing the patient to multiple anesthetics, my colleagues and I prefer to perform multiple and even bilateral procedures at one sitting. A typical patient with a nonfunctional arm, elbow flexion contracture, wrist flexion contracture, and finger flexion contractures might have biceps release, brachialis release, brachioradialis release, superficialis-to-profundus transfer, flexor carpi radialis release, flexor carpi ulnaris release, proximal row carpectomy, and wrist fusion performed at one sitting.

Several techniques are used to avoid wound complications in this patient group. Routine perioperative antibiotic administration with a first-generation intravenous cephalosporin is administered within 1 hour of skin incision and before tourniquet inflation. The antibiotics are continued for 24 hours. Dead spaces created by releases of muscles, particularly in the shoulder and elbow, are drained using a closed suction system. Because this patient group can be intolerant of suture removal, skin closure is ideally performed using absorbable suture.

Fracture Malunion

Fracture malunions are common in the patient with traumatic brain injury and have a multifactorial etiology. The complexity of fractures associated with the initial trauma that caused brain injury may be an inherent risk

Table 35-8

CLASSIFICATION OF DYNAMIC ELECTROMYOGRAPHIC ACTIVITY

Class I	Normal phasic activity
Class II	Premature prolonged activity
Class III	Phasic prolonged activity
IIIA	Mild prolongation activity
IIIB	Moderate prolongation activity
IIIC	Severe prolongation activity
Class IV	Continuous activity
Class V	Stretch response activity
Class VI	Absent activity

From Keenan MAE, Haider T, Stone LR: Dynamic electromyography to assess elbow spasticity. J Hand Surg [Am] 15:607-614, 1990.

factor for malunion. Injuries may also be missed in the initial resuscitation and progress to malunion or nonunion. The prognosis of the brain injury may be so poor that optimal internal fixation of fractures is not initially prioritized. Hemodynamic or pulmonary instability may cause optimal fracture fixation to be delayed or abandoned. Finally, poor patient compliance, agitation, and spasticity may alter the initial reduction. Specific treatment of malunited fractures are discussed in the individual sections that follow.

Heterotopic Ossification

Results of resection of heterotopic ossification are better in patients who have higher cognitive function and the ability to volitionally move the involved extremity. Radiographically immature lesions have a higher rate of recurrence. It may not be feasible or desirable to allow the heterotopic ossification to reach maturity before resection, because while the risk of recurrence is higher, ankylosis of the joint and subsequent contracture worsen the overall functional result. Heterotopic ossification may be detected in its earliest stage of formation with a bone scan.

SHOULDER

The paretic shoulder deserves special attention because it is a common source of pain. A variety of different factors contribute to the painful, immobile shoulder: acute trauma, including rotator cuff injuries and fractures or dislocations; fracture malunion; heterotopic ossification; complex regional pain syndrome; brachial plexitis; inferior subluxation; spasticity with adduction; internal rotation contracture; adhesive capsulitis; and spastic abduction.

Trauma

Shoulder girdle injuries (scapula, clavicle, and acromioclavicular joint) are the most common upper extremity injuries in traumatic brain injury. Most commonly these injuries can be treated nonoperatively; however, patient agitation and muscle spasticity may necessitate open reduction and internal fixation. A malunion of the proximal humerus may result from inadequate closed reduction or failed internal fixation and is difficult to treat because of scar formation, heterotopic ossification, and retraction of the tuberosities. Treatment must include open reduction of the greater tuberosity to prevent subacromial impingement. In three- and four-part fracture malunions, prosthetic replacement is generally indicated (see Fig. 35-3). In a three-part malunion without avascular necrosis of the head, osteotomy and internal fixation may be considered.

Heterotopic Ossification

Heterotopic ossification about the shoulder most commonly appears inferior and medial to the joint on plane radiographs. Computed tomography may be helpful to localize abnormal bone. For resection of anterior heterotopic ossification, a standard deltopectoral incision is used. Release or lengthening of contracted internal rotators can be performed at the same time, without entering the joint capsule. Release

of the pectoralis major may produce a cosmetically unappealing wound contour, but its release is necessary if there is a severe internal rotation and adduction deformity. The wound is closed in layers over a drain. When the heterotopic ossification is located posterior to the joint, a posterior approach is used. Heterotopic ossification commonly forms within or along the teres muscles, and great care must be taken to identify the axillary nerve in normal tissue proximal and distal to the affected area. The nerve is commonly encased within the mass of heterotopic bone and is at risk for injury. After resection for heterotopic ossification, range-of-motion exercises are begun immediately, even if the internal rotators have been released.

Adhesive Capsulitis

Adhesive capsulitis can occur in patients after stroke or brain injury and in those with complex regional pain syndrome. These patients have a characteristically painful shoulder with limited glenohumeral motion. Adhesive capsulitis has three defined clinical stages: the painful stage, the adhesive stage, and the recovery stage. Four arthroscopic stages have been identified (Table 35-9).[57] Stage I consists of a patchy fibrinous synovitis. Capsular contraction, fibrinous adhesions, and synovitis are seen in stage II. Increased contraction and resolving synovitis are characteristic of stage III. Severe contraction is seen in stage IV. The treatment in brain-injured patients is similar to that for the general population: nonsteroidal anti-inflammatory drugs, physical therapy, and intra-articular injections represent the mainstay of treatment. Selected cases may benefit from manipulation under anesthesia.

Arthroscopic capsular release may be performed for adhesive capsulitis that has not responded adequately to nonoperative treatment. Capsular release is performed via a three-portal technique, with a standard anterior port and two posterior ports, one just above and one just below the posterior soft spot. After diagnostic arthroscopy, the posterior superior capsule is released using a straight punch through

Table 35-9
STAGES OF ADHESIVE CAPSULITIS

Stage	Characteristic
Clinical	
Painful	Gradual onset of diffuse pain
Stiff	Decreased range of motion; affects activities of daily living
Thawing	Gradual return of motion
Arthroscopic	
1	Patchy fibrinous synovitis
2	Capsular contraction, fibrinous adhesions, synovitis
3	Increased contraction, resolving synovitis
4	Severe contraction

Data from Harryman DR II: Shoulders: frozen and stiff. Instr Course Lect 42:247-257, 1993; and Mornaghan JP: Frozen shoulder. *In* Rockwood CA Jr, Matsen FA III (eds): The Shoulder. Philadelphia, WB Saunders, 1990, p 837.

the posterior superior portal with visualization by the arthroscope through the anterior portal. The posterior inferior port is established; and with the arthroscope in the superior port, a straight punch is used through the inferior port to release the inferior capsule. Care must be taken to bluntly dissect the inferior capsule away from the underlying tissue to avoid injury to the axillary nerve. Range-of-motion exercises are begun immediately and may be facilitated by a long-acting interscalene block.

Inferior Subluxation

Inferior subluxation of the shoulder is a common occurrence in patients with flaccid paralysis of the shoulder girdle. This subluxation is usually self-limiting but, occasionally, chronic shoulder subluxation is painful. Affected patients typically have little or no use of the involved extremity. They complain of greater pain when sitting or standing if the arm is not supported. Typically, the symptoms are not relieved by either subacromial or intra-articular injections of local anesthetics. The pain may be due to chronic stretch on the shoulder capsule or trapezius muscle or traction on the brachial plexus. When the pain is alleviated by manually reducing the subluxation, treatment should be aimed at reduction of the joint.

On physical examination, patients demonstrate a positive sulcus sign with little to no active motion of the involved shoulder. There is a prominence of the acromion and atrophy of the deltoid. There may be contracture of the shoulder in adduction and internal rotation. Radiographs show inferior subluxation of the humerus on the glenoid (Fig. 35-7). Brachial plexopathy must be ruled out by using diagnostic EMG.

Conservative treatment may include electrical stimulation of the deltoid and supraspinatus muscles if the con-

dition is believed to be transient, but commonly and pragmatically the arm is placed in a sling. This relieves the symptoms by elevating the humeral head in the glenoid. While usually successful in the short run, this is frequently unacceptable to the patient as a permanent solution.

Several procedures have been described to treat paralytic inferior subluxation of the shoulder, but none has gained widespread acceptance. Braun has advocated using the coracoacromial ligament to suspend the humeral head. The lateral portion of the coracoid process together with the coracoacromial ligament is detached and transferred to the humeral head, where it is fixed using a cancellous lag screw. Garland described detaching the proximal end of the long head of the biceps tendon and looping the tendon over the clavicle and securing it back on itself. With time the paretic biceps muscle tends to stretch and the humerus once again subluxates inferiorly. Shoulder arthrodesis has also been performed but is not well accepted by the patient because it produces a rigid joint that interferes with passive positioning, hygiene, and nursing care.

Technique of Coracoacromial Ligament Suspension

The patient is placed in the supine position with a small bolster under the scapula. The arm is then prepped and draped so that the entire arm and shoulder are accessible. A 7-cm incision is made over the deltopectoral interval. The cephalic vein is dissected and preserved. The deltopectoral interval is opened; and if the pectoralis major is contracted, it is released using electrocautery. The clavipectoral fascia is opened, and the conjoint tendon is retracted medially and the deltoid is retracted laterally. If the subscapularis is contracted, it is released superficial to the capsule. The lateral portion of the coracoid process together with the coracoacromial ligament is then predrilled and detached, taking care not to detach the conjoint tendon. The bone plug,

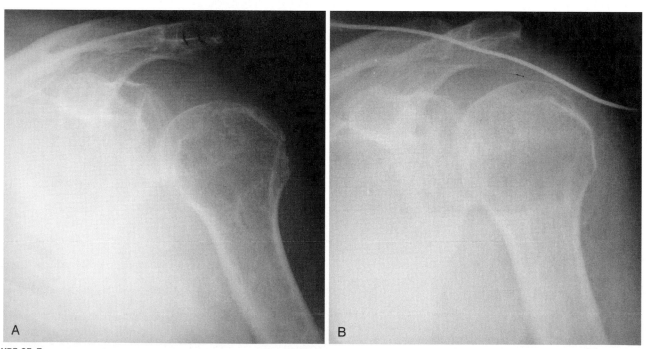

FIGURE 35-7. Anteroposterior radiographs of the shoulder in a patient with painful inferior subluxation before (**A**) and after (**B**) biceps suspension. Note inferior subluxation of the humerus preoperatively with reduction postoperatively.

together with the coracoacromial ligament, is then swung down to the humeral head and fixed to the head of the humerus using a cancellous lag screw. After fixation, the safe zone for passive shoulder range of motion is assessed to avoid tension on the transposed ligaments. Postoperatively, the patient is limited to this range of motion while participating in both activities of daily living and physical therapy.

Author's Preferred Method: The Biceps Suspension Procedure

My preferred procedure is to convert the long head biceps tendon to a proximally based suspensory ligament. This preserves passive shoulder motion while correcting the subluxation. Because only the tendon is used, there is no opportunity for paretic muscle to develop laxity and for the deformity to recur.

The patient is placed in the beach chair position with a small bolster under the scapula. A standard deltopectoral approach is made. If the pectoralis major is causing an adduction/internal rotation deformity, it is released from its insertion on the humerus. The musculotendinous region where the tendon of the long head of the biceps joins the muscle belly is identified. Care should be taken to preserve the musculocutaneous nerve as it enters the medial aspect of

the muscle. The long head of the biceps should be detached at the musculotendinous junction in an effort to obtain the greatest length of tendon. The remaining portion of the long head of the biceps is attached side-to-side to the conjoint tendon medially to preserve elbow flexion and supination strength. The proximal portion of the long head of biceps tendon is then dissected in the biceps groove and rotator interval. If necessary, the subscapularis may be released from its insertion at this time.

Two drill holes are made in the humerus, one on either end of the biceps groove, and then connected using an angled curet to create a tunnel running posterior and parallel to the biceps groove. It is important to direct the biceps tendon in the same direction as the groove. This ensures that the biceps tendon pulls the humeral head proximally and medially during final tensioning of the graft and reduction of the glenohumeral joint (Fig. 35-8). A braided, nonabsorbable traction suture is then placed in the distal portion of the biceps tendon. A wire loop is used to pass the tendon from proximal to distal through the tunnel. The arm is then positioned with the humeral head reduced in the glenoid and the arm in 30 degrees of internal rotation. The suture is then used to attach the distal tendon back to the proximal tendon, thus creating a suspensory loop of biceps tendon. The repair is protected in a sling for 3 months to allow bone-to-tendon healing.

Spastic Abduction

Overactivity of the supraspinatus muscle can cause spastic abduction posturing. The contracture may be fixed but is

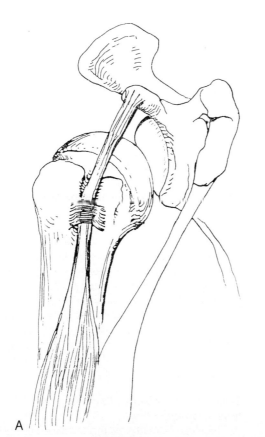

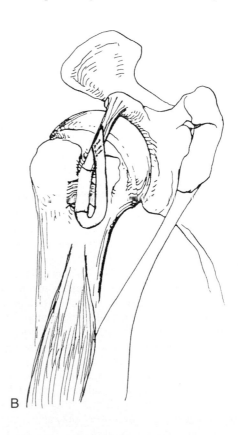

FIGURE 35-8. **A** and **B**, Schematic representation of biceps sling procedure.

more often dynamic and becomes more prominent with ambulation, transfers, or other attempted activities. The affected arm is held in an abducted posture, which causes balance to be impaired while ambulating. Patients complain of bumping into furniture, doorways, and people in crowds. Diagnosis requires examination of the patient at rest and during a variety of activities. It is also helpful to elicit from caretakers or family members any history of activities that trigger this posture. Dynamic EMG confirms that spasticity of the supraspinatus muscle is causing the deformity.

Technique of the Supraspinatus Slide

It is possible to effectively lengthen the supraspinatus and correct a spastic abduction deformity by means of a muscle slide. The patient is placed in the lateral decubitus position with the affected extremity uppermost. An axillary roll is placed in the unaffected axilla to protect the brachial plexus, and all bony prominences are well padded. A 10- to 15-cm incision is made overlying the scapular spine. The trapezius insertion is detached from the spine of the scapula, leaving a cuff of fascia for later reattachment. With a small periosteal elevator, the origin of the supraspinatus is elevated subperiosteally from the medial border of the scapula. The dissection is continued laterally, with care being taken to avoid injury to the neurovascular pedicle at the suprascapular notch. The muscle is allowed to slide laterally. The trapezius is then reattached to the scapular spine. The remainder of the closure is performed in routine fashion. The patient is allowed full, unrestricted postoperative motion.

Spastic Adduction/Internal Rotation

The glenohumeral joint normally functions as a universal joint, enabling the hand to reach an almost spherical volume of locations in three-dimensional space. When patients attempt to reach forward, spastic adductors and internal rotators can severely restrict acquisition of targets in the environment and on the body. The arm is adducted tightly against the lateral chest wall, and shoulder internal rotation causes the forearm to lie against the abdomen. The patient's ability to stabilize, push, or apply force to an object is also compromised. The clinical question is whether the limited forward flexion and external rotation is a result of weakness of the shoulder muscles or the result of inappropriate activity of the shoulder extensor muscles during forward reach. If the limitation of forward reach is caused by restriction of movement by the posterior muscles, then these muscles can be selectively lengthened.

Muscles that often contribute to spastic adduction/internal rotation dysfunction of the shoulder include the latissimus dorsi, the teres major, and the clavicular and sternal heads of pectoralis major and subscapularis. One must also consider involvement of the latissimus dorsi, the teres major, and the long head of the triceps when hyperextension posturing of the shoulder is observed, especially during standing transfers and gait. Antagonistic activity in these muscles may be masking a patient's potential for active flexion. Diagnostic bupivacaine or lidocaine blocks to the thoracodorsal nerve and/or lower subscapular nerve may unmask that voluntary potential. When the pectoralis major is chronically spastic, the musculotendinous insertion

of pectoralis major is prominent and tight. However, the two heads of this muscle may be differentially spastic and EMG recordings from each or diagnostic lidocaine blocks to medial and lateral pectoral nerves may help to distinguish whether one or both heads are pathophysiologically active.

Phenol or botulinum toxin motor point blocks of the pectoralis major muscle are effective in reducing tone and improving shoulder abduction during the physiologic recovery phase. The blocks are placed using surface stimulator guidance. The onset of muscle relaxation with phenol occurs gradually over the first 24 hours and can be expected to last approximately 2 months, during which time an active therapy program can continue. Blocks can be repeated as needed during the period of time in which neurologic recovery can be expected to continue. In addition, blocks of the thoracodorsal nerve can also be performed.

From the perspective of passive function, goals such as skin care and axillary hygiene, spastic adductors, and internal rotators hinder efforts of caregivers to gain access to the axilla to provide needed care. Restricted motion may impair dressing, washing, and bathing and promote skin irritation and maceration. Passive manipulation of the shoulder during personal care may cause pain when motion and contact trigger spastic resistance in reactive muscles. In patients with shoulder contractures who do not have volitional control of their muscles, release of the pectoralis major, latissimus dorsi, subscapularis, and teres major muscles is usually required to relieve the contractural deformity. In patients who have retained volitional control of their shoulder musculature, selective lengthening of these muscles can be performed.

Technique of Shoulder Muscle Release

The patient is placed in a slight beach chair position with a small bolster under the scapula. The arm is then prepped and draped so that the entire arm and shoulder are accessible. An incision is made on the anterior shoulder beginning at the coracoid process and extending distally for approximately 7 cm. The tendinous insertion of the pectoralis major tendon is identified and released near its insertion with electrocautery (Fig. 35-9). The subscapularis is exposed and isolated from the shoulder capsule near its insertion on the humerus. Release of the subscapularis muscle is performed without violating the glenohumeral joint capsule. The joint capsule should not be opened because instability or intra-articular adhesions may result. The latissimus dorsi and teres major muscles are identified through the interval between the short head of the biceps and deltoid musculature. Release of these muscles can then be performed in a nonfunctional extremity (see Fig. 35-9C). A drain should be placed deep into the wound before closure. Postoperatively, an aggressive mobilization program is instituted after skin healing. Gentle range-of-motion exercises are employed to correct any remaining contracture. Careful positioning of the limb in abduction and external rotation is necessary for several months to prevent recurrence.

Technique of Selective Shoulder Muscle Lengthening

An incision is made on the anterior shoulder beginning at the coracoid process and extending distally in the deltopec-

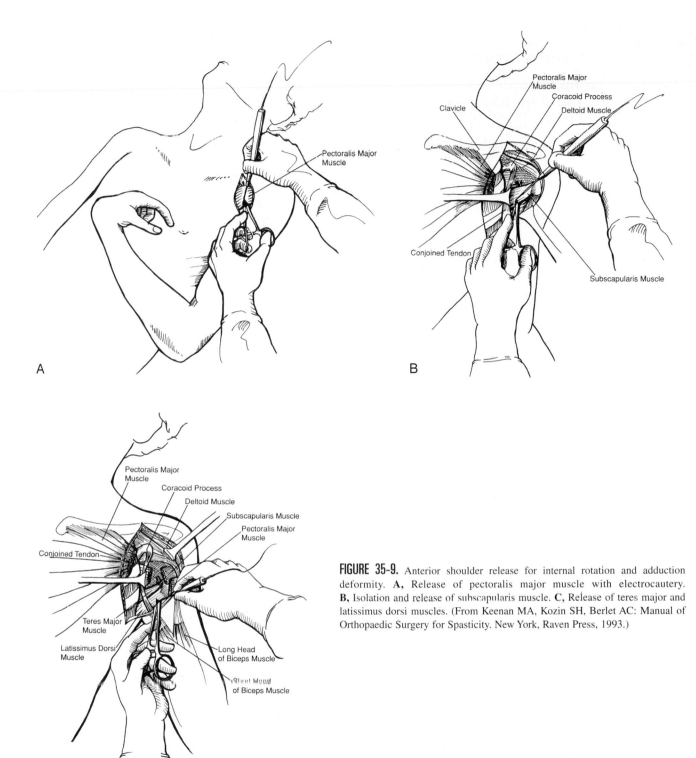

FIGURE 35-9. Anterior shoulder release for internal rotation and adduction deformity. **A,** Release of pectoralis major muscle with electrocautery. **B,** Isolation and release of subscapularis muscle. **C,** Release of teres major and latissimus dorsi muscles. (From Keenan MA, Kozin SH, Berlet AC: Manual of Orthopaedic Surgery for Spasticity. New York, Raven Press, 1993.)

toral groove for approximately 7 cm. The tendinous insertion of the pectoralis major tendon is identified. The pectoralis is lengthened by transecting the tendon where it overlaps with the muscle belly. This junction can be found on the undersurface of the muscle. The tendon must only be transected proximally to avoid complete rupture of the muscle-tendon unit. The amount of spasticity in the muscle ultimately determines the amount that the muscle-tendon

unit will lengthen. A new tendon forms within 3 weeks of the surgery. The latissimus dorsi and teres major muscles are identified through the interval between the short head of the biceps and deltoid musculature and lengthened at their musculotendinous junctions. When the long head of the triceps is dyssynergic, it is also lengthened. The long head of the triceps can be exposed and fractionally lengthened at the muscle-tendon junction on the proximal muscle belly through the same incision. Care must be taken to avoid injury to the brachial plexus. A narrow Deaver retractor can be used to retract the brachial plexus and axillary artery laterally.

After surgery the patient does not need immobilization. Therapy is started on the first postoperative day and consists of active and active-assisted movement of the shoulder. No passive stretching or resistive exercises are permitted until 3 weeks after surgery to avoid overlengthening or rupture of the lengthened muscles.

ELBOW

Trauma

Because of the risk of heterotopic ossification in patients with elbow fractures, stable internal fixation and early motion is recommended for unstable fractures. Heterotopic ossification forms in 90% of fractured or dislocated elbows in head-injured adults. It may form anterior or posterior to the joint (see Fig. 35-2). Because of this, prophylactic treatment with either diphosphonates (20 mg/kg/day) or radiation should be considered. When heterotopic ossification does form, ulnar nerve compression is frequent, particularly when the bone is located medial or posteromedial. Anterior heterotopic ossification occurs roughly one third as often as posterior heterotopic ossification, and posterolateral heterotopic ossification is most frequent. The decision regarding the appropriate approach is based on plain radiographs, computed tomography, location of previous incisions, and the need for nerve decompression. When in doubt, a universal posterior approach allows access to the entire elbow. (Specific approaches and treatment of the stiff elbow with heterotopic ossification are reviewed in detail in Chapter 25.)

Spastic Flexion

During the physiologic recovery phase of brain injury, control of elbow flexor spasticity requires the elimination or decrease of excessive tone in each of the flexor muscles. The brachioradialis muscle has been shown by dynamic EMG studies to be the most spastic of the elbow flexor muscles.[77] The tone may be decreased nonoperatively by chemodenervation of the brachioradialis muscle using botulinum toxin. Spasticity of the biceps and brachialis muscles also interferes with elbow extension, and injection of these muscles with botulinum toxin is also helpful. Active and passive range of motion of the elbow is begun immediately after the blocks. Every attempt is made to incorporate functional activities of the upper extremity into the therapy program. Associated elbow contractures are treated with physical therapy, serial casting, or dynamic splints.

Upright posture favors hypertonia in the "antigravity" elbow flexors of the upper limb. Many patients complain that their elbows persistently "ride up" when they stand up and walk. They also complain that their flexed elbow hooks door frames and other people and that putting on a shirt or jacket is a struggle. Contractures and spasticity impair a patient's ability to reach for objects in the environment or to place them elsewhere or bring them to the body. When neurologic recovery has plateaued, surgical correction of an elbow flexion deformity is performed.

The usual clinical picture is one of cogwheel motion on attempted extension of the elbow. Elbow flexion is relatively normal. Laboratory examination utilizing dynamic EMG helps to confirm the presence of volitional capacity as well as dyssynergy during movement for each of the elbow flexors. Dynamic recordings are obtained from biceps, brachialis, brachioradialis, and lateral, medial, and long head of the triceps. The pattern most commonly seen is that all three heads of the triceps muscle are operating in a normal phasic pattern. The brachioradialis muscle most frequently shows continuous spastic activity. One or both heads of the biceps muscle are also spastic. Less spasticity is observed in the brachialis muscle. Armed with this information a rational surgical plan can be devised to improve elbow control.

Techniques of Selective Elbow Flexor Lengthening

Two different techniques can be used to lengthen the elbow flexors in patients with active function. The technique used is dependent on the amount of static contracture present. When the deformity is primarily dynamic, the biceps can be lengthened at its proximal musculotendinous junction. This allows for immediate mobilization of the elbow. If the static component of the deformity is significant, a "Z"-plasty of the distal biceps tendon is needed. When a "Z" lengthening is performed, the elbow should be immobilized for 4 weeks to avoid rupture.

The Elbow With a Predominantly Dynamic Deformity

Beginning with the biceps, a longitudinal incision is made over the proximal anterior arm starting at the lower edge of the pectoralis major tendon. The muscle-tendon junctions of both the long and short heads of the biceps are exposed. The tendons are sharply transected directly overlying the muscle belly, which allows the muscle-tendon unit to lengthen. Next an incision is made on the lateral aspect of the elbow. The radial nerve is identified and protected in the interval between the brachialis and brachioradialis, and the brachialis muscle is exposed and lengthened over its broad muscle-tendon junction. Through a separate 3-cm longitudinal incision on the dorsoradial aspect of the middle third of the forearm, the distal myotendinous junction of the brachioradialis is identified. The muscle is rolled, exposing its deep surface. The radial nerve is carefully protected, and the tendinous fibers are transected sharply, allowing the brachioradialis to lengthen.

When the muscles have been lengthened with this method, no immobilization is needed. Active range-of-motion exercises are started on the first day after surgery. No resistive exercises are allowed for 3 weeks to prevent overlengthening of the muscles and resultant weakness. Functional elbow flexor lengthening will significantly enhance the fluid control of elbow motion and improve hand placement in properly selected patients.

The Elbow With a Significant Static Deformity

Under tourniquet control a curved incision is made on the volar aspect of the elbow beginning laterally over the origin

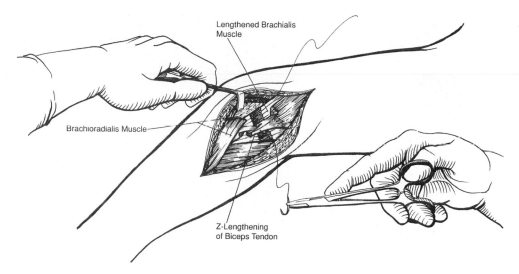

FIGURE 35-10. "Z"-plasty of biceps tendon and fractional lengthening of the brachialis is demonstrated. Also note that the brachioradialis has been released proximally. In a patient with a functional extremity, the biceps is lengthened at the musculotendinous junction and the brachialis is fractionally lengthened through a separate distal incision. (From Keenan MA, Kozin SH, Berlet AC: Manual of Orthopaedic Surgery for Spasticity. New York, Raven Press, 1993.)

of the brachioradialis muscle. The incision passes lateral to the antecubital crease and gently curves anteriorly to the anterolateral aspect of the forearm. Dissection develops the inter-nervous interval between the brachioradialis and the biceps musculature. The radial nerve is identified and protected. If the brachioradialis has been demonstrated by dynamic EMG to be spastic and without any functional capacity, it is transected through its muscle belly proximally using electrocautery. If the brachioradialis has volitional control, then it is lengthened at its distal myotendinous junction through a separate incision on the dorsoradial aspect of the mid forearm.

The lacertus fibrosus is divided and the entire length of the biceps tendon exposed. A "Z" cut is then made for the entire length of the biceps tendon. The biceps is retracted, and the underlying brachialis muscle is exposed. The broad band of tendinous fibers on the anterior surface of the brachialis muscle is sharply transected, leaving the underlying muscle tissue intact. The elbow is then extended, fractionally lengthening the brachialis by approximately 1 cm (Fig. 35-10). The ends of the biceps tendon are then sutured in a lengthened position using a nonabsorbable suture. The subcutaneous tissues and skin edges are closed over a drain.

If preoperative nerve conduction studies have shown an ulnar neuropathy at the level of the elbow, anterior transposition of the ulnar nerve is performed. The skin incision is closed over a suction drain.

Postoperatively the patient is placed in a posterior splint with the elbow in 90 degrees of flexion. The drain is removed within the first 24 hours after surgery. The splint is maintained for 4 weeks, and then a program of active therapy is begun. Night splints are used for 3 additional weeks to protect the biceps tendon repair.

Technique of Elbow Release

In patients with no volitional control of the elbow, persistent spasticity of the elbow flexors causes a myostatic contracture and flexion deformity. This results in skin maceration and breakdown of the antecubital space. This position of severe elbow flexion also predisposes the ulnar nerve to a compression neuropathy.

Under tourniquet control a longitudinal incision is made on the lateral aspect of the elbow beginning over the origin of the brachioradialis muscle. A straight longitudinal incision is preferred to facilitate wound closure as the elbow is extended. Dissection develops the interval between the brachioradialis and the brachialis musculature. The radial nerve is identified and protected. The brachioradialis is detached at its origin using electrocautery. The biceps tendon and lacertus fibrosus are isolated and transected (Fig. 35-11). When the deformity is not severe, the brachialis muscle is lengthened at its myotendinous junction by transecting the tendinous fibers on the anterior surface of the muscle, leaving the underlying muscle intact. The remainder is left to counterbalance the triceps muscle. When the elbow flexion contracture is severe and chronic, it is necessary to completely transect the brachialis muscle using electrocautery. An anterior capsulectomy is usually not needed and should be avoided because of the associated increased stiffness and intra-articular adhesions postoperatively. In very severe contractures, it may be necessary to perform multiple "Z"-plasties of the antecubital skin. If preoperative nerve conduction studies have shown an ulnar neuropathy at the level of the elbow, anterior transposition of the ulnar nerve is performed. The subcutaneous tissues and skin edges are closed over a drain.

Approximately 50% correction of the deformity can be expected at surgery without causing excessive tension on the contracted neurovascular structures. Gradual extension of the elbow with serial casting or physical therapy corrects the residual deformity.

Spastic Extension

Spastic extension of the elbow is much less common than spastic flexion. These patients have frequently had a brain stem infarct or injury. They complain of difficulty reaching their face for activities of daily living. Experience with this is limited, but good results have been reported with surgical lengthening. A "V-Y" triceps plasty allows improved flexion range of motion, at the cost of decreased extension power and extensor lag. This procedure should be used with caution in patients who rely on their arms to assist with ambulation.

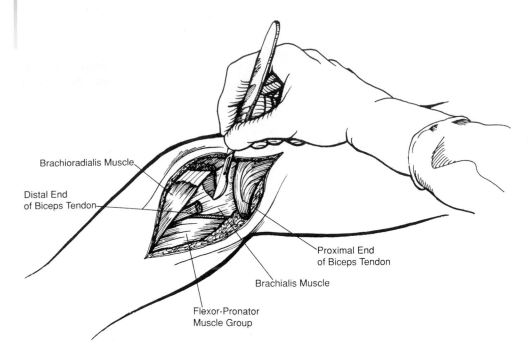

Brachioradialis Muscle

Distal End
of Biceps Tendon

Proximal End
of Biceps Tendon

Brachialis Muscle

Flexor-Pronator
Muscle Group

FIGURE 35-11. Release of the brachioradialis and biceps tendon as well as myotendinous lengthening of the brachialis. (From Keenan MA, Kozin SH, Berlet AC: Manual of Orthopaedic Surgery for Spasticity. New York, Raven Press, 1993.)

Ulnar Neuropathy

Ulnar neuropathy occurs in stroke and brain-injured patients for a number of reasons. Prolonged elbow flexion with traction on the nerve can lead to decreased volume of the cubital tunnel and result in nerve compression. Support of the torso by leaning on a chronically flexed elbow may result in direct compression of the nerve. Heterotopic ossification, particularly in a posterior location, may involve the ulnar nerve causing a neuropathy. The patients are often limited in their ability to complain about ulnar nerve symptoms because of limited cognitive and communicative abilities. The diagnosis is usually suspected because of intrinsic atrophy and confirmed using nerve conduction studies. A 2.5% incidence has been shown in patients with traumatic brain injury at a large brain injury referral center.[78,139]

Treatment is ulnar nerve transposition, often at the same time as elbow flexor lengthenings, flexor releases, or resection of heterotopic ossification. Subcutaneous transposition is preferred to avoid stimulation of heterotopic ossification formation.

FOREARM

Trauma

Nonoperative treatment of both-bones forearm fractures will give predictably unsatisfactory results due to loss of supination and pronation. Open reduction has been reported to result in a 31% incidence of interosseous membrane ossification in brain-injured patients.[41]

For this reason, separate incisions and minimal additional soft tissue dissection are important when performing open reduction and internal fixation of these fractures. The 3.5-mm dynamic compression plates have a lower incidence of synostosis than the 4.5-mm plates in the forearm. Bone grafting should be used only for comminuted fractures, with care to avoid a graft within the interosseous space. Prophylaxis for heterotopic ossification should be instituted unless contraindicated from a medical perspective.

Spasticity

Supination and pronation deformities are commonly associated with elbow spasticity, wrist spasticity, or both. Pronation deformity of the forearm in an upper motor neuron lesion is more common than supination deformity. Many activities of daily living depend on active supination. The use of feeding and grooming utensils and clothes fasteners becomes problematic when supination is restricted by spastic or contracted pronators. Physical examination reveals a fully pronated resting position of the forearm. When passive supination range of motion exceeds the range of active supination, the possibility of pronator muscle dyssynergy during active supination should be suspected. Muscles that potentially contribute include pronator teres and pronator quadratus. Dynamic EMG studies of the pronator teres, pronator quadratus, and biceps greatly augment clinical examination. Both pronator muscles may show varying degrees of volition and spasticity.

During the period of functional recovery, phenol or botulinum toxin may be injected into either or both pronators, depending on clinical and laboratory analyses. In the period of residual deficits, surgical lengthening of pronator teres and pronator quadratus may be performed depending on their individual voluntary capacities. The clinical goal is to improve active supination function by reducing pronator dyssynergy. The possibility of lengthening the pronator teres has long been recognized, but fractional lengthening of the pronator quadratus has been described only recently.[109]

I do not advocate the flexor-pronator slide because it does not target the individual muscles responsible for deformities. When an excessive amount of the pronator teres origin was released or when there was no function in the pronator quadratus muscle, an iatrogenic and less functional supination deformity occurred. When the pronators are contracted and not active volitionally, individual muscle releases may be considered.

Technique of Fractional Lengthening of the Forearm Pronators

The pronator teres is approached in the interval between the mobile wad and the flexor carpi radialis in the mid forearm. Care is taken to preserve the superficial radial nerve and radial artery within this interval. The pronator teres is then identified as it inserts on the radius. Myotendinous lengthening is then performed by cutting the tendinous fibers of the musculotendinous junction and allowing the tendon fibers to slide on the muscle belly, thereby lengthening the muscle-tendon unit. When dynamic EMG has demonstrated that the pronator is spastic but does not have any volitional activity, the pronator is released from its insertion on the radius.

The pronator quadratus is approached via an incision over the volar aspect of the forearm just proximal to the wrist crease. The finger flexor tendons are retracted radially to expose the broad myotendinous junction of the pronator quadratus. The tendon fibers are transected, leaving the underlying muscle fibers intact. The arm is then supinated, separating the ends of the tendon fibers and lengthening the pronator quadratus (Fig. 35-12). When the pronator quadratus is contracted and does not have any functional capacity, it is transected to eliminate it as a deforming force.

Spastic Supination

Spastic supination is a far less common deformity but is also associated with elbow flexion deformities. Supination deformity may be caused by the biceps, supinator, or both. Physical examination supplemented by dynamic EMG may be used to determine the relative contribution of each. Most commonly a supination deformity can be treated by re-routing the direction of pull of the biceps. On rare occasions, supinator release is needed.

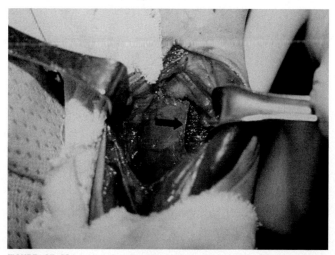

FIGURE 35-12. Intraoperative photograph showing pronator quadratus myotendinous lengthening. The arrow indicates the cut edge of the pronator quadratus tendon.

Technique of Biceps Re-routing

Correction of a supination contracture is done by re-routing the course of the biceps tendon distally around the radius to reposition the forearm in neutral rotation. A curved incision is made on the volar aspect of the elbow. The lacertus fibrosus is released, and the full length of the biceps tendon is exposed. A step cut is made in the biceps tendon as is done for a "Z"-plasty. The distal end of the tendon is then passed around the neck of the radius to rotate the forearm to a neutral rotation position. Care must be taken to avoid injury to the posterior interosseous nerve. The tendon is then repaired using nonabsorbable sutures. It is necessary to protect the repair with a long-arm cast for 6 weeks to allow the biceps tendon to fully heal.

CRITICAL POINTS: BICEPS RE-ROUTING

- Use a two-incision technique.
- Make a second incision on the posterolateral aspect of the elbow.
- Detach the muscles from the lateral surface of the olecranon and retract them laterally.
- Protect the posterior interosseous branch of the radial nerve as it enters the forearm within the substance of the supinator muscle.

Technique of Supinator Lengthening

The supinator is lengthened by elevating it off of its radial insertion. The approach used is a standard anterior approach to the elbow and proximal radius. The supinator is approached in the plane between the brachialis and the brachioradialis. The radial recurrent artery must be ligated to allow exposure of the supinator. The existing supination deformity facilitates exposure of the insertion of the supinator by pulling the posterior interosseus nerve laterally. Nevertheless, extreme care must be taken to visualize and preserve the nerve as it enters the arcade of Frohse. The broad insertion of the supinator is then incised through the periosteum, exposing the shaft of the radius. The supinator is then elevated in a subperiosteal plane. Care must be taken to avoid excessive traction on the posterior interosseus nerve when elevating the supinator. It is also important to understand that the posterior interosseus nerve comes into contact with the radius in 25% of patients. Once elevated, the supinator is allowed to slide. It will subsequently scar down in a lengthened position. The wound is then closed in routine fashion.

WRIST

A flexed wrist is common after traumatic brain injury, but hyperextension deformity may also be seen. Patients complain of difficulty inserting their hand into shirts, jackets, and other narrow openings, and they frequently have pain on passive motion. They may also have symptoms of carpal tunnel syndrome secondary to compression of the median nerve against the transverse carpal ligament by taut flexor tendons (see Fig. 35-4).[84,116] In severe cases, wrist subluxation may be present. Radial or ulnar deviation and a clenched fist are often present as well.

Spastic Flexion

Muscles that potentially contribute to wrist flexion include the flexor carpi radialis (FCR), flexor carpi ulnaris (FCU), palmaris longus (PL), flexor digitorum sublimis (FDS), and flexor digitorum profundus (FDP). Singly or in combination, these muscles may have variable features of spasticity, contracture, and voluntary control. Because they have a larger cross-sectional area, wrist flexor muscles are generally stronger than their extensor counterparts. Despite a net balance of forces favoring flexion, the extent to which a patient may have voluntary control over wrist extensors should be investigated. Dynamic EMG studies and temporary diagnostic motor point blocks are helpful in this regard.

Clinical examination begins by observing "resting" posture of the wrist. The FCR, FCU, or both may bowstring across the wrist, and radial or ulnar deviation suggests their respective involvement. A clenched fist points to extrinsic finger flexors as having a role. If fingernails dig into the palm, the FDP is likely to be involved. If the proximal interphalangeal (PIP) joint is markedly flexed but the distal interphalangeal (DIP) joint is not, involvement of the FDS is likely. Distinguishing between limitations attributable to wrist versus finger flexors is one aim of passive range-of-motion testing. By allowing the fingers to remain flexed in the palm, passive extension of the wrist provides information about wrist flexors. Spastic wrist flexors are strongly resistive to passive extension, range of motion is typically limited, and deviation of the wrist with bowstringing of the FCR or FCU is noted when these muscles are differentially spastic. When finger flexors are also tight, simultaneous passive stretch of the wrist and finger flexors restricts wrist motion more markedly.

Active range of motion of the wrist is similarly tested with the fist closed and the fist open. Observing even a small degree of wrist extension may be important because surgical interventions that alleviate muscle contracture and spasticity on the flexor side may unmask more voluntary extension on the extensor side. When a patient has more overt extension, it may be useful to observe the patient's effort performing repetitive flexion/extension movements of the wrist. Smoothness of motion, speed, effort, decrement in movement amplitude over time, and fatigue may be observed.

Laboratory examination of the flexed wrist deformity includes recordings from the FCR, FCU, extensor carpi radialis (ECR), extensor carpi ulnaris (ECU), FDS and FDP; and additional information is obtained during whole limb movements such as reaching, grasping, and releasing objects. Recordings made during passive stretch of the wrist flexors and finger flexors provide an indication of spastic reactivity. Dynamic EMG findings are not easily predictable from clinical examination. Some patients show extensive activation of wrist extensors during extension and reaching efforts. Nevertheless, the wrist remains flexed because tension in the wrist flexors and finger flexors overcomes extensor forces. Because EMG activity is not correlated with force production, diagnostic nerve blocks are often

helpful in unmasking volitional activity. Temporary chemical "weakening" of a dyssynergic wrist flexor may unmask strength in the wrist extensors sufficient to improve active wrist motion. Blocks are helpful to study the extrinsic finger flexors after dynamic EMG reveals whether the FDS and/or FDP are generating antagonistic activity during wrist extension. Motor point block of the target muscle group or median and/or ulnar nerve blocks at the elbow may be performed to examine for active wrist extension during reach. Combined median and ulnar nerve blocks at or above the elbow will also reveal the presence of muscle contracture.

Spastic forearm flexor muscles causing wrist and finger flexion deformities are treated during the physiologic recovery phase by chemodenervation with botulinum toxin or occasionally using phenol motor point blocks. Because of the large sensory components of both the median ulnar nerves, selective motor point injections of the wrist and finger flexors are performed using surface electrical stimulation for localization. Motor blocks can be supplemented with functional electrical stimulation of the wrist and finger extensor muscles and by casting or splinting techniques. Gentle passive range of motion of the wrist and fingers is performed. When motor control is present, a program of active exercise and functional training is also employed.

When a patient has underlying voluntary control, surgical options for flexed and hyperextended wrists may include myotendinous lengthenings. Selective muscle releases, wrist fusion, proximal row carpectomy, and superficialis-to-profundus tendon transfer may be considered when the goal is to improve passive function only.

When wrist flexion deformities are severe and there is little or no function seen in the hand, release of the wrist flexors is performed. A proximal row carpectomy may be necessary in some patients to correct a fixed deformity. The wrist is then fused to eliminate the need for a wrist orthosis after surgery (Fig. 35-13). Splints tend to be lost by these patients and their caretakers, and gravity alone can cause a recurrence of the flexion deformity. Because the median nerve is frequently compressed in severe deformities and causes a painful neuropathy, a carpal tunnel release is recommended.

Technique of Fractional Wrist Flexor Lengthening
In an extremity with documented volitional control, fractional lengthening of the appropriate wrist flexors is performed. This is done in conjunction with lengthening of the extrinsic finger flexors when indicated. A longitudinal incision is made on the volar surface of the forearm. This incision is extended distally if a carpal tunnel release is necessary. The PL tendon is divided if it is tight. A myotendinous lengthening is performed by transecting the tendinous portion overlying the myotendinous junction. No immobilization is used after surgery. The patient is begun on a program of active exercise immediately after surgery. No passive stretching of the wrist is allowed for 3 weeks. Resistive exercises can be started 6 weeks after surgery.

Technique of Wrist Flexor Release and Wrist Fusion
The patient is positioned supine, and an arm tourniquet is applied. A volar forearm incision is made extending to the transverse carpal ligament. The PL, FCR, and FCU tendons are identified and transected. Care is taken to protect the radial and ulnar artery as well as the median, radial, and

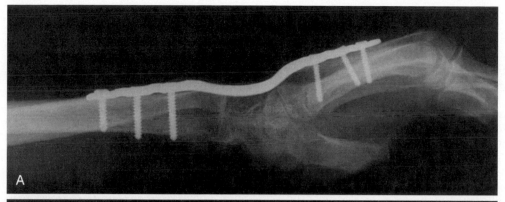

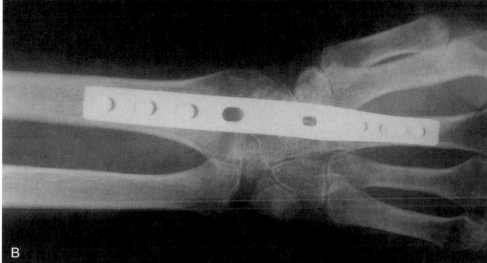

FIGURE 35-13. Postoperative antero-posterior (**A**) and lateral (**B**) radiographs showing the pre-bent titanium wrist fusion plate.

ulnar nerves. Carpal tunnel release is performed. The volar incision is closed in routine fashion.

If wrist fusion is to be performed, the forearm is then supinated and a longitudinal dorsal incision in made to expose the wrist. Lister's tubercle is removed. The capsule and ligaments are divided in line with the third metacarpal, and flaps are raised to expose the carpus. With the use of a high-speed bur the articular cartilage and the subchondral bone of the radiolunate, radioscaphoid, scaphocapitate, lunocapitate, and capitate/third metacarpal joints are removed. Exposure is facilitated by hyperflexing the wrist. The wrist is then positioned such that the wrist is in 15 degrees of extension with the third metacarpal in line with the shaft of the radius. If this position is achieved only with excessive tension on the volar tissues, proximal row carpectomy is performed. The denuded surfaces are then grafted with local autologous bone with or without allograft. The wrist is then stabilized using a pre-bent titanium wrist fusion plate fixed distally to the third metacarpal with 2.7-mm screws and proximally to the radius with 3.5-mm screws. Closure is then performed in a routine manner. The wrist is then placed in a well-padded splint or cast for 6 weeks.

Spastic Extension

Extension deformity of the wrist causes hygiene problems and may prevent release in patients with poor digital extension. Median nerve compression may also be caused by prolonged extension. If median nerve compression is diagnosed, carpal tunnel release is performed.

Technique of Wrist Extensor Lengthening

When volitional control has been demonstrated in the dyssynergic wrist extensors, myotendinous lengthening of the ECU is performed through a short longitudinal incision on the ulnar border of the forearm. The myotendinous junction is identified and the tendinous portion transected, allowing the muscle to stretch. The extensor carpi radialis longus and brevis (ECRL and ECRB) are then identified in a separate longitudinal incision on the radial side of the forearm. Again, the myotendinous junction is identified and the tendinous portion cut, allowing the muscle to lengthen. The incisions are closed in routine fashion. Active motion is begun immediately after surgery.

Technique of Wrist Extensor Release

When no volitional activity is seen in the wrist extensor muscle by clinical examination and dynamic EMG, tendon release with wrist fusion with or without proximal row carpectomy is performed. A midline dorsal incision is made. Dissection is carried out medially and laterally exposing the distal ECRL and ECRB and the distal ECU. These tendons are transected proximal to their insertions. Wrist fusion with or without proximal row carpectomy is performed as described earlier.

HAND

Trauma

Neglected or malunited fractures that occurred concomitantly with brain injury can cause pain and/or dysfunction and may require additional reconstructive treatment. Excessive dorsal angulation, particularly if in the proximal metacarpal, can cause a pseudo claw deformity secondary to relative weakness of the short intrinsic muscles. Grip can be painful, especially with malunions of the index and long metacarpals. Symptomatic patients can be treated with a dorsal closing wedge osteotomy and percutaneous or internal fixation. Rotationally misaligned fractures cause a gap or overlap between fingers and make manipulation of small objects more difficult, particularly in brain-injured patients. Rotational malunions can be corrected by rotational osteotomy and internal fixation.[125]

Spasticity

Preoperative evaluation will allow extremities to be grouped into one of two patterns: those with problems of active function and those with problems of passive function. The criteria for determining which procedures are most appropriate are summarized in Table 35-10. Once it is determined whether active function or passive function releases will be undertaken, specific patterns are identified.

Spastic Clenched Fist

The spastic clenched fist deformity is common in brain injury or stroke involving the upper extremity. This pattern results from unmasking of the primitive grasp reflex. The fingers are typically clasped into the palm. Fingernails may dig into palmar skin and access to the palm for washing may be compromised. When access is chronically restricted, skin maceration, breakdown and malodor occurs. Patients may complain of pain when they or their caregivers attempt to pry fingers open to gain palmar access. Some relaxation of finger tightness may occur if the wrist is positioned by the examiner in extreme flexion. The deformity, however, is often accompanied by wrist flexion as well.

The degree of motor control may be masked by the severe amount of tone present in the finger flexors or by the presence of some element of fixed contracture. Passive range of motion should be established first. Following this the patient is asked to open and close the fingers and to flex and extend the wrist. If no active wrist or finger extension is seen, it is still important to assess whether there appears to be active control of finger flexion. In the continuum of neurologic impairment and recovery, control of wrist and finger flexion is seen prior to active control of extension. A finger is placed in the patient's palm, and the patient is asked to grasp. Often an increase in the pressure of grasp can be felt, indicating underlying muscle control.

An anesthetic block of the median nerve can be performed in the antecubital space to temporarily eliminate flexor tone. A block of the ulnar nerve in the cubital canal can supplement relaxation. With the flexor muscles relaxed the activity of the extensor muscles can be more accurately evaluated.

Muscles that contribute to the clenched fist deformity include the FDS and FDP. If the PIP joints flex while the DIP joints remain extended, spasticity of the FDS rather than the FDP may be suspected. Dynamic EMG studies have shown that the FDS muscles often exhibit a marked degree of spasticity, whereas the FDP muscles may be normal or minimally spastic.[81] Despite the marked increase in tone, the FDS often has some underlying volitional control. Volitional control of the finger extensors is present in 50% of patients with spastic flexion deformities. The intrinsics may also be spastic along with the extrinsics, but an intrinsic-plus posture (i.e., combined MCP flexion and PIP extension) is not seen because spastic extrinsic flexors dominate by flexing the PIP joints. Some degree of contracture of the extrinsics is typical of the chronically clenched fist.

Table 35-10

CRITERIA FOR ACTIVE FUNCTION PROCEDURES VERSUS PASSIVE FUNCTION PROCEDURES

	Active Function	Passive Function
Cognition	Able to obey simple commands	Does not obey commands
	Able to cooperate with postoperative occupational therapy	Uncooperative with occupational therapy efforts
	Able to retain what is taught from one session to another	No retention of information from one session to the next
	Able to assimilate newly taught activities into activities of daily living	Unable to use what was taught in daily activities
Sensation	Intact pain, light touch, and temperature sensation	Absent pain, light touch, or temperature sensation
	Two-point discrimination less than 10 mm	Two-point discrimination greater than 10 mm
	Kinesthetic awareness	Unable to reproduce body positions
Spontaneous Use of the Extremity	Yes	No
Motor Control	Able to move affected extremity volitionally	No volitional movement of extremity
	Palpable movement in involved extremity	No movement palpable in involved extremity
	Electromyogram shows volitional control during manual muscle testing (class I, II, or III) (see Table 35-7)	Continuous, stretch response or absent electromyographic activity during manual muscle testing (class IV, V, or VI)

During the period of motor control/musculoskeletal recovery, focal chemodenervation is a useful intervention. It should also be pointed out that reduction of spasticity in the extrinsics may unmask spasticity in the intrinsics, potentially converting an extrinsic deformity into an intrinsic-plus deformity. Chemodenervation with botulinum toxin is an excellent remedy for treating spasticity of the intrinsics because these small muscles of the hand are readily accessible for injection and require only small amounts of toxin to be effective (see Fig. 35-5).

During the period of residual deficits/remediable function, a variety of treatment options are available. When volitional control is demonstrated in the extrinsic flexor muscles by dynamic EMG, fractional lengthening is indicated. In a hand with skin maceration and malodor from a clenched fist deformity in which no volitional movement is detected, more significant lengthening of the flexor tendons is required. In this situation a superficialis-to-profundus (STP) tendon transfer is performed.

Technique of Selective Fractional Lengthening of Extrinsic Finger Flexors

The surgery is performed through a longitudinal incision on the volar surface of the forearm, commonly at the same sitting with wrist flexor lengthenings (Fig. 35-14). The PL tendon is divided if tight. The lengthening of the individual FDS and FDP tendons is performed by sharply incising the tendon fibers as they overlie the muscle belly at the musculotendinous junction, allowing the tendon to slide distally. The flexor pollicis longus (FPL) tendon is lengthened in an identical manner. This technique allows the tendons to lengthen with minimal scarring. By transecting the tendon over the muscle belly, no sutures are needed. This eliminates scarring from foreign body reaction to suture material. The underlying support and vascularity of the muscle provide an optimal environment for the tendons to heal and reconstitute themselves (see Fig. 35-14). Lengthening of the pronator teres and pronator quadratus is done at this time, also as indicated by the dynamic EMG studies.

Postoperatively a volar wrist splint is applied to prevent hyperextension of the wrist and inadvertent overstretching of the finger flexor tendons. The fingers are not immobilized. The patient is begun on a program of active and active-assisted exercises on the first postoperative day. This immediate active motion allows the flexor tendons to continue to lengthen in the postoperative period as necessary. Ultimately, the amount of flexor lengthening is determined for each individual muscle by its underlying tone and control rather than by the surgeon's "educated guess" of tone while the patient is under anesthesia. Using this technique we have had marked improvement in functional results when compared with our previous regimen of postoperative immobilization.

Technique of Superficialis-to-Profundus Tendon Transfer

In a hand without volitional movement, a superficialis-to-profundus tendon transfer is performed (Fig. 35-15). This provides a more cosmetically pleasing hand position, aids in hygiene by getting the fingers out of the palms, and provides, at best, a mass action grasp pattern and, at least, a passive restraint to extension.

The superficialis-to-profundus tendon transfer is performed through a longitudinal volar incision that may be extended distally to allow release of the carpal tunnel and Guyon's canal. The PL tendon is identified and transected. The four superficialis tendons are sutured together distally using a nonabsorbable suture and then transected. The profundus tendons are sutured together proximally and then cut. The fingers are extended and the distal ends of the superficialis tendons are sutured en masse to the proximal end of the profundus tendons. By suturing the tendons together before transfer, the normal cascade of the hand is maintained.

Several other surgical procedures are routinely done in combination with the superficialis-to-profundus tendon transfer to treat concurrent deformities. A neurectomy of the motor branch of the ulnar nerve is needed to prevent an intrinsic-plus deformity.[82] If an intrinsic contracture is seen at the time of surgery after the superficialis-to-profundus lengthening, then release of the intrinsics is also performed. To prevent a recurrent wrist flexion deformity, fusion of the wrist in 15 degrees of extension provides the most reliable means of maintaining hand position and is now routinely performed. A proximal release of the thenar muscles may be needed to correct a thumb-in-palm deformity. Because the superficialis-to-profundus transfer and wrist fusion are extensive surgery, I prefer to perform the thenar slide procedure at a later time if indicated.

Postoperatively, the wrist and hand are immobilized for 2 weeks in a short-arm splint that includes the fingers and thumb. The wrist is held in 15 degrees of extension and the fingers are immobilized in extension. Gentle range of motion of the MCP joints is started after splint removal. A volar wrist splint is used until the wrist fusion is healed.

Spastic Thumb-in-Palm Deformity

The thumb-in-palm deformity is heterogeneous in appearance and may be secondary to spasticity of multiple muscles including the FPL muscle and the median- and ulnar-innervated thenar muscles.[10,72,101,128] The thumb is held within the palm, the DIP joint of the thumb is commonly flexed, and the thumb is unable to function during key grasp or in three-jaw chuck grasp (i.e., in opposition to the pads of the index and third fingers). In addition, skin maceration and breakdown can occur because proper hygiene is prevented.

Clinically, spasticity of the FPL is indicated by flexion of the IP joint. Some patients may be able to extend the thumb if the wrist is flexed, suggesting that a spastic FPL may be impeding active thumb extension when the wrist is more extended. The thumb-in-palm deformity may result from spastic activity in FPL, adductor pollicis, and/or the thenar muscles (particularly the flexor pollicis brevis). The adduction deformity may be due to spasticity of muscles innervated by the ulnar nerve, median nerve, or, commonly, a combination of both. Adduction of the thumb metacarpal indicates spasticity of the adductor pollicis muscle and possibly the first dorsal interosseous muscle. A quick stretch of the thumb into abduction will often elicit a clonic response. An anesthetic block of the ulnar nerve in Guyon's canal at the wrist will temporarily eliminate intrinsic tone. This will demonstrate the presence of any myostatic contractures and will also confirm that the adductor pollicis was an offending muscle in the deformity. Contracture of the

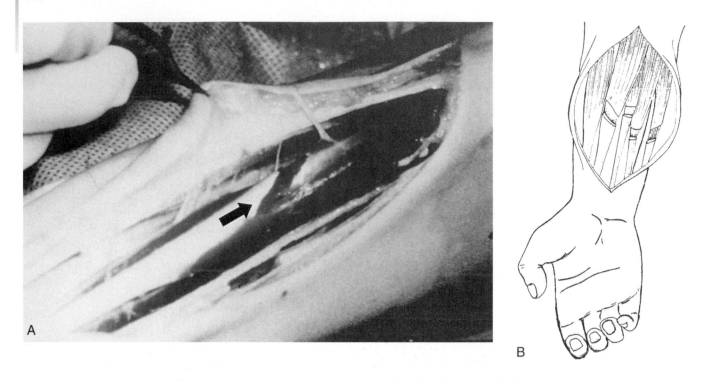

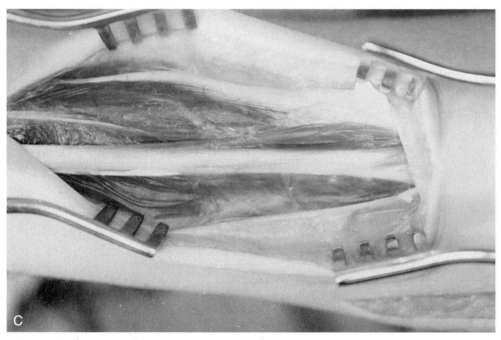

FIGURE 35-14. A, Intraoperative photograph showing myotendinous lengthening of the flexor carpi radialis *(arrow).* **B,** Line drawing showing the site and technique of myotendinous lengthening. **C,** Reoperation in a different patient shows excellent healing of the myotendinous junction, which had been lengthened 2 cm.

skin of the web space and IP joint contracture of the thumb may also develop over time. If some volitional potential in thumb extensors or thumb abductors is present, treatment of spastic FPL and adductor pollicis may facilitate active grasp, usually in the form of a modified type of key grasp. Dynamic EMG and lidocaine blocks are helpful in this regard.

During the period of motor control/musculoskeletal recovery, treatment of spastic muscles by chemodenervation

using botulinum toxin may allow application of hand orthoses for passive or active purposes. I no longer perform phenol blocks of the median or ulnar nerve branches. Casting or splinting may be needed after the block if a contracture is present. Active and passive range-of-motion exercises are performed. Functional training is performed when any motor control is present in the upper extremity.

In the period of residual deficits/remediable function, surgical treatment consists of fractional lengthening of the

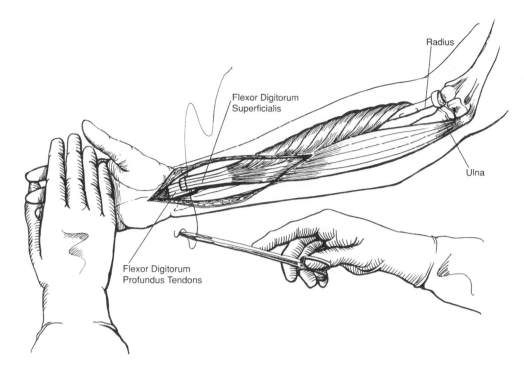

FIGURE 35-15. Superficialis-to-profundus tendon transfer. The four superficialis tendons are sutured together distally and then transected for transfer. The profundus tendons are sutured together proximally and then cut. The fingers are extended and the distal ends of the superficialis tendons are then sutured en masse to the proximal end of the profundus tendons. (From Keenan MA, Kozin SH, Berlet AC: Manual of Orthopaedic Surgery for Spasticity. New York, Raven Press, 1993.)

FPL at the myotendinous junction combined with a thenar muscle slide in which the origins of the thenar muscles are detached from the transverse palmar ligament while preserving the neurovascular pedicle. Surgical lengthening of the FPL is generally performed in conjunction with wrist or digital flexor lengthening. To provide a functional lateral pinch, it is desirable to stabilize the IP joint of the thumb. This may be done using a Herbert screw (Fig. 35-16). A stab incision is made on the tip of the thumb pulp, and, under fluoroscopic guidance, the pilot hole for the screw is passed through the tuft and shaft of the distal phalanx, across the joint, and into the proximal phalanx. The screw is then advanced through this hole, compressing the articular surfaces. In this patient group I have not found it necessary to denude the IP joint surfaces. The thumb is then protected in a thumb spica splint or cast for 3 weeks.

In those cases with a fixed adduction contracture, surgical lengthening of the thenar muscles is indicated. Generally, all of the thenar muscles are spastic or contracted and a proximal muscle slide is required to reposition the thumb and decrease the underlying tone to improve pinch function. Distal releases are to be avoided because these often result in a hyperextension deformity of the MCP joint of the thumb.

Technique of Thenar Muscle Slide

Under tourniquet control, an incision is made along the thenar crease on the palm. The neurovascular structures and flexor tendons are retracted ulnarly. The origins of the flexor pollicis brevis, opponens pollicis, and abductor pollicis muscles are detached from their origins while protecting the recurrent branch of the median nerve. The transverse carpal ligament is preserved, and the carpal canal is not entered. The thumb is extended, allowing the released muscles to slide radially and reattach in an improved position, preserving function and preventing a hyperextension deformity.

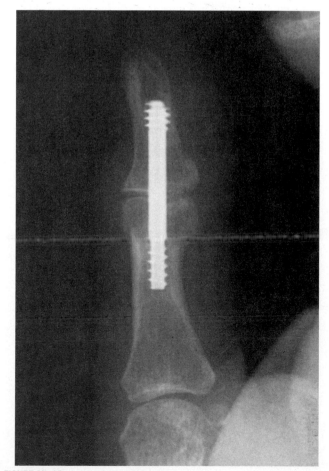

FIGURE 35-16. A thumb IP "fusion" accomplished with a Herbert-Whipple screw without denuding the joint surfaces.

The origin of the adductor pollicis muscle is released from the third metacarpal. Careful dissection to retract the digital neurovascular bundles and flexor tendons to the index and long digits is necessary. The deep palmar vascular arch and deep branch of the ulnar nerve are identified as they penetrate the adductor pollicis muscle between its oblique and transverse heads before adductor muscle release. The neurovascular supply of the adductor pollicis is preserved.

If the first dorsal interosseous muscle is contracted, a release is performed through a dorsal incision along the ulnar margin of the thumb metacarpal while protecting the radial sensory nerve. The origin of the first dorsal interosseous is released from its origin on the base of the first metacarpal. In persistent web space contractures despite appropriate muscle releases, a "Z"-plasty of the thumb web space is indicated.

Postoperatively the patient is immobilized in a thumb spica cast for 3 weeks. Active therapy is initiated after cast removal to optimize functional results.

Deformities From Intrinsic Spasticity

When spasticity of the extrinsic flexors is present, intrinsic spasticity should be suspected,[71,72,79,82,84,86] although intrinsic spasticity and contracture are frequently masked by the presence of extrinsic flexor spasticity or contracture. Extension of the fingers at the MCP joints may be blocked by spasticity of the interossei and lumbrical muscles of the hand. Another manifestation of intrinsic spasticity is the tendency toward swan neck or boutonnière posturing of the fingers. When a release or tendon lengthening of the spastic extrinsic-flexor muscles has already been done, an intrinsic positive deformity of the hand may be unmasked. These hand deformities can be painful and disfiguring.

The degree of tension caused by the intrinsic muscles can be demonstrated by comparing the amount of PIP joint flexion obtained with the MCP joints both flexed and extended. If there is less PIP joint flexion with MCP joint extension, then the intrinsic tendons are tight. This test should be performed both before and after a lidocaine block of the ulnar nerve at the wrist to distinguish between intrinsic tone and contracture.

Boutonnière deformities are commonly associated with intrinsic spasticity. They result from a combination of intrinsic spasticity combined with FDS tone. Swan neck deformities may also result from increased intrinsic tone (Fig. 35-17). The central extensor band is relatively shortened relative to the lateral bands because of tension exerted by the intrinsics and long extensor. In both of these cases care must be taken to distinguish between deformities caused by the intrinsic spasticity, which should improve with treatment, and deformities resulting from traumatic mechanisms such as central slip injury or mallet finger, which will not improve with intrinsic release.

Because it is impossible to fully delineate the relative contributions and balance of spasticity and contracture of the intrinsic and extrinsic muscles by clinical assessment alone, I routinely obtain dynamic EMG studies of the intrinsic muscles before embarking on treatment of hand deformities. This is especially important before considering any surgical intervention.

During the period of physiologic recovery, treatment of spastic muscles by chemodenervation is performed. In the period of residual deficits/remediable function, three treatment options are available. The procedure chosen is based on considerations of contracture and the presence or absence of volitional activity in the intrinsic muscles. When no significant intrinsic contracture is present and dynamic EMG indicates that there is no volitional control in the intrinsic muscles, a neurectomy of the motor branches of the ulnar nerve in the palm is performed (see Fig. 35-5). The sensory branches are left intact to preserve protective sensation in the hand. When a contracture of the intrinsic muscles is present and the dynamic EMG study shows no

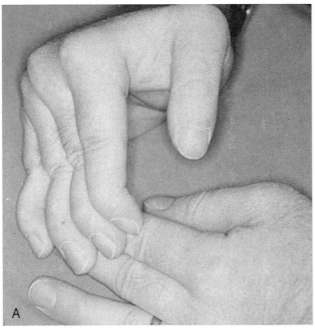
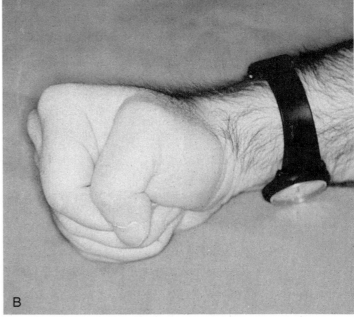

FIGURE 35-17. A, Multiple swan neck deformities of the fingers after traumatic brain injury. B, Note that combined flexion is not lost.

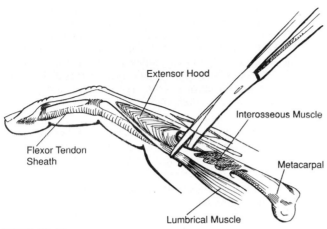

FIGURE 35-18. Isolation and release of the intrinsic interossei and lumbricales muscles. (From Keenan MA, Kozin SH, Berlet AC: Manual of Orthopaedic Surgery for Spasticity. New York, Raven Press, 1993.)

volitional activity, a release is performed of the lateral bands of the extensor hood mechanism at the level of the proximal phalanx (Fig. 35-18). In these cases, neurectomy of the motor branches of the ulnar nerve is done simultaneously to prevent recurrence of the intrinsic-plus deformity from spasticity of the interosseous muscles. When there is either a dynamic or static intrinsic-plus deformity but the EMG demonstrates volitional control, the interossei are lengthened in the palm.

Technique of Ulnar Motor Neurectomy

An incision is made on the palmar surface of the hand radial to the pisiform bone and extended distally for 1 inch. Care is taken to prevent injury to the ulnar artery. The ulnar nerve is exposed, and the motor branches are identified using a nerve stimulator. Generally, two motor branches are seen. The main motor branch lies beneath the sensory branch, and a smaller motor branch can be seen entering the hypothenar muscles. Once identified, the nerves are transected, with care taken to preserve the ulnar artery and the sensory branch of the ulnar nerve (see Fig. 35-5).

Unless combined with other surgery, no splinting or casting is necessary postoperatively. A soft dressing is applied to the hand and active and passive range-of-motion exercises are begun on the first postoperative day. The wound must be observed closely for evidence of infection because patients with flexion deformities of the fingers frequently have poor quality palmar skin secondary to maceration.

Technique of Intrinsic Lateral Band Release

In a hand in which a contracture of the intrinsic muscles is present and the dynamic EMG study shows no volitional activity, lateral band releases are performed (see Fig. 35-18). A midline longitudinal incision is made over the dorsum of the MCP joint and proximal phalanx of each finger. Dissection is carried out both on the ulnar and radial sides of the extensor mechanism. The palmar edge of the lateral bands are identified. The lateral band and oblique fibers of the extensor hood are transected on each side. Care is taken to preserve the transverse fibers of the sagittal extensor hood.

Recurrent intrinsic-plus deformities are common. This is thought to be secondary to residual attachment of the

interossei muscles to the base of the proximal phalanges. To prevent recurrent deformities, it is advisable to perform a concomitant neurectomy of the motor branches of the ulnar nerve in Guyon's canal, as described earlier.

Technique of Palmar Intrinsic Lengthening

In a hand with volitional control of the intrinsic musculature, palmar intrinsic lengthenings are performed. Palmar incisions are made, one between the second and third and one between the fourth and fifth metacarpals. The flexor tendons are retracted. The lumbrical muscles are much too small to lengthen. Dissection is continued to the palmar interossei where a substantive muscle-tendon junction can be found in these bipennate muscles. The tendon is sharply transected within the muscle belly. Postoperatively, the hand is splinted with the MCP joints extended for 2 weeks. Active motion is then started.

Intrinsic-Minus Deformities

A less common deformity pattern is the intrinsic-minus hand. In these patients the intrinsic muscles have normal or weakened tone but there is spasticity of the extrinsic finger flexors. There may be increased tone in the extrinsic extensors as well. This pattern results in a claw hand posture, with hyperextension of the MCP joints and flexion of the PIP and DIP joints. Ulnar nerve compression must be considered as a possible diagnosis. Hyperextension contracture of the MCP joint capsule is common. When present, the contractures require surgical release. Treatment of this deformity may also require lengthening of the extrinsic digital flexors or superficialis-to-profundus transfers, as described earlier. Zancoli capsulodesis may also be required to restore MCP flexion and place the hand in a more functional and cosmetic position.

ANNOTATED REFERENCES

10. Botte MJ, Keenan MA, Gellman H, et al: Surgical management of spastic thumb-in-palm deformity in adults with brain injury. J Hand Surg [Am] 14(2 pt 1):174-182, 1989.

    Spastic thumb-in-palm deformity was surgically treated in 27 adults. At mean follow-up of 39 months, 23 of 27 had a satisfactory correction. Unsatisfactory results included two with inadequate correction and two with overcorrection.

34. Fuller DA Keenan MA, Esquenazi A, et al: The impact of instrumented gait analysis on surgical planning: Treatment of spastic equinovarus deformity of the foot and ankle. Foot Ankle Int 23:738-743, 2002.

    Two surgeons prospectively evaluated 36 consecutive patients with a spastic equinovarus deformity. Each surgeon independently formulated a surgical plan before and after instrumented gait analysis. Overall a change was made in 64% of the surgical plans after the gait study. The frequency of changing the surgical plan was not significantly different between the more and less experienced surgeons. Instrumented gait analysis alters surgical planning for patients with equinovarus deformity of the foot and ankle and can produce higher agreement between surgeons in surgical planning. A muscle-specific approach that identifies the deforming forces will produce the best outcomes when treating the spastic equinovarus deformity.

37. Garland DE: A clinical perspective on common forms of acquired heterotopic ossification. Clin Orthop (263):13-29, 1991.

The clinical courses of heterotopic ossification (HO) as a consequence of trauma and central nervous system insults have many similarities. Detection is commonly noted at 2 months. The incidence of clinically significant HO is 10% to 20%. Approximately 10% of the HO is massive and causes severe restriction in joint motion or ankylosis. The locations are the proximal limbs and joints. Treatment modalities include diphosphonates, indomethacin, radiation, range of motion exercises, and surgical excision.

71. Keenan MA, Abrams RA, Garland DE, Waters RL: Results of fractional lengthening of the finger flexors in adults with upper extremity spasticity. J Hand Surg [Am] 12:575-581, 1987.

The results of fractional lengthening of the finger flexors of 27 patients with upper extremity flexor spasticity of the finger flexors were examined. Patients were divided preoperatively into those with potentially functional hands and those who were nonfunctional based on the presence of motor control and hand sensibility. Postoperatively, all five nonfunctional hands improved in posture, and the hygiene problems resolved. Twenty of the 22 patients with potentially functional hands (91%) improved their spastic hand function score a mean of 3.7 points. Two patients (9%) decreased their spastic hand function score as a result of overlengthening of the finger flexors, with loss of grip strength.

75. Keenan MA, Fuller DA, Whyte J, et al: The influence of dynamic polyelectromyography in formulating a surgical plan in treatment of spastic elbow flexion deformity. Arch Phys Med Rehabil 84:291-296, 2003.

The objective of this study was to determine the influence of motor-control analysis with dynamic EMG on surgical planning in patients with spastic elbow flexion deformity. A prospective observational design was used. Twenty-one patients with spastic elbow flexion deformity were evaluated. Two surgeons each formulated a detailed surgical plan for each individual muscle-tendon unit before and after the patients underwent motor-control analysis in which kinetic and polyelectromyographic data were collected. Fifty-seven percent of the surgical plans were changed after the motor-control study. The frequency of change did not differ by clinical experience. Detailed EMG motor-control analysis alters surgical planning for patients with spastic elbow flexion deformity. Clinical assessment alone does not accurately identify the muscles responsible for the deformity or dysfunction.

79. Keenan MA, Korchek JI, Botte MJ, et al: Results of transfer of the flexor digitorum superficialis tendons to the flexor digitorum profundus tendons in adults with acquired spasticity of the hand. J Bone Joint Surg [Am] 69:1127-1132, 1987.

Thirty-one patients who had transfer of the flexor digitorum superficialis tendons to the flexor digitorum profundus tendons en masse in 34 nonfunctional spastic hands were examined at an average of 50 months postoperatively. All of the patients had had a clenched-fist deformity, with severe hygienic problems of the palmar skin and no active function of the hand. Postoperatively, all of the hands were in an open position, which allowed for good hygiene of the palmar surface.

81. Keenan MA, Romanelli RR, Lunsford BR: The use of dynamic electromyography to evaluate motor control in the hands of adults who have spasticity caused by brain injury. J Bone Joint Surg Am 71:120-126, 1989.

A dynamic EMG analysis of grasp and release, performed on 48 upper extremities of 42 adults who had had injury to the brain causing spasticity, showed volitional motor control of the finger flexors in 80% and active extension of the fingers in 60%. The flexor pollicis longus showed volitional control in 75% of the hands and the extensor pollicis longus showed active control in 50%. The extensor carpi radialis longus acted as an appropriate stabilizer of the wrist in 85% of the extremities.

87. Keenan MACE, Mehta S: Neuro-orthopaedic management of shoulder deformity and dysfunction in brain-injured patients: A novel approach. J Head Trauma Rehabil 19:143-154, 2004.

Shoulder problems are common in patients with traumatic brain injury. Shoulder problems can be classified and evaluated using several different strategies: bony versus soft tissue restrictions, static versus dynamic deformities, traumatic injuries versus impairments secondary to weakness and spasticity, or problems of active function versus problems of passive function. Regardless of the classification system employed, a systematic approach to evaluation and treatment is essential. Shoulder impairments can be corrected leading to significant improvement in functional outcomes.

101. Matev I: Surgery of the spastic thumb-in-palm deformity. J Hand Surg [Br] 16:127-132, 1991.

A 20-year experience with a surgical procedure, previously described, for dynamic correction of spastic thumb-in-palm deformity in cerebral palsy is reported. The procedure includes lengthening of the long flexor of the thumb, proximal thumb intrinsic release, and augmentation of abduction-extension of the thumb. Bone-stabilizing operations are not performed. Fifty-six patients were followed up for an average period of 4 years and 11 months after the treatment (range, 2 to 15 years). Correction of the deformity was recorded in 82% of the patients.

103. Mayer NH: Clinicophysiologic concepts of spasticity and motor dysfunction in adults with an upper motoneuron lesion. Muscle Nerve Suppl 6:S1-S13, 1997.

Spasticity is one component of the upper motoneuron syndrome, along with weakness, and loss of dexterity. Chronic spasticity can lead to changes in the rheologic properties of the involved and neighboring muscles. Stiffness, contracture, atrophy, and fibrosis may interact with pathologic regulatory mechanisms to prevent normal control of limb position and movement. In the clinical examination it is important to distinguish between the resistance due to spasticity and that due to rheologic changes, because the distinction has therapeutic implications.

120. Perry J: Contractures: A historical perspective. Clin Orthop (219):8-14, 1987.

Orthopedic history vividly documents the continuing battle between restoring tissue stability and preserving functional mobility. Prolonged and uninterrupted rest ensures healing. Contractures that permanently limit function are not an uncommon consequence. Hippocrates, Hunter, Lucas-Championniere, and David advocated judicious motion. Timing and the interpretation of the patient's pathologic state have proved to be the critical criteria. Physiologic posturing of inflamed or swollen joints to minimize tissue strain introduces resting positions of 15 degrees plantarflexion at the ankle, and 30 degrees flexion at the knee and hip. These will be perpetuated by contractures if not actively counteracted by timely mobilizing procedures. Each of these joint positions is a serious deterrent to walking without stressful substitutive posturing, and the patient's ability to function is impaired.

121. Perry J: Determinants of muscle function in the spastic lower extremity. Clin Orthop (288):10-26, 1993.

The upper motor neuron lesion that causes hemiplegia impairs the patient's selective control and exposes primitive modes of muscle activation. Dynamic EMG revealed the primitive mechanisms leading to these inconsistencies. The rate of stretch does not differentiate spasticity from contracture, because either a quick or a slow stretch frequently causes a sustained muscle response. Using knee flexion to differentiate gastrocnemius and soleus spasticity is not reliable, because the change in neurologic input with flexion may inhibit the extensor muscle's response to stretch so that the soleus is also relaxed. The change in body position from lying supine to sitting can double the intensity of soleus spasticity, and standing further increases the tone. Primitive patterns of mass extension and flexion, while voluntary, inhibit normal progression during walking. Simultaneous activation of the soleus and gastrocnemius with the knee's quadriceps causes premature ankle plantarflexion as the limb is loaded in stance. The primitive flexion synergy between the hip, knee, and ankle (dorsiflexion) inhibits terminal swing knee extension while the hip remains flexed. Consequently, surgical planning for the hemiparetic limb must rely heavily on gait analysis findings (systematic observation or by instrumentation).

128. Pomerance JF, Keenan MA: Correction of severe spastic flexion contractures in the nonfunctional hand. J Hand Surg [Am] 21:828-833, 1996.

The superficialis-to-profundus transfer has been a time-honored treatment of spasticity in nonfunctional hands, but it does not address the many associated problems. Fourteen patients were treated with 15 procedures (1 bilateral) designed to relieve severe flexion contractures of the hand and wrist over a 3-year period with a single-stage comprehensive surgical correction consisting of superficialis-to-profundus transfer, wrist flexor release, flexor pollicis longus lengthening, wrist arthrodesis, carpal tunnel release, and ulnar motor branch neurectomy or intrinsic release. All preoperative hygiene problems and infections resolved. The comprehensive protocol allowed correction of severe contractures of the hand and wrist by a single operation with improved care and appearance of the hand.

144. Teasdale GM, Pettigrew LE, Wilson JT, et al: Analyzing outcome of treatment of severe head injury: A review and update on advancing the use of the Glasgow Outcome Scale. J Neurotrauma 15:587-597, 1998.

The Glasgow Outcome Scale (GOS), two decades after its description, remains the most widely used method of analyzing outcome in series of patients with severe head injuries. This review considers limitations recognized in the use of the GOS and discusses a new approach to assessment, using a structured questionnaire-based interview. Assignments can be made to an extended eight-point scale (GOSE) as well as the original five-point approach in each case, with a high degree of interobserver consistency. It is concluded that, in its improved structured format, the GOS should remain the primary method of assessing outcome in trials of the management of severe head injury.

149. Waters RL, Frazier J, Garland DE, et al: Electromyographic gait analysis before and after operative treatment for hemiplegic equinus and equinovarus deformity. J Bone Joint Surg Am 64:284-288, 1982.

Gait EMGs were obtained before and after tendon transfer, lengthening, or release in 27 hemiplegic patients with equinus or equinovarus deformities. Abnormal patterns of muscle activity almost always were present preoperatively in the gastrocnemius, soleus, tibialis posterior, flexor hallucis longus, flexor digitorum longus, peroneus brevis, and tibialis anterior muscles in these patients. The surgical procedures to correct the foot deformities altered the gross patterns of activity of most of the muscles operated on by very little. Of particular importance to the surgeon was the finding that the pattern of activity of the muscles whose tendon was transferred, lengthened, or released was not altered after operation. This finding makes the preoperative gait EMG a useful means of determining the appropriate surgical plan, because it is an indication of the type of muscle activity to expect postoperatively.

CHAPTER 36

Tetraplegia

Ann Van Heest

In the United States, spinal cord injuries have an annual incidence estimated at 40 new cases per million people, as reported in 2000.[13] The most common causes are motor vehicle accidents and falls from a height. Fifty-five percent occur in patients 16 to 30 years old, and 80% are males. Most occur in the cervical or lumbar regions, because these anatomic areas have the greatest mobility.

PATHOGENESIS

The cervical spinal cord contains eight cervical segments encased in the seven cervical vertebrae. The bone and ligamentous structure of the cervical spine allows wide range of motion, thus exposing the cervical spinal cord to greater risk of injury. Injury occurs most commonly through bone or disk compression of the cord after fracture and/or dislocation or through traction of the cord with translation due to spine instability with injury, most commonly flexion deformity.[33] Immediate hemorrhage and edema subsides, followed by local reparation and finally scar formation. The area of injured spinal cord can vary in width and length and is termed the *injured metamere*. Nerve function above the injured metamere is normal; nerve function within the injured metamere is absent and the lower motor neuron cannot be stimulated because the anterior horn cell is absent; nerve function below the injured metamere may be stimulated if the lower motor neuron unit is without injury.[14]

The muscles that are innervated above the level of injury will have normal strength. The muscles that are innervated below the level of injury may be flaccid or have some elements of spasticity. The muscles at the level of injury may improve in muscle strength, most commonly within 1 year after spinal cord injury. Ditunno and colleagues[22] and Waters and associates[83] reported upper limb strength recovery rates using manual muscle testing. One third of muscles at grade 0 at 1 month after injury improved to grade 3 at 4

to 6 months after injury, sometimes with improvement seen to 24 months after injury. All upper limb muscles with an initial strength of grade 1 improved to at least a grade 3 at 1 year after injury, with the exception of the triceps. If a muscle was greater than grade 1 at 1 month after injury, then the median time was 6 months for full recovery.

PREOPERATIVE WORK-UP

The hand surgeon is not as concerned with the specific vertebral level of cervical injury as much as the specific strength of each muscle in the upper limb. Classically, tetraplegic patients have been classified by the cervical spine segment injured by fracture or dislocation, and formerly there was an assumption that the level of paralysis and sensory loss coincided exactly with the bony injury, producing a precise transverse spinal cord lesion. Careful examination of patients rendered tetraplegic has shown that (1) there is frequently little relationship between the level of the skeletal lesion and the spinal cord lesion; (2) lesions may be asymmetrical; and (3) there may be unusual patterns of sparing of sensory or motor function. Thus, a more useful classification had to be developed that used spared functions as its basis.[56,60,87,88] The classification (Table 36-1) used in this chapter was developed by an international group of tetraplegic hand surgeons in 1978 in Edinburgh[58] and modified in 1984 at Giens, France.

By using manual muscle testing (Table 36-2), the most helpful evaluation of the tetraplegic patient is to make a working list of what the patient *has* (grade 4 strength or higher), as shown in Table 36-1, and what the patient *needs* (grade 1 strength or lower), as shown in Table 36-3. Lastly, one must determine what muscles are *available* for transfer and which muscles best *match* to the patient's needs using tendon transfer principles of work capacity, amplitude, and direction of pull combined with other surgical adjuncts of arthrodesis and tenodesis.

The author would like to acknowledge **Dr. James House** for his mentorship in tetraplegic hand surgery and his contributions to this manuscript; **Dr. Charles McDowell** for his contributions to the manuscript; **Dr. Michael Keith** for his manuscript review; and **Catherine Girard** for manuscript preparation.

Table 36-1

INTERNATIONAL CLASSIFICATION FOR SURGERY OF THE HAND IN TETRAPLEGIA (EDINBURGH 1978, MODIFIED—GIENS, 1984)

Sensibility		Motor	Description
O or Cu	**Group**	**Characteristics**	**Function**
	0	No muscle below elbow suitable for transfer	Flexion and supination of the elbow
	1	BR	
	2	ECRL	Extension of the wrist (weak or strong)
	3*	ECRB	Extension of the wrist
	4	PT	Extension and pronation of the wrist
	5	FCR	Flexion of the wrist
	6	Finger extensors	Extrinsic extension of the fingers (partial or complete)
	7	Thumb extensor	Extrinsic extension of the thumb
	8	Partial digital flexors	Extrinsic flexion of the fingers (weak)
	9	Lacks only intrinsics	Extrinsic flexion of the fingers
	X	Exceptions	

BR, brachioradialis; ECRL, extensor carpi radialis longus; ECRB, extensor carpi radialis brevis; PT, pronator teres; FCR, flexor carpi radialis.

*Caution: To determine the strength of the ECRB, see text (page 1283).

1. This classification does not include the shoulder. It is a guide to the forearm and hand only. Determination of patient suitability for posterior deltoid-to-triceps transfer or biceps-to-triceps transfer is considered separately.
2. The need for triceps reconstruction is stated separately. It may be required in order to make BR transfers function properly (see text).
3. There is a sensory component to the classification. Afferent input is recorded using the method described by Moberg and precedes the motor classification. Both ocular and cutaneous input should be documented. When vision is the only afferent available, the designation is "Oculo" (abbreviated O). Assuming there is 10 mm or less two-point discrimination in the thumb and index finger, the correct classification would be Cu, indicating that the patient has adequate cutaneous sensibility. If two-point discrimination is greater than 10 mm (meaning inadequate cutaneous sensibility), the designation O would precede the motor group (example, O 2).
4. Motor grouping assumes that all listed muscles are grade 4 (MRC) or better and a new muscle is added for each group; for example, a group 3 patient will have BR, ECRL, and ECRB rated at least grade 4 (MRC).

From McDowell CL, Moberg EA, House JH: The Second International Conference on Surgical Rehabilitation of the Upper Limb in Tetraplegia (Quadriplegia). J Hand Surg [Am] 11:604-608, 1986.

Table 36-2

CURRENTLY ACCEPTED MUSCLE GRADING SYSTEM FIRST DEVISED BY THE BRITISH MEDICAL RESEARCH COUNCIL

Grade	Description
0	No contraction
1	Flicker or trace of contraction
2	Active movement with gravity eliminated
3	Active movement against gravity
4	Active movement against gravity and resistance
5	Normal

From Council Medical Research: Aids to the investigation of peripheral nerve injuries. War Memorandum No. 7. London, His Majesty's Stationery Office, 1943.

Table 36-3

LIST OF FUNCTIONAL NEEDS TO BE ASSESSED AS PART OF THE PREOPERATIVE WORK-UP

What the Patient Needs	Muscles to Be Tested and Graded
Elbow flexion	Biceps, brachialis
Elbow extension	Triceps
Wrist extension	ECRL, ECRB, ECU
Wrist flexion	FCR, FCU
Finger extension	EDC, EIP, EDQ
Finger flexion	FDP, FDS
Thumb extension/abduction	EPL, EPB, APL
Thumb flexion/opposition	FPL, APB, opponens, FPB
Intrinsics	Adductor pollicis, interossei, lumbricals

Example of Preoperative Evaluation

A sample worksheet for preoperative planning of a patient with a C7 injury who presents 1 year after a motor vehicle accident is shown in Table 36-4. First, the physician needs to evaluate general suitability for surgery with regard to the patient's age, occupation, interests, level of education, learning capacity, economic support, family and agency support, personality type, and understanding of what can and cannot be expected from surgical treatment. Next the patient's physical examination would include sensory and motor testing to establish his or her group (0 to 9) using the

Table 36-4
SAMPLE WORKSHEET FOR PREOPERATIVE PLANNING WITH C7 FRACTURE (GROUP 5)

What Muscles the Patient HAS (Muscles Below Elbow With > Grade 4 Strength)	What Functions the Patient NEEDS	What Muscles Are AVAILABLE to Transfer	MATCH Available Muscles and Adjunct Procedures to Functions That Patient Needs	Surgical Plan
BR	Finger extension	BR	BR to FPL (thumb flexion)	Extensor phase (stage 1)
ECRL	Finger flexion	ECRL	ECRL to FDP (finger flexion)	EDC tenodesis
ECRB	Thumb extension and abduction	(PT)[†]	EPL tenodesis	EPL tenodesis
PT	Thumb flexion and opposition (intrinsics)*		EDC tenodesis	CMC fusion
FCR			CMC fusion for thumb positioning	Flexor phase (stage 2)
				BR to FPL
				ECRL to FDP

*Intrinsics reconstructions may be necessary if joint imbalances exist.
[†]Pronator teres may be used for transfer, but strength for manual wheelchair propulsion may be diminished, so it is not a first-choice muscle.

International Classification (see Table 36-1). By establishing which muscles the patient has over grade 4 strength, the group is designated by what the patient *has.* For example, this patient may be a group 5; that is, the patient has grade 4 strength of the brachioradialis (BR), both the radial wrist extensors, the pronator teres (PT), and the flexor carpi radialis (FCR). The next step is to determine what the patient *needs* from Table 36-3. For this patient, there is absent thumb extension/abduction, finger extension, thumb flexion/opposition, and finger flexion, as well as intrinsics. The patient needs to be examined for passive range of motion to evaluate joint/muscle contractures, tenodesis effect, and resting posture of the hand. The hand must have passive mobility or tenodesis ability to achieve what the patient *needs;* for example, if the thumb sits at rest in a fully supinated position and lacks any tenodesis for thumb flexion or opposition, then tendon transfers will be ineffective unless the thumb is repositioned, possibly with a carpometacarpal (CMC) fusion in a key pinch position. The last step is to determine which muscles are *available* for transfer. For this patient, the BR is available because the patient has biceps and brachialis for elbow flexion (no function will be lost by transfer); the extensor carpi radialis longus (ECRL) is available because the patient has extensor carpi radialis brevis (ECRB) for wrist extension. At times, the PT can be used as a transfer as well, but this may result in diminished pronator power (manual wheelchair function). Finally, the muscles available for transfer (BR, ECRL) are matched to the needed functions (thumb extension/abduction, finger extension, thumb flexion/opposition, finger flexion, intrinsics) using principles of tendon transfer surgery (see Chapter 31), combined with other surgical options of arthrodesis and tenodesis. In this example, work capacity is most important for finger and thumb flexion because these functions need strength for grasp and pinch; thus the BR and ECRL would be transferred for finger and thumb flexion for pinch and grip strength. The BR would be transferred to the flexor pollicis longus (FPL) because it has less (and needs less) excursion, whereas the ECRL would be transferred to the flexor digitorum profundus (FDP), which needs greater excursion. Surgical adjuncts will be used to preposition the thumb in key pinch with a CMC fusion and to provide thumb and finger extension through an extensor pollicis longus (EPL) and extensor digitorum communis (EDC)

tenodesis. If necessary, intrinsic reconstruction could be added if joint imbalance exists.

A similar process to that just described should be carried out for each patient to establish an appropriate treatment plan. By evaluating what the patient *has,* what the patient *needs,* what is *available,* and how they best *match* for function, an appropriate patient evaluation can be used to establish an appropriate surgical reconstructive plan.

PERTINENT ANATOMY

Nerve deficits cause a predictable pattern of injury. Injuries of the central nervous system cause a different pattern from a spinal cord injury, a brachial plexus injury, or an isolated peripheral nerve injury. The pattern seen with a spinal cord injury is based on segmental innervation; this concept means that the anterior horn cells in the spinal cord that are injured occur in a predictable pattern from cephalad to caudad position. Motor nuclei form longitudinal columns crossing several segmental levels, in a predictable manner.

Figure 36-1 shows the segmental anatomy that is present based on Zancolli's clinical experience with tetraplegic patients.[87] When a spinal cord injury occurs, the motor nuclei cephalad to the injury will be functional; the motor nuclei at or caudad to the level of the injury will be nonfunctional. The International Classification for Surgery of the Hand in Tetraplegia (ICSHT) groups characterize the most common patterns of presentation, based on strength of muscles below the elbow. Groups are based on the number of muscles (below the elbow) and at least grade 4 strength on manual muscle testing (see Table 36-2) based on segmental innervation patterns of injury.

HISTORICAL REVIEW

Before the 1960s, the poor prognosis and poor survival rate of patients with spinal cord injury precluded the need for upper extremity reconstruction. As the prognosis and medical care of the patient with spinal cord injury improved, so did the surgical advancements in tendon transfer surgery. As shown in Table 36-5, the advancements in tendon transfer surgery, initiated by Sterling Bunnell, were applied to

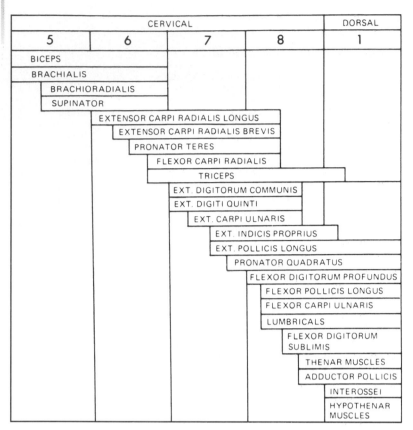

CERVICAL				DORSAL
5	6	7	8	1

(Muscle innervation chart)

- BICEPS (C5)
- BRACHIALIS (C5)
- BRACHIORADIALIS (C5–6)
- SUPINATOR (C5–6)
- EXTENSOR CARPI RADIALIS LONGUS (C6–7)
- EXTENSOR CARPI RADIALIS BREVIS (C6–7)
- PRONATOR TERES (C6–7)
- FLEXOR CARPI RADIALIS (C6–7)
- TRICEPS (C6–8)
- EXT. DIGITORUM COMMUNIS (C7–8)
- EXT. DIGITI QUINTI (C7–8)
- EXT. CARPI ULNARIS (C7–8)
- EXT. INDICIS PROPRIUS (C7–8)
- EXT. POLLICIS LONGUS (C7–8)
- PRONATOR QUADRATUS (C7–8)
- FLEXOR DIGITORUM PROFUNDUS (C7–8–D1)
- FLEXOR POLLICIS LONGUS (C8–D1)
- FLEXOR CARPI ULNARIS (C8–D1)
- LUMBRICALS (C8–D1)
- FLEXOR DIGITORUM SUBLIMIS (C8–D1)
- THENAR MUSCLES (C8–D1)
- ADDUCTOR POLLICIS (C8–D1)
- INTEROSSEI (C8–D1)
- HYPOTHENAR MUSCLES (C8–D1)

FIGURE 36-1. Segmental innervation of muscles of the elbow, forearm, and hand. Although not shown in this figure, the deltoid and the biceps both are innervated from the C5-6 level. Both the deltoid and triceps receive their innervation from a higher level on the cervical cord than the triceps. (From Zancolli EA: Structural and Dynamic Bases of Hand Surgery. Philadelphia, JB Lippincott, 1979.)

the tetraplegic patient by Moberg, Lamb, Zancolli, and Freehafer. Now in the 21st century, patients and physicians have become enthusiastic about the benefits that can be achieved with a well-designed and well-executed surgical plan for upper limb reconstruction in the tetraplegic patient.

INDICATIONS/CONTRAINDICATIONS TO OPERATIVE INTERVENTION

The general goal of surgery is greater independence for the patient, so the main indication for operative treatment remains functional impairment that can be improved through surgical reconstruction.

Specific operative indications include patients with a spinal cord injury, at least 12 months after injury, with a stable motor examination in the upper extremity that leads to functional impairments that could be improved by hand reconstruction. Ideally, the patient is free from contractures, pain, and spasticity; is compliant with the postoperative rehabilitation regimen (with appropriate postoperative support services available); is stable medically, including bowel and bladder function, blood pressure control, without infected decubitus ulcers, and without bladder infection; and is highly motivated to improve hand function.

Two factors have had a uniformly adverse effect on results of surgical treatment: spasticity and psychological problems. Spasticity that cannot be controlled by the patient is a strong contraindication to surgery. Freehafer and colleagues[26] and Moberg stated that some spasticity might be helpful, but judging the degree of spasticity compatible with

CRITICAL POINTS: INDICATIONS/CONTRAINDICATIONS TO OPERATIVE INTERVENTION

INDICATIONS

- Cervical spinal injury with upper limb partial paralysis
- Stabilized motor recovery (12 months post injury)
- Preoperative work-up compatible with functional improvement with surgical reconstruction
- Medically stable (blood pressure, bowel and bladder function)
- Infection free (decubitus ulcers, bladder)
- Full passive range of motion
- Realistic goals with good motivation/desire
- Personal and social stability to carry out rehabilitation and staged procedures (if necessary)

CONTRAINDICATIONS

- Spasticity
- Contractures
- Chronic pain problems
- Psychological instability

Table 36-5
HISTORICAL REVIEW OF SURGICAL RECONSTRUCTION IN THE TETRAPLEGIC PATIENT

Authors	Publication	Importance
Bunnell	*Surgery of the Hand,* 1948 (second edition)	C6/7 treated with tendon transfer/tenodesis
Nickel, Perry, and Garret	J Bone Joint Surg Am 45:933-952, 1963	Development of useful function in the severely paralyzed hand
Wilson	J Bone Joint Surg Am 38:1019-1024, 1956	Providing automatic grasp by flexor tenodesis
Street and Stambaugh	Clin Orthop, 1959[80]	Finger flexor tenodesis
Lipscomb, Elkins, and Henderson	J Bone Joint Surg Am, 1958[54]	Two-stage surgical grasp and release for C6/7 fracture-dislocation patients
Freehafer and Mast	J Bone Joint Surg Am, 1967[25]	First described brachioradialis to wrist extension in "high" cervical injuries
Zancolli	*Structural and Dynamic Bases of Hand Surgery,* 1968	Comprehensive review of anatomic bases of tendon transfers and operative options including two-stage reconstruction for grasp/pinch and release
Lamb and Landry Lamb and Chan Lamb, et al.	Hand, 1971[50] J Bone Joint Surg Am, 1983[49] J Hand Surg [Br] 14:143-144, 1989	Flexor phase surgical technique and results; principles of tendon transfer and results
Zancolli	Clin Orthop, 1975[88]	Surgery with strong wrist extension preserved (97 cases), treated with two-stage reconstructions
Moberg	J Bone Joint Surg Am, 1975[61]	Posterior deltoid to triceps transfer and single-stage pinch tenodesis
Moberg	The Upper Limb in Tetraplegia: A New Approach to Surgical Rehabilitation, 1978	Presented classification based on sensibility and available grade 4 muscles; importance of key pinch position
First International Conference on Surgical Rehabilitation in the Upper Limb in Tetraplegia	Edinburgh, Scotland, 1978, reported in J Hand Surg, 1979	First international classification for surgery of the hand based on sensibility, motors available below the elbow, and hand function
Peckham, et al.	J Hand Surg [Am] 1980[72]	First described use of functional electrical stimulation for restoration of key pinch
Hentz, Brown, and Keoshian	J Hand Surg [Am] 1983[31]	Functional assessment of the upper limb after reconstructive surgery
Second International Conference	Giens, France 1984, reported in J Hand Surg, 1986[57]	Classification modified to present day (see Table 36-1)
Allieu, et al.	Chirurgie, 1986	52 Reconstructions with 28 posterior deltoid to triceps complicated by stretching in 7 cases
Waters, et al.	J Hand Surg [Am] 10:385-391, 1985 J Hand Surg, 1987	Key pinch using BR to FPL and elbow extension transfers to increase pinch strength
House and Shannon House, et al. House	J Hand Surg, 1985[36] J Hand Surg, 1992[34] J Hand Surg, 1997	Opposition transfers vs. fusion for thumb control One-stage key pinch with thumb CMC fusion Intrinsic reconstructions

good results is very difficult; in fact, Moberg noted such an error in his poor result group.[61] Psychological impairment with unrealistic expectations, insufficient motivation to complete the operative and postoperative protocols, and inadequate social support mechanisms should be assessed before surgery. When the psychological impairment is not detected and left untreated, the results of surgery become unsatisfactory. Patients who want to have reconstructive surgery and who are strongly motivated to improve their functional status are more likely to obtain a better outcome. The surgeon and patient must be able to communicate effectively and share *realistic* expectations of the benefits of surgery. Allowing a prospective patient to visit with a

postoperative patient with a similar condition is particularly useful.

TYPES OF OPERATIONS

Three types of surgical procedures are most commonly performed: tendon transfers, tenodeses, and arthrodeses.

Tendon Transfers

To the extent that voluntary muscle control and strength exist, and no essential function will be lost with transfer of the donor muscle, tendon transfers are prioritized because these give active control and strength. However, the primary problem after spinal cord injury is a paucity of available adequate donor muscles for transfer. The available muscles are prioritized first for wrist extension, then for pinch, then for grasp, and finally for release functions. Tendon transfer principles, including donor availability, donor strength, amplitude of excursion, passive mobility of recipient joints, and adequate soft tissue bed for transfer, must be followed (see Chapter 31). The remaining functions that cannot be provided for using tendon transfer are provided through tenodesis and arthrodesis.

Tenodesis

Tenodesis is defined as the resultant movement of one joint produced by motion of an adjacent (usually proximal) joint. The "tenodesis effect" seen in the paralytic hand is that with active extension of the wrist, the fingers and thumb will flex, and with wrist flexion, the fingers and thumb will extend. Although the finger and thumb muscles are paralyzed, the fact that the finger and thumb flexors and extensors cross the wrist joint allows tenodesis movement of the fingers with active movement of the wrist, despite finger and thumb muscle paralysis. Spinal cord injury patients learn to use the tenodesis effect extensively and will commonly have functional but very weak pinch or grasp owing to the tenodesis effect alone. The tenodesis effect can be enhanced surgically without need to transfer an active muscle. Passive tenodesis procedures anchor the paralyzed tendon proximal to the wrist joint to increase digital movement with active wrist movement. Common tenodesis techniques include those for finger extension, finger flexor, thumb extensor/abductor, and thumb flexor, as described later in this chapter. Intrinsic tenodeses are also used to mimic normal function of the intrinsic muscles of the fingers and thumb.

Arthrodesis

Arthrodeses are useful in the thumb to make this multi-articular joint more stable and simpler for the patient to control. The CMC, metacarpophalangeal (MP), and interphalangeal (IP) joints of the thumb are each separately used concomitantly with tendon transfers and tenodesis procedures to provide effective positioning and control of the thumb in producing pinch function. Occasionally, proximal interphalangeal (PIP) joint fusions are used in the fingers, particularly the index finger, if the patient cannot stabilize the digit as a post for pinch. The wrist is never fused because the tenodesis effect would be lost. Surgical techniques for arthrodesis procedures are no different in the paralytic hand, except that the fixation technique chosen should be sufficiently stable to allow some weight bearing in the cast and early mobilization for tendon transfer rehabilitation.

Surgical reconstruction is based on the patient's International Classification group category (see Table 36-1). The International Classification deals only with muscles functioning below the level of the elbow. Thus, elbow procedures will be presented first, followed by procedures used for grasp, pinch, and release organized by the patient's International Classification.

ELBOW EXTENSION TENDON TRANSFERS

For patients lacking active elbow extension, two options exist for reconstruction: (1) deltoid to triceps and (2) biceps to triceps transfers.[81] Active elbow extension assists the patient in reaching objects above shoulder level and improves driving abilities, aids in wheelchair propulsion, permits pressure relief, and facilitates independent transfer.[4,23,76,78] Additionally, active elbow extension provides an antagonist to elbow flexion, which facilitates improved function after hand reconstructions that use the BR as a tendon transfer.[10]

The biceps and the deltoid are innervated from the spinal cord at a higher level than the triceps. The posterior deltoid to triceps transfer has been used extensively over the past 30 years, but, more recently, the medially routed biceps to triceps has become the author's preferred method of treatment.

Posterior Deltoid to Triceps Tendon Transfer

The posterior deltoid to triceps transfer uses the posterior third and the posterior half of the middle third of the deltoid muscle as a donor (Fig. 36-2). An interposition tendon graft is used, and the triceps tendon serves as the insertion. The posterior deltoid is tested before surgery by supporting the limb in 90 degrees of shoulder abduction and palpating the muscle for bulk and selective control while testing strength of shoulder extension. Scapular stabilization and control are also necessary to maximize the effectiveness of the transfer.

The procedure is performed with the patient in a lateral decubitus position with the shoulder forequarter draped free. An incision is made from the tip of the posterior corner of the acromion distally to the deltoid tubercle insertion. Dissection is along the posterior border of the deltoid leading into its insertion onto the deltoid tubercle. The axillary nerve courses about 5 cm distal to the acromion on the deep surface of the deltoid and must be protected as the posterior half of the middle deltoid is dissected with the posterior deltoid and freed from its insertion. A separate incision is made over the distal one third of the humerus to expose the triceps tendon. A subcutaneous tunnel is made connecting the two incisions for placement of an interpositional graft.

Several alternatives exist for the interpositional graft. Moberg[61] originally used toe extensors from the second, third, and fourth toes to allow at least three weaves at each attachment site. Alternative graft materials have included fascia lata,[31] tibialis anterior,[48,52] and extensor carpi ulnaris (ECU).[49] Alternatively, Castro-Sierra and Lopex-Pita[12] have used the central one third of the triceps. In this method, a 1-cm strip from the central one third of the triceps is harvested from its insertion in a retrograde manner (proximally based), mobilizing it sufficiently to graft back to the distal end of the posterior deltoid. Reflecting the central third of triceps with a bone block and internally fixing this to a bone block from the deltoid insertion has also been described.[59]

After the interpositional graft has been placed, the transfer is sewn in place and tensioned with the shoulder in 30 to 40 degrees of abduction and no forward flexion, so that the elbow can flex to 60 degrees with moderate tension. Most commonly, a well-padded long-arm cylinder cast is applied to hold the elbow in about 10 degrees of flexion. The

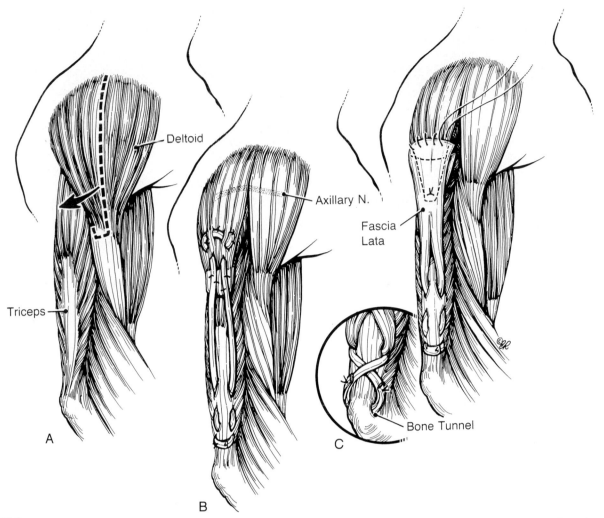

FIGURE 36-2. Deltoid to triceps transfer (Moberg). **A,** The posterior border of the muscle belly is isolated, preserving as much of the tendinous insertion as possible. **B,** Tendon grafts are laced into the distal end of the deltoid muscle belly and triceps aponeurosis. **C,** Fascia lata is used rather than tendon grafts. Direct insertion into the olecranon through a bone tunnel can also be done with either type of graft.

wrist can be left free. Forward flexion and shoulder adduction are avoided during the 6 weeks of cast immobilization. Gentle active exercises are performed to slowly gain flexion for the next 3 months with a rate of 5 to 10 degrees of increased flexion per week.

Posterior deltoid to triceps transfers are compromised by the prolonged shoulder and elbow immobilization required postoperatively, as well as tendon graft elongation over time.[21,63,73,74] Friden and colleagues[27] used intraoperative metal markers at the ends of the tendon grafts and measured an average of 2.3 cm of elongation after 2 years. They changed their postoperative regimen to include longer elbow extension immobilization, and more shoulder abduction positioning was recommended. Follow-up of five patients using this regimen using the same markers averaged 0.8 cm. Elongation of the tendon graft leads to decreased strength over time.

Biceps to Triceps Tendon Transfer

The biceps to triceps tendon transfer is my preferred method for establishing elbow extension (Fig. 36-3). The biceps is used as the donor muscle. To verify that function will not be lost with transfer of the tendon, the strength of the brachialis as an elbow flexor and of the supinator as a forearm supinator needs to be verified before transfer. While holding the forearm in supination, the elbow can be contracted against resistance, instructing the patient in biceps relaxation. This can be verified by palpating the groove between the more tubular biceps anteriorly and the flatter brachialis posteriorly to differentially test strength.

In reviewing the segmental innervations of the upper limb from the spinal cord (see Fig. 36-1) note that the biceps, brachialis, and supinator are all innervated at about the same level. If the patient has strong wrist extension, the spinal cord lesion should be below the innervation level of the biceps, brachialis, and supinator, leaving them strong, yet above the innervation of the triceps, leaving it paralyzed. Additionally, the muscles should be palpated and observed, teaching the patient to differentially relax the biceps and still flex the elbow and supinate the forearm. Such findings on clinical examination verify that transfer of the biceps will not lead to a functional loss. Such verification is imperative before proceeding with this surgery.

The biceps to triceps tendon transfer can be performed using a medial[47,75] or a lateral[24,28,64] routing technique. The

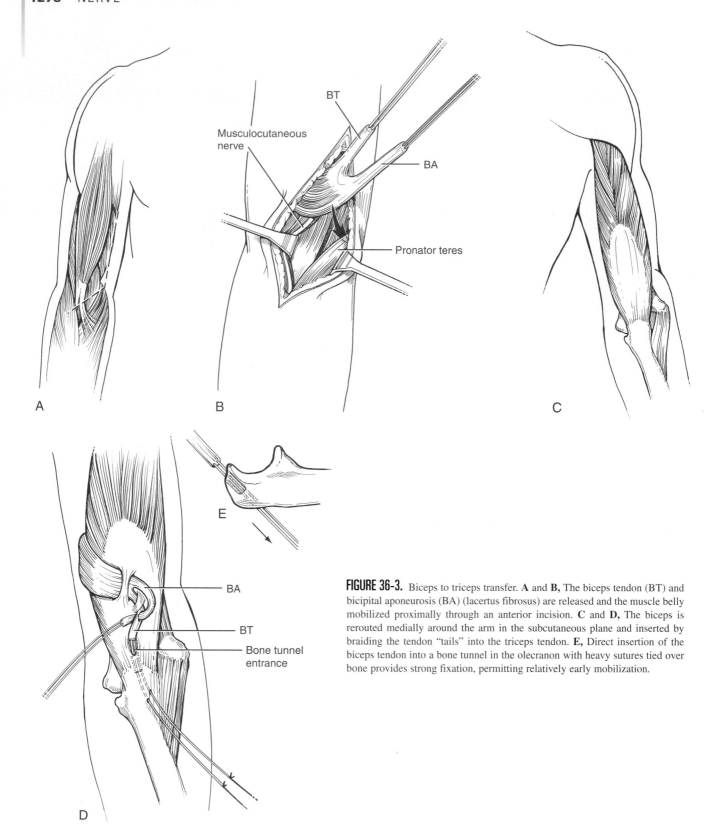

FIGURE 36-3. Biceps to triceps transfer. **A** and **B,** The biceps tendon (BT) and bicipital aponeurosis (BA) (lacertus fibrosus) are released and the muscle belly mobilized proximally through an anterior incision. **C** and **D,** The biceps is rerouted medially around the arm in the subcutaneous plane and inserted by braiding the tendon "tails" into the triceps tendon. **E,** Direct insertion of the biceps tendon into a bone tunnel in the olecranon with heavy sutures tied over bone provides strong fixation, permitting relatively early mobilization.

lateral technique was first described by Friedenberg in 1954[28] and further reported by Zancolli.[86,89] No loss of active elbow flexion was noted, although flexor strength was diminished by 24%. In 1988, Ejeskar[24] reported his results using lateral routing technique in five patients, including the first complication of radial nerve palsy. Because the radial nerve is the only functioning peripheral nerve in these patients, such a complication is devastating and has subsequently been noted by others using the lateral routing technique. Thus, a medial routing is now preferred.

The procedure is performed with the patient in a supine position with a roll under the operative shoulder blade and the limb draped free with a sterile tourniquet used for initial dissection. The incision extends from the mid humerus on the medial side, transversely across the antecubital crease, and distally centering over the biceps insertion on the radial tuberosity.[47] The musculocutaneous nerve is identified and protected as the biceps muscle is dissected free from its medial and lateral fascial attachments and sharply dissected off its insertion on the bicipital tuberosity. The lacertus fibrosus is freed from the forearm fascia during the dissection and is preserved as a second tail of the biceps tendon for subsequent weaving.

A second (posterior) incision is made over the distal one third of the triceps tendon, passing lateral to the olecranon to avoid subsequent olecranon pressure ulceration, and allowing an adequate skin bridge with the medial incision. A subcutaneous tunnel is made medially from the anterior wound to the posterior wound, creating a line of pull that is straight and free for the biceps medial rerouting. The medial intermuscular septum may need to be partially resected. The biceps tendon is passed from the anterior wound, into the posterior wound, superficial to the ulnar nerve. Biceps length will usually allow two or three weaves through the triceps tendon before inserting it into a drill hole in the olecranon. A bone tunnel is created in the tip of the olecranon with a 4-mm (or appropriately sized) drill bit to receive the terminal end of the biceps tendon. A No. 5 nonabsorbable grasping suture is placed into the end of the biceps tendon and passed through the bone tunnel with two small drill holes for passing on a Keith needle, tying the grasping suture over bone.

The transfer is tensioned to allow 60 to 90 degrees of elbow flexion. The lacertus fibrosus is then interwoven through the biceps to triceps weaves to further secure the position. Postoperatively, the elbow is placed in about 30 degrees of flexion in a long-arm cast for 4 weeks. A flexion block splint (hinged elbow orthosis) is then used full time, and 15 degrees of increased flexion is added each week until full flexion and adequate arm control is achieved. Strengthening exercises are then added.

Expected outcome for biceps to triceps transfer is continued improvement in strength over at least 1 year and significant improvement in activities of daily living as arm use increases. Published series[24,46,47,87,89] have reported significant functional improvements for overhead, reaching, and driving activities. No clinical loss of active flexion has been reported, although flexor strength has been diminished by 24%[89] in one series. Mulcahey and coworkers[67] have published a randomized prospective comparison of posterior deltoid to biceps versus biceps to triceps with medial routing tendon transfer. These authors reported that at 2 years, seven of eight arms treated with biceps to triceps transfer had antigravity use of the arm, whereas only one of eight arms treated with posterior deltoid to triceps had antigravity use of the arm.

FOREARM PRONATION

Pronation is important to patients who have active wrist extension only (groups 2 and 3). These patients use the automatic or tenodesis effect for grasp, but if the hand cannot be pronated, gravity cannot be used to provide a tenodesis effect. Those patients using a tenodesis brace need pronation for the same reason.

CRITICAL POINTS: BICEPS TO TRICEPS TENDON TRANSFER

INDICATIONS

- Available biceps for donor (adequate brachialis and supinator strength)
- Full passive range of motion or less than a 30-degree elbow flexion contracture
- Absent triceps function

PREOPERATIVE EVALUATION

- Verify brachialis and supinator strength
- Obtain elbow passive range of motion (splint if necessary)
- General indications/contraindications as listed in the introduction to the chapter

PEARLS

- Medial routing avoids possible complication of radial nerve palsy

TECHNICAL POINTS

- Anterior and posterior incisions with adequate skin bridge

- Mobilize biceps tendon with lacertus fibrosus included
- No. 5 Ethibond grasping suture in biceps tendon
- Straight line of pull around *medial* distal one third of the humerus
- Two to three weaves of biceps tendon into triceps tendon
- Terminal end of the biceps tendon into bone tunnel at tip of olecranon

PITFALL

- Posterior incision over olecranon is potential pressure sore area.

POSTOPERATIVE CARE

- Long-arm cast in 30 degrees of flexion for 4 weeks
- Full-time flexion block splint increasing 15 degrees/wk until full range of motion
- Strengthening at 8 weeks, starting with a powder board to eliminate gravity

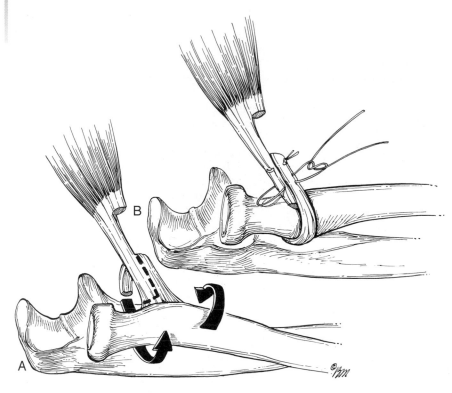

FIGURE 36-4. Zancolli's method for rerouting the insertion of the biceps tendon to provide pronation of the forearm. Half of the tendon is passed behind the neck of the radius (**A**) and then sutured into the remaining biceps tendon (**B**). (From Zancolli EA: Structural and Dynamic Bases of Hand Surgery. Philadelphia, JB Lippincott, 1979.)

Zancolli produced pronation by converting the biceps into a forearm pronator (Fig. 36-4). He rerouted the tendon around the radius, converting the biceps from a supinator to pulling in the opposite direction as a pronator.[88]

GROUP 0

By definition, patients in this group have no muscle groups below their elbow with grade 4 strength (see Table 36-1). Insufficient innervated motors are available for restoration of pinch function without supplemental electrical stimulation,[72] as described later in this chapter. Group 0 patients may be candidates for elbow extension transfers, as already described. Additionally, a few group 0 patients may have both a weak BR and a weak ECRL. Assessing the strength of the BR muscle is difficult and requires an experienced examiner. It is best performed by having the patient flex the elbow against resistance while the examiner evaluates muscle tension by palpitating and trying to deflect the muscle belly. Transfer of the BR to the radial wrist extensors may provide sufficient strength to extend the wrist against resistance; this tendon transfer technique is described below for group 1 patients. The patient would need good elbow extension to serve as an antagonist to the BR transfer to enhance wrist extension function. If sufficient wrist extensor strength were obtained, a wrist-driven hinged tenodesis splint (Fig. 36-5) could be used, or a passive pinch tenodesis reconstruction could be considered as a later reconstruction.

GROUP 1

Patients in this group have BR with grade 4 or greater strength, and all other muscles groups below the elbow have less than grade 4 strength (see Table 36-1). As elbow flexion

is provided by the biceps and brachialis (innervated above the level of the BR as shown in Figure 36-1), the BR is available for tendon transfer to provide wrist extension, which is the most necessary basic function. Lateral key pinch can then be provided by tenodesis using a wrist-driven tenodesis splint as shown in Figure 36-5 or by surgical reconstruction.

Two procedures are necessary for group 1 patients, and both can be done simultaneously, if desired: (1) BR to ECRB for active wrist extension and (2) passive key pinch reconstruction.

BR to ECRB Tendon Transfer (Fig. 36-6)

I prefer the technique described by Freehafer and Mast.[25,26] They make a "utilitarian" incision on the radial side of the forearm near the junction of the proximal and middle thirds. At this site the BR is on the radial aspect of the forearm, the ECRL is dorsal and parallel to it, and the ECRB is on the ulnar side of the longus. The tendons are exposed by opening their sheaths. The BR tendon is dissected off its insertion, preserving sufficient length of the proximal stump so that it can be threaded through the ECRB tendon for a strong tendon juncture. Special care is required to protect the branches of the superficial radial nerve beneath the BR muscle and tendon. Another critical technical detail is adequate proximal dissection of the BR muscle belly. It must be mobilized toward the elbow sufficiently to increase its excursion to 3 cm or more.[45] The BR tendon is passed through a small slit in ECRB tendon, looped back, and sutured back to itself, or alternatively, with two to three Pulvertaft weaves. The BR tendon is usually woven through and sutured only to the ECRB tendon to reduce radial deviation of the wrist. The tension should be set with the elbow at 45 degrees of flexion, with tension sufficient to hold the wrist in 0 degrees. Postoperatively, a long-arm cast is applied in the operating room to hold the elbow in 90

CRITICAL POINTS: BR TO ECRB TENDON TRANSFER

INDICATIONS

- Group 1 patient with > grade 4 strength BR with < grade 4 strength of wrist extension
- Group 0 patient with grade 3 strength BR and < grade 4 strength wrist extension

PREOPERATIVE EVALUATION

- Strength testing (BR, ECRL, ECRB)
- General indications/contraindications as listed in the introduction to the chapter

PEARLS

- Full mobilization of the BR to achieve excursion of 3 cm or more after fascial dissection

TECHNICAL POINTS

- Utilitarian radial side incision extending the proximal incision enough to fully mobilize the BR from its fascial attachments

- BR to ECRB tendon transfer with two to three tendon weaves sewn in place
- Tension so that with 45 degrees of elbow flexion the wrist rests at neutral. With elbow extension, the wrist extends; with elbow flexion, the wrist flexes.

PITFALLS

- Inadequate BR excursion
- Inadequate tendon weaves
- Not too tight and not too loose; if it is not too tight or too loose, it is probably just right.*
- Protect superficial branch of radial nerve

POSTOPERATIVE CARE

- Long-arm cast for 4 weeks.
- Active range of motion with protective wrist cock-up splint for an additional 4 weeks; then strengthening and functional use with night splint if necessary.

---

* Editor's note (DPG): Dr. Van Heest is not being flippant when she gives this advice about tension. Setting the proper tension on any tendon transfer is not only difficult but virtually impossible to teach precisely. There is a "feel" to proper tension that is learned only through experience, and most fellows and residents have a sense of frustration when trying to learn this difficult aspect of surgical technique. Until we have some more accurate biomechanical means to assess tension, her admonition is probably the best we have to offer.

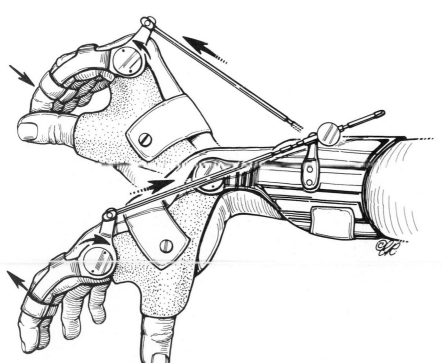

FIGURE 36-5 The wrist-driven flexor hinge splint uses the principle of synergistic action. As the wrist is extended, the fingers are flexed to bring them into contact with the thumb, which is fixed. As the wrist is flexed, the fingers are extended. (Courtesy of T. Engen, MD.)

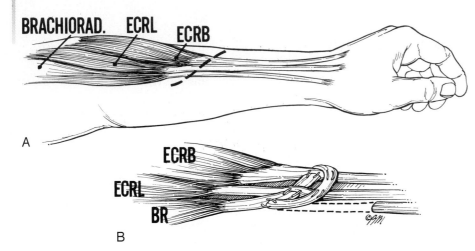

FIGURE 36-6. Brachioradialis (BR) transfer to extensor carpi radialis longus (ECRL) and extensor carpi radialis brevis (ECRB). An important technical detail is that the BR muscle belly must be mobilized completely to the elbow, taking care to protect its nerve supply from the radial nerve. I prefer to weave the BR three times into the wrist extensor (ECRB). Usually the ECRL is not included in the juncture (see text).

degrees of flexion and the wrist in 45 degrees of extension. The cast is removed at 4 weeks, and the active range of motion is started, using a removable splint to support the wrist when the patient is not exercising for an additional 4 weeks. Then strengthening and functional use is advanced with night splinting only if necessary. Transfer of the BR to a weak or nonfunctioning radial wrist extensor should provide adequate strength for the use of a hinged tenodesis splint or surgical reconstruction of a passive pinch function.

Passive Key Pinch Reconstruction

To say that reconstruction of the paralyzed thumb for pinch function is a difficult proposition is an understatement at best. In activities of daily living, lateral key pinch is most useful. Although pulp-to-pulp pinch was described by Bunnell in 1944[11] and referred to by Curtis[17] as an "opponodesis," this procedure has largely been abandoned, because opposition pinch is beyond the scope of restoration in high-level injury.[3,84] Skeletal control of three segmental joints (CMC, MP, and IP) needs to be combined with tenodesis vectors that appropriately position the thumb for effective pinch and release.

Because no additional muscles are available in this group (after BR to ECRB transfer), tenodesis of the FPL is used to produce a weak pinch, motored by active wrist extension (from BR to ECRB transfer). Tenodesis of the EPL is used for release of pinch, activated through passive wrist flexion. Alternatives to passive key pinch tenodesis reconstruction are use of a tenodesis splint (see Fig. 36-5) or functional electrical stimulation (see page 1294).

Mentioned by Bunnell,[11] and popularized by Moberg,[61] the following combination has been recommended for passive key pinch reconstruction:

1. FPL tenodesis to the radius at the proximal edge of the pronator quadratus
2. Kirschner wire fixation of the IP joint to prevent premature and excessive flexion (Froment's sign).

Additional optional steps could include:

1. A1 pulley release to increase FPL flexion axis at the MP joint
2. Tenodesis of the EPB to the dorsal first metacarpal to avoid MP hyperflexion.

This combination is classically referred to as the "Moberg tenodesis pinch" reconstruction as shown in Figure 36-7.

Moberg's procedure has been modified to change the technique for the FPL tenodesis, so that it is divided high in the forearm, delivered into a volar wound over the MP joint through the flexor sheath proximal to the A1 pulley, and rerouted across the palm, deep to the flexor tendons and neurovascular bundles. The FPL tendon is passed proximally via Guyon's canal and is anchored onto the volar aspect of the radius. This change in pull provides a greater

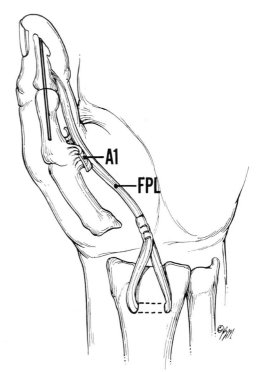

FIGURE 36-7. The classic "Moberg" passive keypinch reconstruction included FPL tenodesis to the radius at the proximal edge of the pronator quadratus and Kirschner wire fixation of the IP joint to prevent premature flexion (Froment's sign). Additional optional steps could include A1 pulley release to increase FPL torque at the MP joint and fixation of the EPB to the dorsal first metacarpal to avoid MP hyperflexion. This classic combination is used very infrequently, because it has undergone many modifications as described in the text. (From Moberg EA: Surgical treatment for absent single-hand grip and elbow extension in quadriplegia. J Bone Joint Surg [Am] 57:196-206, 1975.)

adduction moment arm, in addition to flexion. This modification is termed the *Brand-Moberg tenodesis* but when reviewed by Hentz[32,33] was shown to provide less pinch power than the original Moberg tenodesis.

Alternative techniques for the FPL tenodesis include fixation of the FPL tendon around the distal ulna as a "winch procedure," as described by Brummer.[8] Forearm supination helps activate the tenodesis as it "winds up" the ulna, which pulls the thumb into lateral pinch. This is generally not acceptable because most functional activities are not carried out with simultaneous supination, wrist extension, and thumb pinch; however, for very high level involvement, the tenodesis strength of wrist extension is augmented with the added strength of forearm supination.

Moberg stressed the importance of and described techniques for creating key pinch,[60,61] and Hentz[33] modified Moberg's original tenodesis as follows:

1. Stabilization of the thumb IP joint by pin fixation, fusion, or split FPL transfer (see intrinsic reconstruction section on page 1290 for technique)
2. FPL tenodesis to the distal radius for the correct tension for lateral pinch
3. Stabilization of the MP joint. If greater than 45 degrees of flexion is present, use extensor pollicis brevis (EPB) and EPL tenodesis to the dorsal first metacarpal with a bone anchor suture; if greater than 10 degrees of passive hyperextension is present, use a volar capsulodesis or an MP arthrodesis.

Many authors have reported fairly uniformly good results using this procedure. Results are diminished in group 1 patients compared with groups 2 and 3. Ejeskar[24] reported a typical series with an average final pinch strength of 0.7 kg. However, pinch *power* may be less important than thumb positioning. Because of the common supination posturing of the thumb after a modified Moberg type reconstruction, I prefer a CMC arthrodesis to better control thumb position as described by House[35] in the active one-stage key pinch reconstruction (see later under groups 2 and 3).

GROUPS 2 AND 3

By definition, patients in these groups have BR and wrist extension with grade 4 or greater strength, and all other muscles groups below the elbow have less than grade 4 strength (see Table 36-1). One of the deficiencies in the International Classification is the difficulty present in determining the differential strength of ECRL (group 2) and ECRB (group 3). If the patient has grade 4 or greater strength of the ECRL and grade 0 strength of the ECRB, then significant radial deviation will occur; however, this large difference between ECRL and ECRB strength is uncommon. In my experience, both the ECRL and ECRB show active function, making it impossible to clearly differentiate group 2 (grade 4 or greater ECRL only) from group 3 (grade 4 or greater ECRL and ECRB). If the ECRB is less than grade 4 strength, and the ECRL is transferred, the result is devastating, with functional loss of wrist extension. To avoid this serious complication, I prefer to treat patients in group 2 and 3 identically and not transfer either the ECRL or ECRB. Methods have been described to differentially

test ECRL versus ECRB strength. Mohammed and coworkers[65] described on clinical examination finding Bean's sign: a groove between the ECRL and the ECRB if both are firing at grade 4 or greater strength. Moberg[62] stated that the only way to measure differential ECRB versus ECRL is with surgical exploration; with the use of local anesthesia, a needle is passed through the ECRB tendon and hooked up to a 5-kg weight. If the ECRB can lift at least 5 kg, then the ECRL can be used without risk of loss of wrist extension function. Allieu[2] stated that if PT function is present, then the two radial wrist extensor strengths can be assumed to be intact. Hentz and LeClerq[33] stated that in 25 years they have only had one patient who was treated as a group 3 patient with transfer of the ECRL but was actually a group 2 patient, with resultant loss of wrist extension function. Hentz recommended transfer of the ECRL only if the ECRB is grade 5 strength (not grade 4 strength). Most surgeons recommend using the ECRL for transfer and leaving the ECRB in place, because its insertion is more central.[35,54,87]

Review of the literature shows a variety of options described for group 2 and 3 patients. For the patients in groups 2 and 3, the BR is always available for transfer and has been used in a variety of ways. Street and Stambaugh[80] recognized the value of side pinch or "key grip" in 1959 and, in an attempt to increase the strength of pinch, transferred the BR to the FPL. Moberg reported four patients with BR transfer to FPL, and on comparison he found the FPL tenodesis to be stronger than the transfer. House[34] and Zancolli[88] preferred to stabilize the thumb CMC joint with an arthrodesis to ensure positioning the thumb in some abduction. In most cases, House transferred the BR to the FPL for a one-stage active key pinch reconstruction.

Moberg used the BR to open the thumb-index web space to improve the release phase of the grasp-release sequence. He tested the EPL, EPB, and abductor pollicis longus (APL) at surgery to determine which gave the best abduction and then transferred the BR to that one. He did this operation as a second-stage procedure, following construction of his simple key grip (lateral pinch). He reported that the additional abduction was not as useful for the patient as he had anticipated.[61]

For group 3 patients, Zancolli[87] recommended a two-stage reconstruction. The first stage is (1) extensor tenodesis of the thumb and fingers; (2) intrinsic tenodesis using the "lasso" procedure to reduce clawing; and (3) thumb IP joint fusion. The second stage is (1) ECRL to FDP tendon transfer; (2) BR to FPL tendon transfer; (3) if the thumb MP joint is hyperextended, a volar thumb MP capsulodesis; and (4) if the thumb is in excessive extension, a volar tenodesis of the EPB.

Surgical Technique of Zancolli: Staged Reconstruction for Group 3

Stage 1: Extensor Tenodesis

Zancolli makes an 8- to 10-cm longitudinal incision on the radial side of the forearm and exposes the dorsum of the radius proximal to the extensor retinaculum. A window, large enough to accept the distal stumps of the common extensor tendons (which have been divided just distal to the musculotendinous junction), is made on the dorsum of the radius. Suturing the distal stumps together preserves tendon balance. The ends of the sutures are brought through two drill holes made proximal to the window, drawing the tendon stumps snugly into the bone window. The sutures are tied to each other for fixation. Zancolli sets the tension so that the finger MP joints will be extended to 0 degrees with the wrist in slight palmar flexion. A strip of the APL tendon is freed through the original radial longitudinal incision and is kept small enough to pass it proximally through the tunnel of the EPL around Lister's tubercle and into the window on the dorsum of the radius, where it and the tendon of the EPL are sutured to the bone with wire, as described for the common extensor tendons. This tenodesis will produce thumb extension and abduction. Arthrodesis of the thumb IP joint is done to prevent hyperflexion of the joint and to facilitate side pinch. Additionally, a lasso is performed, as described in the intrinsic rebalancing section (see pages 1289 and 1290).

Stage 2

When scar resolution is complete and the preoperative range of motion is restored, the second-stage operation is done. The same radial lateral incision used in stage 1 is reopened to expose the ECRL and the FDP tendons. The ECRL is detached at its insertion and transferred to the FDP tendons with an end-to-side connection. Tension is set so that the fingers and thumb come together in a lateral pinch with the wrist in approximately 20 degrees of dorsiflexion. The tension is set loosely enough to allow easy release of the fingers during wrist flexion.

The BR is detached from its insertion (leaving a short stump) and dissected well proximally so that maximum excursion can be obtained. The BR is sutured to the FPL, with tension set to achieve lateral pinch with the wrist in approximately 20 degrees of extension and the elbow at 90 degrees (the same as in the ECRL transfer). If the thumb MP joint is hyperextended, a capsulodesis can be performed, by fixing the volar capsule to bone. The flexor tendon sheath is exposed through a transverse incision just proximal to the thumb MP joint flexion crease. The sheath is opened and the FPL retracted away from the volar plate. Care should be taken to protect the digital nerves. A longitudinal incision is made in the volar plate to expose the neck of the metacarpal. Two holes are drilled in the bone to receive a nonabsorbable suture. The volar plate is pulled proximally and sutured against the bone. Tension is set with the MP joint in 10 degrees of flexion.

Zancolli also constructs a volar tenodesis of the EPB tendon if the thumb is in excessive extension and lateral pinch is impaired. Through the radial incision, the EPB tendon is divided as far proximally as possible. The tendon is passed through the FCR tunnel and sutured into the short distal stump of the BR, which was left in place when it was divided for transfer previously. Tension is set to hold the thumb in complete abduction with the wrist in moderate flexion.

Author's Preferred Method of Treatment

For group 2 and 3 patients, I prefer House's one-stage active key pinch reconstruction[34] consisting of (1) CMC fusion; (2) BR to FPL tendon transfer; (3) EPL tenodesis; (4) split FPL transfer for stabilization of the thumb IP joint; and (5) if the index finger does not flex enough to be a base for key pinch, then a lasso procedure.

Surgical Technique of House One-Stage Key Pinch Reconstruction for Groups 2 and 3

In the House key pinch reconstruction,[34] the following surgical components of the procedure are performed.

CMC Fusion

A 3- to 4-cm incision is made centered over the CMC joint in the interval between the APL and the abductor pollicis brevis (APB). After exposure of the joint, a Kirschner wire is placed from the thumb metacarpal to the index metacarpal to "pre-position" the thumb in the desired key pinch position—about 20 degrees of extension, 30 to 40 degrees of palmar abduction, and 10 degrees of pronation. The pulp of the thumb should be able to pinch against the radial side of the index finger at the PIP level. A thin slice of articular cartilage is resected from the base of the thumb metacarpal and the distal trapezium, using a small oscillating saw and taking care to minimize bone stock loss. The Kirschner wire is withdrawn from the index metacarpal, the joint surfaces are firmly opposed, and the Kirschner wire is advanced back into the index metacarpal, securing the thumb position before final internal fixation. After any appropriate positioning adjustments are made, final fixation is secured with a mini-fragment blade plate, as illustrated in Figure 36-8.

BR to FPL Tendon Transfer

The radial side of the forearm is exposed through a utilitarian radial incision from the proximal third of the radius to the radial styloid. The BR muscle is identified and mobilized until 3 to 4 cm of passive tendon excursion is available. The volar compartment is exposed, identifying and protecting the radial artery. The FCR and flexor digitorum superficialis (FDS) tendons and median nerve are gently retracted ulnarly to expose the FPL tendon. The BR is woven into the FPL tendon, beginning the first weave at the musculotendinous junction. Tension is adjusted so that when the elbow is in about 45 degrees of flexion and the wrist is in neutral, the thumb is in neutral. With wrist extension, the thumb should come into a key pinch position. After EPL tenodesis, the thumb should come into extension with wrist flexion. Tenodesis key pinch should also be tested with elbow flexion and extension before final weaving.

EPL Tenodesis

The proximal portion of the EPL tendon is exposed from the utilitarian radial side incision after identifying and protecting the superficial radial nerve. The tendon is divided at the level of the musculotendinous junction. The EPL is left in the third dorsal compartment, and the proximal portion of the tendon is woven through the extensor retinaculum just radial to Lister's tubercle and woven back into itself distal to the retinaculum. This creates an EPL loop around Lister's tubercle, as shown in Figure 36-9; fixation can be augmented with a bone anchor into Lister's tubercle if necessary.

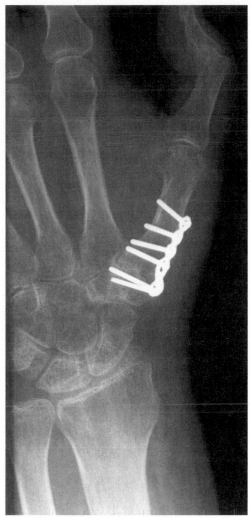

FIGURE 36-8. Mini-blade plate CMC fusion. CMC fusion is best achieved using stable internal fixation; this allows mobilization of the hand when the tendon transfers are ready for active motion at 4 weeks after surgery.

Split FPL Transfer

The split FPL transfer option is used to correct Froment's sign that leads to premature and excessive flexion of the thumb IP joint, which can prevent proper placement of the pulp onto the index finger for key pinch. Surgical technique is described as part of intrinsic rebalancing (see page 1291).

If the index finger does not flex into a key pinch position as part of the hand's natural tenodesis, index finger MP joint flexion can be enhanced through use of a lasso tenodesis. Surgical technique is described as part of intrinsic rebalancing (see page 1292).

GROUPS 4 AND 5

By definition, patients in this group have BR and wrist extension (ECRL and ECRB) as well as PT (group 4) and FCR (group 5) with grade 4 or greater strength, and all other muscles groups below the elbow have less than grade 4 strength (see Table 36-1).

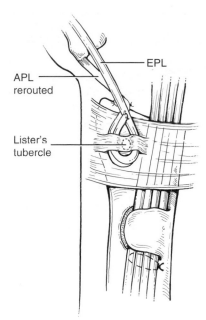

FIGURE 36-9. EPL tenodesis is woven through the extensor retinaculum, around Lister's tubercle, and back onto itself. This loop can be augmented by a bone anchor suture at Lister's tubercle if necessary. APL, abductor pollicis longus.

In patients in group 4, the PT is strong enough to consider for transfer. The PT does provide strong action for manual wheelchair propulsion and should be avoided as a donor for transfer if this action is important to the patient. In its use for reconstruction, Zancolli transferred the PT to the FCR to further enhance the usefulness of the wrist-activated tenodesis or tendon transfer to the FPL operations. House[37] described transferring the PT to the FPL as part of his two-stage reconstruction. His experience since the 1970s is that transferring the PT does not produce a significant loss of pronation (JH House, personal communication, 2003).

In patients in group 5, the addition of wrist flexion strength improves antagonist power for the wrist extension-driven tenodesis function of the fingers. In 1958, Lipscomb and colleagues[54] and, in 1971, Lamb and Landry[50] reported transfer of the FCR in this group. House's method favors leaving the FCR in place to preserve maximum wrist control.

In groups 4 and 5, the BR, ECR, and the PT muscles are available for transfer. The ECRB and the FCR are left in place to preserve good wrist control. Because there are more muscles available in patients in groups 4 and 5, the surgeon most commonly would choose a two-stage reconstruction of grasp (flexor phase) and release (extensor phase), using either of the methods described by House and Zancolli. At the first stage (extensor phase), the thumb is positioned and the extensor tendons are tenodesed. At the second stage (flexor phase), the thumb and finger flexor tendons are activated for grasp and the finger intrinsics are activated for balance. Other options include a simple lateral pinch reconstruction, or a single-stage reconstruction, prioritizing grasp.

The author's preferred method is the House two-stage reconstruction using a thumb CMC joint arthrodesis to place the thumb in optimum position. The first choice for positioning the thumb is arthrodesis of the thumb CMC joint because it ensures a stable and permanent position.

CRITICAL POINTS: HOUSE ONE-STAGE KEY PINCH

INDICATIONS

- Group 1 patients using FPL for passive tenodesis
- Group 2 and 3 patients with > grade 4 wrist extensor strength using BR to FPL for active pinch
- General indications/contraindications as listed in the introduction to the chapter

PREOPERATIVE EVALUATION

- Verify BR and wrist extensor strength
- Evaluate thumb position and index finger position in its "natural tenodesis" pattern to verify that this combination of FPL tenodesis, EPL tenodesis, and CMC fusion will obtain desired thumb position

PEARLS

- Thumb is tensioned so that it "hits" the lateral aspect of the PIP joint of the index finger with wrist extension and opens with wrist flexion providing adequate clearance for release.

TECHNICAL POINTS (INCLUDE EACH OF THE FOLLOWING STEPS)

1. CMC fusion: stable mini-fragment fixation after parallel CMC joint surfaces are prepared positioning the thumb in 40 degrees of abduction, 25 degrees of extension, and 10 degrees of pronation—yet most importantly so that the thumb "hits" the lateral aspect of the PIP joint of the index finger.
2. EPL tenodesis: the EPL is tenodesed around Lister's tubercle, woven through the extensor retinaculum and back through itself, tight enough to allow full thumb opening with passive wrist flexion and full passive thumb flexion with passive wrist extension.
3. BR to FPL transfer (group 2 and 3): full mobilization of the BR tendon with Pulvertaft weaves to the FPL.
4. Split FPL transfer for IP stabilization (see section on Intrinsic Reconstruction).
5. If the fingers do not pull into enough flexion to allow a stable base for key pinch reconstruction, then a lasso procedure may be necessary (see section on Intrinsic Reconstruction on page 1290)

PITFALLS

- Not too tight and not too loose; if it is not too tight or too loose, it is probably just right. (See Editor's Note for Critical Points: BR to ECRB Tendon Transfer, earlier in this chapter.)
- Check thumb position based both on elbow flexion/extension as well as on wrist flexion/extension because the BR is a biarticular muscle crossing both joints.

POSTOPERATIVE CARE

- Thumb spica short-arm cast in neutral to protect from active flexion/extension of the thumb for 4 weeks.
- Active range of motion with protective forearm-based thumb splint for an additional 4 weeks; then strengthening and functional use with night splint if necessary

However, when bilateral reconstruction is performed, a different technique is often used for each thumb.[36] The second thumb has an adduction-opponensplasty transfer (Fig. 36-10) to maximize mobility. One of the available motors (usually BR) is then transferred to the paralyzed FDS graft in the forearm[7,35] to motor the opponensplasty.

Surgical Technique of House Two-Stage Grasp, Pinch, and Release

Stage 1: Extensor Phase (Fig. 36-11)

CMC Fusion

An incision is made over the interval between the APL tendon and the APB, centered over the CMC joint of the thumb. After the superficial radial nerve branches are protected, the trapeziometacarpal joint is exposed through this interval. A pre-positioning Kirschner wire from the midportion of the thumb metacarpal and advanced into the index metacarpal is placed, positioning the thumb for lateral or key pinch in approximately 20 degrees of extension, 40 degrees of palmar abduction, and 10 degrees of pronation. Articular cartilage is resected from the base of the thumb metacarpal and the trapezium. The wire is withdrawn from the index metacarpal to allow firm apposition of the joint surfaces, and the Kirschner wire that had been placed between the thumb and index metacarpals is reinserted into the index metacarpal to further stabilize the thumb ray in an appropriate position. Appropriate orientation and thumb position is confirmed. A mini-blade plate or internal fixation plate is then used for fusion fixation as shown in Figure 36-8, and the stabilizing Kirschner wire can be removed.

EPL and EDC Tenodeses

EPL Tenodesis. The proximal portion of the EPL tendon is exposed from the utilitarian radial side incision after identifying and protecting the superficial radial nerve. The tendon is divided at the level of the musculotendinous junction. The EPL is left in the third dorsal compartment, and the proximal portion of the tendon is woven through the extensor retinaculum just radial to Lister's tubercle and woven back into itself distal to the retinaculum. This creates an EPL loop around Lister's tubercle, as shown in Figure 36-9; this can be augmented in its fixation with a bone anchor stitch into Lister's tubercle if necessary.

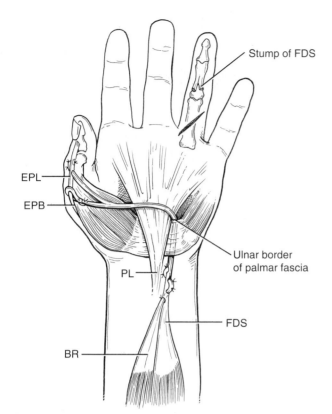

FIGURE 36-10. The "adduction-opponensplasty" is produced by transfer of a motor to the paralyzed flexor superficialis as an "in situ tendon graft" rerouted around a palmar fascial "pulley" to a dual insertion that controls thumb rotation and stabilizes the MP and IP joints for more effective lateral pinch. The BR is usually used as the motor in group 5, and the FCU in group 7 or 8. (Adapted from House JH, Gwathmey F, Lundsgaard DK: Restoration of strong grasp and lateral pinch in tetraplegia due to cervical spinal cord injury. J Hand Surg [Am] 10:22-29, 1985.)

Finger extension is produced by tenodesis of the common extensors to the distal radius or tendon transfer of the BR to the EPL and common extensors. If a tenodesis of the extensor tendons to the distal radius is chosen, the extensor digitorum tendons are exposed through the utilitarian radial side incision. The antebrachial fascia is opened from the proximal edge of the extensor retinaculum to the musculo-tendinous junction. Retracting the extensor indicis proprius (EIP) and the common extensors ulnarward exposes the floor of the fourth dorsal compartment. A 2 × 2-cm flap of periosteum is elevated, leaving it attached on its ulnar side. Next, the common extensor tendons are sutured together with the fingers in balance using nonabsorbable suture. The tendons are secured into a bone window into the metaphysis or onto the radial metaphysis with bone anchor sutures. The periosteal flap is then sewed over the extensor tendons using a 2-0 braided, nonabsorbable suture. The tension is adjusted so that when the wrist is passively flexed to 30 degrees, the MP joints are held at 0 degrees; full finger flexion is possible with full wrist extension.

Option: BR to EPL/EDC Tendon Transfer. One may choose to use the BR for tendon transfer to produce some active thumb and finger extension, provided that the BR is not needed for the flexor phase of the reconstruction. The

BR tendon is exposed through the utilitarian radial side incision. The tendon is divided at its insertion and freed from its investing fascia to the proximal third of the forearm, taking care to protect the superficial radial nerve, lying directly underneath. This extensive mobilization of the BR is required to produce 3 to 4 cm of excursion.

The antebrachial fascia overlying the tendons of the EPL and EDC proximal to the extensor retinaculum is excised. The BR tendon is woven through the EDC, EIP, and EPL tendons, with the tendon weaves sewn proximal to the proximal edge of the extensor retinaculum. Appropriate tension is achieved by having the MP joints of the fingers at 0 degrees while the wrist is passively flexed to 30 degrees and the elbow is flexed to 45 degrees; the MP joints can be passively flexed with the wrist in extension. Furthermore, the thumb should sit against the lateral side of the index finger in a key pinch posture.

Stage 2: Flexor Phase (Fig. 36-12)
If the BR was transferred in the extensor phase, the ECRL is transferred to the FDP for digital flexion, and the PT is transferred to the FPL for pinch. If the BR has not been used, then the ECR is transferred to the FDP and the BR is transferred to the FPL.

ECRL to FDP Tendon Transfer
The same utilitarian radial side incision that was used in the extensor phase is reopened. Through this incision, the FDP and FPL tendons are exposed at and distal to their musculo-tendinous junctions. Dorsally, the ECRL is exposed and divided at its insertion. The ECRL tendon is passed proximally in the wound, and dissected away from the investing fascia to improve its excursion and to create a straight line to its new insertion. The ECRL tendon is woven through each of the profundus tendons and sutured with care to produce balance among all of the fingers. In addition to finger balance, tension should be set by observing finger motion during passive wrist flexion and extension and tested again in varying degrees of elbow flexion. Full extension of the MP and IP joints is possible when the wrist is passively flexed.

BR to FPL Tendon Transfer
The BR tendon is exposed through the same utilitarian radial side incision. The tendon is divided at its insertion and freed from its investing fascia to the proximal third of the forearm, taking care to protect the superficial radial nerve lying directly underneath. This extensive mobilization of the BR is required to produce 3 to 4 cm of excursion. The BR is woven into the FPL tendon and the tension sewn so that the thumb comes into contact with the lateral side of the index finger when the wrist is passively extended to 0 degrees.

Option: PT to FPL Tendon Transfer
The PT is also available for transfer to the FPL. The PT can be harvested from its radial insertion, adding additional length to the tendon by a long periosteal extension. When the tendon-periosteal material is sutured into the FPL, the tension should be set so that the thumb comes into contact with the lateral side of the index finger when the wrist is passively extended to 0 degrees.

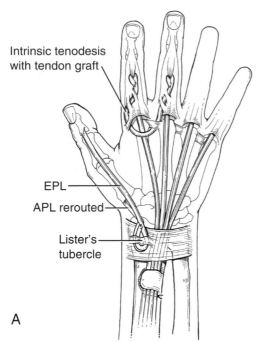
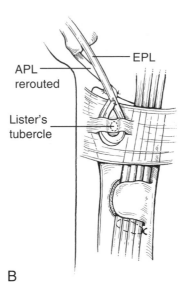

Intrinsic tenodesis
with tendon graft

EPL

APL rerouted

Lister's
tubercle

A

EPL

APL
rerouted

Lister's
tubercle

B

FIGURE 36-11. A, Stage 1 (extensor phase) of House's two-stage reconstruction for patients in group 5. Tenodesis of the EDC is accomplished by fixation of the tendons into a "horseshoe window" in the distal radius with a heavy suture that also balances the relative tension of all four fingers. The EPL and APL (rerouted through the third dorsal compartment) are usually passed around Lister's tubercle and braided together to provide balanced thumb abduction and extension and sutured in a loop around the extensor retinaculum. Intrinsic tenodesis of the index and middle fingers is also performed in this stage with a free tendon graft routed through the lumbrical canals, beneath the deep transverse metacarpal ligament, around the second metacarpal, and braided and sutured into the lateral bands and central slips of each finger. The same technique is used for the ring and little fingers (around the fourth metacarpal) when IP joint extension is inadequate in those digits. **B,** Close-up views of technique. (Adapted from House JH, Gwathmey F, Lundsgaard DK: Restoration of strong grasp and lateral pinch in tetraplegia due to cervical spinal cord injury. J Hand Surg [Am] 10:22-29, 1985.)

CRITICAL POINTS: HOUSE TWO-STAGE GRASP, PINCH, AND RELEASE

INDICATIONS

- Group 4 patients with BR, ECRL, ECRB, and PT strength grade 4/5 or greater
- Group 5 patients with BR, ECRL, ECRB, PT, and FCR strength grade 4/5 or greater

PREOPERATIVE EVALUATION

- Verify muscle strength testing
- General indications/contraindications as listed in the introduction to the chapter

PEARLS

- At least three tendon weaves increases strength at the tendon weave junctions

TECHNICAL POINTS

Flexor Phase

1. CMC fusion for thumb positioning
2. EDC and EPL tenodesis for passive finger and thumb extension

Option: BR to EDC and EPL tendon transfers for active finger and thumb extension

Extensor Phase

1. ECRL to FDP tendon transfer for active finger flexion
2. BR to FPL tendon transfer for active thumb pinch

Option: PT to FPL tendon transfer for active thumb pinch (if BR was used in extensor phase)

PITFALL

- Not too tight and not too loose; if it is not too tight or too loose, it is probably just right. (See Editor's Note, page 1281.)

POSTOPERATIVE CARE

- After each phase, a cast is worn to protect the repairs for 4 weeks
- Active range of motion with protective forearm-based thumb splint for an additional 4 weeks, then strengthening and functional use with night splint if necessary

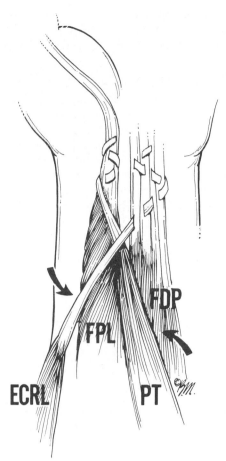

FIGURE 36-12. Stage 2 (flexor phase) of House's reconstruction includes both ECRL to FDP tendon transfer, as well as FPL tendon transfer. Another option would be ECRL to FDP with BR to FPL tendon transfers. (Adapted from House JH, Gwathmey F, Lundsgaard DK: Restoration of strong grasp and lateral pinch in tetraplegia due to cervical spinal cord injury. J Hand Surg [Am] 10:22-29, 1985.)

GROUPS 6 AND 7

Patients in these groups have at least grade 4 strength of the BR, ECRL, ECRB, PT, and FCR. Additionally, at least grade 4 strength of the EDC is present in group 6, and also of EPL in group 7 (see Table 36-1). Because some degree of finger/thumb extension is present for these patients, a separate extensor phase is not required. Reconstruction for these groups of patients consists of a flexor phase only. Because these patients have active unopposed digital extension, they often present with a characteristic "flat hand" appearance[33] without significant digital contraction. Their digital function is not significantly greater than groups 4 and 5, however, because they lack active grasp and release. Additionally, patients at this lower level of spinal cord injury also have stronger shoulder and elbow control, so their ability to position their hand in space is usually excellent. They benefit greatly from grasp and pinch reconstructive surgery.

For the group 6 patients, the finger extensors are strong but EPL function is either absent or too weak to extend the thumb adequately. The EPL can be tenodesed to the dorsal radius or transferred into the digital extensors to improve thumb extension. This can effectively be done in conjunction with the flexor transfers, yet it is also reasonable to divide the operation into two procedures if desired.

For the group 7 patient, both finger and thumb extensors are strong, so the flexor phase alone is performed. Thumb control can be achieved through either CMC fusion or opponensplasty, depending on the thumb's stability and position as well as the patient's desires. Many patients prefer different techniques for each thumb.[34]

Results after surgery in patients in groups 6 and 7 are much better than in higher groups because normal extensor function gives the patient more precise control. Also, better shoulder and elbow control allows these patients better upper extremity use.

Surgical Technique of Group 6 and 7 Reconstructions

The extensor phase for group 6 can be performed simultaneously with the flexor reconstruction (author's preference) or staged. The EPL can be transferred to the common extensors so that active extension of the fingers will produce extension of the thumb, or the EPL can be tenodesed to the dorsal radius as part of the flexor phase. Braiding a half-thickness slip of the EPL tendon through the EDC allows the length-tension relationship of the EPL to remain and ensures that relative tension will be maintained between the multiple EDC and EPL tendons. They are firmly sutured together with three or four horizontal mattress sutures of a nonabsorbable material. If the common extensor tendon to the index finger is small, additional common extensor tendons can be included to produce a strong union. Tension is set with all extensors in the relaxed posture.

ECRL to FDP for Active Finger Flexion
The technique is described under group 4 and 5 reconstruction.

BR or PT to FPL for Active Pinch
The technique is described under group 4 and 5 reconstruction.

Thumb Control Options
Examination for joint instability is essential. The CMC joint can be fused to provide key pinch positioning, as described on page 1284 under group 2 and 3 reconstruction. The MP can be fused if unstable, using a capsulodesis technique or a sesamoid fusion technique as described by Zancolli.[87] The IP joint can be controlled from hyperflexion (Froment's sign) using the "split FPL" technique as described under the intrinsic reconstruction section on page 1290. Additional power and positioning control can be provided by performing an opponensplasty using the BR or PT as a motor, as described under group 4 and 5 reconstruction.

Lasso Procedures
These patients have excellent selective digital control because their digital extensors are intact, but they may also benefit from an active lasso, as described under Intrinsic Reconstruction. Tendon transfer using the BR or PT to FDS can provide a motor to the lasso. This type of tendon transfer strengthens this lasso procedure.

GROUP 8

Group 8 patients have weak finger flexion and lack intrinsic function. Usually, the long flexors to the ulnar digits (ring and small fingers) are stronger than those to the thumb, index, and long fingers.

Flexion of the index and long fingers can be improved or strengthened by connecting all four profundus tendons together. An active motor should be transferred to give independent function of the FPL. Finally, intrinsic balance will need to be assessed and addressed as outlined in the next section. The reconstruction can be performed as a two-staged reconstruction as described by Zancolli[88] or in one stage (author's preference).

Technique for Zancolli's Two-Stage Reconstruction (Group 8)

Stage I: Extrinsic Transfers

FDP Side-to-Side Transfer

The four profundus tendons are exposed by opening the forearm fascia and retracting the median nerve ulnarward with its palmar cutaneous branch and the four superficial tendons. A site in the distal forearm is selected for side-to-side suture of the four profundus tendons. The peritenon is scraped away from the tendons for a distance of 3 cm, and the tendons are sutured together with horizontal mattress sutures using nonabsorbable material. Half of the FDP of the index finger is woven transversely across the other FDP tendons to ensure proper relative tension among the four tendons.[37] The fingers should be evenly balanced during the connection.

BR to FPL Transfer

As described in the previous sections, the BR is transferred directly to the FPL and connected by braiding the tendon of the BR into the tendon of the FPL with the wrist in neutral and the thumb just touching the side of the index finger, with mild tension on the BR.

Stage 2: Intrinsic Reconstruction

Opponensplasty

The opponens transfer can be motored by the flexor carpi ulnaris (FCU), and the palmaris longus can be used as a free tendon graft (if it is not present, a toe extensor or the plantaris tendon may be used) to extend the tendon of the FCU to its insertion into the ulnar side of the base of the proximal phalanx of the thumb. The FCU is exposed through an "L"-shaped incision over its insertion, which is split in half for a distance of 3 to 4 cm proximal to its insertion. One half of the tendon is left attached to the pisiform, and this segment is divided 3 to 4 cm proximal to the insertion. The proximal end of this segment is sutured to the insertion to create a loop. The other half is detached from the pisiform and attached to the proximal end of the free tendon graft using a braiding technique. A subcutaneous tunnel is created from the loop to the MP joint of the thumb. The tendon graft is passed around the loop at the pisiform and through the subcutaneous tunnel to be attached to the tendon of the APB

at the base of the proximal phalanx. Tension is adjusted so that with the wrist in neutral the thumb pulp will just touch the radial side of the index finger.

Zancolli Lasso

As described in the intrinsic reconstruction section (see below), Zancolli[87] recommended transfer of the ECRL to the FDS tendons to produce active control of the lasso intrinsic replacement.

The intrinsic replacement procedure is modified as described by Zancolli by transferring the ECRL tendon to the superficialis tendons in the forearm. After the distal portion of the lasso procedure is complete, as shown in Figure 36-14, then tension is set so that with the wrist in neutral the MP joints of the fingers are at 0 degrees.

GROUP 9

Patients in group 9 have functioning superficialis muscles, as well as all the other extrinsic finger and thumb flexors and extensors, but do not have intrinsic muscle innervation. This is the smallest group in patients with tetraplegia[33] and in many ways can be treated much like a patient with a combined low median and ulnar peripheral nerve palsy. These patients will benefit most from opponensplasty and from intrinsic reconstructions, tailored to the intrinsic imbalance present. The lasso operation, described later, can be expected to be more effective because the superficialis muscles are under voluntary control in group 9 patients.

INTRINSIC RECONSTRUCTION

Tendon transfer surgery in patients with spinal cord injury has focused primarily on reconstruction of extrinsic muscle function for grasp, pinch, and release. After spinal cord injury, loss of intrinsic and extrinsic control leads to varying degrees of muscle imbalance, influenced by the level of motor control, flaccid paralysis, spasticity, and ligamentous laxity, as well as different post-injury splinting protocols. Extrinsic reconstructive procedures refer to the tendon transfers or tenodeses used to restore the functions of muscles originating in the forearm or at the elbow. Intrinsic reconstruction procedures are an adjunct to extrinsic reconstructions and serve to improve the results of extrinsic procedures. Intrinsic reconstructive procedures are tendon transfers or tenodeses designed to improve intrinsic balance in the fingers and/or thumb. Extrinsic reconstructive procedures done *with* intrinsic reconstructions have been shown to have greater final follow-up grip strength than those done *without* intrinsic reconstructions.[55] Intrinsic reconstructions can be done in conjunction with the extrinsic reconstructions or as a separate staged procedure. They need to be tailored to the particular intrinsic imbalance present. In patients with little digital imbalance, the extrinsic reconstruction is performed without concomitant intrinsic transfers.

Patient evaluation needs to include assessment of digital balance. Evaluation of passive motion of the joints is necessary, as is assessment of dynamic deformity and position of the fingers with wrist tenodesis. At the MP joint, lack of intrinsics can lead to MP hyperextension deformities (clawing). At the PIP joint, spasticity of the FDS muscles and/or central slip deficits (stretched or incompetent) can lead to PIP joint flexion deformities.

The most common intrinsic imbalances and their recommended treatments include the following:

1. Hyperflexion of the thumb IP joint (Froment's sign) treated with split FPL transfer
2. Clawing of the digits with MP hyperextension of the fingers and PIP flexion with early digital "roll-up" treated with Zancolli lasso procedure. Intrinsic imbalance can lead to early digital roll-up, which occurs when the distal interphalangeal (DIP) joint flexes before the PIP without MP flexion. Such hand positioning makes it very difficult to grasp large objects. The Zancolli lasso procedure helps initiate MP flexion as the first stage of digital roll-up followed by PIP and DIP flexion, which makes large cylindrical grasp more effective.
3. PIP flexion deformity due to central slip deficiency treated with intrinsic tenodesis free grafts

Hyperflexion of the Thumb IP Joint Treated With Split FPL Transfer

Hyperflexion of the thumb IP joint (Froment's sign) often results after restoration of thumb flexion by tendon transfer to the FPL. Hyperflexion of the thumb IP joint significantly impairs the quality of lateral pinch because the thumb pulp misses the index finger. This can be prevented by arthrodesis of the IP joint or by transferring one half of the FPL to the

EPL distally. This split FPL transfer maintains joint flexibility and is the author's preferred method.

Surgical Technique: Split FPL Tenodesis

The final goal of preventing hyperflexion of the thumb IP joint is best achieved by using Sinclair's[65] method of split FPL distal tenodesis (Fig. 36-13). Sinclair and his colleagues described splitting the FPL through a longitudinal incision over the proximal phalanx. The radial half is detached and transferred subcutaneously to the dorsum, where it is sutured to the EPL, thus equalizing the pull on the volar and dorsal sides of the IP joint. I prefer a zigzag palmar incision to provide access for splitting the FPL, mobilizing it proximal to the oblique pulley, and rerouting it around the proximal phalanx to a longitudinal dorsal incision, where it is inserted into the EPL. The tendon is usually set so that the IP joint rests in about 30 degrees of flexion and contacts with the side of the index finger in an appropriate key pinch position.

Digital Clawing Treated With Zancolli Lasso Procedure

The goal of intrinsic balancing operations is to prevent MP joint hyperextension or clawing of the fingers during the extensor phase of function, that is, when the wrist is flexed.[55] The lasso procedure uses the superficialis to flex the MP joints. For patients with a PIP flexion deformity associated with FDS spasticity, the lasso procedure additionally removes the FDS as a spastic deforming force at the PIP joint and transfers it to a more useful position as an MP flexor. The lasso procedure is recommended during the

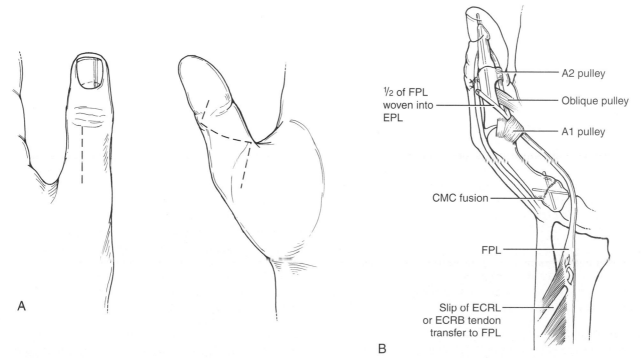

Figure 36-13 The split FPL distal tenodesis: Transfer of the radial half of the FPL to the EPL improves thumb intrinsic balance by stabilizing the MP and IP joints, providing more effective lateral pinch. (Modified from Mohammed KD, Rothwell AG, Sinclair SW, et al: Upper limb surgery for tetraplegia. J Bone Joint Surg Br 74:873-879, 1992.)

CRITICAL POINTS: SPLIT FPL TENDON TRANSFER

INDICATION

- All patients undergoing transfer to the FPL tendon with IP joint flexion of greater than 60 degrees or a Froment sign that precludes effective key pinch positioning of the thumb pulp onto the side of the index finger

PREOPERATIVE EVALUATION

- Joint stability assessment of thumb CMC, MCP, and IP range of motion
- Intraoperative assessment of effect of FPL pull on the thumb pulp in "hitting" the side of index finger as the FPL is tensioned

PEARLS

- Many patients benefit from this procedure as a part of their overall reconstruction.

TECHNICAL POINTS

- Tension can be set to allow some IP joint flexion with FPL activation; yet as the dorsal tenodesis of the split FPL into the EPL tightens, no further flexion will occur.
- The tendon weave can occur over the dorsal proximal phalanx to allow adequate lengths for weaves.

PITFALL

- Not too tight and not too loose; if it is not too tight or too loose, it is probably just right. (See Editor's Note, page 1281.)

POSTOPERATIVE CARE

- Same as the remaining reconstruction: cast immobilization including the thumb IP joint for 4 weeks; splint immobilization that includes the thumb IP joint, along with active range of motion for the next 4 weeks; then strengthening and active functional use with night-time bracing if needed.

flexor phase for groups 3 to 8 in patients with excessive clawing deformity of their digits. It can be performed with a paralyzed FDS tendon as a passive tenodesis or with a tendon transfer into the FDS as an active transfer.

Surgical Technique: Lasso Procedure

A single transverse incision, or separate Bruner incisions, is made across the MP flexion creases; the A1 and A2 pulleys are exposed, protecting the neurovascular bundles. The proximal and distal limits of the A1 pulley are identified at the base of each digit. Tension is applied to each A1 pulley

to be certain that transfer around the A1 pulley will pull the MP joint into flexion; if it does not, the proximal portion of the A2 pulley should be included for looping the FDS transfer; testing whether tension applied produces MP flexion needs to be repeated until the surgeon is certain that the transfer will have the desired MP flexion. Once the surgeon is assured that MP flexion will occur, the sheath is opened transversely at that point. Both slips of FDS are divided as far distally as possible, delivered through the transverse opening in the pulley sheath, then looped back toward the palm (Fig. 36-14). The two slips of FDS are then looped back over the A1 pulley and sutured with an interweave technique into the FDS tendon itself, using 4-0 nonabsorbable material. After the first suture is inserted, appropriate tension is confirmed by observing MP joint motion in response to passive wrist motion. With the wrist extended, the MP joints should flex in a uniform cascade. As the wrist is passively flexed, all MP joints should extend fully but not hyperextend. The same procedure is repeated in each finger.

PIP Central Slip Deficiency Treated With Intrinsic Tenodesis

In patients with a significant PIP joint flexion contracture due to central slip deficiency, an intrinsic tenodesis with a free tendon graft is included in the extensor phase to increase the effect of intrinsic balancing.[55] A free tendon graft is passed volar to the joint axis of the MP joint (using the intermetacarpal ligaments as the proximal anchor) and dorsal to the joint axis of the PIP joint with a direct insertion into the central slip of the extensor tendons. Thus, extension of the MP joint by the extrinsic muscles provides PIP joint extension through a tenodesis effect.

Surgical Technique: Intrinsic Tenodesis (Fig. 36-15)

The intrinsic tenodesis is performed in the extensor phase of reconstruction after tenodesis of the extrinsic finger extensors. The EIP, extensor digiti minimi (EDM), palmaris longus, or toe extensor tendons can be harvested for use as a free tendon graft. For grafting the index and long fingers, a curvilinear incision is made over the dorsum of the index finger metacarpal neck. The EIP can be harvested through this incision, in combination with the forearm incision made for the extrinsic extensor tenodesis. The extensor mechanism is exposed over the index metacarpal. A curvilinear incision is made from the radial midlateral line over the dorsal PIP joint. Subcutaneous dissection is performed to follow the lateral band from the lumbrical canal to the central slip. A tendon passer is gently passed retrograde from the midlateral incision through the lumbrical canal, out the index metacarpal incision along the radial side of the index metacarpal. The tendon graft is threaded through this path (Fig. 36-15). The tendon passer is similarly passed from the long finger midlateral incision retrograde, through the lumbrical canal, volar to the intermetacarpal ligament (deep transverse metacarpal ligament), and ulnar to the index metacarpal neck. The free tendon graft is threaded through this path. The free graft is then woven through the index finger central slip, then tensioned so that the PIP joints are held in nearly full extension when the MP joints are in full extension (i.e., wrist flexion). When this tension is

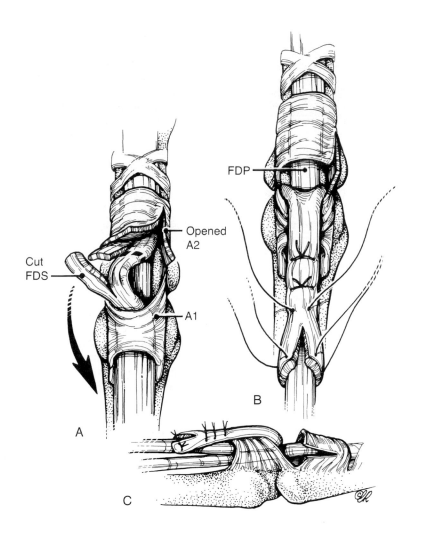

FIGURE 36-14. A to **C,** Zancolli's lasso operation is an intrinsic balancing operation that can be used to improve MP joint flexion, as well as decreasing IP joint flexion deformities with early digital "roll-up." (From Zancolli EA: Structural and Dynamic Bases of Hand Surgery. Philadelphia, JB Lippincott, 1979.)

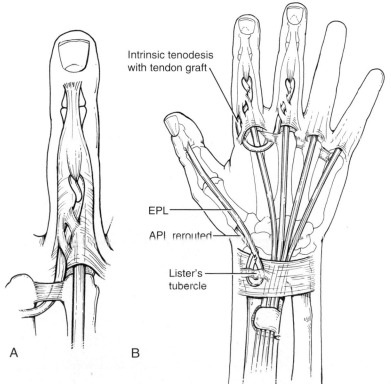

FIGURE 36-15. Intrinsic tenodesis technique. **A,** Close-up view illustrates weaving of the free graft from under the deep transverse metacarpal ligament, in line with the lateral band, and into the central slip. This simulates intrinsic function with the graft volar to the axis of the MP joint for MP flexion and dorsal to the axis of the PIP joint for PIP extension. **B,** Larger view shows the entire free tendon graft, routed from the central slip of the index finger, through the lumbrical canal, beneath the deep transverse metacarpal ligament, around the second metacarpal, back through the long finger lumbrical canal beneath the deep transverse intermetacarpal ligament, routed to the central slip of the long finger. The same technique is used for the ring and little fingers (around the fourth metacarpal) when IP joint extension is inadequate in those digits. (Adapted from House JH, Gwathmey F, Lundsgaard DK: Restoration of strong grasp and lateral pinch in tetraplegia due to cervical spinal cord injury. J Hand Surg [Am] 10:22-29, 1985.)

achieved the remaining free tendon graft end is sewn into the long finger central slip to maintain this tension. When the wrist is in extension and the MP joints are in flexion, passive flexion of the PIP joints should occur without difficulty. The same procedure can be performed harvesting the EDM tendon and using it as a free graft to provide a tenodesis from the central slip of the small finger, along the ulnar lateral band of the small finger, over the small finger metacarpal neck, then volar to the axis of the MP joint under the intermetacarpal ligament, along the ulnar lateral band of the ring finger, and into the central slip of the ring finger.[37]

FUNCTIONAL ELECTRICAL STIMULATION

Application of the use of electric current to muscle stimulation for upper extremity function after spinal cord injury has led Keith and his associates at Case Western University[40-43,69] to the development of a fully implantable functional neuromuscular stimulation (FNS) system that has been approved for use in tetraplegic patients by the Food and Drug Administration (FDA) and its European counterpart, the CE Mark. The commercial version was an eight-channel neuroprosthesis known as the Freehand System (FHS). This technology takes advantage of the existence of muscles that are no longer under cortical control (due to the spinal cord injury) but that remain with spinal reflex arcs intact. Muscles with an intact spinal reflex arc (below the level of the direct spinal cord anterior horn cell injury) can be stimulated to contract with relatively weak electrical currents. Muscle signals, nerve signals, or movements under volitional control (above the level of spinal cord injury), typically from the contralateral shoulder or neck, are used to control the device.

The FHS system provides a means to restore hand grasp and release, pronation, and supination as well as active elbow flexion or extension. Two grasp patterns are typically used: lateral grasp (or key pinch) and palmar grasp (or tip pinch). The neuroprosthesis consists of an implanted eight-channel stimulator/receiver that stimulates electrodes attached to appropriate muscles of the hand and forearm to provide elbow extension, wrist stabilization, grasp, and release. If the specific muscles necessary for the desired function cannot be electrically stimulated, then the neuro-prosthesis can be combined with traditional tendon transfer techniques[39] to transfer muscles that can be stimulated (e.g., ECU) into muscles that had direct injury of the anterior horn cell (e.g., EDC) to provide the desired hand function (e.g., finger extension/release).

The FHS system is indicated for tetraplegic patients for whom standard surgical procedures or orthotic devices cannot provide useful improved function or who have exhausted these options. Most commonly, they are implanted in patients in groups 0, 1, 2, and 3 (see Table 36-1), provided that preoperative assessment identifies key muscles that respond to external direct current stimulation, which with implantation of electrodes can be controlled with the contralateral shoulder to provide grasp and release function.

More than 200 patients have been implanted worldwide with this system,[5,9,16,19,38] including children.[18,20,66,68,77] The functional outcomes from the use of these devices have been well documented by means of subjective patient assessment and objective functional analysis and have been sustained over time.[53,70,71] Patient acceptance has been high. Yet, the device is expensive, the surgical procedure is complex, and its rehabilitation is extensive to meaningfully integrate the device into the patient's daily use. As of 2003, the company producing the device has discontinued its production, limiting FNS to second-generation 12-channel devices with telemetry and myoelectric control only available under research protocols.

CONCLUSION

Hand reconstruction is only one facet of the medical care and support services necessary for rehabilitation after spinal cord injury. Assessment of outcomes for tetraplegic hand reconstruction continues to improve and allow for comparison of interventions.[1,6,29,31,51,65,79,82,85] The most useful evaluation of the tetraplegic patient is to make a working list of what the patient *has* (grade 4 strength or higher), as shown in Table 36-1, and what the patient *needs* (grade 1 strength or lower), as shown in Table 36-3. Lastly one must determine what muscles are *available* for transfer and which muscles best *match* to the patient's needs using tendon transfer principles of work capacity, amplitude, and direction of pull, combined with other surgical adjuncts of arthrodesis and tenodesis. A summary of the most common tendon transfer recommendations[30,44] based on their International Classification is presented in Table 36-6.

Table 36-6
SURGICAL GUIDELINES BASED ON INTERNATIONAL CLASSIFICATION GROUP

Group (see Table 36-1)	Author's Preferred Method of Treatment
Group 1	BR to ECRB FPL tenodesis *Option:* split FPL tenodesis
Group 2	1. BR to FPL 2. CMC fusion 3. EPL tenodesis *Option:* split FPL tenodesis
Group 3	1. BR to FPL 2. CMC fusion 3. EPL tenodesis *Option:* split FPL tenodesis

Groups 4 and 5	House 2 stage
	Extensor phase:
	1. EDC tenodesis (option: BR to EDC)
	2. EPL tenodesis
	   Option: CMC fusion
	   Option: Intrinsic tenodesis
	Flexor Phase:
	1. ECRL to FDP
	2. BR to FPL (option: PT to FPL)
	   Option: Adduction-opponensplasty
	     (BR or PT with FDS graft)
	   Option: Split FPL tenodesis
	   Option: Lasso procedure

Table 36-6

SURGICAL GUIDELINES BASED ON INTERNATIONAL CLASSIFICATION GROUP—cont'd

Group (see Table 36-1)	Author's Preferred Method of Treatment
Group 6	1. ECRL to FDP 2. BR to FPL (option: PT to FPL) 3. EPL tenodesis (option: EPL to EDC) *Option:* CMC fusion or adduction-opponensplasty (BR or PT with FDS free graft). *Option:* Split FPL tenodesis *Option:* Lasso procedure (BR or PT to FDS)
Group 7	1. ECRL to FDP 2. BR to FPL (option: PT to FPL) *Option:* CMC fusion or adduction-opponensplasty (BR or PT with FDS free graft). *Option:* Split FPL tenodesis *Option:* Lasso procedure (BR or PT to FDS)
Group 8	1. FDP side to side 2. BR to FPL *Option:* Opponensplasty (BR or PT with FDS graft) *Option:* Split FPL tenodesis *Option:* Lasso procedure (BR or PT to FDS)
Group 9	

ANNOTATED REFERENCES

10. Brys D, Waters RL: Effect of triceps function on the brachioradialis transfer in quadriplegia. J Hand Surg [Am] 12:237-239, 1987.

     The role of elbow extension in augmenting hand reconstruction surgery is outlined in this important article.

33. Hentz VR, LeClercq C: Surgical Rehabilitation of the Upper Limb in Tetraplegia. London, WB Saunders, 2002.

     This recently published book provides the treating physician with the most comprehensive, yet practical, guide to the assessment and treatment of the spinal cord injured patient. It includes sections on basic science of the injury, rehabilitation principles, and surgical treatment by level of injury—a must-have book.

34. House JH, Comadoll J, Dahl AL: One-stage key pinch and release with thumb carpal-metacarpal fusion in tetraplegia. J Hand Surg [Am] 17:530-538, 1992.

     A classic article that describes the surgical treatment for International Classification groups 1 to 3.

55. McCarthy CK, House JH, Van Heest A: Intrinsic balancing in reconstruction of the tetraplegic hand. J Hand Surg [Am] 22:596-604, 1997.

     A review of the intrinsic reconstruction procedures that can be considered as part of tetraplegic hand reconstruction.

65. Mohammed KD, Rothwell AG, Sinclair SW, et al: Upper limb surgery for tetraplegia. J Bone Joint Surg Br 74:873-879, 1992.

     In this article that summarized an extensive experience in tetraplegia hand reconstructive surgery, the split FPL transfer is discussed.

CHAPTER 37

Pediatric Brachial Plexus Palsy

Peter M. Waters

The focus in this chapter is on the diagnosis, treatment, and long-term expected outcomes of infants and children with brachial plexus birth palsies. Because the type and severity of neural injury vary by infant afflicted, the treatment and outcome are not expected to be the same. For the mild neurapraxic lesion, spontaneous recovery is to be expected over the first several months of life, with complete recovery evident by the first year of life.[69,70,77,172] This is in contrast to the severe avulsion injury that will have a lifetime of disability despite extensive physical therapy and surgical management.[41,68,171,172] Unfortunately at the time of this writing, a severe brachial plexus birth palsy is not a solved problem. Although there have been many advances since Duchenne's (1872)[55] and Erb's (1874)[62] classic descriptions of infantile paralysis, there are many difficult challenges that remain. These include neural injuries that are more severe than can recover spontaneously; more complex and extensive neural injuries than available donor nerve grafts or transfers can repair[110]; and avulsion injuries from the spinal cord that cannot be repaired directly or replaced adequately with nerve transfers. In these circumstances, therapeutic intervention with microsurgical reconstruction of the plexus in the first 3 to 9 months of life* will hopefully improve but not normalize the situation. Further advances in neural repair, regeneration, and growth are necessary to solve this problem. Fortunately, these severe avulsion or axonal disruption injuries have been cited as between 8% and 25% of all brachial plexus birth palsies.[41,68,73,77,145,172] The remainder of birth palsies with an incomplete recovery can be effectively managed with physical therapy and, if necessary, secondary tendon transfers and osteotomies, to improve their situation. The goal of this chapter is to help the reader differentiate infants and children with varying

expected outcomes by spontaneous recovery and guide the decision-making regarding surgical intervention. The present controversies are well described and potential future advances are addressed.

Anatomy

Essential to any discussion regarding the natural history and treatment of a brachial plexus lesion is a thorough understanding of the anatomy (Fig. 37-1). Therefore, a brief review of the pertinent anatomy is described.

The brachial plexus most commonly receives contributions contiguously from the fifth cervical (C5) to the first thoracic (T1) ventral spinal nerve roots. Prefixed cords (22%) receive an additional contribution from the C4 nerve root, whereas the much less common postfixed cords (1%) receive a contribution from T2.[107] The C5 and C6 nerve roots join to form the upper trunk; the C7 nerve root continues as the middle trunk; and the C8 and T1 nerve roots combine to form the lower trunk. Each trunk bifurcates into anterior and posterior divisions. The posterior divisions of all three trunks make up the posterior cord. The anterior divisions of the upper and middle trunks form the lateral cord. Finally, the anterior division of the lower trunk forms the medial cord. The major nerves of the upper extremity are terminal branches from the cords, with the ulnar nerve arising from the medial cord; the radial and axillary nerves from the posterior cord; the musculocutaneous nerve from the lateral cord; and the median nerve from branches of the medial and lateral cords. The other nerves to the upper extremity arise sequentially throughout the brachial plexus and are illustrated in Figure 37-1. Of note, the dorsal scapular nerve

---

*See references 6, 29, 41, 68, 99, 103, 105, 106, 124, and 147.

The author wishes to recognize the work of previous authors **Drs. Robert Leffert, Vincent R. Hentz,** and **Michelle James** for their contributions to *Green's Operative Hand Surgery* and this manuscript. I also wish to recognize the hard work of Ms. Anne Kuo in assisting with the references and illustrations for this chapter.

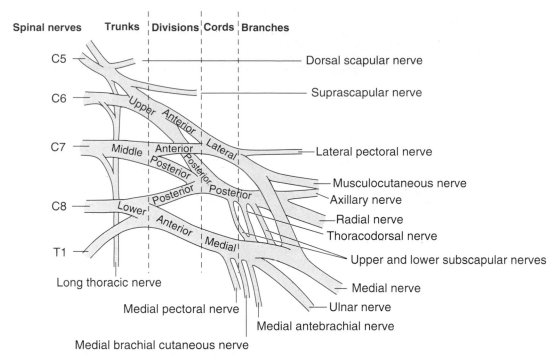

FIGURE 37-1. Normal anatomy of brachial plexus. (Redrawn from Waters PM: Obstetric brachial plexus palsy. J Am Acad Orthop Surg 5:205-214, 1997.)

arises from the C5 nerve root along with a branch to the phrenic nerve; the suprascapular nerve arises from the upper trunk; and the long thoracic nerve arises from the C5 to C7 nerve roots. In addition, the lateral pectoral nerve arises from the lateral cord and the medial pectoral from the medial cord. Finally, the thoracodorsal nerve and the upper and lower subscapular nerves arise from the posterior cord. The sequential peripheral to distal orientation of the brachial plexus is nerve roots, trunks, divisions, cords, and terminal branches. Every muscle in the upper limb is innervated by the brachial plexus.

Surgical exploration and reconstruction of the brachial plexus requires a thorough understanding of the three-dimensional anatomy. As noted, the brachial plexus extends proximally from the C5 to T1 ventral nerve roots of the spinal cord distally to the terminal branches in the upper brachium. In the neck, it is located between the anterior scalene and middle scalene muscles. The plexus extends beneath the clavicle, superficial to the first rib, as it passes into the axilla. It is thus divided into its supraclavicular and infraclavicular portions. It is joined by the major vessels of the arm beneath the clavicle. As it passes beneath the muscles to the coracoid, the plexus surrounds the axillary artery. The relationship of the cords to the artery gives them their appropriate medial, lateral, and posterior designations. Complete exposure of the brachial plexus often requires retraction or an osteotomy of the clavicle, release of the muscular insertions to the coracoid, and release of the clavicular origin of the pectoralis major muscle.

PREOPERATIVE EVALUATION

Brachial plexus birth palsy has an incidence of 0.38 to 1.56 per 1000 live births.[103,109] The difference in incidence may depend on the type of obstetric care and the average birth weight of infants in different geographic regions.[103,139] Perinatal risk factors for brachial plexus palsy include large-for-gestational-age infants (macrosomia),[19,30,115,152] multiparous pregnancies, previous deliveries resulting in brachial plexus birth palsy,[8,147] prolonged labor, breech delivery,[65] assisted (vacuum or forceps), and difficult deliveries.[74,146,162] Delivery by caesarean section does not exclude the possibility of a birth palsy.[12,127,131] Fetal distress may contribute to muscle hypotonia and provide less protection of the plexus from stretch injury during delivery.[154] Mechanically, shoulder dystocia[4,17,88,153] in vertex deliveries and difficult arm or head extraction in breech deliveries increase the risk to neural injury.[65,147] Most commonly, a brachial plexus birth palsy involves the upper trunk (C5 and C6), potentially in combination with an injury to C7; or, less often, the entire plexus (C5 to T1) is injured. On extremely rare occasions, the lower trunk can be most significantly involved (C8 and T1). Injuries are described classically as neurapraxia (Sunderland I), axonotmesis (Sunderland II to IV), neurotmesis (Sunderland V), or avulsion.[158] Mechanically, lesions have been described as stretch (Sunderland I), varying degrees of rupture (Sunderland II to V), and avulsions (Fig. 37-2). Upper trunk extraforaminal ruptures are more common with vertex delivery and shoulder dystocia. The right upper limb is more often involved because of the more frequent left occiput anterior vertex presentation. The C5 and C6 root avulsions are particularly frequent with breech presentation and can at times be bilateral.[65] Entire plexus involvement can be a combination of stretch, rupture, and avulsion injuries and generally involves a more severe injury.[68] Extensive work from Smellie's[148,149] and Duchenne's[55] original descriptions of brachial plexopathy with delivery through the anatomic studies of Stevens[155] and Metaizeau[117] define a mechanical basis for the infantile paralysis.[4] This is the predominant theory regarding the etiology of brachial plexus birth palsies.

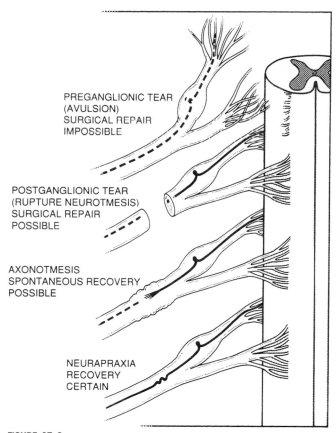

PREGANGLIONIC TEAR
(AVULSION)
SURGICAL REPAIR
IMPOSSIBLE

POSTGANGLIONIC TEAR
(RUPTURE NEUROTMESIS)
SURGICAL REPAIR
POSSIBLE

AXONOTMESIS
SPONTANEOUS RECOVERY
POSSIBLE

NEURAPRAXIA
RECOVERY
CERTAIN

FIGURE 37-2. A severe traction injury to the brachial plexus may cause nerve injuries of varying severity in the same plexus. These include avulsion of the nerve root from the spinal cord (cannot be repaired), extraforaminal rupture of the root or trunk (can be surgically repaired), and intraneural rupture of fascicles (some spontaneous recovery possible).

However, there are rare reports of possible in utero causes of a birth palsy.[68,71,130] It has been postulated that there may be abnormal in-utero forces on the posterior shoulder region and, therefore, plexus, as the fetus passes over the sacral promontory before obstetric manipulation.[66,129] Increased in-utero pressure and traction have been proposed for plexopathies in an anomalous uterus, such as a bicornuate or fibroid uterus.[58,96] These alternative causes become very important elements of debate in a litigious society in which the presence of a brachial plexus birth palsy may result in a malpractice suit against the obstetrician, midwife, labor nurse, and/or hospital participating in the birth of that infant.[95,129]

Diagnosis is made predominantly by physical examination. The differential diagnosis is limited to pseudoparalysis as the result of fracture or, less commonly, infection; central nervous system or cervical spinal cord derangement with peripheral paralysis; or congenital differences of the upper limb that result in limited motion and strength. Because fracture of the clavicle[9] or humerus can occur concomitantly with a birth palsy, radiographs may be clinically indicated. Generally, the diagnosis of a brachial plexus palsy is readily apparent. The spectrum of clinical presentation is dependent on the extent of neural injury and the timing of examination. Recovery is dynamic, and there is an evolution to the clinical examination over the first few weeks and months of life. Patience is required to obtain a reliable examination in an infant. Observation of spontaneous movement, utilization of neonatal reflexes, and stimulated motor activity are necessary for accurate examination. The most important aspect to the examination is to prognosticate recovery.[41,68,70,106,172] Therefore, serial examinations on a 1- to 3-month basis in infancy are critical to predict outcome and indications for surgical intervention.[54]

Narakas[124] and others[24,25,147] have attempted to categorize this clinical continuum into four categorical groups. The mildest clinical group (I) represents a classic Erb (C5 and C6) palsy[62] with initial absence of shoulder abduction and external rotation, elbow flexion, and forearm supination. Wrist and digital flexion and extension are intact. Successful spontaneous recovery is cited as high as 90% in this group.[147] Group II includes involvement of C7 with the additional absence of wrist and digital extension along with C5 and C6 impairment. These infants have the classic "waiter's tip" posture of their hand and wrist. Prognosis is poorer with C5 to C7 involvement. Group III is a flail extremity but without a Horner syndrome. The most severe involvement (group IV) is a flail extremity and a Horner syndrome (ptosis, myosis, enophthalmos, anhidrosis). These infants may have an associated phrenic nerve palsy with an elevated hemidiaphragm.[11] This can be assessed by observation of the abdominal wall for symmetric diaphragmatic movement during respiration or by an expiratory chest radiograph. Phrenic nerve involvement increases the likelihood of an avulsion injury and limited spontaneous recovery.

For prognostic reasons, it is important to determine whether the level of injury is preganglionic or postganglionic.[20,24,50,68] Due to the proximity of the ganglion to the spinal cord and the fact that the motor cell body is in the spinal cord, preganglionic lesions are avulsions from the cord that will not spontaneously recover motor function. By assessing the function of several nerves that arise close to the ganglion, one can often determine by physical examination the level of the lesion. Specifically, the presence of a Horner syndrome (sympathetic chain); an elevated hemidiaphragm (phrenic nerve); winged scapula (long thoracic nerve); and the absence of rhomboid (dorsal scapular nerve), rotator cuff (suprascapular nerve), and latissimus dorsi (thoracodorsal nerve) function all raise significant concern about a preganglionic lesion. Preganglionic lesions can only be reconstructed microsurgically by nerve transfers,[123,125] most commonly with thoracic intercostals[101,111,122] or a branch of the spinal accessory nerve.[100] Postganglionic ruptures have reconstructable proximal and distal nerve beyond the zone of neural injury. Thus, a postganglionic injury is a complex peripheral nerve lesion that can be reconstructed with nerve grafts if necessary.[171]

The majority of obstetric plexus injuries involve the upper trunk.[68,72] The classic Erb palsy involves only C5 and C6 (46%), whereas it is also common to have C5 to C7 involvement (29%).[22,23] The level of injury is usually postganglionic. When the lower plexus is involved, it is more common to have a preganglionic avulsion of C8 and T1. The exception to this situation is an upper trunk lesion seen with a breech delivery. These neural injuries tend to be preganglionic C5 and C6 avulsions from the spinal cord.[65] A true Klumpke paralysis (isolated C8 and T1) is very rare.[10]

Most authors[49,50,72,105] simplify the clinical continuum of recovery of a brachial plexus birth palsy into timing of recovery of specific motor function and use the absence of motor recovery as an indication for surgical intervention. Wyeth and Sharpe, in 1917,[178] advised surgical intervention if there was absence of recovery by 3 months of life. Gilbert and Tassin's[69] classic study concurred with the 3-month time interval and utilized the recovery of biceps function as the key indicator of brachial plexus spontaneous recovery. Waters similarly found biceps recovery statistically reliable.[172] Laurent[106] advised monitoring biceps, triceps, and deltoid function. Clarke's group in Toronto described the timing of return of elbow flexion and elbow, wrist, finger, and thumb extension as discriminators of outcome.[119] Ultimately, though, in difficult cases, Clarke advised isolated elbow flexion recovery at 9 months by his "cookie test" to predict outcome and determine the need for microsurgical intervention.[41] In this test, a positive outcome is if the infant can get a cookie to the mouth with the affected arm.

Defining and grading specific muscle recovery in an infant is difficult. Many centers utilize the Medical Research Council[44] Muscle Grading System to define results. This classifies muscle strength as 0 (no contraction), 1 (trace contraction), 2 (active motion with gravity eliminated), 3 (active motion against gravity), 4 (active motion against gravity and resistance), and 5 (normal power). However, this system requires volitional contraction, which is not feasible in an infant and difficult in a young child. Understanding this, Gilbert and Tassin modified the MRC grading system to a four-grade system of 0 (no contracture), 1 (contracture without movement), 2 (movement with gravity eliminated), and 3 (complete movement against the corresponding weight of the extremity).[70] Gilbert and Tassin also modified Mallet's classification[113] (Fig. 37-3), which assesses more global motor function of the upper trunk as opposed to isolated muscle testing. This system assesses global abduction, global external rotation, hand-to-mouth, hand-to-neck, and hand-to-spine activities on a score of 1 to 5, where 1 is no function, 5 is normal function, and grades 2 to 4 denote progressive strength as depicted in Figure 37-3. The majority of late 20th century papers on the infantile brachial plexus have utilized these two classification schemes to determine results of spontaneous recovery and surgical intervention. More recently, Clarke and colleagues have advocated use of the Hospital for Sick Children (HSC) Muscle Grading System (Table 37-1), a seven-grade system dividing muscle strength into gravity eliminated (grades 0 to 4) and against gravity (grades 5 to 7). This system requires that full active motion with gravity eliminated occur (grade 4) before scoring antigravity muscle strength. All of these grading systems require reliability and validity testing in infants and children. The Mallet, initial Toronto active motion scale,[119] and HSC grading system were recently noted to be statistically reliable in interobserver and intraobserver analysis.[13] As might be expected, intraobserver reliability was higher than interobserver reliability, and less complicated systems (Mallet) had higher reliability than more complicated schemes (HSC). This information is critical for comparison of results and for multicenter study analysis of therapeutic interventions in brachial plexus birth palsy care.

Invasive radiographic studies with myelography, combined CT-myelography, and magnetic resonance imaging (MRI)[1,53,84,120,163,173,174,179] have been used in an attempt to distinguish between avulsion and extraforaminal ruptures.[170]

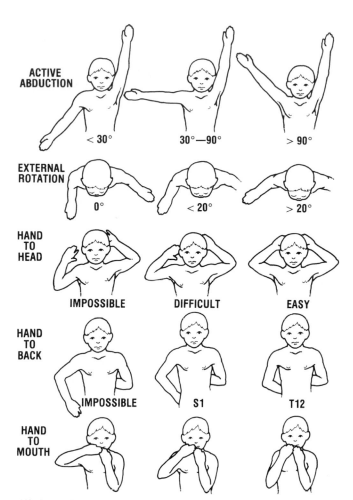

FIGURE 37-3. Mallet's system for grading shoulder function in the child. (From Mallet J: Paralysie obstetricale du plexus brachial: Traitement des sequelle: Primaute du traitement de l'epaule: Method d'expression des resultants. Rev Chir Orthop Reparatrice Appar Mot 58[Suppl 1]:166-168, 1972.)

Table 37-1
MUSCLE GRADING SYSTEM

Observation	Muscle Grade
Gravity Eliminated	
No contraction	0
Contraction, no motion	1
Motion ≤ one-half range	2
Motion ≥ one-half range	3
Full motion	4
Against Gravity	
Motion ≤ one-half range	5
Motion ≥ one-half range	6
Full motion	7

Note: Full active range of motion with gravity eliminated (muscle grade 4) must be achieved before active range against gravity is scored (muscle grades 5 to 7).

From Clarke H: An approach to obstetrical brachial plexus. Hand Clin 4:567, 1995.

Kawai[102] compared all three techniques with operative findings in infants. Myelography had an 84% true-positive rate with 4% false-positive and 12% false-negative rates. The addition of CT with myelography increased the true-positive rate to 94%. The presence of small diverticula was only 60% accurate for an avulsion. However, the presence of large diverticula or frank meningoceles was universally diagnostic. MRI had a true positive rate similar to CT-myelography but also allowed extraforaminal evaluation of the plexus. This permitted evaluation of possible double crush injuries. High spin-echo MRI,[64] MR-myelography, and MR-neurography may improve the resolution of MR analysis.[168] MRI has the potential value of the need for sedation only because myelography requires general anesthesia in an infant.[85] These radiographic studies may improve the quality of preoperative planning, but the final decision regarding the presence or absence of an avulsion injury is still made intraoperatively.

Electrodiagnostic studies with electromyography (EMG) and nerve conduction velocities (NCV) have also been utilized in an attempt to improve diagnostic accuracy of the severity of the neural lesion.[28,141] The presence of normal sensory nerve conduction in the absence of motor nerve conduction is diagnostic of root avulsion. The absence of reinnervation at 3 months is indicative of an avulsion. Unfortunately, the presence of motor activity in a muscle has not been accurate in predicting an acceptable level of motor recovery in that muscle. In an EMG, the presence of reinnervation can at times confuse the clinical picture.[50,71,102] It has been documented that a near-normal EMG can be found in infants with a severe lesion or even root avulsion.[47,147,166,168] There often are significant discrepancies between preoperative EMG, sensory nerve action potential (SNAP), somatosensory evoked potentials (SSEP) testing, and intraoperative surgical findings. A potential source for this is the plasticity of the infantile nervous system.[169] For example, Slooff documented innervation of deltoid and biceps from C7 in the presence of avulsions of C5 and C6.[147,168] At this stage it is clear that neurophysiologic studies may underestimate the severity of injury and falsely provide optimism regarding recovery.[165,166] At present, most centers and brachial plexus microsurgeons still ultimately rely on physical examination to assess recovery and decide on surgical interventions.

NATURAL HISTORY

Despite flaws in methodology or loss of patient enrollment in many of the natural history studies, there is sufficient evidence in several studies* to draw significant conclusions:

1. The majority of brachial birth palsies are transient. Those infants who recover partial antigravity upper trunk muscle strength in the first 2 months of life should have a full and complete recovery over the first 1 to 2 years of life.
2. Infants who do not recover antigravity biceps strength by 5 to 6 months of life should have microsurgical

reconstruction of the brachial plexus because successful surgery will result in a better outcome than natural history alone.
3. Those infants with partial recovery of C5 to C7 antigravity strength during months 3 through 6 of life will have permanent, progressive limitations of motion and strength as well as risk the development of joint contractures in the affected limb. At some point these limitations cross the line from clinical observations to functional impairment with permanent consequences.
4. This is most evident about the shoulder where children with incomplete recovery almost universally develop an internally rotated, adducted shoulder. With the development of limited glenohumeral motion, there is universal increased compensatory scapulothoracic motion. Parents and therapists will often complain about the scapular winging. These patients can have functional limitations for above-shoulder, facial, and occipital region activities.
5. The muscle imbalance of external rotation and abduction weakness and relatively normal internal rotation and adduction strength leads to glenohumeral joint deformity.[132,172] This was described in the early 20th century,[63,142] but more recent studies have defined the risk factors and progressive deformities in more detail with the use of arthrograms,[132,175] CT, and MRI.[173,174]

The glenohumeral deformity is progressive with age and appears very early in infancy. The development of glenohumeral deformity in these children follows a basic pediatric orthopedic principle that muscle imbalance in a growing child will lead to bone and joint deformity. Adapting Severin's classification of hip dysplasia, Waters described various grades of deformity (Fig. 37-4).[174] The deformity evolves sequentially by grade from normal (I) to increased glenoid retroversion (II), posterior glenohumeral subluxation with posterior glenoid dysplasia (III), and development of a false glenoid (class IV) to flattening of the humeral head and glenoid (class V). In addition, on occasion a true infantile glenohumeral dislocation (VI) will occur. Pearl's arthrographic classification was very similar. It is unclear if glenohumeral deformity is reversible with surgical intervention. The factors that influence outcome include degree of deformity, age of patient, and surgical procedure performed. Longitudinal studies are ongoing to assess glenoid remodeling with surgical intervention. It is clear if left alone that the deformity will progress with growth.[174]

In addition to shoulder weakness and contracture, many children develop an elbow flexion contracture associated with antigravity triceps weakness.[16] Most often this is less than 30 degrees and therefore of limited functional consequence. There are individuals with marked weakness of the triceps who develop a more severe contracture that can impede activities of daily living. Limitations of forearm supination are also commonplace and bothersome to therapists and parents alike. This limitation is clinically exacerbated by the presence of limited shoulder external rotation in adduction because these motions are complementary. Finally, there are some rare individuals who have profound permanent loss of hand and wrist function. It is this later group for whom microsurgery clearly offers the best alternative to their poor prognosis with natural history. This is especially true in the patients with an avulsion injury for

---

*See references 6, 20, 29, 69, 76, 77, 83, 126, 151, 168, and 172.

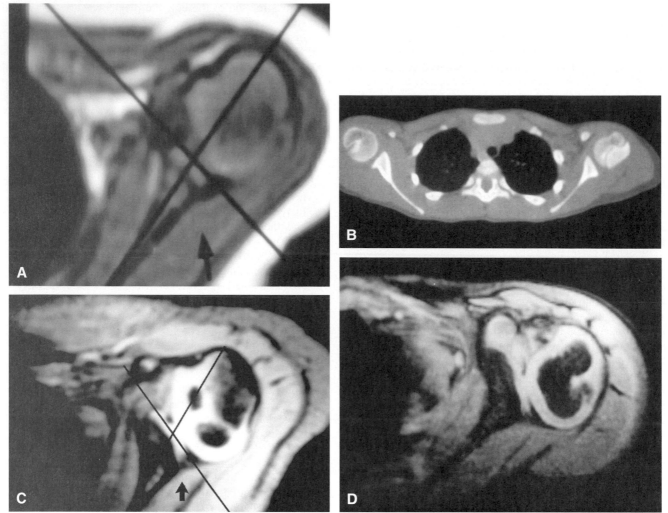

FIGURE 37-4. Radiographic types as determined with use of computed tomographic or magnetic resonance imaging scans. **A,** MR image of a type I (normal) glenohumeral joint (less than a 5-degree difference in glenoid version compared with that on the normal, contralateral side. The bisecting line extending from the spine of the scapula through the humeral head is outlined. The angle in the posterior medial quadrant is indicated by the *arrow.* Ninety degrees is subtracted from this measurement to determine glenoid version. **B,** CT scan of a glenohumeral joint with type II deformity (on the right). The deformity is minimal (more than a 5-degree difference in glenoid version compared with that on the normal, contralateral side and no evidence of posterior subluxation of the humeral head). **C,** MR image of a glenohumeral joint with type II deformity. There is moderate deformity of the glenoid with posterior subluxation of the humeral head (less than 35% of the head is anterior to the scapular line). The scapular line and the tangential line indicating the anterior and posterior cartilaginous margins of the glenoid are shown. The angle in the posterior medial quadrant is indicated by the *arrow.* **D,** MR image of a glenohumeral joint with type IV deformity. There is progressive deformity (a false glenoid) and subluxation. (From Waters PM, Smith GR, Jaramillo D: Glenohumeral deformity secondary to brachial plexus birth palsy. J Bone Joint Surg 80:668-677, 1998.)

whom satisfactory recovery is not possible without surgical intervention. Unfortunately, microsurgery also has limitations to functional recovery in these situations.

The major clinical dilemma presently is to determine if infants without antigravity return of C5 to C7 function at 3, 4, 5, or 6 months of age warrant surgical exploration and neural reconstruction. These infants have varying degrees of rupture (Sunderland II to IV) and their ultimate neuromuscular recovery from spontaneous recovery and tendon transfers has still not been compared with their recovery with microsurgery and tendon transfers. Parents, primary care physicians, and therapists are under significant emotional pressure to do what they believe is best for the affected infant.[171,172] Unfortunately, despite strong opinions and, at times, solicitous pressure from specific medical centers, there are still insufficient data to answer this ques-

tion.[14] Ideally this would be addressed with a prospective randomized clinical trial with sufficient enrollment.[27] At present, too few microsurgeons will participate in a patient randomized trial due to clinical equipoise. The American Society for Surgery of the Hand and the Pediatric Orthopedic Society of North America has sponsored a multicenter randomized trial that is presently underway and it is hoped will further our knowledge base regarding this very important issue.

MICROSURGERY

Without question, the role and timing of microsurgery are the most controversial issues in the care of these infants. The original surgical interventions of the brachial plexus were at the turn of the 20th century with resection of the neuroma and direct repair.[40] Kennedy[104] initially described three cases in 1903, with subsequent reports by Wyeth and Sharpe in 1917 and Taylor in 1920.[159] However, in a report on 1100 infantile brachial plexus patients in 1925, Sever[142] was uncertain of the benefit of surgical intervention. By the 1930s, brachial plexus nerve surgery had fallen out of favor. It was not until the advent of microsurgical advances and the extensive work in the 1970s and 1980s by Narakas,[124] Millessi,[121] Gilbert,[69,70] and others[2,3] in Europe, and comparable work by Kawabata[99] and others in Asia, that brachial plexus microsurgical reconstruction became commonplace. At this stage, it is nearly universal for major medical centers throughout the world to have plastic surgery, neurosurgery, and/or orthopedic surgery subspecialty brachial plexus centers actively performing brachial plexus nerve reconstructive surgery.

The spectrum of nerve surgery includes neurolysis, neuroma resection and nerve grafting, and nerve transfers.[61] Direct repair is rarely performed, owing to the extensive nature of the lesion and inability to obtain a tension-free repair without grafting. Although neurolysis has been performed extensively,[106,145] most centers have abandoned its independent use.[42,68] Clearly there is no role for neurolysis in the presence of an avulsion injury. It has been shown to be no different than natural history in total plexopathy,[33] and the evidence is similar although less conclusive in upper trunk rupture situations. Gilbert strongly states that he sees no role for neurolysis.[68] Laurent advocates its use in conjunction with intraoperative electrodiagnostic studies. If there is maintenance of more than 50% of a muscle action potential across a neuroma in continuity, then Laurent indicates that neurolysis is performed.[106] Otherwise, the neuroma is resected and grafted. However, the recovery of muscle strength results with nerve grafting were more dramatic than neurolysis despite the fact that the preoperative status of the neurolysis patients was better than the grafting patients. Capek and Clarke[33] describe better long-term results after resection and grafting of both conducting and nonconducting neuromas than with neurolysis despite an initial worsening of the situation with resection. Based on the

available information at this time, neurolysis alone should be viewed as having very little therapeutic benefit.

The present microsurgical standard of care is transection of the neuroma and sural nerve grafting in extraforaminal ruptures.[43,49,56,150,160] In the usual upper trunk rupture, sural nerve grafts are performed from the C5 and C6 roots to the most proximal healthy nerve tissue of (1) the upper trunk anterior division/lateral cord/musculocutaneous nerve[41]; (2) suprascapular nerve; and (3) upper trunk posterior division/posterior cord/axillary-radial nerves (Fig. 37-5). In the case of segmental avulsions, nerve transfers,[124,125,128] in conjunction with nerve grafting, are performed utilizing the thoracic intercostals (T2 to T4) and/or a branch of the spinal accessory nerve[5] after it innervates the trapezius (Fig. 37-6). In total plexal avulsions, nerve transfers are the only nerve reconstructive option and may include intercostals,[101,111,122] spinal accessory,[100] phrenic,[80] cervical plexus,[32,140] contralateral C7,[39,78,116] and even the hypoglossal nerve. With breech presentation avulsions of C5 and C6, transfer of a part of the ulnar nerve to the motor branch of the biceps is useful (Oberlin transfer).[128] Carlstedt has done experimental and limited clinical work on direct reimplantation or grafting into the spinal cord,[35,36] but, at present, the risk of cervical instability from the laminotomy and fasciectomy or injury to the nerves to uninvolved limbs does not warrant its use.[36] Gilbert[68] and Slooff[147] advocate that priority be given to microsurgical reconstructions of the hand in infants with extensive avulsions and limited nerve options. Unlike adults, infants with brachial plexopathy may have the potential to regain hand function after nerve grafting or nerve transfers. In each microsurgical case, the plan is individualized depending the extent of injury and available reconstructive options.

Although there is ongoing debate about the timing of microsurgical intervention, the most common criteria utilized in clinical practice as an indication for microsurgery is the absence of return of biceps muscle function associated with (1) total plexopathy and Horner's syndrome or (2) upper trunk lesion. Predominantly, reconstruction is performed between 3 and 9 months of age, although the range of repairs cited in the literature extends from 1 to 24

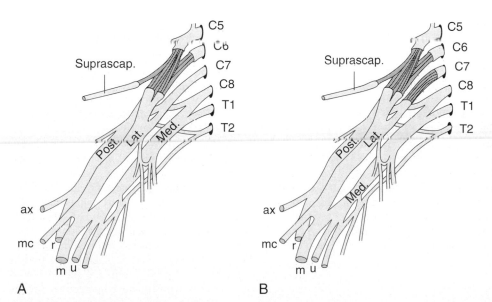

FIGURE 37-5. **A** and **B,** Nerve grafting strategies for upper trunk rupture. (Redrawn from Narakas AO: Obstetrical brachial plexus injuries. *In* Lamb DW [ed]: The Paralysed Hand. Edinburgh, Churchill Livingstone, 1987, p 130.)

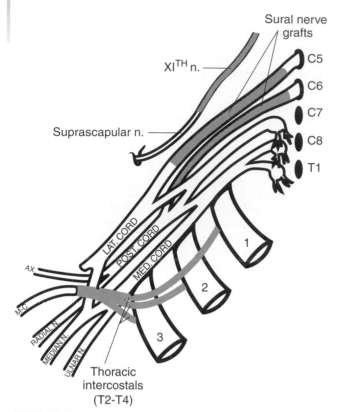

FIGURE 37-6. Nerve grafting strategies for nerve transfers and grafts. (Redrawn from Narakas AO, Hentz VR: Neurotization in brachial plexus injuries: Indication and results. Clin Orthop 237:43-57, 1988.)

months.* The quality of muscle recovery is open to debate, and observer error makes comparative analysis difficult. Gilbert[68] and others[3,24,29,87,97,124,146] advocate for microsurgery when there is absence of antigravity biceps recovery by 3 months of life. The reasons for early intervention include less risk of irreversible loss of motor end plates with prolonged denervation and better parental acceptance of surgical intervention if performed while the limb is still flail or with minimal motion. However, prospective studies by Al-Qattan[6] and myself[172] indicate that recovery of antigravity biceps function by 4 and 5 months of age, respectively, results in outcomes that are equivalent to microsurgery, especially when combined with secondary tendon transfers to improve shoulder external rotation and abduction. Microsurgical results in both these papers resulted in improved function when performed later than 3 months of age. Finally, Clarke[41] advocates microsurgery as late as 9 months in those infants who fail the "cookie test" and thus have less than a grade 6 strength of biceps on the HSC muscle scale.[41] Microsurgical reconstruction at that relatively late time was of positive benefit. Therefore, the motor end plates in infants may be more resilient than those in adults. Ultimately, it is still unknown what is the best time for microsurgical intervention. However, it is clear that there is a marked difference in number of procedures performed depending on the individual surgeon's bias toward timing.

*See references 6, 24, 25, 29, 41, 69, 72, 86, 106, 135, 143, and 144.

The problem with reviewing the results of microsurgery is that very few of these patients have long-term follow-up or microsurgery alone. Gilbert and Tassin's[69,70] original study compared microsurgery with spontaneous recovery. For C5 and C6 lesions, 100% had class III recovery spontaneously, whereas 37% were class III and 63% were class IV with microsurgery. With C5 to C7 lesions, 30% were class II and 70% were class III with observation. With microsurgery, 35% were class II, 42% were class III, and 22% were class IV. Later, Gilbert and Whitaker cited results of Mallet scores of III, IV, or V for abduction at 81% in C5 and C6 reconstructions and scores of III or IV at 64% with total plexus reconstruction at greater than 2-year follow-up.[71] In combination with secondary shoulder reconstructions, at 5 years these results increased to 70% Mallet class IV or V abduction for C5 and C6 lesions. Similarly, with total plexopathy reconstructions prioritizing the hand, at 2-year follow-up there were only 25% grade III or IV shoulder function; 70% with grade III, IV, or V elbow function; and 35% with grade III or IV hand function by Gilbert's new classification scheme.[71] With the addition of secondary shoulder and hand procedures, this increased to 77% in the shoulder and 75% in the hand at 6-year follow-up. Gilbert maintains that microsurgery not only improves function over natural history in selected patients but also increases the possibilities for secondary tendon transfers that will then further improve the clinical situation.

These results, however, are comparable with the limited natural history data available. Benson and colleagues[23] presented data on 142 patients with follow-up to assess the natural history of brachial plexopathy in regard to timing of biceps recovery. Seventy-one patients had full recovery by 6 weeks. The other 71 had recovery of biceps at greater than 6 weeks of age. At final follow-up of the later group, 67% had excellent, 12% had good, 5% had fair, and 10% had poor results by their assessment of shoulder function. Zancolli[184] found that 82% of the affected infants followed from birth had recovery of biceps function, 75% of whom began recovery between months 4 and 5 of life. I addressed the same issue and found that, prospectively, of the 49 infants with no biceps recovery at 3 months, 42 of those infants recovered antigravity biceps function by 6 months.[172] At follow-up at more than 2 years of age, those infants with recovery of biceps between 3 and 6 months had a progressive decrease in Mallet grades for abduction, external rotation, hand-to-mouth, and hand-to-neck activities depending on month of biceps recovery. In those infants with biceps recovery between 3 and 6 months of age, the recovery of function by Mallet class was as follows: global abduction—II (3%), III (52%), IV (46%); global external rotation—II (54%), III (31%), IV (15%); hand to neck—II (39%), III (33%), IV (28%); and hand to mouth—II (33%), III (24%), IV (43%). These results are similar to Gilbert's published microsurgical results.

In addition, in both natural history and microsurgery patients, secondary shoulder transfer and osteotomies significantly improved function. In the subgroup of 20 patients with recovery of biceps between 3 and 6 months of life with shoulder reconstruction, there was an improvement to an average grade IV for all Mallet classes. Therein lies two of the present controversies. How different are patients with microsurgery at 3 months from those who recover biceps between 3 and 6 months and have secondary reconstructions? It is critical to know the answer to this question to resolve if (1) unnecessary surgery is being performed or if (2) some centers are failing to adequately treat these infants by not being aggressive enough with microsurgery at 3 months of life. Furthermore, because the published microsurgery results include secondary procedures, this controversy is presently unresolved because of lack of comparable data. Although there are many believers of the importance of microsurgical intervention at 3 months, at present there are no studies that fully answer these questions. As mentioned previously, there presently is a multicenter international study to address these issues.

Surgical Technique

The extent of surgical exposure is dependent on the level and severity of injury. All microsurgical procedures in infants are performed under general anesthesia without the use of neuromuscular blocking agents. Both lower extremities are prepared for sural nerve grafting. The shoulder girdle, chest, and neck are prepared for brachial plexus exposure and all possible planned nerve grafting and nerve transfer procedures (i.e., intercostals, spinal accessory, partial ulnar nerve,[7,128] contralateral plexus). The infant is supine, head tilted to the unaffected side, with slight "beach chair" position to improve venous outflow from the head.

For upper trunk ruptures, exposure can be performed through a transverse incision in the supraclavicular region. Dissection is carried through the platysma and supraclavicular fascia to the plexus. The omohyoid muscle and, at times, the transverse cervical artery, are transected. The phrenic nerve is identified, usually in a scarred position on the anterior scalene muscle. Following the phrenic proximally leads to the C5 root. The C5, C6, and C7 roots are sequentially exposed between the anterior and middle scalene muscles and labeled with Silastic loops (Figs. 37-7 and 37-8). These muscles are usually fibrotic and adherent to the plexus. A decision is made regarding the integrity of each nerve root. Electrophysiologic studies, inspection of the transected nerve under the microscope, and/or rapid histologic staining may all be factors in the decision making.[112] Generally the roots are intact and there is an extraforaminal neuroma at the junction of C5 and C6 roots to form the upper trunk (Erb's point). Distal dissection beneath the clavicle leads to identification of the cords and major nerves. This includes identifying and protecting the axillary artery. In the infant, often the clavicle can be left intact and mobilized with a Penrose drain for adequate exposure. If necessary, the clavicle can be obliquely transected and repaired with suture through drill holes at the end of the operation. Sequentially, the major nerves are identified. The suprascapular nerve is exposed and labeled with a Silastic loop, usually as it exits the upper trunk neuroma and passes

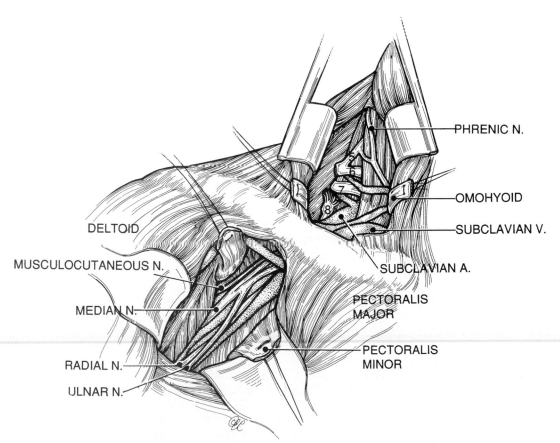

FIGURE 37-7. Key anatomic landmarks include the omohyoid muscle and the pectoralis minor muscle, which are divided between ligatures for later reapproximation. The C8 root is located just above and posterior to the subclavian artery, whereas the T1 root is almost directly posterior to the artery. With dissection of the deltopectoral grove, the lateral cord is the most superficial structure. In this example, the superior trunk and the C7 root are ruptured and the C-8 root is avulsed (note the rootlets attached to the swollen dorsal root ganglion).

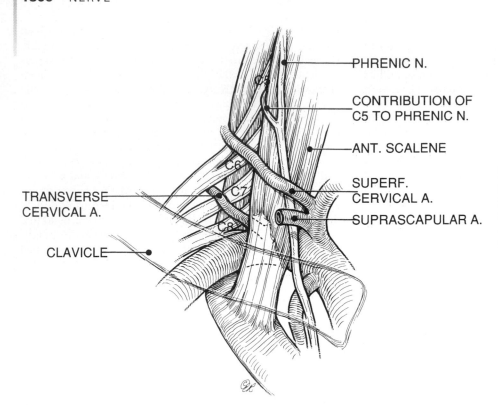

PHRENIC N.

CONTRIBUTION OF C5 TO PHRENIC N.

ANT. SCALENE

SUPERF. CERVICAL A.

SUPRASCAPULAR A.

TRANSVERSE CERVICAL A.

CLAVICLE

FIGURE 37-8. Additional landmarks helpful in identifying the various roots include the phrenic nerve contributions from the C5 root and the transverse cervical (scapular) artery, which frequently crosses over the C7 root.

posteriorly to the suprascapular notch. The musculocutaneous nerve is identified, labeled, and exposed from the lateral cord to the anterior division of the upper trunk until the neuroma is encountered. Similarly, the radial and axillary nerves are exposed and dissected to the posterior cord and posterior divisions of the upper, middle, and lower trunks. The posterior division of the lower trunk is usually intact, but the posterior division of the upper trunk and, at times, middle trunk, are usually encased in the neuroma. Intraoperative evoked potentials and nerve conduction are tested to determine the integrity of the nerve roots proximally and peripheral nerves distally. Some centers still advocate neurolysis if there is generation of at least 50% of a normal action potential across the neuroma with electrical stimulation.[49,106] However, Gilbert,[68] Meyer,[118] Laurent and associates,[106] and Clarke and colleagues[42] have all reported less than desired results with neurolysis. Therefore, transection of the fibrous neuroma proximally and distally and reconstruction of the defect with sural nerve grafts in an end-to-end fashion is almost universally performed. A few centers utilize vascularized grafts.[26] The cable grafts are joined and cut for desired length on the working table with fibrin glue before insertion into the plexal graft sites (Fig. 37-9). Microscopic 9-0 or 10-0 suture is used to approximate the epineural repair, and fibrin glue is again used to consolidate the cable graft repairs (Fig. 37-10).

When avulsions are encountered, more extensive exposure is necessary. This may include modifying the skin incision into a "Z" to expose the infraclavicular area. Each nerve root is assessed closely to determine the viability of the root. This can be a difficult intraoperative decision owing to partial avulsions. Electrophysiologic studies and histologic staining can augment direct microscopic observation. The C5 and C6 roots are usually intact with an extraforaminal rupture. The exception is an upper trunk lesion in a breech delivery in which C5 and C6 are often avulsed. Typically, in severe lesions, C8 and T1 are avulsed. C7 is variable in its integrity. Each case presents a unique intraoperative decision-making challenge. However, there are principles and usual case scenarios with avulsions that can lead to the most optimal results:

1. C5 to C7 nerve roots have extraforaminal ruptures, and C8 and T1 are avulsed. With three nerve roots available for grafting, it is possible to reconstruct the entire injured plexus. In this situation, transection of the C5 and C6 nerve roots to viable nerve and sural nerve grafting are done to the most viable proximal aspects of the suprascapular nerve, the medial, lateral, and posterior cords.
2. C5 and C6 have extraforaminal ruptures, and C7 to T1 have avulsions. This means there is less viable proximal nerve. The hand receives priority with grafting from C5 or C6 to the medial (ulnar and median nerves) and lateral cords (musculocutaneous and median nerves). Spinal accessory nerve transfer[5,134] is usually performed to the suprascapular nerve. Reconstruction of the posterior cord may need to be abandoned or reconstructed with nerve transfers to the musculocutaneous nerve with intercostal and grafting to the posterior cord.
3. C5 is the only viable nerve root. This is the most difficult situation and requires prioritizing an anatomic site. If the elbow and shoulder are chosen, the resultant outcome can be the creation of a Klumpke-type paralysis with shoulder and elbow function but no useful wrist or hand function. In infants, it is advised that the hand be given priority with grafts from C5. A combination of spinal accessory[5,134] and intercostal nerve transfers[124,125] along with C5 grafts is performed to the suprascapular,

CRITICAL POINTS: MICROSURGERY FOR BRACHIAL PLEXUS BIRTH PALSY

INDICATIONS

- Controversy regarding timing of intervention
- Flail extremity, Horner's syndrome at 3 months of life
- Failure of antigravity C5 to C7 function at 3 to 6 months of life: failure of antigravity biceps function most often used as indication in upper trunk rupture

PREOPERATIVE EVALUATION

- Perform careful, repeated physical examinations at 1- to 3-month intervals.
- Use CT-myelography or MRI to assess for avulsion at 3 months if in doubt.
- Electromyography/nerve conduction velocity study can be misleading except for avulsion diagnosis.

PEARLS

- Extensive experience at assessing brachial plexus pathoanatomy is strongly recommended.

TECHNICAL POINTS

- Use "beach chair" position with extensive prepping and draping for complete exposure of brachial plexus and possible nerve transfers.
- Use supraclavicular exposure for upper trunk ruptures. It may be a transverse or a "Z" incision. The transverse incision is more cosmetic.
- Use supraclavicular and infraclavicular exposure for more extensive injuries or avulsions.
- Ligate interfering external jugular vein branches and transverse cervical vessels as necessary.
- Transect omohyoid muscle.
- Mobilize clavicle. In infant, this may be feasible with Silastic tubing; oblique osteotomy may be indicated.

- Identify phrenic nerve and follow proximally to the C5 nerve root.
- Dissect nerve roots from anterior and middle scalene interval. Often fibrotic scar and neuroma are present.
- Identify each individual nerve root in a zone of injury (C5 to C7 in ruptures, C5 to T1 in avulsions) and follow it distally to the neuroma, or identify avulsion levels as appropriate.
- Dissect trunks, divisions, cords, and individual peripheral nerves.
- Isolate neuroma in rupture. Use electrodiagnostics to identify viable proximal and distal nerve conduction.
- Transect nerve and visualize it under the microscope for status of fascicles. If in doubt from microscopic appearance and electrodiagnostics, use histologic evaluation.
- Use sural nerve cable grafts without tension.
- Perform nerve transfers for avulsions. Spinal accessory and/or intercostals are most common.
- Use epineural approximating sutures and fibrin glue for neural repairs.

PITFALLS

- Nerve grafting necessary for partial or complete avulsion injuries
- Inadequate resection of fibrotic nerve
- Neurolysis alone
- Insufficient neural reconstruction for extent of injury

POSTOPERATIVE CARE

- Immobilize shoulder and neck for 4 weeks after surgery.

---

musculocutaneous, and median nerves (Fig. 37-11). Utilization of the contralateral C7 nerve root[39] and even the phrenic nerve may be necessary to maximally reconstruct the plexus.

Author's Preferred Method of Treatment: Microsurgery

As noted, there are limits to the present information available for the clinician to make decisions regarding timing of microsurgical intervention and ultimate outcome of these

patients versus natural history and tendon transfers. Within these limits, I presently care for these infants in the following ways:

1. Observation of all infants with brachial plexus birth palsy who begin to have antigravity biceps muscle recovery in the first 3 months of life. Physical therapy is performed until recovery is complete or plateaus to maintain a full range of motion of all joints of the upper limb, especially shoulder abduction and external rotation.
2. If there is a Horner syndrome and failure of recovery of some antigravity biceps strength by 3 months, surgery is performed at that time. Nerve grafting is performed if there are any intact nerve roots. Nerve transfers are almost always necessary owing to avulsion injuries and

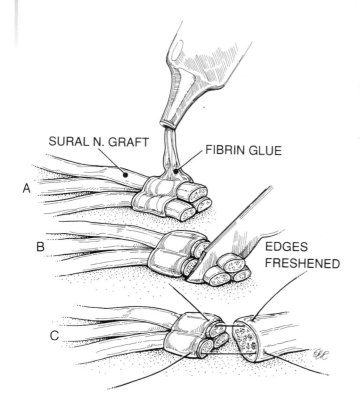

SURAL N. GRAFT — FIBRIN GLUE

A

B — EDGES FRESHENED

C

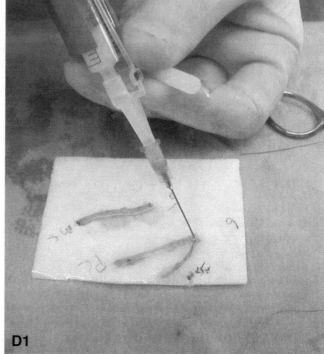

D1

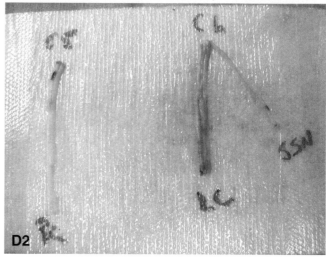

D2

FIGURE 37-9. Tissue adhesives can simplify the approximation of multiple strands of nerve graft proximally to a single large root stump or distally to a trunk or cord. **A,** The graft strands are first glued together. **B,** The graft strands are freshened. **C,** The mass is then approximated to the correct recipient site with a few microsutures passed through the glue and epineurium. Additional glue can be used to reinforce this juncture. **D,** Intraoperative photograph of surgical planning.

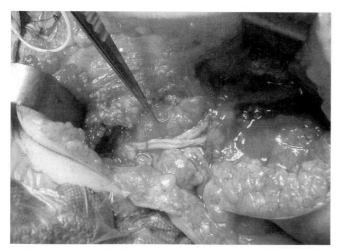

FIGURE 37-10. Intraoperative cable grafts for rupture of upper trunk.

limited viable proximal nerve roots. Transfers of a branch of the spinal accessory nerve, T2 to T4 intercostal nerves, and/or anterior fascicles of the ulnar nerve (requires an intact C8-T1 root)[7,128] are performed as appropriate. The hand, wrist, elbow, and shoulder are prioritized in that order.

3. If there is progressive recovery of wrist extension and finger extension without a Horner syndrome, I wait 5 to 6 months to determine if there will be return of some antigravity biceps function. If there is still no adequate return of biceps function by 5 to 6 months, surgery is performed at that time. Neuroma resection and nerve grafts or nerve transfers are performed based on intraoperative decisions.

4. All nonoperative patients are followed closely for the first 9 months of life to be certain recovery is progressive. In the rare instances of failure of biceps recovery to

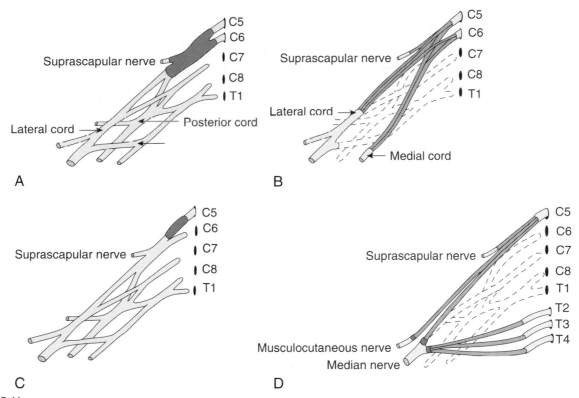

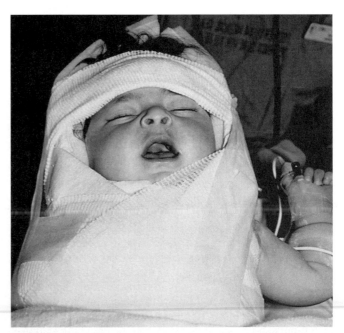

FIGURE 37-11. **A** to **D,** Combination grafting for C5-C7 rupture and C8-T1 avulsion. (From Gilbert A, Hentz VR, Tassin JL: Brachial plexus reconstruction in obstetrical palsy: Operative indications and postoperative results. In Urbaniak JR [ed]: Microsurgery for Major Limb Reconstruction. St. Louis, CV Mosby, 1987.)

AU: Is this the correct credit line?

progress to sufficient antigravity strength by 9 months of life (i.e., a positive "cookie test"), microsurgery is performed.

Postoperative Care

Postoperative immobilization is with a well-padded stockinette sling and swathe that binds the arm to the side. If there is any concern that neck motion will cause undue tension on the neural repairs, the neck is included in the immobilization (Fig. 37-12). Lower-extremity casts or bandages for the sural nerve graft donor sites are removed at 2 weeks after surgery. Arm immobilization is discontinued at 4 weeks. Shoulder and arm range of motion is reinitiated at this time to prevent contracture development. The parents and therapists are informed that improved function will not occur for 6 to 18 months. However, failure to observe progressive recovery of the biceps by 6 to 9 months is of concern. Re-exploration and additional microsurgery may be indicated for the failure of biceps recovery by 9 to 12 months after surgery.

Complications of infection, systemic deterioration, bleeding, or worsening neural condition are rare. At times, a phrenic nerve palsy can recur with a postoperative elevated hemidiaphragm. If this persists and affects respiratory function, a late diaphragmatic plication is appropriate. The major complication of microsurgery is the failure to achieve the desired outcome. It is important for parents to understand that perfect range of motion, strength, posture, and function are rarely achieved with microsurgery.[82] However, improvement from the natural history in all those areas is desired

FIGURE 37-12. Postoperatively, the infant is placed in a prefabricated "clam shell" orthosis that limits motion of the neck, shoulder, and arm.

and possible. Still, between 10% and 20% of ruptured and avulsed patients will not have an optimal result. In addition, even with a positive outcome for arm function and strength, the majority of these patients require secondary tendon transfers to further improve their situation. Finally, the life-long implications for self-esteem, psychosocial well-being, and function in these children are still unclear.[18,37,60]

SHOULDER WEAKNESS AND DEFORMITY

There is frequent shoulder weakness, contracture, and joint deformity in infants and children with brachial plexus birth palsies.[136,137] Even the children with the mildest chronic plexopathy will have some limitation of glenohumeral motion with increased scapular winging. Only those infants who recover antigravity biceps strength in the first 4 to 6 weeks of life will have no asymmetry of their shoulder girdle on long-term examination. The initial trauma of the birthing process may cause muscular injury that leads to myostatic contracture.[182,184] Peri-articular injury can be the result of the same process with resultant glenohumeral capsular and ligamentous tightness. On rare occasions, an infantile glenohumeral dislocaton[57,161] can occur due to the birth trauma. More commonly, abduction and external rotation weakness from a failure of neuromuscular recovery, in conjunction with the muscular and periarticular tightness, leads to an internal rotation and adduction contracture.[94] If the soft tissue contracture and muscle imbalance is allowed to persist, then progressive glenohumeral joint deformity is universal.[132,172,173,177,182] This only worsens the clinical situation of limited motion, strength, and function. The infantile treatment options of physical therapy, splinting, botulinum injections,[138] and surgical interventions are all designed to reverse this process.

Preoperative Evaluation

Recovery of active muscle strength in infants is graded by Medical Research Council grading, Mallet classification, and/or HSC scores. Assessing infants for shoulder function involves observation of spontaneous activity, neonatal reflex activity (Moro, asymmetrical tonic neck, symmetrical tonic neck), and stimulated activity with and without gravity assistance. Passive glenohumeral motion is assessed with scapular stabilization. Internal and external rotation is performed both in adduction and in 90 degrees of abduction while stabilizing the scapula against the thorax. The degree of scapular winging posteriorly with internal rotation, superiorly with full adduction, and into the axilla with full abduction and forward flexion is recorded. It is important to palpate for posterior glenohumeral joint dislocation in the posterior soft spot because it is critical not to miss the rare infantile dislocation. Dynamic instability is assessed by palpation posteriorly while monitoring passive and active range of motion, especially with adduction and internal rotation. Subscapularis tightness is evaluated by measuring the scapular-humeral angle in abduction again with scapular stabilization. Pectoralis major, latissimus dorsi, and teres major tightness are assessed by palpation of the muscles with abduction and external rotation.

Infantile treatment of the shoulder focuses on maintaining a full passive range of motion. It is unclear how long after birth the nerves should be protected with immobilization to lessen recurrent traumatic stretch. However, early motion is important to prevent myostatic and periarticular

contractures. Initially, a gentle home program is begun at 7 to 10 days of life, followed by a formal physical therapy program with home supervision in infants who do not recover rapidly in the first month of life. Full glenohumeral range with scapular stabilization is the goal. Abduction and external rotation splints have been used to improve or maintain range of motion. Compliance can be poor, and Zancolli has expressed concern that these splints may increase the risk of injury to the physis and developing joint.[182,184] Botulinum injections have been used to lessen the contracting muscle forces.[48,138] Post-botulinum splints, spica casts, electrical stimulation, and intensified therapy have all been advised. However, at present there are no data to guide the clinician on the indications and expected outcomes from these various treatments. It is clear, however, that the failure to maintain full passive range of motion of the joint puts the child at risk for the development of glenohumeral deformity.

If the child fails to recover external rotation strength and motion, there will be significant functional consequences.[90] External rotation of the shoulder is necessary to achieve above-horizontal shoulder activity (i.e., reach the hand to the occiput and forehead). Scapulothoracic winging can compensate for limited glenohumeral motion in all planes except external rotation. In this circumstance, the scapula abuts the posterior thorax. This leads to marked limitation of function owing to the inability to appropriately place the hand in space for many activities. In addition, weakness about the shoulder further limits hand use away from the body. The child has difficulty placing and maintaining the hand at a desired location in space due to fatigue. The affected limb will, therefore, most often be used at the child's side or with support from furniture or the ipsilateral leg.

Ultrasound can be used in infancy to evaluate the glenohumeral joint and proximal humerus. Similar to the hip, the joint can be assessed for congruency and dynamic stability by ultrasound. Proximal humeral fractures and glenohumeral joint dislocations can be detected by ultrasound as well. Plain radiographs are not usually helpful in infancy because the secondary centers of ossification are not present from birth to 6 months of life. If there is persistent muscle imbalance with growth, later radiographs will reveal the progressive deformity of the glenoid, proximal humerus, acromion, and/or coracoid.[98] Arthrograms provide a clearer picture of the joint and bony development than radiographs in these infants and children.[132] However, most institutions utilize MRI[81] to assess the cartilaginous surfaces of the glenohumeral joint in young children and CT[89] or MRI to evaluate the joint and bony structures in older children. In infants and young children, MRI requires sedation, while arthrograms have been performed under anesthesia.[132] The glenohumeral deformity progresses from normal (I) to posterior glenoid deformity (II), to humeral head subluxation and further glenoid dysplasia (III), to the development of a false glenoid (IV), to flattening of both the glenoid and the humeral head (V) (see Fig. 37-4). The degree of joint deformity can guide the surgeon in selection of surgical procedure. It is clear that with minimal joint deformity (grades I and II), release or lengthening of contracted muscles and tendon transfers for improved external rotation and abduction have a very favorable outcome.[92,173,174] With more severe deformity of the joint (grade V and advanced grade IV), a humeral derotational osteotomy improves function significantly.[173] The role of arthroscopic débridement and reduction, open reduction and capsulorrhaphy, and glenoid osteotomy are still not well defined.[132,133] The degree of glenoid remodeling possible with a soft tissue procedure is still unknown but age, degree of preoperative deformity, and the type of surgical procedure(s) performed must all be factors. In patients with grade III and grade IV deformity, these issues become very important in the decision regarding timing and choice of surgical procedure(s).

Historical Review

In 1888, Stimson described a posterior dislocation of the shoulder in a child with a brachial plexus birth palsy.[156] Later, Whitman (1905) distinguished between a congenital dislocation and an acquired dislocation associated with a brachial plexopathy.[176] Fairbanks (1913)[63] performed an operative reduction of a dislocation by anterior capsulotomy and subscapularis release. L'Episcopo[108] described the results of tendon rebalancing procedures about the shoulder for obstetric paralysis in the 1930s, initially with the teres major alone and subsequently with the teres major and the latissimus dorsi muscles. Wickstrom defined a high incidence of permanent deficits about the shoulder with joint deformity in a classic article in 1962.[177] Hoffer, Wickenden, and Roper[92] described transferring the latissimus dorsi into the greater tuberosity region to improve not only external rotation but also abduction. Many authors since then have described favorable results with tendon transfers about the shoulder in patients with residual brachial plexus birth palsies.[21,22,38,45,46]

Operations

Indications for surgical intervention about the shoulder include (1) infantile dislocation, (2) persistent internal rotation contracture despite aggressive nonoperative management, (3) limitation of abduction and external rotation function with plateauing of neural recovery, and (4) progressive glenohumeral deformity. The age at intervention is dependent on the problem and its severity.

The rare infantile dislocation is treated as early as it is recognized, hopefully before the glenoid deficiency becomes unreconstructable.[57,161] Ideally this is within the first 3 to 12 months of life. An anterior release of the thickened capsule and middle and inferior glenohumeral ligaments and a débridement of the joint are necessary for reduction of the humeral head. Lengthening of the subscapularis and pectoralis major muscles is often required. A posterior capsulorrhaphy is performed, usually via a second incision. The deltoid is elevated from the spine of the scapula while protecting the axillary nerve, and the latissimus dorsi and teres major tendons are released from their often conjoint insertion onto the humerus. The infraspinatus/teres minor interval is used to expose the joint. The degree of glenoid dysplasia is assessed, and the joint is atraumatically reduced into the deformed glenoid. This may require more extensive release or lengthening of additional myostatic contractures, such as the deltoid. Stability of the joint is assessed. On rare occasions, a glenoid osteotomy to ele-

vate the posterior glenoid, with a posterior acromial bone block or allograft, is necessary to maintain joint reduction and congruency. The posterior capsule is reefed, but not excessively so, because this will limit postoperative glenohumeral motion. The latissimus dorsi and teres major tendons are transferred to the greater tuberosity of the humerus. Postoperative immobilization involves a shoulder spica cast for 4 to 6 weeks.

Carlioz and Brahimi[34] described a subscapularis lengthening for infants who fail to regain passive external rotation in the first 6 to 12 months of life with extensive physical therapy. The subscapularis can be lengthened by an anterior "Z"-lengthening of the tendon; musculotendinous lengthening via a posterior axillary incision; or, as Carlioz and Brahimi[34] described, elevation of the subscapularis off the anterior scapula as a muscle slide. All of these procedures can improve passive external rotation and glenoscapular excursion.

Arthroscopic surgery has been utilized in children with brachial plexopathy and glenohumeral problems.[133] It allows for direct visualization of the joint to assess the degree of deformity and soft tissue contractures. Anterior release of the thickened middle and inferior glenohumeral ligaments can be performed, and the subscapularis can also be released. The joint can be débrided of interposing, intra-articular tissue and synovitis. In an infant, this can performed in a lateral decubitus position with manual traction of the affected limb. The smaller arthroscopic equipment is utilized with standard shoulder arthroscopy techniques. Direct visualization of the joint reduction can be performed and tendon transfers can be performed in the same surgical setting without difficulty. It is too preliminary to know the ultimate role of arthroscopic surgery in these children, but early clinical experience is promising and arthroscopy provides a less invasive form of treatment based on the principles Fairbanks outlined in 1913.

Children who fail to attain active abduction and external rotation are candidates for tendon transfers (Fig. 37-13).* Most commonly this involves transfer of the latissimus dorsi and teres major to the greater tuberosity insertion of the rotator cuff. In children with an associated internal rotation contracture, surgery includes lengthening the pectoralis major, subscapularis, and/or muscular origins from the coracoid as appropriate. Examination of the passive range of motion in the operating room will complete the diagnosis regarding contractures of the pectoralis major, subscapularis, teres major, latissimus dorsi, and coracoid musculature. Surgery is performed in the lateral decubitus position, with care taken to protect the contralateral plexus and peroneal nerve. If the pectoralis major is contracted with external rotation in 90 degrees of abduction, then a small 2- to 3-cm anterior axillary incision is utilized to perform a musculotendinous lengthening. Through the same incision, the origin of the coracobrachialis, short head of the biceps, and pectoralis minor can undergo a musculotendinous lengthening (while protecting the musculocutaneous nerve) if there is a mild elbow flexion contracture. A second small

---

*See references 21, 22, 38, 45, 56, 59, 67, 79, 91, 92, 157, 164, 173, 174, 180, and 182.

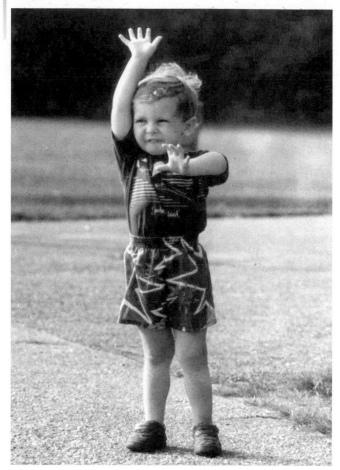

FIGURE 37-13. Clinical photograph of child with limited shoulder external rotation and abduction preoperatively.

posterior axillary incision is made from the edge of the latissimus dorsi inferiorly to the inferior edge of the deltoid posterosuperiorly. In obese or older children, the anterior and posterior incisions can be joined to protect the brachial plexus and improve exposure. The often conjoint insertion of the latissimus dorsi and teres major is isolated and released from the humerus. These muscles can be confused with the more posterior triceps by the uninitiated surgeon. The muscles are mobilized for maximal excursion while identifying and protecting the neurovascular pedicle. The interval between the triceps and deltoid is now exposed. There may be crossing fascial connections between the triceps, latissimus, and axillary skin that need to be released. The greater tuberosity, infraspinatus, and supraspinatus tendons are identified. The axillary nerve and circumflex vessels are identified and protected. The subacromial space is decompressed. The glenoid and posterior humeral head should be easily palpable. If the joint is unstable or subluxed, a decision regarding a posterior capsular shift is necessary. If a capsular stabilization or glenoid osteotomy is appropriate, then joint exposure is performed through a teres minor/infraspinatus interval while protecting both the axillary and radial nerves. If appropriate, the capsule is incised off the posterior glenoid and reefed to improve static stability. Again, it is important to avoid excessive tightening

CRITICAL POINTS: LATISSIMUS DORSI, TERES MAJOR TENDON TRANSFER; SHOULDER MUSCULOTENDINOUS LENGTHENING, PECTORALIS MAJOR, SUBSCAPULARIS

INDICATIONS

- Internal rotation contracture, external rotation weakness of the shoulder
- Minimal glenohumeral deformity
- Functional impairment above the shoulder in external rotation

PREOPERATIVE EVALUATION

- MRI to assess degree of glenohumeral joint deformity

PEARLS

- Standardized MRI is used to assess joint.
- Marked glenohumeral deformity is a contraindication to transfer.
- Assess pectoralis major, subscapularis, biceps tightness, and reducibility of the joint intraoperatively.

TECHNICAL POINTS

- Make axillary incisions: anterior lengthenings, posterior tendon transfers.
- Use anterior musculotendinous lengthening of pectoralis major for adduction and internal rotation contracture with palpable intraoperative tightness.
- Use posterior exposure and release of conjoint latissimus dorsi and teres major tendons.
- Mobilize latissimus and teres while protecting neurovascular pedicle.
- Expose rotator cuff insertion in greater tuberosity in posterior deltoid/triceps interval.
- Protect subdeltoid axillary nerve.
- Assess subscapularis contracture. If humeral-scapular excursion is limited, then lengthen subscapularis.
- Assess glenohumeral joint stability. If necessary, perform posterior capsular reefing.
- Insert latissimus and teres subdeltoid into greater tuberosity and supraspinatus and infraspinatus tendons.
- Reassess axillary nerve to be certain no compression or compromise

CRITICAL POINTS: LATISSIMUS DORSI, TERES MAJOR TENDON TRANSFER; SHOULDER MUSCULOTENDINOUS LENGTHENING, PECTORALIS MAJOR, SUBSCAPULARIS—cont'd

PITFALLS

- Tendon transfer in the presence of significant glenohumeral dysplasia will result in limitations of motion (generally adduction-external rotation).

POSTOPERATIVE CARE

- Immobilize in forward flexion, abduction, and external rotation for 4 to 6 weeks.
- Begin passive and active range-of-motion exercises.
- When out of cast, motion is almost immediately improved.

RETURN TO ACTIVITIES

- After surgery in 2- to 5-year-old children return to full activities can be done shortly after regaining motion.

Surgery is performed with the patient in a "beach chair" position. The entire shoulder girdle region including the scapula is left exposed with prepping and draping. The proximal humerus is exposed in the extended deltopectoral interval. Curvilinear incisions that take into account the expected external rotation of the skin after correction will lessen the risk of unsightly hypertrophic scars. The cephalic vein is protected and subperiosteal exposure of the humerus is performed lateral to the pectoralis major insertion. The transverse osteotomy is performed just proximal to the deltoid insertion. By securing the proximal screws of the plate before the osteotomy, control of the humerus with correction is facilitated. The proximal and distal aspects of the humerus are marked for the desired correction, usually 60 to 90 degrees. It is important to protect the radial nerve during the osteotomy because it lies posterior to the humerus at this level. With derotation, the plate is temporarily fixed to be certain that the hand can reach the mouth, occiput, chest, abdomen, and genitalia. Final internal fixation is then performed (Fig. 37-14). Postoperative immobilization depends on the age of the child and strength of the internal fixation. Of note, the osteotomy can also be performed distally through a medial incision. The principles of planning, osteotomy, and fixation are the same at that level as they are with a proximal osteotomy.

because this will limit postoperative glenohumeral motion. At this stage, a final decision regarding the subscapularis is necessary. If greater than 130 degrees of passive scapular-humeral motion is not possible under anesthesia without scapular winging into the axilla, then a subscapularis lengthening is performed. This can be by any of the three methods described previously. Finally, the latissimus dorsi and teres major tendons are inserted into the supraspinatus and infraspinatus tendon insertions of the greater tuberosity. Periosteal and tendinous sutures are appropriate in the young; osseous suture anchors, avoiding the physis, may be necessary in the older child or adolescent. Postoperative immobilization in appropriate abduction, forward flexion, and external rotation for the procedure performed and the age of the patient is used for 4 to 6 weeks.

If the glenohumeral joint is markedly deformed, a derotational humeral osteotomy is indicated for patients with functional limitations of abduction and external rotation. This is most often needed in teenagers or younger children with advanced-for-age joint deformity. Under anesthesia, a final assessment of the passive range of motion of the joint is performed. Often these children have limited glenohumeral motion owing to their deformity or dislocation. It is critical to understand the range of motion available, because this will ultimately determine the degree of humeral external rotation correction. The goal is to have the hand easily reach the mouth, forehead, and occiput without loss of the ability to reach the genitalia, abdomen, chest, or contralateral hand.

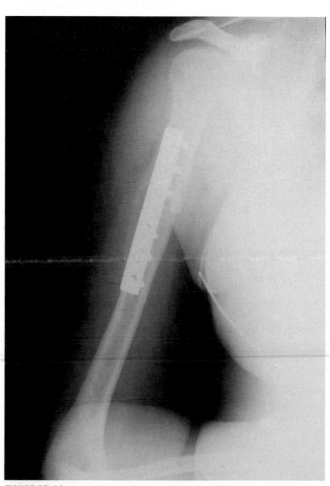

FIGURE 37-14. Postoperative radiograph of proximal humeral osteotomy.

CRITICAL POINTS: HUMERAL DEROTATION OSTEOTOMY

INDICATIONS

- Internal rotation contracture and external rotation weakness of shoulder
- Functional impairment for above-shoulder activities

PREOPERATIVE EVALUATION

- CT of glenohumeral joint. Classify degree of glenohumeral dysplasia.

PEARLS

- Advanced deformity with dislocated and flattened humeral head but compensatory scapulothoracic motion will have functional improvement with osteotomy.

TECHNICAL POINTS

- Locate distal deltopectoral interval.
- Use subperiosteal exposure at level of deltoid insertion.
- Apply plate proximally before osteotomy.

- Mark bone for desired degree of correction before osteotomy.
- Perform a transverse osteotomy protecting the posterior radial nerve.
- Perform temporary fixation distally after external rotation of distal fragment. Check ability to reach occiput, mouth, chest, abdomen, and genitalia. If correction is insufficient or excessive, adjust degree of external rotation before permanent fixation.
- Perform compression fixation distally.

PITFALL

- Failure to control osteotomy and degree of correction

POSTOPERATIVE CARE

- Immobilize the shoulder for 4 to 6 weeks.
- Begin rehabilitation for strength and function.

RETURN TO ACTIVITIES

- After healed osteotomy, full return of strength, and recovery of corrected motion

Author's Preferred Treatment

Infants who present with a brachial plexus birth palsy are examined closely for a dislocation or instability of the glenohumeral joint as well as for contractures about the shoulder. In the presence of an infantile dislocation, an MRI under sedation is obtained to assess the development of the glenoid and the joint alignment. If the patient is young and the glenoid is not severely deformed, either an arthroscopic or an open reduction is performed. A posterior capsulorrhaphy along with latissimus dorsi and teres major tendon transfers are performed at the same surgical setting.

Usually, infants and children with chronic brachial plexus birth palsy will develop an internal rotation and adduction contracture about the shoulder. Ideally, physical therapy instructions for passive range of motion with scapular stabilization are begun in the first few weeks of life in an attempt to prevent contractures and joint deformity. If a contracture develops in the first 1 to 2 years of life that does not resolve with 3 months of supervised therapy, an MRI is utilized to assess the glenohumeral joint. If the joint is normal, then more aggressive therapy, potentially in combination with botulinum injections and splinting program, is considered. At times an isolated scapularis release is performed, but this situation is rare. Unfortunately, joint deformity occurs very often early in life in the presence of muscle imbalance and periarticular contractures. In the presence of mild deformity (types II and III), an anterior release of myostatic contractures and posterior latissimus dorsi and teres major tendon transfers are performed. An

arthroscopic examination and release may be performed initially to improve joint reduction. If the joint deformity is more severe (more advanced type III or type IV), it may be difficult to decide if the joint can be reconstructed. Visualization of the joint, either open or arthroscopically, can aid in this decision. Reduction of the humeral head and stabilization of the joint by an anterior capsule release (arthroscopic or open), posterior capsular reefing, and posterior tendon transfers is preferred. However, to be successful, this requires maintenance of the reduction, acceptable glenohumeral motion, and remodeling of the glenoid. The degree of glenoid remodeling with soft tissue procedures is still unknown. If the joint deformity is too severe at any age (advanced type IV, type V), a humeral external rotation osteotomy is performed. This is done when it is determined that the joint cannot be reconstructed. This is common in adolescent patients with an internal rotation contracture, external rotation limitation, and advanced deformity evident by CT or MRI. A posterior, opening wedge glenoid osteotomy with bone graft is utilized rarely to provide posterior bony stabilization in reconstructable type IV deformities. However, the indications and outcomes from this procedure are still unclear.

Postoperative Care

Infants and young children with open reductions and/or tendon transfers are immobilized in a shoulder spica cast or brace for 4 to 6 weeks. Generally the position of immobilization is forward flexion, abduction, and external rotation with a scapular mold to maintain correction of contractures, reduction of the joint, and protection of the soft tissue repairs. Unrestricted active and passive motion is begun after immobilization. Improved active motion of forward flexion, abduction, and external rotation is expected after tendon transfers.[173,174] Postoperative improvement in external rotation of greater than 45 degrees and abduction of greater than 60 degrees has been reported for these transfers.[92,137] Global improvement in function is also expected by Mallet scores with average preoperative global scores of 9.5 improving to 15.6 postoperatively.[173] In addition, improved hand utilization occurs because the hand can be better stabilized in space without fatigue owing to the active strength of the transfer.

Humeral osteotomies are immobilized with a spica cast in younger children and a sling and swathe in adolescents for 4 weeks. Unrestricted rehabilitation is begun once bony healing occurs. Outcomes for osteotomy are very similar to tendon transfers,[173] with improved range of motion and function expected.[75]

Complications are rare in these operations. Even in situations of marked weakness of the affected arm, the latissimus dorsi and teres major transfers usually provide a positive antigravity result.[173] The status of the glenohumeral joint determines outcome. Preoperative assessment of the joint with an MRI or arthrogram will aid in the process of selecting a specific surgical intervention. If the joint is deformed, there may be continued postoperative restriction of motion with a tendon transfer. This is most common with limited external rotation in adduction. Increased scapulothoracic motion cannot compensate for the limited glenohumeral motion in these planes. A secondary humeral osteotomy with external rotation may be necessary to remedy the marked trumpet posture and inability to externally rotate the arm from an adducted position. This situation could be viewed potentially as a failure of preoperative selection because an osteotomy may have been indicated instead of muscle transfer.

Joint remodeling may be limited with tendon transfer procedures alone. Closed reductions have been described,[91] but follow-up radiographic studies are limited. Open or arthroscopic reductions may improve the potential for joint stabilization and remodeling. Longer follow-up studies are necessary to answer these questions. The risk of long-term pain and disability from a deformed joint is unknown but appears to be much less than a dysplastic hip. This issue is central to many medicolegal disputes regarding the outcome of these children.

ELBOW

Early in infancy, the major issue with the elbow in these children is the failure of return of biceps function for elbow flexion and forearm supination. As mentioned in the preceding sections, this is one of the major indicators for microsurgical intervention in the first 3 to 9 months of life. Fortunately, it is rare to have long-term persistence of antigravity elbow flexion weakness. Failure to recover antigravity biceps strength is a disappointing end result in both the natural history and with microsurgical reconstruction. Failure of biceps recovery by natural history observation may be a failure of surgical decision making, because nerve

exploration and reconstruction might have been appropriate. Late exploration may be indicated and has been performed as late as 22 months of age. With failure of microsurgery, the surgeon needs to determine if re-exploration and neural surgery will have a positive outcome; however, there is a time element to this decision. Too early re-exploration may be unnecessary and harmful; re-exploration too late may be beyond the time that the motor end plates can respond positively to reinnervation. The situation that lends itself best to re-exploration is a missed avulsion injury that was inappropriately grafted, because this can potentially be treated with nerve transfers. This may require the use of unusual transfers such as a contralateral C7, phrenic nerve, or the more common intercostal, spinal accessory, or partial ulnar or median nerve transfers. Review of the literature provides little information on the success of re-exploration of surgical repair of the plexus.

The other options available for failure of biceps recovery include tendon transfers and vascularized muscle transfers.[15,21,22,114] Regional tendon transfers include use of the pectoralis major, latissimus dorsi, triceps, or forearm flexor-pronator muscle origin (Steindler flexorplasty).[167] (see Chapter 38 for a detailed description of these procedures.) The donor muscles must be near normal in strength for successful transfer, and the loss of donor function cannot lead to worsening impairment. All three muscle groups have been used successfully to provide active elbow flexion in this situation.[21,22] The latissimus dorsi and pectoralis major muscles need to be mobilized on their neurovascular pedicles without undue tension. Both are aligned from the proximal coracoid or acromion to the distal native biceps tendon, radial tuberosity, or coronoid. In performing the Steindler flexorplasty, the medial epicondyle, and origin of the forearm flexor, the pronator mass is detached and secured to the central aspect of the distal humerus with a compression screw and washer.[167] Doi has popularized the use of free gracilis vascularized muscle transfers in both failed natural history and microsurgical recovery.[50,52] For elbow flexion, the gracilis is similarly secured proximally at the coracoid or acromion and distally at the native biceps tendon, radial tuberosity, or coronoid[15] (see Chapter 38). Neural connection is necessary via the intercostals, spinal accessory, or ipsilateral or contralateral C7. The information on results in children is limited.

The development of an elbow flexion contracture is common in these children.[16] This is often associated with antigravity triceps weakness and may involve co-contractions. Initial treatment of the elbow flexion contracture is with physical therapy for stretching the biceps, brachialis, and anterior elbow capsule. Night-time splinting may be helpful, although there is limited information to determine its cost-effectiveness. Fortunately, most of these contractures are mild and less than 30 degrees. This mild degree of contracture does not appear to limit activities of daily living. More significant contractures (>60 degrees) may need to be addressed surgically. Anterior release of the capsule with lengthening of the biceps and brachialis has a short-term positive benefit. However, postoperative rehabilitation is extensive; and, in the absence of triceps muscle function, recurrence is high.

There is limited experience with the restoration of antigravity triceps function in these children. Transfer of the posterior deltoid with a graft is the usual procedure for triceps weakness in tetraplegia. In children with a brachial plexus birth palsy, there usually is deltoid weakness that is a contraindication for transfer both because of donor morbidity and failure of sufficient recipient site strength. Use of the latissimus dorsi as a tricepsplasty has been described in a limited study.[21,93] A vascularized transfer of the gracilis to the triceps has been advocated by Doi in adults,[51] but it has not been utilized as commonly in children. More often than not, the triceps weakness and elbow flexion contracture are reluctantly accepted by the surgeon, patient, and family. Restoration of antigravity triceps strength in these children with persistent C7 weakness is an unsolved problem.

FOREARM

Limitation of active supination is very common in children with incomplete recovery of their brachial plexus birth palsy. When combined with an internal rotation contracture and external rotation weakness of the shoulder, this deficiency becomes more obvious. These children posture in pronation and raise their hands toward their mouth with marked abduction and internal rotation with a neutral or pronated forearm (see Fig. 37-13). Correction of the shoulder problem will improve the forearm motion because shoulder adduction, external rotation, and forearm supination are complementary motions. However, in the absence of full biceps strength, there often will be some unresolved supination weakness. Therapy, splints, and electrical stimulation do not seem to resolve this problem. Surgery is rarely indicated for mild supination loss.

It is possible after microsurgery or natural history to attain recovery of C5 and C6 function without more distal recovery. These children appear to have a Klumpke paralysis of sorts. There is functional deltoid and biceps recovery without sufficient radial, median, or ulnar nerve recovery. The child will posture into elbow flexion and forearm supination, often with a marked contracture of both joints. There may be recovery of some active wrist extension and potentially some limited finger flexion. The wrist often is contracted into extension owing to lack of antigravity flexor strength. These children utilize only their forearm for assistive function such as lifting with a flexed elbow. They avoid active use of their hand, often far beyond what one would expect.[181,183] Frequently they are bothered by their unsightly posturing of elbow flexion, forearm supination, and wrist extension. Surgery is indicated for improved elbow extension, forearm pronation, and hand function. The factors determining the type of operation performed include triceps function, passive range of pronation, and status of the distal radioulnar joint. The elbow flexion contracture is addressed with a brachialis musculotendinous lengthening, biceps "Z"-lengthening, and, at times, anterior elbow capsular release. The lack of active pronation is most often addressed by rerouting the biceps tendon so it dynamically pronates rather than supinates. The biceps tendon is wrapped around the radial neck, while protecting the posterior interosseous nerve, so the line of pull of the biceps provides forearm pronation. It is repaired in a "Z"-lengthened position to improve passive extension of the elbow. In the absence of

triceps function, there is a significant concern regarding recurrence of the elbow flexion contracture. The supination contracture can be addressed by interosseous membrane release, forearm osteotomy(ies), or radioulnar fusion. Zancolli advocates an interosseous membrane release,[181] whereas Gilbert performs a radial osteotomy distally along with the biceps rerouting.[68] In severe contractures, osteotomy of both the radius and ulna may be necessary. In the presence of radioulnar joint dislocation, creation of a single bone forearm may be the best solution. The forearm is positioned in neutral to mild pronation (20 degrees) in all these procedures to avoid overcorrection. An active pronation force needs to be provided by either a biceps rerouting transfer or by rerouting the flexor carpi ulnaris to the brachioradialis.[184] Antigravity wrist extension strength must be present preoperatively for the hand to function in a pronated position. The anticipated outcome from these procedures is generally improved utilization of the hand. The patients are often pleased with the cosmetic result owing to a more natural posturing of the arm and hand in social settings.

WRIST AND HAND

Fortunately, the majority of children with a brachial plexus birth palsy have an upper trunk lesion with near-normal recovery of the wrist and hand. The C8 and T1 function often recovers without marked limitation. The C7 functional recovery may be incomplete with some limitation of wrist and finger extension, but frequently there is sufficient compensatory function by tenodesis strength that surgery is not indicated. If not, transfer of the flexor carpi ulnaris to the wrist or digital extensors is appropriate. However, there are rare individuals who have permanent, devastating limitations in the use of their affected hand. The dilemma is that there are few options for improving hand function in these children later in life. There too often are limited donor muscles for active transfer. Generally those muscles available for transfer are weak, and thus wrist stabilization may be necessary for functional transfers to work. This can be achieved with wrist capsulodesis, arthrodesis of the radial epiphysis to the carpus in the skeletally immature patient, or arthrodesis in a skeletally mature person. The results of these procedures show improvement, although rarely to the level of an independent functioning hand. Double free gracilis muscle transfer for prehension in adults with complete avulsion of the brachial plexus has been performed by Doi and coworkers with positive results (see Chapter 38).[50,52] The experience with this technique is more limited in children. It is because of these limited secondary options that Gilbert advocates prioritizing the hand in infantile microsurgery for more severe brachial plexus birth palsies.[68]

Ulnar deviation deformity of the wrist is not uncommon in those children with incomplete recovery of hand and wrist function. The deforming force is an unbalanced extensor carpi ulnaris and/or flexor carpi ulnaris. Transfer of the deforming force to a more central location, usually the extensor carpi radialis brevis, is common. This is usually performed with elbow, forearm, and wrist procedures as noted earlier. Again, there often is improvement in both function and cosmesis. However, it is rare to achieve a desired independence of hand function in these individuals.

ANNOTATED REFERENCES

6. Al-Qattan MM: The outcome of Erb's palsy when the decision to operate is made at 4 months of age. Plast Reconst Surg 106:1461-1465, 2000.

   This study confirms previous studies that early recovery of biceps function in the first 2 months of age leads to full recovery. Biceps recovery between 2 and 4 months of age will result in return of elbow flexion but there may be some residual shoulder weakness. Microsurgery performed for failure of biceps recovery beyond 4 months still improved function.

33. Capek L, Clarke HM, Curtis CG: Neuroma-in-continuity resection: Early outcome in obstetrical brachial plexus palsy. Plast Reconst Surg 102:1555-1562, 1998.

   The authors note improved function 6 to 12 months after resection of both conducting and nonconducting neuromas-in-continuity despite an initial worsening of the clinical situation. This study addresses the role of neurolysis versus resection and grafting of neuromas-in-continuity.

52. Doi K, Muramatsu K, Hattori Y, et al: Restoration of prehension with the double free muscle technique following complete avulsion of the brachial plexus. J Bone Joint Surg Am 82:652-666, 2000.

   Although this is a report on adults, any microsurgeon caring for children with severe brachial plexus injuries should be aware of this work and the results. Free gracilis transfers are utilized in devastating injuries with limited reconstructive alternatives in children.

65. Geutjens G, Gilbert A, Helsen K: Obstetric brachial plexus palsy associated with breech delivery. J Bone Joint Surg Br 78:303-306, 1996.

   Eighty-one percent of the 36 breech delivery infants had an upper trunk avulsion injury rather than the usual upper trunk rupture. Surgical reconstruction will require nerve transfers because grafting will fail.

69. Gilbert A, Tassin JL: Reparation chirurgicale du plexus brachial dans la paralysie obstetricale. Chirurgie 110:70, 1984.

72. Gilbert A, Hentz VR, Tassin JL: Brachial plexus reconstruction in obstetrical palsy: Operative indications and postoperative results. *In* Urbaniek JR (ed): Microsurgery for Major Limb Reconstruction. St. Louis, CV Mosby, 1987.

   The original Gilbert and Tassin in French is expanded and translated in the book chapter for easier English review. The clinical data by Tassin and Gilbert is classic for defining the timing of recovery of biceps antigravity function as an indicator of long-term outcome. The outcome with biceps recovery beyond 6 months was poor and served as the basis for microsurgical intervention. Subsequently, microsurgery was recommended for infants with no antigravity biceps recovery by 3 months of life.

92. Hoffer M, Wickenden R, Roper B: Brachial plexus birth palsies: Results of tendon transfers to the rotator cuff. J Bone Joint Surg Am 60:691-695, 1978.

   Describes transferring the latissimus dorsi and teres major tendons to the rotator cuff. Technique is well described for now-classic operation.

100. Kawabata H, Kawai H, Masatomi T, Yasui N: Accessory nerve neurotization in infants with brachial plexus birth palsy. Microsurgery 15:768-772, 1994.

   A report on 13 spinal accessory nerve transfers at a mean age of 5.9 months with improvement in function. Their indications and surgical technique are described.

102. Kawai H, Tsuyuguchi Y, Masada K: Identification of the lesion in brachial plexus injuries with root avulsion: A comprehensive assessment by means of preoperative findings, myelography, surgical exploration, and intraoperative diagnostics. Neuro-Orthop 7:15-23, 1989.

   This study compares preoperative radiologic studies with intraoperative findings. By comparing myelography, CT-myelography, and MRI with findings by intraoperative electrodiagnostics and surgical findings, it was found that CT-myelography is more diagnostic than myelography alone and comparable to MRI.

104a. Kirkos JM, Papadopoulos IA: Late treatment of brachial plexus secondary to birth injuries: Rotational osteotomy of the proximal humerus. J Bone Joint Surg Am 80:1477-1483, 1998.

   This study confirms other clinical studies that rotational osteotomy of the humerus is effective in improving function in patients with long-standing birth palsies.

106. Laurent J, Lee R, Shenaq S, et al: Neurosurgical correction of upper brachial plexus birth injuries. J Neurosurg 79:197-203, 1993.

   A review of 116 infants with birth palsies. Twenty-eight patients with poor motor recovery at 4 months underwent microsurgical reconstruction. Recovery of biceps, deltoid, and triceps function were used as surgical indicators. With a greater than 50% decrease in amplitude of action potentials of distal muscles, nerve grafting was performed. Nerve grafting results were better than neurolysis results.

119. Michelow B, Clarke H, Curtis C, et al: The natural history of obstetrical brachial plexus palsy. Plast Reconstr Surg 93:675-679, 1994.

   A thorough statistical analysis of the physical examination parameters utilized to predict outcome. When elbow flexion and elbow, wrist, thumb, and finger extension were combined into a test score, the proportion of patients whose recovery was incorrectly predicted was reduced to 5.2%. Microsurgery in this study was performed at a mean age of 12 months.

128. Oberlin C, Beal D, Leechavengovongs S, et al: Nerve transfer to biceps muscle using a part of the ulnar nerve for C5-C6 avulsion of the brachial plexus: Anatomic study and report of four cases. J Hand Surg [Am] 19:232, 1994.

   This describes a useful technique for nerve transfer utilizing a part of the ulnar nerve directly to the motor branch of the musculocutaneous nerve. This is particularly useful with breech presentation avulsion injuries of C5-C6.

162. Ubachs JM, Sloof AC, Pheeters LL: Obstetric antecedents of surgically treated obstetric brachial plexus injuries. Br J Obstet Gynecol 102:813-817, 1995.

   Risk factors are described for brachial plexus birth palsies, noting macrosomia for cephalic presentation and upper trunk ruptures and breech presentation for C5-C6 ruptures. This is a thorough review of a busy clinical service for birth palsies and includes operative indications and results.

172. Waters PM: Comparison of the natural history, the outcome of microsurgical repair, and the outcome of operative reconstruction in brachial plexus birth palsy. J Bone Joint Surg Am 81:649-659, 1999.

   This study confirms Gilbert and Tassin's original work in that (1) biceps is a reliable predictor of functional recovery and (2) there is progressive loss of function with recovery of biceps after 3 months of life. However, those infants with biceps recovery between 3 and 6 months had long-term Mallet scores averaging 4 or greater by either spontaneous recovery or with the addition of secondary tendon transfers. This leaves open to debate the recommendation that microsurgery be performed in all infants without biceps recovery at 3 months of life.

174. Waters PM, Smith GR, Jaramillo D: Glenohumeral deformity secondary to brachial plexus birth palsy. J Bone Joint Surg Am 80:668, 1998.

This study outlines a progressive glenohumeral deformity with persistent muscle imbalance about the shoulder in brachial plexus birth palsies. A categorical CT and MRI radiographic classification is utilized to define this common clinical continuum. Recommendations for tendon transfer, osteotomy, or open reduction are based in part on the status of the glenohumeral joint.

CHAPTER 38

Traumatic Brachial Plexus Injury

Vincent R. Hentz and Kazuteru Doi

In the early 19th century, well before microsurgical equipment and techniques were developed, surgeons published encouraging results of brachial plexus reconstruction.[90] Soon thereafter, others reported poor results and high complication rates,[21] and little else was published regarding reconstruction of the brachial plexus until the 1970s and 1980s, when surgeons began to apply the fascicular nerve grafting techniques described by Millesi to birth and traumatic injuries of the brachial plexus. These pioneers established indications and techniques for plexus reconstruction and reported better recovery in operated patients than in those observed without surgical reconstruction.*

In the late 1980s and early 1990s, advances occurred in diagnostic and surgical techniques. New surgical procedures and experimental nonoperative treatments were introduced. In the late 1990s very aggressive reconstruction, using extraplexal sources for reinnervation of vascularized muscle transfers, were reported. Full recovery of function after brachial plexus reconstruction still remains unachievable but probably not permanently so. The exciting developments of the past several years have considerably improved surgical outcomes, and future directions for research are promising. These developments and directions are discussed later in this chapter.

PATHOLOGY OF THE TRACTION INJURY

Essentially all birth and many traumatic injuries of the brachial plexus are due to traction.[42] Traction injuries of the brachial plexus may be associated with varying amounts of energy imparted to the plexus.[99] Low-energy stretching injuries, not severe enough to cause rupture or avulsion, typically cause more or less reversible injuries, such as neurapraxia[151] (Sunderland degree of injury type I[167]) or various degrees of axonotmesis (Sunderland types II to IV). There is experimental evidence that low-energy injuries may interfere with the microcirculation of the plexus, causing ischemic injury.[92] High-energy injuries are associated with

more significant damage to the plexus, including rupture of a peripheral nerve at any plexus level (Sunderland type V) or avulsion of nerve roots from the spinal cord. When brachial plexus elements are ruptured or avulsed, some spontaneous recovery may occur, but early microneurosurgical reconstruction improves the functional outcome.

The typical candidate for microneural reconstruction is the young man who is thrown from his motorcycle.[20] Although his helmet saves his life, it cannot prevent his shoulder from being driven downward and posteriorly and his neck driven in the opposite direction as he lands. If his shoulder-neck angle is forcibly widened by downward traction of his arm, damage is imparted first to the upper roots and trunk; if the scapulohumeral angle is forcibly widened, damage is imparted first to C8 and T1 roots and the inferior trunk. If the impact is extreme, all levels will sustain damage.[42] Anatomic studies have determined that the supporting tissues anchoring the upper roots to the vertebral foramina are significantly stronger about the C5 and C6 roots than distally.[135] This anatomic arrangement predicts that the more caudal structures of the brachial plexus would suffer more significant injuries than the upper roots, and this is what has been observed clinically. The T1 and C8 roots are more likely to be avulsed from the spinal cord,[78] whereas the C6 and C5 roots are more likely to stretch or rupture in continuity after exiting the neural foramina (Table 38-1). The principal factors determining the extent of injury are the energy of the blow and, to a lesser degree, the direction and the relationship of the arm to the body.

---

*See references 2, 3, 5, 25, 65, 78, 115, 117, 129, 131, 132, 152, and 178.

Table 38-1
OPERATIVE FINDINGS FOR EACH ROOT (114 CASES)

Root	Ruptured	Avulsed	Other
C5	59	14	40
C6	44	35	35
C7	39	53	20
C8	11	67	31
T1	11	61	37

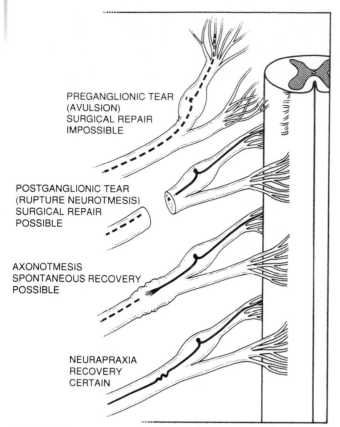

FIGURE 38-1. A severe traction injury to the brachial plexus may cause nerve injuries of varying severity in the same plexus. These include avulsion of the nerve root from the spinal cord (cannot be repaired), extraforaminal rupture of the root or trunk (can be repaired with surgery), and intraneural rupture of fascicles (some spontaneous recovery possible).

Every Sunderland degree of injury, plus root avulsion, can occur in the same patient (Fig. 38-1). For example, the T1 and C8 roots may be avulsed, the C7 root or middle trunk ruptured (Sunderland type V), with the upper trunk remaining intact but with varying degrees of internal damage. Within the upper trunk, some axon populations may be merely contused and other fascicles may have suffered various levels of axonotmesis (Sunderland types II and IV.) In this case, no spontaneous recovery will occur in muscles and sensory end organs innervated by C7, C8, or T1, and varying degrees of spontaneous motor and sensory recovery *may* occur in structures receiving innervation from axons of the upper trunk over widely varying periods of time (a few weeks to a few years), depending on whether the axon must regenerate to the motor end plate or the sensory end organ.

The same high-energy traction injury that damages the vulnerable plexus may also cause other injuries. About 75% of traumatic brachial plexus injuries are associated with head injury, thoracic trauma, or fractures or dislocations of the cervical spine or ipsilateral upper extremity and 20% are associated with vascular trauma.[180] Fractures and dislocations can further damage the plexus.

PREOPERATIVE EVALUATION

History

A good history of the mechanism of injury is helpful in determining the severity of injury. If the injury was associated with high energy, a thorough search for life- and limb-threatening injuries should be conducted. Brachial plexus injury is often underdiagnosed in the presence of head injury or spinal cord injury[66]; the opposite error may also occur when the surgeon focuses on the upper extremity and fails to diagnose a head injury or incomplete spinal cord injury. The patient should be asked about loss of consciousness and paresthesias or weakness in other extremities.

Special Physical Signs

One important indicator of severity of injury is the presence of Horner's sign (Fig. 38-2) on the affected side. This may be present immediately but occasionally is not readily apparent for 3 to 4 days after injury. Horner's sign has been strongly correlated with avulsion of C8 and/or T1 roots[78] and is therefore a poor prognostic sign for spontaneous recovery. Severe pain in an anesthetic extremity indicates some degree of deafferentation of the limb and is strongly correlated with root avulsion injuries and a poor prognosis. When the patient presents with the head shifted away from the injured side, this is evidence of denervation of paraspinous muscles, also strongly associated with severe nerve injury such as root avulsion. Finally, stability of the glenohumeral joint should be assessed. Shoulder dislocation may occur with the same types of trauma that are associated with brachial plexus traction injuries. Inferior or posterior dislocation is uncommon, but they may compound the brachial plexus injury by avulsing the axillary nerve from the deltoid muscle or rupturing it in its posterior course around the humerus.

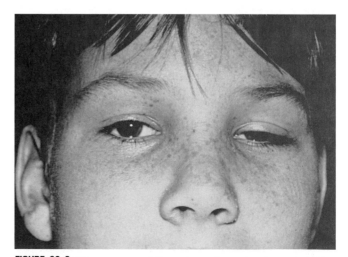

FIGURE 38-2. The presence of Horner's syndrome (ptosis, meiosis, and anhidrosis caused by paralysis of the sympathetic nerves) is associated with avulsion of the C8 and T1 roots.

Neurologic Examination

The examination of a patient with a brachial plexus injury must be carried out in a standardized and minutely detailed manner with the objective of establishing the location of the nerve lesions and their degree of abnormality. Determining the level of the lesion, whether it is intradural or a postganglionic rupture, is more difficult but important in deciding treatment and prognosis.

Algorithm of Decision Making for Level and Degree of Injury

The essential element in diagnosis is the distinction between preganglionic and postganglionic lesions. In preganglionic rupture, the afferent nerve fibers with cell bodies in the dorsal root ganglion do not degenerate. Only efferent fibers to skeletal or smooth muscle undergo wallerian degeneration. It is now of more than academic interest that a preganglionic (or intradural) lesion is diagnosed accurately as either a rupture of the rootlet peripheral to the central transmission zone or a true avulsion from the spinal cord, which is an injury to the central nervous system. Until recently, this distinction could be made only by inspection of the cord or by histologic examination of the tips of avulsed rootlets. Today we have powerful weapons in the form of imaging, electrophysiologic methods, and biochemical assays to make the diagnosis more accurate. From the standpoint of prognosis, distinguishing between preganglionic and postganglionic lesions has meaning; however, from the standpoint of surgical repair, a more detailed classification such as Nagano's zone classification has benefits.[125] Zone II injuries are subdivided into intraforaminal root lesions (IIA) and extraforaminal root lesions (IIB) because the former cannot be repaired but the latter can be. Recently, however, some have suggested a rather aggressive approach in attempting to repair intravertebral lesions via a cervical laminectomy.[29,30]

Physical Examination

The physical examination remains a good means of determining the level of injury and should not be neglected. Acute cases usually present as complete paralysis, and the first physical examination is rarely consistent. Testing should be repeated frequently and at close intervals. Commonly, 3 weeks after injury, when neurapraxia may recover, the definite diagnosis can be made, although the muscle atrophy or motor recovery of paralysis associated with axonotmesis or neurotmesis will be delayed another 3 or 4 months.

Horner's sign, winging scapula, muscular atrophy of parascapular muscles, and causalgia indicate preganglionic injury whereas Tinel's sign in the supraclavicular region, sweating in the palm, and minimal movement of joints may be evidence of postganglionic or distal injuries.

The metameric organization of innervation of the muscles of the upper extremity is well known, and charts of sensory or motor innervation assist the surgeon in predicting the location of nerve lesions (Fig. 38-3). It is not usually necessary to test all individual muscles; rather, it is more helpful to assess functional groups of muscles such as the external or internal rotators of the shoulder or flexors of the elbow. The function of the rhomboids and serratus anterior muscles is an important indicator of the level of injury. The dorsal scapular and long thoracic nerves, which supply these muscles, originate from the roots of the plexus; thus, paralysis of these muscles is typically associated with avulsion of the C5, C6, and C7 roots from the spinal cord. Sensation can be accurately and rapidly assessed by sharp-dull discrimination.

Several systems for recording the results of the examination of the injured brachial plexus have been published. A modification of the format introduced by Merle d'Aubigne is commonly used to record the evaluation of adults with traumatic brachial plexus palsy[132] (see Fig. 38-3). This system helps the surgeon record the examination accurately and thereby enables him or her to detect changes in motor function. Charts that include muscle innervation represent the average situation, and individual variations in plexus anatomy are common. For example, a prefixed plexus receives significant innervation from the C4 root and a postfixed plexus receives innervation from T2. Anatomists have reported that 62% of plexuses are prefixed and 60% are postfixed.[105] Unusual motor and sensory impairment, which is not distributed in the proper territory of cervical nerve root and peripheral nerves, may indicate incomplete nerve injury and some recovery.

Adjunctive Evaluations

Radiography

The same high-energy trauma that causes brachial plexus palsy can also cause spine, shoulder girdle, and upper limb fractures and dislocations. Radiographs of the cervical spine, chest, shoulder girdle, and humerus should be obtained in patients with traumatic brachial plexus palsy. The chest radiograph should include inspiration and expiration anteroposterior views to determine the activity of the diaphragm. A paralyzed diaphragm is an indicator of severe injury to the upper roots of the plexus. The presence of fractures of the transverse processes of the cervical vertebrae is also associated with a high-energy injury. Standard radiography, while necessary, has been supplanted in terms of diagnostic accuracy by more modern imaging techniques and electrophysiologic and biochemical assays. Among these advanced diagnostic techniques, the most useful examinations, such as myelography, magnetic resonance imaging (MRI), spinal evoked potentials and biochemical assay, are briefly described here.

Myelography

Myelography, although an invasive technique, is the most reliable supplemental method for detecting root avulsion. In the past, oil-based contrast material was used with injection performed via lumbar puncture.[185] Recent improvements in myelography with water-soluble contrast material achieve clearer and more reliable visualization of the cervical roots, however.[125] Preoperative myelography can be performed with iotrolan with a concentration of 240 mg/dL by lateral puncture through the interval between the C1 and C2 vertebrae.[54] Root and rootlet lesions are visualized in greater

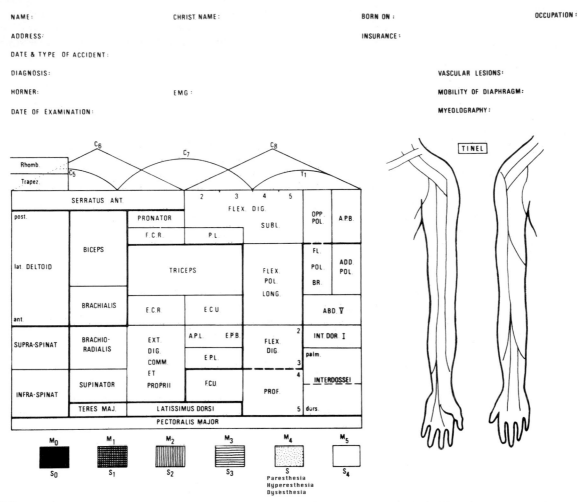

FIGURE 38-3. Motor and sensory findings must be accurately documented preoperatively and postoperatively. Most plexus surgeons use some variation of this format introduced by Merle d'Aubigne to record the data.

detail in myelograms done by a lateral puncture through the C1-C2 interval than by the lumbar puncture technique.

Based on Nagano's modified myelographic classification, myelographic findings are classified into six categories (Fig. 38-4).[125] N is a normal root sleeve shadow. A1 is a slightly abnormal root sleeve shadow with distinct root and rootlet shadow but different from the unaffected side. A2 shows an obliteration of the tip of the root sleeve with visible root or rootlet shadows. A3 is obliteration of the tip of the root sleeve with no root shadow visible. D is a defect instead of the root sleeve shadow, and M is a traumatic meningocele.

Computed Tomographic Myelography (CTM)

Nerve root lesions are well demonstrated in the multiple views possible with a CT scan.[69,106,123,176] After myelography has been performed, CT can be obtained from C4 to T1 with 3-mm axial slices. Additional 1-mm axial slices are obtained when abnormal pathology was detected or a high index of suspicion is present on the initial scan. The scan angle is oriented parallel to the cervical discs.

Diagnosis of root avulsion by CTM is based on the absence of either one (P: partial avulsion) or both ventral

and dorsal roots (A: complete avulsion) or the presence of a meningocele (M: meningocele). When both ventral and dorsal roots are visualized from the spinal cord to the intervertebral foramen on axial slices, it is considered to be intact (N: normal) (Fig. 38-5). Determining the presence of an avulsed or intact root is further aided by comparison with the contralateral intact root. When the root of the intact side cannot be identified, the affected root is classified only by myelography.

Magnetic Resonance Imaging

After the work of Blair and colleagues,[18] many reports of the MRI appearance of the brachial plexus have been published,[33,128,136,138] most using coronal slices of the brachial plexus with T2-weighted imaging. This technique makes it possible to image only traumatic meningoceles and does not give detailed information about the nerve roots. MRI has not been widely used to define lesions at the root level, because myelography and CTM can clearly image root lesions.

Doi and colleagues introduced a new MRI technique with overlapping coronal-oblique slices (OCOS MRI)[54] and concluded that the technique is a reliable and reproducible method for detecting root avulsions by retrospective and

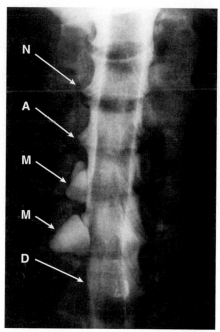

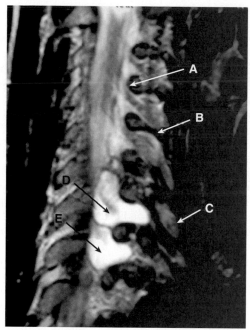

FIGURE 38-4. Myelography obtained in a patient with brachial plexus injury, illustrating the modified classification schema of Nagano and coworkers. N, normal root sleeve shadow; A, abnormal root sleeve shadow, grading from a slightly abnormal (A1) root sleeve shadow to no root shadow visible (A3); D, a defect instead of a root sleeve shadow; M, traumatic meningocele. (From Doi K, Cervical nerve root avulsion in brachial plexus injuries: Magnetic resonance imaging classification and comparison with myelography and computed tomography myelography. J Neurosurg 96:277-284, 2002.)

FIGURE 38-6. An MR image obtained in a patient with brachial plexus palsy, demonstrating normal and abnormal findings of rootlet and ganglion: C5 (a) and C6 (b), normal anatomy (normal ganglion); C7 (c), partial injury (decreased number of rootlets and displacement of the ganglion from the intraforaminal space); and C8 (d) and T1 (e), meningocele (meningoceles and disappearance of the ganglion from the intraforaminal space) (turbo spin-echo T2-weighted imaging [TR 4000 msec; TE 180 msec]). (From Doi K, Cervical nerve root avulsion in brachial plexus injuries: Magnetic resonance imaging classification and comparison with myelography and computed tomography myelography. J Neurosurg 96:277-284, 2002.)

prospective studies. Details of this technique and its application can be found in the Annotated References. Figure 38-6 shows an example of images obtained with this technique.

The corresponding categories of each modality are listed in Table 38-2. A, D, and M in myelography, P, A, and M in CTM, and R, A, and M in MRI all mean avulsion of the roots, although the exact pathologic anatomy of each cate-

gory is different. Patients who are diagnosed to have A and M lesions by the OCOS MRI technique should undergo a primary reconstructive procedure instead of surgical exploration of the brachial plexus.

Sensory and Motor Evoked Potentials
These tests should be carried out after wallerian degeneration is underway (several days to weeks after injury). Several different tests may be helpful in determining the severity of the injury. Standard electromyography (EMG) is not as helpful for severe injuries as sensory evoked potentials, corticosensory evoked potentials, and spinograms.[95] For example, the sensory evoked potential examination may demonstrate that the ulnar nerve conducts a compound

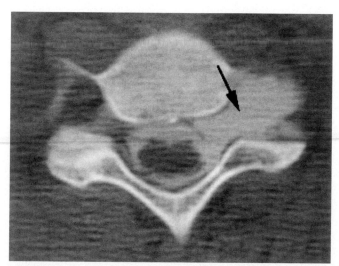

FIGURE 38-5. CT myelogram obtained in a patient revealing a meningocele of the left root *(arrow)*. The right side is normal.

Table 38-2
COMPARISON OF DIFFERENT CATEGORIES OF MYELOGRAPHY, CTM, AND MRI CLASSIFICATION

	Myelography	CTM	MRI
Normal	N	N	N
Avulsion			
Partial	A(A1-A3)	P	R
Complete	D	A	A
Meningocele	M	M	M

action potential in the presence of electrically unexcitable ulnar-innervated muscles and ulnar anesthesia. This is strong evidence that a preganglionic injury, usually root avulsion, exists. In this case, some sensory axons may remain capable of conducting (they have not undergone wallerian degeneration because they are still connected to their dorsal root ganglion cells) but they are disconnected from the spinal cord, and thus the brain. Similarly, when cerebral cortex signals are recorded from scalp electrodes while stimulation is given over Erb's point in the supraclavicular fossa, some roots may still be in continuity with the spinal cord.

The spinogram can determine information about the level of denervation from the paraspinous muscles. Because these are innervated by the posterior primary rami of the plexus, paralysis of these muscles indicates a very proximal injury but does not tell the examiner whether the injury is associated with avulsion, rupture, or axonotmesis.

No single test can tell the surgeon whether the injured plexus requires surgical exploration and reconstruction. All the information gathered must be assimilated and analyzed within the context of the presumed energy of the trauma.

INDICATIONS FOR SURGERY

A sufficient number of reviews of the results of exploration of traction injuries of the brachial plexus have now been published to allow us to assess the indications for and value of plexus reconstruction.* Most of these series attest to the inverse relationship between time interval from injury to operation to outcome and show that in cautious and skilled hands, exploration seldom results in extension of the injury. Even when total palsy exists, less than 20% of patients demonstrate avulsions of all five roots of the plexus[78] (Table 38-3). Thus, the surgeon will usually find a root suitable for repair or grafting. If neurotization (nerve transfer from a plexus or nonplexus nerve source) is performed, then virtually 100% of patients might benefit from microneural reconstruction. When there is a strong suspicion of root avulsion and nerve ruptures, surgical exploration is warranted.

Controversial Indications

Occasionally a patient presents with a partial C8 and complete T1 lesion, with some finger flexors working but with an intrinsic palsy and anesthesia in the C8 and/or T1 distribution. The C8 and T1 nerve roots are so often avulsed from the spinal cord that it is unlikely that a lesion that can be repaired will be found at surgery, and surgical reconstruction at the plexus level is very unlikely to recover intrinsic muscle function in the adult. When the patient with a partial C8 and T1 lesion is older than age 15, we recommend plexus surgery only when he or she is disabled by pain. Exploration may alleviate pain, even if only minimal reconstruction can be performed.[131] If pain is not disabling, we recommend the standard muscle-tendon transfers.

*See references 1, 37-39, 42, 57, 82, 97, 109, 115, 132, 148, 152, and 159.

Table 38-3

FREQUENTLY OCCURRING PATTERNS OF INJURY IN TOTAL PALSY (107 CASES)

C5 ruptured; C6–T1 avulsed	9
C5, C6 ruptured; C7–T1 avulsed	13
C5, C6, C7 ruptured; C8, T1 avulsed	13
All roots avulsed	8
All roots ruptured	6
All roots intact (distal injury)	14

Contraindications

If the surgeon is experienced, risk to intact nerves and other structures is not a contraindication to surgery. Loss of function secondary to nerve exploration is unusual. The surgery, while sometimes lengthy, is not particularly stressful, at least to the patient. There is no hard rule regarding the timing of exploration, but if more than 1 year has passed since injury, plexus reconstruction is contraindicated, except perhaps in the young patient. Advanced age of the patient is not an absolute contraindication to surgical exploration, although, in general, younger patients will have better results; in one large series, none of the patients older than age 40 had a good result from nerve transfer.[159]

TIMING OF SURGERY

Immediate Surgery

Immediate plexus exploration and reconstruction is indicated for a penetrating injury, such as a stab wound, or after an iatrogenic injury, such as injury to the plexus at the time of first rib resection for the treatment of thoracic outlet syndrome. Occasionally, the reconstructive surgeon gets the opportunity to assess the degree of damage to the plexus when emergency vascular reconstruction of an injured subclavian or axillary artery is performed by the vascular surgeons at the time of injury. The vascular surgeon's incisions may be extended as described later, and the plexus surgeon may explore the supraclavicular fossa, map the damage to the plexus, tag damaged nerves with vascular clips, and begin planning for secondary plexus reconstruction. If at all possible, the plexus surgeon should be involved in this emergency procedure, to take advantage of the opportunity to assess nerve damage. In addition, he or she can consult with the vascular surgeon in the dissection of the distal vessel in its intimate association with the components of the plexus and help him or her place vein grafts. With the assistance and guidance of the plexus surgeon, the vascular surgeon can pass the vein graft deep to the injured plexus, keeping it out of the plexus surgeon's eventual path to the plexus, and thus out of harm's way during later nerve reconstruction.

There are many arguments against immediate reconstruction of the plexus in traction injuries, in addition to the diagnostic dilemmas discussed earlier. Most surgeons believe that some period of time must pass to permit the surgeon to be able to delineate injured from noninjured nerve.[2,115,130] If exploration is indicated at the time of injury (high-energy injury causing a total plexus palsy), we prefer to wait 6 to 8 weeks after injury. This waiting period allows time for diagnostic tests and permits the patient to experience the effects of the injury. Because the functional results of reconstruction of severe plexus injuries are, on average, disappointing when compared with the function of the normal limb, the patient who has lived with a flail limb for some time may better accept the ultimate functional limitations of microneural reconstruction. If the initial assessment proves incorrect and the patient begins to recover function in previously paralyzed muscles, then further observation is indicated, unless distal muscles begin to recover in the absence of any recovery in more proximal muscles; this recovery pattern is a strong indication for early exploration. Serial physical examinations are far more valuable than serial EMG examinations, which almost always overestimate the potential for functional recovery.

Early Surgery

Early surgery (6 weeks to 3 months after injury) is indicated for patients who present with total or near-total palsy and for those with an injury associated with high energy, including gunshot wounds. For injuries associated with partial upper level palsy and those associated with lower levels of energy, we prefer to observe the course of recovery for 3 to 6 months, operating when recovery seems to plateau as determined by several successive examinations at monthly intervals. Thus, patients with in-continuity stretch lesions with a reasonable probability of useful spontaneous regeneration will be given enough time to show recovery before exploration. The key to decision making is a careful examination with careful recording of the results by the same observer. The presence or absence of an advancing Tinel sign can be a useful guide; no Tinel's sign in the supraclavicular fossa in a patient with a nearly complete C5 and C6 level palsy is a poor prognostic sign for spontaneous recovery and warrants an early exploration, because C5 and C6 nerve roots may be avulsed. If this is the case, neurotization will be necessary (see later). Easy and noninvasive supplemental tests such as EMG or MRI reinforce the physical examination. If MRI (OCOS) shows root avulsion (A or M in our classification) and EMG of the muscles innervated from the individual roots provides denervation potential, the proper roots should be preganglionic and early exploration of the brachial plexus is recommended. Even by these examinations, whenever preganglionic injury cannot be definitely excluded, myelography and CTM are the next steps of examination. However, EMG and imaging methods are not enough to decide the real state of nerve lesion. Finally, all patients with acute brachial plexus injuries earlier than 6 months after injury who are not rapidly improving should undergo exploration of their brachial plexus and have measurements taken of spinal evoked potentials and choline acetyltransferase activity if possible. If these advanced examinations such as measurements of evoked potentials and biochemical assay are not available to use, compromised decision may select surgical options, although final outcomes should be inferior.

OPERATIVE TECHNIQUE

Patient Preparation and Informed Consent

The surgeon must discuss the expected outcome of surgery in detail and compare it with the expected outcome if surgery is not performed. The patient and family must be made aware of the long period of time necessary for reinnervation of muscles, when essentially nothing happens that the patient can appreciate.

Before surgery, the patient should be taught the exercises necessary to maintain normal passive range of motion rather than depending on the therapist to perform these exercises for him or her. The therapist can record progress, teach, and advise, but the patient must accept responsibility for performing the exercises. If the patient has had a previous subclavian artery reconstruction, a unit of autologous blood should be donated before surgery. The need for intraoperative or postoperative transfusion is rare. Otherwise, no special preoperative preparations are necessary.

Positioning of the Patient and Microscope

If possible, the electrodes for intraoperative corticosensory or spinal evoked potentials are placed before the patient's arrival in the operating room. This permits the neurologist or technician to test the equipment, electrodes, and electrode placement. Once the scalp electrode positions are confirmed, and after induction of anesthesia, we may replace the adhesive-backed electrodes with spiral-barbed electrodes that are less likely to be displaced during movement of the patient's head.

The nature of the case, especially the indeterminate length of the procedure and the need to perform intraoperative stimulation and recordings, is discussed with the anesthesiologist before induction of anesthesia. This allows the anesthesiologist to alter techniques and agents to avoid giving a long-acting paralytic agent and those agents that depress cortical response sufficient to compromise corticosensory recordings. The anesthesiologist is also reminded of the need to reposition the patient's head periodically to avoid causing scalp ischemia and hair loss.

The patient is positioned in the supine position and a small pillow is placed beneath the ipsilateral scapula to bring the shoulder forward. The head is turned to the opposite side and the arm is abducted on an arm board. The ipsilateral or bilateral (if the contralateral C7 nerve root may be transferred) neck, mandible, and hemithorax and the ipsilateral axilla, entire upper extremity, and both lower extremities (for possible nerve grafts) are prepared and draped. The arm is prepared and draped freely so the response to nerve stimulation can be observed and so traction can be applied during the procedure. Muscle relaxant agents should be avoided so that intraoperative electrical stimulation can be performed. The surgeon should be prepared to expose both supraclavicular and infraclavicular portions of the brachial plexus. If nerve grafts are required, sural nerve, radial nerve, or vascularized ulnar nerve is harvested depending on the length and diameter of the nerve graft. All donor nerve can be harvested in the supine position, avoiding the need for positional change during operation.

When intraoperative measurement of spinal evoked potentials is available, the electrode is inserted and placed in the epidural space preoperatively under imaging control. A bipolar microcoagulator, nerve stimulator, magnifying loupes, and operative microscope should be available.

Well-padded tourniquets are placed on both thighs, and both legs are draped free to the tourniquet, in preparation for harvesting sural nerve grafts. A second surgical team available to harvest the sural nerve grafts after the need for them has been established while the plexus surgeons prepare the recipient sites speeds the surgery. Other surgeons have recommended that if the likelihood of using sural nerve grafts is high, the operation should begin by placing the patient in the prone position, harvesting both sural nerves, closing and dressing the leg wounds, and then turning the patient to the supine position and proceeding with the plexus exploration.[64,117] This may be a reasonable way to proceed if a second surgical team is unavailable. To harvest the sural nerve, a combination of vertical and horizontal incisions over the course of the nerve is used, enabling removal of both the sural nerve and its peroneal derived branch.[183] The distal portion of the nerve can be harvested with the patient in the supine position if the hip is flexed and maximally internally rotated. The proximal portion is dissected as the assistant holds the leg elevated, assisting with skin retraction while the surgeon harvests the nerve. The skin wounds are rapidly closed with skin staples, and the legs are wrapped in elastic bandages and slightly elevated before releasing the tourniquets. The surgeons must make certain that the leg tourniquets are deflated after harvesting the nerve grafts.

Surgical Approaches to the Brachial Plexus

There are two main surgical approaches to the brachial plexus, supraclavicular and infraclavicular, using a zigzag skin incision (Fig. 38-7). The classic supraclavicular approach begins at the angle of the jaw and drops vertically to the mid clavicle along the posterior border of the sternocleidomastoid, and the infraclavicular approach begins at the insertion of the sternocleidomastoid medially and extends to the deltopectoral groove laterally. These incisions may be connected if the widest exposure is preferable. However, connecting these incisions increases the risk of scar hypertrophy and recently some surgeons prefer to use separate transverse skin incisions, as described later.

 Authors' Preferred Approaches

We use two basic approaches. For supraclavicular injury, the upper roots are exposed through a transverse cervical skin incision and the lower roots and plexus are exposed through a transverse clavicular skin incision to minimize the operative scar (Fig. 38-8). For infraclavicular lesions the traditional exposure through the transverse clavicular and deltopectoral incisions is utilized.

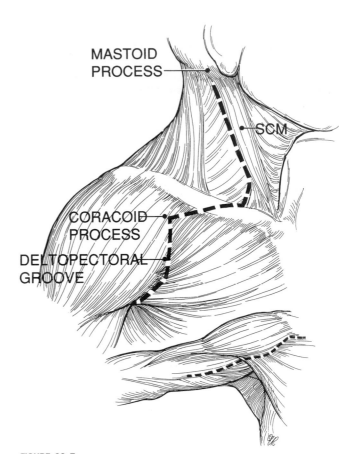

FIGURE 38-7. Classic skin incision for exploration of the entire brachial plexus. This entire incision is used in adult traction injuries to expose the plexus from the vertebral foramen to the branch level.

Supraclavicular Lesions

The upper cervical two roots, C5 and C6, are explored through a transverse cervical skin incision, between the posterior tubercle of the C5 transverse process and anterior tubercle of the C6 transverse process, which can be palpated easily (see Fig. 38-8). The skin incision is infiltrated with a vasopressor agent to decrease bleeding. After the skin incision, the platysma muscle is incised in the same line and the cutaneous branches of the cervical plexus are identified and protected, as is the spinal accessory nerve, which lies beneath the sternocleidomastoid muscle at the apex of the wound. The external jugular vein on the surface of the sternocleidomastoid muscle is dissected and retracted with a tape. Dissection proceeds along the posterolateral margin of the sternocleidomastoid muscle, which is retracted anteriorly. Underneath the sternocleidomastoid muscle the cutaneous branches of the cervical nerves and the supraclavicular nerve (which arises from the C4 cervical root) are traced proximally. The phrenic nerve, which is easily distinguished by contraction of diaphragm following electrical nerve stimulation, is found as it branches from the C4 nerve root and runs distally on the anterior scalenus muscle (Figs. 38-9 and 38-10). The internal jugular vein is protected. Dissection is carried under the anterior scalenus muscle, identifying the palpable posterior tubercle of the C5 transverse process and anterior tubercle of the C6 transverse process. The C5 and C6 nerve roots are identified in this interval, and the condition of these roots can vary considerably depending on the level of injury. If the nerve root exists in situ, it is traced distally to find the level of the lesion and electric stimulation is applied proximal to the lesion. If contraction of proximal muscles such as the rhomboids or serratus anterior occurs, the lesion should be postganglionic and the nerve root can be repaired. If more distal muscles such as the supraspinatus or deltoid contract with electric stimulation of the nerve root, the lesion is infraclavicular. If no muscular contraction occurs, the lesion may be preganglionic or intraforaminal and cannot be repaired. We use intraoperative measurement of spinal evoked potentials and biochemical assay of choline acetyltransferase for definitive diagnosis of the proximal lesions. However, if these techniques are not available, gross diagnosis can be done by electrical nerve stimulation and macroscopic findings of the cut surface of the nerve root.

The lower three cervical roots (C7, C8, and T1) and upper trunk of the brachial plexus are explored through the transverse supraclavicular skin incision. This incision begins at the infraclavicular fossa proximally and runs transversely over the clavicle to the supraclavicular fossa distally along the skin fold. This incision can be connected to the deltopectoral incision for exposure of infraclavicular lesions (Figs. 38-9 and 39-11). The platysma muscle is cut in the same line of skin incision.

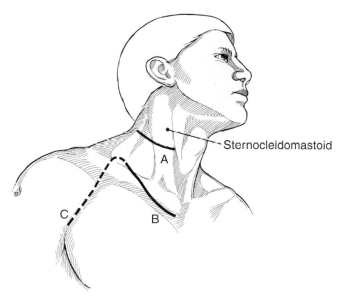

FIGURE 38-8. Skin incision for surgical exploration of brachial plexus. A, Transverse upper cervical skin incision for exploration of C4 to C6 roots; B, transverse lower cervical skin incision for exploration of C7 to T1 roots and infraclavicular lesion; and C, deltopectoral skin incision for exploration of distal lesion.

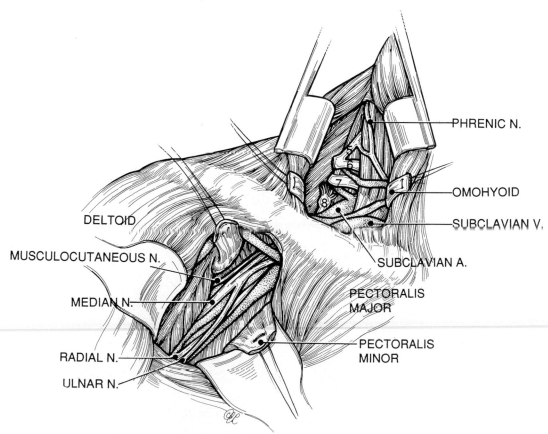

FIGURE 38-9. Key anatomic landmarks include the omohyoid muscle and the pectoralis minor muscle, which are divided between ligatures for later approximation. The C8 root is located just above and posterior to the subclavian artery, whereas the T1 root is almost directly posterior to the artery. With dissection of the deltopectoral groove, the lateral cord is the most superficial structure. In this example, the superior trunk and the C7 root are ruptured and the C8 root is avulsed (note the rootlets attached to the swollen dorsal root ganglion).

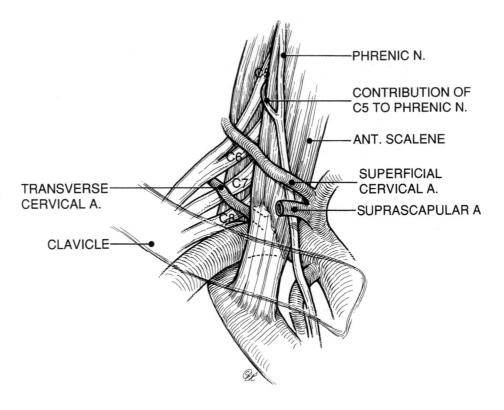

FIGURE 38-10. Additional landmarks helpful in identifying the various roots include the phrenic nerve contributions from the C5 root and the transverse cervical (scapular) artery, which frequently crosses over the C7 root.

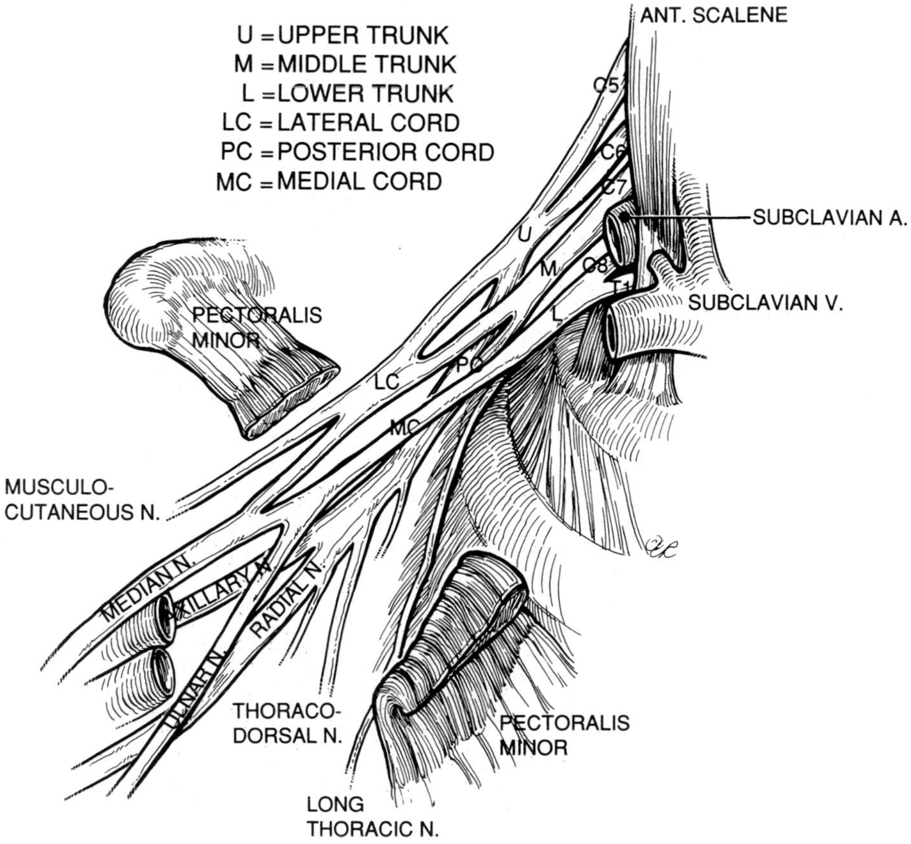

PHRENIC N.

CONTRIBUTION OF C5 TO PHRENIC N.

ANT. SCALENE

SUPERFICIAL CERVICAL A.

SUPRASCAPULAR A

TRANSVERSE CERVICAL A.

CLAVICLE

U = UPPER TRUNK
M = MIDDLE TRUNK
L = LOWER TRUNK
LC = LATERAL CORD
PC = POSTERIOR CORD
MC = MEDIAL CORD

ANT. SCALENE

SUBCLAVIAN A.

SUBCLAVIAN V.

PECTORALIS MINOR

FIGURE 38-11. Exploration of infraclavicular lesions.

MUSCULO-CUTANEOUS N.

MEDIAN N.

AXILLARY A.

RADIAL N.

ULNAR N.

THORACO-DORSAL N.

PECTORALIS MINOR

LONG THORACIC N.

Dissection proceeds into the supraclavicular fossa, identifying and retracting the external jugular vein and supraclavicular nerve. The clavicular head of the sternocleidomastoid muscle is detached from the clavicle. The omohyoid muscle is usually divided, and beneath this the transverse cervical and suprascapular vessels cross the brachial plexus perpendicularly. They may be preserved if necessary; however, they are usually ligated and cut for better exposure of the brachial plexus. Underneath these vessels, the upper trunk of the brachial plexus (if present) is visualized. The suprascapular nerve, arching posteriorly away from the upper trunk, is identified and preserved. The C7 root and the middle trunk are found dorsal and caudad to the C5 and C6 roots between the anterior and middle scalene muscles. The caudal roots course in a more horizontal and less oblique direction than the cranial roots. The C8 and T1 roots are hidden partially behind the arching third part of the subclavian artery. The exposure of the inferior trunk is facilitated by identifying the medial cord through the infraclavicular incision and following it in a central direction. Maximal lifting of the clavicle increases the space for access and may obviate the need for osteotomy. If further exploration of the T1 root is necessary, the clavicle should be predrilled for plating and then osteotomized and retracted. This approach will require the additional infraclavicular incision described later. In total paralysis with postganglionic injury of the C5 root and preganglionic injuries of the other lower roots, a supraclavicular exposure without osteotomy of clavicle is enough to examine the lower roots by division of the scalenus anterior muscle (protecting the phrenic nerve) and mobilization and gentle retraction of the subclavian artery inferiorly.

If the upper roots are avulsed, the rootlets and swollen dorsal root ganglion may be found twisted and lying either behind the clavicle or slightly above it in the region of the C8 root (Fig. 38-12). If the upper roots or superior trunk and/or the middle trunk are ruptured, the distal ends typically lie behind the clavicle. The avulsed (often) or ruptured (infrequently) C8 and T1 structures are usually found much closer to their respective foramina than is the case with C5 or C6.

Any combination of injuries may occur, including avulsion, rupture, and neuroma-in-continuity. Supraclavicular dissection usually allows the surgeon to determine the type(s) of injuries. However, if the supraclavicular findings favor some type of reconstruction by nerve grafting, the surgeon must perform the infraclavicular exploration. Two-level injuries are common, and an untreated distal injury can diminish the results of the surgical treatment of a proximal injury. For example, rupture of the superior trunk is often seen in combination with avulsion of the axillary nerve from the deltoid or rupture of the musculocutaneous nerve at the level of the shoulder.

Infraclavicular Lesions

The infraclavicular approach to the brachial plexus is designed to expose the cords and branches. The skin incision is transverse, running parallel to the clavicle as described earlier and follows the deltopectoral groove, beginning proximally at the clavicle and extending over the coracoid to the axillary crease distally (see Fig. 38-11). The deltopectoral interval is developed, exposing the cephalic

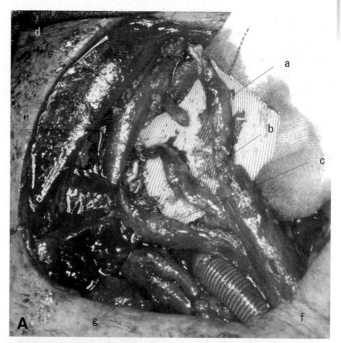

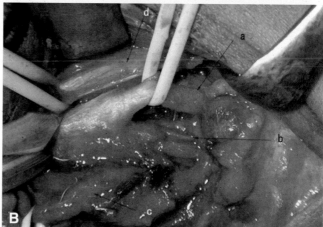

FIGURE 38-12. Operative exploration of the cervical nerve roots. **A,** A 50-year-old man presented with complete avulsion of his left brachial plexus and rupture of the subclavian artery. Note avulsed C5 and C6 roots (a), C7 (b), and C8 and T1 roots (c); the subclavian artery was repaired with a Dacron graft (f). **B,** A 17-year-old man presented with total paralysis of his right brachial plexus and partially innervated supraspinatus muscle: a, C5 root (normal appearance); b, C6 root (neuroma in continuity); c, C7 root (avulsed); d, suprascapular nerve from C4.

vein and thoracoacromial artery and its comitant veins, which are isolated and reflected with a vascular tape if free muscle transfer or vascularized nerve grafting is planned. The clavicular origin of the pectoralis major muscle is detached, and the subclavius is isolated. By elevating the clavicle with a retractor, the infraclavicular brachial plexus is exposed. The lower plexus is explored by detaching the tendinous origin of the pectoralis minor from the coracoid process. The clavipectoral fascia is incised, exposing the lateral cord superficial and lateral to the axillary artery. The posterior cord is slightly lateral and deep to the artery, and the medial cord is medial and deep to the axillary artery. Care should be taken to preserve the medial and lateral pectoral nerves that arise at this level. If there is extensive scarring, exploration should begin as far distally as necessary to locate normal tissue before proceeding proximally. The lateral cord can be identified by following the median nerve from distal to proximal. At this point the musculocutaneous nerve can be seen branching laterally and piercing the coracobrachialis muscle. The medial root of the median nerve is followed to the medial cord, which is then followed distally to the ulnar, medial brachial cutaneous, and medial antebrachial cutaneous nerves. Medial and deep to the axillary artery and vein, coursing laterally, is the radial nerve. It is followed proximally to the posterior cord and axillary nerve, which is seen branching from the posterior cord.

Different anatomic structures can be marked using different-colored vessel loops. We have found it useful to bring a sterilized drawing of the normal plexus (Fig. 38-13) and to make a sketch of the operative findings on this. We use this map to plan the priorities in reconstruction and to describe what reconstruction was performed. It is a mistake to depend on memory to dictate the operative note.

Intraoperative Evoked Potentials

After the plexus is visualized, we perform intraoperative corticosensory or spinal evoked potentials on the nerve roots to determine if they are in continuity with the spinal cord.

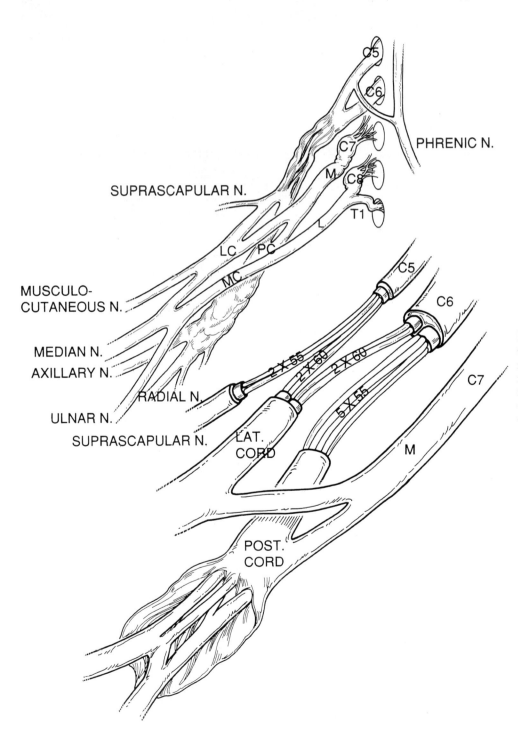

FIGURE 38-13. It is useful to sketch the operative findings and the repair method, detailing the distribution of nerve graft, including the length and number and the source and destination of nerve transfer. (See Fig. 38-11 for explanation of abbreviations.)

The root is placed on electrodes and either 64, 128, or 256 stimulations are performed and averaged (Fig. 38-14). We rely on this examination to differentiate between an avulsion from the spinal cord and a rupture.

Intraoperative electrodiagnosis has included the use of intraoperative somatosensory evoked potential (SSEP), spinal-evoked potential (SpEP) obtained by stimulating the nerve root, nerve action potentials, and eccentric motor nerve-evoked potential obtained by stimulating the cerebral cortex.

Somatosensory Evoked Potentials

In 1947, Dawson showed that after stimulating a peripheral nerve of the upper or lower limb, it was possible to record very low amplitude potentials on the scalp overlying the contralateral cortex.[46] Studies of the SSEP proceeded with the introduction of the first compact computers used in association with electrophysiologic instruments and was utilized for intraoperative electrodiagnosis of root avulsion during brachial plexus surgery.[28,44,86,166]

Intraoperative SSEP recording enables the integrity of the intraforaminal part of the sensory tract to be evaluated. However, not even indirect information can be obtained as to the condition of the anterior motor root. This limitation is important, considering that there are dissociated intra-foraminal lesions of both the motor and the sensory roots. SSEP is easily affected by depth of anesthesia, and technical failures can be problematic. To monitor the depth of anesthesia, simultaneous recording of SSEP after peripheral nerve stimulation in the unaffected upper limb is also recommended. We apply SSEP only to children, in whom recording of SpEPs is difficult because insertion of an epidural electrode is contraindicated owing to the risk of spinal cord injury. In adults, we prefer SpEP for assessment of the proximal continuity of severed roots.

Spinal-Evoked Potentials

SpEP has been used in the past for diagnosis of spinal cord disorders and for monitoring during spinal surgery.[9,157,158,166] These recordings can be made from the spinous processes, interspinous ligaments, ligamenta flava, and intervertebral disks, but none of these provides such a clear potential as SpEP recorded from the epidural space.[44] Kawai and coworkers[88,124] and Sasaki and colleagues[149] introduced SpEP for the accurate diagnosis of brachial plexus nerve injuries.

A catheter with five electrodes is placed in the epidural space with the aid of an image intensifier preoperatively. Stimulation of the median nerve on the uninjured side is utilized as a control, and findings of SpEP amplitudes of greater than 5 μV on the involved side are believed to correlate with an intact nerve root.[76,149] Amplitudes of less than 5 μV but at a detectable level should have correlation of the presence of motor fibers in the root by choline acetyltransferase staining.

Eccentric Motor Nerve-Evoked Potentials

Theoretically, SSEP and SpEP are examinations to confirm proximal continuity of sensory fibers, not motor fibers, and clinically we need information regarding the proximal continuity of motor fibers, that is, motor evoked potentials (MEP). Turkof and colleagues[179] recorded nerve compound action potentials (NCAPs) from surgically exposed spinal nerves with central stimulation. If NCAPs can be recorded, the anterior root is considered to be intact. NCAPs is theoretically an ideal examination of the proximal anterior nerve root. However, the technique is still too sensitive and difficult to standardize. It needs further improvements of instrumentation and technique to find wide application.

Biochemical Examination

Choline Acetyltransferase Activity

Choline acetyltransferase (CAT) is a synthetic enzyme of acetylcholine. CAT is synthesized in the nerve cell body and is transported by axonal flow to the nerve terminals. The activity of CAT is higher in motor fascicles in comparison to sensory fascicles. This has been applied clinically to differentiate between motor and sensory fascicles intraoperatively during nerve grafting procedures[62,89,184] and also to distinguish the availability of the proximal nerve stump as a donor motor nerve during brachial plexus surgery.

After intraoperative measurement of spinal evoked potentials, a 2-mm length of nerve fascicle from the proximal stump of the remaining cervical nerve root is harvested and sent for measurement of CAT activity. This technique requires approximately 60 minutes to perform (from resection of the nerve slices to determination of the final results). Hattori and Doi, in a retrospective study, have found that fascicles with CAT activity above 2000 cpm are of good quality and have intact motor fascicles and can be useful as a donor motor nerve.[73,74] The details of CAT activity measurement can be found in the Annotated References.[72-74]

Authors' Preferred Methods of Treatment

Not every hospital will have the facilities necessary to perform all the advanced techniques just described. At the minimum, however, preoperative myelography or MRI should be performed with subsequent operative exploration and electric stimulation of potentially repairable cervical nerve roots. This approach maximizes the chances of finding nerve roots that can be repaired, because primary nerve repair can achieve a superior outcome to nerve transfer. If the nerve root is classified as N or A1 by Nagano's classification or N in Doi's OCOS MRI classification, it should be explored and examined. If the macroscopic appearance of its cut surface looks normal and if the muscles that are innervated from its proximal branches contract on electric stimulation of the root, the lesion is postganglionic and can be repaired. If no muscle contraction is obtained yet the appearance of the cut surface is normal, the lesion is preganglionic and not a candidate for repair. This type of gross diagnosis may be all that is available but cannot always be reliable or definitive.

Intraoperative Decisions and Priorities of Repair

We have followed the recommendations of Narakas and others in developing a sequence of reconstruction based on

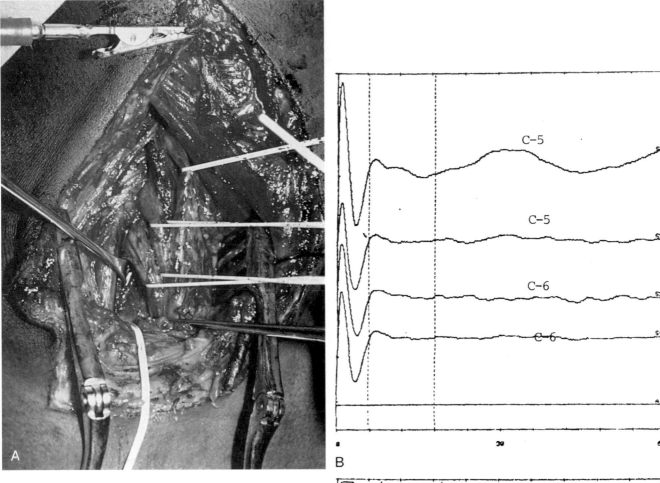

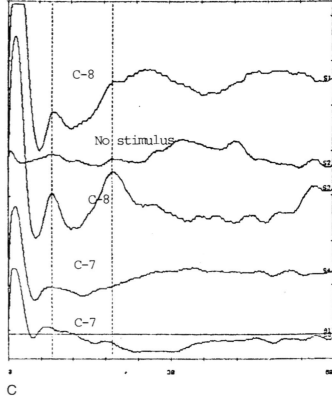

FIGURE 38-14. At exploration, the C5, C6, and C7 roots (marked by Silastic tape) were scarred and stretched (**A**) but in continuity. However, evoked potential studies (**B** and **C**) demonstrated no cortical activity with stimulation of these roots, whereas stimulation of the C8 root gave a large amplitude response. This indicates a probable intraforaminal avulsion of C5, C6, and C7. In this case, no plexoplexal grafting was possible; nerve transfer to several important nerves using extraplexal donor nerves was performed.

Table 38-4
TREATMENT RECOMMENDATIONS IN OBSTETRIC PALSY

Ruptured/Avulsed Roots	Recipient Site	Functional Goal
C5, C6/0	Superior trunk	Shoulder, elbow, wrist control
C5, C6, C7/0	Superior trunk Middle trunk	Above plus Finger extension
C5, C6, C7/C8, T1	Posterior cord Lateral cord Medial cord	Shoulder control Elbow control Finger flexion + ?intrinsics
C5, C6/C7, C8, T1	Lateral cord Medial cord ?Suprascapular n.	Elbow control Finger flexion + ?intrinsics Shoulder control
C5/C6, C7, C8, T1	Musculocutaneous n. Suprascapular n. Intercostal nn. 2–5 to lateral cord	Elbow control Shoulder control Sensation
0/C8, T1	Graft from C6 to medial cord	Finger flexion + ?intrinsics
0/C5, C6	Graft from medial pectoral n. to musculocutaneous n.	Elbow control

functional priorities (Table 38-4). The microneural reconstruction performed depends on the intraoperative assessment of the damage and the following list of priorities. These priorities have been chosen for three reasons: first is functional significance; second is the likelihood of regaining the function by nerve reconstruction (proximal muscles are reinnervated more successfully than distal muscles); and third is the degree of difficulty in achieving the function by secondary surgery.

For the patient with a total brachial plexus palsy, the classic priorities of repair include:

1. Elbow flexion by biceps/brachialis muscle reinnervation
2. Shoulder stabilization, abduction, and external rotation by suprascapular nerve reinnervation
3. Brachiothoracic pinch (adduction of the arm against the chest) by reinnervation of the pectoralis major muscle
4. Sensation below the elbow in the C6-C7 area by reinnervation of the lateral cord
5. Wrist extension and finger flexion by reinnervation of the lateral and posterior cord

However, recent aggressive procedures change those conventional priorities to those as described in the section on nerve grafting.

For the patient with an injury limited to the upper roots (C5, C6), regaining elbow flexion and shoulder stability (numbers 1 and 2 above) are priorities; in addition, we will attempt to help the patient recover wrist extension (number 5). The decisions regarding the rare patient with an injury limited to the lower elements of the plexus have already been discussed.

Nerve Reconstruction

Nerve Grafting

Indications
Exploration of the brachial plexus and supplemental examination such as imaging, electrodiagnosis, and biochemical assay provide the exact lesion of injury, and evaluation of postganglionic injury of cervical roots and a lower lesion of the plexus should take into consideration whether primary repair with nerve grafting or immediate reconstruction such as a Steindler procedure, shoulder arthrodesis, or muscle transfer is planned. This decision is influenced by the age of the patient and time interval between injury and operation. In young patients, less than 3 or 4 months after injury, operative exploration of the brachial plexus and nerve grafting is indicated.[111-115] In patients older than 40 years old, or longer than 6 months after injury even if the patient is young, in whom the chance of nerve regeneration is poor, an immediate reconstruction procedure is the better choice.

Operative Procedure
Exploration of the brachial plexus was described earlier, and each lesion should be meticulously examined concerning the level of the lesion (preganglionic or postganglionic), degree of the lesion (Sunderland's classification; degree 1-5 and mixed lesions),[167,168] and continuity of lesion by macroscopic findings and supplemental electrodiagnosis with nerve action potentials and compound motor action potentials.

When discontinuity of the nerve is found, the decision is to proceed with nerve repair, although the proximal stump should be examined by the electrophysiologic diagnostics, biochemical assay, and imaging described earlier to rule out the more proximal or intraforaminal lesion. Lesions in continuity are treated by microsurgical neurolysis. First, the nerve is liberated from adhesions to neighboring tissue at the level of the epineurium (external neurolysis). Next, electrical stimulation is applied to the proximal side of the lesion, and when no contraction from muscle distal to the lesion occurs or no compound motor action potential can be measured, the lesion is one of discontinuity of the nerve fibers and neurotomy is indicated. When contraction or compound motor action potential are found from the distal muscles to the lesion, internal neurolysis is indicated under the microscope. Longitudinal incisions are made in the fibrotic layers of the epineurium and epifascicular epineurium, and all fascicles are completely separated, removing the surrounding scar tissue. If any fascicles are divided or scarred, they are cut and repaired with interfascicular nerve grafting. There are many occasions when it is difficult to decide whether neurolysis alone or further neurotomy and nerve repair should be selected, especially in the presence of positive contraction of the distal muscles by electric nerve stimulation, because continuity of a few fascicles is not enough to achieve useful function yet will provide muscle contraction. In such situations, the preoperative clinical condition should be considered and when EMG recovery was poor longer than 3 or 4 months after injury, neurotomy and nerve repair are recommended depending on the condition of scar tissue.

Priority of Nerve Repair

In the presence of a partial nerve injury in the distal brachial plexus, division, cord, and branches, when it is a short defect, we prefer to reestablish continuity to all injured parts, using every available donor nerve. For longer defects in the distal plexus and proximal nerve injury at the level of the root and trunk, this approach becomes impossible because there is not enough autologous donor nerve tissue available to restore continuity to all parts of the brachial plexus and the priorities of repair nerve should be considered.

The shorter the length between the site of nerve suture and the neuromotor unit of the target muscle, the better the final outcome. Therefore, the more proximal muscles should be selected as the target muscles for nerve repair. Traditionally, most previous surgeons selected the musculocutaneous nerve as the first priority, followed by the suprascapular nerve and axillary nerve for shoulder reconstruction. The musculocutaneous nerve can be successfully reconstructed by intercostal nerve transfer or by partial ulnar nerve transfer; however, the suprascapular nerve can be repaired only by spinal accessory nerve transfer. The spinal accessory nerve is an important nerve that innervates the trapezius muscle and is useful as a donor nerve for musculocutaneous neurotization or free muscle transfer. We prefer to repair the suprascapular nerve as the first choice, followed by the musculocutaneous. The axillary nerve can be ignored in most severe plexus injuries, because simple axillary nerve palsy does not result in serious paralysis of shoulder function.

The serratus anterior muscle also has a very important function and, if possible, the long thoracic nerve is neurotized. The triceps brachii muscle is also a unique and useful muscle as an antagonist of elbow flexion in reconstruction of distal function and is a potential donor muscle for secondary transfer to the biceps. The radial nerve, especially the branches to the triceps brachii muscle, is the next priority. Attempting to reinnervate the forearm muscles is avoided because the chance of their recovery is minimal and useless for voluntary finger function. Sensory reinnervation of the median nerve can be important in terms of digital sensibility, however.

Selection of Donor Nerves

Conventional fascicular nerve grafts (nonvascularized) are commonly used to repair nerve defects of the brachial plexus; however, a vascularized nerve graft is indicated when the segment to be grafted is excessively long (15 to 20 cm) and when the diameter of the required graft is large.

Conventional Nerve Grafting

Several donor nerves for conventional nerve grafts are used; however, the most commonly used donor nerve for brachial plexus injury is the sural nerve

Sural Nerve. The full length of the sural nerve is harvested from the popliteal fossa to the ankle and is used in nerve grafting for brachial plexus injury where 30 to 40 cm of donor nerve is needed. The sural nerve is harvested in the supine position placing a pad beneath the donor-side buttock to internally rotate the leg, because this nerve is located posteriorly in the calf. Under a field made bloodless by a thigh tourniquet, a small transverse incision is made one fingerbreadth posterior to the lateral malleolus and the sural nerve is found in the subcutaneous tissues adjacent to the lesser saphenous vein. It is transected distally. Gentle traction is applied, and the remaining portion is harvested by making multiple small transverse incisions in the skin proximally. The dissection of this nerve graft must be atraumatic. By applying traction to the free end of the nerve and dissecting carefully surrounding the nerve, each new skin incision can be planned up the leg. As the nerve is located beneath the fascia in the middle of the leg, the fascia is divided to gain adequate length. The sural communicating branch of the peroneal nerve joins the main sural nerve in the midcalf area, and very often the peroneal branch is very small and this branch is divided to mobilize the nerve higher in the leg.

Authors' Preferred Method

Conventional Sural Nerve Graft for Small Segmental Nerve Defects. Most recipient beds for nerve grafting following brachial plexus injury are surrounded by healthy soft tissue, not scarred tissue, and nerve defects less than 10 cm can be successfully repaired with conventional sural nerve grafts. Usually two or three strands are cut and folded and repaired by interfascicular nerve grafting. The authors commonly use this graft between the C5 nerve root and the suprascapular nerve, or in segmental nerve defects of the upper trunk (see Fig. 38-13).

When coapting both nerve stumps with sural nerve grafting, different fascicular patterns are matched individually to lead the generating axons to the proper motor fascicles of the distal nerve. Distally, selection of the proper motor branch will avoid misdirection of the regenerating axon, and the motor dominant fascicles among the proximal stump can be distinguished from the sensory dominant fascicles using electrophysiologic examination such as measurement of spinal evoked potentials, biochemical assay of choline acetyltransferase, and anatomic topography of the fascicles. Epiperineurial sutures between the proximal nerve and each nerve graft and epineurial suture between the distal nerve and each nerve graft are commonly used under microscope magnification using 8-0 to 10-0 nylon sutures.

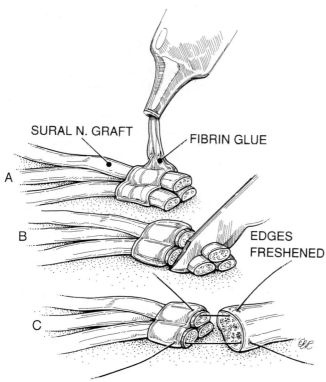

FIGURE 38-15. Nerve repair with tissue adhesive. The graft strands are first glued together (**A**), the graft ends are freshened (**B**), and the mass is then approximated to the correct recipient site with conventional epiperineurial suture (**C**).

Tissue adhesive can simplify the approximation of multiple strands of nerve graft proximally to a single large root stump or distally to a trunk or cord (Fig. 38-15).

Vascularized Nerve Graft

Vascular Anatomy. The ulnar nerve has an extrinsic blood supply consisting of multiple dominant systems: direct branches from the axillary artery, the superior ulnar collateral artery (SUCA), the posterior ulnar recurrent artery, the inferior ulnar collateral artery, and the ulnar artery (Fig. 38-16).[19,22,156,174] When the ulnar artery and its venae comitantes are employed as the dominant source of extrinsic blood supply, only that segment of the ulnar nerve in the forearm and cubital fossa (20 to 25 cm) is harvested, however. The entire length of the ulnar nerve (55.6 cm) will survive based only on the SUCA and its venae comitantes.

The authors prefer the vascular pedicle of the SUCA and its venae comitantes for nerve grafting to the brachial plexus. The SUCA arises from the medial surface of the brachial artery at midhumeral level (14 to 22 cm proximal to the medial epicondyle of the humerus). The SUCA then pierces the medial intermuscular septum and courses posterior to (behind) it distally, joining the ulnar nerve on its posterior surface. It accompanies the ulnar nerve for 4 to 15 cm, giving rise to an average of three arteriae nervorum, which pass directly into the nerve. The SUCA descends between the medial epicondyle and the olecranon and ends deep to the flexor carpi ulnaris muscle by anastomosing with the posterior ulnar recurrent artery and the inferior ulnar recurrent artery. Venae comitantes accompany the SUCA and terminate in the venae comitantes of the brachial artery.

Authors' Preferred Method

Vascularized Ulnar Nerve Graft Based on the Superior Ulnar Collateral Artery and Vein for Repair of Nerve Defects Between C5 Root and Posterior Cord. A vascularized ulnar nerve graft can be utilized to bridge a nerve defect between the ipsilateral C5 root and the posterior cord, accompanying conventional sural nerve grafts between the same C5 root stump and the suprascapular nerve in patients with postganglionic injury of C5 and preganglionic injuries of the other lower four roots of the brachial plexus.

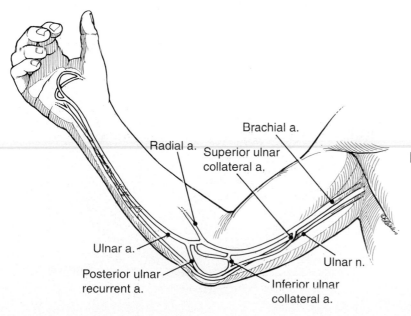

FIGURE 38-16. Vascular anatomy of ulnar nerve.

Through the transverse cervical and clavicular skin incision, the brachial plexus is explored and examined to determine the definite character of the injury. The proximal stump of the C5 root is explored via the transverse cervical skin incision, the suprascapular nerve, and the transverse cervical artery, and a branch of the external jugular vein is exposed via the supraclavicular transverse incision and the posterior cord through the infraclavicular transverse incision. These are identified and prepared for repair.

The entire ulnar nerve is exposed through a longitudinal medial skin incision extending from the axilla to the wrist depending on the length of the nerve needed. First, the ulnar nerve is dissected from the brachial artery (laterally) to approximately the midhumeral level. The SUCA arising from the medial surface of the brachial artery is identified 4 to 14 cm from the cubital fossa. The venae comitantes of the SUCA are similarly identified arising from the venae comitantes of the brachial artery at a similar or more distal level. The SUCA and ulnar nerve are traced through the medial intermuscular septum. Dissection from a proximal to a distal direction to the cubital fossa separates the entire neurovascular pedicle as a single unit. Just proximal to the cubital fossa, where the SUCA and superior ulnar collateral vein (SUCV) diverge medially from the ulnar nerve to form anastomotic networks with the inferior ulnar collateral artery and vein and the posterior recurrent ulnar artery and vein, they are ligated and divided. Leaving a small cuff of surrounding connective tissue, the ulnar nerve is dissected off the medial head of the triceps muscle and from the interval between the medial epicondyle and the olecranon process. The origin of the flexor carpi ulnaris muscle is partially detached, exposing the course of the underlying ulnar nerve. Dissection continues distally into the distal two thirds of the forearm. At this level, the ulnar artery is noted to join the nerve and course distally on its lateral surface. The ulnar nerve is separated from the ulnar artery and its venae comitantes using the bipolar electrocautery unit to coagulate the arteriae nervorum (one to seven in number). Dissection continues to the wrist, where the nerve is sharply transected. Similarly, the nerve is transected proximally in the arm. The ulnar nerve, attached only by the SUCA and

SUCV (Fig. 38-17), is observed for adequate perfusion after deflation of the tourniquet. After several minutes, capillary bleeding can be seen from the cut epineurium both proximally and distally.

The vascular pedicle is clamped and divided, and the graft is transferred to the supraclavicular region and placed between the C5 nerve root proximally and the posterior cord distally in a subcutaneous tunnel between the superior transverse skin incision and supraclavicular transverse incision and clavicle. The SUCA and SUCV are anastomosed to the transverse cervical artery and the branch of the external jugular vein individually, using 10-0 nylon suture. The proximal stump of the graft is sutured to the proximal stump of the C5 root in standard epiperineurial fashion with 8-0 nylon, leaving the space of the stump of C5 root to suture the accompanying conventional sural nerve graft to the supraclavicular nerve. Distally, in the infraclavicular region, the distal stump of the vascularized ulnar nerve graft is connected to the posterior cord, the radial nerve, and axillary nerve in the same fashion (Fig. 38-18). Following this graft, the conventional sural nerve graft bridges between the remnant of the C5 root stump and suprascapular nerve.

Postoperative Protocol. Timing of reinnervation of the target muscles depends on the length of the nerve graft and the distance between the site of nerve suture and the neuromotor units of the muscle. Typically, it takes 3 months before reinnervation of the supraspinatus muscle, 5 to 7 months for the triceps brachii muscle, and 10 months for the deltoid muscle. Visible and palpable muscle contraction are not seen for an additional 2 months, and the strength of the muscle gradually increases afterward.

Complications. Thrombosis of the anastomosed vessels results in necrosis of the nerve graft and limits regeneration of motor axons. If the Tinel sign stops at the proximal suture site of the graft this means that vascular occlusion has occurred. The graft cannot be salvaged at this point, and another reconstructive plan should be considered. Weakness of the target muscles 1 year after surgery is an indication to

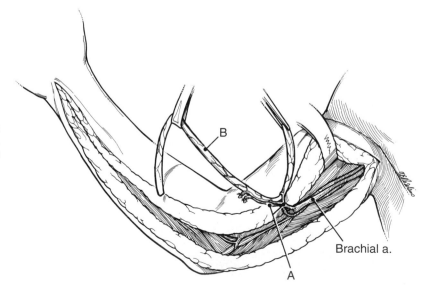

FIGURE 38-17. A vascularized ulnar nerve graft with a pedicle of the superior ulnar collateral artery and vein. *A* points to the segmental vascular pedicle. *B* points to the longitudinal vascularity.

Brachial a.

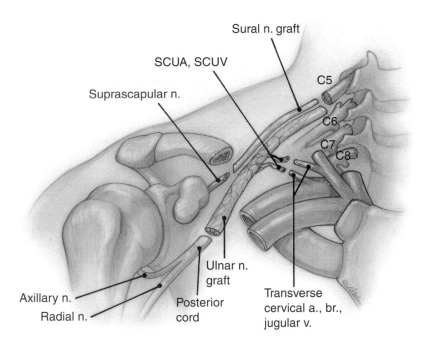

FIGURE 38-18. Vascularized ulnar nerve graft based on the superior ulnar collateral artery and vein for repair of the nerve defect between C5 root and posterior cord with simultaneous grafting of the sural nerve between C5 root and suprascapular nerve.

consider supplemental procedures or changes in the final goal of reconstruction.

Expected Outcomes. Final outcome of shoulder function depends not only on recovery of strength of the supraspinatus muscle but also that of the other muscles, especially the serratus anterior and primary movers such as the deltoid, biceps, and triceps. However, our experience has shown that patients without scapular winging obtain stability and mean movement of 30 degrees of flexion and extension of the scapulohumeral joint. Most patients with M2 power of elbow extension can extend the elbow assisted by gravity, which is enough to contribute to stability of the elbow if free muscle transfer is undertaken.

CRITICAL POINTS: FOR REPAIR OF POSTERIOR CORD FROM C5 ROOT

INDICATION

- Total paralysis with postganglionic injury of C5 and preganglionic injury of other lower four roots in patients who will undergo elbow reconstruction by extraplexus nerve transfer or prehensile reconstruction by free muscle transfer

PEARLS

- Minimal recovery of range of shoulder motion and reliable recovery of shoulder stability and elbow extension should be expected.

TECHNICAL POINTS

- Standard exploration of the brachial plexus and examination
- Preparation of the C5 root, suprascapular nerve, posterior cord and transverse cervical artery, and a branch of the jugular vein
- Ulnar nerve dissection through a longitudinal medial skin incision from axilla to wrist
- Identification of the vascular pedicle of the superior ulnar collateral artery and vein

- Harvest of vascularized ulnar nerve including the vascular pedicle, long enough to bridge the nerve defect
- Division of the nerve and vascular pedicle
- Transfer of the graft and vascular anastomoses of the vascular pedicle to the transverse cervical artery and vein
- Nerve suture between the proximal stump of the graft and C5 root proximally and the distal stump of the graft and posterior cord distally
- Additional conventional sural nerve graft between the remnant of C5 root and suprascapular nerve

PITFALLS

- Small diameter of the comitant vein of the transverse cervical artery
- Inability to monitor the vascular status of the graft postoperatively

POSTOPERATIVE CARE

- Immobilization of upper limb by cast or splint (depending on other reconstructive procedures) and neck collar

Vascularized Radial Nerve Graft

A vascularized radial nerve graft is used in lieu of an ulnar nerve graft in C5 to C8 paralysis, in which the ulnar nerve is working and should be preserved. Contrary to the ulnar nerve, the radial nerve innervates proximal muscles such as the triceps brachii, which may recover after nerve transfer. Therefore, we prefer to use the superficial radial nerve as a vascularized graft and preserve the proximal radial nerve. The diameter of the superficial radial nerve is smaller than that of the ulnar nerve, and the former graft is more adaptable to distal nerve lesions with smaller diameters such as the musculocutaneous nerve.

Vascular Anatomy and Harvest of the Graft. The superficial branch of the radial nerve has an extrinsic blood supply consisting of a single dominant system, the radial artery and its venae comitantes.[155,172,173]

A tourniquet is employed during dissection. A longitudinal lateral skin incision is made in the forearm. Dissection begins in the proximal third of the forearm and antecubital fossa. The brachial artery is identified, as are the origins of the radial artery and venae comitantes. The radial recurrent artery is identified and ligated, as are the inferior cubital artery and septocutaneous perforators.

The superficial branch of the radial nerve is identified and dissected proximally. An intraneural dissection can be performed, separating the donor nerve fascicles from the posterior interosseous nerve. The mesoneurium, containing the arteriae nervorum, is identified. An arcade of vessels on the adjacent muscle is carefully dissected and separated from the extensor muscle mass distal to any recurrent nerve branches. The incision is then extended through the forearm fascia, exposing the lateral intermuscular septum located between the flexor carpi radialis muscle medially and the brachioradialis muscle laterally in the middle third of the forearm. Dissection next proceeds deep to the brachioradialis muscle, which is retracted laterally. The radial artery (medially) and the superficial branch of the radial nerve (laterally) are identified deep in the intermuscular septum. Great care is exercised during this portion of the dissection to avoid injury to the arteriae nervorum. Further dissection of this area is deferred until more distal and proximal dissections of the neurovascular structures are completed. Dissection continues in the distal third of the forearm, separating the radial artery and superficial branch of the radial nerve from the surrounding tissue. The nerve is traced distally to the point at which it penetrates the forearm fascia and divides into two branches.

The radial artery and attached venae comitantes are traced to the wrist, isolated, clamped, and divided. The venae comitantes will be ligated, and the nerve is sharply transected. The neurovascular bundle now remains attached proximally. The superficial radial nerve is divided from the main trunk of the radial nerve.

The tourniquet is released and bleeding from both the proximal and distal nerve segments is observed. After perfusion is confirmed, the vascular pedicle is divided and transplanted to the recipient site. After harvest of the radial artery, one may bridge the gap with an interposition vein graft if perfusion of the hand is in question.

Vascularized Sural Nerve Graft

The sural nerve may also be taken as a vascularized graft, although it is usually utilized in a nonvascularized fashion. The nerve is taken with its vascular supply from the superficial sural artery (SSA) and may be folded with this supply to provide several bundles. This is particularly applicable when placing nerve grafts in a scarred bed. We prefer to use the vascularized sural nerve graft in brachial plexus reconstruction because of its simple design, although the external diameter of the SSA is small and varies between 0.6 and 2 mm, with a mean of 1.2 mm. This graft is also used to repair nerves of small diameter such as the musculocutaneous nerve from the C5 nerve root or the suprascapular nerve from the contralateral C7 nerve root. The reader is referred to the pertinent literature for details of the anatomy and technique.[51,52,154]

Nerve Transfer (Method of Doi)

In the case of complete root avulsion of the brachial plexus, no functioning nerves are available proximally to restore function of the extremity. In these situations, there are no musculotendinous transfers available for restoration of extremity function and an intact extraplexal nerve is transferred and coapted to the distal peripheral nerve of the brachial plexus as a method of reinnervation of a critical sensory or motor territory. The terms *nerve transfer, neurotization,* and *nerve crossing* are all confusedly used for this procedure.

The term *neurotization* is used when a healthy but less valuable nerve or its proximal stump is transferred to reinnervate a more important sensory or motor territory that has lost its innervation through irreparable damage to its proximal nerve. This term originally implied straightforward nerve repair or simple implantation of nerve ends into the muscle to reinnervate denervated muscles.

The term *nerve transfer* is used most frequently in the current literature. *Nerve crossing* is a new technical term that means neurorrhaphy between different nerves and expresses the exact technique. While one of us (Doi) prefers to use the term *nerve crossing,* for purposes of clarity we will use the terms *nerve transfer* and *neurotization* without distinction in this text.

Spinal Accessory Nerve Transfer

Surgical Anatomy. The spinal accessory nerve (cranial nerve XI) innervates the sternocleidomastoid and trapezius muscles. The spinal accessory nerve is formed in the posterior cranial fossa from spinal and cranial nerve roots. After passing through the jugular foramen it divides into an internal branch (containing fibers originating from the "cranial part") that joins the vagus nerve and an external branch consisting of the fibers from the "spinal part"; this portion supplies the sternocleidomastoid and trapezius muscles. After supplying the sternocleidomastoid muscle, the spinal accessory nerve descends obliquely in the posterior triangle of the neck between the superficial and deep layers of the deep cervical fascia. Here it is embedded in loose connective tissue and is in contact with the cervical lymph node chain. The spinal accessory nerve provides two or three branches for the upper part of the trapezius muscle before passing under its anterior edge. Intramuscularly, the nerve follows an oblique caudal course toward the middle and lower parts of the trapezius, giving off branches to the muscle throughout its course.[10] There is great variability in the connections between the spinal accessory nerve and the roots of the cervical plexus.[6,45] Our clinical experience has shown that in two thirds of the patients, after transfer of the terminal branch of the spinal accessory nerve distal to the connection from the cervical plexus, the middle and distal parts of the trapezius were not completely denervated electromyographically.[84]

Dissection and Transfer. Traditionally, the spinal accessory nerve is exposed from the posterior border of the sternocleidomastoid, traced as far as possible to the undersurface of the trapezius, transected, and transferred to the supraclavicular fossa for neurotization.[93,147,159] Although this is the most popular approach to the spinal accessory nerve, there are some disadvantages. First, a large longitudinal scar on the neck is inevitable. Second, after its exit from the sternocleidomastoid, the nerve is extremely vulnerable in the posterior triangle of the neck owing to its superficial location. During this course in the posterior triangle of the neck it gives off small branches to the upper part of the trapezius. Our preferred technique utilizes a transverse incision and makes a less conspicuous scar over the clavicle.[75] When spinal accessory transfer is to be utilized, a second 5-cm transverse incision is made over the neck, which results in an acceptable scar. Moreover, the important branches innervating the upper part of the trapezius are completely preserved with this approach, as dissection at the posterior triangle of the neck is avoided.

Authors' Preferred Method

Proper positioning of the patient on the operating table is very important for this approach. Once the patient is anesthetized, a large folded sheet is placed in the interscapular region and the neck is turned to the contralateral side. This maneuver elevates the shoulder and neck off the table and provides an easy access to the spinal accessory nerve. The use of muscle relaxation is avoided to facilitate use of electrical stimulation to make identification of the spinal accessory nerve easier.

A 10-cm transverse incision is made along the clavicle from the midclavicular to the acromioclavicular joint. The upper part of the trapezius, which is inserted to the clavicle and the acromioclavicular joint, is detached using electrocautery. The detached upper part of the trapezius is retracted posteriorly. The spinal accessory nerve can be found on the anterior surface of the trapezius, but identification of the nerve at this site is difficult because it is embedded in adipose tissue. The landmark to detect the spinal accessory nerve at this site is the transverse cervical artery and vein. These vessels enter the muscle at the base of the neck and then descend vertically, midway between the vertebral column and the medial border of the scapula, accompanied by the spinal accessory nerve.[140] After identification of these vessels, an electrical stimulator is used around the vessels to identify the distal part of the spinal accessory nerve (Fig. 38-19A). Small branches from the cervical plexus are frequently found around the vessels, but the size of these branches is comparatively small and the response of the

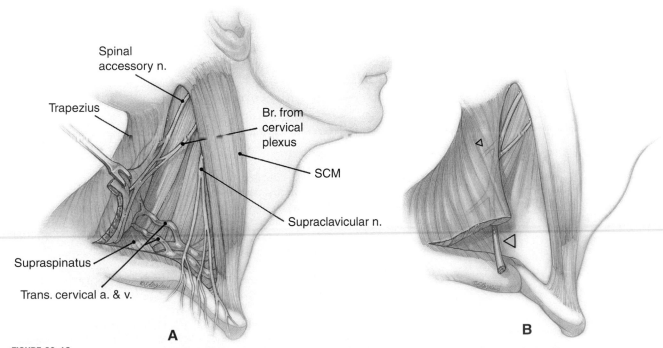

FIGURE 38-19. Harvest of the spinal accessory nerve. **A,** Dissection of the spinal accessory nerve. **B,** Division and transfer of the spinal accessory nerve. *Small arrowhead* is the branch to the upper part of the trapezius. *Large arrowhead* is the terminal branch of the nerve.

trapezius to electrical stimulation is weak. The spinal accessory nerve is always found in the adipose tissue on the anterior surface of the trapezius. A small branch to the upper part of the trapezius should be preserved. The terminal division of the nerve is dissected distally as far as possible, divided, and transferred to the supraclavicular fossa for neurotization (see Fig. 38-19B). The division of the nerve at the level of the scapular spine usually gives enough length to reach the supraclavicular fossa.

Suprascapular Nerve Neurotization. The spinal accessory nerve is the first choice of donor nerve for nerve transfer to restore shoulder function in C5 and C6 avulsion type paralysis in cases less than 6 months after injury. For adequate return of shoulder abduction, it is imperative to preserve serratus anterior function. In C5 to C7 avulsion injuries, the final outcome for shoulder function is poor because of serratus anterior paralysis, even if the reinnervated supraspinatus muscle works well.

The suprascapular nerve innervates the supraspinatus and infraspinatus muscles. The suprascapular nerve branches off the upper trunk about 3 cm above the clavicle, and it is not unusual to find it arising entirely from the fifth cervical nerve. It passes laterally and posteriorly, deep to the omohyoid muscle, to the scapular notch, entering the supraspinatus fossa deep to the superior transverse ligament. The nerve then traverses the fossa deep to the supraspinatus muscle to wind around the lateral border of the spine of the scapula to enter the infraspinatus fossa. Its course renders it particularly vulnerable to traction lesions at the supraspinatus notch and within the supraspinatus and infraspinatus fossae. It is imperative to dissect the suprascapular nerve distal to the supraspinatus notch even when the location of a lesion proximal to the upper trunk is obvious (Fig. 38-20).

When nerve transfer from the spinal accessory nerve is undertaken, the suprascapular nerve is transected just distal to its bifurcation from the upper trunk, transferred, and coapted to it without nerve grafting.

Most authors transect the spinal accessory nerve more proximally, just distal to the sternocleidomastoid muscle,

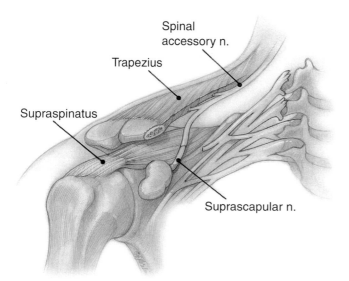

FIGURE 38-20. Spinal accessory nerve to suprascapular nerve transfer.

Spinal accessory n.
Trapezius
Supraspinatus
Suprascapular n.

CRITICAL POINTS: SPINAL ACCESSORY TO SUPRASCAPULAR NERVE TRANSFER FOR UPPER TYPE PARALYSIS

INDICATIONS

- Cases with C5 and C6 avulsion and no winging of the scapula
- Injuries less than 6 months old

PEARLS

- Transfer of only the terminal branch of the spinal accessory nerve
- Easy neurorrhaphy between the spinal accessory and suprascapular nerves without nerve graft
- Transverse inconspicuous linear scar

TECHNICAL POINTS

- Use a transverse skin incision over the distal clavicle and medial acromion.
- Transfer only the middle and distal branch of the spinal accessory nerve.
- Perform direct coaptation to the suprascapular nerve without nerve grafting.

PITFALL

- Poor outcomes with C5 to C7 avulsion and scapular winging

POSTOPERATIVE CARE

- Limitation of excessive movement of neck and shoulder postoperatively
- No special immobilization
- EMG reinnervation occurs 2 or 3 months postoperatively
- Re-education program of reinnervated muscles

---

and use long nerve grafts to connect to the suprascapular, axillary, or musculocutaneous nerve. We do not use a nerve graft while performing spinal accessory nerve to suprascapular nerve transfer, because we transect the spinal accessory nerve distal to the branch to the upper portion of the trapezius as described earlier.

Postoperative Protocol. The postoperative protocol is described previously.

Complications. There are no serious complications in this procedure as long as the proximal branch of the spinal accessory nerve to the upper fibers of the trapezius muscle is preserved. If it is injured, shoulder depression and dysfunction will occur.

Expected Outcome. The standard outcome of spinal accessory nerve to suprascapular nerve for restoration of shoulder abduction is 20 to 80 degrees of range of shoulder abduction (mean, 45 degrees).

In 12 patients who have undergone spinal accessory nerve to suprascapular nerve transfer, 3 patients with C5 and C6 root avulsion obtained more than 90 degrees of shoulder abduction (Fig. 38-21). The abduction and flexion of the shoulder of the remaining 9 patients with C5 to C7 root avulsion was between 20 to 60 and 40 to 80 degrees, respectively. The latter 9 patients underwent multiple muscle transfers secondarily. The serratus anterior muscle also plays a key role. The patients with partially intact innervation of the serratus anterior (from an intact C7 root) or in cases of C5 and C6 root avulsion or postganglionic injury of the upper trunk achieve significantly better range of shoulder abduction and flexion (more than 90 degrees) with control of scapular movement. On the contrary, patients with complete C5 to C7 root avulsion cannot regain such function and need secondary tendon transfers.

Musculocutaneous Nerve Neurotization. We do not utilize the spinal accessory nerve to musculocutaneous nerve transfer, because the musculocutaneous nerve can be neurotized by the other nerves such as intercostals or ulnar nerve in upper or total type paralysis. Others prefer this transfer and report good results.[159] However, there are a few occasions when the spinal accessory nerve is preferred for elbow flexion, that is, when the intercostal nerves are damaged by thoracotomy or chest trauma. This technique and the standard outcomes are briefly described.

Operative Procedure. The musculocutaneous nerve originates from the lateral cord of brachial plexus just distal to the coracoid process. After the musculocutaneous nerve pierces the coracobrachialis muscle, the branches to the biceps enter the muscle at about 12 cm from the acromion. Two types of distribution of motor branches to the two heads of the biceps are found: a common trunk (pattern 1) and two separate nerve branches (pattern 2). A common trunk (median length, 2 cm) arises from the musculocutaneous nerve about 13 cm from the acromion and divides into two branches, one to the short head and another to the long head. There can be intercommunicating nerve fibers between these branches. After traveling a median distance of 1 cm in the short head and 2 cm in the long head, the main branches divide into terminal branches distributed throughout the muscle bellies. The origin of the nerve to the brachialis muscle is found even more distal, about 17 cm from the acromion. Each portion of the separate nerve branches originates from the musculocutaneous nerve at different levels. In those instances the branch to the short head originates proximally 11 cm below the acromion. It also divides on the deep surface of the muscle belly after an average length of 3 cm. The branch to the long head originates about 2 cm distally and ramifies after an average length of 3 cm.

After the dissection of the spinal accessory nerve the musculocutaneous nerve is explored and dissected through a deltopectoral skin incision, beginning at the lateral cord to its branches into the biceps, to unmask any injury to the nerve itself. The spinal accessory nerve is cut distal to the branch of the upper trapezius muscle to avoid total denervation of the trapezius muscle and transferred to the

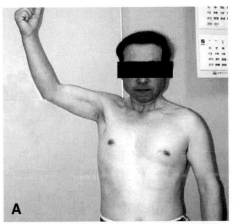
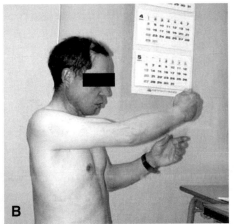
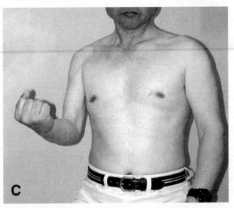

FIGURE 38-21. A 49-year-old man sustained a right brachial plexus injury with C5 and C6 root avulsion. Ninety degrees of shoulder abduction (**A**), 90 degrees of shoulder flexion (**B**), and 0 degrees of external rotation (**C**) were achieved 14 months after spinal accessory nerve to suprascapular nerve transfer.

supraclavicular region. The musculocutaneous nerve is then cut just after it branches to the coracobrachialis muscle. A sural nerve graft 9 to 10 cm long is used to connect the spinal accessory nerve to the musculocutaneous nerve. The nerve graft is usually placed beneath the subcutaneous tissue over the clavicle and connected to the spinal accessory nerve first and then to the musculocutaneous nerve without tension using 9-0 or 10-0 nylon under magnification of operating microscope.

Expected Outcome. By meta-analysis, the typical outcome of transfer of the spinal accessory nerve to the musculocutaneous nerve for restoration of elbow flexion showed that 77% of patients achieved biceps strength of M3 and 29% achieved M4.[110] Results comparing spinal accessory nerve transfer without the use of interposition nerve grafts and intercostal nerve transfers for restoration of elbow flexion were comparable at M3 biceps strength (72% vs. 77%). Intercostal nerve transfers, however, achieved significantly better results relative to spinal accessory nerve transfers in obtaining a biceps strength of M4 (41% vs. 29%; $P<.001$). Many differences in outcome for elbow flexion can occur between cases of complete avulsion of all five roots and upper type paralyses, since in the latter case Steindler's effect of the forearm muscles contributes to elbow flexion.

Functioning Free Muscle Transfer

The spinal accessory nerve can be used as a donor motor nerve for functional free muscle transfer as well. Technical details of functioning free muscle transfer are described below.

Intercostal Nerve Transfer. Intercostal nerves have been widely used for reinnervation of the musculocutaneous nerve,[39,94,117,127] and this donor application has been extended to reinnervation of the triceps, deltoid, free muscle transfer, and sensory restoration of the hand.

Intercostal nerve to musculocutaneous nerve transfer is indicated for reconstruction of elbow flexion in brachial plexus injury with total or upper type paralyses due to a preganglionic lesion, less than 6 months after injury. Postganglionic lesions should undergo nerve repair with nerve grafting for elbow flexion, and delayed cases are candidates for secondary muscle transfer such as Steindler's flexorplasty, latissimus dorsi muscle transfer, or free muscle transfer. Neurotization of the triceps brachii is used as one step in double free muscle transfer for prehensile reconstruction after total paralysis of brachial plexus as described later or sometimes as treatment of co-contraction between the triceps and biceps in obstetric palsy. Historically, neurotization of the deltoid and forearm muscles has been attempted, but the long-term outcomes of these transfers are unreliable and too frequently functionless. The authors do not recommend transfer of intercostal nerves to the axillary, median, ulnar, or radial nerve except for sensory reconstruction by nerve transfer to the median or ulnar nerve.

Candidates for this procedure should have no history of rib fracture, thoracotomy, or chest tube placement in the potential donor region.[175] Although it is possible to use both the sensory and motor fiber components of each intercostal nerve to provide both sensory and motor reinnervation,[38,82] motor reinnervation alone is usually the goal of this neurotization. Direct suture of the third, fourth, and fifth intercostal nerves to the musculocutaneous nerve without nerve graft is performed most commonly. By extending the dissection more anterior, sufficient intercostal nerve length is gained, which permits direct coaptation to the target motor branch, thus minimizing the need for intercalary nerve grafting. There are anthropomorphic differences between various races, and it has been the experience of some authors that direct suture is less often possible in whites, and thus interpositional nerve grafts may be necessary depending on the contours of the patient's thorax.

Surgical Anatomy. Intercostal nerves run within the intercostal space along the pleural side of external intercostal muscles (Fig. 38-22). These nerves pass between the two layers of intercostal muscles inserted on the posterior thirds of the ribs. Just beneath the axilla, they enter deep to the intercostal muscles and run anteriorly between the transverse thoracic muscles and the endothoracic aponeurosis. The lateral cutaneous branch pierces the intercostal muscle toward the skin and divides into a dorsal and a ventral branch. The anterior cutaneous branch pierces the pectoralis major close to the sternum and ramifies into the skin. The more proximal part of the intercostal nerve should be used for transfer, since the motor fiber content of intercostal nerves decreases distally.[63,79]

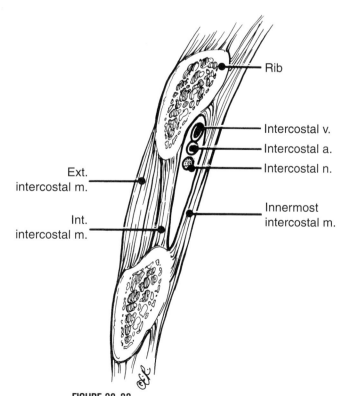

FIGURE 38-22. Anatomy of the intercostal nerve.

Author's Preferred Method

Dissection and Transfer. The third, fourth, and fifth intercostal nerves are explored through a transverse incision placed between the third and fourth ribs extending from the midaxillary line to the costochondral junction. The subcutaneous tissue and underlying pectoralis major and minor muscles are elevated from the distal margin of the muscles so as not to injure the muscles themselves. In the axillary region, the intercostobrachial nerve, a branch of the second intercostal nerve, is identified and protected. Care should be taken not to injure this nerve, because the intercostobrachial nerve is the only sensory nerve remaining after total avulsion of the plexus and may be utilized as a donor nerve for sensory restoration of the hand. The anterior surface of the third and fourth ribs as well as the associated intercostal musculature is exposed from the anterior axillary line to the costochondral junction. When the serratus anterior muscle is functional, the long thoracic nerve and serratus anterior muscle should be preserved. The long thoracic nerve courses down posteriorly to the midaxillary line along with the thoracodorsal vessels. The lateral sensory branch of the intercostal nerve is identified and marked between the serratus anterior muscle after detaching the upper margin of the costal attachment of the muscle along with periosteum from the rib. The midline of the anterior surface of each rib is incised and the lower half of the anterior and posterior periosteum is elevated so as not to injure the pleura. With cephalad retraction of the rib, the upper portion of the intercostal muscle inserting into its inferior margin can be exposed. If exposure is difficult, rib mobilization may be facilitated by circumferential elevation of the periosteum from the rib using a rib periosteal elevator. Osteotomy of the rib is not generally necessary. Occasionally removing a few millimeters of the lower margin of the rib with a sharp

ronguer facilitates exposure of the intercostal nerve. The periosteal sleeve of the rib is then carefully incised on the line where the medial intercostal nerve runs. This can be identified by tracing the lateral sensory branch proximally or finding the flash of bleeding from the intercostal artery and veins. The periosteum is usually torn during the dissection, and the underlying intercostal nerve can be found easily. By gentle spreading of the intercostal muscles, the motor branch of the intercostal nerve can be isolated and traced anteriorly toward the costochondral junction. The motor nature of this nerve branch is confirmed by direct electrical stimulation. The lateral cutaneous sensory branch of the nerve is found at a point between the anterior and midaxillary lines and may be separated from the motor component posteriorly as far as necessary. Anterior dissection of the motor branch is continued far enough to gain the necessary length to reach the target nerves. A similar procedure is then carried out for harvesting the other intercostal nerves as needed for reconstruction. After appropriate dissection, each intercostal nerve is elevated and then passed through the serratus anterior muscle and via a subcutaneous tunnel into the axillary region. Care is taken not to compress the nerve at the corner of the posterior margin of dissection by incising the inferior periosteum. We use the second intercostal nerve and intercostobrachial nerve for sensory reconstruction, if this is indicated, by connecting them to the median or ulnar nerve component of the medial cord. The third and fourth intercostal nerves are used for simple nerve transfer, such as musculocutaneous nerve transfer (Fig. 38-23), and the fifth and sixth intercostal nerves for functioning free muscle transfer, if this is planned. After transferring the intercostal nerves, the dissected periosteum should be sutured tightly so as not to leave a large dead space under the rib.

Neurotization of Musculocutaneous Nerve. At the time of coaptation of the intercostal nerves to the musculo-

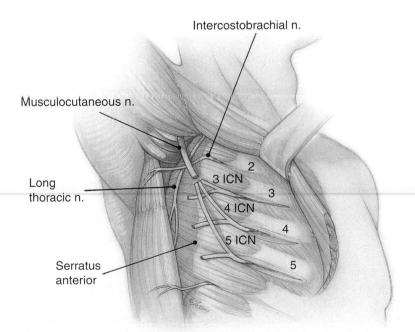

FIGURE 38-23. Intercostal nerve to musculocutaneous nerve transfer. Note the nerve suture site of the intercostal nerves (just distal to the medial cutaneous branch).

cutaneous nerve, the dissection of the musculocutaneous nerve is carried out through the axillary and medial borders of the biceps, beginning at the lateral cord to its branches to the biceps to unmask any injury to the nerve itself. The branch to the biceps is dissected proximal to its branching from the lateral cord, and enough length is harvested so as to reach the transferred intercostal nerves without any tension. Knowing that the intercostal nerves have more motor fiber content in their proximal parts, we prefer to perform coaptation as proximally as possible. Usually we connect the intercostal nerves just distal to the lateral sensory branches. Other authors have described more distal neuror-rhaphy,[137] but the more distal the nerve coaptation is performed, the less the content of motor fibers are present. We prefer end-to-end fascicular suture.

Postoperative Protocol. Chest pain when the biceps is pinched is distinguished at approximately 3 months postoperatively as an early sign of reinnervation. Proximal biceps contraction without elbow joint movement, especially during deep inspiration, is usually recognized by 3 to 6 months postoperatively. Later distal biceps contraction without elbow joint movement and a Tinel sign appears in the lower arm lateral to the biceps tendon (percussion of this area causes tingling in the chest and develops around 12 months postoperatively). Elbow flexion against gravity appears at 12 to 18 months after surgery, and voluntary flexion against weight can be recovered.[39]

A relationship between elbow movement and respiration is observed for 4 to 8 months after motor recovery, and volitional small action potentials synchronized with respiratory movement are noted. After 12 months, patients learn to flex the joint voluntarily without relating it to respiratory rhythm. Twenty-four months after operation, respiratory rhythm still affects the interval of spiked discharge on EMG, but at the 32-month interval, biceps activity was completely distinct from the respiratory cycle. Involuntary muscle contraction still occurs when the patient coughs or sneezes.[127]

Complications. Lack of tension at the coaptation site and proper positioning of the shoulder are imperative to prevent rupture of the nerve repair.

Expected Outcome. Intercostal to musculocutaneous nerve transfers without interposition grafts achieve more than M3 strength in 72% of patients. Only 47% of nerve transfers using interposition grafts for restoration of biceps function achieve more than M3 strength. In a study of 418 patients who underwent intercostal to musculocutaneous nerve transfers without interposition nerve grafts, 59% had two intercostal nerves and 34% had three or four intercostal nerves transferred.[110] Of 15 patients who underwent intercostal nerve to musculocutaneous nerve transfers 66% of them achieved more than M3 strength of elbow flexion (Fig. 38-24). Most authors advocate that the operation

CRITICAL POINTS: INTERCOSTAL NERVE TO MUSCULOCUTANEOUS NERVE TRANSFER

INDICATIONS

- Cases of upper or total type paralysis with avulsion of C5 and C6 roots
- Less than 6 months after injury
- If patients with total paralysis do not want to undergo further complex reconstruction of prehensile function, they are candidates for simple intercostal nerve transfer for elbow flexion.

PEARLS

- Reliable procedure for elbow flexion with experience as long as performed within 6 months after injury

TECHNICAL POINTS

- Expose the third, fourth, and fifth intercostal nerves through a transverse incision.
- Each intercostal nerve dissection and transfer is done without osteotomy of the ribs.
- Proximal dissection of proper motor nerve to the biceps brachii of the musculocutaneous nerve is performed.
- More proximal neurorrhaphy of the intercostal nerves without tension provides a better outcome.

PITFALLS

- Technically demanding neurorrhaphy
- Dehiscence of nerve repair when neurorrhaphy is performed under tension

POSTOPERATIVE CARE

- The arm should be immobilized in the position of 60 degrees of shoulder abduction and 30 degrees of shoulder flexion and not in a position of 0 degrees of shoulder abduction and flexion.

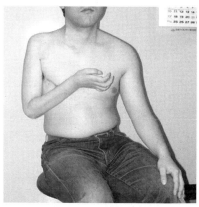

FIGURE 38-24. A 27-year-old man sustained complete avulsion of his right brachial plexus and underwent transfer of the third and fourth intercostal nerves to the musculocutaneous nerve. He can flex his elbow fully 18 months postoperatively.

should be performed within 5 to 6 months after the original trauma and the age of candidates should be younger than 40 years.[39,127]

Partial Ulnar Nerve to Musculocutaneous Nerve Transfer

In place of intercostal nerve transfers for elbow flexion, transfer of a part of the ulnar nerve has gained popularity because of its technical ease and reliability.[59,71,133,134] Recently injured patients with C5 and C6 root avulsion, or sometimes those with C5 to C7 root avulsion within 10 months after injury, are candidates for this procedure. This procedure provides powerful elbow flexion in patients older than 40 years of age in whom intercostal nerve transfers are not applicable. This operation is usually done in conjunction with spinal accessory nerve to suprascapular nerve transfer for reconstruction of shoulder function.

Surgical Anatomy. Anatomy of the musculocutaneous nerve is described earlier in the section on the spinal accessory nerve to the musculocutaneous nerve transfer.

The larger of the two terminal branches of the medial cord of the brachial plexus continues as the ulnar nerve, while the smaller terminal branch forms the medial root of the median nerve. In the axilla and upper arm the ulnar nerve runs inferior and medial to the axillary artery. It passes anterior to the triceps muscle and enters the ulnar groove between the medial epicondyle of the humerus and the olecranon. In the upper half of the arm, the ulnar nerve has 6 to 10 fascicles, each of which contains both motor and sensory nerve fibers. According to Sunderland's intraneural topography,[168] the posteromedial fascicles contain the motor fibers to the forearm muscles and the anterolateral fascicles tend to contain the motor fibers to the intrinsic muscles of the hand. This region of the ulnar nerve has rich interfascicular connections.

Authors' Preferred Method

Dissection and Transfer. Through a longitudinal medial skin incision in the proximal upper arm (Fig. 38-25A), the branch of the musculocutaneous nerve supplying the biceps muscle after it traverses the coracobrachialis muscle is identified (see Fig. 38-25B). After the type of branch (common or separated branches pattern) is confirmed, the branch long enough to reach the ulnar nerve is divided and transferred to ulnar nerve. The ulnar nerve is dissected intra-epineurially and the single posteromedial fascicle, which mostly innervates the flexor carpi ulnaris muscle, equal to the size of branch to the biceps, is selected and transected just proximal to the distal interfascicular connection of the fascicle under magnification of an operating microscope (see Fig. 38-25C and D). One of us (Doi) does not utilize electrodiagnostic means to distinguish the motor fascicles from the sensory fascicles because the fascicles of the ulnar nerve at the upper arm are mixed and all fascicles contain both motor and sensory nerve fibers. One of us (Hentz) prefers to perform microstimulation to avoid inadvertent transfer of the motor fascicle supplying primarily the intrin-

sic muscles. The motor branch of the biceps is sutured without tension to a single or two fascicles of the ulnar nerve in epineural fashion using 10-0 nylon suture (see Fig. 38-25E).

Clinical Application. A partial fascicle transfer of the ulnar nerve is indicated to reconstruct elbow flexion for patients with C5 and C6 root avulsion because the motor nerve fibers of the ulnar nerve originate from the C7, C8, and T1 nerve roots. If this procedure is applied to the patients with C5, C6, and C7 root avulsion, there may be insufficient motor fibers to reinnervate the biceps with maintenance of motor innervation of the ulnar innervated muscles. Previous authors have recommended the application of this technique to C5 and C6 root avulsion cases only; however, we have used it in C5, C6, and C7 avulsion and achieved satisfactory recovery without any sequelae of ulnar nerve palsy.

CRITICAL POINTS: PARTIAL ULNAR NERVE TO MUSCULOCUTANEOUS NERVE TRANSFER IN UPPER TYPE PARALYSIS

INDICATIONS

- For reconstruction of elbow flexion in fresh cases with C5 and C6 root avulsion and sometimes C5 to C7 root avulsion
- Less than 10 months after injury
- Younger than 50 years old

PEARLS

- Technical ease of the surgery
- Reliable recovery
- Limited skin incision and less invasive surgery

TECHNICAL POINTS

- Division and transfer of motor branch of biceps brachii muscle
- Meticulous interneural dissection of ulnar nerve
- Selection of the fascicles for transfer
- Perineurial suture

PITFALL

- Transient ulnar nerve paralysis

POSTOPERATIVE CARE

- No postoperative immobilization by cast or splint
- Arm sling to hold the arm and prevent shoulder subluxation due to accompanying paralysis of shoulder girdle musculature
- Reinnervation 2 or 3 months after surgery

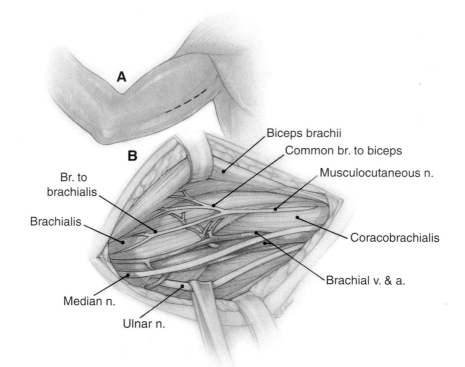

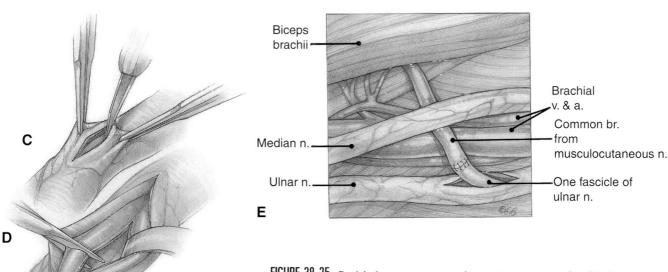

FIGURE 38-25. Partial ulnar nerve to musculocutaneous nerve transfer (Oberlin's method). **A,** Skin incision. **B,** Dissection of the common branch of the musculocutaneous nerve and ulnar nerve. **C,** Epineurectomy of the ulnar nerve. **D,** Interfascicular dissection of the ulnar nerve and division of one or two fascicles for transfer. **E,** Neurorrhaphy between the common branch of the musculocutaneous nerve and a fascicle of the ulnar nerve.

Special Considerations. Patients with weakness and sensory deficit due to ulnar nerve palsy preoperatively are not candidates for this technique.

Postoperative Protocol. Using EMG biofeedback techniques facilitates re-education of reinnervated muscle. When the patient is asked to make a fist in the ulnopalmar flexion position of the wrist, the reinnervated biceps muscle fires easily. In the postoperative rehabilitation period,

patients can learn to flex the elbow while making a fist. Patients can often learn to flex the biceps without wrist flexion after therapy.

Complications. In 10 of our patients who had this procedure, 1 patient complained of transient numbness in the ipsilateral little finger postoperatively and 1 other patient had transient muscle weakness of the ulnar interosseous muscle. However, there were no long-standing sensory or motor deficits of the ulnar nerve. Most patients gained powerful grip and pinch strength during the postoperative rehabilitation program, which included progressive muscle strengthening exercises.

Expected Outcome. Most authors emphasize the quick recovery after this procedure as an important advantage. Most patients have good recovery of biceps contraction after 2 to 5 months. More than 90% of patients achieved biceps strength of Medical Research Council (MRC) grade 3 or better.[98,138] The operative results in the patients with C5 and C6 avulsions were better than those with C5, C6, and C7 avulsions.[134]

Contralateral C7 Root Transfer

The contralateral C7 root transfer is a controversial operation because it is difficult for most surgeons to accept that a normal root can be divided and transferred without any neurologic sequelae. Based on many experiences from China and East Asia, however, it has gained acceptance in other countries. Postoperative complications do occur and when transfer of the contralateral C7 root is being considered, the potential functional outcome should be carefully assessed with reference to its risk-to-benefit ratio.

Surgical Anatomy. Although certain anatomic variability exists, usually the supraclavicular plexus receives contributions from 5 spinal roots: C5, C6, C7, C8, and T1. It is important to remember that each spinal root sends axons to more than one major nerve and, in turn, each major nerve contains axons from more than one spinal root. Accordingly, innervation of the muscles in the upper limb is often multilevel. Although the C7 spinal nerve contributes to the posterior cord and median, musculocutaneous, and ulnar nerves, C7-innervated muscles are cross innervated by other spinal nerves, primarily C6 and C8. Because isolated C7 division does not result in significant loss of any individual muscle function, both the ipsilateral and contralateral C7 nerve roots are a source of axons.[67] The posterior aspect of C7 contains more motor fibers, but both the entire root and its posterior portion have been harvested with similar, albeit transient deficits.

Dissection and Transfer. The contralateral neck and shoulder should be prepared when contralateral C7 root transfer is planned. The plexus is exposed as described earlier, with preservation of the transverse cervical vessels for anastomosis. All five roots of the brachial plexus are explored, and their anatomic configuration is identified to determine the number and contribution of each root. The contralateral C7 root is dissected distally to the level of divisions, and motor function is tested using a nerve stimulator. Elbow and wrist extension has to be observed when the C7 root is stimulated before division of the root. The anterior and posterior divisions of the contralateral C7 root are transected and transferred. The transverse cervical artery and a branch of the external jugular vein are prepared for anastomosis. A subcutaneous tunnel is prepared in the upper chest region leading to the skin incision of the ipsilateral brachial plexus.

The ulnar nerve in the injured arm is harvested as a vascularized graft, as described earlier (see Figs. 38-16 and 38-17). When the median nerve is neurotized by a contralateral C7 transfer, the ulnar nerve can be used as pedicled graft based on the superior ulnar collateral vessels, eliminating the need for vascular anastomosis. If it is to be utilized as a pedicled vascularized nerve, the distal end of the ulnar nerve is cut at the wrist and passed under the skin of the upper chest to the exposed contralateral C7 root. The anterior and posterior divisions of C7 are cut and matched to the distal end of the ulnar nerve. When no bleeding is noted from the distal end of the ulnar nerve, the ulnar artery and veins that had been harvested with the ulnar nerve are connected to the contralateral transverse cervical artery and vein. The proximal end of the ulnar nerve is connected to the target nerve such as the median nerve in the upper arm (Fig. 38-26).

When the ulnar nerve is used as a free vascularized nerve graft, the proximal end of the ulnar nerve is connected to the contralateral C7 root first and the superior ulnar collateral artery and vein are anastomosed to the contralateral transverse cervical artery and vein individually. The distal end of the ulnar nerve is passed into the subcutaneous tunnel in the upper chest region and connected to the target nerve, such as the suprascapular nerve or the posterior cord in the supraclavicular or infraclavicular region (Fig. 38-27).

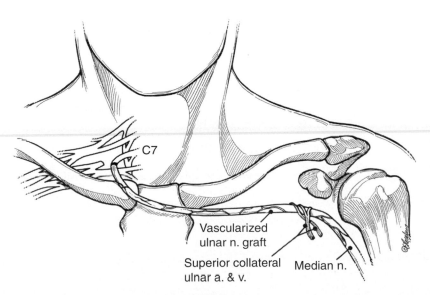

FIGURE 38-26. A contralateral C7 root transfer to the median nerve using a vascular pedicled graft of ulnar nerve based on the superior collateral ulnar artery and vein.

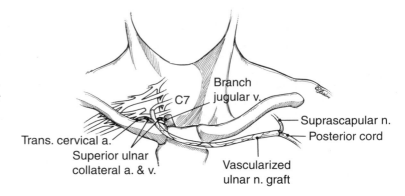

FIGURE 38-27. A contralateral C7 root transfer to the suprascapular nerve and posterior cord using a free vascularized ulnar nerve graft.

All the wounds are closed in layers and the ipsilateral upper limb is immobilized with shoulder abducted, elbow flexed, and neck in neutral position by splints for 3 weeks. Abduction of the shoulder more than 90 degrees should be avoided in the postoperative period.

Authors' Preferred Method

Most authors utilize the contralateral C7 root transfer to repair the median nerve using a vascularized ulnar nerve graft,[67,77,160,182] but we prefer to repair the suprascapular nerve and the posterior cord first as a part of double free muscle transfer procedure for reconstruction of prehension.[77] Results of recovery of motor function after median nerve neurotization with a contralateral C7 root have been less than satisfactory, except in children. Recent work with median neurotization by contralateral C7 root transfer has focused on sensory reinnervation of the hand. When a vascularized ulnar nerve is not used in cases of C5 to C8 root avulsion or in cases of distal ulnar nerve injury, a vascularized superficial radial nerve or sural nerve graft can be utilized.

Postoperative Protocol.   Regeneration of the repaired nerve can be traced by an advancing Tinel sign, and EMG reinnervation of the target muscles will occur depending on the length of the graft and distance from the neuromotor unit of the muscle. After reinnervation, re-education of the muscle starts, using EMG biofeedback techniques. Usually, muscles reinnervated from the contralateral C7 root can be activated by adducting, internally rotating, and extending the shoulder and extending the elbow of the contralateral upper limb. After that, a rehabilitation protocol of strengthening muscle power is added and patients can learn to activate the muscle without assistance of the contralateral limb.

CRITICAL POINTS: CONTRALATERAL C7 ROOT TRANSFER

INDICATIONS

- Very limited in total avulsion or C5 to C8 root avulsion, in which double free muscle transfer for prehensile function is planned
- In cases in which an ipsilateral root is not available for suprascapular nerve repair, especially in children or young adults

PEARLS

- The younger the patient's age, the better the outcome.
- Nerve repair to the median nerve is only for children.
- Reconstruction of proximal function can be done in adults.
- Vascularized nerve graft should be utilized.

TECHNICAL POINTS

- Identify the contralateral C7 root by anatomic relation and electric nerve stimulation.

- Divide the anterior and posterior division of the C7 root.
- Perform nerve graft with vascularized ulnar nerve graft.
- Nerve repair to the suprascapular nerve is the first choice.

PITFALL

- Existence of prefixed and postfixed brachial plexus by examining the corresponding number of intervertebral foramen

POSTOPERATIVE CARE

- Immobilize with shoulder abducted, elbow flexed, and neck in neutral position with splints for 3 weeks. More than 90 degrees of shoulder abduction is avoided postoperatively.

Complications. Liu and associates[101] and Sungpet and coworkers[169] have described in detail the donor arm sequelae after contralateral C7 root transfer in their own 2 and 24 patients, respectively. None of the patients had normal sensation after C7 root transfer. Sensory abnormalities were still present by 1.5 and 2 years in Liu and associates' series but had disappeared within 3 months in all except 1 patient, who experienced sensory abnormality on the tip of the index finger more than 20 months after the operation, in Sungpet and coworkers' experience. Temporary motor deficits always occurred immediately after surgery in shoulder extension and adduction, elbow extension, forearm pronation, wrist extension, and hand movement. Full functional recovery was usually documented within 6 months after surgery. Other reports of contralateral C7 root transfer also confirm the absence of any long-term functional deficits.[67,160,182] This makes cross C7 transfer a viable option in the surgical management of complete unilateral brachial plexus injury.

Anatomic variability, such as a prefixed plexus with significant C4 contribution or a postfixed plexus with substantial T2 contribution (with diminished C5 component) produces considerable paralysis after C7 transfer. Millesi[115] claimed that preliminary ligation of the C7 root before division prevents this complication. We have no experience with this anatomic abnormality, but we recommend exploration of all five roots and examination for the existence of a prefixed or postfixed plexus by normal anatomic relationships and intraoperative electrical nerve stimulation.

The other potential problem with this procedure is the severe pain that may be caused by dividing the contralateral, normal C7 nerve root. This problem has been noted particularly by surgeons in Europe. This appears to be much less common in Chinese and Japanese patients, based on the literature. In the case of American or European patients, it may seem unjustified to subject them to the risk, albeit slight, of significant loss of function in their remaining arm. Informed consent concerning complications of this procedure is extremely important and should be exhaustively discussed with the patient before undertaking it. Despite reports of minimal complications in the literature and our own experience, the possibility of problems in the donor arm exist. Contralateral C7 transfer should not be undertaken without a thorough understanding of the potential risks and complications of this procedure.

Expected Outcome. Most authors recommend repairing the median nerve by contralateral C7 root transfer, but the outcomes have been disappointing and patients achieve only minimal recovery of forearm motor strength and far from functional recovery.[67,160] With the exception of children, we prefer to neurotize the suprascapular nerve or posterior cord, which innervates the proximal musculature of the limb,[77] because the shorter the distance between the site of nerve repair and the neuromotor unit of the target muscle, the better the functional outcome. In our series of eight patients, contralateral C7 transfer was performed to the posterior cord in five patients, the suprascapular nerve in two, the musculocutaneous nerve in two, and the median nerve in only one. All five patients with the posterior cord repair achieved at least M2 recovery of triceps function, which contributed to stability of the elbow joint in reconstruction of prehension by a double free muscle transfer procedure (Fig. 38-28). Each patient with nerve repair of the suprascapular and musculocutaneous nerve also achieved M3 or M2 recovery.

Free Muscle Transfer

Free muscle transfer is a feasible procedure in reconstruction of brachial plexus injury, not only for secondary salvage in delayed or failed cases but also for prehensile reconstruction in recent cases.[53,56] In this section, detailed techniques concerning free muscle transfer for reconstruction of elbow flexion and prehensile reconstruction will be described after a brief discussion of concepts of free muscle transfer and harvest of the donor muscle, since the basic science, anatomy, and principles of free muscle transfer are described by Manktelow and colleagues[103,104] in Chapter 49.

Stability of the Proximal Joints. Because most free muscle transfers in brachial plexus injury are used to move more distal joints, such as the elbow, wrist, and fingers, stability of the proximal joints is imperative to reconstruct distal function effectively.[48] In reconstruction of elbow flexion by free muscle transfer, instability of the shoulder decreases the performance of the transferred muscle even if the muscle recovers strength sufficient to flex the elbow. Shoulder stability should be reconstructed simultaneously or previously by available nerve transfers to the suprascapular nerve and long thoracic nerve if they are paralyzed or secondarily by arthrodesis of the humeroscapular joint when

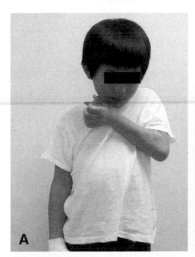
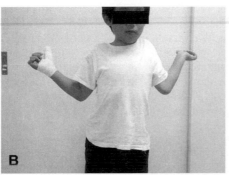

FIGURE 38-28. A 7-year-old boy sustained a traumatic complete avulsion of his left brachial plexus and underwent reconstructive procedures consisting of a contralateral C7 root transfer to the suprascapular nerve and the posterior cord using a vascularized ulnar nerve graft and double free muscle transfer procedure. **A** and **B,** Twenty months postoperatively he obtained prehensile and shoulder function. He can perform external rotation of his left shoulder by the reinnervated infraspinatus muscle, although the serratus anterior muscle remains completely paralyzed, which limits shoulder abduction.

there are no options to restore muscle function. When attempting to reconstruct prehensile function by free muscle transfer, additional procedures to stabilize the elbow and wrist joints are mandatory to achieve useful function.

Antagonist of the Transferred Muscle. Without an antagonist muscle, the functional outcome is unsatisfactory, although the weight of the forearm and gravity work together as an antagonist in reconstruction of elbow flexion by free muscle transfer. For reconstructing finger flexion, supplemental dynamic extension splinting may not be needed on a daily basis. Providing a functioning antagonist is an important requirement before free muscle transfer in the extremity, and double free muscle transfer can solve this problem because dynamic tenodesis is not enough to extend the range of motion of the transferred muscle.

Selection of Donor Muscle. When planning free muscle transfer, selection of donor muscle depends on the type of blood supply to the muscle; the length, volume, and shape of the muscle; the type of muscle fiber architecture; and the contractile capacity of the muscle fiber.

The latissimus dorsi, gracilis, and rectus femoris muscles are all commonly used as donor muscles for free muscle transfer. When reconstruction is planned only for elbow flexion and not for finger function, the ipsilateral latissimus dorsi can be used as a pedicled flap based on its vascular pedicle for this purpose if it is transferred early after injury. Nerve crossing to the thoracodorsal nerve from the spinal accessory nerve or intercostal nerves will be needed if the latissimus dorsi is affected in the brachial plexus injury. If the duration of injury is longer than 1 year, the paralyzed ipsilateral latissimus dorsi will have become atrophic. In this case, the contralateral latissimus dorsi muscle is used as a free donor muscle for functioning free muscle transfer.

The rectus femoris muscle is also a powerful muscle and can be used to supplement elbow flexion. Transient reduction of knee extension occurs after harvest of the rectus femoris muscle. The gracilis may also be used as a donor muscle for elbow flexion, although its power may be weaker than that of the former two muscles.

For wrist and finger function, the gracilis is the best choice of donor muscle, because of the shape of the muscle-tendinous portion and great amplitude of contraction.

Free Muscle Transfer for Elbow Flexion in Delayed Cases

Indication. In complete or upper type of brachial plexus injury, free muscle transfer for only elbow flexion is indicated for patients with absence of available regional muscles of adequate strength for tendon transfer or a time interval of longer than 9 months from injury. The younger the patient, the better is the recovery; and patients older than 2 years of age are candidates for free muscle transfer. Satisfactory results are not usually obtained in patients older than 50 years because of poor reinnervation of the transferred muscles. Other problems such as joint contractures and causalgia may limit the indications for this procedure in older patients as well.

Donor Nerve Selection. The intercostal nerves and spinal accessory nerve are usually used as donor motor nerves for isolated reconstruction of elbow flexion. Selection of the donor nerve depends on the potential for combined reconstruction. When shoulder reconstruction is necessary, the spinal accessory nerve should be left intact for secondary transfer of the trapezius muscle and intercostal nerves should be used. When reconstruction of elbow extension by intercostal nerve transfer is planned, the spinal accessory nerve is a potential choice for a donor nerve.

The most frequently used donor motor nerves are the third to sixth intercostal nerves, as noted earlier. When the intercostal nerves have already been used as donor motor nerves for nerve crossing to the musculocutaneous nerve, more inferior intercostal nerves than those previously taken can be harvested. Fracture of the corresponding ribs may have injured the intercostal nerves, and this should be taken into consideration when deciding to use the intercostal nerves.

The spinal accessory nerve is our donor motor nerve of choice if it has not been used for nerve transfer to the suprascapular nerve. In C5-C6 or C5-C7 paralysis, the ulnar nerve offers an excellent option as a donor motor nerve for innervated muscle transfer.[71]

Operative Procedure. For elbow flexion by free muscle transfer, the nutrient vessels of the transferred muscle are anastomosed to the thoracoacromial artery and the cephalic vein, or to the thoracodorsal artery and vein when the subclavian artery is thrombosed.

Dissection of each donor nerve such as the intercostals, spinal accessory nerve, or ulnar nerve has been already described in the section on nerve transfer.

Anatomy and harvest of the donor muscles is described in Chapter 49,[103,104] but our technique of harvest differs somewhat.[49,70] We make a small proximal skin incision to harvest a skin paddle, while utilizing an endoscopic approach for the remainder of the harvest. This avoids a large incision on the medial thigh and with experience is a straightforward procedure. The reader is referred to the literature for details of this approach.[49,70]

The details of the anatomy and dissection of the latissimus dorsi muscle are contained in Chapters 47 and 49. A few pertinent points for functional transfer of this muscle should be made. During harvesting, the fascial origin of the muscle attached to the posterior crest of the ilium should be included with the musculocutaneous flap to facilitate distal tendon suture. The insertion of the muscle is detached from the humerus, and the neurovascular pedicle is preserved when the ipsilateral latissimus dorsi muscle is being transferred.

Both edges of the latissimus dorsi muscle are sutured to each other, and the muscle is shaped into a tubed muscle flap (Fig. 38-29A). The musculocutaneous flap is placed in the skin defect of the upper arm and forearm. The fascial origin of the muscle is sutured to the biceps tendon when reconstructing elbow flexion, enveloping the tendons with the tubed muscle (see Fig. 38-29B).

Postoperative Protocol. The elbow is immobilized postoperatively for 6 weeks in a position of 100 degrees of elbow flexion and supination of the forearm. After 6 weeks, passive elbow flexion is permitted but extension beyond 30 degrees of flexion is avoided for at least 3 months. Re-

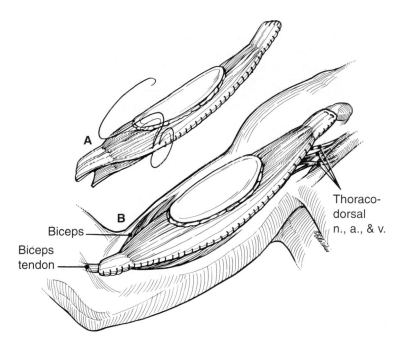

A

B

Biceps

Biceps
tendon

Thoraco-
dorsal
n., a., & v.

FIGURE 38-29. **A,** Both edges of the latissimus dorsi muscle are sutured to each other, and the muscle is shaped into a tubed muscle flap. **B,** The fascial origin of the muscle is sutured to the biceps tendon and the humeral attachment of the muscle is sutured to the coracoid process, keeping the continuity of the thoracodorsal artery, vein, and nerve.

CRITICAL POINTS: FREE MUSCLE TRANSFER FOR ELBOW FLEXION

INDICATIONS

- Delayed cases longer than 10 months after injury
- Failed cases after nerve grafting or nerve transfer
- Patients younger than 40 years old

PREOPERATIVE EVALUATION

- Available donor nerves and recipient vessels for vascular anastomosis
- Stable shoulder joint

PEARLS

- More reliable recovery of elbow flexion by nerve transfer of spinal accessory nerve than by intercostal nerves

TECHNICAL POINTS

- Dissection and transfer of donor nerve
- Dissection and transfer of recipient vessel

- Harvest of donor muscle
- Suture of proximal attachment of the muscle
- Neurovascular anastomoses
- Suture of distal attachment of the muscle in its correct tension
- Suture of tendons in proper tension

PITFALLS

- Suture of tendons in incorrect tension
- Position of immobilization of shoulder

POSTOPERATIVE CARE

- Immobilization of shoulder in 30 degrees of abduction and flexion and 60 degrees in internal rotation with elbow in 100 degrees of flexion supported by a pillow and cast for 6 weeks.

education and strengthening exercises using EMG biofeedback are initiated when evidence of muscle contraction is observed.

Expected Outcome. More than 90% of cases with free muscle transfer for elbow flexion recovered more than 90 degrees of elbow flexion after nerve transfer of the spinal accessory nerve or intercostal nerves.[37,53] Patients older than 40 years old did not recover considerable degrees of elbow flexion in spite of successful reinnervation to the transferred muscle. The final quantitative measurement of

muscle strength showed one- to two-tenths of the mean values of normal elbow flexion more than 2 years after operation.

Free Muscle Transfer for Prehensile Reconstruction After Complete Avulsion of Brachial Plexus. *Rationale for Surgical Approach.* After complete brachial plexus avulsion, several surgical approaches have been developed to restore prehension.[60,61,116,118] In these patients one goal was to restore key pinch in a Moberg-type of simple hand grip reconstruction. However, functioning free muscle transfer failed to achieve reliable activation of the forearm muscles, because finger flexion was weak as it was achieved by the synergistic action of wrist extension.[1,19] Most patients with brachial plexus injury have a normal contralateral upper limb and can perform most of the activities of daily living. This is very different from patients with spinal cord injury. Patients with complete brachial plexus palsy need reconstruction of a few important two-handed activities, such as lifting a heavy box with both hands or holding a bottle while opening its cap. They need a powerful grip independent of the contralateral limb and the use of both hands. Direct activation of finger flexion and extension is imperative for a powerful grip. Weak pinch function by synergistic action was originally designed for patients with spinal cord injury and is useless for patients with brachial plexus injury.[56,57]

Grasp release is also necessary for useful prehension. Release reconstructed by secondary tenodesis of the finger extensor tendons as in a Moberg-type reconstruction will need gravity-aided wrist flexion[118-120,187] and can be accomplished only with the elbow flexed. This synergistic action cannot be accomplished when the elbow is extended. To achieve voluntary finger extension independent of elbow position, a second free muscle transfer is essential.

Stability of the shoulder and elbow joints is necessary for proper transmission of power of the transferred muscle to achieve effective hand function. Double free muscle transfer acts to supplement shoulder stabilization but may not be adequate. Shoulder stabilization can be achieved by scapulohumeral arthrodesis when shoulder instability persists after double free muscle transfer. Stability of the elbow is extremely important for optimal use of the hand in day-to-day activities. Many authors dismiss the significance of elbow stabilization because of the technical difficulty in obtaining this[1,16] and reconstruct finger flexion or extension without providing some form of elbow stabilization. These patients, in spite of achieving powerful wrist extension or finger flexion, cannot use their fingers optimally in daily activities because their elbow is unstable. In addition to finger extension or finger flexion, all the transferred muscles in this double muscle technique simultaneously cause elbow flexion, similar to the transferred brachioradialis muscle in cases of spinal cord injury. In this situation without elbow extensor function, the patient must stabilize the unstable elbow with the contralateral hand, a useless maneuver in daily activities. Reconstruction of elbow extension is imperative whenever prehension is being reconstructed by the transfer of one muscle that moves multiple joints simultaneously.[58] Available intercostal nerves are used to neurotize the triceps brachii muscle via the radial nerve for elbow extension. This enables the patient to stabilize the elbow independently, without the need of the contralateral hand, and use the powerful finger flexion afforded by muscle transfer effectively.

Claw finger deformity frequently develops after reconstruction of finger flexion and extension and should be prevented to achieve useful prehension. A plastic static volar splint that holds the wrist in neutral position and the proximal and distal interphalangeal joints in full extension postoperatively facilitates the development of stabilizing joint contractures and creates a stable wrist and prevents claw finger deformity.

Basic sensory functions such as protective sensation and position sense should be restored when motor function is being reconstructed in a severely paralyzed limb. The supraclavicular or intercostal nerve-crossing procedures provide limited sensibility of the hand after double muscle transfer.

Donor Muscle Selection. The gracilis is the best choice for the donor muscle. The latissimus dorsi muscle, gracilis, and rectus femoris muscles were used as the donor muscles in the initial period of reconstruction by this technique. Long-term results showed that the latissimus dorsi did not provide satisfactory finger function because of adhesion of the muscle to the fabricated pulley system and rupture of its tendon owing to ischemic necrosis of the portion distal to the pulley. The rectus femoris is a bipennate muscle and has reduced excursion, resulting in poor finger function.

Operative Technique. The double free gracilis muscle transfer technique consists of five established but modified reconstructive procedures: (1) exploration of the brachial plexus and repair of the ruptured motor nerves if possible; (2) the first free muscle transfer, neurotized by the spinal accessory nerve, for elbow flexion and finger extension; (3) the second free muscle transfer, neurotized by the fifth and sixth intercostal nerves for finger flexion; (4) a nerve-crossing procedure using the third and fourth intercostal nerves to neurotize the motor branch of the triceps brachii muscle for elbow extension, done simultaneously with the second muscle transfer; and (5) the intercostal sensory rami coapted to the medial cord of the brachial plexus to restore sensibility of the hand. In addition, a sixth set of procedures for secondary reconstruction such as arthrodesis of the glenohumeral joint, carpometacarpal joint of the thumb, and the wrist joint to increase stability may be required. If the strength of the triceps brachii muscle is too weak to stabilize the elbow joint, tendon transfer of the reinnervated infraspinatus muscle may be indicated. Tenolysis of the transferred muscle and tendons also may be necessary.

Timing of the various reconstructive procedures is important and is guided by several criteria. Procedures 1 and 2 are performed at the first stage of the operation, and procedures 3 to 5 are performed at the second stage, usually 2 or 3 months after the first operation. The sixth procedure is done depending on the condition of recovery, approximately 1.5 years after the first stage of the operation.

Brachial plexus exploration is described in detail earlier.

In the first stage, simultaneous elbow flexion and finger extension is reconstructed with a free muscle transfer using the spinal accessory as the motor nerve (Fig. 38-30). The donor gracilis muscle from the contralateral thigh is selected because the orientation and location of its neurovascular bundle matches the site of the donor vessels. The length of the gracilis muscle should be sufficient to span the distance between acromion and mid forearm without tension. This is verified by measuring the length of the gracilis muscle from its pubic origin to tibial insertion. The donor muscle is then harvested from its proximal origin to the distal attachment.

Correct muscle tension is critical for good postoperative function. Before detaching the muscle, the resting length of the muscle is reproduced and black silk sutures are placed on the surface of the muscle at 5-cm intervals, as described by Manktelow and colleagues[103,104]:

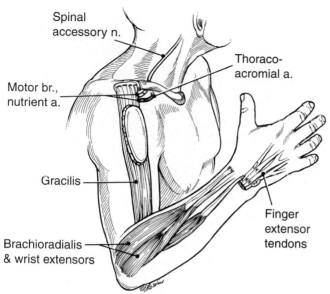

FIGURE 38-30. The initial operative procedure for reconstruction of prehension after complete brachial plexus avulsion is a free muscle transfer to restore finger extension and elbow flexion simultaneously. The gracilis is transferred and innervated by the spinal accessory nerve.

over the anterior part of deltoid and is sutured to the acromion with nonabsorbable sutures or by a soft tissue anchoring system. A simple and straight route for the free muscle is created from its new origin to final insertion to maximize the force of contraction. It is placed on the anterolateral aspect of arm and dorsal surface of forearm. To prevent bowstringing, the free muscle is passed deep to brachioradialis and radial wrist extensor muscles just distal to elbow.

This position of the muscle is optimal for elbow flexion and finger extension; however grip strength may weaken when the elbow is flexed. Correct muscle tension is reproduced in the upper limb before final suturing of the muscle to the finger extensors. The original muscle length is restored by stretching the muscle until the distance between the markers is once again 5 cm. Tension is adjusted with the shoulder in 60 degrees of abduction and 15 degrees of anterior flexion, with the elbow in 150 degrees of flexion and the wrist in neutral with the fingers in full extension. After adjusting the tension, the position of coaption is marked over the tendon of the extensor digitorum communis and the donor muscle tendon. The elbow is then flexed to 90 degrees and with the wrist in neutral and fingers fully flexed the tenorrhaphies between the donor muscle tendon and extensor digitorum communis tendon are completed at the previously marked sites. The appropriateness of tension in the transfer is evaluated by using the tenodesis principle.

The distal portion of the spinal accessory nerve is dissected, divided, and transferred. The motor nerve of the transferred muscle is passed behind the clavicle and coapted to the distal branch of spinal accessory nerve in the supraclavicular area. The nutrient vessels of the free gracilis muscle are then anastomosed to the thoracoacromial artery and vein or to the cephalic vein. The transferred muscle is placed superficially

Finger flexion reconstruction is done by using a second free muscle transfer (Fig. 38-31). It is performed 2 to 3 months after the first operation after improvement in postoperative contracture of the elbow and finger joints. The third to sixth intercostal nerves are dissected as far as the midclavicular line and transferred to the axillary region. The fifth and sixth intercostal nerves are used as the donor motor nerve for the second gracilis muscle transplant. The gracilis is harvested from the ipsilateral thigh, after ensuring

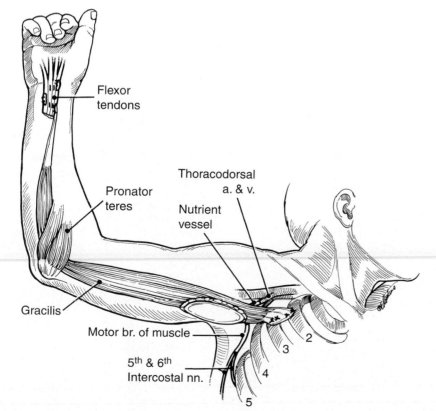

FIGURE 38-31. The second operative procedure for reconstruction of prehension after complete brachial plexus avulsion is a second free muscle transfer to restore finger flexion. The gracilis is transferred and is innervated by the fifth and sixth intercostal nerves.

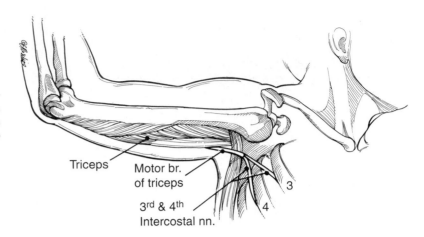

FIGURE 38-32. Intercostal nerve transfer to the motor branch of the triceps brachii. As one step of prehensile reconstruction, the third and fourth intercostal nerves are transferred to the motor branch of the triceps brachii to stabilize the elbow against the antagonist flexors.

that it will reach the mid forearm from the second rib. The proximal end is sutured to the second and third ribs. To activate finger flexion, it is placed on the medial aspect of the upper arm and forearm so as not to be a secondary elbow flexor.

The muscle is passed under the pronator teres and long wrist flexors, just distal to the elbow. The distal portion of the gracilis muscle is tendinous and thin and can easily be passed through the small hiatus deep to the forearm flexor muscles. The distal tendinous portion of the gracilis is coapted to the flexor digitorum profundus tendons. Muscle tension is determined with the principles described earlier. When the tension is adjusted, the shoulder, elbow, and wrist are in the same position as described earlier. The fingers are kept in full flexion. The nutrient vessels of the gracilis are anastomosed to the thoracodorsal artery and vein. The fifth and sixth intercostal nerves are coapted without tension to the motor nerve of the second muscle transplant.

The third and fourth intercostal nerves are coapted to the motor branch of the triceps brachii muscle, to activate the elbow extensors. Coaptation is performed before the second muscle is detached from the thigh (Fig. 38-32).

To restore hand sensibility, the sensory rami of intercostal nerves are sutured to the medial cord of the brachial plexus at the second operation (Fig. 38-33). The sensory-dominant fascicles of the medial cord can be easily distinguished from the motor-dominant fascicles by measuring the sensory nerve action potentials, if available. Sensory nerve fibers do not undergo wallerian degeneration because most dorsal ganglion cells survive after preganglionic injury to the nerve roots.

FIGURE 38-33. A second free muscle transfer and nerve transfers for elbow extension and sensory restoration are simultaneously performed at the second operation.

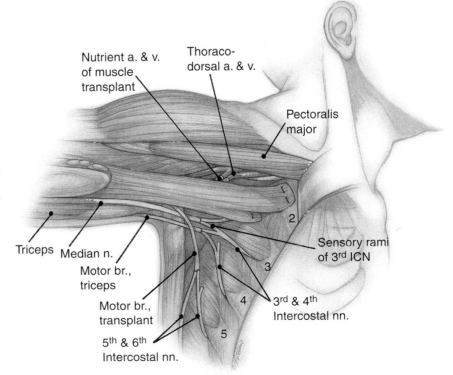

CRITICAL POINTS: DOUBLE FREE MUSCLE TRANSFER FOR PREHENSILE FUNCTION

INDICATIONS

- Total paralysis of the brachial plexus
- Fresh cases less than 6 months after injury
- No injury of subclavian artery, spinal accessory nerve, and intercostal nerves
- Age younger than 40 years

PREOPERATIVE EVALUATION

- Normal function of the trapezius muscle
- Supple joints

PEARLS

- Basic function of upper extremity, prehension, can be restored by this procedure.

TECHNICAL POINTS

- Dissection of donor nerve and recipient vessels
- Harvest of donor muscle
- Suture of the proximal attachment of the muscle
- Nerve suture of the motor nerve of the muscle
- Vascular anastomosis of the nutrient vessels of the muscle
- Suture of the distal tendon of the muscle to the target muscle in proper tension
- Accompanying procedures of nerve transfer for shoulder reconstruction in the first stage and of nerve transfers for elbow extension and sensory reconstruction in the second stage

PITFALL

- Proximal joint stability is imperative to achieve useful recovery.

POSTOPERATIVE CARE

- Immobilization of shoulder in 30 degrees of abduction and flexion and 60 degrees of internal rotation, with elbow in 100 degrees of flexion, wrist in neutral position, and fingers in forced flexion or extension depending on reconstruction supported by a pillow and cast for 4 weeks

Postoperative Protocol. Low-intensity electrical stimulation to the paralyzed target muscles (the two transferred gracilis muscles, the triceps brachii, and the supraspinatus and infraspinatus, if the suprascapular nerve has been repaired) is started during the third postoperative week and is continued until EMG reinnervation is detected in the muscles.

A functional orthosis is used to immobilize the reconstructed upper limb during the early postoperative period. A plastic static splint is used to maintain the wrist in a neutral position and the proximal and distal interphalangeal joints in extension to allow these joints to contract in this position. At the sixth postoperative week, while protecting against overpull at the muscle-tendon suture site of the transferred muscle, passive extension of the elbow is started. Only the metacarpophalangeal joints are moved passively because the transferred muscle is intended to move this single joint to decrease the effect of the claw finger deformity. At the ninth postoperative week, the shoulder pillow orthosis is removed and an elbow sling orthosis is applied to prevent subluxation of the shoulder.

After EMG documentation of reinnervation of the transferred muscle (usually 3 to 8 months postoperatively), EMG biofeedback techniques are started to train the transferred muscles to move the elbow and fingers. Muscular re-education is indicated when patients display minimal active contraction with an identified muscle or muscle group. The initial goal of re-education is for patients to reactivate voluntary control of the muscle. Rehabilitation should continue to master the use of the reconstructed hand in daily activities for at least 2 years after operation.

Complications. Vascular compromise after free muscle transfer is very infrequent, and reinnervation of the muscle occurred in all of our patients except one who had had a previous injury of the spinal accessory nerve. Adhesion of the transferred muscle to the surrounding tissue occurs more or less in all cases. About one third of the patients will need tenolysis. The most important factor that affects the outcome is recovery of the triceps, because, without recovery of elbow flexion antagonists, simultaneous elbow flexion occurred with finger movement (either flexion or extension). If reinnervation of the triceps brachii fails, secondary reconstruction, such as reinnervated infraspinatus or deltoid transfer to the triceps brachii, is recommended to restore elbow stability.

If the glenohumeral joint remains unstable even after recovery of these muscles, glenohumeral arthrodesis should be performed, although it may limit several activities, such as turning over during sleep. Care must be taken to prevent fractures of the proximal humerus after arthrodesis. After recovery of active finger motion, arthrodesis of the thumb carpometacarpal joint may be helpful. In addition, tenodesis flexion of the metacarpophalangeal joint and interphalangeal joint of the thumb and proximal and distal interphalangeal joints of the fingers may augment stable pinch function.

None of our patients had severe causalgia that could not be controlled by the usual analgesics. However, many American and European patients complain of severe pain after brachial plexus injury that cannot be controlled with conventional analgesics. If no sensory recovery from the original nerves of the brachial plexus is anticipated, these patients may be candidates for radiofrequency destruction of the dorsal root entry zone (DREZ lesion) of the affected portion of the spinal cord. Recently, encouraging results with continuous electric stimulation of the spinal cord have been reported.

Expected Outcome. Thirty of 36 patients (Doi) undergoing reconstruction by the double free muscle procedure

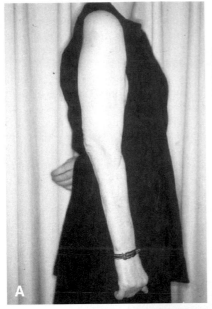

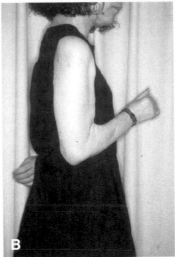

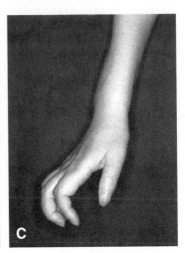

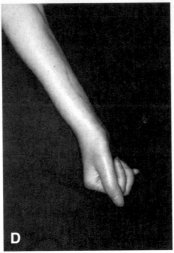

FIGURE 38-34. Postoperative motor function 36 months after the initial procedure in a patient who underwent double free muscle transfer after complete avulsion of the brachial plexus. Elbow extension (**A**), and flexion (**B**) and finger extension (**C**) and flexion (**D**) with the elbow extended. (From Doi K, Sakai K, Kuwata N, et al: Reconstruction of irreparable brachial plexus injuries with reinnervated free muscle transfer. J Neurosurg 85:174-177, 1996.)

and followed up for more than 24 months after the second free muscle transfer (mean follow-up, 40 months) were assessed for long-term outcome of universal prehension, including motion and stability of the shoulder and elbow, voluntary and independent motion of the fingers, sensibility, and activity of daily living functions.[53,55] Functional outcome of prehension according to the authors' classification was excellent in 6 (which implies restoration of more than 90 degrees of elbow flexion, dynamic stability of the elbow while moving the fingers, and more than 60 degrees of total active motion of the fingers), good (same as excellent, except total active motion of 30 to 60 degrees) in 11, fair (total active motion of less than 30 degrees) in 3, and poor in 10. Satisfactory results (excellent and good) were obtained in 17 of 30 patients (56%) (Figs. 38-34 and 38-35).

Half of the patients recovered sensibility of the palm and adequate positional sense. However, protective sensation in the ulnar side of the hand and fingers does not recover in half of the patients. Minor injury and burns can easily occur in these parts of the hand.

Reconstruction of Glenohumeral or Scapulothoracic Function

In total or upper type paralysis, shoulder stability and movement are key requirements for distal function. Even if the distal elbow, wrist, and fingers have normal function, the patient's abilities are limited if shoulder function is impaired. Neuromuscular biomechanics of the shoulder are more complicated than those of the other joints in the upper extremity. In this section, a brief description of the neuromuscular biomechanics of the shoulder and surgical options after brachial plexus injuries is presented.

Neuromuscular Biomechanics of the Shoulder

Elevation of the arm is performed by synergistic motion of the glenohumeral, scapulothoracic, acromioclavicular, and sternoclavicular joints. The former two joints significantly contribute to this motion. The glenohumeral joint has two components of muscles. The rotator cuff muscles control activities of the glenohumeral articulation and include the

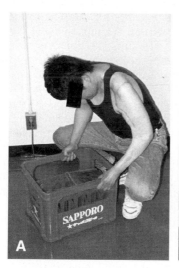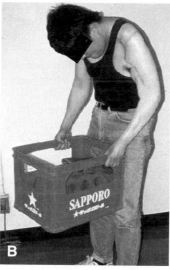

FIGURE 38-35. Postoperative ADL function 20 months after the initial procedure in a patient who underwent double free muscle transfer after complete avulsion of the brachial plexus. **A** and **B,** The patient is shown lifting a 13-kg box with both hands. (From Doi K: Obstetric and traumatic pediatric palsy. *In* Peimer C [ed]: Surgery of the Hand and Upper Extremity. New York, McGraw-Hill, 1996, pp 1443-1463.)

supraspinatus, infraspinatus, subscapularis, and teres minor, which are called the steerers by Saha.[146] The scapulohumeral muscles provide power to the humerus and include the deltoid, the long and short head of the biceps, the coracobrachialis, the long head of the triceps, and the teres major, which are called the primary movers by Saha. Motion of the upper extremity occurs as a result of the coordinated activity of all of these muscles.

In reconstruction of shoulder flexion-abduction the priority of reconstruction is the supraspinatus first and the primary mover second. External rotation of the shoulder is the other important function in daily activities and is performed by the infraspinatus and teres minor.

Scapulothoracic articulation is a critical component of shoulder function. However, it receives far less attention in reconstruction of the paralytic shoulder. The scapulothoracic muscles coordinate scapulothoracic motion and include the rhomboideus major and minor, the levator scapulae, the serratus anterior, the trapezius, the omohyoid, and the pectoralis minor. Disorders of these muscles may manifest as scapular winging or scapulothoracic dyskinesia.

Almost every functional upper extremity movement has components of scapulothoracic and glenohumeral motion. In general, the overall effort to obtain 90 degrees of elevation requires approximately a 2:1 ratio of glenohumeral to scapulothoracic motion. When planning reconstruction of arm elevation, scapulothoracic function should be considered as well as glenohumeral function.

When discussing evaluation of paralysis, the plan of reconstruction, and its outcome, the severity of paralysis and the level of nerve lesion are the most important factors. Most previous reports concerning shoulder reconstruction by multiple muscle transfers after brachial plexus injury do not discuss how to assess these factors. There are significant differences in outcome between the C5, C5 and C6 and the C5, C6, and C7 nerve root injuries and also between the preganglionic and postganglionic injuries of the same nerve root, even after the same reconstructive procedure has been performed. In preganglionic injuries of C5 and C6, the lower parts of the serratus anterior and the latissimus dorsi muscles are working. The remaining innervated part of the serratus anterior stabilizes and moves the scapulothoracic joint and prevents winging of the scapula. The remaining innervation to the latissimus dorsi makes it possible to transfer this muscle to provide external rotation. However, in the preganglionic injuries of the C5, C6, and C7 nerve roots there are no functioning parts of the serratus anterior and the remaining power of the latissimus dorsi is not strong enough to transfer for external rotation. Simple paralysis of the deltoid and supraspinatus after injury of the C5 nerve root or upper trunk is relatively easy to treat by reconstructing the function of the supraspinatus rather than the deltoid. The other primary movers including the long head of the biceps, the triceps, and the pectoralis major work well to substitute for lost deltoid function. In lesions distal to the branching of the suprascapular nerve from the upper trunk, reconstruction can focus on the primary movers by transfer of the trapezius or the long head of the biceps and triceps because the supraspinatus and infraspinatus are still working as "steerers." When discussing the reconstructive procedures described in the following sections, their outcomes should be compared by careful evaluation of the preoperative conditions by focusing on the type of paralysis and level of lesions.

Multiple Muscle Transfer for Reconstruction of Glenohumeral Function

Several procedures involving multiple muscle transfer for reconstruction of glenohumeral function have been utilized classically as combinations of three representative techniques: Saha's, Harmon's, and Bateman's procedures are commonly used, depending on the nature of the paralysis and available donor muscles. First, outlines of the classic three techniques are introduced and the author's preferred method is described in detail.

Saha's Procedure

The three basic functions described by Saha can be reconstructed with available nonparalyzed muscles.[146] The deltoid and clavicular head of the pectoralis major, which are prime movers, are substituted for by the trapezius. The supraspinatus, a vertical steerer, is replaced by the levator scapulae or sternocleidomastoid muscle. The anterior horizontal steerers can be replaced by the pectoralis minor, the upper two fascicles of the serratus anterior, or the residual part of the pectoralis major. The posterior horizontal steerers are replaced by the residual part of the latissimus dorsi or teres major. Either combination of multiple muscle transfers described earlier is selected depending on the type of paralysis and residual power of the transferring muscles.

Saha's multiple muscle transfers can usually be applied to preganglionic injuries of the C5 and C6 and the C5, C6, and C7 nerve roots, in which the vertical steerer (supraspinatus) and most primary movers (deltoid, long head of biceps, and triceps) are paralyzed. The serratus anterior is the important stabilizer and mover of the scapulothoracic joint, and the upper two slips of the muscle may be paralyzed in this situation and thus cannot be used for transfer. Those muscles innervated from extrabrachial plexus sources, such as the trapezius and levator scapulae, are good candidates for transfer. The latissimus dorsi (a depressor or horizontal steerer) may be used, although its power is difficult to evaluate by ordinary manual muscle testing and it may not be strong enough for transfer.

Harmon's Procedure

The multiple muscle transfer, originally described by Harmon, is another reliable procedure for reconstruction of the paralyzed shoulder.[15,68] Transfers performed in combination include transfer of the posterior third of the deltoid muscle to the lateral aspect of the clavicle together with transfer of the tendinous origins of the long head of the triceps muscle and the short head of the biceps muscle to the lateral aspect of the acromion, to aid in abduction. The transfer of the latissimus dorsi and teres major tendons or of the tendinous insertion of the clavicular head of the pectoralis major muscle posteriorly can provide external rotation of the humerus. Multiple options are available.

Bateman's Procedure

The primary indication for Bateman's procedure is axillary and suprascapular nerve palsy.[13] A more extensive paralysis such as the preganglionic injury of the C5 and C6 nerve roots needs additional muscle transfers, as described earlier. Paralysis of the deltoid and supraspinatus is confirmed clinically and by EMG. The trapezius must show full strength against resistance. Passive abduction of 80 degrees is needed to transfer the acromial fragment to the humerus.

 Authors' Preferred Procedure

In brachial plexus palsy, after full neurologic treatment and adequate physiotherapy, secondary surgery may be needed to improve the stability and function of the shoulder. Depending on the type of lesion and the degree of involvement of the arm muscles, good stability and function of the shoulder will help to achieve better use of the elbow and hand, possibly aided by other tendon transfers. According to Saha's theory of biomechanics of the glenohumeral joint, we select the procedure by calculating the number of functional deficits and available muscles for transfer. The priorities of shoulder reconstruction are (1) supraspinatus function as a vertical steerer and elevator, (2) transfers to reconstruct primary movers, and (3) reconstruction of external rotation or of a horizontal steerer. When patients have no subluxation of the glenohumeral joint and the supraspinatus has become reinnervated and is strong enough to work as steerer, either the classic Harmon or Bateman's procedure can be selected. We prefer Harmon's procedure when the biceps and triceps have recovered to M4 and the spinal accessory nerve has been previously used for transfer to the suprascapular nerve. When the strength of the biceps or triceps is insufficient for it to serve as a primary mover, we add a trapezius transfer. When there is no function of the supraspinatus, a modified Saha procedure (in which the primary mover can also be reinforced by a triceps or pectoralis major transfer) provides a satisfactory outcome.

The most common procedure consists of trapezius, pectoralis major, and latissimus dorsi transfer after C5 and C6 root avulsion, in which the lower portion of the serratus anterior is working and controls movement of the scapula. This technique is easily modified to use the other available donor muscles depending on the extent and degree of paralysis.

Operative Procedure. The patient is placed in a lateral decubitus position and a saber-cut skin incision exposes the trapezius and deltoid muscles at their attachments to the acromion, clavicle, and spine of the scapula. The deltoid is released from the lateral third of the clavicle, the acromion, and the lateral half of the spine of the scapula. The root of the acromion is osteotomized, and the lateral clavicle is divided lateral to the coracoclavicular ligaments. The remaining insertions of the trapezius into the clavicle and spine of the scapula are released, and the deltoid is split longitudinally to expose the proximal humerus (Fig. 38-36A).

The posterior third of the deltoid muscle is taken off the scapular spine. The latissimus dorsi tendon is taken off its insertion on the humerus and dissected distally enough to reach the proximal attachment of the infraspinatus, taking care not to injure the thoracodorsal artery, veins, and nerve (see Fig. 38-36B).

Anteriorly, the clavicular portion of the pectoralis major is explored and elevated from the clavicle, with care taken to avoid injury to the neurovascular pedicles. The released clavicular portion of the pectoralis major is turned and placed over the anterior deltoid muscle (see Fig. 38-36C). It is then sutured over these structures to the lateral aspect of the clavicle using suture-anchor kits (see Fig. 38-36D). With the humerus in 100 degrees of abduction, the acromial fragment with its trapezius insertion is transferred and fixed to the humerus as distally as possible, using a 4.5-mm-diameter screw. The released tendon of the latissimus dorsi muscle is sutured under tension to the insertion of the infraspinatus muscle in 90 degrees of external rotation. The deltoid is then sutured over the trapezius, and the skin is closed over two suction drains. Radiographs are taken to assess the position of the screws and the acromial fragment.

Saha described the transfer of the pectoralis minor to replace the subscapularis and transfer of the sternocleido-

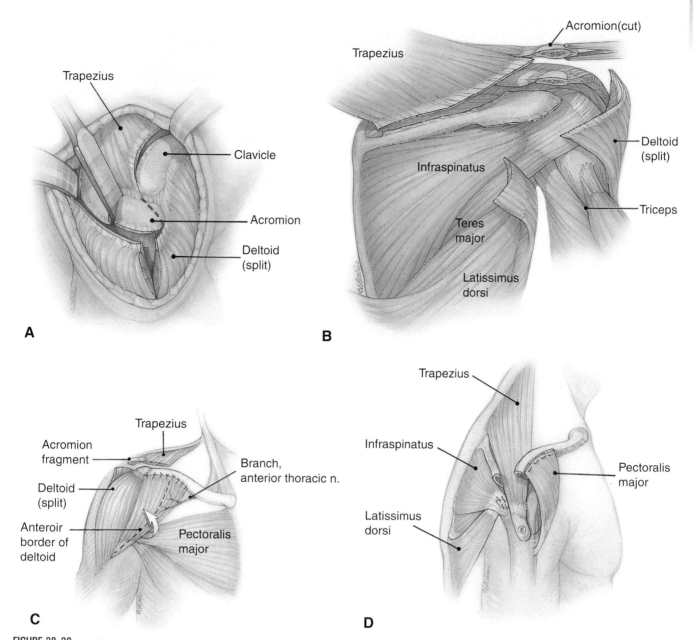

FIGURE 38-36. Multiple muscle transfer for shoulder reconstruction. **A,** Elevation of the trapezius. The root of the acromion is osteotomized. **B,** Elevation of the latissimus dorsi. The humeral attachment of the latissimus dorsi tendon is taken off its insertion on the humerus. **C,** Detachment of the clavicular portion of the pectoralis major muscle which is placed over the anterior part of the deltoid. **D,** Completion of multiple muscle transfer. The detached clavicular portion of the pectoralis major muscle is sutured to the lateral aspect of the clavicle. The acromion fragment with its trapezius attachment is fixed to the humerus as distally as possible, using a screw. The released tendon of the latissimus dorsi muscle is sutured to the insertion of the infraspinatus muscle.

mastoid to act as an elevator. We generally avoid these classic procedures because the pectoralis minor is a small, unreliable muscle to replace the subscapularis and transfer of the sternocleidomastoid is cosmetically unacceptable.

Postoperative Protocol. After the procedure, the arm is immobilized in the individual position described previously for 6 to 8 weeks. Assisted and active exercises for the elbow, hand, and fingers start on the first day, except the elbow, following Harmon's procedure. From the eighth day isometric contraction and electric stimulation of the transferred muscles are begun, but the proper position of

shoulder abduction is maintained during therapy. At 6 weeks a radiograph is taken to certify the location of screws or fixation materials and gradual adduction of the arm is started as an inpatient procedure. The aim is a steady increase in active abduction and forward flexion with an actively stabilized scapula.

The most important key of postoperative rehabilitation is to first strengthen the steerer (supraspinatus muscle), not the primary movers. Otherwise, when the strong primary movers overcome the depressive force of the steerers, superior instability of the humeral head will negate the abduction power of the primary movers.

CRITICAL POINTS: MULTIPLE MUSCLE TRANSFER FOR RECONSTRUCTION OF GLENOHUMERAL FUNCTION

INDICATIONS

- No winging of the scapula (serratus anterior muscle working at least partially)
- Selection of proper procedure depending on available muscles for transfer

PRIORITY OF RECONSTRUCTION

- (1) Horizontal steerer, (2) primary movers, (3) external rotator (anterior, posterior depressor)

PREOPERATIVE EVALUATION

- Manual muscle testing of available donor muscles
- Isolated scapular movement to negate serratus anterior paralysis

PEARLS

- Better functional recovery when both serratus anterior and supraspinatus muscles are working.
- Final range of motion depends on power of primary movers and stability of the glenohumeral joint.

TECHNICAL POINTS

- Saber-cut and additional skin incisions
- Release of trapezius from the clavicle and spine of the scapula with osteotomy of the acromion
- Release of deltoid from the clavicle and scapula
- Detachment of the humeral attachment of the latissimus dorsi and distal release
- Release of the clavicular attachment of pectoralis major and turning over the anterior deltoid
- Suture of the pectoralis major to the lateral portion of the clavicle
- Fixation of the osteotomized acromion with attached trapezius to the humerus as distally as possible using screws in 100 degrees of abduction
- Suture of latissimus dorsi to infraspinatus tendon in 90 degrees of external rotation
- Suture of the released deltoid
- Skin closure

PITFALL

- No satisfactory recovery of shoulder motion without functioning serratus anterior muscle (no scapular winging preoperatively) and vertical steerer of the glenohumeral joint

POSTOPERATIVE CARE

- Immobilization of shoulder and elbow joints in zero position with a splint for 6 to 8 weeks
- Isometric exercise of each transferred muscle commencing at fifth postoperative week
- Gradual increase of range of passive motion and progressive resistance exercise of the muscle

---

Complications. Dehiscence of the suture sites of the transferred muscles is not uncommon, and we have experienced several breakdowns of the suture sites and migration of the screws. We thus recommend splint immobilization for as long as possible (longer than 8 weeks) and gradual adduction of the arm.

Multidirectional instability of the glenohumeral joint may occur after these procedures when the steerers are paralyzed or weak and may require further surgical intervention such as a Bankart procedure or posterior capsuloplasty.

Expected Outcome. Most cases in the literature do not report the state of paralysis in detail, especially in terms of the presence or completeness of paralysis of the serratus anterior muscle and supraspinatus muscle. These two muscles greatly contribute to the final outcome of multiple muscle transfers.

Takahashi and colleagues described nine patients who had reconstruction of shoulder function by Saha's procedure consisting of transfers of the trapezius, pectoralis major, and latissimus dorsi.[171] The mean postoperative range of motion in active forward flexion was 68.3 degrees (range, 60 to 80),

the mean abduction was 55 degrees (40 to 90), and the mean external rotation was 30 degrees (0 to 80 degrees). The patients used their reconstructed limbs in all daily activities but were not satisfied with this small range of shoulder motion. The authors have experienced the same type of results (Fig. 38-37).

The outcomes of shoulder function by Harmon's or Bateman's techniques are variable depending on the preoperative condition and type of paralysis, although the patients with axillary and suprascapular nerve injuries achieved a mean of 120 degrees of flexion and abduction and 30 degrees of external rotation (Fig. 38-38). However, the remaining patients with C5 and C6 or with C5, C6, and C7 root avulsions obtained minimal improvement of shoulder function, consisting of 60 degrees of flexion and abduction and −10 degrees of external rotation.[145] There was no contribution of the reinnervated muscles by intercostal nerve transfer or free muscle transfer as primary movers. When biceps function is lost, the original Harmon's procedure cannot provide satisfactory improvement of abduction and flexion and needs other primary movers such as a trapezius transfer.

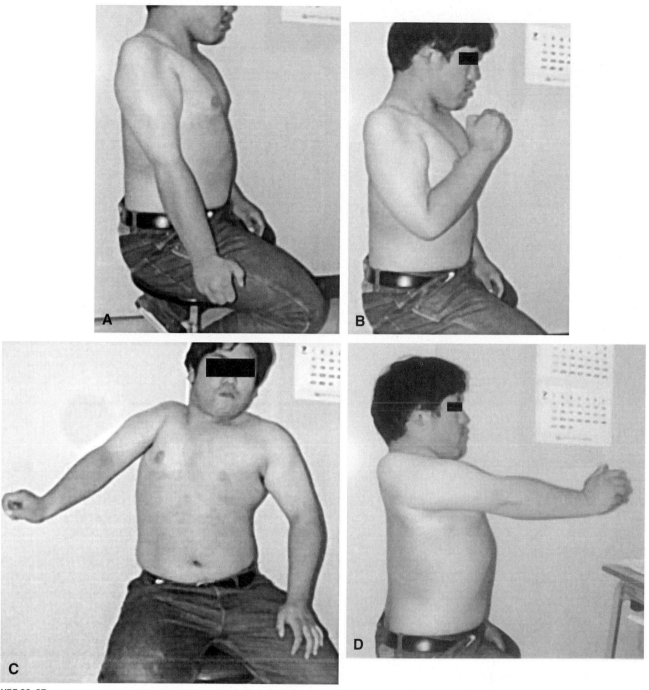

FIGURE 38-37. A 15-year-old boy sustained preganglionic injuries of C5, C6, and C7 roots of his right brachial plexus and had undergone a spinal accessory nerve to suprascapular nerve transfer and third and fourth intercostal nerve transfers to the musculocutaneous nerve 11 months after injury but failed to recover elbow and shoulder function. Subsequently, he underwent secondary reconstruction of elbow and shoulder function. At the initial reconstruction, he underwent a pectoralis major muscle transfer for elbow flexion; and at the second operation, multiple muscle transfers consisting of the trapezius, latissimus dorsi, and triceps brachii were performed. He can flex the elbow fully (**A** and **B**), but shoulder function is unsatisfactory because of posterior instability of the glenohumeral joint and paralysis of the serratus anterior muscle (**C** and **D**).

Shoulder Arthrodesis

Shoulder arthrodesis is a well-established operative procedure that involves fusion of the humeral head to the glenoid. The indications include total paralysis in brachial plexus injuries and upper type paralysis.[12,121,142] We prefer procedures other than shoulder arthrodesis because the decreased arc of shoulder motion after arthrodesis limits use of the reconstructed hand after prehensile reconstruction. Patients also complain of difficulty with turning during sleep. Lastly, fracture of the humerus is not a rare complication of shoulder arthrodesis. Traditionally, the term *glenohumeral arthrodesis* is used; however, some surgeons prefer to include *acromiohumeral arthrodesis. Humeroscapular arthrodesis* is commonly called *shoulder arthrodesis,* and we use that term in this text for simplicity. The contraindications to shoulder arthrodesis include paralysis of the trapezius,

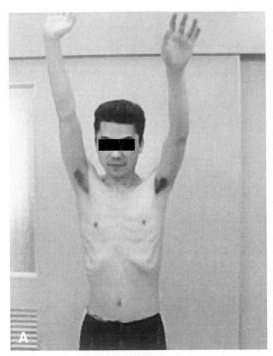 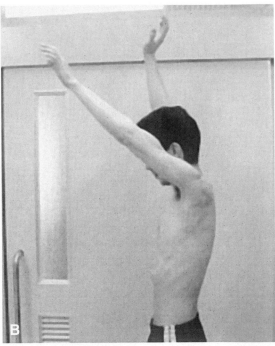

FIGURE 38-38. A 26-year-old man sustained combined paralysis of his left axillary, suprascapular, musculocutaneous, and radial nerves 16 months before operation. At the initial operation, he underwent free muscle transfer for elbow flexion and wrist extension and tendon transfer for finger extension. At the second operation, multiple muscle transfers consisting of pectoralis major, latissimus dorsi, and triceps brachii were performed for shoulder reconstruction. **A** and **B,** He obtained satisfactory function of shoulder, elbow, wrist, and finger function.

levator scapulae, serratus anterior, or rhomboid muscles, because these scapula-stabilizing muscles are required to provide motor function to the extremity. Richards[139] reported that if these muscles are nonfunctional the extremity will be severely impaired despite successful joint fusion.[8,52] However, stability of the humeroscapular joint by shoulder arthrodesis is necessary if the patient is to be able to move the distal elbow and fingers when these are reconstructed by nerve transfer or free muscle transfer, even if paralysis of the serratus anterior muscle produces some instability of the scapulothoracic joint.

The shoulder is a difficult joint to fuse because the humerus has a long lever arm, the area of contact at the glenohumeral joint is small, and paralyzed muscles cannot contribute as a compressive force to aid in the union. The optimum position for arthrodesis of the shoulder is debatable. However, we recommend that for all patients with paralysis of axillary and suprascapular nerves and weak elbow flexors but good scapulothoracic muscles that the glenohumeral joint should be arthrodesed at 80 to 90 degrees of abduction to assist elbow flexion. Patients with total paralysis of the brachial plexus with normal function of the trapezius and serratus anterior muscles should undergo arthrodesis in 30 to 40 degrees of abduction and flexion and 30 degrees of internal rotation. On the other hand, in total paralysis of the brachial plexus with absence of serratus anterior or trapezius function, the joint should be arthrodesed in 20 degrees of abduction, 10 degrees of flexion, and 30 degrees of internal rotation.

Many operative techniques for shoulder arthrodesis have been described.[35,47,76,126]

The AO technique provides rigid internal fixation and good results. However, it carries the risk of increased devascularization and occasional problems from prominent screws and the loosening of the hardware in osteoporotic bone. Fixation by a Rush pin and tension-band wiring provides good shear control and low axial stiffness. Unlike conventional rigid fixation, it maintains axial elasticity, which may accelerate union. It does not affect the growth plate of the proximal humerus in children, can be used in the presence of osteoporosis, and has a high rate of fusion. External fixation has its own complications due to neurovascular injury, pin tract infection, pin loosening, and fractures through pin sites, but it is particularly useful for infected joints. We prefer to use long AO cancellous screws for transfixing both the glenohumeral joints and acromiohumeral joints using additional iliac bone grafts.

Authors' Preferred Method

The operation is performed in the lateral position, and the alignment of the spine should be straight to monitor the optimal position of fusion during surgery. Through the posterior half of the conventional saber-cut incision (taking care not to injure the nerve to any previously transferred muscle), the posterior half of the deltoid is detached from the scapular spine and acromion and retracted distally. All soft tissue under the acromion is removed, and the rotator cuff muscles are also detached from the greater and lesser tuberosity, exposing the joint capsule, glenohumeral joint, and acromiohumeral joint. Articular cartilage from each joint is removed to facilitate contact of the subchondral bone of the humeral head and glenoid cavity. Bone graft from the iliac crest is then inserted under the subacromial space. The glenohumeral joint and acromiohumeral joint are transfixed with long 4.5-mm-diameter cancellous screws in the position of 30 degrees of abduction-flexion and internal rotation. Cancellous bone chips are used to pack the vacant space of both joints.

CRITICAL POINTS: HUMEROSCAPULAR ARTHRODESIS

INDICATIONS

- Failed or neglected cases with glenohumeral instability
- Total or upper type paralysis with or without paralysis of the serratus anterior
- Normal functioning trapezius

PREOPERATIVE EVALUATION

- Good strength of trapezius and rhomboid
- No contracture of scapulothoracic joint

PEARLS

- Provides stability to the shoulder
- Improvement of range of shoulder motion depending on strength of scapulothoracic muscles

TECHNICAL POINTS

- Posterior saber-cut skin incision
- Removal of all soft tissues including rotator cuff in the subacromial joint
- Removal of cartilage of the subacromial and glenohumeral joints
- Iliac bone graft between the acromion and humeral head
- Transfixation of subacromial and glenohumeral joints with AO cancellous screws in the position of 30 degrees of abduction-flexion and internal rotation of shoulder
- Bone chips in vacant areas around the joints
- Skin closure

PITFALLS

- Postoperative fracture of the humerus
- Disability on turning during sleep

POSTOPERATIVE CARE

- Immobilization of the fused shoulder joint for 3 months
- Range-of-motion exercise of the scapulothoracic joint
- Radiographs monthly

Postoperative Protocol. An external splint is used to immobilize the fused joint for 12 weeks. Movement of the reconstructed elbow and distal joints is allowed if possible. Passive and active range of motion of the scapulothoracic joint is initiated, and radiographs are taken monthly until bone union.

Complications. In our experience with 16 patients undergoing humeroscapular arthrodesis, 1 patient needed additional bone graft because of delayed union and 3 patients had humeral fractures. Failure of union may occur after either primary or revision shoulder arthrodesis, but this is rare when current fixation techniques are used.

Expected Outcome. The purpose of shoulder arthrodesis after brachial plexus injuries is to stabilize the humeroscapular joint and to permit the patient to move the upper arm through the scapulothoracic joint using innervated scapular movers. The postoperative range of shoulder movement depends on the residual strength of the parascapular muscles, such as the trapezius, levator scapulae, serratus anterior, latissimus dorsi, and rhomboid muscles.

Previous reports have shown satisfactory outcome of range of shoulder motion, averaging 60 degrees of abduction and flexion,[7,34,40,43,139,141] because most of the patients had normal function of the serratus anterior muscle.

In our 16 patients who underwent arthrodesis of the humeroscapular joint because of shoulder instability after complete paralysis of the brachial plexus, postoperative range of flexion-abduction shoulder motion was 17 ± 3.3 degrees. The arc of shoulder rotation was 35 ± 6.7 degrees, because most had paralysis of the serratus anterior muscle.

RECONSTRUCTION OF ELBOW FUNCTION

Elbow Flexion

Residual paralysis of elbow flexion can be treated by transferring the tendons of innervated muscles or by transplanting the muscles themselves, such as the proximal advancement of the common origin of the forearm muscles (Steindler flexorplasty),[162-164] transfer of pectoralis major,[11,23,32,41,150,177] pectoralis minor,[161] sternomastoid,[27,99] triceps,[31] and latissimus dorsi muscles,[01,96,133,106] and free muscle transfer.

These conventional muscle transfers can be used only in partial paralysis, especially upper type paralysis. Final outcome is greatly affected by the preoperative strength of the donor muscle, because strength of the muscle to be transferred is rarely easy to estimate definitively. In severe brachial plexus injuries there are very few completely normal muscles available for transfer. Many donor muscles are paralyzed partially. Preoperative evaluation of muscle power is difficult, especially for the latissimus dorsi. However, pectoralis major, triceps brachii, and the forearm muscles can be evaluated more accurately.

Another pitfall in selecting a donor muscle for the reconstruction of elbow flexion is considering only stabilization as part of reconstruction. Optimal arm movement of a functional shoulder joint is imperative for the hand to be functional. The latissimus dorsi and pectoralis major muscles should be reserved for shoulder reconstruction, although elbow flexion is the priority of reconstruction because inability to restore elbow flexion obviates the need for shoulder reconstruction.

We recommend free muscle transfer neurotized from a part of ulnar nerve[71] or intercostal nerve for elbow reconstruction as the first procedure of choice in chronic or failed cases of brachial plexus reconstruction. As the second procedure of choice, we prefer a modified Steindler's procedure (described next), and lastly latissimus dorsi or pectoralis major muscle transfer is utilized when they are not needed for reconstruction of movement of the shoulder.

Authors' Preferred Methods

Modified Steindler's Procedure

The procedure that has been used classically to restore flexor function to the elbow paralyzed by any injury is the flexorplasty described by Arthur Steindler in 1918.[100,165] The flexor-pronator muscles arising from the medial epicondyle are transposed to a more proximal point on the humerus, increasing their moment arm for elbow flexion, sufficient to permit active control. Although most patients can flex their elbows through a useful range against gravity, it is rare for them to be able to lift more than 2 kg after such a transfer[91]; nevertheless it is a useful operation.[4,26,107] As with all potential candidates for tendon transfer, the preoperative evaluation of the strength of the proposed donor muscle is critical to the success of the Steindler flexorplasty or any of its variations. Because the muscles originating from the medial epicondyle of the humerus (the pronator teres, flexor carpi

radialis, palmaris longus, flexor carpi ulnaris, and flexor digitorum superficialis) will now serve to flex the elbow in addition to their usual functions, they must have normal or near-normal power to achieve a meaningful result. Patients who already have weak elbow flexion or who can achieve flexion by the so-called Steindler effect preoperatively are most likely to have satisfactory results from surgery. The Steindler effect makes use of contraction of those muscles in a supplementary movement as follows: the patient may achieve elbow flexion by flexing the wrist and fingers and pronating the forearm, usually while the arm is flexed forward in the horizontal plane to eliminate the effect of gravity. Because this is precisely the muscular activity that is enhanced by moving the origins more proximally, it may be used to identify those patients whose muscles are adequate for transfer. Although one may proceed in the absence of a demonstrable Steindler effect, the postoperative result is likely to be barely functional. The modified technique that is preferred is that described by Mayer and Green.[108]

Operative Procedures. The incision begins posterior to the medial epicondyle of the humerus and is then directed proximally and anteriorly for 7.5 cm over the distal upper arm. The incision curves distally over the anterior forearm for 10 cm, following the outline of the pronator teres muscle (see Fig. 38-39A). The skin flap thus formed is retracted gently with the full thickness of subcutaneous tissue, and the incision is then undermined posteriorly to identify the ulnar nerve, which is mobilized from behind the elbow. The articular branch of the ulnar nerve must be sacrificed, but the branches to the flexor carpi ulnaris are preserved and protected as the nerve is mobilized for approximately 5 cm distal to the elbow. The median nerve is then identified after the fascia over the pronator teres has been incised. The branch of the median nerve to the pronator is usually found on the medial side of the median nerve, 2.5 to 5 cm proximal

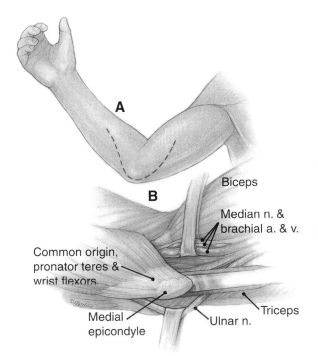

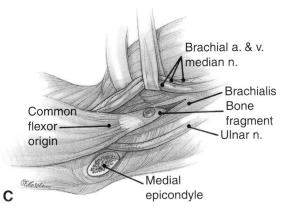

FIGURE 38-39. Authors' preferred Steindler's procedure for reconstruction of elbow flexion. **A,** Skin incision. **B,** The common origin of the pronator and wrist flexor muscles is dissected and detached with a fragment of bone from the medial epicondyle using an osteotome, taking care not to injure the ulnar and median nerves and brachial vessels. **C,** The bone fragment with the common origin of the pronator and wrist flexor muscles is fixed to the anterior surface of the humerus using a screw and suture anchors.

to the elbow, and also must be preserved as the nerve is mobilized. The common origin of the pronator and wrist flexor muscles is dissected from above downward and then detached with a fragment of bone from the medial epicondyle using an osteotome (we prefer 1 cm diameter of bone; see Fig. 38-39B), and the muscles are gently retracted while their nerve supply is protected from injury. Distal stripping of the muscles is continued until, with the elbow acutely flexed to 130 degrees, the bone fragment and muscle origin can be advanced 5 to 7 cm proximally.

Although in the original Steindler technique the transfer was attached to the medial intermuscular septum and fascia, Mayer has utilized bony fixation to the anterior aspect of the humerus. The reasons given for this type of attachment are twofold: (1) the attachment to bone is stronger than to fascia and (2) the more lateral the insertion, the less the pronator effect of the muscles. The original technique had a significant drawback in that with increased tension on the pronator teres, flexion was usually accompanied by marked pronation of the forearm, a functionally compromised attitude for hand function. The median nerve and brachial artery are retracted gently, and the brachialis is incised so that the humerus can be prepared for receipt of the transfer by shaving the cortex of anterior humerus. A screw and commercially available suture-anchor kits are preferred to fix the fragment of the medial epicondyle to the humerus. First, a drill hole is made in the center of the fragment and also in the anterior surface of the humerus. Additionally, two or three suture anchors are inserted into the humerus around the drill hole. The distal portion of the wound is closed before the fragment of the medial epicondyle is secured in its new site. Sutures from the suture-anchor are passed around the fragment, and the screw is passed through the fragment and into the drill hole in the humerus. Anchor sutures are tied with the elbow flexed 130 degrees and the forearm supinated (see Fig. 38-39C). The proximal portion of the wound is closed and the dressing is applied.

Postoperative Protocol. A posterior plaster splint maintains 100 degrees of elbow flexion for 6 weeks. Passive flexion of the elbow, wrist, and fingers commences just after the operation. Active flexion of the wrist and fingers with the elbow in full flexion is started in the third week. Extension of the elbow, wrist, and fingers is allowed from the seventh week after operation. Postoperative rehabilitation and muscle re-education take several months, and no attempt should be made to overcome the last 30 degrees of elbow flexion contracture, because the mechanical advantage in initiation of flexion from a partially flexed position would be lost.

Complications. Most patients with the Steindler's procedure tend to have a residual flexion contracture of the elbow from 30 to 60 degrees of flexion.

Expected Outcome. Recent articles have noted that Steindler's procedure can achieve more than 120 degrees of elbow flexion in more than two thirds of patients and have

CRITICAL POINTS: FLEXOR-PRONATOR MUSCLE TRANSFER (STEINDLER'S PROCEDURE)

INDICATIONS

- Failed or neglected cases of upper type brachial plexus palsy greater than 6 months
- Normal or subnormal power of forearm flexor-pronator muscles
- Good shoulder control

PREOPERATIVE EVALUATION

- Good strength of forearm flexor-pronator muscles

PEARLS

- Reliable recovery of elbow flexion

TECHNICAL POINTS

- Longitudinal curved skin incision from the distal one third of upper arm to the proximal one third of forearm
- Exploration of ulnar nerve
- Identification of the median nerve, brachial artery, and veins
- Release of the proximal portion of forearm flexor and pronator muscles
- Osteotomy of the medial epicondyle of humerus
- Longitudinal split of brachialis muscle
- Subperiosteal dissection and shaving the anterior cortex of humerus
- Drill hole on the humerus to accept the screws
- Transfixation of the fragment of medial epicondyle with forearm muscles to the humerus with a screw
- Additional suture of the fragment to the humerus with suture-anchor kits
- Skin closure

PITFALL

- Flexion contracture of elbow

POSTOPERATIVE CARE

- Immobilization of the elbow in 100 degrees of flexion for 6 weeks
- Passive flexion of elbow, wrist, and finger immediately after operation
- Active flexion of wrist and finger 3 weeks postoperatively
- Passive extension of elbow at 7 weeks postoperatively

emphasized that the modified Steindler flexorplasty is a comparatively simple operation and gives very reliable results.[14,24,36,37,102,181]

We prefer the modified Steindler procedure for the patients who are elderly or those with failed nerve repair such as intercostal nerve transfer or Oberlin's ulnar nerve transfer. We do not use it as the first procedure of choice for the reconstruction of elbow flexion. We have been unable to achieve enough recovery in our patients with this procedure to allow them to lift heavy objects, despite reports to the contrary in the literature. The mean range of elbow motion in our series of five patients is from −40 degrees in extension and 100 degrees in flexion, and the mean power of lifting with the forearm is 2 kg (Fig. 38-40).

Latissimus Dorsi Transfer

The latissimus dorsi is innervated by the thoracodorsal nerve (C6-C8), and in cases of upper paralysis that require reconstruction of elbow flexion, this muscle is usually partially denervated. If the strength of the muscle is enough to supplement elbow flexion, it can be used as a donor muscle. However, definitive evaluation of muscle strength of the latissimus dorsi is difficult because other muscles for internal rotation of the shoulder work together with it. It is also difficult to assess by EMG because the latissimus dorsi is too flat for an electrode to be placed properly. The most accurate assessment is obtained when the examiner is grasping the bulk of the muscle between two fingers and then having the patient try to lift his or her body off the examining table. The fully contracting muscle must be able to resist the examiner from displacing the muscle from its natural course.

Operative Procedure. The basic technique for latissimus harvest is described earlier and in Chapters 47 and 49. The important technical points for pedicled transfer for elbow flexion are described here. After the muscle is harvested, a longitudinal curved skin incision over the coracoid process and in the anterior cubital fossa is done with the patient in the supine position. In the infraclavicular region, the coracoid process is exposed, and in the distal antecubital fossa the biceps tendon is also exposed. A subcutaneous tunnel in the anterior upper arm is made for passing the muscle flap.

Both edges of the latissimus dorsi muscle are sutured to each other, and the muscle is shaped into a tubed muscle flap. The musculocutaneous flap is placed in the skin defect of the upper arm and passed underneath the tunnel. The fascial origin of the muscle is sutured to the biceps brachii tendons, enveloping the tendons with the tubed muscle. The authors prefer to suture the fascial origin of the muscle not to the biceps brachii tendon but to the radius as distal as possible, because the muscle moment arm is greater when it attaches as far from the joint center as possible (Fig. 38-41). The tension when suturing the proximal origin of the latissimus dorsi muscle to the coracoid process is correct when the shoulder is in full adduction and the elbow is in 100 degrees of flexion. This elbow position results in a muscle fiber length somewhat shorter than the normal resting length of the latissimus muscle fibers. The latissimus dorsi muscle should be sutured to the coracoid process using anchor sutures under tension, but the neurovascular pedicle should be without tension. Finally, the overlying skin flap (if transferred) is sutured to the recipient skin edges of the proximal skin incision.

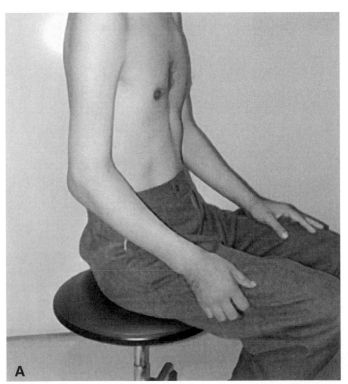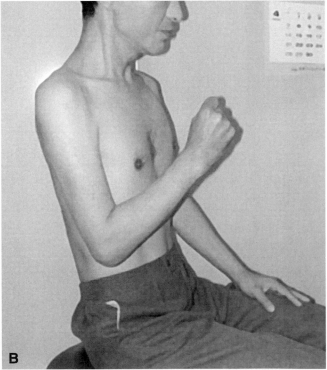

FIGURE 38-40. A 43-year-old man sustained combined paralysis of the right spinal accessory nerve and C5 and C6 nerve roots 2 years ago and underwent Steindler's procedure for elbow flexion. **A** and **B,** Elbow function 6 months postoperatively.

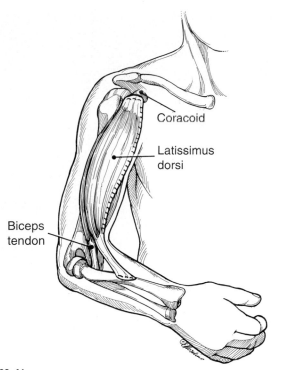

Coracoid

Latissimus dorsi

Biceps tendon

FIGURE 38-41. Diagram of attachment of latissimus dorsi muscle distally to improve moment arm for reconstruction of elbow flexion.

Postoperative Protocol. An abduction pillow holds the position of shoulder in 30 degrees of flexion and abduction with the elbow in 100 degrees of flexion immediately after surgery. This postoperative immobilization should be maintained for 4 weeks. At the end of the fourth week, the splint is removed and active flexion is started, but passive and active extension of the elbow more than −60 degrees is prohibited until the seventh postoperative week. The transferred latissimus dorsi muscle is activated by the patient attempting to extend the shoulder at the beginning of the exercise, but patients will be able to learn how to contract the muscle in any shoulder position. We have found it useful to ask the patient to forcefully cough while he or she holds the transferred muscle with the contralateral hand. Because the latissimus dorsi automatically contracts to stabilize the thorax during forceful cough, it will automatically contract to move the elbow. Biofeedback by means of EMG is useful during the postoperative re-education of the transferred muscle. Later, exercise against resistance will produce powerful flexion of the elbow.

Complications. Weakness of elbow flexion may occur owing to partial paralysis of the latissimus dorsi muscle and poor tension at the muscle attachment sites.

CRITICAL POINTS: LATISSIMUS DORSI TRANSFER FOR ELBOW FLEXION

INDICATIONS

- Neglected cases with C5-C6 type of paralysis greater than 6 months
- Neglected cases with distal type of paralysis of the musculocutaneous nerve greater than 6 months

PREOPERATIVE EVALUATION

- Definite measurement of strength of the latissimus dorsi muscle

PEARLS

- Reliable recovery and satisfactory power of elbow flexion
- Flexion contractures of elbow unusual

TECHNICAL POINTS

- Lateral position
- Longitudinal skin incision along the anterior margin of the latissimus dorsi muscle and accompanying skin flap (if needed)
- Harvesting the entire muscle of the latissimus dorsi from the fascial origin of the ilium to the humeral insertion
- Dissection of the neurovascular pedicle and preservation of continuity

- Transfer of the muscle to the upper arm and closure of skin incision
- Position change from lateral to supine
- Skin incision over the coracoid process, anterior surface of upper arm, and cubital fossa
- Suture of the fascial origin of the muscle to the biceps tendon (or to the radius as distal as possible)
- Skin closure of the distal skin incision
- Suture of the humeral attachment of the muscle to the coracoid process in 100 degrees of elbow flexion
- Skin closure

PITFALLS

- Difficult to estimate the strength of the latissimus dorsi muscle
- Tension at suturing of the muscle

POSTOPERATIVE CARE

- Immobilization of elbow in 100 degrees of flexion and shoulder in 30 degrees of flexion and abduction by a shoulder pillow type of splint for 4 weeks

Expected Outcome. Generally, latissimus dorsi transfer provides the most reliable results, better than Steindler flexorplasties or pectoralis major transfers, as long as the extent of brachial plexus injuries are known, because it is difficult to examine the actual strength of the latissimus dorsi muscle preoperatively. Postoperative range of elbow flexion averages 100 degrees, and patients can lift from 2 to 5 kg based on our experience and that in the literature[83] (Fig. 38-42).

Pectoralis Major Muscle Transfer

Several techniques that use the pectoralis major to restore effective elbow flexion are available. We prefer to transfer all components of the pectoralis major muscle including the sternocostal and clavicular origins and humeral insertion without a fascial graft.[27,153]

Operative Procedure. The procedure is performed with the patient in a supine position and with a flat bolster under the blade of the scapula. The upper limb is draped to allow complete freedom of motion of the elbow and shoulder. A long curvilinear incision is first made from the seventh sternocostal joint cephalad, 2 fingerbreadths inferior to the clavicle. The incision continues laterally to the coracoid process, then distally along the anteromedial aspect of the arm to the level of the axilla with the forearm held in neutral position. The fascia overlying the entire pectoralis major muscle is exposed then by elevating this broad, inferior-based flap to the nipple line (Fig. 38-43A). The deltopectoral groove is delineated carefully and the anterior deltoid and cephalic veins retracted laterally to expose the clavipectoral fascia and the glenohumeral joint capsule,

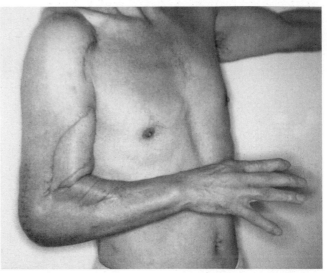

FIGURE 38-42. A 56-year-old man sustained postganglionic injury of C5 and C6 roots of his right brachial plexus 1 year ago and underwent a pedicled transfer of the ipsilateral latissimus dorsi muscle. He could flex his elbow 5 months postoperatively. Note the distal attachment of the muscle to the middle of the radius, not to the biceps tendon.

proximal to the anterior acromion. Depending on the degree of paralysis, the anterior deltoid may or may not have to be detached from the anterolateral clavicular border and the margin of the acromion to allow for sufficient exposure. With the acromion and entire pectoralis major exposed, a second curvilinear incision is made over the antecubital fossa with the transverse limb across the fossa and the

CRITICAL POINTS: PECTORALIS MAJOR MUSCLE TRANSFER FOR ELBOW FLEXION

INDICATIONS
- Neglected cases with upper type of paralysis greater than 6 months
- Neglected cases with paralysis of musculocutaneous nerve greater than 6 months

PREOPERATIVE EVALUATION
- Manual muscle testing of pectoralis major

PEARLS
- Reliable evaluation of muscle power
- Reliable recovery and satisfactory power of elbow flexion

TECHNICAL POINTS
- Supine position
- Curved longitudinal skin incision from the anterior chest to the axilla and upper arm
- Exploration and harvest of the entire pectoralis major muscle
- Transfer of the muscle to the upper arm
- Skin incision over the acromion, upper arm, and cubital fossa
- Suturing of the rectus fascial origin of the muscle to the biceps tendon
- Skin closure of distal skin incisions
- Suturing of the humeral attachment to the acromion under tension
- Skin closure of all skin incisions

PITFALL
- Weak tension when suturing the muscle

POSTOPERATIVE CARE
- Immobilization of elbow in 100 degrees of flexion and shoulder in 60 degrees of flexion and extension by an abduction pillow for 4 weeks

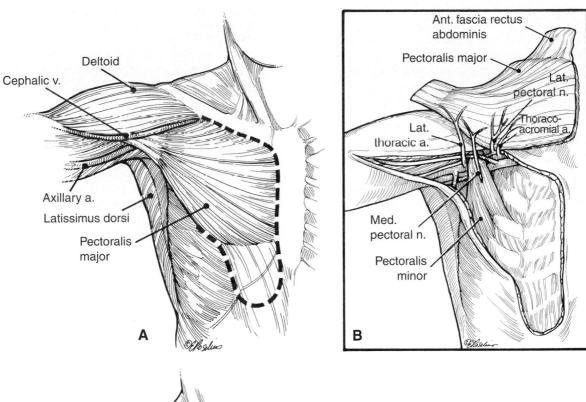

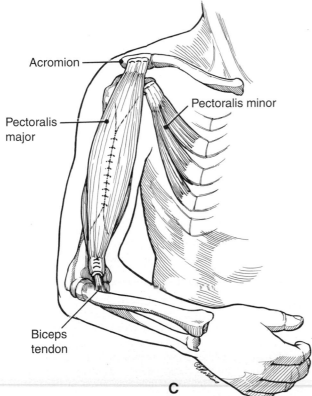

FIGURE 38-43. Authors' preferred pectoralis major transfer for elbow flexion. **A,** The entire mass of the pectoralis major muscle is detached from the clavicle, sternum, and ribs, taking a portion of the anterior rectus abdominis fascia. Note the dotted line indicating the border of transplant. **B,** The entire mass of the pectoralis major muscle with the anterior fascia of the rectus abdominis is elevated based on the branches of the thoracoacromial artery and veins and innervated by the medial and lateral pectoral nerves. **C,** The humeral attachment of the pectoralis major muscle is sutured to the acromion, and the pectoralis major origin with the anterior fascia of the rectus abdominis is sutured to the biceps tendon.

longitudinal limb extending medially and distally 6 cm. The biceps tendon is exposed by dividing the lacertus fibrosus and bicipital aponeurosis. The entire mass of the pectoralis major muscle then is detached from its origin along the medial half of the clavicle and its sternocostal border. With the use of both sharp and blunt techniques, the muscle is elevated with a wide strip of attached anterior rectus abdo-

minis fascia (see Fig. 38-43B).[80] While elevating the pectoralis major from the chest wall and underlying pectoralis minor, meticulous care must be given to preservation of its neurovascular pedicles. The lateral pectoral nerve from the lateral cord of the brachial plexus (C5, C6, and C7) innervates the clavicular and upper sternocostal heads of the pectoralis major, coursing with the large and constant pectoral branch of the thoracoacromial trunk. The medial pectoral nerve (Clark's so-called anterior lateral thoracic nerve) from the medial cord of the brachial plexus (C8, T1) either pierces directly through the belly of the pectoralis minor or passes laterally to it, innervating both this muscle and the inferior third of the pectoralis major. The lateral thoracic artery accompanies the medial pectoral nerve into the lower substance of the pectoralis major. After detaching the humeral insertion of the muscle, the entire muscle mass is then rotated 90 degrees on its two neurovascular pedicles. The origins of the clavicular and sternocostal heads with attached anterior rectus abdominis sheath are rolled into a tube and directed down the arm through an anterior subcutaneous tunnel, exiting through the second incision. The rectus fascial tube is sutured to the biceps tendon, taking care not to kink the neurovascular pedicle. The humeral attachment of the muscle is now directed cephalad and sutured securely to the anterior aspect of the acromion with anchor suture kits, under correct tension with the muscle in 100 degrees of elbow flexion (see Fig. 38-43C). The final position of the transplanted pectoralis major is co-linear with the anatomic origin and insertion of the biceps brachii.

Postoperative Protocol. Postoperative immobilization and rehabilitation after the pectoralis major muscle transfer is the same as that for latissimus dorsi transfer.

Expected Outcome. Most reports in the literature refer to a small numbers of patients, with satisfactory results.[32,80] We have only eight cases in which the pectoralis major muscle transfer was applied to reconstruction of elbow flexion. In six cases more than 100 degrees of elbow flexion and M3 to M4 strength was restored (see Fig. 38-37B and C). The other patient with C5 to C7 paralysis and cervical myelopathy recovered only 60 degrees of elbow flexion. Outcome of elbow flexion after pectoralis major muscle transfer also depends on the degree of paralysis of the pectoralis major, because in all cases it is partially paralyzed by the injury to the plexus.

ANNOTATED REFERENCES

46a. De Jager LT: The functional benefits of reconstructive surgery for complete lesions of the brachial plexus in adults. J Hand Surg [Br] 27:342-344, 1999.

   This short article offers a sober estimation of what can be achieved with surgery in patients with brachial plexus injuries using techniques of nerve repair and neurotization/nerve transfers. It serves as a guideline for what might be the expected results after surgery.

48. Doi K, Hattori Y, Tan SH, Dhawan V: Basic science behind functioning free muscle transplantation. Clin Plast Surg 29:483-495, 2002.

   Free muscle transfers never regain their full strength after microvascular transfer. By utilizing biomechanical advantages such as increasing the muscle moment arm, the power of transferred muscles can be improved for functional purposes. This paper discusses the basic science and biomechanics of functional free muscle transfer.

54. Doi K, Otsuka K, Okamoto Y, et al: Cervical nerve root avulsion in brachial plexus injuries: Magnetic resonance imaging classification and comparison with myelography and computerized tomography myelography. J Neurosurg 96(Suppl):277-284, 2002.

   Previous MRI techniques have not been used widely to define lesions at the root level, because myelography and computed tomographic myelography can clearly image plexus root lesions. To overcome the limitations of MRI, Doi and colleagues introduced a new MRI technique with overlapping coronal-oblique slices (OCOS) MRI.[54] They concluded that the technique is a reliable and reproducible method for detecting root avulsions by retrospective and prospective studies. The reader should be familiar with this technique because it is less invasive than CT myelography.

58. Doi K, Shigetomi M, Kaneko K, et al: Significance of elbow extension in reconstruction of prehension with reinnervated free muscle transfer following complete brachial plexus avulsion. Plast Reconstr Surg 100:364-372, 1997.

   Many authors tend to neglect the significance of elbow stabilization in brachial plexus reconstruction and instead focus their attention on flexion and extension of the reconstructed hand. Despite achieving powerful wrist extension or finger flexion, patients without a stable elbow cannot use their fingers optimally in daily activities. This article emphasizes the significance of elbow extension and introduced the concept of reconstruction of prehension with free muscle transfer.

102a. MacKinnon SE, Novak CB: Nerve transfers: New options for reconstruction following nerve injury. Hand Clin 15:643-666, 1999.

   This paper describes the theory and technique of nerve transfers for reconstruction of function in the upper extremity. Although not limited to lesions of the brachial plexus, it offers a very good discussion of the background of nerve transfers and a good description of the techniques. It is very worthwhile reading for surgeons who operate on the brachial plexus or any nerve problem in the upper extremity.

110. Merrell GA, Barrie KA, Katz DL, Wolfe SW: Results of nerve transfer techniques for restoration of shoulder and elbow function in the context of a meta-analysis of the English literature. J Hand Surg [Am] 26:303-314, 2001.

   The authors of this paper reviewed the results of 1088 nerve transfers from 27 different studies and subjected them to meta-analysis. This paper is probably the best attempt to put together results from different centers that are often difficult to compare. They note that interposition nerve grafts lead to poorer results than direct nerve coaptation. They also give a comparison of results of different donor nerves to restore elbow function.

127. Nagano A, Tsuyama N, Ochiai N, et al: Direct nerve crossing with the intercostal nerve to treat avulsion injuries of the brachial plexus. J Hand Surg [Am] 14:980-985, 1989.

   This paper describes Nagano's classification of root lesions as delineated on myelograms. The reader should be familiar with this classification, and this paper gives a more complete description of this than given in the text of this chapter.

146. Saha AK: Surgery of the paralysed and flail shoulder. Acta Orthop Scand Suppl 97:5-90, 1967.

   When discussing reconstructive procedures for shoulder function following brachial plexus injury, outcomes should be compared by careful evaluation of the preoperative condition focusing on the type of paralysis and level of lesion. However, neuromuscular biomechanics of the shoulder are more complicated than those of the other joints in the upper extremity. Saha studied biomechanics of the paralyzed shoulder in detail. When planning shoulder reconstructive procedures, the surgeon should read his articles, including Acta Orthop Scand 44:668-678, 1973 and Acta Orthop Scand 42:491-505, 1971.

169. Sungpet A, Spuhachatwong C, Kawinwonggowit V: Sensory abnormalities after the seventh cervical nerve root transfer. Microsurgery 19:287-288, 1999.

Previous reports emphasized that using the contralateral C7 nerve root did not result in any permanent sequelae. All of the patients in this article had sensory abnormalities, which has been our experience. Most patients' symptoms will disappear by 6 months post operation, but some patients will continue to have severe pain caused by the damage to the C7 root. The risks of this surgical consequence may not be justified based on the long-term results of this procedure. These authors are among the few who have pointed out the potential problems from contralateral C7 transfer.

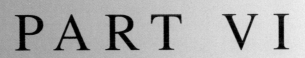

PART VI

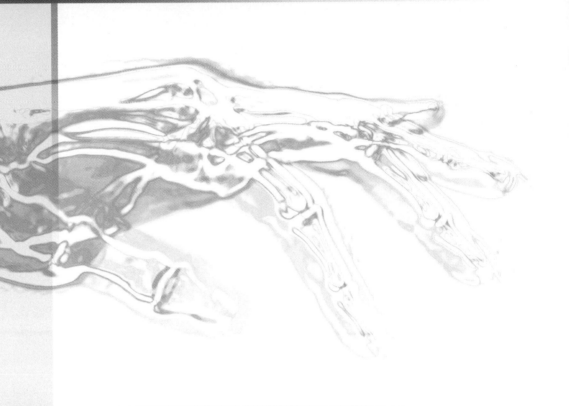

Congenital Disorders

CHAPTER 39

Embryology

Scott H. Kozin

Congenital anomalies affect 1% to 2% of neonates, and approximately 10% of these children have upper extremity abnormalities.[12] The incidence of congenital anomalies has not changed appreciably over the past decade. Congenital limb anomalies are second only to congenital heart disease in the incidence of birth malformations.[3] Most anomalies occur spontaneously or are inherited.[41] Few malformations are attributed to teratogens.[16,29,40] Recent advancements in limb anomalies are directly related to an increased understanding of embryogenesis. Knowledge of hominoid limb development has been greatly expanded by the experimental embryologists. Animal models with similar limb patterning have been used to dissect and manipulate crucial signaling centers that effect limb development and orientation.[32,33,39] Research into gene misexpression and loss-of-function has enhanced our understanding of limb formation.[3,33] The evaluating physician must possess a basic comprehension of embryogenesis and limb formation to comprehend congenital limb anomalies and to communicate relevant knowledge to the family.

EMBRYOGENESIS

Limb development begins with judgments made early during embryogenesis. These decisions affect the position, number, and orientation of the limb. The limb bud is first visualized at 26 days after fertilization when the embryo is about 4 mm in length (crown-rump length).[45,49] The bud rapidly develops through 47 days of life until the embryo length is close to 20 mm. At 52 to 53 days after gestation the embryo is between 22 and 24 mm of length and the fingers are entirely separate.[22] At this point the joints form by condensation of the chondrogen to form dense plates between future bones.[7] Joint cavitation further defines the articulation, although proper joint development requires motion for modeling of the final joint surface. Eight weeks after fertilization, embryogenesis is complete and all limb structures are present.[3,34,39] The majority of upper extremity congenital anomalies occur during this 4- to 8-week period of rapid and fragile limb development. After 8 weeks' gestation, the fetal period commences with differentiation, maturation, and enlargement of existing structures.

The limb bud represents an outgrowth of the mesoderm into the overlying ectoderm. Two sources of cells migrate from their origins into the limb bud.[3,7] The cells from the lateral plate mesoderm become bone, cartilage, and tendon. The cells from the somatic mesoderm form the muscle, nerve, and vascular elements of the limb bud (Fig. 39-1).

There are three spatial axes of limb development: proximodistal, anteroposterior, and dorsoventral.[7] Three signaling centers have been discovered that control these different aspects of limb development: the apical ectodermal ridge (AER), the zone of polarizing activity (ZPA), and the Wnt (Wingless type) signaling center (Table 39-1).[3,34,39] A coordinated effort between the AER, ZPA, and Wnt pathways is necessary for proper limb patterning and axes development.[7,17,27]

Proximodistal Limb Development

The limb develops in a proximal to distal direction, and the progression is controlled by the AER, a thickened layer of ectoderm that forms at the apex between the dorsal and ventral ectoderm and condenses over the limb bud.[7] This signaling center guides the underlying mesoderm to differentiate into appropriate structures.[3,34] Removal of the AER results in limb truncation, and ectopic implantation of the

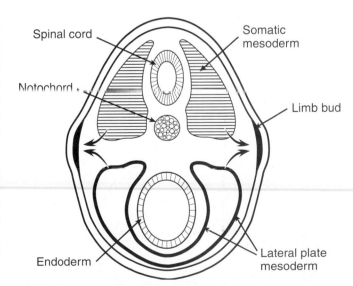

FIGURE 39-1. Axial view of embryo. The lateral plate mesoderm forms the bone, cartilage, and tendon and the somatic mesoderm forms the muscle, nerve, and vascular elements of the limb. (Adapted from Riddle RD, Tabin C: How limbs develop. Sci Am 280:74-79, 1999.)

Table 39-1
SIGNALING PATHWAYS DURING EMBRYOGENESIS

Signaling Center	Responsible Substance	Action
Apical ectodermal ridge	Fibroblast growth factors	Proximal to distal limb development, interdigital necrosis
Zone of polarizing activity	Sonic hedgehog protein	Radioulnar limb formation
Wnt pathway	Lmx-1	Dorsalization of the limb

AER produces additional limb formation (Fig. 39-2).[7,34,49] The secreted proteins within the AER that yield this effect are fibroblast growth factors.[28,46] In fact, removal of the AER can be supplanted by application of fibroblast growth factors (Fig. 39-3). Mice deficient in various fibroblast growth factors have complete transverse limb defects.[11,28,38]

Anteroposterior Limb Development

The limb also develops in an anteroposterior (radioulnar or preaxial-postaxial) direction. The ZPA resides within the posterior margin of the limb bud and functions as a signaling center for anteroposterior limb development.[3,33] This signaling pathway polarizes the limb into a radioulnar axis and governs preaxial-postaxial limb development.[44] The signaling molecule within this pathway is the sonic hedgehog compound.[33] Transplantation of the ZPA or sonic hedgehog protein causes mirror duplication of the ulnar aspect of the limb (Fig. 39-4).[7] The extent of duplication is dose dependent, and greater transference results in more replication.[43] Mutant mice that express sonic hedgehog protein in the anterior limb bud are polydactylous with duplication of their ulnar digits.[21]

Dorsoventral Limb Development

Dorsoventral limb development, or the process of differentiation between the dorsum of the finger with a fingernail and the volar surface abundant with pulp tissue, is not as well understood.[7] The Wnt signaling pathway resides in the dorsal ectoderm and produces a transcription factor, Lmx-1, that induces the mesoderm to adopt dorsal characteristics.[32] In the ventral ectoderm, the Wnt pathway is blocked by a product of the gene Engrailed-1 (En-1). Mice lacking the Wnt pathway have ventralization of the dorsal surface (i.e., biventral limbs with palmar pads on both sides of the foot).[15,30] In contrast, mice lacking En-1 develop dorsalization of the volar surface (i.e., bidorsal limbs).[19]

CLINICAL SCENARIOS

Signaling Center Abnormalities

Certain limb anomalies have been directly related to alterations in these signaling centers. Removal of the AER during embryogenesis yields a truncated limb similar to a congenital amputation.[34] Transplantation of the ZPA or sonic hedgehog signaling molecule to the anterior part of the developing limb bud results in duplication of the elements along the radioulnar axis.[33,34] This misplacement of the signaling center or sonic hedgehog molecule offers a plausible explanation for the rare mirror hand deformity. Lastly, inactivation of the Wnt pathway prevents dorsalization of the mouse limb and results in ventral pads on both sides of the foot.[15,30,32] In humans, loss of Lmx-1 is associated with nail-patella syndrome.[10]

Molecular Abnormalities

Primary axis formation is only one aspect of limb development. Mutations encoding signaling proteins, receptor molecules, and transcription factors can alter normal limb arrangement and yield anomalies. The number of congenital anomalies seen by the practicing hand surgeon identifiable at the molecular level increases each year. Despite the accelerated pace of discovery, only a small number of limb anomalies have been mapped to specific chromosomal segments and are less defined at the molecular level.[3]

The *HOX* and *T-BOX* genes encode transcription factors crucial for limb formation and exhibit some control over upper limb formation.[3,14,24,26,35,47] Abnormalities in *HOX* and *T-BOX* gene production alter limb constitution. The extent

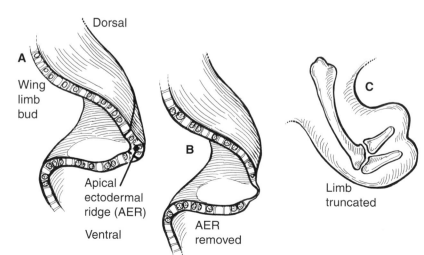

FIGURE 39-2. Removal of the apical ectodermal ridge (AER) from the developing limb bud results in limb truncation. (Adapted from Riddle RD, Tabin C: How limbs develop. Sci Am 280:74-79, 1999.)

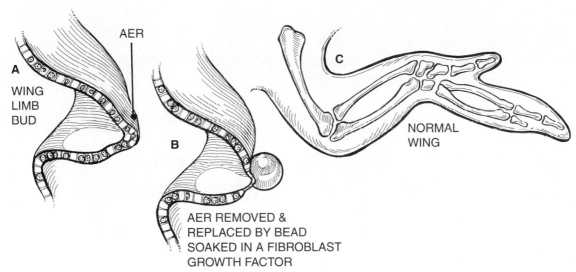

FIGURE 39-3. Removal of the apical ectodermal ridge (AER) and replacement with fibroblast growth factors can result in normal limb formation. (Adapted from Riddle RD, Tabin C: How limbs develop. Sci Am 280:74-79,1999.)

of malformation is related to the number and extent of gene irregularities.[3,9] Mutations within the *HOX* gene locus have been identified as the cause of several types of human differences. Synpolydactyly and hand-foot-genital syndrome have been related to mutations within the *HOX* genes (Figs. 39-5 and 39-6).[13,23,25,48] Madelung's deformity associated with Leri-Weill dyschondrosteosis has also been connected to *HOX* gene defects.[36]

The *T-BOX* genes are a highly conserved family of transcription factors that govern both limb and organ system development.[1,6] Altered expression of T-box products can affect the anteroposterior (i.e., radioulnar) development of the limb. The combination of a cardiac defect and radial deficiency (i.e., Holt-Oram syndrome) has been specifically linked to the production of transcription factor Tbx5.[4,5,18] *T-BOX* gene mutations have also been linked to limb

anomalies associated with a variety of systemic syndromes, including ulnar-mammary syndrome (Tbx3 mutation), which is associated with postaxial limb anomalies.[2,3]

The family of bone morphogenetic proteins is expressed in the developing limb.[7] Cartilage-derived morphogenetic protein appears paramount to digital length during embryogenesis. Deficiencies in a cartilage-derived morphogenetic protein are associated with various forms of brachydactyly. Grebes' and Hunter-Thompson chondrodysplasias are associated with severe brachydactyly and have been directly related to a cartilage-derived morphogenetic protein deficiency (Fig. 39-7).[31,42]

During the period of embryogenesis, additional organ systems are developing and maturing at the same time. The error during limb formation can also disturb formation of these other systems. Certain upper limb anomalies are

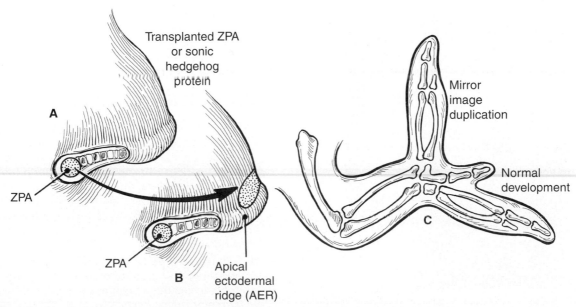

FIGURE 39-4. Transplantation of the zone of polarizing activity or sonic hedgehog protein causes mirror image duplication of the ulnar aspect of the limb. (Adapted from Riddle RD, Tabin C: How limbs develop. Sci Am 280:74-79,1999.)

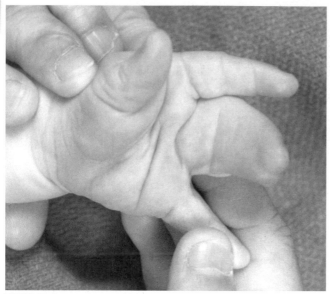

FIGURE 39-5. Child with synpolydactyly, characterized by long/ring finger syndactyly combined with digital duplication within the web. (Courtesy of Shriners Hospitals for Children, Philadelphia.)

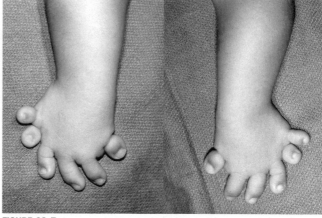

FIGURE 39-7. Hands of a child with Grebes' chondrodysplasia and severe brachydactyly that has been related to a cartilage-derived morphogenetic protein deficiency. (Courtesy of Shriners Hospitals for Children, Philadelphia.)

associated with concomitant systemic disorders (e.g., radial deficiency).[8,20] Other limb anomalies occur in isolation or are combined with other musculoskeletal problems (e.g., ulnar deficiency).[37] The discrimination between anomalies that occur in isolation versus anomalies associated with systemic ailments is mandatory. Many of the systemic illnesses are more important than the limb anomaly and require accurate evaluation to prevent life-threatening consequences.

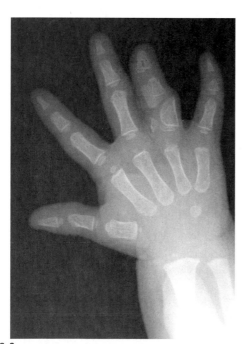

FIGURE 39-6. Radiograph of synpolydactyly reveals concealed polydactyly within the syndactyly. (Courtesy of Shriners Hospitals for Children, Philadelphia.)

CRITICAL POINTS: EMBRYOLOGY

LIMB BUD FORMATION

- Limb bud formation begins approximately 4 weeks after gestation and is complete by 8 weeks. The majority of limb anomalies occur within this time of rapid and fragile limb development.

SIGNALING CENTERS

- Three signaling centers control the spatial axes of limb development. The apical ectodermal ridge (AER) governs proximodistal, the zone of polarizing activity (ZPA) manages anteroposterior (i.e., radioulnar), and the Wnt (Wingless type) signaling center directs dorsoventral limb formation.

MOLECULAR ABNORMALITIES

- The *HOX* and *T-BOX* genes encode transcription factors crucial for limb formation. Mutations within the *HOX* gene locus have been identified as the causes of synpolydactyly, hand-foot-genital syndrome, and Madelung's deformity associated with Leri-Weill dyschondrosteosis. T-box gene abnormalities have been linked to Holt-Oram syndrome and ulnar-mammary syndrome.

- Cartilage-derived morphogenetic protein appears paramount to digital length, and deficiencies have been associated with various forms of brachydactyly, such as Grebes' and Hunter-Thompson chondrodysplasias.

The basic molecular events of hand formation are being discovered at a rapid rate. The complex interaction between signaling centers and the inherent redundancy within the gene pool make definitive determination difficult. In addition, variation in the amount of molecular damage can result in innumerable phenotypes. Application of this material to the clinical setting is a necessary linkage. The National Institutes of Health National Center for Biotechnology Information web site (www.ncbi.nlm.nih.gov) is frequently updated and invaluable when evaluating a child with congenital deficiencies.

ANNOTATED REFERENCES

3. Bamshad M, Watkins WS, Dixon ME, et al: Reconstructing the history of human limb development: Lessons from birth defects. Pediatr Res 45:291-299, 1999.

   Understanding limb development is a daunting task for the hand surgeon. This review article is reasonably easy to read and discusses embryogenesis and developmental programs used to modify the architecture of the hominoid limb. A classification system based on gene and/or chromosome defect is also provided, although the clinical utility of this type of scheme is limited.

7. Daluiski A, Yi SE, Lyons KM: The molecular control of upper extremity development: Implications for congenital hand anomalies. J Hand Surg [Am] 26:8-22, 2001.

   This in-depth review of the molecular control of upper limb development covers the basics of limb formation and signaling pathways. The molecular component of limb formation is detailed with regards to *HOX* genes, secreted factors, and feedback loops. Clinical corollary between specific defects and primary condition is a strong point of this review, along with a detailed bibliography.

21a. McCarroll HR Jr: Congenital anomalies: A 25-year overview. J Hand Surg [Am] 25:1007-1037, 2000.

   This article is a must for the hand surgeon treating children with congenital differences. McCarroll discusses the major advances in the treatment of congenital hand anomalies over the past 25 years and provides personal insight into these difficult problems. The article also provides a glimpse into the future treatment regimens, such as genetic engineering of joints and the field of fetal surgery.

34. Riddle RD, Tabin C: How limbs develop. Sci Am 280:74-79, 1999.

   This article is a concise review of limb embryogenesis, including axes development. The apical ectodermal ridge, zone of polarizing activity, and Wnt pathway are discussed with regard to normal and abnormal limb development. The article provides a resource for families and caregivers.

CHAPTER 40

Deformities of the Hand and Fingers

Simon P. Kay, David McCombe, and Scott H. Kozin

Syndactyly

Simon P. Kay

Syndactyly occurs when the normal processes of digital separation and web space formation fail to some degree. During normal development, the fingers form as condensations of mesoderm within the terminal paddle of the embryonic upper limb. These condensations differentiate into the fingers. Spaces form between the fingers in a distal-to-proximal direction to the level of the normal web space.[53] This process is dependent on the apical ectodermal ridge[34] and the molecular signaling of several cytokines, including bone morphogenetic proteins (BMPs), transforming growth factor-β, fibroblast growth factors (FGFs), and retinoic acid.[14,15,31,47,49] Regulated apoptosis results in individual web spaces consisting of a rectangular fold of skin that slopes 45 degrees in a dorsal to palmar direction from the metacarpal heads to the level of the midproximal phalanx (Fig. 40-1). The third web is slightly narrower than the second and fourth. Failure of normal interdigital necrosis results in syndactyly.

EPIDEMIOLOGY

Syndactyly is a common congenital anomaly of the hand with an incidence of approximately 1 in 2000.[44] It occurs bilaterally in 50% of cases. Between 10% and 40% of cases demonstrate a positive family history that is inherited as an autosomal dominant trait.[26,27] Variable expressivity and incomplete penetrance account for the male predominance (2:1) and the variable phenotype within a family pedigree.

PATHOLOGY

Syndactyly is a variable fusion of the soft tissue and/or skeletal elements of adjacent digits. The conjoined digits may possess anomalies of the nails, the digital neurovascular bundles, and the tendon systems. Syndactyly may be associated with other hand anomalies, such as polydactyly, clinodactyly, symphalangism, and synostosis.

The native skin is inadequate to resurface the circumference of each independent digit as shown by mathematical calculations and clinical experience.[17,25] The abnormal underlying fascia has a continuous thickened lateral digital sheet that spans the length of the syndactyly across the potential interdigital web space. The phalanges may be fused across the web space, particularly at the level of the distal phalangeal tufts. Distal phalangeal fusion results in a synonychia with loss of the paronychial fold and flattening of the nail matrix across the bony mass. Extra phalanges or digits (synpolydactyly) may be contained within the conjoined digital mass (see Fig. 39-5). In simple syndactyly the joints are usually normal. The flexor tendon and extensor

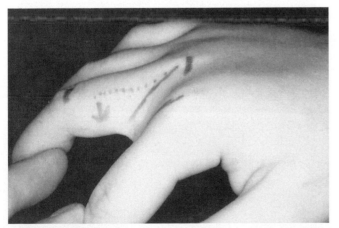

FIGURE 40-1. Normal web of skin slopes 45 degrees in a dorsal to palmar direction from the metacarpal heads to the level of the midproximal phalanx.

tendon mechanisms are usually independent, although they may be deficient or shared between conjoint digits affected by complex syndactyly. The digital neurovascular anatomy is usually normal, although the bifurcation of the common digital structures may be quite distal. With the more complex syndactylies, abnormal anatomy is more common.

CLINICAL FEATURES

Syndactyly is usually noted shortly after birth, unless the anomaly is incomplete and mild. In isolated syndactyly, the long/ring finger web space is most commonly affected (57%), followed by the ring/small finger web space (27%). Thumb/index finger and index/long finger web syndactylies are the least common.[25] In syndromic cases, the thumb/index finger and index/long finger web spaces are more frequently affected.[25,61]

Important features to consider with syndactyly are the web space(s) involved, the extent of the syndactyly, the involvement of the nail, and the presence of other anomalies. Lack of differential motion between the digits may indicate bony fusion and/or an extra digit concealed within the conjoined digits. Examination involves the entire affected upper limb, the contralateral hand, the chest wall, and the feet. Radiographs may reveal skeletal fusion, a concealed extra digit (synpolydactyly), or other bony or articular deformities.

Syndactyly may be associated with anomalies such as amniotic disruption syndrome, symbrachydactyly, cleft hand, or synpolydactyly. Numerous syndromes feature syndactyly as a dominant or minor feature. Syndactyly is also present in some chromosomal abnormalities.

CLASSIFICATION

Syndactyly is described as *complete* if the web space extends to include the fingertip and *incomplete* when the web space occurs anywhere between the normal commissure and the fingertips. *Simple* syndactyly has only skin or soft tissue connections (Fig. 40-2). *Complex* syndactyly is marked by skeletal anomalies. The most common form of *complex* syndactyly is a side-to-side fusion at the distal phalangeal tuft level (Fig. 40-3). The *complex complicated* syndactylies are those with accessory phalanges interposed within the abnormal web space.[26] The incidence of tendon and neurovascular abnormalities increases with the complexity of the syndactyly.

MANAGEMENT

Syndactyly can have cosmetic, functional, and developmental impact on the growing child. The appearance of the hand is altered, particularly complete complicated forms. Syndactyly of the first web space hampers grasp and the development of pinch. Syndactyly of the second, third, and fourth web spaces inhibits independent digital motion. The deleterious effect of syndactyly may increase during growth. Syndactyly between digits of unequal length yields progressive tethering of the longer digit, which deviates toward the

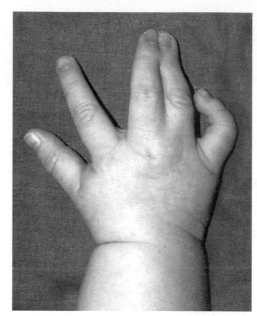

FIGURE 40-2. Simple and complete syndactyly between third and fourth rays.

shorter digits and causes a flexion contracture (Figs. 40-4 and 40-5).

Surgery is indicated for most children. Exceptions to surgery include mild incomplete syndactyly without functional impairment, medical conditions that preclude surgery, or complex syndactylies that risk further functional impairment with attempted separation. On occasion, there are insufficient components in the fused mass to produce independent, stable, and mobile digits. In this situation, the syndactyly is better left alone rather than risk reducing function.

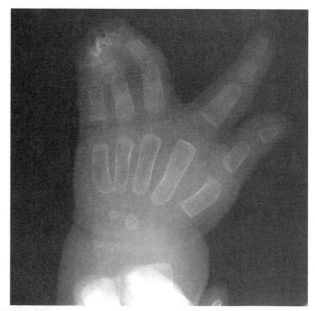

FIGURE 40-3. Radiograph of complex syndactyly with distal skeletal fusion.

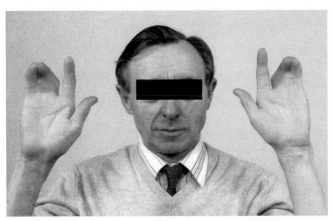

FIGURE 40-4. Fifty-year-old man who never had treatment for bilateral syndactyly. Differential growth has deviated the longer digits.

Several important surgical principles apply to the correction of syndactyly. These include the timing of the procedure(s), the order of release of multiple web space syndactylies, the creation of a commissure, the techniques of separation and resurfacing of the digits, as well as the postoperative dressing and aftercare.

Timing of Surgery

Syndactyly release has been performed in the neonatal period,[37,52] during infancy, or delayed until childhood. Long-term reviews by Flatt[26] and Ger[27] have shown better outcomes with release after 18 months. Many authors, however, prefer to undertake surgery when the patient is approximately 12 months of age to decrease the risk of developing increasing deformity. The goal is to complete all the releases by school age.

Syndactyly involving multiple web spaces requires decision making of the sequence and staging of the release procedures. Only one side of an affected digit should be released at a time to avoid vascular compromise of the skin flaps or digits. Therefore, separation of three or more adjacent digits requires staged procedures. Syndactyly of all web spaces is usually treated in two stages. The first procedure separates the thumb/index finger and long/ring finger web spaces. Three months later, a second procedure separates the index/long finger and ring/small finger web spaces. In addition, the first procedure can be combined with isolated release of the fingertips and distal phalangeal fusions of all the digits to reduce the tethering effect between surgical procedures.[22]

Commissure Reconstruction

A basic tenet of syndactyly release is reconstruction of the interdigital commissure with a local skin flap. These flaps are designed and raised at the beginning of the procedure. A proximally based rectangular flap raised from the dorsum of the syndactyly is the most frequently used method (Figs. 40-6 and 40-7).[4] Several modifications have been proposed, including a trapezoid shape[26] or supplementation with lateral wings,[18,28,50,56] all in an effort to resurface the digits adjacent to the commissure. Many alternative choices for commissure skin are available. Skin from the dorsum of the hand raised as an island flap can be advanced "V-Y" fashion into the web space.[9,55] The palmar surface of the syndactyly alone[6] or in combination with the dorsal surfaces of the syndactyly can be introduced into the web space as apposing triangular flaps.[57]

Commissure reconstruction in incomplete syndactyly may be achieved by deepening the existing web space. This may be accomplished by a simple "Z"-plasty, a four-flap "Z"-plasty, or the double-opposing "Z"-plasty ("butterfly flap") (Fig. 40-8).[54] Other methods include combinations of

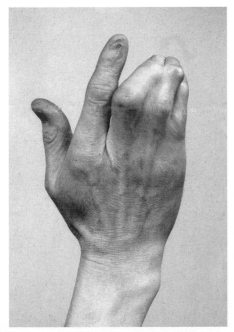

FIGURE 40-5. Dorsal view of right hand with angular deformities of long and ring fingers.

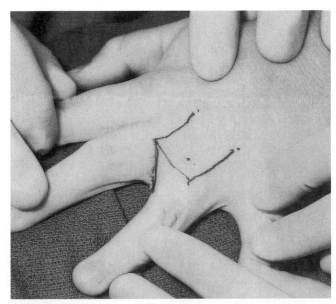

FIGURE 40-6. A proximally based rectangular flap from the dorsum of the syndactyly is the most frequently used method to reconstruct the commissure. (Courtesy of Shriners Hospitals for Children, Philadelphia.)

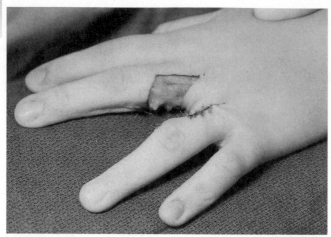

FIGURE 40-7. Dorsal commissure flap inset to reconstruct the web space. (Courtesy of Shriners Hospitals for Children, Philadelphia.)

local flaps, such as the three-flap web-plasty or an "X-M"-plasty.[16]

Syndactyly of the first web space varies in extent. Mild to moderate syndactyly can be treated with a local flap, such as a four-flap "Z"-plasty (Fig. 40-9). Complete syndactyly can be treated by a standard syndactyly release and local commissure flap. Severe syndactyly with marked thumb/index web narrowing may require more skin than is made available by local flaps. In this situation, skin may be imported from the radial border of the index finger as a transposition flap,[27] from the dorsum of the hand after tissue expansion,[10] or as a rotation advancement flap.[8,24] Pedicled or free flaps from distant sites, such as the groin or lateral arm, can also be utilized.[6,43]

Separation of the Digits

Syndactyly release requires careful planning of the skin incisions to maximize use of the available skin and to allow surgical exposure for separation of digits and structures. Incision design must be placed such that scar formation will avoid joint or web space contracture with healing. Numerous patterns of skin incisions have evolved, including laterally based triangular and rectangular flaps.[13,23,40] Cronin's technique of a combination of palmar and dorsal triangular flaps with matched zigzag incisions on both surfaces of the conjoined digits remains the basis of most techniques (Fig. 40-10).[11] Modifications of this pattern have been proposed in an attempt to redistribute the available skin in an asymmetrical manner to avoid skin grafting both sides of the commissure.[4,21,26]

Separation of the digits requires division of fascial interconnections between the digits, with care taken to identify and preserve the individual neurovascular bundles. Bifurcation of the common digital nerve and artery may be distal to the planned position of the web space. Most authors advise ligation of a proper digital vessel.[7] Other authors either curtail the release to this level[26] or reconstruct the vessel to maintain continuity. When multiple digits are released, each digit must have at least one proper artery. Distal bifurcation of the digital nerve is managed by interfascicular dissection and proximal separation.

Resurfacing the Digits

Resurfacing the digits is achieved with local palmar and dorsal flaps supplemented with skin grafts.[17] Full-thickness skin grafts are preferred to split-thickness skin grafts to lessen graft contracture.[12,51,61] Skin grafts are usually

FIGURE 40-8. The double opposing "Z"-plasty or butterfly flap is occasionally useful for mild degrees of web deepening. **A,** The palmar "V" of this flap may be given a stem, converting it to a "Y". **B,** The classic double opposing "Z"-plasty and the flap transfers following mobilization.

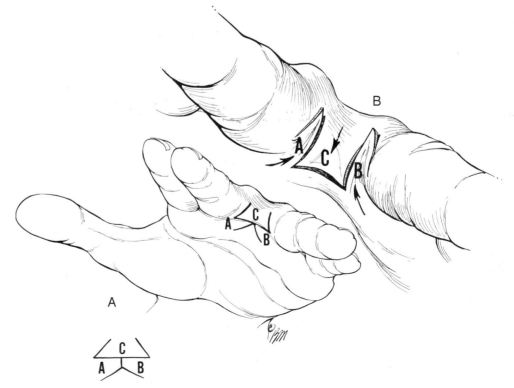

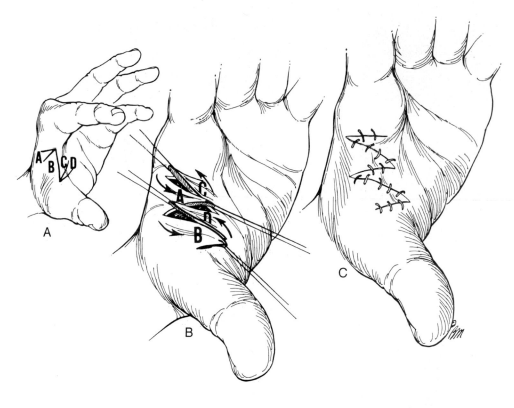

FIGURE 40-9. The standard four-flap "Z"-plasty often used in deepening broader webs such as the thumb web. **A,** The incisions are outlined. **B,** The flaps have been mobilized and crossed. **C,** Closure.

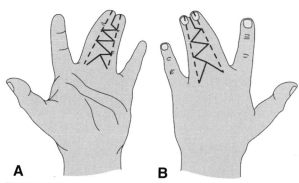

FIGURE 40-10. Cronin's technique of a combination of palmar and dorsal triangular flaps with matched zigzag incisions on both surfaces of the conjoined digits. (From Cronin TD: Syndactylism: Results of zig-zag incision to prevent postoperative contracture. Plast Reconstr Surg 18:460-468, 1956.)

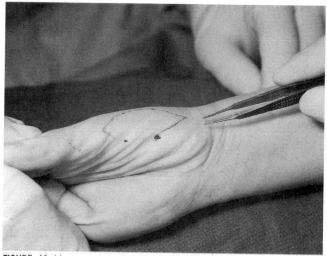

FIGURE 40-11. Full-thickness skin graft harvested from the hypothenar border of the hand for incomplete syndactyly.

obtained from the inguinal donor site.[39] Alternative donor sites include the cubital fossa, the hypothenar border of the hand (Fig. 40-11), or the skin of an accessory digit.[22] The foreskin has been used, although it tends to take poorly and pigments.[26]

Resurfacing the digits without skin graft has been performed to improve overall skin match and to avoid the risk of contracture associated with graft loss.[30] This technique requires reduction of digital diameter via extensive defatting to allow primary coverage while preserving the dorsal venous system.[66] Aggressive defatting, however, carries the risk of vascular injury and may lead to a thin finger after the involution of the fat of infancy.[22] Another option to avoid skin grafting is to import skin from the dorsum of the hand and/or adjacent digits (Figs. 40-12 and 40-13).[28,50] Even more skin can be generated with tissue expanders, although this technique has limited success in

syndactyly.[2] Tissue expansion has also been achieved with transverse soft tissue expansion through the use of a distraction frame.[21]

Paronychial Fold

Release of a complete syndactyly, particularly when associated with distal phalangeal fusion, requires the formation of a paronychial fold. The distal phalangeal tufts may be covered using the procedure described by Buck-Gramcko.[7] Laterally based triangular flaps are raised from the hyponychium of the conjoined digital mass and folded around to form the lateral nail fold (Fig. 40-14). Alternatively, the

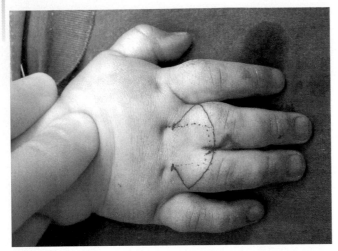

FIGURE 40-12. A triangular lateral extension with the flap can allow direct closure over the dorsum of the finger and can often spare the amount of tissue required in the transverse direction.

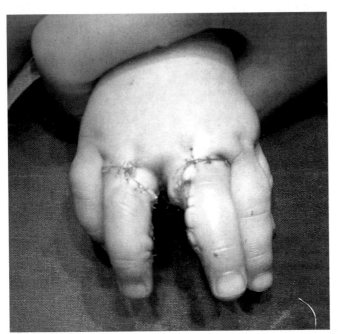

FIGURE 40-13. Postoperative appearance with primary closure of incomplete syndactyly using lateral extension. (Courtesy of Mr. Henk Giele, Oxford, United Kingdom.)

defect may be resurfaced with a skin flap from the conjoined pulp for one of the nail folds and a subcutaneous fat flap from the conjoined pulp covered with a graft for the other nail fold.[7] Distant skin flaps including a thenar flap have been used,[36] but this technique requires delayed division and a second surgical procedure. A composite graft of skin and subcutaneous fat harvested from the toe can also be used to reconstruct the fingertip.[7,42,58]

Outcome

The complexity and technical demands of syndactyly release are often underestimated. An acceptable outcome with independent digits that are freely mobile is usually achieved with simple syndactyly separation. In contrast, the

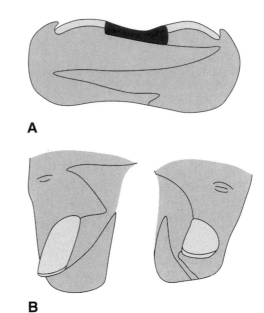

A

B

FIGURE 40-14. A and **B,** Laterally based triangular flaps from the hyponychium of the conjoined digital mass are folded around to form the lateral nail fold. (From Buck-Gramcko D: Congenital malformations: Syndactyly and related deformities. *In* Higst H, Buck-Gramcko D, Millesi H, Lister G (eds): Hand Surgery. New York, Thieme Medical Publishers, 1988.)

outcome after complex syndactyly separation is often limited by associated anomalies and severe skin shortage, which result in diminished mobility.

Complications

Early complications include vascular compromise, infection, wound dehiscence, and graft loss. Defatting and tension-free wound closure are mandatory to prevent dehiscence. Over time, the commissure may advance in a distal direction (web creep) (Fig. 40-15). Poor flap design with

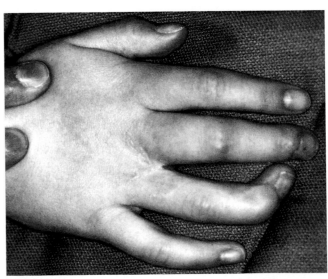

FIGURE 40-15. Ten-year old status post syndactyly release with web creep distal interphalangeal joint instability and angular deformity. (Courtesy of Shriners Hospitals for Children, Philadelphia.)

placement of longitudinal scars at the base of the finger can precipitate web creep. Web creep is also associated with areas of skin graft loss that heal by secondary intention, the use of split-thickness grafts, or the dehiscence of the commissure flap. Joint contractures are a result of scar contracture on the palmar surface of the interphalangeal (IP) joint. This complication may require additional surgery to excise or "Z"-plasty the scar. In the fingertip, inadequate soft tissue bulk and scarring can produce a beaked nail deformity or an inadequate paronychial fold. Lastly, joint instability may occur after separation of complex syndactyly owing to insufficient collateral ligaments (see Fig. 40-15).

Author's Preferred Technique (Complete Syndactyly)

Syndactyly release is performed with the patient under general anesthesia using a pediatric tourniquet and loupe magnification. The groin is preferred as the skin graft donor site to allow full-thickness harvest with minimal morbidity. The graft is drawn in an elliptical fashion to allow primary wound closure and outlined lateral to the femoral artery to decrease the chance of hair growth during puberty.

A dorsal flap is preferred for commissure reconstruction (see Fig. 40-6). The flap begins at the level of the metacarpal heads and encompasses two-thirds the length of the proximal phalanx. On the palmar surface of the dorsal commissure flap a rectangular flap is fashioned to resurface the proximal area of a digit adjacent to the commissure (Fig. 40-16). The proximal transverse incision represents the palmar level of commissure reconstruction, and the distal transverse edge equals the length of the dorsal commissure flap. Subsequently, interdigitating zigzag dorsal and palmar

flaps are constructed distal to the dorsal commissure and palmar rectangular flap (see Fig. 40-10). The dorsal zigzag incision begins at one distal corner of the commissure flap, whereas the palmar incision starts at the opposite corner of the rectangular flap. The dorsal incision extends to the midline of the proximal interphalangeal (PIP) joint of the adjacent finger and back across to the midline of the distal interphalangeal (DIP) joint. At this level, the incision extends distal between the tips of the interconnected digits. The palmar flaps are based opposite the dorsal flaps (mirror images) with the base centered over the opposite PIP and DIP joints to allow for interdigitation. This orientation minimizes the tendency for formation of a flexion scar contracture and maximizes coverage potential. The palmar rectangular flap (opposite the dorsal commissure flap) and zigzag construction is often biased to cover one digit entirely, leaving residual bare areas on the adjacent digit that require skin grafting.

The flaps are elevated by sharp dissection with hemostasis using bipolar electrocautery. Dorsal flaps are elevated first, preserving the paratenon surrounding the extensor tendon. Next, the palmar flaps are raised and the underlying neurovascular bundles isolated. The digits are separated from distal to proximal while protecting the neurovascular bundles. Manual spreading of the digits places the intervening tissue under tension, which facilitates digital separation. The sturdy transverse fascial bands are incised to allow for sufficient proximal placement of the commissure. The transverse intermetacarpal ligament is not divided. The bifurcation between the common and proper neurovascular structures is identified during proximal dissection. A distal split of the digital nerves is easily separated by microdissection. A distal arterial junction requires surgical decision-making, because ligation of a proper digital artery for an acceptable commissure placement is usually required. Selection of the proper digital artery to ligate depends on the status of the proper digital artery on the adjacent sides of the digits being separated. If both digits have intact proper digital arteries on both sides, the smaller artery is usually ligated. However, if one of the digits still requires additional surgery (e.g., staged syndactyly release), then ligation of the larger artery may be considered. If the status of the opposite digital artery is unclear, vascular clamps are applied to the digital arteries and the tourniquet deflated to ensure adequate perfusion of each digit.

Before insetting of the flaps, the adjacent sides of the separated digits are defatted. Defatting decreases the tension across the flaps and improves the overall appearance of the separated digits. The commissure flap is sutured first to assess placement and configuration of the web space. Subsequently, the interdigitating flaps are approximated, avoiding excessive tension. An absorbable 5-0 or 6-0 suture is used for closure. The remaining skin defects are covered with a full-thickness skin graft.

Proper postoperative dressings are an essential part of the operation. The dressings must apply compression across the skin graft sites and protect the separated digits. Nonadhering dressings and moist cotton are placed into the web spaces and reinforced with large amounts of soft gauze. In young children, the compressive hand dressing is reinforced by above-the-elbow plaster immobilization to prevent inadvertent removal. A sugar-tong splint wrapped around the elbow

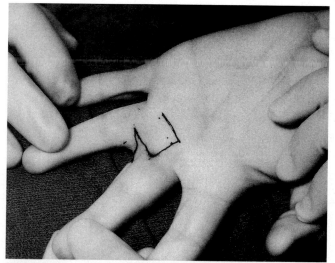

FIGURE 40-16. A palmar rectangular flap to resurface the proximal area of a digit adjacent to the commissure. The proximal transverse incision represents the palmar level of commissure reconstruction. (Courtesy of Shriners Hospitals for Children, Philadelphia.)

and over the hand protects the digits and allows the elbow to be positioned in more than 90 degrees of flexion. The dressings are removed 2 weeks after surgery, and gentle washing and wound care initiated. The wounds are kept covered for an additional week until the scabs desiccate and detach. Normal hand use is encouraged with the dressing removed. Formal therapy is usually not required. Scar massage, silicone gel sheets, or elastomere products can be used to treat areas of hypertrophic scarring.

SPECIAL CASES OF SYNDACTYLY

Acrosyndactyly

Acrosyndactyly is a syndactyly with a fenestration through the web proximal to the distal fusion. It is seen in amniotic disruption sequence, is bilateral in 50% of cases, and is associated with amputations in 50% of patients.[26] The syndactyly can vary from a simple syndactyly to a complex anomaly with distal fusion of multiple digits producing a jumble of fingertips. A distinguishing characteristic of this anomaly is the presence of a sinus tract or cleft from the dorsal to the palmar surface of the conjoined digits (Fig. 40-17).[41] The sinus is variable in size (from a pin tract to a broad passage) and is usually distal to the normal commissure level. The digits distal to the constriction ring may be edematous or atrophic.[3,19,20]

Management is dependent on the severity of the distal deformity and the position and size of the sinus.[26] Mild deformities with well-preserved distal digits can be released with the standard techniques as described previously. The sinus may be incorporated during resurfacing the digit or excised. For more complex deformities, staged release of the fingertips followed by delayed commissure reconstruction is recommended. Staging allows unimpeded growth of the digits. In severe deformities, amputation of atrophic fingertips may be preferred, because the potential for reuniting them with the appropriate digit is limited. In addition to the syndactyly release, associated constriction rings can be managed by excision and "V-Y" plasty.[48]

Apert's Syndrome

Apert's syndrome is the combination of the craniofacial deformity of bicoronal craniosynostosis and midfacial hypoplasia with severe complex syndactyly of the hands and feet.[1] It is due to a mutation of the fibroblast growth factor receptor type 2 gene (FGFR2), which is located on chromosome 10q.[68] Several other acrocephalosyndactyly syndromes have been identified; however, the hand deformities are typically less complex than those of Apert's syndrome.[46] In addition to the characteristic hand deformity, upper limb manifestations include abnormalities of the shoulder and elbow. The development of the glenohumeral joint is asymmetrical with relative overgrowth of the greater tuberosity and a hypoplastic glenoid fossa.[38] Clinically, the shoulder stiffens with growth.[64] Elbow anomalies primarily involve the radiocapitellar articulation. The hand deformities include complex syndactyly of the index, long, and ring fingers and a simple syndactyly between the ring and small fingers. Incomplete first web space syndactyly and radial clinodactyly of the thumb are also present (Fig. 40-18). The fingers are short, and IP joints are stiff in the central rays. There may also be a capitohamate coalition and synostosis between the ring and small metacarpals.[33,63] There is an apparent inverse relationship between the severity of the hand and craniofacial deformities.[64] The hand deformity has been classified according to the involvement of the first web space and conformation of the central mass (Table 40-1).

The management of hand anomalies in patients with Apert's syndrome must be performed in concert with the management of the craniofacial and other associated anomalies. The goal of surgery is to complete separation of the digits and correct the thumb deformity before 2 years of age to allow for growth and the development of function. Surgery to mobilize the small finger by release of the ring and small metacarpals synostosis may be required if the small finger is functional. Surgery is rarely performed about the shoulder and elbow.[64]

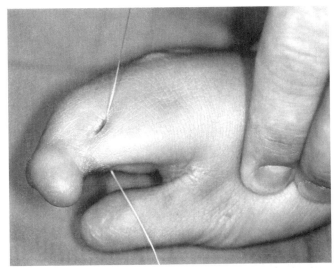

FIGURE 40-17. Acrosyndactyly in amniotic disruption sequence with a sinus tract or cleft from the dorsal to the palmar surface of the conjoined digits.

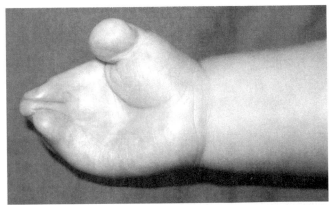

FIGURE 40-18. Complex multiple syndactyly associated with Apert's syndrome. The hand deformity includes complex syndactyly of the index, long, and ring fingers, simple syndactyly between the ring and small fingers, and incomplete first web space.

Table 40-1

CLASSIFICATION OF THE APERT HAND DEFORMITY

Type	First Web	Central Mass	Fourth Web
Type 1: obstetrician or spade hand	Incomplete simple syndactyly	Digital mass flat in palmar plane. Good metacarpophalangeal joint with variable degree of symphalangism at the interphalangeal joints	Incomplete simple syndactyly
Type II: mitten or spoon hand	Complete simple syndactyly	Digital mass forms palmar concavity with splaying of metacarpals proximally and tight fusion of fingertips distally with synonychia of central digital mass	Complete simple syndactyly
Type III: hoof or rosebud hand	Complete complex syndactyly	Thumb incorporated into mass, which is tightly cupped. Synonychia of all digits apart from the small finger. Skeletal abnormalities of index ray. Complicated by paronychial infections and maceration of palmar skin	Simple syndactyly usually with metacarpal synostosis of fourth and fifth metacarpals

From Upton J: Apert syndrome: Classification and pathologic anatomy of limb anomalies. Clin Plast Surg 18:321-355, 1991.

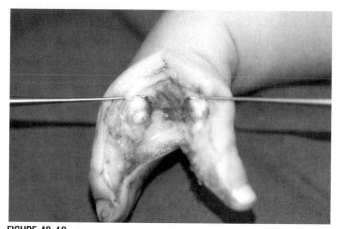

FIGURE 40-19. First web space release with sequential release of the skin and fascia, intrinsic muscle lengthening, and capsulotomy of the CMC joint to position the thumb into abduction.

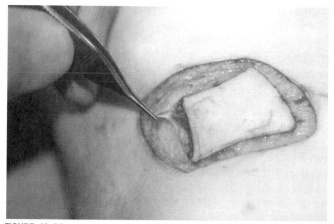

FIGURE 40-20. A free groin flap for severe contracture of the first web space.

Reconstruction of an adequate first web space is the first priority. Sequential release of the skin and fascia, intrinsic muscle lengthening, and capsulotomy of the carpometacarpal (CMC) joint allow the thumb ray to be positioned in 45 degrees of abduction (Fig. 40-19). Minor first web space narrowing can be addressed with local flaps such as a four-flap "Z"-plasty.[57] Considerable narrowing with deficient skin requires a dorsal advancement rotation flap[8,24] or preliminary tissue expansion on the dorsum of the hand.[10] I prefer to use a transposition flap from the radial border of the index finger for incomplete thumb-index finger syndactyly. The index finger flap can lengthen the first web space and be positioned into the thenar crease to correct any associated flexion-adduction contracture. For severe contracture of the first web space, a groin or lateral arm flap is used as a free tissue transfer (Fig. 40-20). Substantial tissue is placed within the first web space, which adds bulk to maintain the abducted position of the thumb (Figs. 40-21 and 40-22). In my experience, the flap caliber of vessels

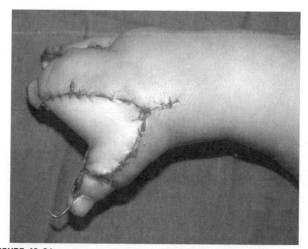

FIGURE 40-21. Restoration of substantial soft tissue within the first web space after free groin flap.

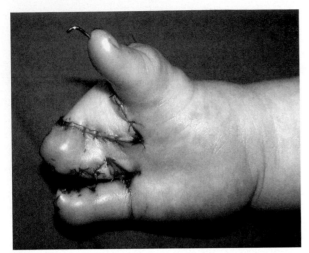

FIGURE 40-22. Another view of restoration of substantial soft tissue within the first web space after free groin flap.

within the first web space is adequate for microvascular anastomosis. The thumb clinodactyly can be corrected with a corrective osteotomy of the phalanx. An opening wedge osteotomy and a bone graft are preferred to lengthen the shortened thumb. Usually there is a resultant skin shortage on the radial aspect of the thumb that can be addressed with "Z"-plasty. Thumb clinodactyly surgery may be combined with the release of the fourth and fifth metacarpal synostosis between the ages of 4 and 6 years.

Release of the finger syndactylies is usually staged.[65] Anomalies of the neurovascular bundles are common. The surgical plan is influenced by the extent of the first web space reconstruction and the status of the index finger. A severely deformed index may be sacrificed if it is unlikely to yield a stable finger of adequate length. More information about the skeleton abnormality can be assessed with three-dimensional computed tomography, which may be combined with the craniofacial imaging.[32] Syndactyly release of the most severe connections may be simplified by releasing the distal osseous union via a fishmouth incision, thereby converting the tight bunched hand into the flat "spade" of the type I deformity. Stabilization in this posture is attained with a transverse Kirschner wire. The syndactyly is then released by standard techniques.[64] I have staged the release of the severely deformed hand by releasing the distal osseous fusion and dividing the common nail plate through dorsal incisions between the distal digits. This converts the complex syndactyly to a simple syndactyly and releases the digits from the osseous tether. The interdigital defects are resurfaced with full-thickness grafts to allow some differential motion between the digits. The grafts generate enough pulp skin to provide adequate pulp and paronychial flaps for the release of the fingers at a later stage.[7]

Surgery to mobilize the small finger may be required if it is functional. Release of the synostosis between the ring and small metacarpals should include fascia or fat interposition to prevent recurrence. Upton's experience suggests that this procedure is best delayed until 5 years of age to decrease the incidence of recurrence.[64] The position of the fifth ray can be improved by release of the CMC joint to allow flexion of the metacarpal. This surgery can be combined with angular correction of the deviated thumb.

Symbrachydactyly

Symbrachydactyly consists of short stiff fingers that are often combined with syndactyly. Symbrachydactyly occurs sporadically and is associated with Poland's syndrome. The anomaly is usually unilateral, and the severity varies from almost complete absence of digits to relatively well-formed short fingers. When the digits are well formed, the syndactyly component requires intervention.[57] The technique may be modified to include division of the transverse metacarpal ligament to increase the mobility and apparent length of the fingers. The commissure should not be placed too proximal between the metacarpal heads at the risk of producing a narrowed, "V"-shaped web space.[26]

Poland syndrome

Poland syndrome has been attributed to disruption of the blood flow in the subclavian artery in the embryo, producing a spectrum of hypoplastic anomalies in the upper limb.[5] The syndrome is defined by the aplasia of the sternocostal head of the pectoralis major; brachydactyly affecting the index, long, and ring fingers; hypoplasia of the hand; and syndactyly of the digits.[35,59] The chest wall anomalies may be extensive and include hypoplasia of the breast, aplasia of the pectoralis minor and latissimus dorsi, and skeletal thoracic wall anomalies. The hand deformity is variable, but the central digits are most commonly affected and are usually shortened secondary to an undersized middle phalanx. The syndactyly is usually simple and either complete or incomplete. Surgical separation follows the timing and technique described previously.

Dystrophic epidermolysis bullosa

Syndactyly in dystrophic epidermolysis bullosa is not truly a congenital anomaly but rather a consequence of the scarring from this blistering condition of the squamous epithelial surfaces. Epidermolysis bullosa (EB) is a rare heterogeneous group of congenital blistering conditions. The skin structure is disrupted by a loss of the normal adhesion between the various lamina of the skin.[45] The variants are classified according to the level and cause of

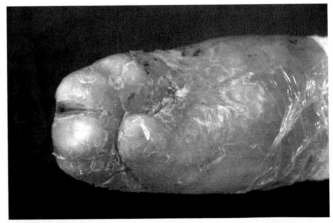

FIGURE 40-23. The hand deformity in dystrophic epidermolysis bullosa with flexion contractures of the digits that have become cocooned into a common mass.

blistering. EB simplex variants blister at the basal keratinocyte level, junctional EB blisters within the lamina lucida of the basement membrane, and dystrophic EB blisters because of abnormal anchoring collagen VII fibrils within the papillary dermis. Dystrophic EB is associated with repeated dermal injury. The inevitable scarring produces syndactyly and contracture in the hands. Autosomal dominant and recessive forms of dystrophic EB have been recognized, with the recessive form being the most severe. Typically, the hand deformity progresses toward flexion contractures of the digits that become cocooned into a common mass (Fig. 40-23). The thumb can be included within the cocoon. The hand problem, however, is only part of a complex condition that requires a multidisciplinary approach to management. Treatment of the hand is based around release and resurfacing of the syndactyly and con-

tractures. Radical release, particularly of the first web space, is recommended to maintain some hand function.[60,62] Syndactyly release is performed with straight-line incisions. The skin deficits can be allowed to heal by secondary intention[57,67] or by using the skin of the cocoon,[69] skin flaps from filleted fingers,[29] or grafts.[45] Split-thickness skin grafts are preferred, although I have successfully used free groin flaps to resurface the vital first web space. Despite initially satisfactory results, recurrence is common, with reoperation rates over 50%.[60]

ANNOTATED REFERENCES

30. Greuse M, Coessens BC: Congenital syndactyly: Defatting facilitates closure without skin graft. J Hand Surg [Am] 26:589-594, 2001.

     Syndactyly was corrected without skin grafts in 16 consecutive patients (24 syndactylies). Digital volume decreased by defatting the full length of the fingers to allow closure of the fingers with minimal tension. Defatting was believed to be the most important determinant of whether the wound could be closed. Results were evaluated after a mean follow-up period of 22 months. Supple and good quality scars were observed in all but 2 patients. The technique remains controversial.

39. Kozin SH: Syndactyly. J Am Soc Surg Hand 1:1-13, 2001.

     The various forms of syndactyly are reviewed and the established principles with regard to timing, technique, and postoperative management are detailed. Technical details are described and highlighted. A classification system is provided to guide management.

52a. Rider MA, Grindel SI, Tonkin MA, Wood VE: An experience of the Snow-Littler procedure. J Hand Surg [Br] 25:376-381, 2000.

     Snow-Littler procedure results are reported in 12 hands with classic central longitudinal deficiency and in 1 hand with symbrachydactyly. No instances of major flap necrosis were seen although two flaps showed tip ischemia. The width of the first web was satisfactory, although four web space revisions were performed. Three derotational osteotomies of transposed index fingers were performed. Improved appearance and function were evident. The Snow-Littler procedure is preferred for the cleft hand combined with thumb/index finger syndactyly.

65. Van Heest AE, House JH, Reckling WC: Two-stage reconstruction of Apert acrosyndactyly. J Hand Surg [Am] 22:315-322, 1997.

     Twenty-eight hands (14 children) with Apert's acrosyndactyly were evaluated and a classification system developed. Type I deformities (7 hands) had minimal angular deformity at the metacarpophalangeal (MCP) joint; two-stage reconstruction created a four-fingered hand. Type IIA deformities (11 hands) had mild MCP joint angular deformity and a more proximal complex syndactyly of the middle three digits; two-stage reconstruction created a three-fingered hand with ray resection of the third digit. Type IIB deformities (7 hands) had pronation of digit 2 superimposed on the thumb and radial angulation at the MCP joint of digit 2; two-stage reconstruction created a three-fingered hand with ray resection of the second digit. Type IIC deformities (3 hands) had supination of digit 4 superimposed on digit 5 with ulnar angulation at the MP joint of digits 4 and 5; two-stage reconstruction created a three-fingered hand with ray resection of the fourth digit. The article offers a management algorithm for Apert's acrosyndactyly to guide the hand type and staging of reconstruction.

CRITICAL POINTS: SYNDACTYLY

- Syndactyly may involve only the soft tissue (simple) or include bony connections (complex).

- Atypical forms of syndactyly are labeled complicated and present as either convoluted soft tissue abnormalities or a hodgepodge of abnormal bones. Many atypical configurations occur in conjunction with a variety of syndromes.

- Mild, incomplete syndactyly that does not interfere with function does not require treatment. In contrast, simple syndactyly of any considerable degree warrants surgical reconstruction of the web space for improved function and appearance.

- Border digits (thumb/index finger and ring/small finger web spaces) have marked differences in their respective lengths and should be separated within the first few months of life. This prevents tethering of the longer digit that results in a flexion contracture and rotational deformity.

- Syndactyly that combines digits of relatively equal lengths (e.g., long/ring finger web space) negates the development of deformity. Separation may be delayed until the child is older and the hand larger to facilitate surgical reconstruction.

- Surgical reconstruction should only include one side of an affected digit at a time to avoid vascular compromise of the skin flaps and/or digit.

- Surgical reconstruction of the commissure must be free of skin graft. Creation of a flap to re-create the commissure avoids interdigital contracture.

- Complex syndactyly is more challenging to treat, especially as the quantity of bony union increases.

Ulnar Polydactyly

Scott H. Kozin

EPIDEMIOLOGY

Polydactyly can occur on the preaxial (radial) and postaxial (ulnar) side of the limb. Postaxial polydactyly is frequently inherited via an autosomal dominant pattern but has a variable penetrance pattern. Postaxial polydactyly is more common in Africans and African Americans. Preaxial polydactyly is more frequent in whites.[2,3] The prevalence of postaxial polydactyly in African Americans is estimated to be 1 in 143 live births. In comparison, the prevalence of postaxial polydactyly in whites is estimated to be 1 in 1339 live births. Postaxial polydactyly in a white individual is often indicative of an underlying syndrome (e.g., chondroectodermal dysplasia or Ellis-van Creveld syndrome) (Fig. 40-24).[3]

CLASSIFICATION AND MANAGEMENT

The supernumerary digit is either well developed (type A) or rudimentary and pedunculated (type B).[3] A small nubbin or scrawny postaxial element (type B) can be safely removed by tying the base of the pedicle in the nursery (Fig. 40-25). Suture or vessel clips can be applied to the base of the digit. The digit will turn gangrenous and fall from the hand.[1,3] A residual bump or nubbin is the most common complication (Fig. 40-26).[3]

A well-developed or near-normal digit (type A) requires operative ablation. The extra digit is removed, and any important functional parts (e.g., ulnar collateral ligament and abductor digiti quinti) are transferred to the adjacent finger.

An elliptical incision around the digit is outlined (Fig. 40-27). The incision is extended in a proximal direction to

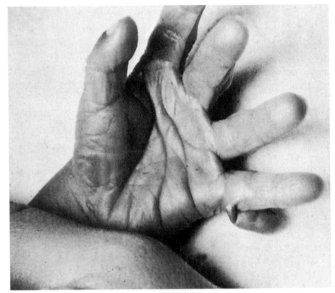

FIGURE 40-25. Postaxial type B polydactyly with rudimentary postaxial element.

allow adequate exposure. Anomalous tendons are removed with the extra digit. The digital nerves are incised, and the digital arteries are coagulated. If the ablated digit contains the abductor digiti quinti, the muscle and tendon to the adjacent digit are transferred to restore digital abduction. The skin is closed with absorbable suture and the limb immobilized in a long-arm cast for 3 weeks to protect any ligament and/or muscle-tendon transfer.

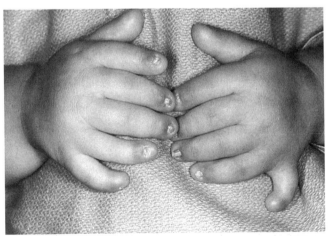

FIGURE 40-24. Postaxial polydactyly in chondroectodermal dysplasia or Ellis-van Creveld syndrome. Dorsal view demonstrates the characteristic nail dysplasia.

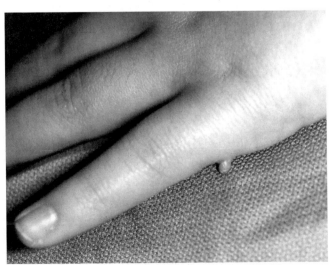

FIGURE 40-26. A residual nubbin after suture ligation of postaxial polydactyly. (Courtesy of Shriners Hospitals for Children, Philadelphia.)

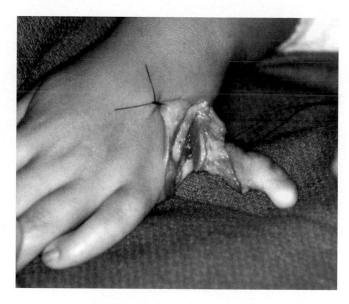

FIGURE 40-27. An elliptical incision around the postaxial digit that is extended in a proximal direction to allow adequate removal of the digit. (Courtesy of Shriners Hospitals for Children, Philadelphia.)

CRITICAL POINTS: ULNAR POLYDACTYLY

- Postaxial polydactyly is frequently inherited via an autosomal dominant pattern but has a variable penetrance pattern. Postaxial polydactyly is more common in African Americans, and preaxial polydactyly is more frequent in whites.
- A small nubbin or rudimentary postaxial element can be safely removed by tying the base of the pedicle in the nursery.
- A well-developed postaxial polydactyly requires operative ablation with transfer of any important parts (e.g., ulnar collateral ligament and abductor digiti quinti) to the adjacent finger.

ANNOTATED REFERENCE

3. Watson BT, Hennrikus WL: Postaxial type-B polydactyly: Prevalence and treatment. J Bone Joint Surg Am 79:65-68, 1997.

A prospective screening program of 11,161 newborns identified 21 infants with postaxial type B polydactyly. Sixteen infants (76%) had bilateral postaxial type B polydactyly. Eighteen infants (86%) had a family history of the anomaly. The racial prevalence was 1 in 143 live births of black infants and 1 in 1339 live births of white infants. The duplicated small fingers were treated in the newborn nursery with suture ligation at the base of the pedicle. No major complications occurred. A residual bump was the most common sequelae, although all of the parents were satisfied with the cosmetic result.

Central Polydactyly

Scott H. Kozin

EPIDEMIOLOGY

Central polydactyly is an extra digit within the hand and not along its borders. Central polydactyly is uncommon compared with border polydactyly.[1] The ring digit is the most common duplication, followed by the long finger, and lastly the index digit.[4] Central polydactyly occurs in isolation or is part of a syndrome, such as Grebes' chondrodysplasia (see Fig. 39-7). The central polydactyly may be hidden within a concomitant syndactyly (i.e., synpolydactyly) (see Figs. 39-5 and 39-6). Identification of synpolydactyly requires careful examination supplemented by radiographic verification. A particular form of central polydactyly (ring finger duplication) combined with syndactyly has familial propagation and has been linked to a gene mutation (*HOXD13*) on chromosome 2.[2]

MANAGEMENT

Treatment depends on the status and extent of the extra digit and the presence or absence of concurrent anomalies, such as syndactyly. A central polydactyly that has a fully formed digit and normal function does not require removal to restore the normal complement of digits (Fig. 40-28). An isolated central polydactyly with limited motion of the extra

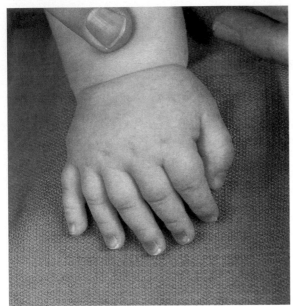

FIGURE 40-28. One-year-old child with central polydactyly consisting of five fingers with full motion and function. (Courtesy of Shriners Hospitals for Children, Philadelphia.)

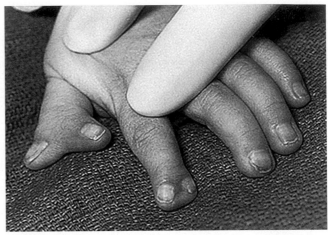

FIGURE 40-30. Partial index finger polydactyly with concomitant thumb duplication. (Courtesy of Shriners Hospitals for Children, Philadelphia.)

digit is treated with ray resection. The span of the hand is maintained by transposition of adjacent digits and/or intermetacarpal ligament reconstruction. Synpolydactyly is treated with syndactyly separation and reduction of the concealed polydactyly. Complete removal of the redundant bones, however, is difficult to accomplish without jeopardizing joint structure or digital circulation. The result is often incomplete resection of the surplus bones that enhances appearance but not motion (Fig. 40-29). Partial central polydactyly is treated with similar principles used to

CRITICAL POINTS: CENTRAL POLYDACTYLY

- Central polydactyly is uncommon compared with border polydactyly.
- Central polydactyly may be hidden within a concomitant syndactyly (i.e., synpolydactyly).
- Synpolydactyly is difficult to treat. Syndactyly separation and reduction of the concealed polydactyly often results in incomplete resection of the extra bones without an increase in motion.
- Central synpolydactyly with complicated connections may be better untreated rather than separated into individual digits with limited motion and instability.

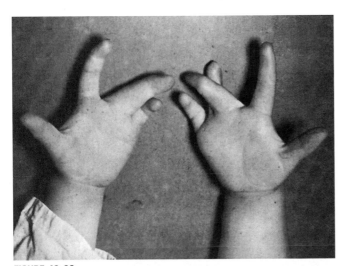

FIGURE 40-29. After release of central synpolydactyly, angular deformity and stiffness may be evident in released fingers. (From Wood VE: Treatment of central polydactyly. Clin Orthop 74:196-205, 1971, with permission.)

reconstruct the duplicated thumb (Fig. 40-30).[1] Creativity and intraoperative flexibility may be required to restore the best functioning digit using components of each part.[1] Multiple surgeries may be required, and the outcome may still be disappointing.[3] Similar to complex syndactyly, duplicated digits with complicated connections may be better left untreated rather than separated into individual digits with limited motion and instability.

ANNOTATED REFERENCE

1. Graham TJ, Ress AM: Finger polydactyly. Hand Clin 14:49-64, 1998.

   This review article on finger polydactyly discusses the incidence, genetics, and inheritance and highlights the principles of management with illustrative case examples.

Mirror Hand

Scott H. Kozin

Mirror hand is a rare congenital anomaly characterized by symmetrical duplication of the limb at the midline. Typically, there is a central digit with three digits on each side that represent the middle, ring, and small digits in mirrored symmetry (Fig. 40-31).[2,6] Despite the seven digits, the thumb is absent. Within the forearm, there are two ulnae and no radius. The ulnae support duplicated ulnar carpal elements. The duplicated ulna has led to the term *ulnar dimelia* (Fig. 40-32).[1] There are many variants, however, that complicate classification and treatment. The notion that mirror hand is a spectrum that culminates in the exceedingly rare anomaly of multiple hands has been presented (Table 40-2).[1,2,6]

The preaxial ulna is often short and the hand positions into radial deviation. The soft tissue anatomy is bizarre and

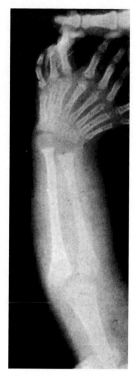

FIGURE 40-32. Ulnar dimelia with two ulnae and no radius articulating with the humerus. One distal ulna is broad, resembling a distal radius. The hand consists of eight fingers.

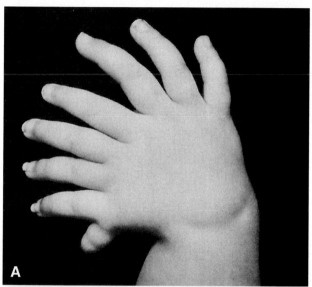

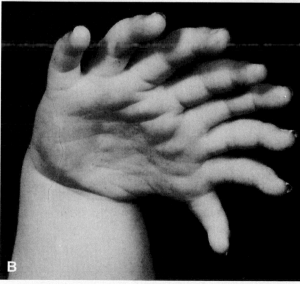

FIGURE 40-31. A and **B,** Mirror hand with eight digits.

Table 40-2
CLASSIFICATION OF MIRROR HANDS

Type	Name	Clinical Features
1	Ulnar dimelia	Multiple fingers with two ulnae Type A: Each ulna well formed Type B: Preaxial ulna hypoplastic
2	Intermediate form	Multiple fingers with two ulnae and a radius
3	Intermediate form	Multiple fingers with one ulna and a radius Type A: Radius well formed Type B: Hypoplastic radius
4	Syndromic form	Bilateral, mirror feet and nasal defects characteristic Type A: Sandrow's syndrome—two ulnae Type B: Martin's syndrome—an ulna and a radius
5	Multiple hand	Complete duplication of the hand including the thumb; forearm normal

Adapted from Al-Qattan MM, Al-Thunayan M, De Cordier M, et al: Classification of the mirror hand-multiple hand spectrum. J Hand Surg [Br] 23:534-536, 1998.

CONGENITAL DISORDERS

complicated. Unpredictable anatomic variations are commonplace. Barton and colleagues[2] have summarized some of the peculiarities.

ETIOLOGY

The etiology has been attributed to replication of the signaling center that controls radioulnar development. The zone of polarizing activity (ZPA) within the posterior margin of the limb bud polarizes the limb into a radioulnar axis and governs preaxial-postaxial limb development.[4] Transplantation of the ZPA or its signaling molecule, sonic hedgehog protein, causes mirror duplication of the ulnar aspect of the limb (see Fig. 39-4).

The examination of the mirror hand begins with an inventory of the number and function of the digits. The amount of wrist, forearm, and elbow motion is recorded. Limited wrist extension is common secondary to concomitant deficiency of the wrist extensor tendons (Fig. 40-33). There is limited forearm and elbow motion, because the presence of two ulnae prevents normal movement.

MANAGEMENT

Treatment is designed to reduce the number of digits to four and reconstruct a thumb from the deleted digits (Fig. 40-34). Selective ablation of the supernumerary digits and thumb reconstruction are the mainstays of surgery. The procedure must reconstruct the first web space and augment the motor function of the preserved thumb via tendon transfer (Fig. 40-35). The principles of pollicization and "spare parts" are used to construct the thumb.[3,5]

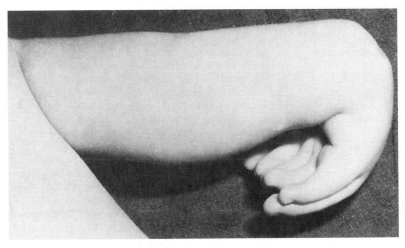

FIGURE 40-33. The absence or paucity of wrist and finger extensors results in severe flexion contracture in many children with ulnar dimelia. (Courtesy of Professor Dieter Buck-Gramcko.)

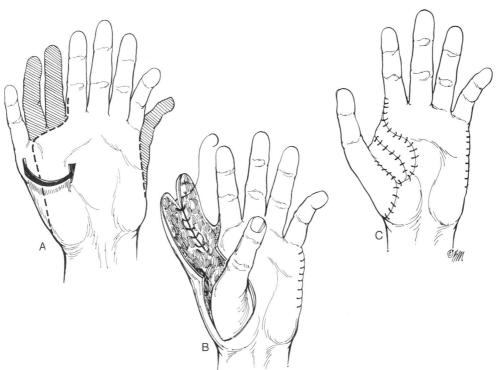

FIGURE 40-34. A to **C,** When eight digits are present, the most preaxial digit may be retained and pollicized whereas the second and third digits are filleted to surface the first web space. Amputation of the most postaxial digit improves the cascade alignment of the four residual fingers.

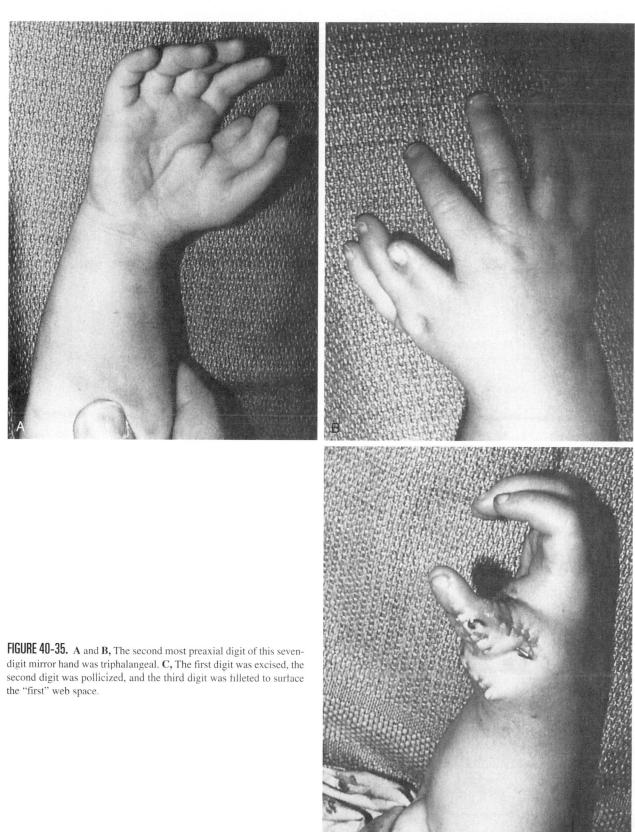

FIGURE 40-35. **A** and **B,** The second most preaxial digit of this seven-digit mirror hand was triphalangeal. **C,** The first digit was excised, the second digit was pollicized, and the third digit was filleted to surface the "first" web space.

CRITICAL POINTS: MIRROR HAND

- Mirror hand is rare and is characterized by symmetrical duplication of the limb at the midline. Typically, there is a central digit with three digits on each side and an absence of the thumb.
- The forearm often has two ulnae and no radius.
- The etiology has been attributed to transplantation or replication of the zone of polarizing activity (ZPA) from the posterior margin of the limb bud into the anterior region.
- Treatment includes reducing the number of digits to four and reconstructing a thumb from the deleted digits.

ANNOTATED REFERENCES

1. Al-Qattan MM, Al-Thunayan M, De Cordier M, et al: Classification of the mirror hand-multiple hand spectrum. J Hand Surg [Br] 23:534-536, 1998.

The article presents an interesting classification of the mirror hand–multiple hand spectrum. Classification begins with classic "ulnar dimelia" and progresses to the rare multiple hand deformity. Intermediate types are included with the duplicated ulna evolving into a radius.

2. Barton NJ, Buck-Gramcko D, Evans DM: Soft-tissue anatomy of mirror hand. J Hand Surg [Br] 11:307-319, 1986.

The article summarizes the soft tissue anatomy of mirror hand. Unpredictable anatomic variations are commonplace. The surgeon must be aware of these anomalies during reconstruction of the mirror hand.

3. Barton NJ, Buck-Gramcko D, Evans DM, et al: Mirror hand treated by true pollicization. J Hand Surg [Br] 11:320-336, 1986.

The article discusses treatment of the mirror hand with reduction of the supernumerary digits and thumb reconstruction using the principles of pollicization and the use of "spare parts." Adequate first web space reconstruction is critical to create a functioning thumb.

Brachydactyly

David McCombe and Simon P. Kay

The term *brachydactyly* describes a short finger where all the elements of the digital skeleton are present but one or more are reduced in size.[9] The description can be extended by specification of the bone involved. *Brachytelophalangy, brachymesophalangy,* and *brachybasophalangy* refer to short distal, middle, and proximal phalanges, respectively. *Brachymetacarpia* refers to shortening of the metacarpal. These specific terms are rarely used anymore, because *brachydactyly* has become the preferred terminology. Brachydactyly may occur in isolation, as part of a complex hand anomaly, as a constituent of a generalized syndrome, or as a consequence of trauma (Table 40-3). The functional and aesthetic aspects of brachydactyly can range from minimal to considerable, depending on the degree of shortening and the status of the remaining digits. The diagnostic aspects and genetic implications are pertinent to the patient and family.

EPIDEMIOLOGY

Brachydactyly, as a feature of congenital hand anomalies, is quite common. Anomalies where brachydactyly is the dominant feature are rare and are typically inherited anomalies with an autosomal dominant pattern of inheritance. Brachydactyly may also occur as a sporadic anomaly or may be part of a systemic syndrome that does not conform to the

classification. For example, short metacarpals are seen with pseudohypoparathyroidism or pseudopseudohypoparathyroidism (Fig. 40-36). Lastly, noncongenital brachydactyly can occur after growth plate injury from trauma, infection, or frostbite.

CLASSIFICATION

Bell's classification is the most widely quoted classification of inherited anomalies that include brachydactyly as the dominant feature. These have been classified by Bell[4] into brachydactyly A to E based on phenotypes expressed within pedigrees. Following the initial description in 1951,[4] the classification has been modified by numerous authors with additions of variants and subclassifications (Table 40-4).[3,12,16,17,24]

PATHOLOGY

Recent research has identified candidate genes for some forms of brachydactyly through pedigree analysis and DNA examination. Various mutations have been identified that affect digital length. Brachydactyly E[23] has been linked to a Glypican 1 gene mutation on Ch2q; brachydactyly B[22] has been associated with mutations of *ROR2*, a tyrosine kinase

Table 40-3
SYNDROMES ASSOCIATED WITH BRACHYDACTYLY

Generalized Brachydactyly	***D Brachydactyly (Stub Thumb Brachydactyly)***
Achondroplasia	Tabatzinik's syndrome
Hypochondroplasia	Rubinstein-Taybi syndrome
Diastrophic dwarfism	Robinow's syndrome
Mucopolysaccharidosis	
Multiple epiphyseal dysplasia	***Brachydactyly with Metacarpal Shortening***
Spondyloepiphyseal dysplasia	Turner's syndrome
Metaphyseal dysostosis	Albright's hereditary osteodystrophy
Peripheral dysostosis	Pseudohypoparathyroidism
Dyschondrosteosis	Pseudopseudohypoparathyroidism
Hereditary multiple exostosis	
Ollier's disease	***Brachydactyly with Short First Metacarpal***
Weill-Marchesani syndrome	Holt-Oram syndrome
Ellis-van Creveld syndrome	Fanconi's anemia
Orofaciodigital syndrome	Progressive myositis ossificans
	Otopalatodigital syndrome
Underdevelopment of Distal Phalanges	Diastrophic dwarfism
Pyknodysostosis	
Cleidocranial dysostosis	***Brachydactyly with Polydactyly***
Fanconi's anemia	Ellis-van Creveld syndrome
Progeria	Orofaciodigital syndrome
Larsen's syndrome	
Keutel's syndrome	***Brachydactyly with Syndactyly***
Pudiger's syndrome	Cornelia de Lange syndrome
Coffin-Siris syndrome	Apert's syndrome
A3 Brachydactyly (Short Middle Phalanx of Little Finger)	***Brachydactyly with Cone-Shaped Epiphyses***
Down syndrome	Trichorhinophalangeal syndrome
Poly X syndrome	Langer-Giedion syndrome
Russell-Silver syndrome	Acrodysostosis
Coffin-Siris syndrome	
Orofaciodigital syndrome (types I and II)	***Miscellaneous***
Otopalatodigital syndrome	Du Pan's syndrome
Thrombocytopenia-absent radius syndrome	Hand-foot-uterus syndrome
Noonan's syndrome	

From Kelikian H: Congenital Deformities of the Hand and Forearm. Philadelphia, WB Saunders, 1974.

receptor gene at Ch9q22; brachydactyly A1[11,15] has been related to nucleotide mutations within the Indian hedgehog gene; and brachydactyly C[8,20] has been associated with mutations in the gene for growth differentiation factor-5.

Deficiencies in a cartilage-derived morphogenetic protein have also been associated with various forms of brachydactyly. Grebes' and Hunter-Thompson chondrodysplasias are associated with severe brachydactyly and have been directly related to a cartilage-derived morphogenetic protein deficiency (see Fig. 39-7).[2,6]

These mutations account for some forms of brachydactyly; however, a variety of additional genetic mutations have yet to be determined to explain the numerous phenotypes.

CLINICAL FEATURES

The severity of the digital shortening is variable. Mild shortening may be apparent only because the normal cascade of the digits is disrupted. The most commonly affected phalanx is the middle phalanx, which is the last component of the digital skeleton to ossify. The small finger and the index are the most commonly affected digits.[9,18] Associated anomalies, such as syndactyly, clinodactyly, and/or symphalangism, also exist and often create a greater functional problem than the brachydactyly (Fig. 40-37).

Careful examination of the remainder of the upper limb, the pectoral girdle, the contralateral upper limb, and the lower limbs is a requisite. Additional limb or chest wall involvement may lead to a diagnosis of a specific form of brachydactyly or a more inclusive anomaly, such as Poland's syndrome. Examination of parents and siblings may reveal further evidence of an inherited anomaly, although the phenotype may not be uniform throughout the affected family members because of variable expression. Traumatic brachydactyly is usually identified via a history of injury and subsequent radiographs that reveal physeal arrest.

MANAGEMENT

The management of brachydactyly depends on the degree of shortening, associated anomalies, and status of the remaining digits. In a complex anomaly, brachydactyly may be a relatively minor component compared with the syndactyly, clinodactyly, and/or symphalangism. As an isolated

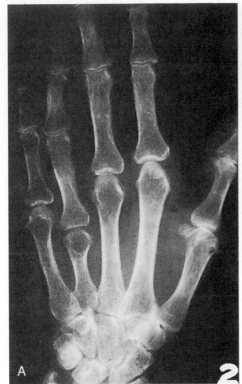

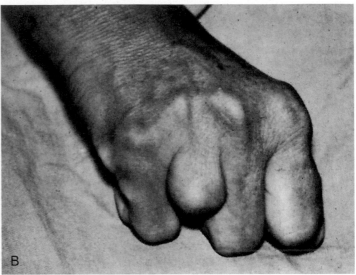

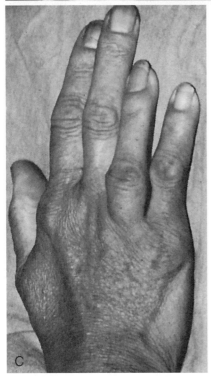

FIGURE 40-36. **A,** In this patient with pseudohypoparathyroidism, only the ring finger is short. **B,** A gap appears when a fist is made. **C,** Instead of a graceful curve of the fingertips, a jagged irregularity appears.

deformity, the indications for intervention are either aesthetic or functional. The appearance of the hand is most affected when there is disruption of the normal cascade of the hand, particularly the central digits (see Fig. 40-36). A short central metacarpal head may be palpable in the palm and interfere with power grip.

Enthusiasm for surgery on the part of the parents, patient, or surgeon must be tempered by potential problems of lengthening, including joint stiffness, contracture, and loss of hand function.[10] Lengthening of the shortened digital skeleton requires osteotomy of the shortened element, distraction to the desired length, and either bone grafting or bone regeneration of the lengthened skeleton. The technique varies with regard to approach, configuration of the osteotomy, and a method of bone lengthening (i.e., immediate lengthening versus gradual distraction osteogenesis).

Table 40-4
MODIFIED BELL CLASSIFICATION OF BRACHYDACTYLY

Type A

A1: Farabee brachydactyly (Farabee, 1903) — *Principal feature:* short middle phalanges (sometimes fused to distal phalanges)
Associated feature: short proximal phalanges of thumbs and great toes

A2: Mohr-Wriedt brachydactyly (Mohr, 1919) — *Principal feature:* short "delta" phalanx deformity—middle phalanges, index fingers, and second toes

A3: Bauer brachydactyly—clinodactyly (brachymesophalangy V) (Bauer, 1970) — *Principal feature:* short rhomboid or "delta" middle phalanx—small finger

A4: Temtamy brachydactyly (Temtamy, 1978) — *Principal feature:* short middle phalanges of index and small fingers.
Associated features: ring finger, middle phalanx, short middle phalanges of toes, and talipes calcaneovalgus

A5: Bass brachydactyly (Bass, 1968) — *Principal feature:* absent middle phalanges, hypoplastic nails in fingers and toes
Associated features: Hypoplastic distal phalanges

Type B

Mackinder brachydactyly (MacKinder, 1857) — *Principal feature:* hypoplastic distal phalanges with absent nails
Associated features: thumbs and great toes may be normal or duplication of distal phalanges
Symphalangism
Syndactyly

Type C

Drinkwater brachydactyly (Drinkwater, 1916) — *Principal feature:* short middle phalanx index and middle fingers. Short "delta" middle phalanx, small finger. Hyperphalangism of index and middle fingers with ulnar deviation of these digits
Associated feature: short metacarpals
Symphalangism

Type D

Breitenbecher brachydactyly (stub thumb) (Breitenbecher, 1923) — *Principal feature:* short distal phalanx of thumb

Type E

Bell brachydactyly (brachymetacarpia/brachymetatarsia) (Bell, 1951) — *Principal feature:* short metacarpals/metatarsals with normal length phalanges
Associated feature: short stature

Subclassified by Hertzog (Hertzog, 1968) — Joint laxity

Type E1 — Short fourth metacarpals/metatarsals

Type E2 — Variable combinations of short metacarpals and phalanges

Type E3 — Variable combinations of short metacarpals with normal phalanges

Other

Pitt-Williams brachydactyly (Pitt, 1985) — Short distal phalanges, ulnar digits, short metacarpals, and normal stature

Sugarman brachydactyly (Sugarman, 1974) — Short proximal phalanges with symphalangism

Smorgasboard brachydactyly (Meiselman, 1989) — Combination of types A2 and D brachydactyly

From McKusick V: Mendelian Inheritance in Man. A Catalogue of Human Genes and Genetic Disorders. Baltimore, Johns Hopkins University, 1994.

The majority of lengthening techniques have used a dorsal approach to the phalanx or metacarpal. Saito and colleagues[21] described a palmar approach for lengthening short central metacarpals to avoid the dorsal scar, although care is required to preserve the deep branch of the ulnar nerve. Most authors achieve lengthening using a simple transverse osteotomy and a distraction frame for lengthening. Single-stage lengthening has been performed using a variety of bony cuts to achieve stability, including step-cut osteotomy,[14] chevron osteotomy,[21] or a dowel-shaped osteotomy (Fig. 40-38).[25] Immediate lengthening of the metacarpal may require soft tissue release, reconstruction of the transverse metacarpal ligaments, and/or advancement of the origins of the interosseous muscles (Fig. 40-39).[5] Intercalary bone graft is usually required and fixation is accomplished with external fixation, Kirschner wires, or internal fixation to stabilize the lengthened skeleton.

The alternative approach is distraction osteogenesis with osteotomy and gradual lengthening using a distraction frame.[19] Alignment is best maintained with two fixation pins on each side of the osteotomy to prevent palmar or dorsal angulation. Dhalla and colleagues[7] described a technique suited to small bones using only one pin on each side of the osteotomy, supplemented with an intramedullary Kirschner

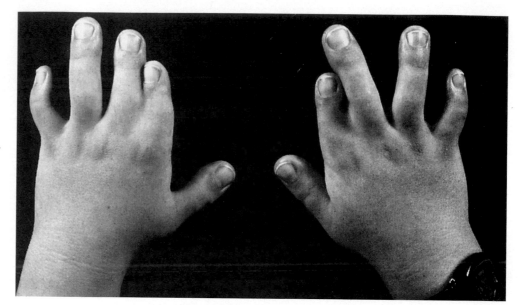

FIGURE 40-37. Bilateral brachysyndactyly.

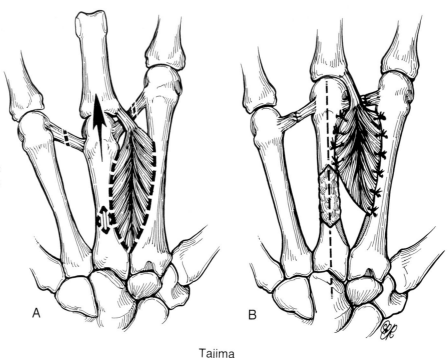

FIGURE 40-38. A and **B,** The chevron-type slot graft used to lengthen the metacarpal, as described by Tajima.

A   B

Tajima

wire to maintain alignment. Advantages of distraction osteogenesis are concomitant soft tissue lengthening and the formation of regenerate bone that negates the need for bone graft. Recent results of distraction lengthening for congenital short digits and metacarpals are positive, with mean gains in length of up to 15 mm without the need for bone grafting.[1,7,13] Distraction osteogenesis, however, is time consuming and requires cooperation of the patient and parents. The external fixation frame is often in place for upward of 4 months to achieve consolidation of the skeleton.

Authors' Preferred Technique

The authors' treatment preference for brachydactyly secondary to short phalanges is to avoid surgery. Hand function is often preserved and lengthening is difficult; it often produces a stiff or contracted digit, and the aesthetic result is usually disappointing. Distraction lengthening in the phalanges has been used in selected cases of shortening com-

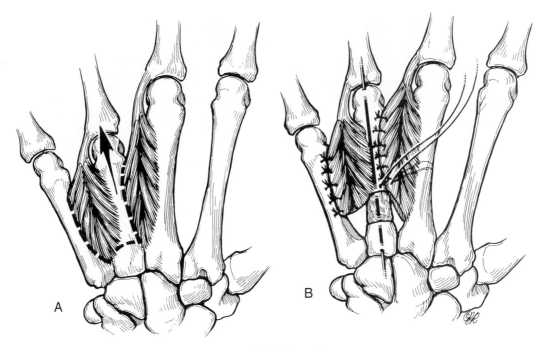

Buck-Gramcko

FIGURE 40-39. **A** and **B,** Buck-Gramcko technique for lengthening a short metacarpal.

bined with an associated deformity, such as angulation. Immediate lengthening combined with angulatory correction is the preferred approach for brachydactyly combined with angulation. An opening wedge osteotomy and insertion of a trapezoidal bone graft restores alignment and achieves length in a single setting. A closing wedge osteotomy should be avoided in a short digit. On occasion, a single flail shortened hypoplastic digit within an otherwise normal or near-normal hand is treated by ray amputation.[9]

For brachydactyly secondary to a short metacarpal, lengthening is often recommended to restore hand contour. The authors' preference is distraction lengthening using an uniaxial distractor. The first stage requires application of the external fixator and osteotomy. Two open or percutaneous pins are placed into the metacarpal on each side of the planned osteotomy site. A dorsal approach is used with the aid of an image intensifier to ensure accurate placement. A distraction frame is applied across the metacarpal. The metacarpal is exposed at the site of osteotomy with retraction of the extensor tendon(s) and cutaneous nerves. A longitudinal incision is made in the periosteum, and subperiosteal dissection is performed to expose the osteotomy site while preserving a sleeve of periosteum. A transverse osteotomy is performed using an osteotome or fine-bladed saw, and the wound is closed. Distraction of the osteotomy site is begun between 4 and 7 days after surgery at a rate of 0.25 to 0.5 mm twice a day. Distraction continues until the desired length is achieved. The frame is not removed until consolidation of the metacarpal is documented on radiograph. If poor quality regenerate bone persists, secondary bone grafting may be required. Throughout the period of distraction and consolidation, the patient requires close supervision by the surgeon and hand therapist to ensure that digital range of motion is maintained. Regular radiographs are required to assess the progress of the distraction and

CRITICAL POINTS: BRACHYDACTYLY

- The functional and aesthetic aspects of brachydactyly are variable depending on the degree of shortening and the status of the remaining digits.
- The most commonly affected phalanx is the middle phalanx, which is the last component of the digital skeleton to ossify.
- Brachydactyly may occur with syndactyly, clinodactyly, and/or symphalangism, which increase the functional problem.
- Enthusiasm for lengthening on the part of the parents, patient, or surgeon must be tempered by potential problems of lengthening, including joint stiffness, contracture, and loss of hand function.

identify potential complications of pin displacement and/or failure of the apparatus.

ANNOTATED REFERENCES

7. Dhalla R, Strecker W, Manske PR: A comparison of two techniques for digital distraction lengthening in skeletally immature patients. J Hand Surg [Am] 26:603-610, 2001.

Twenty metacarpals and 7 phalanges were lengthened in 16 skeletally immature patients (mean age: 7.9 years). Seven digits were lengthened with two fixator half-pins on either side of the osteotomy site (dual half-pin group). Twenty digits were too small to accommodate four half-pins and were lengthened over a longitudinal intramedullary guide wire with one fixator half-pin on either side of the osteotomy site (single half-pin/Kirschner-wire group). The mean total length gained was 14 mm (9 to 23 mm) in the dual half-pin group and 12 mm (6 to 19 mm) in the single half-pin/Kirschner-wire group. Eighteen complications occurred; a greater number of complications occurred in the single half-pin/Kirschner-wire group.

10. Foucher G, Pajardi G, Lamas C, et al: [Progressive bone lengthening of the hand in congenital malformations: 41 cases]. Rev Chir Orthop Reparatrice Appar Mot 87:451-458, 2001.

Callostasis lengthening was used in 31 cases. Ten cases required a second stage with an iliac graft (2 cases), vascularized metacarpal bone graft (1 case), and vascularized (1 case) or nonvascularized (3 cases) toe epiphysis. In the other 3 secondary cases, the distal part of the lengthened index was translocated to the tip of the long finger. Mean lengthening was 2.3 cm (0.9 to 3.5) with a mean treatment duration of 3.8 months (1.5 to 8.2). The complication rate was 32%. There were two complete failures, one extensor tendon tear, three pin tract infections, two delayed unions, two angulations, one callus fracture, one metacarpophalangeal dislocation, and one case of joint stiffness.

13. Kato H, Minami A, Suenaga N, et al: Callostasis lengthening in patients with brachymetacarpia. J Pediatr Orthop 22:497-500, 2002.

Callostasis lengthening to treat brachymetacarpia was performed in six digits in three patients. The patient age at the time of distraction ranged from 10 to 19 years. The period of application of an external fixator averaged 13.9 weeks (range, 10 to 19 weeks). All the metacarpals achieved the target length, and all patients were satisfied with the aesthetic improvement. The length of the metacarpal distraction averaged 15.2 mm (range, 10 to 18 mm). There were no serious complications.

19. Ogino T, Kato H, Ishii S, Usui M: Digital lengthening in congenital hand deformities. J Hand Surg [Br] 19:120-129, 1994.

Twelve hands with congenital short finger in 11 patients were treated with various types of metacarpal bone lengthening. Three patients had brachydactyly, 7 had transverse deficiency, and 1 had constriction ring syndrome. Single-stage lengthening was performed in seven cases, on-top plasty in three cases, and distraction lengthening in six cases. The length gained ranged from 2 to 10 mm in single-stage lengthening, 3 to 17 mm in on-top plasty, and 12 to 30 mm in distraction lengthening. Delayed union and malunion occurred in single-stage lengthening or on-top plasty.

Central Hand Deficiencies

Simon P. Kay and David McCombe

Within the classification of congenital anomalies of the hand is the concept that congenital deficiencies may be either transverse or longitudinal.[44-46] Longitudinal absence includes ulnar, central, or radial deficiency. Central deficiency was initially subdivided into a typical true and an atypical type. True cleft hand, however, is distinct from atypical cleft hand, which is now recognized as part of the teratologic sequence of symbrachydactyly. In contrast to radial and ulnar deficiencies, true cleft hand is not seen in association with proximal deficiencies of the nerves, vessels, tendons, muscles, and bones.

Cleft hand is characterized by a "V"-shaped cleft in the center of the hand, which may or may not be associated with the absence of one or more digits (Fig. 40-40). Multiple digit absence during the clefting process can leave only a single digit remaining, which is invariably the finger on the ulnar border. In contrast, severe ulnar deficiency can result in a single digit that is usually the thumb. Syndactyly of the digits that border the cleft may occur, and the first web space is often abnormal and tight. The cleft can be widened by transverse bones that may occur within the hand that span the cleft.

ETIOLOGY

A wedge-shaped defect of the apical ectoderm of the limb bud is thought to lead to cleft hand. Maisels' centripetal theory proposed a progression of cleft formation from a central soft tissue defect to complete absence of all digits. This hypothesis attempts to explain the progressive spectrum of deformity via "teratologic sequence."[22] In central deficiency, suppression progresses in a radial direction so that in the monodactylous form the most ulnar finger is preserved. In contrast, "atypical" cleft (symbrachydactyly) proceeds in an ulnar direction so that in the monodactylous form the thumb is the last remaining digit. This theory is not based on embryogenesis but does represent the clinical findings.

Several investigators[24,25,28,47,52,53] have suggested that polydactyly, syndactyly, and cleft hand occur from a common mechanism, because all entities can occur within the same hand (Fig. 40-41).[30,31,34] In addition, osseous syndactyly adjacent to the cleft is commonplace. Ogino[32] has produced rats with central polydactyly and/or osseous syndactyly identical to typical cleft hand. The defects are so similar that Ogino believes that polydactyly, syndactyly, and cleft hand should be grouped within the same category. Miura, Watari and Tsuge[24,25,28,47,52,53] have also emphasized the importance of central polydactyly in the etiology of cleft hand. A modified IFSSH classification has been proposed to include a "failure of finger ray induction group" that includes typical cleft hand, central polydactyly, and (bony) syndactyly.

INHERITANCE

Cleft hand is commonly inherited as an autosomal dominant trait and is associated with a number of syndromes (Table

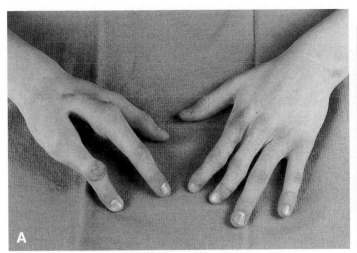
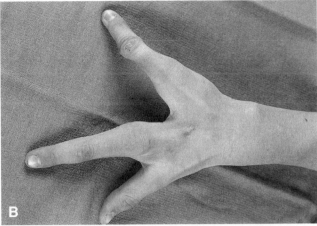

FIGURE 40-40. **A** and **B,** Typical cleft hand with severe suppression of central rays. (Courtesy of Shriners Hospitals for Children, Philadelphia.)

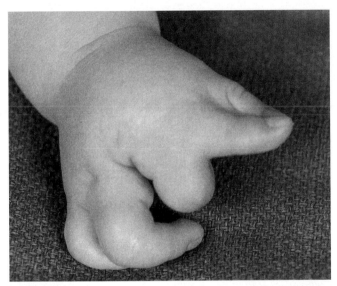

FIGURE 40-41. Central deficiency with six metacarpals and complete thumb-index finger syndactyly. (Courtesy of Shriners Hospitals for Children, Philadelphia.)

40-5). The most common syndromes are split-hand/split-foot (SHSF) and EEC syndrome (ectrodactyly, ectodermal dysplasia, and cleft lip/palate).* SHSF is inherited as an autosomal dominant pattern with variable penetrance. Phenotypic abnormalities occur in 70% of cases that inherit the gene mutation. In the other 30% the presence of the mutant gene cannot be determined by examination alone.

Cleft hand appears analogous to dactylaplasia in mutant mice in which the central segment of the apical ectodermal ridge (AER) degenerates, leaving the radial and ulnar segments intact.[17] A gene in the region of chromosome 3q27 plays a critical role in the formation and maintenance of the AER. Mutations in this gene have been identified in families affected by SHSF syndrome and also in families affected by EEC syndrome.[49,54]

---

*See references 9, 15-17, 21, 36, 38, 41, 49, 54, and 56.

Table 40-5
CONDITIONS THAT MAY FEATURE A CLEFT HAND AND/OR FOOT

Condition	McKusick Number
EEC syndrome	129900
Cornelia de Lange syndrome	122430
Acrorenal syndrome	102520
Focal dermal hypoplasia	305600
Ectrodactyly and cleft palate syndrome	129830
Ectrodactyly/mandibulofacial dysostosis	183700
Ectrodactyly and macular dystrophy	185800

From Buss PW: Cleft hand/foot: Clinical and developmental aspects. J Med Genet 31:726-730, 1994, with permission.

INCIDENCE

The variable expressivity and reduced penetrance cause difficulty in predicting future phenotypes in an affected family. The wide range of phenotypes leads to confusion between cleft hand and other conditions, such as ulnar deficiency and atypical cleft hand (symbrachydactyly). Birch-Jensen[3] estimated the incidence of cleft hand at 1 in 90,000 births. More recent studies estimate a higher incidence, at 1 in 10,000 births.[2,35]

CLINICAL FEATURES

The condition may be unilateral or bilateral and may or may not involve the feet. The extent of cleft hand varies from generation to generation, and the characteristics are described in Table 40-6. Cleft hand is differentiated from symbrachydactyly, previously known as atypical cleft hand, by varying clinical features.[7,8,10,29] The manifestations of cleft hand may vary from only a very minor cutaneous cleft

Table 40-6

COMPARISON OF CLINICAL FEATURES OF TYPICAL CLEFT HAND AND ATYPICAL CLEFT HAND

Typical Cleft Hand	Atypical Cleft Hand (Symbrachydactyly)
Autosomal dominant	Sporadic
One to four limbs involved	One limb involved (no feet)
"V"-shaped cleft	"U"-shaped cleft
No finger "nubbins"	Finger "nubbins" may occur
Syndactyly (especially first web)	

without loss of the finger to a severe form in which only the little finger remains.[8,33] Syndactyly between the digits bordering the cleft is common; the first web space is often narrowed. Duplications can also occur adjacent to the cleft. Within the cleft, metacarpals may or may not be present, and transverse lying metacarpals or phalanges can occur that may further expand the cleft. Phalangeal anomalies often coexist, including longitudinal bracketed epiphyses or double phalanges. Metacarpal anomalies are variable, including absence within the cleft, bifid metacarpals supporting one finger, and duplication. The anomaly is often bilateral, and in the SHSF phenotype it is associated with comparable defects in the feet.[27]

CLASSIFICATION

Multiple classifications exist; the most useful addresses the first web space (Table 40-7).[2,5,8,11,12,23,40,53] This classification acknowledges that more extensive clefts merge with the first web space and produce a wide and competent web.

Table 40-7

MANSKE'S CLASSIFICATION OF CENTRAL DEFICIENCY BASED ON THE THUMB WEB SPACE

Type	Description	Characteristics
I	Normal web	Thumb web space not narrowed
IIA	Mildly narrowed web	Thumb web space mildly narrowed
IIB	Severely narrowed web	Thumb web space severely narrowed
III	Syndactylized web	Thumb and index rays syndactylized, web space obliterated
IV	Merged web	Index ray suppressed, thumb web space is merged with the cleft
V	Absent web	Thumb elements suppressed, ulnar rays remain, thumb web space no longer present

From Manske PR, Halikis MN: Surgical classification of central deficiency according to the thumb web. J Hand Surg [Am] 20:687-697, 1995, with permission.

Continued cleft formation, however, involves the thumb and produces hypoplasia or absence.

INDICATIONS FOR TREATMENT

Flatt[13,14] touted the cleft hand as a "functional triumph, but a social disaster" because many cleft hands, while stigmatizing the child, function very well. A family with one or more generations of cleft hands may avoid surgery for their children, because they perceive function as excellent and cosmetic improvement as marginal. Such opinions require sensitive handling when outlining the indications for surgery and the surgical plan. Surgery should reduce the deformity and/or improve function. Many authors have attested to the psychological consequences of cleft hand, and the moving testimony by Walker[51] highlights the psychosocial complexities faced by families with this condition.

Surgery is considered for a variety of indications: (1) the progressive deformity (deforming syndactyly, transverse bones); (2) the first web space; (3) the cleft; (4) the absent thumb; or (5) the feet. The timing of surgery is debatable, because parents of children with congenital differences are vulnerable during the first few months of life and should not be expected to make complex decisions about care.[6,18] Most parents, however, will accept surgery to prevent worsening of the deformity. Indications for early surgery include the separation of syndactyly between digits of unequal length (especially the thumb and index) and the removal of transverse bones that result in widening of the cleft during growth and progressive deformity. Most of the other surgical procedures are less urgent and may be reserved until the child is between 1 and 2 years of age.

MANAGEMENT

The Progressive Deformity (Deforming Syndactyly, Transverse Bones)

Removal of Transverse Bones
Transverse bones that expand the cleft during growth may occupy the cleft. Removal can prevent progression of the deformity and serve as a prerequisite for closure of the cleft. The transverse bone may originate and insert from either the metacarpal or proximal phalanx. The bone may join the metacarpophalangeal (MCP) joints, and removal requires preservation or reconstruction of the collateral ligaments about the joint. Articular surface resurfacing of the remaining joint may be required.

Syndactyly Release
Syndactyly may affect the border rays of the hand. Early release is indicated to prevent progressive deviation of the longer ray (Fig. 40-42). For patients who require concomitant cleft closure and thumb/index finger syndactyly separation, the cleft skin can be rotated as a random flap into the first web space.

Release of the First Web Space and Closure of the Cleft
The classification proposed by Manske and Hallikis[23] (Fig. 40-43) has focused attention on the importance of the first

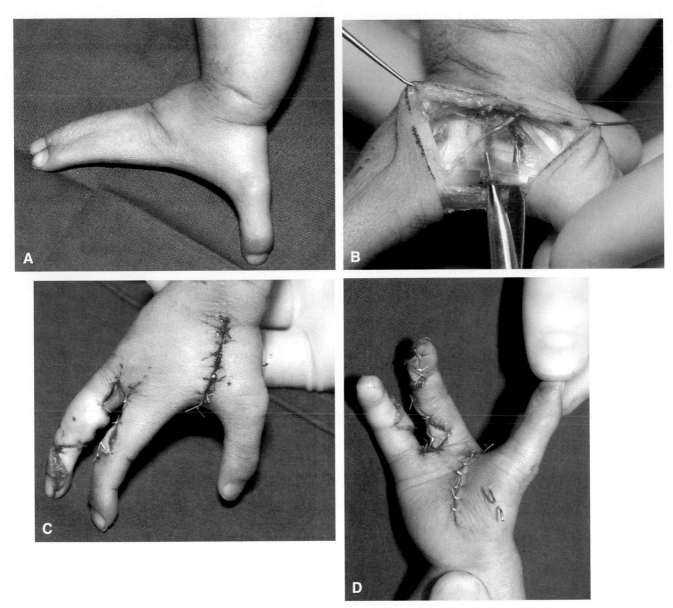

FIGURE 40-42. **A,** Syndactyly of the ulnar rays with merging of the first web space and cleft. There is limited mobility of the thumb via bony fusion across the cleft. **B,** Surgical release of the bone block combined with narrowing of the cleft by excision of bone and division of abnormal tendon connections. **C** and **D,** Skin from the cleft is used as full-thickness skin graft for the syndactyly release.

web space morphology in dictating surgical treatment of the cleft hand. In type IIA cases, the first web space is mildly narrowed and a cleft is present between the index and the ring finger with complete absence of the central ray. Concomitant syndactyly of the ulnar digits is often present. In type IIB hands, the web space was more severely constricted and the cleft element more variable. In type II and III cleft hands with complete syndactyly between the thumb and index finger, simultaneous release of the first web space and closure of the cleft can transfer skin from the cleft to the first web space. Snow and Littler[43] described an elegant technique that has been elaborated on by Flatt (Fig. 40-44).[14] Release of a slightly narrow first web space may require simple skin release from volar to dorsal across the narrowed first web space. Release of complete first web space syndactyly may require formal separation with release of the thick fascia or muscles within the abnormal web space. In cases of index finger/thumb syndactyly, the thumb may be rotated into the plane of the other digits and a rotation metacarpal osteotomy may be required to reposition the thumb.

The cleft incision is designed to re-create the commissure after the cleft is narrowed. For this purpose, a small commissural flap is prepared on one border of the cleft and a recipient defect planned on the other border of the cleft. The rest of the cleft skin is raised as a palmar-based flap and designed to transpose into the first web space. The position and dimensions of the first web space will change after translocation of the index ray. The viability of this palmar flap depends on preservation of the intrinsic blood supply, and dissection must maintain the subdermal plexus. If possible, a digital artery may be included with the flap to transform its blood supply from random to axial. Index finger relocation to the base of the third metacarpal widens the

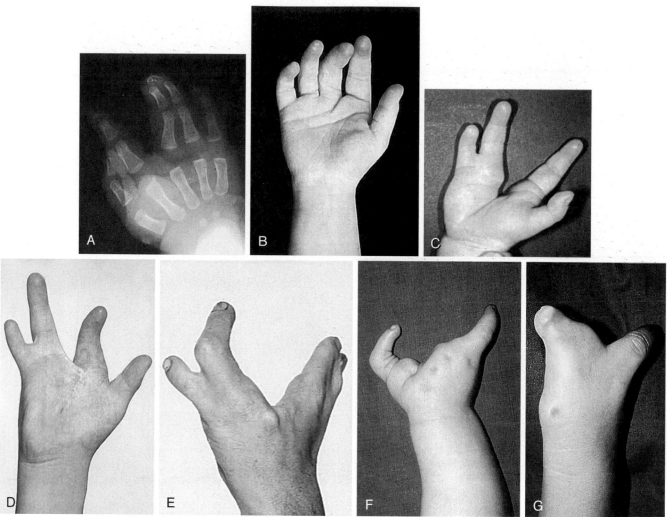

FIGURE 40-43. **A** to **G,** These images illustrate Manske's classification and also some aspects of the teratologic sequence in cleft hand. **A,** Type I hand, with a normal web space between the thumb and index finger. A very minor cleft is present between the second and third rays and syndactyly between the third and fourth rays. **B,** The same hand after correction of the syndactyly alone. No surgical treatment has been undertaken for the commissure between the index and long finger, where a minor cleft remains. The thumb web space is normal. **C,** Type IIa hand, in which the thumb web space is mildly narrowed. Note the suppression of the central ray with a deep cleft and minor syndactyly between the ring finger and the little finger. **D,** Type IIb cleft hand with a severely narrowed first web space, deletion of the third ray, and minor syndactyly between the fourth and fifth rays. **E,** Type III cleft hand (untreated). This adult was born with hands and feet affected by clefting. The thumb and index fingers have untreated syndactyly that completely obliterates the first web space. The central ray is absent, and the fourth ray deviated toward the cleft with minor syndactyly with the fifth ray. **F,** Type IV cleft hand with a merged web space. The two border rays are present, but the index ray and other central rays are suppressed, and the first web space merges with the cleft. **G,** Type V cleft hand. The web space for the thumb and the thumb are absent. The ulnar digits remain, with the third and fourth rays being fused as a single mass and the fifth ray deviated.

first web space and decreases the amount of flap transposition. The index finger must be carefully positioned to prevent malrotation and scissoring during finger flexion.[13] The osteosynthesis at the base of the metacarpal is usually performed with a Kirschner wire and/or interosseous sutures. Mini-plate fixation has been proposed as another option. In those cases without a base of the third metacarpal to receive the index transposition, the cleft may be closed by wedge excision of the index metacarpal or within the carpus to widen the thumb-index web and realign the fingers.

Reconstruction of the intermetacarpal ligament can be used to reinforce the cleft closure and to prevent splaying of the digits. Reconstruction is accomplished using the technique of Saito and colleagues[39] or Ogino,[31] which utilizes the A1 pulleys from the digits (Fig. 40-45). The final stage in cleft closure is creation of a commissure across the cleft. The flaps previously outlined are raised and transposed (Fig. 40-46).[2] The Snow-Littler procedure is not a simple procedure; the planning and execution can be difficult, and the transposed flap may not inset into the correct position. Skin graft supplementation may be necessary. In addition, the flap can undergo partial necrosis, because its length substantially exceeds its breadth. Rider and coworkers[37] have reported a low rate of flap necrosis, but a third of patients required revision, and supplementary skin grafting was required in tight first web spaces.

Miura and Komada[26] have described a simpler technique. The cleft is incised from side to side across its leading edge.

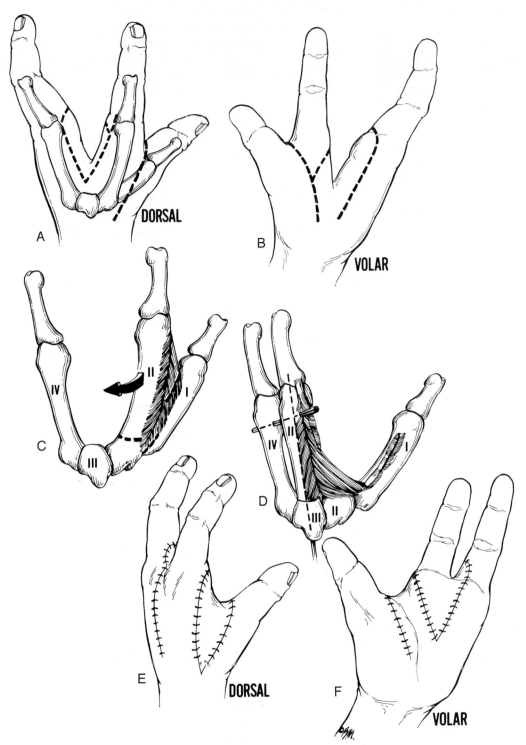

FIGURE 40-44. **A** to **F,** The Snow-Littler procedure. The cleft is raised as a palmar-based flap preserving a small radial flap for the re-creation of the commissure. The first web space is released, which may require a division of the first dorsal interosseous origin and surrounding fascia. The second metacarpal is transposed and fixed to the remnant of the base of the third metacarpal if present. Fixation is achieved by axial and transverse wires, and careful attention must be given to correction of rotation at this point. The palmar flap is then transferred, and the new commissure between the second and fourth rays re-created.

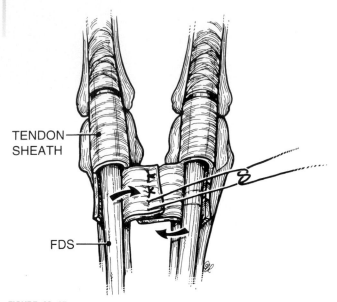

FIGURE 40-45. The deep transverse metacarpal ligament is reconstructed using the flexor sheaths (part of the A1 or A2 pulleys) of the index and ring fingers.

The index finger is raised on its neurovascular bundles and transposed by osteosynthesis with the third metacarpal or by angulation osteotomy. The first web space is re-created by local flap design or "Z"-plasty using the remaining skin (Fig. 40-47).

Ueba[48] also describes a less complicated procedure using transverse flaps from either border of the cleft and transposition of the index digit (Fig. 40-48). The flaps from either side of the cleft are used to resurface the palm, the dorsal aspect of the metacarpal head of the transposed digit, and the ulnar part of the first web space. Ueba[48] also used slips of tendon material to connect the common extensor tendons of the digits bordering the cleft to prevent digital separation during extension. This technique allows a simpler approach to cleft closure but has the cosmetic disadvantage of transferring palmar skin to dorsal and dorsal skin to palmar.

In reality, the surgeon versed in congenital hand surgery will treat type IIB and type III cleft hands on an individual basis borrowing elements of the above technique(s). In cases in which there is a small digital remnant within the cleft, the use of a bilobed flap technique may also transport a large amount of pliable, vascularized skin into the first

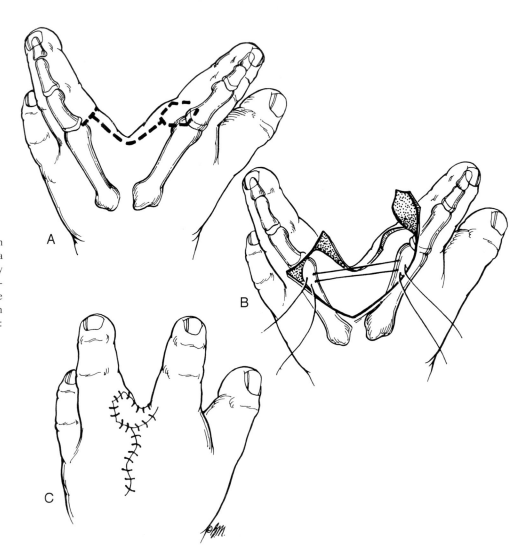

FIGURE 40-46. **A** to **C,** Steps in creating a commissure with a diamond-shaped flap. (From Barsky AJ: Cleft hand: Classification, incidence, and treatment. Review of the literature and report of nineteen cases. J Bone Joint Surg Am 46: 1707-1720, 1964, with permission.)

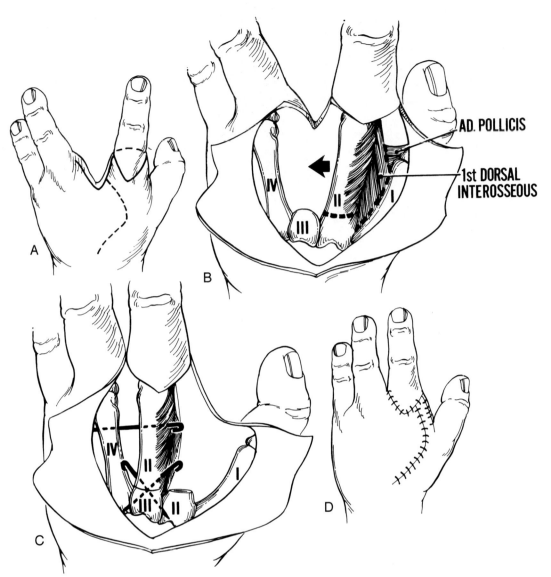

AD. POLLICIS

1st DORSAL INTEROSSEOUS

FIGURE 40-47. Miura and Komada[26] recommended simple transverse incision of the cleft with an ulnar translocation of the radial border ray. The same principle for release of the first web space applies as for the Snow-Littler procedure, but once the translocation has taken place and the new commissural flap is inset, the first web space may be created by simple closure or closure with "Z"-plasties. The axial dorsal incision varies in length and is not an essential component of the skin closure.

web space (Fig. 40-49). In rare cases of drastic skin deficiency within the first web and cleft, distant skin may be required, such as a vascularized forearm flap or a groin flap.

An acceptable outcome is ensured by adherence to the principles of adequate first web release, resurfacing of the first web with pliable tissue, transposition of the most radial finger, re-creation of an intermetacarpal ligament, and re-creation of a commissure about the cleft.

In the type IV cleft hands, the first web space is merged with the cleft and function does not require creation of a first web space. Surgical effort is usually directed toward mobility and/or position of the thumb or ulnar digit to promote pinch and grasp.

In type V cleft hands, there is no cleft or web space and the thumb is very deficient. Surgery for this group is considered next.

Management of the Absence of the Thumb

An absent or deficient thumb (type V cleft hand) requires consideration of creating a radial digit. In certain cleft hands, two digital rays are present and fused and resemble a thumb positioned in the plane of the other digit(s). Separation and rotation of this radial ray may re-create a functional and useful hand but requires distant flap cover for the first web space. Options include free or pedicled flaps from the forearm and groin. Complete absence of a radial ray can only be replaced by free toe transfer. In contrast to microsurgical toe transfer in children for other indications, transfer for cleft hand is fraught with problems.[19,20,50] The available toes may be abnormal or insufficient in number for transfer. In addition, any available toe is replete with abnormal anatomy that makes harvest complicated and limits the ability to drive the transfer secondary to anomalous tendons.

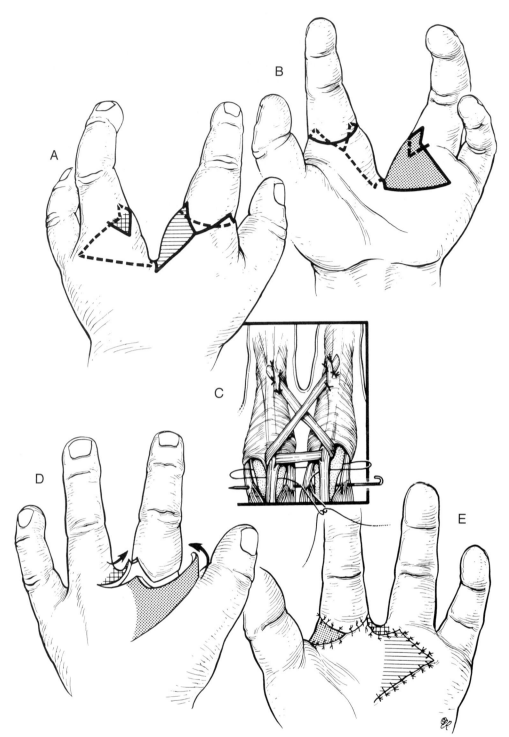

FIGURE 40-48. **A** to **E,** Ueba's technique for treatment of typical cleft hand with one ray suppressed. Ueba used a tendon graft between the extensor tendons of the border digits (**C**), but this is not an essential component of the procedure, and Ogino's method of creation of a transverse palmar ligament (see Fig. 40-45). The disadvantage of this technique lies in the transfer of palmar skin dorsally or radially in the cleft and vice versa.

Experience of such free toe transfers is limited. A child who underwent transfer of the tibial rays of the foot to the hands is shown in Figure 40-50. A number of interesting clinical and anatomic findings were found. First, the flexor and extensor tendons were connected around the distal part of the limb and had adequate excursion after separation.

Second, vessels and cutaneous nerves were readily found on exploration aided by 10-mHz Doppler examination (angiography was not performed in either foot or hand). Last, useful function was achieved despite limited power and range of motion. Prehension provided useful holding and manipulative abilities.

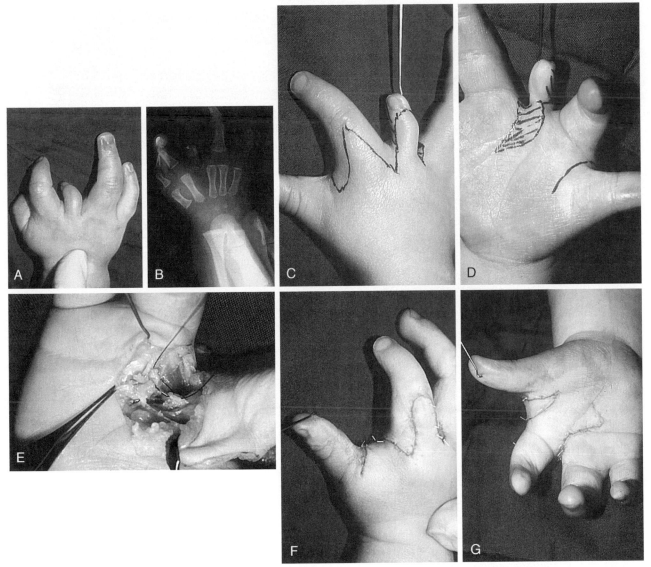

FIGURE 40-49. Clinical photograph (**A**) and radiograph (**B**) of a type IIb cleft hand with a digital remnant in the central cleft and a narrowed first web space. **C,** A bilobed flap has been designed on the dorsum of the hand. The flap from the index finger will now resurface the first web space and in turn be replaced by the flap from the dorsum of the digital remnant to be excised. The flap is not transposed; rather, the index ray is translocated ulnarward. **D,** A palmar view noting the incision for release of the first web space, cross hatching of the area of skin to be excised, and the small radially based flap of Barsky for re-creation of a commissure. **E,** The digital remnant and contents of the cleft have been excised, and the small flaps from the A2 pulleys on either border of the cleft are being sutured together after the technique of Ogino (see Fig. 40-45) to re-create a metacarpal ligament. **F,** The cleft has been closed, the remnant excised, and the flaps transposed to resurface both the first web space and the donor defect from the dorsum of the index finger. **G,** Palmar view.

Surgical Management of the Feet

The foot deformity in cleft hand often parallels the hand deformity.[1,42,55] The hand surgeon may or may not also be involved in the feet, but his or her opinion will be sought at the time of consultation. Blauth and Borisch[4] have classified the foot deformities that occur with cleft formation into six types. Types I and II have only minor abnormalities without absence of metatarsals, whereas the metatarsals are progressively absent in the remaining types. Type VI is the monodactylous cleft foot in which the fibula ray is always the last remaining ray. Whereas the fibula ray is the last ray to be deleted, the ultimate deletion is the status of the great toe ray or tibial ray. It is not uncommon to see patients with great

toe polydactyly and deviation in whom the decision about preservation and correction of the tibial ray is required. In our experience, the fibular ray is always the more important and the tibial ray may be present but may not participate in weight bearing. In those rare cases in which a microsurgical transfer is considered from the feet, it is likely that the feet will also be severely afflicted, with perhaps only two rays remaining. In these cases, reluctance to sacrifice the tibial ray is understandable. Nonetheless, this ray can be transferred, and waiting until the child is of an age to undertake gait analysis is wise.

Rarely is surgery indicated for cleft foot. When it is, it is usually because of difficulty in fitting footwear because of

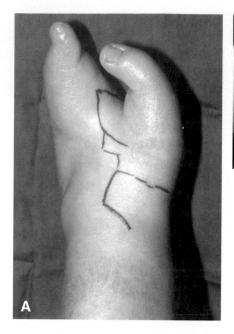

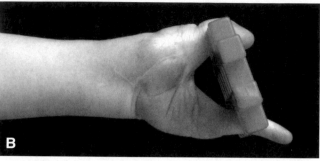

FIGURE 40-50. **A,** Foot of a child with monodactylous cleft hand with a stiff single digit. Only the fibula toe is used in walking, and the tibial toe hinders footwear. **B,** Free toe transfer resulted in two-digit hand with some prehension and function.

either duplication or deviation of the border digits. This may be corrected either by osteotomy or excision of trapezoidal phalanges. Occasionally, as in the hand, resection of a transverse bone may be necessary. The common experience is that despite quite bizarre appearance in the feet, function is remarkably good and gait is rarely considerably impaired.

CRITICAL POINTS: CENTRAL HAND DEFICIENCIES

■ True cleft hand is distinct from atypical cleft hand, which is recognized as part of the teratologic sequence of symbrachydactyly.

■ Cleft hand is commonly inherited as an autosomal dominant trait and is associated with split-hand/split-foot (SHSF) and EEC syndrome (ectrodactyly, ectodermal dysplasia, and cleft lip/palate).

■ Surgery is considered for a variety of indications, including the progressive widening of the cleft secondary to transverse lying bones, a narrowed first web space, and the widened cleft.

■ Indications for early surgery are separation of syndactyly between digits of unequal length, especially the thumb and index, and the removal of transverse bones that results in progressive widening of the cleft.

■ In cases of thumb/index finger syndactyly, the first web space requires reconstruction. The technique depends on the severity of the syndactyly. Complete syndactyly can be released and the cleft closed in a single setting. The skin from the cleft is rotated into the first web space to create supple tissue.

In summary, surgical treatment for children with central deficiency is challenging but can provide good functional and aesthetic results. In more severe forms, ingenuity of the surgeon is required. In these cases, the surgeon must discuss with parents that experience over generations shows that despite the adverse appearance, children will adapt and learn to use their hands in a way that might have been considered impossible when they were born. Surgery should improve appearance and/or function. Surgical correction should be planned according to a schedule that recognizes the urgency of some aspects of treatment and the discretionary nature of others. The overriding determinant of function is the first web space, and this structure is the basis of the most useful classification. Microvascular transfers from the foot can be useful in highly selected cases.

ANNOTATED REFERENCES

9a. Cole RJ, Manske PR: Classification of ulnar deficiency according to the thumb and first web. J Hand Surg [Am] 22:479-488, 1997.

Fifty-five upper extremities with ulnar deficiency were reviewed to evaluate the hand abnormalities. Thumb and first-web abnormalities were noted in 73% of hands. This classification is based on the progressive involvement of the thumb and first web. In type A, the thumb and first web are normal. In type B, the first web space has mild deficiency and the thumb has mild involvement. In type C, the thumb has varying degrees of involvement. The first web has moderate to severe deficiency, including thumb/index finger syndactyly, and is often associated with malrotation of the thumb and dysfunction of the extrinsic tendons. In type D, the thumb is absent.

14. Flatt AE: Cleft hand and central defects. *In* Flatt AE (ed): The Care of Congenital Hand Anomalies, 2nd ed. St. Louis, Quality Medical Publishing, 1994, pp 337-365.

This is a classic single-author textbook on congenital hand anomalies. The chapter on cleft hand delineates the functional triumph of the hand missing part or all of the long ray. Advantages and disadvantages of surgical reconstruction are discussed. Numerous clinical examples are provided, including illustrations.

29. Miura T, Suzuki M: Clinical differences between typical and atypical cleft hand. J Hand Surg [Br] 9:311-315, 1984.

   The authors differentiate the clinical features of the cleft hand from atypical cleft hand (symbrachydactyly). It provides a basis for categorization into different types of embryologic failure.

37. Rider MA, Grindel SI, Tonkin MA, Wood VE: An experience of the Snow-Littler procedure. J Hand Surg [Br] 25:376-381, 2000.

Snow-Littler procedure results are presented for 12 hands with classic central longitudinal deficiency and 1 hand with symbrachydactyly. There were no instances of major flap necrosis, although two flaps showed tip ischemia. The width of the first web was satisfactory, although four web space revisions were performed. Three derotational osteotomies of transposed index fingers were performed in patients. Improved appearance and function were evident. Snow-Littler remains the preferred procedure for the cleft hand combined with thumb-index syndactyly.

Absence of Fingers

Simon P. Kay and David McCombe

Transverse and longitudinal absences are distinguished by the presence or absence of proximal structures. In transverse deficiency, the digit is absent but the proximal supporting structures required to support digital function, such as neurovascular structures and bone, are present to some degree. Examples are symbrachydactyly, amniotic disruption sequence, and idiopathic transverse absence. In longitudinal deficiency, the supporting structures are severely deficient or absent. Examples are thumb absence in radial deficiency, absence of ulnar digits in ulna dysplasia, or central absences in central deficiency.

Reconstruction of transverse absence may be achievable by replacing the distal part (e.g., microvascular toe transfer) and connecting the part to the proximal structure. Reconstruction of longitudinal absence requires replacement of the whole part, such as pollicization for thumb absence.

AMNIOTIC DISRUPTION SEQUENCE

Amniotic disruption sequence (also known as amniotic band syndrome or constriction ring syndrome) is characterized by partial or complete circumferential constrictions around limbs or digits.[94] Consequences include acrosyndactyly of digits, terminal absence, and localized swelling with digital edema distal to constrictions (Fig. 40-51).

Etiology

Streeter,[69,70] in 1930, and others have proposed that this syndrome was caused by vascular disruption in the embryo.[18,80] Others believe that it is due to amniotic disruption with release of amniotic bands that encircle and strangulate limbs or parts of limbs in utero. The limb may also become entrapped within the ruptures of the amniotic wall.[72,73] The most prevalent theory is amniotic disruption based on the appearance of the circumferential constrictions

strangling the digit and the recovery of amputated digits within the womb.

Clinical Features

The condition is caused by mechanical strangulation from the ring constrictions. The constrictions may be circumferential or incomplete and may occur anywhere on the body but are most commonly seen on the limbs. From the hand surgeon's perspective, the most important thing about the transverse absence in amniotic disruption sequence is that the proximal structures of the hand are normal (Fig. 40-52). Pseudosyndactyly may occur with distal digital fusion and a proximal sinus cleft. Occasionally, the digits may have adhesions to nonadjacent digits creating a complicated syndactyly (see Fig. 40-51C). Amputations or absences may occur at any level of the limb and have been described in the head and neck. Lesser constrictions may be responsible for some cases of rare facial clefting.

The digital stumps may exhibit tapering skeletal elements with tight skin cover. Distal edema and threatened viability may be present. Distal to the constriction ring, the skin may be hard and swollen with an uncompressible edema. Nerve palsies have been associated with amniotic disruption sequela and are present at birth (Fig. 40-53).

Classification

Amniotic disruption sequence is classified as a whole entity and subclassified according to limb manifestations (Table 40-8).[63,64] These classifications are not useful for directing treatment but may assist in collaborative research.

Management

Treatment of the Digit or Limb Threatened at Birth

On rare occasions, a proximal ring may cause overt distal ischemia. Surgical release of the constriction may be appro-

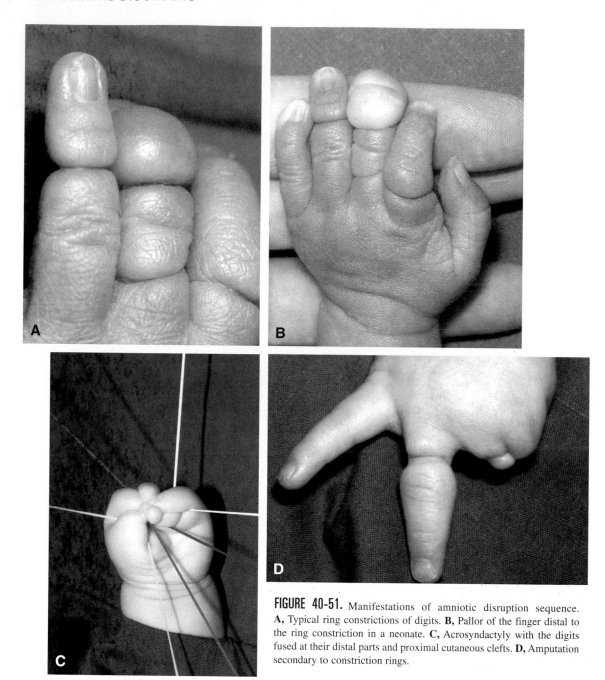

FIGURE 40-51. Manifestations of amniotic disruption sequence. **A,** Typical ring constrictions of digits. **B,** Pallor of the finger distal to the ring constriction in a neonate. **C,** Acrosyndactyly with the digits fused at their distal parts and proximal cutaneous clefts. **D,** Amputation secondary to constriction rings.

priate. Survival of the limb is often questionable, and amputation is usually required.

Nerve Palsies

A peripheral nerve palsy may occur underlying a constriction ring. The value of electrodiagnostic evaluation is questionable.[95] Successful outcomes following decompression of the nerve compression have been described, although the authors and others have seen cases with limited nerve continuity and no improvement after surgery.[21,76]

Constriction Ring

Treatment[46] is aimed at both functional and aesthetic improvement. Simple correction of the skin is not enough. Upton and Tan[78] have shown superior results with inclusion

of the deeper subcutaneous layer during skin repositioning. The mainstays are excision of the ring and subcutaneous tissue combined with "Z"-plasty or "W"-plasty. This technique elongates and reorients the scar to allow relaxation and concealing of the constriction.[21] Previously, circumferential surgery was not recommended at a single setting; however, complete circumferential excision may be safely conducted. An exception to circumferential surgery is two rings that are closely adjacent. In this case, it is prudent to release the bands one at a time.[84]

Acrosyndactyly

Acrosyndactyly secondary to amniotic disruption sequence is separated according to the principles of syndactyly reconstruction (see Syndactyly). Separation requires attention to

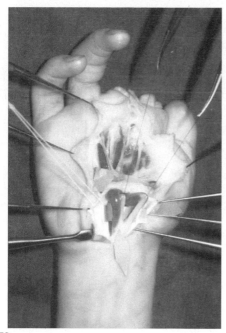

FIGURE 40-52. Normal structures are present, proximal to the constriction ring. The intrinsic muscles, flexor tendons, and neurovascular structures are identifiable.

Table 40-8
CLASSIFICATION OF RING CONSTRICTION SYNDROME

1	Simple constriction rings
2	Rings accompanied by distal deformity, with or without lymphedema
3	Rings accompanied by distal fusion: acrosyndactyly
	(a) Type I Tips are joined
	(b) Type II Tips are joined: webs too distal
	(c) Type III Tips are joined: no web. Complex syndactyly with proximal sinus
4	Amputation

Adapted from Patterson T: Congenital ring-constrictions. Br J Plast Surg 14:1-31, 1961.

the commissure, resurfacing of the digital surfaces, and attention to the nail and pulp. The sinus is usually too distal to incorporate into the skin flaps. Typically, the sinus is excised and any skin available used as a full-thickness graft.[46] Additional attention may be directed toward release of concomitant constriction rings.[25,53] The timing of separation is important, because connected nonadjacent digits are often of unequal length, which creates angulatory deformities during growth. Release of the distal connection is often enough to release the tethering effect. Formal separation and commissure reconstruction may be deferred until the child is older.

Skin Protuberances

Skin protuberances are often present in amniotic disruption sequence. These lumps are present on the dorsum of the fingers and appear firm and edematous. These protuberances may be treated via numerous techniques. "Z"-plasty is often unsatisfactory, and excision is preferred with resurfacing using full-thickness skin grafts (Fig. 40-54).

Digital Absence

Digital absence is common in amniotic disruption sequence. The number of absent digits is variable. The digits appear similar to a transverse absence. The proximal enabling structures are present and may be used to control and drive a transferred digit. The means of reconstructing profound absence of digits is addressed later.

SYMBRACHYDACTYLY

Symbrachydactyly (fused short fingers) describes relatively common patterns of digital loss that have certain characteristics in common but that also have similarities with

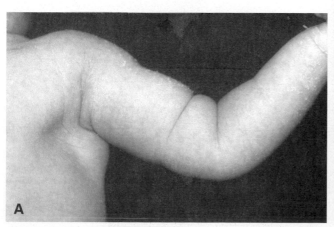
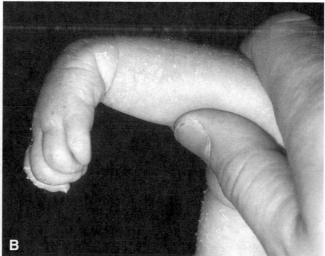

FIGURE 40-53. A, A constriction ring around the arm in a newborn child. **B,** Associated radial nerve palsy.

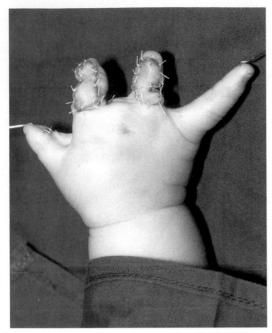

FIGURE 40-54. Dorsal skin lumps are common and can be treated with excision and skin grafting.

Table 40-9
CLASSIFICATION OF SYMBRACHYDACTYLY

1. Triphalangia type	A hand with no missing bone. All four fingers should have three phalanges even though some phalanges (often the middle phalanges) are short.
2. Diphalangia type	A hand in which one phalanx (usually the middle) is missing in one or more digits
3. Monophalangia type	A hand that has a finger or fingers with only one phalanx
4. Aphalangia type	A hand in which all three phalanges are missing in a digit or digits
5. Ametacarpia type	A hand with absence of a metacarpal bone as well as three phalanges in a digit or digits
6. Acarpia type	A hand that has absence of all the digits and partial or complete absence of the carpal bones
7. Forearm amputation type	An arm with absence of the distal portion of the forearm. Usually there are rudimentary digits on the stump.

Adapted from Yamauchi Y: Symbrachydactyly. *In* Buck-Gramcko D (ed): Congenital Malformations of the Hand and Forearm. London, Churchill-Livingstone, 1998, pp 149-157.

simple transverse absence of digits. Blauth and Gekeler[5-7] produced the first useful classification of this condition. This scheme separates symbrachydactyly into four types that represent a continuum of malformation (Fig. 40-55). The dominant characteristic that separates symbrachydactyly from transverse absence is the presence of finger remnants (i.e., nubbins) with nail or nail fold remnants.[11-13,16,20,32,33,54] An alternative classification has been proposed and focuses on the number of phalanges missing (Table 40-9).[98] This scheme also identifies a teratologic sequence passing

from the presence of five digits to complete midforearm amputation.

Clinical Features

Symbrachydactyly occurs sporadically.[54] There appears to be a spectrum of deficiency, beginning with short middle phalanges (type 1), extending to absence of the central rays,

FIGURE 40-55. Types of symbrachydactyly. **A,** Symbrachydactyly with reasonable thumb but absent fingers represented by nubbins with nail remnants. **B,** Complete absence of the fingers that become more pronounced toward the ulnar side of the hand.

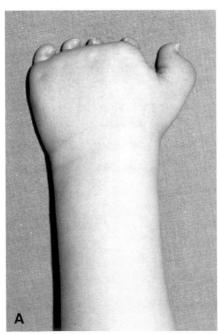

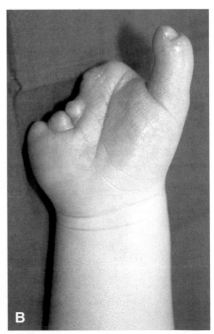

and culminating in absence of the entire hand. The defect is believed to be mesodermal, which explains the remaining distal finger ectodermal structures (pulp, nail fold, and nail). This results in the characteristic nubbins or buds that are the hallmark of symbrachydactyly (see Fig. 40-55).[54]

Symbrachydactyly may occur with Poland's syndrome, which has unilateral hand hypoplasia and absence of shoulder girdle muscles. The sternal head of the pectoralis major muscle is most commonly absent, although considerable chest wall deformity may be present. The correlation between these conditions and other syndromes with similar findings is unknown.[10,20,68,75] Previously, there existed some confusion between oligodactyly (i.e., "few finger form of symbrachydactyly") and cleft hand.[2,55] The central deficiencies form of symbrachydactyly was previously called atypical cleft hand.[50]

Management

Treatment of Short Finger Types (Types 1, 2, and 3)

This group of symbrachydactyly has short fingers with small or absent middle phalanges.[3,23,65] It may be associated with syndactyly, especially of the fifth finger. This fifth finger often deviates in a radial direction. Function is usually excellent, and surgery has little role other than release of syndactyly.

Treatment of the Oligodactylic (Few Fingers) Type (Type 4)

This type of symbrachydactyly is characterized by some degree of absence of the central three rays (see Fig. 40-57). The resultant deformity was originally called the "atypical cleft hand."[2,50] The central rays are represented by nubbins that may contain small remnants of phalanges that articulate with the metacarpal. In the absence of phalangeal remnants, the metacarpals are usually small and may only be present at their bases.

The fifth finger typically lacks a middle phalanx but has a competent metacarpophalangeal (MCP) joint and a variably stable distal joint. The fifth finger is often deviated in a radial direction. This angulation is partly the result of the oblique pull by the extensor tendon, which bridges the "U"-shaped cleft.

The thumb is also variable in form. Generally the thumb is adequate but may have only a single phalanx and a shortened tip. The web space may be narrowed, and the thumb may lack full circumduction at the basal joint. This combination can impair prehension and may warrant treatment.

Treatment of Monodactylic (Single Finger) Type (Type 5)

The hand with this type of symbrachydactyly lacks all fingers and has only a thumb, which is of varying size and quality. A markedly deficient thumb may be present with a very short metacarpal and underdeveloped basal articulation. The digits are represented by metacarpal bases and finger nubbins with nail remnants. These nubbins have vestigial connections via the palmar aponeurotic and retinacular system to the extrinsic tendons. This connection is apparent by the ability of the nubbins to pucker into the palm during hand use. The wrist is usually sufficient for function.

Treatment of Peromelic (Short Limb) Types (Types 6 and 7)

The hand with this type of symbrachydactyly has only nubbins with nail remnants. There is a transverse absence at or about the metacarpal row, although more proximal absences may be seen. Finger nubbins may even be noted on a midforearm stump.

 # Anatomy

Each form of symbrachydactyly occupies a place on the continuum from the normal hand through the various degrees of deficiency to complete absence of the hand. The severity of deficiency correlates with the degree of aberrant anatomy (see Table 40-9). As stated previously, the presence of proximal enabling structures offers hope for reconstruction of functioning digits (Fig. 40-56).

In all degrees of symbrachydactyly, the central rays are the most abnormal. In the mild forms, the skeletal elements are the most affected. The middle phalanges are reduced in size and may be absent. Because mild symbrachydactyly rarely requires surgical exploration, little is known about the aberrant anatomy.

In more severe symbrachydactyly, the central rays virtually disappear and are replaced by finger nubbins with aponeurotic attachments to extrinsic tendons around the end of the hypoplastic metacarpals. The extrinsic flexor tendons often share a muscle belly and may be coalesced into a single tendon mass within the carpal canal. The fifth ray is least affected and shows hypoplasia or absence of the middle phalanx with instability of the distal interphalangeal (DIP) joint. The extrinsic extensor tendon pulls the distal phalanx in a radial direction as it bowstrings across the central defect or "U"-shaped cleft. The extensor tendons along the dorsum of the hand appear quite normal and often have independent extensor indicis proprius or extensor digiti quinti tendons. The thumb is affected in the oligodactylic form with absence of the proximal phalanx and shortening of the pulp and nail. The basal joint shows adequate competent circumduction.

In the advanced monodactylic or single digit form of symbrachydactyly, the anatomy is widely abnormal. Surgical attempts at reconstruction have provided considerable information about the aberrant anatomy. The thumb may or may not have a proximal phalanx. The extrinsic tendons end in a conjoined fashion at the level of the metacarpal end. The aberrant rays may lack even vestigial metacarpals, and the fifth ray is usually represented by a short metacarpal. Flexor tendons are conjoined and end at the tips of the skeletal rays. The flexor tendons attach to the extensors and to the aponeurotic system, which yields a variable amount of movement of the finger nubbins. The extensor tendons are disordered and may be conjoined, although the extensor indicis proprius or extensor digiti quinti are often still distinct. The wrist extensors appear normal. The excursion of the extensor tendons is variable. In general, a wrist and nubbins that are active and mobile correlate with tendons that have some useful excursion. The tendons may be conjoined, and Vilkki[83] has recommended

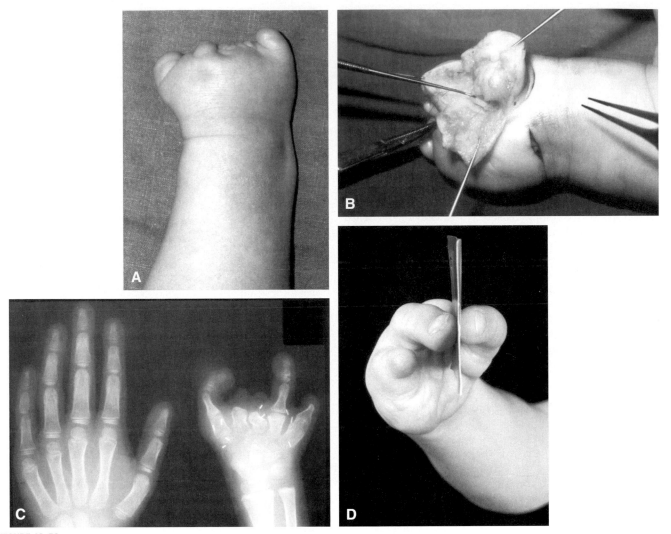

FIGURE 40-56. **A,** Adactylia form of symbrachydactyly with all digits absent and represented by nubbins with small nail remnants. **B,** Exploration revealed useful long flexor and extensor tendons with good excursion. **C,** Radiographs show the placement of a free toe transfer on the metacarpal remnant. Note the presence of a CMC joint in the thumb ray. **D,** Outcome with useful grasp of small and large objects.

exploration into the forearm to divide the donor tendon from any common muscle belly to prevent a quadriga effect.

In the more severe degrees of symbrachydactyly there are no useful intrinsic muscles to the fingers. Nerve abnormalities are common. The radial nerve is almost always present, regardless of the severity. In contrast, the median and ulnar nerves are small and may be absent. The presence of a thumb implies the presence of a median nerve. Rarely, complete absence of all major nerves in the hand may be found.

The peromelic form of symbrachydactyly (types 5 and 6) has severe skeletal absence. There may or may not be a carpal row. The wrist motors may be present. The flexor or extensor tendons of the fingers may be vestigial but have minimal excursion.

ACQUIRED TRANSVERSE ABSENCES IN CHILDREN

Acquired causes of transverse absence are also seen in childhood. Traumatic amputation is prevalent in countries that use child labor in the manufacturing industry. These

injuries may be bilateral and pose extraordinary challenges in reconstruction.[85,90,91] Other traumatic causes include burns, electrocution, thrombosis, and embolism. Lastly, infection may lead to gangrene of the extremities, primarily from meningococcal septicemia.[59,82,96]

Reconstruction for Transverse Absence

Augmentation of Existing Digital Rays

There are three main ways to augment the existing digit or ray in a child. The digit may be lengthened by a bone graft, may be lengthened by distraction, or may have composite parts of another digit transferred to it ("on-top plasty"). Bone grafting is most commonly performed using free phalangeal transfers from the foot.

Free Phalangeal Transfer

In the adult, many surgeons have found that the placement of bone grafts on the terminal part of the skeleton of a digit results in early and complete resorption of that graft. Resorption, however, is not invariably the case in the child. There are many descriptions of enduring transfers of whole or partial phalanges from within either the hand or foot. Some authors have reported poor results in terms of growth using this technique, whereas others have reported improved function.[15,17] Lister[48] and Radocha and colleagues[66] have defined three important conditions for success in these transfers if growth is to be observed: (1) transfer must be done before the age of 15 months; (2) periosteum must be included in the transfer; and (3) collateral ligaments and tendon insertions must be repaired.

In the authors' experience, the earlier the transfer is completed, the better the chance of subsequent growth.[35,71] The inclusion of periosteum allows more rapid revascularization of the free transfer, which may preserve the bone. The role of load across the physis is uncertain, but Radocha and colleagues[66] found unequivocal evidence that attachment of ligaments and tendons to the transferred bone was important. The best growth results in our children have been seen in those cases in which the phalanx was affixed to the proximal skeleton using chondrodesis, presumably increasing the amount of force transduced across the growth plate.

Indications

The surgeon and family must be aware of the other options, including microvascular toe transfer. The phalanges should not be harvested from the second toes unless microvascular toe transfer has been excluded as an option. Free phalangeal transfers are not a simple reconstructive option. A successful transfer grows and adds function, and this result is not inevitable. In addition, the donor site in the foot can be troublesome and a source of morbidity unless properly managed.

The requisite in the hand is a mobile, flexible adequate skin envelope, which is common in transverse absence or symbrachydactyly. The transfers should be planned in patients who can expect to have some functional improvement. The transfers are not indicated in patients who will have no increase in prehensile function. The absence of extrinsic tendon function is a relative contraindication. The parents must be aware of the potential cosmetic side effects for the foot, which are more important in patients undergoing concomitant microvascular toe transfer. Finally, the procedure is relatively contraindicated in the older child; we do not offer this treatment in children older than 15 months of age.

For the most part, whole toe transfers have replaced free phalangeal transfer because of the greater growth, mobility, and stability. The ideal recipient for free phalangeal transfer is a digital ray with a small remnant of proximal phalanx with tendon attachments and a suitable skin envelope. Free phalangeal transfer is especially useful in the thumb in cases of monodactylic symbrachydactyly (Fig. 40-57). In these cases, the fingers can be constructed from two toe transfers (see later), and the free phalangeal transfer augments the length of an otherwise competent thumb.

 ## Authors' Preferred Technique

Preparation of the Hand

Under tourniquet, the empty skin nubbins may be approached either by dorsal or volar longitudinal incision. Skin may be closed using a "Z"-plasty when additional length is required.

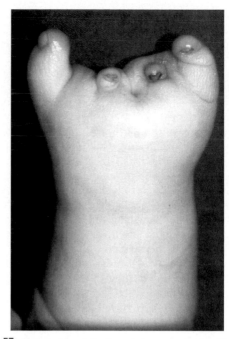
FIGURE 40-57. Image of hand for free phalangeal transfer. The thumb is devoid of skeletal elements despite its appearance.

The nubbin is opened and some fat is removed to accommodate the toe phalanx. Gentle traction on the nubbin with a skin hook reveals the extent of the cavity created for the transfer. The metacarpal head is evaluated and usually has a thin layer of articular cartilage overlying the epiphyses of the metacarpal. The metacarpal head is capped with a coalescence of the flexor and extensor tendons (Fig. 40-58). The authors' preference is to incise this in a cruciate manner and to raise the dorsal and volar capsule with the extensor and flexor tendons. The radial and ulnar parts of the capsule are preserved as collateral ligaments. Each of these elements will subsequently be repaired to the phalangeal transfer.

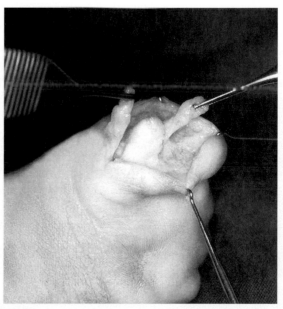
FIGURE 40-58. The flexor and extensor tendons are identified and separated over the metacarpal head.

In those cases with a remnant of proximal phalanx, the procedure is simpler, because the tendons do not require exploration. The end of the residual phalanx is prepared for chondrodesis with the free toe phalanx.

Harvesting the Graft

The toe phalanx is approached through a zigzag incision on the dorsum of the toe. The harvested phalanx is usually the proximal phalanx of the third or fourth toe. The second toe may be preferred in those cases in which microsurgical toe transfer is not being considered. After the dorsal exposure, the extensor apparatus is split in the midline of the digit and the toe phalanx dissected from its surrounding attachments, leaving the periosteum intact. The fibrous flexor sheath is divided laterally on the volar surface, taking care not to injure the flexor tendon. The distal capsular attachments are incised adjacent to the phalanx. The phalanx is harvested with the volar plate and capsular attachments (Fig. 40-59). Frequently, a small cap of the distal portion of the proximal phalanx is retained within the toe.

The donor defect may be closed in a variety of ways. Some have advocated simple longitudinal Kirschner wire fixation, whereas others have recommended suturing the flexor and extensor tendons together to serve as a spacer.[15,17] We prefer harvesting a cylindrical graft from the iliac crest that is capped with epiphyseal cartilage (Fig. 40-60). The graft is placed into the toe with the epiphyseal cartilage directed proximally. The tubular cancellous bone abuts the small fragment of distal toe phalanx that was retained within the foot. The graft and toe construct are fixed with a longitudinal Kirschner wire. The extensor tendons and skin are repaired. This pin is removed 4 to 6 weeks later.[8]

Placement of the Graft

The graft is transferred to the hand. The volar capsular attachments and flexor tendon within the hand are sutured to the volar plate on the free phalangeal graft. The graft is then transfixed with a longitudinal Kirschner wire passed from proximal to distal and exiting through the apex of the skin

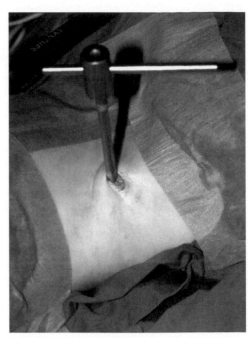

FIGURE 40-60. The bone graft is harvested from the iliac crest using a tubular osteotome and includes the apophysis.

envelope (Fig. 40-61). This wire is then withdrawn, the phalangeal graft then aligned with the metacarpal head, and the wire then advanced to fix the graft in place. The wire should be placed with as little trauma and heat dissipation as possible to avoid physeal plate injury. The collateral ligaments are repaired to the lateral margins of the capsule at the metacarpal head. The dorsal capsule and extensor tendon are repaired to the dorsal capsule of the free phalangeal graft. The skin is closed either with a "Z"-plasty or directly with

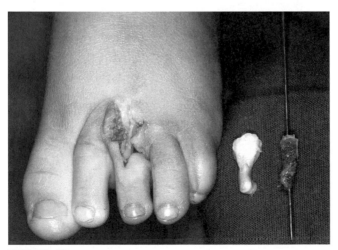

FIGURE 40-59. The proximal phalanx has been harvested from the third toe (preserving the second toe for possible future microvascular transfer). A tubular bone graft has been harvested to replace the phalanx and fixed with a longitudinal wire.

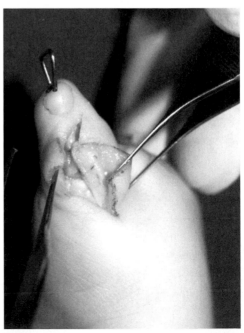

FIGURE 40-61. The toe proximal phalanx in place with Kirschner wire fixation and extensor tendon attachment.

absorbable sutures and the hand immobilized in an above-elbow cast.

Postoperatively, the Kirschner wires in the foot and the hand are removed 4 to 6 weeks after surgery. The parents may move the phalanx gently.

Complications

Complications include skin necrosis and absent growth of the transferred phalanx. Skin necrosis occurs when the transferred phalanx is too large for the skin envelope. Absent growth is more likely in the older child, when the tendons or ligaments are not repaired, or when the periosteum is not included in the transfer. Scarring may occur in the foot, especially when a longitudinal incision is used. Contraction may result in dorsal displacement of the toes that may become unstable. In addition, the donor defect may be worse in cases in which the extensor and flexor tendons have been sutured together as a "spacer." This technique may lead to unstable toes that angulate and override adjacent digits.

Transposition of Rays

This principle involves transposition of rays to allow prehension. In certain hands, the thumb lacks enough excursion to reach the fingers. Transposition of a finger or fingers into a more radial position can allow pinch or grasp. Transposition may be combined with microvascular toe transfer to enhance hand function (Fig. 40-62).

MICROVASCULAR TOE TRANSFER FOR HYPOPLASTIC DIGITS

Single-stage microvascular toe-to-hand transfer is not a new concept.[19] The technique has been primarily utilized in post-traumatic cases in adults. Before the 1990s, relatively few reports dealt with children.[29,30,47,61,62] Lister[47] reviewed 12 toe transfers for congenital deficiency of the thumb and reported good return of sensibility but poor return of interphalangeal (IP) motion. Kay and colleagues[41,42] extended the indications to include reconstruction of the congenital hand with absent thumb or finger and traumatic loss.

Choice of Technique

Many variations of toe transfers have been developed, including the wraparound free flap,[22,31,56-58,60,74,77] the twisted toe transfer,[26-29] the double toe transfer,[34,41,45,62,81] the great toe transfer,[61,79,86] and the trimmed toe transfer.[43,88] Many surgeons believe that the donor defect must be minimized, especially in children. For this reason, we are reluctant to transfer anything other than the second toe. This limits the reconstruction to two digits. These digits can be transferred in separate operations or in the same operation (synchronous bilateral toe transfer). In selected cases when either single or bilateral second toe transfer is not appropriate, transfer of the great toe may be considered with caution. The cosmetic defect is greater and there may be functional consequences. Rarely, a wraparound free flap or partial toe transfer may be used in the older child.

Indications

The indications for digital reconstruction include transverse deficiencies in the thumb and/or fingers. Longitudinal deficiency has been a contraindication because of the deficient proximal structures, such as tendons and nerves. Longitudinal deficiency is usually reconstructed by transfer of adjacent digit. In the monodactylous cleft hand, however, we have found tendons and nerves that are available for transfer. This finding further demonstrates the erosion of the clear distinction between categories of digital absence.

Reconstruction of the Thumb

Traumatic or congenital transverse thumb deficiency is the ideal indication for microsurgical toe transfer. The most important determinant of useful outcome is the presence of a stable and mobile carpometacarpal (CMC) joint (Fig. 40-63).[41,42] The recipient structures vary according to the etiology. The proximal structures are virtually normal in the amniotic disruption sequence. Useful recipient structures are also found in symbrachydactyly or transverse arrest and are more likely to be present when there is a considerable metacarpal remnant. The lack of IP joint motion after transfer reflects the limited amplitude of the extrinsic tendons.[24,47]

Reconstruction of the Fingers

Reconstruction of the fingers is not as common as reconstruction of the thumb. Reconstruction may be indicated after trauma or congenital absence when there is a reasonable thumb present. In such cases, bilateral second toe transfer creates a competent three-digit hand with powerful pinch and grasp. The presence of existing MCP joints enhances surgical outcome. However, absent MCP joints may still provide satisfactory function. Symbrachydactyly with a thumb and a small finger that is short, deviated, and unstable may be a candidate for bilateral second toe transfer to create a more complete hand. Such cases occupy the borderline between the functional and cosmetic indication for toe transfer.[41,42]

The Hand with No Digits

Transverse arrest or severe symbrachydactyly without digits requires reconstruction of the thumb and fingers to create any prehensile function. These cases are challenging, and the outcome depends on the level of absence and the competence of the basal joint of the thumb. A substantial thumb metacarpal remnant may be enhanced by bony augmentation. Even a free phalangeal transfer may be attempted to create an articulated thumb. Successful transfer may change the reconstruction from a hand that requires thumb and finger restoration to one that requires only finger restoration.

If thumb augmentation is not possible, the surgeon may consider one transfer to the thumb and one to the finger rays (Fig. 40-64). Poor or absent basal joint function requires placement of the digits facing each other. The majority of the movement will originate from the IP joints of the thumb and finger. Postoperative motion is often poor and limits the functional benefits of such transfer. If surgery is selected, a decision must be made to position the transfers to touch in

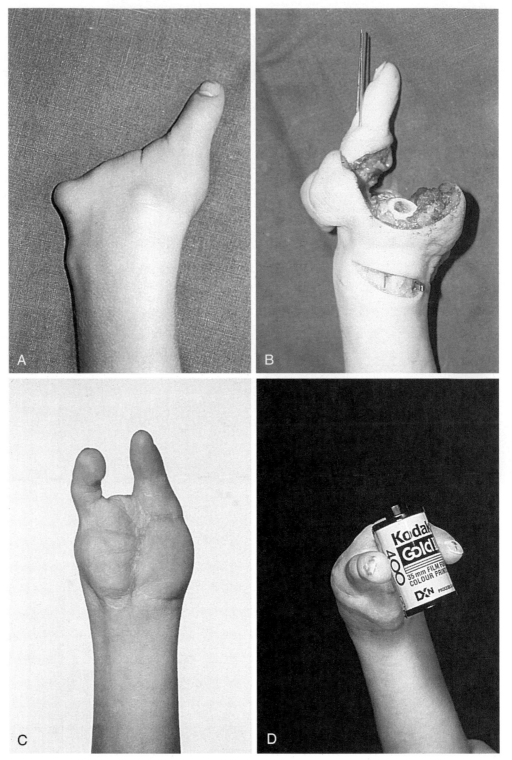

FIGURE 40-62. A, The left hand of a child with congenital digital absence. Although a thumb ray is present, there is no active or passive movement at any level in that ray including the basal joint. The hand has no prehensile function. **B,** Rather than creating a mobile ulnar ray against a static radial ray, it was decided to transfer the existing "thumb" to the ulnar border of the digit as a microvascular pedicle transfer. A single second toe transfer to the radial ray was undertaken at the same procedure creating a thumb. **C,** The postoperative result with the static ulnar ray and the thumb present on the radial ray. **D,** Strong small object pinch and grasp resulted from this combination of transfers.

maximum flexion or to place them more widely apart. The former allows small object grasp, whereas the latter allows larger object acquisition. In our experience, small object grasp is preferred to allow the child to hold fine objects such as paper, buttons, and shoelaces.

In the presence of a reasonable basal joint, a second toe is placed on the thumb and another placed on the third or fourth ray. The transfer may create a composite joint, using one articular surface from the toe and one from the finger. The preferred approach, however, is to perform a chondrodesis or arthrodesis between the base of the proximal phalanx in the toe and the shaft of the metacarpal in the thumb and finger. This technique has the additional benefit of stability and precise orientation of the digit.

Finally, a decision is required regarding the length of the digit to be created. The initial temptation is to create long

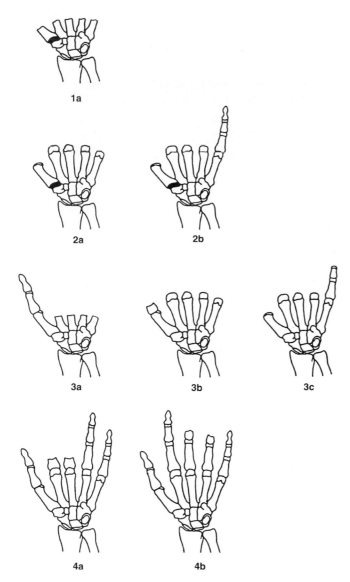

FIGURE 40-63. A simple grouping of common types of congenital transverse deficiency in the hand based on the author's experience of the reconstructive options available and the likely functional outcome.

Group 1a: The absence is at a proximal level through the base of the metacarpal or at the carpometacarpal level. There is no circumduction in the thumb ray, and here bilateral second toe transfers will allow pincer grip between the toe pulps. It is likely that a choice will have to be made between small or large object grasp because the range of motion in the reconstructed toes is unlikely to allow both.

Group 2a: The absences are at the distal level of the metacarpals, and the basal joint of the thumb is competent. A reconstruction at this level with one toe on the first ray and one toe on the fourth ray will allow good small and large object grasp with competent pulp-to-pulp pinch by virtue of the basal motion in the thumb.

Group 2b: The distal metacarpal loss with a poorly competent basal joint but the presence of a relatively normal fifth ray. The mobility in all the joints of the fifth ray including the basal joint means that any reconstruction on the thumb ray will probably allow both small and large object grasp. Single toe transfer to the thumb ray is therefore indicated, and the optional transfer of a further toe to the ring finger ray is unlikely to result in great improvement. One further option in this situation is microvascular pollicization of the fifth ray and a double toe transfer to the hand on the third and fourth rays. This has the advantage of producing a more full hand but retaining and restoring mobility in the first ray.

Group 3a: Proximal metacarpal level in the hand with a competent and strong first ray. Here bilateral second toe transfer on the fourth and fifth rays will produce a strong and competent hand even if relatively little motion is restored in the transferred digits.

Group 3b: Distal metacarpal absence with the presence of a MCP joint in the thumb. If the patient is seen early in life, free phalangeal transfer in the thumb will convert the patient's hand to essentially a group 3a hand and allow bilateral second toe reconstruction in the hand rays.

Groups 4a and 4b: This type of transverse absence is most commonly seen in ring constriction syndrome where the function of the hand is already excellent. Little or no functional improvement will result from microsurgical toe transfers, but there are potentially considerable cosmetic benefits from creating a more full hand. Although the function in the hand itself is already good, good function in reconstructed digits can be expected as a result of the relatively normal structures present proximally in the hand.

digits; however, long digits may look bizarre in a two-digit hand (Fig. 40-65). This altered appearance may be disturbing for the child compared with shorter digits that allow the hand to appear more compact and natural. The physis of the transferred digit is retained for growth, which may require some resection of the thumb metacarpal to coordinate the length of the thumb and finger.

Contraindications

Contraindications to toe transfer are diminishing over time. There are few contraindications from the anatomic point of view. Absence of recipient nerves is a contraindication to surgery. We warn parents that when no recipient nerve is found, surgery will be aborted. An extremely proximal level of transverse absence (e.g., the distal carpal row or radiocarpal level) will produce a disappointing result, and prosthetic alternatives should be considered. Absence or deformities of the toes clearly precludes surgery.

The most considerable contraindications are the psychosocial considerations within the family and competence within the surgical unit. Careful assessment and counseling of the family and child are essential to ensure an adequate understanding of the aims and consequences of surgery, to accept the donor defect, and to manage the consequences of either a successful or an unsuccessful procedure.[4,9,38]

The age of the child is a relative contraindication. Absolute rules about indications and contraindications in respect to age of the child do not exist. We have found no benefit in performing the procedure before 1 year of age, and there may be some disadvantages in terms of ultimate range of motion. There are benefits in completing the surgery before school age, and this reconstruction is rarely accomplished in a single stage. After the age of 6, the child becomes involved in the choice of surgery and is able to take an active part in rehabilitation.

Presurgical Assessment

Angiography is not required unless there is considerable concern about the proximal vasculature. The child must be in good general health. Preoperative assessment by an anesthesiologist is required, because the procedure is lengthy.[97]

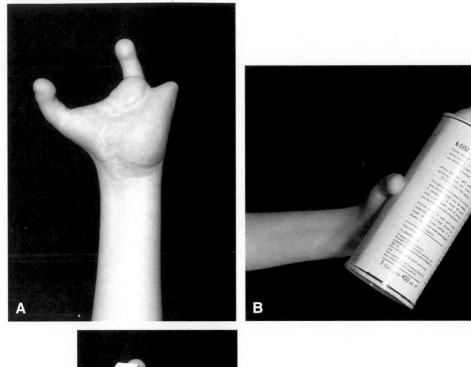

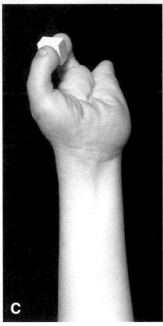

FIGURE 40-64. A, Two simultaneous second toe transfers for symbrachydactyly with absent digits at the metacarpal level. There was a competent thumb basal joint. **B,** Useful large object grasp with considerable power. **C,** Small object pinch as a result of limited circumduction at the thumb basal joint.

Surgical Technique

Hand Preparation

The hand is explored under tourniquet control. The dorsal exposure is via a transverse incision at the wrist crease. This incision avoids unsightly longitudinal or zigzag incisions on the dorsum of the hand. The extensor tendons, veins, and the dorsal branches of the radial or ulnar nerve are identified and marked. Proximal excursion of the extensor tendons is confirmed via traction. The tendon with the greatest excursion is chosen as the donor tendon. When more than one tendon is required, either the extensor indicis proprius or extensor digiti quinti is used in an attempt to achieve some independent function. The venous anastomosis is performed on the dorsum of the hand, and the arterial anastomosis is completed on the palmar surface or in the anatomical snuff-box.

The recipient site skin incisions are planned to result in a transverse scar on the palmar surface and a "V"-shaped scar on the dorsum. This shape allows insetting of a tongue of dorsal foot skin. The level of bony union is identified and marked. The proximal palmar exposure is accomplished via a zigzag incision. The median and/or ulnar nerves are identified at the level of the carpal canal along with the flexor tendons. The ulnar artery, the superficial palmar arch, and the radial artery within the anatomical snuff-box are examined and identified for later use.

Harvesting the Second Toe (Points Relative to Children)

The skin pattern on the toe is designed with reference to the defect in the hand, usually incorporating a "V"-shaped flap

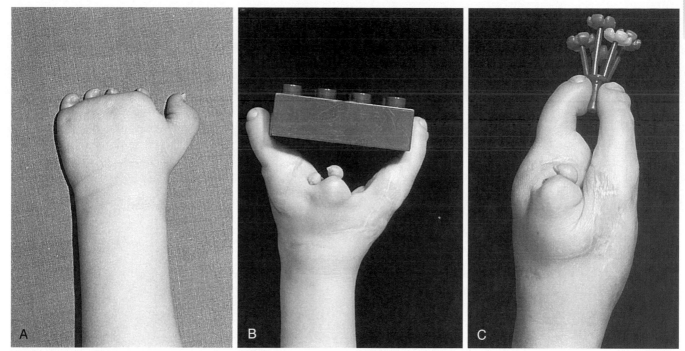

FIGURE 40-65. **A,** Transverse arrest in the hand of a 2-year-old girl. The thumb is absent from the midmetacarpal level distally and is represented by a skin envelope devoid of skeleton. **B,** This child underwent bilateral second toe transfer with one toe to the first and one toe to the fourth ray. An alternative might have been free phalangeal bone graft to the thumb and a double toe transfer to the hand. In this case, the digits have a long, narrow appearance, giving the hand the appearance of clefting. However, large object grasp is successfully created. The child refused removal of the skin bobbles within the cleft. **C,** The same hand exhibits good small object grasp by virtue of the mobility of the basal joint. The length of the digits contributes to their range and power, but they have the disadvantage of poor cosmesis.

of dorsal skin. The harvest begins under tourniquet control using the entire skin incision, including a dorsal linear incision running between the first and second metatarsals. A single dorsal vein is then isolated. In the child, the major veins lie in a distinctly deeper layer of subcutaneous fat than the smaller superficial veins. We have developed a method for defining the vascular anatomy of the toe in a retrograde distal-to-proximal manner.[39,41,42,93] An assistant separates the first and second toes, and the fibular digital artery of the great toe is identified (Fig. 40-66). The artery is traced to its common origin with the second toe vessel. From this bifurcation, both the plantar and dorsal metatarsal arteries may be traced in a proximal direction. This technique facilitates selection of the artery for anastomosis. In two-thirds of cases, there is a sizable first dorsal metatarsal artery for anastomosis and the plantar artery and vessel to the great toe can be divided. The proximal dissection of the dorsal artery is then straightforward.[40] In one third of cases, the plantar artery must be used for anastomosis and the dissection is more difficult. The deep peroneal branch of the anterior tibial nerve is harvested and usually lies closely applied to the vein and first dorsal metatarsal artery. Both plantar digital nerves of the second toe are then dissected in a proximal direction and separated from the adjacent component of the common digital nerve.

The flexor tendons are exposed at the proximal edge of the flexor sheath just proximal to the metatarsophalangeal (MTP) joint. The tendons are retracted and divided deep within the sole of the foot. The bone transection is then performed through the MTP joint. Other authors have preferred to incorporate the MTP joint as a mobile joint. The

tourniquet is deflated, perfusion of the toes is confirmed, and hemostasis is achieved.

Osteosynthesis

After the toe is separated from the foot, the bone is prepared on the back table. When the osteosynthesis is planned at the base of the phalanx, the cartilage is removed until subchondral bone is encountered. In some cases, a composite joint can be formed between the articular surface of the base of the proximal phalanx of the toe and the articular surface of the metacarpal. Longitudinal Kirschner wires are usually preferred. The wires cause little damage to the growing epiphyses, are quick to apply, and are adequate to achieve union in these young hands. Crossed Kirschner wires interfere with the adjacent toes, risk damage to the digital vessels, and do not allow correction of rotation after preliminary placement. Interosseous wire and plates are rarely used because of the proximal growing epiphyses.

Tendon Repairs

The toe is brought into the hand and the extensor tendons are repaired first. The tendons are passed deep to dorsal skin and fat and are repaired at the wrist level. Two extensor tendon repairs are preferred. After extensor tendon repair, any extensor tendon that passes to an absent ray is divided to prevent a tethering or quadriga effect.

The flexor tendon choice is more difficult. In symbrachydactyly or transverse absence, inadequate excursion is common. Unless individual flexor digitorum profundus (FDP) and flexor digitorum superficialis (FDS) tendons are present, only the toe FDP is repaired. An overlapping repair or a

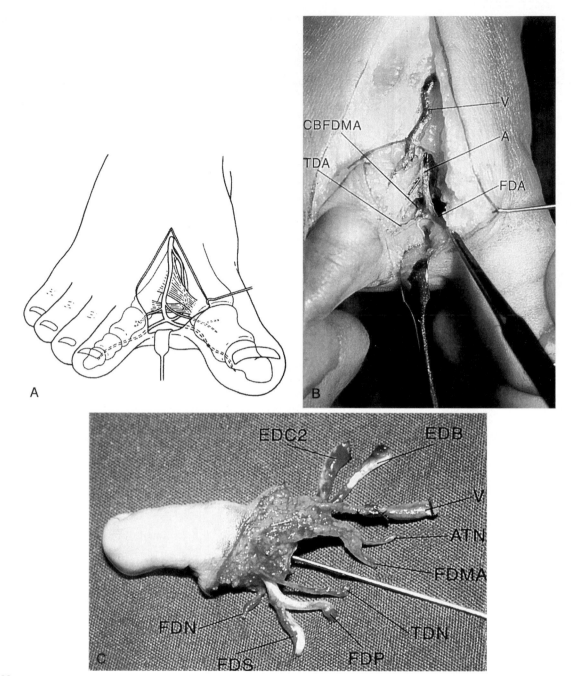

FIGURE 40-66. A, The first web space is approached from distal to proximal. The fibula vessel of the great toe is most easily identified and traced proximally to the communication with the first dorsal metatarsal artery, the first plantar metatarsal artery, and the tibial vessel to the second toe. The exact architecture of the junction between these vessels is variable, but all these named vessels are usually present, although either the plantar or the dorsal may be predominant. The dorsal branches to the toes arise from the dorsal metatarsal artery as shown. **B,** The vessels of the first web space. The fibula digital artery (FDA) of the great toe is clearly seen and when traced proximally leads to the junction between the first dorsal metatarsal artery (A) and the communicating branch for the first dorsal metatarsal artery to the plantar artery arterial system (CBFDMA). At or about the same level, the tibial digital artery of the second toe arises. The dorsal venous network is also clearly seen. **C,** The second toe has been harvested and a Kirschner wire has been introduced through the base of the proximal phalanx in preparation for osteosynthesis. The individually identified structures are noted: the extensor digitorum communis (EDC2) tendon; the extensor digitorum brevis (EDB) tendon; the dorsal vein (V), a tributary of the long saphenous vein; the dorsal digital nerve (a branch of the anterior tibial nerve [ATN]); the first dorsal metatarsal artery (FDMA); the tibial digital nerve (TDN); the flexor digital and profundus tendon (FDP); the flexor digital and sublimis tendon (FDS); and the fibula digital nerve (FDN).

weave is performed. The toe FDS tendon is cut short. The flexor tendon is sutured under slightly less tension than the extensor tendons.

Nerve Repairs

Repair as many nerves as possible. The nerves are coapted under the microscope. The nerve repair should be as proximal as possible to ensure good recipient nerve quality in the hand.

Vessels

A single artery and a single vein are repaired.[37] Other authors have recommended repair of more vessels. Before tourniquet deflation, vessels intended for repair are clamped to ensure that the existing digits perfuse. This perfusion implies safe anastomosis without jeopardizing blood flow to existing digits. The tourniquet is re-inflated and vessel anastomosis is completed. The lumina of the vessels are irrigated with heparin solution. Vein grafts are rarely needed. A warm pack is applied to the limb and the tourniquet is deflated. The transferred digit is observed for 10 or 15 minutes to ensure vascular patency.

Skin Repair

The skin is loosely closed with absorbable sutures at wide intervals to allow blood to ooze from the wounds. No attempt is made to close the wound completely under tension. Most children will require scar revision surgery, so the use of split-skin grafts is encouraged rather than tight closure. The exception to this tenet is the dorsum of the hand. Considerable swelling may create shear forces on the vein and, therefore, skin closure should be complete. The hand is then gently wrapped without compression and a plaster slab applied with the elbow at 90 degrees.

Postoperative Care

The child is admitted to the intensive care unit in a temperature-controlled room for 24 hours after surgery. Core and peripheral temperature, pulse, central venous pressure, and urine output all are monitored. The child is kept relatively sedated and has indwelling regional local anesthetic infusions. The child is discharged to home 3 to 5 days after surgery. Dressings are changed 6 weeks after surgery, usually under general anesthesia. The Kirschner wires are removed and the digits gently manipulated. A thermoplastic splint is fabricated for night time and during challenging physical activity. Parents are instructed in passive and active motion and to protect the insensate digit from harm. The parents are warned that during reinnervation the child will experience uncomfortable dysesthesias that are normal and transient.

Other Indications and Techniques

Another indication for microvascular toe transfer is traumatic loss of digits. Toe transfers have been reported in children for the reconstruction of traumatic defects, including the metacarpal hand.[49,91] In some cases, these defects are bilateral, and the use of a single toe from each foot will not produce adequate reconstruction of function. The use of transfers from the great toe (wrap-around flap or trimmed toe transfer) and the use of monobloc transfer of the second and third toes have been necessary in some of these cases.[49,91]

Transfers from the Great Toe

Transfers from the great toe are favored in adults for certain aspects of hand reconstruction.* In the congenital hand, great toe transfer is seldom indicated because reconstruction can usually be accomplished using the second toe. In some traumatic defects, however, great toe transfer may be necessary. Considerable cosmetic morbidity results from harvesting the whole great toe. Parents are reluctant to allow such harvest. The wrap-around free flap from the great toe contains no epiphysis and is usually unsuitable in the growing child. The wrap-around free flap may be used in the older child or in distal digital injuries with soft tissue avulsion.

The Metacarpal Hand

Loss of most or all of the digits may be a result of trauma. The metacarpals may be spared, and the thumb may or may not escape injury. Adequate function can be expected when the thumb has been amputated distal to the middle of the proximal phalanx and if a portion of the proximal phalanges of the fingers is present. Any more proximal loss usually results in poor function. Such hands are best reconstructed using some form of free toe transfer.[49,91]

Results

The results of toe transfer in children have been reported. Lister[47] reported good recovery of sensibility and function. Poor recovery of IP joint motion was noted. Wei[92] has reported on 45 whole toe or partial toe transfers performed in 28 children treated for traumatic loss. The transfers included six trimmed great toe transfers, two great toe pulp transfers, 24 second toes, 4 combined second and third toes, and five monobloc toe transfers.[85-87,89,92] All but one toe transfer survived transplantation. Good sensory recovery occurred (5-mm static two-point discrimination), and useful recovery of function was observed. Growth continued in the transferred toes.

The senior author initially reported on 66 toe transfers in 40 children.[41,42] All but three children achieved motion in their transferred toes. Mean total range of active motion was 60 degrees and was independent of the number of tendons repaired. The passive range was always greater than the active range. Grasp function was useful and satisfactory in both small and large object grasp in the majority of cases (Fig. 40-67). Sensibility recovery showed two-point discriminations between 4 and 5 mm. Currently, 200 transfers have been performed with the loss of a single partial toe transfer. The thumb ray was the most common recipient, and the fourth ray was the second most common beneficiary.

Additional attention has focused on the psychological aspects of surgery.[42] The vast majority of parents (84%) and

___
*See references 1, 14, 19, 31, 36, 43, 44, 49, 51, 52, 61, 67, 79, 88, and 99.

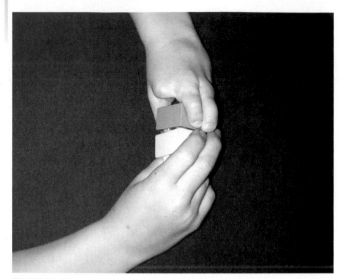

FIGURE 40-67. The results after double synchronous second toe transfer in a child with transverse absence of all fingers but a competent thumb. There was recovery of good sensibility and some prehension.

children (88%) thought the hand was improved after surgery. Only one adult and one child thought the hand looked worse. Scarring was not a dominant complaint of the parents and was virtually ignored by the children. Most parents (80%) believe the hand was incorporated into function most of the time. No adverse effect of toe transfer from the psychosocial viewpoint was found. The impression was that the reconstructive surgery had a positive response on the child and family.

Secondary Surgery

Microsurgery rarely offers a one-stage reconstruction; secondary procedures are common. The need for adjustment of the skin, bone, and tendon transfers is widespread. Procedures include pulp plasty, scar revision, excision of skin graft, and tenolysis. Opposition transfers and rotation osteotomies may also be needed. Secondary surgery is usually deferred for at least 18 months to allow scar maturation, joint motion, and the incorporation of the transfer into use.

CRITICAL POINTS: ABSENCE OF FINGERS

- Symbrachydactyly is a spectrum of deficiency, beginning with short middle phalanges and extending to absence of the central rays, culminating in absence of the entire hand.

- The treatment of symbrachydactyly depends on the degree of digital suppression. Mild forms with a competent thumb and digit(s) require no treatment. Severe forms with an absent thumb or absent fingers may benefit from extraperiosteal phalanx transfer or microsurgical toe-to-hand transfer.

ANNOTATED REFERENCES

15. Buck-Gramcko D: The role of nonvascularized toe phalanx transplantation. Hand Clin 6:643-659, 1990.

   Ninety-seven toe phalanx transplantations were performed in 57 children. Follow-up examinations of 44 patients with 69 transplanted toe phalanges showed 100% take of the bone graft provided it had been unsplit and the periosteal cover undamaged. A joint construction was attempted in 64 digits with variable results. The range of active motion varied between 0 (fusion) and 90 degrees.

35. James MA, Durkin RC: Nonvascularized toe proximal phalanx transfers in the treatment of aphalangia. Hand Clin 14:1-15, 1998.

   This article discusses the indications for nonvascularized toe phalanx transfers. Radiolucency in the region of the transferred physis does not necessarily indicate a functional growth plate. The results of this procedure can be improved by inclusion of the periosteum and collateral ligaments to decrease graft resorption.

41. Kay SP, Wiberg M: Toe to hand transfer in children: I. Technical aspects. J Hand Surg [Br] 21:723-734, 1996.

   Forty children (age range: 9 months to 14 years) with either congenital (85%) or acquired hand deformities underwent reconstruction by microvascular transplantation of one or more toes. Regardless of whether one or two toes were transferred, the children spent on average 9 days in the hospital. No transfers failed, but 75% of the children underwent staged additional surgery to improve appearance and function. Technical considerations are presented.

54. Miura T, Nakamura R, Horii E: The position of symbrachydactyly in the classification of congenital hand anomalies. J Hand Surg [Br] 19:350-354, 1994.

   Clinical features of 53 cases of intercalated hypoplasia and 113 cases of distal aplasia are compared with each other and with 129 cases of syndactyly. Progressive digital loss from missing a single digit to adactyly was reasoned to represent similar deficiencies of varying phenotypes.

66. Radocha RF, Netscher D, Kleinert HE: Toe phalangeal grafts in congenital hand anomalies. J Hand Surg [Am] 18:833-841, 1993.

   Seventy-three toe phalangeal grafts were reviewed to determine the effects of age and operative technique on subsequent growth of the transferred phalanx. Physeal openness rates were 94% for those operated on before 1 year of age, 71% for those 1 to 2 years of age, and 48% for those older than 2 years of age. Mean growth rates were 1.0 ± 0.2 mm, 1.0 ± 0.6 mm, and 0.5 ± 0.5 mm per year, respectively, for these three age groups.

83. Vilkki SK: Advances in microsurgical reconstruction of the congenitally adactylous hand. Clin Orthop 314:45-58, 1995.

   Eighteen microsurgical toe transfers were performed for adactylous hands. The functional results achieved were dependent on the approach and technical features applied. Function was improved significantly by using three-jointed second toes, including the MTP joint. The ability to pinch was restored successfully in 14 of 17 congenitally impaired extremities.

94. Wiedrich TA: Congenital constriction band syndrome. Hand Clin 14:29-38, 1998.

   This is an overview of constriction band syndrome with a discussion of proposed etiologies. The various clinical presentations are addressed and potential treatment options are reviewed.

Clinodactyly

David McCombe and Simon P. Kay

Clinodactyly is angulation of the digit in the radioulnar plane distal to the metacarpophalangeal (MCP) joint (Fig. 40-68). Minor angulation, particularly of the small finger, is common to the point of normalcy. Significant clinodactyly has been defined as angulation greater than 10 degrees.[5] The anomaly arises when the alignment of an interphalangeal (IP) joint is away from perpendicular to the normal longitudinal axis of the finger. The shape of the underlying phalanx is the cause. The abnormal shape develops as result of asymmetrical longitudinal growth.

EPIDEMIOLOGY

The true incidence of clinodactyly is difficult to ascertain, with figures ranging from 1% to 19.5%.[7] Clinodactyly presents most commonly as an isolated radial inclination of the small finger, owing to the middle phalanx adopting a triangular or trapezoidal shape. This form of clinodactyly is inherited as an autosomal dominant trait and is often bilateral (Fig. 40-69).[8,15,22] Expression of the trait is variable, with males more likely to express the phenotype.[22] Clinodactyly is also seen as part of many syndromes and complex hand anomalies.

PATHOLOGY

The longitudinal growth of tubular bones such as the phalanges is generated at the epiphyseal growth plate, with axial alignment maintained by factors intrinsic and extrinsic to the growth plate.[16] An abnormal growth plate secondary to a congenital anomaly or postnatal insult will produce deformation with growth. The growth plate anomaly associated with clinodactyly is the "C"-shaped physeal plate extending along one side of the bone, forming a bracket that

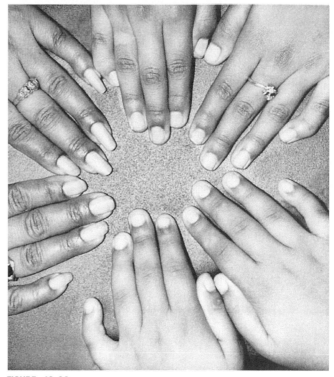

FIGURE 40-69. A family with mother and two daughters exhibiting clinodactyly of the fifth fingers, emphasizing the autosomal dominant transmission in some cases. (Courtesy of M. Patel, MD.)

restricts longitudinal growth. The pathology was described initially by Jones[10] in his description of triangular or "delta" phalanges in severe clinodactyly. Further descriptions have led to new terminology[13,18] (the "longitudinal diaphyseal bracket" or the "longitudinal epiphyseal bracket"), along with recognition of a spectrum of severity and a classification system.[12] When the bracket completely ossifies early, no longitudinal growth is possible and a short, triangular bone, the "delta phalanx," is produced. If the bracket is incomplete or is cartilaginous, some longitudinal growth occurs and the phalanx is trapezoidal and the digit angulated. The "delta phalanx" anomaly, however, does not inevitably produce angulation, because it may be concealed within a complex skeletal mass such as synpolydactyly. The epiphyseal bracket anomaly also occurs in the metacarpals, metatarsals,[9] and elsewhere,[14] although it is believed to occur only in bones that have a secondary ossification center at their base.[13,21] The epiphyseal bracket affects the middle phalanx most commonly, perhaps because this is the last bone to ossify in the digital skeleton.[7,9] The epiphyseal bracket may also occur in the proximal phalanx or within the extra phalanx in hyperphalangism.[20] Acquired causes of clinodactyly include trauma to the growth plate from injury or frostbite, inflammatory arthritis with asymmetrical physeal closure, and tumor within the bone, such as an enchondroma.

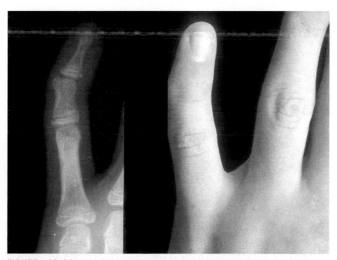

FIGURE 40-68. Radiographs and photograph of left small finger clinodactyly.

Although the skeletal anomaly generates the angulation of the finger, the underlying soft tissues are affected. Severe angulation leads to soft tissue shortening on the concave side of the digit and possible displacement of the extensor mechanism. This soft tissue deformation requires consideration during surgical correction.

CLINICAL FEATURES

Clinodactyly will present either in isolation or as part of a broader anomaly. Isolated, severe clinodactyly may present in the neonate or infant, although most present later as the angulation becomes more obvious with growth. The reason for presentation is usually cosmetic, because compensatory abduction of the small finger will prevent substantial interference with flexion. Thumb clinodactyly may cause functional impairment as seen in the Apert hand.

The radiographic appearance varies with the age of the patient and degree of bony involvement. In the skeletally mature patient, a triangular or trapezoidal bone will be apparent. In the skeletally immature patient, the secondary center of ossification may be malformed, traverse around the base of the phalanx, and travel along the shortened side of the bone. The most severe form of longitudinal epiphyseal bracket forms a "C"-shape as the bracket that unites the proximal and distal growth centers. Clinodactyly can be classified according to etiology[1] or pathology[12]; the most useful classification is that proposed by Cooney (Table 40-10).[4]

MANAGEMENT

The majority of patients with isolated clinodactyly of the small finger present with a cosmetic rather than a functional problem. Surgery should be avoided in these cases, because any improvement in appearance occurs at the risk of scarring and stiffness. Surgical correction is indicated for severe clinodactyly with shortening and angulation or thumb involvement.

Splinting for clinodactyly is pointless. Correction of the skeletal anomaly requires either an osteotomy to realign the digit or resection of the longitudinal epiphyseal bracket to release the longitudinal growth potential of the shortened side of the digit. Realignment of the axis of the digit with an osteotomy may be achieved with a closing wedge, opening wedge, or a combined procedure, the reverse wedge osteotomy. The closing wedge osteotomy (Fig. 40-70) is attractive because of its relative simplicity and reliability[2]; however, in the shortened digit a further loss of length may be unacceptable. An increase or maintenance of length is possible with an opening wedge or reverse wedge osteotomy,[11] respectively. The bone graft requirement for an opening wedge or the more extensive surgery for the reverse wedge, however, are disadvantages.

Corrective osteotomy is indicated in moderate deviation that interferes with function. If possible, correction is best deferred until skeletal maturity to allow ample time for bone growth. In the skeletally immature patient, osteotomy is technically challenging, with risks of incomplete or excess correction or physeal injury with the additional consequences. In severe clinodactyly or thumb clinodactyly, earlier surgery may be required. Corrective osteotomy tries to

Table 40-10
CLASSIFICATION OF CLINODACTYLY

Type	Deformity	Angulation	Associated Deformity
Simple	Middle phalanx	< 45 degrees	
Simple complicated	Middle phalanx	> 45 degrees	
Complex	Bone and soft tissue	< 45 degrees	Syndactyly
Complex complicated	Bone and soft tissue	> 45 degrees	Polydactyly or macrodactyly

From Cooney WP: Camptodactyly and clinodactyly. In Carter P (ed): Reconstruction of the Child's Hand. Philadelphia, Lea & Febiger, 1991.

achieve a single-stage correction. The soft tissue deficit on the concave side may be addressed with a "Z"-plasty (Fig. 40-71).[17,23] In severe angulations, "Z"-plasty may be inadequate and a rotational flap or step advancement flap described by Evans and James[6] may be required (Fig. 40-72). For the severe types, realignment of the extensor mechanism may also be necessary to maintain balance of the corrected digit.[7] Clinodactyly in the triphalangeal thumb or hyperphalangism of the fingers may be addressed by excision of the extra malformed phalanx. Ligament reconstruction or arthrodesis of the adjacent joints is obligatory to restore stability.

An alternative to corrective osteotomy is epiphyseal bracket resection and fat grafting (Fig. 40-73).[19] This procedure is based on the premise that resection of the bracket will allow the normal portion of the epiphyseal growth plate to generate "catch-up" longitudinal growth on the shortened side and produce angulatory correction over 1 to 2 years.

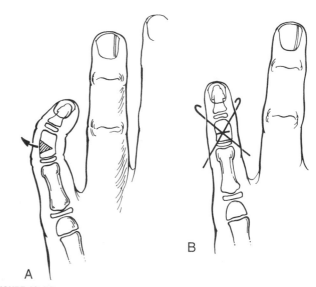

FIGURE 40-70. **A** and **B,** A closing wedge osteotomy through the abnormal middle phalanx can be best accomplished on the convex side of the digit. (Adapted from Flatt AE: The Care of Congenital Hand Anomalies. St. Louis, CV Mosby, 1977, pp 154-163, with permission.)

The procedure is performed through a midlateral incision on the short side of the phalanx. The cartilaginous or bony bracket is resected until metaphyseal bone is exposed from dorsal to volar and the growth plate is defined. The defect created is filled with fat, harvested from the forearm, to fill the dead space and prevent fusion across the growth plate. The procedure is limited to patients with open growth plates and is best performed early, although Vickers has performed the procedure with good results on children with only 1 to 2 years of growth remaining.[20] In a review of this procedure,[3] a group of 23 children with 35 operated fingers obtained a mean correction of 11 degrees after a mean follow-up period of 3.2 years. Further analysis revealed that better results were obtained with surgery before the age of 6. In addition, fingers with angulation greater than 40 degrees had a greater degree of improvement (20 degrees) compared with those with less than 40 degrees of preoperative angulation (7.5 degrees). Bracket resection does not preclude the use of corrective osteotomy for residual angulation and requires minimal splinting or postoperative immobilization.[20]

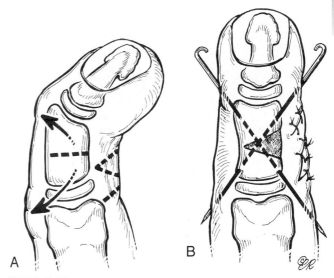

FIGURE 40-71. **A** and **B,** An opening wedge osteotomy will give more length to a digit but requires a soft tissue release, including a "Z"-plasty of the skin.

 Authors' Preferred Technique

The preferred approach for mild to moderate clinodactyly is to avoid surgery. Surgery is especially rejected in the common mild deformity of the small finger. When the angulation is considerable and the phalanx is a "delta phalanx," early epiphyseal bracket resection and fat grafting may be performed. When the patient presents with substantial angulation and is skeletally mature, the decision is based on the configuration of the phalanx. The trapezoidal phalanx tolerates the shortening of a closing wedge osteotomy,

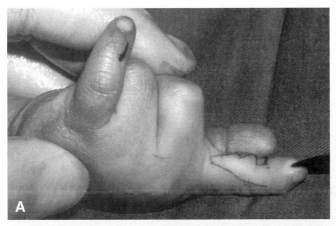

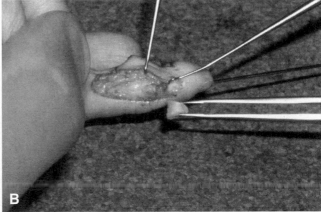

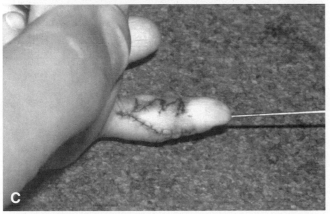

FIGURE 40-72. **A** to **C,** A child with clinodactyly requiring an opening wedge osteotomy to an already short digit. An advancement flap has been used to lengthen the skin that was too deficient in both dimensions to be lengthened with a "Z"-plasty.

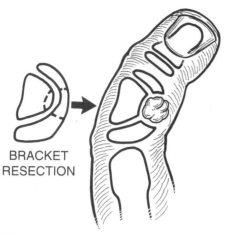

FIGURE 40-73. Bracket resection option for the treatment of clinodactyly caused by a delta phalanx. (Adapted from Upton J: Congenital anomalies of the hand and forearm. *In* McCarthy JG [ed], May JW, Littler JW [eds of Hand Surgery Vols.]: Plastic Surgery, Vol 8, The Hand. Part 2. Philadelphia, WB Saunders, 1990, pp 5337-5340, with permission.)

CRITICAL POINTS: CLINODACTYLY

- Clinodactyly is angulation of the digit in the radioulnar plane distal to the MCP joint.
- Minor angulation, particularly of the small finger, is common to the point of normalcy. Etiology is usually abnormal trapezoidal shape of the middle phalanx that leads to radial deviation of the distal interphalangeal joint.
- Greater angulation may be secondary to a "longitudinal diaphyseal bracket" or the "longitudinal epiphyseal bracket" along the middle phalanx.
- Mild to moderate clinodactyly requires no treatment.
- Substantial clinodactyly requires realignment of the digit via a closing wedge, opening wedge, or the reverse wedge osteotomy. The soft tissue deficit on the concave side must also be addressed.

whereas a triangular bone will benefit from an opening wedge osteotomy. After corrective osteotomy, fixation is achieved with an axial Kirschner wire. The associated soft tissue deficit with severe clinodactyly can be addressed with the bipedicle step advancement flap described by Evans and James.[6] A reverse wedge osteotomy is technically demanding in small triangular phalanges, and a simple osteotomy is preferred with the addition of bone graft. In patients with thumb clinodactyly, a primary corrective osteotomy is performed to produce a well-aligned thumb column rather than rely on gradual correction with growth after bracket resection.

ANNOTATED REFERENCES

6. Evans DM, James NK: A bipedicled neurovascular step-advancement flap for soft tissue lengthening in clinodactyly. Br J Plast Surg 45:380-384, 1992.

   The article describes a bipedicled neurovascular step advancement flap for soft tissue lengthening in clinodactyly. It is applicable in cases with substantial angulations that make "Z"-plasty inadequate.

13. Light TR, Ogden JA: The longitudinal epiphyseal bracket: Implications for surgical correction. J Pediatr Orthop 1:299-305, 1981.

    These authors coined the term *the longitudinal epiphyseal bracket* to describe the anatomy of the abnormal physis. A functioning physis was found along the lateral side of a metatarsal. Histologic sectioning was performed. The bracket was a longitudinal composite of proximal and distal epiphyseal (secondary) ossification centers. Growth within the bracket is unpredictable and dependent on the growth potential within the cells and the bracket morphology. Corrective surgery is recommended based on the orientation of the bracket.

19. Vickers D: Clinodactyly of the little finger: A simple operative technique for reversal of the growth abnormality. J Hand Surg [Br] 12:335-342, 1987.

    Classic article describes a prophylactic procedure for young children with progressive clinodactyly. A midlateral approach along the digit provides exposure to the apex of the longitudinal epiphyseal bracket. The longitudinal portion of the bracket is excised and a fat graft inserted to cover the ends of the split physis. Over time, the digit gradually straightens as growth of the digit occurs through the horizontal portions of the growth plate.

Kirner's Deformity

David McCombe and Simon P. Kay

Kirner's deformity[13] is a specific skeletal deformity characterized by progressive palmar-radial curvature of the distal phalanx of the small finger. It typically develops in adolescence. The deviation occurs in two planes, which is different than single radioulnar plane deviation of clinodactyly.[23]

EPIDEMIOLOGY

Incidence figures range from 0.15% to 0.25% of the population, and females are affected twice as frequently as males.[3,29] The deformity may be inherited as an autosomal dominant trait with incomplete penetrance. The homozygous state is responsible for expression of the deformity in multiple digits and both hands.[28] The deformity occurs sporadically in at least half of the cases.[22]

PATHOLOGY

Kirner's deformity has been attributed to a nontraumatic disruption of the physis of the distal phalanx. The subsequent distal deformity develops secondary to either asymmetrical physeal growth or traction across the damaged physis from the flexor tendon. Other potential contributing factors include an abnormally situated flexor tendon[4] or a normal flexor tendon acting on an abnormal osteopenic distal phalanx.[30] A vascular etiology for the deformity has also been postulated.[24,27]

Kirner's deformity is characterized by distortion and widening of the physeal plate along with curvature of the diaphysis of the distal phalanx. Physeal plate closure is also delayed.[7] Histology of the phalanx demonstrates lysis at the junction of the metaphysis and physis.[6]

CLINICAL FEATURES

Kirner's deformity develops in late childhood or adolescence.[11] Initially, swelling along the dorsum of the distal phalange(s) of the small fingers develops in one or both hands.[1,12,27] There may be some discomfort associated with this stage, but usually the swelling is painless.[5,11] The deformity ensues with the development of the palmar-radial curvature of the distal fingertip (Fig. 40-74), which is marked by the clubbed or beaked appearance of the fingernail. Joint motion at the distal interphalangeal joint is preserved.

The radiographic appearance of the distal phalanx varies with the stage of the deformity (Fig. 40-75).[29] Early in the development of the deformity, the physis is widened, the palmar lip of the epiphysis is lengthened, the metaphyseal margin of the physis is sclerotic and ragged, and the diaphysis begins to curve. Later, the diaphyseal curvature is well established and the epiphyseal plate begins to ossify along its dorsal half. The mature form of the deformity has a completely fused physis and restoration of normal bone density throughout the deformed phalanx.

Kirner's deformity has been seen in cases of Cornelia de Lange syndrome,[10,14,18,25] Silver's syndrome,[20,23,26] Turner's syndrome,[9,15,16,21] and Down syndrome.[30] The differential diagnosis includes traumatic injury to the physis or physeal injury consequent to burns or frostbite. The history, physical examination, and x-ray findings, however, usually enable confident diagnosis.

MANAGEMENT

Kirner's deformity has little effect on function. Musicians and keyboard operators may identify specific problems related to small finger position. The indication for surgery is primarily restoration of the finger appearance. For this reason, the patient must be counseled about the potential risks of surgery and expected results.

Splinting the small finger into extension has been reported as effective in relieving discomfort in the early swelling stage of the deformity,[5] although no benefit in prevention or correction of deformity was obtained. Other

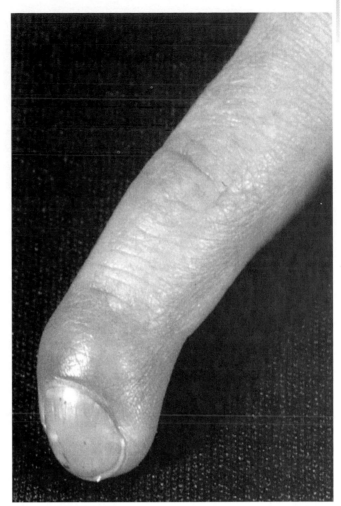

FIGURE 40-74. Kirner's deformity of the small finger.

investigators have reported prolonged serial splinting useful in correcting the deformity if applied in the early stages and before completion of growth.[8,31] If the epiphysis remains open, another option is to perform a dorsal hemiepiphysiodesis[20] or resect a dorsal wedge including the dorsal growth plate[17] to prevent progression of the deformity. For the mature deformity, corrective osteotomies have been used to improve the alignment of the phalanx and corresponding nail growth (Fig. 40-76). The deformity has been addressed with a dorsal closing wedge osteotomy[17] or, alternatively, two or three opening wedge osteotomies of the volar cortex to unfold the phalanx.[2] The technique of distraction lengthening has also been used to correct the deformity.[19]

Authors' Preferred Technique

Splinting can be attempted in the immature patient, although it needs to be rigorously monitored to be effective in preventing or correcting the deformity. Corrective surgery is deferred until the patient is able to participate in the

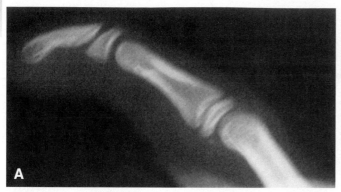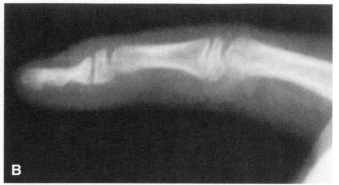

FIGURE 40-75. Preoperative (**A**) and postoperative (**B**) radiographs of Kirner's deformity treated with an osteotomy.

decision-making process, because surgery is primarily for appearance rather than function. The authors' preference is to use volar osteotomies to correct the phalangeal curvature. The nail plate is removed and a radial dorsolateral incision preserving the paronychial fold is used to expose the distal phalanx. The osteotomies are planned distal to the flexor tendon insertion. Two or three are used, depending on the size of the phalanx. The volar periosteum is incised, and the dorsal periosteum is elevated over the site of the osteotomies to act as a hinge for the correction and prevent injury to the nail matrix. The osteotomies are performed with a sharp osteotome. The curvature of the phalanx is corrected, and fixation is accomplished with an axial Kirschner wire. The Kirschner wire is left in place until the osteotomies have healed. The digit is protected with a splint during the healing process.

CRITICAL POINTS: KIRNER'S DEFORMITY

- Kirner's deformity is characterized by progressive palmar-radial curvature of the distal phalanx of the small finger.
- The precise etiology is unknown.
- Radiographs reveal distortion and widening of the physeal plate along with curvature of the diaphysis of the distal phalanx.
- Kirner's deformity develops in late childhood or adolescence with initial swelling along the dorsum of the distal phalanx. Subsequently, palmar-radial curvature of the distal fingertip develops over time.
- Kirner's deformity has little functional effect, and the indications for surgery are limited.

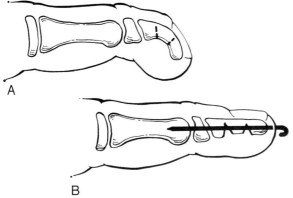

FIGURE 40-76. **A** and **B,** Multiple opening wedge volar osteotomies are used to straighten the distal phalanx over a Kirschner wire. (Adapted from Carstam N, Eiken O: Kirner's deformity of the little finger. J Bone Joint Surg Am 52:1663-1665, 1970, with permission.)

ANNOTATED REFERENCES

2. Carstam N, Eiken O: Kirner's deformity of the little finger: Case reports and proposed treatment. J Bone Joint Surg Am 52:1663-1665, 1970.

   Brief report of two cases treated by two osteotomies through the volar three fourths of the distal phalanx diaphysis. This technique of sequential osteotomies resulted in correction of the radial-volar angulation. The authors remark that correction was done for reasons of cosmesis.

5. Dykes RG: Kirner's deformity of the little finger. J Bone Joint Surg Br 60:58-60, 1978.

   Twelve cases of Kirner's deformity (10 female, 2 male) were reviewed, with an average presentation of about 9 years of age. Four cases occurred in one family. Residual clinical deformity was uniform with few functional problems.

Macrodactyly

David McCombe and Simon P. Kay

Macrodactyly is a descriptive term used for a disproportionately large digit noted at birth or within the first years of life. Both the soft tissue and skeletal elements are diffusely enlarged in the affected digit(s). Several alternative terms have been used, including *megalodactyly,*[7,29] *gigantism,*[8,12] *macrodystrophia lipomatosa,*[24] and *macrodactylia fibrolipomatosis.*[42] *Macrodactyly* is the preferred term that is widely recognized. The most common form of macrodactyly is an isolated anomaly associated with lipomatosis of the proximal nerve. Macrodactyly may also be part of a more diffuse hypertrophy or a component of a broader syndrome. A specific lesion within the digit can also cause disproportionate enlargement of the digit, such as a tumor (soft tissue or bone), vascular malformation, or lymphedema. These cases are not considered true macrodactyly, because the overgrowth is secondary to the specific lesion.[4]

EPIDEMIOLOGY

Macrodactyly is uncommon. In Flatt's series of upper extremity anomalies, the incidence of macrodactyly was 0.9%.[14] Most cases appear sporadically without evidence of inheritance.[3,22,27] Macrodactyly is sometimes a feature of neurofibromatosis (von Recklinghausen's disease), which is an autosomal dominant condition.

PATHOLOGY

The etiology of true macrodactyly is unknown. Potential mechanisms have been postulated, including an abnormal nerve supply leading to unimpeded growth, an increase in blood supply, and/or an abnormal humeral mechanism stimulating growth.[19] The most convincing theory is based on the association between peripheral nerve pathology and macrodactyly, because the most common type of macrodactyly is associated with fatty infiltration and enlargement of the nerve associated with the digit (Fig. 40-77).[1,15,18,34] This lipofibromatosis of the nerve has been alternatively reported as a fibrolipoma,[9,31] lipofibroma,[2,26] or hamartoma. The macroscopic findings are increased amount of subcutaneous fat, an enlarged tortuous digital nerve(s), and skeletal overgrowth in all dimensions. Most macrodactyly occurs in a single digit or in a region innervated by a single nerve. The term *nerve territory oriented macrodactyly* describes this relationship.[22]

Typically, the palmar aspect of the finger is more affected than the dorsum, and the distal finger is more enlarged than the proximal digit. The tendons have a normal appearance, although the flexor tendon sheath may be thickened. Histology of the digital tissues shows thickening of the skin with decreased sweat gland density, abundant subcutaneous fat with increased fibrous stroma, fatty infiltration of the digital nerves with endoneural and perineural fibrosis,[32] and enlarged digital arteries.[34] The bony structure shows wide medullary canals, irregular trabeculae, and thickening of the periosteum.[5,14] Macrodactyly associated with neurofibromatosis is similar, although the plexiform nerve has an increased fibrovascular stroma and nodular appearance rather than fibrolipomatosis changes.

Exostoses and other skeletal deformities may be noted in the enlarged digit. A specific form of the deformity, hyperostotic macrodactyly, is marked by periarticular exophytic osteocartilaginous masses and is typically not associated with enlargement of the associated peripheral nerve.

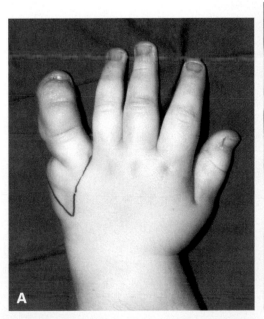
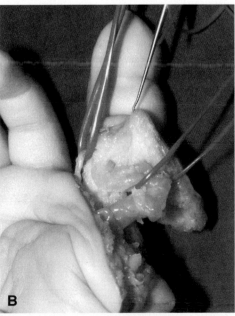

FIGURE 40-77. **A** and **B**, Macrodactyly of the fifth finger associated with lipofibromatous change in the ulnar digital nerve compared with the normal radial digital nerve.

CLINICAL FEATURES

Macrodactyly associated with lipofibromatosis is often noted at birth or develops within the first 3 years of life.[37] The growth of the enlarged digit may be disproportionate *(progressive macrodactyly)* (Fig. 40-78), or the digits may maintain a consistent proportion to the remainder of the hand *(static macrodactyly)*. The anomaly is usually unilateral[14,22] and may affect more than one digit. Multiple digital enlargement is two to three times more common than a single digit.[4,40] The index finger is the most frequently affected digit, particularly in combination with the thumb or long finger.[40] If a patient has involvement of all digits, the remainder of the limb should be examined for hemihypertrophy. Affected radial digits usually deviate in a radial direction. In contrast, affected ulnar digits deviate in a radial direction. Where two digits are involved, the deviation is usually divergent (Fig. 40-79). Enlarged thumbs are typically abducted and extended. Osseous growth and deviation continues until physeal closure; however, soft tissue enlargement may continue into adulthood.[37] The enlarged digits stiffen during growth, which further limits function.

The radiograph reveals an enlarged skeleton with advanced bone age compared with the normal digits (see Fig. 40-79). The phalanges may be trapezoidal with deviation of the digit. Osteoarthritic changes may be noted early with osteophyte development. If angiography is performed, one of the digital arteries is often enlarged.[23] Apart from the obvious digital deformity, soft tissue swelling in the palm may be present along with a compression neuropathy associated with fatty infiltration of either the median or ulnar nerves (Fig. 40-80).[15,24] The thickening of flexor sheath may produce triggering if digital range of motion is preserved. Syndactyly is seen in 10% of cases (Fig. 40-81).[14,40]

Hyperostotic macrodactyly is rare and can be distinguished on clinical examination by nodular enlargement of the digit and profound loss of motion secondary to periarticular osteochondral mass formation (Fig. 40-82). Although unusual, concurrent peripheral nerve lipofibromatosis has been reported with hyperostotic macrodactyly.[26] The radiographic appearance of the periarticular osteochondral masses confirms the diagnosis.

Macrodactyly may also be part of a broader anomaly (e.g., *congenital partial gigantism* or *neurofibromatosis*) or be a component in a syndrome. Gigantism can be diagnosed on the basis of enlargement of the entire limb or body part in addition to the enlarged digit. The gigantism may be *segmental gigantism,*[12] affecting only a part of one limb; *hemihypertrophy,*[32] affecting one side of the body (associated with neurofibromatosis or Klippel-Trenaunay syndrome);

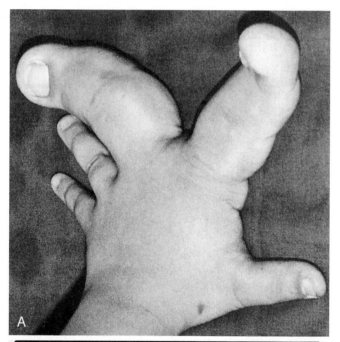

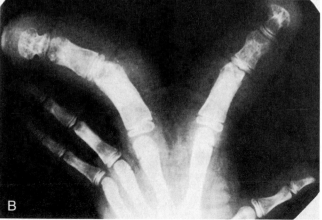

FIGURE 40-79. **A** and **B,** Clinodactyly of two adjacent enlarged fingers. The fingers usually deviate away from each other.

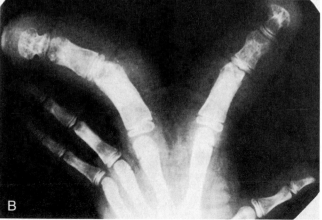

FIGURE 40-78. Progressive type of macrodactyly in a 4-year-old boy. Note that the normal adjacent fingers are crowded away from their normal position by the abnormally enlarged ring finger.

or *crossed gigantism,* affecting regions on both sides of the body.

Macrodactyly associated with neurofibromatosis is diagnosed by the characteristic cutaneous stigmata (pigmented skin lesions, café-au-lait spots, multiple neurofibromas, and pedunculated skin tumors). Syndromes that feature macrodactyly include Ollier's disease (multiple enchondromas), Maffucci's syndrome (multiple hemangiomas and enchondromas), Klippel-Trenaunay-Weber syndrome (cutaneous hemangioma, atypical varicose veins and hemihypertrophy), and Proteus syndrome[39] (hamartomatous dysplasia with features of macrodactyly, pigmented nevi, and subcutaneous hamartomas). Proteus syndrome is extremely variable with regard to phenotype and associated anomalies.

CLASSIFICATION

Flatt's classification[14] is based on the pathologic basis of the deformity (Table 40-11). The original classification has been supplemented by the addition of the type IV group.[38]

MANAGEMENT

Macrodactyly is often a disfiguring anomaly. Patients usually present in childhood, although they may present later with a compression neuropathy secondary to pathologic enlargement of affected nerve(s). Children with macrodactyly are often subject to teasing and have social difficulties. As a consequence, the hand is often concealed and ignored. Indications for surgery include functional and aesthetic rationale. The enlarged digit(s) often obstruct grasp and pinch.

Macrodactyly is extremely difficult to treat. The progressive and diffuse nature prevents complete correction to normalcy. Family and patient must have realistic expectations for treatment and be cognizant of the need for repeated procedures. Available surgical options can be divided into procedures that limit ongoing growth or surgeries that

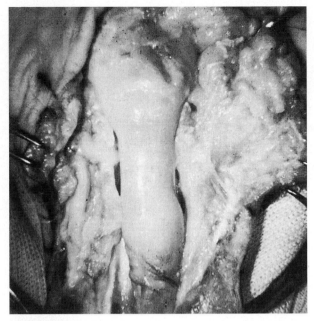

FIGURE 40-80. Median nerve involvement in a patient with macrodactyly of the thumb. This resulted in carpal tunnel syndrome that required decompression.

reduce the size of the digit (Table 40-12). The procedures may be combined at the same time or staged according to the patient's needs. In addition, carpal tunnel or Guyon's canal decompression may be warranted in cases with concurrent compressive neuropathy (see Fig. 40-80).

Limiting Digital Growth

Proposed methods to limit growth include ligation of the digital arteries, compression bandaging, stripping the digital nerves,[35] or resection of the digital nerve.[20] The most reliable

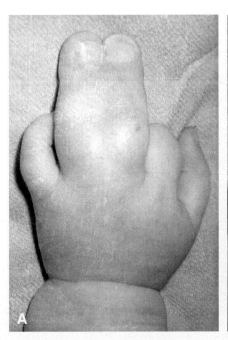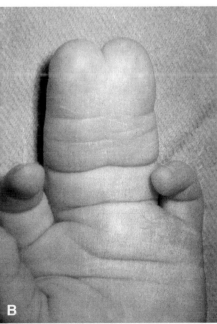

FIGURE 40-81. A and **B,** Macrodactyly with associated syndactyly. This combination occurs in about 10% of patients.

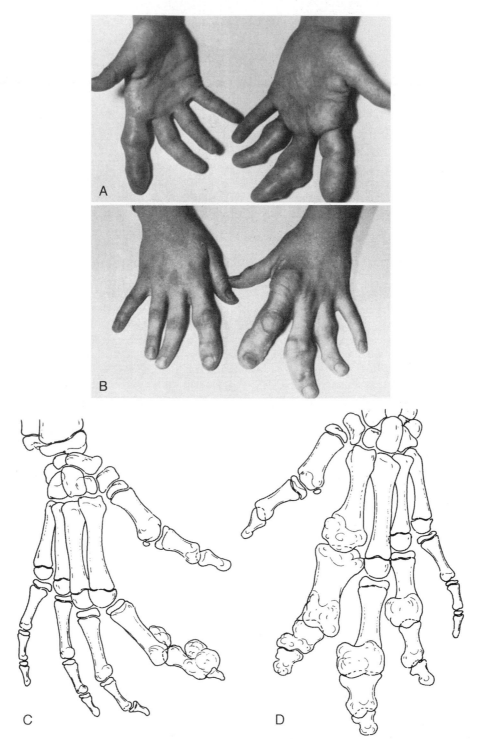

FIGURE 40-82. Hyperostotic macrodactyly. **A,** Palmar view of the hands of a 13-year-old girl with macrodactyly of the right index and middle fingers and left index, middle, and ring fingers. **B,** Dorsal view. **C** and **D,** Tracings of oblique radiographs of both hands. The left second metacarpal head is bulbous. Note that the articular ends of the bones entering into the IP joints of the involved fingers are bulbous. (From Kelikian H: Congenital Deformities of the Hand and Forearm. Philadelphia, WB Saunders, 1974, pp 610-660, with permission.)

method, however, is epiphysiodesis.[20] This may be accomplished by various methods including a burr or drill,[10] resection of the epiphyseal plate,[21] or physeal stapling in larger bones. Epiphysiodesis is performed when the digit reaches adult length of the same sex parent. Digital deviation can be corrected simultaneously by a closing wedge

resection of the physis (Fig. 40-83). Progressive deviation can also be managed by hemiepiphysiodesis on the convex side of the digit, although not as reliably as corrective osteotomy. Percutaneous Kirschner wires are often required to stabilize the phalanx after physeal resection, particularly if combined with a wedge osteotomy. Complications of phy-

Table 40-11
CLASSIFICATION OF MACRODACTYLY

Type I: Gigantism and lipofibromatosis	Associated with enlarged, fat-infiltrated nerves within the digit and extending proximally through carpal tunnel Most common form
Type II: Gigantism and neurofibromatosis	Usually occurs in conjunction with plexiform form of neurofibromatosis and is often bilateral May be osteochondral masses associated with the enlarged skeleton
Type III: Gigantism and digital hyperostosis	Hyperostotic form with osteochondral periarticular masses developing in infancy No significant nerve enlargement Very rare and not hereditary Nodular and stiff digits; may be other skeletal anomalies
Type IV: Gigantism and hemihypertrophy	Rare anomaly without known inheritance pattern or etiology Macrodactyly part of hemihypertrophy All digits involved, but less severe than type I or II Deformity marked by intrinsic muscle hypertrophy or abnormal intrinsic anatomy Presents as flexion contracture, ulnar deviation, and an adducted thumb deformity

Table 40-12
TREATMENT OF MACRODACTYLY

Limiting Growth	Digital nerve stripping Epiphysiodesis

Digit Reduction	Soft tissue debulking
	Skeletal terminalization
	  Reposition nail unit on shortened skeleton
	    Palmar pedicle (Barsky procedure) (Barsky, 1967; Flatt, 1977)
	    Dorsal pedicle (Tsuge procedure) (Tsuge, 1967)
	    Nail island flap (Rosenberg, 1983)
	    Resection of distal portion of nail and pulp
	      Tsuge (Tsuge, 1985)
	      Hoshi (Hoshi, 1973)
	      Fujita (Fujita, 1983)
	      Bertelli (Bertelli, 2001)

Correction of Deviation	Closing wedge osteotomy (combined with epiphysiodesis as required)
Thumb Macrodactyly	Metacarpophalangeal arthrodesis Millesi procedure (Millesi, 1974)
Amputation	Ray amputation (with transposition of digit for central ray amputation)

seal arrest include joint stiffness, excessive bone formation at the site of the physis, or secondary angulation after incomplete physeal destruction.[34] Physeal arrest does not reduce soft tissue growth or the transverse (appositional) growth of the skeleton. Currently, resection and repair or grafting[22] of the tortuous nerve is rarely recommended, because the sensibility of the digit is usually intact.[41]

Reducing the Digit

Debulking the digit can reduce the size of the enlarged digit (Fig. 40-84). Usually, one side of the digit is debulked at a time. The digit is approached through a midlateral incision. Skin flaps are elevated to the volar and dorsal midline, and the neurovascular bundle is dissected from the subcutaneous fat. The fat is resected, and the excess skin is excised. Care must be taken to maintain viability of the undermined skin flaps.[11] An alternative approach is to address the palmar aspect of the finger via a Bruner incision.

Narrowing of the skeleton can be achieved by burring the sides of the phalanges or longitudinal ostectomy. This ostectomy is limited by the attachment of the flexor sheath and has been complicated by hematoma and/or joint stiffness.[14]

Skeletal shortening can be achieved by several techniques. A deviated digit can be shortened and realigned via corrective ostectomy. A trapezoid rather than a wedge resection has been recommended to increase shortening. The amount of resection, however, is limited by the excessive soft tissue.[36]

The simplest procedure is "terminalization" of the enlarged digit, although the loss of the nail may only exacerbate the appearance of deformity. Several techniques attempt to preserve the nail and shorten the digit. Barsky's procedure[4] involves shortening the digit by filleting the distal phalanx, excising the skin over the dorsum of the middle phalanx, and placing the nail on the end of the middle phalanx. Flatt[13] modified this technique by preserving the distal part of the distal phalanx and fusing this to a shortened middle phalanx to reduce the skeleton. Considerable bony shortening (greater than 3 cm) may require concomitant flexor digitorum profundus shortening. The excess palmar skin produced by the shortening can be excised at a second stage.

The use of a palmar pedicle maintains a reliable blood supply and good sensation in the distal finger. In contrast, Tsuge's procedure[35] preserves the nail on a dorsal skin pedicle including the dorsal cortex of the distal phalanx (Fig. 40-85). The digit is shortened with excision of the pulp and the palmar part of the distal phalanx. The nail is fitted into a recess on the dorsum of the middle phalanx. A fold of skin is produced on the dorsum of the digit, which can be

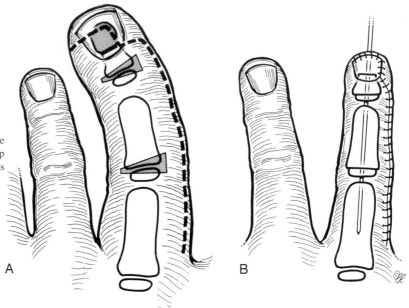

FIGURE 40-83. **A** and **B,** Excision of the epiphyseal plate and partial removal of the bone by osteotomy can stop growth and correct angulation all in one maneuver, as suggested by Tsuge.

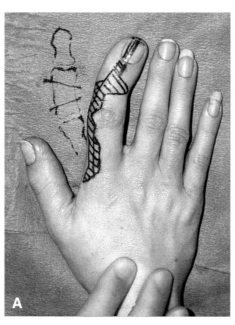
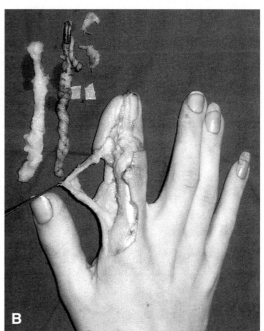

FIGURE 40-84. **A** and **B,** Reduction of the index finger using a combination of angulation osteotomy, resection of skin and fat, debulking of the enlarged digital nerve, and narrowing of the nail bed.

revised with a second procedure. The dorsal pedicle, however, has proven to be unreliable in the fingers but has been used in the toes with success.[36]

Rosenberg's technique[30] transposed the nail farther by raising the nail unit as an island flap on the digital neurovascular pedicle. After excision of the distal phalanx and pulp, the nail unit was repositioned on the dorsum of the middle phalanx.[28]

An alternative to transposing the nail unit onto a shortened skeleton is to reduce the nail and shorten the digit

further with segmental ostectomies along the length of the digit. Tsuge[36] narrowed the width of the nail and distal phalanx by ostectomies and shortened the digit by excision of the metacarpophalangeal (MCP) joint. Hoshi and associates[17] combined soft tissue debulking and skeletal shortening with excision of the tip of the distal phalanx and nail, proximal shortening with distal interphalangeal joint (DIP) arthrodesis and debulking via the convex side of the deviated digit. Fujita and colleagues[16] raised a palmar flap including the radial neurovascular bundle along the length

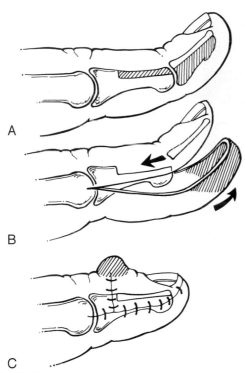

FIGURE 40-85. Tsuge's method for reducing the length of the macrodactylous finger. **A,** The incision is midlateral to the end of the finger. The volar part of the distal phalanx and the dorsal portion of the middle phalanx are removed. **B,** Excess volar skin and soft tissues are removed from the end of the finger. **C,** The dorsal part of the distal phalanx and nail are recessed to fit the middle phalanx. The remaining dorsal excess soft tissue can be removed later.

of the digit, which left the ulnar neurovascular bundle, skeleton, and flexor tendon on the dorsal flap. The ulnar one third and distal end of the palmar flap and the radial one third and the tip of the distal phalanx and nail were excised to match each other.

The thumb can be addressed using similar techniques.[6] Debulking is similar, and shortening can be performed via MCP arthrodesis. Millesi[25] devised a more complicated pattern of reduction osteotomies that preserves joint motion. The nail width and length are reduced, but the central nail is excised. This technique often results in ridging of the nail.

The ultimate reduction procedure is amputation. This procedure is an option for macrodactyly isolated to a single digit or showing progressive uncontrollable growth. Amputation of the thumb should be avoided. Ray amputation of a border digit and transmetacarpal amputation of a central digit and adjacent digit transposition are the procedures of choice.

Hyperostotic Macrodactyly

Loss of motion can be addressed with ostectomy of the osteochondral masses, which may include part of the volar plate. Recurrence is the rule, and arthrodesis is often required after the digit attains adult length. Implant arthroplasty of the MCP joints has been used in select cases.[14]

Hemihypertrophic Macrodactyly

In hemihypertrophic macrodactyly, contracture of the digit(s) is common, which further impairs motion. Contracture release, debulking of the hypertrophic intrinsic musculature, and soft tissue rebalancing has been performed in a limited number of cases. Skeletal correction may also be required.[33]

Authors' Preferred Technique

Macrodactyly is a devastating anomaly for the child and represents a social stigma, focus of anxiety for parents, and a technical challenge for the surgeon. Multiple procedures are required, and the end result may be unsatisfactory. In contrast, ray amputation is a worthwhile procedure and should be considered early, before the patient invests in multiple procedures to salvage a deformed digit with limited function. Most parents with young children find this a difficult decision and prefer digit-preserving surgery. Experienced surgeons, however, will take the time and convey the trials and tribulations with reduction surgery.

The surgical plan is based on digital involvement, size of the digit(s), estimated adult length, degree of motion, and the overall alignment. For digital retention in young children, improving the appearance before school age is indicated. Debulking of subcutaneous fat with isolation of the neurovascular bundle is performed via a midlateral approach (see Fig. 40-84). One side of the digit is debulked at a time with a 3-month interlude. This debulking can be combined with corrective osteotomy for deviated digits.

When the digit has reached adult length, longitudinal growth can be terminated with epiphysiodesis of all the phalanges. A midlateral approach is performed with physeal plate ablation using a blade, curet, or drill. Fluoroscopy guidance is helpful. The physeal plate resection can be configured as a closing wedge osteotomy to correct alignment of the digit (see Fig. 40-83). The skeleton is stabilized with Kirschner wires at each level. The soft tissues can be debulked at this procedure.

If a digit exceeds adult length, a shortening procedure is recommended. The procedure used depends on the location and extent of excess. Minimal shortening can be accomplished by reduction of the distal fingertip pulp and nail using the method of Hoshi.[17] Excessive length requires distal phalanx excision and repositioning of the nail to the dorsum via a nail island flap.[30] For the thumb, MCP joint resection and arthrodesis are preferred. These techniques address digital length and alignment, but excessive soft tissue and nail contribute to persistent disfigurement. This deformity can be addressed with debulking, nail bed excision, and longitudinal removal of bone. The procedures are difficult and limited by the finger's vascularity, joint stability, and flexor tendon integrity. Recurrence is common, and functional deterioration with continued growth is prevalent (Fig. 40-86). At this point, patients often consider amputation, because removal of the digit may actually improve hand function. The aesthetic appearance can be enhanced with adjacent digit transposition.

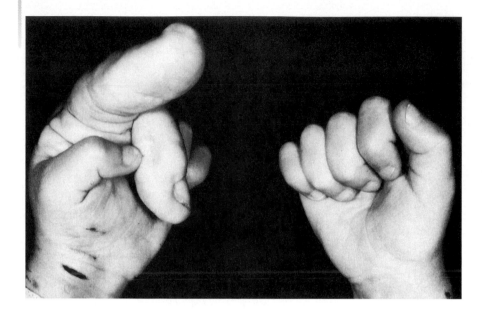

FIGURE 40-86. Unsightly macrodactylous digits that have gradually lost motion and stiffened over time.

CRITICAL POINTS: MACRODACTYLY

- The most common form of macrodactyly is an isolated anomaly associated with lipofibromatosis of the proximal nerve.
- The etiology is unknown.
- Most macrodactyly occurs in a single digit or in a region innervated by a single nerve ("nerve territory oriented macrodactyly").
- Macrodactyly is often noted at birth or develops within the first 3 years of life. The growth of the enlarged digit may be disproportionate *(progressive macrodactyly)*, or the digits may

maintain a consistent proportion to the remainder of the hand *(static macrodactyly)*.
- Macrodactyly is extremely difficult to treat. Its progressive and diffuse nature prevents complete correction to normalcy. Despite multiple surgeries to remove the extraneous tissues, the end result may be unsatisfactory.
- Ray amputation should be considered early in progressive macrodactyly before the patient invests in multiple procedures to salvage a deformed digit with limited function.

ANNOTATED REFERENCES

2. Al-Qattan MM: Lipofibromatous hamartoma of the median nerve and its associated conditions. J Hand Surg [Br] 26:368-372, 2001.

Ten cases of lipofibromatous hamartoma of the median nerve are reported. Six cases had associated macrodactyly. Two cases had associated fatty tumors, and another two had bony tumors. An additional literature review adds to the paper along with a classification of the sites of involvement of the median nerve along with its associated conditions.

20. Ishida O, Ikuta Y: Long-term results of surgical treatment for macrodactyly of the hand. Plast Reconstr Surg 102:1586-1590, 1998.

Retrospective review of 23 patients treated for macrodactyly of the hand. Treatment regimens varied among the patients, and greater than two procedures were performed in 65% of the patients. At final follow-up, the average length of the affected digits was 102% compared with the normal contralateral side. The average circumference of the digits was 121% and 124% at the PIP and DIP, respectively. The average range of motion was 65, 57, and 37 degrees at the MCP, PIP, and DIP joints, respectively. Although difficult to compare treatment regimens, epiphysiodesis/epiphysectomy was effective in the prevention of longitudinal overgrowth of the digits. In contrast, resection of the hypertrophic nerves was unsuccessful in preventing finger overgrowth.

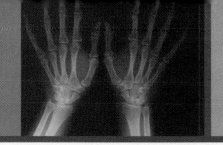

CHAPTER 41

Deformities of the Thumb

Scott H. Kozin

THUMB HYPOPLASIA

Epidemiology

Thumb hypoplasia represents a spectrum of deficiencies from a slightly smaller thumb to a completely absent thumb and is considered part of radial deficiency. Related syndromes or associations warrant consideration and systemic evaluation. The primary concerns are Holt-Oram syndrome, thrombocytopenia–absent-radius (TAR) syndrome, VACTERL association (vertebral abnormalities, anal atresia, cardiac abnormalities, tracheoesophageal fistula, esophageal atresia, renal defects, radial dysplasia, lower limb abnormalities), and Fanconi's anemia.[1,9,15] The Holt-Oram syndrome is inherited as an autosomal dominant syndrome, whereas TAR syndrome and Fanconi's anemia are inherited in autosomal recessive patterns.[1,9]

Classification

The underdeveloped thumb has been classified into five types, which guides treatment recommendations (Table 41-1).[9,12,18]

A type I deficiency represents the least involvement with generalized thumb hypoplasia without discrete absence of structures and good function. A type II deficiency is more involved and is characterized by thumb/index web space narrowing, thenar muscle absence, and instability of the thumb metacarpophalangeal (MCP) joint with a normal articulation (Fig. 41-1). Type III hypoplasia possesses the intrinsic anomalies associated with a type II deformity plus additional skeletal and extrinsic musculotendinous abnormalities (e.g., flexor pollicis longus). Type III anomalies have been further subdivided into IIIA and IIIB, depending on the presence or absence of a stable carpometacarpal (CMC) joint.[18] Type IV deficiency represents a severe expression of thumb hypoplasia and denotes a "pouce flottant" or residual digit (Fig. 41-2). Type V is noted by complete absence of the thumb (Fig. 41-3).[2,10,20]

Clinical Features

The examination varies with the age of the child. A neonate prefers digital grasp and rarely incorporates the thumb into use. Inspection and palpation are the mainstays of the examination. The thumb is inspected for size, consistency,

Table 41-1
THUMB DEFICIENCY CLASSIFICATION

Type	Findings	Treatment
I	Minor generalized hypoplasia	Augmentation
II	Absence of intrinsic thenar muscles	Opponensplasty
	First web space narrowing	First-web release
	Ulnar collateral ligament (UCL) insufficiency	UCL reconstruction
III	Similar findings as type II plus: Extrinsic muscle and tendon abnormalities Skeletal deficiency A: Stable CMC joint B: Unstable CMC joint	A: Reconstruction B: Pollicization
IV	Pouce flottant or floating thumb	Pollicization
V	Absence	Pollicization

and stability. The length is recorded in relation to the adjacent index digit. The status of the intrinsic and extrinsic muscles is assessed. The stability of the MCP and CMC joints is determined by gentle stress (Fig. 41-4). Mild hypoplasia (grades I and II) can be readily distinguished from severe hypoplasia (grade IV). The intermediate hypoplasia

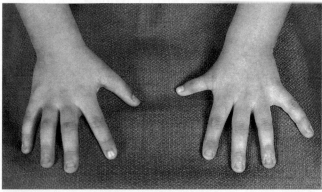

FIGURE 41-1. Type II thumb deficiency on the left hand with thumb/index finger web space narrowing, thenar muscle absence, and instability of the thumb MCP joint. (Courtesy of Shriners Hospitals for Children, Philadelphia.)

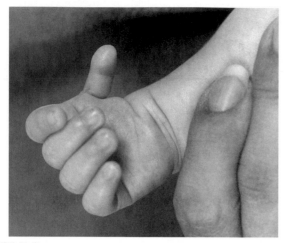

FIGURE 41-2. Type IV thumb deficiency with severe expression of thumb hypoplasia or "pouce flottant." (Courtesy of Shriners Hospitals for Children, Philadelphia.)

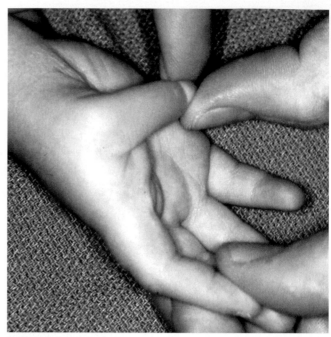

FIGURE 41-4. Instability of the MCP joint associated with grade II and III thumb hypoplasia. (Courtesy of Shriners Hospitals for Children, Philadelphia.)

(grade III) is more difficult to classify and subdivide into its subtypes. Serial examinations may be necessary to differentiate a type IIIA from a type IIIB thumb. This distinction is critical, because the presence or absence of a CMC joint distinguishes a thumb that can be reconstructed from a thumb that is better treated by ablation and pollicization. Radiographs may reveal a tapered metacarpal without a base, which confirms type IIB hypoplasia (Fig. 41-5). Radiographs to visualize the trapezium and trapezoid, however, are not useful, because ossification does not occur until 5 or 6 years of age.[8]

The child often helps discriminate between a type IIIA and a type IIIB deficiency during the development of pinch and grasp. A stable IIIB thumb is incorporated into object acquisition and manipulation activities, whereas an unstable thumb is often bypassed and prehension develops between the index and long digits. The hand responds by widening the index/long finger web space and index finger pronation out of the palm.

Treatment

Type I hypoplasia often requires no treatment.[20] Thumb reconstruction in types II and IIIA requires addressing all elements of the hypoplasia.[7,18] The goal of reconstruction is to provide the hand with the best-functioning thumb unit. Pollicization is the procedure of choice for types IIIB, IV, and V hypoplasia.[2,10,18,20] The timing of pollicization remains controversial, with a trend toward early surgery (6 months

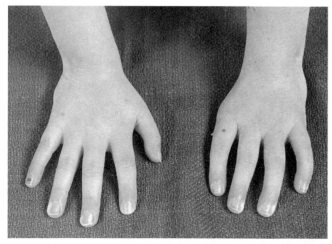

FIGURE 41-3. Type V thumb deficiency is noted by complete absence of the thumb. (Courtesy of Shriners Hospitals for Children, Philadelphia.)

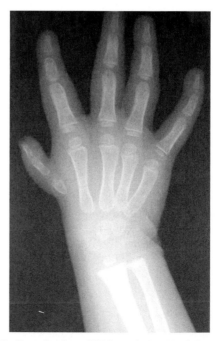

FIGURE 41-5. Radiograph of type IIIB hypoplasia with absence of a CMC joint. (Courtesy of Shriners Hospitals for Children, Philadelphia.)

to 1 year of age). This recommendation is based on pollicization before the development of oppositional pinch. This early intervention avoids the development of compensatory side-to-side pinch pattern between adjacent fingers.

Attempts at microsurgical joint transfer to restore the CMC joint in types IIIB and IV have been reported.[5] Currently, the results appear mediocre compared with index finger pollicization and involve considerable microsurgical expertise.[5,20]

Thumb Reconstruction in Types II and IIIA Hypoplasia

The adducted posture of the thumb is corrected with web space deepening. Mild web narrowing is treated by release of the first dorsal interosseous fascia and some form of "Z"-plasty. A four-flap design is preferred to widen the web and attain a rounded contour (Fig. 41-6).[6,12,26] Moderate web narrowing is managed with release of the first dorsal interosseous muscle from the index metacarpal and a dorsal transposition flap rotated into the web space. The donor defect is closed primarily without the need for skin graft. The MCP joint instability involves the ulnar side. Many of these thumbs have an anomalous connection between the flexor pollicis longus and extensor pollicis longus muscles (i.e., pollex abductus).[4,13,25] The pollex abductus attenuates the ulnar collateral ligament over time and prevents active interphalangeal (IP) joint motion. Treatment requires release of this abnormal connection and repair or reconstruction of the ulnar collateral ligament.[7] Usually, the ligament can be released and advanced in a proximal direction along the metacarpal head.

An opposition transfer, using either the abductor digiti quinti or ring flexor digitorum superficialis tendon as the donor, circumvents the deficient thenar muscles (Fig. 41-7).[11,12,16,22,23] The techniques are similar to standard opposition transfers. During abductor digiti quinti transfer, the ulnar neurovascular pedicle is identified and protected. In addition, the origin of the abductor digiti quinti is released

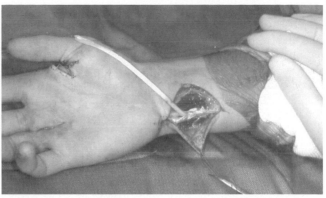

FIGURE 41-7. Ring flexor digitorum superficialis tendon harvested as donor for opposition transfer in type II thumb hypoplasia. (Courtesy of Shriners Hospitals for Children, Philadelphia.)

from the pisiform to increase length of the transfer (Fig. 41-8).

A type IIIA thumb also requires transfers to overcome the extrinsic musculotendinous abnormalities of extensor pollicis longus and/or flexor pollicis longus tendons.[7,18] These extrinsic tendon transfers can be done at the same time of initial thumb reconstruction or delayed until later. Transfer of the adjacent extensor indicis proprius can consistently supplant extensor pollicis longus function.[20,21] Reconstruction of the flexor pollicis longus, however, is more difficult. The flexor tendon sheath may be deficient, which requires pulley reconstruction combined with tendon centralization or tendon transfer.[7,18] Despite valiant surgical efforts, achieving functional IP joint motion remains a challenge.

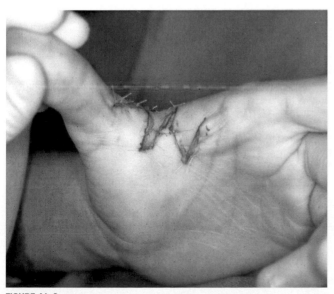

FIGURE 41-6. Four-flap "Z"-plasty for mild web narrowing associated with type II thumb hypoplasia. (Courtesy of Shriners Hospitals for Children, Philadelphia.)

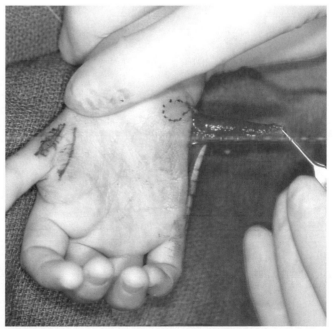

FIGURE 41-8. Abductor digiti quinti transfer requires identification of the ulnar neurovascular pedicle, which is released from the pisiform to increase length of the transfer. (Courtesy of Shriners Hospitals for Children, Philadelphia.)

Pollicization for Types IIIB, IV, and V Hypoplasia
(Table 41-2)

The current technique of pollicization represents a consolidation of contributions from surgeons over the past 100 years.[2,14,17] Pollicization remains a complicated procedure that requires strict attention to detail. A stepwise approach delineates the multiple steps required for completion of the procedure. The procedure begins with the design of the skin incision. Multiple options are available with the goals of creating a thumb with sufficient skin coverage and an adequate first web space that is devoid of scar. The most popular skin incision was developed by Buck-Gramcko,[2] although I

Table 41-2
STEPWISE APPROACH TO POLLICIZATION

Step	Rationale	Technique
Gently exsanguinate.	Visualization of vasculature.	
Incise skin.	Creation of thumb/index finger web space, with provision of adequate exposure to all structures.	Ezaki design.
Isolate palmar neurovascular bundles.	Preservation of sensibility and circulation to index.	Use loupe magnification, meticulous dissection, and direct exposure.
Microdissect common digital nerve.	Mobilization of nerve for pollicization.	Perform intrafascicular dissection.
Ligate proper digital artery to radial side of long finger.	Maintenance of proper digital artery with index and long fingers perfused with ulnar proper digital artery.	Use suture or ligature clip. Ligature clip is preferred to allow visualization throughout the procedure.
Release first annular pulley to index finger.	Prevention of buckling of flexor tendons.	
Elevate dorsal skin with preservation of dorsal veins.	Veins have filled with blood to facilitate identification; preservation of venous egress.	
Free extensor tendons from adjacent structures.	Insurance of appropriate line of pull to index finger pollicization.	
Extensor and flexor tendons are not shortened.	Shorten themselves over time.	
Elevate the first dorsal and palmar muscles from the index metacarpal and MCP joint.	Metacarpal will be excised and muscles advanced to PIP joint.	Use sharp dissection.
Release first dorsal and palmar muscles with a strip of extensor hood.	Tendons are sutured to lateral bands about PIP hood.	
Identify and tag the radial and ulnar lateral bands about the PIP joint.	Identification before bony resection easier and safer. Later transfer of the first dorsal and first palmar tendons, respectively.	Pull on lateral band until desired function is evident and tag band with suture.
Incise intermetacarpal ligament.	Allowance for repositioning of index finger, which has provided additional stability until this point.	
Shorten the index finger by removing the majority of the metacarpal bone, including physis ablation.	Index too long for a thumb; must prevent continued metacarpal growth.	Use fine-bladed saw to cut metacarpal perpendicular to bone through its metaphyseal portion. Make distal cut through physis (epiphysiodesis).
Reposition index MCP joint into hyperextension.	Normal index MCP joint hyperextends and normal thumb carpometacarpal joint does not hyperextend.	Fix the index MCP joint into hyperextension using a nonabsorbable suture placed through the epiphysis and dorsal capsule.
Align the index finger into the thumb position.	Positioning into 45 degrees of abduction and between 100 and 120 degrees of pronation.	Align metacarpal epiphysis to its remaining base. Place nonabsorbable sutures between the metacarpal base and epiphysis.
Perform tendon transfer to restore intrinsic function to the pollicization.	Maximizes function in grasp and pinch.	First dorsal interosseous is sutured into the radial lateral band and the first palmar interosseous is sutured into the ulnar lateral band.

Table 41-2
STEPWISE APPROACH TO POLLICIZATION—CONT'D

Step	Rationale	Technique
Inset skin.	Provides adequate coverage without scar in thumb/index finger web space.	Inset skin along the palmar aspect of the pollicization while avoiding neurovascular bundles. Inset web space skin. Trim any excess skin.
Deflate tourniquet and apply meticulous postoperative dressings.	Ensures circulation, protects pollicization, and decreases chances of inadvertent removal of dressings.	Use bulky hand dressing with long-arm splint.

use a modified design by Ezaki and Carter (personal communication) that allows more glabrous skin along the palmar aspect of the pollicization (Fig. 41-9).

The limb is gently exsanguinated to allow identification of the vasculature. The palmar skin is incised first and the radial neurovascular bundle isolated. Dissection proceeds in an ulnar direction to identify the common digital vessels to the second web space. The proper digital nerves to the ulnar side of the index and the radial side of the long finger are located (Fig. 41-10). These nerves are traced in a proximal direction and further separated by microdissection of the

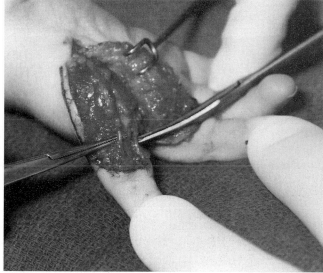

FIGURE 41-10. Identification of the digital nerves to the index finger. (Courtesy of Shriners Hospitals for Children, Philadelphia.)

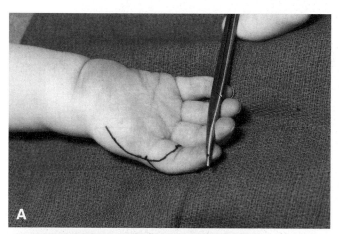

A

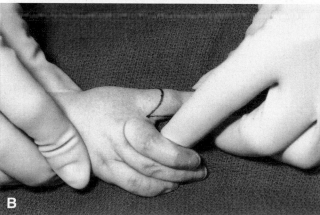

B

FIGURE 41-9. A and **B,** Skin incision for pollicization to allow glabrous skin coverage along the palmar aspect of the pollicized digit. (Courtesy of Shriners Hospitals for Children, Philadelphia.)

common digital nerve to allow tension-free index finger pollicization (Fig. 41-11). Similarly, the proper digital artery to the ulnar side of the index and the radial side of the long finger is isolated (Fig. 41-12). The proper digital artery to the long finger is ligated to allow index finger pollicization based on the radial digital artery and the common digital artery. We prefer to use ligating clips to mark the ends of the artery (Fig. 41-13). The clips remain visible throughout the procedure and prevent inadvertent vessel injury. The common digital artery is traced in a proximal direction. Be aware that the artery may originate from the deep arch, which requires careful dissection to prevent injury.

The index finger's first annular pulley is incised to prevent buckling of the flexor tendons, and the intermetacarpal ligament is isolated for later division (Fig. 41-14). The dorsal incision is then elevated with preservation of as many dorsal veins as possible (Fig. 41-15). The index extensor tendons are inspected and any juncturae tendinum released to promote straight-line pull to the index finger (Fig. 41-16). I do not shorten the extensor or flexor tendons. Next, the first dorsal and palmar interossei muscles are elevated from the index metacarpal and MCP joint (Fig. 41-17). The tendons are traced to their insertion along the extensor hood

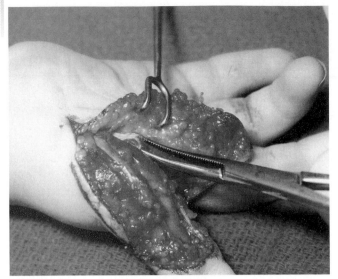

FIGURE 41-11. Dissection of the common digital nerve to allow tension-free index finger pollicization. (Courtesy of Shriners Hospitals for Children, Philadelphia.)

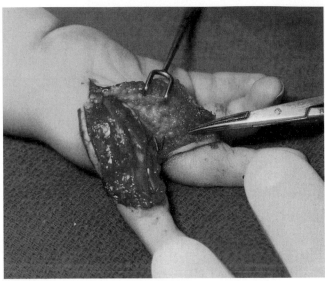

FIGURE 41-13. Ligation of the proper digital artery to the long finger. (Courtesy of Shriners Hospitals for Children, Philadelphia.)

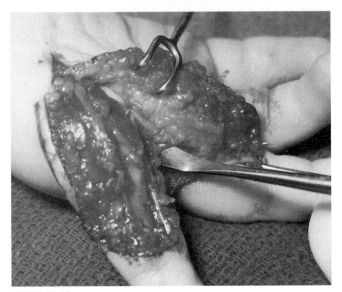

FIGURE 41-12. Identification of the proper digital artery to the radial side of the long finger. (Courtesy of Shriners Hospitals for Children, Philadelphia.)

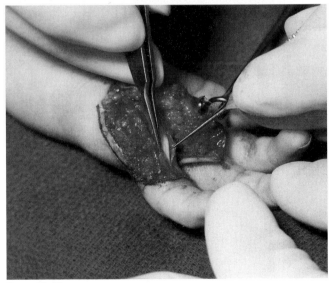

Figure 41-14. Release of the first annular pulley. (Courtesy of Shriners Hospitals for Children, Philadelphia.)

and released with a portion of the hood to elongate the tendons in preparation for transfer. The radial neurovascular bundle must be protected during elevation of the first dorsal interosseous, and the ulnar neurovascular bundle must be safeguarded during mobilization of the first palmar interosseous muscle. Before cutting the bone the insertion sites for the tendon transfers are identified. The extensor hood over the proximal IP joint is exposed by dorsal dissection while protecting the surrounding veins. The radial and ulnar lateral bands are defined and a suture placed for later transfer of the first dorsal and first palmar tendons, respectively (Fig. 41-18).

At this point, important structures have been isolated and prepared for index pollicization. The intermetacarpal ligament is incised to allow repositioning of the index finger. The index finger is shortened by removal of the metacarpal bone, leaving its base and epiphysis. Reverse retractors are placed around the index metacarpal base. A fine-bladed saw is used to cut the metacarpal in a perpendicular direction through its metaphyseal portion (Fig. 41-19). A bone-holding clamp is applied to the diaphysis, and the metacarpal is sharply dissected from proximal to distal to the physeal plate. The distal cut is made with a knife through the physis while protecting the adjacent collateral ligaments

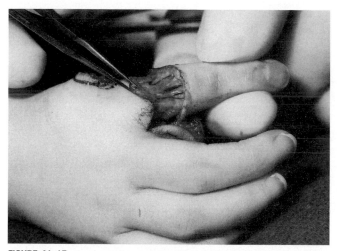

FIGURE 41-15. Preservation of dorsal veins during elevation of the dorsal incision. (Courtesy of Shriners Hospitals for Children, Philadelphia.)

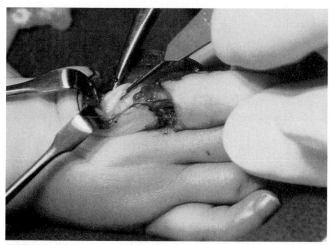

FIGURE 41-16. Dissection of the index extensor tendons to promote a straight-line pull. (Courtesy of Shriners Hospitals for Children, Philadelphia.)

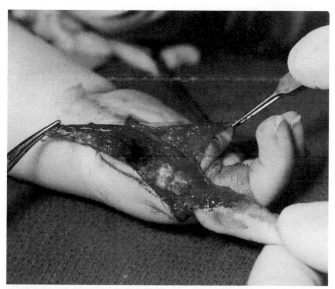

FIGURE 41-17. Elevation of the first dorsal interosseous muscle from the index metacarpal and MCP joint. (Courtesy of Shriners Hospitals for Children, Philadelphia.)

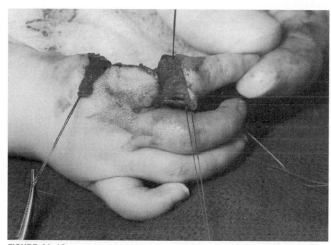

FIGURE 41-18. The radial and ulnar lateral bands are defined with a suture for later attachment. (Courtesy of Shriners Hospitals for Children, Philadelphia.)

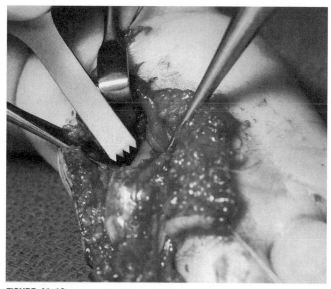

FIGURE 41-19. The metacarpal is cut with a fine-bladed saw through the metaphyseal portion at the base. (Courtesy of Shriners Hospitals for Children, Philadelphia.)

(Fig. 41-20). Physeal ablation (epiphysiodesis) prevents excessive growth of the index pollicization. The resected bone is removed from the surgical field and discarded.

The index finger is freely mobile and can now be situated into a thumb position. The normal index MCP joint hyperextends and the normal thumb CMC joint does not hyperextend, which must be corrected. This conversion should be made before repositioning. Placement of the index MCP joint into hyperextension will prevent additional extension after pollicization. To accomplish this task, the MCP joint is sutured into hyperextension using a nonabsorbable suture placed through the epiphysis and dorsal capsule (Fig. 41-21). The index finger is shortened, and the metacarpal epiphysis is aligned to its remaining base. The index finger must be carefully positioned to replicate the function of a thumb. It is positioned into 45 degrees of abduction and between 100 and 120 degrees of pronation to re-create

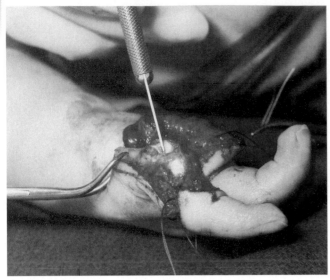

FIGURE 41-20. Distal cut of metacarpal through the physis. (Courtesy of Shriners Hospitals for Children, Philadelphia.)

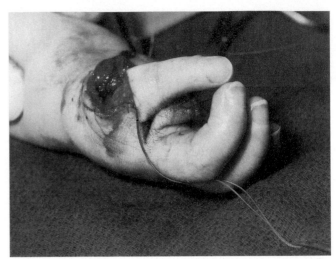

FIGURE 41-22. Careful positioning of the index finger to replicate the function of a thumb with 45 degrees of abduction and between 100 and 120 degrees of pronation. (Courtesy of Shriners Hospitals for Children, Philadelphia.)

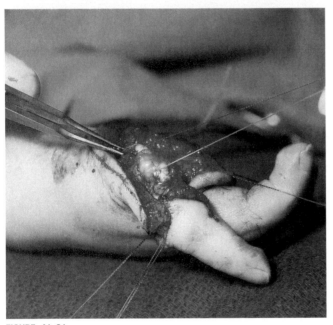

FIGURE 41-21. The MCP joint is sutured into hyperextension using a nonabsorbable suture material placed through the epiphysis and dorsal capsule. (Courtesy of Shriners Hospitals for Children, Philadelphia.)

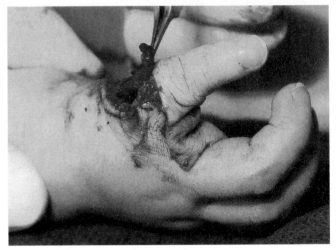

FIGURE 41-23. Transfer of the first dorsal interosseous to the radial lateral band. (Courtesy of Shriners Hospitals for Children, Philadelphia.)

normal thumb alignment (Fig. 41-22). Interosseous nonabsorbable sutures are placed between the metacarpal base and epiphysis after alignment has been established. Additional stability is obtained via tendon transfer of the first dorsal interosseous to the radial lateral band and of the first palmar interosseous to the ulnar lateral band (Fig. 41-23). The skin is initially inset along the palmar aspect of the pollicization with care taken to avoid the neurovascular bundles. The first web space is configured with skin devoid of suture (Fig. 41-24). The dorsal skin is closed last and often requires some trimming to enhance overall appearance.

The tourniquet is deflated after insetting the palmar skin along the pollicization or following complete skin closure,

depending on total tourniquet time, which is usually limited to 2 hours. The circulation usually restores quickly, although vasospasm can result. Warm soaks and patience often lead to resolution. Persistent lack of blood flow requires exploration, although fortunately this is rarely required. The postoperative dressings are crucial and follow standard practice in dressing of the hand. A long-arm splint with the elbow flexed to greater than 100 degrees decreases the chance of inadvertent removal. The arm is elevated to promote venous drainage and is monitored overnight. Although the concern for arterial compromise exists, venous problems are more prevalent.

Results

The results of thumb reconstruction for hypoplasia are uniformly good (Fig. 41-25).[7,12,16,18,22] Comparison among patients and surgeons, however, is complicated by inconsistencies within thumb hypoplasia. All hypoplastic

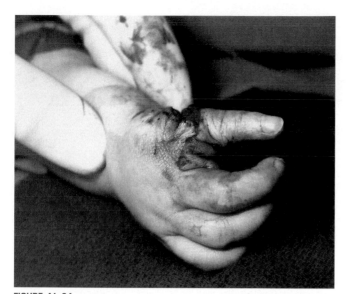

FIGURE 41-24. The palmar skin is advanced dorsal to create a web space devoid of suture. (Courtesy of Shriners Hospitals for Children, Philadelphia.)

thumbs are not equivalent with respect to size, degree of hypoplasia, and anomalous tendon structure. Nonetheless, surgery that addresses each deficient component will result in an improved thumb that better participates in pinch and grasp.

The results after pollicization are directly related to the status of the transposed index digit and surrounding musculature.[3,10,16,19,20,24] A mobile index finger transferred to the thumb position will provide stability for grasp and mobility for pinch (Fig. 41-26). In contrast, a stiff index finger will provide a stable thumb for gross grasp but will not participate in pinch. In addition, the ability to restore intrinsic muscle function is integral for a successful outcome. For these reasons, pollicization of the index finger provides good functional and aesthetic results in patients with isolated thumb hypoplasia and is less reliable in patients with associated radial forearm deficiencies.[10,19,24] Early good results in childhood persist into adulthood.[3]

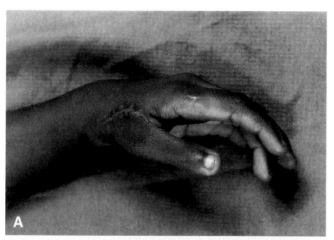

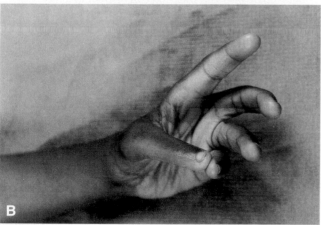

FIGURE 41-25. A and **B,** Function and appearance after web space deepening, ulnar collateral ligament reconstruction, and flexor digitorum superficialis tendon transfer for opposition. (Courtesy of Shriners Hospitals for Children, Philadelphia.)

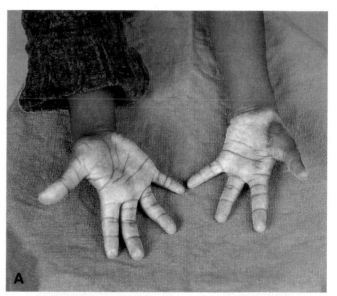

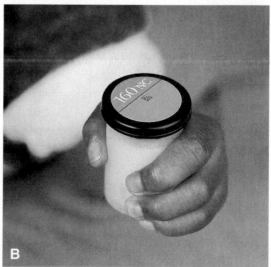

FIGURE 41-26. A and **B,** Two-year old status post left index pollicization with good alignment and grasp. (Courtesy of Shriners Hospitals for Children, Philadelphia.)

Complications

Pollicization is a complicated procedure with multiple potential causes of failure or dissatisfaction. Early complications are related to blood flow. Arterial compromise is a tragedy, and immediate surgical exploration is required. Fortunately, arterial injury is rare, although transient venous problems are common. A "blue thumb" requires additional measures, such as strict elevation, loosening of the dressings, removal of dorsal sutures, and even evacuation of hematoma. Careful postoperative monitoring of the thumb is required until ample arterial inflow and venous outflow is ensured.

Late complications are more prevalent. The short- and long-term results are influenced by multiple factors. Unsatisfactory results require a stepwise approach to analyze the cause of disappointment. An inventory of the perceived troubles yields an algorithm for additional reconstruction to enhance function (Table 41-3).

A common source of error is first web space scarring and/or contracture. An immobile or inadequate web space limits thumb motion and prohibits object acquisition. Resurfacing and/or deepening of the first web space can rectify this problem.

A normal thumb resides just proximal to this joint, and excessive length after pollicization can be a source of discontent. Failure to ablate the index metacarpal epiphyseal plate is a common cause of excessive thumb length (Fig. 41-27).[10] Persistent growth of the metacarpal will elongate the thumb over time. Epiphysiodesis of the metacarpal growth plate and ostectomy will correct excessive thumb length.

Rotational errors are another potential source of dissatisfaction. Rotation of the index finger out of the palm and precise positioning are required to create a usable thumb. At the time of surgery, the correct amount of abduction and rotation is often difficult to judge. Over-rotation and under-rotation of the index finger can occur, which results in a thumb that is poorly aligned for pinch. This malalignment can be corrected by rotational osteotomy to better position the thumb for pinch.

Malposition of the index MCP joint is another source of error. The normal index MCP joint motion is 30 degrees of hyperextension to 90 degrees of flexion. In contrast, the normal thumb CMC joint has no hyperextension. The index

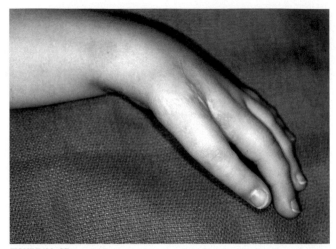

FIGURE 41-27. Excessive length after pollicization attributed to failure to ablate the growth plate and persistent growth. (Courtesy of Shriners Hospitals for Children, Philadelphia.)

MCP joint, therefore, must be positioned in hyperextension at the time of pollicization. Failure to properly position the MCP joint results in a hyperextensible CMC joint that creates problems during grasp. This abnormal posture can be corrected by wedge osteotomy of the bone adjacent to the CMC joint.

Limited motion is another frequent source of concern. As stated earlier, the preoperative status of the index finger directly affects the outcome after pollicization.[10,19,20] A stiff index finger will provide a stable thumb for gross grasp, but oppositional pinch is unlikely. In contrast, a mobile index finger transferred to the thumb position can provide stability for grasp and mobility for fine pinch. The evaluation of a stiff pollicization, therefore, begins with an inquiry regarding the status of the index finger before pollicization. A stiff index finger before pollicization cannot be mobilized by secondary reconstruction, because the inherent capacity for motion is limited. In contrast, a mobile index finger before pollicization can become stiff secondary to a postoperative complication, such as infection or bleeding. In this instance, tenolysis and release of adhesions may enhance movement.

Inadequate intrinsic function can also yield a thumb with limited active motion. Reconstruction of the abductor pollicis and adductor pollicis muscles by transfer of the first

Table 41-3
POLLICIZATION: POTENTIAL SOURCES OF DISSATISFACTION

Type of Failure	Etiology	Treatment
First web space contracture	Insufficient web space reconstruction	Web space deepening via "Z"-plasty or rotational flap
Stiffness	May be attributed to preoperative condition of index finger or secondary to surgical complication	Stiffness before pollicization not correctable. Adhesions can be treated by tenolysis.
Excessive length	Failure to ablate index metacarpal growth plate	Epiphysiodesis and ostectomy of metacarpal
Malrotation	Technical error or loss of fixation during postoperative care	Rotational osteotomy
Lack of opposition	Primary deficiency in intrinsic muscles or inability to reconstruct interossei	Opponensplasty

CRITICAL POINTS: THUMB HYPOPLASIA

- Thumb hypoplasia occurs in varying grades and is most frequently part of radial deficiency.
- The underdeveloped thumb has been classified into five types that guide treatment recommendations. The presence or absence of a stable CMC joint is the deciding factor of retention and reconstruction versus ablation and pollicization.
- Pollicization is the procedure of choice for types IIIB, IV, and V hypoplasia. Attempts at microsurgical joint transfer to restore the CMC joint in types IIIB and IV have been reported; however, the results appear mediocre compared with those of index finger pollicization.
- Results after pollicization are related to numerous factors, including the status of the index digit, the surgical technique, and the ability to restore intrinsic muscle function.
- Early good results in childhood persist into adulthood.

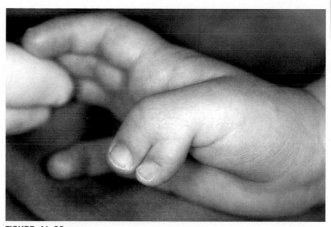

FIGURE 41-28. Type IV duplication with duplicated proximal and distal phalanges that articulate with a bifid metacarpal head. (Courtesy of Shriners Hospitals for Children, Philadelphia.)

dorsal and first palmar interossei has its limitations. Secondary tendon transfer using the abductor digiti quinti or ring flexor digitorum superficialis can enhance opposition.[11,12,16,22,23]

THUMB DUPLICATION

Epidemiology

Polydactyly can occur on the preaxial (radial) and postaxial (ulnar) side of the limb. Preaxial polydactyly is more common in whites, and postaxial polydactyly is more frequent in African Americans.[3,19] Preaxial polydactyly is also documented in high proportions in Native Americans and in many Asian populations.[5,7] Even though preaxial thumb duplication demonstrates a racial predilection toward white children, most cases are unilateral, sporadic, and without systemic problems.[3]

Classification

Thumb duplication has been classified into various categories based on the degree of skeletal replication.[18] In this classification, the extent of duplication is defined and indexed according to whether the components are attached proximally (bifid) or completely separated (duplicated) (Fig. 41-28). The most common type is that of duplicated proximal and distal phalanges that share a common articulation with a bifid metacarpal head (about 50% of cases).[3,18] Various adaptations and modifications have been added to this scheme, but the basic premise remains unchanged.[6,15,20] In addition, variations of duplicated thumb occur that defy classification.

Clinical Features

The diagnosis of thumb duplication is usually straightforward, especially in type IV duplication. A subtle type I or II duplication, however, may not be readily apparent on physical examination and may only be diagnosed by widening of the nail plate (Fig. 41-29). An inquiry regarding family history for thumb duplication is required, because familial transmission may be present. Radiographs are routine and assist in defining the extent of duplication.

The thumb components are palpated for bony elements, assessed for joint stability, and observed for motion. One of the duplicated elements is usually dominant and preferred for use. Serial examinations can be performed because there is no urgency for treatment. Surgery is usually performed between 6 months and 1 year of age, before the development of pinch.

Several investigators have noted that the thumb is not truly duplicated.[3,4,8] Neither component is as robust as a normal thumb. Each thumb is thinner than normal and has diminished mobility. The term *split thumb* seems more appropriate.[3,4] This terminology also makes parents aware that the reconstructed thumb will be smaller in size and girth. The split parts may share bony elements, tendons, ligaments, joints, neurovascular structures, and nails. The surgical goal is to create the best thumb possible. The ideal reconstruction aligns the thumb along a longitudinal axis, stabilizes the joints, balances the motor functions, provides an adequate nail plate without deformity, and restores sufficient thumb size.[1,3,8,10,13] Treatment often requires using portions of each component to construct a properly aligned and functional thumb, so-called spare parts surgery.[1,3]

Treatment

Treatment of types I and II depends on the extent and size of each duplicated part. A subtle type I or II duplication that has a common nail and is well aligned does not require treatment (see Fig. 41-29). Asymmetrical type I or II duplication with distinct components is treated by ablation of the smaller thumb with transfer of the collateral ligament and centralization of the extensor tendon (Fig. 41-30). The skin

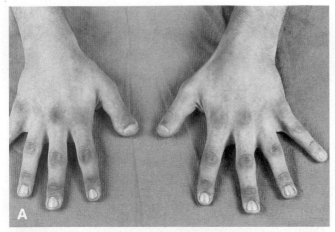

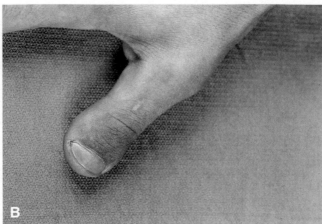

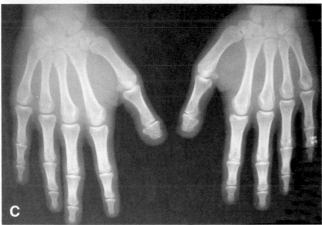

FIGURE 41-29. A, Bilateral subtle type III duplications. **B,** Widened left thumb nail plate. **C,** Radiograph reveals bilateral type I distal phalanx duplications. (Courtesy of Shriners Hospitals for Children, Philadelphia.)

incision is designed to ensure adequate soft tissue coverage of the retained component. Inadequate soft tissue along the side of the retained thumb (e.g., pulp tissue) can be supplanted with a flap from the deleted component. Proximal exposure is obtained by a zigzag approach. The extensor tendon to the lesser component is removed with the digit. The remaining tendon is centralized along the retained component. The tendon can be detached and reattached in the midline, or the eccentric portion can be folded over to the midline.[1,3] The flexor tendon(s) are treated in a similar fashion; however, exposure of the retained flexor system is more limited. The collateral ligament from the deleted component is elevated with an osteoperiosteal sleeve and attached via periosteal suture to the reconstructed thumb (Fig. 41-31).[9] The IP joint is inspected for any articular anomalies, such as a separate facet for the deleted component. This facet is removed with an osteotome to narrow the surface and properly align the joint with the retained component.

Additional extra-articular malalignment may require corrective osteotomy to ensure longitudinal alignment of the thumb. This realignment can been done using a closing wedge osteotomy with a scalpel blade or bone cutter to align the IP joint perpendicular to the thumb axis. A percutaneous Kirschner wire is placed antegrade from the thumb tip across the IP joint. The incision is closed with absorbable sutures, and a long-arm/thumb spica cast is applied. The cast and Kirschner wire are removed 4 to 5 weeks after surgery. A short-arm/thumb spica splint is fabricated, which is removed for therapy and gentle activities. The splint is discontinued 6 to 8 weeks after surgery.

Symmetrical thumb duplication is difficult to treat. Wedge resection of the central portions of bone and nail from each component and approximation of the retained borders can be performed (Bilhaut-Cloquet procedure) (Fig. 41-32). The epiphyses are usually not included in the wedge for fear of growth plate injury. The retained bone is coapted

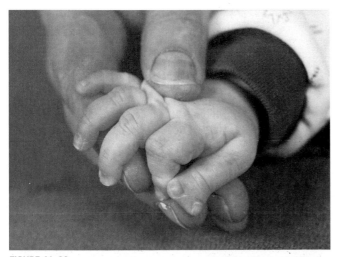

FIGURE 41-30. Asymmetrical type II duplication with distinct components. (Courtesy of Shriners Hospitals for Children, Philadelphia.)

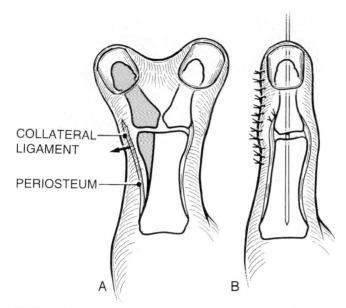

FIGURE 41-31. **A,** When duplication occurs at the joint level, the proximal articular surface needs to be narrowed. **B,** The collateral ligament is elevated from the deleted digit and reattached to the residual digit. The repair is protected by temporary Kirschner wire joint stabilization.

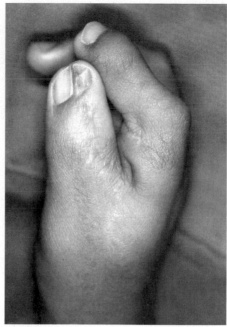

FIGURE 41-33. Eight-year-old status post Bilhaut-Cloquet procedure with nail deformity and IP joint stiffness. (Courtesy of Shriners Hospitals for Children, Philadelphia.)

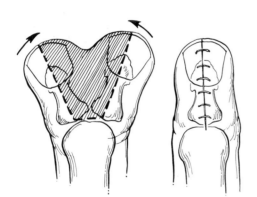

FIGURE 41-32. The classic Bilhaut-Cloquet procedure in which the lateral portions of two distal phalanges are joined in the midline after excision of the excess central soft and osseous tissues.

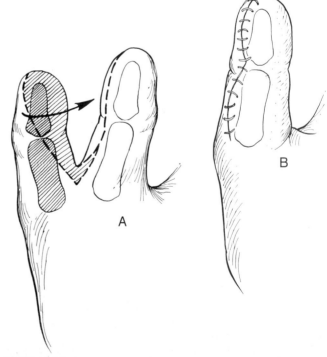

FIGURE 41-34. **A,** Type IV duplication with excision of radial digit. **B,** Soft tissues of the radial and ulnar digits combined.

and secured with suture or transverse Kirschner wire fixation. This operation is difficult, and subsequent nail deformity and IP joint stiffness are common (Fig. 41-33).[2,17]

Types III and IV duplication are treated with selection of a dominant thumb and ablation of the lesser counterpart (Fig. 41-34). This decision is not always straightforward and requires careful examination. If the components are equal, the ulnar thumb is preserved to retain the ulnar collateral ligament for pinch. The soft tissues from the ablated thumb are used to augment the retained thumb (Fig. 41-35). The collateral ligament is retained with an osteoperiosteal sleeve from the deleted thumb and transferred to the preserved thumb (Fig. 41-36).[3,9] The joint surface of the metacarpal is routinely inspected in a type IV duplication for a separate facet that articulates with the deleted component. Removal of this facet with preservation of the collateral ligament via a proximal osteoperiosteal sleeve is necessary. This articular

modification correctly aligns the thumb and prevents progressive angulatory deformity. Additional extra-articular malalignment may require corrective osteotomy to ensure longitudinal alignment of the thumb (Fig. 41-37). This realignment can be done using a closing wedge osteotomy to align the joint surfaces parallel. Tendon realignment is

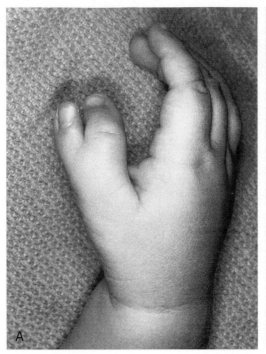

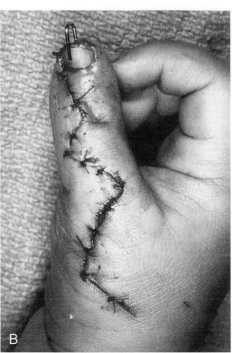

FIGURE 41-35. **A,** In this patient, the soft tissues of the radial and ulnar digits are asymmetrical, adequate peripherally, and hypoplastic centrally. **B,** Zigzag incisions allow coaptation of soft tissues to reconstruct the paronychial border of the nail. (From Light TR: Congenital anomalies: Syndactyly, polydactyly, and cleft hand. *In* Peimer CA [ed]: Surgery of the Hand and Upper Extremity. New York, McGraw-Hill, 1996, pp 2111-2144, with permission.)

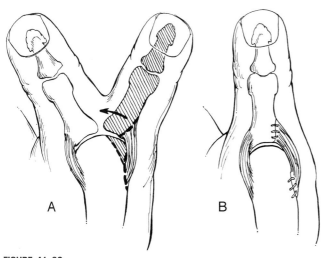

FIGURE 41-36. **A** and **B,** Angular deformity of the residual digit may be corrected by shifting the digit on a smooth common articular surface and creating a snug collateral ligament repair.

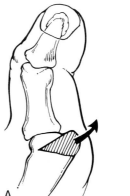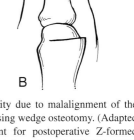

FIGURE 41-37. **A** and **B,** Angular deformity due to malalignment of the articular surface may be corrected by a closing wedge osteotomy. (Adapted from Miura T: An appropriate treatment for postoperative Z-formed deformity of the duplicated thumb. J Hand Surg [Am] 2:380-386, 1977, with permission.)

also necessary to centralize the tendons along the retained thumb (Fig. 41-38). Any thenar intrinsic muscles that are attached to the deleted thumb are transferred to the retained thumb (Fig. 41-39). Typically, the abductor pollicis brevis inserts into the radial thumb and must be detached with an osteoperiosteal sleeve with the radial collateral ligament. This composite is reattached to the retained ulnar thumb via periosteal suture to restore joint stability and abductor function.

A percutaneous Kirschner wire is usually placed antegrade from the thumb tip or positioned in an oblique direction across the MCP joint. The incision is closed with absorbable sutures, and a long-arm/thumb spica cast is applied. The cast and Kirschner wire are removed 4 to 5

weeks after surgery. A short-arm/thumb spica splint is fabricated, which is removed for therapy and gentle activities. The splint is discontinued 6 to 8 weeks after surgery.

Treatment of types V and VI duplication utilizes similar principles with the added complexity of additional intrinsic reconstruction. In addition, the thumb/index finger web space may be narrowed. A concomitant "Z"-plasty or dorsal transposition flap may be required.

Results

The results vary with the degree and complexity of the thumb duplication. Satisfactory results are readily obtainable in types I, II, and IV duplications. Unsatisfactory

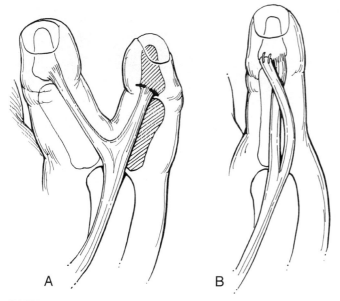

FIGURE 41-38. A, The extensor tendon often bifurcates in a "Y" configuration with one limb inserting on each digit. **B,** The tendon limb inserting on the deleted skeleton is reinserted onto the opposite border of the retained digit to balance extensor tendon forces.

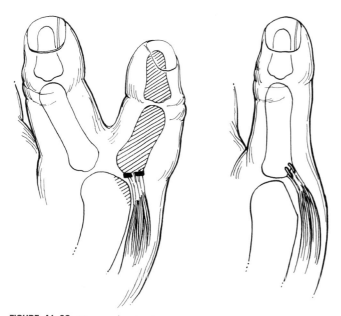

FIGURE 41-39. Thenar muscle detached from the radial component and reinserted on the ulnar component.

results are prevalent in types III, V, VI, and triphalangeal thumbs.[6,14] The acceptable size and girth of the reconstructed thumb is unclear, although estimations range from 25% to 33% less than the normal thumb.[1,16,17]

The Bilhaut-Cloquet procedure is difficult to perform, and its outcome is poorly documented.[2,6,10,17] Subsequent nail deformity and IP joint stiffness is common (see Fig. 41-33). Most authors have either abandoned this procedure or reserve its use for symmetrical distal type I or II duplication.[3,6,16,17]

Complications

The reconstructed thumb is always smaller than the normal. In addition, angulation, joint instability, limited motion, and scar contracture are common problems.[6,14] Reoperation rates between 20% to 25% have been reported.[11,12] More complicated thumb duplications create more postoperative problems. Any offset in bone axis, persistent joint instability, or tendon malalignment will lead to problems. Joint instability and/or imbalanced tendon action will cause thumb deviation and a "Z" deformity over time (Fig. 41-40). The approach to the malaligned thumb is to consider the potential underlying

CRITICAL POINTS: THUMB DUPLICATION

- A supernumerary thumb is not a true duplication, because neither component is as robust as a normal thumb. The term *split-thumb* is more appropriate.

- Thumb duplication has been classified into various categories based on the degree of skeletal replication. The most common type involves duplicated proximal and distal phalanges that share a common articulation with a bifid metacarpal head (about 50% of cases).

- The ideal reconstruction aligns the thumb along a longitudinal axis, stabilizes the joints, balances the motor functions, provides adequate nail plate without deformity, and restores sufficient thumb size. This often requires using portions of each component, so-called spare parts surgery.

- Any residual offset in bone axis, persistent joint instability, or tendon malalignment will lead to thumb deviation and a "Z" deformity over time.

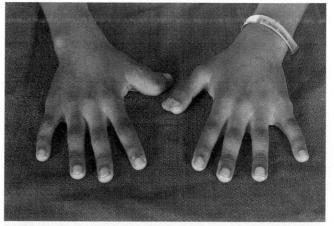

FIGURE 41-40. A 12-year-old with bilateral thumb duplication. Right thumb was reconstructed as an infant and developed a "Z" deformity. Subsequently, the patient and the family elected to forgo left thumb reconstruction. (Courtesy of Shriners Hospitals for Children, Philadelphia.)

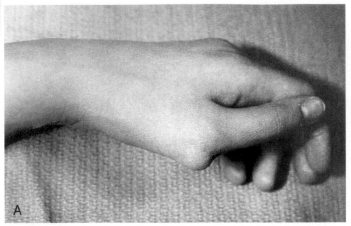 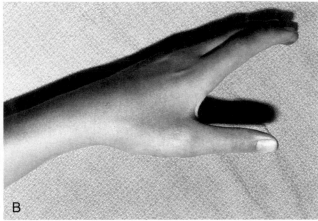

FIGURE 41-41. A, Simple deletion of the radial thumb component results in substantial residual deformity. **B,** Correction of the deformity was accomplished by narrowing the metacarpal head, reconstructing the collateral ligament, and reattaching the median nerve–innervated thenar intrinsic muscles. (From Light TR: Congenital anomalies: Syndactyly, polydactyly, and cleft hand. *In* Peimer CA [ed]: Surgery of the Hand and Upper Extremity. New York, McGraw-Hill, 1996, pp 2111-2144, with permission.)

cause(s).[11,12] Treatment requires restoration of parallel joint surfaces, restitution of joint stability, and realignment of tendon(s).

Poor motion and persistent instability are even more difficult to treat. Joint contracture often results after articular modification followed by subsequent scarring and arthrofibrosis. Limited treatment is available to restore motion. The thumb with preservation of passive motion without active motion, however, may benefit from tenolysis. Persistent instability combined with limited motion requires ligament reconstruction or arthrodesis. In general, arthrodesis or chondrodesis is preferred to reliably restore stability.

Joint enlargement is also a later problem after surgery (Fig. 41-41). This protuberance is usually secondary to inadequate removal of an intra-articular facet. Arthrotomy and removal will rectify this problem. The collateral ligament must be preserved and reattached.

TRIPHALANGEAL THUMB

Triphalangeal thumb may occur as an isolated anomaly, may be associated with a systemic abnormality (e.g., Holt-Oram syndrome or Fanconi's anemia), or may be concurrent with thumb duplication.[2,3] Triphalangeal thumb is also associated with congenital heart disease, including atrial septal defect, patent ductus, anomalies of the coronary arteries, and transposition of the great vessels.

Triphalangeal thumbs can be divided into two distinct forms. The first type has an extra phalanx of variable size within a relatively normal-appearing thumb (Fig. 41-42). The extra phalanx may be triangular, trapezoidal, or rectangular.[5] The second variety has a fully developed phalanx that lies in the plane of the fingers. This form is considered a five-fingered hand and probably represents an absent thumb with index polydactyly (Fig. 41-43).[4] As with most divisions, there are triphalangeal thumbs that appear to be a pedigree of the two types with characteristics of each form.

Both forms of triphalangeal thumbs are inherited as an autosomal dominant trait with variable expressivity and

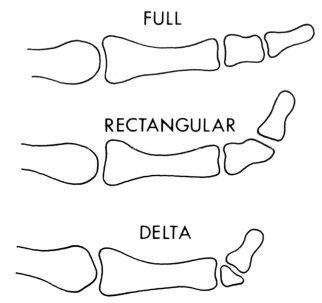

FIGURE 41-42. The three types of abnormal phalanges. (From Wood VE: Treatment of the triphalangeal thumb. Clin Orthop 120:188-200, 1976, with permission.)

high penetrance (Fig. 41-44).[5] Triphalangeal thumb can also occur sporadically.

Management Considerations

The management of the triphalangeal thumb can be divided into individual components. The definitive treatment depends on the type of triphalangeal thumb and the presence or absence of any concomitant anomalies, such as thumb duplication. There are multiple elements of the triphalangeal thumb that may require management, including the length and angulation of the digit, the extra IP joint, the status of the thumb/index finger web space, and the presence or absence of thumb opposition.

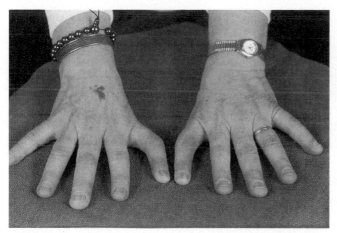

FIGURE 41-43. A fully developed phalanx that lies in the plane of the fingers is considered a five-fingered hand. (Courtesy of Shriners Hospitals for Children, Philadelphia.)

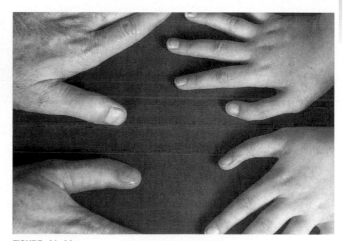

FIGURE 41-44. Father and daughter with bilateral triphalangeal thumbs. (Courtesy of Shriners Hospitals for Children, Philadelphia.)

The timing of treatment also depends on any concomitant anomalies. The goal is to reconstruct a thumb with adequate function before the development of oppositional pinch, which occurs between 12 and 18 months of age. The treatment of minor length discrepancy or angulation can be delayed until later. The proposed plan should be completed to school age.

Treatment

Length and Angulation

The extra phalanx has a variable shape and natural history. The length and shape of the extra phalanx will determine the length and alignment. The growth rate of the extra phalanx is variable, however, and initial treatment consists of observation to assess growth potential. Surveillance also allows assessment of motion at each IP joint, which is an important factor during reconstruction. The extra bone may ultimately be rudimentary, demonstrate little growth, and require no treatment. In contrast, continual or asymmetrical growth will lead to excessive length or progressive angulation, respectively (Fig. 41-45). The angulation is usually in an apex radial direction.

A small, wedge-shaped middle phalanx that causes progressive deviation requires excision with ligament reconstruction. Surgery is best performed at about 1 year of age. A dorsal approach is preferred with a longitudinal incision through the extensor mechanism. The extra phalanx is isolated, and its size is delineated. Osteoperiosteal sleeves are elevated from each side that include the collateral ligaments. The extra phalanx is removed and the collaterals reattached. The distal and proximal phalanges are coapted and secured with a longitudinal Kirschner wire. This wire skewers the phalanges and provides immobilization until ligamentous healing. The incision is closed with absorbable sutures, and a long-arm/thumb spica cast is applied. The cast and Kirschner wire are removed 5 weeks after surgery. A short-arm/thumb spica splint is fabricated, which is removed for therapy and gentle activities. The splint is discontinued 6 to 8 weeks after surgery. This benign-appearing operation can result in multiple problems, including instability, joint

stiffness, and insufficient motion. Lateral pinch should be minimized for the first 3 months to prevent radial deviation at the IP joint.

Extra Interphalangeal Joint

A small, wedge-shaped extra phalanx does not require treatment. The extra joint is of little consequence. A large, wedge-shaped extra phalanx produces excessive length with or without deviation. The phalanx should not be excised, as subsequent instability is common. Fusion of the abnormal phalanx with the distal or proximal phalanx combined with bone removal for realignment is a better option (Fig. 41-46). The joint with the greatest motion is preserved, and the joint with the least movement is fused. The bone reduction both shortens and realigns the thumb, whereas the arthrodesis eliminates the supernumerary joint.

A dorsal approach is preferred with a longitudinal incision through the extensor mechanism. The extra phalanx and adjacent joints are isolated. An arthrotomy is performed at the joint with least motion and is avoided at the joint with maximum motion. The bone is resected from both sides of the joint to shorten and realign the thumb. The bones are coapted surrounding the bony resection. Kirschner wires in a crossed and/or longitudinal direction are used for internal fixation. The extensor tendon is approximated, and the skin is closed with absorbable sutures. Redundant extensor tendons may require shortening. A long-arm/thumb spica cast is applied. The cast and Kirschner wire are removed 5 weeks after surgery. A short-arm/thumb spica splint is fabricated, which is removed for therapy and gentle activities and discontinued 8 weeks after surgery.

Thumb/Index Finger Web Space

A narrow web space hampers thumb function. Mild thumb/index finger syndactyly can be managed by web deepening. A four-flap "Z"-plasty deepens the web and provides a more rounded contour than a two-flap configuration.[7] Moderate involvement requires a local dorsal rotation flap for adequate deepening. A five-fingered hand has no web space. Pollicization provides an opposable digit and a thumb/index finger web space.

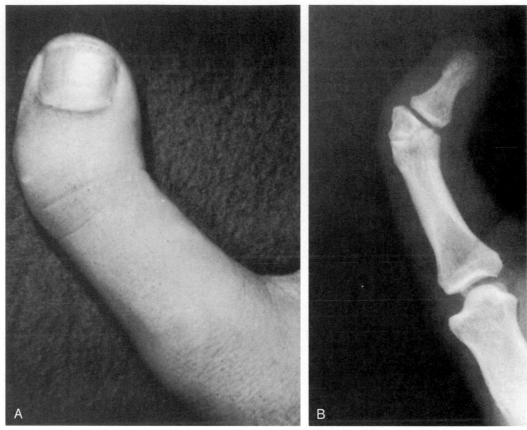

FIGURE 41-45. The clinical (**A**) and radiographic (**B**) findings in a triphalangeal thumb showing a wedge-shaped delta phalanx and ulnar deviation. (**A** from Wood VE: Treatment of the triphalangeal thumb. Clin Orthop 120:188-200, 1976, with permission.)

Absence of Thumb Opposition

Lack of opposition prohibits thumb function. Tendon transfer to restore opposition is required, using either the abductor digiti minimi or flexor digitorum superficialis as a donor (see Thumb Hypoplasia). If the thumb/index finger web space is narrow, concomitant web space widening is required. Joint reduction can be performed at the time of tendon transfer.

The five-fingered hand is hampered by the lack of an opposable digit. Treatment consists of pollicization of the nonopposable radial digit into the thumb position (see Thumb Hypoplasia).[1]

Concomitant Anomalies

A triphalangeal thumb combined with thumb duplication is treated according to the principles of thumb reconstruction (Fig. 41-47).[6] Usually, the dominant component is preserved and the nondominant part deleted with use of any important elements (e.g., collateral ligaments). If the triphalangeal component is preserved, the treatment of the extra phalanx is based on the above guidelines. The treatment of the triphalangeal portion of the anomaly can be performed at the same time as duplication reduction or delayed until later.

A triphalangeal thumb shared with a central deficiency is treated by combining the principles of cleft and triphalangeal thumb reconstruction. The degree of cleft formation and the status of the thumb-index finger web space are critical components. A complete thumb/index finger web syn-

CRITICAL POINTS: TRIPHALANGEAL THUMB

- Triphalangeal thumbs can be divided into two distinct forms. The first type has an extra phalanx of variable size within a relatively normal-appearing thumb. The second variety has a fully developed phalanx that lies in the plane of the fingers and is considered a five-fingered hand.

- The extra phalanx in a triphalangeal thumb may be triangular, trapezoidal, or rectangular. The growth rate of the extra phalanx is variable, and initial treatment consists of observation to assess growth potential.

- A small, wedge-shaped middle phalanx that causes progressive deviation requires excision with ligament reconstruction.

- A large, wedge-shaped extra phalanx requires fusion of the abnormal phalanx with an adjacent phalanx combined with bone removal. The joint with the greatest motion is preserved and the joint with the least movement fused.

- A five-fingered hand is treated with pollicization of the nonopposable radial digit.

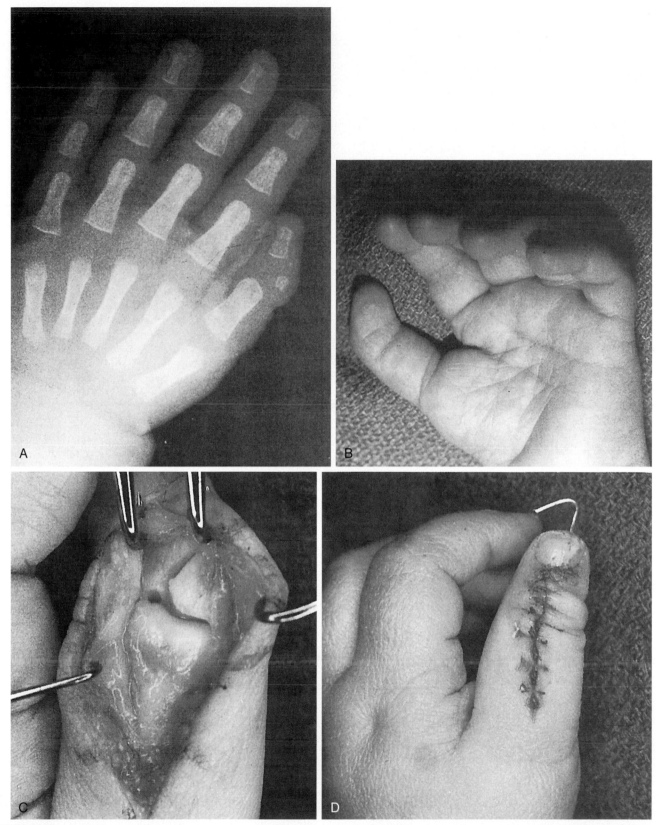

FIGURE 41-46. **A** and **B,** The preoperative radiographs and clinical appearance of a 6-month-old child with a triphalangeal thumb. **C** and **D,** The delta bone was fused to the distal phalanx, considerably improving the appearance of the thumb, seen immediately postoperatively.   *Continued*

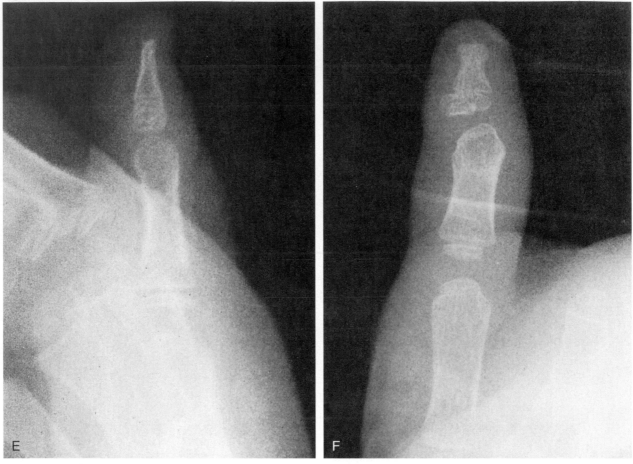

FIGURE 41-46—cont'd. **E** and **F**, Five months after surgery the fusion is complete and the thumb much straighter.

dactyly warrants early thumb separation. The cleft closure and joint reduction are usually performed at a second stage.

TRIGGER THUMB

Trigger thumb is about ten times more common than trigger finger.[1,3] The exact incidence remains unknown. Bilateral

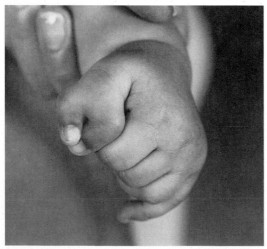

FIGURE 41-47. Triphalangeal thumb combined with thumb duplication.

involvement is present in 25% to 30% of children.[1,5] The term *congenital* is probably a misnomer, because widespread evaluations of newborns have failed to discover a trigger thumb.[5,6] In addition, the term *trigger* is inaccurate, because the vast majority of children present with a fixed flexion deformity of the thumb IP joint (Fig. 41-48).

The precise development of this flexion deformity is often uncertain, because an infant postures with the thumb in flexion.[6] The exact etiology remains controversial; however, nodular thickening of the flexor pollicis longus tendon and/or narrowing of the flexor sheath prevents the flexor tendon from entering into the sheath. Palpation of the nodular thickening of the flexor tendon (i.e., Notta's nodule) is readily apparent just proximal to the A1 pulley and is the indicator of a trigger thumb (Fig. 41-49).[5]

Passive manipulation into extension may produce a noticeable click or pop. Splinting can be used to maintain this position. The role of splinting as definitive treatment is controversial.[4,6] Successful splinting has been reported in 24 of 33 digits with night-time use for an average of 10 months' duration.[4] The natural history is also controversial with regard to spontaneous resolution. Dinham and Meggitt[2] reported that approximately 30% of trigger thumbs diagnosed before 1 year resolve, although this has been questioned.[6] A delay in surgery up to 3 years of age has not been detrimental with regard to contracture or motion.[6] Therefore, a period of observation with or without splinting

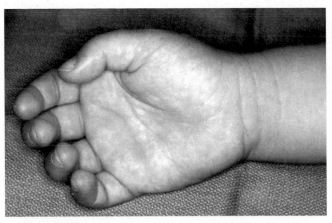

FIGURE 41-48. Trigger thumb with fixed flexion deformity of the IP joint.

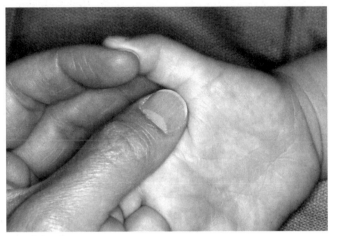

FIGURE 41-49. Notta's nodule is palpated just proximal to the A1 pulley.

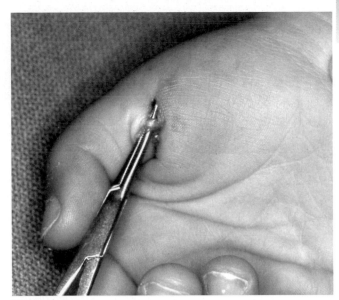

FIGURE 41-50. The radial digital nerve is identified and protected before pulley release.

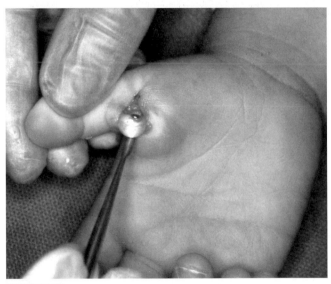

FIGURE 41-51. The flexor pollicis longus is isolated after release of the first annular pulley.

is often recommended for children younger than 1 year of age. Failure to resolve is treated with surgery. A trigger thumb in a child who is older than 1 year of age at presentation or a rigid deformity that cannot be corrected also warrants surgical release.

Surgical Technique

Surgery is performed under general anesthesia and loupe magnification. A tourniquet is used to facilitate dissection. A transverse incision is made over the first annular pulley. Only the skin is incised, and it is spread in a longitudinal fashion through the subcutaneous tissue. The radial digital nerve (Fig. 41-50) is identified and protected, and the first annular pulley is isolated. The pulley is released to expose the flexor pollicis longus (Fig. 41-51). The nodular thickening of the flexor pollicis longus is not addressed. The thumb is fully extended. The wound is irrigated and closed with absorbable suture. A soft dressing is placed around the extended thumb and forearm. The tourniquet is deflated, and the child is awakened. Dressings are removed 1 week later, and the child is allowed to return to normal function.

Release of trigger thumb is uniformly successful, and recurrences are rare.[1-3,6] Persistent triggering is usually secondary to inadequate release of the flexor tendon sheath.

Complications are related to surgical technique and include scarring after poor incision design, tendon bowstringing after release of the oblique pulley, and numbness secondary to digital nerve injury.

Trigger fingers in children are uncommon and less straightforward. The finger is usually not fixed in flexion, and the role of nonoperative treatment is unclear. In addition, the triggering may not respond to release of the first annular pulley. An abnormal relationship between the flexor digitorum profundus and superficialis tendons, proximal decussation of the superficialis tendon, nodular formation within the flexor tendons, and tightness of the second and/or third annular pulleys have all been implicated as potential causes. The surgeon must be prepared to perform a more diligent search for alternative causes when release of the first annular pulley does not resolve the triggering.

CRITICAL POINTS: TRIGGER THUMB

- Trigger thumbs are not "congenital" but rather acquired problems related to a discrepancy between a tight flexor tendon sheath and an enlarged flexor pollicis longus tendon.
- The classic finding is a fixed flexion contracture of the IP joint and a palpable nodule over the flexor pollicis longus tendon.
- Observation and/or splinting can be attempted; however, surgery is the most efficacious treatment that leads to resolution.
- Surgery must identify and protect the radial digital nerve before release of the A1 pulley.

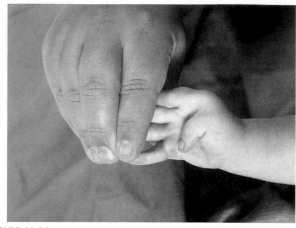

FIGURE 41-53. A type III clasped thumb in a child with arthrogryposis. (Courtesy of Shriners Hospitals for Children, Philadelphia.)

CLASPED THUMB

Congenital clasped thumb refers to a spectrum of thumb anomalies that ranges from mild deficiencies of the thumb extensor mechanism to severe abnormalities of the thenar muscles, web space, and soft tissues. The initial classifications attempted to subdivide into individual types and remain inclusive.[7,8] This scheme has not been useful in the clinical setting. A more practical approach has been proposed by McCarroll[4] and expanded by Mih.[5] A type I clasped thumb is usually supple, with absence or hypoplasia of the extensor mechanism (Fig. 41-52). A type II clasped thumb is complex with additional finding(s) of joint contracture, collateral ligament abnormality, first web space contracture, and thenar muscle abnormality. A type III clasped thumb is associated with arthrogryposis or its related syndromes. In this case, the extensor mechanism may have minimal or no abnormality (Fig. 41-53).

Treatment of the relatively mild type I clasped thumb is discussed here. The more severe type II and III forms are discussed under the congenital contracture section and arthrogryposis.

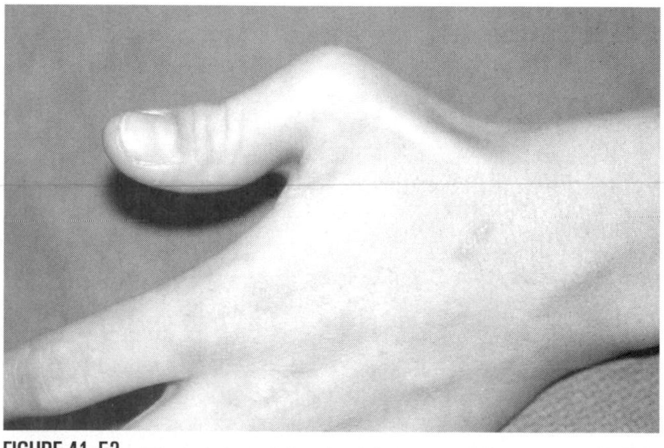

Clinical Features

The diagnosis of clasped thumb is often delayed because an infant frequently holds the thumb within the palm for the first 3 to 4 months. The thumb rests in flexion with an extension lag. Most commonly, the lag is present at just the MCP joint extension, which implies hypoplasia of the extensor pollicis brevis muscle tendon unit (see Fig. 41-52).[1,9] Additional extensor pollicis longus and/or abductor pollicis longus anomalies have also been reported.[5,10] Diagnosis of these deficiencies is based on thumb and joint position. Simultaneous extension lag at the IP joint indicates a concomitant deficiency of the extensor pollicis longus. Concurrent metacarpal adduction implies insufficiency of the abductor pollicis longus.

Treatment

Initial treatment of the type I clasped thumb includes splinting of the affected joint(s) in extension. The goal is to prevent additional attenuation of the hypoplastic extensor mechanism and to allow hypertrophy over time. Full-time splinting for 2 to 6 months has been shown to be effective. Miura[6] reported on 96 hands in 66 patients who underwent splint application. Good results were obtained in 70% of children who were splinted within 12 months of birth. In contrast, splinting was effective in only 21% of children older than 1 year after birth and in none older than 2 years of age.

Surgery is warranted in situations in which splinting has failed or if the child is older than 2 years of age. The degree of impairment, however, must be considered during formulation of a treatment plan. Mild MCP joint extension lag does not hinder hand function and does not always require treatment (Fig. 41-54). Frequently, adolescents are seen with a mild clasped thumb that has never been treated and report no problems.

Considerable lack of thumb extension that interferes with grasp warrants treatment. Any associated thumb MCP joint or thumb-index web space contracture requires treatment (Fig. 41-55). Initially, serial casting or splinting may be tried to stretch the taut skin and correct the contracture.

FIGURE 41-52. A type I clasped thumb with absence of the extensor pollicis brevis tendon. (Courtesy of Shriners Hospitals for Children, Philadelphia.)

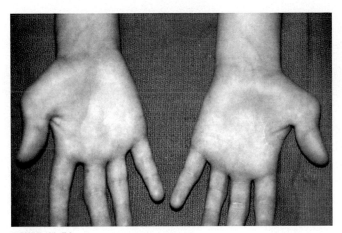

FIGURE 41-54. Adolescent with bilateral untreated clasped thumbs and minimal functional impairment. (Courtesy of Shriners Hospitals for Children, Philadelphia.)

Correction of the residual contracture must be incorporated into the surgical plan. In a type I clasped thumb, skin and subcutaneous tissue release is usually enough to correct the contracture. Thumb/index finger space deficiency is treated with standard techniques of four-flap "Z"-plasty or dorsal rotation flap. Palmar skin deficiency requires a rotational flap into the palmar aspect of the thumb MCP joint.

A second incision is performed over the dorsum of the thumb metacarpal and proximal phalanx. The extensor apparatus is explored. The extensor pollicis brevis tendon is usually present but is small and attenuated. A tendon transfer is performed to augment thumb extensor function.[3] The donor tendons depend on availability and expendability. The extensor indicis proprius tendon is the first choice and may or may not be present.[5,9] Absence of the extensor indicis proprius requires selection of an alternative donor tendon. Options are the flexor digitorum superficialis or abductor digiti minimi muscle.[2,5] The tendon transfer is secured into the attenuated tendon and/or the base of the proximal phalanx. The limb is placed into a long-arm/thumb spica cast with the MCP joint in extension for 4 weeks. The cast is removed, and a short-arm/thumb spica splint is fabricated. Gradual active flexion of the thumb is encouraged. The splint is worn only at night beginning at 6 weeks and is discontinued at 12 weeks after surgery.

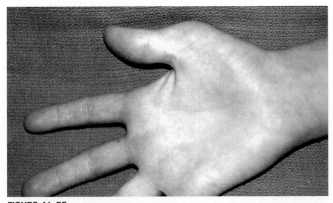

FIGURE 41-55. Clasped thumb with flexion contracture of the MCP joint. (Courtesy of Shriners Hospitals for Children, Philadelphia.)

CRITICAL POINTS: CLASPED THUMB

- Congenital clasped thumb refers to a spectrum of thumb anomalies that ranges from mild deficiencies of the thumb extensor mechanism to severe abnormalities of the thenar muscles, web space, and soft tissues.
- A mild clasped thumb is usually supple, with absence or hypoplasia of the extensor mechanism. An extension lag at the MCP joint extension implies hypoplasia of the extensor pollicis brevis muscle tendon unit. Simultaneous extension lag at the IP joint indicates a concomitant deficiency of the extensor pollicis longus.
- Initial treatment is splinting of the affected joint(s) in extension. Splinting has been shown to be fairly effective in children younger than 1 year of age.
- Surgery is warranted for children who have failed splinting or present at older than 2 years of age and have a functional impairment.
- Surgical goals are to correct any soft tissue contracture and overcome tendon deficiency via tendon transfer.

ANNOTATED REFERENCES

Thumb Hypoplasia

2. Buck-Gramcko D: Pollicization of the index finger: Method and results in aplasia and hypoplasia of the thumb. J Bone Joint Surg Am 53:1605-1617, 1971.

    Classic article details the technique of pollicization. Buck-Gramcko championed the details of pollicization based on extensive experience after the thalidomide disaster.

3. Clark DI, Chell J, Davis TR: Pollicisation of the index finger: A 27-year follow-up study. J Bone Joint Surg Br 80:631-635, 1998.

    Long-term follow-up is reported of 11 patients treated by pollicization of the index finger after 20 to 38 years. Function was excellent in 6, good in 3, fair in 2, and poor in 4; three of the poor results were in patients with radial forearm deficiencies. Ten of the 15 transfers were used as normal thumbs, but in five hands function required trick movements.

10. Kozin SH, Weiss AA, Webber JB, et al: Index finger pollicization for congenital aplasia or hypoplasia of the thumb. J Hand Surg [Am] 17:880-884, 1992.

    Fourteen hands (10 patients) were evaluated after index finger pollicization. Patients with unilateral pollicization averaged 67% grip strength, 60% lateral pinch, 56% palmar pinch, and 39% three-point pinch compared with the normal contralateral hand. Manual dexterity averaged 70% efficiency as compared with normal standards. Fifty-five of the patients, however, used side-to-side pinch when stressed under time. Those patients who used side-to-side pinch averaged 54% performance of normal standards, compared with 93% in patients who used tip-to-tip pinch for prehension.

18. Manske PR, McCarroll HR Jr, James MA: Type III-A hypoplastic thumb. J Hand Surg [Am] 20:246-253, 1995.

Thirteen type IIIA hypoplastic thumbs with narrow thumb-index finger web space, hypoplastic thenar muscles, unstable MCP joint, as well as extrinsic tendon abnormalities were discussed. All had stable CMC joints. Extrinsic tendon abnormalities included absent extensor pollicis longus tendon, absent or aberrant flexor pollicis longus tendon, and a tendon interconnection between the flexor pollicis longus and extensor aponeurosis. Twelve of the thumbs had surgical reconstruction.

20. McCarroll HR: Congenital anomalies: A 25-year overview. J Hand Surg [Am] 25:1007-1037, 2000.

Review article discusses the advances in congenital hand surgery over the past 25 years. Pollicization and the reconstruction of the hypoplastic thumb are detailed with reference to our current state of knowledge, treatment algorithm, and anticipated outcome.

Thumb Duplication

3. Ezaki M: Radial polydactyly. Hand Clin 6:577-588, 1990.

Review article highlights the anatomy, classification, incidence, and surgical treatment. Illustrative cases are presented and surgical techniques discussed. Complications and late reconstruction are briefly mentioned with ample references.

14. Ogino T, Ishii S, Takahata S, Kato H: Long-term results of surgical treatment of thumb polydactyly. J Hand Surg [Am] 21:478-486, 1996.

One hundred thirteen hands with thumb polydactyly were treated and their outcome assessed at an average of 49 months. Radial thumbs were resected in 107 hands and ulnar thumbs in 2 hands. Four hands were treated using a modified Bilhaut procedure. The results were evaluated as good in 97 hands, fair in 12 hands, and poor in 4 hands. The incidence of unsatisfactory results was relatively high in Wassel types 3, 5, and 6 and triphalangeal-type thumb polydactyly. Unsatisfactory outcome was also higher when the ulnar digit was removed.

Triphalangeal Thumb

5. Wood VE: Treatment of the triphalangeal thumb. Clin Orthop 120:188-200, 1976.

Review of the literature and extensive personal experience with triphalangeal thumb. Probably the best overall assessment of the triphalangeal thumb and its associated anomalies.

Trigger Thumb

1. Cardon LJ, Ezaki M, Carter PR: Trigger finger in children. J Hand Surg [Am] 24:1156-1161, 1999.

Review of trigger digits at the Texas Scottish Rite Hospital was reported over a 10-year period. Approximately 90% of children had trigger thumbs. A smaller cohort (16 patients) of trigger fingers was reported in detail. Surgical release of the A1 pulley relieved the triggering in 10 children. The recalcitrant cases required a more diligent search for causation. Various causes were found including a flexor tendon nodule and abnormal flexor digitorum superficialis slip.

6. Slakey JB, Hennrikus WL: Acquired thumb flexion contracture in children: Congenital trigger thumb. J Bone Joint Surg Br 78:481-483, 1996.

Prospective study of 4,719 neonates was done to screen for the presence of a "congenital" trigger thumb. No cases of triggering, locking, nodule formation, or fixed-flexion contracture were noted. A separate cohort of 15 children was treated for trigger thumb. Surgery was performed with release of the A1 pulley. Correction of the flexed posture and resolution of the nodule was achieved in all children.

Clasped Thumb

3. Lipskeir E, Weizenbluth M: Surgical treatment of the clasped thumb. J Hand Surg [Br] 14:72-79, 1989.

Twelve patients (19 hands) with clasped thumb were treated with surgery. The series is divided into three groups. The first group was secondary to hypoplasia of the extensor tendons, and treatment was tendon transfer. The second group was associated with arthrogryposis with contracture of the intrinsic muscles of the thumb and shortening of the skin. Treatment was primarily release of the contracted tissues. The third group was attributed to a combination of skeletal, muscular, and tendon hypoplasia. Associated instability of the MCP joint and adduction contracture of the first ray was universal. Final results were better with isolated extensor tendon hypoplasia and less contracture.

5. Mih AD: Congenital clasped thumb. Hand Clin 14:77-84, 1988.

Review article of clasped thumb provides insight into classification and a treatment regimen and discusses pathophysiology and management options. Surgical approach is preferred to overcome extensor mechanism deficiency.

8. Weckesser EC, Reed JR, Heiple KG: Congenital clasped thumb (congenital flexion-adduction deformity of the thumb: A syndrome, not a specific entity. J Bone Joint Surg [Am] 50:1417-1428, 1968.

A series of clasped thumbs with different underlying problems is presented. Group I was encountered most frequently by weak, attenuated, or absent extensor tendons. The most common anomaly involved the extensor pollicis brevis muscle and tendon. Early splinting of the thumb in extension and abduction resulted in the majority of cases. Delayed immobilization after 2 years of age resulted in a poor outcome.

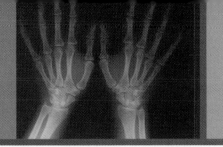

CHAPTER 42

Deformities of the Wrist and Forearm

Michelle A. James and Michael Bednar

Radial Deficiency

EPIDEMIOLOGY

Radial deficiency is a spectrum of malformations affecting the structures of the radial side of the forearm (radius, radial carpus, and thumb), including hypoplasia of the bones and joints, muscles and tendons, ligaments, nerves, and blood vessels.[10,17,27] Radial deficiency is an uncommon condition (approximately 1:30,000 live births),[28] although it is the most common type of longitudinal failure of formation.[12]

CLINICAL FEATURES

Children with radial deficiency should have thorough and serial examinations of both upper extremities. Radial deficiency is frequently bilateral and asymmetrical, and manifestations may be subtle.[22] Radial deficiency is commonly associated with several congenital syndromes (Table 42-1). Therefore, a complete physical examination must be performed and a consultation with a clinical geneticist is recommended.

Children with bilateral and severe radial deficiency have considerable functional impairment owing to thumb dysfunction, wrist instability, and short upper extremities. Performing activities of daily living independently, such as fastening buttons and zippers or accomplishing personal hygiene, is difficult.

RADIOGRAPHY

Radiographs will show the degree of involvement of the radius, carpus, and thumb and are essential to classify the deficiency. Spine radiographs, renal ultrasound, and echo-

Table 42-1
SYNDROMES ASSOCIATED WITH RADIAL DEFICIENCY

Syndrome	Other Anomalies	Inheritance
VACTERL	Spine, renal, gastrointestinal, cardiac	Sporadic
Holt-Oram	Cardiac (septal defects); other upper extremity malformations	Autosomal dominant
TAR	Thrombocytopenia, anemia; radius absent but thumb present	Autosomal recessive
Fanconi's anemia	Pancytopenia	Autosomal recessive
Chromosome aberrations (trisomy 13 and 18)	Multiple	Sporadic
Nager, Rothmund-Thomson, IVIC	Craniofacial	Varies with syndrome

VACTERL, vertebral, anal, cardiac, tracheo-esophageal, renal/radial, limb; TAR, thrombocytopenia–absent-radius; IVIC, Instituto Venzolano de Investigaciones Cientificas.

cardiography are required to assess for associated anomalies. Genetic counseling and testing for Fanconi's anemia is recommended in the absence of an identifiable syndrome, because life-threatening pancytopenia can be treated with bone marrow transplantation.[13,18,21,30]

ASSOCIATED ANOMALIES AND/OR SYSTEMIC CONDITIONS

Radial deficiency is associated with other upper extremity anomalies, including humeral hypoplasia, proximal radioulnar synostosis, congenital radial head dislocation, and finger stiffness. Less common associations include metacarpal synostoses and syndactyly.[10,16] An infrequent finding is contralateral radial polydactyly.[26]

CLASSIFICATION

Bayne and Klug[3] classified radial deficiency into four types based on radiographic severity of the radius deficiency (Table 42-2). James and associates[17] have modified Bayne's classification to include patients with deficiency of the thumb or carpus in the presence of a radius of normal length (Fig. 42-1). This scheme is used in combination with the modified Blauth scheme for classifying thumb hypoplasia.

SURGICAL MANAGEMENT

Indications

Function is impaired by thumb hypoplasia, wrist instability, and forearm length deficit. The appearance of the hand—namely, the radial angulation of the wrist and the short forearm—is often troubling to the family and the older child with radial deficiency. Surgical attempts to improve function and appearance include carpal centralization, forearm lengthening, and thumb reconstruction or index pollicization.

Treatment indications vary with the severity of the deformity and the age of the patient. Children with type 0, 1, or mild type 2 radial deficiencies may require only stretching and splinting. When considerable radial deviation is present, tendon transfers and soft tissue releases are indicated.[24] Severe type 2 radial deficiency is difficult to treat. Lengthening of the radius may be possible or centralization of the carpus on the end of the ulna may be necessary to achieve stability. The wrist instability and radial deviation associated with types 3 and 4 is treated with centralization of the carpus on the end of the ulna. The best results are obtained when aberrant radial wrist extensors are transferred to help maintain the new position and the centralization is done before 1 year of age.[10] Before centralization, serial casting and/or application of a distraction device facilitates stretching of the taut radial soft tissue structures. Use of external distraction has been reported to eliminate the need for serial casting. In addition, diminishing the soft tissue tension will diminish the possibility of any required bony resection during centralization.[20,25,28,31] External distraction is most helpful for older children with untreated type 3 or 4 radius deficiency. A bilobed skin flap may be helpful to redistribute excess tissue from the ulnar to the radial side of the wrist.[8]

With unilateral type 3 or 4 involvement, the affected forearm is usually only half as long as the unaffected side. This length deficit has been surgically addressed with ulnar lengthening using distraction osteogenesis.[1,6,19] Lengthening is usually performed in the older child after centralization.

Vilkki[31] has described the combination of soft tissue distraction and microvascular epiphysis transfer for the treatment of type 4 radial deficiency (Fig. 42-2). Historically, attempts to treat radius deficiency with surgical transfer of nonvascularized growing bone have failed because the graft fails to grow.[2,14] Although Vilkki's early results are promising, the technique is technically demanding and the outcome at skeletal maturity is not yet known.

Table 42-2
MODIFIED BAYNE CLASSIFICATION OF RADIAL LONGITUDINAL DEFICIENCY

Type	Thumb	Carpus	Distal Radius	Proximal Radius
N	Hypoplastic or absent	Normal	Normal	Normal
0	Hypoplastic or absent	Absence, hypoplasia, or coalition	Normal	Normal, radioulnar synostosis, or congenital dislocation of the radial head
1	Hypoplastic or absent	Absence, hypoplasia, or coalition	> 2 mm shorter than ulna	Normal, radioulnar synostosis, or congenital dislocation of the radial head
2	Hypoplastic or absent	Absence, hypoplasia, or coalition	Hypoplasia	Hypoplasia
3	Hypoplastic or absent	Absence, hypoplasia, or coalition	Physis absent	Variable hypoplasia
4	Hypoplastic or absent	Absence, hypoplasia, or coalition	Absent	Absent

Modified from Bayne LG, Klug MS: Long-term review of the surgical treatment of radial deficiencies. J Hand Surg [Am] 12:169-179, 1987; and James MA, McCarroll HR Jr, Manske PR: The spectrum of radial longitudinal deficiency: A modified classification. J Hand Surg [Am] 24:1145-1155, 1999.

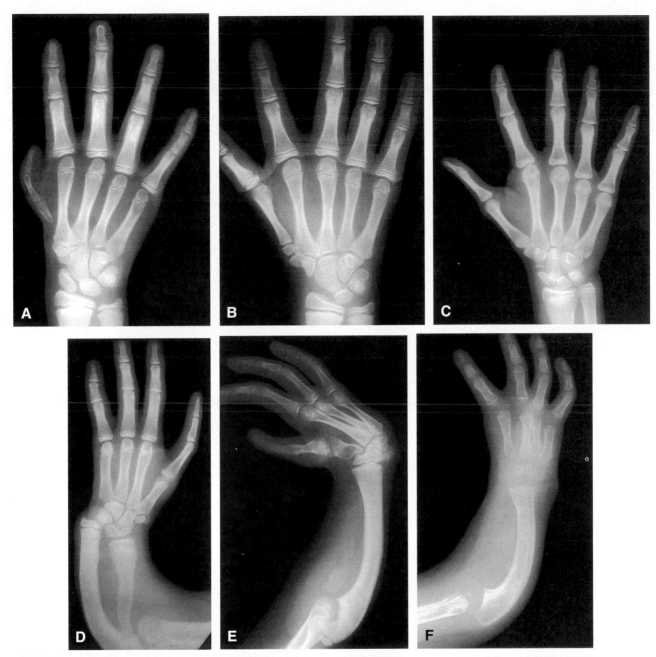

FIGURE 42-1. Types of radius deficiency. **A,** Type N. **B,** Type 0 (absent scaphoid). **C,** Type 1. **D,** Type 2. **E,** Type 3. **F,** Type 4 (post centralization).

Contraindications

Contraindications for centralization include major organ defects that make the anesthetic risk unacceptable, inadequate elbow flexion for the hand to reach the mouth after centralization, and firmly established functional patterns in adults.[10]

Techniques

Preliminary Soft Tissue Distraction

Unilateral and circumferential fixators have been successfully used to distract the radial soft tissues before central-

ization (Fig. 42-3).[20,25,28] The fixator is applied across the wrist using an open technique for pin placement to protect the anomalous anatomy. Gradual distraction is performed until the wrist can be centralized without residual radial deviation after the external fixator is loosened or removed.

Centralization

Although the wrist and forearm are profoundly abnormal in the radial deficient limb, the anomalies are predictable (Fig. 42-4). All of the radial forearm structures are deficient to varying degrees. The radial wrist extensors and extrinsic thumb motors are usually absent or aberrant. The radial nerve is usually absent below the elbow (Fig. 42-5). The

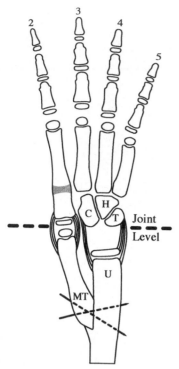

FIGURE 42-2. Free toe transfer to support the radial side of the wrist. The toe proximal phalanx is fused to the base of the second metacarpal, and the proximal metatarsal is affixed to the side of the distal ulna. (C, capitate; H, hamate; T, triquetrum; U, ulna; MT, metatarsal.) (From Vilkki SK: Distraction and microvascular epiphysis transfer for radial club hand. J Hand Surg [Br] 23:445-452, 1998.)

median nerve is always present and often is the most prominent structure on the radial side of the wrist. The radial artery is usually absent.[10,23,27]

The incision begins at the level of the distal end of the ulna just radial to the midline. The incision extends in toward the ulna in a transverse direction and then forms an ellipse to excise excess skin and subcutaneous tissue after centralization. The incision ends at the volar midline. The dorsal ulnar sensory nerve is identified and preserved. The extensor retinaculum is exposed. The extensor carpi ulnaris is identified and detached near its insertion into the base of the fifth metacarpal. The extensor retinaculum is raised as a radially based flap and the finger extensor tendons are identified and retracted in a radial direction. The radial wrist extensors are usually absent or adherent to the dorsal capsule and devoid of proximal musculature. The remnants are isolated and elevated with a piece of dorsal capsule.

The wrist capsule is incised in a transverse direction over the ulnocarpal joint exposing the distal ulna. The carpal bones are often palmar and radial to the distal ulna. The ulna is freed from its soft tissue attachments distal to the physis. The carpal bones are detached from the palmar capsule. The carpus is reduced onto the distal ulna. Failure to achieve reduction requires repeat examination of the radial structures for any persistent taut tissue. In severe cases, adequate reduction cannot be obtained and alternative measures are necessary. Surgical options include carpectomy or limited shaving of the distal ulna epiphysis while avoiding injury to

the growth plate (Fig. 42-6). Another option is application of an external fixator, postoperative distraction, and delayed formal centralization.

The wrist is held reduced by a Kirschner wire placed through the carpus and third metacarpal and into the ulnar shaft (Fig. 42-7). If the ulnar angulation is greater than 30 degrees, a diaphyseal closing wedge osteotomy is performed at the apex of the deformity and is secured with the same Kirschner wire. The wrist capsule is imbricated, and, if present, the radial wrist extensors are transferred into the extensor carpi ulnaris tendon. The extensor carpi ulnaris is advanced and reattached to its insertion or imbricated to increase soft tissue tension on the ulnar side. The retinacular flap is passed underneath the finger extensors to reinforce the wrist capsule. Excess skin and subcutaneous tissue are excised. The skin is closed with an absorbable suture. A long-arm bulky compressive dressing is applied and covered with a long-arm fiberglass cast. The extremity is casted for at least 8 weeks and the pin kept in place for as long as possible. A long-arm orthoplast splint, custom fabricated to maintain wrist position, is worn full time for 3 to 6 months then indefinitely at night time.

Ulnar Lengthening

The principles of distraction lengthening are followed (Fig. 42-8).[6,15,19] A uniplane or multiplane fixator is used, depending on any concomitant angular bony correction. For application of a circumferential frame, two half pins and one transfixion wire are used proximal to the osteotomy. One half pin and two transfixion wires (one in the ulna and one in the metacarpals) are placed distal to the osteotomy. Any residual radial deviation is corrected at the time of fixator application or during the distraction. Acute bony correction can be obtained by a closing wedge osteotomy followed by distraction osteogenesis. Distraction is initiated approximately 1 week after fixator application and is continued at 1 mm per day divided into three increments. Radiographic progress of bony regeneration is followed weekly. The rate of lengthening is slowed if regeneration is lagging. The child and family are taught lengthening techniques and exercises to maintain elbow and digit motion. The ulna can usually be lengthened by 30% to 50%. The fixator is maintained during consolidation of the bony regenerate, which usually takes at least as long as the lengthening phase.

Complications are common, especially pin tract infections that resolve with local care and antibiotics. Osteomyelitis is a rare complication. Finger stiffness may occur during the lengthening process and is treated by slowing the distraction rate and therapy. Delayed consolidation of the bony regenerate is fairly common in congenital shortening. Prolonged external fixation until bony consolidation is required. Occasionally, supplemental bone grafting is necessary.

Authors' Preferred Techniques

Serial casting for preoperative soft tissue stretching is started shortly after birth. The wrist is stretched as close to

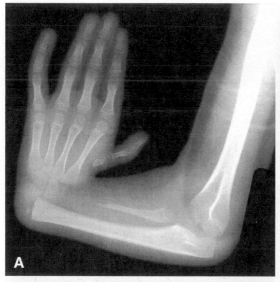

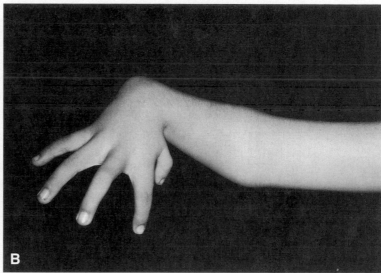

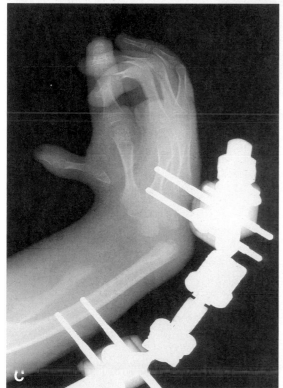

FIGURE 42-3. An 8-year-old child presented with cardiac problems associated with Holt-Oram syndrome that precluded earlier surgery. **A** and **B,** The deformity from his type 3 radius deficiency was too severe for single-stage centralization. **C,** A unilateral fixator was applied across the wrist and gradual distraction was performed by the child.

Continued

neutral as possible, and a long-arm cast is applied. The cast is changed on a weekly basis with further correction each time. If the wrist can be stretched to neutral, a custom fabricated long-arm orthoplast splint is applied. The parents are instructed to continue stretching the wrist several times each day until centralization is performed. In recalcitrant cases, soft tissue distraction is accomplished with external fixation.

Centralization is performed at about 1 year of age. Prolonged pin fixation followed by long-term splinting is necessary to minimize recurrence. Ulnar lengthening is reserved for the mature older child or teenager. Lengthening requires realistic expectations and emotional stamina on the

part of the patient and family. Preoperative counseling and psychological assessment are helpful. The support of a limb-lengthening team, including a nurse, social worker, and occupational therapist, is also essential.

OUTCOME

Long-term follow-up studies report problems with recurrence and stiffness (Fig. 42-9).[7,11] The wrists tend to be either flexible and deviated or stiff and straight (Fig. 42-10). Centralization has been shown to improve the appearance of the extremity but has not been proven to enhance function.

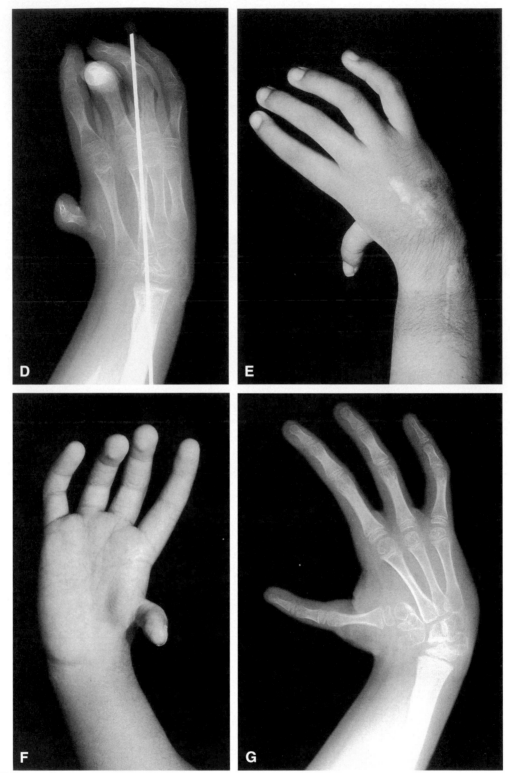

FIGURE 42-3—cont'd. **D** to **F**, After adequate distraction, centralization was performed. **G**, Pollicization was performed 6 months later.

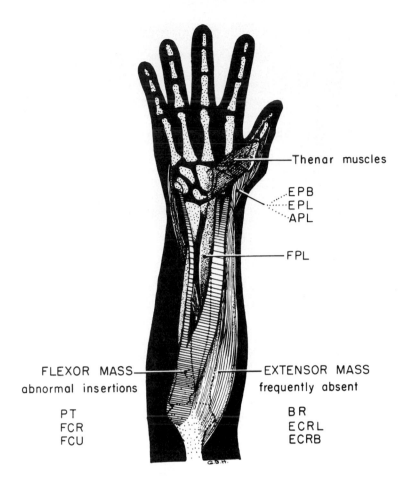

Thenar muscles

EPB
EPL
APL

FPL

FLEXOR MASS
abnormal insertions

PT
FCR
FCU

EXTENSOR MASS
frequently absent

BR
ECRL
ECRB

FIGURE 42-4. Associated muscle deficiencies. The extensor muscles are frequently absent or defective to some extent. The flexor muscles have abnormal insertions. The thenar and thumb muscles are defective in proportion to the thumb deficiency. EPB, extensor pollicis brevis; EPL, extensor pollicis longus; APL, abductor pollicis longus; FPL, flexor pollicis longus; PT, pronator teres; FCR, flexor carpi radialis; FCU, flexor carpi ulnaris; BR, brachioradialis; ECRL, extensor carpi radialis longus; ECRB, extensor carpi radialis brevis.

ARTERIAL ANOMALIES

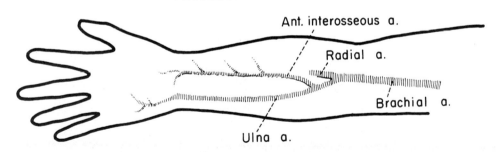

Ant. interosseous a.

Radial a.

Brachial a.

Ulna a.

NERVE ANOMALIES

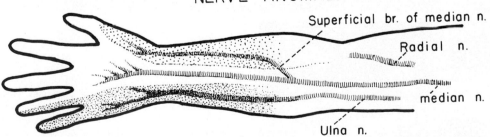

Superficial br. of median n.

Radial n.

median n.

Ulna n.

FIGURE 42-5. Associated neurovascular abnormalities. The radial artery is usually absent. The anterior interosseous artery supplies the radial distribution through the forearm. The superficial radial nerve is absent. The sensory area of the radial nerve is supplanted by the superficial dorsal branch of the median nerve.

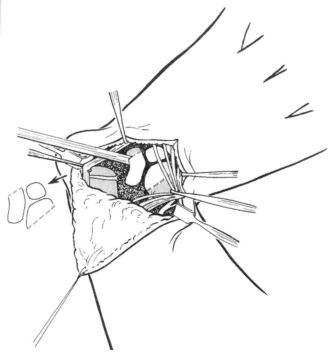

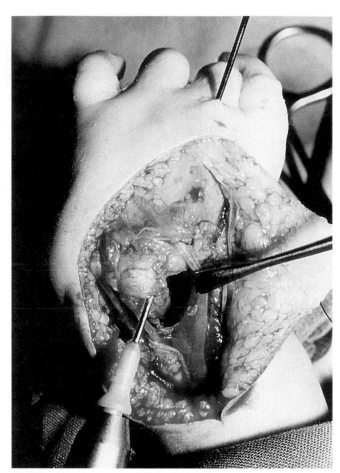

FIGURE 42-6. Centralization: excision of the lunate with partial resection of the scaphoid and triquetrum. It may be necessary to remove all of the central carpal bones in both rows to the bases of the metacarpals. (From Buck-Gramcko D: Congenital malformations. *In* Nigst H, Buck-Gramcko D, Millesi H, Lister GD [eds]: Hand Surgery. New York, Thieme, 1988, vol 1, pp 12.77-12.91, with permission.)

FIGURE 42-7. Placement of Kirschner wire through the carpus and metacarpal.

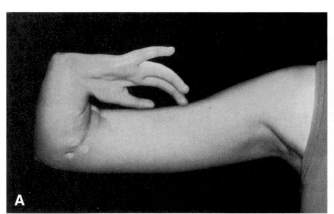

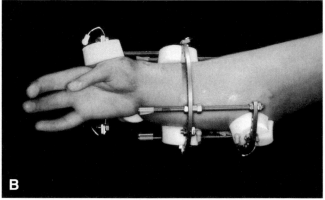

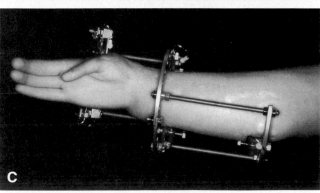

FIGURE 42-8. Twelve-year-old child with right forearm shortening. **A,** Forearm before shortening. **B,** Forearm and hand after carpal wedge osteotomy, ulnar osteotomy, and application of fixator. **C,** Forearm and hand after lengthening period and during consolidation phase.

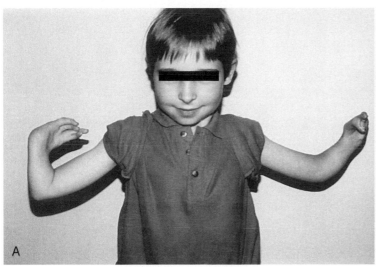

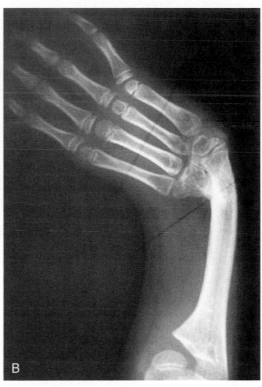

FIGURE 42-9. Recurrence of deformity and shortening after centralization: clinical (**A**) and radiographic (**B**).

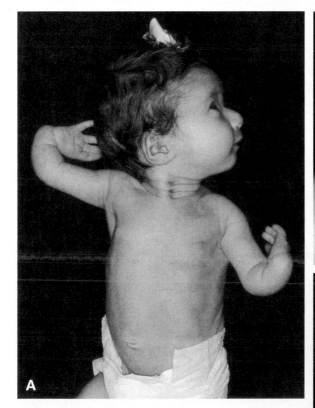

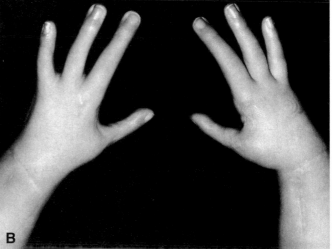

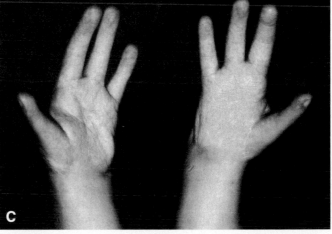

FIGURE 42-10. Preoperative and long-term postoperative follow-up of centralization and pollicization. **A,** Infant with bilateral radius and thumb absence. **B,** Dorsal view of 6-year follow-up. **C,** Palmar view of 6-year follow-up.

Radialization of the ulna has been described to improve the position and lessen recurrence (Fig. 42-11).[4,5] Some experienced pediatric hand surgeons have abandoned formal centralization in favor of soft tissue reconstruction, such as the bilobed skin flap combined with musculotendinous releases and tendon transfers (Fig. 42-12).[9]

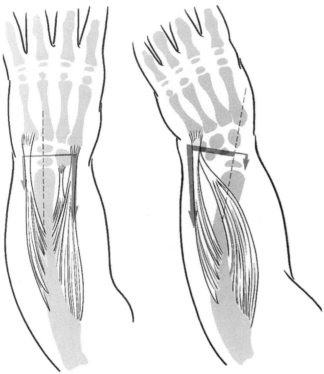

FIGURE 42-11. Improved lever arm after radialization and transfer of radial muscles to the extensor carpi ulnaris. (From Buck-Gramcko D: Congenital malformations. *In* Nigst H, Buck-Gramcko D, Millesi H, Lister GD [eds]: Hand Surgery. New York, Thieme, 1988, vol 1, pp 12.77-12.91, with permission.)

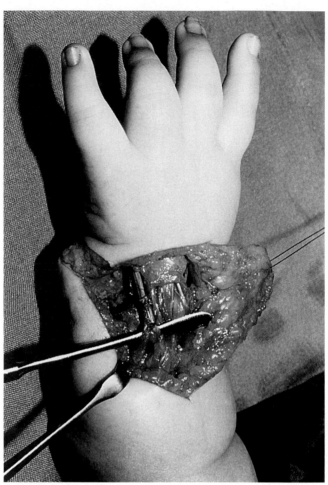

FIGURE 42-12. Transfer of the radial wrist extensors to the extensor carpi ulnaris.

CRITICAL POINTS: RADIAL DEFICIENCY

- Radial deficiency ranges from mild thumb hypoplasia to complete absence of the radius.
- All forms warrant systemic evaluation for syndromes or associations. Holt-Oram syndrome, TAR (thrombocytopenia–absent-radius) syndrome, VACTERL association (vertebral abnormalities, anal atresia, cardiac abnormalities, tracheoesophageal fistula, esophageal atresia, renal defects, radial dysplasia, lower limb abnormalities), and Fanconi's anemia are the primary concerns.
- The most devastating associated condition is Fanconi's anemia. Children with Fanconi's anemia lack signs of bone marrow failure at birth. A chromosomal challenge test, however, is available that allows detection of the disease before the onset of bone marrow failure.
- The basic goals of treatment are to (1) correct the radial deviation of the wrist; (2) balance the wrist

on the forearm; (3) maintain wrist and finger motion; (4) promote growth of the forearm; (5) reconstruct the thumb deficiency; and (6) improve the function of the extremity.
- Passive stretching and splinting of the taut radial structures is initiated in the infant.
- Centralization or radialization combined with tendon transfer is indicated in children with severe radial wrist deviation and insufficient support of the carpus. Thumb hypoplasia is usually addressed at a second stage after wrist centralization.
- Despite numerous technical modifications to preserve alignment, some recurrence of the radial deficiency is universal. Currently, long-term maintenance of the carpus on the end of the ulna without sacrificing wrist mobility or stunting forearm growth remains a daunting task.

ANNOTATED REFERENCES

6. Catagni MA, Szabo RM, Cattaneo R: Preliminary experience with Ilizarov method in late reconstruction of radial hemimelia. J Hand Surg Am 18:316-321, 1993.

Ulnar lengthening was used in five adults with radial deficiency and previous wrist centralization. Indications were either a functional deficit due to the short ulna or poor appearance. All patients had a successful lengthening of the ulna, with a gain in length from 4 to 13 cm; however, the procedures were prolonged (7 to 25 months), and all patients experienced complications.

7. Damore E, Kozin SH, Thoder JJ, Porter S: The recurrence of deformity after surgical centralization for radial clubhand. J Hand Surg [Am] 25:745-751, 2000.

Preoperative, postoperative, and follow-up radiographs were used to determine the initial deformity, amount of surgical correction, and degree of recurrence in 14 children (19 cases of radial deficiency). The average preoperative angulation measured 83 degrees. Centralization corrected the angulation an average of 58 degrees to an average immediate postoperative total angulation of 25 degrees. At the final follow-up examination there was a loss of 38 degrees, and the total angulation increased to an average of 63 degrees.

11. Geck MJ, Dorey F, Lawrence JF, Johnson MK: Congenital radius deficiency: Radiographic outcome and survivorship analysis. J Hand Surg [Am] 24:1132-1144, 1999.

The experience at the Los Angeles Shriners Hospital for Children was reviewed. A cohort of 29 limbs in 23 patients was identified with congenital radius deficiency. Average follow-up was 50 months. Radiographic parameters were assessed using the hand-forearm angle, hand-forearm position, and ulnar bow. The effect of radialization compared with centralization, ulnar osteotomy, age, preoperative deformity, and extent of deficiency was assessed. Radialization was similar to centralization in the final outcome. Ulnar osteotomy was efficacious to correct ulnar deformity. Age, preoperative deformity, performance of an ulnar osteotomy, and deficiency type did not affect the final wrist position. Using revision as the end point, survivorship rate at 5 years was 67%. Significant risk factors for revision included radial or positive hand-forearm angle and young age at the time of the index procedure. This result offers support for the hypothesis that a more ulnar translation and an ulnar angulation of the wrist may reduce the radial lever arm and the incidence of deformity recurrence.

19. Kawabata H, Shibata T, Masatomi T, Yasui N: Residual deformity in congenital radial club hands after previous centralisation of the wrist: Ulnar lengthening and correction by the Ilizarov method. J Bone Joint Surg Br 80:762-765, 1998.

Seven patients with severe congenital radial club hands underwent distraction histiogenesis to correct residual shortening, bowing of the ulna, and recurrent wrist deformity. The mean length gained was 51% of the original ulna. The ratio of the length of the lengthened ulna to the normal side improved on average from 64% to 95%. The length ratio, however, decreased to 83% at the final follow-up. In four patients, the angular deformity partially recurred.

25. Nanchahal J, Tonkin MA: Pre-operative distraction lengthening for radial longitudinal deficiency. J Hand Surg [Br] 21:103-107, 1996.

Twelve patients were evaluated after centralization or radialization for correction of deformity. Five of six limbs were realigned by radialization after preliminary distraction. In contrast, only one of six treated without distraction was capable of radialization. The average improvement in radial angulation in the distraction group was 38 degrees compared with 19 degrees in the nondistraction group.

31. Vilkki SK: Distraction and microvascular epiphysis transfer for radial club hand. J Hand Surg [Br] 23:445-452, 1998.

Microsurgery is presented as an alternative to treat the radial deficient limb. A microvascular joint transfer was used to reconstruct the absent half of the wrist joint, aiming for better movement and stability at the wrist joint with preservation of longitudinal growth. Preoperative soft tissue distraction was used to obtain proper alignment of the hand on the ulna before the second metatarsophalangeal joint with the entire metatarsal bone was transplanted. Twelve cases are reported and the results of the first nine cases are detailed with a mean follow-up of 6 years. Slight recurrence was noted, but continued growth of the transplanted digit was evident. The technique is promising but technically demanding.

Ulnar Deficiency

EPIDEMIOLOGY

Ulnar deficiency occurs approximately once in 100,000 live births and is 4 to 10 times less common than radial deficiency.[22] Ulnar deficiency occurs sporadically and is not associated with systemic conditions that affect children with radial deficiency. Ulnar deficiency, however, is associated with other musculoskeletal abnormalities that warrant careful physical examination supplemented by radiographs.[8]

CLINICAL FEATURES

Unilateral ulnar deficiency is more common than bilateral deficiency.[21] Children with ulnar deficiency have hypoplasia of the entire upper extremity. The elbow is malformed or fused (i.e., radiohumeral synostosis) in the majority of cases.[21] The ulna may be partially or completely absent, and a cartilaginous ulnar "anlage" may be present.[2,3,13-15] The hand and carpus are always affected. About 90% of hands are missing digits, 30% have syndactyly, and 70% have thumb abnormalities (Fig. 42-13).[4,6,11,21]

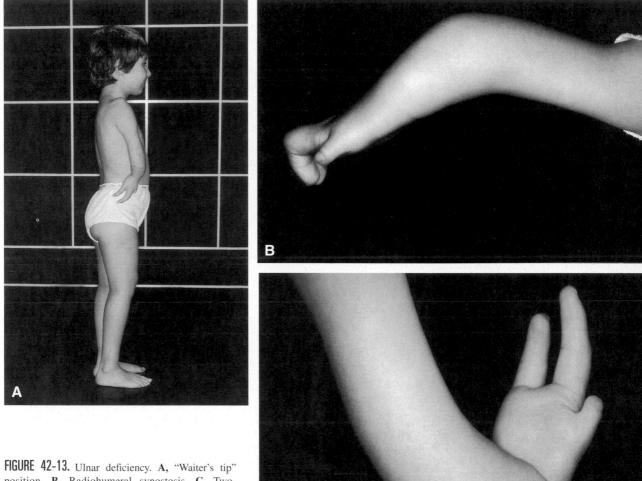

FIGURE 42-13. Ulnar deficiency. **A,** "Waiter's tip" position. **B,** Radiohumeral synostosis. **C,** Two-fingered hand, with hypoplastic thumb.

Children with unilateral ulnar deficiency usually function well.[1,7,19] They are adept at bimanual function but perform one-handed tasks much more slowly on the affected side. Children with radiohumeral synostosis and absent or stiff fingers are more impaired with regard to function.

RADIOGRAPHY

Radiographic imaging is required to determine the extent of deficiency. Radiographs should be taken of both upper extremities and the spine. Subtle anomalies of the spine are common and may be unrecognized on clinical examination.[8]

ASSOCIATED ANOMALIES AND/OR SYSTEMIC CONDITIONS

Ulnar deficiency is most commonly seen with other musculoskeletal anomalies, including proximal femoral focal deficiency, fibular deficiency, phocomelia, and scoliosis.[7,21,22] Ulnar deficiency is rarely associated with anomalies of other organ systems.[11,22]

CLASSIFICATION

Most classification systems are based on elbow and forearm anomalies (Table 42-3).[5,9,14,15,17,21] Ogino and Kato[16] have used hand anomalies as the basis for classification. Cole and Manske[4] have described a classification system based on thumb and first web anomalies and their related treatment (Table 42-4). This scheme can be combined with one of the elbow and forearm classifications.

SURGICAL MANAGEMENT

Indications

Surgical indications for many of the hand anomalies are well established. Hand function is improved by syndactyly

Table 42-3

CLASSIFICATIONS OF ULNAR DEFICIENCY BASED ON ELBOW AND FOREARM ANOMALIES

Characteristics	Kummel (1895)	Ogden, et al (1976)	Riordan (1986)	Bayne (Dobyns) 1993	Swanson, et al. (1984)	Miller, et al. (1986)
Elbow						
Normal/near-normal humeroradial joint	I					
Humeroradial synostosis	II		III	IV	III	D
Radial head dislocation	III					A,B*
Ulnar Length						
Normal-length ulna						
Ulnar hypoplasia		I		I	I	
Partial ulnar aplasia		II	II	II		
Complete ulnar aplasia		III	I	III	II	
Other upper extremity characteristics						
Congenital wrist amputation					IV	
Internal rotation deformity below the shoulder						C†

*B, Radial head dislocation with complete ulnar absence and cubital webbing.
†C, Humeroradial synostosis with variable absence of the ulna and associated internal rotation deformity.
Modified from Cole RJ, Manske PR: Classification of ulnar deficiency according to the thumb and first web. J Hand Surg [Am] 22:479-488, 1997.

Table 42-4

CLASSIFICATION OF ULNAR DEFICIENCY ACCORDING TO THE THUMB AND FIRST WEB

Type	Characteristics
A	Normal first web space and thumb
B	Mild first web and thumb deficiency
C	Moderate to severe first web and thumb deficiency; possible loss of opposition; malrotation of the thumb into the plane of the fingers; thumb/index finger syndactyly; absent extrinsic tendon function
D	Absent thumb

Modified from Cole RJ, Manske PR: Classification of ulnar deficiency according to the thumb and first web. J Hand Surg [Am] 22:479-488, 1997.

release and reconstruction of thumb and first web deficiencies. Procedures include first web space deepening, opponensplasty, thumb metacarpal rotational osteotomy, and pollicization.[2,4]

With marked internal rotation limb combined with radiohumeral synostosis, the child's hand rests on the buttock or flank. This position prohibits hand to mouth activity and placement of the hand on top of the head (see Fig. 42-13A). Over time, children may compensate for this position and obtain adequate function. In recalcitrant cases, external rotation osteotomy of the humerus improves the position of the hand and the overall function of the limb.[7,12,14] A concomitant closing wedge osteotomy has been recommended to place the elbow in flexion. However, children with radiohumeral synostosis have a short upper limb, and they can usually reach their mouth with rotational correction alone. Forearm rotational osteotomy is rarely necessary, even though the forearm is usually supinated.

The indications for surgical treatment of the ulnar deviation of the wrist and forearm instability are less certain. Several authors have reported that ulnar deviation at the wrist is due to tethering by the ulna anlage, a fibrocartilaginous structure occasionally found in the forearm of children with ulna deficiency (Fig. 42-14). The ulna anlage fails to grow with the radius and causes increasing ulnar deviation. Proponents of this theory[3,15] have advocated early excision of the ulna anlage to prevent progressive deformity. More recent reports, however, indicate that increasing ulnar deviation is uncommon and anlage resection should be reserved for documented progression.[7,13,14] The indications for surgical treatment of the forearm are even less defined. Some authors[3] advocate surgical construction of a one-bone forearm to enhance forearm stability. In contrast, others[7] believe that the loss of forearm rotation should not be sacrificed for forearm stability.

Techniques

1. Thumb reconstruction (first web deepening, opponensplasty, pollicization) (see Chapter 41, Deformities of the Thumb)
2. Syndactyly release (see Chapter 40, Deformities of the Hand and Fingers)
3. Excision of ulnar anlage (Fig. 42-15).[7] The ulnar remnant is approached via a longitudinal incision along the ulnar border of the forearm. The ulnar extrinsic flexor muscles are often absent. The anlage will be adjacent to the ulnar neurovascular bundle. The bundle must be protected as

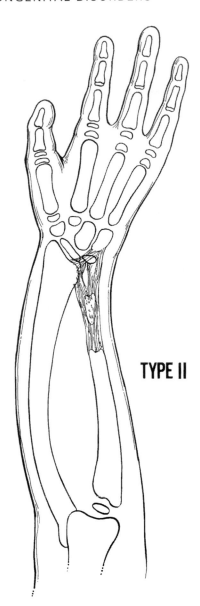

TYPE II

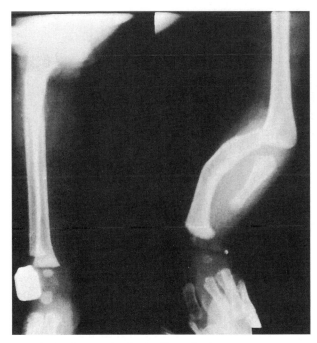

FIGURE 42-14. Ulnar anlage acts as a tethering force on the distal radius and wrist.

the anlage is dissected off its carpal attachment. The entire anlage need not be removed; removal of the distal one third is adequate. The subcutaneous tissue and skin are closed with absorbable sutures and a long-arm cast is applied. The wrist is positioned as close to neutral as possible. Casting is maintained for 6 weeks and is followed by a short-arm splint that is worn at night until skeletal maturity.

4. Rotational osteotomy of the humerus.[14] The distal humerus is approached via a lateral incision. Careful dissection is performed through the subcutaneous tissue. The alignment of the humerus is marked by electrocautery or by inserting parallel Kirschner wires above and below the planned osteotomy site. A transverse osteotomy is made, and the distal fragment is rotated until the hand can be placed in front of the trunk. Tight soft tissues may require bone shortening to prevent a traction injury to neurovascular structures. The osteotomy is fixed with crossed Kirschner wires or a small plate. The subcutaneous tissue and skin are closed with absorbable suture. A well-fitted long-arm cast is applied and attached to the body with a Velpeau-type dressing.

5. Creation of one-bone forearm. This operation is rarely indicated. See Lloyd-Roberts,[10] Spinner and colleagues,[20] or Smith and Greene[18] for details.

6. Forearm lengthening. This operation is also rarely indicated (Fig. 42-16).

Authors' Preferred Technique

Excision of the ulnar anlage is reserved for children with progressive ulnar deviation of the wrist. The anlage may be resected at the same time as hand reconstruction, usually at around 1 year of age. Humeral rotational osteotomy is reserved for children who are unable to obtain adequate function. Surgery is performed after the child is old enough

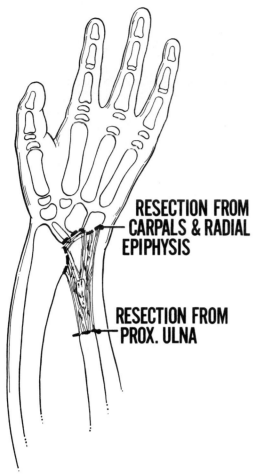

FIGURE 42-15. Excision of the ulnar anlage. This may prevent further ulnar deviation of the hand.

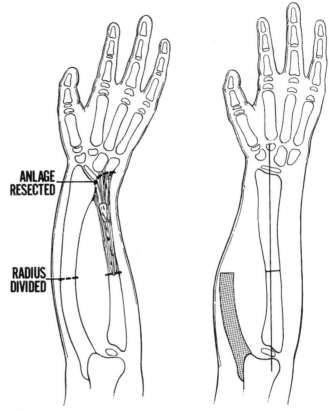

FIGURE 42-16. One-bone forearm technique. The distal ulnar anlage is resected, and the radius is divided as far proximally as possible. The distal radius is aligned with the proximal ulna, and an intramedullary Kirschner wire is used for fixation.

CRITICAL POINTS: ULNAR DEFICIENCY

- Ulnar deficiency is 4 to 10 times less common than radial deficiency and is not associated with systemic conditions as seen in children with radial deficiency.
- Ulnar deficiencies are associated with other musculoskeletal abnormalities that warrant careful physical examination supplemented by radiographs (e.g., congenital scoliosis).
- The forearm is difficult to manage, and treatment should be individualized. Treatment is dependent on forearm stability, available elbow motion, and function. Surgery to restore motion for synostosis across the elbow and/or forearm is unsuccessful.
- Ulnar deficiencies may have thumb anomalies, ranging from a narrow web space to absent thumb, that are a major predictor of function. The thumb deficiency limits prehensile activities and is treated according to similar principles for isolated thumb hypoplasia.

to evaluate his or her ability to perform activities of daily living. This age allows additional determination of the optimum limb position for function.

ANNOTATED REFERENCES

8. Kozin SH: Upper-extremity congenital anomalies. J Bone Joint Surg Am 85:1564-1576, 2003.

This update of congenital anomalies of the upper extremity provides a concise overview for the surgeon who encounters upper extremity congenital anomalies. Emphasis is on accurate diagnosis and thorough evaluation. Specific conditions are highlighted that occur with systemic associations and require extensive work-up versus those isolated anomalies that occur without malformation of other organ systems.

18. Smith AA, Greene TL: Preliminary soft tissue distraction in congenital forearm deficiency. J Hand Surg [Am] 20:420-424, 1995.

Four patients (five limbs) with radial or ulnar deficiency were treated with preliminary soft tissue distraction. Soft tissue distraction was continued in radial deficiency until the hand could be passively corrected, allowing centralization to be accomplished through a single mid-dorsal incision. In the ulnar deficiency, soft tissue distraction was carried out until the cut radius was distal to the partially absent ulna, allowing for the creation of a one-bone forearm. All radial deficiency limbs remained centralized at a mean follow-up period of w14 months.

Madelung's Deformity

EPIDEMIOLOGY

Madelung's deformity is excessive radial and palmar angulation of the distal radius caused by a growth disturbance of the palmar and ulnar portion of the distal radial physis.[11] This growth disturbance may be due to a combination of a bony lesion in the ulnar portion of the distal radius physis and an abnormal palmar ligament tethering the lunate to the radius proximal to the physis (Vickers' ligament).[22] Girls are affected more often than boys. The disorder is usually bilateral, presenting most commonly between the ages of 6 and 13 years.[2,4,6,17,20] The exact incidence of Madelung's deformity is unknown.

CLINICAL FEATURES

The distal ulna of the affected wrist is dorsally prominent, and the distal radius appears to have a dorsal concavity in the lateral view (Fig. 42-17). Ulnar deviation and extension may be decreased. The forearm is shorter than normal. Despite the clinical appearance, there is minimal functional impairment. In advanced cases, however, pain may limit function.

RADIOGRAPHY

Madelung's deformity is characterized by radial and palmar angulation of the distal radius (Fig. 42-18). The ulna is relatively long with a positive ulnar variance.

ASSOCIATED ANOMALIES AND/OR SYSTEMIC CONDITIONS

Leri-Weill dyschondrosteosis (LWD), which has a dominant inheritance pattern with 50% penetrance, is the most common dysplasia associated with Madelung's deformity.[12,19,22]

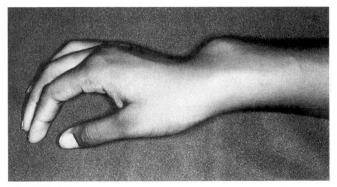

FIGURE 42-17. Clinical appearance of a patient with Madelung's deformity. The hand is palmar and pronated with respect to the long axis of the forearm. The distal ulna appears prominent dorsally.

Recent gene mapping studies have found that mutation of a gene termed the short stature homeobox-containing gene (*SHOX*) is associated with LWD.[7,8,16] The *SHOX* gene associated with LWD is located on the X or Y chromosome.[7,13,15] Histopathologic studies of the microanatomy of the physes and the palmar ligaments of patients with Madelung's deformity and *SHOX* mutations showed a disruption of normal physeal architecture.[13]

Madelung's deformity may also be associated with other syndromes, including nail-patella syndrome (onychoosteodysplasia).[10] Repetitive loading of the wrist in the growing child may cause a partial physeal arrest. The resultant appearance is similar to Madelung's deformity.[3,4]

CLASSIFICATION

There is currently no classification system to describe the severity of Madelung's deformity. Rarely, growth may be disturbed on the dorsal and ulnar physis, causing a reverse Madelung's deformity in which the distal radius is angulated dorsally and radially.[4,22] This type of Madelung's deformity has similar underlying causes.[7]

SURGICAL MANAGEMENT

Indications

No treatment is necessary for the painless deformity. However, physiolysis combined with the release of the abnormal ligament should be considered for asymptomatic, skeletally immature patients. The most common motivation for surgery is appearance. Many patients dislike the distal forearm concavity and dorsal prominence of the distal ulna and request surgical correction.

The recalcitrant, painful deformity is an obvious indication for treatment. Physiolysis combined with the release of the Vickers ligament[1] may reduce pain and gradually improve the deformity during growth.[22] However, most patients do not complain of pain until adolescence, when there is insufficient growth remaining for physiolysis to correct the deformity. In these instances, physiolysis and ligament resection may be combined with a dome osteotomy.[1,9] In the skeletally mature patient with wrist pain, there are multiple options for deformity correction and pain relief, including (1) ligament resection and dome osteotomy[1,9]; (2) radial closing wedge osteotomy and ulnar shortening[6]; (3) radial opening wedge osteotomy[14]; (4) radial osteotomy and distal ulna resection[21,23]; or (5) radial osteotomy and Sauvé-Kapandji procedure.[18]

Techniques

1. Physiolysis (Fig. 42-19).[22] The radius is approached through a longitudinal palmar incision. Exposure pro-

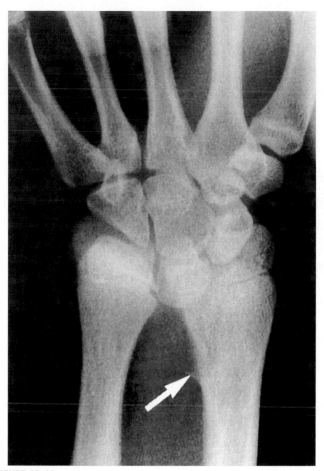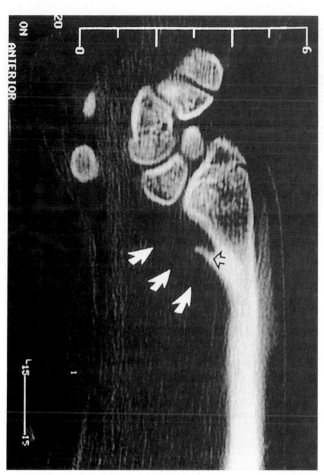

FIGURE 42-18. Radiograph and computed tomographic scan show radial and palmar angulation of the distal radius with a positive ulnar variance. (From Ezaki M: Congenital muscular deformation. In Fleckenstein JL [ed]: Muscle Imaging in Health and Disease. New York, Springer-Verlag, 1996, with permission.)

ceeds ulnar to the palmaris longus and flexor carpi radialis tendons, protecting the radial artery and median nerve. The distal edge of the pronator quadratus muscle is located. A flap of distal radius periosteum that includes Vickers' ligament is raised in a proximal to distal direction. The flap is elevated until the physis is identified, which appears narrow and wavy. The lunate is carefully protected. Any tethering fibrous tissue and bone are removed about the physis. A fat graft may be applied into any physeal defect to inhibit bone formation. The fat graft is held in place by the surrounding soft tissue. The skin is closed with a running absorbable suture. The forearm is immobilized in a bulky compressive dressing with a removable wrist splint. A similar procedure can be done dorsally for reverse Madelung's deformity.

2. Physiolysis and dome osteotomy (Fig. 42-20).[1,9] A longitudinal palmar incision is made starting just proximal to the wrist crease and extending 8 to 10 cm along the radial border of the flexor carpi radialis tendon. The radial artery is protected, and the pronator quadratus is incised near its radial border, leaving a cuff of tissue for later repair. Ulnar reflection of the pronator quadratus reveals Vickers' ligament, which is released from the radial metaphysis and reflected distally. The metaphysis of the

distal radius is exposed. A biplanar dome osteotomy is performed with curved osteotomes. The distal radius fragment is manipulated from an anterior ulnar position to a dorsal ulnar position. The dome shape of the osteotomy makes this complex three-dimensional deformity easier to correct than a simple wedge osteotomy. A Steinmann pin may be used as a joystick to position the distal fragment. The distal fragment is pinned to the proximal fragment after lunate coverage has been achieved. Two parallel pins are inserted from the radial styloid across the osteotomy site. The palmar step-off of the proximal fragment is removed with a rongeur. The dorsal step-off will remodel after the osteotomy heals. The pronator is repaired and the subcutaneous tissue and skin closed with absorbable suture. A long-arm splint or cast is applied. Pins are removed after 6 weeks, and the osteotomy is protected for an additional 4 to 6 weeks in a short-arm cast.

3. Dorsal closing wedge osteotomy of the distal radius and ulnar shortening.[5] The size and shape of the radial wedge osteotomy is planned according to the preoperative radiographs and amount of deformity. The goal is to restore palmar and radial tilt. The osteotomy is performed at the point of maximum angulation. A dorsal or volar approach

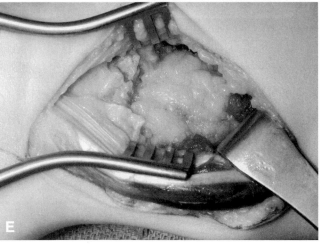

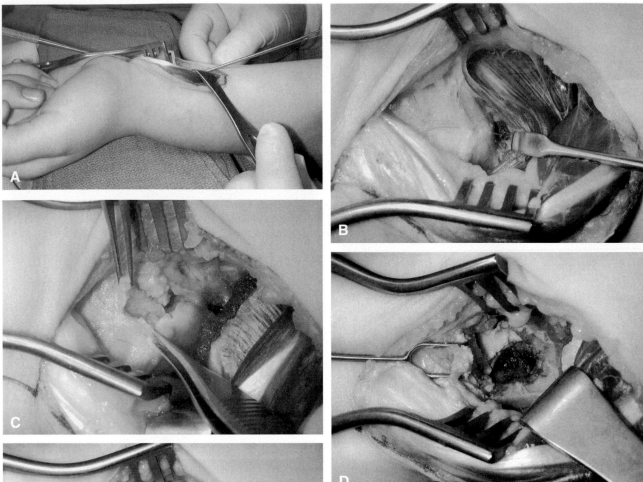

FIGURE 42-19. Eight-year-old with early Madelung's deformity treated with physiolysis and fat grafting. **A,** Palmar approach. **B,** Pronator quadratus retracted. **C,** Vicker's ligament identified (in forceps). **D,** Cavity after resection of bar. **E,** Cavity filled with fat graft harvested from forearm.

may be used. Plate fixation is preferred. The ulna is shortened using standard techniques. The goal is to obtain a neutral or slight minus ulnar variance. Dynamic compression plate fixation is preferred.

4. Radial opening wedge osteotomy. See the work of Murphy and colleagues.[14]

5. Distal radius osteotomy and distal ulnar resection. See earlier for distal radius osteotomy; and see Van Demark and Van Demark[21] or Watson[23] for details of distal ulnar resection.

6. Distal radius osteotomy and Sauvé-Kapandji procedure. See earlier for distal radius osteotomy and Shroven and colleagues[18] for details of the Sauvé-Kapandji procedure.

Author's Preferred Technique

Physiolysis alone may provide satisfactory correction in the young patient with early Madelung's deformity (Fig. 42-21). However, most patients present with considerable deformity and limited growth potential. Physiolysis combined with dome osteotomy is the most common procedure for mild to moderate deformity without distal radioulnar joint (DRUJ) degeneration. Dorsal closing wedge osteotomy of the distal radius and ulnar shortening is an alternative option. Osteotomy of the radius combined with some form of ulnar resection is warranted in the patient with DRUJ arthritis.

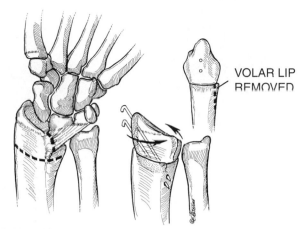

FIGURE 42-20. Technique of ligament release and dome osteotomy. (From Harley BJ, Carter P, et al: Volar surgical correction of Madelung's deformity. Techniques Hand Upper Extremity Surg 6:30-35, 2002.)

OUTCOMES

In most cases, dorsal wrist pain is relieved by distal radius osteotomy and DRUJ pain by ulnar shortening. Both dome and closing wedge radius osteotomies improve appearance by reducing the dorsal concavity associated with Madelung's deformity (Fig. 42-22). Ulnar shortening reduces the dorsal distal ulnar prominence.

CRITICAL POINTS: MADELUNG'S DEFORMITY

- Madelung's deformity is characterized by radial and palmar angulation of the distal radius caused by a growth disturbance of the palmar and ulnar portion of the distal radial physis.
- The growth disturbance may be due to a combination of a bony lesion in the ulnar portion of the distal radial physis and an abnormal palmar ligament tethering the lunate to the radius proximal to the physis (Vickers' ligament).
- No treatment is necessary for the painless deformity. However, asymptomatic skeletally immature patients with progressive deformity should be considered for a physiolysis combined with the release of the abnormal ligament.
- Most patients present in adolescence with limited growth potential and considerable deformity. In these cases, physiolysis and ligament resection are combined with osteotomy to realign the radius.

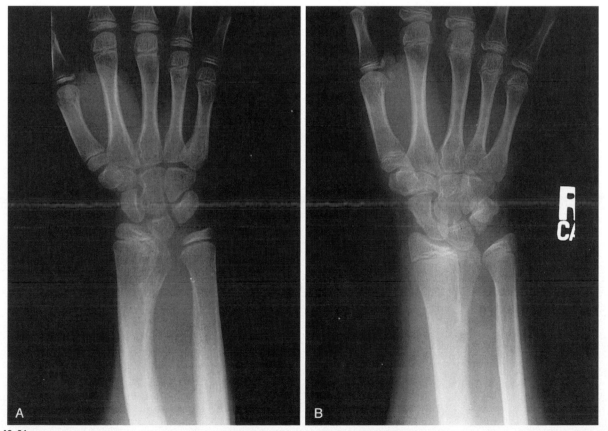

FIGURE 42-21. **A,** Preoperative radiograph showing Madelung's deformity of the right wrist of a skeletally immature girl. **B,** Postoperative films of the same wrist 28 months after physiolysis. Longitudinal growth has been restored, and there has been no increase in deformity.

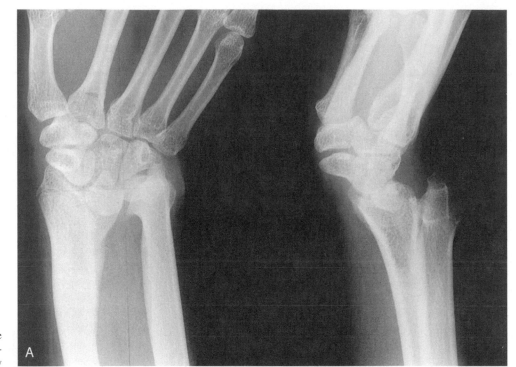

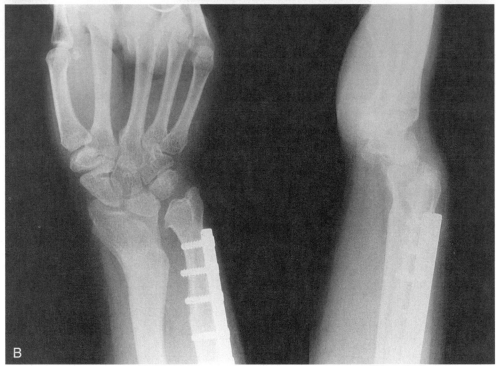

FIGURE 42-22. A, Preoperative Madelung's deformity. **B,** Postoperative correction with a dome osteotomy through the distal radial metaphysis. Additional ulnar shortening was required.

ANNOTATED REFERENCES

1. Carter PR, Ezaki M: Madelung's deformity: Surgical correction through the anterior approach. Hand Clin 16:713-721, 2000.

Review of Madelung's deformity with update on current knowledge and treatment recommendations. Preferred surgical approach consisting of release of Vickers' ligament and/or dome osteotomy is highlighted. Outcome on 23 wrists in 18 patients is reported. Vickers' ligament was found in 21 wrists. Dome osteotomy was performed in 16 of the 23 wrists, and all had relief from pain.

5. dos Reis FB, Katchburian MV, Faloppa F, et al: Osteotomy of the radius and ulna for the Madelung deformity. J Bone Joint Surg Br 80:817-824, 1998.

Prospective study of 18 patients with Madelung's deformity (25 wrists). All were treated by wedge subtraction osteotomy of the radius and shortening of the ulna. Results demonstrate significant improvement in grip strength and range of movement of the wrist and forearm. Pain improved in 80% of the patients, and 88% were satisfied with the appearance. Two had some recurrence due to continued growth of the ulna. The authors recommend that this procedure be delayed until skeletal maturity or combined with epiphysiodesis of the ulna.

13. Munns CF, Glass IA, LaBrom R, et al: Histopathological analysis of Leri-Weill dyschondrosteosis: Disordered growth plate. Hand Surg 6:13-23, 2001.

   Leri-Weill syndrome (LWS) is a dominant skeletal dysplasia with mesomelic short stature and bilateral Madelung's deformity, owing to dyschondrosteosis of the distal radius. LWS results from the loss of one copy of the short stature homeobox genes *(SHOX)* from the tip of the short arm of the X or Y chromosome. *SHOX* molecular testing allowed evaluation of the histopathology of the radial physis in LWS patients with a documented *SHOX* abnormality. A widespread disorganization of physeal anatomy was revealed with disruption of the normal parallel columnar arrangement of chondrocytes. Vickers' ligament was confirmed to blend with the triangular fibrocartilage complex. This histopathologic study demonstrates that the zone of dyschondrosteosis in LWS is characterized by marked disruption of normal physeal chondrocyte processes and that a generalized physeal abnormality is present.

Transverse Failure of Formation

Transverse failure of formation, often inaccurately termed *congenital amputation,* occurs when the upper limb fails to form below a certain level. The most common level of failure of formation is at the proximal forearm or below elbow (Fig. 42-23), followed by transcarpal, distal forearm, and through humerus (above elbow).[29] This condition is almost always unilateral.[18,23]

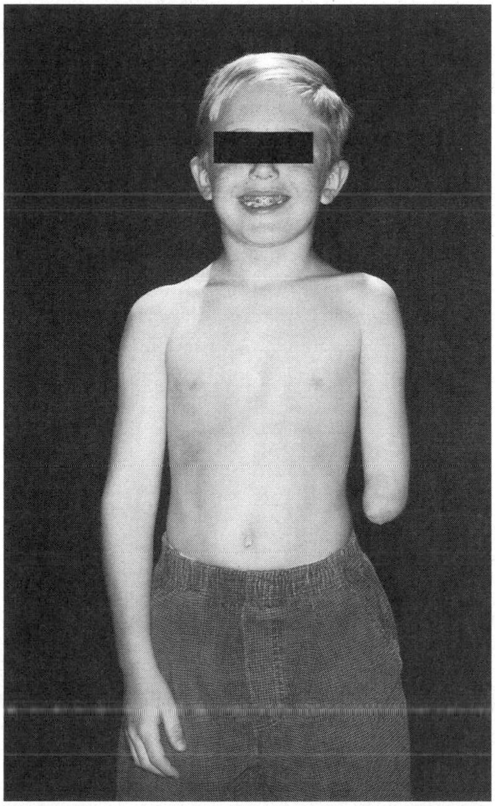

EPIDEMIOLOGY

Transverse failure of formation is sporadic. The most prevalent theory is vascular compromise to the developing limb bud or apical ectodermal ridge (see Chapter 39, Embryology)[3,5,11,15,17,22,28] Risk factors include maternal use of misoprostol (Cytotec), alcohol, tobacco, or cocaine.*

CLINICAL FEATURES

The diagnosis is readily apparent, although there is variability in the length of the below-the-elbow residual limb. The elbow usually has full flexion and extension. Forearm rotation is frequently restricted by proximal radioulnar abnormalities. Finger nubbins are usually present at the distal end of the limb.

   Cognition and developmental milestones are usually normal, except that the child with a very short arm may not crawl. Children with this level of amputation have remarkably few functional deficits.[4] Prostheses are commonly prescribed for unilateral transverse below-elbow deficiency but have not been shown to improve function. A prosthesis is usually prescribed for the child around age 6 months of age or when the child sits independently. A passive hand or mitt is the initial type of prosthesis.[18] Children who wear a prosthesis before the age of 2 years are more likely to continue to use the prosthesis throughout childhood.[23] Between

FIGURE 42-23. A left short, below-the-elbow transverse failure of formation.

the ages of 2 and 3, the child is evaluated for readiness for an active terminal device. A child is probably ready to learn to use an active terminal device when he or she readily bears weight on the passive prosthesis during crawling and uses it for pulling up, balance, and two-handed activities. Active terminal devices may be body powered (cable operated) or powered by electrical signals from proximal forearm muscle contractions (myoelectric) (Fig. 42-24). Each of these prostheses has advantages and disadvantages. The terminal

---

*See references 8, 10, 12, 13, 16, 19, 21, 25, 27, and 30.

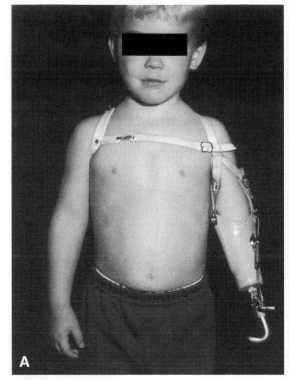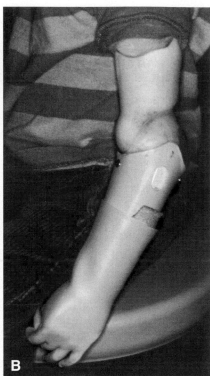

FIGURE 42-24. Terminal devices may vary in design and usage. **A,** Body-powered terminal device to enhance function. **B,** Myoelectric prosthesis.

device may look like a hook or a hand. Most studies comparing performance of body powered and myoelectric prostheses use a hand terminal device, which has some increased resistance to opening. This resistance is easily overcome by the myoelectric motor but may be more difficult with a body-powered prosthesis. In spite of this obstacle, studies have revealed that children perform most tasks faster with the body-powered prosthesis.[9] Furthermore, consistent users of a body-powered prosthesis are more likely to be pleased with prosthetic function.[20] However, parents are often influenced by the "high tech" image of the myoelectric prosthesis. Interestingly, children and adolescents allowed to try different types of prostheses usually choose a passive prosthesis rather than an active one.[7] Appearance may be a stronger motivating factor than function in this population. A prosthesis may enhance unilateral prehension but blocks sensory feedback, which most users find detrimental.[2]

RADIOGRAPHY

Elbow and forearm radiographs should be obtained. Proximal radioulnar joint abnormalities are common, such as synostosis.

SURGICAL MANAGEMENT

Indications

Removal of finger nubbins from the distal end of the amputation stump is controversial. Some parents want their

infant's nubbins removed, but older children with nubbins rarely request this procedure. Children with nubbins use them for sensory feedback and manipulation of small, light objects, so removal is probably not indicated. Nubbins should be removed when they frequently become infected or interfere with prosthetic use.

There have been isolated reports of forearm lengthening for transverse below-elbow deficiency. This procedure has a high complication rate, although the added length may assist with prosthetic fitting for the very short below-elbow deficiency.[1,24]

The Krukenberg procedure is rarely indicated. The radius and ulna are separated and the muscles reattached such that the radius pinches against the ulna. This procedure is most useful for blind bilateral distal forearm amputees, because it provides unilateral prehension with sensory feedback. This operation may occasionally be indicated for a sighted child with below-elbow deficiency and a long forearm who does not have access to prosthetic facilities.[6,14,26] However, the appearance of the Krukenberg forearm is strikingly abnormal and must be discussed with the patient and family.

 Authors' Preferred Technique

The greatest challenge in the treatment of children with transverse failure of formation is helping parents adjust their often unrealistically high expectations of prosthetic technology. Good communication is important, focusing on numerous areas, including the remarkable abilities of the child with or without the prosthesis, the opportunity to try

CRITICAL POINTS: TRANSVERSE FAILURE OF FORMATION

- Congenital transverse deficiency is classified according to the last remaining bone segment. A short below-elbow type failure of formation is the most common transverse deficiency of the upper extremity.

- The residual limb is usually well cushioned with rudimentary nubbins or dimpling often found on the end.

- These anomalies are usually unilateral, sporadic, and rarely associated with other anomalies.

- Prostheses are commonly prescribed for unilateral transverse below-elbow deficiency but have not been shown to improve function.

- A prosthesis is usually prescribed for the child around age 6 months of age or when the child sits independently.

- Children who wear a prosthesis before the age of 2 years are more likely to continue to use the prosthesis throughout childhood.

- Between the ages of 2 and 3 the child is evaluated for use of an active terminal device, which may be body powered or myoelectric.

different prostheses as the child grows, and the need for improved prosthetic technology.[2] In general, children are fitted at 6 months with a passive prosthesis and progress to an active terminal device. Surgery is rarely required.

ANNOTATED REFERENCES

1. Alekberov C, Karatosun V, Baran O, Gunal I: Lengthening of congenital below-elbow amputation stumps by the Ilizarov technique. J Bone Joint Surg Br 82:239-241, 2000.

   Patients with short congenital amputations below the elbow often function as if they have had a disarticulation of the elbow. Six patients underwent lengthening of residual limbs by the Ilizarov technique to improve the fitting of prostheses. The mean lengthening was 5.6 cm (3.4 to 8.4), and in two patients flexion contractures of the elbows were corrected simulta-neously. Additional lateral distraction was used in one patient to provide a better surface on the stump. There were no major complications. All six patients were able to use their prosthesis at the latest follow-up after 39 to 78 months.

5. Burton BK, Schulz CJ, Burd LI: Spectrum of limb disruption defects associated with chorionic villus sampling. Pediatrics 91:989-993, 1993.

   Three hundred ninety-four fetuses and infants were evaluated after undergoing chorionic villus sampling. A total of 13 (3.3%) had major congenital anomalies, including 4 with transverse limb reduction deformities, 3 with cleft lip with or without cleft palate, and 1 each with a nasal encephalocele, large port-wine stain, craniosynostosis, omphalocele with associated defects, ambiguous genitalia, and undescended testes. The limb malformations in the 4 affected infants were all very similar and were comparable to those described by others in association with chorionic villus sampling.

7. Crandall RC, Tomhave W: Pediatric unilateral below-elbow amputees: Retrospective analysis of 34 patients given multiple prosthetic options. J Pediatr Orthop 22:380-383, 2002.

   Thirty-four unilateral below-elbow amputees were retrospectively analyzed in long-term follow-up. All were provided with a variety of prosthetic options, including a "passive" cosmetic upper extremity device. Most of the patients were also fitted with conventional prostheses using a body-powered voluntary closing terminal device (97%) as well as myoelectric prostheses (82%). Patients were considered consistent prosthetic users. Average follow-up was 14 years. Analysis indicated that 15 patients (44%) selected a simple cosmetic "passive hand" as their prosthesis of choice. Fourteen patients (41%) continued as multiple users. Fourteen patients (41%) selected the conventional prosthesis using a voluntary closing terminal device as the prosthesis of choice. Only 5 patients (15%) selected the myoelectric device as their primary prosthesis. The authors conclude that successful unilateral pediatric amputees may choose multiple prostheses on the basis of function and that frequently the most functional prosthesis selected is the simplest in design.

13. Gonzalez CH, Marques-Dias MJ, Kim CA, et al: Congenital abnormalities in Brazilian children associated with misoprostol misuse in first trimester of pregnancy. Lancet 351:1624-1627, 1998.

   Misoprostol is commonly used to induce abortion in Brazil, although it is not very effective. Exposure to the drug in utero can cause abnormalities in the fetus. Forty-two infants exposed to misoprostol during the first 3 months of gestation were born with congenital abnormalities. Seventeen infants had equinovarus with cranial nerve defects. Ten children had equinovarus as part of more extensive arthrogryposis. The most distinctive phenotypes were arthrogryposis confined to the legs (five cases) and terminal transverse-limb defects (nine cases) with or without Mobius sequence.

Congenital Dislocation of the Radial Head

EPIDEMIOLOGY

Congenital dislocation of the radial head (CDRH) is the most common congenital anomaly of the elbow and is usually bilateral.[1,2,8,10,12] CDRH may be sporadic or familial. The etiology of CDRH is unknown. The radial head may be dislocated in an anterior, posterior, or lateral direction (Fig. 42-25). Almquist and coworkers[2] reported that 47% of dislocations are anterior, 43% are posterior, and 10% are lateral.

CLINICAL FEATURES

A delay in presentation is common with CDRH. The lack of forearm rotation is unrecognized until the complexities of daily activities amplify, such as catching a ball or eating soup.[9] CDRH often presents after a perceived elbow injury and may be erroneously attributed to that injury. When unilateral, CDRH may be difficult to distinguish from chronic traumatic dislocation (Table 42-5).[4] The presenting complaint usually involves prominence, restricted elbow extension, and forearm rotation. Elbow "popping" or pain with activity is uncommon before adolescence.[1]

The anterior dislocated radial head is palpable just distal to the cubital fossa. The posterior dislocated radial head is palpable and visible lateral to the capitellum. Posterior CDRH usually impedes terminal extension (≤30 degrees), and anterior CDRH may limit full flexion. Diminished forearm rotation is more prominent with CDRH in both pronation and supination. Slight limitation of wrist motion may be present.[1,2,8,10]

The limitation of elbow and forearm motion rarely causes considerable functional impairment. Certain activities that require the extremes of motion may be limited, such as accepting change and performing push-ups. Older children may develop erosions between the radial head and capitellum, which cause pain and additional motion loss.

RADIOGRAPHY

The diagnosis is usually confirmed by radiography (Fig. 42-26). The radial head fails to align with the capitellum.

Table 42-5
CONGENITAL VS. TRAUMATIC RADIAL HEAD DISLOCATION

Feature	Congenital	Traumatic
Trauma	Sometimes	Always
Radial head	Dome shaped, no central concavity (anterior dislocation) Elongated and narrow (posterior dislocation)	Normal shape with concavity
Bilateral	Common	Rare
Other anomalies	Common	Rare
Ulna	Shortened; possible palmar bow (anterior dislocation) or dorsal bow (posterior dislocation)	Normal
Capitellum	Hypoplastic or absent	Normal

Data from Mardam-Bey T, Ger E: Congenital radial head dislocation. J Hand Surg [Am] 4:316-320, 1979; and Kelly DW: Congenital dislocation of the radial head: Spectrum and natural history. J Pediatr Orthop 1:295-298, 1981.

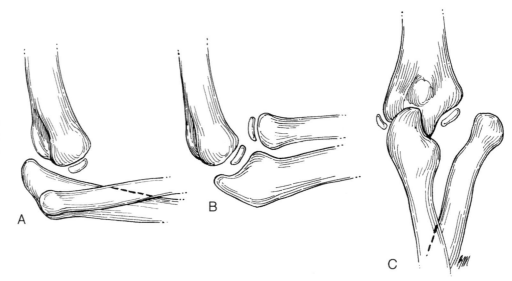

FIGURE 42-25. Congenital dislocation of the radial head. **A,** Posterior dislocation. **B,** Anterior dislocation. **C,** Lateral dislocation.

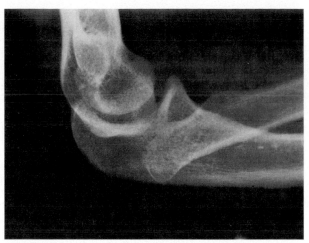

FIGURE 42-26. Radiograph of a congenital posterior dislocation of the radial head.

Additional radiographic findings include dysplasia of the capitellum, abnormal shape of the radial head, and ulnar positive variance.[7,8,10] In the infant, the unossified dislocated radial head may be visualized with diagnostic ultrasound.[3]

ASSOCIATED ANOMALIES AND/OR SYSTEMIC CONDITIONS

CDRH is associated with congenital radioulnar synostosis[11] and numerous syndromes including Klinefelter's, Cornelia de Lange, Ehlers-Danlos, and nail-patella.[1,2,5,8,10,12,13,15]

CLASSIFICATION

CDRH is classified by the direction of the dislocation. Anterior and posterior dislocations are the most common.

SURGICAL MANAGEMENT

Indications

Surgical intervention is seldom necessary in childhood. Most children are asymptomatic and have minimal functional limitations.[5,12] Open reduction of the radial head with reconstruction of the annular ligament has not been consistently successful.[2,11,12,14] In adolescence or adulthood, a dislocated radial head may become painful due to degenerative changes at the contact point between the radial head and the distal humerus. Radial head excision reliably relieves pain, improves appearance, and may improve range of motion.[4,8]

Contraindications

The timing of radial head resection deserves mention. Early head excision before skeletal maturity has been postulated to lead to postoperative elbow deformity with growth. Radial head resection before skeletal maturity, however, has been performed with successful results.[4]

Technique: Resection of the Radial Head (Posterior or Lateral Dislocation)

A longitudinal incision is made over the dislocated radial head. The location of muscle splitting depends on the location of the radial head. A posterior CDRH is approached through the interval between the extensor carpi ulnaris and the anconeus (Kocher approach). In contrast, an anterior CDRH requires a more anterior approach. The capsule is incised with the forearm in maximum pronation. The capsular incision is not extended distal to the radial neck to avoid injuring the posterior interosseous nerve.

Reverse retractors are placed around the radial neck. The radial head is excised with a saw perpendicular to the radial neck. The elbow is moved through a full range of motion to make sure that the proximal radius does not contact the distal humerus. Additional impingement requires further resection. The capsule is closed with nonabsorbable suture. The subcutaneous tissue and skin are closed. The arm is placed in a long-arm splint with the elbow at 90 degrees and the forearm in neutral rotation for 7 to 10 days.

OUTCOME AND COMPLICATIONS

Radial head excision in CDRH reliably results in decreased pain and improved rotation.[4] Complications include regrowth of the proximal radius, postoperative radioulnar synostosis,[4] and cubitus valgus deformity.[7] In one study,[6] however, radial head resection for a variety of indications

---

CRITICAL POINTS: DISLOCATION OF THE RADIAL HEAD

- Dislocation of the radial head is usually bilateral. The radial head most commonly dislocates in an anterior or posterior direction. Lateral dislocation is less common.
- A delay in presentation until 2 to 3 years of age is common, because the lack of forearm rotation is unrecognized until the complexities of daily activities amplify, such as catching a ball or eating soup.
- The diagnosis is usually confirmed by radiography as the radial head fails to align with the capitellum.
- Surgery is seldom necessary in childhood. The limitation of elbow and forearm motion rarely causes considerable functional impairment.
- Open reduction of the radial head with reconstruction of the annular ligament has not been consistently successful.
- In adolescence or adulthood, a dislocated radial head may become painful because of degenerative changes between the radial head and the distal humerus. Radial head excision reliably relieves pain, improves appearance, and may improve range of motion.

(including CDRH) did not cause cubitus valgus in 25 children with an average age of 14 years (range, 5 to 18 years). Other potential complications include posterior interosseous nerve injury, proximal migration of the radius (Essex-Lopresti lesion), and wrist pain.[2,4,8,10]

ANNOTATED REFERENCES

4. Campbell CC, Waters PM, Emans JB: Excision of the radial head for congenital dislocation. J Bone Joint Surg Am 74:726-733, 1992.

    Eight elbows in six patients underwent excision of the radial head for congenital dislocation. Evaluation was performed at an average of 7 years after surgery. The average age of the patients at the time of the excision was 13 years (range, 10 to 15.5 years). The dislocation was posterior in five elbows and posterolateral in three. A small increase of the flexion-extension arc (11 degrees) was noted. The overall increase in the arc of rotation was significant at 53 degrees. Pain in the elbow had decreased, but all patients had minor pain in the wrist. Contrary to previously published data, excision of the radial head for congenital dislocation resulted in an increased range of motion and a decrease in elbow pain.

6. Hresko MT, Rosenberg BN, Pappas AM: Excision of the radial head in patients younger than 18 years. J Pediatr Orthop 19:106-113, 1999.

    The results of excision of the radial head in 25 patients (27 elbows) were evaluated. The patients were younger than 18 years with stiff and painful radiocapitellar joints. The mean age was 14.2 years (range, 4.6 to 17.8 years). Average follow-up was 7.8 years. Results with a postoperative elbow score revealed excellent or good results in 19 of the 27 elbows. Skeletal maturity of the patient did not alter the results. Revision surgery to remove appositional bone growth was required in 6 of the 12 post-traumatic cases and 1 of 15 developmental elbows. Cubitus valgus, wrist pain, and ulnar neuropathy were not clinical problems at follow-up examination.

Proximal Radioulnar Synostosis

EPIDEMIOLOGY

Congenital proximal radioulnar synostosis (PRUS) is an uncommon anomaly caused by failure of prenatal separation of the radius and ulna, which normally occurs late in the first trimester.[20] The incidence of the PRUS is unknown. PRUS may be sporadic or inherited as an autosomal dominant trait, which is more common in some European populations.[5,10,19]

CLINICAL FEATURES

Forearm rotation is absent and the forearm is usually fixed in pronation.[10,26] Forearm rotation must be assessed at the radial styloid and ulnar head to avoid measuring wrist instead of forearm movement. Children with PRUS usually present between 2 and 6 years of age with painless absence of forearm rotation and a slight elbow flexion contracture.[5,21] On occasion, PRUS is not recognized until adolescence.[7] The delay in diagnosis is attributed to lack of forearm rotation requirement in the infant and the use of compensatory shoulder and wrist motion.[5,6,13,18] CDRH often presents after an unrelated trivial trauma, which alerts the parents to the absent forearm rotation. Bilateral involvement is seen in approximately 60% of children, and the forearm is fixed in greater than 60 degrees of pronation in approximately 40% of patients.[18,21]

Initially, a parent or teacher notices that the child has difficulty positioning the hand to catch a ball, drink from a cup, or accept small objects in an open palm. The child tends to hold objects in a backhanded or hyperpronated position. The child may also have trouble with sports that require supination, such as catching a ball, and with midline activities requiring the use of both hands. Children with bilateral involvement and forearms fixed in marked pronation have more functional limitations.

RADIOGRAPHY

PRUS is usually visualized on radiographs (Fig. 42-27). The synostosis is nearly always proximal.[1,20,21] The connection is initially cartilaginous but eventually ossifies and forms a bony connection. The length of the synostosis varies, and a concomitant radial head dislocation may be present.

ASSOCIATED ANOMALIES AND/OR SYSTEMIC CONDITIONS

PRUS is usually an isolated anomaly, although it is associated with other conditions in up to one third of affected children.[21] Other anomalies include thumb hypoplasia, carpal coalition, symphalangism, and clubfoot.[15] Associated syndromes include Apert's syndrome, arthrogryposis, fetal alcohol syndrome, and Klinefelter's syndrome.[12,22-24]

CLASSIFICATION

PRUS is part of a spectrum of anomalies ranging from radial head abnormalities to complete synostosis and culminating in radial head absence.[15,21] The spectrum of variations has not been formally divided into types.

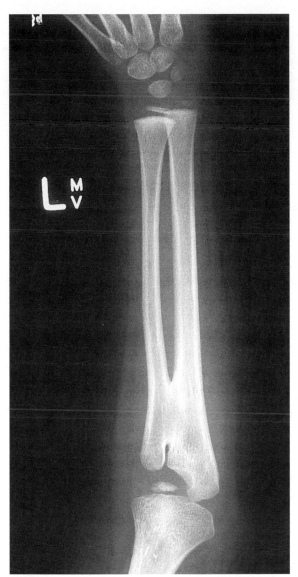

FIGURE 42-27. Congenital proximal radioulnar synostosis with an intact radial head.

SURGICAL MANAGEMENT

Unilateral PRUS usually does not cause considerable functional impairment or require treatment.[1,5] Surgery is not indicated for appearance alone, because the risks outweigh the benefits. Extreme pronation or supination that interferes with function is an indication for surgery. A forearm fixed in greater that 60 degrees of pronation usually warrants correction.[17,21]

Surgery to restore forearm rotation has been uniformly unsuccessful.[16] Recent reports of a free vascularized fascial flap interposed between the separated forearm bones state that it may prevent recurrence, although additional work is required.[8,9] Currently, the accepted surgical treatment is derotation osteotomy through the fusion mass. The osteotomy may be fixed with small Steinmann pins or a plate with screws.[6,16,18,21] Other options include gradual correction using the Ilizarov method for severe deformity, a two-stage osteoclasis without internal fixation, and osteotomy distal to the synostosis.[2,14,17]

The child's preoperative rotational position should be carefully measured and recorded. The optimal rotational position of the forearm is controversial, because the best position varies with the task. Preoperative evaluation by an occupational therapist helps determine the individual child's functional deficits and optimal forearm position. Bilateral recommendations are to place the dominant forearm in 10 to 20 degrees of pronation and the nondominant forearm in neutral rotation. For unilateral PRUS, the forearm is usually placed in 0 to 15 degrees of pronation.[21] A study[4] of the optimal rotational position for a one-bone forearm indicated that 30 degrees of pronation provides the best function for writing and working with small objects using the dominant arm.

The timing of surgery is also controversial. Recommendations vary from prior to school age to waiting for the child to choose his or her intended occupation.[5,21]

Technique: Rotational Osteotomy

A dorsal longitudinal incision is made along the subcutaneous border of the ulna at the level of the synostosis (Fig. 42-28). The fusion mass is identified between the extensor

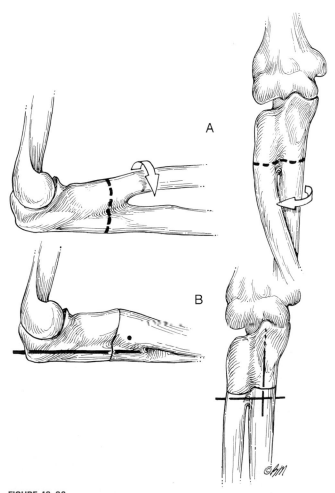

FIGURE 42-28. Rotational osteotomy for PRUS as described by Green and Mital (1979). **A,** The desired position of rotation is attained by the osteotomy through the synostosis mass. **B,** The new position is maintained by one longitudinal Kirschner wire and one transverse Kirschner wire that is incorporated into a cast. This allows the surgeon to control the degree of rotation postoperatively.

and flexor carpi ulnaris muscles. Subperiosteal dissection is performed around the synostosis. A smooth Steinmann pin is placed from a percutaneous position through the olecranon apophysis and into the intramedullary canal of the ulna under fluoroscopic guidance. The pin is positioned just proximal to the planned osteotomy site. A longitudinal mark is made across the osteotomy site to determine rotation. The osteotomy is performed through the fusion mass with an oscillating saw distal to the coronoid process. The forearm is then rotated to the desired position. The osteotomy is transfixed with the longitudinal wire and an additional oblique Kirschner wire. After closing the wound, the arm is placed in a splint or long-arm cast with the elbow flexed to 90 degrees. The patient is admitted to the hospital overnight for strict elevation and neurovascular monitoring. The cast and pins are removed after bony union.

A substantial change in forearm rotation may result in traction injury to the posterior interosseous nerve or compartment syndrome. Methods to diminish neurovascular problems have been proposed, including resection of 5 mm of bone from the osteotomy site and prophylactic forearm fasciotomy.[3,18] Gradual sequential correction of severe forearm malposition may be a better alternative using a two-stage osteoclasis technique.[14,21]

Alternate techniques have been described. Green and Mital[6] use a technique similar to that described above, but the second Kirschner wire is placed distal to the osteotomy in a transverse direction and anchored in the cast. Murase and coworkers[17] have recommended making the osteotomy distal to the synostosis and fixing both bones with longitudinal Kirschner wires.

OUTCOME

Rotational osteotomy for PRUS is a reliable procedure to realign the forearm (Fig. 42-29). Most children and parents note improvement in hand positioning for activities of daily living and midline activities. Rotational malalignment does not recur.[3] Wrist and elbow pain has been reported in adoles-

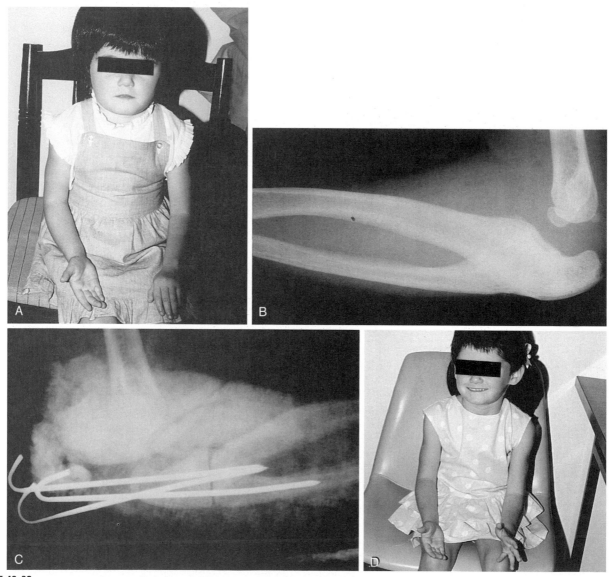

FIGURE 42-29. Rotational osteotomy. **A,** Pronation deformity of the left forearm. The synostosis seen radiographically before (**B**) and early after (**C**) the operation. **D,** Postoperative positions of the forearm in neutral position.

cents after surgical treatment, but there are few reports of long-term follow-up.[11]

COMPLICATIONS

Complications may occur during or after rotational osteotomy.[6,25] The most serious complications are vascular compromise and compartment syndrome, which occur more frequently with rotational position change of greater than 85 degrees. Immediate intervention is required to lessen the correction and to release the forearm fascia.[21] If excessive correction is needed, a two-stage operation is safer. Other complications include posterior interosseous nerve palsy (either due to intraoperative damage or traction from rotational change) and nonunion.[5,14,18,21]

CRITICAL POINTS: PROXIMAL RADIOULNAR SYNOSTOSIS

- In proximal radioulnar synostosis, forearm rotation is absent and the forearm is usually fixed in pronation.

- Children usually present between 2 and 6 years of age with painless absence of forearm rotation and a slight elbow flexion contracture. The delay in diagnosis is attributed to lack of forearm rotation requirement in the infant and the use of compensatory shoulder and wrist motion.

- Proximal radioulnar synostosis is usually visualized on radiographs, although the connection is initially cartilaginous and ossifies over time. The length of the synostosis varies, and a concomitant radial head dislocation may be present.

- Extreme pronation or supination that interferes with function is an indication for surgery. A forearm fixed in greater than 60 degrees of pronation usually warrants correction.

- Surgery to restore forearm rotation has been uniformly unsuccessful.

- Corrective osteotomy through the fusion mass is the preferred surgical treatment to better position the forearm.

ANNOTATED REFERENCES

17. Murase TT, Tada K, Yoshida T, Moritomo H: Derotational osteotomy at the shafts of the radius and ulna for congenital radioulnar synostosis. J Hand Surg [Am] 28:133-137, 2003.

    Correction osteotomy for congenital radioulnar synostosis was performed via combined osteotomy at the distal one third of the radius and proximal one third of the ulna. After intramedullary Kirschner wires are inserted into both bones, the forearm is derotated manually to the position planned before surgery followed by cast immobilization. Four patients with an average age of 3.9 years underwent surgery with this method and were followed up for 45.8 months. All of their forearms were fixed before surgery at over 70 degrees of pronation. The average correction after surgery was 65 degrees, and bone union occurred at 8 weeks after surgery without any complications. The patients' ability to perform daily activities showed a marked improvement after surgery, but there was a 20-degree loss of correction during cast immobilization in one case.

18. Ogino T, Hikino K: Congenital radioulnar synostosis: Compensatory rotation around the wrist and rotation osteotomy. J Hand Surg [Br] 12:173-178, 1987.

    Forty cases of congenital radioulnar synostosis were analyzed for compensatory rotation around the wrist and functional results after rotation osteotomy. The mean pronation of the ankylosed forearm in those who complained of disabilities in daily life was 60.7 degrees and that in patients without complaints was 21.2 degrees. In almost all cases with total ankylosis, the forearm had compensatory movement around the wrist, the mean arc being from 76.3 degrees of pronation to 42.9 degrees of supination. Thirteen limbs in 11 patients treated by transverse rotational osteotomies through the fusion mass were satisfactory after surgery.

Congenital Pseudarthrosis of the Ulna

EPIDEMIOLOGY

Congenital pseudarthrosis of the ulna occurs when a portion of the ulna (usually in the distal third or middle third) fails to form and has been replaced by fibrous tissue (Fig. 42-30).[8] This condition is rare and is usually associated with neurofibromatosis.[17] Neurofibromatosis occurs in approximately 1 in 3000 live births and is the most common single gene disorder.[27] Neurofibromatosis is inherited as an autosomal dominant trait with variable penetrance and has a high rate of spontaneous mutation (up to 50%). Five to 10 percent of people with neurofibromatosis develop a pseudarthrosis, most commonly in the tibia.[11,27]

The etiology of congenital pseudarthrosis is unknown. In the majority of cases, the pseudarthrosis contains fibrous tissue and not a neurofibroma.[10] Pseudarthrosis may occasionally involve both the radius and ulna (Fig. 42-31).[5,23,24]

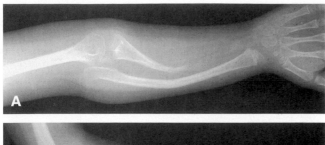

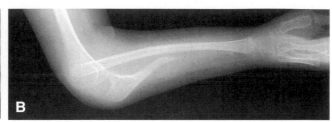

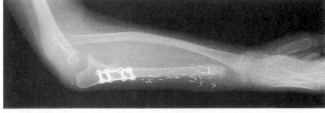

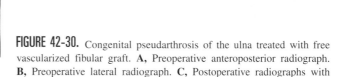

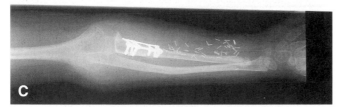

FIGURE 42-30. Congenital pseudarthrosis of the ulna treated with free vascularized fibular graft. **A,** Preoperative anteroposterior radiograph. **B,** Preoperative lateral radiograph. **C,** Postoperative radiographs with healed fibular graft.

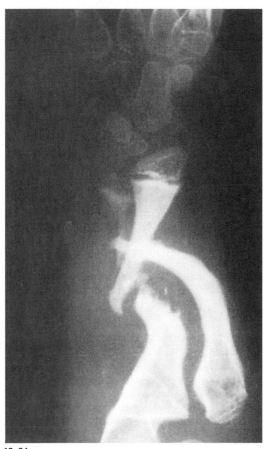

FIGURE 42-31. This child with congenital pseudarthrosis of both bones of the forearm demonstrates the radiolucent defects, very little callus formation, and tapered bone ends. (Courtesy of Louis G. Bayne, MD.)

CLINICAL FEATURES

Congenital pseudarthrosis of the ulna causes a progressive forearm deformity. The forearm is short, and the radius bears the entire load of the forearm. This excessive load yields radial bowing and eventual radial head dislocation.[1,7,17]

Pseudarthrosis of the ulna causes forearm deformity, instability, and weakness. Pain may be present. Diminished forearm rotation is evident, although some degree of rotation is preserved.

RADIOGRAPHY

Radiographs reveal the pseudarthrosis within the ulna. The extent of radial bowing and position of the radial head are additional features to assess (see Fig. 42-30).

ASSOCIATED ANOMALIES AND/OR SYSTEMIC CONDITIONS

Seventy percent of persons with ulnar pseudarthrosis have neurofibromatosis.[9] Familial pseudarthrosis associated with neurofibromatosis has been reported but is unusual.[9]

SURGICAL MANAGEMENT

Indications

The goal of treatment is to obtain union to reduce deformity and instability. Additional challenges are to maintain motion and to preserve the distal ulnar epiphysis. Similar to tibial pseudarthrosis, attempted union with bone grafting and immobilization often results in recurrence.[16,19] Historically, creation of a one-bone forearm was the only option available to restore forearm stability.[8,22,26] External distraction techniques combined with compression across the pseudarthrosis may successfully restore union in tibial pseudarthrosis.[21] This technique is complicated within the paired-bone forearm, because differential lengthening often results in loss of forearm rotation.

Resection of the pseudarthrosis and free vascularized fibular graft transfer to the defect reliably results in union (see Fig. 42-30C). Fibular transfers maintain length and may preserve some forearm rotation.* Although follow-up of a large number of patients to skeletal maturity is pending, this technique is promising.

Preoperative Planning

The donor fibula is contralateral to the ulnar pseudarthrosis to facilitate intraoperative positioning. Radiographs of both forearms and the donor leg are obtained (Fig. 42-32A and B). Preoperative arteriograms of the donor and recipient sites are not essential. The amount of fibular graft needed after pseudarthrosis resection is estimated. A minimum of the middle third of the fibula must be harvested to protect the nutrient artery. At least the middle half of the fibula can

---

*See references 2, 3, 6, 8, 13, 17, 18, 23, 24, 29, and 30.

be harvested without problems. Some reports indicate that the distal 6 to 8 cm of fibula should be preserved to maintain ankle stability.[4,25,28] Recent biomechanical studies indicate that only the distal 10% of the fibula is necessary to preserve ankle stability.[20]

Technique: Free Vascularized Fibular Graft to the Ulnar Pseudarthrosis

Severe soft tissue contracture may require preliminary distraction to allow resection and fibular grafting. Two surgical teams are used to decrease operative time. The patient is placed in a floppy lateral decubitus position with the affected arm along an arm board (see Fig. 42-32C). The ulnar pseudarthrosis is isolated via an incision that exposes the distal ulnar artery and curves along the ulnar forearm (see Fig. 42-32D). The ulnar neurovascular bundle is carefully protected. The entire ulnar pseudarthrosis is resected back to healthy bone at each end (see Fig. 42-32E). The defect size determines the length of fibula resected.

Simultaneously, the fibula is harvested and centered along the length of the bone. The nutrient artery enters the middle third of the medial fibula. A longitudinal incision is made along the subcutaneous border of the fibula. The peroneal and soleus muscles are separated, and the fibular periosteum is left intact. The distal fibula and peroneal vessels are isolated. The distal osteotomy level is selected based on the amount of fibula required and the necessity to preserve ankle stability (see Fig. 42-32F). After distal osteotomy, careful retraction of the fibula exposes the interosseous membrane, which is divided in its distal half.

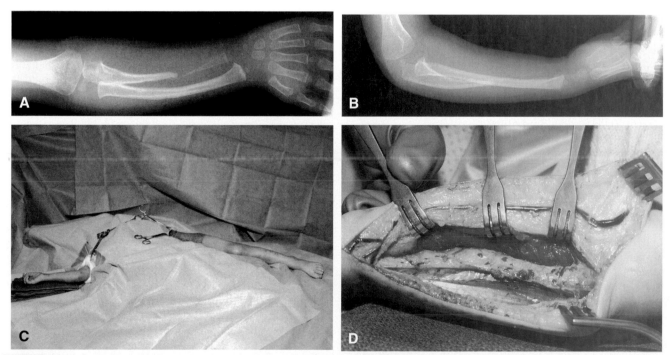

FIGURE 42-32. A 3½-year-old child presented with neurofibromatosis and progressive deformity associated with right congenital pseudarthrosis of the ulna. Left free vascularized fibula was transferred to the right ulna. **A,** Preoperative anteroposterior radiograph shows "sucked candy" appearance of the ulna. **B,** Preoperative lateral radiograph shows radial head has not yet dislocated. **C,** Surgical positioning. The child is in the right semilateral decubitus position. The right arm, left lower extremity, and iliac crest are prepared and draped. **D,** Exposure of ulna pseudarthrosis.   *Continued*

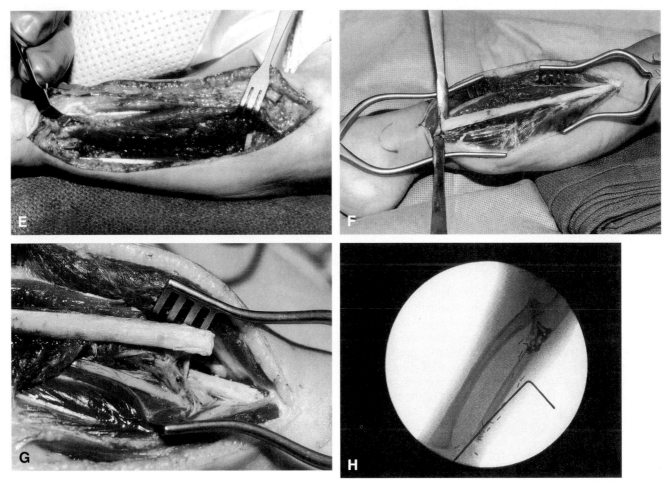

FIGURE 42-32—cont'd. E, Forearm after resection of ulna pseudarthrosis. **F,** Exposure of fibula for graft. **G,** Proximal fibular osteotomy with peroneal vessels exposed. **H,** Postoperative radiograph of forearm with fibular graft in place.

The proximal peroneal vessels and nerve are isolated. The proximal osteotomy is performed while the neurovascular structures are protected. At this point, the fibula segment can be externally rotated and the remaining interosseous membrane divided with preservation of the peroneal vessels adjacent to the middle third of the fibula.

The peroneal vessels are then ligated at the level of the distal osteotomy. The tourniquet is deflated to ensure perfusion to the fibular segment. After the forearm is prepared, the peroneal artery and vein(s) are ligated proximally (see Fig. 42-32G). The graft is passed into the arm and contoured to fit the deficit. A distal tibiofibular synostosis is performed to maintain angle stability. Bone graft trimmed from the fibula or graft harvested from the iliac crest may be placed between the tibia and fibula. One or two syndesmosis screws are used for internal fixation. Placing a screw(s) through the distal tibial or fibular physes should be avoided (see Fig. 42-32H). The leg wound is closed with interrupted subcutaneous sutures and running absorbable skin sutures.

Internal fixation with short plates is used to secure the graft in place before vascular anastomosis. Frequently, a small amount of distal metaphyseal bone remains after resection of the pseudarthrosis, which may preclude plate fixation. Alternative fixation with Kirschner wire fixation is used. An end-to-end or end-to-side arterial anastomosis is performed between the peroneal and ulnar arteries. The peroneal veins are often larger than the venae comitantes and require anastomosis with subcutaneous veins about the forearm. Supplemental cancellous bone graft from the ends of the donor fibula or from the iliac crest can be placed at each end of the fibular graft to enhance union. The wound is closed with interrupted subcutaneous sutures and running absorbable skin sutures. A drain is placed if necessary. Long-arm and long-leg casts are applied.

Postoperative Management

The patency of the anastomosis may or may not be monitored. Monitoring options include fibula harvesting with a skin paddle or implantable flow monitors. Children are kept warm, calm (with sedation if necessary), and at bed rest for 72 hours. Caffeine and cigarette smoke are avoided.

The child is kept non–weight bearing on the affected leg for 6 weeks. Radiographs of both extremities are obtained out of casts at 6 weeks. Long-arm and short-leg walking casts are applied for 4 to 6 additional weeks. Immobilization is discontinued after radiographic union is apparent at both ends of the graft and at the tibiofibular synostosis. Union usually occurs 3 to 6 months after surgery.

OUTCOME

A vascularized fibular graft achieves a higher rate of union than any other operative treatment of ulnar pseudarthrosis other than the one-bone forearm.[29] Unlike creation of a one-bone forearm, vascularized fibular grafting preserves motion. This operation is best performed early to avoid progressive forearm deformity.[29] No published studies have reported follow-up to skeletal maturity.

COMPLICATIONS

Donor site morbidity is a frequent occurrence. Progressive ankle valgus deformity frequently occurs in skeletally immature patients after fibular resection.[12,14,20] This can be prevented or at least minimized by preserving adequate distal fibular length,[20] inserting a distal tibiofibular syndesmosis screw,[12,14,20] and/or creation of a synostosis between the distal tibia and fibula (Langenskiöld procedure).[12,14,20] Distal tibiofibular synostosis is the preferred method of stabilization of the fibula to prevent ankle valgus deformity. Other donor site problems include objective motor weakness, pain, and sensory abnormalities.[15,25]

CRITICAL POINTS: PSEUDARTHROSIS OF THE ULNA

- Congenital pseudarthrosis of the ulna occurs when a portion of the ulna fails to form (usually in the distal third or middle third) and has been replaced by fibrous tissue.
- Congenital pseudarthrosis is rare and is usually associated with neurofibromatosis.
- Etiology of congenital pseudarthrosis is unknown. The pseudarthrosis usually contains fibrous tissue and not a neurofibroma.
- Pseudarthrosis of the ulna causes forearm deformity, instability, and weakness.
- The goal of treatment is to obtain union to reduce deformity and instability.
- Resection of the pseudarthrosis and free vascularized fibular graft transfer to the defect is the preferred technique.

ANNOTATED REFERENCES

3. Allieu Y, Meyer zu Reckendorf G, Chammas M, Gomis R: Congenital pseudarthrosis of both forearm bones: Long-term results of two cases managed by free vascularized fibular graft. J Hand Surg [Am] 24:604-608, 1999.

The clinical and radiographic outcome of two cases of congenital pseudarthrosis of both forearm bones managed by free vascularized fibular grafts was assessed. The follow-up periods were 17 and 13 years, respectively. A 4-year-old girl had reconstruction of both the radius and ulna by a vascularized fibular graft. Pronation/supination was restored to a 110-degree arc. A 17-year-old boy underwent a one-bone forearm procedure using a vascularized fibular graft. A stable forearm was achieved, although there was considerable shortening (15 cm).

11. Crawford AH, Schorry EK: Neurofibromatosis in children: The role of the orthopaedist. J Am Acad Orthop Surg 7:217-230, 1999.

Type 1 neurofibromatosis, also known as von Recklinghausen's disease, is one of the most common human single-gene disorders, affecting at least 1 million persons throughout the world. It encompasses a spectrum of multifaceted disorders and may present as a wide range of clinical manifestations, including abnormalities of the skin, nervous tissue, bones, and soft tissues. Most children with type 1 neurofibromatosis have no major orthopaedic problems. For those with musculoskeletal involvement, the most important issue is early recognition. Spinal deformity, congenital tibial dysplasia (congenital bowing and pseudarthrosis), and disorders of excessive bone and soft tissue growth are the three types of musculoskeletal manifestations that require evaluation.

12. Fragniere B, Wicart P, Mascard E, Dubousset J: Prevention of ankle valgus after vascularized fibular grafts in children. Clin Orthop 408:245-251, 2003.

Ankle valgus after the use of vascularized fibular grafts is a known complication of the donor site ankle in the growing child. This study evaluated the rate of ankle deformities and analyzed the efficiency of two prevention methods. Twenty children were treated for sarcomas of long bones with a mean follow-up of 4.1 years. Ankle valgus was considered if the tibiotalar angle on standing radiographs was 5 degrees or greater in valgus than that of the opposite ankle. The deformity was considered severe if surgery was required. Prevention was done in some patients with a tibiofibular syndesmotic screw or with reconstruction of the fibula using a tibial autograft. Valgus occurred in nine patients (45%) and was severe in five (25%). Valgus prevention with a syndesmotic screw was efficient and lacking in complications, whereas patients with fibula reconstruction had a high incidence of deformity and relevant complications. The authors recommend using a tibiofibular syndesmotic screw in all patients whose growth plates are open.

Elbow and Forearm Deformity Due to Hereditary Multiple Exostoses

EPIDEMIOLOGY

Hereditary multiple exostoses (HME) is an inheritable disorder of enchondral bone growth. HME is inherited in an autosomal dominant pattern with high penetrance[20] and variable expressivity. Cartilaginous exostoses, also called osteochondromas, grow from the physes of long bones and from the pelvis, ribs, scapula, and vertebrae.[1,10,16] Many different names have been used to describe HME, including multiple cartilaginous exostoses, diaphyseal aclasis, dyschondroplasia, hereditary deforming chondrodysplasia, and osteochondromatosis.[10,26] HME is frequently confused with multiple enchondromatosis (Ollier's disease), an entirely different condition.

The prevalence of HME is approximately 1 in 50,000.[20] HME has an equal prevalence in both sexes, although males tend to have more severe involvement.[14] The most common sites of involvement are the knee, humerus, hip, scapula, ribs, distal radius and ulna, ankle, elbow, hands, feet, and pelvis.[21,24] Approximately one half of all patients with HME have forearm involvement.[3,5,10,11,20,25,26]

Genetic studies of families with this condition[4,14,15] have mapped the chromosomal abnormality to at least three different genes. The genes are termed EXT genes and are located on different chromosomes.[8,9] EXT genes are also tumor suppressor genes.[17,24,27,28] On this basis, HME has been classified as a familial neoplastic syndrome.[18]

CLINICAL FEATURES

A clinical "bump search" of all long bones is indicated if HME is suspected, but the diagnosis has yet to be established. Shoulder, elbow, wrist, and digit range of motion should be measured. Radiographs should be obtained of any part of the extremity where osteochondromas are suspected or that have decreased range of motion. Serial measurements of forearm rotation are used to document forearm deformity.

Most exostoses are asymptomatic and do not require removal. Exostoses removed before skeletal maturity may recur. However, exostoses may cause local discomfort, nerve or tendon impingement, decreased range of motion, and longitudinal and angulatory growth abnormalities.[4,16] Growth abnormalities may also occur in HME in the absence of radiologically visible exostoses.[2] Two studies reveal that adults with untreated forearm deformities maintained function and were comfortable with their appearance.[1,22] These reports question the role of aggressive surgical treatment to maintain or improve function.

RADIOGRAPHY

The exostosis may appear sessile (broad based) or pedunculated. More severe angular deformities appear to be associated with a predominance of sessile lesions.[4] Exostoses possess a cartilage cap and are larger than their radiographic appearance.

Magnetic resonance imaging is not routinely obtained but will reveal the size of the cartilaginous cap. It is the imaging technique of choice to evaluate for suspected malignant transformation.

ASSOCIATED ANOMALIES AND/OR SYSTEMIC CONDITIONS

HME is an inheritable condition that occurs with variable expressivity. Multiple exostoses can also occur in other conditions, such as metachondromatosis and the Langer-Giedion syndrome.[14]

CLASSIFICATION

Masada and associates[11,13] developed a classification scheme for forearm deformities based on location of the osteochondromas (Fig. 42-33). This scheme is based on the location of the main forearm osteochondroma, the resultant deformity, and concomitant clinical problems. Type I is the most common form. The main osteochondroma is located in the distal ulna, which causes a short ulna and bowed radius. The radial head remains located within the radiocapitellar joint. In type II, the main osteochondroma is located in the distal ulna, which causes a short ulna and bowed radius. The radial head, however, dislocates from the capitellum (Fig. 42-34). Type II is subdivided into type IIa, with an osteochondroma on the proximal radial metaphysis, and type IIb, with no proximal radial osteochondroma. In type III, the main osteochondroma is located in the distal radial metaphysis and the radius is relatively short.

SURGICAL MANAGEMENT

Indications

Osteochondromas may cause visible deformity, local pain, and growth disturbance. Malignant transformation is uncommon. Local pain is a frequent indication for exostosis removal. Exostoses of the distal radius and ulna may

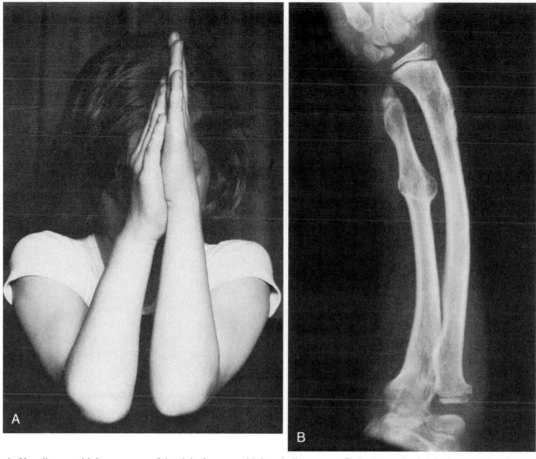

FIGURE 42-33. **A,** Hereditary multiple exostoses of the right forearm with length discrepancy. **B,** Radiograph of right forearm of child (Masada type 1).

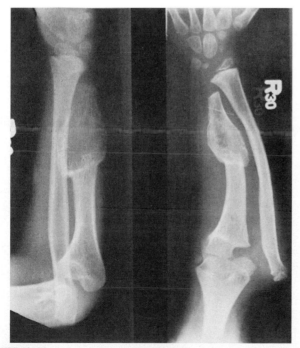

FIGURE 42-34. Radiograph of the hereditary multiple exostoses of the right forearm (Masada type IIb).

impinge on the surrounding cutaneous nerves and tissues. Surgical excision effectively relieves symptoms. An exostosis in the interosseous space may block forearm rotation. Early removal may preserve motion.

Forearm osteochondromas frequently cause a length discrepancy between the radius and ulna.[21] The forearm deformities caused by growth arrest due to HME are complex, and their interrelationships are not well understood. Even when osteochondromas of the distal ulna are not visible on radiography, distal ulnar growth arrest is common. The ulnar physis appears to be more susceptible to growth impairment because it has a smaller cross-sectional area than the radius. The resultant deformity is a length discrepancy within the forearm. The radius becomes longer than the ulna and accepts the entire forearm load. This results in radial bowing, radial tilting, and possible radial head dislocation.[26] The increased radial inclination and lack of ulnar support positions the wrist into ulnar deviation and causes the carpus to "slip" toward the ulna.[3,21] The changes in radius and ulna length and alignment lead to diminished forearm rotation.

Early osteochondroma removal to retard or prevent progressive growth disturbances is controversial.[7,13,16] Hemiepiphyseal stapling of the radial side of the distal radius retards radial growth and allows correction of the radial articular angle and ulnar length discrepancy with growth.[26] Stapling may be performed in conjunction with ulnar lengthening.[7,16] Ulnar lengthening may be performed in a single stage or using gradual distraction osteogenesis. Differential lengthening combined with angular correction can be used to reduce the radial head.[9a] Restoration of normal forearm anatomy may result in spontaneous radial head reduction. Resection of a dislocated radial head is indicated for pain. Resection relieves pain and removes the associated prominence.[1,13] Radial head resection is delayed until skeletal maturity, because removal of the radial head in the growing child may cause cubitus valgus or proximal radial overgrowth.[12] Creation of a one-bone forearm may be used to salvage a severely disorganized forearm.[19]

A late indication for HME is suspected malignant transformation. Symptoms and signs of malignant transformation include local pain and growth of an osteochondroma after skeletal maturity. Radiographic changes include internal lytic areas, erosion or destruction of the adjacent bone, and/ or presence of a soft tissue mass containing irregular calcifications.[24] Malignant transformation, however, is quite rare in the upper extremity.[16,23]

Contraindications

Contraindications to osteochondroma removal are relative. The risks and benefits of surgery need to be considered. Simple procedures, such as removal of symptomatic osteochondromas and dislocated radial heads, may improve appearance and relieve pain. Complicated procedures, such as forearm lengthening, possess considerable complications and require considerable contemplation before recommendation, especially because surgical treatment has not been shown to improve forearm function.

Preoperative Planning

Recent radiographs should be available. Careful preoperative neurologic and range of motion examinations are required before surgery. The patient, parent, and surgeon should agree on exactly which osteochondroma(s) will be removed, because often there are several present.

Techniques

1. Removal of osteochondroma. The osteochondroma is approached through a longitudinal incision centered over the tumor. The most readily available anatomic interval is used for the approach. Usually, the osteochondroma splits the surrounding structures and the approach is straightforward. Nerves and/or vessels may be wrapped around the pedicle of the tumor or flattened over its surface. These neurovascular structures are retracted. The entire tumor is removed, leaving a smooth bony contour.
2. Distal radius hemiepiphyseal stapling (Fig. 42-35). The radial aspect of the distal radial physis is approached through a transverse incision, taking care to avoid injuring the dorsal radial sensory nerve. Under radiographic guidance, three extraperiosteal staples are placed across the distal radial physis. One staple is placed along the radial portion, a second palmar bridging the growth plate, and a third crossing the dorsal aspect.
3. Radial head excision (posterolateral dislocation). See section on resection of the radial head under Congenital Dislocation of the Radial Head.
4. Differential forearm lengthening. This complex operation is uncommon and is beyond the scope of this text. See Dahl's detailed description of planning osteotomies,

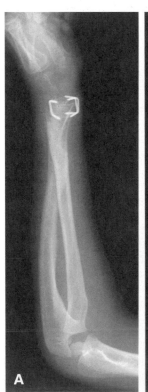
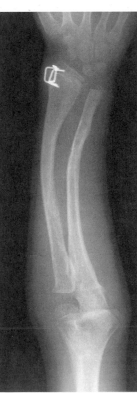
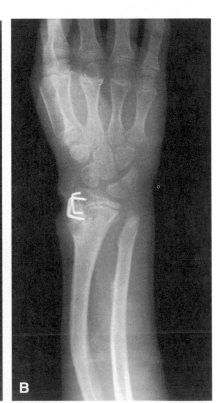

FIGURE 42-35. Distal radius hemiepiphyseal stapling. **A,** Anteroposterior and lateral radiographs after distal radius hemiepiphyseal stapling. **B,** Follow-up radiograph with correction of radial tilt.

designing fixation, ulnar lengthening and angular correction, and radial head reduction.[6]

Postoperative Management

For distal forearm osteochondroma removal and distal radius hemiepiphyseal stapling, a soft dressing and wrist splint for 2 to 3 weeks is adequate immobilization. Radiographs of the distal radius should be obtained twice a year after hemiepiphyseal stapling, and the staples should be removed when the desired amount of radial tilt (usually 20 degrees) is attained.

 Authors' Preferred Technique

Hemiepiphyseal stapling, osteochondroma resection, and radial head removal are simple operations with good results. Forearm rotation should be measured twice a year for children with HME and forearm involvement. Progressive loss of forearm rotation is considered an indication for osteochondroma removal and possible ulnar lengthening.

CRITICAL POINTS: HEREDITARY MULTIPLE EXOSTOSES

- HME is inherited in an autosomal dominant pattern with high penetrance. Cartilaginous exostoses (osteochondromas) grow from the physes of long bones and from the pelvis, ribs, scapula, and vertebrae.
- Most exostoses are asymptomatic and do not require removal. Early removal of osteochondromas to retard or prevent progressive growth disturbances is controversial.
- Large exostoses may cause local pain from irritation of surrounding tissues. Simple removal is recommended.
- Forearm deformities are common in HME and are based on location of the osteochondromas, although the forearm deformities are complex and not well understood.
- Hemiepiphyseal stapling of the radial side of the distal radius retards radial growth and allows correction of the radial articular angle and ulnar length discrepancy with growth.
- Ulnar lengthening may be performed in a single stage or using gradual distraction osteogenesis. Differential lengthening combined with angular correction can be used to reduce the radial head.
- Malignant transformation is uncommon.

OUTCOME

Osteochondromas tend to grow until skeletal maturity. Recurrence is uncommon when resection is performed near skeletal maturity. Hemiepiphyseal stapling can restore radial tilt when performed on the patient with enough remaining growth. Radial head resection reliably relieves pain in persons with radial head dislocation. Differential forearm lengthening may improve appearance, but there is no evidence that function is improved.

ANNOTATED REFERENCES

4. Carroll KL, Yandow SM, Ward K, Carey JC: Clinical correlation to genetic variations of hereditary multiple exostosis. J Pediatr Orthop 19:785-791, 1999.

    HME is an autosomal dominant disorder leading to polyostotic periphyseal osteochondroma formation. These tumorous lesions can cause growth disturbances, painful local symptoms, restriction of joint motion, and neurologic compromise. Malignant transformation has been noted. The reports of the incidence of these complications vary widely in the literature. Recently, genetic lineage mapping disclosed three locations for HME with loci on chromosomes 8, 11, and 19. These three genotypes may result in different phenotypic expression of HME and thus explain the variable manifestations of the disease.

9a. Horii E, Nakamura R, Nakao E, et al: Distraction lengthening of the forearm for congenital and developmental problems. J Hand Surg [Br] 25:15-21, 2000.

    Thirty-five lengthenings of the forearm were performed in 23 patients divided into two groups according to the cause of the shortening. Eleven cases (group A) had congenital dysplasia and 12 cases (group B) had growth disturbances from tumors or infection. The mean amount of lengthening was 27 mm in group A and 25 mm in group B. The mean percentage increase in length was 35% and 17%, respectively. The mean duration of fixation was 159 days and 127 days, respectively. The healing index had a positive correlation with the age at surgery in group A, but not in group B. The main complication was callus deformity after the removal of a fixator, which was especially frequent in group A. To avoid complications, the etiology of shortening and the age of the patient should be considered.

17. Porter DE, Emerton ME, Villanueva-Lopez F, Simpson AH: Clinical and radiographic analysis of osteochondromas and growth disturbance in hereditary multiple exostoses. J Pediatr Orthop 20:246-250, 2000.

    This clinical and radiographic analysis of patients with osteochondromas assessed paired bone length along with exostoses number and dimensions. The local presence of osteochondromas was consistently associated with growth disturbance. In particular, an inverse correlation between osteochondroma size and relative bone length (*P* < .01) was found. These data suggest that the growth retardation in HME may result from the local effects of enlarging osteochondromas rather than a skeletal dysplasia effect. This study provides the clinical rationale for ablation of rapidly enlarging exostoses to reduce growth disturbance.

CHAPTER 43

Congenital Contracture

Scott H. Kozin, Simon P. Kay, John R. Griffin, and Marybeth Ezaki

Arthrogryposis

Scott H. Kozin

Arthrogryposis (also known as arthrogryposis multiplex congenita) is a syndrome of nonprogressive joint contractures that is present at birth.[9] There are multiple forms of arthrogryposis that vary in presentation, severity, and number of involved joints. The joint contractures are secondary to lack of motion during fetal life. Multiple processes can lead to lack of fetal limb movement, including muscle abnormalities, nerve anomalies, a restricted intrauterine space, vascular insufficiency, and maternal illness. The precise cause often remains unknown.

There are many syndromes and genetic conditions that have features of arthrogryposis. A classic example is Freeman-Sheldon syndrome (whistling face syndrome), an autosomal dominant condition affecting the hands and feet with a characteristic facial appearance.[4,8,11,12] Another example is Beal's syndrome, an inheritable condition with contractural arachnodactyly and proximal interphalangeal (PIP) joint flexion contractures.[2,14] The windblown hand (congenital ulnar drift) is probably a variation of arthrogryposis and is often inherited as an autosomal dominant trait[22] (Fig. 43-1). The combination of metacarpophalangeal (MCP) joint flexion and ulnar deviation resembles arthrogryposis. These conditions that assimilate distal arthrogryposis are frequently inheritable but have variable phenotypes within affected families.[1]

CLINICAL FEATURES

Amyoplasia (classic arthrogryposis) is the most common form and is characterized by symmetrical positioning of the limbs. It occurs sporadically.[15] The upper extremities posture with shoulder adduction and internal rotation, elbow extension, forearm pronation, wrist flexion, and hand ulnar deviation (Fig. 43-2; see also Fig. 43-1). The digits are postured in flexion and stiff (Fig. 43-3). The contracted clasped thumb is a common finding in arthrogryposis, which creates functional difficulties with activities of daily living.[3,7]

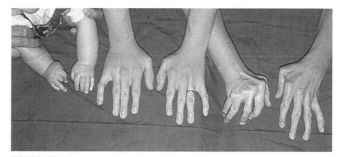

FIGURE 43-1. Three generations of the same family showing features characteristic of windblown hand. On the right, the grandmother's hands have never received treatment and show characteristic features of adduction and flexion contractures at the thumb and ulnar deviation at the MCP joint. Center, the mother's hands were less severely afflicted and show less marked ulnar deviation but flexion contractures of the fingers and adduction contracture of the thumb. The child's hand shows ulnar deviation with the fingers and flexion contractures with adducted flexed thumbs.

Additional clinical features include waxy skin devoid of skin creases, considerable muscle wasting, and a paucity of subcutaneous tissue.

TREATMENT

Goals

The treatment of arthrogryposis is individualized to each child's needs. Upper extremity treatment goals include achieving independent function for self-feeding and peroneal care. A team approach between physicians and therapists facilitates decision making. Adaptive equipment and technology assistance are helpful in maximizing independence. Frequently, upper and lower extremity surgery may be combined to lessen the number of anesthesias.

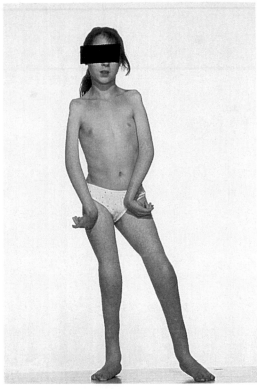

FIGURE 43-2. The upper limb abnormalities in arthrogryposis multiplex congenita in a 9-year-old girl. The shoulders are adducted, the elbows extended, and the wrists flexed with flexion contractures of the thumb and finger. The forearms are held pronated. By contrast the lower limb abnormalities are mild.

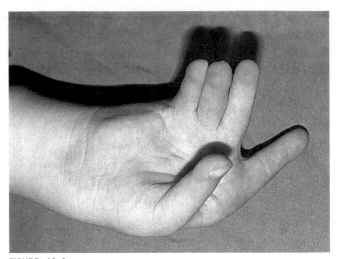

FIGURE 43-3. Typical hand deformity in arthrogryposis with flexion deformity of the fingers and the thumb flexed and adducted.

Nonoperative Management

The mainstays of early treatment are frequent passive movement of all involved joints and judicious use of splints. Static progressive splinting creates a low load and prolonged stretch and may be efficacious for diminishing contractures. An increase in passive motion is beneficial for function and enhances the possibility of surgical reconstruction (Fig. 43-4). Passive stretching, serial casting, and orthotics are most efficacious in distal arthrogryposis.[16] In contrast, the joint contractures in amyoplasia are often rigid and refractory to therapy.

FIGURE 43-4. A and B, Progressive splinting of the elbow in this child with arthrogryposis resulted in a flexible passive range of motion at the elbow that could then accept a muscle transfer.

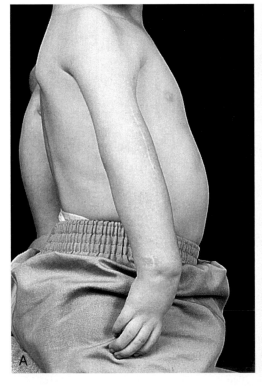

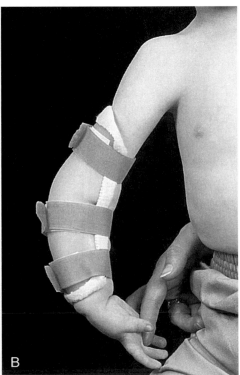

Surgical Management

The timing of surgery is controversial.[7,13] Early treatment has certain advantages and disadvantages. Surgery is usually recommended before school age (4 or 5 years of age) to minimize compensatory movements and maximize mainstream school function.[7] Older children develop adaptive maneuvers to accomplish many daily tasks. These positions may appear awkward but are functional for many activities.[15] For example, tasks are often accomplished with bimanual limb usage that utilizes scissoring of the upper limbs for grasp. Surgical recommendations must consider these adaptive maneuvers and ensure no degradation in function after surgery.

Shoulder and Elbow

The shoulder often has limited motion secondary to undeveloped musculature and capsular contracture. An internal rotation deformity develops over time. No reliable procedures exist to enhance shoulder mobility. Severe internal rotation that prohibits limb function is uncommon and may require treatment. Release of the muscles that rotate the shoulder into internal rotation is often not rational, because children with arthrogryposis frequently use adduction of the humerus against the thorax to hold objects. Osteotomy of the humerus to rotate the arm into a better position is more reliable. Slight internal rotation is preferred to allow hand-to-mouth function and midline use. The osteotomy may be performed anywhere along the humerus.

The elbow is often the most problematic joint in children with arthrogryposis. Lack of flexion is the common impairment, which prohibits hand-to-mouth function and many daily tasks. The first goal is restoration of passive motion. Adequate passive flexion allows the hand to be placed near the face using a tabletop or adaptive equipment. Early efforts to restore passive elbow flexion are critical and emphasized in therapy. Recalcitrant elbow extension requires consideration of surgical release via lengthening of the triceps and posterior capsular release.[7]

A posterior surgical approach is used with a curvilinear incision that extends over the medial aspect of the elbow. The ulnar nerve is isolated and released from the cubital tunnel. The triceps is lengthened using a "V-Y" technique. The triceps is reflected to reveal the posterior capsule, which is divided from medial to lateral. The elbow is flexed with an ultimate goal of greater than 90 degrees of flexion. Unfortunately, less flexion is often obtainable because care is necessary to avoid damaging the distal humerus growth plate. The triceps is approximated in a "V-Y" method. The ulnar nerve is inspected for iatrogenic compression, which requires subcutaneous transposition. The wound is closed and the arm splinted in flexion (at least 90 degrees) for 3 weeks. A splint is fabricated at 90 degrees of flexion, and passive elbow flexion is initiated. Activities that require elbow flexion are encouraged. Some elbow extension strength may return depending on the integrity of the triceps muscle and tendon.

A secondary goal is restoration of active elbow flexion.[17] Passive flexion is a prerequisite to active motion (Fig. 43-5). Posterior release does not result in active elbow flexion. Potential donor muscles for elbow flexorplasty include the pectoralis major, latissimus dorsi, triceps, and flexor-pronator mass.[5,6,10] The available donor muscle must be expendable and possess adequate strength and excursion. The selection of donor is more difficult in children with arthrogryposis. Adequate evaluation of muscle strength and excursion is difficult, and selected transfers may be contraindicated. For example, triceps transfer is contraindicated in children who use upper extremity devices (e.g., crutches) to ambulate. Unfortunately, the results after elbow flexion transfers for arthrogryposis are not as predictable compared with other causes.[17] This inconsistent outcome reflects the lack of passive joint motion, paucity of donor muscles, and the inadequate quality of the donor muscle.

Forearm and Wrist

Forearm pronation and wrist flexion coupled with ulnar deviation are the typical contractures. The amount of contracture and degree of malposition is variable. The wrist position is difficult to overcome because of the rigid volar structures (fascia, ligaments, tendons, skin) and the deficiency in active wrist extension. In addition, carpal coalitions form and fixed bony changes accumulate with skeletal maturity. Persistent wrist flexion recalcitrant to therapy may require surgery to better position the wrist for function.

Numerous surgical procedures have been recommended, including proximal row carpectomy, dorsal wedge osteotomy of the distal radius or midcarpus, distraction histiogenesis, and arthrodesis.[13,18-21] Proximal row carpectomy may be beneficial in young patients with mild to moderate flexion, although the results are often unpredictable.[13,19] In severe deformities, proximal row carpectomy often yields insufficient wrist extension. Long-term follow-up of proximal row carpectomy is disappointing with recurrent wrist flexion and secondary bony changes (Fig. 43-6).[7] Distraction histiogenesis with multiplanar fixation may be used to correct the wrist position. Careful pin placement and a compliant patient are prerequisites to successful correction. Long-term follow-up and outcome are still pending. Arthrodesis eliminates all motion and remains a salvage procedure. Osteotomy is the preferred approach to correct both the wrist flexion and ulnar deviation. The preferred site of osteotomy is the mid carpus. A radial osteotomy may jeopardize the growth plate and is not at the point of maximum deformity, which creates a secondary angulation.

The technique for dorsal wedge osteotomy of the mid carpus requires a volar and dorsal approach.[7] A longitudinal incision is made along the distal third of the forearm (Fig. 43-7). The tight forearm fascia is incised, and the wrist flexor muscles and tendons are inspected. Taut wrist flexors that appear anomalous are incised or lengthened. Taut wrist flexors that appear fairly normal are considered for transfer to the dorsum of the wrist for wrist extension. The extensor carpi ulnaris, however, is the preferred donor tendon to augment wrist extension.

A transverse dorsal incision is designed over the mid carpus with later excision of redundant skin for dermadesis. The extensor carpi ulnaris tendon is released from the small finger metacarpal. The extensor tendons of the fingers are mobilized. The radial wrist extensors are isolated at their insertion, although they are usually adherent to the dorsal capsule and devoid of proximal musculature.

A dorsal capsulotomy is made over the mid carpus. The capsule is reflected to expose the distal edge of the proximal

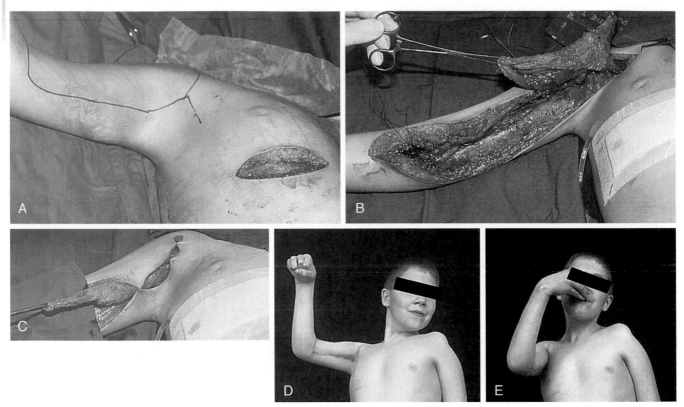

FIGURE 43-5. Pectoralis major transfer. **A,** The pectoralis major muscle is harvested through a short transverse incision overlying the costal margin. An oblique "saber cut" incision is disfiguring and unnecessary. **B,** The donor wound has been closed, the muscle insertion at the humerus divided, and the muscle raised on its neurovascular pedicle. **C,** The insertion of the muscle is now repositioned on the acromion, and the muscle is tubed. The distal origin of the muscle includes the anterior rectus sheath, which provides good tissue for accepting suture material and fixation to the ulna. **D,** Elbow flexion 5 months postoperatively. **E,** The hand can reach the mouth with an elbow that previously had no active flexion. Note some flexion of the shoulder aided by the acromial insertion of the pectoralis major.

row and the distal carpus. A biplanar wedge resection is planned to straighten and position the wrist in slight extension. The wedge is wider at the radial and dorsal margins. The proximal cut is perpendicular to the long axis of the forearm. The distal cut is perpendicular to the metacarpals. Violation of the palmar capsule should be avoided. Preliminary placement of Kirschner wires and use of mini-

fluoroscopy facilitate planning of the wedge. The wedge of bone is removed with a scalpel blade, osteotome, or fine-bladed saw, dependent on the age of the child (Fig. 43-8). The osteotomy site is coapted by wrist extension (Fig. 43-9). Interosseous sutures and/or percutaneous Kirschner wires are used for fixation. If Kirschner wires are used, they are initially passed in an antegrade direction through the

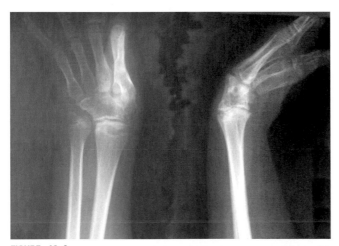

FIGURE 43-6. Status 12 years after proximal row carpectomy with secondary bony changes. (Courtesy of Shriners Hospitals for Children, Philadelphia.)

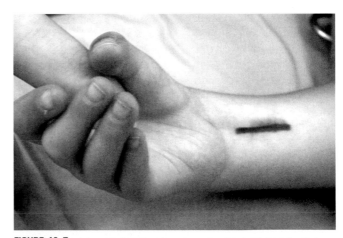

FIGURE 43-7. A longitudinal incision along the distal third of the forearm to release tight forearm fascia and inspect wrist flexor tendons. (Courtesy of Shriners Hospitals for Children, Philadelphia.)

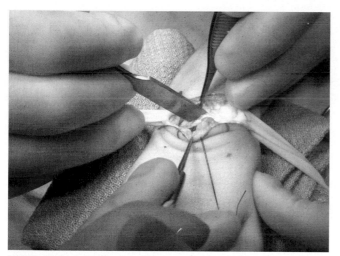

FIGURE 43-8. Osteotome to remove wedge of bone from mid carpus. (Courtesy of Shriners Hospitals for Children, Philadelphia.)

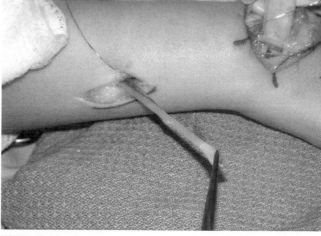

FIGURE 43-10. Mobilization of extensor carpi ulnaris tendon in preparation for transfer to the radial wrist extensors. (Courtesy of Shriners Hospitals for Children, Philadelphia.)

osteotomy site and between the metacarpals and through the skin. The osteotomy is then closed and the wires redirected retrograde across the osteotomy site.

The dorsal capsule is approximated over the osteotomy site. The extensor carpi ulnaris tendon is mobilized through a transverse incision about 5 cm proximal to the wrist (Fig. 43-10). The tendon is passed through a subcutaneous tunnel toward the reflected radial wrist extensors. The extensor carpi ulnaris tendon is woven through the radial wrist extensors as a tendon transfer for wrist extension. If the extensor carpi ulnaris is unavailable, a wrist flexor tendon may be used.

The limb is immobilized in a long-arm splint for 6 weeks. A splint is then fabricated and active motion initiated. If Kirschner wires were placed, they are removed at the time of splint fabrication (Fig. 43-11). The osteotomy site is protected with intermittent wearing of a splint for 3 months.

Thumb and Fingers

The fingers are stiff, fixed in flexion, and positioned in ulnar deviation. Mild to moderate digital overlap may be present during flexion. The degree of stiffness and the available motion varies between involved fingers within the same hand and affected hands among patients. Considerable stiffness and/or angulation create a functional handicap. Unfortunately, surgical treatment to restore supple finger motion is unsuccessful. Osteotomy may be used to realign fingers that are poorly positioned.

The contracted clasped thumb is a common finding in arthrogryposis.[7,12] The thumb may be released from the palm to enhance prehension and function. The treatment algorithm for the contracted clasped thumb is detailed within this chapter.

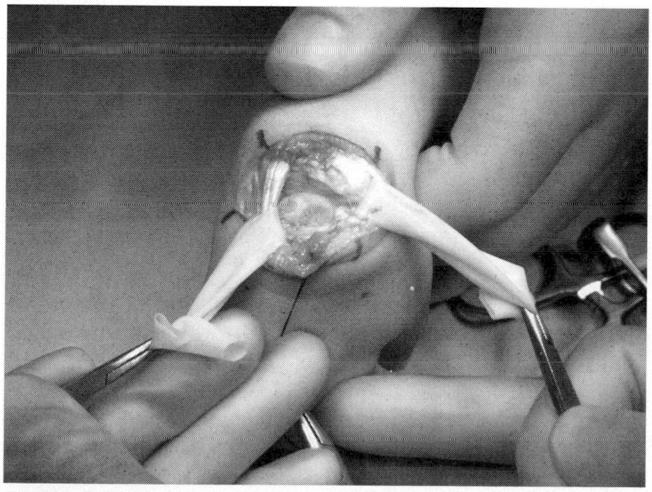

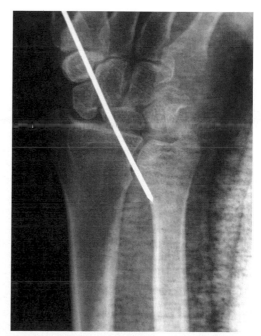

FIGURE 43-11. Postoperative radiograph after Kirschner wire fixation of midcarpal wedge osteotomy. (Courtesy of Shriners Hospitals for Children, Philadelphia.)

FIGURE 43-9. Wedge resection of mid carpus. (Courtesy of Shriners Hospitals for Children, Philadelphia.)

CRITICAL POINTS: ARTHROGRYPOSIS

- Arthrogryposis is a syndrome of joint contractures that are present at birth and nonprogressive. Multiple forms occur that vary in presentation, severity, and number of involved joints.
- Amyoplasia is the most common form, characterized by symmetrical positioning of the limbs with shoulder adduction and internal rotation, elbow extension, forearm pronation, wrist flexion, and hand ulnar deviation.
- Upper extremity goals are to achieve independent function for self-feeding and peroneal care. Early treatment is directed toward methods to enhance passive motion using stretching, serial casting, and splinting.
- The elbow is often the most challenging joint, because limited motion prohibits hand-to-mouth activity. Restoration of passive motion allows limb positioning for this function.
- Persistent wrist flexion recalcitrant to therapy may require surgery to better position the wrist for function. Dorsal wedge osteotomy of the mid carpus is preferred to correct both the wrist flexion and ulnar deviation.

ANNOTATED REFERENCES

7. Ezaki M: Treatment of the upper limb in the child with arthrogryposis. Hand Clin 16:703-711, 2000.

This overview of upper extremity management for the child with arthrogryposis discusses the need to preserve elbow and wrist motion and details the technique of posterior elbow release with tricepsplasty. Particulars of closed midcarpal wedge osteotomy are discussed, along with surgical technique and postoperative management.

15. Sells JM, Jaffe KM, Hall JG: Amyoplasia, the most common type of arthrogryposis: The potential for good outcome. Pediatrics 97:225-231, 1996.

Review of 38 children with amyoplasia describes their birth characteristics, therapeutic interventions, and functional outcomes. Eighty-four percent of the children had symmetrical, four-limb involvement. The children underwent an average of 5.7 orthopedic procedures. They had multiple castings and splintings of their limbs and participated in physical and occupational therapy on a regular basis. By the age of 5 years, 85% were ambulatory and most were relatively or completely independent in their activities of daily living. Most children were in regular classrooms at the appropriate grade level.

17. Van Heest A, Waters PM, Simmons BP: Surgical treatment of arthrogryposis of the elbow. J Hand Surg [Am] 23:1063-1070, 1998.

Results of 18 tendon transfers for elbow flexion in 14 children with arthrogryposis with an average follow-up period of 4 years (range, 1 to 14 years) were reported. The 18 tendon transfers showed 9 triceps to biceps transfers in 9 arms (7 good, 1 fair, and 1 poor), 5 pectoralis to biceps transfers in 4 arms (1 good, 3 fair, and 1 poor), and 4 latissimus dorsi to biceps transfers in 3 arms (2 good and 2 fair).

Camptodactyly

Scott H. Kozin and Simon P. Kay

Camptodactyly is a painless flexion contracture of the proximal interphalangeal (PIP) joint that is usually gradually progressive.[11,33,39] Camptodactyly occurs without intra-articular or periarticular PIP joint swelling. The metacarpophalangeal (MCP) and distal interphalangeal (DIP) joints are not affected, although compensatory deformities may develop. The definition of camptodactyly has been divided to include a reducible or flexible form and an irreducible or fixed type, which creates disparity among reports.[18,21] Different treatment algorithms apply to flexible and fixed deformities.

INCIDENCE

Most cases of camptodactyly are sporadic. However, camptodactyly can be inherited and is considered an autosomal dominant trait with variable expressivity and incomplete penetrance.[39,41] Camptodactyly occurs in less than 1% of the population. Most cases are mild and asymptomatic and probably do not warrant evaluation (Fig. 43-12).[11,17]

Camptodactyly is bilateral in approximately two thirds of the cases, although the degree of contracture is usually not symmetrical. The fifth finger is most commonly involved.[5,33] Camptodactyly may affect other fingers, although the incidence decreases toward the radial side of the hand.

CLASSIFICATION

Camptodactyly has been divided into three categories (Table 43-1; Fig. 43-13).[4,33,40] A type I deformity is the most common form and becomes apparent during infancy. The deformity is usually an isolated finding and is limited to the fifth finger. This "congenital" form affects males and females equally. A type II deformity has similar clinical features, although they are not apparent until preadolescence. This "acquired" form of camptodactyly develops between the ages of 7 and 11 and affects girls more than boys.[17] This type of camptodactyly usually does not improve spontaneously and may progress to a severe flexion deformity.[8,11] A type III deformity is often a severe defor-

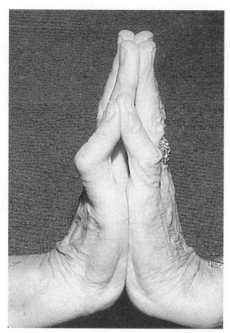

FIGURE 43-12. Bilateral untreated camptodactyly in an elderly woman. Her long-standing deformities were not bothersome to her.

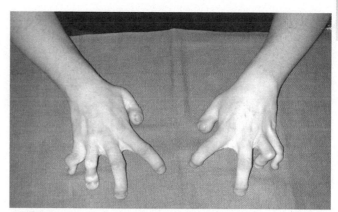

FIGURE 43-13. Severe bilateral hand camptodactyly in a 16-year-old boy with otopalatodigital syndrome.

mity that usually involves multiple digits of both extremities and is associated with a variety of syndromes. The extent of involvement between hands is often asymmetrical. This syndromic camptodactyly can occur in conjunction with craniofacial disorders, short stature, and chromosomal abnormalities (Table 43-2).[11,18,33]

PATHOPHYSIOLOGY

The precise etiology underlying camptodactyly remains unknown. There is no consensus about the pathogenesis of camptodactyly. Almost every structure about the PIP joint has been implicated as the primary cause or a contributing factor (Fig. 43-14).[8,19,21,27,39] Proposed skin and subcutaneous tissue changes include a deficiency or contracture within the dermis and fibrotic changes within the subcutaneous tissue and/or fascia.[22,36] Plausible periarticular alterations consist of contractures of the collateral ligaments and/or volar plate.[10] Possible musculotendinous anomalies involve abnor-

Table 43-1
CATEGORIES OF CAMPTODACTYLY

Type	Occurrence	Characteristics
I	Infant or congenital	Isolated finding and usually limited to the fifth finger
II	Preadolescence or acquired	Often does not improve spontaneously; may progress to a severe flexion deformity
III	Associated with a variety of syndromes	Usually involves multiple digits of both extremities

Table 43-2
GENERALIZED CONDITIONS ASSOCIATED WITH CAMPTODACTYLY

Craniofacial Disorders
Orofaciodigital syndrome
Craniocarpotarsal dystrophy (Freeman-Sheldon syndrome)
Oculodentodigital dysplasia

Chromosomal Disorders
Trisomy 13-15

Short Stature
Camptomelic dysplasia I
Mucopolysaccharidosis
Facial-digital-genital (Aarskog-Scott syndrome)

Others
Osteo-onychodysostosis (Turner-Kieser syndrome)
Cerebrohepatorenal (Zellweger's syndrome)
Jacob-Downey syndrome

malities of the flexor tendons, intrinsic muscles (lumbricals and/or interossei), and extensor apparatus.* Potential abnormalities in the restraining ligaments about the finger include anomalies of the transverse or oblique retinacular ligaments.[27] Plausible bone and joint deformities include atypical configurations of the PIP joint, specifically the head of the proximal phalanx and base of the middle phalanx.[30,36] Even an abnormality within the spinal cord at the eighth cervical and first thoracic nerve segments has been implicated as a potential cause of camptodactyly.[39]

The most prevailing anomalies associated with camptodactyly affect the flexor digitorum superficialis (FDS) and intrinsic musculature (lumbricals and interossei).[8,22,23,35,36,39] In camptodactyly, the FDS has been described as contracted, underdeveloped, or devoid of a functional muscle.[12,22,27,32,34,36,39] The tendon may originate from palmar fascia or the transverse carpal ligament instead of a muscle belly.[8,28,35,39] This abnormal musculotendinous architecture cannot

*See references 5, 16, 19, 20, 22, 23, 25-28, 35, and 39.

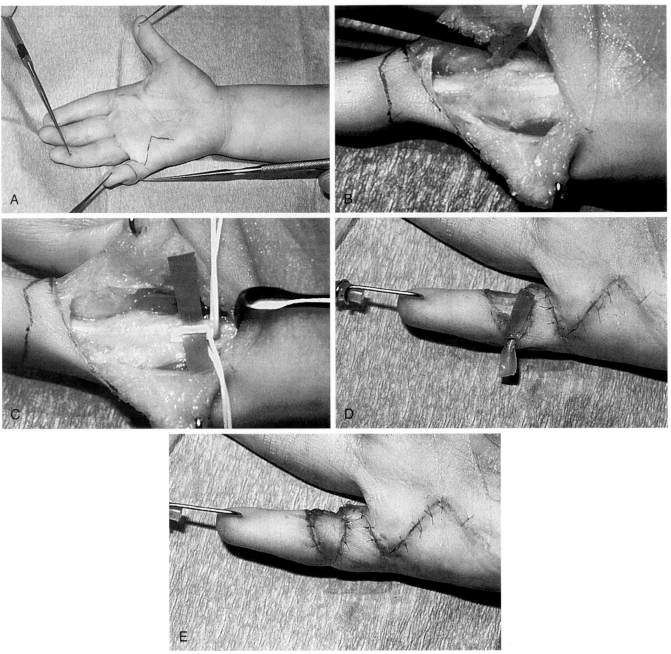

FIGURE 43-14. Surgical exploration of congenital camptodactyly of the small finger in a 4-year-old child. **A,** The extent of the flexion contracture and markings for the surgical incisions. **B,** Exploration revealed an abnormal lumbrical tendon, which has an insertion onto the flexor sheath that has been released. The lumbrical muscle has been released from its abnormal insertion, and retraction here shows a small atrophic tendon passing to the extensor surface. **C,** The flexor superficialis and the profundus tendons have now been explored. The flexor superficialis tendon was found to have no excursion proximally and was subsequently divided. **D,** Some release of contracture has been achieved by the two maneuvers shown in **B** and **C**. Now a tight ulnar band of palmar fascia restricts the joint extension. This is highlighted by the background material and, without magnification, may easily be confused with the digital neurovascular structures. **E,** The fascial hand has been divided, and the only remaining structure that is short and preventing full extension is the skin, which here is replaced with a full-thickness skin graft. This case serves to illustrate that in the established case of camptodactyly multiple structures and tissues may be abnormal.

elongate during the periods of rapid growth associated with infancy and adolescence, which creates a PIP joint flexion deformity.

An aberrant lumbrical muscle has also been implicated as the principal cause of camptodactyly.[18,22,23] In the normal hand, the typical insertion into the extensor apparatus was found in 60% to 72% of specimens, with an abnormal insertion recognized in 17% to 35%. Furthermore, up to 5% of specimens lacked the lumbrical muscle altogether.[2,9,24] In camptodactyly, the lumbrical may have an abnormal origin or insertion, although a constant anomaly has not been reported.[18,22,26] An abnormal origin has been reported from the transverse carpal ligament or from the ring flexor tendons.[26] Abnormal insertions are more common and include an attachment directly into the MCP joint capsule, onto the FDS, into the ring finger extensor apparatus, or within the lumbrical canal.[5,17,22,23] The deficiency of the lumbrical muscles leads to an intrinsic minus deformity, which may lead to camptodactyly. This notion is supported by examination of the active PIP joint extension with the MCP joint positioned in extension and flexion. In flexible camptodactyly, enhanced PIP joint extension during MCP joint flexion is often evident. This finding implies abnormal function of the intrinsic tendons and normal performance of the extrinsic tendons.[17]

Persistent PIP joint contracture will lead to secondary alterations in the surrounding structures. The palmar skin may appear to bowstring across the PIP joint, similar to a pterygium. Abnormal facial bands can form beneath the skin, and secondary changes in the bone and joint configuration of the PIP joint can develop in response to persistent joint flexion.[18,35,36,39]

DIAGNOSIS

The type I camptodactyly presents as a flexion deformity at birth or during infancy.[4,8,19] The type II or acquired form begins with a subtle deformity that is gradually progressive. The contracture often remains mild up to the age of 10, and this small amount of flexion may go unrecognized, which delays evaluation. During the adolescent growth spurt, the PIP flexion deformity may progress up to 90 degrees.[1,36,39] The PIP joint position can progress up until 20 years of age.[39] Pain is not a common complaint but rather the angulation and appearance of the finger area noted. The differential diagnosis includes other potential causes of a PIP joint flexion deformity that are often excluded by an astute history and thorough physical examination (Table 43-3; Fig. 43-15).[3,11,18,29,33,42]

The examination records the active and passive motion of the PIP joint. A flexible deformity is differentiated from a fixed flexion contracture. Active PIP joint flexion is uniformly preserved, and the child should be able to make a full fist. A fixed PIP joint flexion contracture implies shortening and thickening of the flexor tendon sheath, checkrein ligaments, and/or volar plate.[7] The amount of passive PIP joint extension is determined while varying the positions of wrist and MCP joint (Fig. 43-16). Flexion of the wrist and MCP joint can often increase the amount of passive PIP joint extension. This result implies tightness of the extrinsic flexor(s), principally the FDS.

The central slip tenodesis test is useful to determine the integrity of the central slip in a flexible deformity.[37] In a normal hand, simultaneous flexion of the wrist and MCP joints results in complete PIP joint extension. An extension lag during this maneuver infers central slip attenuation that may require augmentation at the time of surgery. Compensatory MCP joint hyperextension frequently develops in response to a PIP joint postured in flexion. Holding the MCP joint in flexion prohibits this abnormal posture. Full active PIP joint extension during MCP joint positioning implies hyperextension of the joint, to be a considerable part of the problem. This assessment is similar to the Bouvier's test for ulnar nerve palsy, which assesses the ability of the extrinsic extensors to achieve active PIP joint extension.[31]

Table 43-3
DIFFERENTIAL DIAGNOSIS OF CAMPTODACTYLY

Diagnosis	Distinguishing Feature
Pterygium syndrome	Multiple pterygia, usually includes the knee and elbow
Arthrogryposis	Multiple joint involvement, waxy skin and underdeveloped musculature, ulnar deviation of the digits
Symphalangism	No active or passive joint motion, absence of skin creases
Boutonnière	History of trauma and pain, joint swelling, reciprocal DIP joint hyperextension
Beals' syndrome	Congenital contractural arachnodactyly, kyphoscoliosis, external ear deformities, flexion contractures of the PIP joint, elbows, knees
Marfan's syndrome	Arachnodactyly without flexion contractures, loose ligaments, eye problems, dissecting aortic aneurysms
Juvenile palmar fibromatosis (mimics Dupuytren's disease)	MCP joint involvement, characteristic skin changes with nodules adherent to dermis
Trigger fingers	MCP joint involvement, palpable click on finger extension
Inflammatory arthritis	Widespread joint involvement, swelling about joints or tendons
Hypoplasia of the extensor tendons or "late extenders"	Usually multiple fingers, unable to fully extend the PIP joint of the involved finger(s), but passive motion is complete

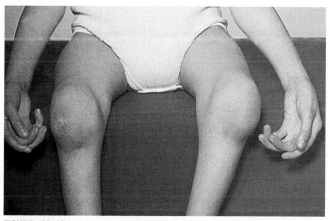

FIGURE 43-15. Beals' contractural arachnodactyly. In addition to the multiple-fingered camptodactyly in association with arachnodactyly there are multiple other joint abnormalities. This child was unable to walk, and the callosities in the knees reflect the fact that these had been his ambulatory weight-bearing surfaces.

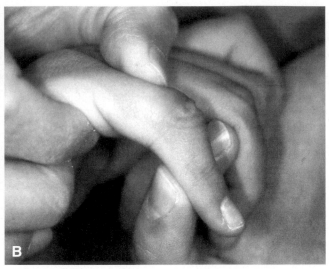

FIGURE 43-16. Amount of passive PIP joint extension is determined while varying the positions of the MCP joint. **A,** PIP joint extension with MCP joint extended. **B,** PIP joint extension with MCP joint flexed. (Courtesy of Shriners Hospitals for Children, Philadelphia.)

The function of the FDS and flexor digitorum profundus to the involved digit(s) must be assessed. The FDS of the small and ring digit can be interconnected (one third of individuals), which prohibits independent PIP joint flexion of the small finger.[36] Therefore, inability to flex the PIP joint of the small finger while holding the remaining digits in full extension may not imply absence of the FDS. The test should be repeated with liberation of the ring finger and similar assessment of active PIP joint flexion. An independent FDS to the small finger is a potential donor for tendon transfer. In contrast, an interconnected FDS must be separated from the ring finger at the time of surgery to be a suitable donor for transfer.

RADIOGRAPHY

Anteroposterior and lateral radiographs are performed to evaluate the PIP joint configuration and the status of the surrounding bones. The lateral radiograph is the most revealing view to assess abnormalities about the PIP joint (Fig. 43-17). In long-standing cases, the radiographs are abnormal with changes about the PIP joint secondary to the prolonged flexion deformity.[6,8,33,36] The proximal phalanx head will often lose its normal convexity and appear misshapen. The flexed middle phalanx base generates an indentation along the palmar neck of the proximal phalanx. The base of the middle phalanx often appears flat and may be subluxated in a palmar direction.

TREATMENT

Indications

Conservatism is the mainstay for treatment of mild camptodactyly. A contracture less than 30 to 40 degrees does not interfere with activity or create a functional handicap.[21,33,35,39] The patient and family should be instructed to accept the deformity and avoid surgical intervention. Static

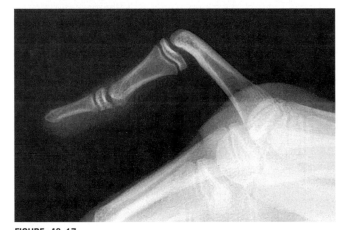

FIGURE 43-17. An 11-year-old child with camptodactyly of the small finger. Note the flattening (chisel shape) on the dorsum of the head of the proximal phalanx, as well as the flexion contracture and the abnormal molding of the base of the middle phalanx with distortion of the articular surface and epiphyseal plate.

splinting at night is recommended to prevent progression (Fig. 43-18).

No improvement or progression of the deformity occurs in 80% of individuals with camptodactyly.[8] Severe involvement hinders activities and warrants treatment, although restoration of full motion is not a realistic goal. Bony changes further downgrade the expectation after surgery.[18]

Nonoperative Treatment

A preliminary period of nonoperative treatment is almost always attempted to resolve or decrease any fixed flexion deformity.[4,15,27,35] Formal therapy is usually required and includes stretching, splinting (static and dynamic), and even serial casting. In infants, the splints must be forearm-based to fit adequately and to decrease the chances of removal.[18] The recommended duration of splint wear per day varies among investigators.[15,27,35] Hori and colleagues[15] used full-

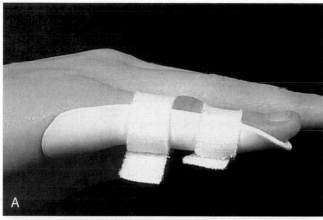

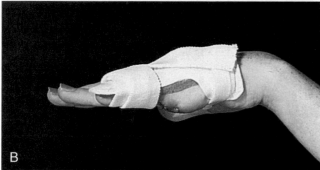

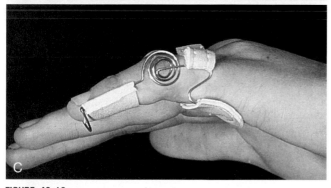

FIGURE 43-18. Splinting for camptodactyly. **A,** In well-corrected cases palmar gutter splints may be satisfactory and are worn at night for maintenance of correction. **B,** Dorsal splints involving the metacarpal area also may be useful in preoperative correction and postoperative maintenance, and in the younger child are more easily retained. **C,** For daytime use in the older compliant child, the standard Capener splint is of value.

time dynamic splinting for "a few months," followed by 8 hours per day after correction was achieved. Miura and colleagues[27] requested full-time splint wear but accepted 12 hours per day in young children. Benson and associates[4] encouraged 15 to 18 hours of splint wear per day in the young infant and 10 to 12 hours per day as the child grew. Irrespective of the initial splinting regimen, part-time splinting needs to be continued for a long period of time. Complete discontinuation of the splint should be delayed until skeletal maturity.[11,15,27]

Operative Treatment

Operative treatment is reserved for a severe deformity that has failed conservative management. Multiple procedures have been recommended. Proposed surgical treatment includes division of some or all offending agents, including fascia, skin, tendons, tendon sheath, capsule, and collateral ligaments[14,23,36,39]; reconstruction or augmentation of the extensor mechanism[17,36,39]; and bony procedures about the PIP joint.[10,30] A global approach that addresses all the potential causes and secondary deformities should be used (see Fig. 43-14).

Surgical Technique

The PIP joint can be approached using a palmar or midlateral incision, depending on the magnitude of the contracture and status of the skin.[17] Local skin rearrangement (e.g., "Z"-plasty) or a supplemental skin graft is required to allow complete PIP joint extension. A palmar longitudinal approach with "Z"-plasty lengthening is used for a mild to moderate flexion contracture.[18,22,36] A full-thickness skin graft is selected for a severe PIP joint contracture. The incision is extended into the palm to the level of the transverse carpal ligament in a zigzag fashion for complete exploration of the digit. Flexible camptodactyly without a fixed PIP joint flexion can be approached with a midlateral incision over the digit combined with a zigzag incision in the palm.

Deeper Dissection

The degree of the PIP joint contracture dictates the extent of release required. A graduated release is performed until adequate PIP joint extension is obtained. Any abnormal fascia and linear fibrous bands are released during exposure of the deeper structures.[18,36] Additional release of the flexor tendon sheath, FDS, checkrein ligaments, collateral ligaments, and palmar plate may be necessary to obtain satisfactory extension.[7,22]

The digit is explored for anomalous structures with detailed examination of the intrinsic muscles and FDS. Any anomalous origin or insertion of the lumbrical and/or interosseous muscle is resected (Fig. 43-19).[18,22,36] The lumbrical should be explored along its entire length to assess for any abnormality. Traction to an anomalous lumbrical muscle will not result in PIP joint extension. The lumbrical may insert into the MCP joint capsule, onto the FDS, or into the ring finger extensor apparatus. An anomalous palmar interosseous muscle can pass into the ring finger, although partial division of the intermetacarpal ligament may be required to completely assess its course.

The FDS is identified proximal to the first annular pulley. Traction is applied to the tendon in a proximal and distal direction to assess its excursion and insertion. Deficient proximal excursion with concomitant inability to flex the PIP joint indicates abnormalities of insertion. This requires release of the FDS through an A3 pulley window. Lack of distal excursion implies proximal pathology and requires excision of the FDS.

Tendon Transfer

Tendon transfer is used in adolescent camptodactyly that is unable to extend the PIP joint when the MCP joint is positioned in flexion. The presence of distal excursion in the FDS makes it suitable for transfer. The preoperative status of the FDS is taken into consideration. An independent FDS to the small finger is transferred without further dissection.

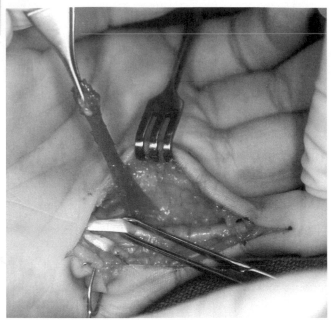

FIGURE 43-19. Resection of an anomalous lumbrical during camptodactyly reconstruction. (Courtesy of Shriners Hospitals for Children, Philadelphia.)

ligament, and into the palm. The tendon is passed through the lumbrical canal and is attached to the lateral band and central slip via a weave technique. The tendon is tensioned with the MCP joint positioned in 30 degrees of flexion and the PIP joint held in full extension.

When the FDS of the small finger is anomalous, a substitute donor for transfer is chosen. The FDS from the adjacent ring finger can also be harvested and passed into the small finger extensor apparatus. The extensor indicis proprius is another alternative.[13] In instances of multi-digit camptodactyly, numerous FDS tendons can be used as donors. The FDS can also be split and transferred into two adjacent digits.[38]

After tendon transfer(s), the skin is closed using a "Z"-plasty or application of a full-thickness skin graft. The arm is immobilized with the wrist in neutral, the MCP joints in 70 degrees of flexion, and the interphalangeal joints straight. Kirschner wire fixation of the PIP joint is controversial. Prolonged wire fixation can lead to loss of finger flexion and restricted grasp. In contrast, no internal fixation can foster early recurrence of the flexion deformity. The choice is usually made at the time of surgery and depends on the degree of preoperative PIP joint contracture and ease of obtaining extension. If Kirschner wire fixation is chosen, the duration is 2 to 3 weeks.

Postoperative Care

Three weeks after surgery, the cast is removed and a thermoplastic splint is fabricated with the wrist in neutral, the MCP joints in 70 degrees of flexion, and the interphalangeal joints straight. Another option is to employ an ulnar wristlet sling that maintains the MCP joint in flexion and encourages PIP joint extension (Fig. 43-21).[38] Therapy is initiated for scar management and tendon transfer train-

However, a dependent FDS must be separated from the ring finger to become a suitable donor for transfer. Failure to achieve independent function is a contraindication to transfer of the small finger FDS.

Transfer of the FDS to the extensor apparatus decreases the PIP joint flexion force and enhances PIP joint extension (Fig. 43-20).[18,22,39] The FDS is transected just distal to the PIP joint through a third annular pulley window and withdrawn into the palm proximal to the first annular pulley. The lateral band and central slip are isolated over the dorsum of the digit. A tendon passer is placed from dorsum of the finger into the lumbrical canal, beneath the intermetacarpal

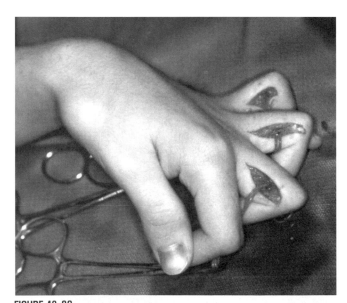

FIGURE 43-20. Transfer of the flexor digitorum superficialis tendons to the extensor apparatus for camptodactyly of the long, ring, and small fingers. (Courtesy of Shriners Hospitals for Children, Philadelphia.)

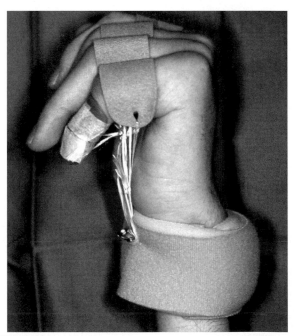

FIGURE 43-21. Ulnar wristlet sling to maintain the MCP joint in flexion and encourage PIP joint extension. (Courtesy of Shriners Hospitals for Children, Philadelphia.)

ing. Six weeks after surgery, light resistive strengthening is started. The splint is removed during the day except during strenuous activity. The splint is discontinued for all activity 12 weeks after surgery, and unrestricted activity is allowed. Prolonged night-time splinting is required to prevent recurrence.[27]

Salvage Procedures

Severe flexion deformity of the PIP joint with secondary bony changes is often not amenable to contracture release and tendon transfer. In these instances, bony realignment is the only method for correcting the excessive flexion. This correction can be made by a dorsal closing-wedge osteotomy of the proximal phalanx or a PIP joint fusion (chondrodesis or arthrodesis). The osteotomy corrects the posture of the finger and shifts the arc of motion. The overall amount of PIP joint motion remains unchanged, which results in loss of full flexion and impaired grasp.[30,33] A PIP joint chondrodesis or arthrodesis sacrifices all motion.

OUTCOME

Camptodactyly is difficult to treat, and inconsistent results have been reported. McCarroll[21] noted different preoperative findings among results after camptodactyly reconstruction. The most notable differences concerned the presence or absence of a fixed PIP joint flexion deformity and the amount of active extension of the PIP joint when the MCP joint is positioned in flexion.

Conservative treatment with splinting and passive stretching has resulted in an improvement in the amount of PIP joint contracture.[4,15,27,35] Formal therapy, a compliant patient, and prolonged diligent splinting are prerequisites. Superior results are obtained in a motivated patient with a mild deformity.[35] Hori and colleagues[15] reported on 24 patients (34 fingers) with small finger camptodactyly who were treated with a splinting regimen. The average follow-up time was almost 4 years. Twenty fingers had "almost" full extension, 9 had improved, 3 were unchanged, and 2 fingers were worse. The average flexion contracture improved from 40 to 10 degrees after treatment.

Benson and coworkers[4] treated 22 patients (59 digits) with a therapy program and reported their results at a mean follow-up of 33 months. Type I camptodactyly (13 patients or 24 PIP joints) improved from a 23-degree flexion contracture to 4 degrees shy of full extension. Type II camptodactyly (four patients or five PIP joints) were relatively noncompliant with therapy and achieved minimal correction. Type III camptodactyly (5 patients or 30 PIP joints) possessed a varied amount of deformity. Twelve PIP joints lacked at least 15 degrees of extension and improved to almost full extension.

Multiple surgical procedures have been reported for camptodactyly. Variable technique and disparate outcome confuse interpretation. Smith and Kaplan[39] performed an isolated FDS tenotomy. The flexion deformity decreased by at least 33% in all fingers without a concomitant loss in finger flexion strength. Jones and associates[17] reported on six patients who underwent FDS tenotomy combined with transfer of the tendon to the extensor apparatus. The residual

average PIP joint contracture averaged 15 degrees (range, 0 to 25 degrees) without mention of any sacrifice in flexion.

Engber and Flatt[8] analyzed the treatment of camptodactyly in 66 patients. Corrective and salvage types of surgery were performed on 24 hands. Twenty hands underwent release of the palmar structures with or without transfer of the FDS. Seven hands improved, 6 remained the same, and 7 worsened after surgery. Slightly better results were noted when the FDS was transferred. Four hands underwent osteotomy or arthrodesis to better align the finger.

Siegert and colleagues[35] reviewed 57 patients with camptodactyly. Multiple digit involvement was common. Thirty-eight fingers were treated with surgery, and 41 digits were treated by therapy. Fifty patients were available for follow-up examination 6 years after treatment. Surgery consisted of release of the contracted structures with or without transfer of the FDS. The results were classified according to the ultimate improvement in PIP joint extension without a simultaneous loss of flexion (Table 43-4). In the operative group, there were 25 poor, 6 fair, 7 good, and no excellent results. The overall improvement in extension was only 10 degrees, and 10 patients lost considerable flexion. An additional 6 patients developed ankylosis of the PIP joint. In the conservative group, there were 6 poor, 8 fair, 27 good, and no excellent results. Seigert and colleagues[35] concluded that camptodactyly is a "long-term and frustrating problem to both patient and doctor."

Ogino and Kato[28] treated 35 cases of camptodactyly over a 14-year period. Surgical treatment was performed on six patients after failure of conservative treatment. The FDS was hypoplastic in five without proximal continuity to its muscle belly. Preoperative active extension deficit averaged 71 degrees; active flexion averaged 93 degrees. At a mean follow-up of 27.5 months, active extension deficit improved to 23 degrees and flexion diminished to an average of 80 degrees. The amount of PIP joint flexion contracture reduced from a mean of 57.5 degrees to 16 degrees.

McFarlane and colleagues[22,23] are strong supporters of abnormalities within the intrinsic system as the principal

Table 43-4

CLASSIFICATION OF OUTCOME AFTER TREATMENT FOR CAMPTODACTYLY

Classification	Criteria
Excellent	Correction to full extension with less than 15 degrees loss of PIP joint flexion
Good	Correction to within 20 degrees of full PIP joint extension or more than 40 degrees of increase in PIP joint extension, with less than 30 degrees loss of flexion
Fair	Correction to within 40 degrees of full PIP joint extension or more than 20 degrees of increase in PIP joint extension, with less than 45 degrees of loss of flexion
Poor	Less than 20 degrees of improvement in PIP joint extension or less than 40 degrees of total PIP joint motion

Adapted from Siegert JJ, Cooney WP, Dobyns JH: Management of simple camptodactyly. J Hand Surg [Br] 15:181-189, 1990.

defect underlying camptodactyly. A series of 53 surgical patients were assessed for preoperative, operative, and postoperative data to evaluate the cause of deformity and results of treatment. An abnormal lumbrical muscle was found in all cases, and FDS anomalies were also found in nearly half the patients. These abnormalities were found to be interdependent, and each had an adverse effect on outcome. Overall, the PIP joint contracture improved from 49 degrees to 25 degrees. The return of finger flexion was protracted, and only 33% of the patients regained full flexion at 1 year. Positive predictors of outcome were a PIP joint contracture less than 45 degrees and independent FDS function.

Smith and Grobbelaar[36] assessed the surgical management of camptodactyly in 16 patients (18 fingers) followed for a mean of 2.8 years. A unified surgical approach was applied to the majority of patients with a graduated release of contracted structures and a thorough assessment for anomalous elements. The results were classified according to Siegert and colleagues[35] with inclusion of parameters for extension and flexion (see Table 43-4). Excellent or good results were reported in 15 fingers or 83% (6 excellent and 9 good). Two fingers were rated as fair, one was rated as poor, and these had preoperative bony deformities.

Koman and associates[19] reported on eight patients seen at birth with severe flexion deformities of multiple digits (27 fingers). This patient population is distinctly different from other reports of camptodactyly because many had associated anomalies. All patients underwent initial hand therapy and splinting. Surgery was performed on 6 children (20 digits) between 13 months and 8.5 years of age. Follow-up on all patients was longer than 2 years. Eight digits had surgery limited to the palmar aspect with release of the contracted structures and lengthening of the FDS. Twelve digits had surgery on the palmar side combined with reconstruction of the extensor mechanism on the dorsal surface. Reconstruction was performed by lateral band realignment and transfer of the FDS. No improvement was noted in the eight digits that underwent an isolated palmar approach. Ten of the 12 fingers that had a combined approach demonstrated less than 20 degrees of residual flexion deformity and a "functional" grasp and release.

COMPLICATIONS

Surgery for camptodactyly is fraught with complications, especially in severe fixed camptodactyly. Release of these rigid fingers can result in injury to the neurovascular structures from laceration, tension during extension of the digit, or subsequent scarring.[35] Skin slough is also more common in digits with considerable contracture. After skin loss, exposure of the tendon may require gallant techniques for coverage, such as a cross finger flap. These complications usually have a deleterious effect on outcome.

Loss of motion after surgery is a major concern. Release of the FDS can lead to scar formation within the flexor sheath. Immediate DIP motion prevents adhesion formation about the flexor digitorum profundus tendon and helps maintain motion.[18] A concomitant PIP joint release further increases the risk of loss of motion. Because lack of full extension is better tolerated than deficient flexion, early mobilization should be used to foster restoration of flex-

ion.[36] Despite early motion of the flexor digitorum profundus and PIP joint, return of flexion is slow and may take 6 to 12 months.[22] Even complete PIP joint ankylosis has been reported after camptodactyly reconstruction.[8,35] This complication is increased with attempts at remodeling the joint surface, which should be avoided.[8]

CRITICAL POINTS: CAMPTODACTYLY

- Camptodactyly is bilateral in approximately two thirds of cases, although the degree of contracture is usually not symmetrical. The fifth finger is most commonly involved.
- Camptodactyly may be diagnosed at birth, observed during preadolescence, or associated with a variety of syndromes.
- The pathogenesis of camptodactyly remains controversial, because almost every structure about the PIP joint has been implicated as the primary cause or a contributing factor. Most cases involve anomalous flexor digitorum superficialis and/or intrinsic musculature (lumbricals and interossei).
- Mild contracture less than 30 to 40 degrees does not interfere with activity and is treated conservatively.
- Severe involvement hinders activities and warrants surgery. A global approach that addresses all the potential causes and secondary deformities is recommended.
- The surgical results are inconsistent, especially in cases with secondary bony changes about the PIP joint.

ANNOTATED REFERENCES

8. Engber WD, Flatt AE: Camptodactyly: An analysis of sixty-six patients and twenty-four operations. J Hand Surg [Am] 2:216-224, 1977.

Analysis of the treatment of camptodactyly in 66 patients. Corrective and salvage types of surgery were performed on 24 hands. Twenty hands underwent release of the palmar structures with or without transfer of the FDS. Seven hands improved, 6 remained the same, and 7 worsened after surgery. Slightly better results were noted when the FDS was transferred. Four hands underwent osteotomy or arthrodesis to better align the finger.

22. McFarlane RM, Classen DA, Porte AM, Botz JS: The anatomy and treatment of camptodactyly of the small finger. J Hand Surg [Am] 17:35-44, 1992.

The authors are strong supporters of intrinsic system abnormalities as the principal defect underlying camptodactyly. A series of 53 surgical patients were assessed for preoperative, operative, and postoperative data to assess the cause of deformity and results of treatment. An abnormal lumbrical muscle was found in all cases, and FDS tendons were also found in nearly half the patients. These abnormalities were found to be interdependent, and each had an adverse effect on outcome. Overall, the PIP joint contracture improved from 49 degrees to 25 degrees. The return of finger flexion was protracted, and only 33% of the patients regained full flexion at 1 year. Positive predictors of outcome were a PIP joint contracture less than 45 degrees and independent FDS function.

35. Siegert JJ, Cooney WP, Dobyns JH: Management of simple camptodactyly. J Hand Surg [Br] 15:181-189, 1990.

Review of 57 patients with camptodactyly. Multiple digit involvement was common. Thirty-eight fingers were treated with surgery, and 41 digits were treated by therapy. Fifty patients were available for follow-up examination 6 years after treatment. Surgery consisted of release of the contracted structures with or without transfer of the FDS. The results were classified according to the ultimate improvement in PIP joint extension without a simultaneous loss of flexion. In the operative group, there were 25 poor, 6 fair, 7 good, and no excellent results. The overall improvement in extension was only 10 degrees, and 10 patients lost considerable flexion. An additional 6 patients developed ankylosis of the PIP joint. In the conservative group, there were 6 poor, 8 fair, 27 good, and no excellent results. The authors conclude that camptodactyly is a "long-term and frustrating problem to both patient and doctor."

The Contracted Clasped Thumb

John R. Griffin and Marybeth Ezaki

Congenital clasped thumb refers to a spectrum of thumb anomalies. The mild form is the simple clasped thumb secondary to absence or hypoplasia of the extensor mechanism. The moderate to severe form is more complex with additional finding(s) of joint contracture, collateral ligament abnormality, first web space contracture, and thenar muscle abnormality. Most are coupled with arthrogryposis or its associated syndromes. In this case, the extensor mechanism may have minimal or no abnormality.

The contracted clasped thumb is a common finding in arthrogryposis.[1,10,12,15] *Arthrogryposis,* a nondiagnostic term meaning stiff joints, includes a large constellation of disorders.[4,6] These include Freeman-Sheldon syndrome (whistling face syndrome), an autosomal dominant condition affecting the hands and feet with a characteristic facial appearance.[5,14,26] Clasped thumbs may also be associated with mental retardation and MASA syndrome, an X-linked syndrome of aphasia and abnormal gait.[2,12,16,19,21,24,29,39] Clasped thumb can also be seen with cleft palate and craniosynostosis, Waardenburg's syndrome, and other syndromes.[6,8,30]

Congenital fixed ulnar deviation and intrinsic tightness of the fingers is referred to as *windblown hand,* or *windswept hand*.[18] Clasped thumb and windblown fingers may occur either alone or together.[26,37] Other descriptive names for congenital clasped thumb include *pollex varus, adducted thumb, persistent thumb-clutched hand,* and the *thumb clasped hand*.[9,12,13,17,20,22,28,34]

CLASSIFICATION

The initial classifications attempted to subdivide into individual types and remain inclusive.[32,33] This scheme has not been useful in the clinical setting. A more practical approach has been proposed by McCarroll[25,26] and expanded by Mih.[27] A type I clasped thumb is usually supple and has absence or hypoplasia of the extensor mechanism. A type II clasped thumb is complex with additional findings of joint contracture, collateral ligament abnormality, first web space contracture, and thenar muscle abnormality. A type III clasped thumb is associated with arthrogryposis or its associated syndromes. In this case, the extensor mechanism may have minimal or no abnormality.

DIAGNOSIS

Congenital contracted clasped thumb is characterized by abnormal anatomy involving skin, extrinsic tendons, intrinsic musculature, and joints to a variable degree.[22] Congenital clasped thumb is a clinical rather than a radiographic diagnosis. Absence of full active extension at the metacarpophalangeal (MCP) joint characterizes all forms. The mildest form (type I) is due to absence of the extensor pollicis brevis (EPB). In this form, the thumb has normal motion at the interphalangeal (IP) and carpometacarpal (CMC) joints. A visible skin dimple often accompanies the absent EPB insertion. Stretching and splinting will often resolve any lack of passive MCP joint extension. The treatment of this type is detailed in an earlier section of this chapter.

As the degree of severity increases (types II and III), contracted clasped thumbs display further extrinsic tendon agenesis and/or tightness. The thumb/index finger web space and the volar skin along the flexor surface are insufficient. There is progressive thenar and adductor muscle contracture, which narrows the thumb/index finger web space and flexes the MCP joint flexion. Active thumb extension is always decreased, and passive range of motion deteriorates with increasing anomalies.

The contracted clasped thumb exists on a spectrum, with gradations in level of severity. It is useful to further subdivide contracted clasped thumb into three grades of anatomic deficiency: mild, moderate, and severe. In the mild type there is isolated extensor tendon agenesis. Passive thumb abduction and MCP joint extension is normal. Extension of the digits may also be compromised (Fig. 43-22).[25,26,41] The moderate form lacks full passive range of motion and has a combination of deficits: thumb MCP joint flexion contracture, skin deficiency, and joint abnormalities (Fig. 43-23). Passive extension at the MCP joint or abduction of the CMC joint is not possible. Passive IP joint extension is preserved. The severe clasped thumb lacks passive motion at the CMC, MCP, and IP joints (Fig. 43-24). These thumbs often demonstrate true thenar and adductor deficiency combined with extrinsic flexor tightness. Although there is a spectrum of moderate and severe clasped thumb, the characterization of the deformity is helpful in planning reconstruction and in anticipating outcome.

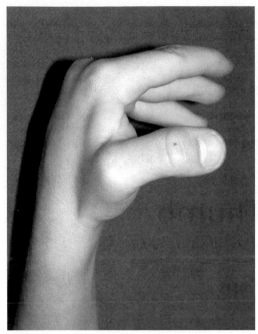

FIGURE 43-22. Mild form of contracted clasped thumb with absence of extensor pollicis brevis and common digital extensors as part of distal arthrogryposis.

TREATMENT

Goals and Timing

The primary treatment goal for the child with a clasped thumb is to restore the ability to grasp by bringing the thumb out of the palm. Repositioning the thumb will also enhance pinch and dexterity. Surgical procedures that have been effective in treatment of other conditions associated with contracture are incorporated in the reconstruction of the clasped thumb.*

Initial treatment should consist of frequent stretching and splinting to take advantage of the plasticity of the infant's skin. During this time, the components of the deformity can be assessed and a plan for additional treatment formulated. The reconstruction of a clasped thumb is an elective procedure and can await growth to minimize anesthetic risks and make the handling of the tissues easier.

There are four main components that require discrete treatment: (1) intrinsic muscle contracture and deficiency, (2) deficiency of the thumb skin and soft tissue envelope, (3) extrinsic tendon deficiencies, and (4) stiff and abnormal joints. Reconstruction should address each of these components at the initial surgical procedure.

Reconstructive Strategy

Skin Envelope

In contracted clasped thumb, the skin will need to be augmented. The surgeon must determine in which plane(s) the soft tissue is deficient (Fig. 43-25). Deficiency can involve the plane defined by the thumb and index metacarpals. This is seen as a thumb/index finger web space contracture. A separate component of the deficiency may involve the plane defined by the flexion arc of the thumb. Combined soft deficiencies involving both planes are most common.

The mild *isolated* thumb/index finger web space deficiency can be addressed with a four-flap Z-plasty that simultaneously deepens and widens the web space. This flap is only effective in those thumbs with no skin constraint on the palmar aspect because the Z-plasty shifts palmar skin

---

*See references 7, 11, 23, 27, 31, 35, 36, 38, 40, and 41.

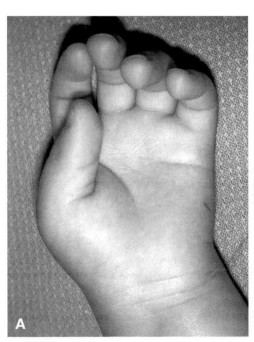
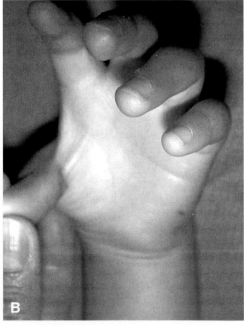

FIGURE 43-23. A and **B,** Moderate clasped thumb showing resting posture and deficiencies in skin and soft tissue envelope in thumb index web and thumb coronal plane.

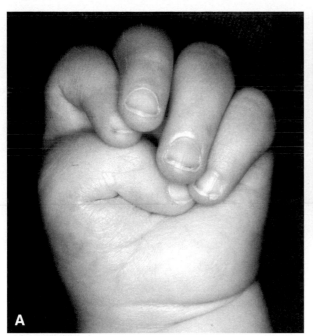

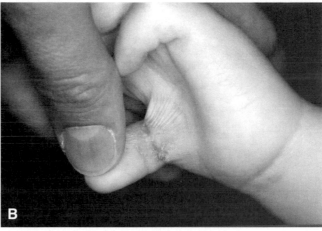

FIGURE 43-24. **A** and **B,** Severe clasped thumb with marked soft tissue deficiency in both thumb/index finger web and flexor aspect of thumb.

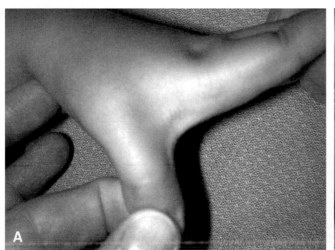

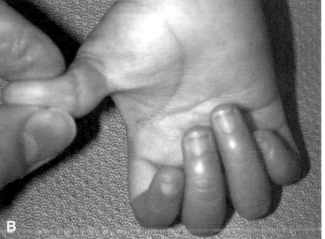

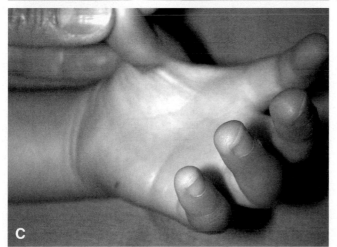

FIGURE 43-25. Primary planes of skin deficiency. **A,** Thumb/index finger web space deficiency. **B,** Thumb palmar or flexion plane deficiency. **C,** Deficiency in both thumb/index finger web and palmar aspect of thumb.

into the web, and this may exacerbate a palmar deficiency. If the skin is deficient in both planes, additional skin will need to be moved onto the palmar aspect of the thumb and into the thumb/index finger web space (see Figs. 43-23 and 43-24). This can be accomplished by local soft tissue rearrangement or by pedicled or free tissue transfer. Full-thickness skin grafts are less satisfactory over the palmar neurovascular structures at joint creases and should be avoided. Split-thickness skin grafts should not be used.

Intrinsic Muscles

Contracted thenar muscles pull the thumb ray across the palm. In addition, any intrinsic muscle that crosses the MCP joint causes flexion at that joint. The strategy that corrects this component incorporates function-sparing contracture releases performed in conditions such as spasticity and ischemic contractures (i.e., muscle origin slide). The skin incision to expose the taught muscles will also release the skin contracture and can be incorporated into planned soft tissue coverage. The tendons of insertion of the intrinsic muscles are left intact to minimize scarring about the MCP joint. The innervation is spared to preserve some function.

Extrinsic Tendons

Abnormalities in the extrinsic tendons include both contracture of the flexor pollicis longus and absence, hypoplasia, or attenuation of one or both extrinsic extensors. The function of flexor pollicis longus muscle varies widely from normal to absence with an atretic or adherent tendon. Preservation of some continuity of the tendon may be accomplished by a long "Z"-lengthening of the tendon in the forearm.

Preoperative assessment of tendons available for transfer is possible in the older child. Exploration of the tendons at the time of reconstruction will be more accurate in the infant. The common digital extensors and the extensor indicis proprius are often deficient in the child with the contracted clasped thumb and cannot be relied on for tendon transfer. Extensor digiti minimi may be available as an option to augment thumb extension (Fig. 43-26).

Joint Stability

The CMC joint is usually not a problem once the contracted muscles have been released. The MCP joint often will need tendon transfer for active extension or stabilization. Static stabilization of the MCP joint at a neutral position is difficult to achieve with soft tissue procedures and is best attained after sufficient ossification to allow a growth-sparing fusion (i.e., chondrodesis).

Surgical Treatment

The precise procedure selected depends on the severity of deformity. Each element of the contracted clasped thumb must be addressed at the time of surgery.

Intrinsic Muscle Contracture—Thenar Muscle Origin Release

Release of the origins of the thenar musculature from the transverse carpal ligament will bring the thumb metacarpal out of the plane of the hand (Fig. 43-27). The release is done stepwise through an incision that parallels the thenar crease. Access to both heads of the adductor pollicis as well as all

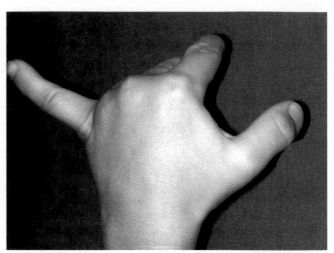

FIGURE 43-26. The extensor digiti minimi may be available for tendon transfer when the thumb and common digital extensors are absent.

the thenar musculature is possible through this approach. The palmar fascia and the fibrous origin of the thenar musculature are thickened. The palmar cutaneous branch of the median nerve and the thenar motor branch are identified and protected. The muscle origin of the short abductor muscle and the flexor pollicis brevis are carefully dissected from the transverse carpal ligament, leaving the ligament intact. The synovium and fibrous tunnel surrounding the flexor pollicis longus tendon mark the dorsal and radial limits of the superficial thenar muscle release. The deep fibers of the short flexor and opponens pollicis are reached by retracting the flexor pollicis longus tendon.

Distal to the motor branch of the median nerve, the radial digital nerve of the index finger is identified. The small motor branch to the index lumbrical muscle is protected as well. By ulnar retraction of the lumbrical, the transverse and oblique heads of the adductor pollicis are visualized. The fatty raphe between the two muscular heads contains the terminal branch of the ulnar nerve that innervates the adductor muscle and the deep palmar arch. These neurovascular structures should be identified and preserved.

While protecting the motor branch to the adductor with gentle retraction, the transverse head of the muscle is released from the periosteum of the third metacarpal with scissors. The maneuver is then repeated for the oblique head as well.

At this point, the thumb should demonstrate considerable improvement in passive abduction and extension at both the CMC and MCP joints. An advantage of thenar and adductor origins release includes preservation of MCP joint stability, because the muscle insertions are intact. Leaving the innervation intact also preserves some function because the muscles can function from their advanced origins. The skin defect within the palm can be covered with a transposed flap from the index finger, or it can be left open to heal by secondary intention.

Skin

Skin incisions are selected to allow access to the thumb, to release the skin contracture, and to prepare for insetting of donor tissue. Access to the thumb index web space may be

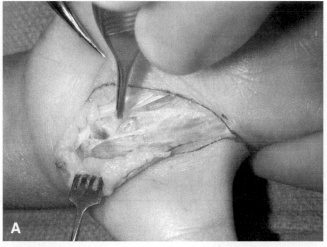

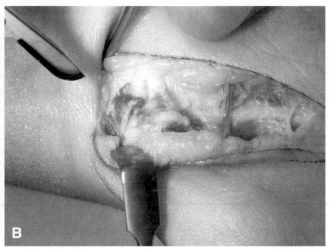

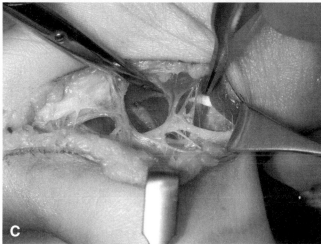

FIGURE 43-27. Release of the origins of the thenar musculature. **A,** Palmar incision and release of fascia. **B,** Release of muscle origin from transverse carpal ligament. Note preserved recurrent motor branch of median nerve. **C,** Exposure of both heads of adductor pollicis.

through a four-flap Z-plasty[3] or through a modified Z-plasty that incorporates a dorsoradial flap from the index finger. A releasing incision may also be needed on the palmar aspect of the thumb MCP joint.

For contracted clasped thumbs that have a single plane of skin web deficiency, standard single or four-flap Z-plasty is useful.[3] For the more typical thumbs with deficient skin in both planes, it is often possible to resurface both of these with a single rotational flap from the radial aspect of the index finger (Fig. 43-28). This flap effectively augments the first web contracture and allows radial abduction of the thumb. The donor defect is closed primarily. The flap is then rotated in a volar and proximal direction to resurface the skin deficiency in the thumb/index finger web or on the flexor aspect of the thumb.

Treatment of Extrinsic Tendon Deficiencies

Although a one-stage approach to the clasped thumb is optimal, it may be necessary to defer extrinsic extensor tendon reconstruction to a second stage. Release of contracture may be sufficient to bring the thumb out of the palm. Inspection of the extensor apparatus at the time of thenar and web release allows planning for later options, which may include joint chondrodesis.

Isolated absence of the EPB usually will not require tendon transfer, and thumb function is sufficient. Absence of

CRITICAL POINTS: CONTRACTED CLASPED THUMB

- The contracted clasped thumb is a common finding in arthrogryposis and may occur with windblown fingers.
- The thumb/index finger web space and the volar skin are insufficient. A thenar and adductor muscle contracture is present that narrows the thumb/index finger web space and flexes the MCP joint.
- The primary treatment goal for the clasped thumb is to restore the ability to grasp by bringing the thumb out of the palm.
- Initial treatment is frequent stretching and splinting.
- Surgery is usually required and must address each element of the problem: (1) intrinsic muscle contracture and deficiency, (2) deficiency of the thumb skin and soft tissue envelope, (3) extrinsic tendon deficiencies, and (4) stiff and abnormal joints.

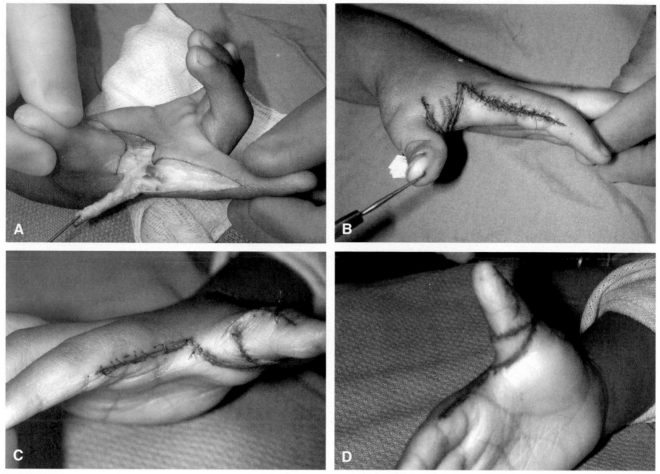

FIGURE 43-28. Dorsoradial rotation flap from index finger. **A,** Radial flap elevated before insetting into palmar defect. **B,** Radial flap donor site and rotation to palm. **C,** Radial flap transposed onto thumb. **D,** Radial flap covering palmar aspect of MCP joint.

both thumb extensors is best reconstructed with a tendon transfer. Transfer of the extensor indicis proprius is preferred. Alternatively, the extensor digiti minimi is more commonly present, although it may not be sufficiently robust. Transfer of the extensor digitorum communis (EDC) to the index finger combined with transfer of a slip of the index EDC to the adjacent long EDC is another option. Transfer of the flexor digitorum superficialis is another option. Anomalies of the flexor digitorum superficialis muscle, however, are common in arthrogryposis and its related conditions.

Treatment of MCP Joint Flexion Contracture

For the majority of clasped thumbs, release of the soft tissue contracture will allow MCP joint passive extension. If a tendon is available to transfer for extension, the joint may function adequately over time. Secondary contracture, however, results from lack of extension combined with growth. Symptomatic recalcitrant MCP joint flexion often requires chondrodesis or arthrodesis.

ANNOTATED REFERENCES

1. Bennett JB, Hansen PE, Granberry WM, Cain TE: Surgical management of arthrogryposis in the upper extremity. J Pediatr Orthop 5:281-286, 1985.

Twenty-five patients underwent 56 operative procedures to correct upper extremity deformities due to arthrogryposis multiplex congenita. Twenty procedures were performed on the thumb. Seven isolated thumb/web space deepening procedures without flap coverage were performed. Only one achieved a good result. Seven thumbs underwent web deepening, adductor release, and coverage. Four had good result with increased span of grasp. Six underwent similar procedures combined with MCP joint fusion. All six obtained stable thumbs with improved grasp. The article highlights a global approach to the contracted clasped thumb in arthrogryposis with attention to each part of the deformity.

32. Tsuyuguchi Y, Masada K, Kawabata H, et al: Congenital clasped thumb: A review of forty-three cases. J Hand Surg [Am] 10:613-618, 1985.

Forty-three patients (75 hands) with congenital clasped thumb were evaluated. Three groups were identified: group I, 14 patients (24 hands) without contracture; group II, 14 patients (21 hands) with contractures of the palmar side; and group III, 15 patients (30 hands) with arthrogryposis multiplex congenita. Forty-two hands were managed with splinting alone, 16 hands with surgery, and 17 hands without treatment. The mean follow-up was almost 3 years. All group I patients showed good response to splinting. In groups II and III, 10 patients (16 hands) with severe deformity without a response to splinting were treated by release of the palmar soft tissues, skin grafts, and reconstruction of the extensors. Satisfactory results were obtained in 12 of 16 hands.

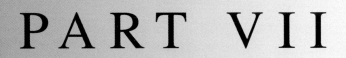

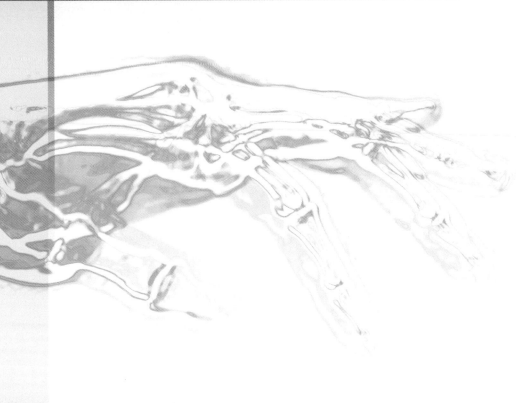

PART VII

Bone and Soft Tissue Reconstruction

CHAPTER 44

Principles of Microvascular Surgery

William C. Pederson

The term *microsurgery* was coined in a paper on experimental anastomosis of 1- to 2-mm vessels at the American College of Surgeons meeting in 1960 by Jacobson and Suarez.[209] The first clinical case of arm replantation was reported 3 years later by Chen and coworkers in the *Chinese Medical Journal*,[71] but this paper was not widely available outside China. Malt and McKhann reported two clinical cases of arm replantation in the *Journal of the American Medical Association* in 1964[266] (they performed the first case in 1962 but waited 2 years to publish it). Although Kleinert and colleagues proved the efficacy of digital vessel repair in their paper in the *Journal of Bone and Joint Surgery* as early as 1963,[231] it was not until 1968 that Komatsu and Tamai reported the first successful replantation of a completely amputated thumb in the English literature in *Plastic and Reconstructive Surgery*.[234] In 1969, Cobbett detailed the first successful toe-to-hand transfer in a human in the *Journal of Bone and Joint Surgery*.[81] The application of microsurgery to upper extremity reconstruction reached a pinnacle when Manktelow gave his paper on "Functioning Free Muscle Transfer" at the American Society for Surgery of the Hand meeting in 1982, which received an unprecedented standing ovation. It may not have been appreciated by the audience at the American College of Surgeons meeting in 1960, but Jacobson's presentation had changed the practice of hand surgery forever.

Microsurgery today cannot rightly be called a specialty, because the techniques it involves cross the boundaries of many surgical specialties—from obstetrics to otolaryngology. The variety of forums in which the early reports were presented attest to this fact in the application of microsurgery to the upper extremity. Nonetheless, sophisticated repair and reconstruction of the upper extremity is difficult, if not impossible, to accomplish without the application of knowledge gained from training in microsurgery. Many excellent hand surgeons do not consider themselves microsurgeons, yet they apply techniques learned in the microsurgery laboratory to areas as diverse as vascularized bone transfer and nerve repair. This chapter deals with the basic principles of microvascular surgery as applied to the hand and upper extremity.

BASIC MICROVASCULAR TECHNIQUES

To the uninitiated, the perceived difficulty in anastomosing vessels with a diameter of 1 mm or less is monumental. This feeling arises from frustration experienced during surgical procedures on small structures without the aid of magnification. In fact, anyone with reasonable technical ability can perform microsurgery, given three prerequisites: (1) suitable magnification, (2) appropriately sized instruments and suture material, and (3) initial training and subsequent practice to establish the hand-eye coordination and experience needed to handle delicate tissues, instruments, and sutures in a variety of laboratory and clinical situations. Although practice is essential, these techniques, once learned, should become more or less natural and can be applied in a number of ways to the practice of hand surgery.

Instrumentation

Magnification
Loupes

Magnifying loupes or surgical telescopes are widely used for magnification, and low-powered loupes are generally worn for most types of hand surgery. "Wide-field" versions are available from several manufacturers, and numerous combinations of magnification, focal length, depth, and size of field are available.

These can be mounted to glasses or headbands, and the wearer's eyeglass prescription can be ground into the lenses. In the wide-field versions, slightly higher magnification of 3.2× to 4.5× can be used comfortably, with working distances of 10 to 20 inches, depending on the surgeon's preference. For general use and to avoid neck pain, the usual

The author would like to acknowledge William F. Sanders, MD, for his contributions to the previous two editions of this chapter.

working distance is about 16 inches. A magnification of 2.5× is widely used by many hand surgeons, but those actively engaged in specific microsurgical techniques should consider having a pair with higher power (3.5× to 4.5×). These higher-power loupes (in the 4.5× range) are used by some microsurgeons for microneurovascular dissection and repair in areas in which the microscope may not comfortably reach (the axilla and brachial plexus, specifically). These higher-power loupes are much heavier than the lower-power ones and are usually much more comfortable mounted on a padded headband rather than eyeglasses.

Some microsurgeons now advocate the use of loupes for all microsurgery (including free tissue transfer),[341,364] but I believe that the microscope affords better visualization, particularly if an assistant is used. Experimental studies have confirmed that suture placement is more precise with the higher magnification afforded by a microscope.[338] Although loupes up to the range of 8× are available, I have found that the level of magnification coupled with unavoidable random head motion makes these extremely difficult to adjust to. Loupes cost in the range of $800 to $3000, but for the surgeon who does microsurgery on a routine basis the expense is easily justified (Fig. 44-1).

Operating Microscope

The operating microscope has evolved rapidly to keep pace with developments in the field of microsurgery; complex, tedious, and lengthy procedures demand an instrument that is "user-friendly" and versatile. Several manufacturers now produce top-quality instruments designed for extremity microsurgery to include the following essentials (Fig. 44-2A):

- A double-headed system allowing the surgeon and assistant to share the same operating field
- Foot-controlled magnification (zoom) and focusing
- Interchangeable eyepiece and objective lenses to match the working distance and magnification range to the clinical situation

- A fiberoptic light source (updated versions are available to provide constant illumination to the field as magnification changes)

Although not essential, motorized "X-Y" axis control is an extremely helpful and time-saving feature, especially during long procedures. This allows the surgeon to move the microscope over the operative field without moving the patient or having to look away from the field. Beam splitters for attachment of a third viewing post and/or photographic equipment are available. Cameras and color video systems can be attached and operated remotely; the latter is especially useful for teaching and for allowing the operating room personnel to observe the procedure (see Fig. 44-2B).

Both ceiling and floor mounts are available; however, floor-mounted microscopes are more versatile and have wider applications. The fact that the microscope can be rolled does not mean that it should be frequently moved from place to place, because it is a fragile instrument and is easily damaged. It is best to keep the microscope in the operating room in which it is primarily used, or at least close by. A handle (or handles) on the head of the microscope with covers that can be steam sterilized is very valuable to allow the surgeon to move the head of the scope out of the way during the procedure, if necessary. Covers should also be available for the knobs controlling the eyepiece adjustments. While some surgeons insist on placing a sterile cover over the microscope, I believe that this is unnecessary if handle covers are available. Placing a drape over the entire microscope takes time and makes use of the microscope cumbersome.

The hand surgeon using the microscope should be thoroughly familiar with the scope and its mechanics; it is surprising how poor an understanding most operating room personnel have of this type of equipment. Before any operative procedure, the workings of the microscope should be thoroughly examined by the operating surgeon. The status of the light source (is the bulb burned out?; are the cables

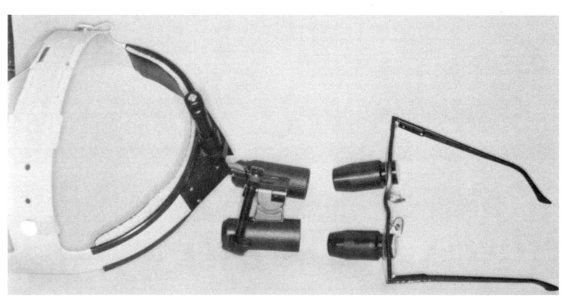

FIGURE 44-1. Surgical telescope. On the left is an adjustable 4.0× headband version. On the right is a pair of 4.5× loupes fixed to the surgeon's prescription eyeglasses. These units are expensive, but the adjustable type has the advantage of use by different members of the microsurgical team.

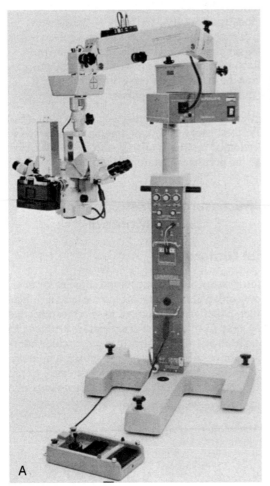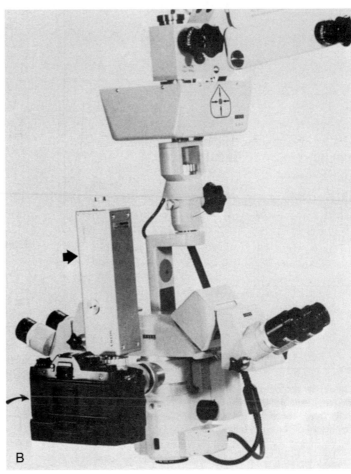

FIGURE 44-2. A, A Zeiss microscope with foot control of focus, zoom, and X-Y movement. Voice-operated controls are also available. **B,** Double heads for the surgeon and assistant, with eyepieces that can be inclined and attachments for video *(straight arrow)* and still photography *(curved arrow)* documentation, are optimum; simpler versions will suffice. (From Zeiss, Inc., with permission.)

broken?), the foot pedal (focus and zoom), and the suspension system must be checked before starting the operation. It is usually best to set the zoom at its lowest power and the focus to its midpoint. The counterbalancing system (if present) and the adjustments on the arm should be checked to make sure that the head of the microscope will stay in place over the operative field. Zeroing the diopter adjustment on the eyepieces and setting the width (interpupillary distance) of the binocular for the surgeon and assistant before starting will save intraoperative time. One does not want to discover that the microscope is nonfunctional after the hand has been dissected out and is ready for the microsurgical portion of the procedure.

Arm, Table, and Chair Positioning

As pointed out by Acland and others, the most important factors in avoiding fatigue, frustration, and tremor are positioning and comfort.[10,182] To that end, multiple (and often conflicting) recommendations have been made in the literature regarding types of seating, table design and height, and microscope design. In fact, they are all interrelated, and each surgeon must devise a system that matches his or her needs and personal desires to the clinical situation. This can be accomplished by experimentation and an understanding of equipment interrelations (Fig. 44-3). Another factor to con-

sider is tremor-inducing drugs such as caffeine and/or nicotine. It has been experimentally shown that caffeine increases random hand motion in individuals not used to its effects.[20] However, no correlation with increased hand motion was found in surgeons who routinely drink coffee. Thus, a surgeon who normally drinks coffee should not be affected adversely in the microsurgical arena by a usual morning cup (or two).

The most comfortable position for sitting for long periods is with the feet flat on the floor and the hips and knees at approximately right angles. The height of the chair is therefore determined by the habitus of the surgeon. Chairs with armrests and backs are available, and in protracted procedures (multiple digital replantations) these can decrease fatigue.

The most effective *working height* is one that places the surgeon's elbows at or near 90 degrees when the forearm and hands are supported to minimize tremor. This implies that the *table height* should be less than the *working height* by a distance equal to the table padding, drapes, and thickness of the extremity being operated on. A bit of experimentation will show that this leaves a relatively short distance between the thighs and the forearm in which to place the hand table. It should therefore be thin and free of large braces projecting downward, yet it must be very stable to

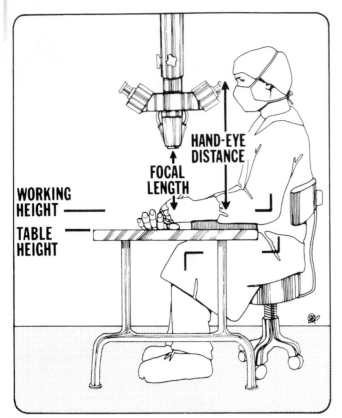

FIGURE 44-3. In the optimal situation, the surgeon is comfortably seated over a stable hand table. The comfort level of the surgeon depends on his or her own habitus, the focal length of the objective lens, and the height of the hand table, as described in the text.

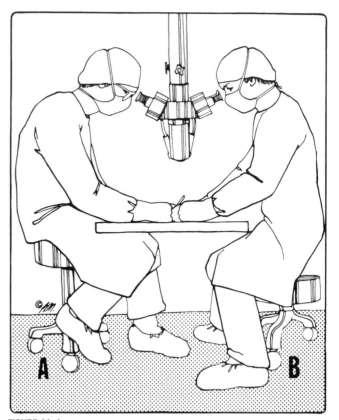

FIGURE 44-4. Incorrect position rapidly leads to fatigue, poor coordination, and poor results. In **A,** the chair is too high, causing back and arm strain; in **B,** the seat is too low and the arms are unsupported.

minimize vibration. I find that many of the standard, commercially available hand tables are not suitable for microvascular surgery for various reasons, including inadequate stability, too small a working surface, and inability to lower the table to an acceptable working height.

Once these factors are determined, the distance from the working height to the microscope eyepieces should be equal to the vertical distance from the surgeon's eyes to the hands (hand-eye distance). The surgeon can vary this distance by flexing or extending the spine from its most comfortable position or by bending the elbows; the former quickly leads to fatigue, but the latter is useful within a limited range (Fig. 44-4). If the hands are not in an optimal position or the area of anastomosis is elevated off the table, the hands and forearms should be supported with stacks of surgical towels or extra drapes. This is essential to prevent gross tremor from interfering with precision anastomosis. The level of tremor increases as the level of lack of support increases up the arm. An unsupported hand will lead to a relatively small tremor, whereas unsupported forearms will lead to a rather gross tremor.

The distance from working height to eyepieces can be varied easily in only two ways. First, if adjustable-incline (versus fixed-incline) eyepieces are available, the angle can be adjusted to meet the surgeon's eye level. Second, the focal length of the objective lens can be changed. There is a common misconception that focusing will vary this distance, but focusing merely places the objective lens at the correct distance above the working height. Selecting the

appropriate focal length objective lens will therefore place the eyepieces at the correct height.

Magnification is determined by the combination of objective lens, magnification changer, and eyepieces, as shown in the following formula:

$$Mt = Fb/Fo \times Me \times Mc$$

where Mt is total magnification, Fb is the objective tube focal length, Fo is the objective lens focal length, Me is the eyepiece magnification, and Mc is the magnification factor of the zoom apparatus.[24]

Various objective lens focal lengths are available, depending on the manufacturer; these range between 125 mm and 450 mm in most instances. I find a 175- to 250-mm objective lens most useful for hand surgery. Eyepieces of $10\times$ or $12.5\times$ are most commonly used, but $20\times$ eyepieces are occasionally needed for repair of small digital vessels in children and for microlymphatic surgery, even though this means a resultant decrease in field size. The size of the field is inversely proportional to magnification, and one should use the zoom control freely. Intimal inspection and suture placement are done under maximum magnification, whereas dissection and suture tying require less magnification and a wider field of view.

A few words of caution are necessary:

1. The working height can vary significantly between a digital vessel repair and a free flap anastomosis on an obese lower extremity, and this may require a change in

the objective lens. If one needs to have the head of the microscope farther from the operative field, an objective lens with a longer focal length should be utilized (i.e., 250 mm).

2. Contamination of the surgical field by contact with the microscope during use is more likely with a short focal length objective lens, and practice is required to avoid this problem.

3. Eyepieces on some microscopes have an annoying habit of "backing out" slightly from the eyepiece holder, leading to focusing difficulties. This is a common cause of calls to the repair service but is easily corrected by the surgeon. Always check to ensure that the eyepieces are firmly seated.

4. Most microscopes will remain in focus at all magnifications (parfocality), but only if the diopter setting of each eyepiece matches the surgeon's vision. The eyepieces of most modern microscopes are adjustable to any diopter setting. If the surgeon wears eyeglasses, it is a simple matter of setting the proper diopter adjustment on the eyepiece to match his or her correction. Alternatively, one's correction can be determined by an ophthalmologist or optometrist. Although not practical for all surgeons, the wearing of contact lenses rather than glasses will obviate this problem.

For further in-depth information regarding the field of microsurgery, the history and development of the microscope, and correction of problems arising with its use, the reader is referred to the pertinent literature.[10,62,208,305,308,355,386]

Microsurgical Instruments and Suture Material
Essential Features
A confusing array of instruments and supplies for microsurgery is now available, and choosing instruments is difficult for the beginner. Experience is required to select features that will be of value or to justify the cost of a special instrument. Essential features in all microsurgical instruments include fine tips to spread, hold, or cut delicate tissue and suture; a nonreflective surface; and comfortable handles that close easily to prevent fatigue.[305] Most microsurgeons learn with No. 3 and No. 5 jeweler's forceps and short scissors and needle holders. Many modern instruments are longer (16 to 18 cm) than in the past and counterbalanced. These are much easier to use than older, short instruments because they rest in the first web space and their increased weight is equalized by the counterbalancing. Likewise, many older instruments are flat, whereas many modern instruments have rounded handles. This rounding allows much more precise and easy manipulation of the instruments with the fingers, which are essential and frequent motions in microsurgery. I prefer the round instruments for clinical use for this reason. Combined and double-ended instruments may decrease operative time, but they require increased closing pressure and are cumbersome.[173,312] With experience, most microsurgery can be done with a surprisingly few instruments and most surgeons will become proficient with a reasonably small set (Fig. 44-5).

A dedicated storage and sterilization case to protect these delicate instruments during use and between cases is mandatory. Although some operating room purchasing agents may believe that the added expense of a case for microinstruments is not justified, this is unreasonable and can lead to rapid destruction of a several-thousand-dollar set of instruments if they are simply thrown in a standard instrument tray.

The best way to clean microinstruments is submersion for 30 minutes in a hemolytic enzyme solution (Hemosol). Saline solutions used in the operating suite will rust even resistant metals; water should therefore be used to rinse the instruments, and they should be dried completely before storage. Only specially trained operating room personnel

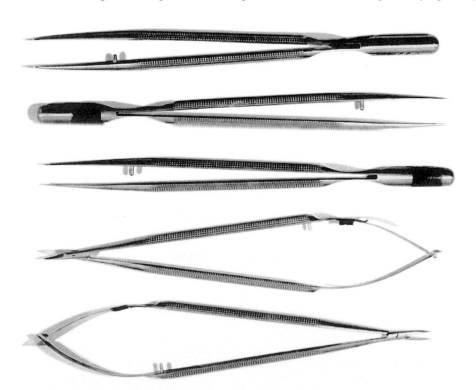

FIGURE 44-5. A simple, standard set of microsurgical instruments. These 18-cm-long instruments are well balanced and the handles are round for improved fine movement. From the top this set includes a dilator, two pairs of pickups, a pair of curved scissors, and a curved needle holder. Nearly every type of microsurgery can be performed with this simple set.

should clean and handle the instruments to prevent damage.[6,9] The cost of replacing several microinstruments after rough handling by inexperienced personnel is usually enough to convince operating room supervisors of the necessity to have the instruments handled by only a select group of people.

Forceps

Forceps of varying designs are always used during microsurgical procedures. Adventitia forceps having a small-toothed end are useful during the initial dissection of small vessels and nerves and for repair of tendons under loupe magnification. Smooth-tipped forceps are used the most in microsurgery and can range from a 1-mm wide tip to very fine tips for vessel dilation (Fig. 44-6). Only the tips meet, and they are easily damaged. Several pairs should be available, because frequent replacement is needed. As noted previously, I prefer the more modern instruments with longer, rounded handles to the short jeweler's forceps for clinical microsurgery.

Tying forceps have a broader grasping area and blunter tips than jeweler's forceps. These types of forceps are the most popular in use today. Whereas they may be utilized for dissection when grasping the vessel, there is a "tying platform" at the tips that affords an area to grasp the suture.

Scissors

Straight and curved scissors are available, both with blunt or sharp tips. Blunt, curved designs are most useful for dissection of vessels and nerves. Straight scissors are used for circumcision of adventitia and freshening the ends of vessels and nerves. Straight scissors with serrated blades for sectioning nerves are also available. A single pair of curved scissors with sharp tips can be used for most dissection and suture cutting, and one can safely perform most microsurgical techniques with this single pair of scissors (see Fig. 44-5).

Dilators

Dilators are available in several styles. Spring-type dilators are similar to forceps but have very fine externally polished jaws for dilation of the vessel end before anastomosis. They are especially useful once clamps have been applied to the vessel where the longer straight dilators cannot be used. These instruments have the finest tips of all microsurgical forceps and can come in handy for use as forceps when working on very small, fragile vessels (digital veins in a child) (see Fig. 44-6B). They must be used with care and will not adequately stabilize the needle without damaging their tips. They are easily bent and usually need to be frequently replaced, because repair of these instruments is difficult, if not impossible.

Straight constant-diameter (lacrimal) dilators can be used to relieve spasm occurring along a vessel, and tapering dilators are used to enlarge a vessel to correct size discrepancy. A set of coronary artery dilators is also useful in a complete set of microinstruments. These instruments have a blunt-ended tip, and the shaft can be bent to allow placement of the dilator in the vessel at unusual angles. Although they do not come in a size appropriate for the smallest vessel, they are very atraumatic and are useful for 2- to 3-mm vessels.

Small Fogarty catheters (in the 2-French range) can be used to dilate and clear thrombus from vessels of larger diameter proximal to the mid palm. This instrument should be inflated with air and not water, and great care must be taken to avoid damage to the intima of the vessel. One should be experienced in the use of Fogarty catheters before their application to microsurgery. Hydrostatic dilation is not recommended,[333] because it can cause severe damage to the vessel wall as a result of potential high pressures generated with a hand-held syringe.[318]

Clamps

To perform an anastomosis, blood flow through the vessel must be temporarily occluded. Vascular clamps accomplish this, and selection of the correct clamp is important to minimize damage to the vessel wall (Fig. 44-7). In general, clamps are divided into use on veins or arteries. Venous clamps require less closing pressure because of veins' thin walls, whereas arteries require slightly more force. Some companies have addressed this problem of different closing pressures by designing the jaws differently. In this instance, the venous clamp has a flat jaw all the way to the end. The arterial clamp, on the other hand, has a very small lip at

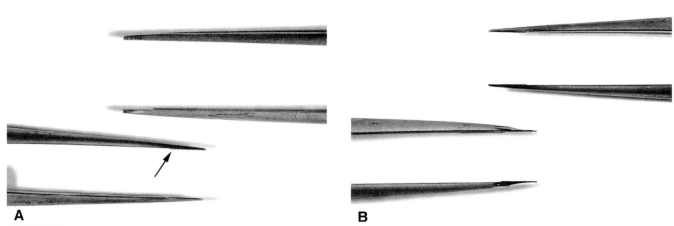

A   **B**

FIGURE 44-6. Types of microsurgical pickups. **A,** Standard pickups *(top)* and pickups with tying platform for grasping the suture *(arrow, bottom).* **B,** Pickups with tying platform *(top)* and dilators with delicate tips for placing inside vessels *(bottom).*

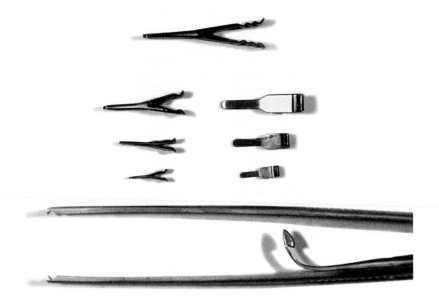

FIGURE 44-7. Various clamps for microsurgery. The larger clamp at top is applied with the fingers, and the smaller clamps below are applied with the instrument at the bottom.

its tip, which keeps the clamp from crushing the vessel wall (Fig. 44-8)

For very small vessels (in the 1-mm range), the closing pressure of the clamp should not exceed 30 g/mm[2].[387] Sets of clamps are available that match the closing pressure to the size of the vessel (0.3 to 0.9 mm, 20 to 30 g; 1.0 to 1.9 mm, 30 to 50 g; 2.0 to 4.0 mm, 70 to 90 g). A variable pressure clamp is also available,[300] but the closing pressure of this clamp is hard to "feel," and damage to the vessel is common. Less traumatic clamp design is important in achieving high patency rates.[107,198,371,373,387] Dual clamps allow tension-free approximation of the vessel edges before anastomosis.[7] The double clamp designed by Ikuta[201] is widely applicable to a number of vessels, from larger arteries (brachial) to small veins on the dorsum of the finger. This clamp has a spring-loaded adjustment that allows for adjustment of the closing pressure. It should be tightened just enough to keep the clamp from coming off the vessel. Single clamps are necessary where space is limited and in other special situations.[1] I believe that although double clamps do have a place, they are often cumbersome to use and get in the way. For this reason, I prefer whenever possible to use two single clamps placed on the vessels to be sewn.

Microsized rubber vessel loops are also available and useful in areas where clamp application is difficult, but these can cause difficulties in anastomosis of smaller vessels. The vessel loops are often placed too tightly around the vessel, which can lead to damage and/or significant spasm at the site of placement. Likewise, they tend to cause a "fluting" of the intima, which can make anastomosis very difficult. I prefer to use loops only as a backup device when larger vessels are used for anastomosis. Such a case would be the repair or anastomosis to the brachial artery, where vessels loops can be placed at a distance from the site of anastomosis.

It has recently been appreciated that the standard reusable microvascular clamps can have a marked increase in their closing pressure after simply undergoing steam sterilization.[132] This is probably lessened by placement of the clamps in an instrument oil soak or instrument "milk" before sterilization. This problem can be avoided by the use of disposable clamps. These are available in a number of sizes and configurations and have carefully controlled closing pressures.[413] The downside of these clamps is that they are relatively expensive, but they can be gas sterilized and used again if necessary.

Background

Thin sheets of plastic background material (available in several colors) are used by some surgeons to enhance the surgeon's view of the vessel and sutures and to isolate the vessel from the surrounding tissue and blood. Models with a mechanism for suction incorporated into the sheets have been introduced. Background material, improperly placed, can be more trouble than it is worth, however. If background is used, it should be helpful and not a hindrance. The smallest piece that will help visualization should be used, but it should be cut so that the edges do not interfere with tying of the sutures. Background that is poorly trimmed and thoughtlessly placed often leads to the vessel's lying in a pool of blood in the background with edges that stick up and

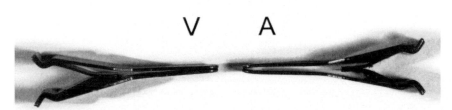

V   A

FIGURE 44-8. A venous and arterial clamp. The venous clamp (V) is flat all the way to the tip of the clamp. The arterial clamp (A) has a slight lip on the end of the clamp that prevents crushing the thicker arterial wall. While a venous clamp will occlude an artery, it may crush the vessel. On the other hand, the arterial clamp will not hold a vein.

make tying the suture difficult. I prefer to avoid its use whenever possible.

Irrigation

Frequent irrigation of the vessel with heparinized saline or lactated Ringer's is necessary during anastomosis to remove small clots and visualize the lumen. Although lactated Ringer's appears to be the least damaging to the vessel experimentally, heparinized solutions are more commonly used and may prevent sticking of the suture to the tissue.[11,52,253,275,330,368] Continuous irrigation systems are available that utilize a pressure pump over a bag of heparinized saline with an irrigating tip.[61] These systems have a simple button valve in the handle and allow the placement of a gentle flow of heparinized saline with a touch of the button. This prevents the need for changing syringes when empty. The tip of the irrigating device should be smooth and blunt, and several commercial types are available (see Fig. 44-9A).[124] I prefer to irrigate with a 3- to 5-mL syringe and a 24-gauge Angiocath. This (or any) irrigation tip should probably never be placed in the lumen of the vessel, because damage to the intima can result.

Other syringes and tips should be available for irrigation of the vessel with lidocaine or other pharmacologic substances to decrease spasm. Once the vascular anastomoses are complete, warming the digit or flap can be helpful. Solutions for this purpose can be kept warm in an inexpensive plastic thermos bottle, which can be gas sterilized for this purpose (see Fig. 44-9B). Warm solution should *never* be placed on tissue without blood flow (an amputated digit or flap), because warmth increases metabolic demand and can decrease the tolerance to ischemia.

Needle Holders

Needle holders are available with straight or curved tips, and a simple, curved nonlocking needle holder will be most often used. Special designs with tips in various planes relative to the handle are helpful in performing end-to-side anastomoses and in difficult situations encountered in free tissue transfer. As noted previously, a needle holder that has rounded handles and is longer allows more precise balance and utilization. Although some surgeons prefer locking needle holders, these instruments have little place in microneurovascular surgery. The force necessary to lock and unlock the instrument can cause significant damage to the vessel if the needle is in place in the vessel wall. Some needle holders are available with "concavo-convex" jaws, which have a slight curvature in the plane in which the needle is grasped. This causes a curved needle to "snap" into the correct position when it is grasped and avoids straightening

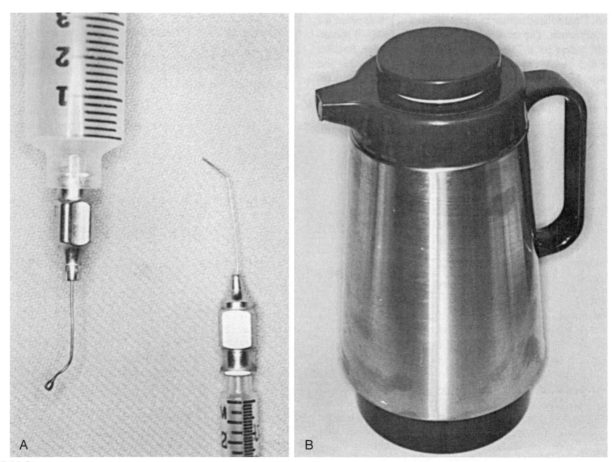

FIGURE 44-9.   Irrigation. **A,** A large syringe and blunt tip for heparinized Ringer's solution is shown on the left; on the right there is a modified 30-gauge needle and tuberculin syringe for lidocaine irrigation. **B,** Gas-sterilized thermos for maintaining warmed irrigating solutions.

of the needle when grasped. A needle holder designed by Dr. Marko Godina is available that has a cutting surface on the proximal surface of the jaws. This is intended to allow a surgeon without assistance to cut his or her own sutures, but in practice this instrument becomes dull quickly and only cuts sutures with difficulty.

The choice of needle holder is usually based on the size of the needle utilized. Some "standard" microsurgical needle holders are too large to use a 50-mm needle, and an instrument with smaller tips will be necessary. Most experienced microsurgeons will become accustomed to a single needle holder, however, and find it useful for nearly all anastomoses.

Accessory Instruments

Several other types of instruments are helpful, including (1) small vascular hemoclips for clamping vessel branches during initial dissection, (2) a bipolar coagulator with both standard and microtips, (3) small absorbent cellulose sponges ("eye" sponges) for removing blood and irrigation fluid from the field, and (4) an instrument demagnetizing coil, which is necessary to prevent attraction of the needle and suture to the instruments.

Suction is occasionally helpful, but it must be used with extreme caution to prevent damage to vessels, suture, and surrounding structures.

Suture ligation is safe at any distance from the parent vessel, and bipolar coagulation is safe as close as 2 mm.[309] Although widely used clinically, hemoclips have a high experimental failure rate as a result of loosening.[78] If used on an appropriately sized branch, however, this is usually not a problem. The time they save over suture-ligating small vessels is usually worth the small risk of their coming loose, however.

Sutures

Microsuture is available from several manufacturers in multiple combinations of material, suture size, and needle configuration. Unsterilized suture for laboratory use can be obtained at less expense. The most widely used suture is 9-0 monofilament nylon on a 100-μm curved needle. Whereas straight needles have been used in the past, they are rarely used today. This suture-needle combination can be used for almost all free tissue transfers and many microneurovascular repairs in the hand. Repair of digital vessels usually requires the use of a smaller suture-needle combination, such as 10-0 nylon in the 75-μm range.

Smaller suture and needle combinations (10-0 and 11-0 on 30-μm and 50-μm needles) are available, but frankly these smaller needles are so fragile that only the most experienced microsurgeons using the very best instruments can avoid damaging the needle on the first throw. The consideration of suture-needle size combination is an important one, because a "large" 130-μm needle is roughly four times the size of a 9-0 suture (which is 35 μm in diameter). Use of a 10-0 suture (25 μm diameter) with a needle of this size is irrational, because the suture has to "plug" a needle hole that is five times larger. For this reason, the smaller needles should be used with smaller sutures, but the smallest needle practical for the average microsurgeon is in the 75-μm range. For repair of larger vessels and nerves, larger combinations are available (Fig. 44-10A).

Microsurgical needles either are tapered or have cutting edges only at the tip to prevent damage to the fragile vessel wall. Needles are designated as straight or curved, by wire diameter in microns, and by chord length (see Fig. 44-10B).

The most common suture material utilized in microsurgery is nylon, which has appropriate characteristics in terms of reactivity and knot-holding ability. Polypropylene

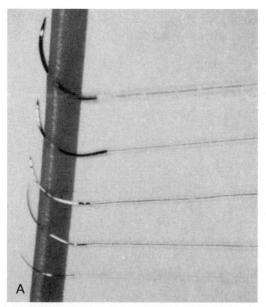
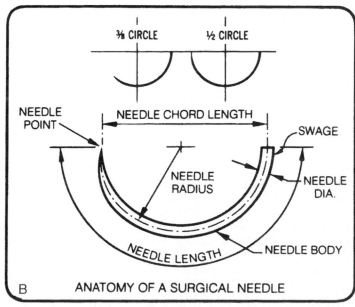

FIGURE 44-10. **A,** Suture material *(top to bottom):* 9-0 nylon, 130-μm needle; 10-0 nylon, 100-μm needle; 10-0 nylon, 75-μm needle; 10-0 nylon, 50-μm needle; 11-0 nylon, 30-μm needle. **B,** Microsurgical needles are designated by diameter and chord length. (Courtesy of Ethicon, Inc.)

is preferred by macrovascular surgeons, because it has excellent tissue reactivity characteristics and slides through the vessel wall very easily. This makes running anastomoses easier as the suture does not bind to the tissue. Polypropylene is available in 9-0 and 10-0 suture for microsurgery, but at this size it loses some of its desirable characteristics. It has a tendency to fray and stretch more than nylon, but it does offer advantages if used with care for continuous-sutured anastomoses.

Laboratory

Microsurgery cannot be learned without a practice laboratory.[150] The surgeon who is forced to do so alone will have to acquire a microscope, instruments, laboratory space, animal models, and someone to care for them.[100] Many hospitals have older operating microscopes suitable for animal use that are sitting about unused. Drug companies, veterinary schools, research facilities, and medical schools may have laboratory space and animal care facilities. A mini-laboratory may be constructed in the office or home.[378] In some cases, a microsurgical laboratory may be already in operation, and permission can usually be obtained to use the facility. Physicians trained in microsurgical techniques may be willing to instruct the neophyte and may have access to practice facilities. Several basic laboratory manuals have been published.[10,16,29,30,64,356] Many of these are out of print but should be available in a complete medical library.

Almost all training programs in hand surgery have access to a microsurgical laboratory, as do most orthopedic and plastic surgical residencies. If a surgeon has had little exposure to microsurgery in his or her training and desires to become competent in microsurgical techniques, the best way to begin is to register for one of the many short, intensive training programs offered.[17] These vary in length from a few days to a few weeks and have many advantages. Everything needed is provided, there are few outside distractions, and "one-to-one" instruction is available so that good habits and techniques are learned from the start. The student also has the opportunity to observe the setup of the laboratory, which will facilitate organizing his or her own laboratory for continued maintenance and improvement of acquired skills. Merely taking a 2-week course in technique does not make one a competent microsurgeon, however. Regardless of one's technical expertise, the techniques of microneurovascular surgery are the easy part. A surgeon should not undertake complex microsurgical reconstruction in the upper extremity "solo" without some experience gained during residency or fellowship.

The first step is to become familiar with the microscope and to adjust the table, chair, and microscope to the surgeon's individual comfort. For those with refractive errors, the eyepieces can be set so that glasses are not needed. In clinical practice, however, those who require glasses should consider wearing them, because manipulating objects out of the field of the microscope can be difficult. I find that removal of the protective eye cups provides a much wider field of vision; they can be replaced after use to protect the eyepieces. The interpupillary distance is adjusted, and coordinated use of zoom, focus, and "X-Y" axis control is then mastered. It is important to adjust the microscope so that it remains parfocal (in focus throughout the entire magnification range) according to the manufacturer's instructions. Once comfortable with the microscope, the student should practice holding and manipulating the instruments without tremor and then master the handling of fine suture material. This is an important step that if well learned will make later exercises much easier. Acland and others have described the intricacies in minute detail, and these references should be read carefully.[5,10,29] For the sake of brevity, they are not reproduced here. Once these are learned, the student is ready for a nonanimal model.

Nonanimal Models. The initial exercise is to suture a slit in a thin piece of rubber or latex. These practice cards can be constructed easily or bought commercially.[23,29,31,247] A nonsterile rubber glove stretched over a Petri dish makes a convenient and cheap model to practice on initially.

A fresh leaf can also be used in a similar manner. It is friable and nonelastic, and technical errors will become readily apparent. This model best demonstrates the tissue damage produced by crude technique.[29,223] Small silicone tubing can be used to simulate vessel anastomosis, and umbilical vessels, easily obtained from obstetric or pathology departments, are a challenging model.[146,277] One company produces a "practice rat," which consists of a silicone tube partially embedded in a soft rubber compound. This allows the student to practice dissecting the vessel from the surrounding tissue and is more lifelike than a loose piece of tubing. I have found this device to be very helpful in training residents on the rudiments of microsurgical technique. One center uses cold-stored vessels harvested from animals used in other experiments after they have been sacrificed.[228] Although not applicable to all microsurgical laboratories, this approach gives the closest approximation to practicing on live animals.

With the ongoing problems related to animal research, attempts have been made to utilize virtual reality simulation for the teaching of microsurgery.[57,240] These simulators at present are problematic and are very expensive. Most teaching programs now utilize nonanimal models of anastomosis until the student is quite facile with the standard technique of microsurgery, which reduces the number of animals necessary to gain the requisite skill.[102,118,195,283] To date, however, there is no replacement for experience gained from live animal microsurgery if one is going to extrapolate that experience to patients.[259,283]

Animal Models. After familiarization with the microscope, instruments, and basic techniques, arterial and venous anastomosis and neurorrhaphy are then learned on animal models. Several are available, with the rat being most widely used for study of basic techniques in the United States.[113,147,320] The rat femoral and carotid arteriovenous systems are easily accessible with the animal anesthetized and held supine to a board. These vessels approximate the size and consistency of digital vessels in the human. Rats are relatively inexpensive and easy to maintain and should be housed in an approved animal care institution. Many techniques can be practiced and refined in rats, including end-to-end and end-to-side anastomosis and dealing with size discrepancy in vessels.[97,158,161,170] The rabbit ear has been used as a model for digit revascularization and replantation,[160]

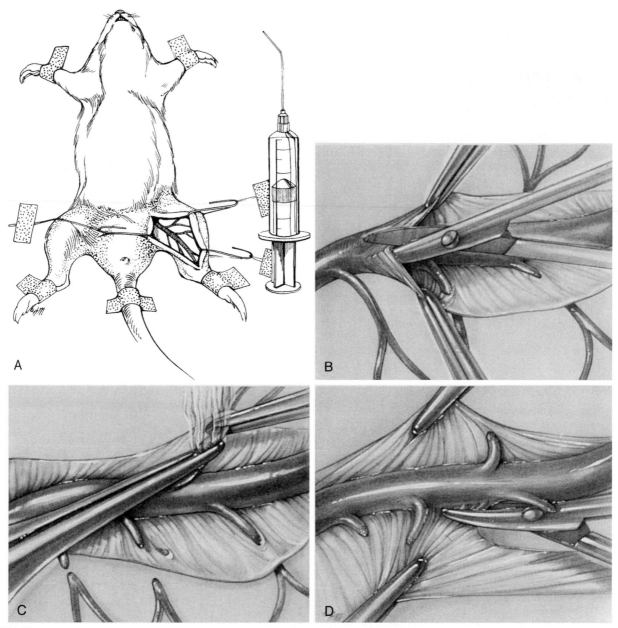

FIGURE 44-11. Animal preparation (rat femoral vessels). **A,** Nembutal (50 mg/mL) is administered intraperitoneally (0.6 to 1.0 mL/100 g body weight). The groin is shaved with clippers, and the animal is taped on a board with all four legs secured. The skin is prepped with povidone-iodine and the groin incised longitudinally. Sutures or bent paper clips secured to the board with tape can be used to provide self-retaining skin retractors. Blunt dissection can be used through the fat layer. The irrigation setup uses a blunt-tipped needle and heparinized Ringer's lactate (200 U/mL). **B,** After dissecting through the fat layer, the adventitia is sharply divided using traction-countertraction and blunt-nosed scissors, keeping close to the femoral artery. **C,** Branches of the artery are cauterized with the bipolar coagulator. Large branches should be cauterized and divided several millimeters from the main vessel, whereas smaller vessels can be transected close to the main vessel. **D,** The artery is dissected from surrounding tissue by pulling the adjacent tissue slightly and sharply cutting with scissors close to the artery. The artery is supported by surrounding tissue; the wall of the artery is never grasped directly with forceps. The basic principles of microdissection include traction and countertraction to place moderate tension on the structure and then sharp dissection of the layers under direct visualization.

and the rabbit femoral and superficial epigastric systems are also used in many laboratories for practice purposes. Larger animals (cats, dogs, and primates) are useful for research in free tissue transfer. These larger animals (particularly dogs) allow practice in more clinically applicable techniques, such as free transfer of soft tissue and bone flaps.[359]

The exact mechanics for animal model anesthesia and preparation are beyond the scope of this chapter, because some attention to detail is required to ensure survival during the procedure. The most complete description of these techniques is by Seaber.[354] Several laboratory manuals also include abbreviated descriptions of animal models.[10,29,30,64]

Basic Techniques

Essentials for a Patent Anastomosis

CRITICAL POINTS: PARAMETERS FOR SUCCESS IN MICROSURGERY

- You must be in a comfortable position.
- Arms, forearms, and hands must be adequately supported.
- Height of chair and height of microscope should be set for comfort.
- Vessels should be out of zone of injury.
- Vessel to be sewn should be under no tension.
- Take your time to do it right the first time; don't be in a hurry.

Once the animal has been prepared and the vascular structures have been exposed, the microscope is then positioned. There are several essential requirements to ensure an anastomosis with long-term patency, whether in the laboratory or clinical situation:

1. Atraumatic dissection and handling of the vessel must be meticulous, with tying or coagulation of branches as necessary.
2. The vessel wall and intima at the site of anastomosis must be normal when visualized under high-power magnification; if not, it is imperative that the vessel be resected back to normal tissue.
3. Adequate flow must then be demonstrated from the proximal vessel.
4. The anastomosis must be performed without tension, and vessel mobilization or grafting may be needed to ensure a tension-free anastomosis. The incidence of early and late failure is increased by tension on the anastomosis.[407]
5. Meticulous attention to detail is required in completing the anastomosis. Adequate removal of local overhanging adventitia (which is intensely thrombogenic),[76] followed by suture placement, without grasping the intima, to produce a nearly leak-proof anastomosis is required. The most common technical error is inadvertent suturing of the back wall, and this may be prevented by several techniques described later in this chapter.

Figure 44-11 illustrates these principles in the preparation of rat femoral vessels.

End-to-End Anastomosis Technique

Once the vessel has been prepared and adequate proximal flow ensured, the anastomosis is performed. Overzealous "cleaning" of adventitia is to be avoided, because this weakens the vessel at the anastomotic site and can lead to false aneurysm formation.[109] Only enough adventitia should be removed so that it is not an impediment to suturing the vessel and cannot get caught in the lumen. If proximal flow is impaired, gentle dilatation with a lacrimal dilator and application of local vasodilating agents (lidocaine and the like) may improve flow. Allowing the vessels to

CRITICAL POINTS: PLACING THE SUTURE IN THE VESSEL

- Clear the tail of the suture away from you.
- The needle should be perpendicular to the jaws of the needle holder.
- The needle should enter the vessel wall perpendicular to the axis of the vessel wall.
- The needle is passed through the vessel wall with a push down and roll movement.
- Don't pull up on the needle as it passes through the vessel wall.
- Follow the curve of the needle as it is pulled out of the vessel wall.
- The second pass (from inside out) is similar to the first.
- Make sure you have included the intima, then pass the needle.
  - Work perpendicular to the vessel wall.
  - Push and roll; do not pull up.
  - Follow the curve of the needle as you pull it through.

rest undisturbed for several minutes and warming of the tissue may also aid in decreasing spasm. The basic anastomosis procedure described next is a summation of the techniques most widely recommended by several noted authors.[10,29,56,64,172,184,308,309,356]

The clamps are adjusted so that no tension exists on the anastomosis site (Fig. 44-12A-C). The artery is divided cleanly, and the adventitia is trimmed (see Fig. 44-12D-F). The lumen is gently dilated (see Fig. 44-12G and H). Overzealous dilation is to be avoided, because this can damage the fragile vessel wall. The vessel is now ready for anastomosis (Fig. 44-13). Only the adventitia is picked up in the forceps, and the sutures are placed atraumatically. Intraluminal counterpressure with the forceps is useful, but the intima and vessel edge should never be grasped with the forceps.

Corner sutures 120 to 180 degrees apart (Fig. 44-14A) are first placed. In arteries, the suture bite should be one to two times the thickness of the vessel wall. In veins, a width of two to three times the wall thickness is used (Fig. 44-15A). One of the most common mistakes made early on is to approach the vessel wall with the needle tip parallel to the vessel wall. If the needle is placed with the tangent of the tip of the needle at anything less than 90 degrees to the vessel wall, inversion with exposure of the adventitial surface to the flow of blood may result. Although proper needle placement is awkward at first, the needle should be rotated backward with the needle holder to ensure that the suture *everts* the vessel wall rather than *inverting* it (Fig. 44-16).

One important factor in avoiding leaks is to minimize trauma to the vessel wall from placing the needle. For this reason, the novice should remember that the needle is curved and not straight (in most instances). Therefore, the

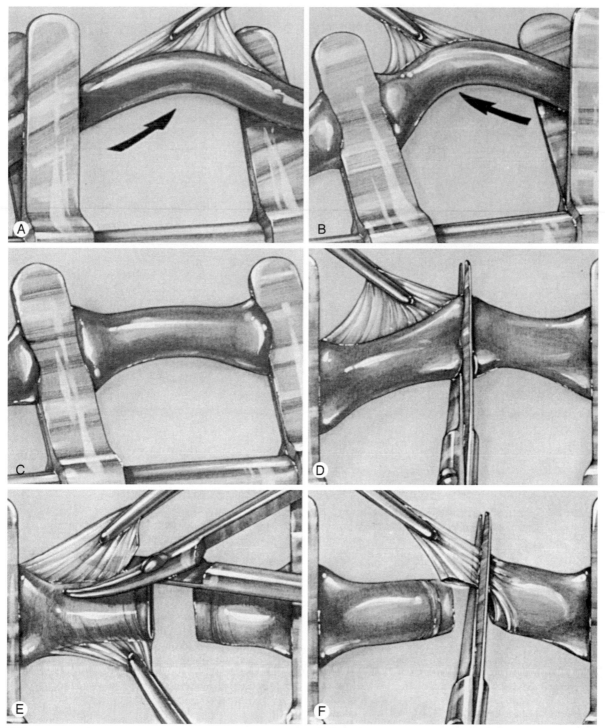

FIGURE 44-12. Technique of arterial anastomosis. Steps in preparation of the vessel ends. **A** to **C,** The vessel is placed in the clamps so there is moderate slack. **D,** The artery is cut clearly with sharp scissors in a single motion. **E,** There will be adventitia in and around the lumen. This must be carefully removed without touching the vessel itself. Only the loose adventitia should be grasped; it is cut cleanly, close to the artery. **F,** The adventitia is pulled and sharply trimmed along the cut edge of the artery ("circumcised"). The extent of adventitia removed should be confined to all loose strands around the end to provide a clear view of the vessel wall and keep any material out of the lumen. Both ends should be thus prepared, switching instruments to accomplish this. **G,** The lumen is gently dilated first with a small, angled dilator and then (**H**) with a pencil dilator. The intima is carefully inspected under high power for any loose material or defects. **I,** The vessel is now ready to be sutured. The adventitia has been cleaned off and the vessel dissected sharply back to good intima. Normal intima can be seen in the lumen of the vessel, and overhanging adventitia has been sharply dissected.   *Continued*

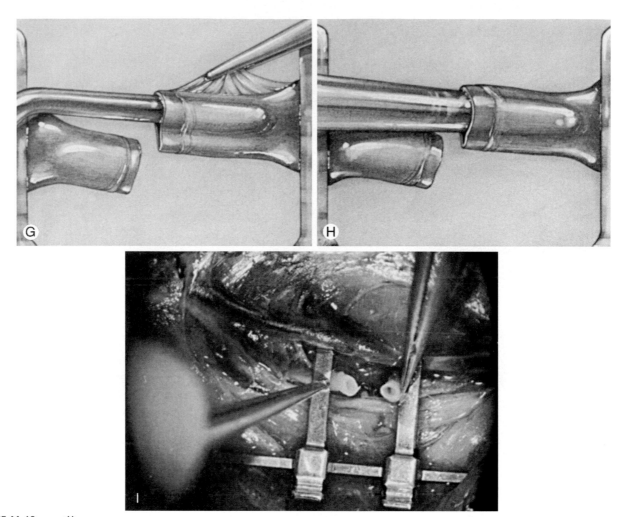

FIGURE 44-12—cont'd. G, The lumen is gently dilated first with a small, angled dilator and then (**H**) with a pencil dilator. The intima is carefully inspected under high power for any loose material or defects. **I,** The vessel is now ready to be sutured. The adventitia has been cleaned off and the vessel dissected sharply back to good intima. Normal intima can be seen in the lumen of the vessel, and overhanging adventitia has been sharply dissected.

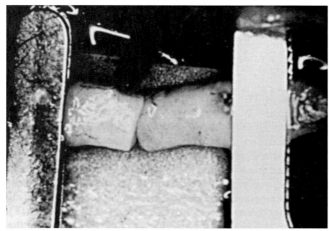

FIGURE 44-13. Close-up view of an 0.8-mm vessel showing the vessel in the clamp. The ends come together easily without tension, even with no sutures. Note that the adventitia has been trimmed back so that there is no adventitia overhanging the lumen.

needle should be pulled through the vessel wall *following the arc of the needle* to avoid trauma to the wall. Pulling the last half of the needle through in a straight motion tears the vessel wall and creates a larger, oblique hole rather than a clean, round one. As the suture is pulled through the vessel wall, care should be taken to guide the leading and following suture with the instruments such that the suture is pulled smoothly through the vessel wall. Suture forcibly pulled through the wall against resistance will tend to "cut through," leading to endothelial damage. I prefer to use a surgeon's knot for the first throw, but the suture should be gently tightened until the vessel walls just meet. Overtightening the suture will invert or tear the vessel wall, exposing thrombogenic surfaces to the lumen.[37,370] Overtightening also results in direct narrowing of the lumen as the tissue is distorted. A square knot and third throw are then completed, again avoiding overtightening.

There are two options for retrieving the needle. First, it may be carefully placed in the field of view before tying the knot and then picked up for the next stitch. The second

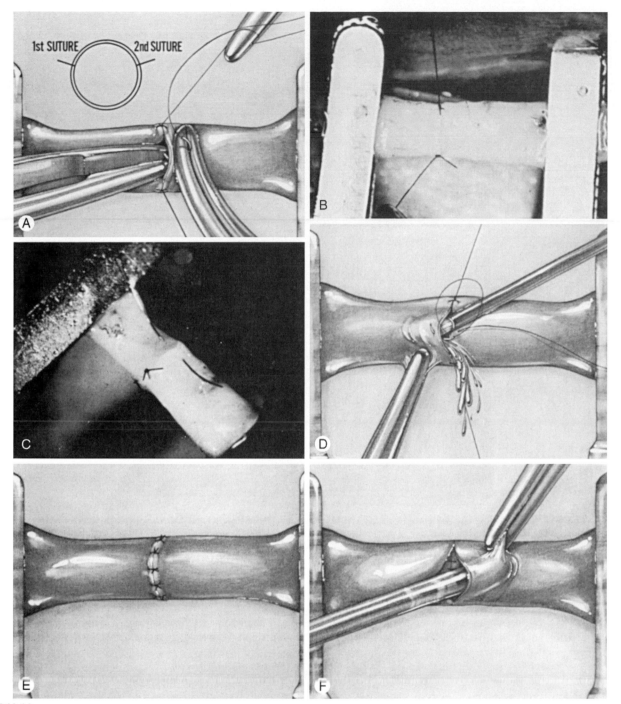

FIGURE 44-14. Suture placement. A minimum of four sutures are placed for 0.5-mm vessels or less and six to eight sutures for 1.0-mm vessels. The number of sutures also depends on the thickness of the wall; more sutures are needed for thin-walled vessels and veins. **A,** Sutures should be evenly placed, with the initial two corner sutures placed 120 degrees apart. This allows the back wall to fall away from the front wall, minimizing the tendency to catch the back wall with the front wall sutures. **B,** The ends of previously placed sutures are used to elevate the front wall of the anastomosis. **C,** The needle is placed through one side of the vessel and visualized in the gap to ensure that the back wall has not been penetrated. **D,** The needle can then be put through the other wall separately or passed through both the vessel ends simultaneously. The correct maneuver in each case is the one that is least traumatic and gives the greatest view of the needle at all times. Angled probes or the irrigating tip can be used to visualize the vessel during placement. **E,** The front wall completed. **F,** The clamp is turned and inspection is made of the lumen to make sure that none of the anterior wall sutures have caught the posterior wall.

Continued

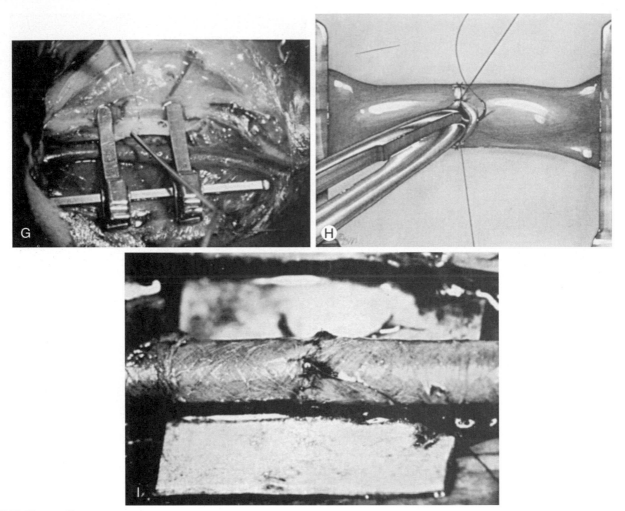

FIGURE 44-14—cont'd. G, The sutures are well placed around the anterior wall, and the vessel will come together nicely. There is no tension. **H,** The final suture. Care must be taken not to catch the back wall. The best way to prevent this is to show the tip of the needle in the gap. Alternative methods for last suture placement are described in the text. When the clamps are released, no major gaps allowing blood to squirt more than 1 to 2 inches should exist. If gaps are present, additional sutures should be added. An ooze of blood is normal and will cease. **I,** A completed anastomosis.

method is to pull the needle and attached suture out of the field, tie the knot, cut the suture, and then pull on the trailing end while guiding the suture with forceps to retrieve the needle. I prefer the latter method, because less suture material is present in the field to interfere with tying the knot. The surgeon must always hold the suture near the vessel with forceps when releasing the needle from the needle holder. If this is not done, the needle or suture may stick to the instrument and be pulled out of the vessel.

One or more sutures are then placed between the corner sutures. The last suture placed in either the front or back wall is critical, because it is difficult to visualize the lumen and prevent inadvertent suturing of the opposite wall. If the corner sutures are placed 120 degrees apart, the back wall will tend to fall away and thus be protected (asymmetrical biangulation technique).[309] The vessel is then rotated 180 degrees by flipping the vessel clamp or previously placed "corner" sutures. The back wall is then sutured; and as each suture is placed, the lumen is irrigated and gently dilated with the forceps to ensure that the back wall is not caught up in one of the sutures.

Placement of the final suture is critical, and several techniques can be used to avoid suturing of the opposite wall.

1. The neighboring two sutures can be left long, and traction can be placed on them to isolate the intervening vessel wall for placement of the final suture.
2. One of the sutures on the opposite wall to the final suture can be grasped to pull the far wall away from the final suture.
3. The needle can be passed through one side of the anastomosis, brought out through the defect, and then used to gently pick up and evert the adjacent wall as it is placed.
4. A two-suture technique can be used in which the first needle is passed through both sides but not pulled through. The second stitch is then placed and tied, and the first suture is then pulled through and tied.[68,130]
5. A modification of the Harashina procedure is often very useful (Fig. 44-17).[166] The last two sutures are placed as if one were performing a continuous running suture. The loop between the sutures is left large instead of being tightened down and is then cut with the suture scissors,

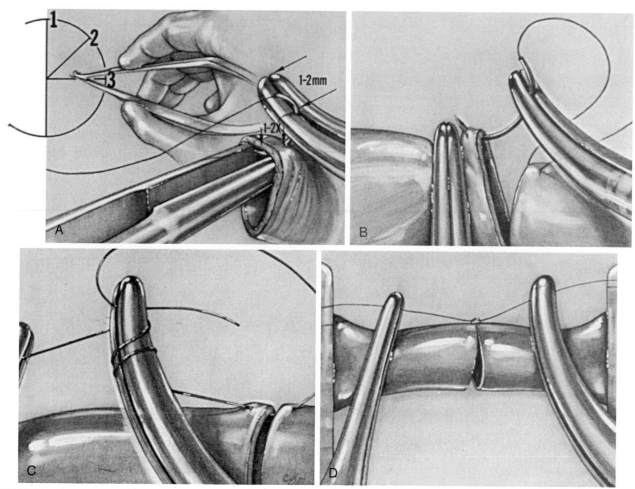

FIGURE 44-15. Suture technique. **A,** The needle driver is held like a pencil, resting comfortably on the long finger and held gently with the thumb and index finger. If one draws a circle with a bisecting line, the straightest line usually gives the most comfortable needle-passing direction (most commonly, position 3 or 2). The needle is passed parallel to the vessel axis, with the forearm perpendicular to the axis of the vessel. The needle is held 1 to 2 mm from the tip of the needle driver. Needle bites should be placed back from the cut edge a distance equal to one to two times the wall thickness in arteries and two to three times that in veins. The tip should pass perpendicular (at right angles) to the surface of the vessel. Care should be taken to pass the needle cleanly, without any pulling or trauma to the vessel wall. The needle is pushed into the wall, using the forceps inside the vessel to provide counterpressure to complete penetration. **B,** In passing through the second wall, the forceps are used outside the wall to provide counterpressure. The suture is pulled carefully through the vessel until 1 to 2 cm of suture material is left on the short end. **C,** The needle is carefully laid either in the microscopic field or on a white lap pad directly in front of the operator. Under the microscope, a surgeon's knot is laid squarely, using the needle driver and tying forceps or two pairs of tying forceps. **D,** The knot is tightened carefully under the microscope to bring the edges together without the suture cutting through. The first tie alone should bring the edges together; if not, then excessive tension on the vessel exists. A total of three knots is laid squarely. One end is cut 1 mm from the knot, and the other is left long for retraction.

leaving two sutures in place and ready for tying. This conserves suture and motion and minimizes the number of needles, instruments, and sutures in the operative field. It also may be the best alternative for the microsurgeon working alone.[383]

The clamp is then released, and the flow is observed under the microscope. Oozing from the anastomosis is normal, but pulsatile bleeding must be controlled by placement of additional sutures. It is usually best to avoid "oversewing" a vessel with too many sutures, because this can lead to the placement of multiple back-wall sutures. Probably the safest way to avoid suturing the back wall is to place sutures in questionable areas after the vessel is full of blood. This must be done expeditiously, however, because platelet thrombi

can form rapidly at the site of significant leaks and may propagate within the lumen. Brisk flow usually occurs through a well-performed anastomosis, but occasionally vessel spasm severely limits flow. If this appears to be the case, apply local vasodilating agents, warm the area if possible, and avoid manipulating the vessel for 15 to 20 minutes.

Patency Test

Assessment of anastomotic patency may be done in several ways.[3,95] In clinical situations, return of color to and capillary oozing or venous bleeding from the revascularized tissue signal a competent arterial anastomosis. If the tissue becomes engorged after a period of arterial flow, the vein may be occluded. Direct inspection of both arterial and venous anastomoses under the microscope may reveal signs

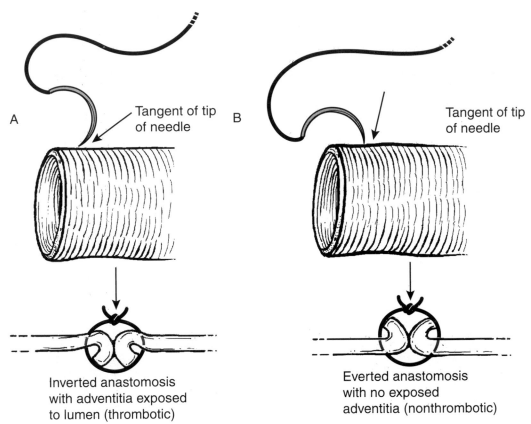

Inverted anastomosis
with adventitia exposed
to lumen (thrombotic)

Everted anastomosis
with no exposed
adventitia (nonthrombotic)

FIGURE 44-16. A, Improper placement of the needle results in inversion of the vessel wall with potential exposure of adventitia to the lumen. **B,** Proper alignment of the needle will place the suture so that it will evert the vessel wall.

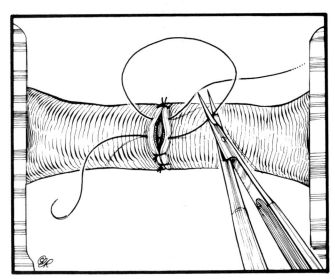

FIGURE 44-17. Modified Harashina procedure. Both sutures are placed as for a running technique, and the loop is then cut as shown, leaving two sutures ready to be tied.

of patency. Arterial patency is indicated by nicely dilated vessels showing pulsatile elongation ("wriggling") or expansile pulsation. Gently lifting the vessel distal to the anastomosis by placing forceps underneath it will demonstrate the "flicker" of blood flowing across this area, but it is easily visible only in thin-walled vessels.

The empty and refill patency test is traumatic and should be performed as gently and infrequently as possible.[184] Two pair of smooth forceps are used to occlude the vessel distal to the anastomosis. The more "downstream" forceps is then moved gently approximately 1 cm down the vessel, creating an empty segment between the two forceps. The proximal compression is then released, and rapid filling of the empty segment indicates patency of the anastomosis. This test is useful for either arteries or veins and for any size vessel (Fig. 44-18).

Veins

Rat vein anastomosis is very difficult because (1) these vessels are extremely friable and thin walled, (2) it is difficult to separate the adventitia from the vessel without damage, and (3) the lumen tends to collapse. Performing the anastomosis under fluid or with copious irrigation to "float" the lumen open is often necessary. Clamps tend to tear the vein and must be used with extreme care or not at all (Fig. 44-19). Fortunately, veins encountered in replantation and free tissue transfer in humans are more substantial, but they still retain some of the characteristics previously mentioned and require more careful handling and additional sutures to prevent intraluminal collapse of segments of the vessel wall.

Tremor

Tremor is a problem with all microsurgery. Very few surgeons are tremor-free, but most good microsurgeons can control it. One must make sure that the hands and arms are

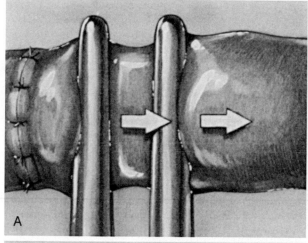
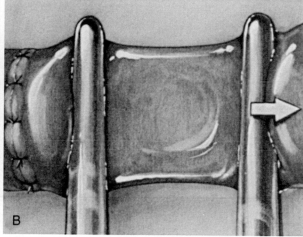
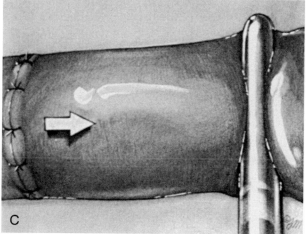

FIGURE 44-18. The patency test is performed using two blunt-tipped tying forceps distal to the anastomosis. **A,** The proximal forceps remains stationary while the second forceps pushes the blood distally and stops, remaining closed. **B,** The proximal forceps is then opened while the distal remains closed. **C,** If the anastomosis is good, there will be immediate filling of the segment. Any delay in filling usually means that there is a problem with the anastomosis.

supported and that the shoulders are relaxed to decrease tremor. The "lathe-rest" principle of supporting one instrument with the other is often useful to control tremor if this is a problem. The frustration that can be experienced in dealing with fine suture and tenacious tissues in vivo defies description. Acland has addressed the handling of suture material in these circumstances, and his article is required reading for microsurgeons who wish to minimize their frustration.[5]

CLINICAL MICROVASCULAR TECHNIQUES

The ability to perform a technically adequate vessel anastomosis in the laboratory does not guarantee success in clinical situations such as replantation and free tissue transfer. Many other factors may influence the eventual outcome, and the surgeon will need to favorably influence as many of these as possible (Table 44-1). This section and the following one on physiology and pharmacology address these problems.

Presentation, Access, and Size Discrepancy

Many difficulties may be encountered in moving from a totally controlled laboratory setting to a clinical situation, including the following:

1. Difficulty in orienting the vessels for ease of anastomosis
2. Limited access to the vessels in a deep wound
3. Vessel size discrepancy
4. Inability to rotate the clamp holding the vessel for suturing of the back wall
5. Difficulty in becoming comfortable in a position appropriate to suture the vessels

It is frequently impossible to significantly change the presentation of the vessels. Anticipating such situations, one should practice anastomoses in the laboratory with the vessels oriented at various angles between horizontal and vertical. The important factor in suturing vessels in different presentations is to remember to move the position of your hands to allow precise suture placement. Sometimes one's entire arm position must be changed to appropriately place the suture, but awkward hand positioning can lead to damaging the vessel, and the surgeon must be comfortable enough with his or her technique to sew with the hands in the proper relationship to the vessel.

The use of "human" retraction is to be avoided whenever possible while suturing vessels or nerves under the microscope. It is hard enough to sew vessels in some situations without the added distraction of an assistant holding a retractor and constantly moving. Exposure is paramount, and one should endeavor to gain sufficient access so that self-retaining retractors are adequate to maintain the field. In

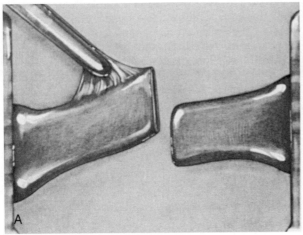

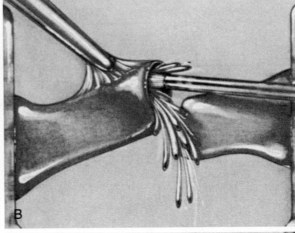

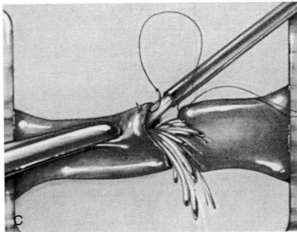

FIGURE 44-19. Technique of vein anastomosis. **A,** Veins are thinner, flatter, and more difficult to anastomose. Although the basic technique is somewhat similar to that for arteries, there are some differences. **B,** Veins can be more easily sutured by using Ringer's solution to float or irrigate the vessel open. Special care must be taken to prevent adventitia from blocking the lumen while suturing and to avoid catching the back wall. **C,** Somewhat deeper bites must be taken equal to two to three times the thickness of the vessel wall. Generally, more sutures must be taken to prevent large gaps and to prevent collapse of the wall.

Table 44-1

MAJOR FACTORS THAT INFLUENCE FAILURE AFTER MICROSURGERY IN EXPERIMENTAL ANIMALS

Technical	*Postoperative Care*
Both walls sutured together	Infection
Traumatic vessel handling	Acidosis
Apposition of vessel edges	Environmental factors
Disproportional vessel size	Transplantation
Tension at suture line	Cold
Excessive clamp pressure	Limb position
Kinking of vessels	
Reperfusion	
No reflow	
Blood turbulence	
Spasm	
Hypercoagulability	
Acidosis	
Cold	
Hypovolemia	
Circulating constrictors	

From Seaber AV: Laboratory design in preparing for elective microvascular surgery. Hand Clin 1:233-245, 1985.

some situations, direct access to the injured vessels may be nearly impossible. A prime example of this is in thumb revascularization or replantation. To approach the volar vessels in the thumb, the forearm must be severely pronated or supinated, and it is extremely difficult to maintain this position and perform the anastomosis. In such a situation, an alternative approach such as grafting of the volar vessels before bone fixation[66] or interpositional vein grafting to a more accessible dorsal vessel (e.g., the radial artery) should be considered. This type of problem is an example in which experience is essential to avoid frustration. Limited access to deeply placed structures may be improved by extension of the surgical incision to provide a more open wound or by placing moist sponges beneath the vessels, lifting them out of the wound. Alternative anastomosis techniques (end-to-side or backwall-first) may be useful in this situation.

Vessel Size Discrepancy

Several solutions have been proposed for vessel size discrepancy. A difference of 2:1 or less may be handled by gently dilating the smaller vessel and not dilating the larger one. With a difference of more than 2:1, however, alternative techniques are preferred. Vein grafts are more distendable than arteries and are very useful to match vessels of varying diameters.[43] It should be noted, however, that successful anastomoses between arteries and vein grafts of diameter discrepancies of up to 5:1 have been reported experimentally with 96% patency rates.[346] The primary message from this study is to place enough sutures accurately to bring the two ends into perfect approximation.

End-in-end and spatulation techniques have been described for differences in size up to 3:1.[54,75,126,170,365,404-406] If the smaller vessel empties into the larger one, the smaller end may be telescoped inside the larger vessel (end-in-end or sleeve technique). This is safest if flow proceeds from the smaller vessel into the larger one. Cutting one or both vessel walls longitudinally and repair by triangulating the corners as is often used by vascular surgeons may be helpful (spatulation technique). Cutting the vessel ends obliquely at varying angles may also be used to change the effective diameter.[32] This method has been described with mathematical precision.[54] Another recent technique involves spatulation of both vessel ends and then suturing them together with only four sutures at the corners. The authors report acceptable patency rates with this technique.[390]

Although they are not necessary in the majority of cases, the accomplished microsurgeon should be familiar with these techniques to use if a large discrepancy is encountered.[260] This is more likely in the case of free transfer rather than replantation or revascularization. One should also remember that end-to-side anastomosis can be used for virtually any size discrepancy problem. When using any of these techniques, it must be remembered that any rapid change in size or direction of the vessel will produce turbulence and increase the chance of thrombosis.

Excessive tension at the suture line is a common cause of both immediate and delayed anastomotic failure. The surgeon should anticipate this problem and use an interpositional vein graft rather than attempt an end-to-end anastomosis that is under tension. This technique is addressed more fully in the section on vein grafting. Likewise twisting of the vessel at or near the site of anastomosis can lead to thrombosis. Whereas experimental work shows that a small amount of twist does not lead to an increased thrombosis rate,[206] the surgeon should make every effort to prevent twisting of the vessel at or near the anastomosis.

Alternative Anastomosis Techniques

Four alternative techniques are frequently used clinically in situations where presentation of the vessels is not optimal for standard end-to-end anastomosis. These are the (1) back wall–first technique, (2) "flipping" of a mobile vessel, (3) 180-degree vertical technique, and (4) end-to-side technique.

Author's Preferred Technique: Back Wall–first Technique (One-Way-up Technique)

The back wall–first technique, also known as the "one-way-up technique," is most useful with vessels of approximately equal size when one or both presenting ends cannot be rotated within a double clamp. This most commonly occurs when the repair is made close to a parent trunk or large branch that cannot be sacrificed. I actually prefer this technique for most anastomoses, because I think that double clamps get in the way. With some practice, this "freehand" anastomosis is not difficult and has the added advantage that one is not likely to suture both walls together. In performing any anastomosis, the most difficult suture should always be placed first, and so I prefer to begin the anastomosis on the posterior wall at the point farthest away from the surgeon. Interrupted sutures are placed sequentially toward the surgeon until the back wall is completed, and then the front wall is repaired. The knots are, of course, placed outside the lumen. The initial suture is left long to aid in traction and rotation of the vessel (Fig. 44-20). Back wall–first repair can also be done by adding sutures alternately to either side of the first suture until the anastomosis is completed.[175,196,301,414] This technique is arguably one of the safest, because the entire inside of the anastomosis can be visualized until the very last few sutures are placed.

CRITICAL POINTS: BACK WALL–FIRST TECHNIQUE

- Begin with the first suture in the middle of the back wall of the vessel.
- Each succeeding suture is placed alternatively on either side of the previous suture.
- Work your way around to the front.
- The last suture is placed 180 degrees from the first.
- This avoids having to turn the vessel, and the inside of the anastomosis is visible until the last suture.

"Flipping" Technique

In many situations, one vessel end is freely mobile and can be "flipped" end-over-end to repair the back wall. Examples are listed below:

1. Vein grafting, where the first anastomosis can be completed in this manner and the second by standard technique.
2. Free tissue transfer, where the flap may be freely mobile if it is revascularized before insetting. Extreme care must be used when handling and insetting the flap to avoid damage to the anastomosis by tension or kinking of the pedicle when using this technique.

This technique is useful when a vessel presents for anastomosis in such a manner that double clamp placement and rotation are difficult. I have found this useful in vein grafting patients with retrocarpal thrombosis of the radial artery,[280,334] where the distal anastomosis is done on a vessel presenting "end-up" toward the surgeon between the two heads of the first dorsal interosseous. A single clamp is placed on the distal vessel and the vein graft, and the front wall is com-

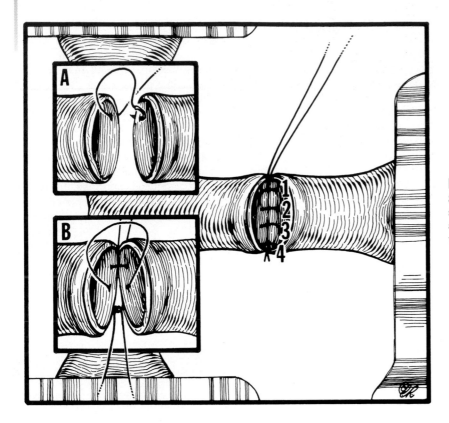

FIGURE 44-20. A and **B,** The back-wall-first technique. Suturing begins at the point farthest away from the surgeon and progresses toward the surgeon. The knots are placed outside the lumen. This method is useful when rotation of the vessel is limited.

pleted (Fig. 44-21A). The vein graft is then flipped end-over-end and the back wall repaired (see Fig. 44-21B and C).

180-Degree Vertical Technique

In the modification of the standard approach, the first two sutures are placed 180 degrees apart rather than the standard 120 degrees. Although this technique contradicts the traditional approach of vascular surgeons (i.e., the "triangulation technique"), it is favored by many experienced microsurgeons, particularly in Japan.[169,200] This is one of my favored approaches, because it allows turning the vessel even if there is little room for this in the field. In this approach, the first suture is placed directly opposite to the surgeon, in the midportion of the back walls of the vessels being anastomosed. The second suture is then placed 180 degrees from the first suture in the midportion of the front wall. These two sutures are cut long, and they can then be used to turn the vessel 90 degrees in either direction to facilitate placement of the remaining sutures (see Fig. 44-22).

End-to-Side Technique

The end-to-side technique is a standard procedure that is taught in all microsurgical laboratory courses and has been studied experimentally.[15,93,133,161,299] If only a single vessel maintains the viability of an extremity it cannot be sacrificed as the donor vessel for an end-to-end anastomosis, and an end-to-side repair must be used. This method is also useful if there is a large size discrepancy between the vessels to be anastomosed. Some believe that this technique offers superior patency rates over end-to-end anastomosis.[15,142] Theoretically, this is because of the propensity of the arterial wall to retract and constrict (due to the muscularis) when cut circumferentially. Making an arteriotomy divides the circu-

lar muscular layer of the artery, thus effectively "holding open" the anastomotic site. Others have believed that flow through an end-to-side anastomosis is superior to that of an end-to-end, but several studies have shown that flow rates are equivalent.[93,299,328] I believe that the technical difficulty of end-to-side compared with that of end-to-end anastomosis may outweigh these theoretical benefits in inexperienced hands.

The arteriotomy into the donor vessel is the most critical (and irreversible) step in the procedure. Creating a clean arteriotomy for making an end-to-side anastomosis is perhaps the most difficult maneuver in microsurgery. One should master the technique in the laboratory on vessels of varying diameter and wall thickness before using it in clinical practice.

The arteriotomy may be done by excising a "wedge" of vessel wall with straight scissors, as described by Godina,[142] or begun with a microknife and enlarged carefully to an elliptical or circular defect with microscissors. Special arteriotomy clamps are available, but these also require practice to achieve consistent results. If not applied properly, the arteriotomy clamp causes irreparable damage to the vessel wall, which then must be repaired (potentially with a vein patch graft). Another technique for performing an arteriotomy is to grasp a small full-thickness bite of the vessel wall with a suture. This suture is then pulled up to tent the vessel wall, and a curved pair of microsutures is placed under the suture, cutting a clean hole in the vessel at the site of the suture.

Some have suggested that a simple straight incision into the larger vessel is sufficient for end-to-side anastomosis,[12] but I prefer to cut out a segment. This makes for an easier anastomosis because it is much more difficult to grab the

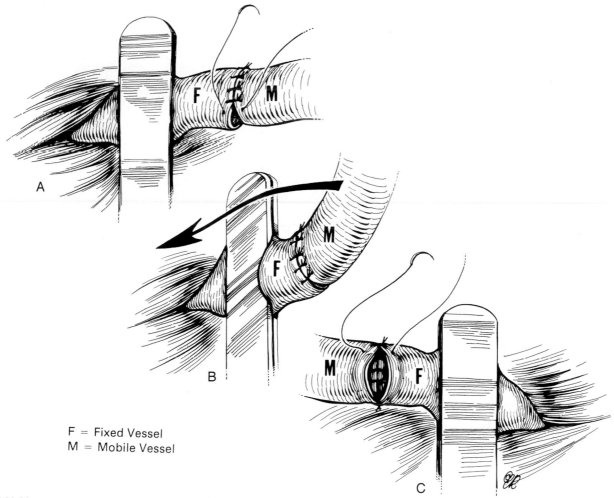

F = Fixed Vessel
M = Mobile Vessel

FIGURE 44-21. A to **C,** "Flipping" a mobile vessel. When the free flap, digit, or vein graft is attached to the mobile vessel, it can be "flipped" to expose the back wall for repair if rotation of the vessel is difficult.

back wall. Likewise, the hole in the larger vessel tends to hold the anastomosis open. An ideal way to perform an arteriotomy is with a small vascular punch.[164] This device is used by the cardiac surgeons for proximal anastomoses of vein grafts to the aorta. The smallest commercial size available is in the 2.4-mm range, but it will produce a very clean arteriotomy for anastomosis, and I prefer this technique in larger vessels.[316]

The arteriotomy should approximately match the size of the vessel to be anastomosed. The angle of takeoff from the larger vessel should theoretically be 90 degrees. In clinical practice, however, the angle of takeoff may need to be modified depending on the lie of the vessels relative to the flap or the necessity to make an oblique cut on the smaller vessel. Oblique cuts through a vessel wall may produce a fragile tip of tissue with the intima and media at different levels, which is weak because of interruption of the circular fibers of the vessel wall. In most cases, the front wall is first repaired and then the back wall is sutured (Fig. 44-23), assuming that the recipient vessel can be flipped. Using one of the techniques mentioned for placement of the last suture is especially important in completing the anastomosis. An end-to-side anastomosis is probably more easily performed using the back wall–first technique if the donor vessel is deeply placed and mobilization of the recipient vessel is difficult

(Fig. 44-24). End-to-side anastomoses are also very amenable to the continuous suture technique.

CRITICAL POINTS: END-TO-SIDE ANASTOMOSIS

- Begin by lining up vessels for anastomosis.
- Choose a site on the vessel to be sewn to.
- Make an arteriotomy with microscissors or a micro knife.
- Begin with back wall.
- Continue to work your way around to the front.
- Be careful at the corners (the "heel" and "toe" of the anastomosis)—avoid back wall suture; this area is also prone to leaks.

Continuous Suture Technique

Macrovascular and cardiac surgeons routinely perform vascular anastomoses with a continuous (running) suture of polypropylene. This technique has not found wide application in microvascular surgery, but this is probably related

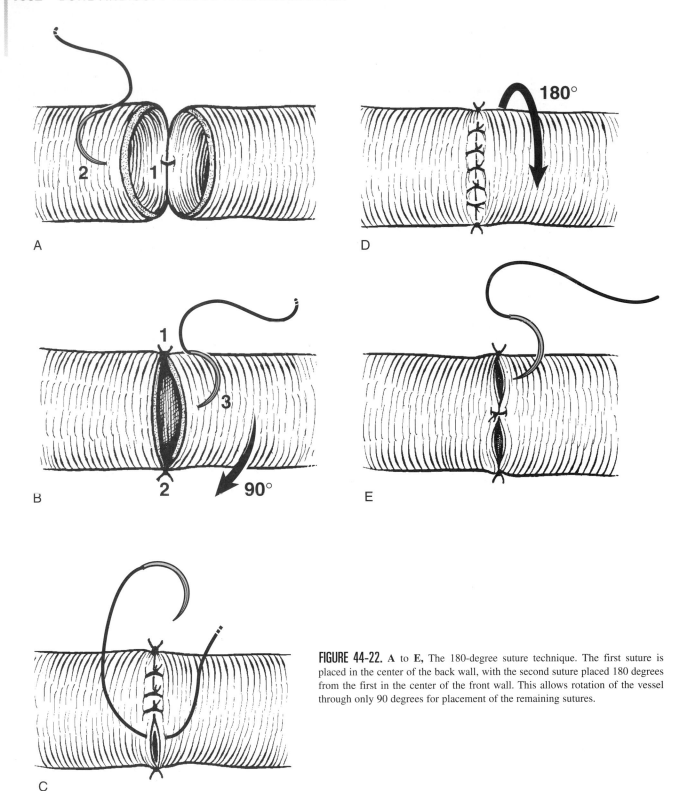

FIGURE 44-22. **A** to **E,** The 180-degree suture technique. The first suture is placed in the center of the back wall, with the second suture placed 180 degrees from the first in the center of the front wall. This allows rotation of the vessel through only 90 degrees for placement of the remaining sutures.

to the orthopedic (rather than general surgical) background of many microsurgeons. A number of studies comparing interrupted versus continuous suture technique in microsurgery have been performed, with no clear advantage of interrupted over continuous suture technique.[13,72,122,138,165,246,391,402] The primary problem with this approach in very small vessels is the potential for creating a "purse-string" constriction

at the site of anastomosis. This can be circumvented by not running a single suture all the way around a single end-to-end anastomosis. In one report a so-called combined technique of running a portion of the vessel and interrupting the last portion was used.[255] These authors found a decreased time for anastomosis with no increase in thrombosis rate. The other problem encountered with the continuous tech-

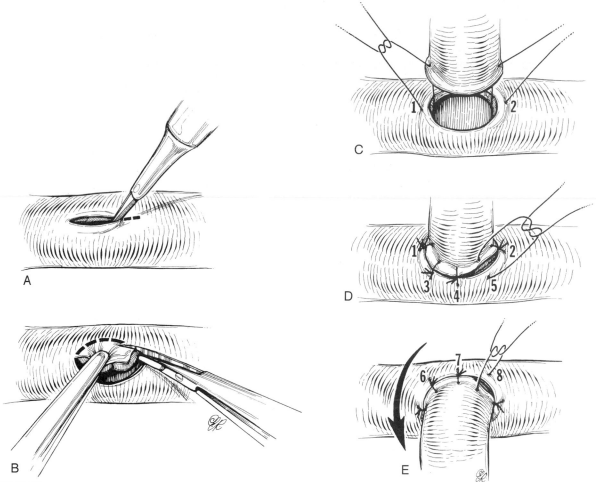

FIGURE 44-23. Standard end-to-side technique. **A** and **B,** The creation of the arteriotomy is critical and irreversible. **C** and **D,** The near side is sutured first, the recipient vessel is mobilized, and (**E**) the far side is then sutured. Care must be taken not to suture the opposite wall of the donor vessel.

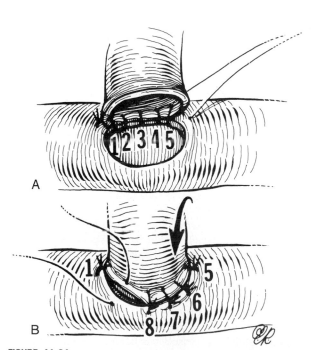

FIGURE 44-24. An optional end-to-side technique. The far side can be sutured using the back-wall-first technique (**A**) and the near side then completed (**B**).

nique in microsurgery is the use of nylon suture, which tends to have more adherence to the vessel wall than polypropylene. This results in difficulty in pulling the continuous suture tight after it is placed, potentially leading to a loose and leaky anastomosis. Although polypropylene is available in 9-0 and 10-0 sizes, it is difficult to work with at this size and is generally inferior to nylon.

I routinely perform continuous anastomoses of microvessels using a modification of the 180-degree technique previously discussed. In this approach, the first two sutures are placed but each suture with needle is left in place. These sutures are then each "run" around one half of the circumference of the vessel. Tension must be kept on the suture after each throw is placed by a following assistant. If this is not done, care must be taken to tighten each loop of the suture before tying, or leaks will result. The learning curve of this technique is rather steep; however, with experience it can provide a very rapid and safe anastomosis.[90]

Sleeve and Cuffing Techniques

In an attempt to decrease the time necessary for anastomosis, several authors have proposed the use of "sleeve" or end-in-end techniques.[245,405,406] In this approach, one vessel is "telescoped" or "sleeved" into another and can be held in place by as few as two sutures. Although this has been applied to either end of the anastomosis, most authors familiar with this technique believe that it should only be used when the upstream vessel (from which blood flows) can be telescoped into the downstream vessel (into which blood flows).[169] If performed in this fashion, the sleeve technique has equal patency rates with standard techniques[416] and is particularly useful if there is a marked size discrepancy between the two vessels undergoing anastomosis. I use this technique on occasion when a vein graft is being placed into a larger, distal artery. The vein graft is telescoped into the artery and held in place distally with two sutures.

A variety of techniques that add an external "cuff" around the anastomosis have been proposed.[281] This cuff can be a slightly larger segment of vein graft[176] or some type of nonbiologic tubing.[278,303] The idea behind this is to decrease the time of vascular repair by using fewer sutures on the anastomosis itself, using the cuffing material to stop leaks. This technique has been proven efficacious when suturing very small vessels (in the 0.5-mm range) to avoid damage to the vessel ends.[298] In most clinical situations, however, this approach is cumbersome, and the time saved by placing fewer sutures is lost by having to harvest a vein graft and fiddling with placing it around the anastomosis.

Non-suture Techniques

Mechanical Devices

The idea of taking the "human factor" of technical error out of vascular anastomosis has been around for quite some time. Lapchinsky developed a complex machine to anastomose larger vessels and used this successfully in autogenous canine limb replantations as early as 1960.[242] Nakayama and colleagues later reported on a ring-pin stapling device for the revascularization of transplanted intestine for esophageal replacement.[297] This instrument was further refined by Inokuchi, which permitted its use in vessels down to the 2-mm range.[204] This idea lay fallow until the 1980s, when Ostrup further refined the ring-pin coupler into what is known as the UNILINK system.[39,311] This device is now commercially available in the United States and is utilized by a number of microsurgeons, especially for venous anastomosis.

The ring-pin technique involves passing each end of the vessels to be anastomosed through a ring that has matching sets of pins and holes. The vessel ends are then everted over the corresponding pins, and a device operated by a thumb nut then pushes the two rings together. This theoretically produces a "perfect" anastomosis, with total eversion of the edges and exact intima-to-intima contact.[47,48,117] This instrument has been shown to provide rapid microvascular repairs in experienced hands, with published reports of 2 to 3 minutes per anastomosis.[311] It has been used successfully in microvascular surgery in the hand for vascular repairs and reconstruction.[306] Reported vascular complication rates are comparable to hand-sewn anastomoses in experienced hands.[360]

The downside of this technique is that it works less well in arteries than in veins, because the thicker arterial wall often lends itself poorly to eversion through the rings. It has found wide application in some surgeon's hands for venous anastomosis, however.[101,302] End-to-side anastomosis *can* be performed with this device[98]; it lends itself poorly to this

technique, however.[40] This problem has been addressed by modifying the device to make it more applicable to end-to-side anastomosis,[221] but no commercial application is available. This device has also been used in replantation of fingers, but I have some concern about the presence of the rings in the thin soft tissue of the digits. Experimental work is being done on developing an absorbable ring, which may obviate this concern.[215,326] Although the use of the UNILINK system may have application in free flap transfer and larger vessels of the upper extremity, I believe that the surgeon should be well versed in standard techniques of microvascular anastomosis before attempting use of this device.

The use of staples for microanastomosis has been proposed.[36,239] The original technique required two stay sutures and continuous eversion of the vessel wall. Successful application of this technique in clinical cases of free flap transfer has been reported,[50,411] with rapid anastomosis times (12 minutes). These authors have noted that this technique could not be used in thickened arteries, however. Work on instrumentation and technique with the use of staples is continuing and may prove clinically feasible in the future.

Lasers

The medical community continues to look for applications for the laser beam, and microsurgery has not escaped this quest. In 1979, anastomosis of vessels with the neodymium:yttrium-aluminum-garnet laser was first performed experimentally.[210] A number of centers have experimented with laser repair of vessels in the microsurgical range.[327,349,357] The promise of laser anastomosis is that it avoids the use of suture material, which must, of necessity, be present in the lumen of the vessel (and thus can promote thrombosis). An unresolved problem with laser anastomoses is that they have a tendency to develop pseudoaneurysms with time.[271] Likewise, several stay sutures must be placed before "welding" the vessel with the laser,[137,382] which cancels out some of its benefits. One group has reported the use of a biodegradable protein "glue" for anastomosis that is activated by the laser.[265] Although the results of this technique were acceptable, there has been no clinical application to date. The cost of the equipment and learning curve place laser-assisted microanastomosis in the realm of the research laboratory at present, and I doubt that this technique will ever eclipse standard suture techniques. This is mirrored by a decreasing number of reports in the recent literature of laser-assisted anastomosis.

Glue

The ability to make a leak-free anastomosis is an intriguing one, and this is where interest in tissue adhesives for microanastomoses was born. Fibrin "glue" has been used in microneural anastomoses for a number of years, particularly in Europe.[293] The problem with the use of fibrin in vessels is the potential to increase thrombogenicity at the site, thus leading to occlusion of the anastomosis. One study found that the patency rate of an anastomosis treated with fibrin glue was inversely proportional to the concentration of the thrombin in the sealant.[268] The use of standard cyanoacrylate glues ("super glue") on vessels has been tried, but with less than optimal results.[152] This is primarily due to toxicity that causes thinning of the vessel walls and the resulting formation of aneurysms. Different formulations of the cyanoacrylates (2-octyl cyanoacrylate) have been tried experimentally and have been found to be less toxic and have reasonable patency rates.[19,162] Non-cyanoacrylate glues have been tried and found to be less toxic than the cyanoacrylates, without causing vascular damage or thrombosis.[108] The use of glues for anastomosis remains experimental but may find some application in the future, especially for providing a completely sealed anastomosis.

The attainment of the "perfect" anastomosis, which requires little skill, is rapidly performed, and is nonthrombogenic, remains elusive. With the notable exception of the pin and ring device, none of the other sutureless techniques has found wide application in microsurgery. The sutured anastomosis remains the benchmark for microvascular anastomosis, despite over 40 years of research into other potential techniques. For this reason, the application of microsurgery to clinical situations still requires extensive training, regular practice, and experience for successful outcomes.

Revision of the Failed Anastomosis

Failure of blood to flow across an anastomosis is usually caused by one of three factors: (1) technical errors with the anastomosis, (2) poor flow from the proximal vessel due to undetected damage more proximally or vasospasm, or (3) a clot or thrombus at the anastomotic site or in an area where a clamp was applied.

Small nonoccluding platelet thrombi occur at every anastomosis and are necessary to seal the suture line. If blood flow is allowed to continue undisturbed, these will usually not progress to occlude the lumen. It has been experimentally determined that the first 30 minutes are the most critical for thrombus formation as regards occlusion of the lumen.[51] Damage to the endothelium from excessive clamp pressure, poor technique, or contamination of the intraluminal blood with thromboplastins from the wound area may, however, result in an occluding thrombus. If blood flow across an anastomosis must be occluded for any reason, the suture line should be bombarded with heparinized solution immediately after occlusion and before flow is restored. Systemic heparin will also protect the anastomosis if reapplication of clamps is necessary.[119,127]

Adequate proximal flow is absolutely necessary for successful anastomosis, and performing vascular repair of a vessel in which the status of flow is unknown is a recipe for disaster. For this reason, I prefer to perform anastomosis without the tourniquet inflated, so that the amount and quality of inflow can be ascertained. *Just because an artery is pulsating with a vascular clamp in place does not mean there is adequate flow at the site chosen for anastomosis.* Brisk bleeding from the end of the vessel must be demonstrated before anastomosis. If bleeding is not adequate, a small clot may be present or the vessel may be in spasm. In the worst case, the vessel is damaged and will have to be resected farther back before anastomosis.

Determining the patency of an anastomosis can present problems even for experienced microsurgeons. Partial thrombi at the site of repair may cause intermittent flow, with a normal patency test distally. If the patency test reveals slow filling of the distal vessel, whether it is arterial or venous, the anastomosis should be taken down and examined. Although the idea of removing a few sutures to inspect

the intima and remove clot seems appealing, I believe strongly that any microanastomosis that is questionable should be completely revised. Inspection of the resected site of anastomosis should always be performed, both for purposes of determining the cause of thrombosis and for avoiding similar problems in the future.

One should attempt to discern the cause of failure and proceed accordingly. If there is sufficient vessel length, reanastomosis can be performed; if not, a vein graft is inserted. Poor proximal flow that does not respond to local vasodilators and warming may require proximal exploration of the vessel, dilatation along a proximal length of vessel sufficient to relieve vasospasm, and/or treatment with local or intra-arterial vasodilators.[199,408] In some cases, a vein graft from an adequate donor vessel more proximally may be required.

CRITICAL POINTS: REVISION OF THE FAILED ANASTOMOSIS

- Heparinize patient if not already heparinized.
- Take anastomosis down and inspect it carefully for technical errors (e.g., back wall suture, adventitia in lumen, tears in intima).
- Revise anastomosis, carefully keeping original problem in mind.
- Trim area of vessel previously sewn.
- May need to add a vein graft if vessel now too short.
- Take your time and do it right to prevent re-thrombosis.

Vein Grafts

One of the most critical essentials of microvascular surgery is that there not be excessive tension on the anastomosis.[345] Experimental studies have shown a high incidence of aneurysm formation and thrombosis in vessels sutured under tension.[37,345,370,407] Both veins and arteries have been used for interpositional grafts in microsurgery, but venous grafts are the most readily available and may have the highest patency rate.[44,67,294,353] There has always been some concern that two anastomoses (as when a vein graft is used) may be inherently more prone to thrombosis than a single anastomosis (direct repair). If a primary repair is done under tension, however, there is no question that a vein graft is superior. Reports of clinical series show that long vein grafts do not increase the likelihood of flap loss, other than from the standpoint of the difficulty of the reconstruction in these instances.[222] Likewise, most authors believe that the advantages of using a vein graft in a difficult situation far outweigh the potential disadvantages.

Although dorsal hand veins are commonly used in digital replantation and revascularization, they are larger than the digital vessels. The small volar subcutaneous veins just proximal to the wrist are long and straight with matching diameter and have few major side branches. The dorsal hand veins and the cephalic vein near the wrist are appropriately sized for palmar and forearm vessels, as is the lower saphenous vein above the ankle for free flap pedicles. The saphenous is very different than upper extremity veins, however, and this should be taken into account if it is selected. It has a very thick muscular wall and can present problems with spasm. It is not an appropriate graft in most instances distal to the wrist. It should be noted that vein grafts that are larger than the diameter of the artery needing grafting usually do not present problems, but experimental work has shown that a significantly smaller vein graft (<50% diameter) leads to higher thombosis rates.[178]

All vein grafts should be marked and reversed when used in arterial reconstruction, because it has been shown that even the smallest digital vessels contain valves.[43,292] Most authors recommend completion of both anastomoses before removal of the clamps to prevent thrombosis at the site of the first repair. The anastomoses should be briskly irrigated with heparinized solution before removal of the clamps. Vein grafts always seem to elongate after reperfusion, and a determination of the required length of vein graft to bridge a defect requires considerable experience. If the graft is too short, tension will be present at the anastomoses; if too long, retraction of the arterial ends with concomitant narrowing or kinking of the elongated graft may occur.[353] When possible (i.e., in elective procedures), the defect to be grafted should be measured before excision and the vein graft measured and marked before harvesting. Measuring the vein graft in situ (to match the arterial defect) before it is divided is probably the best way to avoid making it too short or too long. Another technique is to complete the proximal anastomosis first and allow blood to fill the graft. This technique will usually make the vein graft assume its natural length, and it can be trimmed appropriately once filled with arterial pressure. While this theoretically may increase the chances of thrombosis of the proximal repair, this rarely occurs in clinical practice. Experimentally, the graft can be up to 35% longer than the replaced segment without kinking.[353] Another option is to fill the vein with heparinized saline and clamp it at both ends after harvesting. The vein is then anastomosed just beyond the clamps while it is still distended with saline. This technique prevents kinking and may prevent later spasm owing to the hydrostatic dilatation.[314]

For reasons of potential twisting of the graft and appropriate trimming, I always perform the proximal anastomosis first and then allow the vein graft to perfuse with arterial blood. If the distal end is kept clamped for a short period, the graft will "unwind" and extend to its full length once distended with arterial pressure. Once the appropriate lie and length of the graft have been determined, a microvascular clamp can be replaced upstream from the proximal anastomosis. The vein graft is then flushed with heparinized saline and the distal anastomosis performed. I have frequently used this technique and have not found thrombosis of the proximal anastomosis to be a recurrent problem, despite fears to the contrary.

Prosthetic Grafts

Although adequate prosthetic vessels exist for the macrovascular surgeon, the use of vascular prostheses smaller than a diameter of approximately 6 mm remains problematic.[177,191]

Some series have reported high patency rates with small prostheses,[94,192,286] but in general the long-term (more than 3-week) patency rates are less than with autogenous vein grafts. At the microvascular level, all prostheses tried up to this time have had very high thrombotic rates at the site of anastomosis with standard techniques.[65,191,235,286,294] One of the primary problems presented is in the anastomotic site.[191,192,235] This problem is ameliorated somewhat by using a sleeve technique (see previous discussion) between the prosthesis and the native vessel,[34,144,336] but long-term patencies are relatively poor. Although these problems will probably be worked out in the future, at present there is no suitable prosthetic vessel replacement for microsurgical use.

Venous Drainage

Inadequate venous drainage is a common problem in digital replantation and is occasionally seen in free tissue transfer as well. Venous drainage of the digits has been studied in great detail, and an understanding of venous anatomy may allow location of additional veins for anastomosis.[262,292,412] Transfer of veins dissected from adjacent areas or digits may be helpful. In situations in which adequate venous drainage cannot be established or congestion appears late, several means of augmentation of venous drainage have been described.

The medicinal leech, *Hirudo medicinalis,* has become widely utilized to compensate for poor venous outflow, particularly in cases of replantation.[129,153,238,399] Leeches are quite effective in removing venous blood by feeding and by oozing that occurs later from the powerful anticoagulant (hirudin) they inject locally.[35,189,254,258,269] Medical grade leeches are available within 24 hours from New York for use in the United States or from Great Britain for use in Europe. The primary problem with leeches is the presence of the saprophytic organism *Aeromonas hydrophila* in their gut, which can cause infection. This has primarily been seen in cases of necrotic tissue at the site of leech application.[104,403] Prophylaxis with a third-generation cephalosporin is appropriate to decrease the risk of infection.[258] Leeches may have some place in salvaging a replanted digit but are not adequate in the face of a failing flap. Too much blood is present in a flap for any number of leeches to drain the excess in the face of a patent arterial anastomosis. *Leeches should not be substituted for an appropriate return to the operating room to revise the venous anastomosis if it is occluded.*

Survival of replanted digits without venous anastomosis has been reported by anticoagulation with heparin and allowing open drainage of the part.[128,347,412] Blood loss with this technique can be substantial,[205] and the risks of transfusion must be weighed against the functional need for the amputated part. Venous drainage can also be augmented by removal of the nail and heparinization as reported by Gordon and associates.[148] Blood loss is less with this technique, and survival rates above 70% have been reported. Others, including myself, have been unable to achieve even the reasonable success rates reported using these techniques; my failure rate approaches 100%. Milking the replanted digit of venous blood may also be effective, and an automatic milking apparatus has been constructed from readily available parts.[237] In replantation, Smith and associates reported that if both digital arteries are available, one may be used to construct an arteriovenous anastomosis to decompress the digit if venous drainage is absent.[369]

Despite the method used, if the part survives, venous congestion usually disappears between the fifth and seventh days. The exact mechanism for this is unknown, but presumably some type of collateral vascular channel is reestablished.[148] The time required for reestablishment may vary by the type of tissue (skin, subcutaneous, muscle), and late loss of the pedicle in free tissue transfers has been reported.[123]

Maintaining Flow

Once the anastomoses are completed, what additional steps can be taken to improve or maintain blood flow? Both pharmacologic and nonpharmacologic methods have been suggested, but none will substitute for a technically adequate anastomosis of normal vessel ends without tension. Measures used empirically often have some basis, and others have been studied clinically or in the laboratory.[145] The first opportunity to protect the anastomosis is during the procedure. Meticulous hemostasis will prevent hematoma formation.[342,348] Fasciotomy after a long ischemic interval in limb replantation will prevent constriction due to postoperative swelling. Warming the amputated part or flap will reduce vasospasm and increase flow.[25]

The wound is closed in such a way that the vessels are not kinked or compressed and so that later swelling or hematoma does not compromise the lumen. Veins, being low-pressure systems, are more prone to these problems, and many clinical failures have been attributed to venous compromise. The wound may be left partially open, as in the midlateral incision used for replantation, or loosely closed over drains if adequate skin is available. If not, local flaps, primary skin grafting, or other biologic dressings may provide coverage without constriction. It is always better to place a small nonmeshed skin graft over the vessels than to occlude them with skin closure. I agree strongly with Scheker, who advocates monitoring the revascularized part during closure to avoid pedicle compression.[352] Drains should be soft and pliable (Penrose or silicone) and should not be placed directly against the vessels so that their suction or removal does not cause vasospasm, thrombosis, or necrosis of the vessel wall (all of which I have seen). They may be sutured in place with 6-0 plain suture to prevent migration but still allow later removal.

The dressing has several functions: it protects and immobilizes the extremity and should provide gentle compression to control edema. Soft padding is placed between digits after wound coverage with noncircumferential dressings. Dressing removal may cause pain and secondary vasospasm. I prefer not to change or manipulate the dressing for at least 5 to 7 days postoperatively, if possible. Therefore, in cases in which dressing change is required in the early postoperative period because of excessive bleeding (usually seen with heparinization), the possibility of infection, or for secondary skin grafting, I remove the dressing in a warmed operating suite with the patient under long-acting axillary block or general anesthesia.

Because venous congestion seems more common than problems with adequate arterial inflow, elevation is usually prescribed. Less elevation or even a dependent position helps arterial inflow but increases the risk of edema and venous congestion.

Several studies have looked at the timing and cause of flap loss after microsurgery, and the microsurgeon should be aware of some of these data.[167,315,362] Most flaps that are lost have their initial problem in the first several hours after surgery. It is obvious that problems in the early postoperative period (first 12 hours) are primarily due to technical difficulties at the anastomosis. Thrombosis of an intact anastomosis can also occur during this time period as a result of compression from a hematoma. After this initial period, few flaps are lost until the period of 8 days to 2 weeks. At this stage, anastomotic thromboses that occur are generally due to an abscess around the pedicle. Experimentally, 75% of anastomoses performed in the presence of a staphylococcal infection thrombose.[263] Even a distant infection can lead to anastomotic thrombosis, and studies have documented a microvascular thrombosis rate of approximately 20% in the presence of distant infection.[263,279]

Postoperative Measures

Once the dressing is applied, most measures are directed toward prevention of vasospasm. Of the factors influencing blood flow through a revascularized part, several are under sympathetic control (Fig. 44-25).[321] The following measures appear to be widely recommended by most microvascular surgeons[116,174,291,329,410]:

1. Bed rest or limited moving of the patient for 3 to 5 days
2. Room warmed above 78°F (replants and toe transfers only)
3. Private room; limiting of visitors and telephone calls to decrease emotional stress
4. Adequate analgesia
5. Prohibition of smoking, caffeine, and chocolate because they may cause vasoconstriction

Vascular thrombosis, if it occurs, is most likely in the first 12 hours after completion of the anastomosis, as noted previously. For this reason, I advocate close examination of the flap during the initial 10- to 12-hour postoperative period by an experienced observer, usually a member of the surgical team. After this point, hourly checks by the nursing staff (with routine physician rounds) are probably adequate.

Fluid administration lowers blood viscosity and maintains cardiac output to provide adequate arterial inflow.[24,99,376] Vasopressor agents are contraindicated. Oxygen administration, during periods of postanesthesia respiratory depression, and transfusion to maintain adequate hemoglobin levels will improve oxygenation of the revascularized part.[60] Although practiced by many microsurgeons, subjecting the patient, staff, and surgeon to a room of semi-tropical temperature is usually cruel and unusual punishment. Flaps placed on the body surface are much more sensitive to the patient's core temperature than the ambient temperature. Replanted digits and transferred toes may be very sensitive, however, to acute changes in temperature. Although it is wise to place patients in the immediate postoperative period in a warm room after replantation or toe transfer, the temperature can probably be "normalized" for comfort after the patient is awake and stable.

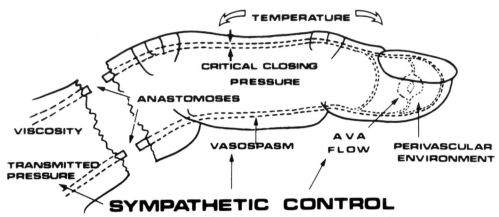

FIGURE 44-25. Factors influencing flow through replanted or revascularized tissues include (1) technical perfection of microvascular anastomoses; (2) intra-arterial pressure transmitted to the distal tissues (which falls with decreasing vessel size and extremity elevation); (3) vasospasm, which may be neurogenic (mediated through sympathetic pathways that control vessel caliber and status of arteriovenous anastomoses) or autonomous (mediated by vessel wall catecholamines); (4) alterations in the perivascular environment (pH, electrolyte concentration, blood outside vessel wall, etc.); (5) ambient temperature (direct vessel effect as well as neurogenic influence); and (6) blood viscosity. The influence of soft tissue edema is significant in the critical closing pressure, that is, an intravascular pressure lower than vessel wall tension and extramural pressure. Note the factors that are under sympathetic control. (From Phelps DB, Rutherford RB, Boswick JA Jr: Control of vasospasm following trauma and microvascular surgery. J Hand Surg [Am] 4:109-117, 1979, with permission.)

In microvascular procedures in the upper extremity, I frequently use an indwelling brachial sheath catheter placed by the anesthesiologist.[203] This catheter can be used for operative anesthesia and maintained for 3 to 5 days postoperatively. The catheter is attached to a bupivacaine (Marcaine) pump that maintains a continuous axillary block in the postoperative period. This technique has also been reported using a catheter placed in the supraclavicular area with good results.[232] I use this primarily for its sympathectomy effect, but it has the added benefit of significantly reducing pain in the operated limb in the postoperative period. One report has noted a decrease in flow to the revascularized tissue if the block is placed after vascular anastomosis, which was believed to be the result of a vascular steal phenomenon.[392] For this reason, the block or catheter should be placed before performing the anastomosis (at the beginning of the case).

Although endothelial regeneration begins immediately, experimental studies have shown that as many as 21 days may be required for complete regeneration at the site of repair.[358,387] Exposed sutures may not be totally covered with endothelium for up to 5 weeks, and therefore I believe that some care should be exercised for up to 3 weeks. I ask that the patient abstain from caffeine and/or smoking for this period to avoid problems with vasospasm.

Failure of Reperfusion

Crush and Avulsion Injuries

Failure of blood flow through an anastomosis may be immediate or delayed. If proximal blood flow was verified, the repair was technically well performed, and vasospasm has been treated, brisk flow usually occurs. If not, the problem is probably to be found in the revascularized part. Immediate failure of flow may be due to unrecognized vessel damage more distally, which should be identified and corrected with a vein graft. It is also important to make sure

that the anastomosis was not made distally to a vein instead of an artery.

In replantation, injury to the amputated part may be of such severity and extent that, perhaps, disseminated coagulation occurs in the distal vessels and capillary network. Soft tissue damage occurring to an amputated part after it is off may not be obvious until it is revascularized. Crush and avulsion injuries may produce sufficient intimal damage to massively activate the cascade mechanism by activation of factor XII.[86,141,381] If this occurs, significant flow does not occur into the revascularized part after revascularization. Milking the amputated part before revascularization, or perfusion with fibrinolytic agents, free radical scavengers, or oxygenated blood substitutes, might help (theoretically), but in our experience these digits are usually not salvageable.

Reperfusion Injury (No-Reflow Phenomenon)

Occasionally, after a well-performed anastomosis, arterial inflow can be demonstrated by initial bleeding from the revascularized part and patency tests may indicate patency but venous return is sluggish or absent.[273] Gradual cessation of flow then occurs, the distal bleeding ceases, and the arterial anastomosis fails. This is termed the *no-reflow phenomenon,* which was first described after revascularization in the cerebral circulation[18] and later in experimental flaps by May.[115,273] Experimental studies have shown a 50% incidence of failure due to no reflow after 4 hours of warm ischemia time in rat hind limbs; ongoing arterial obstruction, arteriovenous shunting, and alterations of the clotting mechanism were suggested as possible factors.[415] Other more likely possibilities include (1) edema and swelling of the vascular endothelium and parenchymal cells with resultant narrowing of the capillary lumen, (2) disseminated intravascular thrombosis, and (3) loss of physiologic integrity of the venule or capillary wall.[115,273]

Whether prior perfusion with various solutions significantly affects the rate of ultimate survival in experimental situations is as yet undetermined.[69,225,275] However, perfusion with oxygenated fluorocarbon, Collins solution, or hemoglobin perfusion solution,[374] combined with hypothermia, has been shown experimentally to markedly lengthen the allowable ischemic interval.[379,389] Perfusion with heparinized saline and/or lactated Ringer's has been shown to be detrimental to most ischemic tissues, however.[69,168,339] Raising a flap some time before the actual transfer (flap delay) increases the time it may remain devascularized without demonstrating the no-reflow phenomenon.[395] Alpha receptor hypersensitivity to circulating catecholamines may play a role,[80] and the delay phenomenon may some day be explained by a better understanding of no-reflow problems.[80,197,396]

Other research has implicated reperfusion injury and the production of free radicals as the cause of the no-reflow phenomenon. During prolonged ischemia, adenosine triphosphate is broken down to hypoxanthine, and xanthine oxidase is formed by the action of a protease in response to the low oxygen tension produced by ischemia.[236] When reperfusion occurs, the presence of molecular oxygen allows hypoxanthine conversion to xanthine and superoxide radicals (oxygen free radicals). The oxygen free radical may react further with water to produce hydrogen peroxide, and hydrogen peroxide may then also react with other oxygen radicals to form highly reactive hydroxyl radicals (OH). During normal metabolism, superoxide dismutase (SOD) is present in sufficient quantities to scavenge these free radicals and prevent damage, but after long periods of ischemia this system is overloaded by excess free radicals.

Pharmacologic manipulation to prevent or reverse this injury is being explored.[74,197,202,236,267,295,366,400] Tissue damage from reperfusion may be decreased by blocking the conversion of hypoxanthine to xanthine or by providing excess SOD to scavenge the oxygen free radicals. Allopurinol blocks the former reaction and has been shown experimentally to exert a protective effect.[202] SOD and other free radical scavengers are still investigational drugs and are not available for clinical use. Some centers, however, routinely give allopurinol after replantation in an attempt to provide some protection. I have not adopted this treatment because of the potential side effects of this drug.

Unfortunately, at the present time there is no satisfactory treatment for failure of reperfusion and these digits or flaps are usually lost. Treatment of the revascularized part with fibrinolytic agents (urokinase, streptokinase) has been suggested in these situations.[87,324] Improvement in flow has been demonstrated in ischemic flaps[88,324] and in hand ischemia secondary to distal arterial occlusion.[212] Human recombinant tissue plasminogen activator has been used effectively for partial flap salvage more recently.[21] However, an experimental study designed to test the effect of intravascular fibrinolysis on small vessel thrombosis showed no effect in vessels with an internal diameter of 0.8 to 1.5 mm.[89]

Monitoring Techniques

Loss of the revascularized tissue may occur in the postoperative period as a result of loss of the arterial inflow and/or venous drainage. After replantation, there is a failure rate of 15% to 25%. In free tissue transfer, to achieve a 90% to 95% success rate, up to 20% of patients will have to be reoperated on for revision of the anastomosis.[257] Considering the investment of time, surgical risk, and money in microsurgical procedures, an objective means of monitoring is highly desirable.[376] The ideal monitoring system should:

- Be safe, reliable, inexpensive, and noninvasive
- Provide continuous monitoring and rapid indication of impaired perfusion
- Distinguish between arterial and venous obstruction
- Be able to monitor all types of tissues
- Be easily interpreted by nursing personnel

One must remember that the most reliable monitor of the adequacy of perfusion is an experienced observer. No machine to date has been found to be foolproof, and all data from such instruments require at least some interpretation by the observer.[317] One study that evaluated clinical monitoring classified changes in tissue perfusion into stages, based on capillary refill time, color, and bleeding from a needle stick to the tissue.[139] The percent loss of the revascularized tissue increased as the clinical situation (stage) worsened, which is what one would expect. The surgeon should be thoroughly familiar with whatever monitoring device is chosen, however, and the personnel should have an understanding of how it works and its foibles. Biomedical technology has produced several instruments for monitoring the vascularity of tissue, but unfortunately no one instrument is optimum for all clinical situations.

End organ systems such as replanted digits can be adequately monitored using temperature probes, and this technique is widely used. The equipment is relatively inexpensive, the minimum temperature associated with viability is generally accepted as 30°C, and interpretation by nursing personnel is straightforward.[261,375]

Monitoring free tissue transfers surrounded by or buried in other well-vascularized tissue cannot be done adequately by temperature measurement. The transfer will assume the temperature of its surroundings and thus may remain warm even if nonviable. More sophisticated monitors are therefore required.[179-181,185,216,229] Transcutaneous oxygen, laser Doppler, pH monitoring, and photoplethysmography have all been used for clinical monitoring by various centers, and the choice of monitoring technique depends on the surgeon. The recent development of a small implantable Doppler probe that can be placed on either the artery or vein at a point beyond the anastomosis has proven an excellent monitoring system for free tissue transfers (Fig. 44-26).[229,409] This probe has a few problems associated with its use but will rapidly recognize any loss of flow. I now utilize this type of monitoring on all free tissue transfers.

Parameters of Success

With experience, microvascular surgery should provide reliable restoration of flow to severed parts and/or free tissue transfers. The results of the surgery should no longer hinge solely on the ability to keep the tissue alive. Unfortunately, even after nearly 40 years of experience with microsurgery, success rates have not reached 100%, nor are they likely to as long as there is a human element involved (both on the part of the surgeon and the patient). Few studies have looked at a large number of patients prospectively in terms of what factors portend success or failure in microvascular surgery. Recently, however, Khouri undertook a prospective study involving 23 experienced reconstructive microsurgeons in a

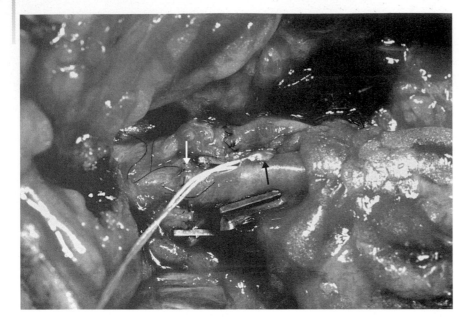

FIGURE 44-26. Implantable Doppler probe on vessel after anastomosis. *Black arrow* points to Doppler probe, which is contained in a thin silicone sheath that is placed around the vessel distal to the arterial anastomosis in this case. *White arrow* points to anastomosis between recipient artery and flap artery.

worldwide survey of this sort.[227] Many of his findings are not surprising, but a few should be noted.

A total of 496 microvascular free flap transfers were included in the study, with a flap failure rate of 4%. Ten percent of the flaps required re-exploration for postoperative thrombosis, and there was an 8% intraoperative thrombosis rate (exclusive of the postoperative thromboses). Very few factors had a statistically significant effect on success or failure of the procedure. The only technical factor with a positive effect (increased success rate) was the anastomosis of more than one vein per flap. The only factor with a negative effect (decreased success rate) was the use of an interposition vein graft. Whether this means that two anastomoses are more risky than one is not clear; this relationship may in fact be due to the increased complexity of procedures requiring vein grafts (with resultant increase in flap loss). Each of the centers used a variety of different protocols in terms of pharmacologic treatment of these patients, yet none of these protocols showed a statistically better flap survival rate. It is interesting to note that the routine use of intraoperative heparin (either as a bolus or a drip) was associated with an increase in flap failure.

These data seem to confirm two points: (1) even with experience, microvascular anastomosis is not successful 100% of the time; and (2) good surgery is more important than pharmacology in terms of a successful outcome.

Organizing a Microsurgical Service

Replantations and free tissue transfer can be tedious and demanding procedures and for many reasons are best performed using a team concept. As the team members work together and learn their respective tasks, less time will be wasted and frustration will be minimized. The reader contemplating such an undertaking is referred to guidelines for organizing a microsurgical team.[58,134,151,285,307]

PHYSIOLOGY AND PHARMACOLOGY OF THE MICROCIRCULATION

Physiology of the Microcirculation

Basic Mechanisms

Poiseuille's law states that fluid flow through a vessel (F) is proportional to the pressure gradient (ΔP/L, change in pressure over length), the radius (r), and the fluid viscosity (η), as shown below[276]:

$$F\alpha(\Delta P/L)(r^3/\eta)$$

Therefore, pressure decreases with decreasing vessel size. Extremity elevation also decreases pressure distally by a hydrostatic effect. Therefore, to increase flow one must (1) increase vessel radius (diameter), (2) decrease the viscosity, and/or (3) increase ΔP/L. This is a factor that can be increased by increasing the perfusion pressure and/or decreasing the vessel resistance.

Smooth muscle in the walls of arteries, arterioles, and temperature-regulating arteriovenous anastomoses (arteriovenous shunts) is under sympathetic control.[25,274] Sympathetic stimulation reduces skin and digital flow, whereas sympathectomy markedly increases flow. Other than agents affecting the clotting mechanism, most adjunctive drug therapy is aimed at producing a chemical sympathectomy, which increases the vessel diameter and decreases the peripheral resistance.[276,397]

In addition, local mechanical factors are important. External pressure on the vessel wall from tight dressings, hematoma, or edema may exceed the "critical closing pressure," especially in the venous system (see Fig. 44-25).[321] Tissue anoxia and decreased perfusion lead to increased capillary permeability and tissue edema, and a vicious circle akin to that seen in compartment syndromes may occur. Both dextran and heparin appear to lower viscosity—dextran by hemodilution and its "anti-platelet clumping effect" and heparin as a result of surface binding to red blood cells. Adequate hydration of the patient is also important, not only to prevent peripheral vasoconstriction but also to lower blood viscosity.[24,99] Maintenance of cardiac output and prevention of shunting to the central circulation will keep the perfusion pressure adequate. Although not a substitute for a perfect anastomosis of undamaged vessel, pharmacologic manipulation of the microcirculation may at times be an important adjunct. Its importance increases in traumatic situations where damaged vessels may be present. The reader in this area will be confused by the multitude of postoperative regimens advocated by various authors, and only through an understanding of the physiology of the microcirculation and clotting mechanisms can one critically assess these recommendations.

Hemostatic Mechanisms

Three major mechanisms function to repair vascular injury. Eventual vessel patency or lack thereof is determined by the net result of the interaction of these three mechanisms: (1) formation of a platelet clot, (2) formation of a fibrin clot, and (3) fibrinolysis.

Drugs commonly used after microvascular surgery may affect one or more of these mechanisms and be helpful or detrimental, occasionally both, as we shall see when discussing aspirin. Several feedback systems prevent extension of the repair process beyond the site of injury.

Platelets

Formation of a platelet clot at a site of vessel injury occurs before a fibrin clot and is most likely to block a small vessel repair.[70,213,226] Endothelial damage exposes collagen and subendothelial factor VIII (von Willebrand factor) polymers (synthesized by endothelial cells), which attract and bind platelets. Once platelets adhere, they change in shape from disks to spheres and release their granule contents locally and into the vessel lumen (release phenomenon). These granule contents are rich in adenosine diphosphate, a potent platelet aggregating agent that causes further platelet aggregation and absorption of fibrinogen from plasma.[287,398] The result is a platelet plug, rich in fibrinogen and ready for conversion into a fibrin thrombus by the action of thrombin. Both thrombin (from the cascade coagulation pathway) and epinephrine (stress hormone) enhance platelet aggregation and the release phenomenon. Epinephrine is also a potent vasoconstrictor.

Endothelial cells also synthesize and release into the vessel lumen prostaglandin I_2 (PGI_2), a vasodilator that exerts a protective effect by limiting excess accumulation of platelets on damaged subendothelial structures. PGI_2 synthesis from arachidonic acid requires the enzyme cyclooxygenase. Aspirin inhibits formation of PGI_2 by acetylating the active site on this enzyme and thus may have a negative effect on patency, but this effect is dose related (Fig. 44-27).[70,125,287,288]

Platelets are derived from megakaryocytes that surround bone marrow sinuses. There are 150,000 to 350,000 platelets in a microliter of blood, and the average platelet survives for up to 10 days. Platelets have no nucleus or DNA, and therefore no metabolic means to synthesize proteins. If they are altered biochemically by drug treatment that renders them incapable of aggregation, they remain ineffective during their life span. The blood level of aspirin attained from a single dose as low as 3 mg/kg (2.5 to 3.5 grains a day) will acetylate the cyclooxygenase present in the platelet wall, preventing formation of endoperoxides prostaglandins G_2 and H_2, and thus thromboxane A_2. Drugs containing an imidazole group block thromboxane production more directly. Thromboxane A_2 potentiates release of platelet granules, induces further platelet aggregation, and is locally vasoconstrictive. Blocking thromboxane A_2 production will limit platelet aggregation and release phenomena (Fig. 44-28).[125,135,288] Therefore, many microsurgeons recommend a low dose of aspirin after microvascular repair to inhibit thromboxane A_2–induced platelet aggregation. Higher doses may be harmful, however, because they block the beneficial effects of PGI_2.

Figures 44-27, 44-28, and 44-29 should be referred to as an aid in understanding the mechanism and/or site of action of any drug that has an anticoagulant effect on the microcirculation. As new drugs are reported, one should attempt to place them appropriately in this scheme as well.

Cascade Pathway

The coagulation proteins in the classic cascade clotting mechanism are labeled with Roman numerals: factors I (fibrinogen), II (prothrombin), and VII through XIII. Activated forms are indicated by the additional suffix "a" (e.g., cleavage of prothrombin [factor II] to the active enzyme thrombin [factor IIa]). The liver synthesizes and secretes all the coagulation proteins. Endothelial cells (including the vascular endothelium) also synthesize and secrete a polymer of factor VIII, bound to von Willebrand factor.[287] The net result of activation of the cascade system is the generation of thrombin, which converts soluble fibrinogen into insoluble fibrin, forming a "red clot." Thrombin is generated by two different sequences known as the intrinsic and the extrinsic pathways (see Fig. 44-29).

In the intrinsic pathway, all needed coagulation factors are present (intrinsic) in normal blood. Vascular endothelial disruption exposes charged subendothelial molecules, and factor XII is attracted to the site of damage, where it is activated. The coagulation cascade is then locally activated.

The extrinsic pathway is initiated by leakage into the bloodstream of phospholipoprotein membranes from disrupted tissue cells, which are normally extrinsic to the circulation. These substances activate factor VII and initiate the cascade. The extrinsic path is probably more rapid in vivo.

Once formed, thrombin splits fibrinogen into fibrin polymers, which link with each other and with aggregated platelets to form a thrombus at the site of injury. When a thrombus is formed, the portions of the thrombus projecting into the vessel lumen that are not necessary for repair of the endothelial injury may be degraded by fibrinolysis, restoring the vessel lumen.

Excessive formation of intravascular thrombin is prevented by inhibition of various coagulation factors and thrombin itself by antithrombin and protein C, which are present both in blood and on endothelial cells. Thrombus formation is normally restricted in this way to the site of vascular injury and does not progress to completely occlude

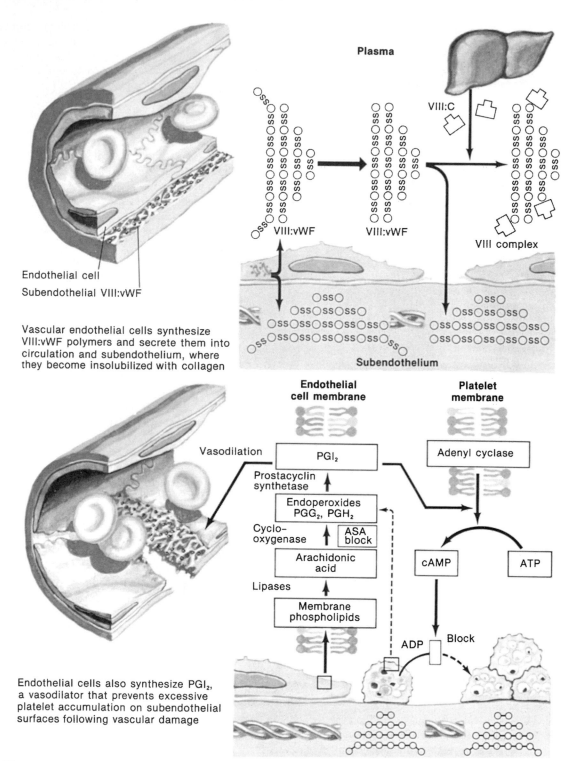

FIGURE 44-27. Vascular endothelial function. (From Moake JL, Funicella T: Common bleeding problems. CIBA Clin Symp 35:2-32, 1983, with permission.)

the lumen. Abnormalities of the clotting mechanism may predispose a patient to thrombosis.[83,140,194,244,282,313,384]

Hypercoagulability

Patients with one of the previously mentioned abnormalities of the clotting mechanism can present formidable problems for the reconstructive microsurgeon. If a patient develops problems with recurrent thrombosis after microvascular anastomosis, he or she should certainly receive a work-up

for one of the hereditary thrombotic disorders. These include deficiencies of antithrombin, protein C, and protein S.[42] The microsurgeon should also be aware that certain disease states carry an increased risk of hypercoagulability, among these cancer[154] and premature atherosclerosis.[252] One study found abnormal protein C levels in 70% of a group of cancer patients undergoing free flap reconstruction, but this had little effect on flap loss.[26] Four of seven cancer patients in another study were found to have the parameters of hyper-

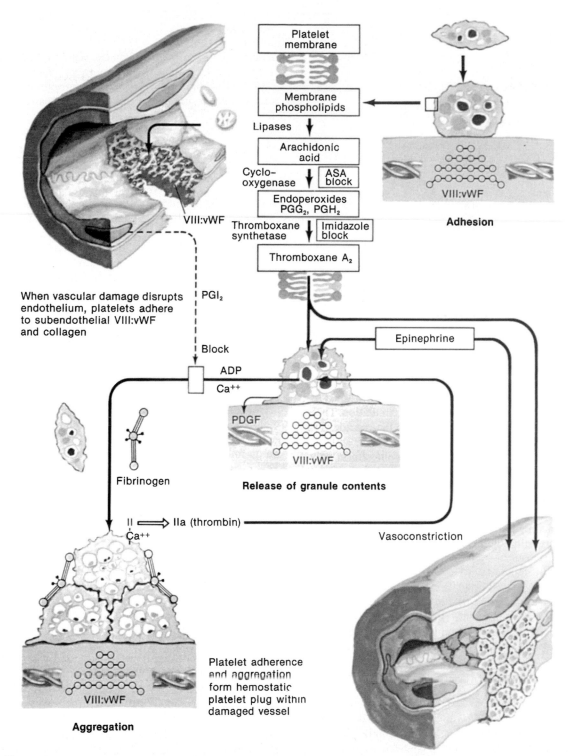

FIGURE 44-28. Platelet adhesion, release, and aggregation. (From Moake JL, Funicella T: Common bleeding problems. CIBA Clin Symp 35:2-32, 1983, with permission.)

coagulability on preoperative laboratory examination, but with appropriate antithrombotic management there were no flap losses.[310] Another group of patients who are frequently hypercoagulable (which is often overlooked) is people with type II diabetes. These patients often have elevated levels of lipoprotein(a), which is associated with a hypercoagulable state.[290] Some microsurgeons routinely screen diabetics for elevated lipoprotein(a) levels before attempting microvascular reconstruction. Heparin and/or long-term oral anti-

coagulation will ameliorate most thrombotic episodes in these patients.[385] Our personal microvascular experience with several patients found to have hypercoagulable states (after failed microvascular procedures) has been dismal, which has been the anecdotal experience of several colleagues as well. Individuals with recognized hypercoagulability should probably not be considered candidates for elective microvascular reconstructive surgery, because they may present insurmountable problems with vascular thrombosis.

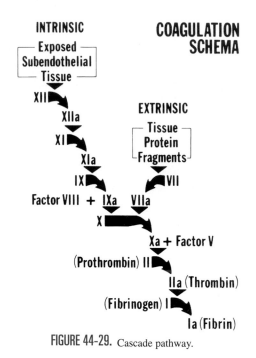

COAGULATION SCHEMA

INTRINSIC

Exposed Subendothelial Tissue

XII
XIIa
XI
XIa
IX

EXTRINSIC

Tissue Protein Fragments

VII

Factor VIII + IXa   VIIa

X

Xa + Factor V

(Prothrombin) II

IIa (Thrombin)

(Fibrinogen) I

Ia (Fibrin)

FIGURE 44-29. Cascade pathway.

Fibrinolysis

Once bleeding is controlled and repair of the vessel wall has begun, the fibrin meshwork is lysed by plasmin. Plasminogen is absorbed onto fibrin from the blood plasma and activated to plasmin by hydrolytic enzymes derived from disrupted tissue lysosomes. In addition, the endothelium has inherent fibrinolytic activity that decreases progressively during ischemia, reaching a minimum after 6 hours of ischemia. After restoration of flow, up to 96 hours is required before this inherent fibrinolytic activity returns to normal levels.[207]

Urokinase (of renal origin) and streptokinase (a bacterial enzyme) do not directly lyse fibrin polymers but instead activate circulating plasminogen by exposing active enzyme sites.[85,87,89,212,226] Recombinant human tissue plasminogen activator acts in a similar fashion to these agents and is utilized more commonly today.[22] The possible clinical use of these agents is discussed later.

Pharmacology of Selected Drugs

The timing and route of administration of pharmacologic agents are important to achieve maximum benefit. The stress of anesthesia and surgery causes epinephrine to be released into the circulation, thus increasing the possibility of thrombosis. Prophylactic adjunctive drug treatment should therefore be considered. Although re-endothelialization begins immediately, some form of anticoagulant therapy should be continued for at least 3 to 5 days until the endothelium regenerates and covers the anastomotic site.[77,289,358] Diurnal variations in coagulability also occur and may affect the outcome of microvascular procedures.[186] The reader should be aware that the recommendations that follow regarding individual drugs are in most cases based on firm theoretical considerations but that supporting experimental data or controlled clinical trials are in most cases lacking.

Anticoagulants

Heparin

Heparin is a complex substance with multiple actions in vivo. Most important to the microvascular surgeon is the preferential binding to vascular endothelial cells that replaces the normal negative charge lost in areas of endothelial damage. This high concentration in the area of damage also inhibits platelet aggregation, decreases fibrinogen clotting, and activates local antithrombin III. Systemic heparin also has two direct effects on the blood itself: activation of serum antithrombin III and lowering of blood viscosity.[110,114,226,340] When sharply divided vessels are repaired, the patency rate using systemic heparin as an adjunct is probably no greater than that for untreated controls.[110,226] However, another laboratory study designed to test the efficacy of systemic heparin after crush and avulsion injuries showed dramatic improvement in the patency rate after repair of traumatized vessels.[86] Also, in a retrospective study of replantation failures, 20% occurred within 4 hours of discontinuing systemic heparin.[186] This same study suggested that full heparinizing doses were required and that "low-dose" regimens were ineffectual. However, low-dose regimens and heparin analogues with less effect on overall clotting are attractive from the standpoint of bleeding complications. Studies of a continuous low-dose infusion of heparin in the postoperative period have demonstrated improved flap survival rates with no increase in bleeding complications. Full heparinizing doses usually require transfusion and repeated dressing changes.[205]

Although heparinization is probably not needed in replantation of sharp amputations or uncomplicated free tissue transfer, it should be strongly considered in problem cases such as avulsion or crush injury, which would be expected to expose multiple areas of endothelial injury.[86,141,381] Patients demonstrating a tendency to hypercoagulability and thrombosis requiring anastomotic revision should also be protected.[119] In patients who are hypercoagulable, a full heparinizing dose of 40 units/kg of body weight should be given before completion of the anastomosis and release of the clamps. If there has simply been a thrombosis of an anastomosis intraoperatively, a smaller dose (in the 1500- to 2000-unit range) should be given to avoid bleeding complications. Heparin is also important as a local anticoagulant in irrigating solutions.[368] Complications of heparin include bleeding and heparin-induced thrombocytopenia and thrombosis.*

Hirudin

Hirudin is an isopolypeptide produced naturally in small amounts by the medicinal leech *Hirudo medicinalis*. Its existence and effects have been appreciated for many years, especially in relation to the use of leeches for venous congestion in microsurgery (see earlier). Hirudin is a direct inhibitor of thrombin. It is not inactivated by platelet factor 4 and may be more effective in the presence of platelet-rich thrombus.[155] It is available as a recombinant product in the form of desirudin and lepirudin.[270,304] It has found application primarily in the management of patients with

*See references 14, 33, 38, 79, 82, 136, 159, 220, 243, 323, 335, 368, and 377.

heparin-induced thrombocytopenia (HITT), who require anticoagulation but are severely allergic to heparin.[155,156] Although it has not been reported in the literature, I have utilized lepirudin in a case of free tissue transfer in a patient who suffered from HITT. After thrombosis of the arterial anastomosis with two revisions, lepirudin was utilized systemically and as an irrigant solution in lieu of heparin. No further problems were encountered and the flap went on to total survival. Further study of this agent and its use in microsurgery may prove its usefulness

Acetylsalicylic Acid (Aspirin)

Aspirin is widely used after microvascular procedures because of its antiplatelet effect. Administration of a single dose as low as 3 mg/kg will inactivate circulating platelets by acetylating the enzyme cyclooxygenase present in the platelet wall.[125] Arachidonic acid cannot be metabolized to prostaglandins G_2 and H_2, and thromboxane A_2 cannot be formed. Thromboxane A_2 is necessary for the release phenomenon that leads to platelet aggregation (see Fig. 44-28). However, aspirin also blocks the synthesis of PGI_2 in the vessel wall. PGI_2 has several beneficial effects, including local vasodilatation and blockage of platelet aggregation (see Fig. 44-27).[288] Fortunately, vascular endothelium has the ability to resynthesize cyclooxygenase (the platelet cannot). Also, the effect of aspirin is dose related. The average dose required to inhibit 50% of platelet aggregation is 3.2 mg/kg, but 4.9 mg/kg is needed to inhibit PGI_2 production by the vessel wall.[70] Because of this differential effect, a small dose of aspirin is theoretically indicated. The recommended dose is 3 mg/kg (2.5 to 3.5 grains) daily. A secondary platelet release phenomenon (which is not blocked by aspirin) may be stimulated by thrombin and high collagen concentrations and may explain the lack of bleeding problems noted when aspirin is given after trauma.[226,398]

Dipyridamole is an aspirin analogue, also with antiprostaglandin effects. Its metabolism has not been as well studied, and it probably does not offer any significant advantage over aspirin, except possibly a concomitant vasodilatory effect. It appears to be rarely used by microsurgeons at this time.

Dextran

The mechanism of action of dextran is not well understood, but it appears to have both antiplatelet and heparin like effects. Although it has been widely used in microsurgery because of its presumed lower incidence of side effects, good statistical evidence to support its clinical use is lacking.[343] Pharmacologically, it is classified as a plasma expander, and it is indicated for prophylaxis of deep vein thrombosis and pulmonary embolism in patients undergoing procedures known to be associated with a high incidence of thromboembolic complications. Rare allergic reactions caused by hypersensitivity to dextran have been reported, and infrequent fatal anaphylactic reactions have also been reported.[149,190,211] Most of these reactions occur in patients not previously exposed to intravenous dextran and occur early in the infusion period. A solution known as dextran 1 has been introduced as a pretreatment to decrease the incidence of adverse reactions. The indication for its use is prophylaxis of severe anaphylactic reactions associated with intravenous infusion of clinical dextran solutions. This drug binds to polysaccharide-reacting antibodies that cross-react with clinical dextran and thus prevents the allergic reaction. The dosage in adults is 20 mL (150 mg/mL) intravenously over 1 to 2 minutes, given 1 to 2 minutes before the intravenous infusion of clinical dextran solutions. The dose in children is 0.3 mL/kg. The administration of clinical dextran should then be started within 15 minutes.[204]

The complication of dextran allergy is extremely rare; and in personal experience with well over 500 patient applications, I have never seen this complication. Osmotic complications, although uncommon, nonetheless can occur with greater frequency in certain patients.[171] I have had experience with several patients who developed pulmonary edema and/or renal shutdown after several days of continuous infusion of dextran, and this has been reported by others.[230,394] These were usually patients with marginal renal function to begin with or some underlying cardiac or pulmonary disorder. The use of dextran is likewise contraindicated in children, because it has been documented to cause an increase in bleeding problems in younger patients.

Many surgeons routinely use dextran after elective or traumatic microvascular procedures. The recommended dose in the adult is 500 mL of dextran 40 in normal saline given over 5 to 6 hours once daily for 3 to 5 days. Other microsurgeons instead administer the 500 mL of dextran slowly over a 24-hour period. Because the peak antithrombotic effect of dextran is present 4 hours after infusion, the initial dose should be started before beginning the anastomosis for maximum effect.[59,226] *Because of its lack of proven efficacy and potential complications, I do not use dextran routinely anymore in microsurgery.* I have not noted any increase in anastomotic thrombosis with its discontinuation.

Prostaglandins

Certain prostaglandins might be useful for preventing primary platelet aggregation. They have been studied experimentally both as local and systemic agents.[70,112,226,251,351] Experimentally, prostacyclin has been shown to decrease platelet aggregation at a microsurgical anastomosis.[27,92,111,131] There have been a few clinical case reports of the use of this agent in cases of recurrent thrombosis of an anastomosis.[331] Other experimental work has shown that platelet deposition at the site of anastomosis is not dependent on this pathway, however.[332] The usefulness of these agents has yet to be proven in microsurgical reconstruction.

In summary, the most widely used drug regimen seems to be aspirin and dextran. In situations where damaged vessels are presumed or known to be present, such as crush and avulsion injuries, heparin is often added and continued until the endothelium regenerates. Endothelial regeneration begins very early, and for small areas coverage may be completed quickly. In cases with more severe trauma, such as the crush and avulsion type, as long as 5 to 7 days may be required to seal the endothelium and the anastomotic site. The complications of heparinization, including bleeding and hematoma formation, have been previously discussed. At present, however, unless there are severely diseased or damaged vessels or an intraoperative thrombosis, I use only intraoperative heparinized irrigation and postoperative aspirin therapy in routine microvascular cases.

Vasodilators

Topical and Intra-arterial Agents

Vasodilatation may be accomplished by topical, intra-arterial, or systemic drug administration. Topical vasodilators are applied directly onto the vessels during dissection or after repair. Lidocaine is the most commonly used agent, but probably in strengths too low to have much beneficial effect. Concentrations of 4% to 20% are recommended based on experimental studies, but above a concentration of 10% there can be problems with toxicity.[45,46,284,325,408] I generally use a 4% solution, which is readily available in most operating rooms. Magnesium sulfate, chlorpromazine, sodium nitroprusside, and certain prostaglandins have also been used as local agents.[2,4,8,63,251,272,284,303] In rare instances, pathologic vasoconstriction that threatens viability of the revascularized tissue may occur and may be refractory to methods previously mentioned. Under these circumstances, papaverine may be injected into the distal vessel, which may release the vasospasm. Intra-arterial injection of tolazoline, nitroglycerin, reserpine, or guanethidine may also be helpful in these situations.[199,226] Reports of clinical use of these agents are sparse, and these reports should be referred to regarding the dosages and method of administration.

Pharmacology of Systemic Agents

The terminal arteries and arterioles of the peripheral circulation contain significant smooth muscle in their walls and are innervated by adrenergic fibers of the sympathetic nervous system. These adrenergic fibers release norepinephrine, which acts on the α-adrenergic receptors of vascular smooth muscle. Cutaneous (skin) vessels of the extremities respond only to changes in the basal tone of the sympathetic system; there are no direct vasodilatory fibers. Therefore, vasodilatation of skin vessels can be accomplished only by a reduction of sympathetic nervous system discharge. Skeletal muscle, on the other hand, also has β-adrenergic receptors and, thus, sympathetic dilator control. Both lowered body or blood temperature and anxiety can cause pronounced vasoconstriction mediated through the hypothalamic axis.[25,276,321]

There are several levels at which sympathetic tone can be blocked or decreased (Table 44-2). The site of action of the various vasodilators is shown in Figure 44-30. A warm, calm environment will decrease central stimulation and the level of norepinephrine released,[25,276,321] as will a stellate block, peripheral nerve block, or sympathectomy.[393] Inhibition of the amine pump and depletion of the norepinephrine precursors will also decrease production of this neurotransmitter. Reserpine blocks the storage granule transport system, and guanethidine replaces norepinephrine in the storage vesicles.[226] Bretylium prevents release of the neurotransmitter. Phenoxybenzamine and prazosin bind to receptor sites, and nifedipine blocks the effect of norepinephrine on the smooth muscle by blocking the calcium channels.[91,233] Patients requiring chronic hemodialysis may develop secondary hyperparathyroidism and hypercalcemia, and parathyroidectomy in these patients may improve peripheral blood flow.[49,84,344,417]

Several systemic vasodilator agents have been tried in microsurgical situations to improve tissue perfusion. No clear indications exist stating when to employ these agents or whether their effect is statistically significant.[121,157,187,188,224,225] Isoxsuprine, terbutaline, and prazosin have each

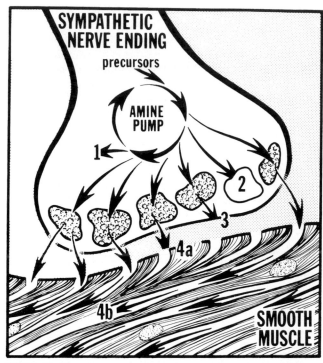

FIGURE 44-30. Methods of decreasing sympathetic tone. (1) Stop production of neurotransmitter; (2) decrease neurotransmitter available in vesicles; (3) block release; (4) block α-adrenergic receptor (4a) or calcium channel blocker (4b).

been discussed in the literature and in some instances recommended for use as peripheral vasodilators. However, these drugs do not appear to be widely used by microsurgeons at the present time. For further information about their effects and possible use in these situations, the reader is referred to the pertinent literature.[73,120,186,350]

Phenoxybenzamine (Dibenzyline) is a long-acting α-adrenergic blocking agent that increases cardiac output. It increases blood flow to the skin and has been used to treat vasospastic disorders such as Raynaud's syndrome and frostbite sequelae and to improve the survival of marginal tissue of pedicle flaps.[121,224,296,401] Orthostatic hypotension is

Table 44-2

METHODS OF DECREASING SYMPATHETIC TONE

1. Stop production of neurotransmitter.
   a. Decrease central stimulation (warm and calm environment).
   b. Perform proximal stellate block or sympathectomy.
   c. Inhibit amine pump.
   d. Deplete precursors.
2. Block storage granule transport system (reserpine) or displace transmitter from axon terminal (guanethidine).
3. Block vesicle release (bretylium).
4. Block receptor uptake or effect of neurotransmitter.
   a. Block α-adrenergic receptor (prazosin, phenoxybenzamine).
   b. Block calcium channels of vascular smooth muscle (nifedipine).

Data from references 233 and 274.

the most common side effect. The initial dose is 10 mg/day orally, which may be increased as tolerated. In the supine patient after flap transfer or replantation, 10 or 20 mg orally two or three times a day is usually well tolerated as long as the patient is supine.

Nifedipine (Procardia) is a calcium channel blocker that is probably the drug of choice for cold intolerance after successful digit or extremity replantation. It is often effective if taken just before cold stress. It is available in an extended-release form and can be given as an initial dose of 30 mg, usually at bedtime. Up to 60 mg/day may be required to relieve symptoms. It is usually well-tolerated but must be used in caution in smaller individuals and those with low blood pressure.

Chlorpromazine (Thorazine) has a wide variety of actions including α-adrenergic blockade, anti-inflammatory properties, antiplatelet effects, and cell membrane stabilization. All these actions aid in increasing the tolerance of tissue to ischemia.[63,226] In extremely large doses, chlorpromazine consistently prevents or diminishes flap necrosis in experimental animals.[41] I routinely use this agent after replantation and free flap surgery. However, no clinical studies after replantation or free tissue transfer are available. The recognized sedative effect of chlorpromazine is probably also beneficial; the recommended dose is 25 mg orally or intramuscularly every 6 to 8 hours. This agent should be used with caution in elderly patients or those with respiratory problems.

Fibrinolytic Agents

Urokinase, streptokinase, and tissue plasminogen activator (t-PA) have been recommended as being possibly beneficial in salvaging a failing replant or tissue transfer. Life-threatening allergic reactions and bleeding complications may occur, and an experienced hematologist should probably be consulted for management of these medications. Treatment must be administered early if it is to be effective, and salvage of failing replants has been reported using these techniques (Russell RC, personal communication, 1987). Likewise, these agents have been shown to be of benefit in cases where flow cannot be established into a replanted digit or flap.[21,143] In these cases, there has probably been distal embolization of clot, which the thrombolytic agent dissolves, allowing restoration of flow. These drugs must generally be administered by intra arterial catheterization, and the literature should be consulted regarding the dose and route of administration.[87-89,207,212,226,337] Local use of t-PA in replantation has been advocated, both for arterial and venous thrombosis.[22]

Research is being done to identify drugs that are more specific in their effects on the microcirculation. This may some day allow protection of the anastomosis without the threat of bleeding complications.[70,213,214]

RESEARCH AND NEW TECHNIQUES IN MICROVASCULAR SURGERY

As one might expect in such a rapidly expanding area, today's laboratory experiment often becomes tomorrow's clinical technique. Many imaginative ideas have been published that fall into this category. Mentioning these will hopefully prevent this chapter from being outmoded before it is even published.[256,361]

Several major areas of research are evident in a review of the recent literature, and each seeks to address a current clinical problem. Alternative anastomotic techniques attempt to decrease operative time and provide a more "perfect" anastomosis.[163,383] Vessel elongation by tissue expansion has been studied.[372] Gene therapy has been utilized to decrease the thrombogenicity of the anastomosis[363] and prosthetic grafts have been lined with genetically modified endothelium to improve patency rates of these grafts.[96]

The last edition of this chapter noted that vascularized allografting and transplantation of extremity parts might some day be feasible. Nerve allografts have now been utilized successfully in cases where the nerve gap exceeded available autologous grafting material.[264] Nerve allografts present a unique situation in that immunosuppression may be discontinued after the patients' axons have regenerated across the length of the allograft.[193] As of this writing, two hand transplants have been performed in the United States and a number overseas.[105,217,319,322] These procedures have instigated a great deal of worldwide controversy and debate, with reasoned voices on both sides of the issue.* Whereas the functional results have been acceptable in many cases, patients undergoing this procedure have suffered a number of sequelae, including repeated episodes of rejection, diabetes, and the need for late amputation of the transplanted hand.[106,217,249,388] Most would agree that composite tissue transplantation (including hand transplantation) should become an accepted procedure in the future, but more work needs to be done in terms of allograft rejection and its treatment to decrease the potential complications of these procedures.[28,55,218,219,248]

Vascularized allografting of various tissues and transplantation of extremity parts may some day be feasible when immunologic responses can be more predictably controlled with less toxic drugs and if problems associated with nerve regeneration can be overcome.[15,67,68,131,280,281,295,299]

ANNOTATED REFERENCES

10. Acland RD: Microsurgery Practice Manual. St. Louis, CV Mosby, 1980.

    Anyone undertaking learning microsurgery needs a manual. Acland's is one of the standards and should be available in medical libraries. This is the place to start to learn the techniques of microsurgery.

81. Cobbett JR: Free digital transfer: Report of a case of transfer of a great toe to replace an amputated thumb. J Bone Joint Surg Br 51:677, 1969.

    This is one of the first reports of a microvascular tissue transfer. Although it is obviously of historical interest, it makes good reading. There were problems with the initial toe transfer, and it is clear from reading this paper that the surgeons involved were not quite sure whether to go back and try and revise the anastomosis or not. It gives an interesting look back at the early days.

---

*See references 53, 55, 103, 183, 218, 219, 241, 248-250, 367, and 380.

90. Cordeiro PG, Santamaria E: Experience with the continuous suture microvascular anastomosis in 200 consecutive free flaps. Ann Plast Surg 40:1-6, 1998.

    Although not utilized widely, the continuous suture technique of microvascular anastomosis has many proponents. This paper discusses the technique and its application to a large series of free flaps.

118. Fanua SP, Kim J, Shaw Wilgis EF: Alternative model for teaching microsurgery. Microsurgery 21:379-382, 2001.

    This paper discusses the use of non-animal models for teaching in microsurgery. The authors began training residents in microsurgery using surgical gloves and small-diameter medical grade tubing. They found that this decreases the number of animals needed for microvascular training and that these models were effective in the early stages of training.

142. Godina M: Preferential use of end-to-side arterial anastomosis in free flap transfers. Plast Reconstr Surg 64:673-682, 1979.

    This is another paper by one of the pioneers of microsurgery, Marko Godina. He makes the case that end-to-side anastomoses are safer than end-to-end ones because the muscular layer is interrupted during arteriotomy, which decreases the risk of spasm.

229. Kind GM, Buntic RF, Buncke GM, et al: The effect of an implantable Doppler probe on the salvage of microvascular tissue transplants. Plast Reconstr Surg 101:1268-1273, 1998.

409. Wise JB, Talmor M, Hoffman LA, Gayle LB: Postoperative monitoring of microvascular tissue transplants with an implantable Doppler probe. Plast Reconstr Surg 105:2279-2280, 2000.

    These two papers discuss the use of the implantable Doppler probe in microsurgery. The implantable probe is the only direct way to evaluate flow distal to an anastomosis. This has become the standard monitoring technique for free tissue transfers.

259. Livingston CK, Ruiz-Razura A, Cohen BE: Guidelines for a successful microsurgery training center and research fellowship. Plast Reconstr Surg 104:1555-1558, 1999.

    This editorial discusses what is needed to establish a training facility for microsurgery and microsurgery fellowships. The authors note that one of the biggest hurdles is funding and discuss the approach to this. This is a very good review for anyone contemplating starting such a laboratory.

354. Seaber AV: Laboratory design in preparing for elective microvascular surgery. Hand Clin 1:233-245, 1985.

    This paper from the long-time director of the Duke University microsurgical laboratory is valuable for those just starting. It goes over how to set up a microneurovascular practice laboratory and is worthwhile reading for anyone undertaking such an endeavor.

364. Shenaq SM, Klebuc MJA, Vargo D: Free tissue transfer with the aid of loupe magnification: Experience with 251 procedures. Plast Reconstr Surg 95:262, 1995.

    This paper describes microsurgery done only with loupe magnification. This approach is particularly applicable in areas where it is difficult to get the head of the microscope (as in the axilla). These authors show that with experience, microvascular anastomosis can be safely done with high-powered loupes.

CHAPTER 45

Replantation

Richard D. Goldner and James R. Urbaniak

Although experimental replantation of amputated limbs of animals was performed successfully at the turn of the century,[18,47] clinical accomplishment of limb replantation was not realized until the 1960s. In Boston in 1962, Malt and McKhann successfully replanted the completely amputated arm of a 12-year-old boy.[66] In 1968, Komatsu and Tamai, of Japan, reported the first successful replantation of an amputated digit by microvascular technique.[57] During the following 20 years, microsurgical centers around the world reported impressive series of successful replantation with viability rates greater than 80%.* Successful replantation of digits and hands has been made possible by the development of an operating microscope with improved magnification, focus, and lighting; ultrafine nonreactive suture material; precision microcaliber needles; and a variety of microsurgical instruments.[1,11,24,77,119,120]

A knowledge of certain terms concerning amputation is essential for surgeons who perform replantations to enable universal comparison of results. *Replantation* is the reattachment of a part that has been *completely* amputated—no connection exists between the severed part and the patient. *Revascularization* is the repair of a part that has been *incompletely amputated*—some of the soft tissue (e.g., skin, nerves, or tendons) is intact. Vascular repair is necessary to prevent necrosis of the partially severed extremity. The distinction between replantation and revascularization is important when discussing the methods and especially the results of reattachment of amputated parts. The viability rates of revascularization are generally better than those of replantation because adequate venous drainage often remains intact in the former.[94] Although revascularization procedures may be easier and require less operative time than replantation, incomplete amputations with a crush-avulsion injury may be even more difficult because two teams cannot work simultaneously on separate parts to débride nonviable tissue and shorten bone to allow repair of healthy structures.

PATIENT SELECTION

Our criteria for proper patient selection for replantation are based on our team's experience with replantation of over 2000 body parts. Even with this knowledge, the decision to replant an amputated part is not always easy.[55] Factors that must be considered include the predicted morbidity to the patient, the expected chance of survival and functional outcome of the replanted part, and the total cost incurred by the patient or third-party payer. For replantation to be chosen, the anticipated function should be equal to or better than that achieved with revision of the amputation or with prosthetic replacement, although appearance is also a factor. Moreover, success in tissue viability should not be misconstrued as success in useful function of the replanted body part. Patients with guillotine-type amputations are ideal candidates;

CRITICAL POINTS: REPLANTATION INDICATIONS AND CONTRAINDICATIONS

INDICATIONS

- Thumb
- Multiple digits
- Partial hand (amputation through the palm)
- Almost any part in a child
- Wrist or forearm
- Elbow and above elbow (sharply amputated or moderately avulsed
- Individual digit distal to the flexor digitorum superficialis (FDS) tendon

CONTRAINDICATIONS

- Severely crushed or mangled parts
- Amputations at multiple levels
- Amputations in patients with other serious injuries/diseases
- Amputations in patients with severely arteriosclerotic vessels
- Amputations with prolonged warm ischemia
- Amputations in mentally unstable patients
- Individual finger amputations in an adult at a level proximal to the FDS insertion (particularly in index or small fingers)

*See references 9, 50, 54, 59, 64, 71, 72, 92, 98, 100, 101, 110-112, 130, and 137.

however, this type of amputation is uncommon. Most limbs are amputated by crushing or avulsing injuries, which makes surgical repair more difficult and lowers the percentage of viability.[2,21,129]

Good candidates for replantation are those with the following amputations: (1) thumb, (2) multiple digits, (3) partial hand (amputation through the palm), (4) almost any upper extremity part of a child, (5) wrist or forearm, (6) elbow and above elbow (only sharply amputated or moderately avulsed), and (7) individual digit distal to the FDS insertion.

Each of the aforementioned is not necessarily an absolute indication for replantation. However, if other factors are favorable, an attempt at reattachment should be performed.[32,44,54,69,72,82a,101,110] Replantation should be considered in most cases of thumb amputation[28,73,89,127] (Fig. 45-1). Even avulsion injuries requiring thumb shortening, metacarpophalangeal (MP) joint fusion, and vein and/or nerve grafting are often functionally and cosmetically superior if successfully replanted than if treated by alternative methods of reconstruction.[8,10,39,95,132]

Our patients with replanted thumbs and good sensibility tended to perform better in tasks requiring fine dexterity than did those with amputation/revision. The patients with amputation/revision often had stronger pinch than did those with replantation, although they had more difficulty holding certain objects. Function decreased in both groups with injuries proximal to the proximal third of the proximal phalanx.

The function of thumbs amputated through the interphalangeal (IP) joint depended on the extent of injury and the patient's motivation.[39]

Individuals with multiple-digit amputations are candidates for replantation. In some instances, only the least damaged digits can be replanted, and these digits are often shifted either to the most functional positions or to the least injured parts of the hand[93] (Fig. 45-2). If both the thumb and index finger have been amputated completely in a crushing injury and the distal portion of the thumb has irreparable distal vessels, the amputated index finger should be attached to the thumb stump. This shifting will result in excellent thumb function and cosmetic acceptability.

Successful replantation at the level of the palm (Fig. 45-3), wrist (Fig. 45-4), or distal end of the forearm generally provides better function than would be achieved with a prosthesis.[40] Sensibility, although decreased, is usually adequate and extrinsic muscles provide sufficient grasp and release even though intrinsic function is often poor.[130a]

In some individuals, replantation at the humeral level provides useful hand function, whereas in others it may permit conversion of an above-elbow amputation to a more functional below-elbow level. Judgment is required when deciding whether to replant an extremity amputated through the proximal forearm muscles or through the elbow or shoulder joints themselves.[22a] Muscle necrosis and subsequent infection can complicate replantation through the

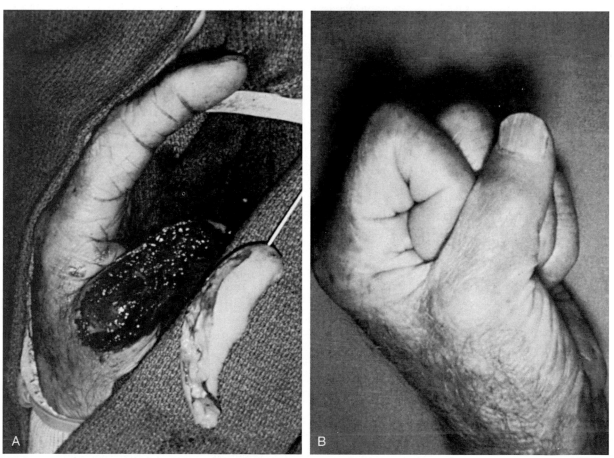

FIGURE 45-1. **A,** Oblique complete amputation of the thumb of a 66-year-old man. An intramedullary pin has been inserted in the amputated thumb for skeletal fixation. Vein grafts were necessary to salvage this thumb because of the oblique injury along the entire neurovascular bundle. **B,** The thumb 4 months after replantation with good range of motion of the MP joint and protective sensation.

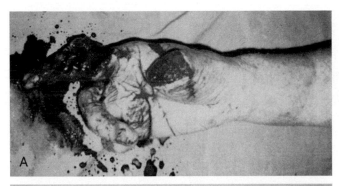

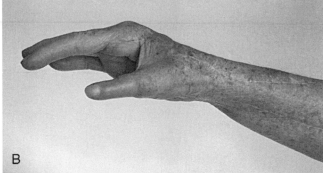

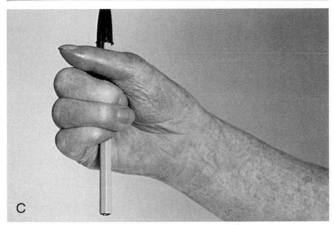

FIGURE 45-2. **A,** This 61-year-old woman's thumb was completely amputated and destroyed by a machine. Her index finger was incompletely amputated. In view of the flexor tendon lacerations and open fracture of the PIP joint in addition to a lacerated radial digital nerve and artery, reconstruction of the index finger would have resulted in a poorly functioning digit. **B** and **C,** Replantation of the index finger in the thumb position resulted in good hand function and appearance.

humerus, and the surgeon must be selective in deciding to attempt replantation at this level[37,40,82,133] (Fig. 45-5).

Replanted digits distal to the FDS insertion function well. Although the distal interphalangeal (DIP) joint is often fused, proximal interphalangeal (PIP) and MP joint motion is excellent. Sensibility is good, digit length is maintained, the cosmetic results are pleasing, operative time is usually less than 4 hours,[19,30,41,65,98,117,135] and painful neuromas are avoided (Fig. 45-6).

The level of the digital amputation is an important determinant for deciding on the replantation. Amputations distal to the IP joint of the thumb or the DIP joint of the fingers can be replanted successfully if dorsal veins can be located in the amputated part. In general, at least 4 mm of dorsal

skin proximal to the nail plate must be present on the amputated digit for realistic venous reconstruction to be possible. If replantation is elected in more distal amputations, volar veins, if present, may be anastomosed successfully. Other salvage methods to achieve venous outflow in replantations distal to the distal digital joints are discussed in the section on technique.

Replantation of nearly all amputated parts should be attempted in healthy children. Epiphyseal growth continues after replantation, sensibility is usually good, and useful function can be anticipated, although the range of motion is often decreased.*

Types of injuries that are not considered to be favorable for replantation are (1) severely crushed or mangled parts, (2) amputations at multiple levels,[5] (3) amputations in patients with other serious injuries or diseases, (4) amputations in which the vessels are severely arteriosclerotic, (5) amputations with prolonged warm ischemia time, (6) amputations in mentally unstable patients, and (7) individual finger amputations in an adult at a level proximal to the FDS insertion, particularly if involving the index or small fingers.

These contraindications to replantation are not absolute. In severe avulsion injuries, some parts can be salvaged successfully with the use of vein grafts to replace the injured vessels,[8,10,95,126] but there is no method of replacing the most distal vessels in an amputated part. In older patients, the arteries at the amputation site should be examined for arteriosclerosis, which frequently precludes functional patency in small vessels after anastomosis.[109] Preexisting medical conditions may preclude the patient's withstanding the blood volume changes that occur with major limb replantation and may even prevent the patient from tolerating the anesthetic required for a lengthy operative procedure.

If the warm ischemic time is greater than 6 hours for an amputation proximal to the carpus or 12 hours for the digits, replantation is not usually recommended. In addition, if the cold ischemic time is greater than 12 hours for a proximal amputation, replantation is not generally performed.

Because it has no muscle, an amputated digit may be preserved at 4° C for 24 hours before replantation is performed.[125] This usually applies only to digital amputations where preservation of muscle tissue is not necessary, although a successful hand replantation has been reported after 54 hours of cold ischemia.[123]

Mentally unstable patients are not uncommon in the group who have their upper extremities severed. However, a patient's mental stability is frequently difficult to ascertain during the limited preoperative evaluation period. If the amputation was purposefully self-inflicted, replantation would probably result in a less than optimal outcome.

In general, in adults, an isolated finger amputation proximal to the FDS tendon insertion should *not* be replanted. Special considerations (e.g., certain musicians who must have 10 digits and individuals whose major concern is appearance) do influence the decision. However, our long-term evaluations have demonstrated that useful function will not usually occur.[38,42,119] Even with the index finger replanted at the base, the patient will usually bypass the replanted digit.

---

*See references 4, 6, 20a, 23, 27, 34, 88, 103, 113, 115, and 138.

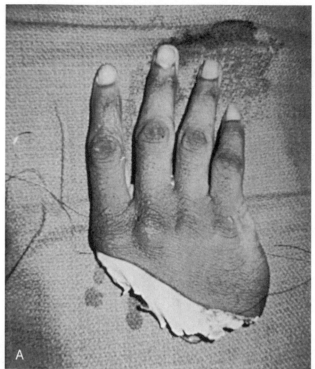

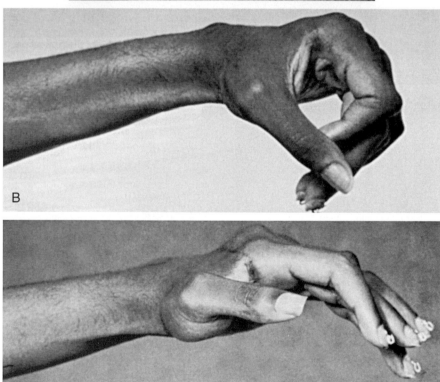

FIGURE 45-3. **A,** Complete amputation through the mid palm of the hand of an 18-year-old boy. Nine months after successful replantation the amount of (**B**) flexion and (**C**) extension is seen. This young man eventually obtained 8-mm two-point discrimination in all replanted digits.

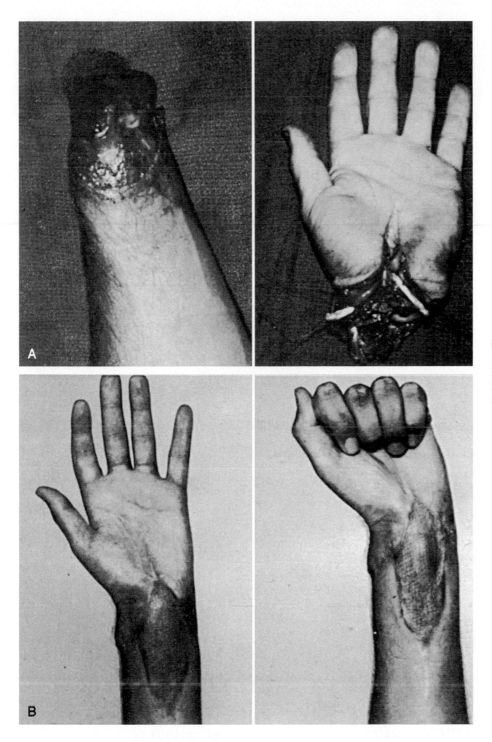

FIGURE 45-4. **A,** Complete amputation through the wrist of a 21-year-old man. **B,** Three years after successful replantation, the amount of digital flexion and extension is seen.

Age is not necessarily a barrier; we have performed replantations in patients who were 10 weeks to 76 years old. The decision cannot be made until the status of the vessels of the amputated part is studied carefully under the operating microscope.

Treatment of complete ring avulsion injuries remains controversial. There are several classifications of ring avulsion injury, but that described by Urbaniak and coworkers is used most commonly.[114]

Class I: Circulation is adequate. Standard bone and soft tissue treatment is sufficient.

Class II: Circulation is inadequate. Vessel repair preserves viability. (Other authors have subdivided class II injuries to distinguish between those in which digital arteries are compromised but bones, tendons, nerves, and veins are intact; those in which circulation is inadequate and bone, tendon, or nerve injury exists[53,76]; and those in which only venous compromise exists.[128])

Class III: Complete degloving or complete amputation.

Complete amputations (class III), especially those proximal to the FDS tendon insertion or those with complete degloving of the ring finger, have the worse prognosis for

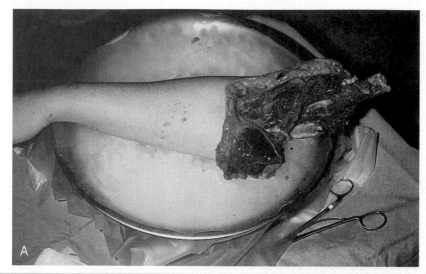

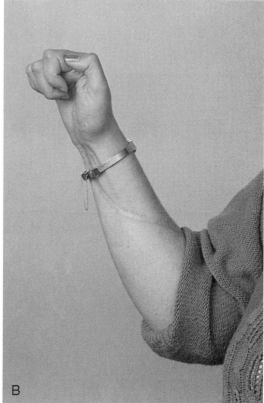

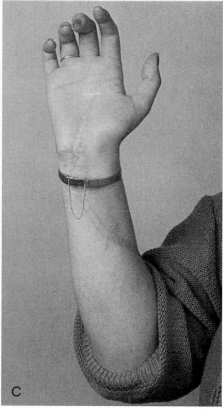

FIGURE 45-5. **A,** This complete humeral amputation occurred in a motor vehicle accident and was this 25-year-old woman's only injury. Two years after replantation she had functioning biceps and triceps, protective sensation in her hand, (**B**) good extrinsic flexion, and (**C**) good extrinsic extension, although intrinsic function was poor. (From Goldner RD, Nunley JA: Replantation proximal to the wrist. Hand Clin 8:413-425, 1992, with permission.)

replantation and are often best managed by surgical amputation of the digit. However, if the amputation is distal to the FDS insertion, the PIP joint is not damaged, and the proximal phalanx is not fractured, vein and nerve grafts can be used to salvage a functional digit.[1b,7,53,76,105]

Usually the patient and family desire a replantation and expect a miraculous result. The surgeon should explain to the patient the chances of success of viability, anticipated function, the length of surgery and hospitalization, and the amount of time lost from work in comparison to amputation/revision.[63,67a]

Individuals whose digits are not able to be replanted may choose to have prostheses fabricated to improve the appearance and sometimes function of their digits. Restorations of extremely proximal digit amputations dislodge easily and are not particularly functional. Distal restorations that cover an almost complete digit decrease sensibility distally. These factors contribute to the two thirds of patients who do not choose to wear their prostheses[59a] (Fig. 45-7).

INSTRUMENTS

Microsurgical instruments and materials are described in detail in Chapter 44; thus only the equipment essential for replantation surgery is emphasized here. Replantation surgeons need not have a vast amount of expensive equipment, but they must have the proper instruments that must be

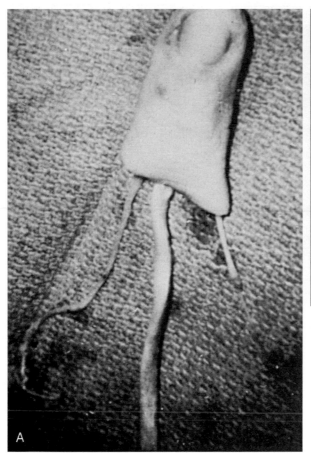

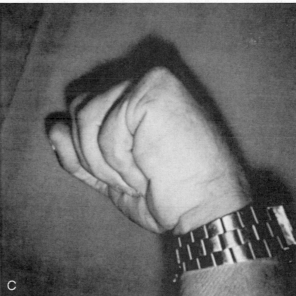

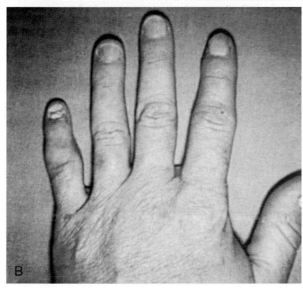

FIGURE 45-6. **A,** Complete amputation by an avulsion injury to the small finger in a 35-year-old man. The amputation was distal to the superficialis insertion. The avulsed digital nerves are apparent, as well as the flexor profundus tendon. **B,** Six months after replantation, the little finger has full extension at the PIP and MP joints. The distal joint was fused. **C,** Full flexion enables the patient to touch his palm. The patient obtained 14-mm two-point discrimination.

maintained in fine functioning order, which is not always easy.[12,77]

Surgical loupes or telescopes with 3.5× to 4.5× magnification are used for the initial exploration and dissection of amputated parts and the injured extremity. An operating microscope, preferably a diploscope, with magnification at least to 20× is essential. The ideal microscope should have a beam splitter in the double head that allows the surgeon and the first assistant to see the same microfield, in addition to foot control for zoom magnification, focusing, and horizontal XY movement. The microscope should be used for repair of any vessels distal to the elbow.

To a degree, the choice of microsurgical instruments depends on the individual surgeon's preferences. All the instruments should be at least 10 cm long to allow the handles to rest comfortably in the thumb/index finger web. Fine spring-loaded (nonlocking handles) needle holders and scissors are helpful. Jeweler's forceps, small-tipped tying forceps, a microtipped dilator (lacrimal duct dilator), and a micro irrigator (30-gauge needle attached to a plastic syringe)

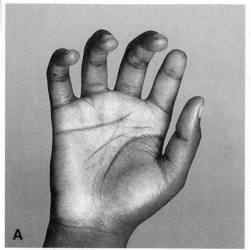 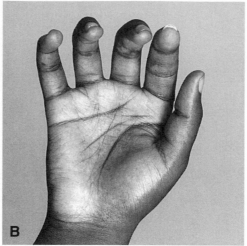

FIGURE 45-7. **A** and **B,** This 19-year-old student sustained complete amputation of her index, long, and ring fingers, just distal to the PIP joints. Long and ring fingers were replanted, but the index finger was too badly damaged and was revised. She was unhappy with the appearance of the amputated index finger and this photograph demonstrates her hand before (**A**) and after (**B**) fitting with a custom-made prosthesis.

Table 45-1

APPROPRIATE NEEDLE AND SUTURE SIZE FOR MICROVASCULAR REPAIRS IN THE HAND

Location	Needle Size μm)	Suture Size
Wrist and forearm	130	8-0, 9-0
Palm	100	9-0, 10-0
Proximal digit	75	10-0
Distal digit	50	11-0

are other essentials. The microclips should have less than 30 g of closing pressure to minimize intimal damage. Two clips mounted on a sliding bar provide a convenient method of approximating the vessel ends without undue tension. The less complex, the better the microclip.

Small silver vascular clips (hemoclips) are used to tag the microvessels and nerves in the initial débridement. A small-tipped bipolar cautery is important for isolating and mobilizing the vessels to be repaired. A small piece of blue or yellow rubber balloon serves as background material to diminish eye fatigue in the longer procedures. Actually, a yellow background is preferred, particularly when the lighting is diminished.

The level of the amputation determines the choice of suture and needle size for the vascular repair. Table 45-1 provides suggestions for needle and suture size at the various levels of the hand and wrist.[111] The most commonly used suture is 10-0 nylon on a 75-μm needle. The use of smaller suture and needles is more difficult and fatiguing. Proximal to the elbow, 8-0 nylon may be used.

Monofilament nylon is preferred over polypropylene and polyglycolic material because nylon is easier to handle and knot. Naturally, smaller sizes of needles and sutures are used in children.

WHO SHOULD PERFORM REPLANTATIONS?

Achievement of survival and useful function in the replantation of upper extremity amputations is difficult. Although the initial survival of the replanted part depends on patent

microvascular anastomoses and immediate postoperative care, the ultimate function and acceptability are dependent on the total performance of the tendon, nerve, bone, and joint repairs. Therefore, the replantation surgeon must first be a thoroughly trained and accomplished hand surgeon, second be a competent microsurgeon, and third have the knowledge for a predictable outcome of the part selected for reattachment.

Surgeons who engage in microvascular replantation should be able to consistently achieve a 90% patency rate in 1-mm vessels in the animal laboratory. The operating theater is not the setting for practice. Although possible, it is very difficult for a microvascular surgeon functioning independently to maintain a high success rate in replantations. The concept of a well-integrated team seems to be essential if a continued high degree of viability and ultimate function is to be realized.[81,83a,110] A replantation team should be available around the clock every day. Reattachment of a single uncomplicated digit may be performed within 3 or 4 hours by an experienced microsurgeon or team, but reattachment of multiple digits may require 15 or more hours. Such emergency procedures may be extremely disquieting to the routine clinical or surgical schedule of the surgeon. The availability of an adequate number of proficient microsurgeons enables relatively rested surgeons to perform efficiently. In addition, many replants survive because of meticulous and intelligent postoperative management, which may mean return-ing some patients to the operating room for re-exploration and revision.

PREPARATION OF THE AMPUTATED PART FOR TRANSPORTATION

There are two methods of preserving the amputated part: (1) wrapping the part in a gauze moistened with Ringer's lactate or saline solution and placing the bundle in a specimen container or plastic bag that is then placed on ice or (2) immersing the part in one of these solutions in a plastic bag or specimen container and placing the bag or container on ice. The amputated part should not be placed directly on ice and should not be frozen. Whichever method the replantation surgeon selects, clear and concise instructions about management of the amputated part must be given to the referring physician. We prefer the immersion method for the following reasons: (1) the part is less likely to become frozen ("frostbitten"), (2) the part is less likely to be strangled by the wrapping, (3) the instructions are easier to explain to the primary care physician, and (4) maceration secondary to immersion is not a problem. In our laboratory we have proved that by using either method of preserving amputated animal parts for 24 hours, equal viability rates of replantation can be achieved.[125]

The tissues will survive for approximately 6 hours if the amputated part is not cooled. If the part is cooled, it may survive 12 hours, or even longer if it is a digit because the digit has no muscle tissue. Transportation of the patient and amputated part should be as rapid as possible, but successful replantation of digits may be achieved in those that have been without a blood supply for 24 to 30 hours if they are properly cooled.

INITIAL SURGICAL MANAGEMENT

When the patient with an amputated part arrives in the emergency department, the replantation team divides into two subteams in an effort to save time. One team transports the amputated part to the operating room, where it is cleansed with Hibiclens and sterile Ringer's lactate solution. The amputated part is placed on a bed of ice covered with a sterile plastic drape. If there are multiple amputated digits, these are cooled by keeping them under ice packets until they are required for reattachment. Radiographs of the amputated parts are obtained.

With the use of operating loupes or an operating microscope (depending on the size of the amputated part), the part is débrided carefully and the nerves and vessels are identified and tagged with small silver vascular clips (hemoclips). Tagging of the vessels and nerves will prove to be very helpful and timesaving when working in a bloody field later. Failure to label these structures, particularly in multiple amputations, can result in extreme frustration of the surgeon in the later stages of reconstruction when the fatigue factor influences the surgeon's proficiency.

Longitudinal midlateral incisions on each side of the digit provide the most rapid and best exposure of the nerves and vessels (Fig. 45-8). The incisions are placed slightly toward the dorsum to permit reflection of both the dorsal and palmar skin flaps so that the arteries, nerves, and veins can be located with ease. The digital nerves and vessels should be dissected free under magnification for 1.5 to 2.0 cm and then labeled. Further débridement is continued after the neurovascular bundles have been isolated. The dorsal veins are identified by reflecting the entire dorsal fold of skin and searching in the subdermal tissue (see Fig. 45-8). In the amputated part, searching for veins may be delayed until after one arterial anastomosis, which makes veins easier to identify by good back-bleeding.

Appropriate bone trimming and shortening are performed on the amputated part. Retrograde insertion of one or more intramedullary Kirschner wires in the amputated part is performed so that the part is ready for immediate reattachment. Mini plates and screws can be used if their application can be achieved without damaging dorsal veins and soft tissue.

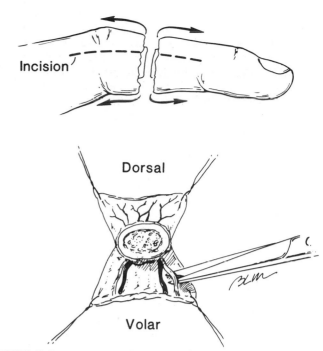

FIGURE 45-8. Midlateral incisions are preferred for an amputated digit and stump. The incisions are made slightly toward the dorsal side so that both the dorsal and volar skin can be reflected to locate the arteries and veins with ease.

During this initial period, the other subteam assesses the patient with a routine physical examination, complete blood cell count, activated partial thromboplastin time, and radiographs of the injured extremity. Depending on the age and health of the patient and the severity of the injury, chest radiography, electrocardiography, blood chemistry analysis, urinalysis, and blood typing and crossmatching are performed. Administration of intravenous fluids is begun, and the patient is given intravenous antibiotics and tetanus prophylaxis. An indwelling urethral catheter is inserted if a long procedure is anticipated.

Most replantations should be performed under a regional block with the local anesthetics bupivacaine (Marcaine) or ropivacaine.[45] An indwelling axillary catheter can be inserted for a continuous block. General anesthesia is usually required for children younger than 10 years of age and for major limb replantation.

Peripheral blood flow to the injured limb is enhanced by the sympathetic block provided by regional anesthesia and by maintaining a warm body temperature.

Under tourniquet ischemia and magnification, while one team prepares the amputated part the other team débrides the stump and identifies and tags the nerves and vessels in a manner similar to that used on the amputated part. The veins on the stump are often particularly difficult to locate in the digit. Their identification requires patience, experience, and meticulous dissection inasmuch as successful replantation depends on skillful anastomosis of an adequate number of veins.

It is useful to find one good vein in the subdermal layer and then use this vein as a guide to the others by reflecting the incised skin and searching in the same subdermal plane of the initially located vein. Another method is to continue

CRITICAL POINTS: REPLANTATION

INDICATIONS/CONTRAINDICATIONS

- See Critical Points box, p. ***.

PREOPERATIVE EVALUATION

- Level of injury and number of digits
- Type of injury (sharp vs. crush vs. avulsion)
- General condition/stability of the patient
- Radiographic evaluation of amputated part and residual limb
- Patient's vocation, avocations, expectations

PEARLS

- Take amputated part to operating room before patient to begin identifying vessels and nerves and débriding.
- May insert distal fixation in part.
- Keep part cool on ice in sterile container.
- Plan to vein-graft arteries early if any question of injury.
- Avoid tension on skin closure.

TECHNICAL POINTS/SEQUENCE OF REPLANTATION

- Locate and tag vessels and nerves (6-0 Prolene or hemoclips).
- Débride soft tissues after identification of vessels and nerves.
- Shorten and fix the bone.
- Repair the extensor tendons.
- Repair the flexor tendons.
- Anastomose the arteries.
- Repair the nerves.
- Anastomose the veins (two for every artery repair).
- Obtain skin coverage.

PITFALLS

- Make absolutely sure that vessel for anastomosis is undamaged or stretched (perform a vein graft if any question).
- Shortening of bone may allow primary vessel repair.
- Avoid tight wound closure or tight dressing.

POSTOPERATIVE CARE

- Keep patient warm.
- Watch volume status; keep blood pressure and urine output at adequate levels.
- Heparinize if crush, avulsion, or if problem with blood flow in operating room.
- Monitor with temperature and close observation.
- Monitor digital temperature and observe capillary refill, color, turgor for signs of arterial insufficiency or venous congestion.

---

to dissect the initial vein proximally until branches to other veins are located.

TECHNIQUE AND SEQUENCE OF SURGERY

The operative sequence of replantation varies slightly with the level of the amputation (digit and hand versus areas proximal to the wrist) and the type of injury (clean cut, crush, or avulsion). Because digital, partial-hand, and hand replantations are much more common than more proximal replantations, the sequence of the surgery is described for digit and hand replantation first and variations in technique are described later.

The operative sequence for digital and hand replantation is as follows:

1. Locate and tag the vessels and nerves.
2. Débride.
3. Shorten and fix the bone.
4. Repair the extensor tendons.
5. Repair the flexor tendons.
6. Anastomose the arteries.
7. Repair the nerves.
8. Anastomose the veins.
9. Obtain skin coverage.

Location and tagging of the vessels was described in the section on initial management. It is extremely important to isolate these vital structures carefully before any débridement. Magnification is mandatory to obtain optimal débridement. The surgeon's haste to reestablish blood flow must not result in inadequate wound débridement. Any potentially necrotic tissue, particularly muscle, must be excised.

All severed structures that can be repaired are reconnected during the replantation procedure. In addition to the tissues already mentioned, periosteum, joint capsule, ligaments, and the lateral bands are repaired when possible. Accurate and complete primary repair results in optimal hand function. Repair of all structures provides effective stabilization and allows early mobilization of the reconstructed hand. It is much easier to repair these tissues primarily rather than subject the patient to additional surgery at a later date. In delayed repairs, there is always the concern of injuring the repaired major vessels.

In multiple-digit replantation, the overall duration of surgery is decreased by using a "structure-by-structure" repair technique as opposed to a "digit-by-digit" technique. Instead of completing all aspects of the replantation of one digit before replanting the subsequent one, digits are approached by repairing the same anatomic structure on each digit to be replanted before repairing the next structures.[17]

Bone Shortening and Fixation

Bone shortening and fixation are critical aspects of replantation.[118,131] Sufficient bone must be resected to ensure the approximation of normal intima in the vascular anastomoscs. The connection of arteries, veins, and nerves must never be performed under tension. Therefore, the bone ends must be shortened sufficiently to obtain easy approximation of these vital structures. In addition, bone shortening allows easier and important dorsal skin coverage of anastomosed veins. The amount of bone resected depends on the type of injury. In an avulsion or crush injury, a greater amount of bone must be resected until normal intimal coaptation is possible without tension. In the digit, it is usually necessary to resect 0.5 to 1.0 cm of bone; and in amputations proximal to the hand, it is frequently necessary to resect 2 to 4 cm of bone. Even more bone may need to be resected in an avulsion injury.[3]

Some replantation surgeons have emphasized that bone shortening is rarely necessary and recommend vein grafting when there is considerable intimal damage.[108] However, it is our opinion that in replantation, bone shortening should initially be chosen over vein grafting, because one easy anastomosis is more favorable than two. Also, in an injury where vessels require vein grafting because of extensive damage, there is frequently concomitant damage to the nerves and other soft tissue structures, which likewise need

to be shortened. In addition, a shortened replanted digit, which usually has a restricted active range of motion, is generally less obvious and less likely to "get in the way." We hasten to add, however, that we do not hesitate to perform vein grafts when they are indicated, for example, when bone shortening may result in the loss of a potentially functional joint or during certain revascularization procedures. It is easier, quicker, less frustrating, and more reliable to perform a vein graft initially than it is to redo a difficult anastomosis that is not flowing well. Again, any anastomosis performed under excessive tension is unlikely to remain patent.

In thumb amputations, the major portion of the bone shortening should be on the detached part so that a maximal amount of bone is preserved on the stump to ensure good bone stock should the replantation fail. However, sometimes this is not possible if an attempt is made to save joint function.

Numerous methods of bone stabilization have been suggested[14,46,96a,104]: (1) one or two longitudinal intramedullary Kirschner wires, (2) a longitudinal intramedullary Kirschner wire plus a short oblique Kirschner wire to prevent rotation,[104] (3) crossed Kirschner wires, (4) intraosseous wiring,[43,60] (5) an intramedullary screw or peg, and (6) a small plate with screws.[78]

All these methods may be used to stabilize amputations through the diaphyseal or metaphyseal areas and the joints (Fig. 45-9). Certain methods of fixation are preferred at different areas.

We prefer single or double axial Kirschner wire fixation when possible in digital bone fixation at the middle or distal phalanx. This is the most universal and easiest method (see Fig. 45-9A). A motorized drill is paramount for accurate and careful pin placement. A drill guide or sleeve is frequently

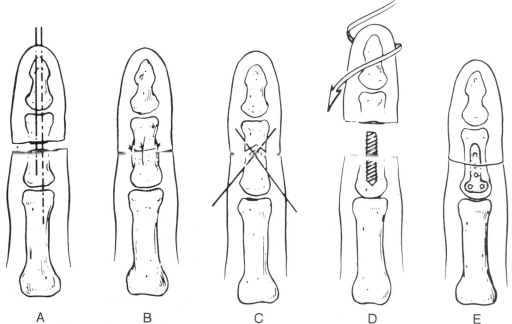

FIGURE 45-9. Methods of bone fixation in digital replantation. **A,** A single intramedullary Kirschner wire is usually adequate. A second Kirschner wire *(dotted line)* may be inserted if the amputation is close to the joint or if rotation is a problem. The second, longer Kirschner wire may be removed early to begin motion at the joint that it previously crossed. **B,** Intraosseous wiring may be used to allow early motion. This method is more often used in a metaphyseal region. **C,** A chevron-type fusion is often used for primary fusion at an amputation through a joint. **D,** A bone screw is inserted into the amputation stump, the screw head cut off, and the digit literally "screwed on." **E,** A mini-plate and screws provide stability to allow early joint motion. The mini-"H"-plate is preferred by us when this type of fixation is used.

useful as a retractor of the surrounding soft tissue near the bone ends. We have experi-mented with all of the aforementioned methods of bone fixation in more than 2000 replantations but usually prefer single or double axial Kirschner wire fixation for the follow-ing reasons: (1) the technique is simple and quick, (2) less bone exposure is required, (3) less skeletal mass is needed for fixation, (4) rotational deformity of the replanted digit is easily corrected if needed, and (5) reshortening after fixation is facilitated if further shortening is indicated for nerve, vessel, or skin approximation.[46,118]

Crossed Kirschner wires or intraosseous wiring is our choice for replantation at the proximal phalanx level when it is undesirable to place a pin across the PIP joint.

Crossed Kirschner wires are our preferred choice for arthrodesis at a joint level. A chevron-type bone cut or a cup-and-cone configuration can be used for stabilization (see Fig. 45-9C). Care must be taken if using crossed pins to avoid damaging a repaired neurovascular bundle by twisting it with the pins or by tethering the vessel or the protective retaining ligaments over the protruding ends of the pins.

Intramedullary screw fixation is possible for thumb MP stabilization in a complete amputation at this level (see Fig. 45-9D). The technique is rapid and provides immediate stability. Both ends of the medullary canals are drilled and tapped before inserting a cortical screw with the head removed. Because joints other than the thumb MP joint are usually arthrodesed in some flexion, the screw method has limited use. The disadvantage of intramedullary screws or pegs is that they are difficult to remove from replanted fingers that become infected. Herbert screw fixation has been used for replantations at the distal joint level. However, its use is not recommended in contaminated wounds.

Intraosseous wiring through four drill holes at 12, 3, 6, and 9 o'clock in each end of the bone permits two strands of 24-gauge wire to be placed perpendicular to each other (see Fig. 45-9B). This method, although requiring additional bone exposure and precise technique, does provide stability and is suggested for replantations at the metaphyseal level to allow early motion with less chance of angulation and nonunion.[131]

Mini plate and screw fixation is gaining popularity in digit and hand replantation. We have used the mini-"H"-plate for immediate stability.[78] These methods require more time and bone exposure, with possibly further damage to soft tissue, particularly the dorsal veins. In major limb replantation we prefer plates and screws because of the rigid fixation.

Even an experienced hand and replantation surgeon has a difficult time obtaining proper alignment when reattaching multiple digits. The relationship of the digits must be checked frequently in flexion and extension. Care should be taken to achieve anatomic alignment and correct rotation of the replanted parts.

There are special indications for primary implant arthroplasty in replantation. An example might be replantation of one or more fingers that have been cleanly amputated through the PIP joint in a piano player. Because the hazard of infection is increased, only plain silicone implants should be used. Actually, experienced hand surgeons will find that it is technically easier and quicker to perform a silicone implant arthroplasty than a primary fusion. However, the indications for this implant are not common.

Extensor Tendon Repair

After bone fixation, the extensor tendon should be repaired for further stabilization. Usually two horizontal mattress sutures of 4-0 polyester are sufficient. In amputations through the proximal phalangeal region, repair of the lateral bands of the extensor tendon is extremely important if optimal extension of the distal joints is to be expected.

In some severe avulsion injuries, no extensor tendons are available for repair. In these situations, IP joint arthrodesis or extensor tendon grafting as secondary procedures are necessary.

Flexor Tendon Repair

Primary flexor tendon surgery should be attempted in most replantations because secondary repair involves returning to areas of tremendous scarring around repaired nerves and vessels. Secondary flexor tendon surgery in replanted digits usually requires two-stage silicone rod procedures in digits other than the thumb. In ragged or avulsion injuries, we do not advocate extensive dissection or lengthy incisions to retrieve or reconstruct the avulsed tendon as a primary procedure.

We prefer to use the Tajima suture method for primary flexor tendon repair in replantation[99] (Fig. 45-10). Routinely, the flexor tendons are repaired after the bone is stabilized, prior to microsurgical repair of digital arteries and nerves. However, if the flexor tendon transection occurs in the proximal portion of the digit, it may be expeditious to insert the sutures into the free flexor tendon ends (Tajima's method) but to not coapt the tendon ends until after the vascular and nerve repairs have been accomplished on the flexor surface. This sequence of repairs has the advantage of allowing the digit to be held in full extension for better exposure for nerve and vascular repairs on the flexor surface of the hand. When multiple tendons, such as in the palm or wrist, are to be repaired, sutures are placed in all the proximal and distal tendon stumps before any knot tying.

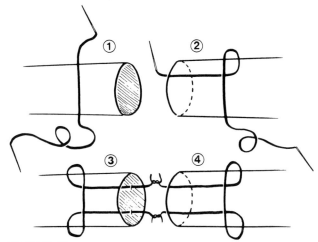

FIGURE 45-10. The Tajima-type flexor tendon suture is preferred because the suture may be inserted in both ends of the tendon and actual connection of the tendons may be subsequently performed at the ideal time, depending on the level and neurovascular structures involved.

After appropriate match-up is ensured, the tendon ends are all connected by securing the knots.

Some of the primary repairs of flexor tendons in replantation may require subsequent tenolysis. If secondary repair of the flexor tendons is necessary, it can be safely performed 3 months after replantation. As mentioned, the two-stage silicone rod method is then usually indicated. Delayed "Z"-lengthening of the flexor pollicis longus at the wrist with advancement distally has been successfully used in some of our replantations of avulsed thumbs,[116] but primary repair is the rule if possible.

Arterial Repair

Microvascular techniques have been described thoroughly in Chapter 44, so only important related points will be emphasized in this section. The arteries are anastomosed after bone fixation and extensor and, usually, flexor tendon repair. In a digit, we attempt to repair both digital arteries when possible; and in a partial-hand or wrist amputation, we repair all arteries that can be restored. Some microsurgeons recommend repairing only one digital artery to save time; however, we stress repairing both, even in multiple-digit amputations, to increase the survival rate.

Arterial repair should not be attempted until spurting blood flow occurs from the proximal vessel. If pulsating proximal arterial flow is not evident, steps to induce flow include (1) relief of vascular tension or compression, (2) proximal resection to healthy vessel walls, (3) warming of the operating room and patient, (4) adequate hydration of the patient (crystalloid and/or blood, when indicated), (5) elevation of the patient's blood pressure, (6) irrigation of the proximal vessel with warm lactated Ringer's solution, (7) external application or gentle intraluminal flushing with papaverine solution (1:20 dilution), (8) checking with the anesthesiologist about a metabolic problem that could incite vasospasm (e.g., acidosis[26]), (9) being certain that the tourniquet is not inflated, and (10) wait!

The severed artery must be resected until normal intima is visualized under high-power magnification; only normal intima is reconnected (Fig. 45-11). If this cannot be achieved, an interpositional vein graft is used (Fig. 45-12). The two most critical factors in achieving successful microvascular

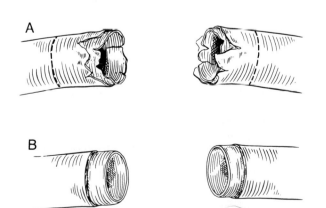

FIGURE 45-11. **A,** Damaged microvessels must be sharply incised back to completely normal intima. **B,** The intima should be evaluated under the highest possible magnification through the operating microscope.

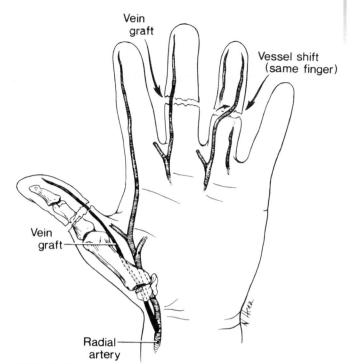

FIGURE 45-12. Three methods of making up a gap in the microvessel: (1) In a completely amputated thumb, an *interposition vein graft* may be used from the ulnar digital artery of the amputated thumb in an end-to-side manner into the radial artery at the wrist. (2) A *vein graft* may be used to bridge the gap. (3) The proximal radial digital vessel has been *shifted* to the distal ulnar digital vessel in the complete replantation. This method is particularly useful in ring finger avulsion injuries.

anastomoses are the skill and expertise of the microsurgeon and easy coaptation of normal intima to normal intima.

In many avulsion or crushing injuries, undamaged arteries may be shifted. For example, in a ring finger avulsion injury, the proximal ulnar digital artery may be attached at the distal radial digital artery if these are the ends that are least traumatized. This shifting principle is most often used when one of the distal vessels is nonsalvageable. In the past, during replantation of an avulsed thumb we often shifted the radial digital artery of the index finger to replace the severely damaged princeps pollicis artery. This practice has been discontinued for three reasons: (1) scar contracture of the thumb/index finger web space, (2) frequent small size of the radial digital artery, and (3) concomitant damage to the radial digital artery of the index finger and the princeps pollicis artery.

Some authors have recommended transposition of vascular pedicles[59,109] and even neurovascular pedicles to replant avulsed thumbs, but we believe that the use of vein grafts is easier, quicker, and more reliable.

For replantation of thumbs we prefer to use an interposition vein graft from the ulnar digital artery of the amputated thumb to the first dorsal metacarpal artery on the dorsum of the hand or in an end-to-side fashion into the radial artery at the wrist (see Fig. 45-12). For expediency, the reversed vein graft is often anastomosed to the ulnar digital artery of the detached thumb before bone fixation.[16,132]

Interposition vein grafts are used in approximately 20% of our replantations to obtain reapproximation of the healthy arteries and veins. The volar aspect of the wrist contains several veins 1 to 2 mm in diameter that are ideal for replantation of digits. In fact, if there is any indication that vein grafts may be needed, one of our initial steps is to harvest the veins from the wrist and store them in lactated Ringer's and papaverine solution. This preparatory procedure is done with loupe magnification, before using the operating microscope; it requires only a few minutes and will save time and eliminate potential frustration later. Two easy anastomoses are quicker and more likely to be successful than one difficult anastomosis under tension.

A pneumatic tourniquet may be used safely for each vascular anastomosis. If the microvascular anastomosis technique is skillfully performed, tourniquet ischemia will not diminish the patency rate. The tourniquet should be released at the conclusion of each anastomosis. The tourniquet may be inflated and deflated many times during the procedure to allow a considerable decrease in operating time and blood loss. If hemorrhage is not excessive or obscuring the visual field, a tourniquet is not used.

Because all available microclips do produce some amount of vessel wall damage, their application time should not exceed 30 minutes. Just before beginning the first anastomosis, we recommend a bolus of 3000 to 5000 U of intravenous heparin. Subsequent doses of 1000 U of heparin every hour or so may be repeated in procedures involving crush or avulsion injuries. The dosage is adjusted for children and the bleeding tendency of the patient as determined by clinical appraisal.

Vein Repair

An attempt should be made to anastomose two veins for each artery, although this is not always mandatory.[58a,67] It may be necessary to mobilize or "harvest" veins to achieve this ratio (Fig. 45-13). The greatest error in vein repair is attempting the anastomosis under tension. This is never necessary. If harvesting of veins does not allow coaptation without undue tension, the surgeon should proceed immediately with a vein graft. The surgeon's time and frustration will be diminished and the patency rate increased.

Many recognized replantation surgeons repair veins before arteries to decrease blood loss and maintain a bloodless field for better vision.[22,72,81] However, by judicious use of the tourniquet, the artery may be repaired first and a dry field maintained. This provides the advantages of earlier revascularization and allows easier detection of the most functional veins by their spurting backflow. In addition, if the veins are repaired first, especially in an avulsion injury, and subsequent arterial anastomosis fails to show adequate arterial inflow, the surgeon has wasted valuable time on a nonsalvageable part.

If replantations are attempted at the level of the base of the nail plate or even more distally, locating the dorsal veins in the distal stump is not usually possible. If surgical reattachment of the distal amputation is believed to be indicated (e.g., a musician's fingertip or the tip of a dominant thumb), adequate venous drainage may be achieved by at least six methods: (1) repair of the volar veins (if present), although these are smaller, have thinner walls, and are more difficult to repair than dorsal veins; (2) anastomosis of one distal

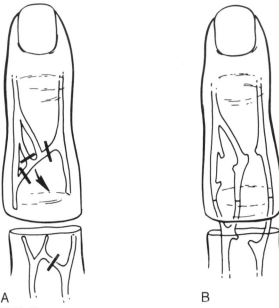

FIGURE 45-13. **A,** The mobilization or "harvesting" of veins is a very useful method of obtaining ease of approximation for vein reconstruction in a complete amputation. **B,** An attempt should be made to repair three veins on each digit replantation.

digital artery (which has backflow) to a proximal vein (creation of an arteriovenous fistula)[97]; (3) removal of the nail plate and subsequent scraping of the raw nail matrix with a cotton applicator every 1 to 2 hours to encourage bleeding, with a heparin-soaked pledget applied afterward to foster continuous venous oozing; (4) transverse stab incision on the periungual area of the tip of the digit with application of heparin to maintain external bleeding[1a,44a]; (5) use of medical-grade leeches; and (6) periodic digital massage of the replanted fingertip, which enhances venous outflow but is usually unsuccessful in maintaining viability of the replanted tip if it has to be continued for more than 48 hours.

Medical-grade leeches are readily available and may be placed on the surface of the failing part when venous congestion occurs.[13,58] The leeches become engorged in 15 to 30 minutes and then detach from the digit. However, they secrete a local anticoagulant, hirudin, that allows the incision to bleed for 8 to 12 hours and thereby prevents congestion. When the bleeding stops, a leech is again applied to the fingertip. Sometimes leech treatment is required for 5 to 7 days.

Leeches will not remain on avascular tissue and can infect the patient with *Aeromonas hydrophila,* identified from wound smears as a gram-negative anaerobic rod.[62] This bacterium is endosymbiotic with the leech in that it inhibits the growth of other bacteria and produces digestive enzymes, including amylase, lipase, and proteolytic hemolysin, that are essential for the breakdown of red cells and hemoglobin. Suppression of leech enteric bacteria by antibiotic administration to the patient may be an effective method to avoid *Aeromonas hydrophila* infection.[59b] Treatment of *Aeromonas* infection consists of early surgical débridement and antibiotic treatment with aminoglycosides, tetracycline, trimethoprim-sulfamethoxazole (Septra), third-generation cephalosporins, or aztreonam.[13]

Venous Flaps

It is important to cover the dorsal veins with skin to prevent desiccation of the venous wall. Split-skin, full-thickness skin, or a local rotational skin flap may be used for coverage. If there is a deficit of veins in addition to skin, the defect may be covered with a venous flap.[31,51,75,106] This flap may be based on a proximal venous pedicle from an adjacent digit or harvested as a free tissue transfer from the volar aspect of the wrist or dorsum of the hand. This composite flap provides skin coverage as well as serves as a vein graft. If skin coverage is needed in addition to an arterial graft, the vein and its overlying skin may be reversed and used for digital artery reconstruction.[75] Unfortunately, none of these methods is totally reliable.

Nerve Repair

Because the bone has usually been shortened in replantation, nerve repair is generally not difficult, because there is no tension at the suture line. The microscope is used for careful fascicular (or bundle) alignment of the injured nerve. Even with the aid of the microscope, it is sometimes difficult to determine how much nerve to resect in severe avulsion injuries. However, in almost all replantations, primary nerve repair should be done.

Primary nerve grafts are performed when end-to-end repair is not possible. The medial antebrachial cutaneous nerve is ideal as a donor for digital nerve grafting.[80] This nerve is located one fingerbreadth medial and two fingerbreadths distal to the medial epicondyle of the elbow and lies superficial to the muscle fascia. In multiple-digit amputations, nerve grafts may be obtained from the discarded digits.

We have noted no statistical difference in nerve recovery in our replants with secondary or primary repair.[35]

The peripheral nerves are repaired with 8-0 to 10-0 monofilament nylon by epineurial repair after fascicular alignment is determined. In the digital nerves only two or three sutures are necessary; more sutures are used in proximal injuries.

Skin Coverage and Dressing

Meticulous hemostasis is obtained after all the structures have been repaired and revascularization of the replanted part has been ensured. The skin is loosely approximated with a few interrupted nylon sutures. All damaged skin that may become necrotic is excised, and no tension should be placed on the skin during closure. Frequently the midlateral incisions of the digit are not closed to allow for decompression of the digital vessels. The vessels should be covered without constriction from the overlying skin or sutures. A local flap or split-thickness skin graft may be necessary, even for digital vessel coverage. Fasciotomies are indicated if the slightest indication of compression or constriction is present. The wounds are covered with small strips of gauze impregnated with petrolatum. Care must be taken in the placement of these strips so that they are not continuous in a circumferential manner.

The upper extremity is immobilized in a bulky compression hand dressing with plaster splints that extend above the elbow to prevent slippage. Each step of the dressing is carefully designed to prevent circumferential constriction.

POSTOPERATIVE CARE

Postoperative management is extremely important in achieving a high success rate in replantation.[37] Despite a technically successful replantation, vascular insufficiency may develop postoperatively but can frequently be corrected if detected early. Postoperative care may be categorized into three segments: (1) routine precautions, (2) procedures for difficult replantation, and (3) reversal of a failing replant.

Routine Postoperative Precautions

The hand in bulky compression dressing is usually elevated by a foam rubber cradle boot or a rope attached to the dressing. The elbow should rest on the bed. If arterial inflow is diminished, the hand may be lowered. If venous outflow is slow, the hand needs additional elevation.

The use and type of anticoagulants are certainly a controversial topic (see Chapter 44). Some surgeons use none (or perhaps only aspirin and dipyridamole [Persantine]), and some use all or various combinations of those discussed here.[24,54,71,81,82a,100,102,110] We prefer the use of some type of anticoagulation in all our patients. In clean-cut amputations and in replantations in which the anastomoses are technically easy and the blood flow immediately brisk, heparin is generally not indicated. In these patients we use aspirin (325 mg/day), dipyridamole (50 mg three times per day), and dextran 40 (20 mL/hr). Additional medication may include chlorpromazine (Thorazine; 25 mg three times per day). Chlorpromazine is useful as a peripheral vasodilator and tranquilizer to diminish vasospasm secondary to anxiety.

If the injury is of the crush or avulsion type, intravenous heparin, 1000 U/hr, is used for 5 to 7 days. The dosage of heparin is regulated according to the activated partial thromboplastin time, which is maintained at one and one-half times normal. If bleeding into the dressing occurs, the dosage is diminished and the dressing changed to prevent constriction by a "blood cast." Heparin prophylaxis is not used in amputations proximal to the wrist level.

Color, pulp turgor, capillary refill, and warmth are all useful aids in monitoring the replant, but quantitative skin temperature measurements have proved to be the most reliable indicators.[86,96] The digital temperature is monitored with a digital thermometer and small surface probes. If the skin temperature of the replanted part drops below 30° C, poor perfusion of the replanted part is certain, and a cause for the compromised circulation must be found and corrected if possible. Of course, the ambient temperature influences interpretation of the recordings. Other methods of monitoring include transcutaneous oxygen measurements, laser Doppler flowmetry,[48] and fluorescein perfusion. These methods are sensitive indicators but are more complex and expensive and require more technical expertise by nursing personnel than does temperature monitoring.

The patient's room should be maintained comfortably warm, and cool drafts should be avoided. The patient is not permitted to smoke[7a,122] or drink caffeine. The patient is kept at bed rest for 2 to 3 days, and then activity is permitted in accordance with the patient's course, desires, and personality. Antibiotics are administered for 1 week.

Procedures for Difficult Replantations

Often the surgeon can predict which replantation is going to have postoperative problems with circulatory perfusion and a decreased chance of survival. Examples are replantations in children younger than 10 years of age, crush and avulsion injuries, ring avulsions, poor proximal flow evident before the anastomosis, and intermittent or inconsistent distal flow despite a technically good anastomosis. In these situations, extra postoperative efforts are advisable to enhance the survival rate.

Intravenous heparin in the dosage previously advised is particularly beneficial in these difficult replants. Insertion of a silicone catheter (No. 5 silicone ureteral stent) adjacent to the median or ulnar nerve (depending on the digits replanted) will permit a continuous regional block to be administered with ease.[83] We recommend 5 mL of bupivacaine (Marcaine) (0.25%) every 6 to 8 hours to provide a continuous sympathetic block for vasodilation. We also advise the use of an indwelling silicone catheter in children because our success rate for viability is lower than that in adults.[115]

The brachial plexus catheter can be inserted before heparin is administered and can provide continuous anesthesia during and after replantation. The continuous block promotes vasodilatation and also alleviates pain in incomplete amputations.

Reversal of Failing Replants

If the reattached part appears in jeopardy (detected by skin temperature, color, pulp turgor, and/or capillary refill), immediate rectifying action must be taken. The dressing should be inspected for any constriction. Sutures causing constriction can be removed. Depression or elevation of the hand may improve vascular flow, depending on whether the problem is arterial or venous. An intravenous bolus of heparin (3000 to 5000 U) will frequently stimulate recovery.[76a] A stellate block or brachial block (if no regional indwelling catheter is present) should be considered as a means of relieving vasospasm unless anticoagulation drugs have been administered. If the patient complains of pain, intravenous narcotics are helpful and should in fact be given before inspecting the dressing. Chlorpromazine may be given to allay anxiety and decrease vasospasm. The surgeon should be certain that the patient is adequately hydrated and that the hematocrit is appropriate. There is no conclusive evidence that the microvessel patency rate is influenced by a normal or low hematocrit, but a near-normal hematocrit is suggested.[69]

The environment of the patient's room may need to be altered, for example, increasing the temperature or removing smokers or other agitating factors. All efforts should be made to calm the patient, especially a child, because pain, fear, and anxiety may instigate unwanted vasospasm.

If the replanted part is perfusing well after the replantation procedure, and if a careful and intelligent postoperative program is instituted, it is rarely necessary to return the patient to the operating room for re-exploration. If this decision is made, however, it must be carried out within 4 to

6 hours of the loss of adequate perfusion. Seldom have we found re-exploration to be of benefit if the exploration occurs more than 1 or 2 days after the replantation. Re-exploration with correction of the problem (redoing the anastomosis, removal of a thrombus, or vein grafting of a previously unrecognized damaged vessel segment) is most effective when acute cessation of arterial inflow is diagnosed.

CRITICAL POINTS: MANAGEMENT OF THE FAILING REPLANT

- ■ Inspect dressing for any constriction.
- ■ Remove too tight sutures.
- ■ Administer heparin (3000 to 5000 U) intravenously.
  Follow with heparin drip (1000 mL/hour) and monitor PTT.
- ■ Perform stellate ganglion or axillary block if patient is not anticoagulated.
  May utilize indwelling axillary catheter
- ■ Administer chlorpromazine to allay anxiety and decrease vasospasm.
- ■ Warm room; decrease anxiety-provoking stimuli.
- ■ Evaluate hydration status; check hematocrit.
  Transfuse for hematocrit less than 25 to 30 if vascular flow is questionable.
- ■ Apply leeches (for venous occlusive problems only).

MAJOR LIMB REPLANTATION

Most amputations of the upper extremity occur at the digit or hand level, so the emphasis on replantation has described reattachment at these levels. Replantation of limbs amputated at or proximal to the wrist level involves similar principles with minor modifications. Because more muscle mass is involved, the duration of avascularity of the detached part is more critical.

Whereas a digit may be successfully replanted 24 hours after amputation, an arm amputated at the elbow is in jeopardy if it has been avascular for 10 to 12 hours, even if it has been properly cooled. Extensive muscle débridement, both on the detached part and the stump, is essential to prevent myonecrosis and subsequent infection, which is a problem in major limb replantation but infrequent in digital reattachment.[49] Bone shortening enables adequate débridement in addition to soft tissue approximation.[3,40]

In replantations proximal to the metacarpal level, immediate arterial inflow is necessary to prevent or diminish myonecrosis. Therefore, after initial débridement and rapid bone stabilization, at least one artery must be anastomosed, and then the surgical sequence is similar to that for digital replantation.

A Sundt shunt or a ventriculoperitoneal shunt (Fig. 45-14) is used to obtain rapid arterial inflow from the proximal vessel to the amputated part.[79] This connection is performed before bone fixation if the duration from amputation to arrival in the operating room is longer than 4 to 6 hours.

Sundt and loop carotid endarterectomy shunts are used for 3- to 4-mm vessels, and Ludenz peritoneal shunts are used for 2.5- to 3-mm vessels (Heyer Shulte Corp, Goleta, CA).

Several authors have recommended perfusing the amputated limb with either venous blood[20b] or with University of Wisconsin (UW) cold storage solution to extend the duration of tissue preservation and to improve the quality of the tissues preserved.[57a]

Stable fixation is necessary, but the method must be rapid. We prefer rigid plate-and-screw fixation of the long bones and crossed Steinmann pin fixation at the joint level. Adequate bone shortening must be carefully planned relative to the type of injury and tissue damage. The working premise is to convert the revascularized limb to a fractured extremity with peripheral nerve injury.

Arterial repair should be performed before venous repair because rapid systemic return of lactic acid and other noxious catabolites can be detrimental to the patient.[126a] We have found it beneficial to give intravenous sodium bicarbonate to the patient before the venous anastomoses. If a stent is inserted initially to reestablish arterial flow, or if the arteries are repaired first, significant bleeding can occur from the unrepaired veins and transfusions will be required.

Extensive fasciotomies are always indicated in major limb replantation. The two most common causes of failure in major limb replantation are myonecrosis with subsequent infection and failure to provide adequate decompression of the restored vessels. Exposed vessels may be covered safely by meshed split-thickness skin grafts. Other areas may be covered in a few days. If a vein graft is required in an area of soft tissue

loss, it is prudent to place the graft in an "extra-anatomic" position to achieve adequate soft tissue coverage.

In replanted digits we usually do not change the dressing for 2 weeks for fear of producing harmful vasospasm. However, in major limb replantation, the limb must be examined in the operating room under anesthesia (regional or general) within 48 to 72 hours to evaluate the condition of the muscle tissue. Any necrotic tissue must be further débrided to prevent infection.

Anticoagulants are not used in major limb replantation. Nevertheless, great care must be taken to maintain the patient's blood volume and pressure inasmuch as blood loss before and during the operative procedure is often underestimated. Postoperative temperature monitoring is reliable in these replants also.

EXPECTATIONS AFTER REPLANTATION

By applying the principles described in this chapter, an experienced and proficient microsurgeon should be able to achieve at least an 80% viability rate in complete replantations.

Nerve recovery is comparable to that of repair of an isolated severed peripheral nerve. Two-point discrimination for replanted thumbs has been shown to average about 11 mm (9 mm in cleanly amputated thumbs and 12 mm in avulsion injuries). The average two-point discrimination for replantation of sharply amputated fingers was 8 mm, whereas that of crush/avulsion injuries was 15 mm. Recovery is better in children and patients with distal amputations.[36]

Active range of motion depends on the level and the extent of injury. PIP joint range of motion was 35 degrees after replantation of single digits proximal to the FDS insertion.

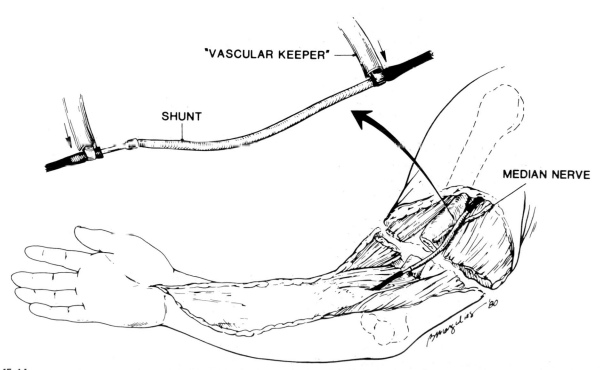

FIGURE 45-14. A Sundt shunt or a ventriculoperitoneal shunt is used to obtain rapid arterial inflow from the proximal vessel to the amputated part.[79]

Average PIP joint motion for digits replanted distal to the insertion of the FDS tendon was 82 degrees.[119]

Cold intolerance is present in most replanted digits[3a] (in addition to those amputated and not replanted[60a]) and may or may not improve after 2 years.[85] Cold intolerance and a normal thermoregulatory response return as this sensibility recovers.[56]

The appearance of the replanted part is usually better than the appearance of either an amputation/revision or a prosthesis.

The best results are obtained in replantation of the thumb,[39] the hand at the wrist or distal forearm level,[81a] and the finger distal to the insertion of the FDS.[41,119]

ANNOTATED REFERENCES

3a. Backman C, Mystrom A, Backman C, Bjerle P: Arterial spasticity and cold intolerance in relation to time after digital replantation. J Hand Surg [Br] 18:551-555, 1993.

This report contradicted what had been taught previously—that cold intolerance generally disappears after 2 years. The authors studied 10 patients after replantation at 2 weeks, 1 year, and 3 years. They measured finger systolic pressure at different finger temperatures and found that those patients with higher arterial pressures had less symptoms. They concluded that those patients with more cold intolerance have a higher degree of vasospasm after replantation. They noted that while cold intolerance will usually decrease in the first 2 years after replantation, it rarely disappears completely.

7a. Betancourt FM, Mah ET, McCabe SJ: Timing of critical thrombosis after replantation surgery of the digits. J Reconstr Microsurg 14:313-316, 1998.

This review of critical thromboses in 76 digits in 63 patients brings out some important points. These authors found that the type of injury had no bearing on the timing of thrombosis. The highest rate of critical thrombosis after replantation occurred in the first 3 days after surgery, but some risk was noted for up to 2 weeks. It was noted that smokers had a higher rate of late failure, which may be related to resumption of smoking after discharge.

20a. Cheng GL, Pan DD, Zhang NP, Fang GR: Digital replantation in children: A long-term follow-up study. J Hand Surg [Am] 23:635-646, 1998.

This paper reviews a rather large experience with digital replantation in children, with an average of 11 years of follow-up. They found excellent motion with normal two-point discrimination in 88%. They also noted 93% normal bone growth in this series of patients. This paper provides proof of the efficacy of replantation in children.

39. Goldner RD, Howson MP, Nunley JA, et al: One hundred eleven thumb amputations: Replantation versus revision. Microsurgery 11:243-250, 1990.

This review compared the results of thumb replantation in 69 patients with revision amputation in another 42. Range of motion of the replanted thumbs averaged 42% of the normal side, with only 21% having 7 mm or less two-point discrimination. Despite enthusiasm for thumb replantation, the authors found that measured lateral pinch and work simulator assessment of pinch was better in the revision group. Jebsen testing revealed that replanted thumbs were slightly better, but neither group functioned as well as normal controls.

82a. Pederson WC: Replantation. Plast Reconstr Surg 107:823-841, 2001.

This review paper presents a reasonable overview of the current state of replantation. It also covers the subject of replantation of parts other than hands and digits.

83a. Pomerance J, Truppa K, Bilos ZJ, et al: Replantation and revascularization of the digits in a community microsurgical practice. J Reconstr Microsurg 13:163-170, 1997.

This paper reviews the results of replantations performed in a community private practice. The authors present very good results but note that this is only possible with an experienced surgeon and "team" approach. One must have the support of other surgeons and the hospital to successfully carry out replantation outside of the medical center setting.

126a. Waikakul S, Vanadurongwan V, Unnanuntana A: Prognostic factors for major limb re-implantation at both immediate and long-term follow-up. J Bone Joint Surg Br 80:1024-1030, 1998.

The authors present their experience with 186 major limb replantations, from the upper arm to the midpalmar level, with a minimum of 2 years of follow-up. The authors note that the degree of injury at the amputation stump and to the amputated part were good predictors of the success rate and final outcome. They also noted that the potassium level in the venous effluent from the replanted part was the best objective measure of potential success. They state that with a level of more than 6.5 mm/L 30 minutes after reperfusion that replantation should be aborted.

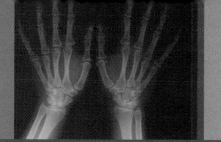

CHAPTER 46

The Mangled Upper Extremity

Nicholas B. Vedder • Douglas P. Hanel

PRINCIPLES

Mangling injuries of the hand and upper extremity are, by definition, devastating injuries that involve multiple critical structures of the fingers, hand, and/or arm and nearly always lead to significant disability, both directly and through their psychosocial impact. These injuries have a dramatic impact on the patient's livelihood and on his or her ability to carry out activities of daily living. Because the forces involved in producing mangling injuries of the upper extremity are often great, serious injury to other organ systems and other areas of the body are often also present and nearly always take precedence over the extremity injury in management.

CRITICAL POINTS: GOALS IN TREATING MANGLING INJURIES OF THE UPPER EXTREMITY

- Preserve life.
- Preserve tissue.
- Preserve function.
- Reconstruct and restore function—of the extremity and the patient.

Mangling injuries generally include all or nearly all of the major functional systems of an extremity, including skin/soft tissue, vascular, nerve, muscle/tendon, bone, and joint (Fig. 46-1). It is because of this multi-system injury, involving all or nearly all layers of the extremity, that ultimate function is so much at risk. Despite the best attempts at reconstruction, scar will form from the skin down through the bone, compromising the function of all structures involved and the extremity overall. Peacock elegantly described this as the "one wound/one scar" concept (Fig. 46-2).[79,80] This variable involvement of multiple tissue layers and critical, interdependent structures and systems, and the disabling result of the "one wound/one scar" concept led to the concept of "combined injuries" described by Büchler and Hastings.[15] The eventual impact of the scarring process must, therefore, be kept in mind throughout the planning

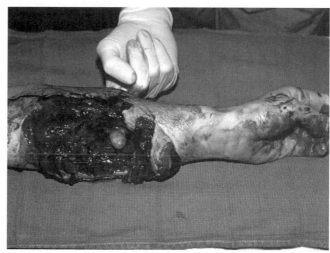

FIGURE 46-1. A mangling injury typically involves all or nearly all of the major functional systems of the extremity, including skin/soft tissue, vessels, nerve, muscle/tendon, bone, and joint.

and reconstruction. Minimizing the negative effects of this process dictates the following general principles in the management of mangling injuries:

- Complete débridement of devitalized tissue
- Restoration of good vascularity
- Rigid skeletal fixation, while minimizing additional soft tissue injury
- Stable, vascularized soft tissue coverage

By following these principles, one can allow early mobilization of the extremity, thereby minimizing the impact of "one wound" scarring and maximizing ultimate motion.

The multi-systemic nature of mangling injuries demands knowledge and expertise in multiple disciplines related to trauma and reconstruction, including trauma surgery, orthopedic surgery, vascular surgery, and plastic surgery, and often benefits from a multi-specialty team approach. Because of the diverse nature of mangling injuries, no two cases are alike and, in general, there is no single "preferred approach" but rather a set of principles that guides the surgeon through the application of multiple approaches and techniques, addressing each of the involved systems while keeping in mind the impact of individual treatment decisions on the

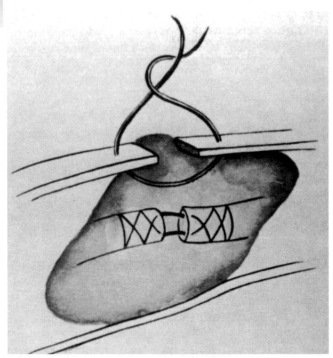

FIGURE 46-2. The "one wound/one scar" concept described by Peacock. Despite the best attempts at reconstruction, scar will form, from the skin down through the bone, compromising the function of all structures in between and the extremity overall. (From Peacock EE Jr, VanWinkle WJ: Surgery and Biology of Wound Repair. Philadelphia, WB Saunders, 1970.)

CRITICAL POINTS: FACTORS NECESSARY TO OPTIMIZE ULTIMATE FUNCTION

- Careful and complete evaluation of the injury, addressing all functional systems
- Formulation of a comprehensive reconstructive plan, tailored to the patient's needs
- Thorough but careful wound débridement of all devitalized tissue
- Meticulous operative reconstruction, often including secondary procedures
  - Restoration of good vascularity
  - Rigid skeletal fixation, while minimizing additional soft tissue injury
  - Stable, vascularized soft tissue coverage
- Comprehensive rehabilitation of the extremity and the patient

comprehensive reconstructive plan and the ultimate outcome. Many of the specific operative approaches are detailed elsewhere in this textbook; therefore, in this chapter we concentrate on principles, judgment, and timing. This chapter is an outgrowth of two chapters in the previous edition of this text, "Open Injuries of the Hand" and "Combined Injuries" to which we refer the reader as excellent resources on the topic of mangling injuries of the hand,[12,15] as well as several other excellent reviews.*

Sometimes, amputation is the most appropriate reconstruction, and the choice between amputation, partial amputation, and salvage with reconstruction requires looking into the "crystal ball" 6 to 12 months in the future, trying to predict the patient's overall function with different treatment choices and then formulating a comprehensive reconstructive plan that includes both short-term and long-term objectives. Optimal management of the mangled extremity is, therefore, one of the most challenging aspects of hand surgery, requiring a broad knowledge and facility with various techniques, and the judgment and experience to know when and how to apply them. It is a true test of one's mastery of the "art" of hand surgery.

MECHANISMS AND PATHOPHYSIOLOGY OF INJURY

A wide variety of mechanisms can produce mangling injuries, including industrial, agricultural, motor vehicle, power tool, explosive, and firearm mechanisms. Most mangling injuries involve some component of crush injury, whereby multiple tissue layers and anatomic systems are injured or destroyed. Certainly, crushing and blast injuries, with their extensive tissue destruction and associated late scarring, are far more difficult to reconstruct and portend a poorer outcome than sharp injuries. As a result of the immediate and delayed tissue necrosis with crushing injuries, infection risk is increased and often compromises the reconstructive plan. Degloving or avulsion injuries are also often mangling in that they involve amputation or partial amputation of one or more critical tissue layers: skin, vessel, nerve, tendon, and/or bone. Abrasion and burn injuries, depending on the extent and the depth of involvement, can also be significant components of mangling injuries.

It should be obvious that mangling injuries frequently result in severe wound contamination, depending on the environment and specific mechanism by which they occur. Farming injuries in particular are usually associated with major contamination, requiring more extensive and often serial débridement and irrigation and special consideration in planning antibiotic management.[37] The combination of a contaminated injury environment with deep, open tissue crushing and devascularized tissue is a dangerous scenario for major, life-threatening infection if not recognized and appropriately managed.

A constant element in most mangling injuries is tissue devascularization, which can occur at multiple levels. Crushing, avulsion, degloving, or blast injuries can disrupt major vessels or the branching, perforator vessels to muscle and skin or can produce endothelial injury that results in thrombosis of large and small vessels, including the microcirculation. Crushing can also cause direct cell disruption and tissue necrosis. Different tissues are more or less susceptible to crushing, with vessels, fat, muscle, and skin being the most severely injured with crushing, in that order. Nerve is unique in that it is often the last structure remaining

---

*See references 3, 9, 19, 23, 32, 40, 41, 74, 76, 86, 89, and 103.

physically "intact" after a crush or avulsion injury, yet axons themselves are quite susceptible to crush or stretching, leading to a difficult dilemma in distinguishing neurapraxia from axonotmesis in the early stages. Tendon, ligament, and bone tend to be more resistant to crushing/avulsing forces; nevertheless, partial injuries of tendon and ligament can result in significant scarring and functional impairment that can only be minimized by early recognition with early and aggressive mobilization.

The metabolic changes after ischemia or traumatic flap elevation are numerous and extreme. Ischemic tissue undergoes a conversion to anaerobic metabolism with a rapid depletion of levels of oxygen, glucose, and adenosine triphosphate, along with a concomitant increase in levels of carbon dioxide and lactic acid. Prostacyclin and thromboxane levels are significantly elevated.[26,51] Associated with the conversion to anaerobic metabolism is the markedly increased production of toxic superoxide radicals.[2,50,51,66] These toxic oxygen radicals can cause direct cytotoxicity, but probably more importantly they are a trigger for local acute inflammation, adherence and accumulation of leukocytes, and endothelial injury, with the subsequent cellular events leading to microvascular shutdown. Levels of the body's key protective enzyme, superoxide dismutase (SOD), are decreased in ischemic tissues as the enzyme is consumed in converting superoxide to oxygen in a tissue-protective mechanism.[69] With reperfusion or reoxygenation, toxic metabolites, including superoxide and hydroxyl radicals, are produced, with subsequent tissue injury through two key mechanisms. The first is by direct reaction of superoxide radical with the endothelial membrane, causing lipid peroxidation, disruption of membrane proteins, increased cell permeability, and, consequently, cytoplasmic swelling and dysfunction. The second mechanism is by the chemotactic property of oxygen metabolites, primarily superoxide anion, which causes neutrophil migration into the reperfused area, with the neutrophils actually causing the tissue destruction.

There is evidence that, frequently, a significant proportion of the tissue damage triggered by ischemia may be a consequence of events associated with reperfusion of ischemic tissues, that is, "reperfusion injury."[97] The rapid intravascular accumulation of neutrophils can lead to progressively decreased perfusion, which may manifest as the "no-reflow" phenomenon[59] or, more precisely, a "diminishing-reflow" phenomenon associated with ischemia and reperfusion.[99] Crushed tissue and traumatically created tissue flaps are a model of "gradient" ischemia, in that tissue is progressively ischemic from the base of the normally perfused tissue out toward the ischemic tip with an "ongoing" ischemia-reperfusion injury present. In this setting, too, neutrophil-mediated injury appears to play a major role in tissue necrosis.[98]

There are several mechanisms whereby activated polymorphonuclear leukocytes may cause injury in the setting of ischemia-reperfusion. First, adherent, activated polymorphonuclear leukocytes can cause direct endothelial injury, resulting in loss of vascular integrity, edema, hemorrhage, and thrombosis (Fig. 46-3). Another possible mechanism involves microvascular occlusion and further ischemia resulting from adherence and accumulation of aggregates of polymorphonuclear leukocytes within the vessel lumen. This progressive, inflammatory-mediated injury is largely

Rolling – Activation – Adherence – Injury

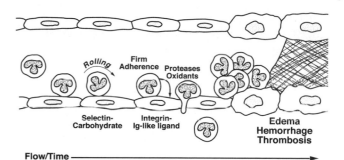

FIGURE 46-3. Diagram of the sequential events that occur at a site of neutrophil-mediated microvascular injury. There is initial selectin/carbohydrate-mediated rolling along the surface of the endothelium and tethering of neutrophils where local agonists then stimulate integrin-mediated firm adherence, leading to neutrophil-mediated endothelial injury with loss of vascular integrity, edema, hemorrhage, and thrombosis. Another mechanism involves microvascular occlusion and further ischemia resulting from adherence and accumulation of aggregates of neutrophils within the vessel lumen. (©2003, Nicholas B. Vedder.)

responsible for the "zone of injury" phenomenon associated with mangling injuries.

The concept of the "zone of injury" is another constant element of mangling injuries. This concept recognizes that the extent of tissue injury associated with a major injury force often extends well beyond the area of initial injury. The combination of local and regional ischemia, in addition to injury-induced inflammation and the resulting ischemia, all combine to extend the zone of tissue necrosis. The zone of tissue injury and late scarring often extend well beyond the area of initial injury. The extent of the zone of injury depends primarily on the force of the original injury. This is a critical concept in the management of mangling injuries because it nearly always precludes immediate or one-stage reconstruction and dictates prudent re-evaluation and re-débridement of the wound 24 to 48 hours after injury before definitive closure can be considered. The zone of injury and related inflammatory response are also important in planning vascular reconstruction in mangling injuries, because reconstructions performed inside the zone of injury are subject to direct and inflammatory-mediated endothelial injury, leading to thrombosis of the vascular reconstruction.

INITIAL EVALUATION

Because mangling injuries of the hand and upper extremity are often associated with significant injury force, it is not uncommon for the patient to have other significant and potentially life-threatening injuries. The mangling extremity injury, although often the most obvious, graphic, and visually compelling injury, is rarely life threatening. As always, one must look beyond the obvious extremity injury and evaluate the patient carefully for other serious injuries. The standard Advanced Trauma Life Support (ATLS) approach to any injured patient must be followed, with immediate attention to the ABCs (airway, breathing, circulation), followed by primary and secondary surveys of the injured patient.[1]

History

As always, the key components of the medical history focus on the "when," "where," and "how."[12] The time of injury is critically important, especially when dealing with devascularizing injuries. Bone, integument, and muscle have, in order, decreasing tolerance to ischemia, with muscle able to survive only 4 to 6 hours of ischemia, even with the normal tissue cooling that occurs after ischemia.[96] In addition, the longer the duration from time of injury, the greater the risk of infection, with delays greater than 6 to 12 hours precluding primary closure or coverage. If ischemia is present, the temperature of the tissue during the ischemic period is critical, because extremity tissues devoid of muscle can be successfully revascularized after 12 to 24 hours, if kept cool. In fact, successful digit replantation has been reported at 94 hours.[102]

The "where" of an injury is also important. Farming injuries, for example, tend to be highly contaminated, requiring more than the usual amount of aggressive débridement, and often preclude primary closure. The presence of caustic industrial chemicals or other contaminated substances can also affect treatment choices. The social and economic aspects of the injury environment must also be weighed in planning treatment. A patient living in an area remote from appropriate medical facilities may not be able to follow through with the complex rehabilitation program required for a complex reconstruction and may be better served with more straightforward reconstructive options.

Finally, the "how," or mechanism of injury, can help reveal the force of the injury and the extent of tissue necrosis or "zone of injury" to anticipate and to address in treatment. Sharp injuries tend to involve a limited zone of tissue injury and are, therefore, easier to manage, unless the sharp injury is tangential in nature. High-velocity, high-pressure, crushing, or avulsion injuries have a much broader zone of injury and require a modified approach to treatment, with more extensive débridement, thorough evaluation of adjacent tissues, removal of foreign bodies, and assessment and treatment of compartment syndrome.

The patient's overall health and comorbidities must be carefully evaluated in planning any type of complex or lengthy reconstructive procedure. The patient's age and the presence of cardiovascular disease, pulmonary disease, bleeding tendencies, or diabetes can greatly increase the risk of perioperative complications or even mortality and should cause the surgeon to consider simplifying the method of reconstruction or at least modifying the perioperative treatment plans. Smoking or the use of other vasoactive drugs such as cocaine is generally a contraindication to any type of complex microvascular reconstruction.

Perhaps the most important aspect of the history is determining the patient's functional needs and goals. The patient's age, occupation, socioeconomic environment, and social support mechanisms should all be considered in formulating a treatment plan. Both the risks that the patient is willing to accept and the costs in terms of financial, emotional, and time must be considered. The patient's willingness to endure a protracted reconstructive course and to follow through with the necessary hand therapy are important issues. A self-employed farmer, without workers' compensation insurance, will likely be interested in reconstructive options that return him or her to work expeditiously, providing durable function suited for heavy work, without multiple complex reconstructive procedures. An office worker or technology professional may have very different goals and may be more willing and economically able to undergo multiple complex reconstructive procedures to restore optimal digit function allowing fine manipulation, keyboarding, and so on. Again, the hand surgeon must make decisions based on his or her knowledge and experience to try to predict the patient's ultimate function with the available reconstructive options and try to select the most appropriate options for that particular patient. Both the patient and the patient's family must be involved in this discussion, although this is often difficult to do when the patient has just suffered a mangling injury and often the surgeon must use his or her best judgment at the time, taking into account all of the known variables.

Examination

Examination of the patient with a severely mangled extremity injury that is wrapped in blood-soaked bandages is often difficult in the emergency department, and definitive evaluation frequently must wait until the patient is in the operating room. Nevertheless, assessment of major structure injuries, in particular vascular status, is important in determining the urgency of definitive treatment and also important in being able to discuss treatment options and prognosis with the patient and family. Usually, a general assessment of vascular status, sensibility, and muscle-tendon unit function as well as radiographic evaluation can and should be performed in the emergency department. Preliminary evaluation will also allow adequate preparation of the operating room, including microsurgical equipment and supplies, implants and fixation devices, traction and radiographic devices, and so on.

The most important system to evaluate is the vascular system of the extremity. Compromised vascularity of the digit or extremity, depending on the duration of devascularization, can dictate whether the digit or limb can be salvaged, whether fasciotomy is required, and the urgency of initiating treatment. Assessment of vascular status is best performed by direct inspection of the affected tissues and comparison to adjacent or similar well-vascularized tissues on that patient. Although nail bed capillary refill is traditionally considered a good indicator of peripheral perfusion, in fact this is a very unreliable indicator of perfusion. A completely devascularized digit can have what appears to be intact capillary refill beneath the nail bed when in fact stagnant blood is merely being pushed to the sides with compression, then moving back to the center with release of pressure on the nail bed. A far more reliable area to assess digit perfusion is the dorsal paronychial tissue on the sides of the nail, which should be pink, and spongy, with good turgor, compressing with pressure and refilling with release (Fig. 46-4). A pink color that returns within 1 to 2 seconds after pressure and release indicates healthy tissue, whereas a pale color without capillary refill or turgor can represent arterial insufficiency. A dusky color with exceptionally brisk refill can represent venous congestion. Probably the most

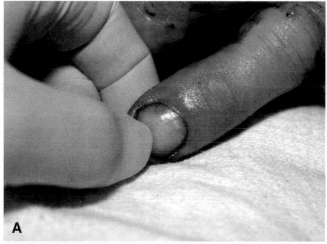

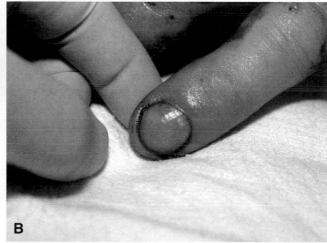

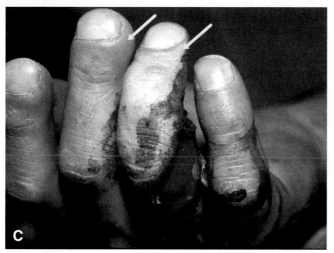

FIGURE 46-4. A completely devascularized digit can have what appears to be intact capillary refill beneath the nail bed when in fact stagnant blood is merely being pushed to the sides with compression (**A**), then moving back to the center with release of pressure on the nail bed (**B**). A far more reliable area to assess digit perfusion is the dorsal paronychial tissue on the sides of the nail, which should be pink, and spongy, with good turgor, compressing with pressure and refilling with release (**C,** long finger, *arrow*), whereas a devascularized digit's paronychial tissue will be pale, flat, and without turgor (**C,** ring finger, *arrow*).

reliable clinical indicator of tissue vascularity is the color of the blood that oozes from the tissue after sticking it with a needle or scalpel. Bright pink oozing reflects a healthy tissue, whereas dark purplish oozing reflects compromised perfusion, if it is sluggish, or venous insufficiency, if it is profuse. Obviously, this should not be performed in sensate tissue of an awake patient but it is often useful in the anesthetized patient.

For assessing the status of the major vessels of the upper extremity and even the digital vessels, the hand-held Doppler device is very useful. The standard Allen test, performed by compressing either the radial or ulnar artery and listening for a signal over the palmar arch or the most distant digital artery, can help determine whether either the radial or ulnar artery has antegrade flow and whether the palmar arch is intact. Angiography has little role in mangling injuries of the forearm, hand, or fingers. In any mangling or crushing injury, a high index of suspicion for compartment syndrome must be maintained. The diagnosis and treatment of compartment syndrome is covered in Chapter 56, but it is worth reinforcing the importance of recognizing the intense pain of compartment syndrome and, in particular, pain with passive stretch of muscle-tendon units. When suspected, the diagnosis is best confirmed with direct pressure measurement of the muscle compartment, usually with a hand-held

device specifically designed for this purpose. The presence of compartment syndrome and attendant tissue ischemia dictates emergent decompression in the operating room.

Although obvious deformity, crepitus, or tenderness on examination can suggest underlying skeletal injury, the evaluation of the skeletal system is generally performed radiographically. In most instances, standard plain radiographs are sufficient, taking care where possible to ensure that emergency splints or traction devices do not obscure the underlying bones or joints. Sometimes, additional views are needed, such as oblique views to evaluate articular congruity or stress views to evaluate ligament injury, such as a clenched-fist view to evaluate intercarpal ligamentous integrity. In questionable cases, comparison views with the contralateral extremity, if uninjured, may be necessary. In the case of most mangling injuries, advanced imaging techniques such as computed tomography (CT) or magnetic resonance imaging (MRI) are rarely indicated, although sometimes, if the patient is stable, CT of suspected carpal injuries or intra-articular displacement can be useful. If amputated parts are involved and replantation is to be contemplated, radiographs should be obtained of the amputated parts. And, as always, the joint proximal and the joint distal to the area of injury must be evaluated (Fig. 46-5). Ligamentous injuries can be identified by tenderness to

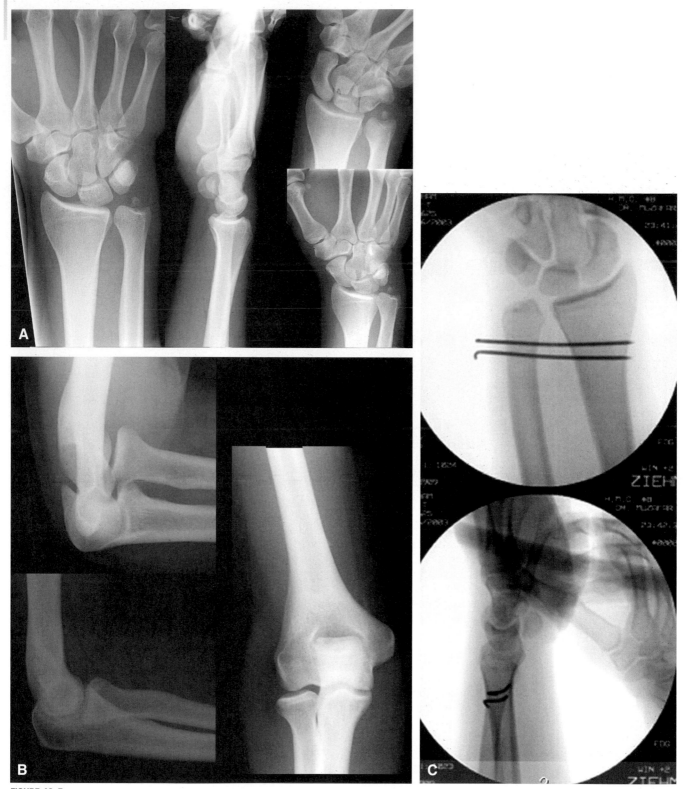

FIGURE 46-5. The importance of obtaining radiographs that include the entire extremity, including a joint above and below the obvious injury, is illustrated in this case of a 22-year-old man who sustained multiple injuries resulting from a motor vehicle accident. **A,** Radiographs were taken after the patient complained of wrist pain. There is an ulnar styloid fracture and subluxation of the distal radioulnar joint (DRUJ). **B,** Elbow radiographs showed no obvious pathology. **C,** The DRUJ was transfixed with Kirschner wires. *Continued*

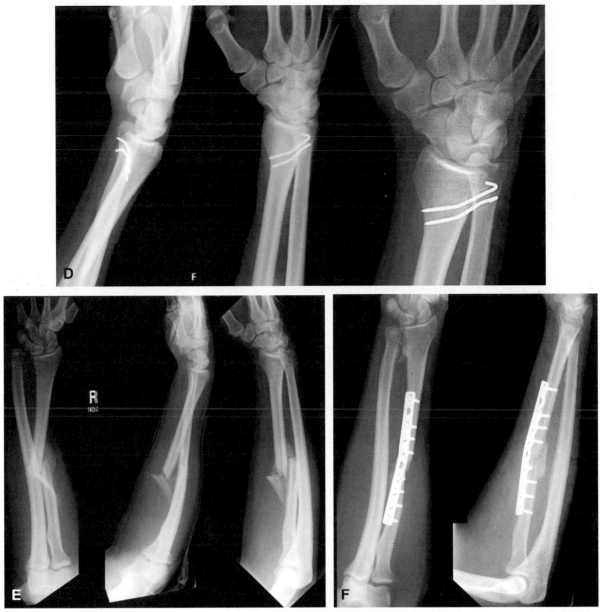

FIGURE 46-5—cont'd. D, Within 3 weeks the Kirschner wires bent. **E,** The fixation wires were removed, full-length forearm radiographs were obtained, and the culprit, a Galeazzi fracture, was identified. **F,** Restoration of the radius and soft tissue reconstruction of the DRUJ resulted in 80 degrees of pronation and 60 degrees of supination).

palpation or to stress. Stability to stress should also be re-evaluated under anesthesia to remove any confounding effect of involuntary muscular splinting.

Evaluating muscle-tendon unit injury is best performed by having the patient actively flex and extend the digits and wrist. In the presence of pain, and especially with underlying skeletal injury, this examination can be difficult to interpret. For the individual digits, noting aberrations in the normal resting cascade can indicate injury to the underlying flexor muscle-tendon unit. This simple observation can be performed even in the comatose patient, as can evaluation of tenodesis tendon function, by passively flexing and extending the wrist and observing the normal cascade of digit flexion with wrist extension and digit extension with wrist flexion (Fig. 46-6). In the end, though, with most mangling injuries, definitive evaluation of tendon injury must wait for careful examination in the operating room.

Nerve injury is evaluated by examining both motor and sensory function. The motor function of the median radial and ulnar nerves is evaluated by testing both extrinsic and intrinsic muscle function. Three simple maneuvers test motor integrity: (1) resistance against palmar abduction of the thumb reflects the median nerve–innervated abductor pollicis brevis function; (2) resistance against flexion of the metacarpophalangeal (MCP) joint of the small finger reflects the ulnar nerve–innervated flexor digiti quinti function; and (3) resistance to extension of the MCP joint of the index reflects the radial nerve–innervated extensor digitorum communis and extensor indicis proprius. Accurate sensory examination is much more difficult, especially in

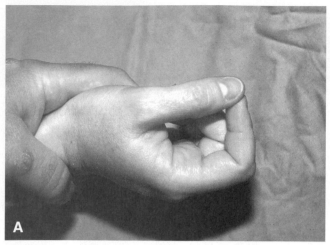
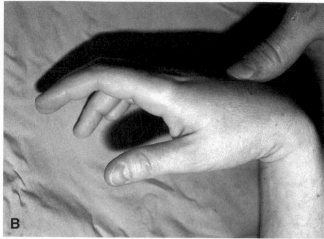

FIGURE 46-6. Evaluation of tenodesis tendon function by passively extending (**A**) and flexing (**B**) the wrist while observing the normal cascade of digit flexion with wrist extension and digit extension with wrist flexion.

the presence of severe injury. By using light touch and, if questionable, pinprick testing, a reasonable assessment can nevertheless be obtained. If the injury is in the palm or digits, specific attention should be addressed to digital nerve function, whereas if the injury is more proximal, attention should be addressed to the independent areas of sensory function, that is, the volar aspect of the index or middle finger for median, the volar small finger for ulnar, and the dorsum of the first web space for radial.

With sharp or penetrating injuries, if you "think the nerve is probably OK," it usually is not. An equivocal examination usually indicates an underlying injury that warrants exploration, whereas a normal sensory examination, with the patient not looking, usually indicates an intact nerve. With blunt or blast injuries, however, nerve contusion and neurapraxia with the nerve in continuity is not uncommon. The threshold of suspicion to explore a nerve in the presence of sharp or penetrating injury should, therefore, be much lower than with blunt or blast injuries.

Laboratory studies should be obtained at this time, including a complete blood cell count, platelet count, electrolyte levels, and any other tests appropriate to the clinical situation, such as blood gas analysis, toxicology screen, or amylase evaluation. In addition, if there has been significant bleeding or significant bleeding is anticipated with surgery, blood for type and crossmatch should be obtained at this time.

GOALS OF TREATMENT: BIOMECHANICS OF THE INJURED HAND

In developing a treatment plan for mangling injuries of the hand and upper extremity, the surgeon must keep in mind the basic seven functions of the hand: precision pinch, opposition pinch, key pinch, chuck grip, hook grip, span grasp, and power grasp. Depending on the severity of injury, some of these functions may not be restored. The basic units that comprise hand function are (1) an opposable thumb; (2) the index and long fingers, serving as the stable fixed unit of the hand for fine manipulation and power pinch; (3) the ring and small fingers, serving as the mobile unit of the hand for

grasping functions; and (4) the wrist. Restoring these units, therefore, should be the general goal of reconstruction, with restoration of an opposition digit and a stable opposition post being the bare minimum.[73] Preservation of length should be a goal, but only functional length should be preserved, not stiff, insensate, potentially painful units with unstable coverage. Durable, stable soft tissue coverage is a necessity, as is at least protective sensation. Without these, chronic breakdown, infection, and failure of the reconstruction can be expected. Not all patients are best served by complex digit reconstruction, especially if the digit is going to be stiff or painful. Sometimes, a prosthesis customized to the patient's occupation is the best option (Fig. 46-7). Highly functional, durable, mechanical prostheses, as well as advanced myoelectric prostheses allow for excellent return of function and are discussed in Chapter 55.

Amputation/Skeletal Contribution

According to the American Medical Association's (AMA) *Guidelines for Evaluation of Permanent Impairment,*[25] the thumb comprises 40% of hand function; the index and middle fingers, 20% each; and the ring and small fingers, 10% each. These contributions should be kept in mind when deciding between reconstruction/replantation versus amputation. In the case of mangling injuries, however, these relative contributions do not always apply. For example, with the loss of the three central digits, the small finger assumes effectively 50% of hand function. As discussed previously, the surgeon must use his or her best knowledge, experience, and judgment in an effort to predict the patient's ultimate function with amputation versus reconstruction and with the various reconstructive options. The factors of patient age, health, drug or nicotine use, occupation, and willingness and ability to undergo complex or multistaged reconstructive procedures and rehabilitation must be taken into account. The topics of amputation, replantation, and thumb reconstruction are covered elsewhere in this text, and the reader is referred to those sections for more detailed coverage of those topics.

The thumb is, of course, the most important digit to preserve or reconstruct. The issues related to thumb ampu-

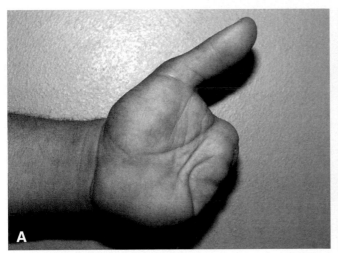
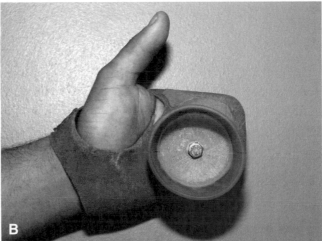

FIGURE 46-7. **A** and **B**, Sometimes, a prosthesis customized to the patient's occupation is the best option, as in this forklift driver.

tation are discussed in Chapter 53 and vary depending on the level of injury. Interphalangeal (IP) joint motion and the distal phalanx are of relatively lower importance to preserve, compared with multiplanar carpometacarpal (CMC) motion and, to a lesser extent, MCP motion.[67] The ability to bring the thumb out of the plane of the hand and into a position of opposition is a key function that must be restored. If the thumb cannot be preserved, consideration should be given to primary pollicization.[55]

The index finger is also important to preserve, because of its independent profundus flexion and its ability to abduct for precision pinch functions. Without good proximal interphalangeal (PIP) function and sensibility, however, the index is often bypassed in favor of the middle finger and can be more of a hindrance than a help.[30,73,94] Amputation at or proximal to the PIP level leaves only intrinsics for flexion, which is then limited to about 45 degrees. The long and ring fingers are important primarily for grip and grasp functions, although either can take over pinch functions for the radial digits if they are lost. Solitary loss of the ring finger probably results in the least-associated functional deficit of all digits.[94] The small finger, although it has the least flexion strength, is actually quite important to hand function in that it defines hand width for grip functions, use of tools, and so on. An important component of this is the significant CMC motion of the small finger that comes into play with terminal grip.

With amputation at the proximal aspect of the middle phalanx (P2), PIP, or especially MCP level, ray amputation also needs to be considered. Although ray amputation is usually aesthetically preferable to a partial finger amputation, function can suffer. For the index finger, power grip, key pinch, and supination strength are diminished approximately 20% and pronation strength is diminished approximately 50%.[75] There is also a fairly high rate of dysesthesia after ray amputation, further arguing against its routine application.

The loss of an isolated digit other than the thumb rarely results in significant compromise of hand function; and as Brown has noted, patient motivation is more important to regaining function than the actual digits lost.[11] The loss of multiple digits, however, is common with mangling injuries

and often does result in significant functional deficits. Maintaining or reconstructing at least the thumb and one opposing digit is a minimal requirement for any type of pinch or grasp. Retaining or reconstructing an additional adjacent digit can, nevertheless, add significant function by providing lateral stability to the radial digit for power pinch and can allow three jaw chuck pinch.

Joints

The choice of whether to salvage or fuse a joint is another, often difficult, decision. This decision is best made by assessing the potential loss of function from a given fusion or set of fusions versus the risks of limited motion, pain, instability, or late arthrosis with reconstruction. Whenever anatomic articular congruity and ligamentous stability can be restored, reconstruction is usually worthwhile. When this cannot be achieved, the potential loss of function needs to be assessed. In general, distal interphalangeal (DIP) fusions of the digits or IP fusion of the thumb are well tolerated with limited loss of function. PIP joint motion is much more important to preserve. Littler has described the PIP joint as the "functional locus of finger function."[62] Not only are fingers with fused PIP joints of little use for grip or grasp, they often get in the way and are easily injured, because they do not follow the normal arc of the other fingers. An additional problem, although less so with the index finger, is a quadriga effect that can occur when profundus excursion is impaired with arthrodesis. Although delayed arthroplasty can be considered, in the presence of combined injuries involving the joint, nerve, and soft tissue, if the PIP joint cannot be primarily reconstructed, serious consideration should be given to amputation, especially in the ulnar two digits.

The MCP joint is perhaps the most important joint in terms of function for the index through small fingers, contributing 77% of the total arc of finger flexion.[62] Most activities, however, do not require full arc of MCP motion and in fact as little as 35 degrees of motion can be acceptable, if that arc is within the key functional range and the joint is stable.[5] To that end, stable but markedly limited MCP motion, even arthrodesis, is far superior to an unstable, painful MCP joint (Fig. 46-8).

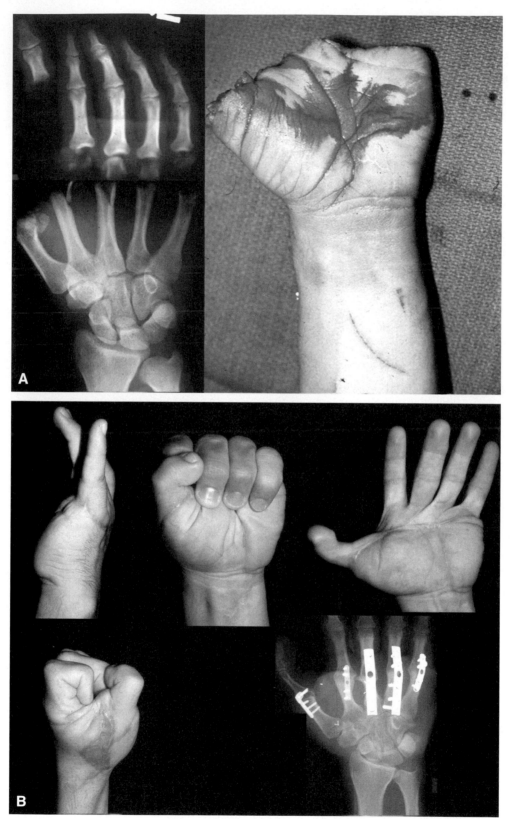

FIGURE 46-8. **A,** A five-digit amputation resulted from a saw accident in this 18-year-old young man. **B,** Treatment consisted of primary arthrodesis of the finger metacarpophalangeal joints and replantation of the index, middle, ring, and small fingers. The thumb could not be replanted. Six months after injury the thumb was reconstructed with a second toe to hand transfer. Hand motion is demonstrated 1 year after injury.

The decision to perform partial or total wrist fusion is seldom made in the acute setting, unless there is extensive, nonreconstructable loss of articular surface. Usually, this decision is deferred until late function and pain can be better assessed, at which time elective arthroplasty or arthrodesis can be performed. Studies have shown that as little as 5 to 10 degrees of flexion and 30 to 35 degrees of extension are needed for most activities of daily living.[14,78] When wrist-level amputation is required, preservation of some wrist motion can be incorporated into a mechanical prosthesis and preservation of an intact distal radioulnar joint can significantly improve pronation and supination under load. The functional benefit of preserving the distal radioulnar joint, although attractive in theory, has never been proved in practice.

Tendons

Preserving and reconstructing skeletal length and joint motion is of little use without a mobile muscle-tendon unit to move it. The extensor tendon mechanism, especially over the digits, because of its complex balanced "shroud" mechanism and limited excursion is susceptible to minor changes in length with repair, as well as adhesion formation and underlying skeletal injury.[29] Intrinsic function is also easily compromised in mangling injuries, especially crush and blast injuries with multiple metacarpal fractures. Fibrosis and contracture leading to significant disability is common. Because of the overlap in function and transmission through the juncturae tendineae, extrinsic extensor tendon injuries tend to be more forgiving, especially if a limited number are involved. Although not ideal, complete loss of the extrinsic extensors with associated reconstruction of dorsal soft tissue coverage in the presence of intact intrinsics is tolerated quite well. In this setting the ensuing deep cicatrix formation allows adequate MCP flexion and extension through scar tenodesis. This combined with intact IP function results in good overall hand function.[84]

Preserving or reconstructing flexor tendon function in the mangled hand is obviously important but often difficult to achieve. It is often difficult to restore independent sublimis and profundus function, and often the pulley systems are ruptured. To prevent bowstringing, the A2 and A4 pulleys must be preserved or reconstructed.[49,60] Given the limited tolerances within the flexor pulley system it is sometimes best to repair only one tendon, usually the profundus tendon. This is especially true if repairing both tendons would lead to adhesions and limited excursion. Two other complications of profundus injury must also be kept in mind and avoided: quadriga and lumbrical-plus deformity. Lumbrical-plus deformity occurs when the cut and unrepaired profundus retracts, increasing tension on the lumbrical and resulting in paradoxical extension with digit flexion. This is avoided by either repairing the profundus or, as with amputations, suturing it without tension to the flexor sheath. Quadriga primarily affects the middle through small fingers and is a result of these tendons arising from a common muscle belly. If one profundus becomes adherent in a lengthened position or is repaired with significant shortening, it can prevent full flexion of the remaining digits.

Soft Tissue Coverage and Nerves

Providing durable, stable, pliable soft tissue coverage, with at least protective sensation in the areas of functional contact has long been recognized to be the most important factor in determining outcome after mangling injuries.[10,35] Stability of the soft tissue coverage is often overlooked in the quest to provide bulk, padding, and durability. Stability is especially important on the volar aspects of the hand and digits. A bulky, mobile flap subject to shear with tangential load leads to poor grip function. One can imagine how difficult the simplest of tasks would be if a small water balloon were strapped to one's palm. For this reason, we favor fascia flaps or thin muscle flaps that are skin grafted, as opposed to thick fasciocutaneous or musculocutaneous flaps, especially on potentially friction-dependent weight-bearing surfaces.

Restoring protective sensation, that is, 7 to 15 mm of two-point discrimination, to the volar weight-bearing surfaces of the hand is critical. According to the AMA's *Guides to the Evaluation of Permanent Impairment,* more than 15 mm of two-point discrimination is considered functionally insensate.[25] Nerve repair, whether primary or delayed, is an essential component to reconstruction of the mangled hand.

EVOLUTION IN THE TREATMENT OF MANGLING INJURIES

Historically, the primary method of treating mangling injuries has been amputation. Surgeons long ago learned that without effective treatment, devascularized, contaminated, or crushed tissues, along with open fractures often led to limb- and life-threatening infections; and only with early and thorough débridement with amputation could this be avoided. With the advent of antibiotics and with advances in anesthesia and surgical care, more aggressive salvage efforts were undertaken. In the 1950s there was a tendency to treat mangling injuries with minimal débridement and a goal of preserving length. The early enthusiasm for the role of antibiotics in surgical patients was tempered by studies showing a failure of antibiotics to significantly alter the rate of postoperative infection.[71] Burke's classic studies finally demonstrated the critical importance of early administration of antibiotics and their significant efficacy when administered before wound inoculation.[18] In the 1970s, the concept of delayed closure to reduce infection risk was popularized and incorporated into the treatment of mangling upper extremity injuries.[21] In the 1980s, management of mangling injuries became increasingly aggressive, combining thorough débridement with revascularization, early reduction and fixation of fractures, and early, vascularized soft tissue coverage with flaps.[4,46] The identification of and growing experience with reliable axial pedicle flaps and microsurgical free flaps provided a wide range of new opportunities in salvaging mangled extremities (see Chapters 47 and 48). Godina's work showed that with a radical débridement and early microsurgical soft tissue reconstruction within 72 hours, infection risk, morbidity, and time to healing were all dramatically improved.[36] Included in Godina's series and reinforced by other centers was the concept of complete reconstruction, including soft tissue reconstruction with free tissue transfer in a single emergent setting.[61,90] This radical and still controversial approach (controversial even between the two authors of this chapter) was viewed as a natural progression in the advances in microvascular surgery used in replantation and the salvage of devascularized tissues (see Chapters 44 and 45).

The treatment of the skeletal component of mangling injuries has undergone a parallel evolution over the past several decades. Although the use of external fixation devices remains a mainstay in the treatment of comminuted open fractures, the development of small, strong, low-profile internal fixation devices, when combined with early vascularized soft tissue reconstruction, has revolutionized the treatment of complex open skeletal injuries.[33] Before the advent of modern internal fixation, most complex hand injuries were treated with prolonged immobilization with the expected results of severe stiffness and tendon adhesions. Concomitant with the development of early rigid internal fixation was the concept of primary flexor tendon repair and early mobilization popularized by Kleinert and colleagues.[58] Improved fracture fixation and early mobilization after tendon repair dramatically improved the outcome of severe hand and upper extremity injuries.

Advances in the treatment of skeletal injuries have prompted independent advances in the repair of vascular and peripheral nerve injuries using microvascular techniques, allowing salvage and reconstruction of mangling injuries that in the past would have certainly led to amputation. Taken together, the advances in antibiotics, microsurgery, skeletal reconstruction, soft tissue reconstruction, and nerve reconstruction have dramatically expanded the possibilities of limb salvage. The critical task of the hand surgeon, however, is to know when to employ these techniques versus when to choose amputation or partial amputation to achieve the best long-term function for the patient.

RECOMMENDED APPROACH TO TREATMENT

Emergent Treatment

By far the most important aspect of treating a patient with a mangling extremity injury is to evaluate the patient for and treat other life-threatening injuries before proceeding to the evaluation and treatment of the extremity injury. Once the patient has been stabilized and attention can safely be turned to the extremity, the most emergent aspect of treatment is controlling ongoing hemorrhage. This is best done by applying direct pressure to the bleeding area long enough to allow the effects of reflex vasoconstriction and thrombus formation to effectively control bleeding. Sometimes, a compressive dressing held on by an elastic bandage is necessary. In rare circumstances, when direct pressure is ineffective, it may be necessary to temporarily inflate a proximal blood pressure cuff as a tourniquet until the area of bleeding can be identified and controlled. It must be kept in mind, however, that tissue distal to the injury may have already been subjected to a period of ischemia and that further complete ischemia will compromise the ability to salvage the limb. Because of the many critical structures running through the extremity, in particular nerves and arteries, it is important never to blindly clamp bleeding areas and to use clamps only on a specific, well-visualized vessel, being careful not to include any adjacent nerve.

If either the brachial artery or both the radial and ulnar arteries are transected or thrombosed, and if extensive skeletal stabilization is going to be required, especially if ischemia has already been present for some time, a vascular shunt should be placed as an initial step.[39,70] This should be performed before operative débridement or skeletal fixation to reperfuse the tissues and remove the time pressure, allowing meticulous débridement and appropriate skeletal fixation and tendon repair before definitive revascularization. A standard carotid vascular shunt usually works very well for the brachial, radial, or ulnar arteries. Before inserting the shunt, any thrombus or debris should be removed from the proximal and distal segments with a No. 2 Fogarty catheter to prevent distal embolization after restoration of flow (Fig. 46-9).

As noted earlier, cooling the tissue is the most effective way to prolong the length of time that tissue can be ischemic yet still remains viable. When tissue is amputated, including digits, limbs, or other potentially revascularizable tissue, it should be wrapped in saline gauze, placed in a plastic bag or container, and placed on ice until it can be revascularized. All intact skin bridges should be left intact. There are often critical draining veins within the skin bridge that can provide adequate venous drainage, obviating the need for venous reconstruction at the time of revascularization. In this case, the ischemic digit or limb should simply be wrapped with moist gauze or a moist towel, if the patient is not suffering from hypothermia. Gross skeletal deformity due to either fracture or dislocation compromises distal circulation and should be reduced, when possible. If any tissue flaps have been traumatically elevated, they should be gently placed back into anatomic position without any tension or kinking to optimize circulation. It is, of course, important to document the motor and sensory examination before local, regional, or general anesthesia.

With any open wound, the patient's tetanus prophylaxis status should be reviewed and the appropriate prophylaxis given, according to the standard guidelines (Table 46-1).[86]

CRITICAL POINTS: EMERGENT TREATMENT

- Evaluate and treat other life-threatening injuries (the trauma "ABCs").
- Control hemorrhage by direct pressure—do not blindly clamp.
- Reduce gross skeletal deformity.
- Administer tetanus prophylaxis and antibiotics.
- If a major limb is ischemic, place temporary vascular shunt.
- Cool devascularized tissue; leave skin bridges intact.

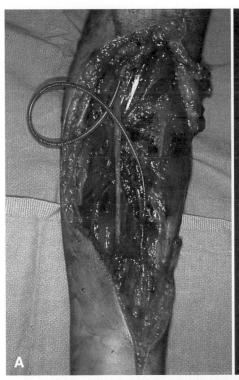

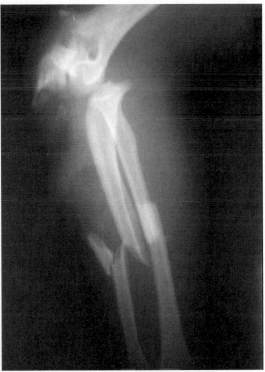

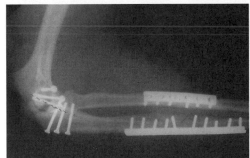

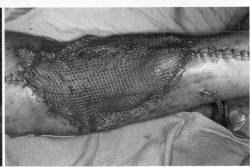

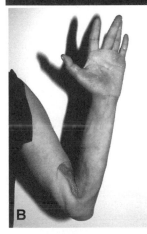

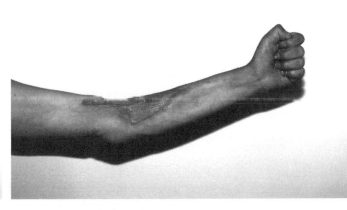

FIGURE 46-9. This 24-year-old man sustained a combined complex injury from a rollover motor vehicle crash. In addition to his open fractures were forearm muscle and skin avulsions and transection of the brachial artery. This accident occurred in a rural area, 6 hours from the nearest trauma center. **A,** The surgeon removed gross debris and reconstructed the artery with a vascular shunt and then transported the patient to our facility. Further treatment consisted of débridement, skeletal fixation, revascularization with vein grafts, and soft tissue reconstruction with a rectus abdominis free muscle flap and split-thickness skin grafts. **B,** Photographs taken 1 year after injury. Forearm rotation is limited to 90 degrees, shared equally by pronation and supination.

Appropriate intravenous antibiotic prophylaxis should be started at this time. In most instances, a first-generation cephalosporin is adequate because the most common infective organism in open hand injuries is *Staphylococcus aureus.*[27,47,91,92] With agricultural or other highly contaminated injuries, additional gram-negative coverage should be given, such as with an aminoglycoside.

OPERATIVE TREATMENT

Débridement/Wound Excision

The initial débridement is perhaps the single most important step that determines the functional outcome of mangling injuries. Performing it properly requires experience and

Table 46-1
CURRENT GUIDELINES FOR TETANUS PROPHYLAXIS

General Principles
1. Active immunization against tetanus with tetanus toxoid markedly reduces the incidence of this disease and resulting death.
2. Recommendations for tetanus prophylaxis are based on (a) the condition of the wound, especially its susceptibility to tetanus, and (b) the patient's immunization history.
3. Regardless of the active immunization status of the patient, all wounds should receive immediate surgical treatment, using meticulous aseptic technique, to remove all devitalized tissue and foreign bodies. Consideration should be given to leaving tetanus-prone wounds open. Such care is an essential part of prophylaxis against tetanus.

WARNING:
4. The only contraindication to tetanus and diphtheria toxoids for the wounded patient is a history of neurologic or severe hypersensitivity reaction to a previous dose. Local side effects alone do not preclude continued use. If a previous systemic reaction to horse serum is suspected to represent allergic hypersensitivity, postpone immunization until appropriate skin testing is performed.

If contraindication to a tetanus toxoid-containing preparation exists, consider passive immunization against tetanus for a tetanus-prone wound.

Wound Classification

Clinical Features	Tetanus-Prone Wounds	Non–Tetanus-Prone Wounds
Age of wound	>6 hr	≤6 hr
Configuration	Stellate wound, avulsion	Linear wound, abrasion
Depth	>1 cm	≤1 cm
Mechanism of injury	Missile, crush, burn, frostbite	Sharp surface (e.g., knife, glass)
Signs of infection	Present	Absent
Devitalized tissue	Present	Absent
Contaminants (e.g., dirt, feces, grass, saliva)	Present	Absent
Denervated and/or ischemic tissue	Present	Absent

Immunization Schedule
Obtain a history of tetanus immunization from medical records so that appropriate tetanus prophylaxis can be accomplished. Individuals with risk factors for inadequate tetanus immunization status (e.g., immigrants, rural or urban poor, elderly without known interval booster shots) should be treated as unknown.

History of Adsorbed Tetanus Toxoid (Doses)	Tetanus-Prone Wounds		Non–Tetanus-Prone Wounds	
	*Tt**	*TIG*	*Tt**	*TIG*
Unknown or <3	Yes	Yes	Yes	No
≥3[†]	No[‡]	No	No[§]	No

Tt, Tetanus toxoid adsorbed (for adult use); TIG, tetanus immune globulin (human).

*For children younger than 7 years old, DPT may be considered.

[†]If only three doses of fluid toxoid have been received previously, a fourth dose, preferably an adsorbed toxoid, should be given.

[‡]Yes, if more than 5 years since last dose.

[§]Yes, if more than 10 years since last dose (more frequent boosters are not needed and can accentuate side effects).

Disposition
Give each patient an appropriate written record describing treatment rendered and providing instructions for follow-up with regard to wound care, drug therapy, immunization status, and potential complications. Arrange for completion of active immunization.

Give every wounded patient a wallet-size card documenting immunization dosage and date received.

Modified from Ross SE: Prophylaxis against Tetanus in Wound Management. Chicago, American College of Surgeons, Committee on Trauma, 1995.

judgment. It should not, therefore, be left to the junior resident to perform. If the initial débridement is inadequate and nonviable tissue is left behind, the result will be infection, further tissue loss, and potential loss of limb or life that might otherwise be prevented. As Pasteur described, and reinforced by the work of Dellinger and colleagues, "It is the environment, not the bacteria, that determines whether a wound becomes infected."[27] Because there is little in the hand and upper extremity that is not functionally important, some argue for conservative initial débridement, allowing marginal tissue to "declare itself" over time. We strongly disagree with this approach. Marginally viable tissue leads to further toxic insult of adjacent tissues as well as systemic complications. Instead, we favor aggressive débridement of marginally vascularized tissue, especially muscle. The only two exceptions to this approach are (1) if revascularization is going to be performed, final débridement should await definitive revascularization, and (2) in the case of pure skin flaps that are critical for coverage of vital structures, the downside sepsis risk in waiting 24 to 48 hours for demarcation of viability is small. Nevertheless, if skin does not bleed, or only oozes dark blood at the time of initial operation, it should be débrided. The concept of débridement in the presence of mangling injuries, therefore, should actually be thought of as "wound excision," creating a healthy soft tissue bed for reconstruction.[43]

Unless prolonged muscle ischemia has already occurred, initial débridement is best performed under tourniquet control. This will allow the safe visualization and preservation of critical structures, specifically major nerves and vessels. Using loupe magnification, all foreign material should be carefully removed, along with clearly devitalized skin, subcutaneous tissue, and muscle. Frayed tendon should only be débrided of loose strands, leaving any potentially structural portions intact. Unless clearly destroyed, nerves should be left intact and adherent foreign material carefully removed. The ends of transected major nerves should be tagged with suture if primary repair is possible or with metal vascular clips if delayed nerve grafting will be necessary, because this will help later identification of the nerve ends, either directly or radiographically. Similarly, transected ends of major vessels to be repaired, that is, radial, ulnar, anterior interosseous, palmar, or digital, should be clamped with spring-loaded microvascular clamps. Smaller branches should be ligated with either suture ties or vascular clips, which we prefer because they are less likely to become a nidus for infection. Nonstructural bone fragments that are not attached to soft tissue should be saved for keying reduction. Attached and potentially viable fragments should be saved, along with structurally important fragments. The remaining bone should be curetted to remove contamination and allow anatomic reduction. The wounds should then be irrigated with a pulse-lavage system if large or with bulb/syringe irrigation if small. The mechanical débridement achieved by scrubbing with a sterile gauze sponge during irrigation is very important.

At this point, the tourniquet should be released and areas of significant bleeding either cauterized or ligated with vascular clips. Any tissues, particularly muscle, that are not pink and bleeding should be débrided down to healthy bleeding tissue. Sometimes it is necessary to reinflate the tourniquet briefly for further débridement. We have not found cultures taken at the time of initial débridement to be of much clinical value.[27] If the wound is heavily contaminated or if there are remaining critical areas where viability is not certain, then planning a repeat débridement in the operating room in 24 to 36 hours is in order. This is especially true of severe crush injuries.

The débridement phase is when the decisions regarding replantation, amputation, partial amputation, or reconstruction must be made, again by looking into the "crystal ball" to predict ultimate function with the various options, relying on the principles described previously for guidance. If amputated tissues have been recovered and on initial inspec-

tion are believed not to be appropriate for replantation, they should, nevertheless, be saved because they could be useful as "spare parts" later in the operation—either as vascularized or nonvascularized grafts: bone, tendon, nerve, or skin.[13] The technical details of different types of amputations are described in Chapter 55. For the digits, if less than a functional amount of the proximal phalanx remains, we will often perform a ray resection or, in the case of the middle finger, index to middle transposition, at the time of initial operation.[44] If the remaining ray will not contribute to function, its removal can often help in achieving primary soft tissue closure, removing the skeletal components, saving the vascularized soft tissue portions, and creating a "fillet flap." This is also the point to pause and plan the reconstruction, both the steps to be performed in the current operation as well as what future operations may be required. After débridement, reconstruction should then proceed beginning with skeletal reconstruction and working from the base up to the skin.

CRITICAL POINTS: DÉBRIDEMENT

- Excise wound.
- Perform aggressive débridement of marginally vascularized tissue, especially muscle.
- Save critical structures: nerve, tendon, and arteries.
- Begin with tourniquet; release; re-inflate for further débridement.
- Tag nerves and arteries.
- Vascularized bone: save for incorporation; devascularized bone: save for keying reduction, then discard.
- Use pulsed lavage.
- Decide about replantation, amputation, partial amputation, or reconstruction (the "crystal ball").
- Perform amputations as part of débridement; save vascularized soft tissue for coverage/closure.
- Save "spare parts" for later use in primary reconstruction.

Skeletal/Joint Reconstruction

The goal of skeletal reconstruction is to restore length, alignment, and stability, along with anatomically smooth and stable articulations so that the complex flexion and extension units of the forearm and hand can produce the key motor functions of the hand outlined previously. This must be achieved while at the same time adhering to principles that optimize fracture biology and promote rapid and stable fracture healing. Because the surrounding tissues become rapidly firmer and less pliable in just a matter of days after injury and because tendon gliding and joint motion require early mobilization, the optimal time to achieve anatomic reduction and stable fixation is with the initial operation or, at the very least, within the first week.

Achieving adequately stable fixation to allow early motion is especially important in mangling injuries where the only chance to overcome the inevitable scar formation around the joints and muscle-tendon units is through early passive and active motion. With the exception of cases with severe contamination, skeletal fixation is generally best performed at the initial operation. The vascularity of the hand and upper extremity is excellent and allows for a far more aggressive approach to fixation than in the lower extremity. The methods of fixation for humerus, forearm, wrist, hand, and digit fractures and dislocations are well covered in other chapters. With open mangling injuries, the wounds often dictate the approach and every attempt should be made to not create additional, unnecessary soft tissue injury in gaining adequate exposure for fixation. Even with good fracture exposure, intraoperative radiographs or fluoroscopy should always be used to confirm reduction and fixation.

Before proceeding with skeletal fixation, the critical decision must be made whether to restore anatomic length or shorten the bone as part of fixation. When concomitant nerve and/or arterial injury is present, skeletal shortening can allow for débridement and primary repair of nerves or arteries, whereas maintaining length may dictate nerve or vessel grafting with an increased risk of complications either from vascular thrombosis or loss of axonal regeneration across a nerve graft. In the case of severe comminution at the fracture site, shortening can also allow primary bone fixation, obviating the need for bone grafting. Shortening can similarly facilitate tendon repair and soft tissue reconstruction. In general, 1 to 1.5 cm of shortening is well tolerated in the phalanges and metacarpals and up to 4 cm in the forearm without significant loss of function. It must be kept in mind, however, that muscle sarcomeres have a limited capacity to shorten in response to skeletal shortening and there is a risk of loss of either flexor or extensor function with significant skeletal shortening when tendon shortening is not also part of the repair.[8]

Intra-articular fractures must be assessed to determine whether they are reconstructable or whether primary or secondary fusion is more appropriate. In general, if 50% to 75% of the articular surface remains and is capable of supporting the joint without resulting in bone-bone contact, an attempt should be made at joint salvage. Depressed articular fragments should be elevated, and every attempt should be made to achieve a smooth anatomic surface. If the articular fragments are sufficiently large, small reconstruction screws provide excellent stable fixation. Often, however, multiple Kirschner wires are required for small yet functionally important articular fragments. The mini condylar plates can be very useful for articular reconstruction.[45,77] If the joint is unstable, an attempt at ligament repair or reconstruction should be made, preferably with adjacent tissue, although sometimes "spare parts" tendon or palmaris graft can be used, as described in Chapter 9. Joint stabilization can also be assisted with transarticular Kirschner wires that are removed after several weeks once the surrounding ligamentous tissues have become stable. Carpal fractures and dislocations should be reduced and pinned with multiple Kirschner wires and ligaments reattached with bone anchors, as described in Chapters 14 and 17.

Fractures of the shaft of radius and/or ulna are best treated with 3.5-mm dynamic compression plates. Fractures of the distal ulna or ulnar styloid associated with instability of the distal radioulnar joint should be treated with Kirschner wire and tension band wire reconstruction as described in Chapter 15. Fractures of the distal radius require first an anatomic reconstruction of the articular surface, then often either dorsal or volar buttress plating as described in Chapter 16. When metaphyseal comminution is present, or with multiple carpal fractures or dislocations, the risk of shortening over time is great. External or internal spanning fixation, from the radius to the second or third metacarpal, can provide excellent stable fixation that will allow early motion and does not carry the infection, tendon adhesion, and other risks associated with the use of an external fixator.[17] We prefer internal spanning fixation, using a plate that is left in situ for 3 to 4 months while the metaphysis and articular surface completely heal (Fig. 46-10). This plate can be both applied and removed with minimal soft tissue dissection, using only a proximal incision of the radius and a distal incision over the metacarpal. In this way, severe metaphyseal comminution can be reconstructed using ligamentotaxis, leaving the periosteum intact and avoiding the depressing scenario of "a bag of bones" spilling out on to the operating table. We find that the Synthes 2.4-mm mandibular reconstruction plate with locking screws works well for this purpose. It can be inserted through a tunnel between the second and fourth dorsal compartments using three and four locking screws on both the radius and the metacarpal. Similarly, it can be removed through fairly small proximal and distal incisions, without reopening the entire area. Whenever possible in such cases, the articular surface should be anatomically reduced through indirect techniques, under fluoroscopic guidance.

Because of the length and narrowness of the plate, some external support in the form of a cast or rigid splint is required while the plate is in place. We have found that this approach provides stability and maintains length better than an external fixator, is much less cumbersome, and has fewer problems related to pain, irritation, and infection of fixator pins.

The specific treatment of carpal, metacarpal, and phalangeal fractures and dislocations is covered in their respective chapters. Again, the focus with mangling injuries is to provide sufficiently stable fixation to allow early motion. In the carpus this is usually achieved with cannulated compression screw fixation, and in the metacarpals and phalanges this is done with mini-plate and screw fixation where possible. Kirschner wires, nevertheless, still do have a role, especially in reconstructing articular fragments and in fractures around the joints where it is not technically possible to perform plate and screw fixation. When Kirschner wires are used, and are expected to remain in place beyond 4 weeks, we cut them below the skin surface with the plan to remove them through a small operation at a later stage in an attempt to reduce the complications of pin irritation and infection. In the metacarpals and phalanges, achieving accurate rotational correction is, as always, paramount. Kirschner wires can be helpful in providing provisional fixation so that rotational deformities can be evaluated and corrected before definitive fixation. In cases of severe diaphyseal comminution, cerclage wires can hold the "barrel staves" together and prevent collapse. Kirschner wires should be thought of as "internal splints" rather than

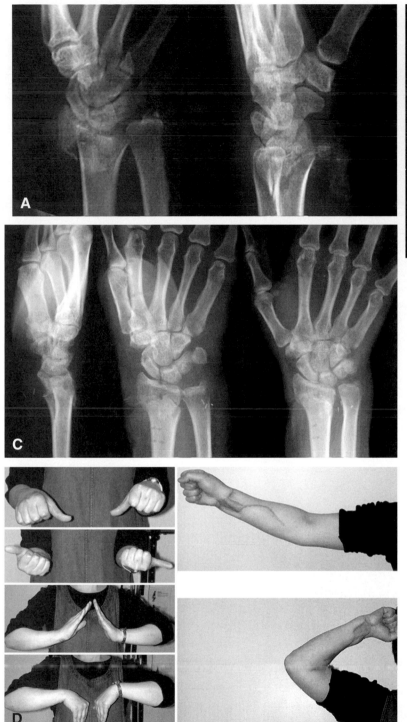

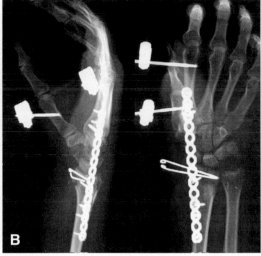

FIGURE 46-10. **A** to **D,** Internal spanning fixation from the radius to the second metacarpal can provide excellent stable fixation that will allow early motion. The plate is left in situ for 3 to 4 months while the metaphysis and articular surface completely heal. A 2.4-mm locking mandibular reconstruction plate was used in this case of severe crush/degloving injury. The plate can be both applied and removed with minimal soft tissue dissection, reconstructing severe metaphyseal comminution using ligamentotaxis and indirect techniques.

rigid fixation. Even crossed Kirschner wire constructs are unstable to horizontal or rotational deformation. Unless numerous crossed wires are used in a single bone (which carries the risk of tendon, ligament, or soft tissue impingement), rigid stability to allow early motion will be difficult to achieve. One trick that should be kept in mind with Kirschner wires is using them as both provisional fixation and as a drill for later screw exchange. In this way, Kirschner wires can be placed under fluoroscopic guidance and the resulting fixation checked both clinically and radiographically. The individual Kirschner wires can then be replaced with screws with minimal soft tissue exposure. The diameter of a 0.045-inch Kirschner wire is 1.1 mm, which is the core diameter of a 1.5-mm screw. Similarly, the diameter of a 0.062-inch Kirschner wire is 1.5 mm, which is the core diameter of a 2.0-mm screw.

Like Kirschner wires, external fixation still does have a role in mangling injuries. In some cases, it is not possible to achieve rigid internal fixation because of comminution or internal fracture anatomy. In these cases, the use of an external fixator either across the wrist (Fig. 46-11) or across an MCP or IP joint is the best option. The mini external

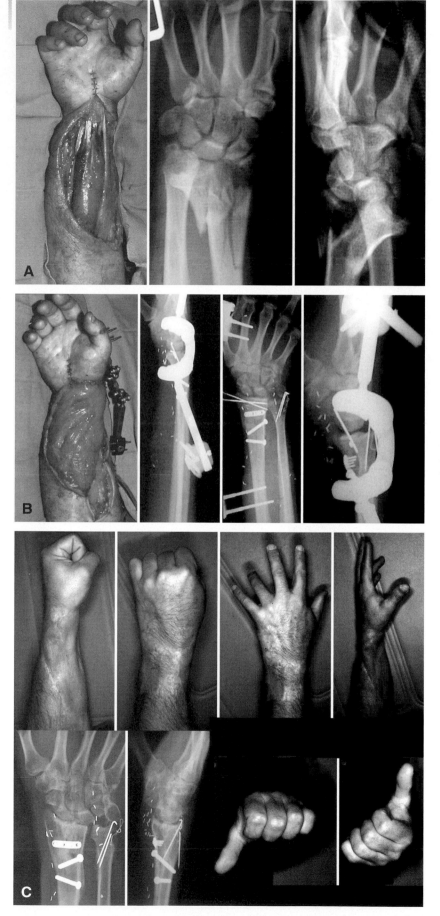

FIGURE 46-11. **A** to **C,** In some cases it is not possible to achieve rigid internal fixation, owing to comminution or internal fracture anatomy. In this case an external fixator across the wrist was used successfully.

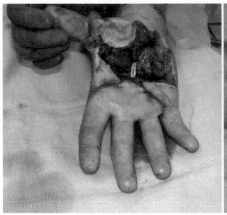 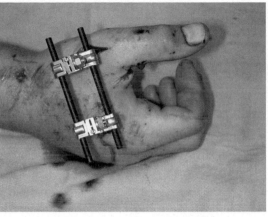

FIGURE 46-12. Use of a mini external fixator to maintain the first web space after a mangling injury to the palm and thenar area.

fixator is also very useful in maintaining the first web space after crushing or mangling injuries to prevent the development of an adduction contracture (Fig. 46-12). The tendency to develop an adduction contracture in the presence of a mangling or crushing injury is so strong that we recommend either a temporary external fixator construct or pinning across the trapeziometacarpal joint in most cases. Although Ilizarov distraction-lengthening techniques could be used for severe, complex upper extremity injuries, we have not found this technique of much use in the forearm or hand.

CRITICAL POINTS: SKELETAL RECONSTRUCTION

- Attempt fracture visualization with minimal dissection and minimal periosteal stripping.
- Restore length for optimal muscle-tendon unit function versus shorten for primary closure/skeletal/nerve repair.
- Perform accurate anatomic reduction with special attention to articular surfaces.
- Use stable, low-profile, minimally invasive fixation and begin early motion with fracture healing
  - Radius/ulna: 3.5-mm LCDC plating versus spanning plate to second or third metacarpal if severe comminution
  - Wrist: fracture fixation: compression screw versus Kirschner wires; repair/reconstruct ligaments, Kirschner wire stabilization
  - Metacarpals: prefer mini-plate fixation for early motion; minimize joint/tendon interference
  - Maintain first web space with external fixator or thumb CMC pinning.
  - Phalanges: mini-plate versus Kirschner wires versus tension band wiring
  - Skeletal defects: shorten versus primary bone graft versus antibiotic spacer/delayed bone graft

When skeletal defects remain, bone grafting will need to be performed. Unlike the lower extremity, the abundant vascularity of the upper extremity will often allow primary bone grafting unless there is significant contamination, poor soft tissue coverage, or compromised adjacent tissue vascularity. We have come to favor cancellous allograft in most cases, unless autograft is simple to harvest from adjacent bone such as the radius for wrist or hand defects. If the wound and/or coverage are deemed unsuitable for primary bone grafting, antibiotic-impregnated polymethylmethacrylate beads or spacers can be used to fill the defect until definitive bone grafting is performed, usually after the soft tissues have healed. These beads are available commercially or can be made by mixing 1 g of tobramycin and 1 g of vancomycin with the polymethylmethacrylate and forming small beads on a length of 1-0 or 2-0 braided suture. Alternatively, a custom block can be fashioned to fit the defect and secured as part of the fracture fixation. After wound stabilization and maturation the spacers are replaced with bone graft (Fig. 46-13).

Tendon Repair/Reconstruction

After skeletal stabilization, the next step is tendon repair. Unless ongoing ischemia is critical, performing tendon repair before vascular repair can reduce the chance of disrupting the vascular repair with the maneuvers involved in repairing the tendons. The details of tendon repair and reconstruction are covered in Chapters 6 and 7. We would like to emphasize that the best outcomes from primary tendon repair are in the setting of sharp lacerations with minimal soft tissue injury, which is rarely the case with mangling injuries. If primary repair can be performed without significant shortening or contracture, flexor tendons should be repaired with four core sutures to allow early postoperative motion, as well as epitendinous sutures in zone II. With mangling injuries in zone II, we generally repair both the flexor digitorum sublimis and flexor digitorum profundus tendons. The exception to this is when repairing both tendons compromises gliding through the A2 pulley, resulting in limited PIP motion. In this situation we only repair the profundus tendon. In mangling injuries, if tendons are transected, the ends are often frayed and with substance missing. Repair may only be possible with concomitant skeletal shortening or with tendon grafting, either

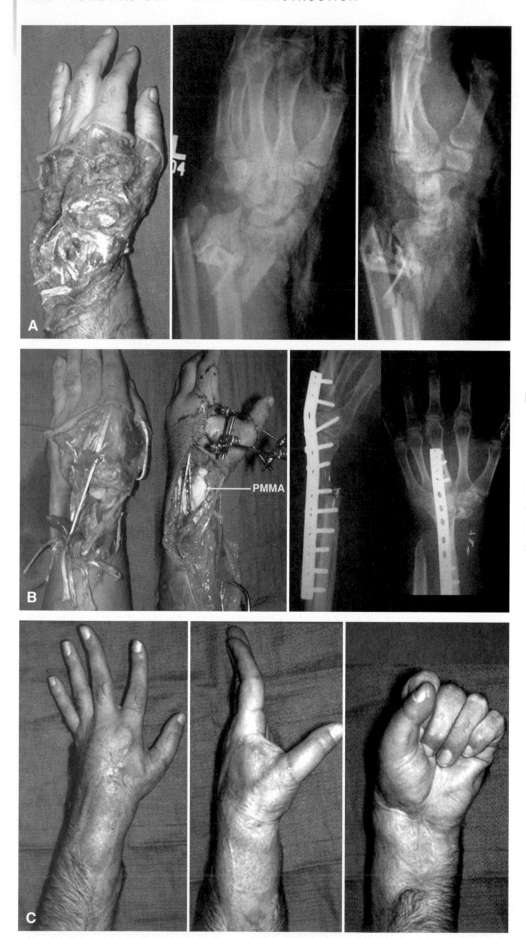

FIGURE 46-13. **A,** This injury resulted from a rollover car accident. **B,** After débridement, skeletal length was restored with a 3.5-mm plate. A block of polymethylmethacrylate (PMMA) was incorporated in the distal bone defect *(arrow)*. Soft tissue coverage was provided by a split latissimus dorsi free flap and skin grafts. Four months after injury the PMMA block was replaced with an 8-cm allograft fibula bone graft. **C,** Functional result 1 year after injury.

acute or delayed. Acute tendon grafting is possible, but it requires an excellent soft tissue bed, stable skeletal fixation, and an intact pulley system so that an immediate passive or active tendon rehabilitation protocol can be started postoperatively.[90] Usually, however, if primary repair cannot be performed, staged tendon grafting should be planned. At the time of definitive soft tissue closure, Silastic tendon spacers should be placed to allow secondary reconstruction. If the critical A2 or A4 flexor pulleys are disrupted, they should be reconstructed with spare parts tendon, fascia, or a portion of the extensor retinaculum as described in Chapter 7. Mangling injuries to extensor tendons, especially on the digits, present some of the greatest challenges in reconstruction. In the digits, the extensor tendon mechanism is a finely tuned, balanced "shroud" mechanism with tight tolerances that reacts poorly to injury or adhesions. The lumbrical and interosseous muscles, which comprise the intrinsic extensor mechanism of the hand, are very susceptible to crushing or mangling injuries. In most circumstances, the scarring and contracture of these intrinsics after injury is the most significant problem; therefore, débridement of crushed, devascularized, and severely injured intrinsics is warranted at the time of initial operation.

In tendon injuries proximal to flexor zone II or extensor zone V, primary tenodesis or tendon transfer should always be kept in mind. Side-to-side tenodesis of either profundus flexor or extensor tendons proximal to the MCP level can restore excellent function. If the flexor pollicis longus can only be repaired with significant shortening and flexion, transfer of the ring sublimis tendon should be considered. Sublimis transfer to other profundus tendons should also be considered in similar circumstances. Any late intrinsic deficiency is best treated by delayed intrinsic tendon transfer. Complete destruction of either flexor or extensor muscle-tendon unit function is best treated by delayed tenodesis, tendon transfer, or free muscle transfer reconstruction as described in Chapters 31 through 33 and 49.

CRITICAL POINTS: TENDON REPAIR/RECONSTRUCTION

- Débride crushed intrinsics to prevent contracture.
- Use four core, locking sutures, plus fine epitendinous suture if zone II.
- Repair both flexor digitorum sublimis and flexor digitorum profundus unless gliding is compromised, then just flexor digitorum profundus.
- Repair/reconstruct A2 and A4 pulleys.
- For tendon rods, use two-stage reconstruction if primary repair is not possible.
- Consider primary tenodesis/tendon transfer.
- Late reconstruction: tendon graft, transfer, tenolysis, functional free muscle transfer.

Vascular Repair/Reconstruction

Optimal revascularization of the mangled extremity is without question the most important aspect of reconstruction. In most cases, to avoid injury to a fragile vascular reconstruction, vascular reconstruction should be deferred until after débridement and skeletal and tendon reconstruction. If, however, major arterial disruption has occurred, rendering the limb ischemic, a temporary vascular shunt should be placed as an initial step, as described previously. If possible, it is helpful to dissect out the injured vessels, identify the ends, and place microvascular clamps across the ends while still under tourniquet control. The actual vascular reconstruction can then be performed after the tourniquet is released. The most important factor in determining success or failure of the vascular reconstruction is ensuring that the vascular anastomosis is performed with uninjured vessel on both sides of the anastomosis and using careful technique, as described in Chapter 44. With mangling injuries, this usually involves trimming the injured vessels back until healthy, uninjured intima can be seen with magnification. Once this is done, it is frequently difficult to achieve a tension-free primary repair. This situation can be addressed in several ways. Sometimes it is possible to ligate and divide small side branches near the ends to allow sufficient mobilization for primary anastomosis. Sometimes, an adjacent joint can be safely flexed to allow a primary repair. This is especially true if flexion is required for concomitant primary nerve repair. In most cases, however, reversed vein graft is required.

Just as it is important to perform the microvascular anastomoses outside of the zone of injury, if vein graft is required, it is also important to harvest vein from outside the zone of injury. Reasonable places to harvest vein graft from the upper extremity, only if uninjured, include the dorsum of the hand or the dorsal or volar forearm. Distant sites include the leg (saphenous) or foot. The dorsal veins of the foot are a good source of vein graft with a reasonable size match for reconstructing the digital vessels in the palm or digits. If the palmar arch needs to be reconstructed, it is sometimes possible to find a venous network on the dorsum of the foot that, when reversed, can provide multiple outflow tracts for the common digital vessels (Fig. 46-14).[43] To reconstruct the brachial, radial, or ulnar arteries, the saphenous, lesser saphenous, and cephalic vein are good choices. For all vein grafts, it is important to remember that the grafts must be reversed to retain antegrade flow with, rather than against, the venous valves. It is also important to minimize damage to the vein during its harvest and to ensure that all small side branches are ligated either with small hemoclips or with bipolar electrocautery.

Once the vessel ends have been identified, clamped, and trimmed back to healthy vessel, the vessels should be cleared of thrombus proximally and distally. With the major vessels this is usually done with a No. 2 Fogarty catheter or in the case of digital vessels by simply milking out the clot and removing it with irrigation and microvascular forceps. The vessels are then irrigated proximally and distally with 10 U/mL heparin saline using a blunt irrigating cannula. If vein graft is to be used, it should first be pre-dilated so that the proper length of vessel can be determined. One of the most common errors in vein grafting is using too long a

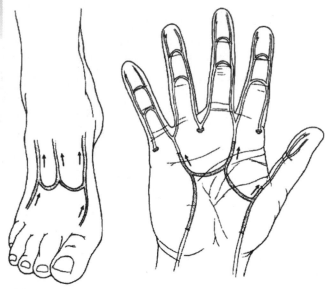

FIGURE 46-14. Venous network on the dorsum of the foot that, when reversed, can provide multiple outflow tracts for the common digital vessels. (From Gupta A, Wolff TW: Management of the mangled hand and forearm. J Am Acad Orthop Surg 3:226-236, 1995.)

piece of vein graft for the defect, resulting in redundancy, kinking, and thrombosis. Pre-dilation is performed by first reversing the graft then placing a microvascular clamp on the outflow end of the vessel. The vessel is filled with heparin saline equivalent to systolic arterial pressure to reproduce the state of the vessel once arterialized. The point of the vein graft that will be used for the proximal anastomosis is cut with microvascular scissors, and a microvascular anastomosis is performed as described in Chapter 44. Using mild tension on both the distal arterial segment and the vein graft to stimulate the state of the vessels under pressure, the point along the vein graft for the distal anastomosis is identified and cut. If a long piece of vein graft is used, it is often helpful to determine the final length by releasing the proximal clamp, allowing the graft to fill with blood under systolic pressure with a distal clamp in place and to assume its eventual length. The graft can then be marked and cut to the proper length for the distal anastomosis. The distal anastomosis is performed using double microvascular clamps to take the tension off the anastomosis during its creation. The clamps are released and flow is established through the anastomoses. Any areas of leakage are addressed with additional sutures at this point, and any previously unidentified cut side branches are ligated.

If multiple levels of vascular injuries are involved, the proximal reconstruction should be performed first, followed by the more distal reconstructions. In the case of palmar arch or common digital artery injuries, it is not always necessary to reconstruct every common digital vessel, because one common digital artery can adequately perfuse two digits. Reconstructing the common digital artery to the index/middle finger and to the ring/small finger is all that is required, in addition to the thumb, of course. Whether to reconstruct either the radial or ulnar artery when the other is intact or whether to reconstruct one or both if both are injured is a matter of debate. Some studies have suggested

only a 50% patency rate if the other vessel is open and uninjured and have suggested that the functional outcome is the same with ligation or repair of a single vessel.[34,53] There is some evidence, however, that with microsurgical repair, patency can be much higher.[87] In the case of most mangling injuries, to maximize flow to all injured tissues through all side branches available and because of thrombosis risk in the other vessel, we generally favor reconstructing both the radial and ulnar arteries, if feasible. The same holds true for digital artery injuries.

It is uncommon to require venous reconstruction except in cases where there is circumferential or near-circumferential transection or crush injury to the subcutaneous venous drainage system of either the digit or forearm. In such cases, the same principles that apply to arterial reconstruction also apply to venous reconstruction. In these cases, the repairs must be performed using an uninjured vessel and may require the use of vein graft. Once the arterial, and if necessary, venous reconstructions have been completed, it is important to monitor their patency continuously throughout the remainder of the operation. Should thrombosis occur, it is important to address this quickly before the thrombus propagates distally. The most common cause of thrombosis in these situations is either technical error in performing the anastomosis or error in judgment with inadequate resection of damaged vessel. In both cases, re-resection of the vessel ends is almost always indicated in revising the anastomosis after thrombectomy. Anticoagulation is generally contraindicated in mangling injuries of the arm and forearm, although it could be considered if injury is confined to the hand or digits. Clinical trials of anticoagulation in microsurgery have failed to demonstrate a consistent benefit.[56,57]

CRITICAL POINTS: VASCULAR REPAIR/RECONSTRUCTION

- Perform after skeletal/tendon repair unless critical ischemia is present (temporary shunt).
- Dissect vessels/microvascular clamp under tourniquet control.
- De-clot with Fogarty catheter proximally/distally.
- Trim vessel ends to healthy, uninjured vessel.
- Irrigate/fill with 10 U/mL heparin solution; then clamp.
- Perform vascular repair with microscope, outside of zone of injury if possible.
- If inadequate length: ligate/divide some side branches; flex joints; reverse vein graft.
- Perform vein graft: vein outside of zone of injury; pre-dilate; reverse (valves).
- Repair/reconstruct both radial and ulnar arteries when possible.
- Perform venous reconstruction only if all or nearly all venous outflow is missing.

Nerve Repair/Reconstruction

Nerve repair usually follows skeletal, tendon, and vascular reconstruction in that order, because it is less urgent than vascular reconstruction and the delicate techniques involved can easily be compromised by the more aggressive maneuvers involved in skeletal and tendon reconstruction. Again, the details of nerve repair and reconstruction are covered elsewhere in the text (see Chapters 30 and 38). As noted previously, it is important to distinguish between neurapraxia, axonotmesis, and neurotmesis in deciding on the appropriate treatment for nerve injury. In nearly all cases involving mangling injuries, if the nerve sheath is in continuity, it is best left alone to see if function will return later. In the case of neurotmesis involving digital nerves or major nerve trunks, primary end-to-end epineurial repair should be performed. Is important that the repair be tension free, because a repair under tension will lead to nerve ischemia or physical gapping, either of which will impair nerve regeneration. Nerve repair should be performed with the aid of the operating microscope to properly align major nerve fascicles, to properly place the sutures in the epineurium, and to control the tension when tying the sutures to achieve proper axon-to-axon apposition without bunching. With traumatic nerve transections and especially with crush or avulsion injuries, it is critically important to trim back crushed or injured nerve endings before performing the repair. Again, this is performed with the aid of the operating microscope to determine when soft, healthy fascicles have been reached. After trimming, it is sometimes necessary to dissect the nerve proximally and distally, without sacrificing critical side branches, to achieve a tension-free repair.

If a primary, tension-free nerve repair cannot be achieved in the acute setting and if the gapping is less than 1 to 2 cm, a nerve conduit can be used to bridge the gap as described in Chapter 30.[64,101] If the remaining gap is longer, however, either delayed nerve grafting or, in the case of a motor nerve deficit, tendon transfer or nerve transfer should be performed. In nearly all cases, if a functional nerve is to be sacrificed for nerve grafting, we prefer to perform this as a secondary procedure so that healthy nerve endings with soft, viable fascicles can be ensured, and the risk of graft loss due to wound contamination and infection is limited.

Soft Tissue Coverage

Achieving a healed wound with stable, durable coverage and with vascularized tissue over critical structures is key. Soft tissue coverage is the last, and in many ways the most important, step in the treatment of mangling injuries of the upper extremity because it determines the environment in which all other repaired and reconstructed structures will heal and ultimately function. In addition, the coverage should be low profile, supple over mobile areas such as joints and tendons, and with minimal shear characteristics on the volar aspect of the hand and fingers where friction is required for function. Ideally, coverage over the volar tips of the digits should be sensate. Often, it is impossible to achieve all these goals with a single method of reconstruction and either some compromise or some combination of methods must be employed.

Although achieving early wound closure is desirable to reduce infection and optimize healing and motion, with severe crush or mangling injuries and in particular in the presence of significant contamination, it is often prudent to delay definitive coverage until a stable wound has been achieved. This will sometimes require serial débridements separated by 24 to 48 hours. In nearly all cases, however, we strive to have definitive coverage by 7 to 10 days, even though some smaller, noncritical wound(s) may remain at that point. During the intervening period before definitive coverage, it is imperative that the wound and all vital structures remain moist. As swelling develops after injury, there is a clear tendency for wounds to enlarge, making closure progressively more difficult. There are two techniques that we find helpful in controlling this situation. The first technique involves using rubber bands or vascular surgical "vessel loops" in a criss-cross fashion with staples along the wound edge to create a "corset effect" that brings the wound together without creating ischemia (Fig. 46-15). This will also allow for a certain degree of limb swelling without creating a compartment syndrome and will naturally bring the wound edges together as the swelling diminishes.

The other method employs negative pressure therapy, using the wound VAC. Negative pressure therapy has a number of salutary effects, including removing exudate, decreasing edema, closing dead space, promoting wound

---

CRITICAL POINTS: NERVE REPAIR/RECONSTRUCTION

- Repair/reconstruct the nerve as the last step before soft tissue coverage.
- Trim clearly crushed nerve to healthy fascicles.
- Perform epineural repair with microscope.
- Use fascicular and surface anatomy for proper alignment.
- Perform tension-free repair.
- If nerve gap: free minor branches; flex joint; use nerve conduit for short gap; use nerve graft for larger gaps.

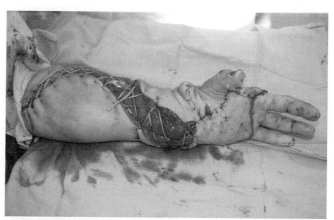

FIGURE 46-15. Using vascular surgical "vessel loops" in a criss-cross fashion with staples along the wound edge to create a "corset" effect brings the wound together without creating ischemia.

contraction, marsupializing the wound edges, and promoting granulation. In essence, it acts as a "mechanical myofibroblast." The wound VAC has revolutionized the approach to soft tissue coverage in complex lower extremity defects, allowing wounds to contract and granulate to the point where they can be covered with a simple skin graft, rather than a complex flap. In the upper extremity, however, because of the importance of maintaining the gliding motion of muscles and tendons, prolonged application of the wound VAC and skin grafting can lead to an inferior outcome compared with early coverage with a supple, vascularized flap. Nevertheless, it does have an important role in the soft tissue reconstruction of mangled upper extremity injuries. When used judiciously and for limited periods of time, it can dramatically improve the wound environment and decrease the size requirements for flap coverage. Details on the use of this device are provided with the device; and because the device can change, the reader is referred to the device manufacturer's instructions for details. Trimming the sponge to a size slightly smaller than the wound helps to shrink the size of the wound with suction. In addition, we find it helpful to staple the edges of the wound to the sponge to hold it in position relative to the wound when applying the seal. Closed negative pressure therapy should not be used, however, in the presence of severe contamination, infection, or significant bleeding. It should also be used with caution in the setting of vascular repair or reconstruction. Because it is a closed system, it is important to change the sponge every 2 to 5 days, or more frequently depending on the level of contamination. In some cases, if the fascial coverage of critical structures is preserved, the wound VAC alone can obliterate dead space and produce a wound that can be skin grafted, while preserving vascularized gliding tissue over critical structures (Fig. 46-16).

In planning soft tissue reconstruction, it is important to keep in mind the concept of the "reconstructive ladder" as originally described by Mathes.[68] This concept implies that the simplest method of coverage appropriate to the situation should be employed.

The reconstructive ladder generally follows the progression:

1. Primary closure
2. Wound contraction ("secondary intention")
3. Skin graft
4. Flap (local—distant—free)

Given the unique functional requirements of the upper extremity, including joint motion and tendon/muscle gliding, the simplest soft tissue reconstruction is not always the most appropriate. The decision often involves making judgments regarding ultimate functional goals and balancing these with the complexity of the reconstruction required to achieve this. If the area in question has exposed "white structures," that is, tendon, nerve, bone, or ligament/ joint, some form of a vascularized soft tissue reconstruction will be required. If, however, critical functional structures are not involved, then a simpler form of reconstruction can be employed.

Whenever possible, primary closure or delayed primary closure (5 to 7 days after injury) should be performed. In doing so, it is critically important to close the wounds loosely so that tension does not lead to ischemia of the wound edges with subsequent dehiscence or ischemia of the underlying structures owing to increased compartmental pressure. It is far better to have small gaps that heal secondarily than to have a large dehiscence or, even worse, to induce necrosis in marginally vascularized skin that would otherwise survive. This is especially true in the case of traumatically elevated flaps. In these cases, it is always best to simply lay the skin down and at most tack it in place loosely rather than stretch it back to its original position, thereby creating ischemia and necrosis in a large area of the flap, resulting in a defect much greater than one that would be left by simply laying the flap down (Fig. 46-17). If the wound edges cannot be closed primarily, it is certainly reasonable to allow the wound to close secondarily by wound contraction if the remaining defect is less than 1 to 2 cm and if there are no vital structures or motion areas such as joints or web spaces left exposed. Many fingertip injuries and amputations heal best with wound contraction, because adjacent, sensate skin comes together to provide coverage, as opposed to insensate grafts or flaps.

For larger noncritical defects a skin graft may be required. Skin grafts can consist of autograft (from the patient), allograft (from a human skin bank), or xenograft (usually pig skin). Xenograft is used primarily as a "biologic dressing" and will usually not revascularize. Allograft can revascularize and "take," but it will be rejected after the first week or so. It is useful in promoting vascular ingrowth into a wound bed and to prepare the wound bed for later autografting. If an allograft can "take," one can be fairly confident that an autograft will do well and that the wound bed is healthy. Autografts can be either full thickness or split thickness. Split-thickness grafts, because they are thinner and more easily revascularized from the bed, will "take" better than full-thickness grafts, are more resistant to infection, and will do better with a marginal wound bed. Full-thickness grafts will contract less, be more durable and flexible, and have better sensation. They are, therefore, preferred for areas prone to shear and load, such as fingertips, the palm, web spaces, and areas over joints. Split-thickness grafts can be either meshed or unmeshed. Meshed grafts will have fewer problems with seroma, hematoma, and infection and will, therefore, have better "take." Their appearance is not as nice, however. In all cases, maintaining contact between the graft and the bed is imperative for inosculation (ingrowth of vessels into already existing vascular channels) and neovascularization (new vessel formation) to occur. During the first 24 to 36 hours the graft must survive on diffusion, sometimes referred to as "serum imbibition"; however, without revascularization after that point, the graft will not survive. Anything that disturbs the revascularization process, such as hematoma, infection, or shear, will prevent proper engraftment. The best way to achieve successful engraftment is with a moist, compressive dressing or bolster over the graft to provide both pressure and immobilization. We prefer a first layer of fine mesh gauze, followed by a layer of gauze soaked in Sulfamylon solution, which has the added benefit of decreasing the local bacterial level, promoting graft "take." For split-thickness grafts in the extremities, the wound VAC is very effective at optimizing graft-bed contact and graft "take."

Donor sites for split-thickness grafts include the lateral thigh, hip, buttock, scalp, or nearly anywhere. The medial

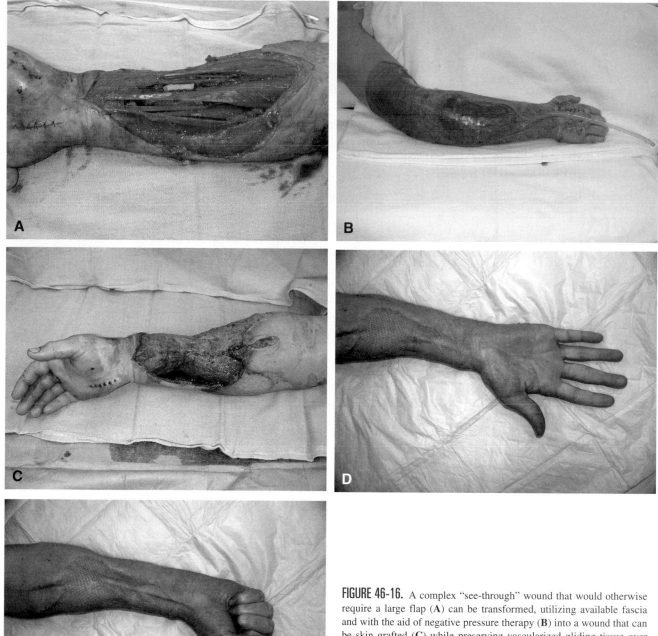

FIGURE 46-16. A complex "see-through" wound that would otherwise require a large flap (**A**) can be transformed, utilizing available fascia and with the aid of negative pressure therapy (**B**) into a wound that can be skin grafted (**C**) while preserving vascularized gliding tissue over critical structures (**D** and **E**).

thigh should be avoided because the skin is much thinner and a full-thickness wound can develop from harvesting skin there. Generally, skin in adults should be harvested at 0.0010- to 0.0012-inch thickness. Full-thickness skin can be harvested from an elliptical excision in the groin crease, the abdomen, or the hypothenar aspect of the hand, which provides thick, glabrous skin. The volar wrist crease can be used, but we avoid this because the resulting scar may be mistaken for scar from a suicide attempt.

For complex wounds, including those with exposed "white structures" over joints or web spaces or those at risk of compromising function due to scarring or contracture or vascularized soft tissue, a flap is required. A flap is simply tissue that contains its own blood supply, as opposed to a graft, which requires revascularization from the bed. Because they remain viable, flaps tend to remain soft and supple while providing vascularity to otherwise devascularized areas. Flaps are mainly classified based on their

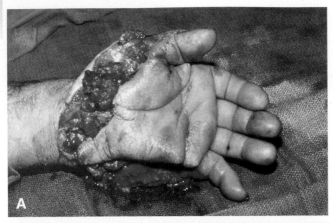

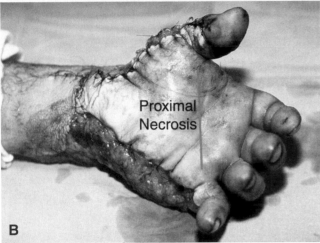

Proximal
Necrosis

FIGURE 46-17. **A** and **B,** With traumatically elevated flaps, "lay it, don't stretch it." It is always best to simply lay the skin down and at most tack it in place loosely rather than stretch it back to its original position, thereby creating ischemia and necrosis of a large area of the flap, as shown in this case.

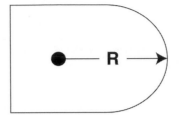

A. Viable random flap

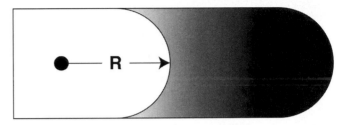

B. Extended random flap with distal necrosis

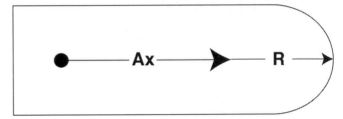

C. Axial flap with viable distal random component

FIGURE 46-18. The importance of axial perfusion of a flap is illustrated. Panel A shows the reliable perfused area of a flap based on purely random perfusion (R) from the vascular pedicle *(black circle).* Panel B shows a random flap designed beyond the limits of reliable random perfusion, resulting in distal flap necrosis. Panel C shows the benefit of designing a flap based on an axial pedicle. The length of reliable flap perfusion includes the same length of reliable random perfusion (R) *plus* the length of the axial pedicle (Ax). (©2003, Nicholas B. Vedder.)

vascular supply as either random or axial. Flaps that are designed based on an axial nutrient vascular system will be much more reliable than flaps that are not. Random flaps are those not based on a dominant nutrient vascular system but instead are supplied by flow through the subdermal and/or subfascial plexus. As a result, random flaps are much less reliable than axial flaps and their length is limited to a short distance from the pedicle origin. The portion of an axial flap that extends beyond the axial vessel is random (Fig. 46-18). An axial flap that is transplanted from its origin and then connected to a new blood supply elsewhere in the body microsurgically is a free flap. Flaps can then be further classified based on the tissue they contain (e.g., cutaneous, fascial, fasciocutaneous, muscle, musculocutaneous, osteomusculocutaneous).

In general, random flaps have little role in the reconstruction of mangling defects of the hand and upper extremities. The exception is in the treatment of fingertip or small digit injuries or in treating small defects over critical structures such as the median nerve at the wrist or exposed vascular repair. In most situations, robust and reliable axial flaps from outside of the zone of injury are required. The various flap choices and the technical details of their transfer

are well described in Chapters 47, 48, and 49. We will, therefore, simply point out some of the "workhorse" flaps that we regularly rely on for different areas of the hand and upper extremity in the setting of mangling injuries.

Fingers, Hand, and Wrist

There are a number of local random and axial flaps described in Chapters 47 and 55 that are suitable for covering fingertip and finger defects as well as digit amputation stumps.[35,83] The Moberg advancement flap, cross-finger flap, flag flap, and other axial intrinsic flaps are suitable for isolated digit defects. For severely crushed digits, removing the crushed skeletal component and converting the area to a fillet flap can often provide the necessary vascularized tissue for covering critical defects. If multiple digits are involved, sometimes employing the Millard "crane principle" and burying the digits in the abdominal fat for 2 weeks and then removing them can result in enough vascularized soft tissue coverage to allow skin grafting (Fig. 46-19). This approach

CRITICAL POINTS: SOFT TISSUE COVERAGE

- Coverage over joints and tendons should be well vascularized, low profile, and supple.
- Coverage over volar pressure-bearing surfaces should be sensate and have minimal shear characteristics.
- Delay definitive coverage until stable wound; repeat débridements if needed.
- Provide definitive coverage by 5 to 10 days; keep moist in interim.
- Control wound size: vessel loop weave versus negative pressure sponge.
- Realize that negative pressure therapy is contraindicated if infection or bleeding is present.
- Cover "white structures" (tendon, nerve, bone, or ligament/joint) with vascularized soft tissue (flap).
- Do not stretch traumatically elevated flaps to original position; simply lay them in place.
- Know that most open fingertip injuries without exposed bone will heal secondarily.
- For larger, noncritical defect: use split-thickness skin graft (use full-thickness graft if small, if subject to pressure/shear, or if motion is critical).
- For complex wounds with exposed "white structures": use flap.
- We prefer axial flaps; include fascia if possible; consider fascia-only flap plus split-thickness skin graft.
- For fingers/hand/wrist: use Moberg, cross-finger, intrinsic flaps, crane, radial forearm, groin.
- For radial forearm flap: consider fascia only plus split-thickness skin graft; stay deep during dissection; use effluent venous anastomosis.
- For groin flap: include sartorius fascia to prevent pedicle kinking; protect lateral femoral cutaneous nerve; delay for 2 weeks; divide/inset at 3 weeks; multiple thinning stages; continue motion to decrease stiffness.
- For forearm: groin flap, gracilis free, latissimus free, lateral arm free, anterolateral thigh fascia or fasciocutaneous free
- For elbow/arm: brachioradialis (antecubital defect), latissimus—pedicle or free

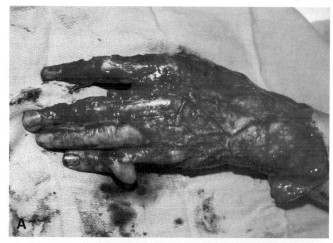

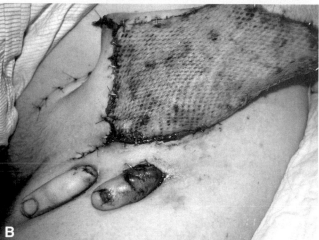

FIGURE 46-19. **A** and **B,** Applying the Millard "crane principle" by burying the digits in the abdominal fat for 2 weeks then removing them can result in enough vascularized soft tissue coverage to allow skin grafting. In this case, the crane principle is combined with a groin flap for the volar hand.

contains a thick, fatty layer that allows tendon gliding beneath it and forms an excellent foundation for secondary reconstructions, including tenolysis, tendon transfers, and toe-to-hand transfers. The disadvantage is that unless it is performed as a free flap, which is technically very difficult owing to the small pedicle vessel size, it requires that the hand be attached to the groin for least 2 weeks, which is both awkward and makes effective hand therapy difficult. The other disadvantage is that it is very thick and bulky and usually requires multiple, staged defatting procedures. It can, nevertheless, produce excellent results (Fig. 46-20).

The other upper extremity workhorse flap is the radial forearm flap, based on the radial artery and perforating vessels coming up in the septum between the brachioradialis and flexor carpi radialis. Preserving these perforators during dissection is critical, and dissection must always focus on staying deep, below the artery and its veins. If it is transferred based on reversed flow through the radial artery from the ipsilateral arm, it has the advantage of confining the surgical defect to that one extremity. It is, of course, critical to first confirm that the remaining ulnar artery and the palmar arch are intact by preoperatively performing an Allen test with the Doppler device. The disadvantage of this flap is

is primarily applicable for dorsal defects and not palmar defects with exposed flexor tendon or digital nerves.

For larger defects, a regional or distant axial flap is required. The tubed groin flap is a reliable axial flap that can cover a large defect. It is certainly an upper extremity "workhorse" flap. In addition to being large and reliable, it

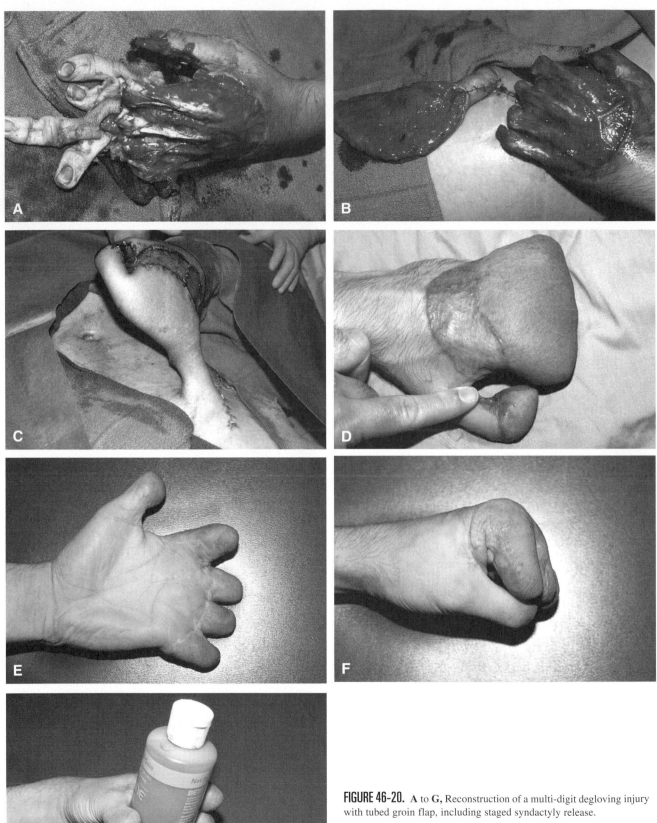

FIGURE 46-20. **A** to **G,** Reconstruction of a multi-digit degloving injury with tubed groin flap, including staged syndactyly release.

that the donor site on the forearm and the palmar arch must not be significantly involved in the zone of injury.

When it is taken as a fasciocutaneous flap, unless the cutaneous component is very small, the forearm donor site morbidity can be significant, both functionally and aesthetically. It is very important to design the flap on the proximal volar forearm, allowing direct closure over the flexor tendons and skin grafting the donor site only over proximal muscle. Because it, like the groin flap, is a fasciocutaneous flap, its bulk can often hinder function and requires defatting. This can also be a significant problem on the palmar aspect of the hand and digits where firm attachment of the skin to the base is required for grasping and friction-based functions. For these reasons, we usually transfer the radial forearm flap as a fascia-only flap with skin grafting on the fascia, leaving the thick skin and fat layer in the forearm. This provides well-vascularized gliding coverage that is both thin and functional (Fig. 46-21). It provides excellent resurfacing for both palmar and dorsal hand and digit defects and can reach even the tips of the fingers (Fig. 46-22). The forearm donor defect is then simply a straight-line scar. The entire width of the forearm fascia can be taken on the radial artery, but even so there is significant contraction and shrinkage when the flap is finally transferred. If the flap is harvested as fascia only, it is very important to leave the network of small fascial vessels on the surface as well as a thin stippling of fat when dissecting the forearm skin and subcutaneous tissue off of the fascia. Even though the flap will usually survive from reversed flow through both the artery and veins, we find it beneficial, whenever possible, to microsurgically anastomose an effluent vein from the tip of the flap to a dorsal hand vein. The other reversed flow flap of the forearm to consider is the posterior interosseous flap, which can also be taken either as a fasciocutaneous or a fascia-only plus skin graft flap. In our experience, this is a much less reliable flap, especially in a mangled extremity.

If a larger piece of fascia is required than can be harvested with the radial forearm, the anterolateral thigh fascia free flap, based on the descending branch of the lateral circumflex femoral artery, is an excellent choice (Fig. 46-23). It is, of course, transferred as a free flap, usually end-to-side into either the radial or ulnar artery or end-to-end into the princeps pollicis artery, and carries the attendant microsurgical risks. It, too, can be taken as a fasciocutaneous free flap, but the bulk is usually detrimental in the hand and wrist unless it is used for reconstructing the forearm.

The lateral arm free flap, either as a fascia plus skin graft or fasciocutaneous flap, can provide more tissue than the radial forearm flap and can be harvested out of the zone of injury. Like the radial forearm flap, the surgery can be confined to one extremity, yet it relies on microsurgery, and the donor defect, even if it can be closed primarily, is very noticeable (Fig. 46-24).

Forearm

Forearm defects requiring vascularized coverage usually require a fairly large flap. Although a groin flap can be used, a free flap is usually more appropriate. While narrower defects can be reconstructed with a free gracilis muscle flap,

for larger defects we usually turn to the latissimus muscle free flap. Again, to reduce bulk and minimize donor site morbidity, we use a muscle-only flap with skin graft rather than a fasciocutaneous flap. Even though it is muscle and not fat, it provides good coverage for tendon and joint gliding and is easily re-elevated for secondary procedures. If a larger fasciocutaneous flap is desired specifically for the purpose of tendon gliding, then either an anterolateral thigh fasciocutaneous flap or a scapular or parascapular fasciocutaneous flap can be used (Fig. 46-25).

Elbow and Arm

For defects around the antecubital area, such as exposed vascular or nerve reconstructions, the proximally based brachioradialis muscle flap is an excellent choice with minimal donor morbidity (Fig. 46-26). For larger defects around the elbow and even extending to the proximal third of the forearm, the latissimus dorsi muscle can be transferred as a pedicle flap and skin grafted. By detaching its insertion from the humerus, significant additional length can be achieved, but it is important to ensure that the proximal pedicle is not stretched or kinked. Although tunneling the flap subcutaneously down the arm has been described, we believe that the risks of vascular compromise favor opening the posterior arm and skin grafting over the muscle, which can later be revised (Fig. 46-27).

Composite flaps and "spare parts" surgery can also play a role in soft tissue reconstruction of mangling injuries. Even though an amputated part or segment of tissue may be deemed not replantable or functional, portions of it may still be useful in reconstruction. The residual nonfunctional proximal phalanx of the index finger can, for example, be transposed to provide additional sensate length to an injured thumb (Fig. 46-28). The palmar skin of the hand, based on either the radial or ulnar artery, with either the median or ulnar nerve and its branches can be used as a vascularized, sensate pedicle flap or free tissue transfer. "Spare parts" surgery may be one of the very few indications for an "emergency" free flap in the setting of a mangling injury.[76] Similarly, skin or skin and radius bone, based on the radial artery, can be used as a composite flap, either as a reversed-flow pedicle flap or as a free tissue transfer. And, of course before discarding amputated tissue it should always be evaluated for potential use as free graft tissue, either defatted skin, nerve, bone, or tendon.

POSTOPERATIVE CARE/REHABILITATION

Early institution of an appropriate and well-planned therapy and rehabilitation program is critical to achieving optimal functional outcome. As mentioned previously, injured tissues rapidly become less pliable in just a matter of days after injury; therefore, optimizing tendon gliding and joint motion requires early, protected mobilization.[22] Edema formation can significantly limit joint mobility, which, if uncorrected, can result in permanent joint contractures. The hand should always be splinted postoperatively in the "safe" position, with MCP joints flexed to prevent shortening of the MCP collateral ligaments, leading to MCP extension contracture, and with the IP joints in extension (Fig. 46-29).

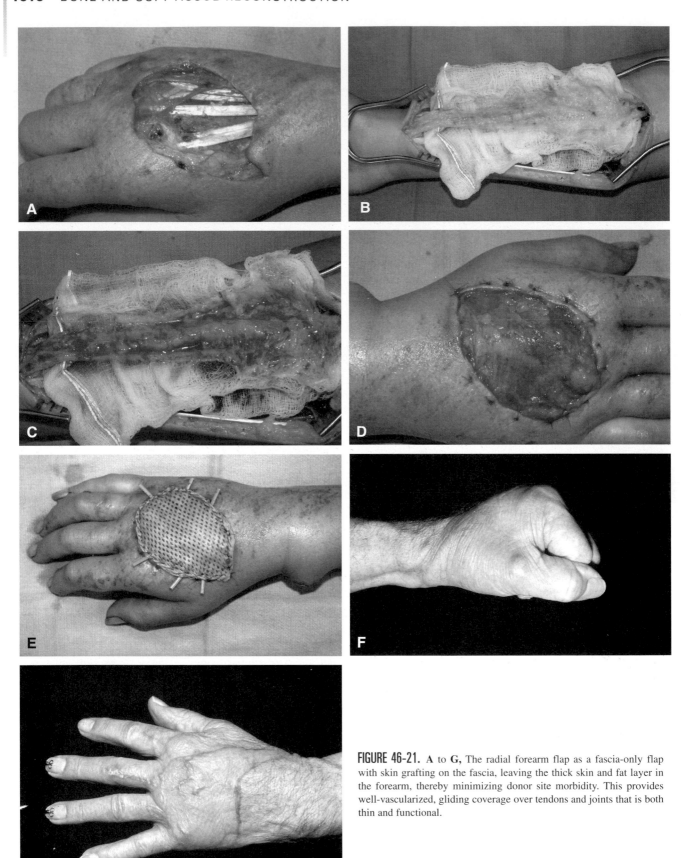

FIGURE 46-21. A to **G,** The radial forearm flap as a fascia-only flap with skin grafting on the fascia, leaving the thick skin and fat layer in the forearm, thereby minimizing donor site morbidity. This provides well-vascularized, gliding coverage over tendons and joints that is both thin and functional.

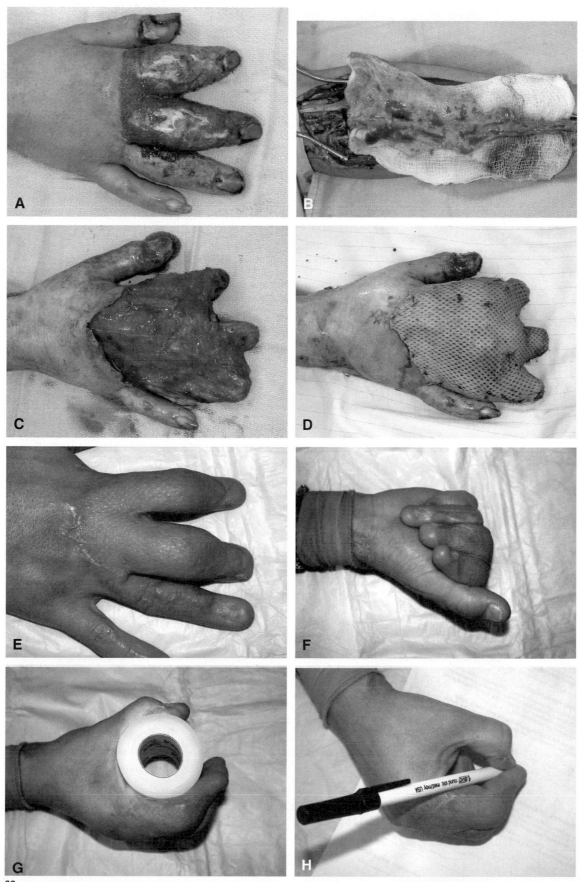

FIGURE 46-22. **A** to **H,** The radial forearm flap as a fascia-only flap with skin grafting can even reach the fingertips, as in this case with severe deep contact burns and exposed interphalangeal joints.

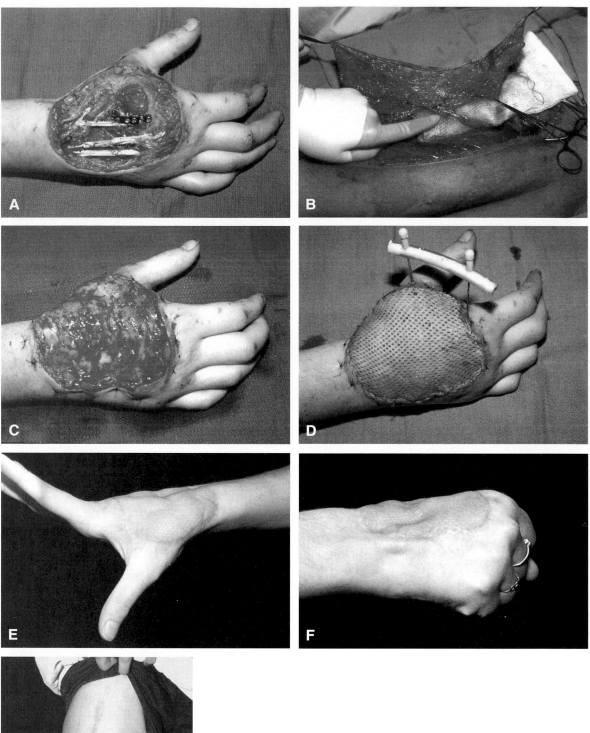

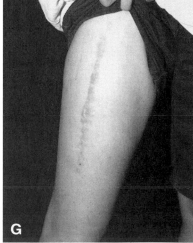

FIGURE 46-23. **A** to **G,** The anterolateral thigh fascia free flap, based on the descending branch of the lateral circumflex femoral artery (see **B**) provides a very large, well-vascularized piece of fascia for covering large defects. When covered with a split-thickness skin graft, it provides thin, pliable coverage with minimal donor site morbidity.

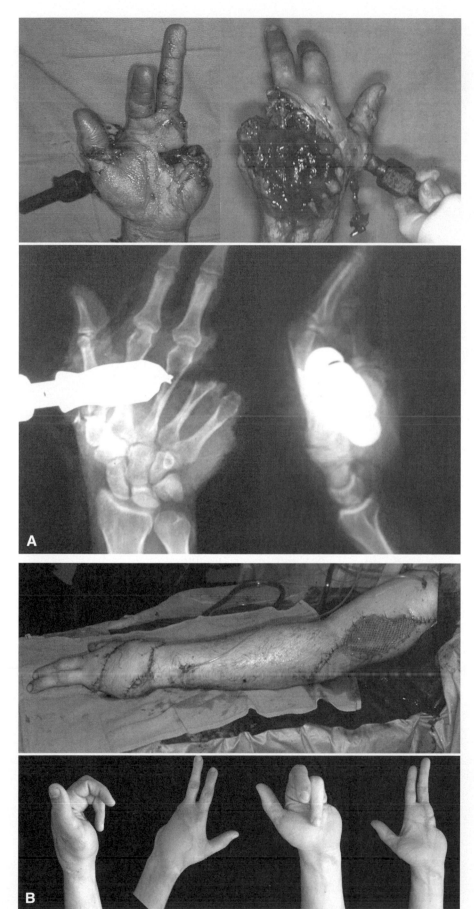

FIGURE 46-24. **A** and **B,** A severe mangling injury to the hand and wrist reconstructed with a free lateral arm fasciocutaneous flap.

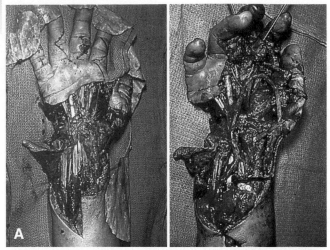

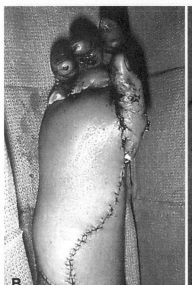

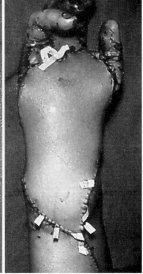

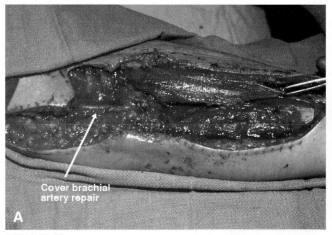

FIGURE 46-25. **A** and **B,** This farmer's hand was caught in a fertilizer spreader. Reconstruction consisted of débridement, skeletal stabilization, and soft tissue coverage with a scapular free flap.

Whenever possible, initial skeletal and tendon reconstruction should be performed in a stable enough fashion to allow early mobilization. Conversion to a thermoplastic splint within the first several days after injury can facilitate both wound care and hand therapy. With most mangling injuries, immediate active motion after tendon repair is usually contraindicated, although passive motion can be started immediately. With nerve injuries, blocking splints can be fashioned to prevent tension across the repair while allowing motion in the direction of the nerve. Hypersensitivity is very common after crush and mangling injuries and should be treated by early desensitization therapy.

If a skin graft is used, it is important to prevent motion or shearing beneath the graft for the first 5 to 7 days to allow inosculation and "take" of the graft. Otherwise, we favor liberal washing and soaking of wounds, rather than keeping them wrapped in occlusive dressings where pus can accumulate and infection result. The exception to this is VAC therapy, which effectively removes serum and exudate. It should be changed every several days, however.

CRITICAL POINTS: POSTOPERATIVE CARE/REHABILITATION

- Splint wrist neutral-extended; MCP flexion; IP extension (minimize contractures; optimize function).
- Prevent early shear of skin grafts/flaps.
- Begin early motion to optimize gliding/motion.
- Control edema.
- Utilize desensitization.
- Use goal-based therapy.
- Do not overlook psychosocial issues/therapy.

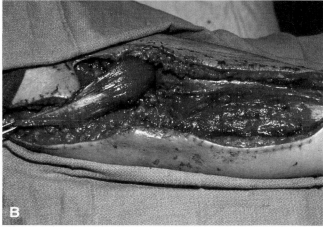

Cover brachial artery repair

FIGURE 46-26. **A** and **B,** For defects around the antecubital area, such as exposed vascular or nerve reconstructions, the proximally based brachioradialis muscle flap is an excellent choice with minimal donor morbidity.

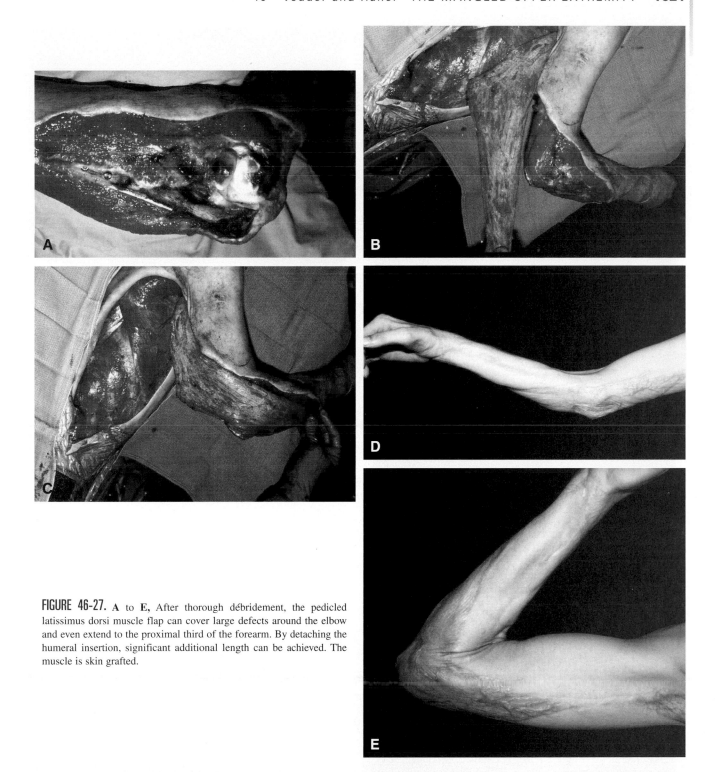

FIGURE 46-27. **A** to **E,** After thorough débridement, the pedicled latissimus dorsi muscle flap can cover large defects around the elbow and even extend to the proximal third of the forearm. By detaching the humeral insertion, significant additional length can be achieved. The muscle is skin grafted.

SECONDARY PROCEDURES

Mangling injuries often require secondary reconstructive procedures to achieve optimal form and/or function. The planning for these secondary reconstructive procedures is best made at the time of the initial operation, again "looking into the crystal ball" and having a vision for the future function of the extremity.[88] The goal of secondary procedures is to improve motion, sensibility, and durability. Some of these have been mentioned previously, including

bone grafting, nerve grafting, joint replacement, tenolysis, and contracture releases. In general, secondary procedures should be delayed until the soft tissues have matured and softened, which often takes 3 to 6 months. The exception to this, however, is bone or nerve grafting, which should be performed earlier. Some secondary procedures require postoperative immobilization and should be performed first, whereas others require mobilization postoperatively and should, therefore, be performed at a separate stage. All secondary procedures require stable, soft, well-vascularized

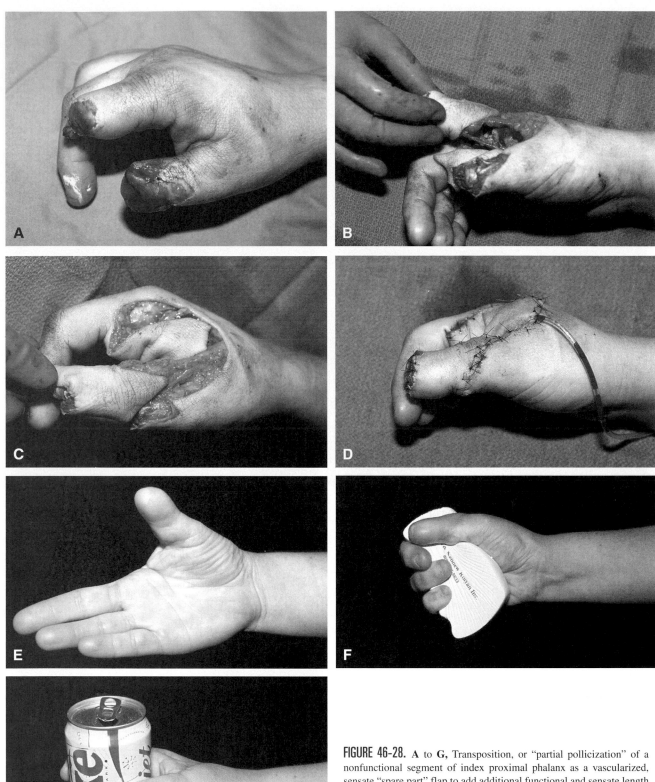

FIGURE 46-28. A to **G,** Transposition, or "partial pollicization" of a nonfunctional segment of index proximal phalanx as a vascularized, sensate "spare part" flap to add additional functional and sensate length to a partially amputated thumb.

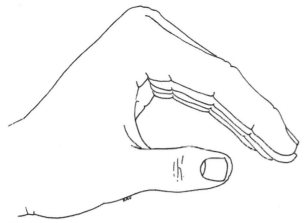

FIGURE 46-29. The hand should always be splinted postoperatively in the "safe" position, with metacarpophalangeal joints flexed to prevent shortening of the metacarpophalangeal collateral ligaments, leading to metacarpophalangeal extension contracture, and with the interphalangeal joints in extension.

soft tissue coverage. This may require secondary flap reconstruction. In rare cases, tissue expansion techniques can be used.[65] In our experience, however, tissue expansion in upper extremity reconstruction is associated with an extremely high complication rate.

If bone grafting is not performed at the initial operation, we perform it as soon as the wounds have healed and crusts have fallen off, to minimize infection risk, generally in 4 to 6 weeks. As mentioned previously, we favor cancellous allograft in most cases, unless autograft is simple to harvest from adjacent bone such as the radius for wrist or hand defects. In cases in which the tissue vascularity is questionable or in cases of nonunion, cancellous autograft, usually from iliac crest, is indicated. For defects larger than 6 cm, vascularized bone grafting is indicated. The possible sources for this and techniques are well described in Chapter 50 and include fibula, iliac crest, rib, and the second metatarsal. Our preference is free fibula because of its

length, minimal morbidity, ease of dissection, and large peroneal vascular pedicle. Structural allograft can also be considered, but only as a secondary procedure in a mature, well-vascularized tissue bed. With all bone grafting, ensuring adequate soft tissue coverage and tissue vascularity as well as good postoperative immobilization are all keys to achieving bony union (Fig. 46-30; see also Fig. 46-13).

Corrective osteotomies for functionally significant malunion and the treatment of nonunion should be performed in the initial series of secondary procedures. These usually involve either metacarpal or phalangeal osteotomies to correct digit crossover, distal radius osteotomy to correct dorsal tilt or shortening, or ulnar-shortening osteotomy to correct ulnar impingement. Details of these procedures are covered in previous chapters.

Nerve grafting for the purpose of restoring motor function should also be performed early, because the degree of functional return is inversely related to the delay from the time of injury.[93] Nerve grafting to restore sensory function, however, can be delayed. Again, the techniques for nerve grafting are well described in Chapter 30. When nerve grafting is not feasible, the decision must be made whether some other form of a sensory or motor reconstruction is required. Again, this depends on the patient's functional needs and a balance between these needs and what can reasonably be expected with additional procedures. For motor reconstruction, tendon transfers should be considered. The indications and techniques for these are well described in Chapters 31 to 33. When inadequate motor units remain to allow tendon transfer for basic functions such as composite flexion or extension, functional free muscle transfer using the innervated gracilis muscle should be considered. This is covered in Chapter 49. In the areas critical for sensation, specifically the ulnar tip of the radial digit (usually thumb) and the ulnar tip of the primary opposing ulnar digit (usually index or middle), sensory reconstruction may be required. If sensation is absent and cannot be reconstructed with nerve grafting owing to lack of sensory organelles in the reconstructed soft tissue coverage,

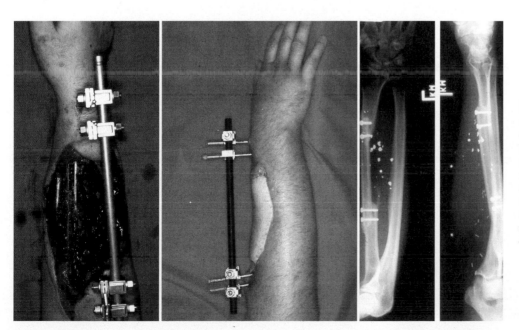

FIGURE 46-30. A close-range gunshot wound resulted in loss of 12 cm of radius, the radial artery, superficial branch of the radial nerve, and the skin defect seen here. After débridement, the radius was stabilized with an external fixator and the bone and skin defects were reconstructed with an osteocutaneous fibular graft. The radiographs on the right were taken 4 months after reconstruction.

then transfer of vascularized, innervated glabrous skin can prevent recurrent ulceration and improve tactile-dependent hand function. The most common indication for sensory reconstruction is when the digit is resurfaced or reconstructed with flap tissue such as radial forearm or groin flap. If the middle or ring fingers are uninjured, the ulnar pulp can be transferred based on the ulnar digital nerve, artery, and periarterial veins, covering the donor defect with a full-thickness skin graft, as described in Chapter 53. Critical to this procedure is ensuring that adequate perivascular tissue is taken along with the pedicle to allow adequate venous drainage, as well as ensuring that the palmar arch and distal arterial system are intact (Fig. 46-31). If pedicle neurovascular island transfer is not possible, then a free tissue transfer of the lateral great toe pulp, along with the lateral digital nerve and vessels can be performed. The technique and dissection are similar to the toe wraparound procedure described in Chapter 52, only in this case a small 1.5 to 2-cm piece of glabrous skin can be used, allowing primary closure of the donor defect (Fig. 46-32).

Amputation neuromas are a common and severely disabling complication after mangling injury. Neuromas are differentiated from normal hypersensitivity after injury by the fact that a symptomatic neuroma is well localized to the nerve stump and does not improve with desensitization therapy, whereas hypersensitivity should improve with desensitization. Treatment involves resecting the neuroma and burying the nerve stump in well-padded, vascularized soft tissue, where it will not be subject to pressure irritation, as described in Chapter 30.

When MCP or IP joints are destroyed as a result of mangling injury or when attempts at their initial reconstruction result in post-traumatic arthrosis, the usual treatment is either arthrodesis or amputation. In rare circumstances, however, when soft tissue coverage is soft, supple, and well vascularized, arthroplasty can be considered. The indications and procedure details of arthrodesis and arthroplasty are covered in Chapters 13 and 27. Post-traumatic arthrosis of the radiocarpal joint, on the other hand, especially in patients who use their hands actively, is best treated with wrist arthrodesis, as described in Chapter 13.

Tenolysis, capsulotomy, and contracture release play important roles in secondary reconstruction after mangling injury.[54,95] Differentiating joint contracture from tendon adhesion is sometimes difficult, and they often occur in concert (see Chapter 11). Although the lack of active motion relative to available passive motion is a reflection of tendon adhesions, sometimes what appears to be joint contracture with a clear block to passive motion can also be due to tendon adhesions. Both need to be addressed at the time of

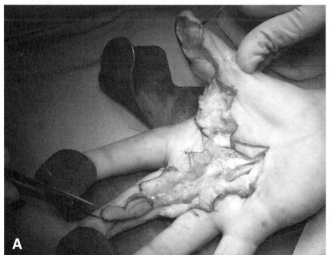

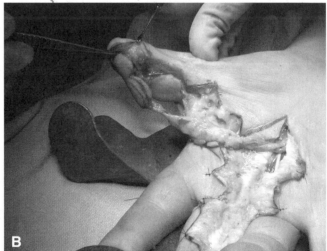

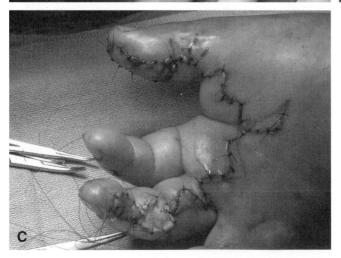

FIGURE 46-31. A to **C,** Neurovascular island flap from ulnar side of middle finger to the volar thumb to restore thumb sensation after replantation of thumb avulsion that had no reconstructable digital nerves. It is critical to ensure that adequate perivascular tissue is taken along with the pedicle to allow venous drainage.

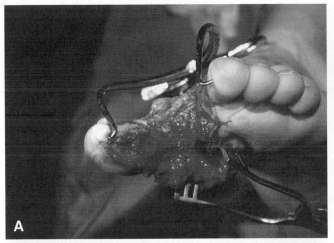

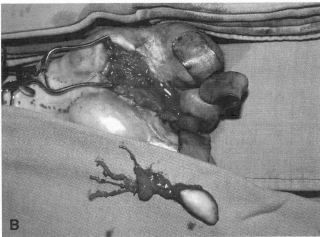

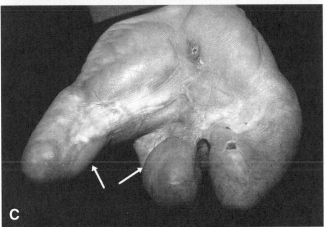

FIGURE 46-32. **A** to **C,** If pedicle neurovascular island transfer is not possible, a free tissue transfer of the lateral great toe pulp, along with the lateral digital nerve and vessels, can provide sensate tissue for critical areas of contact. In this case, functional, sensate pinch is achieved between the residual thumb and middle finger with bilateral lateral great toe pulp neurosensory free flaps (**C,** *arrows*).

secondary operation. If release will result in a coverage defect that will require either skin graft or flap reconstruction (if vital structures are left exposed), this will require postoperative immobilization and should, therefore, be incorporated in the "early" set of reconstructive procedures. Common areas of contracture after mangling injuries include the MCP, IP, and wrist joints, as well as the CMC joint of the thumb. Details of treating these are covered in Chapter 11. For the thumb CMC joint, it is very important to treat both the skin contracture in the underlying adductor muscle contracture and to immobilize the joint in both radial and palmar abduction, using either buried Kirschner wires across the CMC joint or a mini external fixator for a period of at least 6 weeks.

Tenolysis and capsulotomy require early postoperative active and passive mobilization and should, therefore, only be performed at a separate stage after completing any secondary procedures that require postoperative immobilization and after the overlying soft tissues have matured and softened. There is no fixed time that dictates how long one should wait before performing these procedures; instead, the timing should be dictated solely based on the character of the soft tissues. If both flexor and extensor tenolysis and joint releases are required, it is best to begin with the dorsal side first, with aggressive postoperative active and full passive flexion and extension. Flexion contractures and flexor tenolysis can then be performed at a second stage, again followed by aggressive active and passive immediate

postoperative mobilization. Attempting to address both the dorsal and volar problems in one stage carries a significant risk of disabling postoperative edema, pain that prevents adequate mobilization, recurrent stiffness, and risk of vascular compromise, especially in the digits.

CRITICAL POINTS: SECONDARY PROCEDURES

- ■ Procedures requiring immobilization (do first)
  - • Bone grafting
  - • Corrective osteotomies
  - • Joint reconstruction
  - • Nerve grafting
  - • Sensory reconstruction
  - • Tendon transfers
  - • Functional muscle transfer
  - • Soft tissue reconstruction
  - • Toe transfer
- ■ Procedures requiring mobilization (do second)
  - • Tenolysis
  - • Capsulotomy
  - • Contracture releases

COMPLICATIONS

Complications encountered in reconstruction of the mangled extremity are the same as those encountered in the various component parts of the reconstruction: skeletal, vascular, nerve, tendon, and soft tissue. Complications specific to the mangled extremity mostly revolve around failure to recognize and properly address the extent of the zone of tissue injury. Failure to adequately débride devitalized tissue, especially deep muscle, can have devastating consequences, including myoglobinemia, hyperkalemia, necrotizing soft tissue infection, limb loss, generalized sepsis, and death. For this reason, a "second look" débridement 24 to 48 hours after the initial injury and sometimes even a third débridement is important. Tissue that may not initially appear devitalized may become so due to the inflammatory response to injury during this period. Thrombosis of a vascular reconstruction is another complication that may be related to failure to recognize the zone of injury. If soft tissue infection develops, it is important to provide wide, open drainage and débridement to arrest the progression. Even though coverage issues can become a problem, they can always be dealt with later. Osteomyelitis is a challenging complication after mangling injury and can be due to either inadequate bony débridement at the time of the initial injury, inadequate vascularized soft tissue coverage, or percutaneous fixation devices. Treatment involves complete débridement of the devitalized, infected bone down to healthy, bleeding bone, with vascularized soft tissue coverage. Often, a temporary spacer consisting of antibiotic-impregnated methylmethacrylate can be placed after débridement and coverage, allowing delayed bone grafting.

Other common complications include hypertrophic scarring, joint contractures, tendon adhesions, neuromas, and soft tissue ulcerations, all of which are addressed in the previous section on secondary procedures. In the end, one must recognize that these are very high risk cases, that complications are not infrequent, and that they need to be anticipated, quickly identified, and appropriately treated before a "snowball effect" develops, leading to a poor outcome.

EXPECTED OUTCOMES

"Expected" outcomes after mangling injury are very difficult to quantify because no two injuries are the same in terms of their magnitude, location, or involved structures. Although quantitative outcome measurements such as active range of motion, grip strength, pinch strength, sensibility, and so on are all important components, the most important outcome measure is the degree to which the patient incorporates the reconstructed hand into daily activities and is able to resume a normal life. Important contributors to this outcome include not only biomechanical and sensibility factors but also appearance and psychological factors associated with mangling injury and the degree to which the patient is able to adjust to the altered function and appearance. Very often the degree of the injury and the functional loss do not correlate with the psychological impact on the patient. Sometimes a single-digit injury can be more devastating to a patient than a mangling injury involving the entire forearm. Post-traumatic stress disorder is well described in patients following mangling injuries of the upper extremity.[42,72] This is particularly a problem in work-related injuries, when merely revisiting the site of injury can elicit severe symptoms and can be a significant impediment to returning to work. Enlisting the assistance of rehabilitation psychologists early after injury is very important when signs of emotional stress are noted. Sometimes more extensive psychological or psychiatric evaluation is needed, and patients may benefit from antidepressant or anxiolytic therapy.

Of all the factors that contribute to the outcome of a mangling injury, the nature and degree of the soft tissue injury have the most impact. The success of skeletal, nerve, tendon, and joint reconstruction all depend on the overlying soft tissue injury and the quality of its reconstruction, as does the final appearance. For this reason, it is critically important to make soft tissue reconstruction a high priority item in both the initial treatment and secondary reconstruction of mangling injuries.[63]

As noted previously, the success of any reconstruction must be judged against the results of amputation with or without prosthesis. A wide array of outcome scores exist for major extremity trauma.[28,31,52,82] There are also a number of outcome scores specifically designed to address the upper extremity, including the Hand Injury Severity Score (HISS), Hand Function Score (HFS), Disabilities of Arm, Shoulder, and Hand (DASH), and the Michigan Hand Questionnaire (MHQ).[20,24,48,100] Although outcome studies of lower extremity salvage have shown equivocal benefit for complex reconstruction versus amputation and prosthesis,[6,7] it has long been believed that because of the complex mechanical and sensory functions of the hand, nearly any sensate function is preferable to a prosthesis.[9,16,38,81] This has not been definitively shown, however. No scoring system exists that reliably predicts outcome in a way that allows it to be used as the sole discriminator in choosing salvage versus amputation in the upper extremity. Experience and clinical judgment are still key.

CONCLUSION

The treatment of mangling injuries to the upper extremity is among the most challenging facets of hand surgery. Achieving good outcomes requires intimate knowledge and expertise in all aspects of hand surgery and the ability to evaluate, synthesize, and prioritize a wide variety of treatment options in developing a comprehensive treatment plan that may require multiple staged procedures and rehabilitation protocols over many months. Because the initial operation sets the stage for all that will follow, it is important at that point to be able to look into "the crystal ball" many months into the future and envision the patient's overall function with different treatment choices to formulate a comprehensive reconstructive plan that achieves both short- and long-term objectives. Critical aspects of successful reconstruction include complete débridement of devitalized tissue, restoration of good vascularity, early rigid skeletal fixation while minimizing additional tissue injury, and, most importantly, stable, vascularized soft tissue coverage. The important goals of treatment are to preserve life, preserve viable tissue, preserve function, and reconstruct and restore function of the extremity, allowing the patient to incorporate the reconstructed hand into daily life and to resume normal activities. Achieving these goals in the presence of a mangling injury is the ultimate challenge for the multidisciplinary reconstructive hand surgeon. It is a true test of one's mastery of the "art" of hand surgery.

ANNOTATED REFERENCES

4. Beatty ME, Zook EG, Russell RC, Kinkead LR: Grain auger injuries: The replacement of the corn picker injury? Plast Reconstr Surg 69:96-102, 1982.

   This is a classic article from Southern Illinois University that reports on many aggressive microvascular techniques and approaches that were put to use in the management of mangling farm injuries. The authors point out the frequently multiple-level injuries due to this mechanism. Twelve amputations or devascularizations were reattached or revascularized successfully. Heavy contamination was addressed by aggressive, serial débridements before coverage. They conclude that early aggressive surgical treatment can restore a high level of function.

10. Brown JB, Cannon B, Graham B, Davis WB: Restoration of major defects of the arm by combination of plastic, orthopedic and neurologic surgical procedures. Plast Reconstr Surg 4:337-340, 1949.

    A classic article by several of the "founding fathers" of the specialty of plastic surgery, describing the critical importance of quality soft tissue coverage in determining the reconstructive outcome from severe combined injuries of the upper extremity.

15. Büchler U, Hastings H III: Combined injuries. *In* Green DP, Hotchkiss RN, Pederson WC (eds): Operative Hand Surgery, 4th ed. Philadelphia, Churchill Livingstone, 1998, vol 2, pp 1631-1650.

    As broad as the topic of mutilating hand injuries is, there are a number of book chapters that deserve reading and re-reading. One such chapter is that referenced here. In contradistinction to the broad swath approach that we have presented, Büchler and Hastings emphasized the geometric impact of combined system injuries on the reconstruction and the expectations for mutilating hand injuries. To us, the approach, no matter from which direction, is the same: débridement, skeleton stabilization, tendon repair, revascularization, neurorrhaphy, and finally soft tissue coverage. Büchler and Hastings present a series of solutions, "a field guide," based on the anatomic regions exposed.

19. Burkhalter W: Mutilating injuries of the hand. Hand Clin 2:45-68, 1986.

    No one wrote more about war-related mutilating injuries of the hand than W. E. Burkhalter. His Vietnam experience carried over into his leadership of the University of Miami's Orthopaedic Surgery program. His experience and the common sense he derived from it are displayed in this article. Initial operative care of mutilating injuries is discussed as well as reconstructive procedures for partial hand amputees, including digital transposition and bone grafting.

21. Campbell DC 2nd, Bryan RS, Cooney WP 3rd, Ilstrup D: Mechanical cornpicker hand injuries. J Trauma 19:678-681, 1979.

    This is one of the early articles describing the modern approach to mangling upper extremity injuries, focusing on mechanical cornpicker injuries between 1962 to 1975. The importance of multiple, repeated débridement and the relative lack of importance of antibiotics are highlighted. The authors point out that the average length of disability after these mangling injuries is nearly 6 months, with nearly all patients experiencing some permanent disability.

27. Dellinger EP, Miller SD, Wertz MJ, et al: Risk of infection after open fracture of the arm or leg. Arch Surg 123:1320-1327, 1988.

    This is a seminal study addressing the infection risks associated with open extremity fractures, examining 240 patients admitted for operative treatment of an open fracture of the arm or leg. By stepwise multivariate logistic regression, the most significant risk factors were the grade of the fracture, internal or external fixation, and fractures of the lower leg—all related to local wound characteristics. The authors conclude that the most important interventions to prevent infection involve local wound care and that there is little or no relation between the timing of antibiotic administration or duration of antibiotic therapy and infection risk.

33. Freeland AE, Lineaweaver WC, Lindley SG: Fracture fixation in the mutilated hand. Hand Clin 19:51-61, 2003.

    Of the many stages in reconstruction of the mutilated hand, débridement and skeletal reconstruction provide the foundation of rehabilitation. Aggressive débridement prompts one to answer the question, "Should this hand or finger be salvaged and if the answer is yes, where best to start"? In this article the authors support the concept that in digits that have three or more systems injured, strong consideration should be given to amputation. By ascribing to this philosophy, our patients avoid prolonged and impaired recovery of the remainder of the hand. The one exception to the "three-system rule" is the thumb. Every effort should be made to preserve the thumb and its function by repair or reconstruction. The authors further opine that aggressive and thorough débridement allows internal fixation without increasing the risk of infection. They recommend anatomic restoration of the joint surfaces but note that anatomic reconstruction of the nonarticular skeleton is not essential as long as the fingers do not impinge or overlap during flexion and extension. Rigid fixation in the form of plates is most helpful, but severe comminution and fracture fragment size often require the use of external fixation, interosseous wires, and Kirschner wires in lieu of plates and screws.

36. Godina M: Early microsurgical reconstruction of complex trauma of the extremities. Plast Reconstr Surg 78:285-292, 1986.

    With this article, Marco Godina established the bench mark to which we all aspire when using free tissue transfer to reconstruct mangled extremities. By following over 500 cases, he thought that patients were generally affected by the time between injury and the time of free tissue transfer. Three general groups were identified: group 1 underwent free-flap transfer within 72 hours of the injury, group 2 between 72 hours and 3 months of the injury, and group 3 between 3 months and 12.6 years, with a mean of 3.4 years. The results were analyzed with respect to flap failure, infection, bone-healing time, length of hospital stay, and number of operative procedures. The flap failure rate was lowest in group 1 (0.75%) and highest in group 2 (12%). Postoperative infection occurred in 1.5% of group 1, 17.5% of group 2, and 6% of group 3. Bone-healing time was 6.8 months in group 1, 12.3 months in group 2, and 29 months in group 3. Relative to mangled hands, this article drives home the benefit of early aggressive débridement, skeletal stabilization, and soft tissue reconstruction.

43. Gupta A, Wolff TW: Management of the mangled hand and forearm. J Am Acad Orthop Surg 3:226-236, 1995.

The authors present methods they found useful in the reconstruction of mangling hand injuries. Emphasis is placed on assessment of the pathophysiologic condition, careful inventory of the injured structures, and early aggressive wound excision and reconstruction. The importance of vascular restoration, stable skeletal fixation, and provision of adequate skin cover are stressed. In addition to describing their treatment approach, the authors emphasize the need for expert rehabilitation, including physical and psychological counseling.

46. Hentz VR, Chase RA: The philosophy of salvage and repair for acute hand injuries. In: Wolfort FG (ed): Acute Hand Injuries: A Multidisciplinary Approach. St. Louis, CV Mosby, 1979.

A classic article describing the multiple factors that are factored into the decision whether to amputate or salvage and reconstruct severe hand injuries.

56. Khouri RK, Cooley BC, Kunselman AR, et al: A prospective study of microvascular free-flap surgery and outcome. Plast Reconstr Surg 102:711-721, 1998.

This is by far the largest prospective study of the risk of thrombosis in free flap surgery, including 23 centers and 493 free flaps. The overall incidence of flap failure was 4.1%. Reconstruction of an irradiated recipient site and the use of a skin-grafted muscle flap were the only statistically significant predictors of flap failure. Postoperative thrombosis requiring re-exploration occurred in 9.9% of flaps with an incidence significantly higher when the flap was transferred to a chronic wound and when vein grafts were needed. With multivariate analysis, many factors were found to not have a significant effect on flap outcome, including recipient site; indication for surgery; extremes of age; smokers or diabetics; end-to-end versus end-to-side anastomosis; irrigation of the vessel without or with heparin; and a wide spectrum of antithrombotic drug therapies.

61. Lister G, Scheker L: Emergency free flaps to the upper extremity. J Hand Surg Am 13:22-28, 1988.

This 31 case series demonstrates that if strict technical principles are followed and if there is a strong enough team of surgeons and assistants, then spectacular results can be achieved. As impressive as these results are, the single most important message in the article is the authors' discussion of whom they would *not* recommend for primary closure. These include patients with broad crush injuries and patients in whom they could not determine whether they had successfully removed all doubtfully viable tissue. In such cases, repeat débridement was recommended every 48 hours until coverage could be obtained.

Even today immediate internal fixation and primary closure of open fractures remains controversial; when this article appeared 16 years ago it was considered by many to be blasphemy. Of the chapter authors, NVB believes there is no role for immediate free tissue transfer, whereas DPH believes that as long as the surgical team performing the soft tissue reconstruction is not exhausted the effort results in less surgical intervention and a shorter hospitalization.

73. Moran SL, Berger RA: Biomechanics and hand trauma: What you need. Hand Clin 19:17-31, 2003.

This article serves as an outstanding source of biomechanical principles and guidelines that can help the surgeon evaluate the patient with severe hand and upper extremity injuries. Through knowledge of these basic hand biomechanics, the surgeon can assess more accurately what functions can best be optimized by balancing the functional loss or benefit from amputation, fusion, tendon injury, and reconstruction.

76. Neumeister MW, Brown RE: Mutilating hand injuries: Principles and management. Hand Clin 19:1-15, 2003.

This is the introductory chapter in an excellent compendium addressing mutilating hand injuries. This overview is based on the authors' extensive experience with mutilating hand injuries, mostly from farm machinery in the heart of rural Illinois. The core objectives in the treatment of mutilating hand injuries are highlighted: ensure patient's survival, limb survival, and ultimately limb function. They point out the critical role of aggressive débridement, skeletal stabilization, revascularization, replantation, or the use of spare parts at the initial procedure.

88. Russell RC, Bueno RA Jr, Wu TY: Secondary procedures following mutilating hand injuries. Hand Clin 19:149-163, 2003.

This is an excellent description of the many secondary procedures that are often required to achieve optimal functional outcome after mangling injuries and to provide stable wound coverage, restore sensation, achieve bony stability, increase range of motion, and allow prehension. The staging and timing of these procedures are nicely described.

CHAPTER 47

Skin Grafts and Skin Flaps

Skin Grafting

Earl Z. Browne, Jr. and William C. Pederson

The skin is the largest organ of the body and serves a number of vital functions. It functions as a semipermeable membrane and a barrier to toxic material and microbes, but it also contributes to homeostasis through temperature regulation and sensibility. This latter function—perception of stimuli—is most important in the hand, especially on the palmar surfaces of the fingers.

All skin is composed of a thick layer of dermis covered by epidermis. The epidermis constitutes only about 5% of the thickness of the skin, and the thickness varies considerably depending on the area of the body.[7,93] The skin on the palm and back is quite thick, whereas the skin of the inner arms and thighs is relatively thin. Skin in infants and elderly patients is always thinner than that in adults. The quality of skin depends to a great extent on the epidermal appendages contained in the dermis, which also vary a great deal from area to area.[18] This is especially true for the skin of the palmar and plantar areas, which contains no hair or sebaceous glands but is the almost exclusive domain of Meissner's and Vater-Pacini sensory end organs.[63] It is reasonable to think of the epidermis as the barrier and the dermis as the functional portion of the skin.[36,54]

One must also consider the hand as an organ and think of the skin as an envelope enclosing a multitude of tendons, nerves, vessels, bones, and joints. For the hand to function properly, this skin envelope must be elastic and nonadherent, contain as many of the appropriate appendages as possible, and be large enough to allow freedom of motion. The palm skin must also be thick enough to withstand the pressure and friction caused by grasp and pinch.

When considering the replacement of hand skin, as is done in skin grafting, one must keep these principles in mind. It is convenient to divide the hand into dorsal and volar surfaces, each having different basic requisites. Dorsal skin must be thinner, more elastic, and loose enough to not restrict flexion and must serve as a barrier to cover tendons and joints. Volar skin must be thicker and tougher while still being loose and elastic enough to allow motion, but above all it must retain its function of sensibility. It is usually possible to adequately replace dorsal skin by grafting while this may not be possible with volar skin.

HISTOLOGY OF SKIN

Figures 47-1 and 47-2 depict the major differences between dorsal and palmar hand skin. Common to both is the irregularity of the border between the basal layer of the epidermis and the dermis, at whose juncture are located the dermal papillae and the epidermal rete ridges. Both also contain intraepidermal nerve endings terminating in Merkel's cell/neurite complexes and sweat ducts extending out from glands located in the base of the dermis and subcutaneous fat.[74] Although not shown in Figures 47-1 and 47-2, a network of blood vessels and sensory and autonomic nerve fibers in the dermis is shared by all skin.

Figure 47-1 depicts dorsal hand skin, which is similar to skin found anywhere else on the body. The basal layer of the epidermis is continuous with the hair sheaths and sebaceous glands. Hair follicles lie at different depths and are surrounded by a network of fine nerve endings.

Figure 47-2 depicts the palmar hand skin. The papillae and ridges are deeper and the keratin layer is considerably thicker than in dorsal hand skin. Most significant, however, are the absence of pilosebaceous structures and the presence of specialized encapsulated nerve endings. Meissner's corpuscles are present in dermal papillae, and Vater-Pacini corpuscles are present in the deep dermis. These latter structures are also found along nerve trunks, joints, and other areas but exist in the skin almost exclusively in digits and the genital area.

SUBSTITUTION BY SKIN GRAFTS

Because it is similar to the skin of most other areas, dorsal hand skin can usually be adequately replaced by a skin graft. No matter how thick the graft is, however, palmar skin

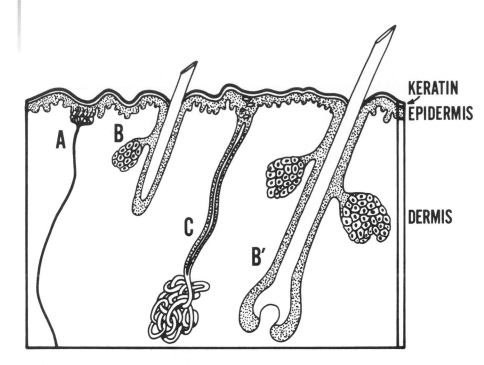

FIGURE 47-1. Dorsal hand skin is similar to skin of the rest of the body in that it has hair and sebaceous glands. **A,** Merkel's cell/neurite complex. **B** and **B′,** Hair follicle and sebaceous apparatus. **C,** Sweat gland.

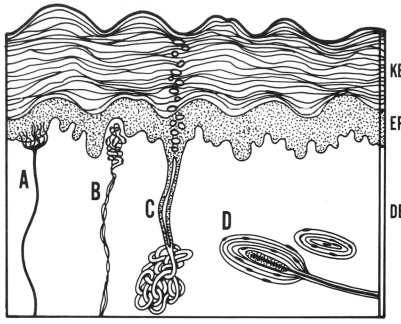

FIGURE 47-2. Palmar hand skin. There are no pilosebaceous structures present. Meissner and pacinian corpuscles exist almost exclusively here. **A,** Merkel's cell/neurite complex. **B,** Meissner's corpuscle. **C,** Sweat gland. **D,** Vater-Pacini corpuscle.

cannot be fully substituted by ordinary grafts because the special dermal neural mechanoreceptors will be absent. Only glabrous skin will provide these, and, unfortunately, not much of this type of skin is available for grafting.[69]

When a split-thickness graft is removed, healing of the donor area occurs by epithelialization from hair follicles and very little dermal regeneration occurs. The deeper the graft, the better the quality of the skin, but the less there is left behind at the donor site to aid in healing.[8,87] Also, a deeper graft increases the chance of reinnervation of Merkel's complexes and restoration of sensibility in the recipient site.[2,39] Thick nonglabrous grafts will transfer hair follicles, however, and result in unwanted hair growth if placed on palmar surfaces.[96] In addition to poor return of sensibility,

grafts on palmar areas do not provide the vascularized subcutaneous tissue necessary to cover tendons and nerves. In general, palmar grafts should be considered a compromise and are usually only indicated in release of flexion contractures in areas not requiring critical sensibility.

RESPONSE TO INJURY

Any injury that results in the loss of a full-thickness segment of skin initiates the process of wound contraction.[1,5,34,76] Although beneficial in helping to minimize defects in other parts of the body, this process of gradual shrinking of the wound edges can be disastrous in hand wounds (Fig. 47-3).

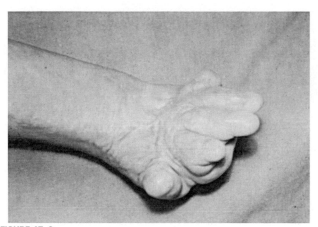

FIGURE 47-3. End result of uninhibited wound contraction of the dorsum of the hand.

It appears that fibroblasts migrate into the base of the wound and differentiate into so-called myofibroblasts.[43,76] These cells have the ability to contract, and the network of these cells and collagen fibers that forms in the base of the wound is responsible for pulling the wound edges together.[42,67] It has been shown that contraction can be temporarily halted by treatment of the wound with smooth muscle relaxants.[75] This process is not altered by epithelialization and appears to continue unchecked until the tension in the wound equals the tension in the stretched skin.[9,84] Once the contraction process has begun, it is not altered to any extent by split-thickness skin grafting.[33,38,85]

In a series of experiments by Stone and Madden, wounds in animals were treated with immediate grafting, delayed grafting, and immediate and delayed grafting with splinting.[95] They concluded that immediate grafting with split-thickness skin did not significantly affect wound contraction. However, immediate grafting and splinting with a compressive dressing for 7 days did significantly inhibit wound contraction. On the other hand, delayed grafting had no effect on wound contraction no matter what adjunctive therapy was used. Splinting, although effective with immediate grafting, was ineffective in preventing contraction when used with delayed grafts.

It is generally believed that the condition of the wound is the main determinant in the result of skin grafting.[31] Even full-thickness skin grafts can be found to contract if wound contraction has already begun.[6,38,85] Rudolph has found that the application of split-thickness skin does not seem to have as much effect on the differentiation of fibroblasts into myofibroblasts as does a full-thickness graft.[83] He has shown in animal experiments that wounds mature much more rapidly after the application of full-thickness grafts than after split-thickness grafts. The amount of actin and fibronectin found in rat wounds that were allowed to heal secondarily was compared in wounds with split-thickness grafts and those with full-thickness grafts. The thicker the graft, the less matrix protein present, which correlated well with the extent of wound contraction that occurred.[100]

This is important in considering the source of a graft for palmar wounds. The Shriners Burn Institute has compared the results of split-thickness and full-thickness grafts for coverage of deep palmar burns. Normal range of motion was found in over half of the full-thickness group, and only a fourth needed reconstructive procedures. In contrast, normal range of motion was present in only a fourth of the split-thickness group, and two thirds required reconstructive procedures.[89]

EFFECT OF INFECTION ON WOUND HEALING

A great deal of bacteria is normally present on the skin. It has been estimated that about 1000 organisms per gram of tissue are normally present in hair follicles, crevices, and recesses of the skin. This number of organisms does not seem to be significant in affecting wound healing.[60] However, when contamination of the wound takes place, much higher levels are present. Surface bacteria, which can easily be removed, do not appear to be important in skin grafting if the wound is carefully prepared before surgery. On the other hand, penetration of the bed of the wound is of great significance.[64] It has been established that 10,000 organisms per gram of tissue is a fairly critical level of contamination.[53] Wounds that contain fewer organisms than this do not commonly become infected. In a series of skin grafts applied to contaminated wounds, Krizek and colleagues[60] have shown that no matter what technique was used to prepare the bed of the wound for grafting, a bacterial count of greater than 10,000 organisms resulted in a successful skin graft take of only 19%. If the count was less than 10,000 organisms, however, there was a 94% successful take.

VASCULARITY OF THE WOUND

After application of a skin graft to the wound, the graft first survives in a precarious fashion, apparently nourished by transudate from the wound. This has been referred to as "plasmatic circulation."[30] It is imperative that the graft become vascularized for ultimate survival, however, and anything that acts as a barrier to this process will cause loss of the graft.[11,24,26] The most potent of all barriers is blood, and hematoma will kill a graft even in the absence of infection.[32]

The actual process of vascularization is not altogether clear, but it is certain that this process must begin within a few days if the graft is to survive.[13-15] Whether coaptation of the cut vessels in the graft to the vessels in their recipient bed (the process of inosculation) occurs to any extent is disputed.[29] It appears that the more important process is the ingrowth of capillary buds into the skin graft from the edges of the wound and, more importantly, from the bed of the wound.[11,27,28,45] For this process to take place, there must be a vascularized bed containing the necessary fine network of capillaries from which budding will take place. Grafts will not take on denuded bone or tendon, and skin grafts are not satisfactory coverage for vital structures.

TIMING OF GRAFTING

From the previous discussion it is obvious that grafting the wound as soon as it is clean enough and after the fine network of vessels has been established is ideal (Fig. 47-4). In this way, contamination of the wound and establishment

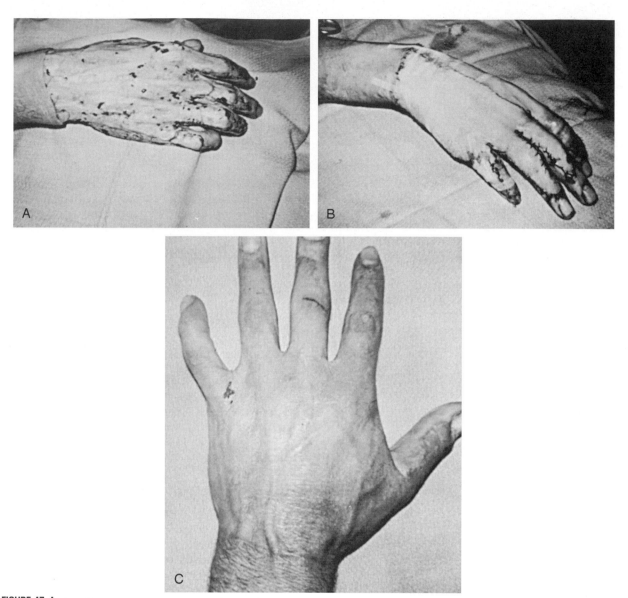

FIGURE 47-4. **A** to **C,** Expected result of immediate grafting and splinting when resurfacing a hypertrophic burn scar of the dorsum of the hand.

of a large milieu of myofibroblasts are avoided. In general, immediate débridement and grafting are often possible, and no more than 2 or 3 days should be allowed to pass for the purpose of establishment of a good bed. The principle of allowing a healthy bed of granulation to develop is no longer considered correct, and it should be replaced with the concept of early grafting[56] (Fig. 47-5).

Bacterial Content Determination

If it appears that the wound may be infected, determination of the bacterial content is necessary. Rather than rely on a wound swab to determine the presence of bacteria, which may yield a false-positive result, it is important to know whether the bed of the wound has become colonized with pathogenic bacteria. A useful method of determining this is by performing a wound biopsy. To do so, the surface of the wound is cleaned to prevent contamination, and a segment of tissue weighing about 1 g is removed. This can be done conveniently with a punch biopsy. A colony-count culture

can be obtained from the biopsy material, or a more rapid determination can be made by crushing the tissue and examining it microscopically. It has been said that bacterial presence greater than 1 per high-power field roughly corresponds to a critical level of 10,000 organisms.[60]

Temporary Storage of Skin Grafts

At times the wound may not seem to be ideal to receive a graft because of infection, bleeding, or poor vascularity. It is often convenient to remove skin from the donor site at the time of surgery for wound preparation to avoid another anesthetic and operation. In this way the skin can be stored while the wound is being prepared by soaks or periodic bedside débridement to reach an ideal state.

There are very convenient methods for storing such skin grafts if they are removed. One is simply to replace the skin on the donor site from which it was removed. The graft will begin to take and will remain well nourished and viable. If this technique is used, it is necessary to remove the graft

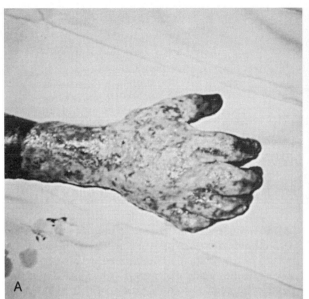
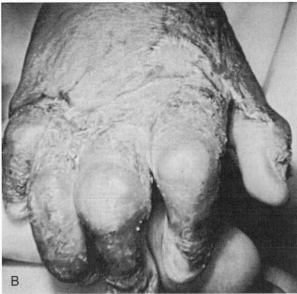

FIGURE 47-5. **A** and **B,** Expected result of grafting a bed of exuberant "granulation tissue." In reality, this is a chronically infected mass of fibrotic tissue. Poor take of the graft occurs, and wound contraction progresses to contracture, as in this patient.

before significant tensile strength has occurred. This may be done by injecting a solution of saline and local anesthetic between the graft and the donor site, and the graft can be placed on the recipient site at the bedside.[90]

Another technique is to store the skin graft in tissue culture medium during this interval. A common practice is to wrap the skin graft in a saline-soaked sponge and store it in the refrigerator. This is effective for a few days, but seldom can the graft remain viable for more than a week. It has been shown that by storing the graft in tissue culture medium with various additives, the viability of the graft can be markedly prolonged. Hurst and associates[55] have demonstrated that the use of McCoy's 5-A medium containing amino acids and vitamins can allow skin grafts to be stored successfully for up to 30 days. The method of preparing the medium and storage of the grafts is described in detail in their article. This is an excellent method for 10 days to 2 weeks, but after that time the quality of the skin does not seem to be as good as the quality of a freshly harvested graft.

TYPES OF GRAFTS

The two primary types of skin graft are split-thickness and full-thickness grafts. While other differences were discussed earlier, the main clinical difference in these grafts is in the way in which they are harvested. Split-thickness skin grafts are harvested with a knife or dermatome, and only the superficial layer of the skin is taken. The donor site of a split-thickness graft will heal on its own from propagation of epithelial cells from the deeper skin appendages (hair follicles and sweat glands.) Full-thickness grafts are harvested with an incision with a knife and involve taking the entire layer of skin down to the subcutaneous fat. These donor sites must be closed as with an incision; otherwise the patient is left with a wound.

The standard thickness for harvesting split-thickness skin grafts is in the range of 0.015-inch thick. Split-thickness skin grafts may be taken as either "thin" grafts (0.008 to 0.010 inch) or "thick" grafts (0.016 to 0.020 inch). Thicker split grafts have the theoretic advantage of potentially less contraction, because they contain more dermis. The downside of these types of grafts is that the donor site may have difficulty healing, and this can lead to worse scarring. One prospective study of the differences between standard and "thick" split grafts in the hand found no advantages in terms of range of motion, appearance, or patient satisfaction.[68]

Although it is true that full-thickness grafts afford better protection, hold up better, establish better sensibility, contain more epidermal appendages, and contract less than split-thickness grafts, thick grafts are not always desirable. There are several disadvantages to thick grafts. Full-thickness grafts do not take as readily as split grafts. It is generally accepted that this is due to the greater distance through which the capillary buds must migrate to reach the cellular layer of the skin, thus affecting survival.[24,26,27] A full-thickness graft requires a much better bed on which to be placed, and the graft is much more prone to infection.

In addition, the availability of skin must be considered. It is not always possible to sacrifice enough skin to afford the luxury of full-thickness grafting, and split-thickness grafts must often be substituted. In general, full-thickness grafts should be used only in situations in which the quality of the skin and the tendency to less contracture are crucial. As a rule, these conditions are necessary only on palmar skin grafts, and the greater level of return of sensibility is an added bonus under these circumstances. Dorsal wounds can generally be treated very adequately with intermediate split-thickness grafts.

Skin Substitutes

There have been many attempts in recent years to develop skin substitutes. Autogenous epithelial cells have been cultured and placed on a variety of collagen matrices and used as skin grafts. These have been of great value in the treatment of massive burns, but the take of the graft is not equal to that of standard autografts and the quality is not predictable.[17,91,107] Cultured epithelial autografts remain extremely expensive and afford very poor coverage, particularly in the hand. These grafts can be cryopreserved, but take has not been as good as that of fresh epithelial sheets.[44]

Work continues on the goal of providing skin coverage without the need for a donor site, particularly in terms of reconstruction of the dermal layer.[10,49,57,73] Several products now exist that provide a collagen matrix to act as a layer of dermis when placed on a vascularized wound.[49,72,79] The primary problem with these dermal substitutes is that they generally have to be applied 1 or 2 weeks before coverage with a split-thickness graft to allow for revascularization of the collagen matrix,[79,104] thus necessitating two operations. Some authors have noted no statistically significant long-term difference in elasticity, scar contracture, and patient satisfaction in patients treated with dermal substitutes plus split-thickness skin grafts versus split-thickness skin grafts alone.[99] The advantage of these dermal substitutes in coverage of the hand remains to be proven.

Skin Thickness

When determining the thickness of a graft to be removed, the skin thickness of the donor area must be considered. Epidermis and dermis vary according to age and sex, as well as location.[7] It is said that the epidermis ranges from 20 to 1400 μm in thickness and the dermis from 400 to 2500 μm.[93] When considering donor sites, however, there is only a practical range of 25 to 80 μm of epidermis and 500 to 1800 μm of dermis. In relation to dermatome settings, these values translate to 0.001 to 0.003 inch of epidermis and 0.020 to 0.070 inch of dermis.

In general, the epidermis is quite thin in infants and reaches a maximum thickness at puberty; it then becomes thinner with age until it is almost as thin in old age as it was during childhood. There is very little difference in epidermal thickness between sexes. The dermis, however, remains relatively thin in youth; it reaches its maximum thickness at about the fourth decade and subsequently becomes thin again in old age. There is a marked difference between sexes, with male dermis being significantly thicker than female dermis.

The skin of the trunk and dorsal and lateral surfaces of the extremities is the thickest. Skin thickness may range from 0.020 to 0.025 inch in a small child to 0.100 inch on the anterior of the abdomen in an adult man. In general, most donor sites cannot be expected to be much thicker than about 0.060 inch in a man and about 0.040 inch in a woman.

SPLIT-THICKNESS GRAFTING

Historical Perspective

There are several names commonly associated with skin grafts.[82] Although Reverdin was not the first to successfully perform grafting, in 1872 he drew attention to the technique by successfully performing small pinch grafts, primarily of the epidermis, measuring 1 to 2 mm in diameter.[80] In 1874 Thiersch extended the application of this type of graft by

using large sheets of thin skin grafts to cover wounds.[97] These grafts were generally somewhat thicker than the Reverdin grafts. The term *intermediate split-thickness graft* was first applied by Blair and Brown in 1929.[16] The full-thickness graft is generally thought of as a Wolfe graft, even though his work in 1875 was not the first of its type.[108]

Choice of Donor Sites

Removal of a skin graft is a morbid procedure. Although regeneration of the epidermis will occur, it appears that loss of the dermis is irretrievable.[86] The thicker the skin graft, the poorer the quality of the donor site after healing. Therefore, the thickness of the desired graft must, to a certain extent, determine the location of the donor site. The thicker portions of the body, such as the posterolateral aspects of the trunk and thighs, afford the best chance of good healing when a thick graft is desired.[7] The thinner areas, such as the inner aspect of the thigh, are generally unsuitable for donor sites (unless they are absolutely necessary) because of the poor quality of healing of the donor site and the tendency of the skin graft to hyperpigment in its new area.[65,71] So that morbidity and subsequent scarring are prevented, a reasonable guideline for graft thickness is offered in Table 47-1.

Most wounds are best covered by grafts approximately 0.015 inch in thickness. These are generally considered to be grafts of intermediate thickness, although this term was originally applied to grafts removing 25% to 75% of the skin thickness.[16] Thinner grafts of 0.010 to 0.012 inch may be best for wounds where graft survival is at risk. Grafts greater than 0.018 inch are seldom indicated because of donor site morbidity. If thicker skin is desired, it is best to use a full-thickness graft.

If possible, a graft should be taken from an area that is easy to care for during the healing process. No one likes to have to lie or sit on a donor site, and donor areas that cross intertriginous areas are very unsuitable because of the constant cracking and subsequent drainage with motion of the area. In women and children, it is desirable to remove the graft from the lateral aspect of the upper thigh or buttocks or perhaps the lower portion of the abdomen so that the donor site can subsequently be covered by a bathing suit or some other article of clothing. It is important to remember that the thicker the skin graft, the more hair follicles are transferred in the graft; thus whenever possible, a relatively hairless area should be selected as a donor site for the hand.[101]

Table 47-1
GUIDELINES FOR APPROPRIATE THICKNESS OF SKIN GRAFTS

Infants	Never over 0.008 inch
Prepubertal children	If > 0.010 inch necessary, remove from lower abdomen or buttocks
Adult males	0.015 inch from thighs, 0.018 inch from abdomen or buttocks
Adult females	Try never to use inner thigh; if > 0.015 inch, use lower abdomen
Elderly adults	Treat like children's skin

Freehand Grafts

Pinch or Reverdin grafts are almost never used in hand surgery. If a very small defect is present, however, a pinch graft can be taken by raising up an area of anesthetized skin with a skin hook. It is very convenient to anesthetize the skin with an intradermal injection of lidocaine for this purpose. This not only affords anesthesia but also thickens the skin so that a tangential cut will remove relatively more epidermis and minimize the effect of removing a divot. A piece 1 to 2 mm in diameter can then be removed with a No. 15 knife blade. Most wounds of this size will heal by themselves as rapidly as a graft will take, and grafting such small wounds is rarely indicated.

A larger piece of skin can be removed with a No. 10 knife blade by dissecting superficially just under the surface of the skin. It is convenient to make a very shallow incision in skin that has been distended with intradermal lidocaine before beginning the tangential dissection. In this way the appropriate depth and width of the graft can be selected. The blade is then placed into the depth of the incision, and with a back-and-forth sawing action, parallel to the skin, the desired size of graft can be removed. It is possible to remove a reasonably uniform piece of skin up to about the size of a dime with this technique (Fig. 47-6).

A much more satisfactory method of freehand grafting is made possible by using the Webster skin graft knife. This is a metal handle containing a groove into which a single-edged Weck blade is inserted. The instrument can be used in the same fashion as the knife blade and handle, but it is possible to remove a much larger piece of skin.

A modification of this knife is known as the Goulian knife set.[47] There are a number of depth gauges available that can be fitted over the blade (Fig. 47-7). These gauges vary in thickness from 0.004 to 0.030 inch. By placing the gauge next to the skin, the appropriate depth and angle of cut are automatically established. Because this instrument tends to take a rather thick graft, we prefer to use the 0.010 guard to avoid a too-thick graft. A strip of skin 2 cm or so in width can easily be removed, and with practice a long strip can be taken (Fig. 47-8). This instrument has the advantage of removing a strip of skin of relatively uniform thickness.

Although it is very convenient to remove skin from the upper inner aspect of the forearm because it is in the opera-

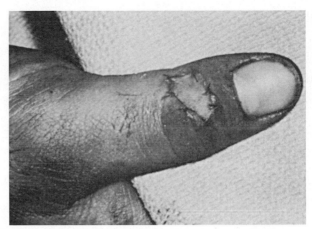

FIGURE 47-6. A freehand graft used to replace a small area of dorsal skin avulsion.

tive field, this is, in practice, a very poor procedure. The skin of the forearm is relatively thin in this area,[93] and often the scar is less than satisfactory. These scars are very obvious to both patients and casual observers, and often women will complain more of the donor site scar than the recipient area. It is preferable to remove these grafts from areas of thicker skin, where the scar will not be so readily apparent.

Types of Dermatomes

Brown Dermatome

The Brown dermatome was the first automatic dermatome to be developed and is available in both electric and air-driven models.[12] As with all modern powered dermatomes, the Brown dermatome has the advantage of rapid removal of large pieces of skin graft, and the instrument is fitted with a disposable blade and both depth and width of graft can be adjusted (Fig. 47-9). This instrument is relatively finicky compared with other, more modern powered dermatomes and has largely been supplanted by them. The technique of taking a skin graft with the Brown dermatome is similar to that of other powered dermatomes (Fig. 47-10). One must remember, however, that it is definitely more difficult to take a "good" graft with the Brown dermatome than the more modern instruments.

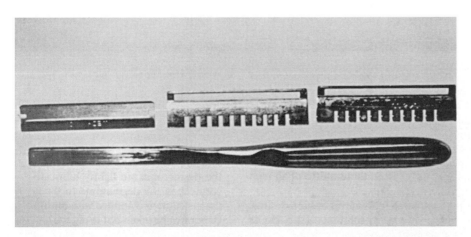

FIGURE 47-7. The Goulian skin graft knife set before assembly. Depth gauges of many thickness make it possible to remove a graft of uniform thickness.

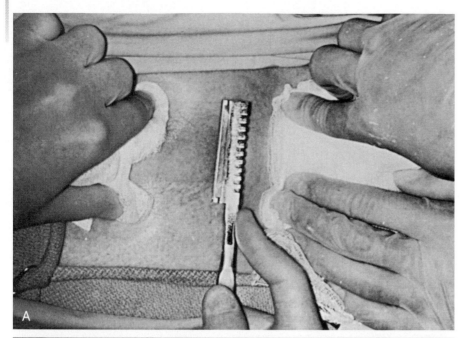

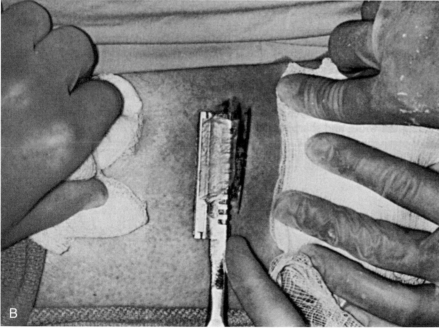

FIGURE 47-8. A, Goulian dermatome placed with the depth gauge next to skin. **B,** A strip of skin removed with back-and-forth sawing action.

Padgett Electric Dermatome

The Padgett dermatome is also motorized and uses a disposable blade with a cutting action similar to that of the Brown dermatome. The variable depth gauge on the side of this instrument is much more accurate than the one on the Brown dermatome. Three plates determine the width of the graft. After determination of the desired width, the blade is fitted on the machine and the appropriate plate placed over the two screws and screwed down tightly (Fig. 47-11). To put the blade on, it is necessary to first slip the base of the blade under the two projecting metal pieces and snap it down so that the hole in the blade fits onto the projection of the drive shaft. The appropriate graft thickness is selected by moving the blade up and down by using the depth gauge on the side of the machine.

The skin is surgically prepped and then cleansed with saline before taking the graft. The skin should be lubricated so that the dermatome will slide easily and not skip. Either mineral oil or a surgical soap solution can be utilized for this purpose and is placed both on the skin and the flat surface of the instrument that is in contact with the skin. The dermatome is placed flat on the donor site and traction is held behind the dermatome. It is not necessary to stretch the skin in the direction in which the dermatome will be advanced (Fig. 47-12). It is very easy to remove a piece of skin with this dermatome, and very minimal pressure should be exerted on the donor area. A common mistake is to dig the edges of the dermatome into the skin and press too hard, which creates an improper cutting angle. As the dermatome is advanced, the skin may be lifted up to check the thickness,

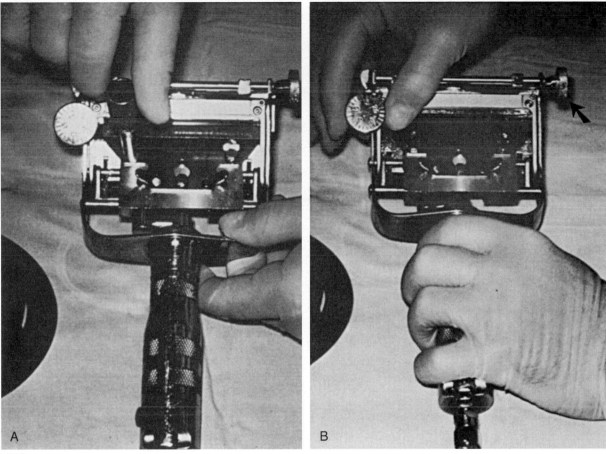

FIGURE 47-9. The Brown dermatome. **A,** The blade is fitted in position and securely tightened. **B,** Skin graft depth is adjusted by the knob on the left, and graft width is adjusted by the knob on the right *(arrow).*

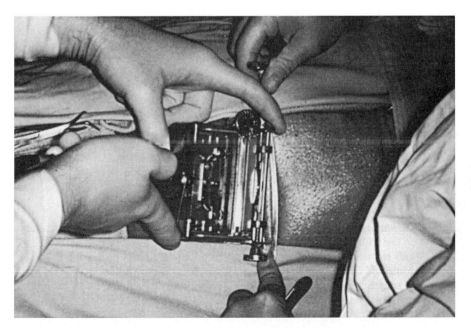

FIGURE 47-10. Traction is held in front of the dermatome with a flat object as the instrument is advanced. Countertraction is maintained behind the advance.

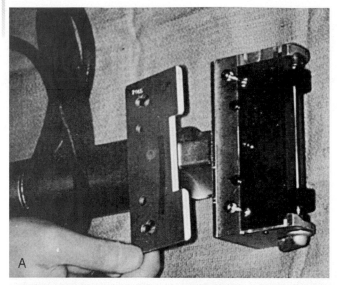

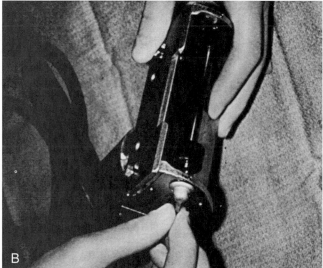

FIGURE 47-11. The Padgett electric dermatome. The width is determined by plate selection (**A**), and the depth is determined by gauge adjustment (**B**).

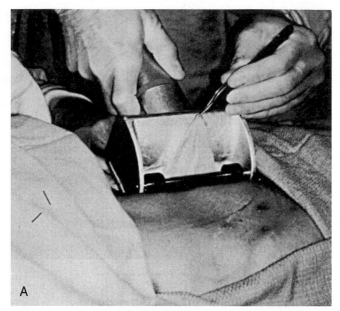

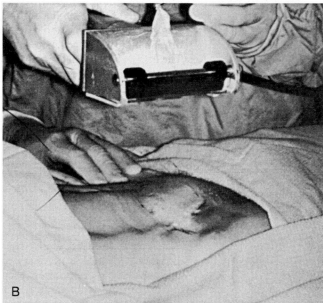

FIGURE 47-12. As the dermatome is advanced, traction behind the machine is maintained. The graft is lifted by the surgeon (**A**) and severed simply by lifting upward (**B**).

if desired. This is not necessary, however, and in general, a very uniform piece of skin is removed with the Padgett electric dermatome. This is probably the best instrument to use to take a skin graft if one is not experienced in this area.

Zimmer Air Dermatome

A similar instrument has been produced by Zimmer and is used in the same fashion as the Padgett electric dermatome (Fig. 47-13). A special disposable blade is made to fit the dermatome and snaps easily onto the reciprocating post. The width gauges are then fitted in place and screwed down in the same fashion. As seen in Figure 47-14, there are four fixed widths; the narrowest one is very useful for taking small grafts such as would be placed on one finger. Unfortunately, the largest one is a little too wide to fit into the standard skin mesher, but a graft that wide is rarely required for hand surgery anyway. The thickness of the graft is adjusted by a gauge on the side of the instrument in the same fashion as the Padgett dermatome, and the technique of skin harvest is identical.

Although this is an instrument comparable to the Padgett electric dermatome, there are some potential advantages. Because it is air driven, the handle is smaller and lighter, thus making its use a little more effortless. Also, it can be autoclaved repeatedly, which makes it available for more than one case per day. We have found it best to gas-sterilize the Padgett dermatome to minimize the repair rate. The choice of utilizing the Padgett vs. the Zimmer dermatome is one that should be based on the experience of the user.

Davol Dermatome

The Davol dermatome consists of a disposable head fitted onto a motorized handle similar to that of an electric toothbrush (Fig. 47-15). There is a sterile plastic bag into which the handle is dropped, and the bag is sealed with a twist tie. The head is fitted onto the handle, with care taken to align

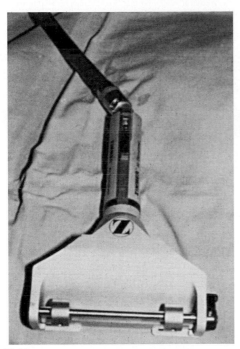

FIGURE 47-13. The Zimmer air dermatome assembled for use. The adjusting gauge is on the right side.

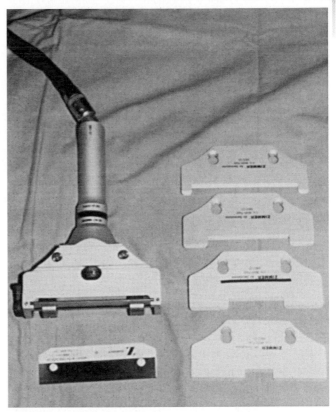

FIGURE 47-14. The undersurface of the Zimmer air dermatome showing the disposable blade, which is fitted over a reciprocating post and covered by a plate to select the desired graft width.

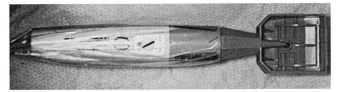

FIGURE 47-15. The Davol dermatome. The disposable head is fitted onto a handle similar to an electric toothbrush handle.

the dot on the head with the dot on the handle. The blade is then powered by turning the handle on with the switch on the side of the handle. Skin is removed in a fashion similar to the procedure for the Brown and Padgett dermatomes.

The head is preset at 0.015 inch, and the width is constant at about 2 cm. Although the depth of the blade cannot be varied, it is possible to remove a thinner piece of skin by pressing the blade down lightly. It is also possible to accomplish the same effect by distending the skin with an intradermal injection of local anesthetic.

The advantage of this dermatome is that it allows removal of a small piece of skin with a minimal amount of trouble in setting up instruments. It also has the dubious advantage of disposability, but it is necessary to keep the battery handle charged. One must be careful to examine the blade before using the instrument because sometimes this can be crooked and cause the blade to cut much deeper on one side than on the other. This problem is easily avoided by centering the blade before using it.

It is also possible to cut too deeply, especially along the edges of the blade, if the machine is pressed down too hard into the skin at an acute angle. It is important not to expect too much from this instrument, and it should not be used to harvest large or thick pieces of skin.

Drum Dermatomes

There are two types of drum dermatomes, the Padgett (Fig. 47-16) and the Reese; they are manual but do allow the surgeon to remove a large piece of skin of variable depth and width. These instruments depend on the use of glue or specially designed tape that causes the skin to stick to the surface of the drum so that the cutting blade can slide back and forth and remove a piece of skin that remains adherent to the drum.[78] Since the advent of good power-driven dermatomes, drum dermatomes are probably of more historic

interest than practical value. They do offer one outstanding advantage under certain circumstances, however, in that a piece of skin can be removed from any region of the body, even in areas that are ordinarily very difficult to remove grafts from, such as over the rib cage. It is almost impossible to remove a good piece of skin from this area with the motor-driven dermatomes. However, a very satisfactory piece of skin of uniform thickness can be removed from virtually any part of the body with the drum because it lifts the skin to be cut in the air rather than pressing it down over an uneven surface. Drum dermatomes may also be used to take skin from an avulsed piece of tissue, as in the case of a degloving injury where a graft for coverage can be taken from the avulsed tissue.[22]

The successful use of drum dermatomes requires patience and experience. These instruments can also be very dangerous in that the blade can swing around the handle and can cause a deep laceration of the user's wrist. For these reasons, application of these dermatomes should probably

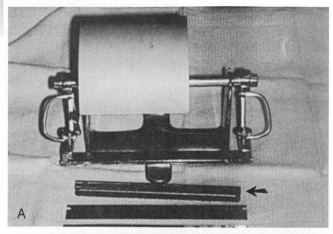

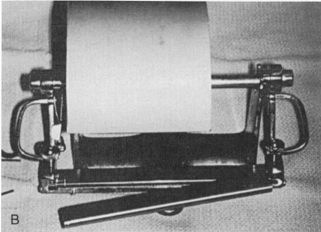

FIGURE 47-16. **A,** The Padgett drum dermatome. **B,** The shim (*arrow* in **A**) is first placed in the handle, followed by the blade, and secured by the guard.

be confined to those with direct experience in their use. The advent of powered dermatomes has largely relegated the drum dermatome to history, as noted earlier.

Mesh Grafting

At times the condition of the wound cannot be made optimal for grafting. The risk of infection or hematoma may be so great that the chance of survival of a sheet of autograft would be small. In these instances, it is often wise to use a piece of skin that has been meshed so that many perforations are present through which blood or exudate can escape.[66,92] An instrument has been devised that will automatically make these perforations. The skin can then be expanded so that the interstices allow drainage and then rapidly become epithelialized (Fig. 47-17). This method of grafting has wide application in the treatment of burns and large, contaminated wounds.[46,55,66]

It must be remembered, however, that only the portion of the wound that has skin applied to it is being grafted and the interstices of the mesh are left open and allowed to epithelialize. The quality of the graft will not be as good as that of a sheet of skin, and the tendency toward contraction and poor cosmetic results is greater. If meshed grafts of this nature are placed over flexion creases, joint contractures are likely to occur.[23] These factors can be limited somewhat by

---

CRITICAL POINTS: SPLIT-THICKNESS SKIN GRAFTING

INDICATIONS

- Simple wound with good underlying soft tissue bed
- Marginal wound with plan for more complex reconstruction at a later time

PREOPERATIVE EVALUATION

- Inspection of wound (for adequate vascularity)
- Possibly quantitative wound cultures

PEARLS

- Avoid a too-thick graft.
- Small grafts may be taken with freehand knife or Weck dermatome.
- Mesh or "pie-crust" graft to avoid fluid collection underneath.

TECHNICAL POINTS

- Recipient site should be very clean and débrided back to viable tissue *everywhere.*
- Avoid air or fluid pockets underneath graft (mesh or pie-crust).
- Graft must be held in place well to avoid moving against wound bed.
- Avoid removing dressing for at least:
  - 3 days if question of wound cleanliness.
  - 5 to 7 days if wound very clean.
- Place bolster for graft in a concave surface.

PITFALLS

- Early infection (usually strep or pseudomonas) which destroys graft
- Early motion which keeps graft from adhering

POSTOPERATIVE CARE

- Immobilize for at least 2 weeks.
- Change dressing if signs of drainage, etc.
- Avoid shearing force on graft for a minimum of 3 weeks.

---

compression, and it is imperative to treat wounds grafted in this fashion with long-term compression, such as can be obtained by use of the Jobst pressure glove.

Although not specifically evaluating hand grafts, el Hadidy and colleagues[39] evaluated the results of meshed versus nonmeshed grafts in burns. As expected, the results of either graft in late excision were significantly worse than the results in early excision, but the meshed grafts contracted more in both groups. In addition, there was a difference in the amount of growth that occurred in the two groups. With

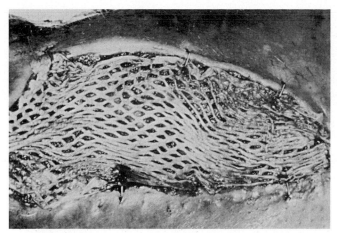

FIGURE 47-17. Meshed skin in place on a suboptimal wound.

early excision, nonmeshed grafts grew back to a size of 91% as compared with 78.5% in the meshed group.

Meshed grafts are often placed on a wound without the graft "expanded," which prevents collection of fluid under the graft but avoids the necessity for skin to grow over the open interstices. Whereas using a meshed graft in this way inevitably leads to more scarring than a nonmeshed graft, the functional differences are usually minimal. The advantages of meshing a graft usually outweigh the disadvantages. Nonetheless, split-thickness skin grafts are usually reserved for coverage of the dorsum of the hand, whether meshed or not. When the dorsum of the hand is covered with a muscle or fascial flap, it is certainly acceptable to place an expanded meshed split-thickness graft over the flap. It is sometimes convenient to use a mesh graft as a "temporary" biologic dressing, however, until a later resurfacing procedure can be done as part of the reconstruction.

Preparation of a Meshed Graft

After the graft is taken, it is spread out onto the surface of a plastic carrier, which is provided with the dermatome (Fig. 47-18). The "dermacarrier" plastic board has angled troughs cut in it that dictate how much the graft will expand. The various boards are marked and allow expansion from anywhere from 1.5:1 to 9:1, but sizes larger than 1.5:1 have very large holes that are not practical for hand surgery. Grafts thicker than 0.015 inch in thickness will not feed well into the meshing machine, and thus grafts thicker than this do not mesh well. After the graft has been carefully spread out onto the surface of the carrier, it is then fed into the lower end of the machine and run through the mesh by using the hand crank.

An alternate method of meshing skin grafts is one that provides multiple holes for drainage but does not allow for expansion. Instead of placing the graft on the mesh card and feeding it through the mesher in the usual fashion, the mesh card can be divided into sections and these pieces then placed side by side rather than end on end. If the graft is then placed on these lined-up pieces of mesh card, the result is skin passing through the mesher at a 90-degree angle from the direction that it would ordinarily go through (Fig. 47-19). This procedure makes a multitude of little punctate holes rather than slits, and when the graft is placed on the wound there are multiple very fine drainage holes

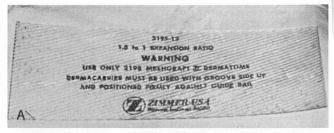

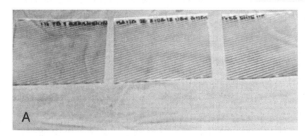

FIGURE 47-18. Skin mesher. Skin is placed on the special carrier (**A**) and passed through the cutting blades by turning a crank (**B**).

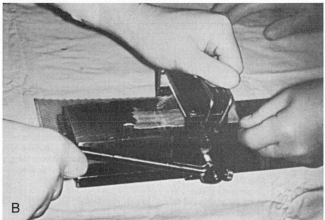

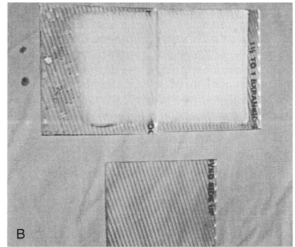

FIGURE 47-19. Method of dividing (**A**) and realigning (**B**) a mesh card to pass it through the mesher at a 90-degree angle from the usual orientation.

present but minimal if any expansion (Fig. 47-20). Skin meshed in this fashion is not as effective when placed on a suboptimal wound, but the cosmetic effect is probably superior, and it is probably a better graft to place over flexion creases to minimize contraction. It is absolutely critical

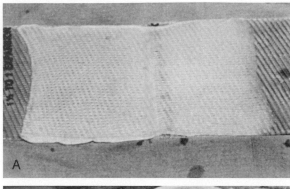

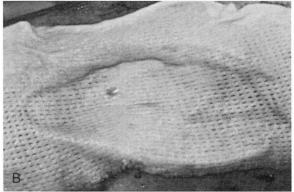

FIGURE 47-20. When the skin is passed through the mesher in this fashion, multiple small drainage holes are created (**A**), but expansion is then minimal (**B**).

that the card be fed through the mesher with the grooved side up, however. If the skin is inadvertently placed on the wrong side of the mesh card and then passed through the dermatome, the result will be multiple strands of "spaghetti" that are unusable.

FULL-THICKNESS GRAFTS

Full-thickness grafts transfer all the skin appendages and nerve endings except the sweat glands located in the subcutaneous tissue and some of the Vater-Pacini corpuscles of the palmar and plantar skin.[63] This thickness is an advantage for the restoration of sensibility and quality of coverage. These grafts must always be taken from relatively hairless areas to minimize subsequent hair growth in the recipient area. Good donor sites for this type of skin are in the lower and lateral abdominal areas. It is possible to obtain good-quality, relatively hairless skin here, and the area is loose enough to allow a large piece of skin to be removed with no subsequent defect after wound closure.[84] Smaller pieces can be removed from the extremity being operated on, and this is often very convenient inasmuch as the area has been prepared along with the operative site. The medial upper arm offers a good choice for full-thickness grafts from the upper extremity, and large pieces of skin may be taken in older patients. If skin is harvested from the posteromedial aspect of the arm, the scar is usually not objectionable. The volar wrist crease and antecubital fossa are often described as good choices for full-thickness skin grafts, but these areas should be avoided owing to potential scarring. Scars on the volar wrist crease

can also be interpreted as a sign of a prior suicide attempt. For coverage of the palmar surface of the fingers, glabrous full-thickness grafts may be taken from the hypothenar eminence. A fairly large graft can be taken from this area with minimal scarring and morbidity. The arch of the foot can also be utilized for harvesting a full-thickness graft for palmar coverage,[70] but the potential morbidity of this donor site should be remembered. In instances in which sensibility is critical, such as in the fingertips, a fairly large piece of "fingerprint" skin can be obtained from the hypothenar area (Fig. 47-21). Small glabrous full-thickness grafts can also be taken from the lateral surface of the great toe.[106] Glabrous full-thickness grafts have the added advantage of transferring skin of a more similar nature, that is, skin containing Meissner's corpuscles, thereby potentially restoring better sensibility.

Most full-thickness grafts will be placed on the palmar aspect of the hand; however, the surgeon must remember that there is a marked difference in pigmentation of the palmar skin in black patients, and nonglabrous donor sites should be avoided if possible. In dark-skinned patients, full-thickness grafts for placement on the palmar fingers or in the palm should be taken from the hypothenar area of the hand or from the previously mentioned foot donor sites.

Technique of Obtaining a Full-Thickness Graft

After the appropriate size has been determined, an ovoid of skin is excised from the predetermined area with the axis in the direction of minimal tension. The wound is then closed in standard fashion. Most donor sites for hand coverage will be small, and primary closure can be performed easily without undermining of the edges. Because there will be a moderate amount of tension on the edges, it is probably best to close the wound with buried subdermal sutures and a subcuticular suture to minimize the crosshatching that might occur with ordinary cutaneous sutures. The wound can then be dressed with sterile skin closure strips only.

It is necessary to remove all fat and subcutaneous tissue from the undersurface of the graft because they will other-

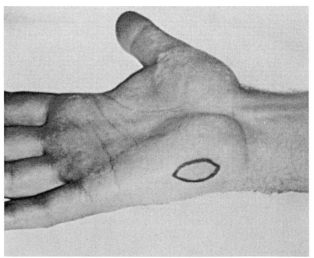

FIGURE 47-21. The hypothenar donor area provides a source of "fingerprint" skin.

wise act as a barrier and prevent vascularization. If desired, this can be done at the time of removal of the graft by very carefully excising only the skin and lifting it off its bed of subcutaneous tissue by dissecting sharply with a scalpel in the subdermal plane. The graft can be rolled over a finger as it is taken, and, with appropriate tension, most of the underlying subcutaneous fat can be removed. Once the graft is excised, the remaining subcutaneous tissue is removed. This is easily done by draping the graft around the surgeon's nondominant index finger while holding tension with the ends of the graft in the other fingers. The remaining fatty tissue is then removed with small curved scissors. The normal tendency is to remove portions of the dermis as well, which can actually lead to creating a "thick" split-thickness graft and lead to more contracture. The final result in terms of quality of the graft will be better if the subdermal areolar tissue is left with the graft. The fat can also be removed by placing small mosquito hemostats on the very tips at each end of the graft and draping the skin over a finger or the thumb while keeping tension on both hemostats (Fig. 47-22). If some tension is maintained, it is very easy to snip away the fat in this fashion.

If more than one piece is needed, as would be necessary if several contractures were being released, it is sometimes difficult to determine exactly how much skin will be required. It is particularly frustrating to go through all the time and trouble to remove a piece of skin and close the wound only to find that one does not have enough skin to adequately fill the defect. Templates can easily be made by using the paper in which gloves are wrapped. If a piece of the glove paper is pressed into the depth of the defect before the tourniquet is released, there is usually enough blood and fluid present to stain the paper so that the appropriate shape can be cut out. It should then be fitted into the defect to make sure that it is the appropriate size. When there is more than one template, they can be put together appropriately so that one large template can be used to excise enough skin to fill all the defects (Fig. 47-23). The resultant large piece of skin can then be used to fill the defects one at a time by sewing one edge of the graft into the largest defect, trimming it to fit, and repeating this process for all the subsequent defects.

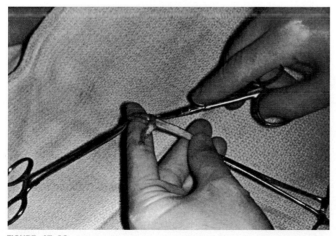

FIGURE 47-22. Technique of removal of subcutaneous tissue from the undersurface of a full-thickness graft.

CRITICAL POINTS: FULL-THICKNESS SKIN GRAFTS

INDICATIONS

- Wounds with very good bed in an area where better coverage is desired
- Management of scar contraction in palmar surface

PREOPERATIVE EVALUATION

- Wound bed vascularity
- Lack of infection in wound bed

PEARLS

- Avoid grafts from wrist crease and antecubital fossa.
- Graft from medial upper arm or groin.
- Don't "defat" graft so much that it becomes a split-thickness graft.

TECHNICAL POINTS

- Place lidocaine (without epinephrine) under skin to be taken first.
- Defat skin graft as you elevate it.
- Take an ellipse that can be closed primarily at donor site.
- Suture graft into defect exactly, trimming as necessary.
- Avoid straight suture lines along web spaces, etc.
- Utilize a "tie-over" bolster for almost all full-thickness grafts.
- Leave in place with extremity immobilized for at least 2 weeks.

PITFALLS

- Infection under grafts
- Motion of graft before revascularization
- Defatting graft too much and making it into a split-thickness graft

POSTOPERATIVE CARE

- Bolster and immobilize for at least 2 weeks.
- Begin motion carefully.
- Consider compression garment/silicone sheeting early to prevent hypertrophy.

CHOICE OF GRAFT

As previously indicated, a thicker graft contracts less, holds up better, and regains better sensibility than a thinner one. In general, split-thickness grafts should not be used on palmar surfaces of the hand unless there is no other choice or the

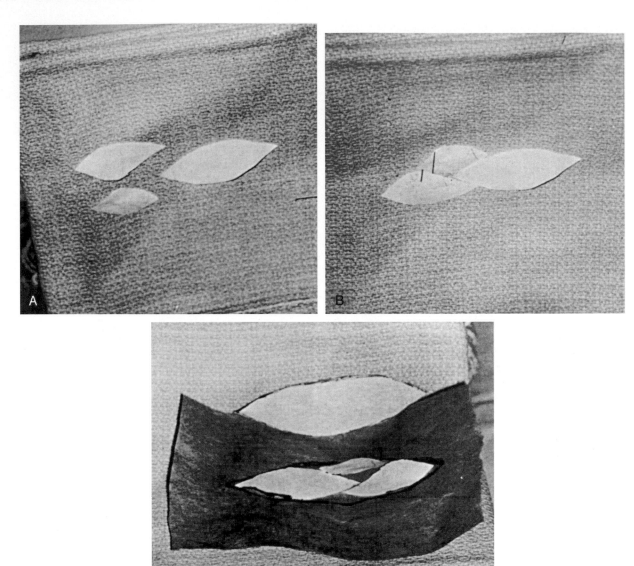

FIGURE 47-23. Method of determining the adequacy of skin to fill multiple defects. A template is made of each defect (**A**) and combined (**B**) to form one template large enough to provide sufficient skin (**C**).

coverage is considered to be temporary, with secondary resurfacing to be followed at a later date. If split-thickness grafts are to be used, they should be relatively thick and long-term compression with a Jobst glove should be used.

Full-thickness grafts are seldom indicated on the dorsal surface of the hand. The need for coverage is not as critical on the dorsum, and split-thickness grafts are generally satisfactory. In addition, the convexity of the dorsum and the subsequent greater tension on the wound edges with motion in the postoperative period appear to allow split grafts to be used with less contraction than would be the case on the concave palmar aspect. The general rule is that a sheet of graft of good-quality skin approximately 0.015 inch thick, if placed on a well-vascularized bed early in the evolution of the wound, will heal so well that it is difficult for a casual observer to know that a graft has been done (see Fig. 47-4). If the bed is not ideal, it makes no difference what kind of graft is used because the result will always be less than

satisfactory (see Fig. 47-5). Large areas of bare tendon, bone denuded of periosteum, and nerves and vessels bowstringing in the wound should never be covered with a graft; in such instances, coverage should be obtained by the use of a flap[27] (see later in this chapter). Very small areas of exposed tendon can sometimes be covered successfully with a full-thickness graft if the surrounding bed is good. This is due to the presence of the capillary bed in a full-thickness graft, which will allow vascularization of small areas of graft that are not over areas with adequate vascularity (assuming that the rest of the graft becomes vascularized).

PREPARATION OF THE RECIPIENT SITE

The recipient bed should be débrided so that all necrotic material and granulation tissue are removed. The bed of the wound should contain only a fine lacy network of capillaries. Often after débridement of a wound or removal of a thick scar for resurfacing purposes it is not possible to obtain an adequate bed for grafting. If it is not possible to obtain adequate hemostasis by coagulating bleeding points after release of the tourniquet, it is best to reinflate the tourniquet, wash away all the blood with saline, and dress the wound with fine mesh gauze and a dressing that will afford light compression and splinting before releasing the tourniquet again. If desired, rubber catheters can be incorporated into the dressing just above the fine mesh gauze so that antibiotic solutions can be instilled periodically to keep the dressing and the wound moist. After waiting 48 to 72 hours, the dressings can be removed while irrigating copiously, and healthy tissue with a fine network of blood vessels will be found. If grafting is to be done for release of contracture, it should always be remembered that the cardinal principle of contracture release is to re-create the original defect before attempting to fill up the hole.[27]

FILLING THE DEFECT WITH THE GRAFT

In general, a graft on a convex surface can be placed on the wound with normal tension and held in place in whatever fashion is desired. The convexity will tend to hold the graft in place; and by securing it to the edges of the defect, the tendency toward shearing will be minimal. One must always remember that the secret to grafting is the amount of dermis that is placed into the wound and that it is a mistake to stretch a graft too tightly for compression of the wound. This will result in thinning of the dermis by stretching, with less net dermis being grafted, which will lead to a poorer result. The graft itself will not cause pressure on the bed inasmuch as any amount of fluid will easily lift the graft up no matter how tightly it is stretched. Compression must come from external dressings. Any blood present under the graft should be irrigated out with saline (Fig. 47-24).

Sheets of skin placed on the hand, whether split thickness or full thickness, should be carefully tailored to the defect.

If the margin of the skin graft lies in a line that is likely to cause a scar contracture (particularly in the palm), darts should be made in the hand skin along this line and the graft fitted into these.[48] These small darts break up the scar and can prevent a linear scar contracture from occurring later on.

Grafts on the dorsum of the hand may be held in place with sutures or skin staples.[19] Meshed split-thickness grafts are usually easiest to hold down with metal skin staples. After closure is completed, the graft is covered with a compressive dressing and splint (Fig. 47-25). Meshed grafts should be kept moist and are usually covered with some type of nonadherent gauze covered with moistened gauze. The gauze is soaked with a solution of antibiotic saline that is used for irrigation in the operating room. Some advocate the use of catheters placed under the dressing to allow periodic instillation of antibiotic solutions, especially in the presence of infection.[51] Many types of nonadherent dressings exist, and most contain some type of petroleum solution that is not water soluble. Scarlet red gauze has been used by many years by some surgeons and has been thought to increase the rate of healing.[41]

Grafts placed on a concave surface must always be held securely in place. They will have a natural tendency to "tent" over the wound and float up off the wound as serum collects under them. One excellent method of preventing this is the use of a bolster or tie-over dressing. In this technique, grafts are placed into the concavity and sutured around the edges with strands of suture that are left long

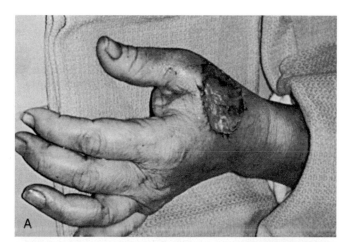

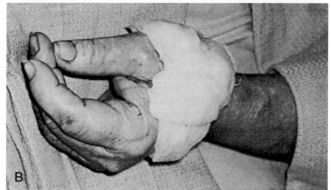

FIGURE 47-25. Grafts on a convex surface (**A**) will tend to stay in place with minimal shearing force. A compressive dressing (**B**) and splint are sufficient.

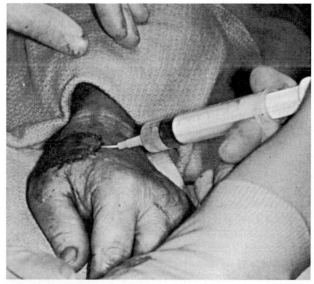

FIGURE 47-24. All blood must be irrigated out from beneath a graft. This can be done with saline from a syringe and flexible catheter.

(Fig. 47-26). After the completion of suturing, the graft is covered with scarlet red or a similar gauze and the concavity filled with wet cotton. The ends of the sutures are then tied over the dressing to make a package that will hold the graft in place and prevent shearing, minimize serous accumulation, and optimally cause some pressure on the base of the wound. This is an especially good dressing for a full-thickness graft. This bolster dressing can be used anywhere desired, but its use is difficult on a convex surface because the sutures tend to pull the graft up from the edges of the defect. If it is believed that the graft needs to be examined early, rather than tying the sutures as shown in Figure 47-26, they can be temporarily secured. One way of doing this is by passing the long ends of the thread through a shortened, disposable syringe cylinder and holding them in place in proper tension by then placing the piston back into the syringe cylinder. This allows the threads to be loosened and the dressing removed, replaced, and secured again by the syringe.[4]

Reston foam also can be used as a skin graft dressing. A piece of nonadherent gauze is placed over the graft, a piece of Reston foam is cut large enough to cover the gauze, and the foam is simply stapled down to the skin defect edges. This holds the graft and dressing in place without other sutures or dressings, provides compression and protection from shearing, and is quick and cost effective.[105]

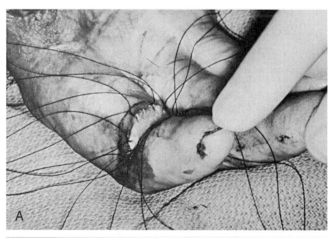

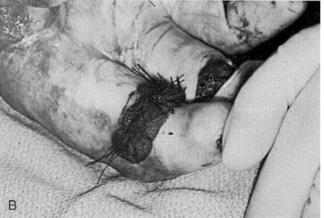

FIGURE 47-26. A full-thickness graft in a concave surface being held into the depth of the defect by a tie-over dressing. The ends of the sutures are left long (**A**) and tied together over a bolus of gauze and cotton (**B**).

With full-thickness grafts in the hand, we prefer to tailor the graft to fit the defect exactly and then suture the margins in place with running 4-0 chromic sutures. The subgraft area is then irrigated with a mixture of thrombin solution and antibiotic solution that is then forced out by manual pressure on the graft. A bolster of nonadherent gauze covered with wet cotton balls is placed over the graft and held in place with several polypropylene sutures placed in the surrounding skin and tied over the cotton.

Many surgeons now utilize vacuum sponge devices to bolster skin grafts.[25,88,94] This technique has the advantage of removing exudates from the wound and is very effective in terms of holding the graft down while it is becoming revascularized. This technique has limited application in skin grafts in the hand, with the exception of large wounds, however.

POSTOPERATIVE CARE

There are two schools of thought in caring for skin grafts.[20,21,27,33,62,77,84] Some surgeons like to look at the grafts within 24 hours so that if a hematoma is present, it can be evacuated. The other group says that doing this might disturb a graft that is getting along well and that a hematoma could be stirred up at that time. In addition, it is almost never possible to put on as good a dressing as the one put on at the time of surgery.

If it is anticipated that hematoma or seroma collection might be a problem, the dressing should be removed at 24 hours and the wound inspected periodically. If fluid collects under the graft, it should be evacuated by stabbing the graft with a No. 11 knife blade and gently rolling the graft with a cotton-tipped applicator to remove the fluid. Care should be taken to roll and not rub, because rubbing can cause shearing of the graft from the bed.

If there is really no reason to suspect that either of these problems will arise, the wound can be monitored just as any other wound would be. As long as there is no drainage, foul smell, fever, or other cause for concern, the splint and dressing can be left undisturbed for 7 to 10 days. After that, the dressing can be removed; and if healing appears to be satisfactory, early guarded motion may begin.

It must be remembered that a skin graft is just like any other wound; that is, there is very little tensile strength present until enough collagen deposition has occurred to cause the wound to be strong. Therefore, even though the graft may be well vascularized at this stage, it will be very prone to injury from shearing forces for another 10 days. If blisters develop, motion should be stopped and the graft adequately protected for a few more days.

Small areas of graft loss several millimeters in diameter will generally fill in satisfactorily without excessive scarring, especially if compression with a Jobst support is used.[40] Larger areas of loss should be débrided and regrafted. After the take is judged to be satisfactory, the grafts should be kept lubricated with a moisturizing lotion or cream.

Because an open wound continues to contract even after it is covered by a skin graft, there is always the concern of scar contracture limiting motion. The elastic compression garment has been the standard of aftercare of grafts to minimize this effect.[102] The principle of this technique is to

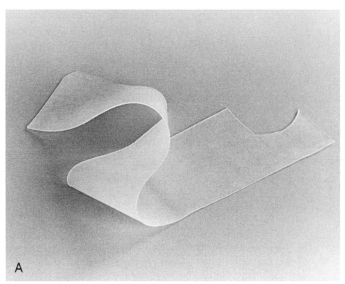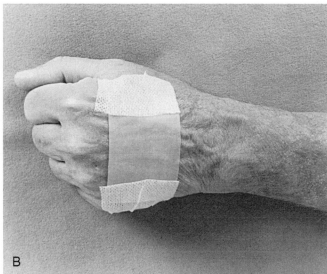

FIGURE 47-27. **A,** Silicone sheeting used to control scarring. **B,** Thin, pliable sheet taped in place over a scarred or grafted area.

provide sufficient compression to exceed capillary pressure to the graft and thus inhibit fibroblasts.[58] To facilitate even pressure, a silicone insert is generally placed over the graft or scar under an elastic glove for the hand.[98] More recently, it has been found that the use of silicone alone will inhibit scar formation, and the effect of mechanical pressure may not be the causative factor.[3] It may be that many types of occlusive dressing on the scar bed will modify the wound, and various materials used in an occlusive fashion have been shown to cause cytokine alterations in wounds.[81] One of the easiest to use is silicone sheeting. Sil-K (Degania Silicone, Israel) is one of the most applicable to grafted skin.[61] It is a thin, pliable membrane that can be cut to size and simply taped over the scar (Fig. 47-27). This product, as opposed to gel, stays relatively clean and can be washed and used over and over again. The patient should use this material as much as possible, at the least sleeping every night with it taped in place. If use of silicone sheeting is begun shortly after the skin graft has been judged to have taken well, significant reduction in scarring can be achieved.

CARE OF THE DONOR SITE

Full-thickness sites require no special care and should be treated like any other wound. Split-thickness grafting, however, is a very morbid event, and the patient should be told before grafting that the donor site will probably cause a great deal more discomfort than the grafted area.

A donor site is just like a skinned knee. The sooner it dries out and forms a scab, the quicker it will become asymptomatic. This obviously is a factor of depth inasmuch as a thinner graft will heal much more rapidly than a thick graft. If a thin scab forms on the surface of the donor site, it will generally separate in about 14 days.

There are many of ways of treating donor sites that involve the application of every known kind of dressing or medication.[50,52,59,87] The longer it takes for the wound to become dry and the thicker the resultant eschar, however, the more morbidity the patient will suffer. Whatever tech-

nique leads to rapid drying of the donor site will usually result in the best healing. The "old" technique of leaving the donor site totally open probably works the best but can be quite painful in the immediate postoperative period. Many surgeons utilize an occlusive adherent plastic dressing to cover their split-graft donor sites,[35,37] but this technique suffers from fluid collection under the plastic and an increased risk of infection at the donor site. This approach has the advantage of decreasing pain in the postoperative period, but the benefits are outweighed by the potential problems.

The donor site is covered immediately with a single layer of fine-mesh gauze, which is then sprayed with thrombin solution. This is covered with a warm, moistened sponge, which is left until the operation is over. At this time the sponge is removed with the fine mesh gauze left in place. There will usually be no further bleeding at this point unless the fine mesh gauze is removed. The local area is cleansed and an appropriately sized occlusive plastic dressing placed. The plastic is removed at 2 to 3 days and the fine mesh gauze left in place to dry onto the wound. This area is then dried out by the nursing staff or patient with a bare-bulb light or hair dryer. This approach makes use of the benefit of decreased pain at the donor site from the occlusive dressing for the first couple of days but allows the donor site to then dry out before infection can become established. Once the donor site is dry, there is usually very little further pain. The scab formed with the fine mesh gauze will usually separate in 2 to 3 weeks.

OUTPATIENT SURGERY

Traditionally, skin grafts have been done as inpatient procedures with the patient kept at bed rest to protect the graft from bleeding and shear effect. In this new era of managed care, this will no longer be possible, so ways to perform quicker and less expensive surgery, preferably under local anesthesia, will be desirable.

One approach is to use lateral femoral cutaneous nerve block for anesthesia of the donor site. This nerve passes under the inguinal ligament and provides sensibility to most of the lateral side of the thigh, the perfect donor site. Enough skin can easily be obtained with this block to surface the entire dorsum of the hand.[103] There is some variability in the course of the nerve, but with practice it can almost always be blocked. The usual landmark is two fingertips inferior and two fingertips medial to the anterior superior iliac spine in the average adult. About 10 mL or so of anesthetic should be injected in a fanlike fashion while making sure to place half of it deep to the underlying fascia lata. No infiltration of the skin of the thigh is necessary, which makes harvesting of a large graft much less morbid. Also, if a longer-lasting anesthetic agent is used, the patient has no trouble getting up and walking out.

Although the Unna boot dressing was developed to heal leg ulcers by compression and the drying action of the paste, those same properties make it an ideal support for skin grafts. The Medicopaste bandage (Graham Field, Inc., Hauppauge, NY) can be rolled right over a skin graft to keep it compressed in a bacteriostatic environment. The dressing can be left on for a long time to maintain compression and is, of course, ideal for a graft on an edematous leg because it allows early mobilization. Sanford and Gore, however, have reported the use of this dressing to facilitate outpatient skin grafting of hands.[86] Sixteen burned hands were treated by outpatient débridement, skin grafting, and Unna boot dressing. When the patients returned on the fifth postoperative day, there was 95% take of all grafts, with no infections. This allowed the shifting of fairly extensive débridement and skin grafting to the outpatient setting.

ANNOTATED REFERENCES

Skin Grafts

5a. Banis JC: Glabrous skin grafts for plantar defects. Foot Ankle Clin 6:827-837, 2001.

While not having to do with the hand directly, this article covers all of the right reasons for utilizing glabrous skin to replace glabrous defects. Dr. Banis notes that utilizing glabrous skin grafts to reconstruct glabrous defects leads to a better quality of skin at the recipient site with less breakdown, less scarring, and a more cosmetic appearance.

17. Boyce JC, Goretsky MJ, Greenhalgh DG, et al: Comparative assessment of cultured skin substitutes and native skin autograft for treatment of full-thickness burns. Ann Surg 222:743-752, 1995.

This paper discusses the outcomes in 17 patients with full-thickness burns treated with either native skin grafts or artificial skin with autologous fibroblasts and keratinocytes. While the authors noted no differences in qualitative outcome after 1 year, there were significant differences in scarring, pigmentation, and need for regrafting between the two groups. This paper should be read by those with early enthusiasm for these very expensive skin "substitutes."

25. Chang KP, Tsai CC, Lin TM, et al: An alternative dressing for skin graft immobilization: Negative pressure dressing. Burns 27:839-842, 2001.

This paper reports on the early use of negative pressure dressings for new skin grafts. This has come to fruition with the use of the vacuum devices for management of new grafts, which may be the state of the art for dressing new skin grafts today.

57. Jones I, Currie L, Martin R: A guide to biological skin substitutes. Br J Plast Surg 55:185-193, 2002.

This paper gives a good introduction and description of the new skin substitutes that are available. It reviews the makeup of these new substances along with their cost and potential application. It also includes a section on technologies that are in the works and may become available in the future.

96. Terzis JK: Functional aspects of reinnervation of free skin grafts. Plast Reconstr Surg 58:142-156, 1976.

This early work provides documentation of the rate and quality of reinnervation of full-thickness skin grafts. It has particular application to grafting in the hands and fingers where innervation is so important.

Skin Flaps

William C. Pederson and Graham Lister

Because scar limits the motion that is essential for function in many areas of the upper extremity, every effort must be made to achieve primary wound healing to avoid healing by secondary intention, which involves significant scar formation. Skin defects that are the result of injury or surgery should therefore be closed directly or covered with imported skin. In certain situations, free skin grafts will suffice. In others, free grafts may not "take" or may, by their necessary adhesion to underlying tissue, be unsuitable. "Take" of a skin graft requires that the bed on which it is placed have a blood supply adequate to revascularize the free graft. This blood supply is not present when bare bone, cartilage, or tendon is exposed in the wound. "Take" requires firm adhesion of the graft. This is not acceptable when further surgery is planned beneath the new skin cover, for example, when tendon grafts will be necessary after an avulsion injury of the dorsum of the hand. It is also not suitable where the firm adhesion of the graft prevents mobility of the skin envelope

We thank Danny Smith, formerly of Louisville and now of Salt Lake City, and Grace von Drasek Ascher, medical illustrator of Louisville Hand Surgery, for their hours of work on the figures in this section of Chapter 47. The copyright to much of the artwork is held by Louisville Hand Surgery, which we thank for permission to publish it here.

over underlying structures, for example, where a graft on a fingertip is adherent to bone. Shear forces applied in daily use will cause intermittent avascularity of the skin and eventual breakdown. A similar mechanism of breakdown may occur when grafts have been placed over the convex aspect of joints. Flexion renders the graft taut and avascular. That along with normal trauma results in ulceration. To a degree that is inversely proportional to its content of dermis, a free skin graft will contract during the first 6 months after its application to the extent that its location permits. Thus, on the dorsum of the hand, which is subjected to repeated stretching by normal use, less contracture occurs than on the flexion aspect of a joint. In the latter location, only full-thickness grafts with perfect take are suitable. In any circumstances in which free grafts do not provide the best skin, flap coverage is indicated.

TYPES OF FLAPS

A flap is skin with a varying amount of underlying tissue that is used to cover a defect and that receives its blood supply from a source other than the tissue on which it is laid. The part of the flap that provides the blood supply is termed the *pedicle*. A *graft* is a piece of tissue that does not have an intrinsic blood supply and must be revascularized by the underlying tissue bed. Table 47-2 lists the various flaps discussed in this chapter.

Random-Pattern Flaps

The manner in which the skin receives its blood supply has been studied by many anatomists. Recently, Lamberty and Cormack[180] again described angiotomes in the upper limb, these being areas of skin with a known single arterial supply. The constancy of these arteries has been confirmed by Doppler studies in patients[331] and volunteers.[127] Taylor and associates[330] studied the venosomes and reported that venous territories correspond closely to recognized areas of arterial supply. Pearl and Johnson[259,260] showed that this supply may

be present in four vascular layers or strata: subdermal, subcutaneous,[210] fascial, and muscular. The blood supply of a flap may come not from a single arteriovenous pedicle but from the many minute vessels of the subdermal or subcutaneous plexus. Such a flap is termed a *random-pattern flap*.[222] Although the shape of a random-pattern flap need not be quadrilateral, it is usually conceived as such, and it is raised by incising three of the four sides. The fourth constitutes the pedicle, or base, of the flap. The side opposite the base is called the free margin. Because the adequacy of the subdermal plexus varies from location to location, the area of skin that can be supported by the vessels of the pedicle also varies. As a general rule, a random-pattern flap with a length not exceeding the width of the pedicle (in other words, a rhomboid) is considered to be reliable with respect to blood supply. This is the 1:1 rule. It does not always apply, however. For example, it is too cautious for the face and too bold for the foot. Observation of this rule and the need to protect the pedicle from undue distortion that would impair blood flow through the subdermal plexus clearly limit the range of applications for the random-pattern flap.

The relatively inadequate blood supply of a random-pattern flap may be enhanced by a "delay" procedure[86,220,338] and will often allow a flap larger than the 1:1 rule to be rotated. In a delay procedure, the margins of the flap are incised and the incisions are sutured. This causes enhancement of the vascularity via the pedicle by interrupting that blood supply to the skin of the flap through the incised margins. The optimal time of delay has been shown to be around 10 days. During that time, both arteries and veins that were random become enlarged and oriented parallel to the axis of the pedicle. They are therefore better able to support the flap when it is transferred.

Axial-Pattern Flaps

When a flap receives its blood supply from a single, constant vessel, it is termed *axial pattern*. Such a single vessel is materially larger than those of the subdermal plexus. For example, the superficial circumflex iliac artery that supplies

Table 47-2
TYPES OF FLAPS

	Random	Axial
Local	Transposition	Axial flag
		FDMA
		SDMA
		Reversed dorsal metacarpal
	Rotation	Advancement—V-Y (Moberg)
		Advancement—rectangular
	Regional	Cross-finger
	Thenar	Neurovascular island
		Fillet
		Scapular
		Forearm
		Reversed PIA
		Latissimus
Distant	Infraclavicular	Groin
	Cross-arm	

FDMA, first dorsal metacarpal artery; SDMA, second dorsal metacarpal artery; PIA, posterior interosseous artery.

the groin flap (see following description) has an average diameter of 2 mm, or five times that of the largest subdermal vessel. Although Poiseuille's law of flow in rigid tubes cannot be applied precisely to blood vessels, it indicates that flow would be approximately 625 times greater through the axial vessel of the groin flap than through a subdermal vessel. The area of skin supplied by such an axial vessel is termed a *vascular territory.*

Where the vascular territories of two axial pedicles meet is termed a *watershed,* and the small arteries that cross it, *choke vessels.* In these areas, veins have no valves and can be said to allow blood to oscillate between territories. Occlusion of one of the two pedicles results in a shift of the watershed toward the site of occlusion, extending the vascular territory of the other, open pedicle. In raising an axial-pattern flap, it is safe to increase the length of the flap beyond the known vascular territory by the amount that would constitute a random-pattern flap. That is, a safe axial-pattern flap equals the normal vascular territory of the flap with a 1:1 extension on the distal portion of the flap.

The vessel of an axial-pattern flap may be purely cutaneous (Fig. 47-28A), supplying skin alone and proceeding directly to it. The superficial circumflex iliac artery to the groin flap is such a vessel. In reaching its cutaneous territory, the axial vessel may first supply fascia. In such circumstances, the vessel commonly reaches the fascia by

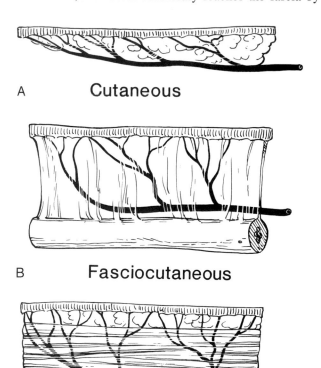

A **Cutaneous**

B **Fasciocutaneous**

C **Musculocutaneous**

FIGURE 47-28. Axial-pattern flaps are either cutaneous (**A**), fasciocutaneous (**B**), or musculocutaneous (**C**) depending on the source of the major portion of their blood supply. Fasciocutaneous vessels commonly run in intermuscular septa and therefore supply the periosteum of underlying bone. The flap can be taken with a segment of that bone where necessary. (From the Christine Kleinert Institute for Hand and Microsurgery, Inc., with permission.)

running in an intermuscular septum. Because this is attached to bone, a segment of bone may be taken with skin and be vascularized by the same pedicle. Axial flaps whose vessels first pass through fascia are termed *fasciocutaneous* (see Fig. 47-28B). As with the musculocutaneous flap, fascia may be transferred without skin but not skin without fascia. Such a flap is the lateral arm flap supplied by the posterior radial collateral artery. The axial vessel may first supply muscle (see Fig. 47-28C). The secondary vessels to the overlying skin are multiple,[24] so the muscle must be taken with the skin to ensure survival of the skin, but the muscle may be transferred without skin. Such flaps have been called *musculocutaneous, myocutaneous,* and *myodermal.* An example of this type of flap is the latissimus dorsi flap, supplied by the thoracodorsal artery.

Axial-pattern flaps clearly have several advantages over random-pattern flaps. The 1:1 ratio can be disregarded in flaps with an axial vessel. Axial pattern flaps have a blood supply superior to that of random flaps. It has been shown experimentally that axial-pattern flaps resist infection better than do random ones.[258] Because axial flaps can be made longer, they can cover a larger primary defect. In addition, the flap tissue adjacent to the pedicle need not be applied to the defect, permitting much more freedom of movement of the part to which the flap is attached. This bridge segment between the primary and secondary defects may be sutured free edge to free edge, creating a tube that closes off all exposed subcutaneous tissue: a tube pedicle. A further advantage of the axial-pattern flap is that the pedicle can be made much narrower, even to the point of reducing it to the (neuro)arteriovenous bundle itself, in which event it is called an island pedicle flap. This permits much more movement of the flap than is possible with a wide skin pedicle. Finally, with the advent of reliable microvascular technology, the pedicle can be divided and anastomosed to vessels adjacent to the primary defect: the so-called free flap.

The disadvantage of an axial-pattern flap is that its vascular pedicle must always be preserved at the time of elevation of the flap; at that first stage it cannot be thinned to the same degree as a random-pattern flap that depends on the subdermal vessels. The vascular advantages of the axial flap are lost if the pedicle is divided in the process of thinning the flap. Indeed, in those instances in which skin from the bridge segment is to be used on an area adjacent to the primary defect, it is prudent to divide the artery in the pedicle 1 week before complete detachment. This constitutes a delay of sorts, because it promotes increased blood flow across the inset wound into the primary defect.

STAGING OF FLAPS

Flaps that come from skin adjacent to the primary defect are called local and require only one operative procedure for their completion. Flaps that come from elsewhere on the limb and commonly require two stages are called regional flaps. Those from other parts of the body are called distant flaps. With the exception of free flaps, all distant flaps require at least two stages for completion. In the first, the flap is raised and applied, attached, or inset. In the second, the pedicle is divided and the free margins inset. In certain instances in which the blood supply is doubtful after division of the pedicle, the final inset may be left until a third stage. This may be necessary if the most distant portion of the divided pedicle has questionable vascularity (as in a pedicled groin flap transfer).

Preparation of the Wound for Flap Transfer

The wound to which a flap is to be applied is called the *primary defect*, or *recipient site*. This may be simply the wound created by trauma or a wound created by excision of a lesion. However, the skin margins are rarely perfect in a traumatic injury and generally the wound margins should be excised back to healthy skin before flap transfer. Similarly, it is important to re-create the original defect in secondary reconstruction and all scarred skin should be excised so that the flap will be sutured to healthy margins. A pattern of this final primary defect may be taken for future use. This is easily done by marking the margins with ink and taking an imprint of this with a pliable, nonporous material (e.g., a piece of Esmarch bandage), the surface of which has been moistened with alcohol. The wound from which the flap is taken is termed the *secondary defect*. The secondary defect may be closed directly, as in a groin flap, or may require application of a skin graft, as in a cross-finger flap. The region from which a skin graft is taken is called the *donor site.*

RAISING A FLAP

Between the vascular strata defined earlier (subdermis, subcutaneous tissue, fascia, and muscle) lie relatively avascular planes. It is in these planes that the dissection of the elected flap should proceed. It is evident that to attain these planes it is necessary to cut through the vessels of the more superficial strata. Thus, in raising a fascial flap, one must first incise the subdermal and subcutaneous plexus and then the fascia. Only when the surgeon has cut through the peripheral ramifications of the vessels from which the flap obtains its blood supply is he or she in the correct plane. To be one plane too superficial results in division of the vessel, or branches of the vessel, supplying the flap. To be one plane too deep results in a time-consuming, often bloody, and entirely unnecessary struggle.

Applied tension plays a major role in flap dissection. Once the marginal incision has been carried down to the correct plane for dissection, skin hooks or stay sutures are applied to the corners of the flap. Firm upward traction away from the bed displays the plane for dissection. Often this contains only loose areolar tissue that can be stroked away with a knife. Care must be taken not to create a "cave" beneath the flap, that is, a central recess between two marginal pillars of unincised skin, muscle, or fascia. No tension can be applied to the tissues in such a cave, and dissection therein may result in damage to the pedicle. Rather, the marginal pillars are incised progressively in such a way as to avoid caves and permit tension to be applied evenly, thereby protecting the pedicle. Tension on a flap lifts the pedicle off the floor of the secondary defect, on which the knife is dissecting, into the roof formed by the inclined vascular stratum. If dissection proceeds far enough, a point will be reached where the pedicle emerges through the floor to gain

the roof. At that point, the surgeon decides whether to proceed. To do so requires dissection of the pedicle. All progress thus far is best made with a scalpel. A scalpel is the instrument of choice both to incise the vascular strata and to dissect the planes, provided that appropriate tension can be applied to the tissues. Cutting with a knife is a result of two opposing forces: the pressure applied to the knife and the resistance offered by the tissues. The traction applied to a flap produces, and varies, that resistance. It therefore plays a primary role in determining which tissue is cut and which is not. This is why the blade must always be equally sharp and why the assistant who holds the flap must do so at the same tension first applied by the surgeon. If the assistant cannot do so, the surgeon must apply the necessary tension by grasping and lifting surrounding tissues with dissecting forceps as he or she proceeds.

Scissors provide both the pressure and the resistance required to cut tissue. They are required when the surgeon cannot efficiently control the relationship between tissue tension and knife pressure. When scissors are introduced closed into the tissues and then opened under gentle pressure to clear planes, they can be both precise and innocuous. They create and enter caves, defining structures to be preserved and those to be divided. When scissors are introduced open and then closed to cut, they are less precise than a knife and can do harm in the hands of even the most experienced surgeon. It is therefore important when using scissors that the surgeon see both surfaces of the tissue to be divided so that he or she is confident what tissues are included between the jaws of the scissors. This often requires that closed-to-open scissor dissection proceed until the instrument can be seen through the tissue to be cut. Such scissor dissection is required as a vascular pedicle is mobilized. Although it has been shown that metal clips are not secure and that bipolar coagulation may harm the pedicle,[282] both are routinely used in dissecting the pedicle. The clips must be applied with sufficient force to ensure that they will not slip. When dividing small vessels between surgical clips, it is helpful to leave a small amount of tissue surrounding the vessels. This approach gives adequate tissue purchase for the clips so that they do not fall off. The setting on the control box of the coagulator must be of adequate temperature to allow coagulation and sealing of the vessel. The pedicle (i.e., the main vessel) is insulated by holding the branch with smooth forceps between the pedicle and the point of coagulation.

LOCAL FLAPS

Because they have identical or similar qualities to the skin lost, local flaps are the most desirable means of providing cover for a defect.[194] They are, however, severely limited in their availability. This is because there is relatively little skin on the hand and because much of it must remain inviolate to preserve function. The skin of the webs, for example, should never be used for flaps, nor should areas of daily contact. Some skin, such as that of the palm, will not move to the extent necessary for most local flap design. The surgeon must carefully weigh these considerations in selecting a flap. "Lines of maximum extensibility"[195] around which the flap should be planned are selected by pinching the skin (Fig. 47-29). These are the lines along which skin is most

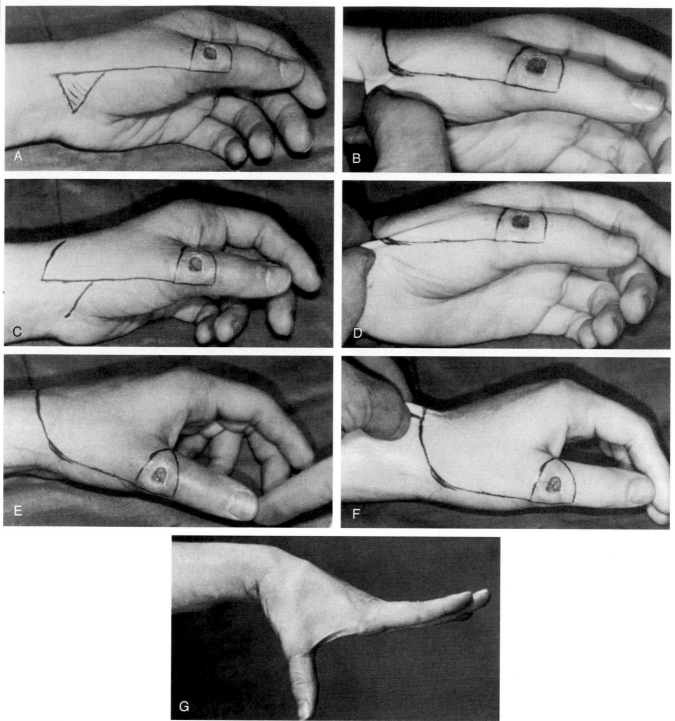

FIGURE 47-29. Testing for maximum extensibility in choosing the best area from which to obtain tissue to close the ulcer on the dorsal aspect of the thumb. **A and B,** The use of the Burow's triangle with a sliding transposition flap would require tissue to be available in the longitudinal axis on the palmar surface of the wrist. **C and D,** If it were elected to use a "Z"-plasty to advance the tissue by the lengthening of the central limb, then tissue would need to be available around the circumference of the wrist, since lengthening of the central limb requires shortening of the transverse axis. **E and F,** If a rotation flap were selected, then tissue would be required on the opposite aspect of the rotation flap from the defect, that is, in the circumference of the wrist on its dorsal aspect. **G,** A rotation flap was selected and satisfactory healing achieved.

available and therefore pinches up more easily. This should be done with the hand in various positions to ensure that function will not be impaired. For example, the skin of the dorsum appears superfluous in extension but not in flexion.

There are three types of local flap: transposition, rotation, and advancement. In the advancement flap, the pedicle is

that side of the flap opposite the primary defect. In transposition and rotation designs, the flap moves laterally relative to the pedicle to cover the defect. These two differ in that the transposition flap leaves a secondary defect that is closed either directly or by application of new skin cover, whereas the rotation flap leaves no secondary defect, the flap skin being stretched to close the primary defect. This is achieved by differential suturing, in which a slightly smaller amount of the flap edge than of the edge of the bed is included between each two adjacent sutures, thereby advancing the flap. Transposition and advancement flaps may be random or axial pattern in design. The vascular basis of the axial pattern may be simply a subcutaneous pedicle rich in small vessels[82] or, more reliably, a single known vessel. The advantage of the axial pattern, apart from its potentially larger area and greater reliability owing to superior circulation, is the fact that its pedicle can be reduced to the vessels alone, giving greater mobility. In the advancement flap, this simply permits more advancement, a gain that can be measured in millimeters. In the axial-pattern transposition flap, however, the gain in mobility is limited only by the length of pedicle that can be developed. The longer the pedicle, the more the flap becomes a vascular island flap rather than a simple transposition. The distinction between a long axial transposition flap and a vascular island is arbitrary. For the purposes of this chapter, a flap is classified as a vascular island when the pedicle is the proper digital artery or larger.

Transposition Flaps

Random Pattern

The theory behind transposition flaps has been analyzed in some detail.[193] There are two basic types of random-pattern transposition flap.

Type I: Transposition Leaving a Secondary Defect Requiring Skin Cover

The basic design of this first type and the problems likely to be encountered in its use can be illustrated by using an equilateral model (Fig. 47-30). The first step in planning

such a flap is to triangulate the primary defect, either in fact or conceptually. In the equilateral model (FLA in Fig. 47-30[1]), one side of the defect is extended by its own length (to P). From the end of that extension, another line of equal length (PS) is drawn parallel to the nearest side (AF) of the primary defect. The end of that line (S) is the most important in the whole design and is called the *pivot point*. As the flap is raised and transposed, it is this point around which the flap moves into the primary defect. By measuring from the pivot point to the far corner of the defect (S to L) and then to the diagonally opposite corner of the flap (S to A), one determines the amount the flap must stretch to cover the defect. The latter dimension (SA) is consequently called the *critical line*. In the simple equilateral model, the critical line would have to stretch by 75% of its original length to achieve closure of the primary defect (see Fig. 47-30[2]), which is beyond the physical capabilities of normal skin.[183] Several solutions are available. Making the flap wider (at the line AP) will decrease the stretch on the flap as the flap becomes wider (see Fig. 47-30[3]). Making the flap longer (at FA and SP) will decrease tension after transposition, but this is at the expense of a narrower flap (>1:1 ratio) and with an increasing dog-ear at the point of rotation.[190] If an extension cut is made (to E in Fig. 47-31), the critical line is lengthened and the stretch on the flap decreased. A back-cut at the base of the flap can be made (SB in Fig. 47-32) that will reduce the stretch in the critical line. This can compromise the vascularity of the flap if not done carefully, however.

Type II: Transposition With Direct Closure of the Secondary Defect

In this second variety of transposition flap, the flap passes across a "promontory" of normal, undisturbed skin (RMI in Fig. 47-33) to gain the primary defect. If the secondary defect is then covered with imported skin, the same rules apply as in type I, with the pivot point and the critical line playing identical roles to those described earlier. If, how-

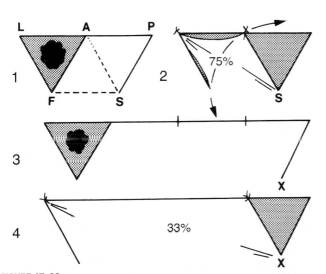

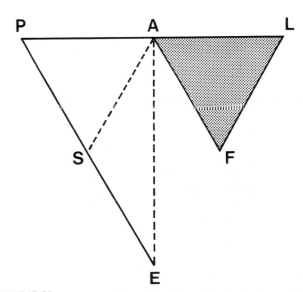

FIGURE 47-30. Transposition flap. In this equilateral model (1), all lines are equal in length. S is the pivot point and SA the critical line, because this is the skin that will have to stretch as the flap is transposed (2) into the primary defect. The lengthening on the critical line in an equilateral design is 75%. One device to reduce the stretch on the critical line is to make the flap wider. If, as here, the flap is three times as wide (3), the stretch required in the critical line (4) is 33%. (Modified from Lister GD: The theory of the transposition flap and its practical application in the hand. Clin Plast Surg 8:115-128, 1981.)

FIGURE 47-31. Extension cut. An extension cut has been made here from S to E of the same length as all other lines in this design. The resultant stretch required in the critical line, now EA, is 16%. (Modified from Lister GD: The theory of the transposition flap and its practical application in the hand. Clin Plast Surg 8:115-128, 1981.)

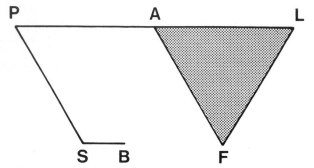

FIGURE 47-32. Back-cut. By moving the pivot point S toward the primary defect by the incision SB, the stretch on the critical line is progressively reduced. This back-cut also reduces the circulation to this random pattern flap. (Modified from Lister GD: The theory of the transposition flap and its practical application in the hand. Clin Plast Surg 8:115-128, 1981.)

ever, the secondary defect is closed directly, other factors become important. The pivot point of such a flap must be sutured to the tip of the promontory between the primary and secondary defects. To achieve this, either the pivot point or the promontory, or both, must move. The key to the planning of such a flap is to ensure that such approximation is possible. In this design of transposition flap, little or no stretch occurs in the flap itself. The critical line is of no consequence. The most disciplined and geometric examples of this second type of transposition flap are the flaps of Limberg and Dufourmentel.[195] In both, the original defect is rhomboid and therefore equilateral. The transverse diagonal of the Limberg flap defect is equal to any of its sides. To create the flap, the transverse diagonal (HM in Fig. 47-33[1]) is produced in either direction by an equal distance (MI). The second side of the transposition flap (ID) is then drawn parallel to either of the two sides of the primary defect (MO or MR), with which the last line is in contact. It follows that there are four potential sites where the flap can be created for this single defect. Unlike that of the Limberg, the transverse diagonal of the defect of the Dufourmentel flap can be of any length. To design the flap, both the transverse diagonal and one or the other of the adjacent sides are produced (GT to G' and NT to N' in Fig. 47-33[3]). The resulting angle between these lines is bisected by the first side of the flap (TX), which is equal in length to any one of the sides of the basic design. From its end, the second side of the transposition flap (XC) is drawn parallel to the longitudinal axis of the defect (UN) and of equal length to the first side. As with the Limberg, there are four possible flaps for each defect. In both the Limberg and Dufourmentel designs, the surgeon has two choices to make. The first is to choose the orientation of the defect, if it is to be created by excision. This may be determined by the shape of the lesion, for appropriate tumor clearance should be taken while discarding as little normal skin as possible. The second is to choose among the four flaps available for that defect. One or more may not be available because the skin is unsatisfactory or because it is of functional importance. Otherwise, the surgeon should select the flap that permits the most easy approximation of the pivot point to the promontory (D to M in Fig. 47-33[1] and C to T in Fig. 47-33[3]). This selection can be made by simply pinching the skin to find the line of maximal extensibility. If the

primary defect is to be created by the surgeon, the flap can be planned in reverse by placing both the pivot point and the tip of the promontory on that line. Once the flap has been raised, approximation of the pivot point to the promontory both places the flap in position and closes the secondary defect.

All random-pattern transposition flaps are variants of one of these two basic designs or a combination of the two. In the first, there is little local skin to spare and the elasticity of the skin along the critical line is important. In the second, slack skin allows movement of the pivot point to the promontory, and little stretch of the flap is required. In many flaps, both elasticity and movement of the pivot point play a role.

Variants of Type I

The Gibraiel flap,[110] described previously as a simple rotation flap, is a pure variant of the type I transposition flap and is so presented by the original author, moving skin from the lateral aspect of the digit to the flexor surface. There is little or no movement of the pivot point, and a full-thickness graft is applied to the secondary defect. In the "sliding" flap described by Smith[307] to cover the dorsal aspect of the proximal interphalangeal (PIP) joint, the defect is not triangulated. Rather, the apex (F in Fig. 47-30) is left curvilinear so that the resultant dog-ear permits movement of the joint.

The "cocked-hat" flap,[13] attributed to Gillies,[273] is a more complex variant used to lengthen the thumb. A dorsal transverse incision at the base of the shortened thumb permits dissection of the skin cover of the entire thumb on a palmar pedicle. The flap is transposed on this pedicle, a bone graft of the maximal length that the flap will accommodate is inserted, and a skin graft is placed on the secondary defect. (This is not an advancement flap, because the pedicle is not on the opposite side of the flap from the defect, and movement is achieved by pivoting around the pedicle and not by stretching or elongating it.)

Variants of Type II

"Z"-Plasty. The "Z"-plasty is a form of type II flap in which the flap and the promontory of skin form the two transposition flaps.[101] Conversely, the rhomboid flap may be considered a specialized "Z"-plasty, with the "Z" being formed by the sides of the triangular flap and one contiguous side of the primary defect (e.g., RMID in Fig. 47-33[1]). The sides of a standard stereometric as opposed to planimetric[279] "Z"-plasty should always be of equal length, but the angles vary according to the needs of the situation and the local skin topography. The angles of the design may also differ. As the angles increase, so does the lengthening that occurs along the line of the central limb of the design when the flaps are transposed.[160] The commonly used 60-degree "Z"-plasty theoretically results in 75% lengthening along the line of the central limb (Fig. 47-34). The skin that is introduced into the line of the central limb is derived from the transverse axis of that line. Said another way, skin must be available lateral to the central limb before a "Z"-plasty can be used. If sufficient skin is not present for one large "Z"-plasty, multiple "Z"-plasties can be used in series (Fig. 47-35), because the longitudinal gain is

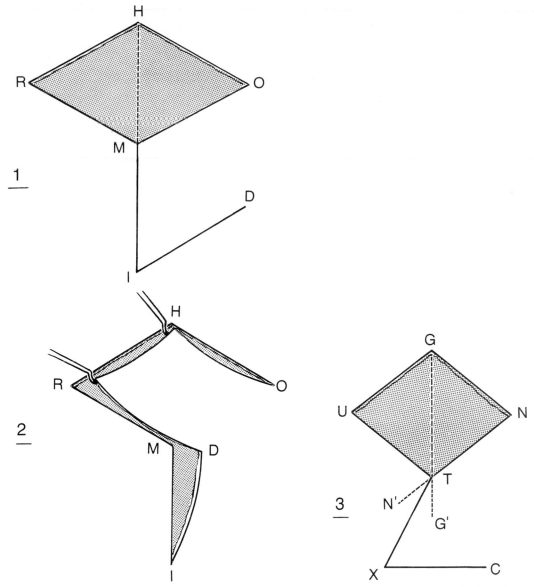

FIGURE 47-33. Rhomboid flap design. **1,** In the Limberg design, all dimensions of the rhomboid that form the primary defect HOMR are equal, including the transverse diagonal HM. This has been extended by the same length to I and the line ID drawn parallel to MO. **2,** The flap is transposed by moving the pivot point D to the promontory M. If this can be achieved, the flap will fit. **3,** In the Dufourmentel flap, the transverse diagonal can be of any length. The transverse diagonal GT and one of the adjacent sides NT are extended to G′ and N′, respectively. The angle that they form is bisected by a line of equal length to one of the sides of the primary defect TX. XC is then drawn parallel to the longitudinal diameter diagonal UN. Transposition is performed by approximating the pivot point C to the promontory T. (Modified from Lister GD: The theory of the transposition flap and its practical application in the hand. Clin Plast Surg 8:115-128, 1981.)

aggregate whereas the transverse loss is not. The following are important points in technique (Fig. 47-36):

1. The angles and limbs should be measured with a ruler and protractor (see Fig. 47-36A and B). When this is not done, mistakes are made, the most common being to cut the angles at 45 degrees but believing them to be 60 degrees.
2. The incisions of the "Z"-plasty should be cut and tested in sequence (see Fig. 47-36C and D).

First, the central limb and one side limb are incised. The flap created is raised and carried across the central limb with a skin hook. If the side limb cut on the flap can be brought by at least half its length across the central limb (see Fig.

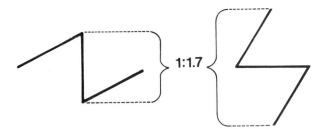

FIGURE 47-34. Standard 60-degree "Z"-plasty. Here all limbs of the "Z"-plasty are of equal length, and the angles between the limbs are 60 degrees. When the flaps are transposed, the lengthening that is achieved along the line of the central limb is 70% to 75% of its original length.

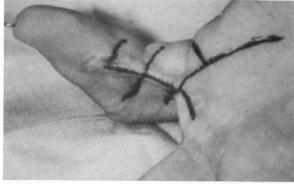

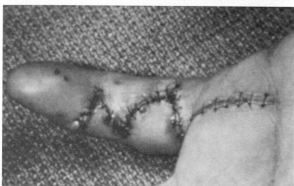

FIGURE 47-35. Multiple "Z"-plasty. Considerable lengthening is required in this scar, and therefore three "Z"-plasties have been planned in series. The resultant lengthening will be along the line of the central limb. The shortening will be one third of that lengthening and be distributed evenly along the transverse axes of the three "Z"-plasties. In the second figure, it is seen that only two of the "Z"-plasties were cut on the finger, and the necessary lengthening was achieved. (Modified from Lister GD: The theory of the transposition flap and its practical application in the hand. Clin Plast Surg 8:115-128, 1981.)

CRITICAL POINTS: "Z"-PLASTY

INDICATIONS

- Scar contracture, especially on volar surface of fingers
- Minimal web space contracture

PREOPERATIVE EVALUATION

- Must examine surrounding skin for elasticity and scars
- Generally should not "Z"-plasty grafted skin

PEARLS

- Central limb of "Z" goes along line of scar
- Lateral limbs should be designed in areas with loose skin
- Limbs should be 60 degrees to central limb
  - Tendency is to make them 45 degrees
- Avoid sewing the flaps back where they came from

TECHNICAL POINTS

- Central tight scar should be excised.
- Tips of small flaps should not be grasped with forceps.

- Base of flap should be thicker than tip when elevating.
- Cut only enough skin so that flap will transpose without tension.
- Avoid placing sutures in midportion of flap.
- "Tip" suture (half-buried horizontal mattress) for tip of flaps.
- Only use enough sutures to hold flaps in place.

PITFALLS

- Poor design
- Flaps with scar at base
- Undermining base of flap so that it is thinner than tip
- Suturing flaps under too much tension

POSTOPERATIVE CARE

- If flaps fit easily, immobilization may not be necessary.
- Massage and stretching are begun when area is healed.

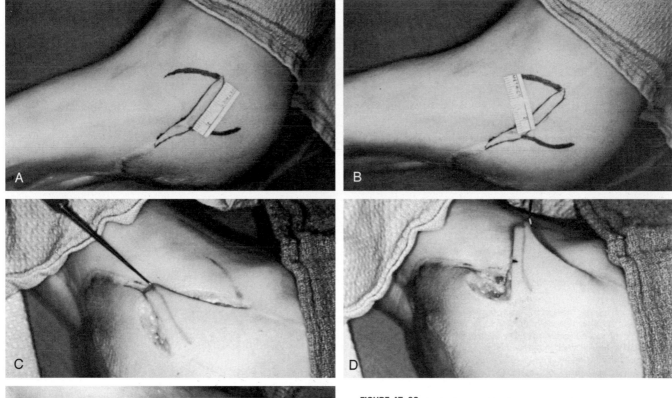

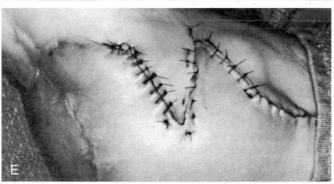

FIGURE 47-36. In designing this 60-degree "Z"-plasty, all measurements are equal; that is, the initial central limb of the "Z" (**A**) is the same length as each of the side limbs but is also the distance (**B**) between the tip of one of the side limbs and the end of the central limb from which the other side limb originates. This will create a 60-degree "Z"-plasty. The first flap has been cut (**C**) and is transposed across the central limb (**D**). The center point of the side limb has been marked with a tick on its margin. It can be seen that this can be carried with comfort well across the central limb. The initial design is therefore satisfactory and can even be made larger if wished. **E**, The flaps are transposed and sutured into position without problems.

47-36D), there is sufficient tissue transversely, and the design was well chosen (see Fig. 47-36E). If it goes farther, a larger "Z"-plasty would work if more lengthening is required. Such a larger design can be made simply by lengthening both initial cuts and testing again. If this first flap can be carried less than halfway across the central limb, the design was too ambitious and must be modified. Because only two limbs have been cut, this modification can be done relatively easily by shortening both the proposed central limb and the as yet uncut second side limb. The excessively long first side limb is simply shortened with one or two stitches.

Four-Flap "Z"-Plasty. To gain greater lengthening along the central limb, the angles of the "Z"-plasty may be increased. When 120-degree "Z"-plasty flaps are transposed, the resultant central limb lengthening is theoretically 164%. However, flaps with angles much over 60 degrees are difficult to transpose; the pivot points cannot be brought to meet the promontories. This difficulty can be overcome by dividing each flap into two (Fig. 47-37). For example, in the split 120-degree "Z"-plasty described 75 years ago by Limberg,[190] four 60-degree flaps are created. Once again, the

design is best created by repeatedly using a ruler and protractor or, better still, calipers set to the same length, nine times in all. Such four-flap "Z"-plasties are applicable only in very acute contractures, often in the first web. The angle at which the dorsal skin meets the palmar at the web—the ridge angle—must not exceed 30 degrees, or the flaps will not move sufficiently.

Other Types. Further combinations and extensions of the type II design include the two- and three-flap rhomboid,[141] the double-"Z" rhomboid,[62,64] and the interdigital butterfly flap.[297] The latter consists of two opposed "Z"-plasties with a small intervening "Y-V" advancement flap. The "butterfly" is related to the "seagull,"[310] also described for web release.

Departing from the rigid discipline of geometric design but adhering to the same principles, free-hand transposition flaps of random-pattern design in which the secondary defect is closed directly are also of type II. Such are the flaps designed in a digit to be transposed from dorsal or lateral to palmar, as described by Green and Dominguez[119] and by Ogunro.[249] These may be used to close defects caused by either injury or surgical release of scar contractures.

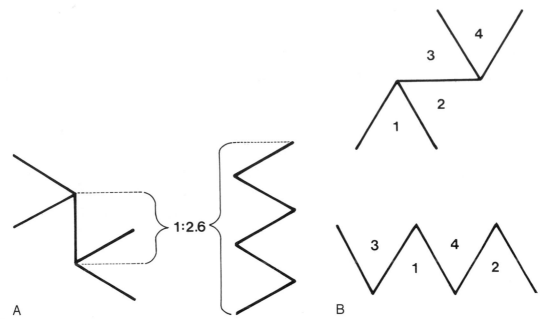

FIGURE 47-37. Four-flap "Z"-plasty. **A,** In the four-flap "Z"-plasty, all measurements are equal; that is, each limb of the design is of equal length but so also are the distances between any two adjacent points in the design. When the flaps are transposed, the two 120-degree angles are closed. As a result, the distance between the points at either end of the initial central limb is some 264% of its original length. **B,** The transposition that is achieved is shown by numbering the flaps. It will be seen that the two 120-degree angles are closed, putting 2 in the right-hand incision and 3 in the left-hand incision and interdigitating flaps 1 and 4.

Because it is possible to bring the pivot point to the promontory tip, there is little or no tension on the flap itself.

Flaps With Both Type I and Type II Features

In these flaps, some movement of the pivot point occurs, but there is insufficient skin available to allow complete closure of the secondary defect, which itself requires imported skin cover. For this reason the flap is stretched to reach the primary defect, and measurement of the critical line as it is before and as it would be after transposition remains an important part of the planning of the flap. The potential movement of the pivot point and the resultant reduction in the stretch required of the critical line can be assessed by applying traction to a skin hook impaled in the proposed location of the pivot point.

Flaps of this type include flaps from the dorsum of the digit to the palmar surface used in releasing Dupuytren's contracture,[124] flaps from the lateral aspect of the digit to resurface the dorsal aspect of the PIP joint after burns (as described by Lueders and Shapiro[205]), and flaps used in release of adduction contractures of the first web space and derived from the dorsum of the index finger[315] and the dorsum of the thumb.[289,324] In the latter two designs, the first web is released through a single incision traversing the web and continuing around on to the dorsum of the web to run just to the radial side of the second metacarpal. The pivot point of the proposed flap is then selected: in the thumb, on the radial side just proximal to the metacarpophalangeal (MP) joint (Fig. 47-38); or on the index finger, to the ulnar side of the neck of the second metacarpal (Fig. 47-39). Moving the pivot point with a hook as described earlier, the length of the critical line as it will be after transposition is then measured from the pivot point to the proximal, palmar end of the releasing incision. In so doing, care must be taken

to follow the edge of the wound in the web and not to go directly across the defect dorsal to palmar. This length is then transferred to the donor digit. If that length cannot be accommodated because the digit proximal to the nail bed is too short, then the distance by which it fails is the amount by which the flap will have to stretch. Devices such as the back-cut and extension-cut can be used, as described for type I.

Types I and II Used in Combination

Two combinations have been described to resurface the stump of an amputated thumb. Argamaso[5] used a radially based type I transposition and covered the defect with a transposition flap from the dorsum of the index finger, as described earlier. Winspur[347] used an ulnar-based transposition advancement, preserving both neurovascular bundles. He moved the tissue and deepened the first web space by a simple "Z"-plasty designed with the central limb along the margin of the web.

Axial Pattern

Vessels that serve to enhance the vascularity of transposition flaps have been isolated at the level of the distal and proximal phalanges. Dorsal digital branches of the digital artery and nerve at the level of the distal phalanx were first described by Holevich.[134] They form the pedicle for dorsolateral flaps transposed to cover digital pulp defects as described by Flint and Harrison,[89] Lesavoy,[186] and notably Joshi.[152-155] Pho[264] demonstrated similar vessels arising from the radial digital artery of the thumb and used flaps based on those vessels and the radial digital nerve and artery to resurface the pulp of the thumb. He states that skin can be taken from the MP joint out to within millimeters of the nail fold but advises that a skin bridge be retained until tourniquet release demonstrates satisfactory flow.

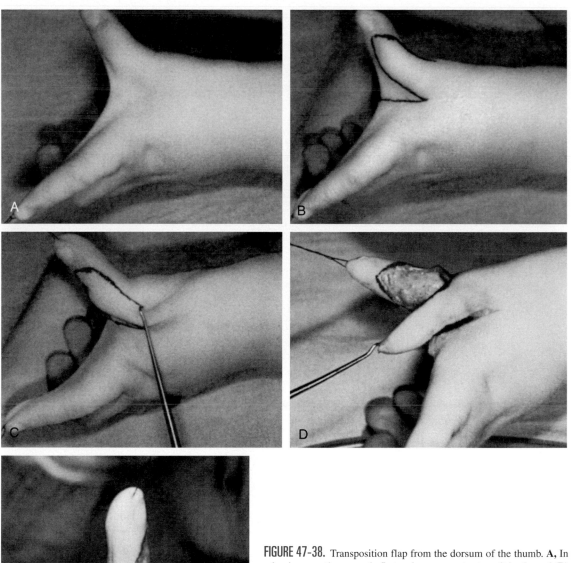

FIGURE 47-38. Transposition flap from the dorsum of the thumb. **A,** In releasing an arthrogrypotic first web space contracture, it is planned (**B**) to incise down the center point of the web both dorsally and on the palmar aspect, where the incision will be carried across the palmar aspect of the MP joint to release the flexion contracture of the thumb. **C,** By moving the pivot point with a hook and measuring from this point to the far side of the flexion surface of the thumb (i.e., the end of the planned releasing incision; see **E**) and then measuring from the pivot point to the tip of the flap, it can be appreciated that some, but not much, stretch will be required in the flap. **D,** The flap is raised and (**E**) transposed into position, widening the web space and also covering the release of the flexion contracture. The secondary defect is covered with a full-thickness skin graft.

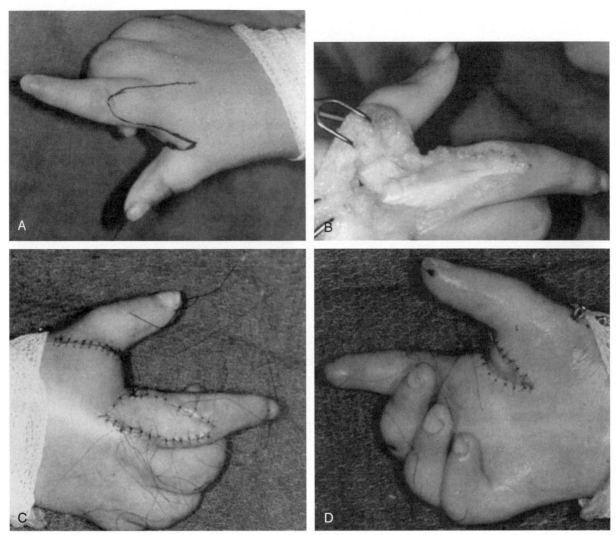

FIGURE 47-39. Transposition flap from the index finger. **A,** The flap is drawn out in combination with releasing the first web space in a patient with arthrogryposis. **B,** Incision and raising of the flap reveals tight bands in the first web space, which are released. **C,** The flap has been transposed and a thick split-thickness skin graft applied to the secondary defect. **D,** The thumb has been pinned in abduction, and the flap can be seen to reach to the level of the superficial palmar arch.

In 1973, both Vilain and Dupuis[343] and Iselin[143] described a flag flap raised on the dorsum of the middle phalanx and so called because the pedicle, narrowed by a generous backcut, was further mobilized by parallel incisions resembling the pole of a flag. No arterial pedicle was described for this flap; however, it is undoubtedly based on the dorsal branches of the palmar digital arteries.

The skin of the dorsum of the proximal phalanx, especially of the index and middle fingers, has been shown to receive axial flow from the branches of the first and second dorsal metacarpal arteries, vessels that are present in 90% and 97% of hands, respectively.[80] Both of these vessels arise from the radial artery or its communications with the dorsal carpal arch, the posterior interosseous artery, the deep palmar arch, and the ulnar digital artery of the thumb. Stated more simply, both vessels arise from arteries around the base of the second metacarpal. They pursue courses either immediately above or immediately below the fascia of the interosseous muscles. At the web space, the second dorsal metacarpal artery has a constant anastomosis with the palmar metacarpal artery, which is doubly significant in flap

design. This communicating vessel must be divided if a longer arc of rotation is to be achieved on a proximally based flap, and it also serves as the axial vessel of reversed dorsal metacarpal flaps.[211,267] According to the dissections of Johnson and Cohen,[148] the branches of these vessels supply the dorsal skin no further than the PIP joint. The venous drainage of these flaps is excellent, being through either end of the proximal venous arcade, which is of very large caliber[237] (Fig. 47-40). These dorsal vessels form the axial basis of four distinct flaps: the axial flag flap, the first dorsal metacarpal artery (FDMA) flap (or kite flap), the second dorsal metacarpal artery (SDMA) flap, and the reversed dorsal metacarpal flap. Those proximally based on the first dorsal metacarpal artery can readily transfer sensibility by incorporating the branches of the radial nerve to the dorsal skin.

Axial Flag Flap
This simple flap requires no pedicle dissection, because it is based on the web space of the donor finger. The dorsal metacarpal artery has been shown to be reliably present in

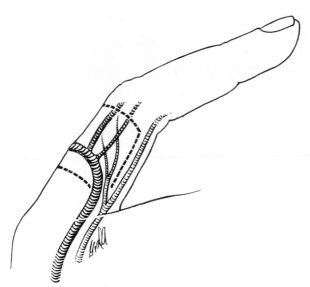

FIGURE 47-40. Axial flag flap. The axial flag flap receives its blood supply from a dorsal digital artery that originates either from the proper digital artery to that finger or from an extension of the dorsal metacarpal artery. Drainage is through the proximal venous arcade to the web space veins. (Modified from Lister GD: The theory of the transposition flap and its practical application in the hand. Clin Plast Surg 8:115-128, 1981.)

the second interspace, and less so in the others, but flag flaps can be safely raised from any of the webs. Because the pedicle need only be as wide as the vessels, the mobility in this flap is its single major advantage. From the dorsum of the middle finger, for example, it can be rotated to cover the dorsum of either the proximal phalanx of the index finger or the MP joint of either the index or middle finger (Fig. 47-41A). It can also, by being passed through the web

space, cover the palmar surface of either proximal phalanx of either MP joint (see Fig. 47-41B). Before commencing elevation of the flap, the presence of the vessel can be confirmed by Doppler examination.[127] As with the cross-finger flap, the entire skin of the dorsum of the selected proximal phalanx is raised (Fig. 47-42), from midlateral line to midlateral line, and from the proximal extension crease of the PIP joint distally to the level of the free margin of the web proximally. As with all random flaps, the plane of dissection is beneath the subcutaneous vascular stratum, leaving the loose paratenon on the extensor hood. The donor site will usually require a skin graft.

The Kite Flap (First Dorsal Metacarpal Artery)

This is an island pedicle flap proximally based on the first dorsal metacarpal artery and veins.[90,91] The skin flap is generally designed on the radial side of the distal portion of the second metacarpal and/or MP joint. With its pedicle fully dissected, it can reach the dorsum of the thumb to about the IP joint. The course of the vessel should be checked with a Doppler probe before elevation, but it runs over the first dorsal interosseous muscle from the radial artery as it courses distal to the anatomical snuff-box. The flap is elevated from distally to proximal. The skin incision is taken to the level of the fascia, and a wide swath of tissue is taken along the course of the artery to prevent damage to the draining veins. If a sensory flap is desired, the branch(es) of the superficial radial nerve to this area of skin may be taken with the pedicle. The fascia is carefully lifted off the first dorsal interosseous muscle to near its base to allow rotation of the flap on its pedicle. Once an adequate pedicle has been lifted, the flap can be taken under a skin bridge of the proximal thumb to reach the defect. The donor site will require closure with a skin graft.

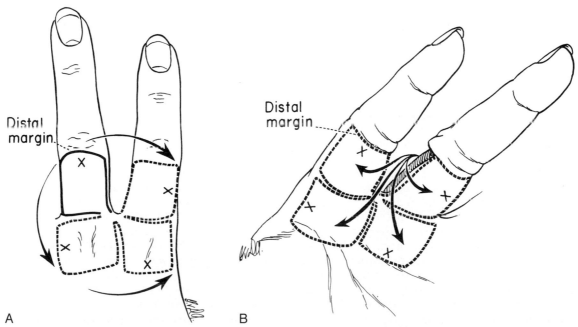

FIGURE 47-41. **A,** An axial flag flap raised on the dorsum of the middle finger can be rotated to cover defects on the proximal phalanx of the index finger or over the MP joint of either of those two digits. **B,** By carrying the flap through the web space, it can reach defects on the palmar surface of the MP joint of either the index or middle finger. (Modified from Lister GD: The theory of the transposition flap and its practical application in the hand. Clin Plast Surg 8:115-128, 1981.)

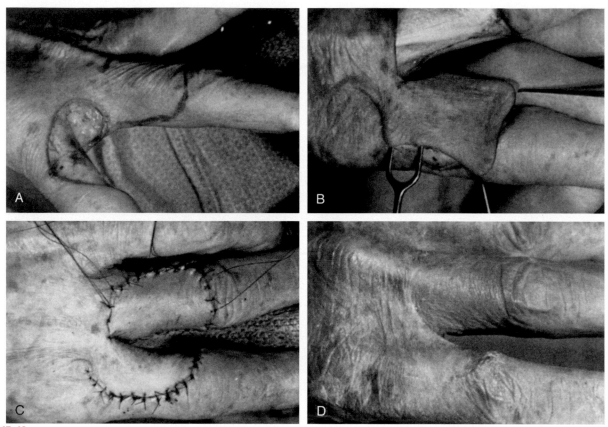

FIGURE 47-42. Axial flag flap. **A,** After resection of a squamous cell carcinoma that was adherent to the underlying digital nerve, and after nerve grafting, cover of a defect on the dorsal and ulnar aspects of the index finger is achieved by use of an axial flag flap. The pedicle is left relatively wide, but it can be reduced down to the vessels alone, as shown in Figure 47-72. **B,** The flap transposes with ease. **C,** The secondary defect is covered with a full-thickness skin graft. **D,** The result.

This flap also may be raised distally based on the perforator near the radial base of the second metacarpal.[92] The arc of rotation of this flap will allow coverage of the index finger to near the distal interphalangeal (DIP) joint. The donor site may be closed primarily (in smaller flaps) or with a skin graft.

The Second Dorsal Metacarpal Artery Flap

This flap is based on the second dorsal metacarpal artery and venous system in the second interspace. It may be proximally based for coverage of an adjacent dorsal finger or distally based. If it is raised on its proximal pedicle, the rotation point is based near the base of the second metacarpal. The skin off the dorsum of the middle finger proximal phalanx can be raised based on these vessels and transferred to the dorsum of the index MP joint for coverage.[108] The presence of the vessel is confirmed before elevation with a Doppler device. The dissection proceeds from distally and laterally. The tissue of the second intermetacarpal space is carefully dissected off the interosseous muscle to include the fascia. The dissection is continued proximally, and great care must be taken to prevent damage to the pedicle. The donor site can be closed with a full-thickness skin graft.

The reverse[211,267] dorsal metacarpal flap is raised in similar fashion but from the dorsal skin of the hand, using the communication between dorsal and palmar metacarpal arteries as the axial vessel. The proximal limit of this flap is the confluence between the extensor indicis proprius and extensor digitorum communis to the middle finger.[90] This flap is raised from proximal to distal and is based over the second intermetacarpal space. Its arc of rotation is generally limited to about the level of the PIP joint based on the pedicle in the second web space. Some authors have successfully transposed this flap more distally, however.[352] The donor site can sometimes be closed primarily or may require a skin graft.

Digital Artery Island Flaps

The digital artery island flap is based on the radial or ulnar digital artery of the finger. It is a distally based flap and has been described for repair of fingertip injuries.[169,175] Flow depends on the integrity of the palmar digital arch that lies beneath the palmar plate, and drainage depends on retrograde flow in the fine veins around the artery. It has the advantage of confining the reconstruction to the injured finger: This flap is most useful in the middle or ring fingers, because the digital vessels are codominant in these fingers and loss of one is unlikely to cause problems with later flow. The index and little fingers, in contrast, may have very small vessels on their radial and ulnar sides, respectively, which theoretically could lead to problems with cold intolerance after flap harvest.

When used for fingertip coverage, a pattern is made of the defect first and is used to draw an outline of the proposed flap near the base of the involved digit, centered over the digital vascular pedicle. The majority of the flap is taken from the lateral side of the finger, however, to avoid loss of the important palmar skin near the MP joint crease. The anterior border of the flap is incised down to the level of the tendon sheath. The distal portion of the incision is made along the midaxial line. The digital bundle is identified, and the digital vascular pedicle is dissected free from the digital nerve. The veins present the greatest challenge in dissection of this flap, because they are quite small and easily damaged. They may be entwined around the digital nerve and must be carefully removed, using bipolar cautery on a low setting to control branches. The vascular pedicle should not be skeletonized but rather taken with a small amount of surrounding tissue, again to avoid damaging the veins. This dissection is carried to a level just proximal to the DIP flexion crease, at which level there is usually adequate pedicle to allow easy rotation of the flap to the fingertip defect. The skin incision is carried all the way out to the tip, and the pedicle is carefully placed in this incision. If fascial fibers cause kinking of the pedicle, they must be released, but, again, damage to the venous structures in the pedicle must be avoided. The donor site is covered with a small split-thickness skin graft, usually taken from the medial upper arm.

This flap has several advantages over other pedicle flaps for fingertip coverage: damage is confined to a single finger, the finger may be mobilized sooner, and the cosmetic defect is minimal. We limit its use to the middle and ring fingers for the reasons outlined earlier, however. It provides an excellent option for coverage when one is presented with a significant loss of the palmar pulp of the distal finger, however.[92]

Rotation Flaps

All rotation flaps are random pattern. As with the basic transposition flap, the surgeon designs a rotation flap by triangulating the primary defect. Unlike the two basic designs of transposition flap, there is nothing geometric about the rotation flap. The base of the defect—the side opposite the angle that is to be closed—is extended in the direction from which the surgeon has determined that tissue is available. The line is continued in a gentle curve until the surgeon deems that, by differentially suturing the wound, the flap can be advanced to cover the defect. This determination is arbitrary and therefore requires experience; however, there are some general rules that can help. First, the flap should be made as large as is reasonably possible. Not only does this provide more tissue to stretch into the defect, but it also makes the differential suturing easier, more even, and therefore more acceptable aesthetically. Rotation flaps are almost always designed too small by those with little experience. Second, the availability of tissue should be checked in that area where two further devices may relax a tight flap, which is at the end of the flap incision and on the side of the incision opposite to the primary defect. It can be called the "critical area" (and is that surrounding 2X in Fig. 47-43). If skin is available there and the simple rotation flap does not move adequately, one of two steps can be taken. A back-cut can be made on the flap side of the incision at its far end and at right angles to it (see Fig. 47-43). The back-cut is opened fully, that is, to 180 degrees, and is sutured to the critical area previously shown to have some

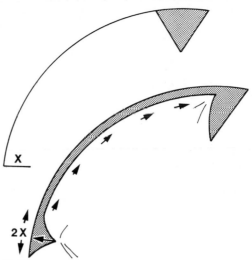

FIGURE 47-43. Rotation flap. The primary defect is triangulated and necessary gain is achieved by differential suturing of the two flap margins. Where the gain achieved is insufficient and there is skin available in the "critical area," that is, the area under 2X, a back-cut X may be cut that will lengthen the margin of the flap. (Modified from Lister GD: The theory of the transposition flap and its practical application in the hand. Clin Plast Surg 8:115-128, 1981.)

loose skin. By opening the back-cut thus, the length of that side of the rotation flap has been increased by twice the length of the back-cut. It follows that if the back-cut is made half the length of the base of the triangle that is the primary defect, no differential suturing will be required to close the defect. This is attractive, but the surgeon must remember two things: the back-cut reduces flap circulation as it is directed across the pedicle, and tissue must be available in the critical area to advance into the back-cut. The alternative step is the use of a Burow's triangle (Fig. 47-44). A Burow's triangle is normal skin that is excised to facilitate movement of a flap. In the case of a rotation flap, the triangle is excised from the critical area. Closure of the triangular defect moves the rotation flap toward the primary defect. If a Burow's triangle is made as large as the primary defect, no differential suturing or stretching will be necessary. Two rotation flaps, one concave and the other convex, are moved equal distances in opposite directions.

A final solution to problems that arise in moving a rotation flap is to incise a generous back-cut and skin graft the resultant defect, that is, convert it to a type I transposition flap. Multiple rotation flaps are uncommon but have been described to move skin from the dorsum of the wrist into the first web space.[88]

Advancement Flaps

In an advancement flap, the leading edge of the flap is drawn directly away from its vascular base to cover the primary defect. In the simplest design, the primary defect is considered as a rectangle. The two short sides of the rectangle are produced as the lateral incisions of the advancement flap until the surgeon deems that, by differential suturing, the flap can be advanced into the defect. A simple advancement flap for use in thumb tip amputation was described by Moberg[233] (Fig. 47-45), which in fact is a bipedicled flap

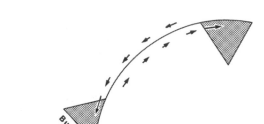

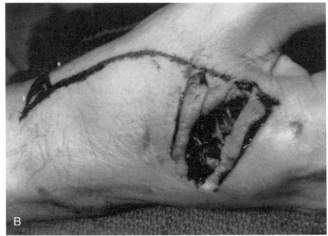

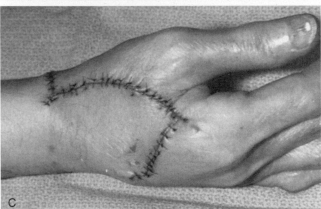

FIGURE 47-44. A, Another device for assisting in movement of a rotation flap is to excise the critical area as a Burow's triangle and thereby rotate both the flap and the adjacent skin. **B,** An irregular saw injury to the dorsum of the hand has created a skin loss that has been triangulated. A rotation flap was designed and a Burow's triangle excised over the region of the snuffbox. **C,** The flap in place. (**A** modified from Lister GD: The theory of the transposition flap and its practical application in the hand. Clin Plast Surg 8:115-128, 1981.)

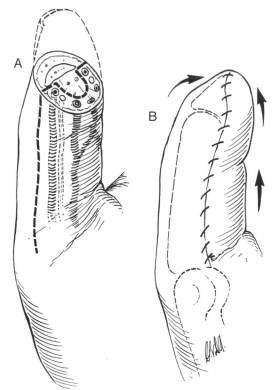

FIGURE 47-45. Moberg advancement flap. **A,** Most useful for amputations distal to the thumb interphalangeal joint, the Moberg advancement flap is composed of the entire palmar skin of the thumb, including the neurovascular bundles. **B,** Flexion of the interphalangeal joint assists in coverage of the defect by the advancement flap. (Modified from Lister GD: The theory of the transposition flap and its practical application in the hand. Clin Plast Surg 8:115-128, 1981.)

(based on the two neurovascular bundles of the thumb.) This is reserved for amputations through the distal phalanx, because flexion of the IP joint may be required to assist in closure of the defect. The two parallel incisions to create the flap are made just dorsal to the two neurovascular bundles of the thumb, which are carefully preserved throughout dissection. The flap is then elevated from the flexor tendon sheath. Because the bundles are included in the flap, there is theoretically no limit to the length of the flap but customarily the base is placed at the MP joint skin flexion crease. If difficulty is encountered in advancing the flap over the thumb tip, four tactics are available. First, the IP joint can be flexed

and, if necessary, pinned in flexion, thus moving the primary defect into the flap. This procedure may cause fears of later problems with extension, but they are unfounded unless the joint is arthritic or has been injured. Second, the lateral incisions can be extended toward the palm, yielding a greater length over which skin can be advanced. The defects on either aspect of the base can then be closed with two small rotation flaps.[68] Third, two Burow's triangles can be excised to assist in advancement, one from either side of the base of the flap, provided that tissue is available (Fig. 47-46). Fourth, because there are two vascular bundles in the base of the flap, the skin of the base can be incised to create an island (Fig. 47-47). A full-thickness graft is applied to the secondary defect overlying the neurovascular bundles and tendon sheath. Posner and Smith[265] reported 22 Moberg advancement flaps with no slough or flexion contracture and normal two-point discrimination. This advancement is usually safe in the thumb, for the dorsum is well perfused by dorsal branches from the radial artery. If the base of the flap is too proximal, however, necrosis of a portion of the distal thumb skin can occur. The dorsal neurovascular branches of the digital vessels can be preserved on one or both sides of the flap, which will obviate any vascular problems of the distal dorsal skin. This will decrease the length that the flap can be advanced, however.

A similar procedure has been reported in the finger,[248,311] but greater care must be exercised here, or loss of the dorsal

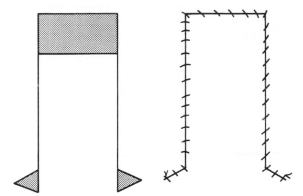

FIGURE 47-46. Advancement flap. If a defect can be considered as a rectangle, an advancement flap can be designed by extending the two short sides of the rectangle. The advancement movement can be assisted also by excision of two Burow's triangles on the outer aspect of the design. (Modified from Lister GD: The theory of the transposition flap and its practical application in the hand. Clin Plast Surg 8:115-128, 1981.)

skin may result. Macht and Watson[206] reported 69 cases with no skin necrosis either palmar or dorsal, two-point discrimination within 2 mm of normal, and a maximum flexion deficit of 5 degrees. However, they emphasized the importance of maintaining the dorsal branches of the proper digital arteries as noted earlier. Increased padding of the pulp with a free dermal graft placed beneath the palmar advancement flap has been advocated by Arons.[6]

"V-Y" Advancement

Commonly used to repair fingertip amputations, the "V-Y" advancement may be single midline (Atasoy[9]) or double lateral (Kutler[174]). Which one is used, and whether the technique is appropriate at all, is determined by examining the primary defect. The great majority of fingertip amputations are best managed by allowing secondary healing to occur. Even if a small portion of the bone is exposed, it can be trimmed back. Allowing secondary healing and wound contraction pulls normal pulp skin into the defect and is usually superior to a badly scarred tip resulting from ill-advised local flaps. If more tissue has been lost from the palmar than from the dorsal surface (Fig. 47-48C), a local palmar flap is unlikely to provide the necessary cover and a cross-finger or thenar flap may be required. If the loss is equal (see Fig. 47-48A) or greater on the dorsal aspect (see Fig. 47-48B), a "V-Y" flap can be used, provided the skin from which it comes is not also damaged. Whether a single midline or double lateral is used depends on whether there is more skin in the midline or laterally.

There are three facts to remember if a "V-Y" flap is to be raised successfully.[346] First, more problems arise through inadequate than excessive mobilization: the flap should advance easily into position (Fig. 47-49). Second, only nerves and vessels need be kept intact.[21] Third, the nerves and vessels in the pulp are slender, are elastic, and will not resist appreciably the movement of the flap; a corollary of this rule is that any tissue that does offer firm resistance can be divided with impunity. The apex of the "V" in a single midline advancement[9,336] for most fingertip amputations worthy of reconstruction (i.e., at or distal to the midportion

of the nail) should be at the distal digital crease. In the rare case in which length is deemed sufficiently important to justify a "V-Y" advancement in more proximal amputations, the apex can be placed more proximally. The base of the triangle, which lies on the free distal margin, should be as wide as the nail bed but no wider or the tip will have a flattened appearance. The incisions are made through the skin with a knife, carrying it to bone at either end of the base where there are periosteal attachments but no vessels. These periosteal attachments should be divided. The deep surface of the flap is freed completely from the underlying tendon sheath as far as its apex. The skin and subcutaneous tissue 6 or 7 mm on either aspect of the apex are incised down to the sheath. With skin hooks on one lateral margin of the flap distracting the flap away from the digit (see Fig. 47-49A), the lateral subcutaneous tissues that contain the pedicle of the flap are spread apart with microscissors. With the use of loupe magnification, any restraining bands are accurately defined and divided, remembering that nerves and vessels will not resist gentle traction.[299]

(An anatomic point should be made here. The veins that accompany the artery of the digital neurovascular bundle are at different levels and of differing, smaller calibers. Therefore, in dissecting a neurovascular bundle for any form of island flap in the digit, no attempt should ever be made to define the artery and nerve independently, for such skeletonization will serve only to damage the veins and thereby seriously impair flap drainage.)

The flap should then advance easily into place (see Fig. 47-49B and C). If it does not, and firm resistance is encountered, one of the fibrous septa must still be intact and must be divided. This process is repeated until the flap moves easily. If the distal end of the flap fails to easily reach the nail bed, it is better to place a small split-thickness skin graft over the raw distal edge of the flap rather than close it too tightly. Closure of the flap is begun at the apex, creating the vertical stem of the "Y" and so advancing the flap. The flap can be inset with the tourniquet inflated, and on completion and after tourniquet release, color usually returns to the flap. If it does not, time and warmth in the form of hot packs should be permitted to play their valuable role for 20 timed minutes. If there is still inadequate flow, the most distal suture(s) in the vertical limb of the "Y" should be released, which usually produces the desired effect.

Although greater palmar loss than dorsal usually contraindicates such palmar "V-Y" advancement flaps, Furlow[100] has shown good results with V-Y "cup" flaps. He sutures the two distal angles of the triangle together after mobilizing the flap, which forms a cup that fits over the tip.

The lateral or Kutler[174] "V-Y" advancement flap[98,299] (Fig. 47-50) is raised in identical fashion to the midline "V-Y", with the exception that there is only one neurovascular bundle to be protected in each flap. These flaps tend to lead to a scarred fingertip, however. Oblique "V-Y" advancement flaps have also been described.[342] "V-Y" flaps need not be based on a single known pedicle such as the proper digital artery and nerve. They can be raised on a pedicle of subcutaneous tissue, relying on random vessels contained therein. In such flaps, the pedicle is made as wide as possible. Such "V-Y" flaps have been described for closure of defects and release of contractures.[245]

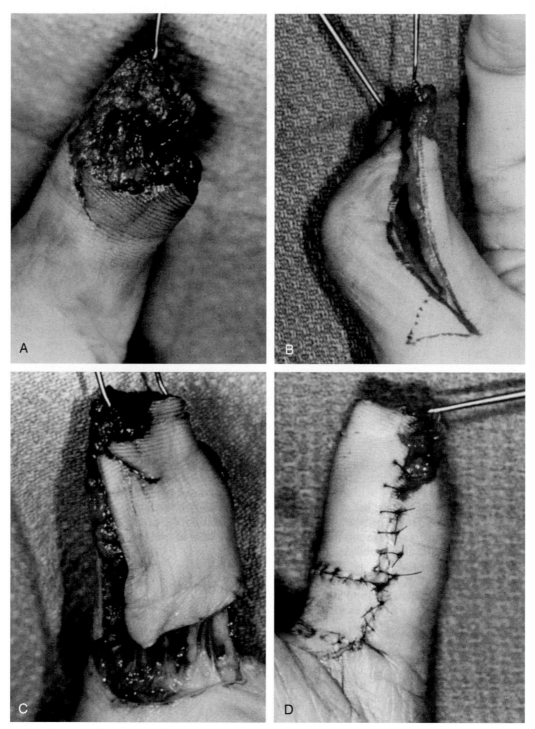

FIGURE 47-47. A, A full-thickness defect of the thumb is to be closed by a Moberg advancement flap. **B,** When the flap is mobilized and the thumb flexed fully, it is seen that the flap will cover the defect, but only with some tension (note that a potential Burow's triangle has been marked out at the base of the flap). **C,** To release the tension, the flap has been divided across its base and the neurovascular bundles carefully preserved. **D,** The flap has been sutured in place and the secondary defect covered with a full-thickness skin graft.

Regional Flaps

Regional flaps derive from tissues not immediately adjacent to the primary defect but from its vicinity. Thus most regional flaps in the hand are raised from another part of the hand. They are both random and axial pattern with respect to their blood supply. In regional flaps, the merit of the axial design is apparent, for all require only one surgical procedure,

whereas regional flaps of random design require at least two. At the first operation, the flap is raised and applied to the primary defect. At the second, the pedicle is divided and inset.

Random-Pattern Regional Flaps

The cross-finger and thenar flaps are random-pattern regional flaps. Both are used in the repair of fingertip

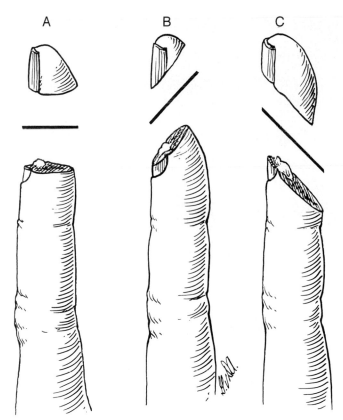

A   B   C

FIGURE 47-48. Suitability for coverage with local flaps is determined by looking at the angle of amputation. Amputations that are transverse (**A**) or have more dorsal loss (**B**) can be treated by local flaps. Where the loss is more palmar (**C**), palmar flaps have been described (see text) but regional flaps are more reliable. (Modified from Lister GD: The theory of the transposition flap and its practical application in the hand. Clin Plast Surg 8:115-128, 1981.)

defects, in particular, those with bone exposed and with more loss of palmar tissue than dorsal. The choice between the two is dictated for many surgeons by the sex and age of the patient. For them, the thenar flap is reserved for young females, because it often requires somewhat more flexion of the injured finger than does the cross-finger flap and therefore carries a greater theoretic risk of persistent joint contracture. The joints in such a patient are likely to be more supple than in her older male counterpart, and she is also more likely to find the secondary defect resulting from a cross-finger flap unacceptable. Whereas the thenar flap is used solely for fingertip injuries, the cross-finger flap and its variants are used also for defects of the dorsal and palmar aspects of all digits.

Cross-Finger Flap

Although the cross-finger flap has several variants, which are outlined later, the basic design is for loss of palmar digital tissue and is fashioned on the dorsal aspect of the middle phalanx of the adjacent finger.[157] For pulp loss, the middle finger is used for the index finger, but otherwise the donor finger is that radial to the injured one. Flaps to and from the thumb are discussed later. The cross-finger flap can be tailored to fit a pattern of the primary defect. The margin of the defect that is adjacent to the donor finger is designated "the hinge" (AB in Fig. 47-51A). It corresponds closely to

the base of the flap, which is also called a hinge (A'B' in Fig. 47-51B). It is similar to the pivot point of transposition flaps, in that it is a fixed reference around which tissues move. It differs in that it is a line rather than a point. A pattern of the primary defect is made and turned through 180 degrees around the hinge and applied to the dorsum of the donor finger. By adjusting the position of the hinge, the necessary flap can be derived entirely from the skin of the dorsum of the middle phalanx. The flap to be raised is then outlined to include not only the necessary flap but also all the skin of the dorsum of the middle phalanx, from midlateral line to midlateral line and from the proximal extension crease of the DIP joint to the distal extension crease of the PIP joint. In marking the hinge, it should be recalled that in all random-pattern flaps, the direction that they face can be altered by extension cuts. Thus, in the cross-finger flap, a proximal transverse incision that extends more palmar than the distal transverse incision will cause the deep surface of the flap to face proximally; one in which the distal cut extends more palmar will face distally. The former is more often required, causing the flap to fit well to an amputation stump (Fig. 47-52). The latter is needed only in longer, more palmar defects when considerable flexion of the injured finger is necessary.

The flap margins are incised. Immediately beneath the skin, multiple longitudinal veins are encountered. These are coagulated and cut to reach the correct plane, which lies immediately superficial to the extensor tendon. Once the veins are divided, the flap is raised with ease, because only loose areolar tissue lies in the plane of dissection. The flap is hinged away from the donor site and applied to the primary defect to check the fit. If the pedicle is kinked to reach the defect, this can often be eliminated by extending either the proximal or distal transverse cut of the flap. When the flap does not fold easily away from the donor finger, Cleland's ligament may be restraining it. The ligament can be incised to permit easier folding of the flap. The vessels to the flap penetrate the more superficial part of the ligament and may be damaged unless care is taken to incise it at its depth, against the skeleton.

Once the flap has been raised satisfactorily, a pattern of the full-thickness graft required for the secondary defect is taken. The tourniquet is released at this juncture, and hemostasis is achieved. During this process, the full-thickness graft to cover the secondary defect is obtained. This is commonly taken from the same limb, usually the inner aspect of the upper forearm or arm. This practice is unacceptable in all except perhaps an older working man in whom scars may be of little consequence. In the young and especially the female, the infliction of a wound in any of these sites is to be condemned. Rather, the grafts should be taken from the inguinal region. Before puberty, the skin that has the potential of bearing pubic hair can be avoided by staying at least 1 cm lateral to the femoral pulse.

As in all flaps, it is desirable to close all raw surfaces. When one considers the hinge of the cross-finger design, the only free edge to which the skin graft can be sutured is the hinge margin of the primary defect, which is inaccessible after the flap has been sutured in place, lying as it does between the fingers. To overcome this difficulty, the skin graft is first laid on the primary defect, as if it were intended to use it to cover the primary wound rather than the flap

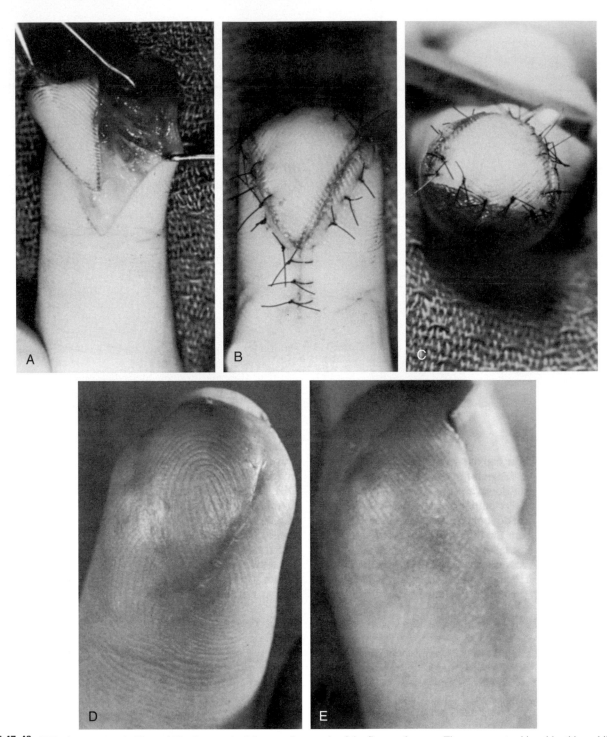

FIGURE 47-49. V-Y advancement. **A,** The mobilization required down to the vessels of the flap can be seen. The movement achieved by this mobilization is sufficient to permit easy suture (**B**) over the amputation (**C**). **D** and **E,** The result at an early stage.

already raised. The graft is then sutured to the hinge margin of the primary defect (see Fig. 47-51C). It will be appreciated that there are now two "flaps," the cross-finger and the graft, with contiguous hinges. If both are swung 180 degrees around their hinges, the flap will come to lie on the primary defect and the graft on the secondary defect (see Fig. 47-51D and E). One last time, the positioning of the flap is checked. If the flap has been well chosen, any kinks can be eliminated by lengthening the extension cut. The flap

can now be inset and sutured into position, trimming as necessary. The skin graft is sutured to the secondary defect. The circulation to the flap should be good, although a little blanching around the margins is common and acceptable. If the flap appears very pale and has been designed and raised correctly, it may be that the recipient finger is extending, thereby exerting undue pressure on the flap and its pedicle. This can be overcome by flexing the recipient finger until circulation returns and then maintaining the position by

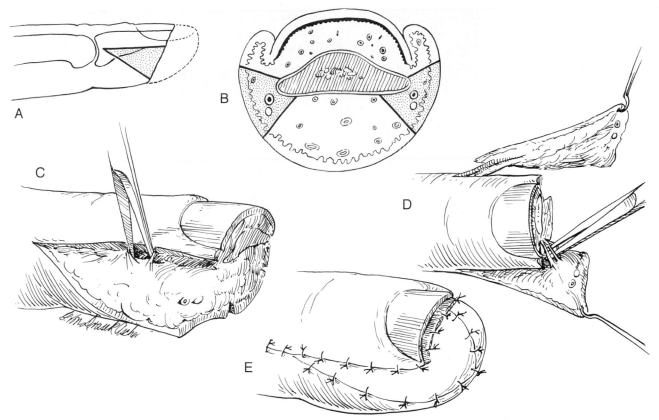

FIGURE 47-50. Kutler double lateral V-Y advancements. **A,** The advancement flaps are designed over the neurovascular pedicles and carried right down to bone (**B**). The fibrous septa are defined and (**C**) divided, permitting free mobilization (**D**) on the neurovascular pedicles alone. The flaps then advance readily to the midline (**E**). (From the Christine Kleinert Institute for Hand and Microsurgery, Inc., with permission.)

inserting a suture or Kirschner wire between the fingers, usually transfixing the middle phalanx of the injured finger and the proximal phalanx of the donor.[157] This is rarely necessary.

Reversed Cross-Finger Flap. Primary defects on the dorsum of the finger cannot be covered by a standard dorsal cross-finger flap as described earlier. They can be treated with a flap taken from the palmar surface, but the skin is rather unsuitable, and the secondary defect would be in a more significant area functionally than the primary defect— never a satisfactory solution. In such circumstances, a reversed cross-finger flap should be used.[8] This is designed on the dorsal aspect of the middle phalanx of the adjacent finger, as with the standard flap, the hinge being adjacent to the primary defect (Fig. 47-53A). The first step, however, is to raise a full-thickness skin graft from the donor site, commencing the elevation at the hinge and leaving it attached on the opposite margin of the design. This is done at the level of the deep dermis above the layer of subcutaneous veins, below the hair follicles, and requires a scalpel (see Fig. 47-53B). The underlying subcutaneous tissue is then raised in the same manner as for the standard cross-finger flap, with its hinge adjacent to the defect (see Fig. 47-53C). When this flap is swung through 180 degrees around the hinge, its superficial surface lies on the primary defect and the deep surface becomes superficial. A full-thickness skin graft is harvested and laid on the flap, and both are sutured to the margins of the primary defect. The

full-thickness graft previously raised from the donor finger is sutured in place to cover the secondary defect (see Fig. 47-53D).

Innervated Cross-Finger Flap. Cohen and Cronin[56] described a technique for innervation of the standard cross-finger flap. The dorsal branch of the proper digital nerve of the donor finger, on the side away from the injured finger, which supplies the dorsum of the middle phalanx, is divided proximally in the course of raising the free margin of the flap. It is then joined to the proper digital nerve of the injured finger on the side opposite the donor digit. Thus the ulnar dorsal digital branch of the middle finger would be joined to the radial digital nerve of the index finger. Although it is attractive theoretically, one is deterred from incorporating this additional complexity by the excellent sensory results of the standard cross-finger flap. Kleinert and colleagues[168] reported 70% of patients as having two-point discrimination of less than 8 mm in standard cross-finger flaps. Johnson and Iverson[149] noted that all their patients had better sensation than that present in an area equivalent to the donor site in the opposite hand, and Nicolai and Hentenaar[247] reported that 53% had two-point discrimination within 2 mm of that of the same pulp in the opposite hand.

For resurfacing the thumb, a cross-finger flap from the dorsum of the proximal phalanx of the index finger can be innervated by transposition of the radial nerve supplying that skin.[2,106,230] Before this flap is used, the radial nerve

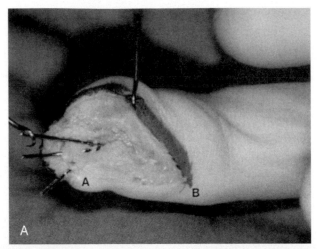

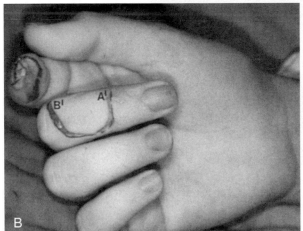
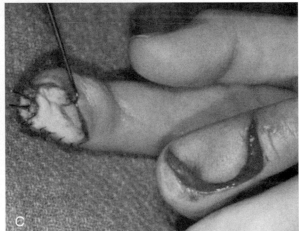

FIGURE 47-51. Cross-finger flap. **A,** The primary defect has been created in an attempt to release a severely hooked nail that the patient wishes to keep. The "hinge" of the primary defect is marked AB. **B,** The cross-finger flap has been raised from the dorsum of the adjacent middle finger. Its hinge is marked A′B′. **C,** The full-thickness skin flap is sewn initially to the hinge of the primary defect. *Continued*

should be blocked at the wrist to delineate its dermatome. The flap is raised with either a proximal or a radial base, taking care to preserve the branches of the radial nerve. At the time of division, the radial nerve branch is isolated and dissected back through an incision extending proximally to a point close to the snuffbox. An adequate length of nerve is dissected free so that it can be transposed to a second incision made on the dorsum of the thumb to the proximal edge of the previously transposed flap. This technique is not of value in providing coverage when almost all the thumb length has been maintained, because sensation in such circumstances often deteriorates with use. This is presumably because of the tension exerted on the transposed nerve with extension and abduction of the thumb. As with the innervated cross-finger flap, results must be compared with those reported for standard flaps. With the radial nerve–innervated flap, Bralliar and Horner[27] reported 64% of patients with two-point discrimination of less than 15 mm, results that are poorer than those reported for standard cross-finger flaps.

Cross-Thumb Flap. Cross-thumb flaps[7] are indicated when the primary defect is on the radial aspect of the index finger or in pulp injuries of that digit when the normal donor finger for a routine cross-finger flap, the middle, is injured

or absent (Fig. 47-54). The cross-thumb flap is invariably taken from the dorsal aspect of the proximal phalanx of the thumb with a proximal pedicle. The flap is raised and applied in the same manner as a standard cross-finger flap, except that it is necessary to apply the full-thickness graft to the secondary defect before suturing the flap in place (see Fig. 47-54).

Thenar Flap
The thenar flap was first described by Gatewood.[105] The procedure has been much criticized because of joint contracture and tenderness of the donor site, but it received strong support from Beasley.[19] His description places the thenar flap high on the thenar eminence in a position almost identical to that illustrated by Gatewood. In a series of 150 cases, Melone and associates[226] showed only 4% persistent PIP joint contracture and 3% hypersensitivity of the palmar scar. With respect to the likelihood of joint contracture, simple observation shows that the PIP joint of the injured finger is flexed almost equally when either a cross-finger or a properly designed thenar flap is applied.

The injured finger is flexed to meet the thenar eminence with the thumb abducted so that the point of contact is adjacent to the MP crease of the thumb. The palmar, proximal margin of the primary defect is marked on the thenar

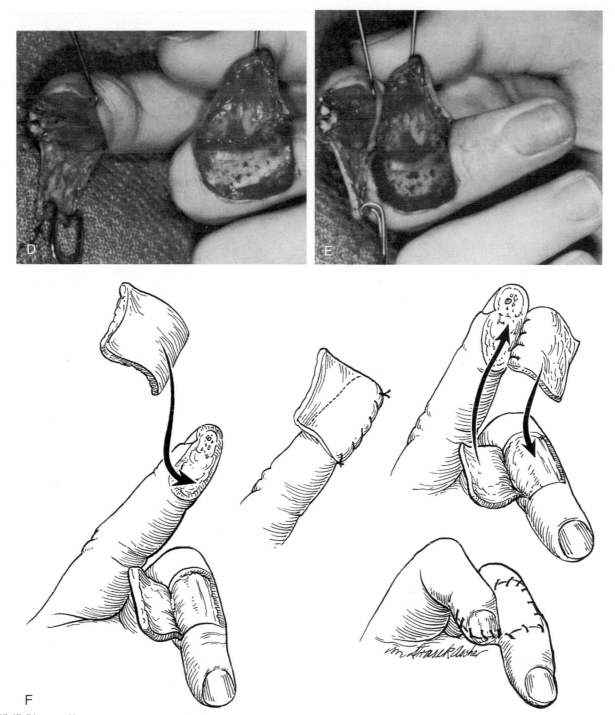

FIGURE 47-51—cont'd. Cross-finger flap. **D** and **E,** The two "flaps" are now swung outward. It can be seen that this approximates the flaps to the defects with full closure of the bridge segment. **F,** The procedure is diagrammed. (**F,** From the Christine Kleinert Institute for Hand and Microsurgery, Inc., with permission.)

eminence and serves as the marking for the hinge of the intended thenar flap, which is customarily based on the radial (proximal) aspect of the thumb. The flap is marked out distal to that base (Fig. 47-55B). The flap should be a little longer than the length of the defect from palmar to dorsal margins. It should also be wider than the primary defect by 50%. The flap is raised at the level of the underlying thenar muscle so as to include as much subcutaneous tissue as possible (see Fig. 47-55C). The only potential hazard is damage to the radial digital nerve of the thumb,

which should be sought and protected. A full-thickness graft is applied to the secondary defect (see Fig. 47-55D), and the flap is sutured to the primary defect. In so doing, the distal end of the flap should not be sutured to the nail bed but should be left a little long (see Fig. 47-55E). This excess can be trimmed after division of the flap, re-creating the hyponychium of the finger. The pedicle of the flap as described is proximal, but it may be ulnar for predominantly ulnar defects[15] and radial for radial ones. Dellon[69] suggested a distal pedicle, which he called a "proximal inset thenar

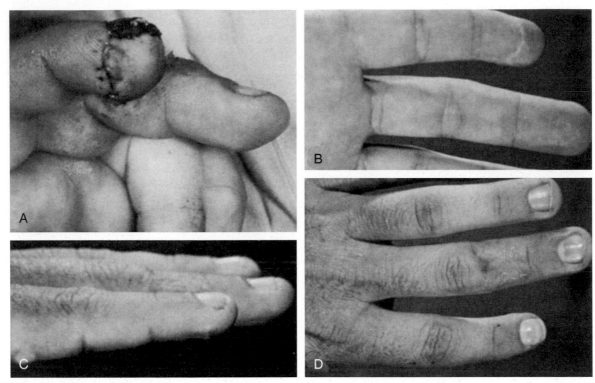

FIGURE 47-52. Cross-finger flap to an amputation. **A,** The orientation of the flap on the tip of an amputation has been achieved by making the proximal cut in the donor finger significantly longer than the distal cut, thus causing the flap to face proximally. **B** to **D,** The result.

flap," believing that this design had the potential to cover a larger defect and to close the secondary defect primarily. He reported six cases, but his claims were refuted by Beasley in discussion.

Division of Random Regional Flaps

Flatt[87] recommended that thenar flaps be divided at 2 weeks. To divide them earlier invites necrosis, although some surgeons test and divide these flaps as early as 7 days.[167] To do so later than 2 weeks might be expected to increase the incidence of joint stiffness, but avoidance of flaps that place the finger at risk mitigates this problem. We prefer to divide most regional flaps at between 2 and 3 weeks. The decision whether to divide a flap is predicated on the apparent healing of the margins to the defect. If healing appears to be delayed, early division may lead to partial or total loss of the flap. Division is usually performed under local infiltration anesthesia. The pedicle may be inset or not, but Beasley[19] and Dellon[69] emphasized the possibility of necrosis if too vigorous dissection is done at this stage. Immediate mobilization is mandatory, and the one benefit of regional over local anesthesia is that the joints can be taken gently through a full range of motion under its protection.

Axial-Pattern Regional Flaps

Regional flaps applicable to the upper extremity that have a known pedicle are the neurovascular island flap, the fillet flap, and those axial cutaneous, fasciocutaneous, and musculocutaneous flaps that may be used in the upper extremity.

Neurovascular Island Flap

Hailed by Hueston in 1965 as "the most important development in hand surgery in the past decade,"[137] the neuro-

vascular island flap was first described in the English literature by Littler.[200,201] The technique was initially popular because it had the potential of transferring sensibility to the functionally significant pulp of the thumb from a less important part of the hand, such as the middle or ring finger. However, after Hueston's comment and Tubiana and DuParc's 1961 report of 10 cases with almost normal two-point discrimination,[340] there were four adverse reports in the decade commencing in 1966[172,219,241,272] expressing dissatisfaction on the grounds of high or absent two-point discrimination, cold intolerance, hyperesthesia, and failure of reorientation. There has been much debate on this latter score, about whether it can happen and, if so, how often. That it can happen has been demonstrated by elegant cortical mapping studies in primates.[50] That it occurs in 25% of patients was shown by both Murray and associates[241] and Henderson and Reid.[129] To overcome this problem, European surgeons[348] divided the nerve of the flap at the time of transfer and sutured it to that of the thumb. This seemingly attractive solution has two potential hazards. First, dissecting in the pedicle may impair the venous return of the flap (see later). Second, a painful neuroma may remain on the unsatisfied nerve of the pedicle, as it may, of course, on that of the thumb if this division and resuture are not done. Both possible neuromas can be eliminated from the thumb by dissecting the nerve in question in the palm, dividing it, and turning it back into the carpal tunnel, where it will be protected from contact. The tide of adverse comment was turned in 1985 with a paper from Markley,[209] who pointed out several important technical reasons for the previous poor results, reporting no loss of two-point discrimination in his cases. Henderson and Reid[129] reported an average of 9 mm in 20 cases, and in 12 cases done by the

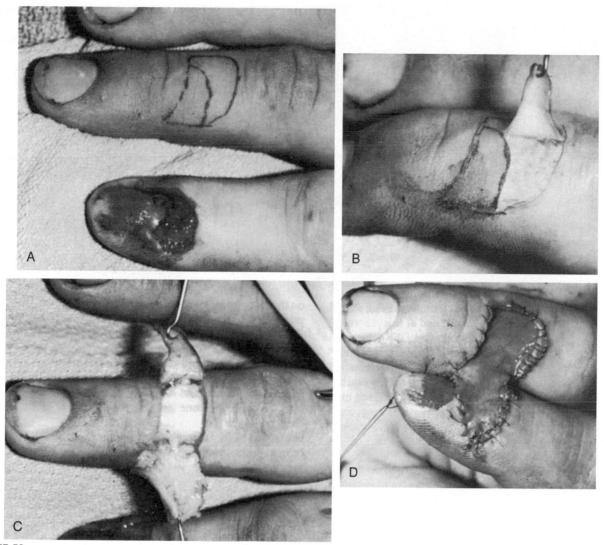

FIGURE 47-53. Reversed cross-finger flap. **A,** A dorsal defect, including the proximal nail fold, was inflicted on the index finger by a router. A flap has been drawn out that includes a segment of skin to replace the superficial surface of the nail cul-de-sac. **B,** The reversed cross-finger flap is begun by raising a layer of skin at the subdermal level based on the aspect of the design opposite to the injured finger, leaving skin on the portion that will form the cul-de-sac when the flap is turned over. **C,** The remainder of the flap is raised as for a cross-finger flap, the hinge being adjacent to the primary defect. **D,** Both the primary and secondary defects are covered together with a thin full-thickness skin graft.

authors over 3 years ending in 1980, two-point discrimination ranged from 3 to 10 mm, with an average of 6.4 mm.

The major indication for neurovascular island transfer is damage to the thumb sufficient to produce a scarred tender pulp, anesthesia, or relative ischemia. Stated conversely, a neurovascular island pedicle can provide robust padding, good sensation, increased blood flow, or any combination of the three. The flap may be taken from any digit, with preference being given to one that is in other respects unsatisfactory but that contains an intact neurovascular pedicle. For example, a digit that is being considered for ray amputation owing to lack of motion or previous partial amputation may be an excellent donor. Otherwise, either neurovascular island from the third web space is selected. Our preference is for the ulnar aspect of the middle finger, because it is longer and makes less contact in normal handling than does the radial aspect of the ring finger. Before surgery, the flow to the hand must be assessed by Doppler imaging. Not only

is good flow necessary in both vessels of the proposed donor digit to supply both the flap and that finger, but it is also essential in the contralateral vessel of the digit adjacent to the flap pedicle, because the other vessel to that digit will be divided in the course of raising the pedicle. Thus, in taking an island flap from the ulnar aspect of the middle finger, flow must be present in the ulnar proper digital artery of the ring finger, as well as in the radial proper digital artery of the middle finger (Fig. 47-56).

The operation is commenced by creating the primary defect on the thumb (Fig. 47-57A). The margins of the defect are undermined quite generously to accommodate the pedicle of the intended flap. In particular, the proximal margin is elevated, and there the distal end of the tunnel from the palm through which the pedicle will pass is made as large as possible by scar excision and blunt scissor dissection toward the palm. The digital nerves are dealt with appropriately. If one digital nerve is to be joined to the nerve

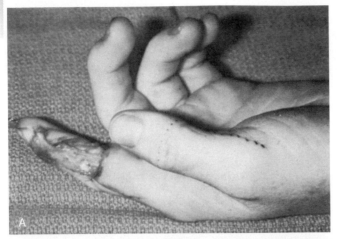

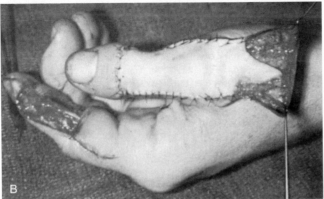

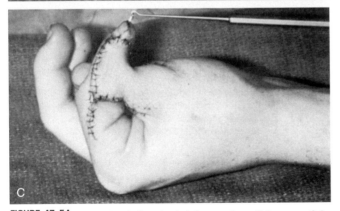

FIGURE 47-54. Cross-thumb flap. **A,** A defect on the radial aspect of the index finger is to be covered by a proximally based cross-thumb flap. **B,** The secondary defect is covered with a split-thickness skin graft that also covers the bridge segment. This must be done before (**C**) suturing the flap into position.

of the flap, as in the European technique, the ulnar digital nerve is selected and prepared, if it is in good condition. If the nerves are not to be used and have been the source of discomfort, they are dissected proximally to the muscle bellies of the flexor pollicis brevis and there transected. A pattern of the defect is then taken, making it sufficiently generous to accommodate the unusual bulk of the pedicle and pulp tissue that will be transferred. The pattern is then applied to the ulnar aspect of the middle finger, carrying the distal point out to or even beyond the tip of the digit onto the radial aspect. When necessary, the flap can extend as far

proximally as the web.[137] The proximal incision is then marked out in the midlateral line as far as the web and into the palm as a zigzag as far proximal as the distal margin of the flexor retinaculum (see Fig. 47-57B). The initial dissection is performed in the palm to ensure that there are no anomalies of the vascular tree. If any are found that preclude transfer, the procedure is abandoned in most instances for some better alternative, although the transfer can be done on the metacarpal artery arising from the deep palmar arch.[291] Where the anatomy is normal, the dissection can proceed into the finger. An important point should be made with respect to the dissection in the finger. The veins that accompany the nerve and artery are not the main drainage of the pulp and, as such, are small, irregular, and unpredictable. To ensure their survival and therefore that of the flap, the pedicle in the finger as far proximal as the bifurcation of the common digital artery must be raised as a monobloc of fatty tissue containing all the unidentified elements of the pedicle (see Fig. 47-57C). Thus, once the incision is made in the side of the finger, the palmar skin is raised off the subcutaneous tissue to almost the midline of the finger. At that point, the subcutaneous tissue is incised down to the tendon sheath and then lifted off the sheath, proceeding dorsally until the skeleton of the finger is reached. There it meets the plane of dissection of the dorsal edge of the incision. Blunt scissor dissection now separates the bloc of pedicle tissue from the skeleton, and a vessel loop of soft rubber can be passed around it. Gentle traction away from the skeleton displays the branches of the vessels and nerve to the flexor tendons and IP joints, which can be divided. With dissection in the finger completed, further progress is made proximally by isolating (see Fig. 47-57D) and ligating the branch of the common digital artery to the ring finger. There is commonly a communication from the metacarpal artery to the bifurcation of the common digital, and this also must be sought and ligated.

The proper digital nerves of the third web space are split from each other in the substance of the common digital nerve (see Fig. 47-57E). It is also possible in this way to preserve the dorsal digital branches of these nerves. The vessel loop previously passed around the pedicle is moved proximally as dissection proceeds, lifting the pedicle from its bed and preventing unnecessary dissection within the pedicle itself, which could harm the veins. The proximal advance is halted only at the superficial palmar arch. Mobilization proceeds this far for two reasons. First, it gives the maximal pedicle length, of importance for reasons discussed later. Second, it allows the surgeon to study the relationship of the pedicle to the intact digital nerve to the ring finger. In some instances, if the pedicle is passed directly to the thumb, it would be kinked by that nerve to a degree that might impair the circulation (see Fig. 47-57F). This potential problem can be eliminated simply by passing the entire neurovascular island beneath that digital nerve before its transfer to the thumb (see Fig. 47-57G and H).

The tunnel to the primary defect is now prepared by blunt scissor dissection in the subcutaneous plane superficial to the palmar fascia. It is made sufficiently wide to permit the withdrawal of the scissors from the primary defect to the palm with the tips open 2 cm. Should the margin of the palmar fascia offer a potential hazard to the pedicle, it is divided transversely. A 1-inch Penrose drain is passed from the palmar wound to the primary defect, leaving a generous length lying across the ulnar border of the hand. A partial cut is made in the drain close to the palmar wound, and a hemostat is passed through it and along the drain, to emerge at its ulnar end (see Fig. 47-57I). A stay suture of 4-0 nylon is placed through the tip of the island flap, which can now finally be raised from its bed. By leaving it in place throughout the dissection, the risk of torsion or traction on the pedicle is minimized. Such risks not only would damage the vascular supply but also might contribute to reduced digital nerve function with the loss of fine sensibility referred to earlier. When the flap is being taken mainly to provide better sensibility or blood supply and little skin is required or has been taken, the palmar aspect of the incision is undermined to the midline, both to ensure inclusion of all branches of nerve and artery and to facilitate direct closure of the donor pulp. The flap is raised with a scalpel kept close to the skeleton, coagulating the many branches of the digital artery in so doing. Once freed from the finger, the flap is immediately put inside the Penrose drain by placing the stay suture of the flap in the hemostat previously inserted into the drain and withdrawing the hemostat from the drain. The flap is thereby carefully introduced into the Penrose. This can now be pulled out of the tunnel into the primary defect, maintaining

traction on the stay suture to prevent the flap from being extruded from the ulnar end of the drain (see Fig. 47-57J). Once the flap is in place, the drain can be discarded.

An important test is now performed (see Fig. 47-57K). With one stitch securing the flap in position in the primary defect, the thumb is fully abducted and extended. With the thumb in this position, the pedicle is checked at the proximal end of the palmar wound for any evidence of tension or kinking. If the steps outlined earlier have been followed, this should not exist. If it does, it should be eliminated, because traction on the nerve with increasingly vigorous use after full healing is the only likely explanation of the phenomenon of decreasing two-point discrimination reported by some authors.[172,252] The flap is now sutured into position, before release of the tourniquet. All hemostasis should have been achieved in raising the flap, and further attempts after release of the tourniquet may damage the pedicle. The tourniquet can now be released, and flow to the flap should be immediate. If it is not, the pedicle is inspected in the palm for any obvious kinks, and hot packs are applied for 10 minutes. If flow is still unsatisfactory, release of a few marginal sutures may improve it. This should not be necessary, however, if the technique has been followed. During the waiting period, a full-thickness graft is harvested for the

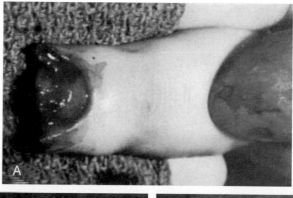

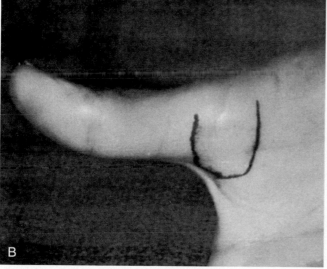

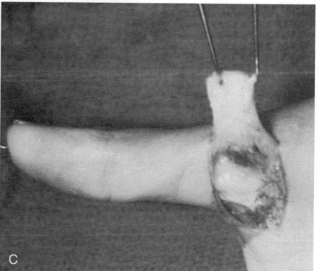

FIGURE 47-55. Thenar flap. **A,** An amputation in a girl of the tip of the index finger in which approximately one half of the nail bed remains with good bony support is an appropriate indication for a thenar flap. **B,** The finger has been carried to the thumb, and the proximal margin of the primary defect has been used as the proximal marking of a proximally (radially) based thenar flap. This is designed in the region of the MP crease of the thumb. **C,** The flap is raised taking care to avoid damage to the digital nerves but carrying as much subcutaneous tissue as possible.   *Continued*

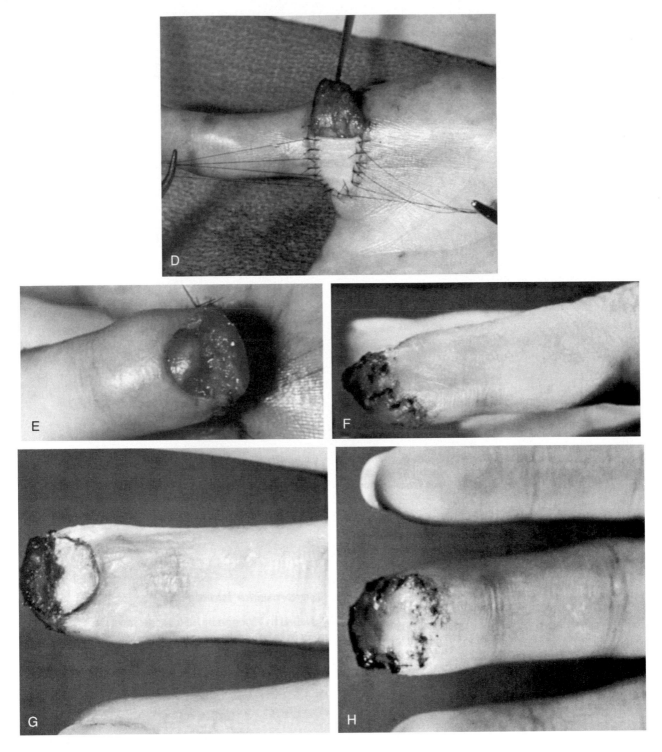

FIGURE 47-55—cont'd. Thenar flap. **D,** The secondary defect is covered with a full-thickness graft. **E,** The flap is sutured in position, but the free margin is left a little long to support the advancing nail. **F to H,** The early result shows good contour of the tip with satisfactory support for later nail growth.

secondary defect (see Fig. 47-57L to N). Postoperative care includes early institution of sensory rehabilitation[67,70] of the island transfer.

Rose[281] described a modification of the Littler flap in which the skin island is taken from some juncture along the course of the neurovascular pedicle, not necessarily the pulp. Dissection is similar, except that the nerve is left in place. This method is useful for small, difficult defects that

do not require innervation, only cover. Rose described six cases with a maximum flap dimension of 5.5 × 2.5 cm. The secondary defect is covered with a full-thickness graft.

Fillet Flap

Fillet flaps are developed from a well-vascularized digit that is otherwise worthless owing to extensive injury to skeleton, nerves, or tendons and commonly to all three.[40,41,257] The

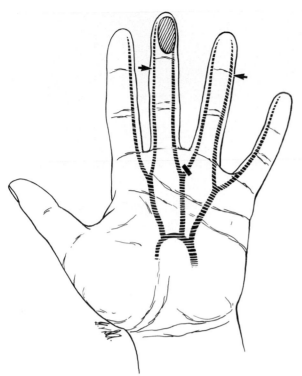

FIGURE 47-56. Neurovascular island flap: preliminary evaluation. It is necessary to ensure by Doppler studies that flow exists not only in the vessel that will supply the flap and in the vessel that will maintain the donor digit after the flap has been raised (*left arrow*) but also in the contralateral digital artery of the adjacent finger (*right arrow*) because the ipsilateral vessel will be divided (*bar*) in mobilizing the pedicle. (From the Christine Kleinert Institute for Hand and Microsurgery, Inc., with permission.)

technique of filleting a finger requires that the skeleton and tendons be removed, preserving all other soft tissues on one or both vascular pedicles. Because the circumference of a finger at the free edge of the web is equal to the distance from the web to a point just proximal to the nail fold, a fillet flap as described here is roughly a square, the sides of which are equal to that measure. The difficulties in planning to use such a flap are, first, determining whether it can reach the presenting primary defect, and, second, incising it to ensure that it does. Measuring the distance from the web of the digit to be sacrificed to the nearest point of defect provides only a rough guide, particularly in the secondary situation in which scar in the soft tissues of the digit reduces their elasticity significantly.

In preparing to fillet a finger, the patency or occlusion of the two proper digital vessels is determined. With this knowledge, the surgeon then plans the longitudinal incision in the digit by visualizing how the flap will first open in a lateral direction and then fold over proximally into the defect. For example, if the middle finger is to be filleted for a defect on the dorsum of the hand, the incision in the finger should be on its radial aspect if that defect is predominantly to the ulnar side of the third metacarpal, on the ulnar if the defect is radial. A further consideration when middle or ring fingers are to be sacrificed is whether the adjacent ray—index or small finger, respectively—is to be transposed into the defect left by the ray ablation (Fig. 47-58). If it is, then the fillet flap is best reduced to an island flap by appropriate excision of palmar skin. Although technically more demand-

ing, this gives a more mobile flap and a more pleasing final result. Once these decisions have been made, the appropriate longitudinal incision is made down to the skeleton. At its distal end, a circumferential incision is made around the finger at a point 5-mm proximal to the nail fold. This means discarding the pulp tissue, because its bulk makes it rather unsatisfactory cover for its new location. At the proximal end of the longitudinal incision, its continuation depends on whether the metacarpal of the digit is to be resected and an adjacent digit transposed. If the metacarpal is not to be resected, a transverse incision is made over the dorsum of the finger so as to create a hinge along the side of the finger opposite the incision. All dorsal veins are ligated with the exception of that end of the proximal venous arcade that corresponds to the hinge. This single vein alone gives excellent venous drainage. If it is intended to transpose a digit, thereby making the fillet an island flap, the incision is again circumferential at the level of the proximal digital crease, that is, at the free margin of the web. A further incision is made in a zigzag manner proximally into the palm, through which the necessary neurovascular bundle is dissected exactly in the manner described in the section on Neurovascular Island Flap. This is always done before the skeleton is removed, because dissection of supported tissues is easier. To remove the digital skeleton, skin hooks are applied to the margins of the longitudinal incision distally, and the soft tissues are peeled off the underlying extensor tendon, bone, and flexor tendon sheath. The deep branches and tributaries of the vessels are ligated as this is done. The flap can now be opened and folded onto the primary defect. The necessary movement of the flap is more readily obtained if the injury to the donor digit is fresh and if the fillet has been raised as an island. Now, for the first time, the surgeon can really judge whether the flap will fit the primary defect. If it is too small, other solutions must be added. If it is too large, but the defect is deep, the excess should not be discarded; rather, it should be de-epithelialized and turned in to fill the depths of the wound. If the hole in the depths of the wound is caused by a segmental bony defect, a portion of phalanx can be taken as a vascularized bone graft with the fillet flap.[104]

Axial Cutaneous Flap

The scapular flap,[76] commonly used as a free flap, can reach the upper extremity as an island and has been described for use after the release of burn contractures of the axilla.[72] This flap has some utility in reconstruction of the scarred axilla but suffers from the potential to be bulky when placed in this position. This can be obviated by making sure the fascia of the flap is tacked deep into the axilla and can also be improved by later thinning of the flap. The scapular flap will cover the superior shoulder as well if taken as a long "parascapular" flap. It has little value as a pedicle flap in coverage of the elbow and lower arm, because the pedicle is not lengthy and the flap will not reach these areas.

Fasciocutaneous Flap

Regional fasciocutaneous flaps have been described from the forearm to the peri-olecranon region[35] and from the medial arm for release of axillary and elbow burn contractures.[34] However, the major fasciocutaneous flaps of the upper extremity are the lateral arm flap; the radial artery

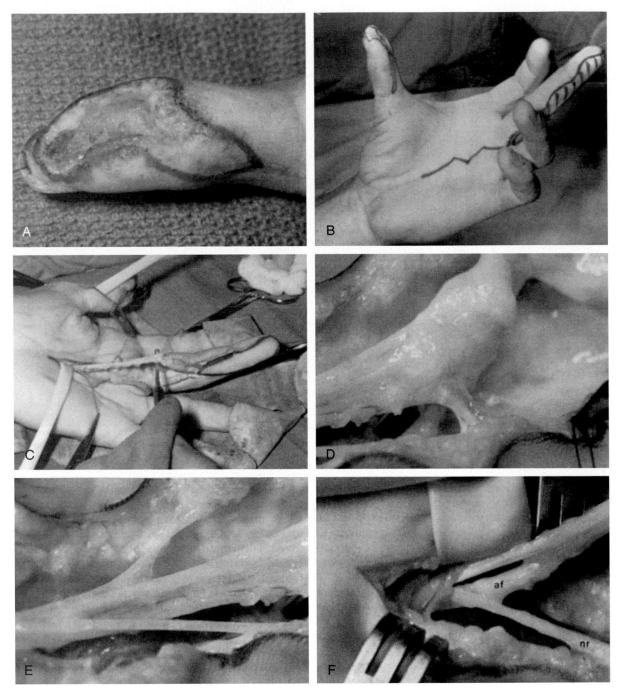

FIGURE 47-57. Neurovascular island flap. **A,** A defect of the thumb caused by a paint injection injury is anesthetic, adherent, and painful. The pattern of the neurovascular island replacement has been marked out. **B,** Here in another patient, again with an adherent and painful scar of the thumb, a long neurovascular island has been marked out not only to replace soft tissue but also to increase the blood supply to this relatively avascular thumb. A long flap has been marked out on the ulnar border of the middle finger and the proximal incision marked on the palm of the hand. **C,** The neurovascular island is shown here at a later stage in dissection to emphasize the manner in which the pedicle should be dissected in the substance of the finger, that is, with a significant surrounding fatty cover that contains the small veins important for drainage. **D,** The proper digital artery to the adjacent ring finger is displayed for division. **E,** The common digital nerve is split as far proximally as the superficial palm or arch. **F,** When the flap is carried over toward the thumb, it can be seen that the artery (af) passes around the proper digital nerve to the ring finger (nr) and may be kinked by it.   *Continued*

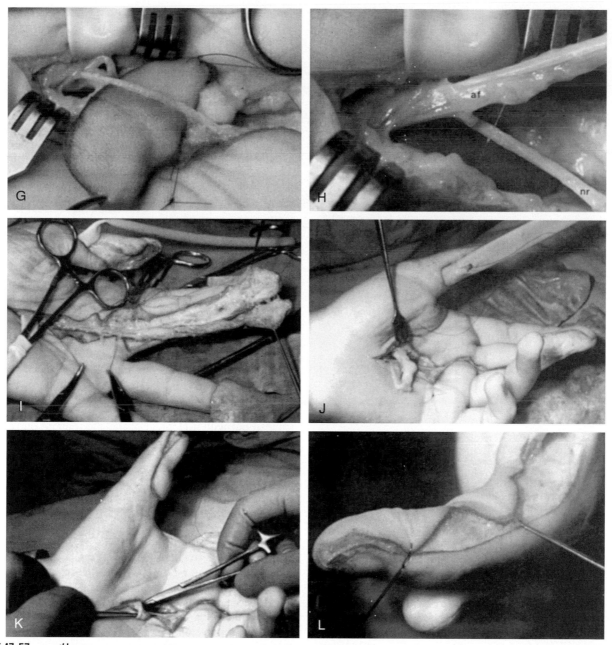

FIGURE 47-57—cont'd. Neurovascular island flap. **G,** The flap is therefore passed beneath that proper digital nerve to the ring finger and (**H**) the vessel (af) released from this kinking (nr) digital nerve to ring finger. **I,** A Penrose drain is placed in the tunnel prepared out to the thumb. A small incision is made in the drain, and a hemostat is advanced through that incision to the ulnar end of the drain. The flap is now released from the tip of the middle finger and placed immediately into the Penrose drain by drawing the stay suture out with the hemostat. **J,** The flap can now be drawn through the tunnel in the Penrose without torsion on the pedicle. **K,** With the flap in place and the thumb fully extended and abducted, the pedicle is checked in the palm to ensure that it is under no tension and is not kinked. **L,** In narrow neurovascular flaps, the donor defect can be closed directly at the pulp, with skin grafts being required more proximally.

Continued

forearm, or "Chinese," flap; the ulnar artery flap; and the posterior interosseous artery flap.[239,312,353] The lateral arm flap is primarily utilized as a free flap for hand coverage, but a small area of the elbow can be covered by a distally based flap[52,176,341] (see later section on elbow coverage). This procedure can give an unsightly scar and also lead to numbness in the proximal forearm. By contrast, the reversed radial artery flap, with its potential area of much of the forearm skin and a pedicle located at the anatomic snuffbox, is capable of covering almost any defect in the hand.[18,314]

Radial Artery Forearm Flap. The radial forearm flap represents one of the best flaps for coverage of hand defects. Based on its distal pedicle, it can cover nearly any wound of the hand and can import a variety of tissue, including skin,[116] fascia,[46] tendon,[271] and bone.[213] It has been called a

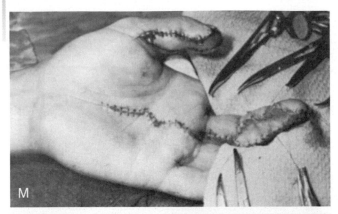

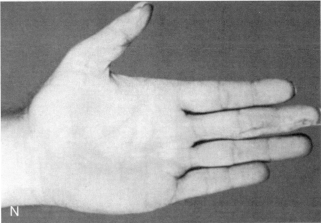

FIGURE 47-57—cont'd. Neurovascular island flap. **M,** In larger defects, a full-thickness or split-thickness graft is applied to the secondary defect. **N,** The result.

"reconstructive chameleon" because of its versatility.[165,246] It can also be based proximally and utilized for elbow coverage[224,300,334] (see later). The two primary disadvantages of this flap are the necessity for harvesting the radial artery and the poor cosmesis of the donor site, particularly in younger patients. One study noted that the radial artery was the dominant vessel to the hand in 12%,[238] and acute ischemia[150] and cold intolerance[135] have been reported. The absolute need for reconstruction of the radial artery after harvest is not known, although some have suggested this to decrease the incidence of cold intolerance.[225] In personal experience with several hundred radial forearm flaps (both pedicled and free), we have seen only two patients who required vein grafting of the radial artery who had a normal Allen test before the procedure. This experience is borne out by several studies,[139,277] with one group noting that while flow to the hand was initially decreased, this improved over time to normal levels via the remaining circulation of the ulnar artery.[142] Although functional problems are minimal, the cosmesis of the donor site remains problematic.[121] If the donor site requires skin grafting, it remains ugly, particularly in younger patients.[139,277,294] Proposals to improve this include suturing the superficialis muscle over the flexor carpi radialis tendon to improve skin graft take[170,326] and various local flaps to avoid the need of a skin graft.[4,138] In many instances, the cosmetic defect can be minimized by

taking a fasciosubcutaneous flap only.[255] This modification is discussed later.

The radial artery (Fig. 47-59) pursues a relatively superficial course in the forearm from its source at the division of the brachial artery to the point where it passes deep to the tendon of the abductor pollicis longus to reach the anatomical snuff-box. In the proximal forearm, it lies on the superficial surface of the pronator teres, just beneath the anterior margin of the muscle belly of the brachioradialis. Leaving the pronator teres, it comes to lie in turn on the radial head of the flexor digitorum superficialis and the flexor pollicis longus, here being palpable through the skin. Throughout its course, the artery gives branches to a plexus of vessels in the overlying deep fascia, and this plexus supplies the skin of the anterior and radiodorsal surfaces of the forearm. By similar fascial branches it also supplies the periosteum of the distal half of the radius between the insertions of pronator teres and brachioradialis. This allows construction of osteocutaneous flaps where desired.[22,94] The artery is accompanied by two or more venae comitantes. The multiple anastomoses between these veins permit reversal of flow in the venae comitantes without valvular obstruction.[191] Thus the artery and veins can be divided proximally, and no venous engorgement will result (valvulotomy has been described to enhance flow[261]). The minimal precaution that should be taken before raising a forearm flap is a timed Allen test[107] to ensure that flow is present and adequate through both vessels. The course of the radial artery is mapped out with a Doppler probe and marked on the skin, as is the course of the major veins in the region of the flap. With the use of a soft inelastic material, the distance from the radial styloid to the closest margin of the primary defect is measured and transposed to the forearm to determine the location of the distal edge of the flap outline. The pattern of the primary defect is drawn out proximal to this point, remembering to place proximal pattern to distal flap, because the flap will be reversed on its pedicle. The margins of the flap are then incised. A straight incision is extended distally from the flap margin over the course of the radial artery. The skin margins adjacent to the flap are elevated from the underlying deep fascia. We prefer to begin the dissection along the ulnar border of the flap and to continue all the way under the vessels before beginning the radial-side dissection. Once the skin has been elevated for 1 cm or so from the flap margin, the deep fascia is incised all around the flap, thereby gaining the plane of dissection. The flap is now raised by dissecting in the loose areolar tissue beneath the deep fascia. In larger flaps, some intermuscular deep extensions may be encountered, which should be incised. In the pedicle forearm flap described here, it is less likely that the secondary defect will lie distally over the wrist tendons than when it is used as a free flap. Nonetheless, whenever tendon is encountered in elevating the flap, care must be taken to preserve the overlying epitenon. Once the flap has been raised across the flexor carpi radialis from the ulnar margin, traction reveals the radial artery and its venae comitantes (Fig. 47-60). Multiple small branches to the muscles must be divided as the dissection proceeds from the ulnar side. Once the underside of the pedicle is freed up, the radial dissection is begun. From proximal to distal, the fascia and septum are carefully dissected off the brachioradialis muscle and tendon. Great care must be taken here to avoid

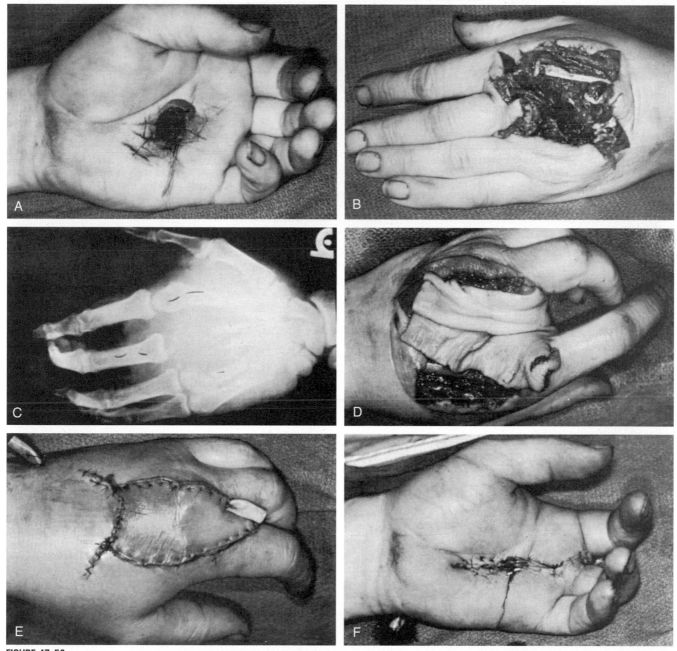

FIGURE 47-58. Fillet flap This patient sustained a gunshot wound of the palm of the nondominant hand (**A**) at close range, producing a large dorsal exit wound (**B**) and destroying the metacarpal of the middle finger (**C**). As the extensor tendons were also disrupted and the flexor tendons heavily contaminated, it was deemed appropriate to sacrifice the middle finger, which was well vascularized. **D,** The resultant fillet flap is seen after its initial dissection, laid onto the dorsum of the hand. Immediate transposition of the index onto the middle metacarpal was undertaken with reduction of the fillet flap to a neurovascular pedicle. **E and F,** The closure of dorsal and palmar wounds.

dividing the perforators to the skin as they run along the brachioradialis. While both the aforementioned muscles are retracted away from each other, the lateral intermuscular septum in which the artery runs is incised parallel and deep to the radial artery. The pedicle is now dissected distally, and the entire pedicle with its surrounding fascia should be taken together. No attempt should be made to separate the veins from the radial artery. The radial artery can now be ligated proximally and the flap transposed to the primary defect (Fig. 47-61), passing it through a tunnel beneath intervening intact skin where it is present, using

the technique described in the section on neurovascular island flaps.

Once the flap is in place, the previously proximal radial artery in the flap, now distal, can be anastomosed either immediately or at a later procedure to supply more distal tissues, such as a devascularized finger or a toe transfer.[93,208] The forearm flap can be used for forearm defects, provided that their location is appropriate (Fig. 47-62). In such cases, one or more superficial veins can be rejoined proximally to make venous drainage more efficient.[112] The quality of circulation in the hand can be evaluated once the flap is raised

CRITICAL POINTS: RADIAL FOREARM FLAP

INDICATIONS

- Wounds of dorsal hand, forearm, or elbow
- For acute coverage of trauma or tumor resection

PREOPERATIVE EVALUATION

- Allen's test and Doppler examination to ascertain adequacy of ulnar artery flow to hand
- Forearm skin without injury or scar (where flap is to be designed)

PEARLS

- For distally based flaps, design pedicle to allow room for rotation
- Dissect pedicle out as a unit, without separation of artery and veins
- Begin dissection on ulnar side of flap

TECHNICAL POINTS

- Take skin, subcutaneous tissue, and fascia off muscle.
- Great care must be taken to elevate flap off of brachioradialis tendon to avoid injury to perforators.

- Identify and protect radial nerve under brachioradialis and distally.
- Avoid separation of artery and venae comitantes.
- With exposure of flexor carpi radialis tendon, suture superficialis muscle over this to improve skin graft take at donor site.
- Avoid kinking pedicle with distal rotation.
- If tunneling flap under intact skin bridge, make sure this is very loose.

PITFALLS

- Elevating fascia with perforators away from skin when dissecting over brachioradialis tendon
- Kinking pedicle with distal rotation
- Loss of skin graft at donor site due to flexor carpi radialis and brachioradialis tendon exposure

POSTOPERATIVE CARE

- Immobilize wrist, MP joint and PIP joint for 2 to 3 weeks for skin graft take.
- Motion may begin after graft has taken.

---

and the tourniquet let down. If it is necessary to reconstruct the radial artery, the gap between the end of the radial artery proximally and the radial artery at the pivot point adjacent to the anatomical snuff-box is measured. A vein graft of that length is harvested from the cephalic vein and interposed end to end proximally and end to side distally, using standard microsurgical techniques.

The secondary skin defect is closed with a split-thickness skin graft. Generally, take of the graft is improved if the tendon of the flexor carpi radialis tendon is covered with some of the flexor pollicis longus and/or superficialis muscle bellies.[170,326] This is cosmetically unsightly, but it rarely causes the problems of distal edema that were feared when this flap was first used. The poor appearance of the secondary defect can be eliminated by raising the flap as fascia alone. In this instance, the fascia is raised alone without the overlying skin. The area of fascia necessary to cover the soft tissue defect is marked on the forearm, adequately proximal to allow rotation of the pedicle (Fig. 47-63A). The skin is elevated off the fascia in the manner of a full-thickness graft, but care must be taken to avoid damage to the underlying fascia. Once the skin is elevated, the dissection deep to the fascia proceeds as described earlier for the standard radial forearm fasciocutaneous flap (see Fig. 47-63B and C). The radial artery with its fascia is then rotated into the defect. The fascia is usually covered with a full-thickness skin graft. This type of flap affords appropriately durable and thin coverage of the hand and avoids the need for skin grafting of the donor site. Although there has been some question about

the efficacy of graft take over fascial flaps, our experience and that from reported series has been reasonable.[147]

Ulnar Artery Forearm Flap. Like the radial artery flap, the ulnar artery flap can be based proximally to cover defects around the elbow[111,146] or distally for hand cover.[120,189,288] First described in 1984,[198] it has gained less popularity than the radial artery forearm flap, despite offering the advantages of less hairy skin and a less obvious secondary defect, which, having more muscle and less tendon, should take skin grafts more readily. The donor site of this flap can often be closed primarily, particularly in older patients who may have excess skin on the ulnar border of the forearm. This flap is particularly useful in the management of distressing chemotherapy burns to the dorsal hands in elderly women. In this group of patients, a large flap can be taken to cover the dorsal hand with primary closure of the donor site in most instances. This flap may also be used as a free flap to the hand in appropriate circumstances.[171]

Dissection is similar to the radial artery forearm flap, except that the vascular septum from artery to skin lies between the flexor carpi ulnaris and flexor digitorum muscles and that care must be taken not to harm the ulnar nerve lying immediately deep to the vessel. If taken very proximally on the arm, the septum can be tenuous, with very small perforators, but the flap is very reliable in my experience. Owing to the proximity of the dissection to the ulnar nerve (and possibly devascularization of the nerve with flap harvest), most patients experience a period of ulnar nerve

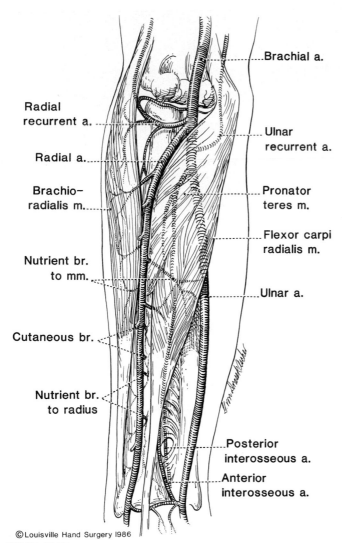

Radial recurrent a.

Radial a.

Brachio-radialis m.

Nutrient br. to mm.

Cutaneous br.

Nutrient br. to radius

Brachial a.

Ulnar recurrent a.

Pronator teres m.

Flexor carpi radialis m.

Ulnar a.

Posterior interosseous a.

Anterior interosseous a.

©Louisville Hand Surgery 1986

FIGURE 47–59. The course of the radial artery is superficial throughout much of the forearm, lying just beneath the margin of the brachioradialis on the pronator teres and the flexor digitorum superficialis. The cutaneous branches supply the overlying skin and nutrient branches of the radius. (From the Christine Kleinert Institute for Hand and Microsurgery, Inc., with permission.)

dysesthesia postoperatively. This generally resolves in a few months.

Reversed Posterior Interosseous Artery Flap. In 1986 the anatomic basis[263] and clinical application[356] of a flap based on the posterior interosseous artery (PIA) was first reported. Initially used as a proximally based flap to cover the elbow,[243] its popularity has increased since description of more detailed anatomy and also because of its use as a reversed flap.[17,60,73,126,355]

The PIA arises in the anterior compartment from the common interosseous artery, which also gives rise to the anterior vessel. The PIA immediately passes dorsally through the interosseous membrane some 6 cm distal to the lateral epicondyle emerging just below the distal edge of the supinator. Throughout its course, it lies between the extensor carpi ulnaris and the extensor digiti minimi, initially lying on the abductor pollicis longus muscle belly in close approximation to the posterior interosseous nerve. Some

2 cm proximal to the ulnar styloid, it has an anastomosis with the anterior interosseous artery, then passes on to the dorsum of the carpus, where it anastomoses with branches of the radial artery. Throughout its course, the PIA gives septocutaneous perforators that supply the skin over the dorsum of the forearm.

To raise the flap, a line is first drawn from the lateral epicondyle to the distal radioulnar joint. A point on this line 2 cm proximal to the ulnar styloid is marked, which represents the pivot point of the distally based flap. Measurements are taken from this point to the proximal and distal edges of the primary defect. These represent the distances from the pivot point along the line initially drawn at which the distal and proximal margins of the flap outline, respectively, are marked. The radial margin of the flap and a distal extension to the distal radioulnar joint are incised. The distal extension can be made 1 cm radial to the previously made surface marking of the PIA.[33] The flap is raised, and the fascia over the extensor digiti minimi is incised 5 mm radial to the thick fascial septum. While the muscle is being retracted radially, the posterior interosseous artery, its branches, and the anastomosis to the anterior interosseous artery distally are dissected, taking care to preserve the perforating vessels to the skin. Provided no anomalies are encountered, a similar skin and fascial incision is now made on the ulnar aspect over the extensor carpi ulnaris, which is again mobilized by division of the muscular branches of the PIA. Most authors suggest keeping a segment of dorsal forearm fascia intact with the septal vessels distally, which may contain veins to improve venous outflow in the distally based flap. The relationship of the motor branch of the extensor carpi ulnaris to the PIA and its most proximal relevant perforator (MPRP)[33] must now be inspected, because if it passes superficial to the PIA and the MPRP is the major septocutaneous perforator, which it may be,[60] the surgeon may decide to divide and repair the nerve, as recommended by Büchler and Frey[33] in that circumstance. This anatomy is one of the primary factors that mitigate against the choice of this flap. The potential morbidity of dividing and repairing the posterior interosseous nerve in a flap that often has questionable viability makes this flap often less than an ideal choice. Once the pedicle and flap have been fully mobilized so that they are attached only by the proximal and distal vascular connections, there is merit in placing a microvascular clamp on the PIA proximal to the MPRP and releasing the tourniquet. If flow is good, ligation can replace the clamp, and the flap can be turned into place on the hand.

The reach of the flap has not been clearly defined. It can certainly reach the first web space and the MP joints. Büchler and Frey[33] have taken the flap to the PIP joint, but they reported a 21% incidence of partial necrosis. Although statistical analysis of their results indicated that this necrosis was not related to pedicle length, this incidence of partial flap loss is higher than that encountered in other series, with only one case of remediable venous congestion of 32 flaps performed. Nonetheless, this flap remains problematic in most hands regardless of the length of the pedicle. Despite enthusiasm for this flap, Brunelli reported a 14% incidence of at least partial necrosis of 113 posterior interosseous flaps.[32] Another more recent report found anatomic variations in 24% of 88 flaps elevated, which led to inability to harvest the flap in 5 (6% of cases).[344] This same group noted

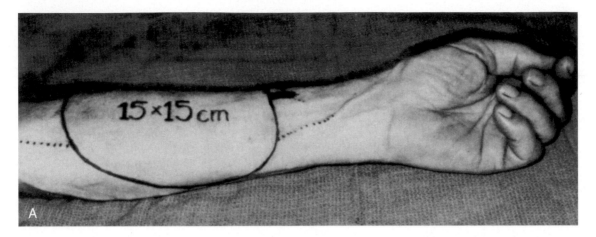

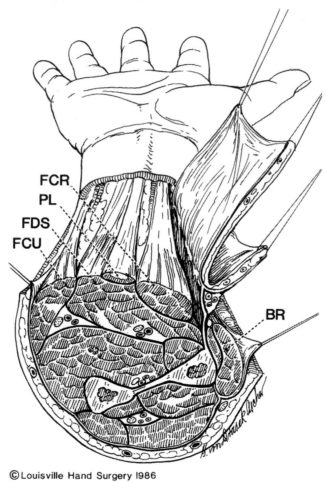

© Louisville Hand Surgery 1986

B

FIGURE 47-60. Radial forearm flap. **A,** The marking for a radial forearm flap is shown (to be used here as a free flap). **B,** Incision of the fascia lifts the entire flap off the underlying muscles of the forearm. (**B,** from the Christine Kleinert Institute for Hand and Microsurgery, Inc., with permission.) *Continued*

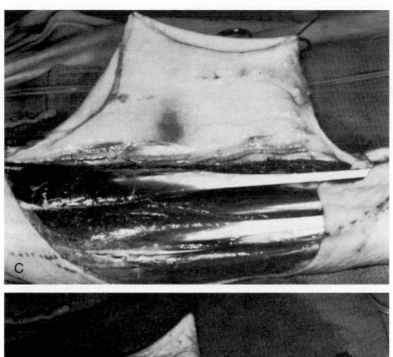

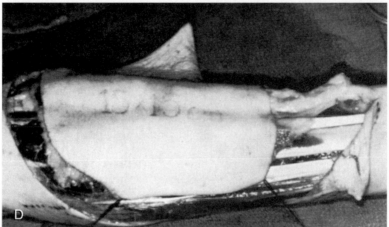

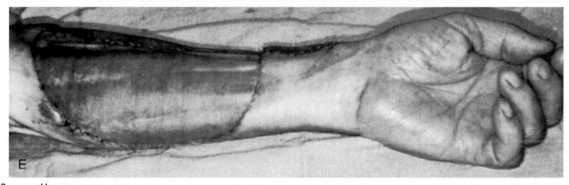

FIGURE 47-60 —cont'd. Radial forearm flap. **C,** Clinical photograph of **B**. These are seen from the ulnar aspect. The radial artery and its venae comitantes run at the lower margin of the flap (**D**). The flap and (**E**) the secondary defect covered with a split-thickness skin graft.

variable degrees of flap necrosis in 13% of cases. For these reasons, this flap should not be attempted without knowledge of both the anatomy (and its variations) and an acceptance of a rather high rate of either partial or complete flap failure.

Musculocutaneous Flap

The blood supply of muscles has been classified into five types[215]:

Type I: One vascular pedicle (e.g., tensor fascia lata)
Type II: One dominant plus other minor (e.g., gracilis)

Type III: Two dominant (e.g., gluteus maximus)
Type IV: Several, equal, segmental (e.g., sartorius)
Type V: One dominant plus peripheral (e.g., latissimus dorsi)

In types I, II, and V, one so-called dominant pedicle[218] is capable of supporting the entire muscle if the others are ligated. Theoretically, therefore, any muscle in the upper extremity that belongs to one of these three types can be transposed on its pedicle. Several have been described: coracobrachialis to the axilla[132]; deltoid to the shoulder[123]; brachioradialis,[177] extensor carpi radialis longus,[250] and flexor carpi ulnaris[163] (Fig. 47-64) to the elbow; flexor

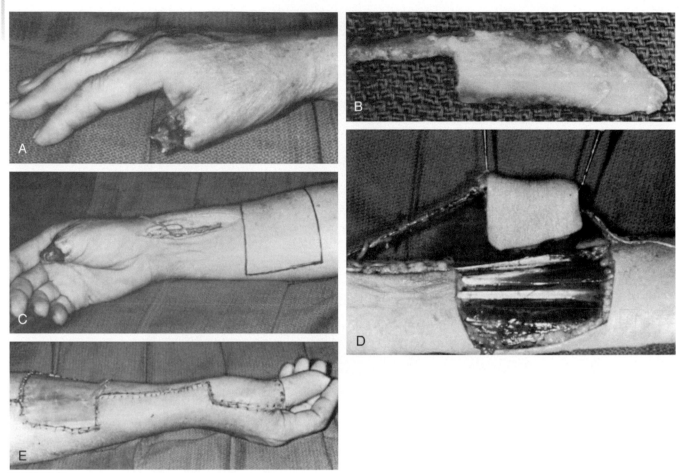

FIGURE 47-61. **A,** This patient suffered an amputation of the thumb in a roping injury. **B,** The thumb is lengthened using a corticocancellous iliac crest bone graft. **C,** A radial forearm flap has been marked out and the radial artery dissected. **D,** The flap is raised on its pedicle. **E,** The flap has been transposed and sutured in position and the secondary defect closed with a split-thickness skin graft.

digitorum superficialis to the antecubital fossa[133]; extensor carpi ulnaris and flexor digitorum profundus to the proximal ulna[54]; pronator quadratus[71] and abductor digiti minimi[228,276] to the wrist; and the first dorsal interosseous to the first metacarpal[215] and to the third metacarpal.[204] Because the majority of these lie beneath a well-vascularized deep fascia, most have been used as muscle flaps to which split-thickness skin grafts have been applied. These flaps have limited value, because they all eliminate a functioning motor. Furthermore, their contour is good only when the defect has a volume similar to that of the muscle belly. The function of the transposed muscle can be preserved where necessary[42,214] provided the correct tension is maintained.[99] The fascia overlying a muscle, if it is thick, has a rich plexus supplied through vessels of the intermuscular septa. In the absence of a direct axial cutaneous vessel, that plexus supplies the overlying skin, which is therefore best raised as a fasciocutaneous flap, leaving the muscle in place. Where the fascia is thin or absent, the supply to the skin comes more from small branches that perforate the muscle; Olivari[251] described 27 such vessels in the latissimus dorsi. In this case, the muscle and the skin overlying it can be moved efficiently as a block to provide skin cover and, where needed, function. Whether the cover achieved is better when the muscle alone is moved and then skin grafted, or when a musculocutaneous flap is used, is still a matter of debate,[242] but most believe today that musculocutaneous flaps are generally too bulky.

Two muscles in the type V classification have been used in this manner to the upper extremity, the pectoralis major and latissimus dorsi. As with other type V muscles, the main vascular pedicle of the pectoralis major—the pectoral branch of the acromiothoracic axis supplemented by the lateral thoracic artery[97,274]—enters close to its insertion. There are numerous small vessels entering the periphery or origin of the muscle, notably from the internal mammary artery. Unlike all the regional axial muscle flaps listed earlier, the pectoralis is left attached at its insertion and released from its origin. It can be split longitudinally to cover two adjacent defects.[234] The pectoralis muscle without skin—in one series, with the addition of pectoralis minor[337]—has long been used for restoration of elbow flexion lost as a result of nerve injury[30,48] or arthrogryposis.[10,78] With an island of overlying skin, it has been used as an axial regional flap for reconstruction of the axilla[96] and shoulder.[77] However, the secondary defect, even when it can be closed directly, is entirely unacceptable to women and largely so to men. Because all primary defects in the upper extremity that can be reached by the pectoralis can be covered with ease and with a much more acceptable donor site by the latissimus dorsi flap, the latter is preferred in virtually all cases.

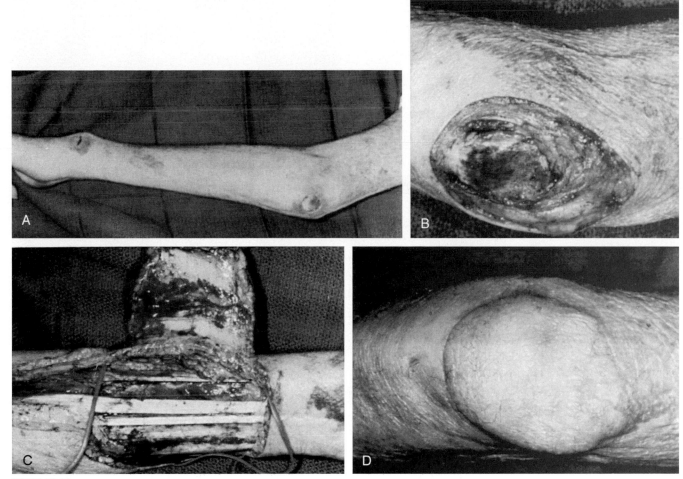

FIGURE 47-62. This patient with scleroderma has undergone more than 20 operations in an attempt to close the ulcerating olecranon bursa (**A**). Pseudotumor resection of the olecranon bursa together with underlying bone yields a clean defect (**B**). A radial forearm flap is raised and transposed on its proximal pedicle (**C**), producing a flap that healed satisfactorily and has remained so (**D**).

Latissimus Dorsi Flap. The wide arc of rotation around its pedicle makes the latissimus currently popular for reconstruction of the breast, the abdominal wall, the head and neck,[25] and the shoulder.[55,77,227] The diameter of the artery (1 to 2.5 mm) and the length of the pedicle (11 cm)[14] have made it the most robust and therefore most popular tissue for free transfer, especially to the extremities.[113] Functional transposition of the latissimus dorsi to restore lost biceps function has been known to the orthopedic surgeon for over 30 years.[295,327,358] Its use to restore both function and skin cover[29,182,318] and to restore cover alone[1,303] is a more recent development.

The latissimus dorsi arises from the lower six thoracic vertebrae, from the thoracolumbar fascia, and from the posterior part of the iliac crest. From this extensive origin the muscle fibers converge to wrap around the lower border of the teres major and end in a quadrilateral tendon that inserts into the intertubercular sulcus of the humerus. Together with the teres major, it forms the posterior axillary fold. Furnas and Furnas[102] reported one patient in whom the lower part of the muscle was absent but its anterior border felt quite normal preoperatively. Its main blood supply derives from the vessel popularly known as the thoracodorsal artery, which is the continuation of the subscapular artery after it

gives off its circumflex scapular branch some 2 cm distal to its origin from the axillary artery (Fig. 47-65). The thoracodorsal artery gives a variable number of branches to the chest wall, notably one to the serratus anterior, before reaching its hilum on the latissimus dorsi some 11 cm from the axillary artery.[14] Immediately distal to the hilum, the artery divides into two branches in 94% of specimens.[335] The upper branch runs parallel to and 3.5 cm from the upper margin of the muscle; the lateral runs parallel to and 2.1 cm from the lateral margin of the muscle. This arrangement permits the surgeon to split the muscle longitudinally when a narrow flap is required.[335] One might suppose that absence of the artery would preclude use of the latissimus dorsi flap, and routine angiography to ensure its presence has been suggested.[283] However, this need was disputed[74] in the belief that previous injury to the vessel served as a delay. Certainly, if the serratus branch remains intact, it has been shown that collateral circulation is established and the flap can be safely transposed.[85] This would, however, severely limit the reach of the flap when it is taken to the arm and carries the risk of kinking the pedicle. The muscle can also be used in "reverse,"[322] based on the vessels of the T9, T10, and T11 intercostal spaces but rarely to the upper extremity. Any significant defect of the upper arm and elbow can be covered

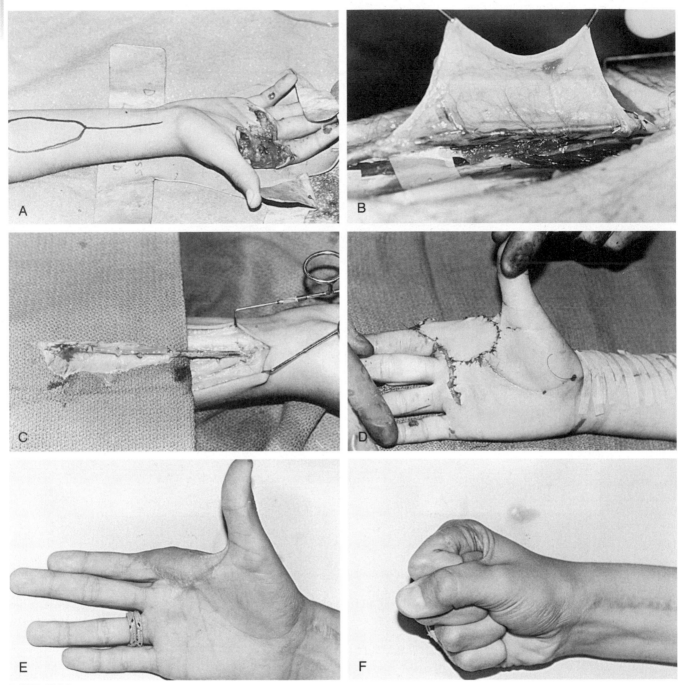

FIGURE 47-63.   The radial forearm fascial flap. **A,** Palmar defect from a shotgun injury with the area of fascia to be harvested outlined on the forearm. **B,** Fascia elevated off the muscle. Note the rich vascularity of the fascia. **C,** The fascia with its radial vascular pedicle after harvest. **D,** Fascia placed in the palmar defect and covered with a full-thickness skin graft. **E** and **F,** Late result with stable coverage and good motion. Note the forearm scar from primary closure of donor site.

with a pedicle latissimus dorsi flap (Fig. 47-66), and it has been transferred successfully to the forearm.[207]

The patient is placed in the lateral position with padding beneath the torso sufficient to protect circulation to the arm on the operating table.[103] When the latissimus dorsi is to be transposed to a defect in the upper extremity, the involved limb, together with the entire ipsilateral hemithorax and distally to the iliac crest, is prepared and draped. The axilla can be displayed by wrapping the forearm with soft padding and then applying upward traction to a ceiling fixture to

achieve 100 degrees of abduction, or a similar position can be less satisfactorily achieved by taping the forearm to a sterile Mayo stand. In either case, there is considerable danger of brachial plexus neurapraxia with consequent paresis[202] and performing the entire dissection with the arm in a single fixed position is to be condemned. Checking the radial pulse regularly is no guarantee that all is well. If the surgeon believes that this dissection requires the arm in a fixed position, plexus injury can be avoided only by a strict practice of returning the limb to the patient's side for 5

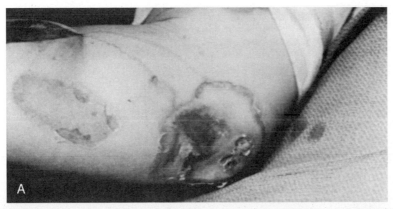

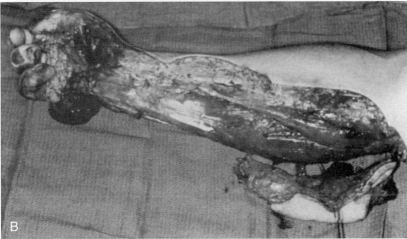

FIGURE 47-64. A, A full-thickness thermal burn is located over the cubital tunnel. **B,** The flexor carpi ulnaris has been destroyed in its distal portion by the same thermal injury. It is possible therefore to transpose it on the proximal ulnar artery, which was thrombosed distally, to cover the defect in the region of the olecranon and medial epicondyle after primary excision of the burn.

minutes every hour, monitored by the anesthesiologist. We prefer to avoid placing the arm in a fixed abducted position and simply have an assistant hold the arm abducted with periodic relaxation of the patient's shoulder (and the assistant). A zigzag incision is made in the axilla, avoiding the hair-bearing area, extending down along the anterior border of the muscle. Through this incision, the anterior border of the latissimus is located and sharply freed up. Once the anterior border is freed up, the submuscular dissection is done easily in the areolar plane next to the chest wall. The thoracodorsal vessel can best be found where it approaches the muscular hilum. This is approximately at the nipple line in a man or a child. With good retraction and light, the vessel can be traced proximally, identifying first the serratus branch and then the circumflex scapular artery. These are ligated and divided. If they are not, they tether and kink the pedicle after transposition. The most proximal extent of the dissection constitutes the pivot point or axis of the flap.

At this juncture, the distance from this pivot point to the proximal margin of the defect in the limb is measured and transposed to the anterior border of the latissimus dorsi previously marked. This second point represents the proximal edge of the proposed flap. With the use of a pattern of the primary defect, the flap can now be marked out over the posterolateral thorax. The anterior margin is incised, and the anterior border of the latissimus is elevated with the overlying skin. The inferior border of the flap can now be raised by incising through skin, subcutaneous tissue, and muscle, using cutting cautery for all but the skin. The benefit

of doing so is that the latissimus dorsi can now be swung away and posterior from the trunk, permitting a clear view of the vascular tree of the thoracodorsal artery. Where a narrow flap is all that is needed, the lateral branch is located and the posterior border of the flap is incised as was the inferior border, while carefully avoiding that lateral branch. The upper (situated also medial and posterior) branch is ligated and divided. The thoracodorsal artery is now dissected off the latissimus dorsi, working from the axilla distally as far as possible without injury to it or its muscular branches. The proximal margin of the flap can now be incised in a similar manner to the inferior (or distal) and posterior, while retracting the pedicle anteriorly and so protecting it from harm. Raising the flap in this manner rather than taking the whole muscle, as was done in the past, yields a flap tailored exactly to the primary defect.[114] In particular, it avoids both a bulky proximal portion to the flap and the difficult task of separating latissimus dorsi from teres major. The bulk proximally was not only unsightly but also difficult to fit into the upper arm. This is particularly so in the common circumstance in which the flap is to be passed beneath an intact skin bridge. The flap can now be passed to the primary defect and sutured in place. The secondary defect is always closed directly, for a skin graft in this location presents many difficulties in terms of graft take and wound care. Seroma formation is common,[269] and prolonged suction drainage is indicated. More tissue is available for superior to inferior closure than in the line of the trunk. Small defects are therefore best closed transversely.

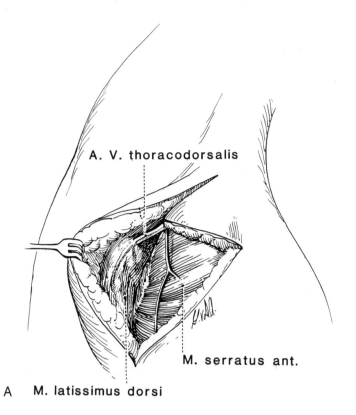

A. V. thoracodorsalis

M. serratus ant.

A M. latissimus dorsi

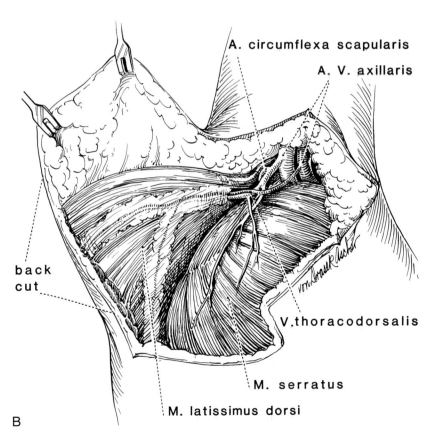

A. circumflexa scapularis

A. V. axillaris

back
cut

V. thoracodorsalis

M. serratus

M. latissimus dorsi

B

FIGURE 47-65. The vascular pedicle of the latissimus dorsi flap is displayed here in the course of its dissection. The subscapular artery arises from the axillary artery and soon gives off the circumflex scapular, which passes between the teres major and the latissimus dorsi. **A,** The next branch to arise is that to the serratus. The thoracodorsal artery passes beneath the epimysium of the latissimus dorsi and there divides into two branches. The upper branch runs parallel to and 3.5 cm from the upper margin of the muscle, the lateral parallel to and 2.1 cm from the lateral margin of the muscle. **B,** The first, distal cut of the flap has been made through skin and muscle.

Continued

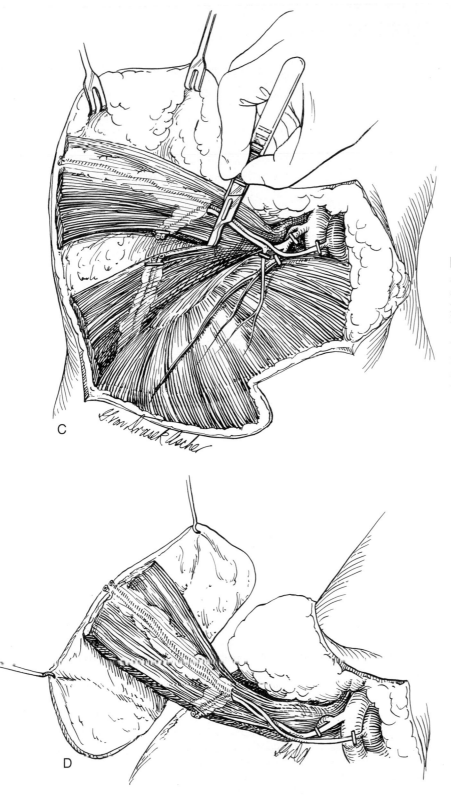

C

D

FIGURE 47-65—cont'd. C, The lateral or anterior portion of the muscle is being used alone in designing this small flap. The posterior or upper branch of the thoracodorsal has therefore been divided and the muscle is split either with a knife, as shown here, or better with cutting diathermy through both muscle and skin as required. **D,** The proximal margin of the flap has been divided here through skin and will then be divided through muscle just proximal to the point at which the thoracodorsal artery passes beneath the epimysium of the latissimus dorsi. In this way a thin, well-tailored latissimus dorsi is created. (The clips shown here on the artery and vein of the pedicle would not, of course, be applied in using the latissimus as a regional flap.) (Modified from Godina M: The tailored latissimus dorsi flap. Plast Reconstr Surg 78:295-299, 1987.)

CRITICAL POINTS: LATISSIMUS DORSI PEDICLED FLAP

INDICATIONS

- Coverage of upper arm, elbow, proximal forearm
- Functional reconstruction of elbow flexion or extension

PREOPERATIVE EVALUATION

- Presence and function of latissimus (especially for functional reconstruction)
- Absence of scars in axilla (axillary dissection, mastectomy, thoracotomy)

PEARLS

- May take skin paddle for coverage or place skin graft over muscle
- If not needed for functional coverage, should cut thoracodorsal nerve to prevent muscle from pulling loose with movement
- Should leave artery and vein in pedicle together in areolar tissue to avoid kinking of vein
- Should divide tendon from humerus to obtain the most length
- Distal muscle possibly not viable, especially if overstretched

TECHNICAL POINTS

- Elevate skin from muscle with knife or cautery.

- Identify pedicle running under proximal portion of muscle.
- Deep surface can usually be elevated with finger dissection.
- Divide distal muscle with cautery once pedicle is identified.
- Dissect pedicle carefully with muscle flipped over.
- Ligate or clip the large paraspinous perforators (not cautery).
- Once pedicle is identified and isolated, divide muscle proximally.
- If taken under an intact skin bridge to the defect, tunnel must be adequate to prevent pressure on muscle.
- Avoid suturing the muscle too tightly distally.

PITFALLS

- Damage to pedicle during dissection
- Passing the muscle under a too-tight skin bridge
- Suturing the muscle under too much tension

POSTOPERATIVE CARE

- Place large drains in donor site for 5 to 7 days (seromas common).
- Immobilize shoulder and elbow for 2 to 3 weeks.
- Begin gradual mobilization.

Larger defects may require transposition of loose tissue from the waistline anteriorly, using a rhomboid design (type II transposition flap; see Fig. 47-33). No significant loss of function has been shown following use of the latissimus dorsi.[178]

DISTANT FLAPS

Distant flaps come from body parts outside the upper extremity. Both random- and axial-pattern varieties exist. All distant flaps require a period of attachment between the operated limb and the donor part. They therefore all require at least two stages: attachment and division. When the blood supply to a random-pattern flap is doubtful, preliminary delay and later inset operations may be necessary, making four operations in total. Distant random-pattern flaps were formerly the routine method of providing skin cover to the hand where free grafts would not suffice,[31,38] but the necessary hospitalization time was long and the outcome unpredictable.[323] When these factors—attachment, multiple stages, prolonged hospital stay, and doubtful result—are considered together, it is readily understood why the random-pattern distant flap has been largely superseded by the axial-pattern distant flap and it, in turn, by free microvascular flap transfer. There are, however, still indications for the use of both

types of conventional distant flaps. The axial flaps all have defined territories based on pedicles that run in the vascular strata previously defined. The need to ensure that the vessel is included in the flap restricts the surgeon's ability to invade its vascular territory too boldly in trying to harvest a flap for a small defect, and the license to thin an axial flap is strictly controlled by the need to preserve the nutrient vascular plane. It follows that for small defects or for ones requiring thin skin, distant axial flaps, either conventional or by free transfer, are unsuitable. Normally, local or regional flaps satisfy the need, but where they are not suitable or available, distant random-pattern flaps are still required. Such a circumstance may arise in loss of palmar skin, circumferential avulsion of soft tissue from the thumb, and small but significant defects (e.g., when bone is exposed on the dorsum of the thumb) in a hand already extensively injured.

Conventional distant axial flaps are indicated in quite different circumstances. They are the most reliable form of coverage when microsurgical expertise is not available. When it is, free flap transfer is the method of choice, not only because it eliminates the problems of attachment and multiple procedures detailed earlier but also because it ensures a permanent, vigorous blood supply to the injured area. It may be difficult, however, to transfer much spare soft tissue with a free flap. Thus, if it is intended at a later stage to transfer the index finger by pollicization[317] or toes from

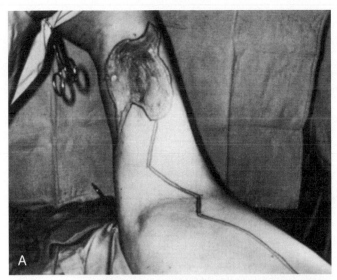

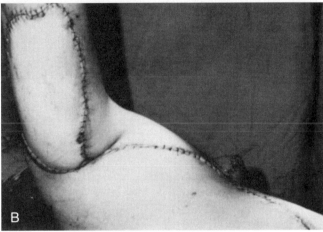

FIGURE 47-66. Latissimus dorsi pedicle flap. **A,** A forearm defect resulting from a gunshot wound is covered with a large latissimus dorsi pedicle flap (**B**).

the foot to restore an amputated thumb or fingers, a conventional axial-pattern flap should be used for skin cover. Its tube pedicle can provide the additional skin necessary to cover the proximal portion of the later digital transfer. In one series, 77% of toe transfers required preliminary groin flaps.[106] The presence of such additional skin allows a minimum of skin to be taken from the foot, so that closure there can be achieved entirely with local skin, a desirable objective. In the case of toe transfer, the use of a conventional flap has the additional benefit over free flap transfer of preserving the vessels of the hand untouched for the later anastomosis to those of the toe. As experience in microvascular surgery increases, this consideration becomes less valid.

Random-Pattern Distant Flaps

Because the blood supply of the random-pattern flap derives from the subdermal or subcutaneous plexus, it can be raised at any site on the body. This apparent freedom is severely restricted by considerations of suitability, availability, positioning, and appearance. To give extreme examples, scalp skin is not suitable, penile skin is not available, leg skin would not be comfortable, and neck skin is not cosmetically

acceptable. Indeed, when all factors are weighed, few donor sites remain. In the male patient, any site on the torso or the other uninjured arm may be used if no better alternative is available. In the female, only the inguinal region, where the defect can be closed directly and concealed beneath a two-piece swimsuit, is universally acceptable. In practice, this means that random-pattern flaps are rarely used in females, except to transfer thin skin from the region of the iliac crest. In some instances, this type of flap may be indicated despite the donor site and circulatory difficulties. These would include suture of cutaneous nerves in the flap to branches of the radial nerve in the defect to reinnervate a thumb reconstruction,[75] the use of double flaps to cover both dorsal and palmar wounds[232] and to create a new first web,[231,343] and the use of several interdigitating flaps to resurface multiple finger injuries.[140]

With the advent of regional axial-pattern flaps (i.e., the radial forearm flap) and the availability of the axial groin flap, there is in fact little application for these flaps today. The donor defects are generally quite ugly, particularly from the chest, even in male patients who usually find these sites marginally acceptable. For these reasons, we believe that these are generally not only a secondary choice for coverage but should be considered as a last resort. For further information on these types of flaps, the reader is referred to prior editions of this text.[199]

Axial-Pattern Distant Flaps

The concept that a large vessel supplying a block of tissue ensures good perfusion is simple. That concept was recognized in 1863 by Wood,[349] who emphasized the importance of including the superficial inferior epigastric artery in a flap to release a burn contracture in a child. This vessel was the basis of the flap used in the first modern description of an axial-pattern flap in 1946 by Shaw and Payne.[298] The same flap has since been described by various authors under different names, including the Shaw flap,[12] the abdomino-hypogastric flap,[292] and the superficial inferior epigastric artery flap.[131,321] The use of a large abdominal flap based on both superficial inferior epigastric arteries and both superficial circumflex iliac arteries for large upper extremity defects has been reported by Kelleher and coworkers.[162] Despite the successes reported by all these authors, neither this hypogastric flap nor other axial flaps from the torso, such as the transverse rectus[36] and thoracoumbilical flaps,[26] have achieved the popularity enjoyed by the groin flap.[95,221]

Groin Flap

The groin flap is an axial-pattern flap of the cutaneous variety (Fig. 47-67). Its axial vessel is the superficial circumflex iliac artery,[309] which is a relatively constant vessel, being present in 96% of a series of angiograms.[158] The vessel arises from the femoral artery in the femoral triangle, which forms a vascular "hub,"[329] because the axes of several flaps converge here. The superficial circumflex iliac artery emerges from the triangle by passing over the medial border of the sartorius immediately after giving off a deep muscular branch. Initially below the deep fascia, the vessel emerges through that fascia as it crosses the sartorius. It passes laterally, parallel to and some 2 cm below the inguinal ligament. At a point below the anterior superior iliac spine, the

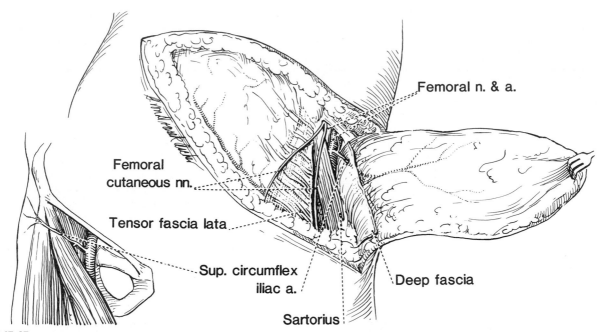

FIGURE 47-67. Groin flap. The groin flap is based on the superficial circumflex iliac artery, which runs parallel to and approximately 1 inch inferior to the inguinal ligament. It emerges through the deep fascia as it crosses the sartorius and breaks up into branches at the level of the anterior superior iliac spine. When the flap is raised, the lateral femoral cutaneous nerve should be preserved or, in certain instances (see text), divided and repaired. The fascia that is divided at the lateral margin of the sartorius can be seen. (From the Christine Kleinert Institute for Hand and Microsurgery, Inc., with permission.)

vessel divides and supplies the skin immediately below the iliac crest. The vascular territory of the superficial circumflex iliac artery therefore ends at some point lateral to the anterior superior iliac spine. Common wisdom and practical experience dictate that the flap can safely be extended beyond the spine by a distance at least equal to the width of the flap. The venous drainage,[262] which is as important as the arterial supply,[306] and the lymphatic outflow[51] of the flap have both been studied in detail. The report by Penteado[262] gives details of venous variations in the femoral triangle that are important to the microsurgeon; a surgeon intent on using the flap as an axial pedicle need only know that all drainage of this region is to the femoral triangle and therefore will lie within the pedicle. Commonly, no reinnervation of the flap is attempted, but Joshi[155] pointed out that the lateral cutaneous branch of the subcostal or 12th thoracic nerve consistently crosses the iliac crest 5 cm posterior to the anterior superior iliac spine. This can be dissected, divided, and sutured to any available cutaneous nerve ending in the hand. The groin flap can provide skin cover for any defect on any aspect of the hand or of the forearm in its distal two thirds.[43] It can safely be made wide enough to replace massive loss, with the only drawback being that the widest secondary defect that can be readily closed directly is 12 cm. For defects on both aspects of the hand, the flap can be split longitudinally or used in conjunction with a hypogastric flap,[308] a tensor fascia lata musculocutaneous flap,[345] or a contralateral groin flap.[128] Where a relatively large block of bone is required in the hand in the depths of a soft tissue defect, the iliac crest (Fig. 47-68) immediately beneath the flap can be taken as a vascularized composite extension.[37,83,275]

In planning the groin flap, a pattern of the primary defect should be made first. It is next decided from which direction the flap should approach the defect. For example, for defects primarily on the dorsal aspect of the wrist, the flap pedicle could lie to either the radial or the ulnar side. Time should be taken with this decision, for the obvious choice is not always the correct one. Factors to be considered are the precise location of the defect, the resulting configuration of the tube pedicle, the freedom of pronation and supination of the forearm, and the patient's comfort and exercise postoperatively. The major fact to be appreciated with respect to the configuration of the pedicle is that it will do well if it is stretched gently and will do poorly if it is kinked; flaps always perfuse more satisfactorily on a convex surface than on a concave one. To take another example, a defect on the dorsal aspect of the hand extending on to the radial border might be best approached by a pedicle around the ulnar border, because full pronation and supination would place little stress on the suture line and would not kink the pedicle. The previously prepared pattern can be extended with a portion to represent the pedicle so that various approaches and positions can be tested. Once the approach and eventual position have been chosen, that edge of the primary defect that will be closest to the pedicle will be known. The original pattern should be laid on the skin immediately below and behind the anterior superior iliac spine, because the more medial, inguinal portion of the flap will largely be used to construct the tube.

A few words about constructing the tube are appropriate at this juncture. Two extreme possibilities should be considered. If a flap is not tubed at all, its distal and lateral margins can be made to fit precisely to the primary defect. The other margin of the defect, adjacent to the pedicle, has to be left unsutured, but the eventual contour of the flap to the hand is excellent, without revision. At the other extreme, if the flap is raised as a rectangle and tubed throughout its length, it

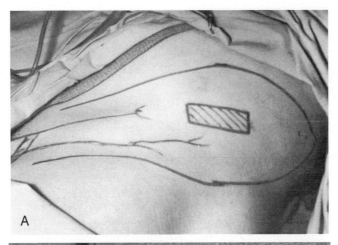

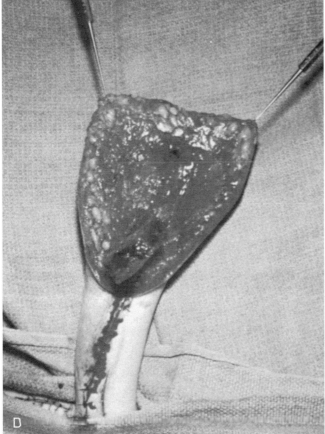

FIGURE 47-68. Groin flap with iliac crest. **A,** The groin flap has been marked out with the inguinal ligament and the expected course of the superficial circumflex iliac artery. A monobloc of iliac crest has been taken with the groin flap, and it can be seen to be bleeding well in the distal portion of the tube (**B**). (This is the same patient as shown in Figure 47-74.)

edges of the flap come to meet the edge of the proximal half of the defect. After division of the flap, there will be too much skin at the proximal margin, which will require excision as dog-ears at the time of division or at a later stage. The surgeon's ability to tube the groin flap depends on the width of the flap but also on its thickness. Because its axial vessel emerges through the deep fascia, the flap cannot be thinned appreciably in the part to be tubed, except at the margins. Thus, in choosing the width of the flap, the surgeon must pay heed not only to the width of the primary defect but also to the weight-height ratio of the patient. If this is high, the flap will be thick and must therefore be wide. Skin grafts may be necessary to close the secondary defect.

Once all these factors have been considered and the patient is prepared and draped, the midline of the flap is drawn out 2 cm inferior and parallel to the inguinal ligament. In children, this vessel can be located by measuring below the inguinal ligament by a distance equal to the breadth of the child's index and middle fingers. In most patients, the circumflex iliac artery can be identified in approximately the midanterior thigh with a pencil Doppler device, which aids in centering the flap. The elected width of pedicle to be tubed is measured out as far as the anterior superior iliac spine, and the distal, lateral margin of the flap is made to conform to the distal half of the pattern of the primary defect. The part of the flap to cover the primary defect can be wider than the pedicle. There must be a limit to the extent by which it can be wider, but this is not a problem in normal practice. The entire margin of the flap is incised down to the superficial surface of the deep fascia. The distal edge of the flap is placed under tension, and the subcutaneous plane is developed with a knife as far as the anterior superior iliac spine, making sure not to create a cave beneath the midportion of the flap. At this point, the flap is laid in a cephalad direction and retraction is applied to the inferior incision. The deep fascia is incised at the level of this inferior incision and retracted toward the abdomen to reveal the sartorius, the tensor fascia lata lateral to it, and the intervening intermuscular septum. While the surgeon maintains traction on the flap cephalad and away from the thigh, the deep fascia is divided in the line of the fibers of the sartorius from inferior to superior and, at its lateral border, just medial to the septum between tensor and sartorius. As this incision in the deep fascia proceeds, the subcutaneous plane previously developed laterally is advanced to meet it. The superficial circumflex iliac artery will be seen in the deep fascia as it is lifted from the sartorius. Incision of the fascia proceeds cephalad beyond the artery as far as the origin of the sartorius from the anterior superior iliac spine. Here the flap is drawn in the opposite direction, caudad, to facilitate dissection of the upper margin. The upper incision, if carried down to the external oblique aponeurosis, will, in the majority of cases, divide a significant artery. This may cause alarm, but it should not, for this is the superficial inferior epigastric artery, which must be cut. Furthermore, its division indicates that the relevant vascular stratum has been cut and the level of dissection is now in the correct plane. The flap is retracted caudad off the aponeurosis until the level of the anterior superior iliac spine is reached. The incision previously made in the sartorius fascia is located and turned medially to free the deep fascia of the thigh from the inguinal ligament. In the course of this

could cover a circular defect, but it would approach the defect perpendicularly and would be most difficult to inset after division. Because the first (untubed) flap is unacceptable because of the open wound, poor flap fixation to the defect margins, and difficulties with postoperative exercise, and the latter is unacceptable because of contour, a compromise must be sought. The distal margin of the flap is cut to conform to the edge of the distal half of the defect. When this design is tubed, the distal few centimeters of the lateral incision, the lateral cutaneous nerve of the thigh will be encountered. Care must be taken not to injure this, because meralgia paresthetica may result.[236] Although this nerve usually passes deep to the vessel of the flap, in which case it can be freed by dissection, on occasion, it or one of its usual two branches may be superficial and is therefore more likely to be injured and also more likely to kink the vessel of the flap. Any such branches superficial to the artery are divided, placed deep to the vessel, and repaired. All fascial incisions are now completed.

It is possible to raise a groin flap without ever dividing either the fascia or the vessel. However, the consequences may be dire, for the superficial circumflex iliac artery is tethered by the intact fascia. The relaxed and redirected flap pulls on the vessel and may kink it severely (Fig. 47-69). Herein lies the explanation for necrotic edges on otherwise well-designed and well-executed groin flaps. The fascia must *always* be incised.

Applying upward traction to the flap, the fascia is dissected from the underlying fibers of the sartorius, paying heed to the vessels, which can usually be seen through the elevated fascia. In preparing a pedicled groin flap, dissection can cease at the medial border of the sartorius. In dissecting for free tissue transfer, or where the flap is to be taken to the opposite hand, the pedicle is dissected farther, using scissors and forceps. The main hazard is the muscular branch of the superficial circumflex iliac artery. This is isolated by retracting the sartorius laterally with instruments on either side of the pedicle, caudad and cephalad. Once dissected free under loupe magnification, the muscular branch is divided. The vessel can then be freed as far as its origin.

The flap can now be thinned. This is done by having an assistant hold the flap vertically with hooks or stay sutures and proceeding with curved tenotomy scissors and forceps. Using the scissors with the concave surface uppermost, the surgeon can thin the flap quite radically at the margins by trimming away fat. In the midline of the flap, the surgeon must be more cautious, or the pedicle may be damaged. Lobules of fat can be lifted with forceps and trimmed away, between periphery and midline, but the deep fascia that has been lifted *must not be transgressed.* Therefore, any fat that lies between it and the skin must be left alone. If there is a significant amount, it makes the tube necessarily bulky.

Closure commences at the lateral end of the secondary defect. It may be difficult, *but the surgeon should not undermine the margins in an attempt to facilitate closure.* Such action only increases the area of the potential dead space and does little to relax the skin. Instead, the surgeon should flex the thigh, take up a heavy suture, and proceed with the knowledge that closure is always possible if the defect was 12 cm or less when first outlined (Fig. 47-70). (The tension created will inevitably result in postoperative inflammation along the closure. Do not remove sutures for an inflamed wound. To do so would open the entire cavity created by the closure. If this then becomes infected, as is almost inevitable, one has created a disaster akin to a bedsore.) Closure of the secondary defect could continue medially all the way to the pedicle. However, a more comfortable closure is achieved if, in the last few centimeters, the flap is resutured whence it came (Fig. 47-71). Where these three suture lines meet, the tubing of the flap commences. This should be easily achieved, provided the width

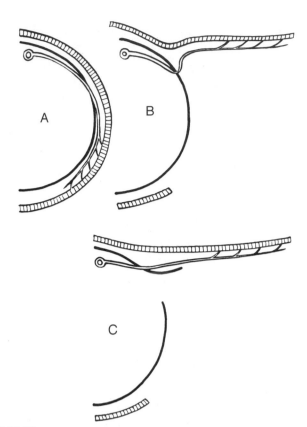

FIGURE 47-69. **A,** In cross-sectional diagram, the course of the superficial circumflex iliac artery is shown. The black line represents the deep fascia, and it can be seen that the superficial circumflex iliac artery pierces that fascia. **B,** If the flap is raised without dividing the fascia, the vessel is restrained and kinked by that deep fascia, reducing significantly the blood flow to the flap. **C,** If the fascia is divided, as recommended, at the lateral margin of the sartorius, this kink in the vessel is eliminated.

has been well tailored to the thickness. If it has not, further marginal thinning should be done. The tube is closed with interrupted sutures. The closure continues until the portion of flap remaining open for the defect is clearly too small. That is, the tube is closed too far. The reason for this is that once the flap is sutured to the hand, it is simple to release sutures from the tube but very awkward to insert them. The limb is now brought to the flap, the planned posture adopted, any minor adjustments made, and the flap sutured in place. It is good to begin this at the center point of the distal margin of the flap and then proceed progressively around both margins alternately toward the pedicle. In this way, little or no distortion is applied to the flap. With each stitch, the skin of the flap is stretched slightly to reproduce tension similar to that present in the margin of the defect. Whether this has been done correctly can be determined by looking at the wound edges between each stitch: neither should sit above the other.

On completion of application of the flap, the involved limb is immobilized. It has been suggested that this be done with external fixation between the iliac crest and the radius,[79,244] but this is not necessary and is disadvantageous if it limits motion of the hand throughout the period of flap attachment. Temporary control can be achieved by placing rolled bandages between the limb and the torso and then

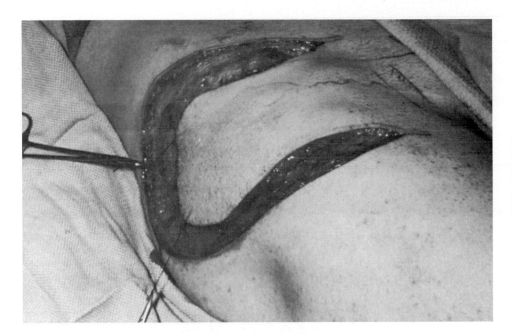

FIGURE 47-70. A groin flap here has been raised, and the size of the resultant secondary defect can be seen. The stay sutures have been kept in place to support the flap during the thinning process (see text). (This is the same patient shown in Figure 47-73.)

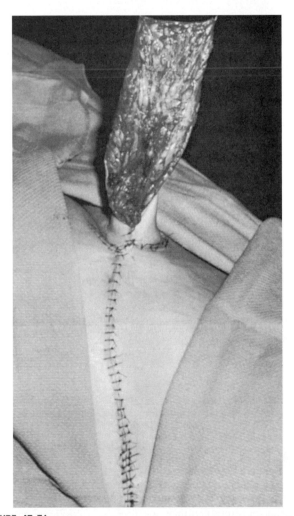

FIGURE 47-71. Closure of the secondary defect. Direct closure of the secondary defect should in all instances be attempted. The junction of the secondary defect and the tube is shown. It is important not to close the secondary defect too far medially or kinking in the base of the tube may result.

strapping the arm in place with tape from the abdomen, around the arm, to the back. The intent of this strapping is to control the arm in such a way that the flap is not kinked; indeed, it is held under gentle traction.

Care must be taken that the flap is not disrupted during recovery from anesthesia. Aside from the surgeon being present during this critical phase, another useful maneuver is to have the anesthesiologist do a brachial block just before awakening the patient. This minimizes stress on (and possible disruption of) the flap suture line during the occasionally turbulent immediate postanesthetic phase.

Once the patient is fully recovered from anesthesia, on the first or second postoperative day, all restraints are removed, and the patient is placed in charge of his or her own flap. Clear instructions are given to maintain a little traction and avoid kinking the flap. The patient is shown how to exercise all joints. By depressing the shoulder and carrying the hand toward the umbilicus, the elbow can be flexed to 90 degrees. By elevating the shoulder and carrying the hand toward the knee, it can be fully extended. Full pronation and supination, flexion and extension of the wrist, and motion of all the digital joints can be attained, and should be, every waking hour. It is in this respect that the axial flap with its tube pedicle is incontestably superior to even the best-designed random-pattern flap. Patients can be dressed soon after surgery by wearing either jeans or trousers with a pocket removed and a fastening incorporated in the waistband above the pocket.

The groin flap can be used in young children[216] with no increased incidence of flap avulsion during the postoperative period. Unless unforeseen circumstances are encountered, the complete survival of the groin flap can be predicted[197] with sufficient confidence that the practiced exponent should not hesitate to undertake extensive reconstruction in the bed of the primary defect, including joint replacement and tendon graft.[316]

Problems with circulation are understandably more likely to arise after division of the pedicle,[351] because the flap,

CRITICAL POINTS: PEDICLED GROIN FLAP

INDICATIONS

- Wounds of hand and/or forearm
- Especially when later toe transfers are to be considered

PREOPERATIVE EVALUATION

- Absence of scars in groin in area of flap to be raised
- Doppler superficial circumflex iliac artery 2 cm below inguinal ligament

PEARLS

- Center flap over "Dopplered" vessel (2 cm below inguinal ligament).
- Make flap longer than needed to allow some elbow/shoulder motion.
- Tube excess flap at base.
- Suture flap into as broad an area as possible of the wound to increase revascularization.

TECHNICAL POINTS

- Begin dissection laterally, stay out of deep iliac fat.
- Once over muscles, stay right on muscle.
- Vessel may often be identified in depths of flap visually.
- Take fascia of sartorius to avoid damage to vessel.
- Stop dissection just at medial edge of sartorius.

- Safely thin fat from margins of flap.
- Close donor site securely *before* insetting flap into defect (flex hip).

PITFALLS

- Damaging vessel with elevation (too superficial dissection)
- Making flap too small (no pedicle for tubing)
- Dehiscence of flap from wound in recovery room
- Dehiscence/infection of donor site

POSTOPERATIVE CARE

- Carefully protect flap until patient is fully awake so as to avoid dehiscence.
  - Suture hand to abdominal wall with large suture.
  - Strap arm around torso.
- Remove protection once patient is fully awake.
- Encourage as much motion of elbow and shoulder as possible.
- Divide flap in 3 to 4 weeks.
  - Must have healing of margins of flap to defect of hand
  - May perform delay procedure of flap before division
- At time of division, if proximal flap (at site of division) is dusky, do not attempt closure (débride nonviable tissue after demarcation and close).

previously nourished by an axial vessel, is now dependent on flow across the wounds of attachment. The optimal time at which to perform the division varies considerably, as shown by fluorescein studies.[217] The first requirement for safe division is perfect healing of the wound of attachment. The second requirement is that the wound of attachment be long when compared with the area of flap skin required on the hand. This is not so, for example, when much or all of the tube pedicle is required for later use. Division of such a flap should be preceded by a delay procedure. The third requirement is that the surrounding skin of the limb be supple and unscarred. If all these requirements are met, the flap can be safely divided at 3 weeks and inset. If one or more are not met, then one or more of the following steps should be taken. First, wait. No harm comes from a longer attachment. Second, test the flow. This is done by placing a rubber tourniquet around the tube pedicle and testing whether flow to the flap remains good. Flow can be assessed by the use of systemic fluorescein or by injecting atropine into the flap and measuring the time until the onset of visual disturbance. It may also be assessed by the simple clinical test of sticking a needle into the flap or observing whether reactive hyperemia develops in the flap after 20 minutes of occlusion. Third, if the flap is divided, and bleeding from the

flap on the hand is poor, do not inset it, but simply wrap the hand and return 1 week later. Fourth, and this is our routine practice when the tube pedicle is needed to cover a later digital transfer, perform a delay procedure. This is done under local anesthetic and consists of making an incision halfway around the tube pedicle, through which all deep soft tissue in the tube is divided. The wound is then closed and the flap divided completely and with confidence 1 week later.

Authors' Preferred Methods of Treatment: Defects of the Hand and Forearm

We are firmly committed to the belief that definitive skin cover at the time of injury is preferable to delayed closure, provided only that débridement is adequate.[113] As is evident from the earlier account of local, regional, and distant flaps, all with both random and axial designs, we have a rich storehouse from which to select that skin cover. If one has microsurgical training, to that store must be added all the free tissue transfers described elsewhere in this book. However, for younger surgeons, these riches may be a source of confusion, causing them to make less than the best choice or, worse, to disregard or remain ignorant of the older techniques in favor of the more complex and more expensive, but more exciting, free skin transfers.[20] In an attempt to offer guidance, we approach the matter of skin cover not from the viewpoint used throughout this chapter, namely, which flaps are available, but rather by the nature of the presenting skin defect (Table 47-3). We have assumed in all that follows that the possibility of a free skin graft has been weighed and rejected. We look at defects on the fingers separately from those on the thumb, and palmar defects apart from dorsal defects. Dorsal defects can be subdivided further into small and large. All small dorsal defects we manage by transposition or rotation flaps taken from either the adjacent dorsal skin or the lateral aspect of the fingers.

Palmar defects distal to the PIP joint are most commonly fingertip injuries.[117,141] The great majority of these injuries can be managed by allowing secondary healing; however, in such injuries in which more skin is lost dorsally or the amputation is transverse, "V-Y" advancement flaps (see earlier) may be indicated. When more is lost from the palmar surface, a regional flap is required. In patients who have sustained an injury to the middle or ring finger, the digital artery island flap is the best option. This has advantages over either a thenar flap or a cross-finger flap. With injury to the index or little fingers, one of the other regional flaps should be selected. In patients younger than 40 years of age (this can be adjusted to circumstance and physiologic condition, which we judge by whether the PIP joints can be hyperextended), the digit can safely be immobilized in flexion for the necessary 14 days. In women who may be dismayed by the secondary defect of a cross-finger flap, we use a thenar flap; in men, who tend to be less supple, we use the cross-finger flap. In those older than 40, if the digit is of considerable functional importance, for example, the thumb or a finger where others have been lost, a neurovascular island flap is justified, taken either from the toe or from the ulnar aspect of the middle fingers. When the digit is of less importance, we explain the thoughts outlined earlier to the patient and recommend revision of the amputation. If he or she balks, we proceed as if the patient were younger than 40, knowing that he or she understands the potential problems. On the dorsal aspect of the finger distally, if the defect is sufficiently large that we cannot use a local flap, a reversed cross-finger flap is indicated. Defects around the PIP joint

Table 47-3
AUTHORS' PREFERRED METHODS FOR SPECIFIC SITUATIONS

	Palmar	Dorsal-Larger Defects

Distal to PIP joint	Loss more dorsal: V-Y advancement
	Loss more palmar: middle/ring—digital artery island flap
	<40
	  Female: thenar
	  Male: cross-finger
	>40
	  Important: neurovascular island
	  Not important: revise amputation
		Reversed cross-finger

PIP joint	Cross-finger	Reversed cross-finger

Proximal phalanx	Small defect: transposition from lateral aspect
	Large defect
	  Palmar alone: cross-finger
	  +Lateral
	    Index/middle: axial flag
	    Ring/small: vascular island
		Reversed cross-finger

MP joint	Index/middle: axial flag Ring/small: vascular island	Index/middle: axial flag Ring/small: vascular island

Metacarpus or several fingers syndactylized	Worthless digit: fillet
	Small defect:
	  Vascular island
	  SDMA
	Large defect: (free lateral arm)
	  Forearm fascia + skin graft
		Worthless digit: fillet
		
		(Free lateral arm)

Thumb	Loss more dorsal: V-Y advancement
	More palmar:
	  <2/3 pulp: Moberg
	  >2/3 pulp
	  (Neurovascular island from toe)
	  Neurovascular island
	  No donor digit, no micro skills
	  FDMA or SDMA
		FDMA from index
		Forearm (preferable PIA)
		No donor digit, no vessel
		  Male: infraclavicular
		  Female: iliac

we cover with cross-finger flaps: conventional for the palmar surface, reversed for the dorsal.

Small defects on the palmar aspect of the proximal phalanx, such as are produced in releasing burn contractures, require transposition flaps from the lateral or dorsal aspect of the finger, as described by Green and Dominguez[119] and by Harrison and Morris,[124] respectively. Larger defects that are confined strictly to the palmar surface can be covered with an extended cross-finger flap. For defects that extend onto the lateral aspect to any great extent, we find it difficult to use a conventional cross-finger flap for cover and fear problems with kinking of the pedicle. In such circumstances, the axial flag flap is ideal for defects on the index and middle fingers. However, the vessel of the flag flap is not always reliable in the third and fourth web spaces. We listen for it there with a Doppler device. If a vessel cannot be heard, we take a vascular island from the adjacent digit, as described by Rose.[281] For dorsal defects over the proximal phalanx, we prefer an axial flag flap in those digits with a demonstrable vessel, because the quality of the skin is identical to that lost. In others, the reversed cross-finger flap is adequate.

Palmar defects around the MP joint, as with palmolateral defects of the proximal phalanx, do well with an axial flag flap, taking care to ensure that the injury did not damage the pedicle. When the vessel cannot be heard, we employ a vascular island. Dorsal defects should be treated similarly. Thus, for example, for full-thickness loss over the middle MP joint, we might use an axial flag from the proximal phalanx of the index finger; for loss over that of the ring finger, an SDMA flap or a vascular island from the small finger might be used.

Injuries over the metacarpus are to the palm or dorsum of the hand. Although skin loss from several adjacent digits over the proximal phalanx can usually be covered by multiple local and regional flaps (Fig. 47-72), on occasion, this is not possible, and they should be considered as one large defect and managed as if at the metacarpus. The defects on the digits are temporarily made one by suturing their adjacent margins, thereby creating a syndactyly, which is later divided. Small defects in the palm can be covered with an SDMA flap or a vascular island. This may be in the form of a fillet flap when a vascularized digit is deemed of no functional value. This solution is also applicable to dorsal defects, a situation most commonly encountered in gunshot wounds. For larger defects on either aspect of the metacarpus, we use a free lateral arm flap: fasciocutaneous when its subcutaneous layer is not too thick and fascial when it is. If

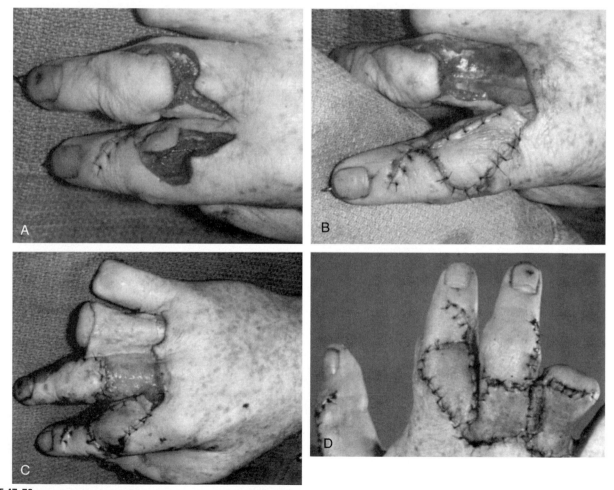

FIGURE 47-72. Multiple flaps. **A,** Defects on the index and middle fingers resulting from the management of multiple nonunions after an injury involving a fan. **B,** The defect on the index finger has been closed by use of an axial flag flap from the middle finger. **C,** The resultant defect in the middle finger has been closed using a reversed cross-finger flap from the ring finger. **D,** The viability of all flaps 1 week later.

microsurgical expertise is not available, a pedicled fascial radial forearm flap (covered with a full-thickness skin graft) can be used for palmar defects. For most defects of this location and size, we adopt a reversed radial forearm flap, using the fascia alone or an ulnar artery flap when the cosmetic defect of a fasciocutaneous flap would be distressing (see Fig. 47-63). For dorsal defects of the metacarpus, a forearm flap is similarly appropriate, the reversed posterior interosseous artery flap being preferred to the radial artery flap, provided that the vessel is present. For coverage of larger wounds in the hand, and in the absence of microsurgical skills, we believe that the groin flap remains an excellent choice for skin cover (Fig. 47-73). This flap has none of the potential cosmetic and vascular problems that exist with the forearm flap. In our practices, however, the groin flap is now reserved for those circumstances in which later microsurgical reconstruction is planned and we know

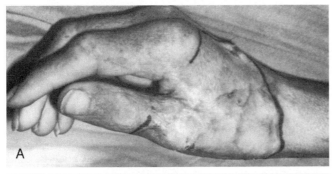

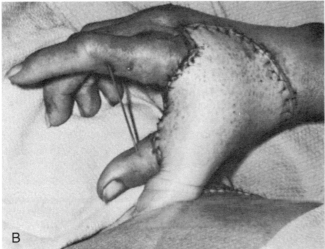

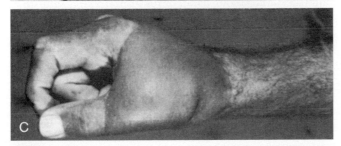

FIGURE 47-73. Groin flap. **A,** A defect on the dorsoradial aspect of the hand. **B,** A pedicle groin flap in position. Note the kinks in accordion-like fashion at the base of the tube. These kinks are dangerous and must be eliminated in later positioning. **C,** The result.

that the skin of the tube will be needed to give additional cover (e.g., a later toe transfer) (Fig. 47-74).

For dorsal defects on the thumb, we raise an FDMA flap from the dorsal aspect of the proximal phalanx of the index finger. When that is not available, owing to the extent of injury, we use a reversed PIA flap; if no vessel can be found, we use a radial forearm skin or fascial flap. Tip amputations in the thumb with more loss dorsally require a "V-Y" advancement. Those with loss that is more palmar but is less than two thirds of the pulp are ideal for a Moberg advancement or some variant thereof. When the entire pulp is lost, we replace it with a neurovascular island flap, preferably as a microvascular transfer from the toe. We would rarely perform a pedicled transfer from a suitable finger. If no donor digit is available, usually when an island transfer is judged unsuitable for a particular patient, an FDMA or SDMA flap must be used.

Circumferential degloving injuries of the thumb require immediate cover with either a pedicled axial groin flap or an immediate great toe wraparound flap. We usually will perform a groin flap before any type of toe transfer, to avoid having to take too much skin from the foot. Toe-to-hand transfer and pollicization both require more skin than that needed simply to cover the primary defect on the thumb. Degloving of a single finger, in the presence of other normal digits, requires amputation. When several digits have been degloved, we cover them all with a tube pedicle groin flap. Thereafter, for short stumps, we remove the skin of the flap and skin graft the soft tissue over the stumps. In longer fingers, we leave the flap in place and the digits are used as a mitten. These can be separated only if the blood supply is improved. We have done this by transferring a neurovascular island, either from the foot or from the thumb, if an arteriogram shows the presence of two sufficiently long digital vessels in that digit.

For defects of the wrist, forearm, and elbow, we prefer free tissue transfers, because the patient is not immobilized and a permanent pedicle is provided to the skin cover. We use the lateral arm flap for small defects, the scapular flap for medium, and the tailored latissimus flap for large. When these are not indicated or available, the groin flap can reach defects of both dorsal and palmar aspects as far proximally as the midpoint of the forearm. The pedicled latissimus dorsi flap can reach the elbow with ease and the forearm with difficulty. Defects of the proximal half of the forearm, where no local flaps suffice, can be covered with a pedicled rectus abdominis muscle flap, or, better, a latissimus dorsi free muscle flap.

The first web space is the remaining specialized region worthy of mention. Contracture here is common, both of congenital and traumatic origin, and the solutions are numerous.[198] We release relatively long yet tight first web contractures, which are composed of normal skin, with a simple 60-degree "Z"-plasty or some variant thereof. When the web is shorter and the tight web margin produces an acute ridge angle, a four-flap "Z"-plasty works well. In other circumstances, when the skin is scarred or the adduction contracture is severe, skin must be brought into the web space by transposition from the dorsum of the thumb or index finger or by rotation from the dorsum of the hand. When these do not suffice or the donor sites are themselves scarred, other skin must be used. It is important that this skin

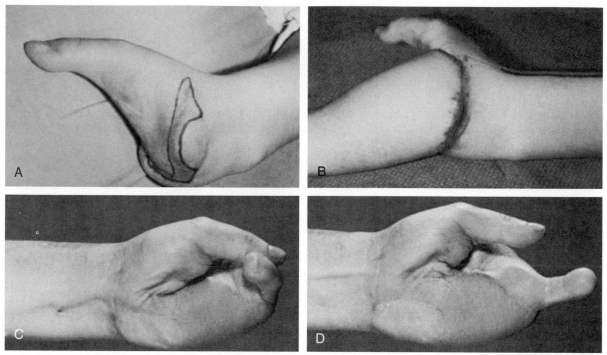

FIGURE 47-74. A, After a bomb explosion, this patient lost all digits from his dominant left hand, together with the metacarpus. **B,** The metacarpus was replaced with a vascularized iliac crest bone graft in conjunction with a groin flap (see Fig. 47-68). **C** and **D,** A long tube pedicle was retained to provide all cover necessary for transfer of a toe to the finger position.

be as thin as possible, for it is pointless to dig a hole—the web space—and promptly fill it with a fat flap. Therefore we favor a reversed forearm flap, preferably the PIA or the radial forearm. The lateral arm free flap also works well to fill a severely scarred first web.

CHEMOTHERAPEUTIC EXTRAVASATION SKIN LOSS

The injury that created the primary defect is of significance mainly when its nature makes it difficult or impossible to define the extent of eventual skin loss. One instance of clinical significance is the chemical injury resulting from extravasation of chemotherapeutic agents,[296] of which the most common is doxorubicin (Adriamycin). Identification of the agent in the tissues has been the subject of some debate.[57,63] However, all are agreed that wide excision of all potentially damaged tissues should be undertaken. A period of observation before applying definitive skin cover has been recommended.[192] The cover eventually chosen should be robust. In this situation, we prefer the ulnar forearm flap for the reasons outlined earlier. If this is unavailable, free tissue transfer is probably the procedure of choice.

POSTOPERATIVE CARE

Postoperative care is directed toward the comfort of both patient and flap and is the responsibility of a team of trained, trusted nurses. The comfort of the patient is pursued through the usual channels and should not be neglected because of concern for the flap. It is important that the patient be up and about as soon as possible, preferably starting on the first postoperative day. All joints are mobilized. Comfort of the flap is achieved mainly by avoiding kinks in its pedicle. This is ensured by correct positioning of the involved upper limb and of the patient. Once the correct position is attained, other patient positions that similarly avoid kinking should also be sought. If conscious, the patient is shown which part of the flap to inspect for kinking and which positions are acceptable. The earlier the patient takes charge of the flap, the better. If the patient is not conscious, the position must be maintained by strapping. Skin-to-skin contact produces maceration and the chance of consequent infection. Therefore, padding is used to ensure that all skin surfaces are exposed to air. A routine of wound cleansing is established, using hydrogen peroxide followed by a thin smear of antibiotic ointment. This routine has many benefits. It eliminates a nutritious medium for bacteria. It ensures that color assessment is neither obscured by blood staining nor impaired by vivid contrast within the observer's visual field. It permits assessment of the rate of bleeding from the wound, in itself a valuable index of venous insufficiency. Finally, it has an inestimable effect on the morale of the patient who can see the wound.

Flap Failure

Flaps fail for a number of reasons, some of which are still debated.[164,305] Therefore, having made the patient and the flap comfortable, the nurse observes the flap regularly to ensure its continued good health. There are several steps in this process.

1. *Observe the color of the flap.* Difficult to learn and impossible to convey adequately, color assessment remains a mainstay of care. The lighting must always be good. The observer can start by neutralizing his or her color perception by looking for 10 seconds at an area of normal skin, similar to the flap. He or she then assesses the flap. The random- and axial-pattern flaps differ in their color. A healthy random-pattern flap is pink. If arterial supply is inadequate, it becomes pale with a faint blue-gray tinge. If venous drainage is occluded, it is first an angry red and then progressively purple-red and purple-blue. The axial-pattern flap, especially the groin flap, is pale to a degree that makes the novice nervous. It is not a pure white, as can be detected by comparing it with a sheet of white paper, but rather a very pale pink. Changes in a failing flap are much more rapid and dramatic in the random than in the axial pattern. Within 48 hours, the failed portion of a random-pattern flap becomes cyanosed and then blistered, and the margin between the part that will fail and that which will survive is represented by a clear line. The sick axial flap at first assumes a waxy pallor (white tinged with yellow or brown) that differs from its healthy pink pallor by a margin so subtle that only the experienced are pessimistic. The failed margin then becomes indurated and may blister, but doubts concerning the extent of loss persist for as long as a week.
2. *Observe the refill after blanching by fingertip pressure or by running a blunt point across the flap.* If refill after blanching is slow and the flap is pale, arterial insufficiency is the likely cause. Very slow refill may be seen in a flap with no flow whatsoever, owing to the movement of stagnant blood by surrounding tissue pressures. If it is too swift and the flap has a bluish hue, venous outflow is impaired. This may be caused by kinking and should be corrected. Kinking of a flap pedicle is similar to strangulation of bowel. In both cases, the pressure is not high enough initially to occlude the arterial flow, but it impedes the venous drainage. The occluded area therefore becomes engorged, and tissue tension rises to a point at which arterial inflow is finally arrested and the tissue dies in engorgement.[339]
3. *Measure the temperature of the flap.* This may be done with the dorsum of the middle phalanx of the observer, comparing the flap with tissue adjacent both to the pedicle and to the primary defect. A marked difference is a significant index of impaired flow. When there is little or no difference, it cannot be concluded that the flap is undoubtedly well, however, because the warmth may be largely or entirely transmitted from the underlying bed.
4. *Stick the flap and adjacent tissue with an 18-gauge needle or a No. 11 scalpel blade. Take care to go to the same depth, and observe the bleeding.* Although this cannot be done repeatedly, it is permissible when the first three clinical tests leave serious doubt. A healthy flap should yield blood of the same color as the control and should bleed just a little longer. If no bleeding occurs or

does so only briefly, arterial inflow is inadequate. If the blood is darker and bleeding persists much longer, there is venous congestion. For the same reason, persistent bleeding from the marginal wounds of a flap indicates venous inadequacy.

Many more complex tests of flap viability have been introduced. They fall into three broad categories: detection of an alteration in local tissue constituent, observation of the presence in the flap of systemically administered agents, and monitoring of pulsatile flow within the flap. These generally have little application in pedicled flaps, because problems with pedicled flaps are more usually due to poor design, which is not amenable to surgical intervention. Although a pedicle flap can certainly undergo kinking or can be sutured in so that flow is compromised, these problems are usually apparent very early on and can be addressed. In most cases, however, there is little need to monitor pedicled flaps—they will either survive or they won't, primarily depending on the appropriateness of their design. A few problems can be seen later on however, and their management is discussed next.

Salvage of a Failing Flap

What actions can be taken to salvage a failing flap?

1. *Seek and eliminate any kinks in the pedicle.* Multiple small kinks produce an accordion-like appearance and are equally as harmful as one large obstruction. Flaps do best if they lie on a convex surface and are gently stretched, thereby eliminating all possible occlusion and reducing edema to a minimum. This should be explained to the patient at an early stage so that he or she can take care of the flap.
2. *Check the patient's general condition.* Hypotension, cardiopulmonary impairment, or a low circulating volume as revealed by urinary output may all affect oxygenation of the flap. Cold extremities may be caused by circumstances as grave as advanced shock or as simple as a low room temperature. Both should be evaluated and corrected.
3. *Look for signs of hematoma and evacuate any if found.* Whenever the possibility of hematoma exists, the surgeon should have inserted a drain underneath the flap. Ensure that the drain is functioning. If no drain is present, the flap is swollen and discolored, there is persistent serosanguineous oozing from the flap wounds, and edema is revealed by pitting on pressure, a hematoma is likely. This has been shown to cause loss of a flap, but it can be saved by evacuation of the hematoma.[240] The use of a Penrose or a small, flat Silastic drain often allows expression of the hematoma via the drain site at the bedside (if it has not been sutured too tightly), which can improve a potentially bad situation. If the hematoma is larger, it should be evacuated in the operating room as a formal procedure.
4. *Look for unduly tight stitches and release them.* This should be done only by the operating surgeon, because only he or she knows their significance.
5. *Reposition the patient.* Determine in particular whether elevation or dependency of the limb improves the flow. If it does, make the patient comfortable in this new position.

There are as many publications in the literature concerning methods of enhancing flap survival as there are of monitoring it, possibly more. They appear to be equally fruitless. Once again, they fall into three main categories: alteration of the environment, physical applications, and administration of drugs. Many of these pharmacologic treatments are discussed in Chapter 44. In the end, the surgeon is left with the knowledge that the only way to ensure that a flap will survive is to follow simple rules: assess the primary defect carefully, select the correct flap for that defect and execute it properly, and train nurses who can be trusted to protect and care for the work.

Coverage of the Elbow

Milan V. Stevanovic, Frances Sharpe, and William C. Pederson

Soft tissue defects about the elbow leaving exposed bone, joint, nerves, or tendon are disabling injuries. Loss of muscle or tendon substance or nerve injury can result in functional impairment at the elbow. Because local tissue may be involved in the zone of injury, it is useful to be familiar with several options for treating soft tissue loss about the elbow. The type of coverage should be appropriate for the size and etiology of the defect. Many of the flaps discussed in the previous section can be utilized for elbow coverage and their application is discussed here.

The elbow is a difficult joint to rehabilitate, even after minor trauma (see Chapter 25). Functional rehabilitation becomes more difficult with a wider zone of injury, increased edema, and structural injury or loss. The elbow joint in particular does not tolerate prolonged periods of immobilization. The goals in treating soft tissue defects is to provide wound closure, decrease the risk of infection, decrease tissue edema, and allow early mobilization and rehabilitation of the elbow. Early reconstruction of all injured structures will maximize functional recovery.[304,320] This section addresses the treatment of large soft tissue defects that cannot be addressed by skin grafts or local random fasciocutaneous flaps. The role of prophylactic tissue transfer in addressing the soft tissue envelope of the elbow is also discussed.

PREOPERATIVE EVALUATION

The preoperative evaluation of the patient is dependent on the etiology of the defect, the size of the wound, and what structures are exposed. Evaluation of structural or functional loss, including bone, ligament, tendon, and nerve, is important in the ultimate selection of soft tissue coverage. The presence of infection or contamination will affect the timing of coverage. Associated injuries, especially those involving the ipsilateral shoulder, should be carefully evaluated because this may affect donor site selection. Thus, the most critical part of the preoperative evaluation is a good history that includes mechanism of injury, etiology of the defect, preexisting medical conditions, previous injuries, and a thorough physical examination of the patient.

In the traumatic elbow defect, a better evaluation of the defect can be done at the time of the initial surgical treatment. The extent of the structural injury can be more accurately assessed, and the soft tissue reconstruction can be better tailored to those losses. Intraoperative evaluation of the ligamentous stability of the elbow is best done with fluoroscopic examination while the patient is under general anesthesia.

Additional studies include laboratory evaluation for any signs of infection. For open wounds, post-débridement cultures should be obtained. Radiographs of the elbow and adjacent joints are important in trauma. Angiographic evaluation is indicated for defects in which coverage with free vascularized tissue may be necessary. For defects from nontraumatic etiology, radiographs of the elbow alone are sufficient. In the case of tumor, the imaging studies ordered by the oncologist should be reviewed. Particular attention to the MRI is important in anticipating the structural and functional losses that will be expected from the resection. Whenever possible, reconstruction of all defects, including bone, ligament, tendon, or nerve, should be done simultaneously with soft tissue coverage.

 Anatomy

The elbow is a naked joint. It is well protected only anteriorly. The posterior and lateral structures are covered only by a thin mobile fasciocutaneous layer. The olecranon is covered by a bursal sac with overlying thick durable and pressure-resistant skin. The stability of the elbow joint is highly dependent on its ligamentous integrity and its bony congruity. Detailed anatomy of the elbow joint is described in Chapters 20 to 22.

TYPES OF OPERATIONS

It is useful to have several reconstructive options available for the treatment of soft tissue loss about the elbow. The particular method of coverage should be tailored to the size and etiology of the defect, in addition to the general health and needs of the patient. Donor site considerations have been discussed in the earlier sections. Whatever the selected donor site, it should ideally allow early motion at the elbow.[23,300]

The majority of patients have defects associated with trauma, post-traumatic or post-surgical infection, or chronic infection. In the setting of acute trauma, wound coverage is ideally completed in the first 48 to 72 hours. Patients requiring immediate soft tissue coverage of a defect about the elbow are less common. This group includes those patients undergoing tumor resection, patients requiring an endoprosthesis or allograft replacement, patients with clean sharp injuries, or patients with poor but intact soft tissue envelope or an unstable scar who require revision elbow surgery combined with soft tissue augmentation.

Patients with grossly contaminated wounds with positive post-débridement cultures should be managed with serial débridements, intravenous antibiotics, and antibiotic bead pouches. It may require 2 to 6 weeks of antibiotic therapy until cultures are negative. Positive cultures after antibiotic therapy and serial débridement necessitate further investigation for possible osteomyelitis, pyarthrosis, distant site of infections, or systemic immunocompromise. Patients with chronic infection and osteomyelitis require a tumor-surgery type resection of bone and affected structures and negative cultures before soft tissue coverage.

Local Random Flaps

The types of local cutaneous flaps include the triangulation of adjacent parallelogram, "Z"-plasty, or double rhomboid "Z"-plasty. The double rhomboid "Z"-plasty helps to decrease tension along the line of closure of the donor site and at the flap corners. These flaps may have some applicability in closure of an unstable scar of the posterior elbow but do little to import well-vascularized tissue into a problem area.

Axial Fasciocutaneous Flaps

Several pedicled axial fasciocutaneous flaps have been described from the upper extremity that have utility in elbow coverage.[3,35,59,180,181,185,253] These flaps can be harvested quickly and use similar textured skin for covering the defect. Island pedicle flaps from the forearm and upper arm can also be utilized for elbow coverage. Examples of these include the lateral arm flap, the posterior interosseous flap,[53,58,59,61,122,159,256,302] the ulnar artery flap,[146] and the radial forearm flap.[325,332,334]

Radial Forearm Rotational Flap

The radial forearm flap[332] is the most versatile rotational flap for elbow soft tissue reconstruction. The flap provides thin durable coverage, which can be a sensate flap when used for elbow coverage. A large skin flap can be harvested alone or with vascularized tendon and/or bone graft.[130,325] Alternately, vascularized fascia alone can be taken as free or rotational tissue.[144] The long pedicle provides a wide arc of rotation, allowing for easy circumferential coverage of the elbow.

A large skin flap can be harvested from the volar aspect of the forearm, from the antecubital fossa to the wrist joint. The flap dimensions depend on the size of the forearm. Most forearms will accommodate a 6 × 15-cm donor area. The flap is supplied by perforating branches of the radial artery. These septocutaneous branches arise principally in the distal half of the artery and are capable of supplying the entire skin of the volar surface of the forearm. The venous drainage of this flap occurs through both a deep and a superficial system. For a proximally based rotational flap, as would be used for elbow coverage, venous drainage relies on both the deep and superficial systems. The disadvantages of this flap include the loss of the radial artery and the potential for cold intolerance. A painful, noncosmetic scar at the donor site and tendon adhesions at the donor site can occur.

SURGICAL TECHNIQUE

The flap is designed on the volar aspect of the forearm. The flap size and design depend on the size and shape of the defect to be covered (see Fig. 47-60). The position of the skin island on the forearm depends on the location of the defect. It should be positioned sufficiently distal to allow the skin island to be rotated to the area needing coverage. The details of dissection are discussed earlier, with the only difference for elbow coverage being that the pedicle is raised proximally for rotation to cover the elbow. Depending on the distance to the defect, the radial artery and its venae comitantes can be traced proximally as far as the bifurcation of the brachial artery to allow a greater arc of rotation. The flap is inset into the defect in a standard manner (Fig 47-75; see also Fig. 47-62).

A composite vascularized flap can also be harvested, as a tendinocutaneous graft or osteotendinocutaneous flap. The brachioradialis, flexor carpi radialis, and palmaris longus can be utilized either alone or in combination for triceps tendon reconstruction or augmentation or for a vascularized medial or lateral ligament reconstruction.[332] The donor site is managed with a skin graft as described earlier.

Lateral Arm Flap

The lateral arm flap is a fasciocutaneous flap that has more frequently been used as a free tissue transfer (see Chapter 48) or as a proximally based rotational transfer for coverage of the shoulder. It has also been used as a source of composite tissue, including vascularized tendon from the lateral triceps and/or bone from the lateral humerus with the fasciocutaneous tissue.[115,136] As a free flap or an antegrade-based rotational flap, it is based on a branch of the profunda brachii, the posterior radial collateral artery, which travels along the intermuscular septum. The interconnection of this vessel with more distal vessels of the radial recurrent artery allows this same territory of skin to be harvested as a reverse pedicle flap, which can be used for more distal coverage about the elbow.[28,173,185,212,328,354] The use of a reverse pedicled lateral arm flap was first described by Maruyama in 1986.[212] There have been few clinical series describing this distally based pedicle flap for soft tissue coverage about the elbow.[3,52,61,185,341] Although the reverse lateral arm flap has been described as an islandized flap, it is much safer to incorporate the skin over the lateral epicondyle to accommodate the superficial position of the distally based vascular network.[328]

There are several advantages to this flap. It has a better blood supply than other described local fasciocutaneous flaps. There is no associated functional impairment, and no

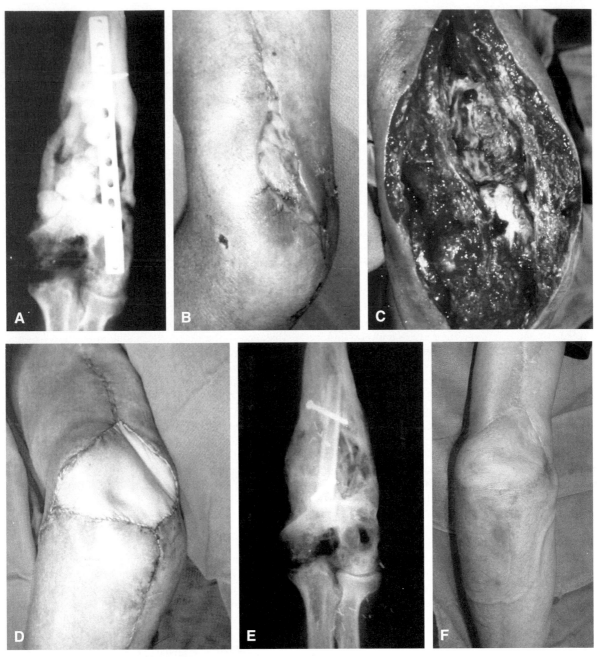

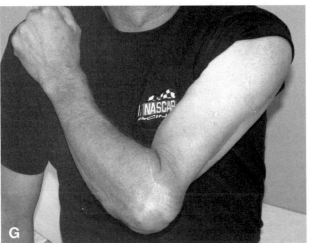

FIGURE 47-75. A 36-year-old truck driver involved in a roll-over motor vehicle accident sustained a severely crushed supracondylar left humerus fracture. Open reduction and internal fixation was performed. The fracture did not heal and deep infection ensued. A total of seven procedures had been performed before presentation to our department. The patient underwent a staged reconstruction. After removal of hardware and control of infection, soft tissue coverage was achieved using a rotational radial forearm flap. After 6 weeks of intravenous antibiotic therapy, the patient was returned to the operating room for bone reconstruction using a vascularized free fibula graft. **A,** Initial presentation radiographs of the distal humerus. Partial hardware removal and placement of tobramycin antibiotic beads had been done before presentation. **B,** Skin appearance at the posterior distal humerus. Wound dehiscence and soft tissue loss resulted from chronic infection. **C,** Soft tissue defect after débridement. **D,** Soft tissue defect covered with a radial forearm rotational flap. **E,** Radiographic appearance 6 months after vascularized free fibula grafting of bony defect of the distal humerus. **F,** Soft tissue appearance 6 months after vascularized free fibula grafting. Patient lacked 15 degrees of extension. **G,** Elbow flexion at 6 months after vascularized free fibula grafting. Flexion was to 105 degrees.

major blood vessel is sacrificed. There are several design variations of the flap, all of which are based on the blood supply from the posterior radial collateral artery (a branch of the profunda brachii), which anastomoses with the radial recurrent artery (the first branch of the radial artery in the cubital fossa). These include a "V-Y" advancement flap, a rotation-advancement flap, and a complete island flap. Reported disadvantages include an unsightly donor site scar and a bulky flap that may require later debulking.

The skin territory supplied by the branches of the profunda brachii extends from the lateral insertion of the deltoid to the lateral epicondyle of the humerus.[122] The flap size can be as large as 8 × 15 cm. When the donor site is larger than 5 cm in width, the donor site cannot be closed primarily and skin grafting is required to cover the larger defect (Fig. 47-76). The donor site scar is often cosmetically unacceptable and is now less commonly used. The posterior brachial cutaneous nerve is sacrificed in the dissection, leaving a sensory deficit on the posterolateral elbow. When used as a free tissue transfer, this nerve can be included in the flap and used to provide a sensate free-tissue transfer. Variations in vascular anatomy have been reported. The most common anomaly is duplication of the posterior radial collateral artery.[159,184]

The flap is outlined, centering the skin paddle over the lateral intermuscular septum (see Fig. 47-76). The posterior radial collateral artery can be located with a Doppler probe. It is mandatory to identify this before the dissection if there has been any previous elbow trauma or surgical procedure. Angiography may be necessary to identify the vessel. The dissection of the flap begins posteriorly, sharply incising the skin down to the deep fascia overlying the triceps muscle. The fascia is divided in line with the skin incision, and the fascia is tacked to the subdermal layer. The fascia is dissected off the muscle belly of the triceps, continuing to the intermuscular septum. The posterior radial collateral artery is identified along the intermuscular septum and mobilized away from the radial nerve, which lies immediately anterior to the posterior radial collateral artery. Muscular branches from the intermuscular septum into the triceps are ligated. The anterior dissection is then carried out in the same fashion, including the fascia covering the biceps, brachialis, and brachioradialis. The dissection is carried to the intermuscular septum, again ligating muscular branches from the septum into the brachialis. The intermuscular septum is included in and critical to the flap because this contains the perforating cutaneous branches. At the cephalad portion of the incision, the posterior radial collateral artery is divided. The intermuscular septum is also divided at this level and sharply elevated from the humerus to the level of the lateral epicondyle, taking care to include the pedicle of the radial recurrent artery within the flap (see Fig. 47-76B). This is best done by leaving a 3- to 4-cm skin bridge over the lateral epicondyle and elevating this skin bridge in the subfascial plane. The flap is now ready to be rotated and inset into the area of soft tissue defect (see Fig. 47-76C).

Although this flap is better suited for cases of tumor, traumatic defects of the anterior and posterior elbow can be easily covered with this flap, provided that the donor vessels are not included in the zone of injury. If the donor site cannot be closed primarily, a split-thickness skin graft should be used to cover the donor site.

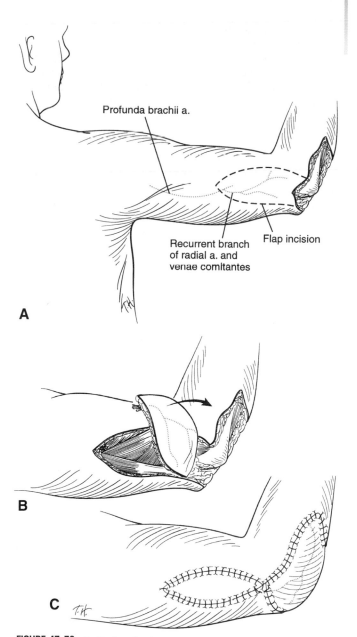

FIGURE 47-76. **A,** Outline for the reverse lateral arm flap. **B,** Elevation of the flap. **C,** Flap insertion with skin graft at donor site.

Distant Pedicle Flaps: Two-Stage Flaps (Temporary Pedicle Flaps)

Distant pedicled flaps are one of the most reliable means of achieving coverage of large soft tissue defects, when recipient vessels are not available, or when the patient is a poor candidate for other types of reconstruction. These flaps rely on the vascularity of the recipient tissue bed and do not bring a permanent independent blood supply to the defect. They have been reported to cover defects as large as 22 cm long.[36] Although seldom used, they remain an important reconstructive option in select patients. The main limitations of these flaps are related to the prolonged immobilization required for two-stage procedures. This prolonged immobilization can significantly compromise functional recovery. Increased difficulties are encountered not only with stiffness and contracture at the elbow and shoulder but also with edema and stiffness of the hand and fingers.

Distant pedicle random pattern flaps from the chest wall or upper abdomen have been largely replaced by the use of axial patterned flaps. Because of the random pattern of vascularity, the length of these flaps usually is limited to 10 cm, requiring close approximation of the arm against the chest. Flap division is performed at 3 weeks.[161]

Distant pedicle axial patterned flaps from the abdomen also have been described.[36,65,84,161,188,290] The thoracoepigastric flap is a fasciocutaneous flap, designed along the internal mammary and superior epigastric arteries. The flap is anteriorly based and is oriented with its superior border along the inferior mammary crease. Because it is anteriorly based, it is best used to cover anterior soft tissue loss around the elbow. The flap is limited to approximately 25 cm in length (not to extend posterior to the posterior axillary fold). Widths less than 8 to 10 cm usually can be closed primarily.[65,188,218] The external oblique fasciocutaneous flap provides a thin, posteriorly based flap. The flap size is limited to 6 to 8 cm in width (to allow primary closure of the donor site) and 16 to 18 cm in length. The blood supply is through segmental vascular pedicles entering the lateral aspect of the external abdominal oblique muscle, sending perforators into the fascia and subcutaneous tissue layers. Usually two pedicles are incorporated into the flap, which can be divided at 2 to 3 weeks. Because of its posteriorly based pedicle, it is well suited to cover defects along the posterior aspect of the elbow.[84] The transverse rectus island flap has been more recently described for elbow joint salvage. A musculocutaneous flap based on the superior epigastric artery is harvested. The fasciocutaneous portion of the flap is inset, providing the soft tissue coverage. The rectus muscle acts as a leash for the pedicle, allowing a greater pedicle length and arc of rotation.[36,290]

Local Muscle Pedicle Flaps

Local muscle rotational flaps can be used to cover small defects about the elbow where there is exposed nerve, vessel, tendon, bone, or implant. Their arc of rotation generally allows for coverage of anterior and posterior wounds. Several local muscle rotational flaps have been described in small series, often only as case reports.[133] These include the brachioradialis,[133,177,179,280] the extensor carpi radialis longus,[145,250] the anconeus,[293] and the flexor carpi ulnaris.[133,223] The brachioradialis and the extensor carpi radialis longus also have been used as musculocutaneous flaps.

These local flaps are limited to relatively small defects. When not released from the proximal origin, the arc of rotation and ability to achieve posterior coverage is reduced. These muscles often lie within the zone of injury, limiting their use in these situations. The functional deficit at the donor site is not trivial, especially when using the flexor carpi ulnaris, which is the strongest flexor and ulnar deviator at the wrist.

Flexor Carpi Ulnaris Flap

The flexor carpi ulnaris muscle for use as a rotational flap has been well described in anatomic studies.[133,256] Its clinical use has been described principally in case reports.[223] This flap has been described as both a muscle rotational flap and a musculocutaneous flap. As the dominant wrist flexor and

ulnar deviator, it should not routinely be sacrificed and in general should only be used when other alternatives do not exist. The principal indications for use of the flexor carpi ulnaris muscle include coverage of the anterior elbow joint, coverage of neurovascular structures or arteriovenous shunts, and coverage of vascular prosthetic grafts. The use of this muscle for soft tissue coverage is better indicated in patients with diabetes and/or end-stage renal disease.

The flexor carpi ulnaris is the ulnarmost structure of the superficial flexors of the forearm. It has two heads of origin, the ulnar and humeral. The humeral origin is on the medial epicondyle. The ulnar origin arises from the proximal posterior border of the ulna. The flexor carpi ulnaris inserts distally on the pisiform. The dominant pedicle is the posterior ulnar recurrent artery. This branch of the ulnar artery is given off near the level of the bicipital tuberosity of the radius and enters the flexor carpi ulnaris muscle approximately four fingerbreadths below the medial epicondyle. The length of the pedicle is 2 to 3 cm, with a diameter of 1 to 2 mm. One to two minor pedicles are present distally. These are also branches of the ulnar artery. These minor branches can be sacrificed when the muscle is used as a rotational flap. The muscle is innervated by branches of the ulnar nerve given off below the medial epicondyle. When harvested as a musculocutaneous flap, the overlying skin paddle is supplied by the medial antebrachial cutaneous nerve. The average muscle belly measures 5 cm in width by 20 cm in length. The muscle belly extends to the distal third of the forearm, around 7 to 8 cm proximal to the wrist crease. Based on the dominant pedicle, this muscle can be rotated to cover the anterior surface of the elbow. The posterior surface of the elbow can also be reached, although with greater difficulty (Fig. 47-77).

The patient is placed in the supine position. The arm and shoulder girdle are included in the surgical preparation. A sterile tourniquet is used on the proximal arm. The surgical incision is made along a line drawn between the medial epicondyle and the forearm. The middle third of this line is incised, and the musculotendinous junction of the flexor carpi ulnaris is identified. The muscle is cut at the musculotendinous junction and elevated from distal to proximal. The skin incision is tailored proximally to fit the area of soft tissue deficit. The muscle is mobilized proximally until the length is sufficient to cover the defect. The pedicle does not need to be dissected. The muscle is inset into the defect, and a split-thickness skin graft is used to cover the exposed muscle belly.

The flexor carpi ulnaris can also be harvested as a musculocutaneous flap. The area of donor skin lies along the mid forearm overlying the flexor carpi ulnaris muscle belly. A skin paddle up to 6 × 10 cm can be harvested together with the muscle, provided that the fasciocutaneous perforators are intact. The skin paddle can be islandized on its perforators to allow greater versatility of coverage. However, this large skin defect can result in poor cosmesis at the donor site. In general we prefer to use muscle alone and use split-thickness skin graft to cover exposed muscle belly.

Brachioradialis Flap

The brachioradialis rotational flap has been described in case studies for use of coverage about the elbow.[177,179,280] It is best suited to cover small defects along the anterolateral or

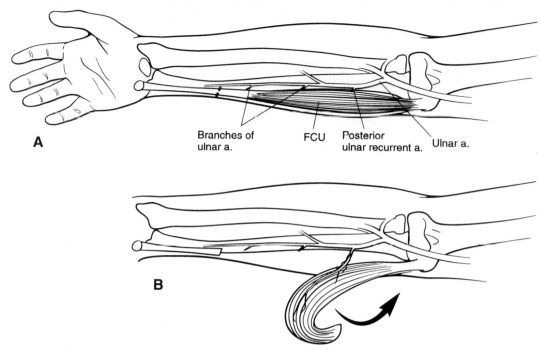

FIGURE 47-77. **A,** Anatomic position of the flexor carpi ulnaris (FCU) and its dominant pedicle, the posterior ulnar recurrent artery. **B,** Flexor carpi ulnaris elevated and ready for rotation.

posterolateral border of the distal arm and proximal forearm. It can be sacrificed with minimal donor site morbidity or functional loss. The muscle has been described as a muscle or musculocutaneous flap. The cutaneous territory lies on the proximal radial forearm between the lateral epicondyle and mid forearm and is supplied by perforating musculocutaneous vessels from the underlying muscle. We prefer not to use this as a musculocutaneous flap, because this commonly results in a bulky disfigured appearance to the forearm. The brachioradialis should not be sacrificed in the absence of the dominant elbow flexors.

The brachioradialis is the most superficial muscle on the lateral side of the forearm. At its origin, it lies between the brachialis and triceps muscles. It arises from the upper two thirds of the lateral supracondylar ridge of the humerus and from the anterior aspect of the lateral intermuscular septum. The muscle inserts on the radial styloid. The muscle belly extends to the mid forearm, at which point it becomes a thin flat tendon. It acts as a weak elbow flexor, with its strongest action when the forearm is at mid pronation. It can initiate both pronation and supination. It is innervated by a branch of the radial nerve, which is given off above the elbow joint. The dominant pedicle is a branch of the radial recurrent artery, close to its origin from the radial artery. The pedicle length is approximately 3 cm, with a diameter of 1 mm. Minor pedicles arise more distally as branches from the radial recurrent artery but are smaller and less consistent (Fig. 47-78).

A sterile tourniquet is used for the dissection. The skin incision is made along a line drawn from the lateral epicondyle to the radial styloid. The initial incision begins proximally and extends to the mid forearm. Branches of the lateral antebrachial cutaneous and dorsal antebrachial cutaneous nerves lie on the superficial surface of the muscle belly. These are identified, preserved, and mobilized with the skin flaps. The muscle is exposed both dorsally and volarly and then traced to its musculotendinous junction. The superficial radial nerve and the radial artery are located just volar and deep to the brachioradialis. These should be identified and protected through the remainder of the dissection. The muscle is released just distal to the musculotendinous junction, leaving a small cuff of tendon to use for insetting the flap. Several small muscle perforating branches from the radial artery can be safely ligated. This will increase the arc of rotation as the muscle is mobilized proximally. The radial recurrent branch of the radial artery is given off near the bicipital tuberosity of the radius. It is not necessary to identify the dominant pedicle or to release the origin of the brachioradialis. The muscle is rotated to cover the area of soft tissue defect. A subcutaneous tunnel may be useful to reach the defect. However, this may compress the muscle flap. In general, we prefer to extend the surgical incision and skin graft over exposed muscle belly.

Anconeus Flap

The anconeus is a small triangular muscle crossing the lateral elbow. Its function is still debated, although it seems to play a role in elbow stabilization.[16,293] Owing to its small size, this muscle is rarely used for elbow defects. Schmidt and colleagues described three areas of coverage that include the lateral radiocapitellar joint, the distal triceps tendon at its insertion, and the olecranon. The anconeus can be expected to reliably cover a 5- to 7-cm² defect. It can be harvested without measurable functional deficit.

The muscle origin is located on the posterior aspect of the lateral epicondyle of the humerus. It inserts on the lateral aspect of the olecranon and the adjacent posterolateral olecranon. The muscle size along its maximum dimensions is 3 to 4 cm × 8 to 10 cm. The muscle is supplied through two constant arterial pedicles, the medial collateral artery

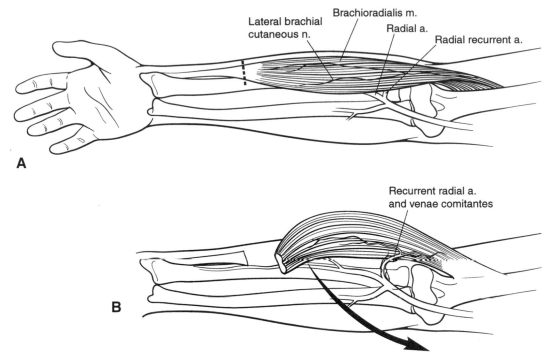

FIGURE 47-78. A, Anatomic position of the brachioradialis muscle and its dominant pedicle, a branch of the radial recurrent artery. **B,** Brachioradialis elevated and ready for rotation.

and the recurrent posterior interosseous artery, which anastomose within the muscle belly. The medial collateral artery is a terminal branch of the profunda brachii. It always travels with the radial nerve branch to the anconeus and enters the muscle on its proximal deep surface. From an arterial standpoint, the anconeus can be mobilized on either its proximal or distal pedicle. However, mobilization on the distal pedicle (recurrent posterior interosseous artery) requires sacrifice of the nerve.

The skin incision is centered over the lateral epicondyle and extends obliquely to the lateral border of the olecranon, near the distal insertion of the anconeus. The antebrachial fascia is exposed, and the interval between anconeus and flexor carpi ulnaris is opened. The dissection of the anconeus must be carried to its most distal insertion, which lies approximately 10 cm from the lateral epicondyle. The tip of the anconeus is subperiosteally elevated from its insertion along the inferior border of the ulna, with attention to preservation of the radiocapitellar joint capsule. The recurrent posterior interosseous arterial pedicle is ligated, and the muscle is mobilized to its origin. The origin can also be released to increase the arc of rotation on its proximal pedicle, the medial collateral artery. If the muscle origin off the lateral epicondyle is released, the proximal pedicle (medial collateral artery) should be identified and protected. Split-thickness skin grafting is used to cover any exposed muscle.

Distant Muscle Pedicle Flaps: One Stage

The latissimus dorsi rotational flap is the only distant pedicled muscle rotational flap that provides coverage of moderate to large soft tissue defects about the elbow.* It has been shown in a cadaveric study to consistently provide

soft tissue coverage on average 6.5 to 8 cm distal to the olecranon. When released from its humeral insertion, an additional 2 to 3 cm of distal coverage often can be achieved.[156] The muscle and its neurovascular pedicle lie well away from the elbow and are generally outside of the zone of injury. Because this is a one-stage procedure, rehabilitation can be started within the first week of reconstruction.

Latissimus Dorsi

The latissimus dorsi is the most versatile muscle both as a rotational muscle or musculocutaneous flap or as a free tissue transfer. It has been widely described for rotational coverage of the arm, shoulder, neck, thorax, and gluteal regions.[39,66,156,207,218,229] Use as a rotational flap for elbow coverage has been described in small case reports, in cadaver dissections,[156] and in small clinical series.[125,278,320] In anatomic dissections, Jutte and coworkers described the ability of the latissimus to cover the olecranon. With the latissimus insertion intact, in all cadavers, the latissimus reliably reached the olecranon. On average, the latissimus was able to reach 6.3 to 8.4 cm distal to the olecranon when transposed posteriorly or anteriorly, respectively.[156] In clinical cases, reliable coverage up to 8 cm distal to the olecranon has been reported.[320] The pedicled latissimus should not be used when there is an ipsilateral shoulder injury or weakness. Donor site morbidity includes seroma formation at the donor site, mild generalized weakness about the shoulder girdle, and mild decrease in the total arc of shoulder motion. The functional deficits are tolerated well by patients.[178,285]

---

*See references 39, 44, 47, 66, 125, 156, 229, 235, 254, 266, and 287.

The majority of the technique is described earlier, with a few caveats for coverage of the elbow and proximal forearm (see Figs. 47-65 and 47-66). As noted previously, release of the humeral insertion of the latissimus allows greater mobilization of the muscle. Even when greater mobilization is not required, we still release 80% of the insertion when covering the elbow. This changes the muscle resting length and reduces muscle contraction that might disrupt the muscle after it is inset. The remaining intact 20% of the insertion helps prevent traction injury to the pedicle. If the latissimus is to be used as a functional transfer, the release of the insertion is performed close to the bony insertion of the latissimus on the humerus.

The muscle can now be rotated on its pedicle to cover defects on any surface of the elbow. The pedicle should not be twisted, and there should be no tension on the pedicle at the time of insetting. During transposition, we do not recommend tunneling of the latissimus under a subcutaneous bridge. This can compress the muscle and or pedicle, leading to myonecrosis.[268] The latissimus is inset below the subcutaneous tissue. The muscle fascia is tacked to the subcutaneous tissue layer beginning proximally to prevent traction on the pedicle. Periodically during insetting, the color of the venae comitantes is monitored. Any change or darkening of the venous return suggests possible venous obstruction proximally. This may be caused by kinking of the pedicle at the axilla. After the muscle is completely inset, a Doppler probe is used to check the patency of the vessel in full elbow extension and at 90 degrees of elbow flexion. If the pulse is completely obliterated at 90 degrees of flexion, the muscle is stretched too far distally and should

be re-inset. Exposed muscle is covered with a split-thickness skin graft (Fig 47-79). If the latissimus has been harvested as a musculocutaneous flap, the skin paddle is inset to cover the area of skin defect. After application of the dressing, the arm is placed in 30 to 40 degrees of shoulder abduction and 40 to 60 degrees of elbow flexion. In this position, swelling about the axilla will be less likely to cause compression of the vascular pedicle. Gentle passive range of motion may be initiated at 1 week.

If the latissimus is to be used for functional reconstruction, before releasing the muscle origin or insertion, the resting length of the muscle is marked by placing the arm in full flexion and placing marking sutures in the muscle belly at 5-cm intervals, starting from the muscle insertion and measuring toward the origin. When the muscle is inset for functional reconstruction, the resting length must be restored. This is done by insetting the muscle such that the marking sutures placed at the time of harvesting the muscle are restored to 5-cm intervals. For reconstruction of elbow flexion, the latissimus is inserted into the residual stump of the biceps. Resting length is restored with the elbow in full extension, and the elbow is immobilized in approximately 90 degrees of elbow flexion. When reconstruction is done for elbow extension, the muscle resting length is restored with the elbow in maximum flexion. Excess muscle at the distal end is débrided. It is better to harvest a skin paddle with the latissimus when performing a functional muscle transfer. This tissue provides a better gliding surface for the muscle than a split-thickness skin graft. Any remaining exposed muscle is covered with split-thickness skin graft. Postoperatively, the elbow is immobilized in maximum

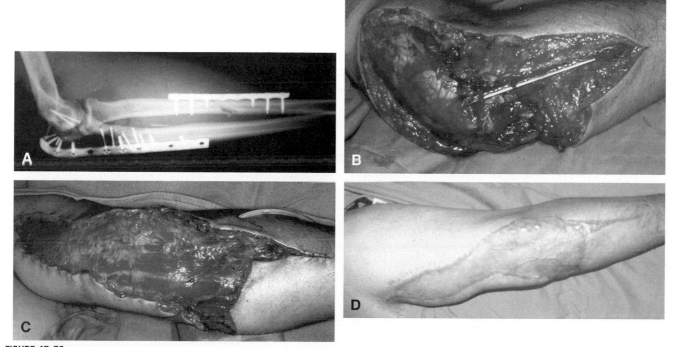

FIGURE 47-79. A 40-year-old man sustained a severe open fracture-dislocation of the elbow. A large soft tissue defect was present, leaving exposed bone and joint. After irrigation and débridement, open reduction and internal fixation was performed of the radius, ulna, and capitellum. The following day, the patient underwent repeat débridement, primary bone grafting, and soft tissue coverage with a latissimus dorsi rotational flap. At 3-month follow-up, his range of motion was from 15 to 105 degrees. **A,** Radiographic appearance immediately after fixation. **B,** Soft tissue defect after second débridement. **C,** Soft tissue defect covered with rotational latissimus dorsi muscle flap. **D,** Soft tissue appearance at 3-month follow-up.

extension. The period of immobilization for a functional reconstruction must be for a minimum of 8 weeks, followed by a gentle program of remobilization.

Free Tissue Transfer

When local rotational flaps or distant one-stage pedicle flaps are not suitable for soft tissue reconstruction, free tissue transfer should be considered. Free tissue transfer may provide the best functional and cosmetic outcome and can be performed as a single-stage reconstruction, allowing early rehabilitation of the elbow.[151,254,270,286,301]

Selection of the donor site depends on several factors. These include the size and location of the defect, any underlying structural or functional deficit, the presence of exposed or prominent implants, and the general health status of the patient. For example, functional morbidity at the donor site is more critical in the polytrauma patient, who is already functionally compromised. Many options for free tissue transfer exist; these include fascial, fasciocutaneous, muscle, musculocutaneous, and osteocutaneous flaps.

Fascial free flaps can be used for defects that do not require the filling of a dead space. The most commonly used fascial flaps include the temporoparietal fascia, radial forearm fascia, and parascapular fascia.

Several fasciocutaneous flaps are available, some of which already have been described. These include the lateral arm flap,[313] radial or ulnar forearm flap,[203,312] groin flap, scapular and parascapular flaps,[284] and medial and lateral thigh fasciocutaneous flaps.[11] The lateral arm and radial and ulnar forearm flaps can be taken as sensory flaps, which can be important in providing protective sensation over areas subject to pressure breakdown. Despite this advantage, these flaps have some donor site morbidity with complaints of chronic aching, dysesthesias, and poor cosmetic appearance.[118,325,333]

Muscle free flaps can be used to cover large defects about the elbow. When covered with split-thickness skin graft taken as a sheet (nonmeshed), they have excellent cosmetic results both at the donor and recipient sites. They also provide a rich and independent blood supply, improving vascularity, promoting healing, and reducing the risk of sepsis. Several donor muscles are available. Selection of the donor muscle depends on the size of soft tissue defect, requirements to fill dead space or cover implants, need for functional reconstruction, and patient comorbidities. Options include the latissimus dorsi, serratus anterior, rectus abdominis, and the gracilis. The most commonly used flaps are the latissimus dorsi and the rectus abdominis. This is based on their limited donor site morbidity, vascular reliability, and accessibility. Disadvantages of muscle flaps include longer and more complex surgery, functional loss at the donor sites, and risk of flap failure. The risk of flap failure is especially important in the patient with multiple injuries, where every functional unit should be preserved.

Composite free flaps can be useful in providing soft tissue coverage in conjunction with reconstruction of structural or functional losses. Both the composite lateral arm flap and the composite radial forearm flap can include both vascularized tendon and bone along with the fasciocutaneous graft.[58,115,136,184] Larger bone defects can be reconstructed with the vascularized osteofasciocutaneous free

fibula graft.[45,319] For more information on the various flaps described, see Chapter 48.

 Authors' Preferred Methods

Indications

Soft tissue coverage about the elbow is indicated for cases of soft tissue loss associated with exposed bone, joint, implant, tendon, or neurovascular structure. Soft tissue defects associated with a functional loss at the elbow can be simultaneously managed with a single procedure that will provide coverage and restore function.

Prophylaxis

There are a few clinical situations in which we believe the use of supplemental soft tissue coverage may be beneficial, even though primary skin closure can be achieved. These cases include severely contused skin directly overlying hardware or prostheses or when the quality of tissue is thin, scarred, or poorly compliant. This may occur in the multiply operated elbow, in which the subcutaneous tissue has become progressively thinner and less mobile, or in cases of previously irradiated tissue. The pedicled latissimus dorsi is an excellent donor for prophylactic soft tissue augmentation. The use of the latissimus as a prophylactic rotational muscle about the elbow is similar to the use of the prophylactic gastrocnemius rotational flap for reconstructive procedures about the knee.[320] Providing a muscular soft tissue envelope at the elbow reduces the risks of tissue breakdown over prominent bone or implants; promotes bone and tissue healing by improved vascularity; and reduces risks of deep infection by improved vascularity and improved tissue durability overlying the implants and improved antibiotic delivery.[39,113,187,284,286]

Technique Selection

The method of coverage depends on the size and location of the defect. These considerations are listed earlier in this chapter. We have found the pedicled radial forearm flap an extremely reliable and easily performed procedure for coverage of small to medium-sized wounds. This flap has also been very useful for augmenting the soft tissue envelope. The pedicled latissimus dorsi muscle flap is best used for coverage of large wounds. The advantages of muscle coverage include better filling of dead space and improved vascularity. This makes it more suitable in treating a previously infected tissue bed.

Postoperative Management/Expectations

The details of flap management in the postoperative period are outlined next. A few points about elbow coverage should be emphasized. After the initial 2 to 3 days of flap monitoring, the patient may be discharged home. The postoperative care beyond this window for flap complications in elbow coverage is dependent on the underlying bone, joint, or nerve injury.

The elbow joint is very prone to develop postinjury or postsurgical stiffness and contracture. Early mobilization is crucial to maximize final outcome with respect to regaining range of motion. Management of these potential problems is discussed in the Elbow section.

Complications

Minimal weakness and shoulder girdle stiffness have been associated with the latissimus dorsi as a donor. This diminishes over time in most patients.[178,285] Axillary scarring with contracture can occur. A straight-line incision about the axilla and the cephalad portion of the latissimus should be avoided. Overstretching of the latissimus dorsi muscle to achieve more distal coverage can result in tip necrosis of the flap, requiring additional surgical débridement and often some form of additional soft tissue coverage.

When a free tissue transfer is required, we recommend the use of a latissimus donor site in young women, because the rectus abdominis may be needed for breast reconstruction in the future. Young males may be more predisposed to develop a postsurgical hernia with the use of a rectus abdominis free flap. Meticulous closure of the rectus sheath, with mesh augmentation when necessary, reduces but does not eliminate this risk.

Results

Results for soft tissue coverage procedures for the elbow are limited and principally are case reports. Success rates for rotational muscle and musculocutaneous flaps in the extremities range from 80% to 100%.[11,125,229,287,318,320] Two series of the use of a pedicled latissimus flap for soft tissue coverage about the elbow have been published, reporting a success rate between 85% to 100% for flap survival.[125,278,320] When used for functional reconstruction, restoration of grade M3 to M5 muscle function has been reported.[44,47,81,109, 266,318,357] Survival of free tissue transfers ranges from 80% to 95%.[49,166,350] Khouri and coworkers reported on 493 free tissue transfers, reporting an overall flap failure rate of 4.1%. They also reported a 9.9% incidence of postoperative thrombosis requiring a return to the operating room for re-exploration.[166]

ANNOTATED REFERENCES

23. Bishop A: Soft tissue loss about the elbow: Selecting optimal coverage. Hand Clin 10:531-542, 1994.

     This well-written review article provides a comprehensive review of techniques of soft tissue coverage. It also provides a useful algorithm for selecting the most appropriate treatment for the size and nature of the injury.

92. Foucher G, Khouri RK: Digital reconstruction with island flaps. Clin Plast Surg 24:1-32, 1997.

     This *Clinics* article provides a very good overview of digital coverage with island flaps from the hand. It is particularly valuable in its description of the many permutations of digital artery island flaps for pulp reconstruction.

110a. Gilbert A, Masquelet AC, Hentz VR: Pedicle Flaps of the Upper Limb. Boston, Little, Brown, 1990.

     This work, although another textbook, provides a complete review of the theory and practice of the larger regional flaps to the arm and hand. It is essential reading for anyone who deals with wounds of the upper extremity.

133. Hodgkinson D, Shepherd G: Muscle, musculocutaneous, and fasciocutaneous flaps in forearm reconstruction. Ann Plast Surg 10:400-407, 1983.

     Four separate cases of upper extremity coverage are presented using local rotational muscle flaps. The surgical technique and a discussion of the donor muscle are provided. Brachioradialis, flexor digitorum sublimis, and flexor carpi ulnaris are described for coverage of the elbow.

156. Jutte D, Rees R, Nanney L, et al: Latissimus dorsi flap: A valuable tool in lower arm reconstruction. South Med J 80:37-40, 1987.

     A clinical series of three patients who underwent pedicled latissimus dorsi muscle flaps for soft tissue reconstruction at the elbow is presented. The strength of the article is in the 30 cadaver dissections performed to identify the average length of distal coverage which could be achieved with a pedicled flap. On average, the latissimus could be transposed to 8.4 cm and 6.5 cm distal to the tip of the olecranon and was reliable for anterior and posterior coverage, respectively.

187a. Levin LS, Germann G (eds): Local flap coverage about the hand. Atlas Hand Clin 3(2), 1998.

     This entire volume is an excellent overall reference covering the anatomy, theory, and application of local and regional flaps to the hand. It is well illustrated and written by several authors with a great deal of experience.

212. Maruyama Y, Takeuchi S: The radial recurrent fasciocutaneous flap: Reverse upper arm flap. Br J Plast Surg 39:458-461, 1986.

     This is the first English language article describing the reverse lateral arm flap based on the radial recurrent vessels. The anatomy of the flap is reviewed and three cases are presented.

320. Stevanovic M, Sharpe F, Thommen V, et al: Use of the pedicled latissimus dorsi rotational flap for coverage of soft tissue defects at the elbow. J Shoulder Elbow Surg 8:634-643, 1999.

     This article presents a large clinical series of latissimus dorsi pedicle flaps used to cover soft tissue defects of the elbow. The surgical technique is well described. Complications and techniques to minimize these complications are reported. The role of prophylactic soft tissue coverage is introduced, similar to the use of a prophylactic gastrocnemius flap for patients with poor soft tissue envelope around the knee at the time of knee arthroplasty.

332. Timmons M: The vascular basis of the radial forearm flap. Plast Reconstr Surg 77:70-91, 1986.

     A detailed anatomic injection study identifying the principal arterial and venous supply of the radial forearm flap. The study is based on injection studies of ink, latex, or barium sulfate in 56 cadaver arms. This provides excellent anatomic support of the use of the radial forearm flap as well as supporting harvest of an osteo or osteotendinous fasciocutaneous flap.

334. Tizian C, Sanner F, Berger A: The proximally pedicled arteria radialis forearm flap in the treatment of soft tissue defects of the dorsal elbow. Ann Plast Surg 26:40-44, 1991.

     One of the largest series on use of the pedicled radial forearm flap to treat soft tissue defects of the elbow. Fourteen patients are reviewed. All cases resulted in stable soft tissue coverage, leaving a supple tissue envelope allowing full range of motion. Only one patient experienced delayed wound healing at the donor site.

CHAPTER 48

Free Skin and Composite Flaps

Neil F. Jones and Graham D. Lister

In contradistinction to a split-thickness or full-thickness skin graft, a flap receives its blood supply from a source independent from the underlying bed on which it is laid. An "axial pattern" flap derives its circulation through an inflow artery and an outflow vein, which is termed the *vascular pedicle.* When this pedicle of an axial pattern flap is divided, the flap becomes a "free" flap. Alternative terms include *microsurgical free flap, microvascular flap,* or *free tissue transfer.* A free flap is any segment of skin, fascia, muscle, bone, or composite combination of some of these tissues that is completely detached from its donor site and then transferred to a distant site with immediate restoration of its blood supply by microvascular anastomoses of its inflow artery and outflow vein to recipient blood vessels in the vicinity of the defect. Almost 30 years ago the first successful free tissue transfers[57,59] were allied to a new understanding of the axial pattern of certain vascular territories. Published review articles have since attested to the rapid and continuing growth in the number and variety of such free tissue transfers, throughout the body[56,210,267,344] and specifically to the upper extremity.*

INDICATIONS

The general indications for flap coverage (detailed in Chapter 47) are (1) a defect with exposed joint cartilage or bone devoid of periosteum or tendon devoid of paratenon that cannot support the neovascularization of a skin graft and (2) any specific location in which a skin graft might be subject to exposure and repeated ulceration or impair later reconstruction.

But why use a free flap, which is the most complex technique in the reconstructive hierarchy? Local or regional flaps to the hand have a distinct advantage in that they provide skin of similar color, texture, and thickness and do not require a donor defect elsewhere in the body. However, they are limited in their size and availability. The larger the primary defect created by injury or excision, the less local

skin remains to provide flap cover. Even when there is sufficient area, the thickness required to fill a defect is often lacking. Furthermore, raising a local flap inflicts additional injury on the traumatized limb. The resultant compound wound may further impair hand function more than would the initial defect.

If not local flaps, are there disadvantages to distant pedicle flaps? Distant pedicle flaps (e.g., the groin flap) can provide sufficient tissue in all but the most massive defects. However, circumferential defects are difficult to cover; the hand must be dependent during attachment; positioning may be uncomfortable; lack of exercise may result in more joint stiffness; the flap may be avulsed by the young or the uncooperative patient; and the thickness of the tube presents a later problem of inset and contour. Most importantly, a pedicled flap is no longer supported by its vascular pedicle after division and the flap becomes like a parasite, obtaining nutrition from the underlying scarred bed. In contrast, a free flap has a permanent vascular pedicle. While the contention that a flap brings new blood supply to relatively avascular tissue is fallacious, certainly at the time the flap is applied and probably in the long term, there is merit in the fact that it will not place additional vascular demands on the area of the defect, further compromising the limb. There is a strong similarity between tissues adjacent to a major wound and those that have been irradiated. The advantage of a "permanent pedicle, blood-carrying flap" in coverage of radiation ulcers was shown many years ago.

Free flaps offer an attractive alternative to the limitations of conventional techniques of skin coverage. They are now available in virtually any size and thickness and may be cut to fit the defect with incomparable precision and readily embrace the entire limb. They do not compound the local wound. They permit elevation of the limb and early mobilization and are relatively unaffected by random movement in the infant or disoriented patient.

CONTRAINDICATIONS

Free tissue transfer in its early years was a lengthy, unpredictable undertaking. In one series of over 500 cases

---

*See references 22, 35, 40, 41, 58, 60, 77, 88, 110, 122, 164, 173, 176, 233, 240, 294, 311, 328, 329, and 342.

performed in Ljubljana between 1976 and 1983, only 12 of the first 100 free flap procedures took less than 6 hours to complete.[92] By contrast, 92 of the last 100 were finished in less than 6 hours, 24 of them in less than 4. The failure rate in the first 100 was 26%, in the last 100, 4%. Similar survival rates have been reported from other centers. Free tissue transfer is now a relatively rapid and highly reliable procedure when performed by an experienced team.

Free flaps are equally successful in both pediatric and elderly patients.[29,50,67,269,317] The youngest patient on whom the authors have performed a free tissue transfer was 9 months; the oldest, 87 years. Both have done well with no complications attributable to their ages.

INADEQUATE DÉBRIDEMENT

Free flaps will not help heal unsuitable wounds. Adequate débridement and preparation is mandatory (see later). In an emergency situation, especially in crush injuries, the wound may be so ill defined that radical débridement might needlessly destroy vital structures that otherwise may potentially survive and continue to function. In these circumstances, débridement of unquestionably dead and contaminated tissue should be followed by the application of wet dressings or, perhaps better, copious application of a petrolatum-based ointment such as Neosporin. At a second look within 72 hours, it may be possible to create a clean wound by further débridement, to which an "early" flap can be applied. If doubt remains much beyond 72 hours and further serial débridements are necessary, the chance of infection beneath the flap rises 12-fold.[92] Split-skin grafts should therefore be employed wherever possible after the last, final débridement. Secondary flap reconstruction is left until the wounds have healed.

The corollary to this approach provides the rationale for an "emergency free flap."[22,40,41,92,176,194] The initial injury or subsequent débridement may expose vital tissues that will not (or should not) support a skin graft: bare bone, cartilage, ligament or tendon, and exposed vessels or nerves.[60] A flap will therefore be required at some stage. Even with the wettest of wet dressings, exposed bone and tendon continue to desiccate, die, and eventually have to be excised. It follows therefore that with exposure of such important but poorly vascularized structures, emergency or early flap coverage is mandatory to preserve function.

POOR LIMB FUNCTION

Free tissue transfer should not be used to salvage a limb with insufficient potential for eventual function. Such function can only be attained by an acceptably sensate hand with mobile joints controlled by sufficient musculotendinous units. In complex injuries, the potential salvage of a limb can often only be assessed by an experienced hand surgeon—consideration has to be made between the three options of primary amputation, radical débridement and emergency free flap coverage or serial débridements and secondary free flap coverage.

CLASSIFICATION

The recognition that free tissue transfers were successful, and that theoretically any vascular territory or angiosome could be transferred on its axial pedicle, led to a renaissance in studies on the vascular anatomy of the skin and underlying muscles[18,297,298] and the development of a wide armamentarium of potential free flap donor sites. Only those flaps that have stood the test of time or are currently evolving as potential free flaps for use in the upper extremity are included in Table 48-1.

AXIAL PATTERN FLAPS

The customary division of axial pattern flaps into "cutaneous," "fasciocutaneous," and "musculocutaneous" has been outlined in Chapter 47 and is reiterated here for convenience.

Cutaneous Flap

The vessel of an axial flap may be purely cutaneous (see Fig. 47-28A), proceeding directly to and supplying skin alone. Free flaps based on these cutaneous vessels are termed *free cutaneous* or *free skin flaps.*

Typical free cutaneous flaps used for reconstruction of the upper extremity include the dorsalis pedis flap,[183,196,291,347] the groin flap,[47,48,104] and the first web space neurosensory flap.[191,211]

Fasciocutaneous Flap

The axial vessel may first supply fascia before reaching its cutaneous territory (see Fig. 47-28B). The vessels commonly reach the fascia by running in an intermuscular septum. Because this is attached to bone, a segment of bone may be taken as a composite flap with the overlying skin and be vascularized by the same pedicle, for example, the fibular osteocutaneous flap. Axial flaps whose vessels first pass along the fascia are termed *fasciocutaneous flaps.* Just as with the musculocutaneous flap, fascia may be transferred alone without the overlying skin[276] but skin cannot be transferred without the underlying fascia.

Typical fasciocutaneous flaps used for coverage of the upper extremity include the radial forearm,[214,278,334] ulnar forearm,[46,180] and lateral arm flaps.[142,143,144,279] Pure fascial flaps include the radial forearm fascial flap, the lateral arm fascial flap,[37,283,343] the dorsal thoracic fascial flap,[53,128,152] the serratus fascial flap,[25,75,201,263] and the temporoparietal fascial flap.[23,316]

Muscle Flap

The axial vessel may first supply muscle (see Fig. 47-28C) with multiple secondary perforators supplying the overlying skin. The muscle must be harvested with the skin to ensure survival of the overlying skin, but the muscle may be transferred itself without the overlying skin.

More recently, "perforator flaps" have been developed in which a specific muscle perforator is dissected in continuity

Table 48-1
POTENTIAL FREE FLAP DONOR SITES

Classification	Flap	Artery	Composite Tissues	References
Cutaneous	Deltoid	Posterior circumflex-humeral	Sensory: axillary nerve	Franklin et al,[82] 1980 Hahn et al,[101] 1990
	Dorsalis pedis	Anterior tibial-dorsalis pedis artery	Bone: 2nd metatarsal Tendon: extensor tendons Sensory: superficial peroneal nerve	McCraw and Furlow,[196] 1975 Ohmori and Harii,[224] 1976 Robinson,[246] 1976 McCraw,[198] 1977 Man and Acland,[183] 1980 Takami et al,[291] 1983 Zuker and Manktelow,[347] 1986
	Groin	Superficial circumflex ilac artery Deep circumflex iliac artery	Bone: iliac crest	Smith et al,[274] 1972 Harii et al,[104] 1975 Ohmori and Harii,[225] 1975 Serafin et al,[264] 1976 Baudet et al,[15] 1976 Shah et al,[266] 1979 Acland,[2] 1979 McConnell et al,[195] 1980 Chuang et al,[47] 1989 Chuang et al,[48] 1992 Taylor et al,[246] 1979 Taylor et al,[247] 1979 Minami et al,[204] 1989
	Scapular	Transverse branch of circumflex scapular artery		
	Parascapular	Descending branch of circumflex scapular artery	Skin: dorsal back Bone: lateral border scapula	Santos,[257] 1980 Hamilton and Morrison,[102] 1982 Mayou et al,[193] 1982 Gilbert and Teot,[89] 1982 Barwick et al,[13] 1982 Swartz et al,[287] 1986 Burns and Schlafy,[27] 1986 Jin et al,[128] 1989 Thoma and Heddle,[251] 1990 Park and Shin,[185] 1991 Nassif et al,[218] 1982 Fissette et al,[76] 1983
Anterolateral	Thigh	Descending branch of lateral circumflex femoral artery	Sensory: medial and lateral cutaneous nerves of thigh	Baek,[9] 1983 Song et al,[280] 1984 Zhou et al,[346] 1991 Pribaz et al,[239] 1995
	First web space–toe pulp	Dorsalis pedis artery		May et al,[191] 1977 Morrison et al,[210] 1978 Strauch and Tsur,[282] 1978 Minami et al,[205] 1984 Ikuta,[122] 1985 Koshima et al,[160] 1988 Kato et al,[141] 1989 Morrison,[212] 1990
Fascial-fasciocutaneous—	Radial forearm	Radial artery	Sensory: medial and lateral antebrachial cutaneous nerves Bone: radius Tendon: palmaris longus	Yang et al,[334] 1981 Muhlbauer et al,[175] 1982 Song et al,[278] 1982 Partecke and Buck-Gramcko,[232] 1984 Braun et al,[21] 1985 Emerson et al,[73] 1985 Mahaffey et al,[182] 1985

Continued

Table 48-1

POTENTIAL FREE FLAP DONOR SITES—cont'd

Classification	Flap	Artery	Composite Tissues	References
Fascial-fasciocutaneous—cont'd				Timmons et al,[308] 1986 McGregor,[199] 1987 Swanson et al,[286] 1990 Sanger et al,[256] 1994
	Ulnar forearm	Ulnar artery		Lovie et al,[180] 1984 Christie et al,[46] 1994
	Posterior interosseous	Posterior interosseous artery		Tonkin and Stern,[312] 1989 Shibata et al,[270] 1992 Shibata et al,[271] 1995 Chen et al,[38] 1996
	Anterior interosseous	Anterior interosseous artery		Shibata and Ogishyo,[273] 1996
	Lateral arm	Posterior radial collateral artery	Sensory: posterior cutaneous nerve of arm Bone: humerus Tendon: triceps	Matloub et al,[185] 1983 Katsaros et al,[142] 1984 Scheker et al,[258] 1987 Waterhouse and Healy,[320] 1990 Yousif et al,[343] 1990 Katsaros et al,[143] 1991 Katsaros et al,[144] 1991 Gosain et al,[98] 1992 Teoh et al,[302] 1995
	Fibular osteocutaneous	Peroneal artery	Bone: fibula	Fukui et al,[85] 1989 Yoshimura et al,[340] 1989 Wei et al,[322] 1986
	Plantar	Medial plantar artery		Morrison et al,[208] 1983 Ibaraki and Kanaya,[120] 1995 Ishikura et al,[125] 1995 Ninkovic et al,[220] 1996
	Saphenous	Saphenous artery from descending genicular artery	Sensory: saphenous nerve	Acland et al,[3] 1981
	Temporoparietal	Superficial temporal artery		Smith,[276] 1980 Brent et al,[23] 1985 Upton et al,[316] 1986 Hing et al,[114] 1988 Chowdary,[45] 1989 Rose and Norris,[250] 1990 Chowdary et al,[44] 1990 Hirase et al,[115] 1990 Hirase and Kojima,[116] 1994
Musculocutaneous	Gracilis	Medial circumflex femoral artery		Harii et al,[105] 1976 Giordano et al,[90] 1990 Jones and Thorvaldsson,[132] 1990
	Latissimus dorsi	Thoracodorsal artery		Watson et al,[321] 1979 Maxwell et al,[186] 1979 Takayanagi and Tsukie,[293] 1980 Chaikhouni et al,[33] 1981 Harii et al,[103] 1981 May et al,[189] 1981 Bailey and Godfrey,[10] 1982 Gordon et al,[96] 1982 Salibian et al,[254] 1983 Stern et al,[281] 1983 Lassen et al,[169] 1985 Nielsen et al,[219] 1985 Godina,[93] 1987 Elliott et al,[72] 1989

Continued

Table 48-1
POTENTIAL FREE FLAP DONOR SITES—cont'd

Classification	Flap	Artery	Composite Tissues	References
Musculocutaneous—cont'd	Rectus abdominis	Deep inferior epigastric artery		Pennington et al,[234] 1980 Taylor et al,[296] 1984 Meland et al,[200] 1989 Press et al,[238] 1990 Foulkes et al,[81] 1991 Rao and Baertsch,[242] 1994
	Rectus femoris	Branch of profunda femoris artery		Schenck,[260] 1978
	Serratus anterior	Thoracodorsal artery	Bone: rib	Takayanagi and Tsukie,[292] 1982 Harii et al,[106] 1982 Logan et al,[179] 1988 Whitney et al,[327] 1990 Brody et al,[24] 1990

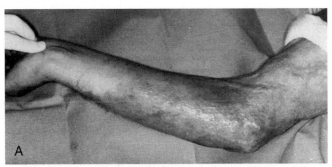
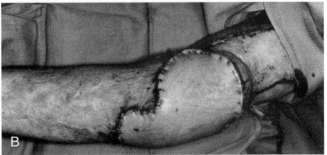
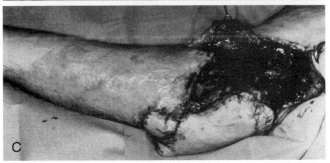

FIGURE 48-1. A, This patient had suffered 40% burns and required replacement of the skin over the extensor surface of the elbow together with excision of heterotopic bone. **B,** A free groin flap was harvested and inset into the defect. Although the extensile incision to dissect the recipient vessels had to be made in scar tissue, no "pseudopod" of the flap had been planned to relieve tension over the pedicle. The crease just proximal to the flap above the Penrose drain bodes ill for later circulation. **C,** The flap subsequently developed venous engorgement, and at exploration extensive hematoma, arising from the congested flap, can be seen in the wound.

between the overlying skin and the main axial vessels that the skin component of a musculocutaneous flap can be transferred without the bulk of the underlying muscle based purely on this single muscle perforator.[6,149,150,151,158]

Flaps containing muscle and skin are termed *musculocutaneous* or *myocutaneous flaps,* whereas transfer of the muscle alone is referred to as a *free muscle flap.* Useful muscle and musculocutaneous flaps for reconstruction of the upper extremity include the latissimus dorsi,[96,189] serratus anterior,[24,179,327] rectus abdominis,[81,200,234,238,2] and gracilis muscles.[90,132]

In certain cases free muscle flaps can be reinnervated by coaptation of their motor nerve to a recipient motor nerve in the forearm to restore otherwise irretrievable motor function (see Chapter 49).[105,260,281] Bone and nerve can also be transferred on their vascular pedicle (see Chapter 50). Apart from these "pure" tissue flaps, composite transfers usually containing two tissue components have been described: skin-bone (osteocutaneous),[95,223,245,255,290,299,302,322] skin-nerve (neurosensory),* and skin-tendon (tendocutaneous).[86,111,121,268,300,318]

These composite flaps have very specific indications: osteocutaneous flaps such as the fibular osteocutaneous flap[322] and the deep circumflex iliac artery osteocutaneous[204,299] flap may be occasionally indicated for reconstruction of combined bone and soft tissue defects of the upper extremity; the radial forearm with palmaris longus tendon[110,237,244] and the dorsalis pedis flap with vascularized long extensor tendons[31,268,318] may be very occasionally indicated for reconstruction of a combined skin and extensor tendon defect due to a dorsal degloving injury of the hand; and the neurosensory flaps[141,185,198,211,282] may be specifically indicated for restoring sensation to an important tactile area of the hand, or the nerve within the flap itself can be used as a vascularized nerve graft[157,249,295] and possibly provide more rapid return of sensation in the distal extremity.

---

*See references 85, 141, 157, 185, 191, 198, 211, 224, 282, and 295.

Venous Flaps

"Venous" flaps* and "arterialized venous" flaps[42,64,117,123,124,138,217,222] have provoked sporadic interest during the past decade.

In a pure venous perfusion flap, a small flap of skin and subcutaneous tissue containing a superficial vein that projects a few millimeters both proximally and distally beyond the flap is harvested from the flexor surface of the distal forearm. The flap is then reversed and can be used for simultaneous coverage of a defect over the dorsal aspect of the fingers or hand as well as restoration of venous outflow by anastomosis of both the proximal and distal ends of the vein to a vein proximal and distal to the defect.[39,78,117,314]

There are two types of "arterialized venous flaps." In the first type, the flap inflow vein is anastomosed to a digital artery and the outflow vein is anastomosed to a vein proximal to the defect, in essence creating an arteriovenous fistula. The second type of "arterialized venous flap" can be used for simultaneous coverage of a defect over the palmar surface of a digit as well as restoration of a segmental defect in the digital artery[117] by repair of the proximal and distal ends of the vein to the digital artery to create a "flow-through" flap. Clinically, "arterialized venous flaps" have survived better than pure "venous" perfusion flaps. The largest successful surviving "venous" perfusion flap measured 10×8 cm, so it is unlikely that these flaps survive purely as a composite graft. Until the hemodynamics are more fully understood, pure "venous" flaps should only be considered for coverage of small dorsal or palmar defects of the fingers requiring simultaneous restoration of venous outflow or arterial inflow.

PREOPERATIVE ASSESSMENT AND PREPARATION

Complete examination of any limb on which surgery is being considered is mandatory. Where free tissue transfer is proposed, particular attention should be paid to the wound itself, the bony skeleton, the vascular anatomy, and any structures that may require simultaneous repair or reconstruction.

Tissue Defect

Preliminary examination of the wound should be directed toward those factors that will influence flap selection: size, depth, and special needs. In the fresh wound, the area may have been reduced somewhat by approximation, but the surgeon should remember two facts. First, one of the major benefits of importing additional tissue is that tension, with all its adverse effects of delayed wound healing, edema, and limitation of early motion, can be eliminated completely. Second, depending on the flap selected, additional area is required to accommodate the bulk of the flap itself. This bulk has its merits, because it serves to fill dead spaces in the wound. In the old wound that is to be excised, the full extent of excision should ideally include all scar, with the incision being made in adjacent normal tissue throughout. If this is impractical, for example, in extensive healed burns, the

excision should include not only ulcerated skin but all the skin that is immobile owing to fixation to deep tissues. It should be recognized that the size of flap required will be considerably larger than the area of skin excised, because of scar contracture affecting the surrounding tissues. For this reason, as emphasized below, the final pattern for the flap should not be made until after wound excision. In those cases in which some scar tissue has to remain on the limb, the surgeon must realize that its lack of elasticity may prevent closure of contiguous incisions, such as that over the pedicle, and make allowances for that fact by planning for "pseudopods" on the flap to close such extensile incisions (Fig. 48-1).

Radiographs, CT, MRI, and Bone Scans

The bony skeleton should be fully evaluated by radiography and, if necessary, computed tomography (CT). Rigid fixation is an essential prerequisite, not only because a rigid skeleton supports the soft tissue reconstruction but also because motion at unstable fractures creates a dead space in which infection can develop. In chronic wounds the presence and extent of any osteomyelitis can be assessed by "four-phase" technetium-99m bone scan and indium-111–labeled leukocytes or magnetic resonance imaging (MRI) with gadolinium enhancement.

Angiography

The vascular anatomy of the limb should be evaluated by the surgeon by palpation of the brachial, radial, and ulnar pulses and also by using a hand-held Doppler pencil probe, making sure to determine the direction of flow and any possible occlusion in the radial-ulnar arch system by selective occlusion. Blood flow distal to the wound in the recently injured limb should be assessed both before surgery and after fixation of any fractures. If blood flow is deemed to be inadequate, revascularization should be considered, either by an interposition vein graft or by using a "flow-through" flap,[207,221,232,258,332,338] such as the radial artery of the radial forearm flap.[19,139,232] In old injuries, information regarding the vascular anatomy should be obtained by noninvasive vascular studies and transfemoral angiography. Whereas some concerns have been expressed in the past[188] regarding the possible adverse effect of angiographic dye injection in the days immediately preceding free tissue transfer, the authors have routinely obtained such studies during the 48 hours before surgery without adverse effect.[190] Magnetic resonance angiography (MRA) and CT angiography are promising newer noninvasive techniques that may eventually supercede the need for invasive angiography of the recipient limb. Angiography of the flap donor site is not necessary, except possibly for some partial and total toe transfers. Instead the surgeon should examine all potential flap donor sites to ensure that there are no previous scars that might compromise harvesting the flap.

Patient Preparation for the Operating Room

As with all free tissue transfers, the patient should be brought to the operating room well perfused.[330] To this end, the patient should be kept warm during the night pre-

---

*See references 8, 34, 39, 78, 84, 137, 203, 304, 314, 339, and 345.

operatively and intravenous fluids should be commenced at midnight at a rate that ensures a urinary output of more than 100 mL/hr in the adult patient at the beginning of surgery. Similarly, the operating room must be kept at a temperature above 70° F. Some surgeons use aspirin or heparin on a routine prophylactic basis, but this is not our custom.

The use of two surgical teams, one to harvest the flap and the other to prepare the recipient site, is common practice and provides the opportunity for the shared experience of two microsurgeons. However, the anecdotal experience of several microsurgeons suggests that little or no time is saved by using two teams and the incidence of complications may be somewhat higher than when one microsurgeon carries the responsibility for the entire procedure.

OPERATIVE TECHNIQUE

Wound Débridement

A wound that is to be covered by a free flap should lie over a stable skeleton. It should not contain any tissue that remains contaminated or has a compromised blood supply. The defect should present as flat a bed as possible for application of the flap. These prerequisites are achieved by rigid fixation and radical débridement (Fig. 48-2).[108] Such

débridement may be performed with confidence only in the knowledge that good soft tissue cover is available. Similarities to tumor surgery exist in that resection of a malignancy with adequate clear margins is best achieved by the surgeon who knows he can close the resulting defect. As with cancer ablation, radical débridement demands incision through normal tissue. This should be done under tourniquet control, otherwise the bleeding from muscle and viable soft tissue will conceal the lack of bleeding from tissues that are not viable. If a major vessel has to be repaired, tissues distal to the arterial injury will be better perfused after the vascular repair and therefore débridement should be performed after reperfusion.

In severe limb trauma, adequate bone shortening can sometimes facilitate approximation of muscle and soft tissue, as in macroreplantation. In these cases, débridement must precede the arterial anastomosis. Those tissues that remain viable can be demonstrated by cannulating the distal end of the vessel to be repaired and perfusing the ischemic part with heparinized saline. Weeping of this fluid will indicate potential viability; absence of this weeping fluid indicates inevitable ischemia.

When immediate flap coverage is planned,[22,40,41] contaminated bone can be retained, scrubbing it vigorously and using burrs and rongeur to remove contamination. Even free fragments can be similarly treated and used as bone grafts,

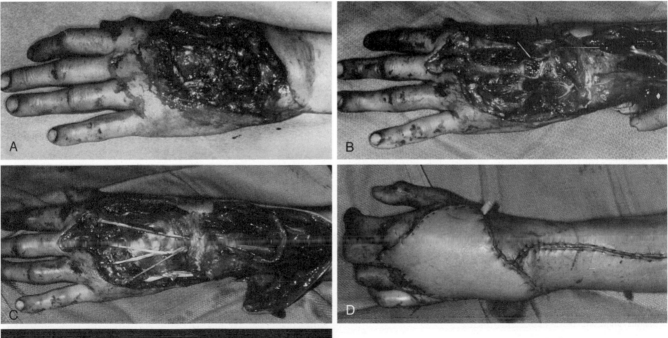

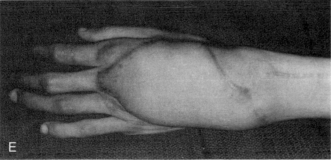

FIGURE 48-2. A, This patient sustained a rollover injury of the left hand with a fracture of the distal radius. **B,** After radical débridement and rigid internal fixation, the sharply excised dorsal carpus is exposed. The carpus was stabilized with Kirschner wires and the distal radius fracture was treated with a T-plate. **C,** Immediate reconstruction of the dorsal capsule using fascia lata and the extensor tendons using tendon grafts has been performed. **D,** A tailored free latissimus flap has been applied, which healed satisfactorily (**E**).

CRITICAL POINTS: WOUND DÉBRIDEMENT

- Wound should be debrided as if it were "tumor resection."
- All foreign material must be removed.
- All nonviable tissue must be removed.
  - Neurovascular structures should be spared.
  - Débride back to bleeding tissue.
  - Remaining muscle should contract with stimulation.
- Size of débridement should not be predicated on size.
  - Free flap can cover almost any defect in the hand or arm.

but only if they are rigidly fixed and are covered with well-vascularized soft tissue. In late cases, in which osteomyelitis has developed, two criteria are used for assessing bone viability. The "paprika" sign denotes the punctate bleeding that occurs when cortical bone has been burred back to the level at which there is adequate perfusion. The presence of adherent periosteum is usually indicative of viable bone, and therefore bone should be resected through adjacent, adherent periosteum.

All marginally viable skin should be removed with the exception of highly specialized areas such as the fingertip or palm. If marginal tissue is retained, such skin may harbor infection and will certainly heal with profuse scarring. When débridement appears adequate, tissue samples are taken from several points in the wound for rapid Gram stain and quantitative cultures.[22] Such tissue samples are only necessary in open wounds and where there has been previous infection. They are taken from tissues that are considered clinically to be noninfected at the end of adequate débridement and therefore serve to draw attention to inadequate débridement; they also identify the probable organism in the event of later infection.

After débridement the wound may be uneven. Additional excision of vital but nonessential tissue is justified to create a flat wound surface. Close contact between flap and bed is thus assured, eliminating dead spaces that may later become the site of infection or fibrosis. The only exceptions to the rule of radical débridement are longitudinal vital structures that carry promise of function: intact tendons or nerves and major vessels carrying flow. These should be retained and cleaned with the help of magnification.

Skeletal Stabilization

Once débridement is complete, rigid skeletal fixation should be applied. Compression plates are preferred for the radius and ulna, low profile mini-plates for the metacarpals, and type A intraosseous wiring or 90-90 intraosseous wiring for the phalanges. External fixation is employed for bony segmental defects. Small defects can be reconstructed primarily with cancellous bone grafts, whereas large defects can be obliterated either with the muscle component of the free flap

or a temporary antibiotic-impregnated methylmethacrylate spacer, pending later definitive bony reconstruction.

After radical débridement of chronic osteomyelitis, secondary cancellous bone grafting should be delayed until 6 weeks after application of the flap, provided that soft tissue healing is uneventful.

Skin Pattern

The skin margins should be freshened and made even by excising any redundant promontories and peninsulas of no functional importance. A pattern of the defect is then taken using any suitable material, such as a piece of an Esmarch bandage that has been moistened with alcohol (see Fig. 48-18C) or the paper of a glove wrapper.

Recipient Vessels

Invariably an additional incision will be required to expose the recipient vessels. In the extremities, closure of the wound over the free flap pedicle may cause impairment of flow to the flap. If this possibility has not been anticipated and a tongue or "pseudopod" of flap has not been incorporated, it may become necessary to apply a split-thickness skin graft over the pedicle. In situations in which no extension of the flap is planned, a zigzag incision is used to expose the recipient vessels with a 60-degree angle between each limb. This not only improves exposure but also permits closure of the wound as a series of "V-Y" advancements, thus increasing the circumference of the limb and avoiding any possibility of vascular compromise of the flap.

With the use of loupe magnification, the recipient vessels are dissected in a preliminary manner, meaning that the vessels are exposed but are not prepared definitively for the microvascular anastomoses. This is for two reasons: the precise location of the anastomoses can only be determined with the flap sutured in place, and the care required for preparation is best achieved under relatively higher magnification under the operating microscope.

Avoiding the Zone of Injury

The key to dissection of the recipient vessels is that exploration should proceed from normal tissue toward the wound, not in the more obvious centrifugal fashion, working outward from the wound. This is especially true in reconstruction of chronic wounds, because the inflammation and subsequent fibrosis that follows the original injury spreads farthest from the wound along the vascular planes. If the surgeon dissects outward from the wound, stopping when the vessels clearly improve, the point at which one stops will be closer to the wound than if one dissects toward the wound, stopping when the vessels clearly deteriorate. The distance between these two stopping points may be small, but it is highly significant, because the vessels still contain scar that is scarcely evident to the examiner but that makes them friable and inelastic. This causes problems in performing the anastomoses, and secondly the vessels may fail to dilate in response to increased flow—this is especially significant in the venous outflow of a free flap.

If prior examination has shown that only one artery to the limb is patent, that artery should be inspected with particular care for the presence of (1) large and expendable side branches to which an end-to-end anastomosis could be performed and (2) atherosclerosis. The latter may be seen as irregular, transverse striations on the vessel or felt as unusual hardness in the vessel wall detected with the touch of either the gloved finger or a jewelers forceps. If atherosclerosis is detected in a single artery extremity in which an end-to-side anastomosis would normally be the technique of choice, the surgeon may elect to perform two end-to-end anastomoses by resecting a segment of the vessel and incorporating a "T" junction in the flap pedicle (see Fig. 48-11).[177]

Pedicle Length and Accessibility

As a final step, the length of vascular pedicle required between the point selected for the anastomoses and the closest margin of the defect should be measured. This should be done before the precise location of the flap on the donor site has been drawn and dissection of its pedicle completed. Pedicle length can be increased by extending the dissection of the pedicle farther than is customary, often with increasing difficulty.[206] In some flaps, the pedicle can be relatively lengthened by moving the skin pattern of the flap away from the vascular pedicle but keeping the majority of the skin paddle within the vascular territory.[2,20]

In those circumstances in which the selected flap does not have a long enough pedicle, three solutions exist. First, choose a different flap. Second, harvest a vein graft. Third, create a temporary arteriovenous fistula using an interposition vein graft between the recipient artery and vein or a recipient shunt by anastomosing a long length of a recipient vein end to side into the recipient artery.[254] However, a recipient shunt should only be considered when the recipient vein is situated away from the recipient artery and when it continues distally into the limb away from the wound and remains unscarred and of good caliber. This last solution is attractive not only when the selected flap pedicle is going to be too short but also when the selected recipient artery is relatively deep and inaccessible and when there are two experienced microsurgical teams. When the intended end-to-side arterial anastomosis is deep and somewhat inaccessible, the additional presence of the flap in the way will make it even more difficult to see and do. Use of a temporary arteriovenous or recipient shunt can improve visibility and move the two end to end anastomoses of the flap to a more accessible location. When there are two teams, the team dissecting the recipient site will always complete its task before the team raising the flap. The whole operation will be accelerated if the recipient team performs the more time-consuming end-to-side anastomosis of the interposition vein graft or recipient vein to the recipient artery.

Raising the Flap

With knowledge of the anatomy of the selected flap, a template of the defect can be positioned on the skin in such a way as to optimize the desired thickness of the flap and the necessary pedicle length. It is usually prudent to maximize the length of pedicle, since the microsurgical anastomoses can be moved more proximally away from the wound. A loose pedicle will also facilitate end-to-side anastomoses. Only one flap margin should be incised initially with an extension over the presumed course of the pedicle. The vascular pedicle can be visualized and dissected through this incision. In those rare cases in which the pedicle is found to be anomalous or absent, this initial incision can be closed without compromising the circulation to the skin.

Between the vascular strata—subcutaneous tissue, fascia, and muscle—lie relatively avascular planes. It is in these planes that the flap should be elevated. To reach these planes, it is necessary to cut through the vessels of the more superficial strata. For example, in harvesting a fascial flap, the surgeon must first incise the subdermal and subcutaneous plexus and then the fascia and elevate the fascial flap in the plane beneath the fascia but superficial to the muscle. To be one plane too superficial would result in division of the vessel supplying the flap. To be one plane too deep would result in a time-consuming, often bloody dissection.

Application of tension plays a major role in flap dissection. Once the marginal incision has been carried down to the correct plane for dissection, skin hooks should be applied to the corners of the flap. Firm upward traction away from the bed will display the plane for dissection. Often this plane only contains loose areolar tissue that can be stroked away with a knife. Tension on the flap lifts the pedicle off the floor of the secondary defect, on which the knife is dissecting, into the roof containing the vascular stratum. Care must be taken not to create a "cave" beneath the flap, that is, a central recess between areas of unincised skin, muscle, or fascia. When closed scissors are introduced into the tissues and then opened under gentle pressure to clear planes, they can be both precise and innocuous. They create and enter "caves," defining structures to be preserved and those to be divided. When scissors are introduced open and closed to cut, they are less precise. It is therefore important when using scissors that the surgeon see both aspects of the structure to be divided so as to be confident what tissues are included between the jaws of the scissors.

Dissection of the Pedicle

Unrecognized damage to the vascular pedicle during dissection is one of the major causes of postoperative complications after free tissue transfer, often resulting in poor perfusion to the flap or culminating in thrombosis at the anastomosis. Any problem in the entire vascular tree either affecting arterial inflow or venous outflow may eventually result in anastomotic thrombosis. Meticulous dissection of the pedicle therefore plays a paramount role in achieving a successful outcome. Hemostasis must be perfect during dissection of any flap, because it is hazardous to achieve once the anastomoses have been completed. Although it has been shown that metal clips are not secure and that bipolar coagulation may harm the pedicle,[251] both are routinely employed in dissecting the pedicle. The clips must be applied with sufficient force to ensure that they will not slip. If bipolar coagulation is being used, the pedicle should be insulated by holding the side branch with smooth forceps between the pedicle and the point of coagulation.

On completion of the dissection of the pedicle, the flap should be allowed to perfuse after bathing the pedicle with either 2% lidocaine (Xylocaine) or papaverine, before dividing the pedicle and transferring the flap to the recipient site.

Flap Insetting

The flap is placed into the defect, checking that the end of the pedicle comes to lie approximately at the predicted site of the anastomoses. The flap can either be sutured definitively into place or temporarily stapled into position. With definitive insetting, the completed anastomoses will be less likely to be at risk during final wound closure. Furthermore, the edema that will inevitably occur in the flap after reperfusion will be controlled and should not produce such swelling as to make complete closure of the flap impossible.

Once the flap is in place, the microscope is introduced, the pedicle is approximated to the recipient vessels, and the site of the anastomoses is selected. If the venous repair lies at some distance from the arterial, this is the stage when the surgeon can most safely separate the vein and artery within the pedicle. The recipient vessels should be dissected circumferentially over sufficient distance to allow easy rotation to bring their back walls forward. When an end-to-end anastomosis is to be performed, the recipient vessel should only be dissected over a length necessary to accommodate a microsurgical approximator clamp. The techniques of microvascular anastomosis have already been described in Chapter 44.

Both the arterial and venous anastomoses should be performed before removing the clamps from either vessel. Whichever anastomosis is more difficult is performed first.

If a monitor such as a photoplethysmograph or a laser Doppler is to be used, the sterile probe should be sutured to the flap and connected before the microsurgical clamps are removed (see Figs. 48-4C and 48-8C). In this way reperfusion of the flap can be charted, as can any changes that occur during wound closure.[259,289] If there is any persistent accumulation of blood in the wound that cannot be controlled—usually from scar or bone—then a drain or drains should be inserted (see Fig. 48-4C). Suction can be applied but only very carefully, because however far from the pedicle the drain lies the two may come together with disastrous consequences.

Dressings

No dressings should be applied to the flap surface, so that the flap can be easily observed at all times. The incisions can be covered with Neosporin ointment and a thin strip of nonadherent gauze. To protect the limb during sleep a cast should be applied, leaving a generous window for inspection. A surgical glove is turned inside out to close the fingers and packed with gauze sponges. The glove is laid over the flap, cast padding is applied to the whole limb including the glove, and a plaster of Paris cast is made. Once the cast is dry, the prominence created by the packed glove is removed with a saw, rather like opening a boiled egg, and the glove is removed, so that the flap is protected yet always visible.

POSTOPERATIVE CARE AND MONITORING

Postoperative care should be directed toward the comfort of both patient and flap and should be the responsibility of a team of trained, trusted nurses. The comfort of the patient is pursued through the usual channels and should not be neglected due to concern for the flap. It is important that the patient be up and about as soon as possible, preferably starting on the first postoperative day. All joints not included in the cast should be mobilized.

Several different anticoagulants such as intravenous dextran 40, intravenous heparin, subcutaneous low dose heparin, and oral low dose aspirin are used prophylactically by many surgeons to prevent thrombosis of the microsurgical anastomoses. There are no prospective controlled trials to confirm the efficacy of any of these anticoagulant regimens and occasionally their disadvantages outweigh the theoretical benefits. One of the authors (NFJ) uses a 40-mL bolus of dextran 40 just before release of the microsurgical clamps followed by a continuous intravenous infusion of 25 mL of dextran 40 per hour for 5 days (based on a 70-kg adult patient) together with aspirin, 325 mg orally daily. The other author (GDL) does not use any anticoagulant therapy after routine free tissue transfer.

Routine wound cleansing should be accomplished using hydrogen peroxide followed by a thin smear of antibiotic ointment. This routine has many benefits: it eliminates a nutritious inoculum for bacteria; it ensures that color assessment is neither obscured by blood staining nor impaired by vivid contrast within the observer's visual field; it permits assessment of the rate of bleeding from the wound, in itself a valuable index of venous insufficiency; and it has an inestimable effect on the morale of the patient who can see the healing wound.

Monitoring

The nurse should observe the flap regularly, usually every hour for the first 48 hours to ensure its continued viability. Clinical evaluation of the flap is based on several criteria.

Color

Although difficult to learn and impossible to convey adequately, color assessment still remains the mainstay of clinical assessment.[112] The lighting must obviously be good. The observer's color perception can be neutralized by first looking at an area of normal skin for 10 seconds and then comparing the color of the flap.

A healthy free flap, especially the groin flap, is pale to a degree that makes the novice nervous. It is not pure white, when comparing it with a sheet of white paper, but rather a very pale pink. If arterial inflow is inadequate, a flap will become paler with a faint blue-gray tinge. If venous drainage is compromised, the flap will at first become an angry red and then progressively purple-red and purple-blue (Fig. 48-3A). The unperfused free flap at first assumes a waxy pallor—that is, white tinged with yellow or brown—that differs from its healthy pink pallor by a margin so subtle that only the experienced are pessimistic. The margins of the failing flap then become indurated and may blister, but doubts concerning the extent of loss may persist for several days.

Capillary Refill

Capillary refill may be assessed after blanching by fingertip pressure or by running a blunt point across the flap. If the refill after blanching is very slow and the flap is pale, arterial insufficiency is the likely cause. If capillary refill is too swift

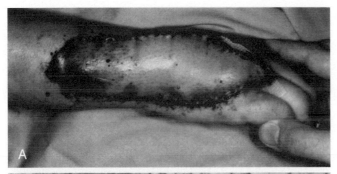

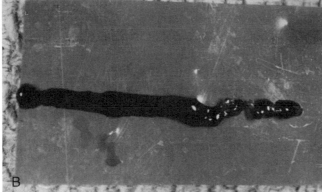

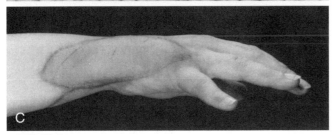

FIGURE 48-3. **A,** This lateral arm flap on the ulnar aspect of the hand is clearly in serious venous embarrassment, with significant discoloration of the proximal end of the flap, which is to the left of the figure. **B,** Exploration revealed thrombosis of the vein of the flap, and thrombectomy resulted in a satisfactory salvage of the entire flap (**C**).

and the flap has a bluish hue, then venous outflow is impaired. Little stock can be placed on this test in isolation because entirely stagnant blood will move around in the tissues in response to pressure, although more slowly than one would see in a healthy flap.

Bleeding

Although the color and capillary refill of a flap can be assessed on a regular protocol, bleeding from the flap should only be evaluated if there is any suspicion of impending compromise to the perfusion of the flap. The flap and adjacent tissue can be punctured with an 18-gauge needle or a No. 11 scalpel blade and the resultant bleeding compared. A healthy flap should produce bright red blood of the same color as the control and should bleed just a little longer. If no bleeding occurs or if the flap only bleeds very briefly, arterial inflow is inadequate. If the blood is dark red or purple and bleeding persists much longer, venous congestion should be suspected. Persistent dark red bleeding from around the margins of a swollen flap is almost pathognomonic of venous occlusion.

Other Monitoring Techniques

Many techniques for postoperative monitoring of free tissue transfers have been developed and evaluated in experimental free flap models.[1,68,107,197,243,307] Several of these techniques have been used in large clinical series.* There have been no prospective clinical trials of any monitoring technique, and there is still no consensus as to which will eventually become the standard accepted method.[134]

An ideal monitoring technique should provide a continuous recording of flap perfusion or flap metabolism, with immediate detection of arterial or venous occlusion. It is important that the criteria indicative of arterial or venous occlusion be easily interpreted by nursing personnel or junior medical staff. Finally, an ideal system should allow monitoring of both visible and "buried" types of free tissue transfers.[134]

Several techniques are currently used:

- Photoplethysmography[259]
- Differential surface temperature monitoring[146,172]
- Doppler surface monitoring[277]
- Laser Doppler[71,109,127,284,285]
- Implantable Doppler probes[63,154,288,289,315]
- Implantable pH electrodes[243]
- Implantable oxygen electrodes[1]
- Pulse oximetry[133]

Photoplethysmography has been shown to indicate early signs of compromised flap perfusion owing to excessive tension during skin closure.[259] Photoplethysmographic waveforms can even be transmitted by telephone to a remote monitoring station[131] to allow the surgeon at home to interpret any abnormal waveforms, so that the nursing personnel can be advised whether the waveform is normal or whether the flap should undergo re-exploration.

A surface temperature probe can be used to compare the relative difference in temperature between the flap and a second control temperature probe on adjacent normal skin.[172] Differential surface temperature monitoring has been evaluated retrospectively in a large series of 600 free tissue transfers.[146] A difference between the differential surface temperature measurements at two points in time of greater than 1.8° C has been shown to be diagnostic of arterial or venous occlusion.

The characteristic arterial pulsation of either a free skin flap or a free muscle flap resurfaced with a split thickness skin graft can be heard with a hand-held pencil 8-MHz Doppler probe.[277] The best arterial Doppler signal on the surface of the flap is marked by a suture and the arterial signal monitored both during closure and every hour postoperatively for the first 48 hours. Augmentation of the venous "hum" can also be produced by compression of the flap tissue, thereby confirming the patency of venous outflow. The laser Doppler flowmeter[71,109,127,284,285] has been used for postoperative monitoring of free skin flaps and musculocutaneous flaps and free muscle flaps resurfaced with split-thickness skin grafts.

An implantable 20-MHz ultrasonic Doppler probe can be used for continuous monitoring of the patency of the arterial anastomosis and will provide instantaneous detection of an

---

*See references 71, 109, 127, 146, 172, 259, 277, 284, 285, 288, and 289.

arterial occlusion.[63,154,289] However, this technology also requires further refinement, both with regard to positioning the probe on the arterial wall and recognition of a venous occlusion.[288]

Paradoxically, because of the ever-increasing success rates of free tissue transfers, it will become more and more difficult to document scientifically the value of any postoperative monitoring technique. One of the authors (NFJ) uses Doppler surface monitoring of the arterial pulsation with a hand-held Doppler probe every hour for postoperative monitoring of free skin, muscle, and osteocutaneous flaps and a pulse oximeter for postoperative monitoring of toe-to-hand transfers.[100,133] An audible alarm can be set to detect the lowest acceptable level of oxygen saturation or loss of the arterial pulse rate, and this obviously reduces the frequency of nursing vigilance. Loss of the arterial pulse is indicative of arterial occlusion in a toe transfer, whereas the oxygen saturation falling below 90% is suggestive of venous occlusion. The other author (GDL) routinely uses photoplethysmography.[259]

SAVING THE FAILING FLAP

Vascular Failure

What actions can be taken to salvage a failing free flap?

1. The patient's general condition—hypotension, cardiopulmonary impairment, or a low circulating volume, manifest by a low urinary output—may all adversely affect oxygenation of the flap. A cold vasoconstricted extremity may be due to circumstances as grave as advanced shock or as simple as a low room temperature. Both should be evaluated and corrected.
2. Look for any unduly tight dressings or sutures. Remove the cast and all the dressings down to the flap. Cut any tight sutures.
3. Reposition the patient's arm; in particular, determine if elevation or dependency of the arm improves flap perfusion. If it does, make the patient comfortable in this new position.
4. Look for signs of hematoma and evacuate the hematoma. If the flap is swollen or edematous and discolored and there is persistent serosanguineous fluid oozing from the flap margins, then a hematoma should be strongly suspected. A flap hematoma has been shown to cause loss of a flap, which can be potentially salvaged by evacuation. A few sutures along the flap margin opposite the entrance of the vascular pedicle into the flap should be cut immediately. This may allow some dissipation of the pressure induced by the hematoma, but formal evacuation of the hematoma should be done in the operating room as soon as possible after the hematoma is detected (see Fig. 48-1C).

If none of these maneuvers rapidly improves the appearance of the flap, the patient should be returned to the operating room immediately for exploration of the pedicle, because if done quickly this can be very successful (see Fig. 48-3).[112] The situation is almost always worse than it appears.

Initially only the incision that provides access to the pedicle is reopened. If all the sutures around the flap are removed, the edematous flap will be very difficult to control during inspection of the pedicle and impossible to replace back into the primary defect with the precision achieved in the first surgery.

Any hematoma should be gently removed with warm irrigation and the gloved finger. Suction should only be used with extreme care.

The pedicle and recipient vessels proximal to the anastomoses should be examined for obvious kinks, occlusions, or thrombosis. The point of occlusion in a vein will usually be obvious, the upstream segment being turgid, the downstream collapsed. Arterial occlusion is usually less evident and can be detected by lack of a pulse on palpation or with a sterile Doppler probe. Arterial flow by the "milking" or "sweeping" test should not be tested until a microsurgical clamp has been placed across the artery downstream distal to a side branch through which emboli, which would otherwise wash into the flap microcirculation, can be safely diverted. After placement of the clamp, the side branch can be opened to determine the presence or absence of flow across the anastomosis.

Do not hesitate to open an anastomosis between clamps to assess flow and if necessary redo the anastomosis. If clot is present in a patient with a normal clotting mechanism, remember that blood flow only stops if arterial inflow is poor, if "runoff" through the flap is impeded, or if the anastomosis was technically imperfect. If the anastomosis looks good, inspect downstream for an unrecognized injury to the pedicle. If none is found and inflow through the recipient artery is strong, then excise the anastomosis and do it again. There is usually enough redundancy in the recipient artery and arterial pedicle to allow a second end-to-end anastomosis. If not, a short interposition vein graft may be necessary. Revision of an end-to-side anastomosis is more difficult unless a "T" graft[91,177] has been or can be harvested (see earlier). With a "T" graft three cuts and three anastomoses can save the situation.

Do not hesitate to excise a redundant segment and perform another anastomosis.

The patient should be kept in the operating room for a period of time after re-exploration and revision of the anastomoses to ensure that further thrombosis does not occur.

Other Salvage Techniques

There are as many publications in the literature concerning experimental methods of enhancing flap survival[145] as there are of monitoring, possibly more, but there are no prospective clinical trials documenting the efficacy of any pharmacologic agent to enhance flap survival. However, medicinal leeches and various thrombolytic agents may play an occasional role in the salvage of a failing free flap, either as an adjunct intraoperatively, during re-exploration of the microsurgical anastomoses, or if the patient or the flap is not deemed suitable for surgical re-exploration.

Leeches

It is well established that leeches can be used to salvage a failing replanted digit,[162] if venous outflow is compromised, or if a suitable vein is not available for anastomosis. In an extension of this technique, leeches have been used to relieve venous congestion in pedicle flaps and free flaps.[14,55,62,162,325] The success of flap salvage after leech therapy has been reported as high as between 60% and 70%. Just as in the replant situation, there is one report of a successful free flap performed with only an arterial anastomosis.[174] Leeches provided venous drainage of the flap for 8 days until neovascularization was reestablished.

Hirudo medicinalis may ingest an amount of blood almost ten times its own weight; however, the therapeutic effect of leeches is not due to the volume of blood ingested but due to continued bleeding from the bite after detachment of the leech. Several pharmacologically active substances are secreted by the leech, including hyaluronidase, an antihistamine, a vasodilator, and hirudin, which is the most potent natural anticoagulant known. Hirudin is a 65-amino acid polypeptide with a molecular weight of 9000 daltons and inhibits the conversion of fibrin to fibrinogen.

The most significant risk of leech therapy is infection[62,202,326] with *Aeromonas hydrophila*, which may cause a major necrotizing soft tissue or muscle infection with an incidence estimated between 7% and 20%. Consequently, it may be prudent not to use leeches for a failing free muscle flap. *A. hydrophila* infections may be prevented or treated secondarily with a second- or third-generation cephalosporin or an aminoglycoside antibiotic. The second major risk of prolonged leech therapy is blood loss and the eventual need for blood transfusion. Leeches must also be prevented from "wandering" or attaching to normal better perfused tissues.

Thrombolytic Agents

Several thrombolytic agents have been used for the treatment of various arterial and venous thromboses, including myocardial infarction, pulmonary embolism, deep venous thrombosis, and thrombotic-embolic problems in the upper and lower extremities. However, there are only a few reports of thrombolytic therapy for salvage of a failing free flap.[7,30,54,83,94,175,261,265]

Heparin may prevent anastomotic thrombosis by blocking the conversion of prothrombin to thrombin and by decreasing platelet adhesiveness. Systemic intravenous infusion of heparin is sometimes used by some microsurgeons to prevent thrombosis of the arterial and venous anastomoses in replanted or revascularized digits, especially when these injuries have been associated with a crushing mechanism or after repeated revision of the anastomoses. However, systemic heparin may be complicated by bleeding and the development of hematomas. Local infusion of heparin through a tiny silicone catheter inserted into one of the venae comitantes of a free gracilis muscle flap was successful in preventing thrombosis of a revised end-to-side anastomosis of the other venae comitantes. Heparin was infused at a rate of 250 U/hr for 6 days, and the flap was successfully salvaged after the revision venous anastomosis without inducing systemic anticoagulation.[192]

Streptokinase is an enzyme isolated from group C β-hemolytic streptococci that converts plasminogen into the enzyme plasmin, which in turn sequentially degrades fibrin in a thrombus.[241] Successful salvage of a failing free flap due to either arterial or venous thrombosis has been reported, either by infusion of streptokinase into the totally isolated free flap[261] or by selective arterial infusion of streptokinase into the flap by direct arterial puncture proximal to the

arterial anastomosis using a fine 30-gauge needle.[175] By avoiding return of streptokinase to the systemic circulation, very high doses of intra-arterial streptokinase infusion can be used, up to 60,000 U in 1 hour.

Urokinase is a naturally occurring enzyme derived from human kidney cells and probably has significant advantages over streptokinase.[265] Unlike streptokinase, urokinase does not cause allergic reactions and can be used at very high concentrations with less risk of hemorrhage and without inactivating plasminogen. One of the authors (NFJ) has successfully salvaged two failing radial forearm flaps and one failing toe transfer due to venous thrombosis or combined arterial and venous thromboses by expedient re-exploration and intra-arterial infusion of urokinase into the recipient artery proximal to the arterial anastomosis. Serletti and associates[265] reported the successful salvage of five failing free flaps owing to thrombosis of the venous anastomosis by infusion of 250,000 U of urokinase over 30 minutes through a 25-gauge catheter inserted into the recipient artery proximal to the arterial anastomosis.

There are two case reports of the use of an intravenous infusion of tissue plasminogen activator (t-PA)[7,83] in conjunction with an intravenous infusion of heparin to successfully salvage a free flap compromised by a presumed arterial thrombosis. The optimal dose of t-PA to achieve therapeutic thrombolysis has not been determined.

CRITICAL POINTS: THE FAILING FREE FLAP

NONOPERATIVE MEASURES

- Check volume status of patient, oxygenation, etc.
- Release or remove constricting dressings.
- Reposition the patient's arm (up or down).
- Release sutures at margin of flap to release pressure and/or hematoma.

OPERATIVE MEASURES

- Return to operating room for exploration.
  - Remove hematoma.
  - Check status of vessels (e.g., clot, kink).
  - Open vessel between clamps (avoid distal embolization of clot).
  - Revise anastomosis.
  - Add vein graft if necessary.
  - Observe closely in operating room after revision for re-thrombosis.

OTHER MEASURES

- Leeches for venous congestion (not in place of return to operating room for revision of clotted anastomosis)
- Anticoagulation (heparin)
- Thrombolytic agents
  - Streptokinase/urokinase/t-PA for distal clot

Intravenous infusion of t-PA was begun at 12 mg/hr but was discontinued after 15 minutes because of hemorrhage from the flap donor site. Finally a multicenter, randomized phase II study investigated the use of recombinant human tissue factor pathway inhibitor (rhTFPI, SC-59735) as an antithrombotic additive to irrigate the microsurgical anastomoses in free flap surgery. Although low-dose rhTFPI at a concentration of 0.05 mg/mL was associated with fewer flap failures than high-dose rhTFPI or the standard heparin irrigation, this was not statistically significant. However, the incidence of postoperative wound hematomas was significantly less using low-dose rhTFPI compared with the standard heparin irrigating solution.[147]

INFECTION

Should infection develop beneath a flap it should be treated just like any wound infection. In a patient who is not compromised systemically, infection invariably means inadequate débridement of the original wound or failure of perfusion of part of the flap. Antibiotics may be used as a supplement, but expeditious surgical exploration is the best guarantee of flap survival. If exploration is delayed, thrombosis of the pedicle may result in complete loss of the flap. The flap should be elevated on the side opposite the pedicle and reflected to the extent necessary to reveal the source of infection. If this is an infected hematoma, then evacuation with subsequent catheter irrigation for 2 days should suffice. Any suspicious areas of infection in the bed or in the flap itself should be radically débrided, followed once again by catheter irrigation for 2 days.

SPECIFIC FREE FLAPS

Lateral Arm Flap

First described by Song and associates,[279] the lateral arm flap and its vascular anatomy were popularized by Katsaros and colleagues.[142-144,262] In many respects, it is ideal for upper extremity reconstruction because it can be harvested from the same limb using the same tourniquet.[258,320] The flap can be made as small as 10 cm² (Figs. 48-4 and 48-5) and as large as virtually the entire circumference of the upper arm or extended onto the proximal forearm. It is thin, is pliable, and can be innervated. A segment of vascularized humerus (up to 10 cm long and 25% [1.5 cm] of the circumference) can also be harvested with the flap,[302] as can a vascularized segment of triceps tendon.[98]

For special contouring, the flap can be divided along the midline of its long axis or transversely from side to side, provided that the lateral intermuscular septum is preserved. This permits the proximal and distal portions to be laid side by side to cover a wider defect or to be placed on both sides of a hand that has sustained a major penetrating wound or requires coverage of both the palmar and dorsal aspects of the thumb/index finger web space (Fig. 48-6). One drawback, which precludes its use in some young female patients, is that the secondary defect is very noticeable, whether it is closed directly or with a skin graft. Another is that the flap may be bulky: in one series of lateral arm flaps

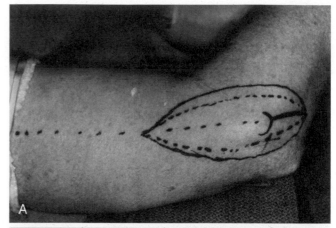
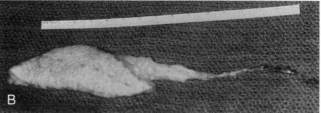
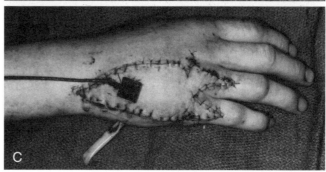

FIGURE 48-4. Lateral arm flap. **A,** The deltoid tubercle and the lateral epicondyle have been marked and joined with a dotted line that traverses the figure from left to right. The skin incision is marked with a dotted line, and the intended incision of the fascia is marked with a solid line. **B,** The distal location of the flap provides a long pedicle. **C,** The lateral arm flap has been inset to cover the lateral aspect of the dorsum of the hand and also the proximal portions of the ring and small fingers. The anastomosis to the ulnar artery was performed proximal to the wrist.

used for reconstruction of the upper extremity, 50% were considered bulky by the surgeon and required defatting.[99] These two disadvantages of the lateral arm skin flap can potentially be avoided by harvesting only lateral arm fascia[283,343] and covering this lateral arm fascial flap with a split-thickness or full-thickness skin graft.

Anatomy

The arterial supply to the lateral arm flap is the posterior radial collateral artery, one of the two terminal branches of the profunda brachii artery. The profunda brachii arises from

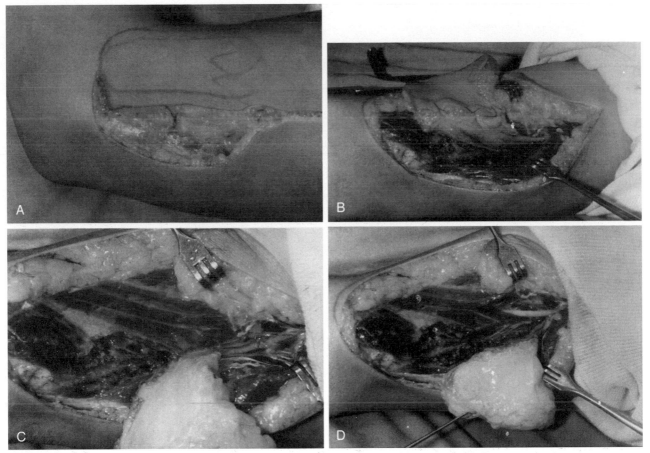

FIGURE 48-5. Lateral arm flap dissection. **A,** The posterior incision has been made, and the fascia overlying the triceps is seen. This must be divided to gain the correct plane for further dissection. **B,** The dissection has been completed to the point of raising the lateral intermuscular septum from the underlying bone. The humerus can be seen in the distal third of the wound with the muscles of the mobile wad anterior and the triceps posterior to it. The sutures between the fascia and the skin prevent any shearing force between these structures. **C,** On close-up, the humerus is seen more clearly. The oozing is from the muscular branches that have been divided. The more proximal course of the pedicle is seen to the right of the incision. **D,** The pedicle has been dissected more proximally, and the radial nerve is now clearly seen as the white structure passing forward between the brachialis and the brachioradialis.

the brachial artery in the distal axilla and accompanies the radial nerve in the spiral groove until both penetrate the lateral intermuscular septum, just distal to the deltoid insertion. Here the artery divides, with the anterior radial collateral artery continuing with the radial nerve anterior to the brachioradialis origin from the humerus and the posterior radial collateral artery passing posterior to the origin of the lateral intermuscular septum. The vessel comes to lie closer to the humerus and supplies bone via the overlying periosteum as it proceeds down to the lateral epicondyle, to which it is adherent.

Between the point at which it leaves the radial nerve and the lateral epicondyle, the posterior radial collateral artery provides branches to bone, to muscles in both anterior and posterior compartments, and to the fascia and overlying skin. The main branches to fascia and skin therefore arise between these two points, which roughly demarcate the lower half of a line between the deltoid tubercle and the epicondyle.

The posterior radial collateral artery anastomoses distally with a rich vascular plexus composed of the olecranon anastomosis and branches of the radial recurrent artery, so that the territory of the lateral arm flap can be extended up to 12 cm below the lateral epicondyle onto the proximal forearm.[20,52,163,168] Alternatively, only the proximal forearm skin can be harvested, thereby increasing the length of the posterior radial collateral artery pedicle.

The artery of the flap is usually accompanied by two venae comitantes and by two nerves, the posterior cutaneous nerve of the arm and forearm and both branches of the radial nerve. The posterior cutaneous nerve of the arm can be used to innervate the flap, whereas the posterior cutaneous nerve of the forearm should be preserved but can be harvested with the flap as a vascularized nerve graft.[185] If the flap is designed on its distal skin territory as the lateral arm/proximal forearm flap, the posterior nerve of the forearm is used to innervate the flap.

Operative Technique

A sterile tourniquet is applied high on the upper arm after preparation to the axilla. A line marking the lateral intermuscular septum is drawn from the deltoid tubercle to the lateral epicondyle and defines the midline axis of the flap (see Fig. 48-4A). The flap template is laid over this line marking the septum and, in most instances, should be centered over the distal half of the line, although if a longer pedicle is required, the template can be moved more distally until it is centered over the epicondyle (see Fig. 48-4B). If

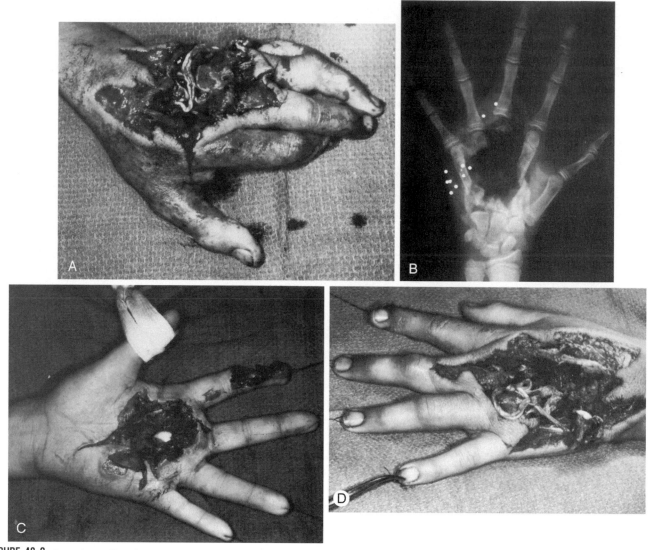

FIGURE 48-6. Lateral arm flap. **A,** A 14-year-old right-handed youth sustained this close-range shotgun injury to his left hand. **B,** Radiograph shows significant metacarpal loss. Distraction displayed the (**C**) palmar and (**D**) dorsal defects.   *Continued*

more skin cover over the pedicle is desired, the template should be moved proximally.

The skin is incised around the posterior margin of the flap and the incision extended proximally along the axial line as far as the deltoid tubercle. The incision is carried down to fascia. The posterior edge of the incision is elevated with skin hooks and the dissection continued posteriorly superficial to the fascia until the midline of the triceps tendon is reached. The fascial vessels can be clearly seen running over the tendon (see Fig. 48-5B). The fascia is incised along the midline of the tendon and elevated from the tendon and muscle by dissecting in an anterior direction with the fascia elevated under some tension, at the same time retracting the triceps muscle in a posteromedial direction. The fascia and skin can be sutured to one other using the long ends of the ties as stay sutures. The dissection proceeds easily, with few if any small vessels to cauterize, until the septum is approached, at which point the flap vessel will be seen with its muscular branches diving into the triceps. Stop the posterior to anterior dissection at this point.

The anterior margin of the flap and the underlying fascia over the brachialis and brachioradialis muscles should now be incised. The fascia here is more flimsy than that posteriorly but can be readily defined and managed in precisely the same way as previously described for the posterior portion of the flap, dissecting this time in a posterior direction beneath the fascia until the muscular vessels are encountered. The distal margin of the flap should now be raised, dissecting right up against the aponeurosis of the extensor origin in a proximal direction until the epicondyle is reached. The fascia here is very ill defined. There is no need, however, to incise the aponeurosis as one is tempted to do, only a need to dissect hard against it up to the epicondyle.

After raising all three margins, the flap can be elevated away from the lateral humerus. The assistant should retract the anterior and posterior muscle bellies away from the septum. With traction applied to the flap in an upward direction with the nondominant hand, the surgeon should now elevate the septum from the periosteum of the humerus with a knife or bipolar cautery, taking care to ensure that all periosteal and muscular branches are cauterized. Although

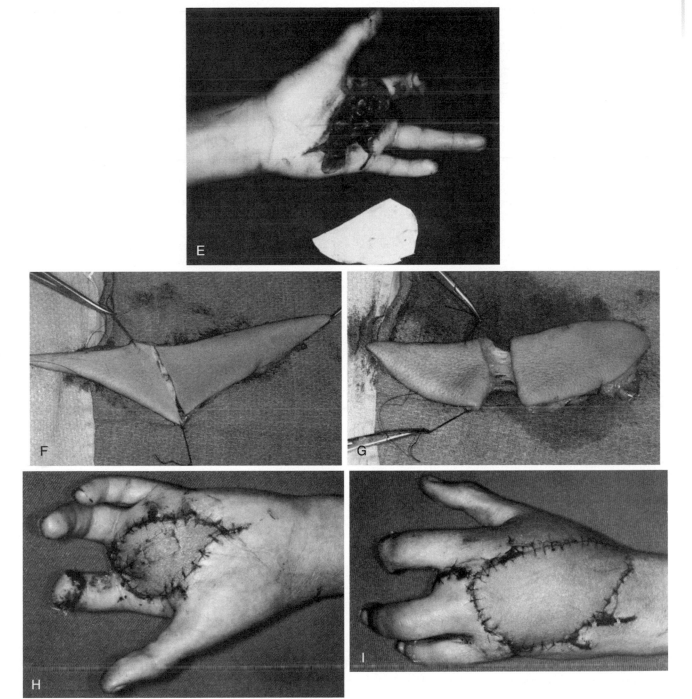

FIGURE 48-6—cont'd. E, The middle finger was nonviable and had no metacarpal. It was therefore amputated and the index finger was translocated into the position of the middle metacarpal. Length was restored by inserting the middle phalanx from the middle finger as an intercalated bone graft. The bony defect in the ring metacarpal was restored by using the proximal phalanx from the middle finger in a similar fashion. Significant palmar and dorsal defects remained. **F,** Patterns were taken and placed end-to-end in designing a lateral arm flap taken from the same arm. **G,** After the lateral arm flap was raised, it was divided transversely through skin and subcutaneous tissue down to the level of the intermuscular septum containing the pedicle. The vessels of the flap were then anastomosed to the radial artery and cephalic vein, placing the proximal portion of the flap on the dorsal defect and the distal portion of the flap on the palmar defect. The intervening pedicle was accommodated between the heads of the ring and now translocated index finger. **H** and **I,** Complete viability of the flap 14 days postoperatively when the patient started on a passive and active exercise program.

initially difficult, the further proximal one proceeds, the more easily the flap is raised (see Fig. 48-5C and D).

When the radial nerve is first seen leaving the field anteriorly between the brachialis and brachioradialis muscles, those vessels passing forward with it should be ligated and the dissection pursued as far proximally as necessary to achieve a pedicle length of approximately 6 cm (see Fig. 48-5D). The two posterior cutaneous nerves will be encountered here: the deeper posterior cutaneous nerve of the forearm can be dissected out of the septum to avoid anesthesia in the forearm; the more superficial posterior cutaneous nerve of the arm can be divided high and later used to innervate the flap. The more proximal the dissection proceeds, the more difficult it becomes, because one is now pursuing the profunda brachii in the spiral groove beneath the lateral head of the triceps. This requires strong retraction with heavy rakes. A further impediment is the overlying tourniquet, but to release it at this stage will only make the situation worse. If necessary, an additional 6 to 8 cm of pedicle length can be gained by splitting the lateral and long heads of the triceps to expose the entire length of the profunda brachii vessels in the spiral groove. A tunnel can then be developed beneath the lateral head of the triceps, and either the flap can be delivered proximally through this tunnel or the pedicle can be divided and the pedicle vessels delivered distally.[206] This extended pedicle also increases the mean diameter of the artery from 1.50 up to 2.45 mm.

The authors adopt the convention of placing metal clips on the veins and silk ligatures on the artery, thus avoiding any potential confusion later. It is customary to release the tourniquet after dissection of a free tissue transfer has been completed to reperfuse the flap before dividing the pedicle, but the lateral arm flap is an exception. It is completely reliable and the inevitable bleeding from adjacent muscles will obscure the important step of dividing the pedicle at its highest point.

The secondary defect can be closed directly if the flap is less than 6 to 8 cm wide, but otherwise a split-thickness skin graft is applied with confident expectation of full take, because the bed is well vascularized. The only complications associated with the harvest of a lateral arm flap are permanent hypesthesia in the distribution of the posterior cutaneous nerve of the forearm if it is divided and temporary radial nerve palsy. The authors have never encountered this serious problem in their practice, but it has been reported after an Esmarch bandage was used as a tourniquet or when careful monitoring of cuff pressure was not the rule.[99]

Scapular Flap

 Anatomy

This cutaneous flap consists of the vascular territory of the cutaneous branch of the circumflex scapular artery.[13,89,102,257] The circumflex scapular artery is the first branch of the subscapular artery, arising 2 cm from the origin of the subscapular artery from the axillary artery. The external diameter of the circumflex scapular artery is 1.72 mm.[193] The circumflex scapular artery passes posteriorly through the triangular space between the long head of triceps laterally, the teres major inferiorly, and the subscapularis mediosuperiorly. It then divides into a number of branches deep to teres minor. The cutaneous branch continues posteriorly between the teres minor above and the teres major below. It then turns sharply medially over the lateral border of the scapula and divides into two: one branch runs transversely, superficial to the deep fascia overlying the teres minor and the infraspinatus, and the other branch runs obliquely downward parallel to the lateral border of the scapula. Flaps based on the transverse branch of the circumflex scapular artery have by convention been described as scapular flaps, whereas those based on the descending branch are described as parascapular flaps (Fig. 48-7B).[218]

Injection studies have shown that the vascular territory includes all of the skin inferior to the scapular spine, extending medially toward the spine and laterally over the deltoid. The lateral border of the scapula can be harvested with either the scapular or parascapular flaps as a vascularized bone graft[287] and could potentially be considered as an option for simultaneous reconstruction of a combined dorsal hand defect and underlying metacarpal bony defect.[61] A combined scapular osteocutaneous flap and latissimus dorsi flap can also be harvested on their common vascular pedicle.[74,87]

Operative Technique

The patient is placed in the lateral position with padding beneath the opposite axilla. The arm that is uppermost

---

CRITICAL POINTS: LATERAL ARM FLAP

INDICATIONS

- Soft tissue defects of the hand (smaller areas)
- Defects of the first web space

PREOPERATIVE EVALUATION

- Doppler examination of the pedicle

PEARLS

- Sterile tourniquet is placed as high as possible.
- Center of flap is line from deltoid tubercle to lateral epicondyle.
- Avoid damage to radial nerve with pedicle dissection.

TECHNICAL POINTS

- Begin dissection posteriorly on skin.
- Elevate skin and fascia toward bone.
- Elevate anterior skin and fascia.
- Dissect pedicle off of humerus distal to proximal.
- Artery can be quite small; vein is fragile.
- Beware of radial nerve running with pedicle proximally.
- It may be necessary to remove tourniquet to get added length on pedicle as it comes around humerus.

PITFALLS

- Elevating skin and fascia without vessels
- Injury to radial nerve

DONOR SITE MANAGEMENT

- Small defects (<7 cm) can be closed primarily.
- Others will need skin graft.

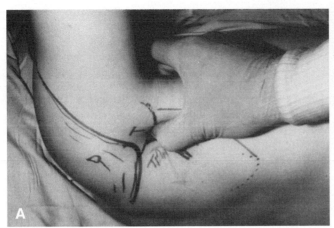
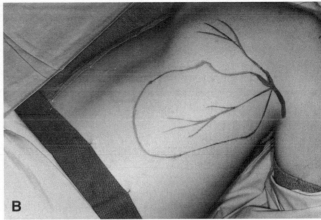

FIGURE 48-7. Scapular flap. **A,** Using the finger and thumb to grip the posterior axillary fold, the triangular space is readily detected lying between the triceps (T), the teres minor (TMn), and the teres major. **B,** With a pencil Doppler probe the transverse and descending branches of the circumflex scapular artery can be traced. In this patient, a parascapular flap is to be harvested based on the descending branch of the circumflex scapular artery.

should be prepared and draped with stockinette, so that the arm can be abducted as required. With the arm abducted, the triangular space through which the pedicle passes can be convincingly palpated by gripping the posterior axillary fold between the finger and thumb (see Fig. 48-7A). The defect into which the thumb intrudes is formed by the teres major, the deltoid, and the combined scapula and teres minor.

A sterile Doppler probe is used to trace the cutaneous vessels across the back, and the axis of the transverse and descending branches should be drawn. The flap template should now be placed over either axis, taking into account the orientation of the pedicle to the primary defect and the laxity of the skin with regard to primary closure. A trans-

verse scapular flap may extend medially as far as the spine and can be extended farther across the midline or laterally over the deltoid if required.[306] Scapular and parascapular flaps should not be designed more than 10 cm wide, because it will be impossible to directly close the secondary defect, and this is not a good site for a skin graft.

The margins of the flap are incised down to the thick fascia overlying the infraspinatus. The plane superficial to this deep fascia is well defined and relatively avascular. The flap can be swiftly raised proceeding from medial to lateral for a scapular flap or from inferior to superior for a para-scapular flap. As the triangular space is approached, the cutaneous branch of the circumflex scapular artery can be

CRITICAL POINTS: SCAPULAR FLAP

INDICATIONS

- Moderate sized soft tissue defects of upper extremity
- Defects with bone loss (with vascularized lateral border of scapula)

PREOPERATIVE EVALUATION

- Doppler the pedicle as it comes out of the triangular space.
- Mark lateral border of scapula, teres major, and teres minor.

PEARLS

- A very large "parascapular" flap can be taken to cover very large defects.
- This flap is useful for bone loss in the mid hand (multiple metacarpals).

TECHNICAL POINTS

- Flaps should be designed over Doppler-defined vessel.

- Avoid flaps wider than 10 cm because this is difficult area for a split-thickness skin graft to take.
- Raise skin with fascia from medial to lateral (scapular flap) or inferior to superior (parascapular flap).
- Watch for multiple branches in triangular space from pedicle to muscles and lateral scapula.
- Pedicle can be lengthened by taking portion of subscapular vessels.

PITFALLS

- Dissection should proceed with caution when approaching triangular space.

DONOR SITE MANAGEMENT

- Limit flap to 10 cm width and close primarily over drains.
- Skin grafting this donor site is unwise.

displayed by transilluminating the flap. The triangular space should be approached by splitting the aponeurotic teres minor away from the muscular teres major. As dissection proceeds into the space the surgeon should be very careful, because there are several large, short, and comparatively fragile branches that supply the muscles and lateral border of the scapula. The assistant should apply traction to the borders of the space, so that the surgeon can visualize and ligate these branches.

To obtain the longest possible pedicle, the incision should be extended into the axilla. The thoracodorsal artery should be located on the undersurface of the latissimus dorsi muscle and traced proximally so that the "T"-bifurcation of the subscapular artery into the thoracodorsal and circumflex scapular arteries can be completely defined. Either the circumflex scapular artery can be divided just distal to the thoracodorsal artery, or the subscapular artery can be divided just below its origin from the axillary artery, thereby incorpo-

rating the "T"-junction that will facilitate two end-to-end anastomoses rather than an end-to-side anastomosis using the circumflex scapular artery. A pedicle some 15 cm in length from axillary artery to flap can be achieved (Fig. 48-8).

After completion of the dissection, the secondary defect can be closed primarily. This should be done with strong sutures, because dehiscence can occur with abduction of the shoulder. A "fascial" version of the scapular flap has been described with the advantage that its width can be greater than 10 cm and that the donor scar is less likely to widen and become hypertrophic.[128,152,336] Strictly speaking, this scapular fascial flap should probably be termed a *subcutaneous* flap or *adipofascial* flap. If the surgeon has decided that a fascial flap is the optimal flap, the scapular fascial flap may be a better selection in men to avoid the potential alopecia seen after harvesting a temporoparietal fascial flap, but it requires a change from the lateral position to supine during surgery.

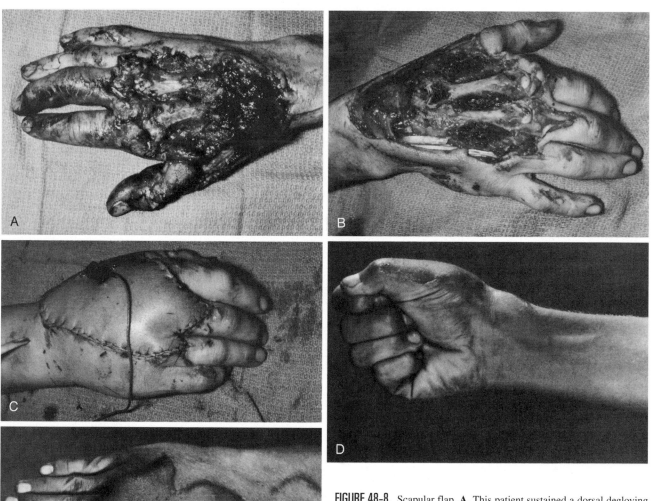

FIGURE 48-8. Scapular flap. **A,** This patient sustained a dorsal degloving injury with loss of the skin and extensor tendons together with associated fractures when he was thrown from a motorcycle. **B,** After radical débridement, which exposed the carpus and metacarpals, Silastic rods were inserted primarily and the entire defect (**C**) covered with a free scapular flap. **D** and **E,** The flap healed without complication, and after replacement of the Silastic rods with extensor tendon grafts, the patient regained satisfactory finger flexion and extension.

Latissimus Dorsi Musculocutaneous and Muscle Flaps

The latissimus dorsi was first described as an axial pattern regional flap for breast reconstruction by Tansini in 1906.[187] It was used only sporadically until Olivari[227] reintroduced it for coverage of radiation defects of the anterior chest wall in 1976. The muscle is supplied primarily by the thoracodorsal artery from which perforators pass through the muscle to supply the overlying skin as a musculocutaneous flap (Fig. 48-11C). The diameter of the thoracodorsal artery (1 to 2.5 mm) and the length of the pedicle (11 to 16 cm) have made it the most robust and therefore popular flap for free tissue transfer, especially to the extremities (Figs. 48-10 and 48-11).[33,186,189,219,293,321]

Harvested as a free muscle flap (see Fig. 48-13),[10,96] the latissimus has the advantages of draping easily into the interstices of a complex convoluted wound and of easy closure of the donor defect. Minor disadvantages include the appearance of the split-thickness skin graft on the muscle and the decreased perfusion in the most distal part of the muscle. The musculocutaneous flap has the advantages of appearance and excellent flow (see Fig. 48-10). If the defect contains deep isolated pockets within the wound, these can be filled with a combined serratus anterior and latissimus dorsi muscle flap (Fig. 48-12).[87,106,230]

Anatomy

The latissimus dorsi muscle arises from the lower six thoracic vertebrae, from the thoracolumbar fascia, and from the posterior iliac crest. From this extensive origin the muscle fibers converge to wrap around the lower border of the teres major and end in a quadrilateral tendon that inserts into the intertubercular sulcus of the humerus. Together with the teres major it forms the posterior axillary fold.

The blood supply of the muscle is supplied primarily by the thoracodorsal artery, which is the continuation of the subscapular artery after it gives off its circumflex scapular branch some 2 cm distal to its origin from the axillary artery. The thoracodorsal artery provides a variable number of branches to the chest wall, notably one to the serratus anterior muscle, before reaching the hilum of the latissimus dorsi muscle some 11 cm from the axillary artery (see Fig. 47-65).[12] Immediately distal to the hilum the artery divides into two branches in 94% of specimens.[310] The upper branch runs parallel to, and 3.5 cm from, the upper margin of the muscle; the lateral branch runs parallel to, and 2.1 cm from, the lateral margin of the muscle. This arrangement allows the surgeon to split the muscle longitudinally as a hemi-latissimus muscle flap when a narrow flap is required[72,309] with the additional advantage of preserving the thoracodorsal nerve innervation to the remaining muscle (Fig. 48-13).

Preoperatively, it may be of some benefit to have the patient abduct the arm against resistance and tattoo four or five points along the posterior axillary fold with methylene blue and a hypodermic needle.

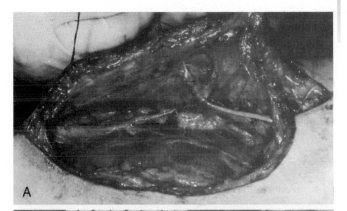

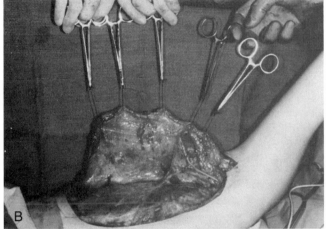

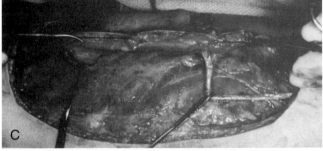

FIGURE 48-9. Latissimus dorsi flap dissection. **A,** After the initial incision has been made, sutures are passed through the skin and anterior margin of the latissimus dorsi muscle. These sutures are used to retract the muscle and display the neurovascular pedicle. The thoracodorsal nerve and beneath it the thoracodorsal vessels are seen running from the axilla toward the left of the figure where they turn toward the upper margin of the latissimus dorsi muscle and its hilum. **B,** By dividing the distal margin of the muscle, the vascular anatomy can be better displayed. The thoracodorsal artery is seen to give off the serratus anterior branch, which passes from the pedicle down to the chest wall in the lower portion of the figure, where the serratus anterior muscle can be seen. **C,** By distal traction on the pedicle using a vessel loop, the retrograde flowing branches of the thoracodorsal vessel can be clearly seen. These vessels that flow in a cranial direction can be safely ligated. The proximal margin of the tailored latissimus flap has only been incised through the skin. Once the vessels previously mentioned have been divided, this incision will be carried directly through muscle.

Operative Technique

The patient should be placed in the lateral position with padding beneath the torso sufficient to protect circulation to the contralateral arm on the operating table. Easy exposure to the axilla is provided by wrapping the forearm with soft padding and then applying upward traction to a ceiling

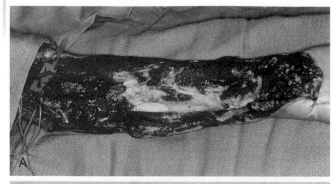

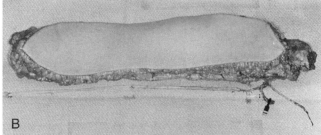

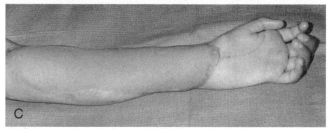

FIGURE 48-10. Latissimus dorsi musculocutaneous flap. **A,** This 9-year-old girl sustained a degloving injury of the entire volar forearm including the median and ulnar nerves, the radial and ulnar arteries, and most of the flexor musculature. **B,** A very large contralateral right latissimus dorsi musculocutaneous flap was harvested with dissection of the vascular pedicle all the way to the origin of the subscapular artery from the axillary artery. A long interpositional vein graft was anastomosed end-to-end to the circumflex scapular artery. The subscapular artery was anastomosed end-to-end to the stump of the radial artery at the elbow and the interpositional vein graft was anastomosed end-to-end to the distal ulnar artery to augment the vascular supply to the hand as well as providing soft tissue coverage of the forearm. The thoracodorsal nerve was coapted to the stump of the anterior interosseous nerve, and the distal latissimus muscle fascia was sutured to the flexor digitorum profundus tendons at the wrist to act as a functioning free muscle transfer. **C,** The latissimus dorsi musculocutaneous flap provides a very satisfactory appearance to the reconstructed forearm 1 year postoperatively.

fixture to achieve 100 degrees of abduction. A similar position can be achieved, although less satisfactorily, by taping the forearm to a sterile Mayo stand. In either case there is considerable danger of a brachial plexus neurapraxia with consequent paresis.[178] Checking the radial pulse regularly is no guarantee that all is well. This complication can only be avoided by a strict practice of returning the arm to the patient's side for 5 minutes every hour, a practice that should be monitored by the anesthesiologist.

An inverted "L"-shaped incision should be made skirting the axillary hair-bearing area and extending down toward the previously tattooed points marking the posterior axillary fold. Through this incision, the anterior border of the latis-

simus is located and everted using retractors or heavy stay sutures placed in the muscle margin (see Fig. 48-9).

The thoracodorsal pedicle can best be found where it approaches the muscular hilum. This is approximately at the nipple line in the male or the child. With good retraction and light, the vessel can be traced proximally, identifying first the serratus branch, a branch to teres major, and then the circumflex scapular artery. These should be ligated and divided.

With a template of the primary defect, the cutaneous component of the flap can now be marked out over the posterolateral thorax, distal to the level of the hilum, which has already been identified. The flap template can be designed either anterior or posterior with respect to the anterior border of the muscle. Placing the skin pattern more posteriorly gives more muscle to fold into a deep defect, whereas moving the skin pattern anteriorly, relative to the muscle, produces a thinner flap.[93] The flap margins are incised and extended down to the underlying muscle with cutting diathermy. Depending on the requirements for extra muscle anterior or posterior to the skin flap, either the anterior or posterior margins of the incision will need to be elevated off the latissimus dorsi muscle. After the anterior border of the muscle is elevated off the underlying serratus anterior muscle, the entire muscle and skin flap is dissected in an anterior to posterior direction (see Fig. 47-65). Care should be taken to ligate any large secondary perforators entering the muscle posteriorly. The requisite amount of muscle is cut with the diathermy and the flap swung superiorly away from the trunk to allow clear definition of the proximal thoracodorsal artery. Careful isolation of the thoracodorsal artery and its two venae comitantes up to their origin from the subscapular artery and vein completes the axillary dissection (see Fig. 48-9B and C).

If an end-to-side anastomosis is to be performed or if the flap is being transferred into an atherosclerotic vessel or into a single vessel limb, it may be advantageous to take the subscapular artery and as much as needed of the circumflex scapular artery as a "T" segment (see Fig. 48-11B and C). By interposing the subscapular-circumflex scapular portion of the "T" segment into the atherosclerotic vessel, a difficult end-to-side anastomosis is avoided. By saving the "T" segment of the subscapular/thoracodorsal/circumflex scapular arteries and performing the end-to-side anastomosis using the thoracodorsal artery, the "T" segment can be used later to salvage the end-to-side anastomosis should it be required.[177]

Dorsi Musculocutaneous Flap

If only a narrow flap is needed, the lateral branch of the thoracodorsal artery should be located and the posterior border of the flap incised as was the inferior border, while carefully avoiding that lateral branch. The superior (situated also medial and posterior) branch should be ligated and divided. The thoracodorsal artery should now be dissected off the latissimus dorsi, working from the axilla as far distally as possible. The pedicle can be made longer by dividing muscular branches that turn in a cranial direction toward the axilla in the muscle (see Fig. 48-9C).

The proximal margin of the flap can now be incised in similar manner to the inferior (or distal) and posterior, while

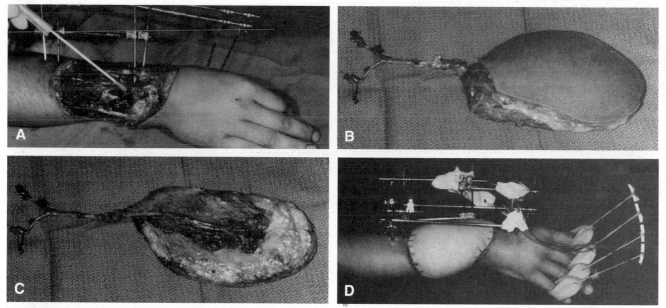

FIGURE 48-11. Tailored latissimus dorsi flap. **A,** After radical débridement and external fixation of a high-velocity gunshot wound, specimens are taken for Gram stain and quantitative culture. **B,** The long pedicle and limited bulk of the tailored latissimus dorsi musculocutaneous flap is displayed. **C,** The small portion of latissimus muscle required to vascularize this musculocutaneous flap is demonstrated. The "T"-segment obtained by harvesting both the subscapular and the circumflex scapular arteries in continuity with the thoracodorsal artery can be seen to the left side of the figures. **D,** The tailored latissimus dorsi musculocutaneous flap has been anastomosed to the ulnar artery in the mid forearm. An extension outrigger has been fitted to allow immediate motion. (B and C From Lister GD, Arnez AO: The Anterior T and Y grafts. Plast Reconstr Surg 88:319-322, 1991, with permission.)

CRITICAL POINTS: LATISSIMUS DORSI MUSCLE FLAP

INDICATIONS

- Large and small defects of the hand and arm
- Complex defects requiring more tissue
- Untidy wounds after débridement or management of osteomyelitis

PREOPERATIVE EVALUATION

- Presence of scars or a prior mastectomy with axillary dissection may contraindicate use (pedicle may have been damaged or ligated).

PEARLS

- "Best" free flap in most hands
- May take a portion of the muscle or "tailor" flap to defect
- Seroma common in donor site

TECHNICAL POINTS

- Approach muscle from anterior border first.
- Elevate muscle and identify pedicle with branch to serratus.

- Once pedicle is identified, elevate muscle off of chest wall.
- Once an adequate portion of muscle is elevated, divide distally and medially and continue dissection.
- Carefully dissect pedicle in axilla.
- Abduction of arm helps with pedicle dissection.
- Pedicle may include the subscapular branch from axillary artery.

PITFALLS

- Damage to pedicle may occur during dissection.
- Do not divide any branch until proximal main pedicle is identified.
- Seroma may occur at donor site.

DONOR SITE MANAGEMENT

- Primary closure is performed over drains.
- Leave drains in until patient is moving around.
- Morbidity from loss of muscle is minimal.

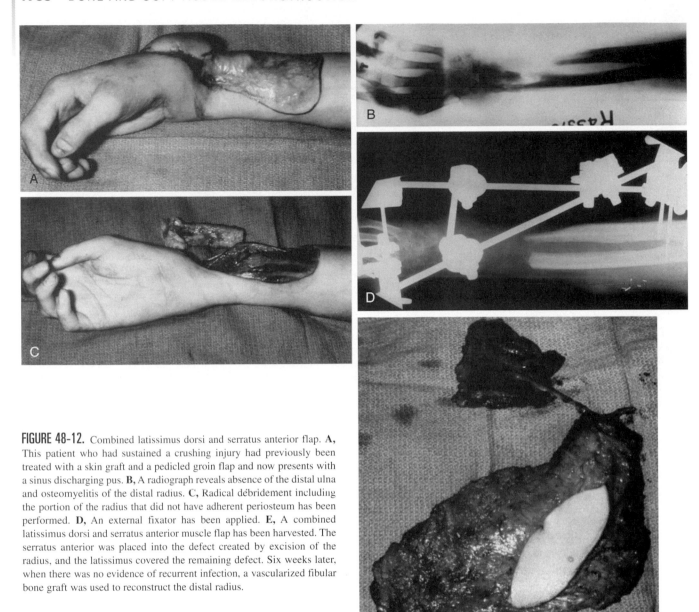

FIGURE 48-12. Combined latissimus dorsi and serratus anterior flap. **A,** This patient who had sustained a crushing injury had previously been treated with a skin graft and a pedicled groin flap and now presents with a sinus discharging pus. **B,** A radiograph reveals absence of the distal ulna and osteomyelitis of the distal radius. **C,** Radical débridement including the portion of the radius that did not have adherent periosteum has been performed. **D,** An external fixator has been applied. **E,** A combined latissimus dorsi and serratus anterior muscle flap has been harvested. The serratus anterior was placed into the defect created by excision of the radius, and the latissimus covered the remaining defect. Six weeks later, when there was no evidence of recurrent infection, a vascularized fibular bone graft was used to reconstruct the distal radius.

retracting the pedicle anteriorly and so protecting it from harm. Raising the flap in this manner, rather than taking the whole muscle as in the past, provides a flap tailored exactly to the primary defect (see Fig. 48-11).[93] Use of the tailored flap avoids the bulky proximal portion of the latissimus muscle that was inevitable when the whole muscle was taken. Recently Angrigiani and coworkers[6] have described harvesting the latissimus dorsi skin flap without the underlying muscle based on a single muscle perforator.[149-151]

The donor defect should always be closed directly, because a skin graft in this location presents a very difficult nursing problem. Large defects may require transposition of loose tissue from the waistline anteriorly, using a rhomboid design (see Chapter 47). Suction drains should be left for several days because this donor site is associated with a higher incidence of seroma formation. No significant loss of function has been shown after use of the latissimus dorsi.[167]

Serratus Anterior Muscle Flap

The serratus anterior free muscle flap has been popularized by Buncke as the flap of choice for small to moderate-sized soft tissue defects in the upper extremity.[24,179,292,327] It is a remarkably reliable free muscle flap because of its consistent long vascular pedicle and large-diameter vessels and is associated with minimal donor site morbidity.[97]

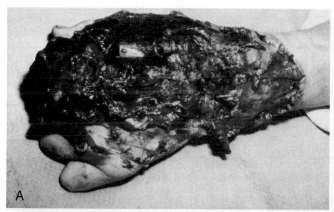

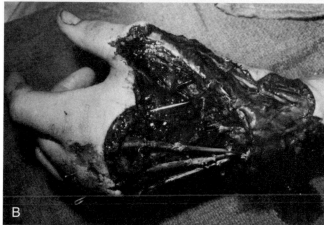

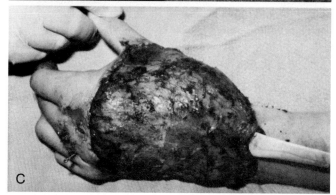

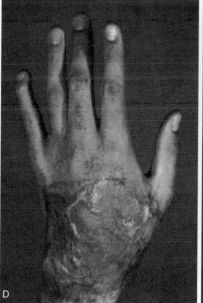

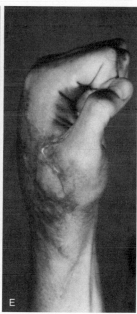

FIGURE 48-13. Latissimus dorsi muscle flap. **A,** This patient sustained open fractures of the metacarpals together with loss of extensor tendons and dorsal skin and damage to the princeps pollicis artery in a rollover injury. **B,** Immediate reconstruction was performed using an intercalated bone graft, plate fixation, and maintenance of the first web space using a "W" wire. The extensor tendons were grafted. **C,** The entire reconstruction was covered with a hemi–latissimus dorsi free muscle flap. **D and E,** The muscle was covered with a skin graft. One year later the patient had a satisfactory range of motion without further reconstruction.

Anatomy

The serratus anterior muscle arises from the first nine ribs medial to the anterior axillary line and inserts into the medial border of the scapula. The lower three slips of the muscle arising from the seventh, eighth, and ninth ribs are supplied by a large branch of the thoracodorsal artery, whereas the upper six slips are supplied by branches of the lateral thoracic artery (Fig. 48-14A). This dual vascular supply allows elevation of the lower three slips of the muscle while still preserving the vascular supply to the upper two thirds of the muscle. If necessary, a very long vascular pedicle, up to 15 cm in length, can be obtained by dividing

the thoracodorsal artery and vein distal to the origin of the branch to the serratus muscle and elevating the thoracodorsal pedicle all the way up to its origin from the subscapular artery and vein just as in the dissection of the latissimus dorsi vascular pedicle (see Fig. 48-14B). The serratus muscle is innervated by the long thoracic nerve that lies directly anterior to the vascular pedicle on the chest wall. Under magnification, the branches of the long thoracic nerve to the lower three slips of muscle can be dissected. This ability to separate the motor innervation and blood supply to the lower three slips of the serratus muscle while still preserving the motor nerve and blood supply to the upper six slips minimizes the morbidity of harvesting the entire serratus muscle. In a series of 100 consecutive

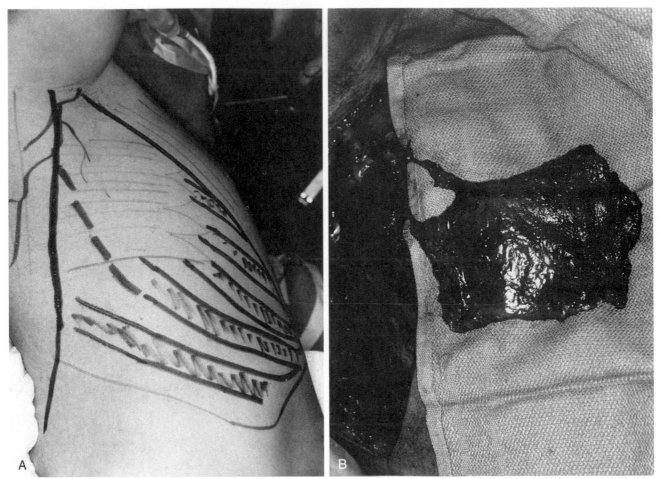

FIGURE 48-14. Serratus anterior muscle flap. **A,** Preoperative marking of the midaxillary incision used to harvest a right serratus anterior muscle flap. The serratus branch from the thoracodorsal artery passes anteriorly down to supply the lower three slips of the muscle. **B,** This small muscle flap can be isolated on a very long vascular pedicle by dividing the thoracodorsal artery and vein distal to the origin of the serratus branch and mobilizing the thoracodorsal artery and vein all the way proximally to their origin from the subscapular artery and vein.

serratus anterior free muscle flap transfers, winging of the scapula did not occur and all patients retained full range of motion of the shoulder.[327] Occasionally, this separate motor nerve to the lower three slips can be reinnervated as a functional free muscle transfer for functional restoration of thenar muscle loss.

Operative Technique

The patient is placed in the lateral position with the arm included in the operative field. Through a long midaxillary incision, the anterior border of the latissimus dorsi muscle can be elevated and retracted to reveal the thoracodorsal vessel pedicle and its branch to the serratus muscle (see Fig. 47-65B). The small vessel branches to the upper six muscle slips can be divided, but all vessel branches to the lower three slips are preserved. With the use of loupe magnification, the nerve branches to the lower three slips are carefully divided from the main branch of the long thoracic nerve. Starting inferiorly and working in a superior direction, the lower three slips of the serratus muscle are divided at their origin from the seventh, eighth, and ninth ribs and elevated in the loose areolar plane between the muscle and

the chest wall, taking care not to penetrate the intercostal muscles and pleura. Posteriorly, the insertion of the three slips into the scapula is divided. This allows the vascular pedicle to be lifted off the upper six slips of the muscle, and the pedicle can then be easily mobilized up to its origin from the thoracodorsal artery and vein. If a long vascular pedicle is not required, the muscle is allowed to perfuse and then the pedicle is divided just distal to its origin from the thoracodorsal vessels. If a longer vascular pedicle is required, the thoracodorsal vessels are divided distal to the origin of the serratus vessels and the entire thoracodorsal-subscapular system dissected up to their origin from the axillary artery and vein (see Fig. 48-14B). If the serratus muscle is also to be used as a functioning free muscle transfer, interfascicular dissection will allow the branches to the lower three slips to be split off from the main long thoracic nerve for several centimeters as a separate group fascicle.

Hemostasis is achieved over the lower chest wall. The distal stump of the lower three slips of the serratus muscle attached to the angle of the scapula can be resutured to the remaining upper six slips of the serratus muscle and the incision then closed directly over a suction drain.

Rectus Abdominis Muscle Flap

The rectus abdominis muscle flap is a distant second choice for coverage of large soft tissue defects of the upper extremity compared with the optimal choice of the latissimus dorsi muscle flap.[81,118,200,234,238,242] The rectus abdominis muscle is long and thin and can therefore be considered for coverage of longitudinal defects of the dorsal or palmar surfaces of the forearm and wrist and may be spiraled in "barber pole" fashion around the radial or ulnar borders of the forearm. This muscle has two vascular pedicles: the superior epigastric artery and the deep inferior epigastric artery arising from the external iliac artery. As a free flap for upper extremity reconstruction, it is isolated on the inferior pedicle, the deep inferior epigastric artery, and two accompanying venae comitantes. The vascular anatomy is very reliable with a pedicle length of 5 to 7 cm and an arterial diameter of approximately 2.5 mm. The muscle can be harvested through a paramedian or transverse Pfannenstiel abdominal incision. A longitudinal or transverse ellipse of overlying skin perfused by musculocutaneous perforators can be incorporated in a rectus abdominis musculocutaneous flap, and this has become the optimal choice for microsurgical breast reconstruction. However, for upper extremity reconstruction, the rectus abdominis is usually harvested as a muscle flap and resurfaced with a split-thickness skin graft. One advantage of the rectus abdominis muscle flap is that it can be harvested with the patient in a supine position, compared with the lateral position used for harvesting a contralateral latissimus dorsi muscle flap. Relative disadvantages include the shorter length of vascular pedicle and the possibility of abdominal bulging or even a hernia of the lower abdomen after harvest of the rectus muscle.

An intriguing potential spinoff is the use of a flap of posterior rectus sheath and peritoneum supplied by the deep inferior epigastric vessels[253] to provide a gliding peritoneal surface for coverage of exposed extensor tendons in dorsal hand degloving injuries.

Massive defects of the upper extremity have been reconstructed using a combination latissimus dorsi and rectus abdominis musculocutaneous flap based on the intact vascular pedicle of the thoracodorsal vessels and microsurgical anastomoses of the deep inferior epigastric vessels to the radial or ulnar arteries at the wrist.[229]

Groin Flap

 Anatomy

The groin flap (Fig. 48-15A) is an axial pattern cutaneous flap. Its axial vessel is the superficial circumflex iliac artery,[274] which is a relatively constant vessel, present in 96% of a series of angiograms.[140] The vessel arises from the femoral artery in the femoral triangle, which forms a vascular "hub"[296] for the axes of several flaps that converge here (see Fig. 47-67).

The superficial circumflex iliac artery emerges from the femoral triangle by passing over the medial border of the sartorius immediately after giving off a deep muscular branch. Initially below the deep fascia, the vessel emerges through the fascia as it crosses the sartorius. It passes laterally, parallel to, and 2 cm below the inguinal ligament (see Fig. 48-15A).[47,225] At a point below the anterior superior iliac spine, the vessel divides and supplies the skin immediately below the iliac crest. The vascular territory of the superficial circumflex iliac artery ends at some point lateral to the anterior superior iliac spine. Practical experience has demonstrated that the flap can be safely extended beyond the anterior superior iliac spine by a distance at least equal to the width of the flap.[2]

The venous drainage,[235,275] which is as important as the arterial supply, and the lymphatic outflow[51] of the flap have both been studied in detail. Penteado[235] has described the variations in venous anatomy in the femoral triangle that are important to the microsurgeon. Usually the groin flap is not reinnervated, but Joshi[135] has pointed out that the lateral cutaneous branch of the subcostal or 12th thoracic nerve consistently crosses the iliac crest 5 cm posterior to the anterior superior iliac spine. This nerve could potentially be dissected, divided, and sutured to any available cutaneous nerve in the hand.

The groin flap can be designed up to 12 cm wide and still allow primary closure of the donor defect (Fig. 48-16D). If a relatively large block of bone is required in the hand in association with a soft tissue defect, a segment of vascularized bone can be taken from the iliac crest immediately beneath the flap (see Fig. 48-15B).[28,95,245,290]

A planning template of the defect should be laid on the skin immediately below the anterior superior iliac spine. This allows a relatively long vascular pedicle by incorporating the more medial inguinal dissection (see Fig. 48-15C).

Operative Technique

See also discussion in Chapter 47.

The midline axis of the flap should be drawn 2 cm inferior and parallel to the inguinal ligament. The lower margin of the flap is incised down to the superficial surface of the deep fascia. The deep fascia should be incised and retracted proximally to reveal the sartorius, the tensor fascia lata lateral to it, and the intervening intermuscular septum. While maintaining traction on the flap superiorly and away from the thigh, the deep fascia should be divided in a superior direction in the line of the fibers of the sartorius and at its lateral border just medial to the intermuscular septum.

The superficial circumflex iliac artery will be seen in the deep fascia as it is lifted from the sartorius. Incision of the fascia proceeds beyond the artery as far as the origin of the sartorius from the anterior superior iliac spine. Once it has been confirmed that the vessel is present, the remainder of the incision outlining the upper margin of the flap is made. As the upper incision is carried down to the external oblique aponeurosis, a significant artery passing superiorly will be encountered in the majority of cases. This should not cause alarm, because this is the superficial inferior epigastric artery, which must be divided. Furthermore, division of the superficial inferior epigastric artery indicates that the level of dissection is now in the correct plane.

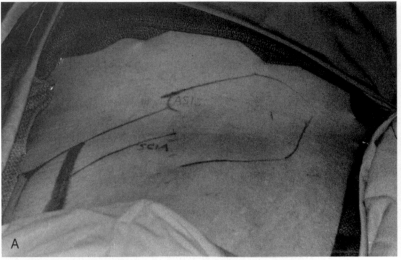

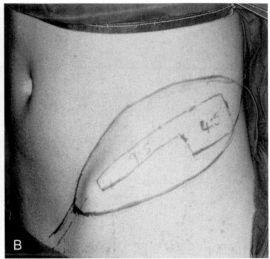

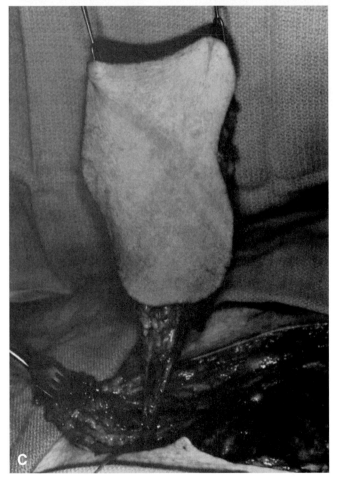

FIGURE 48-15. Groin flap. **A,** The superficial circumflex iliac artery pedicle of a free groin flap lies 2 cm below and parallel to the inguinal ligament passing from the pubic tubercle to the anterior superior iliac spine. **B,** Vascularized bone from the iliac crest can be incorporated into a free groin flap but is better based on the deep circumflex iliac artery rather than the superficial circumflex iliac artery. **C,** The long pedicle that can be achieved in harvesting a free groin flap is demonstrated.

The flap is retracted inferiorly off the external oblique aponeurosis until the level of the anterior superior iliac spine is reached. The incision made previously in the sartorius fascia is located and turned medially to free the deep fascia of the thigh from the inguinal ligament. In the course of this incision, the lateral cutaneous nerve of the thigh will be encountered. Care must be taken not to injure this nerve; otherwise, meralgia paresthetica may result.[213] Whereas the nerve usually passes deep to the flap vessels and can be freed by dissection, on occasion it or one of its usual two branches may be superficial to the vessels. In this situation, the vascular pedicle should be dissected medially, divided, and passed beneath the nerve.

By applying upward traction to the flap, the fascia can be dissected off the underlying fibers of the sartorius muscle as far as its medial border, paying careful attention to the vessel, which can usually be seen passing down through the superficial fascia to lie on the muscle itself. The main hazard

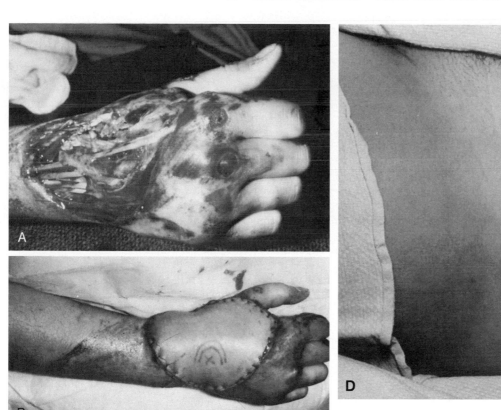

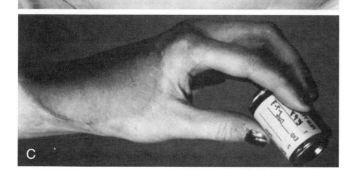

FIGURE 48-16. Groin flap. **A,** This patient degloved the dorsum of her hand against the road surface with exposure of the carpus and loss of the extensor pollicis longus and wrist extensors. Primary transfer of extensor indicis proprius to extensor pollicis longus was performed. The wrist extensors were restored, and the carpus was closed. **B,** The entire reconstruction was covered with a free groin flap. **C,** Full function was achieved and no further reconstruction was required. **D,** The acceptable scar that can be achieved after direct closure of the donor site of a free groin flap.

to further dissection of the pedicle is the muscular branch of the superficial circumflex iliac artery. This should be isolated by retracting the sartorius laterally with instruments on either side of the pedicle, superiorly and inferiorly. Once the muscular branch has been dissected free under loupe magnification, it can be divided. The superficial circumflex iliac artery can then be mobilized all the way to its origin from the femoral artery. If the vessel is of small caliber, a cuff of the femoral artery can be taken. This is especially advantageous if an end-to-side anastomosis is to be performed. The venous drainage of the flap will be encountered as the medial border of the flap is incised. All veins emerging from the flap should be preserved and traced medially. They will usually join before draining into the termination of the long saphenous vein, providing at most two veins, of suitable caliber, for anastomosis.

The flap can now be thinned by having an assistant hold the flap vertically with hooks or stay sutures and the surgeon using forceps and curved tenotomy scissors with their concave surface uppermost. The flap can be thinned quite radically at the margins by trimming away fat. In the middle of the flap, the surgeon must be more cautious; otherwise the pedicle may be damaged. Lobules of fat between the flap margins and midline can be lifted with the pickups and trimmed away. The deep fascia that has been lifted must not be transgressed—any fat that lies between it and the skin must be left alone.

Closure should commence at the lateral end of the donor defect. It may be difficult, but the surgeon should not undermine the margins in an attempt to facilitate closure. This only increases the area of potential dead space and does little to relax the skin. Rather, the surgeon should flex the thigh and use heavy sutures, knowing that primary closure is always possible if the width of the flap was less than 12 cm when first outlined. The tension created will inevitably result in postoperative inflammation along the suture line. Even if this inflammation becomes pronounced, do not remove sutures! To do so would open the entire cavity and if this becomes infected, as is almost inevitable, one has created a disaster similar to a pressure sore.

Radial Forearm Flap

The radial forearm flap[21,73,80,214,278,334] certainly offers unrivaled quality of thin, mobile skin, similar in its characteristics to the skin over the dorsum of the hand. Most dorsal and palmar defects of the hand can be covered by a pedicled reverse radial forearm flap (see Chapter 47), but occasionally the size and the shape of the defect may necessitate using a free radial forearm flap either from the contralateral forearm (Fig. 48-17) or even from the ipsilateral forearm. In any of these variations, the radial forearm flap depends on the presence of good flow through the ulnar artery and the palmar arches into the digital vessels. The radial artery may occasionally be the only patent vessel to the hand when there has been a penetrating or crushing injury to the forearm or palmar surface of the hand. Even when it is not, the radial artery has been shown to be the dominant vessel in 12% of hands. Harvesting a radial forearm flap may potentially result in acute ischemia of the hand[129] or postoperative symptoms of cold intolerance.[21] However, digital temperature and Doppler flow studies have shown that loss of the radial artery does not cause any significant compromise to the circulation of the hand.[155] Therefore, most surgeons no longer reconstruct the radial artery with a reversed interposition vein graft. The appearance of the donor defect, which has to be skin grafted, remains the major drawback of this flap for some surgeons.

Anatomy

The radial artery pursues a relatively superficial course down the forearm, from its origin at the bifurcation of the brachial artery to just distal to the radial styloid where it passes deep to the abductor pollicis longus and extensor pollicis brevis tendons through the anatomical snuff-box (see Fig. 47-59). In the proximal forearm it lies on the superficial surface of the pronator teres, just beneath the medial margin of the muscle belly of the brachioradialis. More distally, it comes to lie in turn on the radial head of the flexor digitorum superficialis and the flexor pollicis longus, where it is palpable through the skin. The artery is accompanied by two venae comitantes.

Throughout its course the artery gives off branches to a plexus of vessels in the overlying deep fascia, which supplies the skin of the anterior and radiodorsal surfaces of the forearm (see Fig. 47-60B). Similarly, deep fascial branches also supply the periosteum of the distal half of the radius between the insertions of pronator teres and brachioradialis. This allows a segment of vascularized bone to be harvested from the radius up to 10 cm in length and up to 30% of the cross-sectional area of the radius as an osteocutaneous flap.[16,79]

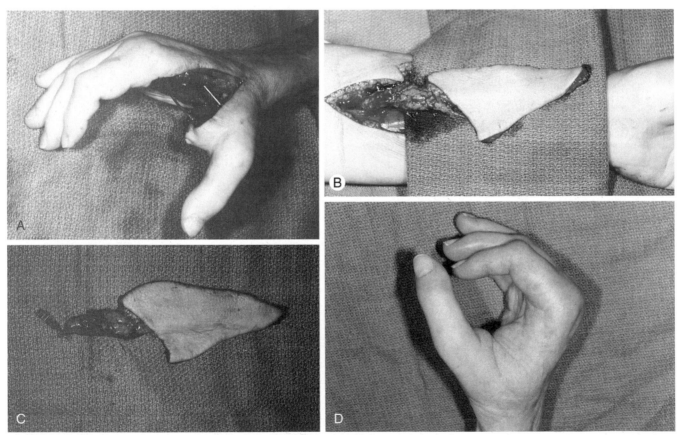

FIGURE 48-17. Radial forearm flap. **A,** This woman sustained a severe crushing injury of her right dominant forearm and required fasciotomies and vein graft revascularization, but unfortunately she developed a severe adduction contracture of the thumb/index finger web space. A reverse radial forearm flap was not an option for coverage of the radical web space release, because the forearm had been skin grafted. **B** and **C,** A contralateral radial forearm flap was therefore used. **D,** This provided thin pliable skin for the widened thumb/index finger web space.

The minimal precaution that should be taken before raising a forearm flap is an Allen test to ensure that flow will be adequate through the remaining ulnar artery. Noninvasive vascular studies to determine arterial dominance are probably unnecessary.

Operative Technique

The course of the radial artery should be mapped out with a Doppler probe and marked on the skin, as should the course of the largest superficial vein in the forearm proximal to the flap (see Fig. 48-18C).

The pattern of the defect is placed on the forearm with the marked course of the radial artery close to the radial border of the template. The radial artery should not be used as the mid axis of the flap; otherwise, if the flap extends around the radial border of the forearm, the skin grafted defect becomes much more noticeable. The flap is usually designed over the middle or distal thirds of the forearm. However, if the radial artery is to be used in a "flow-through" situation to reconstruct an associated arterial defect in the wound (see Fig. 48-18),[20,232] the length of radial artery required proximal and distal to the flap to restore arterial inflow to the distal limb will predetermine the proximal-distal location of the flap on the forearm.

If pedicle length is not a consideration, the flap can be raised with its distal margin 3 to 5 cm proximal to the wrist crease. This avoids skin grafting over the more distal flexor tendons, especially the flexor carpi radialis, and the chances of the skin graft not taking over this critical area are reduced.

The margins of the flap are incised as well as a short longitudinal incision extending distally from the flap margin over the course of the radial artery. The skin margins adjacent to the flap are elevated from the underlying deep fascia. In elevating the radial edge, the cephalic vein should

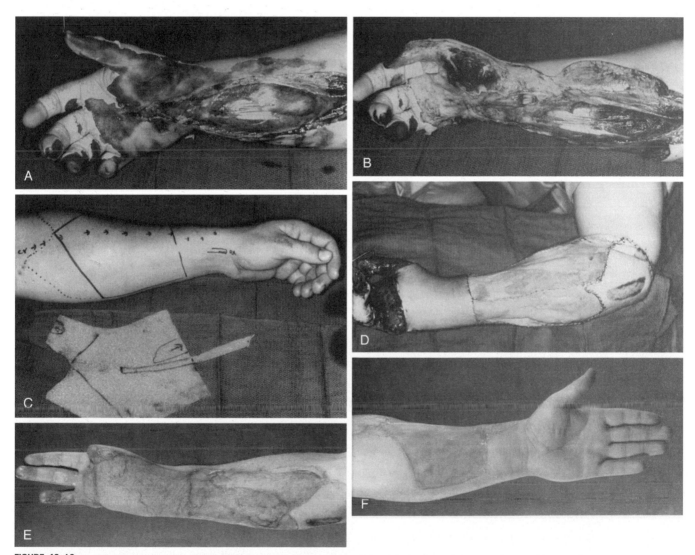

FIGURE 48-18. Radial forearm flap. **A,** This extensive thermal crush injury of the right hand required extensive débridement (**B**) with excision of the thrombosed ulnar artery, the small finger, the flexor retinaculum, and the distal portion of the flexor carpi ulnaris. Circulation to the digits was deemed to be marginal. **C,** A contralateral left radial forearm flap was designed based on the radial artery (RA) and the cephalic vein (CV). The flap was to be applied in retrograde fashion to provide not only cover for the structures of the carpal tunnel but also to restore blood flow to the superficial palmar arch from the proximal ulnar artery. Fascial extensions of the radial forearm flap to be used to cover the palm of the hand are shown in a dotted outline. A pattern has been taken with plastic foam. **D,** The appearance immediately after application of the radial forearm flap, skin grafts, and a transposition flap of the flexor carpi ulnaris. **E,** The result before thumb reconstruction. **F,** The defect of the donor forearm covered with a split-thickness skin graft. (From Chick LR, Lister GD, Sowder L: Early free-flap coverage of electrical and thermal burns. Plast Reconstr Surg 89:1013-1019, 1992.)

be identified and preserved, because very occasionally it may be needed to reconstruct the radial artery. Great care should be taken to preserve branches of the superficial radial nerve. Once the skin has been elevated for 1 cm or so from the flap margin, the deep fascia should be incised all around the flap, thereby gaining the plane of dissection.

The deep fascia can with benefit be sutured to the skin at several points around the flap. This serves to prevent shearing between the two during elevation of the flap. If the ends of these sutures are left long, they can be grasped with hemostats to provide the necessary tension during dissection.

The flap is now raised by dissecting in the loose areolar tissue beneath the deep fascia. Wherever a tendon is encountered in elevating the flap, care must be taken to preserve the overlying paratenon.

Once the flap has been raised from the ulnar margin across to the flexor carpi radialis tendon, traction on the muscle in an ulnar direction will reveal the radial artery and its venae comitantes. Similarly, dissection from the radial margin of the flap will reveal the vessels as the fascia is lifted from the brachioradialis. This muscle conceals the artery beneath its anterior border, the more so the farther proximal the dissection. Strong traction on the brachioradialis in a radial direction and dissection hard against the muscle and tendon is required. Distally, the two venae comitantes are ligated and divided. The radial artery is also divided between a ligature proximally and a microvascular clamp distally. Working from the radial and ulnar aspects, the lateral intermuscular septum containing the radial artery and venae comitantes can be visualized at all times and the portion of the septum passing inferiorly from the artery

down to the flexor pollicis longus and radius can be divided to allow elevation of the vascular pedicle in continuity with the overlying flap. Small perforating vessels passing downward to supply the radius and flexor pollicis longus muscle can be coagulated. Dissection now progresses in a distal to proximal direction, and the vascular pedicle is elevated in the plane between the flexor carpi radialis and brachioradialis muscles. A longitudinal or gently curving incision proximal to the skin flap allows elevation of the proximal radial artery and any subcutaneous veins, if necessary, all the way to the bifurcation of the brachial artery just distal to the antecubital fossa. Occasionally, the two venae comitantes can be traced via a communicating branch into the superficial venous system so that a single large cubital vein can be used as the proximal venous anastomosis.[305] The tourniquet is deflated, and this should reveal immediate reperfusion of the flap and of the hand.

The microvascular clamp is then removed from the distal stump of the radial artery, and this allows subjective evaluation of retrograde flow from the radial artery provided by inflow through the ulnar artery and palmar arches. If this flow is adequate, the distal radial artery is ligated. The proximal radial artery and venae comitantes, or superficial vein are ligated and divided in the antecubital fossa and the flap transferred to the recipient defect.

The radial artery is reconstructed only if there is poor retrograde flow through the distal stump of the radial artery after release of the tourniquet. If this is necessary, either the cephalic vein if it has not been incorporated in the flap or the greater saphenous vein can be harvested, reversed, and used as an interposition vein graft with two end-to-end anasto-

CRITICAL POINTS: RADIAL FOREARM FREE FLAP

INDICATIONS

- Soft tissue defect of hand
- May provide fascia, skin, tendon, and bone if needed
- Wound with need for distal revascularization (flow-through flap)

PREOPERATIVE EVALUATION

- Allen test for patency and adequacy of ulnar flow to hand
- Scars on forearm from prior injury or surgery

PEARLS

- "Best" flap to place on hand but potentially ugly donor site cosmetically
- May use as fascia-only flap to avoid skin graft on forearm

TECHNICAL POINTS

- Design flap 3 to 5 cm proximal to wrist if possible.
- Do not center flap on radial artery but may take most of skin from volar forearm as long as arterial septum is in flap.

- Take pedicle as a "unit"; do not divide veins from artery.
- Preserve cephalic vein; avoid damage to branches of radial nerve.
- Dissection over brachioradialis tendon must be done very carefully to prevent damage to perforators into skin.
- May include palmaris longus in flap if tendon reconstruction is required.

PITFALLS

- Damage to superficial radial nerve branches
- Division of septum when dissecting from radial side

DONOR SITE MANAGEMENT

- All but very small flaps will require skin graft.
- Flexor carpi radialis tendon may be covered with superficialis muscle pulled up and over.
- Split-thickness graft is fine; donor site is somewhat better with full-thickness graft.
- Use splint until graft has taken.

moses to the proximal and distal ends of the radial artery. If bone has been taken from the radius in its distal third for a radial forearm osteocutaneous flap, contour can be restored by transposing the pronator quadratus muscle on the anterior interosseous vascular pedicle. Any exposure of the flexor carpi radialis tendon is covered by imbrication of the flexor digitorum superficialis muscle. The margins of the flap donor defect are sutured to the underlying muscles to provide a shallow contour over which a nonmeshed split-thickness skin graft is placed (see Fig. 48-18F).[11,199,286,308] Some surgeons believe the donor defect to be cosmetically unsightly, but most patients are not embarrassed by the appearance of their forearm in long-term follow-up. The appearance of the donor defect can potentially be eliminated by raising the flap as fascia alone as a radial forearm fascial flap (see Fig. 47-63). However, this has the disadvantage that split-thickness skin grafts may not "take" completely over a fascial flap and may not be sufficiently robust to provide coverage of the primary defect.

Anterolateral Thigh Flap

After the vascular anatomy of the anterolateral thigh flap was first described by Song in 1984,[280] it has been increasingly used over the past decade for microsurgical reconstruction in China and Japan[126,158,165,181,323] but has not really achieved the same popularity in North America and Europe. A large skin island over the anterior and lateral aspect of the thigh can be harvested supplied by either the septocutaneous or musculocutaneous perforators of the descending branch of the lateral circumflex femoral artery. Potentially this flap can be harvested as a sensate flap by including the lateral femoral cutaneous nerve of the thigh.

The flap is designed over a line drawn between the anterior superior iliac spine and the midpoint of the lateral border of the patella with the patient in a supine position. The main cutaneous perforators are detected with a pencil Doppler probe and are centered primarily within a 3- to 5-cm radius of the midpoint of this longitudinal axis. The descending branch of the lateral circumflex femoral artery passes downward in the fascia between the rectus femoris and the vastus lateralis muscles. Either the descending branch of the lateral circumflex femoral artery or the lateral circumflex femoral artery trunk itself may serve as the vascular pedicle with a length of 8 to 12 cm. The medial margin of the skin flap is incised down through the deep fascia overlying the rectus femoris muscle, and the intermuscular space between the rectus femoris and vastus lateralis muscles is exposed. If septocutaneous perforators from the lateral circumflex femoral artery are found, the flap can be harvested as a septocutaneous flap. However, if septocutaneous perforators are absent, the flap is harvested with a small cuff of vastus lateralis muscle as a musculocutaneous flap or as a perforator flap by intramuscular dissection of the musculocutaneous perforators.

Specifically for upper extremity reconstruction, the anterolateral thigh flap can be thinned to a thickness of 2 to 4 mm,[153] and extra fascia can be harvested to wrap around exposed tendons.[215] The anterolateral thigh flap has numerous advantages compared with other free flaps for upper extremity reconstruction: a large skin paddle of up to 20 × 15 cm even for thinned flaps; a long vascular pedicle;

the possibility of restoring sensation by incorporating the lateral femoral cutaneous nerve; harvesting part of the vastus lateralis muscle to fill any dead space; and the ability to harvest the flap simultaneously in a supine position and minimal morbidity at the donor site because the donor site can be closed directly if the width does not exceed 6 to 8 cm (otherwise a split-thickness skin graft is necessary). Potential disadvantages of the anterolateral thigh flap include a lateral thigh scar, especially if a skin graft has to be used (this may preclude its use in women); lateral thigh skin may be quite hairy in men; patients may complain of decreased sensation over the lateral thigh; and the variability of the vascular anatomy may be disconcerting. However, it is likely that in the future the anterolateral thigh flap may become one of the top choices for reconstruction of extensive defects of the upper extremity.

Temporoparietal Fascial Flap

The ultra-thin and highly vascular tissue of the temporoparietal fascia is ideal for coverage of small defects of the hand and wrist* when a skin graft would be preferable to a bulky flap but the recipient bed is poorly vascularized, such as in circumstances where periosteum has been stripped to expose bone or where tendons have been denuded of paratenon.

Anatomy

The temporoparietal fascia is the superior extension of the submuscular aponeurotic system (SMAS), which supports the muscles of facial expression. It is located between the scalp and the fascia overlying the temporalis muscle and is supplied by the superficial temporal artery and vein, which emerge from beneath the parotid gland in front of the ear to pass superiorly into the temporal and parietal scalp (Fig. 48-19A).[23] The superficial temporal artery measures 1.8 to 2.2 mm in diameter in front of the ear and provides a pedicle length of 4 to 5 cm. The superficial temporal vein lies posterior and superficial to the artery and gives off multiple branches to the subcutaneous tissue of the scalp. Most temporoparietal fascial flaps have not exceeded 13 cm in length and 9 cm in width (see Fig. 48-19B). The superficial and deep fascias investing the temporalis muscle are vascularized by the deep middle temporal branch of the superficial temporal artery, and consequently this fascia can also be transferred together with the temporoparietal fascia to provide a "double" fascial flap[116] that can be used to envelope exposed flexor or extensor tendons and preserve gliding.[17]

The auriculotemporal nerve follows the course of the superficial temporal vessels and is divided during flap dissection. A segment of the outer table of the skull vascularized by the temporoparietal fascia has been reported for craniofacial reconstruction, but vascularized bone transfer to

---

*See references 23, 44, 45, 114, 115, 216, 247, 250, 316, and 319.

the hand using the temporoparietal fascial flap has not been described.

Operative Technique

The patient is positioned supine with the head turned to the side. The contralateral side of the head is used to allow simultaneous donor and recipient site dissection (two-team approach). The vascular axis of the superficial temporal artery is determined either by palpation or by using a pencil Doppler probe. A 1- to 1.5-cm strip of scalp is shaved over this vascular axis beginning just above the ear. Narrow temporoparietal flaps can be harvested through this single incision, but for larger flaps an inverted "L"- or "T"-shaped extension may be required within the hair-bearing scalp skin (see Fig. 48-19A). The preauricular part of the incision extends down to the earlobe. The temporoparietal fascia can also be harvested endoscopically.[49] The superficial temporal artery and vein are identified in front of the ear and traced in a superior direction. The vessels are fragile, and great care must be taken in bipolar coagulation of all the small branches. Scalp flaps are then elevated in the plane between the subcutaneous tissue and the temporoparietal fascia. The

proper plane is sometimes difficult to find, but the hair follicles should be kept in the subcutaneous tissue of the elevated scalp flaps. Dissection continues anteriorly and posteriorly from the incision but should not be extended too far anteriorly from the axis of the superficial temporal artery because of injury to the frontal branch of the facial nerve. The superficial temporal vessels lie above or within the fascia, whereas the motor branches of the facial nerve lie below the fascia. A nerve stimulator may be helpful in identifying these facial nerve branches at the level of the zygoma and lateral orbital rim. The template of the recipient defect is either centered over the axis of the superficial temporal vessels or positioned a little more posteriorly, again to avoid damage to the frontal branches of the facial nerve. The superior and posterior margins of the outlined fascial flap are then incised to enter the loose areolar plane between the temporoparietal fascia and the fascia overlying the temporalis muscle. The anterior margin of the flap is incised in a distal to proximal direction up to the point where the frontal branch of the superficial temporal artery passes anteriorly to the forehead. After division of this branch, further dissection proceeds just anterior to the superficial

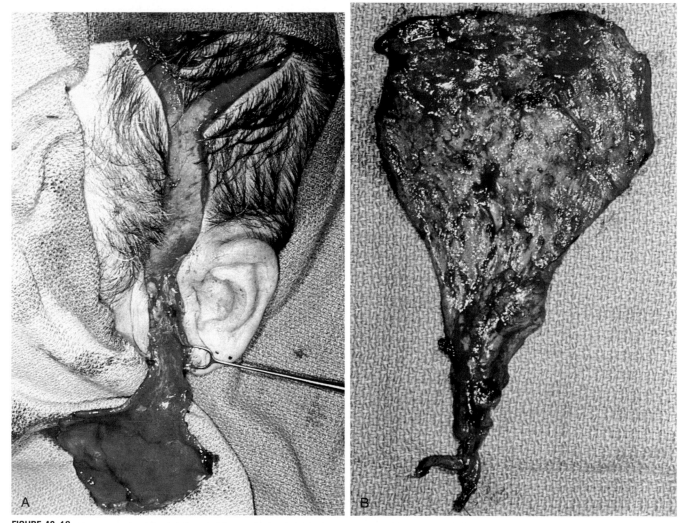

FIGURE 48-19. Temporoparietal fascial flap. **A,** The temporoparietal fascia can be harvested through a preauricular incision extending up into the temporal hair-bearing scalp as a "Y" or "T"-shaped extension. **B,** This thin fascial sheet can be used to wrap around exposed tendons to preserve their gliding and can then be covered either primarily or secondarily with a skin graft.

temporal vessels to taper the pedicle down to the axial vessels at the top of the ear. The temporoparietal fascial flap is now completely isolated as an island based on the vascular pedicle in front of the ear. Additional length to the vascular pedicle can be obtained by more proximal dissection, but this may be both tedious and bloody because of large branches from the artery and vein. After ligation of the superficial temporal artery and vein, the fascia is transferred to the hand and covered with either a split-thickness or full-thickness skin graft.

After hemostasis of the scalp incision has been achieved, it is closed over a small suction drain. The preauricular incision is closed with fine 5-0 nylon sutures, and these are removed within 5 days to prevent conspicuous scarring. The temporoparietal fascia probably produces one of the most inconspicuous donor sites of any free flap, but alopecia may sometimes occur.[336] Patients may occasionally have diminished sensibility within the distribution of the auriculotemporal nerve, but this is usually not painful.

CRITICAL POINTS: TEMPOROPARIETAL FASCIA FLAP

INDICATIONS

- Need for thin soft tissue coverage in hand
- Potential need for "gliding" surface over tendons

PREOPERATIVE EVALUATION

- Doppler examination/palpation of temporal artery

PEARLS

- This offers a very thin flap for reconstruction, particularly on the dorsal hand over and around the extensor tendons.

TECHNICAL POINTS

- This tissue lies directly underneath the hair follicles, and getting in the right plane can be difficult.
- Elevate scalp carefully off of fascia; beware of vein branches into scalp.
- Superficial and deep fascia may be taken.
- Artery and vein are small and fragile.
- Avoid deep dissection proximally in parotid to prevent damage to facial nerve!

PITFALLS

- Alopecia common, particularly around scar
- Damage to thin-walled veins when elevating flap

DONOR SITE MANAGEMENT

- Close primarily over drain.

Sensory Flaps From the First Web Space of the Foot

Either the great toe or the second toe can be transferred for reconstruction of the thumb or fingers (see Chapter 52), but for reconstruction of digital pulp defects or crucial areas of the hand that require sensation there is unanimity regarding the appropriate donor site, namely, the first web space of the foot. Depending on the requirements of the primary defect, this flap may vary from a single pulp alone[26,156] to the fibular aspect of the great toe together with all or part of the nail[159,160,212] combined with the tibial aspect of the second toe.[141,191,205,211,282] Such sensory flaps can be used to reconstruct critical areas of the hand, including pulp defects of the thumb and fingers, pulp defects of adjacent digits, and the thumb/index finger web space.

 Anatomy

All the tissues in the first web space of the foot are supplied by the lateral digital artery to the great toe and the medial digital artery to the second toe, which arise from a variable "arterial complex" in the web.[333] This "arterial complex" receives its blood supply from two sources: the first dorsal metatarsal artery (FDMA) arising from the dorsalis pedis artery, and the common first plantar digital artery (FPDA) arising from the plantar arch (Fig. 48-20A). This common plantar digital artery is supplied not only by the posterior tibial artery but also by the dorsalis pedis artery through a communicating branch that passes downward through the first intermetatarsal space at the point where the FDMA arises from the dorsalis pedis artery, a point designated as "X."

The two feeding arteries and two digital arteries have a varying relationship in the first web space, hence the choice of the term *arterial complex*. The four vessels may come together at one junction with no true common digital artery intervening. The common digital artery, by contrast, may be very long, especially in those cases in which the FDMA pursues a deeper course by diving through the interosseous muscles to enter the plantar compartment of the foot more proximally, instead of pursuing its more common route along the dorsal surface of the interosseous muscles. The "arterial complex" may sometimes give two branches, one each to the first and second toes, leading the unwary to ligate the unwanted one, only to find that a larger, major vessel to the toe to be harvested arises from the apparent proper digital artery to the other at a point distal to the ligature. There may also be other variants of the complex.

The nerve supply to the first web space likewise comes from two sources: (1) the lateral digital nerve to the great toe and the medial digital nerve to the second toe, both originating from the common plantar digital nerve and (2) from the deep peroneal nerve dorsally (see Fig. 48-20B).

Operative Technique

In replacing the pulp of an important digit, such as an avulsed thumb, the fibular aspect of the great toe offers the

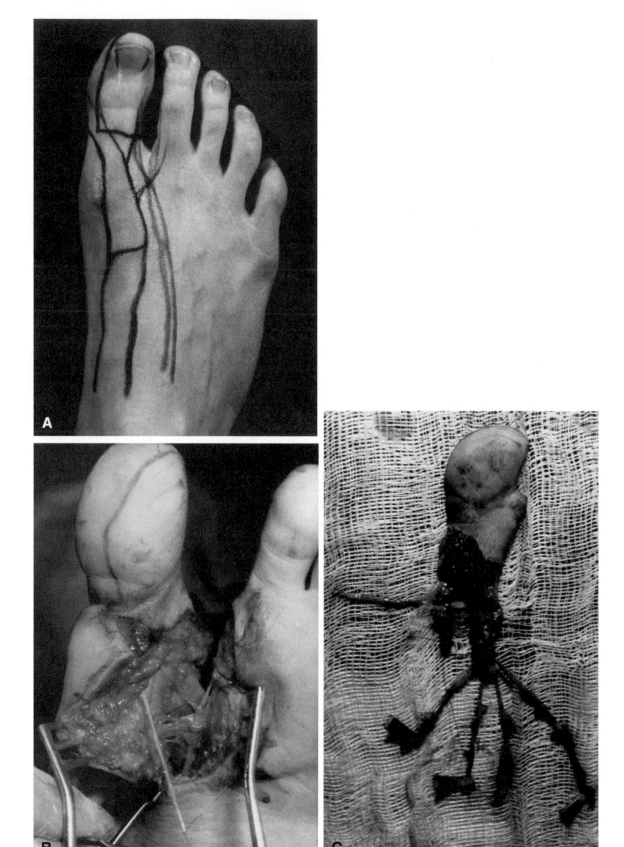

FIGURE 48-20. Sensory flap from the first web space of the foot. **A,** Using a pencil Doppler probe, the first dorsal metatarsal artery has been marked *(double pale line).* The major veins have been marked after temporary elevation of the tourniquet *(dark lines).* **B,** Dissection of the first web space. The plantar digital nerve to the fibular aspect of the great toe has been divided and marked with a suture. **C,** After dissection, the veins and first dorsal metatarsal artery (FDMA) are marked with microvascular clamps.

ideal donor site, having an identical structure to that lost (Fig. 48-21). Preparation for harvest commences with examination of the foot with a pencil Doppler probe directed at the FDMA as it leaves the dorsalis pedis artery to pass distally. It is possible to make some estimate of the depth of the vessel by angling the probe in different directions. Detection of a pulse even from various acute angles suggests that the vessel lies superficial in the most common dorsal location.

The venous drainage on the dorsum of the foot should be mapped out before exsanguinating the limb and inflating the tourniquet (see Fig. 48-20A). There are, in fact, two venous systems on the dorsum of the foot. One drains the medial aspect of the great toe and metatarsal region and lies superficial to the second, larger system, which forms an arch extending from side to side across the dorsum of the foot

and drains into the greater saphenous system. The deeper system is less pronounced on inspection but clearly has larger caliber veins and should be selected for harvest.

The incision should be marked out on the dorsum of the foot overlying the first interosseous space but providing access to the most promising vein and passing distally to reach the outline of the flap, which should be marked on the fibular aspect of the great toe. A second incision extends proximally from the flap on the plantar surface of the foot between the weight-bearing areas of the first and second metatarsal heads.

Only the distal portion of both dorsal and plantar incisions should be opened initially, sufficient to dissect the contents of the web space. Although there are some fibrous septa in the web, the tissue is relatively loose. The most distal structure of importance in the web is likely to be the

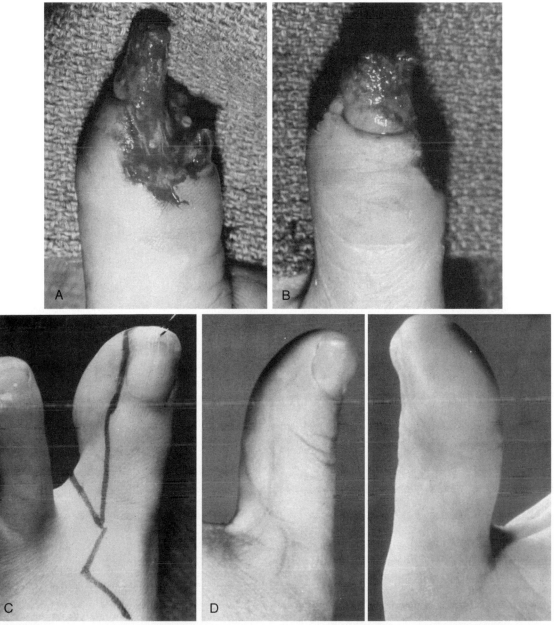

FIGURE 48-21. Sensory flap from the first web space of the foot. **A** and **B,** Palmar and dorsal views of the defect resulting from avulsion of the pulp of the dominant thumb. **C,** The partial toe flap designed on the fibular aspect of the left great toe. **D,** Postoperative result.

arterial complex, because the venous drainage lies more dorsally. Loupe magnification and delicate scissor dissection are required immediately.

Once an artery is encountered (and it may lie as far as 1 cm proximal to the free margin of the web), it should be dissected distally into both toes and proximally on to the dorsal and plantar aspects, until all the ramifications of the "arterial complex" are displayed and understood. If the dorsal artery appears large and seems to communicate with the FDMA, it should be chosen, because it is both easier to visualize and provides a longer pedicle. The dorsal incision is extended proximally and the medial flap reflected until a suitable vein is located over the first metatarsal. The vein need not be dissected distally all the way to the flap, because it will probably have several fragile tributaries. Instead, the medial dorsal flap, which will remain on the foot, should be dissected off the venous system on the dorsum of the great toe. A monobloc of subcutaneous tissue between the toe flap and the selected vein can then be taken by cutting down on to the extensor tendons on either side of the venous pedicle and elevating it by bipolar dissection directly off the extensor tendons. This relatively bulky tissue will be readily accommodated by the loose skin of the thumb/index finger web space.

The more proximal the arterial anastomosis is made in the hand, the easier will be both access and the anastomosis. Therefore, a long pedicle is desirable, another reason for preferring the FDMA and its extension back to the dorsalis pedis artery. The vein is dissected proximally, until sufficient length is obtained to reach a good caliber vein in the hand. If the vein is from the deeper dorsal system, as it should be, it, or one of the large veins with which it communicates, will give a large and fairly constant branch that passes through the proximal part of the first intermetacarpal space adjacent to the communicating branch from the dorsalis pedis artery to the plantar arch. The surgeon should look for this juxtaposition, because it leads directly to the arterial tree, which is much less evident than the venous system. The artery is firmly adherent to surrounding tissue and lies deep to the musculotendinous junction of the extensor hallucis brevis, which passes from proximal lateral to distal medial between the arterial and venous systems. The tendon can either be preserved or divided to improve access, because it is of little functional importance.

Having located the dorsalis pedis artery at the previously defined point "X," a decision should be made as to the length of pedicle required to reach the ideal site in the hand for the arterial anastomosis. A branch of the radial artery just distal to the anatomical snuff-box, between the bases of the first and second metacarpals, is best for the thumb.

Regardless of whether it is deemed necessary to harvest part of the dorsalis pedis artery, the somewhat tedious dissection of the communicating branch should be performed, because it reveals the origin of the FDMA. This artery should be followed distally to the point where it was seen in the earlier web dissection. An alternative and perhaps more simple approach is to dissect the FDMA in a distal to proximal direction from its initial identification in the web space to point "X."[324] This may be simple or difficult, depending on the depth of the vessel in the interosseous muscles. Delicate dissection is required, because the FDMA has a variable number of narrow, short, friable branches. The

communicating branch should now be divided and dissection of the dorsalis pedis artery continued as far proximally as is necessary.

In the rare circumstances in which the FDMA is unsatisfactory, the surgeon will have to decide whether to pursue the shorter common plantar digital artery to the great toe/second toe web space, hoping to achieve a sufficiently long pedicle, or whether to harvest an interposition graft, either arterial from the subscapular, superficial temporal, or interosseous systems[91,177] or venous from the saphenous system. This will depend to some degree on the availability of a second surgical team.

During this dissection of artery and vein, the surgeon will encounter the deep peroneal nerve, which lies just superficial to the artery. The branch of the deep peroneal nerve passing to the great toe should be dissected distally, splitting it from the other branches, and transected with sufficient length so that it can be coapted to the "unsatisfied" radial digital nerve of the thumb ("unsatisfied" since the lateral plantar digital nerve of the great toe will be harvested and sutured to the more important ulnar digital nerve of the thumb).

Whether the FDMA is adequate and whether a vein graft is required, the plantar incision should now be opened. Surgical access can be facilitated by externally rotating the patient's hip, flexing the knee, and tilting the table as far toward the operative side as necessary to afford a comfortable view of the operative field. Initially, the incision should be made only long enough to obtain the necessary length of the lateral digital nerve of the great toe, the length required having been first determined from dissection of the ulnar digital nerve in the thumb. In contrast to the vessels, the lateral digital nerve should be as short as possible to allow early return of sensibility. Nothing of significance lies between the plantar skin and the neurovascular bundle of the first web space, nestling between the flexor tendon sheaths, but the intervening tissue is thick and tough, containing fat and fibrous septa more impenetrable than that encountered in the palm. Dissection can be accelerated by locating the neurovascular bundle in the web space, following it proximally centimeter by centimeter and cutting boldly through the dense plantar subcutaneous tissue only when the bundle has been defined and protected. This technique is similar to that employed in preserving the facial nerve during superficial parotidectomy.

Once sufficient nerve has been exposed, the proper digital nerve should be mobilized as far distally as the proximal edge of the flap. The nerve should then be split proximally from the common digital nerve for the required length while drawing the proper digital nerves apart with nerve hooks (see Fig. 48-20B). If the plantar artery is dominant, the incision should be extended in the stepwise manner described, as far proximally as is necessary for the required pedicle length. The vessel should be left intact for reperfusion after the tourniquet is deflated.

The pulp flap, which has been left undisturbed throughout the previous dissection, can now be elevated. If pulp alone is to be taken, the pattern should be outlined almost to the lateral eponychial fold, leaving only a 1- to 2-mm rim. The dorsal and plantar margins of the flap should be incised directly down to the underlying distal phalanx. The already dissected artery, vein, and nerves should be retracted away from the skeleton with a vessel loop so that the flap can be elevated from proximal to distal beneath these protected structures, using bipolar cautery to raise the flap directly off the underlying bone and collateral ligament of the interphalangeal joint.

If the nail plate is to be incorporated with the pulp flap,[212] the dorsal cortex of the distal phalanx beneath the nail should also be harvested by making a coronal cut, which avoids the vessels passing through the rima ungulae, the aperture that lies between the neck of the phalanx and the lateral interosseous ligament. Access for this cut is made through the distal part of both the plantar and dorsal incisions.

CRITICAL POINTS: FIRST WEB SPACE AND TOE PULP FLAPS

INDICATIONS

- Loss of thumb or digital pulp
- Reconstruction of sensation in other complex reconstructions

PREOPERATIVE EVALUATION

- Perform Doppler examination of first dorsal metatarsal artery web space.
- Mark superficial veins on foot before tourniquet elevation.

PEARLS

- Use fibular aspect of great toe for thumb pulp.
- Inspect vascular anatomy first dorsally and in web.

TECHNICAL POINTS

- Dissection may be done proximally to distally or vice versa.
- Arteries are deep to veins in first web space.
- Proper dorsal digital vessels may branch proximal to web.
- Dissection of vessels in web space must be done very carefully to avoid damage and/or later spasm.
- Base the flap on dorsal side (first dorsal metatarsal artery) if available.
- Flap may need to be based on plantar artery if dorsal artery is small, and this may require vein grafting to reach recipient vessels.

DONOR SITE MANAGEMENT

- Close dorsal foot wound.
- Use a split-thickness skin graft for toe donor site with bolster dressing.
- Place foot in walking cast with toe pad for protection.

The most distal attachment of the flap can be left attached, the tourniquet released, and reperfusion confirmed without the risk of torsion of the pedicle, which might occur if the flap was totally detached. Once all is seen to be well, the artery and vein can be ligated and the flap transferred to the hand (see Figs. 48-20C and 48-21). Closure is achieved by suturing the access incisions and applying a split-thickness skin graft to the secondary defect. If the graft is secured in place with a bolster dressing, the patient can ambulate on the first postoperative day. A walking cast is desirable to ensure undisturbed healing of the foot.

Authors' Preferred Method: Flap Selection

Soft Tissue Defects Alone

The selection of local, regional, distant, or free flaps for coverage of specific defects of the upper extremity has been detailed in Chapter 47. In choosing a specific free flap, the following factors should be considered: the health, comfort, and cosmetic[313] demands of the patient; the size, thickness, and special needs of the defect; and the skill and experience of the surgeon. Patients with respiratory problems require full lung expansion after long surgical procedures. Therefore, latissimus dorsi or scapular flaps from the chest wall should probably be avoided in these circumstances. For the upper extremity wound in the multiple trauma patient, other injuries may dictate a period of prolonged bed rest. Flaps from the back might create a nursing problem. In these patients, the forearm flap[21,73,182,214,278] may be an appropriate substitute for medium to large defects. Female patients in particular are likely to be distressed enough by the primary wound without adding a disfiguring scar on the upper arm, forearm, or over the scapula. Although attempts have been made to improve the secondary defect of such flaps by prior tissue expansion,[166] the free groin flap[15,48,104,195,225,264,266] remains the optimal choice where cosmesis is a consideration (see Fig. 48-16D).

Large defects involving the entire anterior or posterior surface of the forearm require a latissimus dorsi flap.[10,70,169,186,219,293,321] Whether this should be harvested as a musculocutaneous flap[33] or a muscle flap resurfaced with a split-thickness skin graft[96] is a matter of debate. Godina believed that perfusion of the distal part of the muscle was superior when a skin island was included. He also demonstrated that the latissimus dorsi musculocutaneous flap could be accurately tailored to fit virtually any defect.[93]

Medium-sized defects can be covered with the tailored latissimus dorsi musculocutaneous flap,[93] which offers a long pedicle without the disadvantage of the bulky portion of the muscle close to its insertion (see Fig. 48-2). The scapular flap[13,89,102,193,218,257] offers remarkably tough skin with no underlying muscle (see Fig. 48-8). The flap is therefore well suited for large dorsal or palmar defects of the hand and wrist,[27,76,231] except in the overweight patient, where such a flap would be very thick.

Small defects for which no local flap is available or suitable can often be covered with either a lateral arm free flap[142-144,258,320] or a fascial flap. The lateral arm flap can be made small enough to provide coverage of one phalanx in a single finger (see Fig. 48-4). It can also be contoured to be thick in a slim patient or thin in the obese patient. Thickness is achieved by harvesting a larger area of fascia than of skin and folding the fascia into the primary defect; thinness is achieved by taking fascia alone without skin[37,343] and later applying a split-thickness skin graft. Free fascial flaps based on the temporoparietal fascia,* radial forearm fascia, dorsal thoracic fascia,[53,128,152,336] and serratus fascia[25,75,201,230,263] can also provide coverage of small defects in the hand and fingers. These fascial free flaps can be covered by a split-thickness skin graft primarily, but skin graft "take" may be better if the skin graft is applied a few days later. Free fascial flaps have also been advocated for coverage of small wounds with exposed flexor or extensor tendons or even to wrap around the tendons to maintain their gliding function and prevent their adherence to exposed bone.

Composite Defects

Traumatic injuries and surgically created defects of the upper extremity frequently involve the underlying tendons, sensory nerves, and bony skeleton. Even though one-stage reconstruction of all the tissue components of a composite defect would be ideal, composite reconstruction of associated defects of bone, tendon, artery, and nerve is only indicated occasionally.

In the future, it may become possible to prefabricate composite flaps consisting of the exact requirements of each tissue component required to reconstruct a specific defect.[148,209]

Bone

See also Chapter 50.

Vascularized bone that can be included in an overlying free flap as an osteocutaneous flap includes the iliac crest with the groin flap,[95,204,223,245,290,299] the lateral border of the scapula with the scapular flap,[184,287] a rib with the serratus anterior muscle flap,[119] the radius with the radial forearm flap,[16,79] the second metatarsal with the dorsalis pedis flap,[223] the humerus with the lateral arm flap,[142,302] and the fibula with the fibular osteocutaneous flap.[322] Small bone defects can be reconstructed with conventional nonvascularized bone graft, either as a corticocancellous block for structure or as cancellous chips. This can be performed primarily at the same time as free flap coverage of the defect or secondarily once the soft tissues have healed. Large segmental defects of the humerus, radius, and ulna or composite soft tissue and bony defects are best reconstructed with the fibular osteocutaneous flap.[5,25,66,69,170,236,341]

Tendon

Vascularized tendon grafts can be transferred with the dorsalis pedis flap[4,31,43,86,196,268,291,318] or the radial forearm flap.[110,237,244] Such tendinocutaneous flaps may occasionally be indicated for one-stage reconstruction of a degloving injury of the dorsum of the hand with loss of skin and extensor tendons. The donor defect in the foot is trouble-

some after harvest of a dorsalis pedis flap. There is also no evidence that extensor tendon function is any better than with conventional tendon grafting as a secondary procedure beneath a healed skin flap.

Artery

Arterial reconstruction in the upper limb can also be performed using the same arterial system that supplies the free flap. Thus the subscapular artery system has been used to restore arterial continuity via the circumflex scapular branch, while the thoracodorsal branch supplies the overlying latissimus flap. The distal end of the inflow artery to a flap can also be anastomosed to a distal vessel in the limb as a "flow-through" flap to restore flow to the distal limb. The radial artery of the radial forearm flap has been used in such a "flow-through" fashion to replace segmental defects of the radial or ulnar artery and so restore flow to the hand.[19,139,232] Similarly, the continuation of the posterior radial collateral artery supplying a lateral arm flap to cover a defect over the anatomical snuff-box and first metacarpal can be anastomosed to a digital artery to restore flow to the thumb.[207,258] The peroneal artery of the fibular osteocutaneous flap,[221] the medialis pedis free flap,[332] and a flap harvested from the amputated upper extremity[338] have also been reported as "flow-through" flaps.

Sensation

Modest sensibility can be restored to some free flaps by coapting the sensory nerve of the flap, such as the superficial peroneal nerve of the dorsalis pedis flap,[198,224,246] the posterior cutaneous nerve of the arm of the lateral arm flap,[185] the medial or lateral antebrachial cutaneous nerves of the radial forearm flap, and the T12 branch of the groin flap[135] to a sensory nerve in the vicinity of the defect. No such donor sensory nerves exist for the scapular or latissimus flaps.

However, for restoration of critical sensation in the thumb or fingertips, a free neurovascular flap from the fibular aspect of the great toe and the tibial aspect of the second toe is the optimal choice (see Fig. 48-21).[141,191,205,211,248,282]

CONCLUSION

The practicing hand surgeon should have a limited repertoire of highly reliable free flaps that can be used to reconstruct the majority of defects encountered in the upper extremity. The lateral arm flap or various fascial flaps can be used for reconstruction of small defects; the scapular, tailored latissimus or radial forearm flaps for medium-sized defects, and the latissimus muscle flap for large defects. A contralateral radial forearm flap is especially indicated for coverage of the forearm or wrist if reconstruction of a segmental radial or ulnar arterial injury is also required. The free groin flap, although more difficult to dissect, should be considered if cosmesis of the donor site is especially important. The fibular osteocutaneous flap is the optimal choice for composite reconstruction of associated bone and soft tissue defects of the upper extremity. Finally, the fibular aspect of the great toe or the tibial aspect of the second toe or the entire first web space flap is the preferred sensory flap for reconstruction of the thumb or finger pulp for restoration of critical areas of sensibility in the hand.

---

*See references 23, 44, 45, 114, 115, 216, 247, 250, 316, and 319.

ANNOTATED REFERENCES

54. Conrad MH, Adams WP Jr: Pharmacologic optimization of microsurgery in the new millennium. Plast Reconstr Surg 108:2088-2096, 2001.

    This paper provides an overview of the use of heparin, dextran, streptokinase, urokinase, and tissue plasminogen activator in microsurgery.

57. Daniel RK, Taylor GI: Distant transfer of an island flap by microvascular anastomoses. Plast Reconstr Surg 52:111-117, 1973.

    The original historic description of the first free flap transfer.

89. Gilbert A, Teot L: The free scapular flap. Plast Reconstr Surg 69:601-604, 1982.

    Describes the anatomy and clinical applications of the free scapular flap.

92. Godina M: Early microsurgical reconstruction of complex trauma of the extremities. Plast Reconstr Surg 78:285-292, 1986.

    Describes the philosophy, organization, and results of immediate radical débridement of severe traumatic injuries of the upper and lower extremities and emergency free flap coverage.

96. Gordon L, Buncke HJ, Alpert BS: Free latissimus dorsi muscle flap with split-thickness skin graft cover: A report of 16 cases. Plast Reconstr Surg 70:173-178, 1982.

    This paper describes the evolution of the free latissimus dorsi musculocutaneous flap by only harvesting the latissimus dorsi muscle as a free muscle flap and then covering it with a split-thickness skin graft.

134. Jones NF: Intraoperative and postoperative monitoring of microsurgical free tissue transfers. Clin Plast Surg 19:783-797, 1992.

    A review article describing the various techniques for intraoperative and postoperative monitoring of the viability of microsurgical free tissue transfers.

142. Katsaros J, Schusterman M, Beppu M, et al: The lateral upper arm flap: Anatomy and clinical applications. Ann Plast Surg 12:489-500, 1984.

    Provides a description of the anatomy and dissection and gives clinical examples of the free lateral arm flap.

162. Kraemer BA, Korber KE, Aquino TI, Engleman A: Use of leeches in plastic and reconstructive surgery: A review. J Reconstr Microsurg 4:381, 1988.

    Provides a review of the biology and use of leeches in reconstructive microsurgery.

176. Lister G, Scheker L: Emergency free flaps to the upper extremity. J Hand Surg [Am] 13:22-28, 1988.

    The definitive paper detailing the indications for emergency free flaps after débridement of severe injuries of the upper extremity.

191. May JW, Chait LA, Cohen BE, O'Brien B: Free neurovascular flap from the first web of the foot in hand reconstruction. J Hand Surg [Am] 2:387-393, 1977.

    Describes the arterial and neural anatomy of the first web space of the foot as the basis for free flap transfers of the sensate first web space flap, as well as partial toe transfers.

233. Pederson WC: Upper extremity microsurgery. Plast Reconstr Surg 107:1524-1536, 2001.

    A condensed review article of the various free flaps used for reconstruction of the upper extremity.

257. Santos LF: The scapular flap: A new microsurgical free flap. Rev Bras Cir 70:133-141, 1980.

    The original description of the anatomy and dissection of the free scapular flap with clinical examples of its use.

274. Smith PJ, Foley B, McGregor IA, Jackson IT: The anatomical basis of the groin flap. Plast Reconstr Surg 49:41-47, 1972.

    The key paper for understanding the anatomy and dissection of the groin flap, either as a pedicled flap or free flap.

278. Song R, Gao Y, Song Y, et al: The forearm flap. Clin Plast Surg 91:21-26, 1982.

    The original description of the anatomy and surgical technique for dissection of the radial forearm flap or "Chinese" flap.

316. Upton J, Rogers C, Durham-Smith G, Swartz WM: Clinical applications of free temporoparietal flaps in hand reconstruction. J Hand Surg [Am] 11:475-483, 1986.

    This paper describes the anatomy and surgical dissection of the temporoparietal flap and introduces the concept of fascial flaps possibly providing a better gliding surface for coverage of exposed tendons.

322. Wei FC, Chen HC, Chuang CC, Noordhoff MS: Fibular osteoseptocutaneous flap: Anatomic study and clinical application. Plast Reconstr Surg 78:191-199, 1986.

    Describes the anatomy and dissection of the fibular osteocutaneous flap and examples of its use for reconstruction of composite bone and soft tissue defects of the upper and lower extremities.

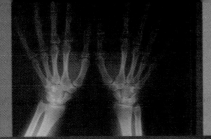

CHAPTER 49

Free Functioning Muscle Transfers

Ralph T. Manktelow and Dimitri J. Anastakis

Most of the muscles of the body have been assessed for their usefulness as free tissue transfers, and many have now been identified as readily expendable and suitable for microvascular transfer. These muscles usually have large, long, predictable neurovascular pedicles that provide a vigorous blood supply and are reliable free tissue transfers. Free muscle transfers have been found to be useful both for soft tissue coverage and as functioning contracting muscles for reconstruction of the extremities.

Functioning muscle transfer is a procedure that involves microneurovascular transfer of a muscle from one location to another (Fig. 49-1). Viability of the transferred muscle is maintained by microvascular anastomoses between the muscle's artery and vein and a suitable artery and vein in the recipient area. Reinnervation and active muscle contraction are produced by suturing a motor nerve in the recipient area to the motor nerve of the transferred muscle. For example, when a muscle is transferred into the flexor aspect of the forearm it is sutured to the flexor digitorum profundus tendons to produce finger flexion. This operation results in the transfer of a viable muscle that is under voluntary control

and will provide the patient with a functional grasp and pinch mechanism.

In 1970, Tamai and coworkers established the applicability of the procedure of transplantation of functional skeletal muscle in experimental animals.[41] In 1976, Harii and associates[16] used the gracilis to replace the muscles of facial expression in a long-standing case of Bell's palsy. In the same year, a surgical team at the Sixth People's Hospital in Shanghai transferred the lateral portion of the pectoralis major muscle to the forearm to replace finger flexor musculature destroyed by Volkmann's ischemic contracture.[40] We have experience with 62 functioning muscle transfers to the upper extremity. The techniques that have evolved on the basis of this experience are described in this chapter. We have also acquired considerable experience in the use of microvascular muscle transfers in patients with brachial plexus injuries. This is a challenging problem because of the lack of innervation. Doi, Akasaka, and Chuang and their colleagues have used the intercostal nerves and the accessory nerve to reconstruct this difficult injury.[1,2,6,9,10,15]

GENERAL PRINCIPLES

This procedure is applicable to patients who have sustained a major loss of skeletal musculature in the upper extremity resulting in a significant functional deficit that cannot be adequately reconstructed by a simpler procedure. Functioning muscle transfer is a complex procedure and should not be used when simpler, satisfactory techniques are available. If a tendon transfer can provide an adequate result, it should be used. The most common causes of muscle loss have been direct muscle trauma, Volkmann's ischemic paralysis, electrical burns, post-replantation gas gangrene, long-standing nerve injury, and muscle excision for tumor.[19,25,28] For a muscle transfer to provide useful grip function, a number of conditions must be satisfied. Good range of passive joint movement and adequate hand sensibility are prerequisites. There must be a mechanism for finger and thumb extension to enable the grasp mechanism to be usable. Intrinsic muscle function should be present. In addition, the recipient of

FIGURE 49-1. Intraoperative view of the right flexor aspect of a forearm that sustained a traumatic forearm injury with loss of the flexor digitorum profundus and sublimis and the flexor pollicis longus. All structures in the forearm and the gracilis muscle have been prepared for transfer.

Table 49-1
GUIDELINES FOR PATIENT SELECTION

Available, undamaged motor nerve, artery, and vein at the site of muscle transplantation

Adequate skin coverage for the distal half of the muscle

Supple joints and gliding tendons

Good hand sensibility and intrinsic function

Adequate antagonist muscle function

Good patient motivation

No simpler solution for the patient's problem

a muscle transfer must have the patience to wait for reinnervation and the persistence to pursue a postoperative muscle-strengthening program (Table 49-1).

Functioning muscle transfer in the upper extremity has been used for the replacement of long finger flexor function, long finger extensor function, biceps reconstruction, triceps reconstruction, and deltoid reconstruction. Of these five applications, the most common is for long finger flexor function (Fig. 49- 2). In all of these locations, the gracilis muscle has been the most commonly used because of its functional and anatomic fit to the defect, ready availability, reliable vascular and neural pedicles, ease of elevation, and insignificant functional loss after removal from the leg.[27]

APPLIED MUSCLE PHYSIOLOGY

An individual muscle is made up of many muscle fibers. Each of these fibers or cellular units is 1 to 40 mm in length and composed of many myofibrils that lie parallel to each other and are enclosed in sarcolemma. Each myofibril is composed of a hexagonal arrangement of thin actin and thicker myosin fibers that lie adjacent to each other.[4] The configuration of muscle fibers is either strap, pennate, or a combination of the two. In a strap muscle the fibers lie parallel to the long axis of the muscle. This is important from a functional standpoint. Strap muscles have a potential range of excursion that is directly proportional to overall muscle length. The maximal potential contractile force of a strap muscle can be estimated by measuring the cross-sectional area of the entire muscle. In mammals, this maximal tension has been calculated experimentally to be 4 kg/cm.[2,4]

A pennate muscle has much shorter muscle fiber units. These muscle fiber units are attached to a central or lateral tendon. The overall length of muscle contraction is proportional to the length of these short muscle fibers rather than the overall length of the muscle itself. If a muscle fiber unit in a pennate muscle is 6 cm, the overall muscle contraction capability is slightly more than 50% of this, or just over 3 cm. Although the overall muscle length may be as long as 30 cm, the entire muscle will only shorten a maximum of approximately 3 cm. If this 30-cm muscle unit were a strap muscle such as the gracilis, the contractile capability would be in excess of 15 cm (Fig. 49-3). However, the pennate muscle is correspondingly more powerful in its contraction inasmuch as the aggregate cross-sectional area of the pennate muscle fibers is considerably larger than those in a comparably sized strap muscle. The practical solution to muscle selection for clinical application is provided by selecting a strap muscle with a large cross-sectional area.

Muscle contraction is a dynamic process of sliding the adjacent thick and thin actin and myosin fibers together into an overlap. The force of muscle contraction is directly proportional to the extent of overlap of the thick and thin fibers. Thus, at maximal extension when there is little overlap, muscle contraction is weak. With shortening of the muscle and increasing overlap between the actin and myosin fibers, the strength of muscle contraction becomes progressively greater until there is complete overlap. This is the peak of the length-tension curve. With further contraction there is crumpling of the myosin fibers, less area of overlap, and considerably less force of contraction (Fig. 49-4). The force of contraction is also aided by elasticity within the connective tissue network that surrounds the muscle fibers. This force of elasticity creates significant tension within a muscle when it is in its fully extended position and plays a significant part in creating the contractile force of the muscle (Fig. 49-5).

In experimental muscle physiology, the total range of contraction of a single muscle fiber is up to 65% of its fully stretched length.[4] However, in an intact muscle, this fully stretched fiber length is limited by the connective tissue network that surrounds each muscle fiber and limits its extension.

When a muscle contracts, the force of contraction depends on the number of individual muscle fibers that respond to neural stimulation. The contraction of a muscle fiber is an all-or-none phenomenon. When a weak muscle contraction is required, only a few muscle fibers are acti-

FIGURE 49-2. **A,** Postoperative view of a patient who has received a gracilis transfer to his right forearm. The muscle provides full finger flexion. The bulk of the forearm is similar to that of his left forearm. **B,** The muscle allows full finger extension.

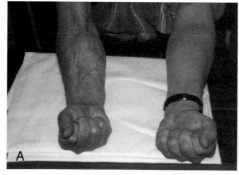
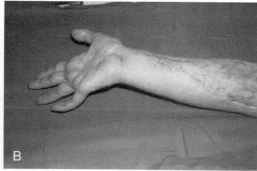

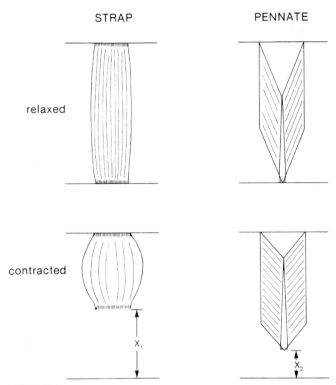

STRAP   PENNATE

relaxed

contracted

X_1

X_2

FIGURE 49-3. Schematic representation comparing contraction in strap and pennate muscles. Note the marked difference in muscle excursions X_1 and X_2 with 50% shortening of the muscle fibers in each muscle.

vated. However, with strong muscle contraction, most of the fibers respond.

In our laboratory, experimental microneurovascular muscle transfer in dogs resulted in muscles in which the force of contraction varied from 35% to 120% of the control muscle in the normal limb.[21] The factors responsible for the range in results were not apparent, but we were impressed with the potential of obtaining a normally functioning muscle after transfer.

Our clinical experience with relatively crude measuring techniques applied to in vitro testing in the human gracilis muscle has demonstrated a shortening comparable to the experimental findings. The gracilis is mostly a strap muscle with an average muscle fiber length of 24 cm. The muscle fibers insert sequentially into its tendon, with the posterior fibers being shortest and the anterior longest. Because of this sequential insertion, the individual fibers in the average muscle have a length of 16 to 30 cm. Adult human gracilis muscles, when stimulated to maximal contraction, shorten 12 to 16 cm when measured from the physiologic, fully extended muscle length (Fig. 49-6). In view of the length-tension curve, it would seem reasonable to assume that a useful range of powerful muscle excursion of the gracilis is less than the maximal excursion but likely to be at least 8 to 10 cm.

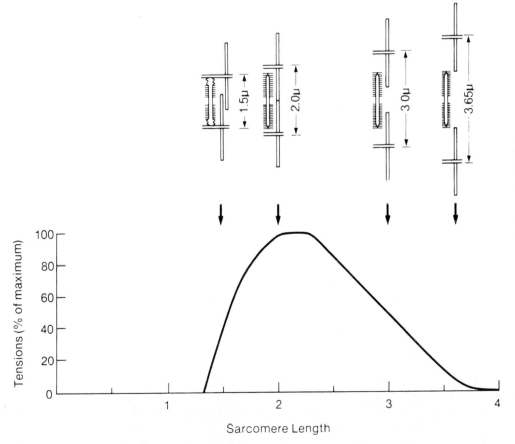

FIGURE 49-4. Length-tension curve of a single muscle fiber during active contraction. Above the curve is a schematic representation of the actin and myosin (with bars) fibers at various stages of contraction. At a sarcomere length of 3.65 μm there is no overlap of actin and myosin fibers and no active contraction. Note that the maximal overlap occurs at 2.0 μm, which represents maximal tension. (Adapted from Carlson FD, Wilkie DR: Muscle Physiology. Englewood Cliffs, NJ, Prentice-Hall, 1974, with permission.)

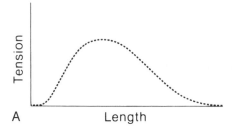

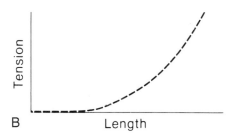

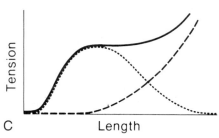

FIGURE 49-5. **A,** Length-tension curve of a single muscle fiber during active contraction. **B,** Length-tension curve of a resting whole muscle being passively stretched. This resting tension curve varies considerably for different muscles depending on the extent of the connective tissue framework with the muscle. **C,** The total tension developed by a whole muscle under tetanic stimulation *(solid line)* is the sum of the forces produced by active contraction and passive stretching. (Adapted from Carlson FD, Wilkie DR: Muscle Physiology. Englewood Cliffs, NJ, Prentice-Hall, 1974, with permission.)

MUSCLES AVAILABLE FOR FREE FUNCTIONAL MUSCLE TRANSFERS

Gracilis

The gracilis is the most suitable muscle for functional muscle transfers. The cutaneous flap, based on the gracilis muscle, is quite reliable in the proximal half of the muscle. A single constant perforator usually exits from the muscle at the level of the dominant vascular pedicle. In most patients, the medial thigh fat is very thick and creates a very thick, bulky cutaneous flap. In many coverage situations it is preferable to transfer the muscle without a skin paddle and apply a split-thickness skin graft directly to the muscle. The donor site scar is excellent because it lies in the upper half of the medial aspect of the thigh. For functioning muscle transfer, this is the preferred muscle for upper extremity reconstruction.

 Anatomy

The gracilis is a superficial muscle located on the medial aspect of the thigh.[17,23] It is a strap muscle that is broad proximally and tapers distally. Its tendon of origin is from the body of the pubis and the adjacent ramus of the ischium. The belly of the muscle lies just posterior to the adductor longus and sartorius muscles and ends in a well-defined tendon that inserts into the medial shaft of the tibia just below the tibial tubercle (Fig. 49-7). In the distal thigh the tendon lies just posterior to the sartorius tendon and anterior to the semitendinosus.

There are two or three vascular pedicles. The proximal pedicle is the dominant one and will reliably perfuse the muscle. It lies under the adductor longus and takes origin from the profunda femoris artery. This dominant proximal artery is 1 to 2 mm in diameter and 6 cm in length and enters the muscle 8 to 12 cm from the muscle's origin. There are two venae comitantes, each measuring 1.0 to 4.0 mm in diameter. In one of our cases, the superior pedicle was a double pedicle with two arteries and four venae comitantes and it appeared that the circulation proximal to the pedicle was dependent on one artery and the circulation distal to the pedicle dependent on the other artery.

There is a single motor nerve, a branch of the obturator, that is composed of two or three fascicles. The nerve enters the muscle immediately proximal to the vascular pedicle and lies under the adductor longus. With nerve stimulation the adult gracilis muscle will shorten more than 50% of its extended length for a functional contraction of 12 to 15 cm. In over 20 operative procedures, the fascicles of the motor nerve were teased apart and each fascicle separately stimulated. By using a nerve stimulator with frequency and voltage control, it was usually possible to separate the muscle into longitudinal, separately functioning neuromuscular territories. Ninety percent of the time a single fascicle will control the anterior 20% to 50% of the muscle, and the remaining portion of the muscle is controlled by the remaining fascicles. This functional separation is quite useful when the muscle is used to provide independent thumb and finger flexion (Fig. 49-8).[26]

Muscle fiber anatomy has been studied by Fish in our laboratory. In the proximal three fifths of the muscle belly, the muscle fibers are parallel in a strap muscle configuration. In the distal two fifths, the muscle fibers insert in a sequential fashion into the tendon located in the posterior border of the muscle. The posterior muscle fibers are shorter and insert distally; the longer anterior muscle fibers insert more proximally.

The function of this muscle is to flex, medially rotate, and adduct the thigh. Removal of the muscle results in no apparent functional deficit in the leg.

Technique of Preparing the Gracilis Muscle

The entire thigh and knee are prepped and draped free. The procedure is done with the surgeon standing on the side of the table opposite the donor leg with the knee and hip flexed and the hip externally rotated and abducted.[23]

A straight line is drawn between the tendon of the adductor longus and the tibial tubercle. The gracilis muscle lies posterior to this line.

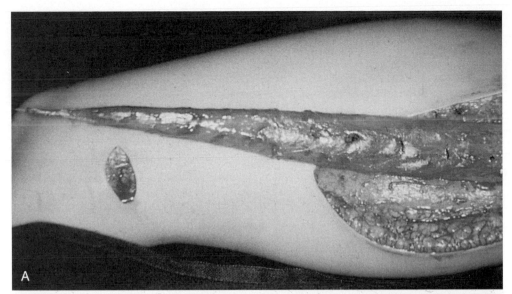

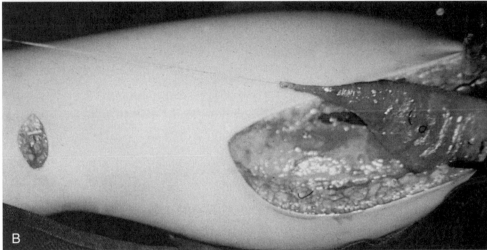

FIGURE 49-6. **A,** Gracilis muscle dissected free from the right thigh while still attached to its origin and neurovascular bundle. **B,** With stimulation of the muscle's motor nerve, the muscle shortens 15 cm (between 50% and 60% of its physiologic extended length).

If the surgeon intends to use the muscle without a cutaneous flap, an incision is made 2 cm posterior to the upper border of the gracilis in its proximal half of the thigh. The incision should be in the midline of the thigh where it is least visible. The dissection is carried through the deep muscular fascia, and the gracilis is separated from the surrounding musculature. The key landmark during the dissection is the easily palpable adductor longus tendon. The adductor longus is retracted superiorly to expose the neurovascular structures that enter the gracilis on the deep aspect of the anterior margin. Arterial and venous side branches to the adductor magnus and longus are divided to develop a long pedicle. Dissection is carried proximally and distally along the muscle. The secondary pedicles to the distal portion of the muscle are located on the anterior margin, and they are divided. The tendon is divided through a transverse incision in the distal thigh. The origin is then divided and the muscle is now dependent on its single vascular pedicle. It is left intact until the recipient site is prepared for transfer. The adequacy of muscle perfusion will be apparent from the color of the muscle. On occasion, the distal few centimeters of muscle will not be perfused and will need to be resected.

If a myocutaneous flap is required, the skin flap must be outlined over the proximal portion of the muscle. A per-forator is always present opposite the dominant pedicle. Our experience with free myocutaneous transfers has shown that the cutaneous portion of the flap is unreliable 15 to 20 cm distal to the pubic tubercle. The flap is quite reliable in the transverse dimension and can be taken wider than the underlying muscle. After the skin flap has been cut, the dermis is tacked anteriorly and posteriorly to the gracilis fascia. This will prevent shearing of the cutaneous flap and damage to the perforating vessels (Fig. 49-9).

Latissimus Dorsi

The latissimus dorsi is a very dependable muscle for free tissue transfers. It can be removed and produce only minimal weakness; however, those who use their arm vigorously in work or for activities such as tennis, skiing, or throwing notice a decrease in strength. The entire muscle or just a small portion of it can be transferred either with or without a cutaneous paddle.[29] The thoracodorsal artery provides a reliable, large-diameter, long pedicle. Frequently, only a small strip of the anterior muscle margin is transferred with a larger paddle of overlying skin to provide aesthetic skin coverage. However, if a large skin flap is removed and the donor site cannot be closed directly, the grafted donor site is

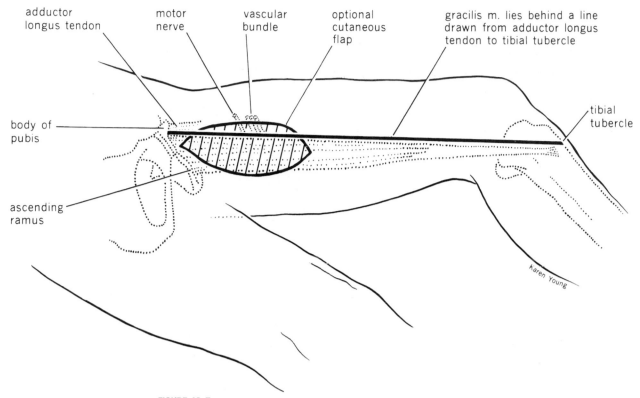

FIGURE 49-7. Anatomy of the gracilis muscle and cutaneous flap (see text).

cosmetically unsatisfactory. For direct closure, a maximal skin flap width of 10 cm is feasible. For larger soft tissue defects, the muscle is usually used as a muscle-only transfer, with a skin graft applied directly to the muscle. Because the thoracodorsal artery also supplies the serratus anterior, both of these muscles can be taken to cover two separate soft tissue defects. Alternatively, the latissimus dorsi can be split longitudinally into two separate, but attached muscle segments with the expectation of good vascularity in each segment.[42] The thoracodorsal artery usually splits at the vascular hilum into a superior transverse branch and an anterior inferior branch. The thoracodorsal artery enters the deep surface of the muscle 8 to 12 cm from its insertion, 2 cm from the anterior margin. The thoracodorsal artery is 1.5 to 3.0 mm in diameter. On its way to supply the latissimus dorsi muscle, it gives off a number of branches to the chest wall, including a branch to the serratus anterior. The two venae comitantes usually join to form a single vein as they approach the axilla. This vein varies in size from 3.0 to 5.0 mm. The nerve to the latissimus dorsi follows the course of the thoracodorsal artery. There are two or three fascicles with the cross-sectional area of approximately 2 mm. The nerve may be separated into two functionally separate divisions in 80% of the muscles. One division supplies the lateral portion of the muscle and the other, the medial portion.[1]

PREOPERATIVE PLANNING

The optimal muscle for the recipient area is selected on the basis of the anatomic and functional requirements of the recipient area and the patient's concern about the resulting functional and cosmetic defects (Table 49-2).

A "pure" motor nerve must be selected to provide good reinnervation. For replacement of finger long flexor musculature, the preferred motor nerves are the anterior interosseous nerve, branches of the median nerve that had innervated the superficialis muscle, or branches of the ulnar nerve that had innervated the flexor digitorum profundus. For the dorsal (extensor) aspect of the forearm, motor branches of the radial nerve are used. The motor component of the musculocutaneous nerve is used for biceps reconstruction, and the motor component of the axillary nerve is used for deltoid reconstruction. For triceps reconstruction, proximal branches of the radial nerve are used. It is important to be sure that there is a healthy, undamaged motor nerve available that has a cross-sectional area approximately equal to that of the motor nerve of the muscle to be transferred. Good muscle function cannot be expected without a technically sound microneural repair to an undamaged recipient motor nerve.

From the history and physical examination it is usually possible to determine which motor nerve branches in the upper extremity are likely to be present and undamaged. If there is significant doubt about the availability of a good motor nerve, the surgeon should carry out an exploratory operation and nerve biopsy to assess the status of the motor nerve branches before the muscle transfer. Neurohistologic examination will indicate the adequacy of the motor nerve branches for neurotization of the muscle.

The upper extremity is assessed for its ability to accept a free flap. A preoperative angiogram is required when the arterial pattern in the arm is not clear from the clinical assessment. Arterial anastomoses in the upper extremity may be end to end or end to side. In the proximal forearm, small branches such as the ulnar recurrent and anterior

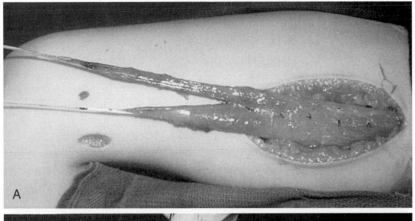

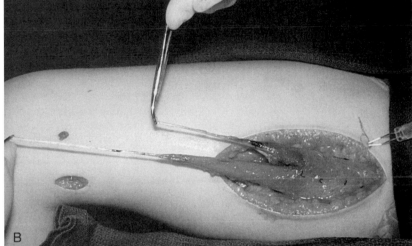

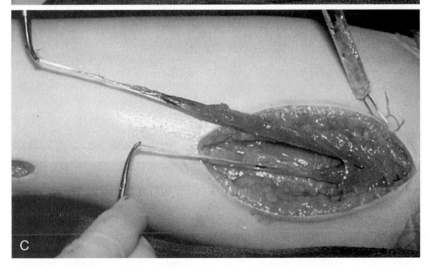

FIGURE 49-8. A, The distal muscle belly and attached portions of tendon of a gracilis muscle are split longitudinally. The location of the split is determined by stimulating each fascicle of the motor nerve and observing the portion of muscle that contracts. This allows the creation of two separately controlled neuromuscular units. **B,** Stimulation of one fascicle produces contraction of the anterior portion of the muscle *(top part of the picture)*. **C,** Stimulation of the remaining fascicles produces contraction of the posterior portion of the muscle *(bottom part of the picture)*.

interosseous arteries are available as end-to-end sources of arterial input. Both the radial and the ulnar arteries are available depending on the extent of injury and provide excellent vessels for end-to-side anastomoses. Within the palm the common digital arteries and the palmar arch are available. On the dorsum of the hand just proximal to the first web space is the radial artery in a very accessible location. This is often the location of choice for arterial repair in free tissue transfers to the digits and thumb. In the upper arm, end-to-side anastomoses are possible to the brachial or axillary artery. However, the thick wall in the vessels makes the repair more difficult than when using smaller vessels, which may be used for end-to-end anastomoses. Useful arteries in the upper arm are the thoracodorsal, anterior and posterior humeral circumflex, profunda brachii, and branches of the acromiothoracic. When the presence or condition of a suitable artery is unclear from the clinical examination, an arteriogram is required.

Either superficial or deep veins can be used for anastomoses. Superficial arm veins are more useful than superficial leg veins, which have a tendency to spasm. However, the superficial veins may have been damaged by

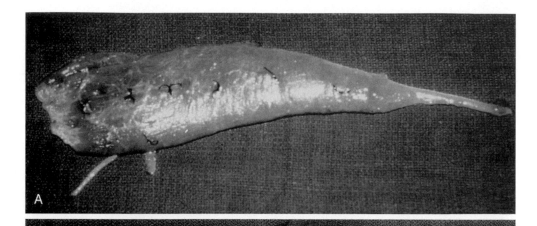

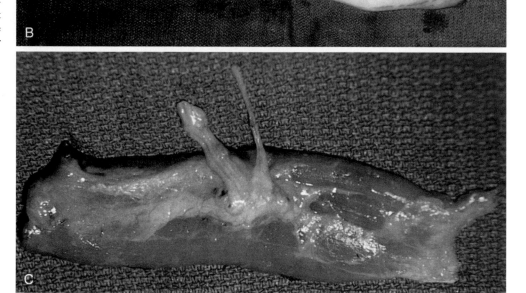

FIGURE 49-9. **A,** Superficial aspect of the gracilis muscle. The motor nerve enters diagonally at the lower left, and the vascular pedicle is adjacent to the nerve. **B,** A myocutaneous gracilis transfer with skin centered on the proximal "safe" portion of the muscle. Note the long length of available tendon. **C,** A 2 × 10-cm segment of the gracilis muscle centered on the neurovascular pedicle, suitable for coverage of small soft tissue defects.

Table 49-2
GUIDELINES FOR MUSCLE SELECTION

Suitable neurovascular anatomy

Adequate strength and range of muscle excursion

Suitable gross anatomy to fit the defect (muscle length, location of neurovascular bundle, and tendon availability)

Ability to be removed without leaving a significant functional or cosmetic donor defect

previous intravenous medication. In the upper arm, the deep veins and venae comitantes are particularly suitable for anastomoses.

In upper extremity transfers, the surgeon must be particularly careful that all factors affecting peripheral perfusion are being considered. Blood volume and pressure must be maintained and the patient warmed to support the peripheral as well as the core body temperature and to prevent peripheral vasospasm.

If local skin is not available for muscle coverage, a skin flap should be provided. This skin flap can be a local or distant flap that is usually applied before the muscle transfer, or it can be a cutaneous flap that is carried with the transferred muscle. Flap coverage must be available for the distal half of the muscle to allow muscle gliding and to cover the muscle insertion.

In our initial experience with the gracilis muscle we raised this as a myocutaneous flap to provide good skin coverage on the forearm. We found that the skin coverage over the gracilis was reliable for its proximal 40% but unreliable distal to this. However, the skin flap tended to be far too bulky for the patient's satisfaction, and we have stopped using this as a myocutaneous flap. Because the critical area for good skin coverage is the distal half of the forearm and the cutaneous flap will rarely reach this area reliably, other techniques should be provided to obtain good skin coverage under which the tendons can glide and, if necessary, neurolysis can be carried out. The proximal half of the muscle belly can be covered with a split-thickness skin graft if necessary. This will not affect the muscle's excursion. Skin flap coverage over the musculotendinous junction in the distal portion of the muscle is very important for tendon gliding. Local flaps from the forearm, developed by the insertion of tissue expanders, are tedious and require great care but may provide a useful solution. Occasionally, a distant flap such as an abdominal or groin flap or free tissue transfer will be used as a preliminary procedure to cover the distal half of the forearm.

MUSCLE TRANSFER FOR FINGER FLEXION

Indications

Microvascular muscle transfer is indicated when the finger flexor musculature is absent because of direct injury or loss through tumor excision. The most common injuries are trauma directly to the muscle and ischemic necrosis secondary to compartment syndrome. If the extensor musculature is intact, transfer of the extensor carpi radialis longus (ECRL) may be a preferred procedure because it is quicker and simpler and provides good functional recovery in a shorter time. However, our experience with gracilis transfer is that it provides greater excursion and strength than an ECRL transfer. Finger joint mobility, the presence of undamaged tendons in the hand, intrinsic muscle function, a mechanism for finger extension and wrist stabilization, good skin coverage in the distal forearm, and an undamaged motor nerve are important prerequisites for this transfer.

Preparation of the Forearm

The intended position of the muscle in the forearm is anticipated and the known location of the neurovascular hilum is matched to the expected position of the neurovascular structures in the forearm. The incision must allow good exposure of the neurovascular structures and flexor tendons and provide flap coverage of the tendon-muscle junction in the distal forearm. While one team is raising the muscle, the second team prepares the forearm. This prepares for the repair of all the structures that are involved in the transfer. For neurovascular structures, proximal-to-distal dissection going from undamaged tissue to damaged areas is safest. In a scarred forearm, this preparation requires meticulous dissection to prevent inadvertent damage to important structures. If exposure of the anterior interosseous artery or nerve is required, the pronator teres, if present, is temporarily separated from its insertion and preserved. The medial epicondyle and its surrounding fascia are exposed in anticipation of suturing the origin of the transferred muscle. The flexor digitorum profundus tendons are identified and their gliding capability is tested.

A two-team approach is used in all upper extremity reconstructions. Simultaneous preparation of the muscle and recipient area for the transfer results in decreased operating time.

Muscle Transfer

After the muscle's separation from the donor site it is left attached to the vascular pedicle to allow observation of the muscle's perfusion. This can be evaluated by observing the color of the muscle.[24]

The muscle is positioned in the arm so that the motor nerve repair can be done as close as possible to the muscle. Tacking sutures are placed between the muscle and its bed so that it will not move during neurovascular repair.

Important technical considerations in muscle transfer (for the upper extremity) include

- Revascularization
- Nerve repair
- Balanced profundus tendon fixation
- Positioning of the muscle at optimal tension
- Adequate flap coverage

Revascularization

While the muscle's origin is held to the medial epicondyle, the insertion is stretched toward the hand and relaxed to simulate finger extension and flexion. Movement of the pedicle is observed relative to the intended site of anastomosis to be sure that with muscle excursion the anastomosis will not be stretched.

Microvascular anastomosis depends on a technically good repair in a normal vessel. If a vessel is lying in an area of previous trauma, it must be used with caution. The vessel must be examined under the microscope and the wall of the vessel scrutinized for scarring, intimal dissection, or evidence of any other abnormality. Vessels that have been in a zone of inflammation and injury for a prolonged period acquire a whitish layer of visible scarring in the adventitia. These vessels are very prone to spasm when they are divided in preparation for anastomosis. A good spurt of blood from the cut artery must be present before doing the microvascular anastomosis. If the cut vessel tends to go into spasm, it must be resected back to a level where there is a good spurt. An end-to-side repair is more reliable if the repair needs to be carried out in a zone of injury because this technique decreases the chance of spasm. Venous return can be adequately handled by one venous anastomosis if the vein is larger than the artery or by anastomosis of two veins if they are on the small side. It is probably of no consequence whether the artery or the vein is repaired first, although our custom is to anastomose the vein first and then the artery. The muscle will become pink and bleed from all cut areas on completion of the arterial anastomosis. The distal few centimeters of the gracilis muscle will usually take 5 minutes or more before they completely "pink" up. Any distal musculature that does not pink up should be removed. Often a short portion of the distal muscle will be removed because the length of muscle is excessive. Because the gracilis tendon extends proximally into the muscle, the excess distal muscle can be removed and cut fibers reattached to the intramuscular portion of the tendon without affecting function.

Reinnervation

The motor nerve repair is placed as close as possible to the muscle's neurovascular hilum to minimize the duration of denervation. Because the gracilis motor nerve has at least

60% fatty connective tissue, a fascicular repair is done with 11-0 nylon to ensure good apposition of the fascicles.

Balanced Tendon Fixation

When a single muscle is used to provide finger flexion, all of the fingers should flex together to provide even contact with the object being gripped. The profundus tendons are sutured in side-to-side fashion to each other in a balanced position, with each digit slightly more flexed than the adjacent radial digit. The transferred tendon will then produce mass flexion of the fingers in a balanced grip position.

When the muscle is going to produce thumb as well as finger flexion, the flexor pollicis longus should be sutured to the finger flexors in a position that has some slack so that the fingers will begin to flex before the thumb moves. In this way, the thumb will come to rest on the radial side of the index and provide useful key pinch rather than flex into the palm. If the gracilis is going to be used for independent finger and thumb movements, the muscle must be split into two separate neuromuscular territories and innervated with two nerve branches that have separate function, preferably thumb and finger flexion functions.[24,26,27]

Muscle Positioning for Optimal Tension

The flexor digitorum profundus tendons are sutured into the distal portion of the muscle or its tendon at a tension that is designed to provide optimal grip strength, a full range of finger flexion, and good muscle balance with the intrinsic and extrinsic extensor musculature. If the extensor and intrinsic musculature is intact, the fingers will rest in a position of function when the muscle has been attached to the flexor digitorum profundus tendons.

We have developed a measuring technique that allows the muscle to be inserted at optimal tension. The technique is dependent on two assumptions: (1) a muscle's most powerful contraction begins near this maximal range of excursion, and (2) if a muscle is chosen whose normal physiologic range of excursion is equal to or greater than that required in the forearm, full range of finger movement will probably be produced.

The technique begins while the muscle is still in its normal site. The muscle is stretched to its maximal physiologic extension (e.g., full thigh abduction and knee extension for the gracilis), and markers are placed along the surface of the muscle every 5 cm (Fig. 49-10A). It can be assumed that the muscle can be safely stretched to this resting, extended length when it is transferred. When the muscle is revascularized and the origin attached to the common flexor origin, the muscle is stretched distally so that the markers are spaced 5 cm apart when the fingers and wrist are fully extended (see Fig. 49-10B). In this position of maximal finger extension and muscle stretch, the flexor tendon stumps are placed beside the distal portion of the transferred muscle and adjacent positions are marked on the flexor tendons and on the tension of the transferred muscle. This marks the point at which the tendon-to-tendon repair should be done. With the wrist and fingers in flexion, tendon-to-tendon muscle fixation is accomplished without tension on the transferred muscle. The profundus tendons to all four fingers are woven into the transferred muscle or its tendon at the position marked. In a muscle that does not have a tendinous portion such as the pectoralis major or the

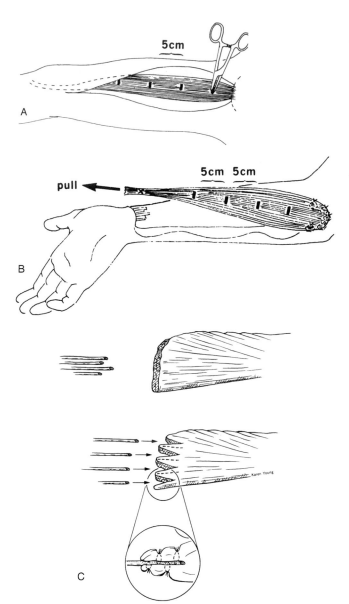

FIGURE 49-10. **A,** Technique of creating optimal tension in the transplanted muscle. The gracilis is stretched to its physiologic maximal extended length by abducting the thigh and extending the knee. Suture markers are applied every 5 cm on the surface of the muscle. **B,** The fingers and wrist are placed in full passive extension and the gracilis is stretched distally until the suture markers are 5 cm apart. Marks are then placed opposite each other on the profundus tendons and the gracilis tendon to locate the points at which the tendons should be sutured together. **C,** Technique used to attach four profundus tendons to the muscle termination (origin) of the pectoralis or latissimus dorsi muscle.

latissimus dorsi, the profundus tendons are inserted into the muscle as shown in Figure 49-10C. This measuring and marking procedure ensures that the muscle will allow full finger and wrist extension and provide a full range of finger flexion within the most powerful range of excursion of the muscle. This technique is used in all muscle transfers. It is particularly valuable if the extensor musculature is not intact.

Flap Coverage

Skin flap coverage must be obtained over the musculotendinous junction and the distal portion of the muscle. This may be carried out with a local flap from the forearm, which can be developed by the insertion of tissue expanders before muscle transfer. If a myocutaneous flap is chosen, it is usually too bulky but it does provide a cutaneous portion that acts as an indicator of the vascularity of the underlying muscle. Occasionally, a distal flap such as an abdominal or groin flap will be used to cover the forearm. A split-thickness skin graft can be applied directly to the proximal half of the muscle without affecting its function and with good aesthetic effect.

Postoperative Management

If a thrombosis does occur and is recognized, it is necessary to return the patient to the operating room, revise the anastomosis, and obtain an intact circulation within 3 to 4 hours or severe ischemic damage to the muscle can be expected. However, it is unlikely that the diagnosis of thrombosis can be made quickly enough to enable such a rapid revision to be accomplished. It is thus imperative that the vascular anastomoses be done as nearly perfect as technically possible. If postoperative thrombosis is recognized, it is preferable to replace the muscle with another one rather than revascularize a muscle that has sustained a damaging period of 4 or more hours of ischemia. Our preferred monitoring technique is direct observation of a small area of exposed muscle. Usually this is possible because the proximal muscle belly has been covered with a skin graft.

The most important aspect of management in the immediate postoperative period is to maintain a normal circulation with good peripheral perfusion. An adequate volume of intravenous fluids is given, and urine output is monitored. The wrist and fingers are pointed in moderate flexion to relax the junction between the flexor tendons and the transferred muscle. Inasmuch as the muscle is flaccid because of denervation, the amount of tension is not excessive for the tendon repairs.

A program of passive stretching of the wrist and fingers is begun 3 weeks postoperatively. The program is designed to obtain full passive muscle extension and overcome any tendency to myotonic contracture. Also, passive stretching improves tissue gliding at the muscle-tendon junction in anticipation of the development of reinnervation and active contraction. This program has resulted in a low incidence of tendon adhesions requiring subsequent tenolysis. After the development of spontaneous contraction of the muscle, the patient is encouraged to attempt active flexion frequently throughout the day. When a good range of movement develops, a program of graduated resisted grip exercises is begun and continued until maximal function is obtained.

We do not believe that electrical muscle stimulation is helpful for the development of a good functional result. However, active use of the muscle once innervation occurs is extremely important, and patients who follow a regular exercise program will have the best functional result. The exercise program should be pursued for at least 1 year after the development of a useful range of muscle movement. Incorporation of the exercise program into activities of daily living and work-stimulated activities is important to maintain the patient's level of interest and enthusiasm and to provide a variety of resisted activities.

MUSCLE TRANSFER FOR FINGER EXTENSION

Indications

Microneurovascular muscle transfer is a complex procedure that should not be considered for finger extension unless tendon transfers are not available. It is common that a patient who has sustained a severe extensor compartment injury will also have a flexor compartment injury. This double injury may preclude tendon transfers from the flexor side. Four of our patients had severe flexor and extensor compartment injuries and required two microneurovascular muscle transfers, one for finger flexion and one for finger extension. In this situation, wrist stabilization must be carried out. This can be done by tenodesis of the ECRL and extensor carpi ulnaris tendons to the radius. This will provide a stable wrist for finger flexion. Tenodesis is not usually required to facilitate finger extension. Alternatively, wrist fusion will give a stable base for finger flexion.

The gracilis muscle is an excellent choice to provide finger and thumb extension. It has adequate excursion and strength and is a good anatomic fit to the extensor side. Additional procedures may be necessary if intrinsic function is not present because the provision of long extensor function in the absence of intrinsic function will produce a clawing type of hand. A full range of finger extension and thumb abduction and extension should be possible with this transfer.

Preparation of the Forearm

The most critical decisions involve selection of the motor nerve and vessels for repair in the recipient site. The posterior interosseous nerve is the nerve of choice for finger extension. The most appropriate site to identify and carry out the nerve coaptation is after the nerve has passed through the supinator. At this point nerve fibers supply finger extension as well as thumb extension and abduction. Some fibers also supply the extensor carpi ulnaris, which is not a desirable innervation for this transfer. If the posterior interosseous nerve is identified proximally before it passes through the supinator, it may be difficult to determine which portions of the nerve pass to the finger extensors and delineate them from branches to the wrist extensors. It is particularly useful to identify the nerve distal to the supinator if there are remnants of finger extensor muscles remaining. It is then possible to select appropriate portions of the nerve-by-nerve stimulation.

Arterial repair may be awkward. The arteries on the extensor aspect of the forearm are usually inadequate for anastomoses. We have used the radial artery as an end-to-side repair or the radial recurrent branch of the radial artery. Routing of the gracilis artery to the radial artery can be either under or over the extensor carpi radialis brevis and longus and the brachioradialis. The deep location is preferred because it is better protected than when lying on the surface. Nevertheless, there is a risk of compression if an adequate-size tunnel is not provided. A superficial or deep vein in the forearm is usually used for venous outflow.

Preparation of the forearm involves identification and preparation of the artery, vein, motor nerve, and all tendons for insertion. In a scarred forearm, preparation is easiest when working in a proximal-to-distal direction along the damaged structures and going from normal to abnormal tissue.

Muscle Transfer

Before separation of the muscle from the forearm, marks are placed at 5-cm intervals when the muscle is in its maximal extended position as described for the flexor transfer.

After transfer to the arm, the muscle is loosely sutured in its expected location and routing of the vascular pedicle is carefully planned so that there will be no compression, kinking, or other obstruction (Fig. 49-11). The origin of the muscle is sutured to the lateral epicondyle and common extensor fascia. The tendon of the gracilis is pulled distally until suitable functional tension has been achieved and the position of the vascular pedicle is evaluated. After anastomosis of the artery and vein to recipient vessels in the forearm, the motor nerve is coapted to the selected portion of the posterior interosseous nerve.

Usually the muscle will provide finger extension and also abduct and extend the thumb. The extensor digitorum communis (EDC) tendons for all four fingers are first woven together so that they extend all fingers equally and symmetrically. The extensor pollicis longus (EPL) tendon is rerouted so that it will both abduct and extend the thumb. This involves withdrawing the tendon at the level of the thumb metacarpophalangeal joint and joining and tunneling it along the radial aspect of the first metacarpal. The soft tissues will form a constraining pulley-like system that will keep the tendon in position. Traction on the end of the tendon will produce both thumb extension and abduction of the first metacarpal if properly rerouted.

After revascularization and secure fixation of the origin, the gracilis muscle is stretched distally until the markers are spaced 5 cm apart, which is its maximal extended length. The wrist and fingers are placed in maximal flexion. With the fingers and hand held in this position and the muscle stretched out to its maximal extended length, the extensor tendons and the gracilis tendon are marked on adjacent surfaces to indicate the point of desired tendon repair. With the wrist and fingers in extension, tendon-to-tendon repairs are then done between the gracilis tendon and the mass of EDC tendons. The EPL tendon is then woven into this mass. The tension of the EPL can be tested by manual traction on the gracilis tendon and evaluation of all fingers and the thumb for balanced extension. The fingers should sit in the position of function or in a slightly extended position after tendon repair.

It is acceptable to skin graft the proximal half of the muscle belly. This will not inhibit movement of the fingers and, aesthetically, is preferable to the bulky cutaneous flap that can come with the gracilis. However, the distal half of the muscle belly and extensor tendon repairs must be covered by good skin flap coverage to allow gliding of the muscle-tendon unit.

Postoperative Management

The wrist is splinted in extension for 10 to 14 days. A program of active and passive wrist, finger, and thumb exercises is then begun. The purpose of these exercises is to prevent joint stiffness and finger and gracilis tendon adhesions. Once innervation has provided a useful range of finger extension, an exercise program against resistance is commenced. This usually begins 6 or more months after surgery.

Clinical Experience with Muscle Transfers to the Forearm

The long finger flexors have been reconstructed in 14 patients, long finger flexors and extensors in 4 patients, and the long finger extensors alone in 1 patient. The etiology of muscle loss in this group included Volkmann's ischemic contracture in 11, traumatic muscle loss in 6, electrical burn injury in 1, and mixed motor paralysis after excision of an astrocytoma (C2 to T1) at a young age.

Pretransfer Abnormalities and Operative Procedures

The typical free functioning muscle transfer patient usually has multiple pretransfer abnormalities such as nerve loss, joint contractures, and tendon adhesions. As such, this group of patients often requires pretransfer procedures to prepare the arm for free muscle transfer. Nerve grafting was the most commonly performed procedure.

Technical Aspects

Muscle transfer operative data are presented in Table 49-3. The gracilis muscle was most commonly used to restore function in both the upper and lower arm groups. The pectoralis major and latissimus dorsi were used in three early cases. The gracilis was inserted into the flexor digitorum profundus alone in 13 of 19 cases and into the flexor digitorum profundus and the flexor pollicis longus in 6. The gracilis was inserted into the EDC and EPL in all cases of extensor reconstruction.

Secondary Reconstruction

The long finger flexor reconstruction group required the most secondary procedures. Seven of 19 patients required secondary procedures, including tenotomy, capsulotomy, tendon transfer, tenolysis, digital fusion, and metacarpophalangeal capsulodeses.

Postoperative Results

More than half of patients were able to close their fist completely to touch the proximal area of the palm (Fig. 49-12). Tip-to-distal palmar crease distances ranged from 0.5 to 4 cm. Grip strength ranged from 14% to 81%, with overall mean grip strength of 38.1% when compared with the opposite normal extremity. Pinch strength ranged from 0% to 70%, with overall mean pinch strength of 37.8% when compared with the normal extremity. The severity of pretransfer upper extremity injury appears to be a significant factor affecting the outcome. Two major factors that may decrease the functional usefulness of the hand are the absence of intact intrinsic function and the absence of good supination and pronation. Protective sensation was present in all patients and did not appear to be a factor limiting functionality.

Improved motor strength (or grip) was noted in male patients who had extensive weight training during their rehabilitation period and in those patients who worked as

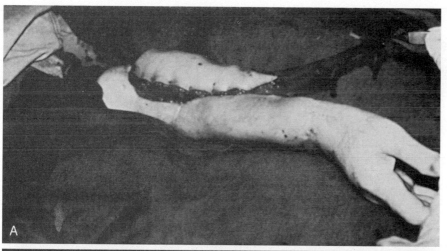

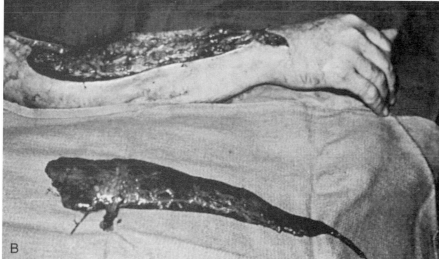

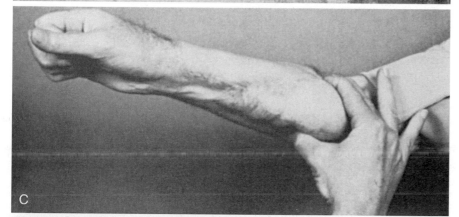

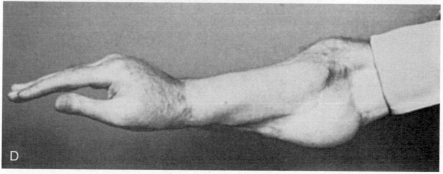

FIGURE 49-11. A patient with loss of flexor and extensor musculature secondary to a crush injury of the forearm. **A,** A gracilis myocutaneous flap to the flexor digitorum profundus was used to restore flexion. **B,** A second gracilis muscle transplantation (done 1 year later), before insertion as a replacement for the extensor digitorum communis, extensor pollicis longus, and abductor pollicis longus. **C,** Active flexion. The examiner's fingers demonstrate the bulk of the gracilis muscle transferred to the flexors (innervation by the anterior interosseous nerve). **D,** Active extension through the second gracilis transplant innervated by the radial nerve.

Table 49-3
OPERATIVE DATA: MUSCLES TRANSFERRED, RECIPIENT NERVE, AND VESSELS

Reconstruction	Muscle	No.	Recipient Motor Nerve	No.	Recipient Artery	No.	Recipient Vein	No.
Deltoid	Gracilis	8/8	Axillary	7/8	Deltoid	2/8	Vena comitans	5/8
					Thoracodorsal	3/8	Cephalic	2/8
					Posterior humeral	1/8	Subcutaneous	1/8
					Circumflex scapular	1/8		
			Musculocutaneous	1/8	Brachial	1/8		
Biceps	Gracilis	6/6	Musculocutaneous	2/6	Thoracodorsal	2/6	Vena comitans	2/4
			Intercostal	4/6	Branch of axillary	1/6	Cephalic	1/4
					Deltoid	1/6	Thoracodorsal	1/4
					Posterior circumflex	1/6		
					Subclavian	1/6		
Triceps	Gracilis	1/1	Axillary	1/1	Circumflex humeral	1/1	Vena comitans	1/1
Flexors	Gracilis	13/14	Anterior interosseous	14/14	Radial	7/14	Vena comitans	9/14
	Pectoralis major	1/14			Brachial	3/14	Subcutaneous	4/14
					Anterior interosseous	2/14	Cephalic	1/14
					Ulnar	2/14		
Flexors and extensors	Gracilis and gracilis	2/4	Anterior interosseous Posterior interosseous	4/4	Radial	3/4	Vena comitans	2/4
	Latissimus dorsi and gracilis	1/4	Anterior interosseous Posterior interosseous		Ulnar recurrent	1/4	Subcutaneous	2/4
	Pectoralis major and gracilis	1/4	Anterior interosseous Posterior interosseous					
Extensors	Gracilis	1/1	Posterior interosseous	1/1	Radial recurrent	1/1	Subcutaneous	1/1

heavy laborers. Some patients who used their upper extremity in heavy work described fatigue in the transfer muscle.

MUSCLE TRANSFER FOR BICEPS RECONSTRUCTION

Indications

The indications to perform muscle transfer for biceps reconstruction are primarily for patients who lack elbow flexion and for whom local transfers are not available. Useful local transfers for elbow flexion include the latissimus dorsi and the pectoralis major. The transfers are simpler than microneurovascular muscle transfers. They are fairly reliable and provide an early return of function.

Donor Nerves

Of the donor nerves available for biceps reconstruction, the musculocutaneous nerve is usually used in cases in which biceps and brachialis muscle loss has occurred. More commonly, loss of biceps function is being reconstructed in patients with brachial plexus lesions. As such, the availability of a donor nerve can be severely restricted. The most suitable donor in such cases continues to be the intercostal nerves. There is a long history of using the intercostals for brachial plexus reconstruction with good results.

Intercostal Nerves

Typically, the second to fourth intercostal nerves are used as donor nerves for biceps reconstruction. In our experience, we have found these intercostal nerves best suited in terms of anatomic position for direct coaptation to the nerve to the gracilis.

The intercostal nerves travel in the intercostal space inferior to the intercostal artery and vein. The nerves run between the intercostalis intimi and the internal intercostal muscles. Each nerve divides into a motor branch, a lateral sensory branch to the chest wall, and a collateral branch that travels along the upper border of the rib below. Each intercostal nerve ends in anterior cutaneous branches that supply the anterior chest or abdomen. The motor branch is usually deep to the sensory branch and can be followed beyond the midclavicular line. There can be up to three nerve branches in the intercostal space.

Motor Axon Counts

The intercostal nerves contain between 1200 and 1300 myelinated fibers.[7,13,31]

Surgical Exposure/Harvesting

We use an anterior thoracic exposure to facilitate direct suture of the intercostal nerves to the gracilis recipient nerve. A semicircular incision is extended from the usual

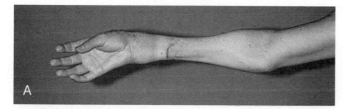

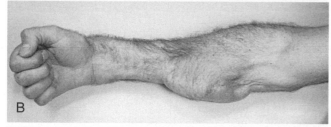

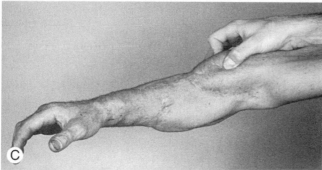

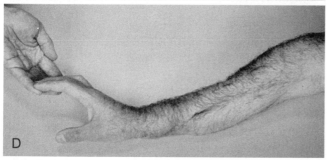

FIGURE 49-12. A, Preoperative view of the right forearm of a 22-year-old man who sustained a crushing injury with loss of all flexor and extensor forearm musculature except for the extensor carpi radialis longus and the brachioradialis muscles. **B,** Flexion of the fingers and thumb after pectoralis major transplantation to motor the flexor digitorum profundus and the flexor pollicis longus. Note the bulging muscle contraction in the proximal forearm. Grip strength is 53 lb. **C,** Extension of the fingers and thumb is provided by a gracilis muscle transplantation to the dorsum of the forearm. Adhesions at the wrist prevent full finger extension. **D,** Relaxation of the pectoralis muscle allows full passive extension of the wrist and fingers.

upper arm incision at the anterior border of the axilla onto the chest wall (Fig. 49-13). The incision is placed so that access to the second to fourth intercostal nerves is possible up to the midclavicular line. The superficial muscular layer in the intercostal space is incised near the lower border of the rib, and then dissection is carried deeper until the nerve is identified. The nerve may be located between the intercostalis intimi and the internal intercostal muscles. The nerve may lie in close relationship to the parietal pleura. Care must be taken not to perforate the pleura during dissection. Intercostal nerves 2 to 4 may be directly coapted to

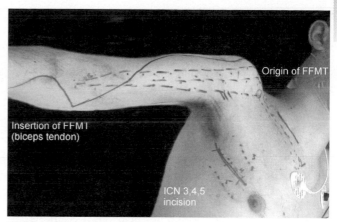

FIGURE 49-13. Intraoperative view of all surgical markings during a planned free muscle transfer for biceps reconstruction.

the gracilis recipient nerve in the upper arm without a nerve graft.

Contraindications

Phrenic nerve palsy is a relative contraindication to using the intercostal nerves for biceps reconstruction with free muscle transfer. Intercostal nerves can be used even when the ribs have been fractured but dissection may be difficult.

Intercostal nerves must not be used when the patient suffers from Brown-Séquard syndrome because they are nonfunctional. Brown-Séquard syndrome is present in 5% of complete palsy cases.[3]

Preparation of the Arm

The recipient area is prepared as described for the forearm, with preparation of the vessels, nerves, and sites of origin and insertion. The skin flaps should be elevated in such a way that closure of skin flaps can be provided to cover at least the distal half of the muscle belly and the area of tendon coaptation so that there will be good gliding.

The recipient area is evaluated for the repair of all neurovascular structures. For elbow flexion reconstruction, vessels are usually readily available either through direct anastomosis to the brachial artery or to branches such as the profunda brachii, the humeral circumflex arteries, and the ulnar recurrent artery. Venae comitantes are usually available. The acromion and distal end of the clavicle are prepared for attachment of the origin of the muscle. This attachment can be provided by sutures placed through the thick periosteum and scar tissue present or by anchors placed in the bone. The biceps tendon is prepared for attachment of the gracilis tendon.

The gracilis muscle is best reinnervated with the motor portion of the musculocutaneous nerve. Approximately 50% of the cross-sectional area of the musculocutaneous nerve is sensory. This nerve is a particularly large one, and it would not be possible to coapt the gracilis motor nerve to the entire nerve in the hope that sufficient motor branches will be picked up. It is necessary to identify the motor component of the musculocutaneous nerve to obtain good innervation. This can be done by identification of branches that lead to remnants of the biceps and brachialis. With total muscle loss this is not possible. In this situation, the technique of awake nerve stimulation or histochemical staining is very helpful.

Awake Nerve Stimulation

Awake nerve stimulation can be used to identify the sensory and motor components of a mixed nerve. With the patient awake, the sensory fascicles of a mixed nerve are stimulated and the patient will identify discomfort in the region of the innervations of the sensory fascicles. When the motor portion of a mixed nerve is stimulated, the patient will experience a deep, discomfort-type sensation localized to the region of the muscle belly that the nerve used to supply. This is a technically demanding procedure requiring the use of a microbipolar electrical probe with a nerve stimulator that has variable frequency and voltage controls. The surgical procedure involves separating the groups of fascicles in the nerve under general anesthesia and then awakening the patient. For the musculocutaneous nerve there will usually be four groups of fascicles. Each group of fascicles should be labeled with fine sutures so that it can be identified later.

With the patient awake after anesthetic reversal, each group of fascicles is stimulated with the microbipolar stimulator at variable voltages. The voltage is adjusted throughout the testing procedure in keeping with the patient's response and to prevent undue discomfort. The patient is asked to identify the presence of sensation, the type of feeling produced, and the anatomic location of the feeling and whether the feeling is deep or on the surface. Sensory fascicles produce a sense of discomfort, often burning, that is localized to the skin of the area usually supplied by the nerve. The motor fascicles, when stimulated, produce a deeper aching sensation that is anatomically localized by the patient to the region of the muscle belly that the nerve used to supply.

Muscle Transfer

For biceps reconstruction, the muscle is loosely tacked in the appropriate position by attaching the gracilis origin to the acromion and lateral portion of the clavicle. The muscle is then stretched distally until the previously placed markers are 5 cm apart, and the location of the vascular pedicle and nerve is evaluated. The vessel anastomoses and nerve coaptation are then done. The nerve coaptation is performed with the repair as close as possible to the muscle belly.

Insertion of the gracilis tendon into remnants of the biceps tendon is done at tension sufficient to produce the most effective muscle function. This is carried out by extending the elbow and the shoulder and then stretching the gracilis muscle until the markers are 5 cm apart. Adjacent points on the biceps tendon and the gracilis tendon are marked, and then the elbow is flexed and the repairs carried out at the point of the marks with an interweaving suture technique.

Postoperative Management

The elbow is placed in flexion and a Velpeau dressing is applied to the arm after closure of the wound; this position is maintained with a sling for approximately 3 weeks. A gentle stretching program involving active and passive exercises is carried out to obtain elbow extension and shoulder extension. Once reinnervation has occurred, a daily exercise program is begun. When the intercostal nerves are used, initially the patient will activate the transfer by taking a deep breath. However with the passage of time the patient will develop the ability to activate the muscle by thinking about flexing the elbow rather than breathing. The muscle is strengthened by an exercise program using weights held in the hand while flexing the elbow.

Clinical Experience

Preoperative Assessment

Biceps function has been reconstructed in six patients. In this group, absent elbow flexion was due to musculocutaneous nerve loss (two cases), muscle loss (one case), polio (one case), and brachial plexus injury (two cases). Brachialis function was absent in all cases. The hand was abnormal in three patients. One patient had only partial right intrinsic hand function and required a wrist tenodesis (ECRB to the radius) and exploration of the right brachial plexus at the time of muscle transfer. The second patient required a tendon transfer to restore active middle finger extension. The third patient had a C8 to T1 root avulsion injury and flail arm.

Postoperative Results

Three of the six patients who underwent biceps reconstructions had full active elbow flexion (M4) and were able to flex their elbows with an average weight of 5 kg held in the hand. One patient had only palpable contraction of her biceps. One patient was only 1 month post transfer. There were no cases of elbow joint flexion deformity (Fig. 49-14).

MUSCLE TRANSFER FOR TRICEPS RECONSTRUCTION

The surgical technique for muscle transfer to replace the triceps is similar to that for biceps reconstruction except that the gracilis muscle is attached to the lateral aspect of the scapula, usually in the region of the glenoid fossa, and is inserted into remnants of the triceps tendon or directly into the olecranon itself. Innervation is through branches of the radial nerve, and revascularization is into any available vessels in the area or directly to the brachial artery and axillary vein.

The only patient who underwent triceps reconstruction was able to extend his elbow fully with a force of M4.

MUSCLE TRANSFER FOR DELTOID RECONSTRUCTION

Indications

Deltoid reconstruction by muscle transfer has been successfully used to provide shoulder flexion and abduction.

Many patients who have had a complete loss of deltoid function, either through axillary nerve injury or through actual loss of the muscle itself, will still be able to abduct and flex the shoulder by using the supraspinatus muscle and secondary shoulder muscles, including the pectoralis major, biceps, and coracobrachialis. However, this ability is variable, and some patients will have very limited ability to flex the shoulder. Loss of shoulder flexion is a major functional deficit. Without shoulder flexion it is not possible to position

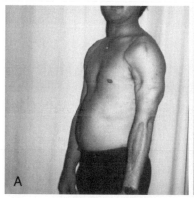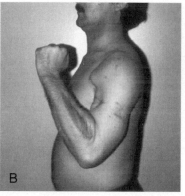

FIGURE 49-14. A, Postoperative view of patient who sustained a crushing injury to his left arm with loss of the biceps and brachialis. **B,** Flexion of the elbow to 120 degrees after gracilis transfer using the motor component of the musculocutaneous nerve. The patient can flex to 120 degrees while holding a 7.5-kg weight in his hand.

the hand in front of the body, which is required for many hand functions.

Preparation of the Upper Arm

The most critical structure to be evaluated will usually be the motor nerve. The axillary nerve is a mixed nerve that combines motor and sensory portions and it will be necessary to identify the motor portions. This can be done by using awake nerve stimulation as previously described for biceps reconstruction. In patients who have long-standing axillary nerve paralysis, secondary to shoulder dislocation, the nerve will be found to be ruptured with a large neuroma present. For revascularization, the thoracodorsal artery is particularly useful because a long pedicle can be developed and brought to the muscle without difficulty. The venae comitantes are available for venous outflow.

The incision is planned to allow access to all structures to be repaired. The acromion and distal end of the clavicle are used for the origin of the muscle, and the insertion is usually into the humerus directly or remnants of the deltoid insertion on the anterior portion of the humerus.

To identify the axillary nerve, the tendon of insertion of the pectoralis major muscle can be divided. This should be divided 1 cm from the humerus so that suture repair of the tendon can be carried out later. This allows an anterior approach to the posterior cord and axillary nerve.

Muscle Transfer

The muscle is loosely sutured in position with the origin firmly fixed to the acromion and clavicle by sutures or anchors. After anastomosis of the artery and the vein, the motor nerve is coapted. The muscle is then stretched until the marks are 5 cm apart, the shoulder is extended, and the position of the gracilis tendon is noted on the humerus. This point on the tendon will be the point at which fixation to bone should be accomplished. A hole can be drilled through the humerus and the tendon passed through it and back on itself to be woven into itself. Usually a small portion of the distal part of the muscle will need to be removed to allow good fixation. If the distal portion of the muscle is removed, the cut muscle ends should be reattached to the remaining intramuscular portion of the tendon. As in all microvascular transfers, skin closure should be done with care to ensure that pedicle kinking or compression does not occur.

Postoperative Management

The arm is placed in a Velpeau dressing after surgery with the elbow in flexion and kept in this position with a sling for 3 weeks. A muscle-stretching program is then begun to recover full active and passive shoulder motion. Once reinnervation has occurred, a resisted exercise program is started to build muscle strength.

Clinical Experience

Preoperative and Technical Aspects

The anterior deltoid has been reconstructed for shoulder flexion in eight patients (Fig. 49-15). The etiology of muscle loss was related to tumor resection in three, late recognition of axillary nerve avulsion secondary to shoulder dislocation in four, and idiopathic isolated deltoid paralysis in one. Preoperatively, all eight patients had atrophy or absence of the deltoid, weak shoulder flexion, and decreased sensation in the distribution of the axillary nerve. The supraspinatus muscle and secondary flexors of the arm were normal in each patient but provided only weak shoulder flexion. All patients in this group lacked active shoulder flexion above the horizontal plane and were unable to stabilize their flexed shoulder in space. Four of the eight patients had chronic subluxation of the glenohumeral joint and complained of shoulder pain before muscle transfer. In all patients, the remaining upper extremity was normal. The decision to reconstruct shoulder flexion was based on the need to flex the arm to and above the horizontal plane. The tendon of the gracilis muscle was directly sutured to the insertion remnant of the deltoid in five cases, and in three cases the tendon was passed through a hole in the humerus. To identify motor fascicles, awake nerve stimulation was used in all deltoid reconstructions in all 7 cases where the axillary nerve was used. The gracilis was reinnervated with the branch of the musculocutaneous nerve supplying the brachialis muscle in one case. The recipient artery and veins used are listed in Table 49-3.

Results

One patient had no active muscle contraction. Seven patients had useful flexion of the shoulder from 60 to 170 degrees and could maintain the humerus in front of the body. Before surgery, four of the eight patients complained of chronic shoulder pain, probably caused by chronic subluxation of

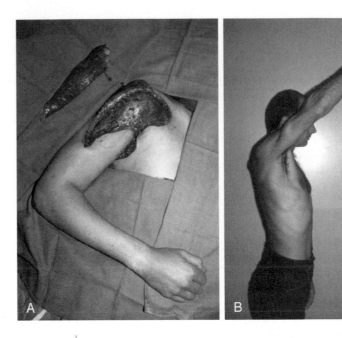

FIGURE 49-15. A, Intraoperative view of a patient who sustained rupture of the axillary nerve secondary to dislocation of the shoulder. The gracilis muscle is transferred to the anterolateral aspect of the shoulder. **B,** The patient can flex his shoulder to 140 degrees after gracilis transfer.

the glenohumeral joint secondary to deltoid paralysis. All four patients noted a significant decrease in shoulder pain after muscle transfer. This was probably due to suspensory function of the gracilis.

CORTICAL PLASTICITY AND MOTOR RELEARNING

We now know that neuromuscular injuries have a profound effect on the human brain. The sensorimotor cortex shows changes after neuromuscular injury, repair, and rehabilitation. Twenty years ago, we thought differently: adult cortical maps were believed to be static. That view has since been replaced by the concept of cortical plasticity, which asserts that the human cortex can change and adapt in response to new conditions and experiences. It is now clear that cortical plasticity occurs in the primary motor (M1) and sensory (S1) cortex in response to a variety of experiences, from learning a new piano piece to losing a leg in an accident. Plasticity contributes in some still-mysterious way to patients' abilities to acquire and use newly reconstructed movements. A better understanding of the mechanisms underlying cortical plasticity holds with it the possibility of establishing more effective recovery strategies after neuromuscular injury in humans.

Research in primates and humans has confirmed that the cortex has the capacity for adaptive and maladaptive change after amputation, deafferentation, and central lesions. Adaptive brain changes in cortical representations have been observed in association with motor skill learning[20,33,35,36] and the practice of basic movements.[8] For our purposes, perhaps it is even more important that adaptive changes in the adult human M1 are now seen as occurring in response to nerve transection, repetitive stimulation, focal cortical lesions, and the practice of object retrieval tasks.[11,12,18,32,34,39] M1 can preferentially allocate an area to represent the particular motor output sources that are proportionally most used.

Animal and human studies emphasize several different entities leading to adaptive or maladaptive brain changes, including amputation and deafferentation, motor skills training, and central lesions. Amputation studies have shown the capacity of surviving motor and sensory representations to "invade" a deafferented zone.[14,30,37,38]

It is well-known that a large region of the sensorimotor cortex is dedicated to the hand and upper extremity. Our group has been studying the cortical changes that occur in a variety of upper extremity conditions, including thumb amputation and toe transfers,[22] upper extremity paralysis reconstruction with free functioning muscle transfer,[5] and, more recently, peripheral nerve lesions. In our study of free muscle transfer patients, transcranial magnetic stimulation (TMS) was used to study nine patients who had motor function restored using a free functioning muscle transfer. (One patient was also studied with functional magnetic resonance imaging [fMRI]). TMS showed that the motor threshold and short interval intracortical inhibition were reduced on the transplanted side while at rest whereas they were not reduced during muscle activation. The difference in motor threshold decreased as time passed following the surgery. Mapping of the cortex with TMS showed no difference in the location and size of the representation of the reconstructed muscle in the motor cortex compared with the intact side or to normal subjects. One patient had a biceps reconstruction by free muscle transfer innervated by the intercostal nerves. Both TMS mapping and fMRI showed that by 6 months the upper limb area of the cortex now controlled biceps function rather than the trunk area of the motor cortex.

Our study demonstrated the existence of plasticity in cortical areas that projected to functionally relevant muscles. We learned that changes in the neuronal level are not necessarily accompanied by changes in motor representation. Brain reorganization may involve multiple processes that are mediated by different mechanisms, and this reorganization continues to evolve long after the initial injury.

Finally, and most importantly, we can now postulate that central nervous system plasticity after neuromuscular injury may have functional relevance.

Advances in our understanding of the mechanisms underlying cortical plasticity promise to help us establish effective recovery strategies after neuromuscular injury in humans. The modulation of cortical excitability may be a promising means of facilitating plasticity and thereby improving final functional outcome in patients undergoing reconstructive microsurgery.

CRITICAL POINTS: FUNCTIONING MUSCLE TRANSFER TO THE EXTREMITIES

INDICATIONS

- Severe injuries with loss of key muscles or muscle groups
- No simpler method such as a tendon transfer is available.

MUSCLE SELECTION

- Muscle must fit the recipient area and have a good anatomic match for the origin, insertion, and neuromuscular structures.
- Muscles that have been used include the gracilis, latissimus dorsi, and the tensor fascia lata.

AREAS OF APPLICATION

- Long finger flexors
- Long finger extensors
- Elbow flexion
- Elbow extension
- Shoulder flexion

TECHNICAL POINTS

- Revascularization
- Nerve repair
- Balanced tendon attachment if multiple tendons are being motored by one muscle transfer
- Location of optimum tension
- Good flap coverage to allow muscle tendon gliding

POSTOPERATIVE CARE

- A period of 2 to 3 weeks of splinting is needed.
- Passive muscle extension is obtained by mobilizing the involved joints.
- When active muscle flexion occurs, a resisted exercise program is required to maximize muscle strength.

ANNOTATED REFERENCES

2. Akasaka Y, Hara T, Takahashi M: Free muscle transplantation combined with intercostal nerve crossing for reconstruction of elbow flexion and wrist extension in brachial plexus injuries. Microsurgery 12:346-351, 1991.

   The initial use of free muscle transfers innervated with intercostal nerves was for biceps reconstruction. Akasaka and colleagues have taken this one step farther and used the muscles in a more distal location for wrist extension as well as elbow flexion.

4. Carlson FD, Wilkie DR: Muscle Physiology. Englewood Cliffs, NJ, Prentice-Hall, 1974.

   Although this book is quite dated, its information on the muscle physiology is still very applicable. It identifies the physiology of a single muscle fiber contractile excursion, length tension curves, and the way that actin and myosin interact during contraction.

5. Chen R, Anastakis DJ, Haywood CT, et al: Plasticity of the human motor system following muscle reconstruction: A magnetic stimulation and fMRI study. Clin Neurophysiol 114:2434-2446, 2003.

   Clinicians have long interpreted some of the changes that take place after neurologic injuries as evidence of cerebral plasticity or cerebral cortical reorganization. With the use of the fMRI and transcranial magnetic stimulation, cortical reorganization can be studied. This article points out the cortical changes that take place when the movement of elbow flexion becomes separated from respiration and can be independently controlled by the patient. The cerebral cortical center that controls elbow flexion has taken over and through influencing parts of the respiratory center now controls elbow flexion.

6. Chuang DC, Epstein MD, Yeh MC, Wei FC: Functional restoration of elbow flexion in brachial plexus injuries: Results in 167 patients (excluding obstetrical brachial plexus injury). J Hand Surg [Am] 18:285-291, 1993.

   This is one of the largest series that assesses different techniques of elbow flexion reconstruction for patients with brachial plexus injuries.

8. Classen J, Liepert A, Wise SP, et al: Rapid plasticity in human cortical movement representation induced by practice. J Neurophysiol 79:1117-1123, 1998.

   The learning process has been shown to be associated with modifications of the organization of the adult motor cortex with changes occurring within days to weeks.

10. Doi K, Sakai K, Kuwata N, et al: Double free-muscle transfer to restore prehension following complete brachial plexus avulsion. J Hand Surg [Am] 20:408-414, 1995.

    This is pioneering work. It involves double free muscle transfers to provide multiple functions. However, the use of one transfer to control two joints such as elbow flexion and wrist extension is controversial because some antagonistic control is necessary to stabilize the proximal joint.

16. Harii K, Ohmori K, Torii S: Free gracilis muscle transplantation with microvascular anastomosis for the treatment of facial paralysis. Plast Reconstr Surg 57:133-143, 1976

    Harii carried out the first known microvascular muscle transfer using the entire gracilis for treatment of the lower face in facial paralysis. Current techniques use the gracilis muscle but only a small segment of muscle, which is discreetly placed in the cheek providing an acceptable aesthetic result along with adequate facial movement.

17. Hollinshead WH: Anatomy for Surgeons. Philadelphia, Harper & Row, 1982, pp 325-326.

This is a superb but out of print anatomy text for surgeons. The feature of particular value is a thorough discussion of the anatomic variations of each structure under examination.

21. Kuzon WM, Fish JS, Pynn BR, McKee NH: Determinants of contractile function in free muscle transfers. Am Coll Surg Forum 35:610, 1984.

The researchers outlined their experience with functioning free muscle transfer of the gracilis muscle in a dog and their assessment of various factors including ischemia time and muscle tension on the eventual functional result.

23. Manktelow RT: Gracilis. *In* Microvascular Reconstruction: Anatomy, Applications and Surgical Techniques. Heidelberg, Springer-Verlag, 1986.

This chapter provides a thorough outline of the functional anatomy of the gracilis muscle.

24. Manktelow RT: Functioning muscle transplantation. *In* Microvascular Reconstruction: Anatomy, Applications and Surgical Techniques. Heidelberg, Springer-Verlag, 1986.

The technical aspects of functioning muscle transfer are outlined in a step-by-step fashion for the transfer of the gracilis muscle to the forearm for long finger flexor reconstruction.

25. Manktelow RT, McKee NH: Free muscle transplantation to provide active finger flexion. J Hand Surg [Am] 3:416-426, 1978.

This paper outlines the case study of the first North American free muscle transfer for long finger flexion.

26. Manktelow RT, Zuker RM: Muscle transplantation by fascicular territory. Plast Reconstr Surg 73:751-755, 1984.

The authors have identified separate neuromuscular territories within each muscle. Each territory is controlled by a separate fascicle of the motor nerve. Independent and separate neurorrhaphies to each of these fascicles will enable a single muscle to have independent functions. This is useful in muscle transfer to the forearm to provide independent finger and thumb flexion.

28. Manktelow RT, Zuker RM, McKee NH: Functioning free muscle transplantation. J Hand Surg [Am] 9:32, 1984.

This outlines the authors' experience with a small series of cases using functioning free muscle transfer for upper extremity reconstruction.

33. Nudo RJ, Milliken GW: Reorganization of movement representations in primary motor cortex following focal ischemic infarcts in adult squirrel monkeys. J Neurophysiol 75:2144-2149, 1996.

While specific movements are lost when a portion of the motor cerebral cortex is damaged, these movements are once again learned as adjacent areas of the cerebral cortex appear to take over the functions of the primary center that has been lost through vascular injury.

36. Pascual-Leone A, Nguyet D, Cohen LG, et al: Modulation of muscle responses evoked by transcranial magnetic stimulation during the acquisition of new fine motor skills. J Neurophysiol 74:1037-1045, 1995.

The investigative technique of transcranial magnetic stimulation allows activation of the primary motor cortex and the modulation of various motor activities. This may evolve to therapeutic benefit, particularly in nerve and tendon transfers.

40. Sixth People's Hospital, Microvascular Service, Shanghai: Free muscle transplantation by microsurgical neurovascular anastomoses. Clin Med J 2:47, 1976.

One of the first cases of functioning muscle transfer for long finger flexor reconstruction was done in China in 1973. The lateral portion of the pectoralis major was transferred to replace forearm flexor musculature in a patient with Volkmann's ischemic contracture.

41. Tamai S, Komatsu S, Sano S, et al: Free muscle transplants in dogs with microsurgical neurovascular anastomoses. Plast Reconstr Surg 46:219-225, 1970.

Tamai was the first person to demonstrate experimentally in the dog that microneurovascular muscle transfers could function. He showed active contraction and EMG evidence of muscle activity.

CHAPTER 50

Vascularized Bone Grafting

Allen T. Bishop

Bone grafts have been used since the first decade of the 20th century to fuse joints and repair defects.[35] The desirability of a living bone graft was recognized by several early investigators who used pedicled fibular grafts for tibial defects as early as 1905.[37,116,267] A pedicled cross-leg flap with bone was described by Farmer for tibial pseudarthrosis in 1952, and the concept of pedicle grafting has been widely developed in recent years using rib, clavicle, iliac crest, scapula, radius, greater and lesser trochanter, medial femoral condyle, pisiform, second metacarpal, and humerus.*

The use of free living bone transfers awaited the development of techniques and instruments for microvascular anastomosis pioneered by the work of Jacobson and Suarez in 1960.[120] With appropriate microsurgical instruments and techniques, development of free vascularized bone grafts was rapid. This included the first free bone transfer of an osteocutaneous composite rib flap by McKee in 1970.[172,173] Clinical reports of vascularized grafting followed with use of rib, fibula, and iliac crest.[34,82,279,282,283] The first vascularized fibula transfer was done by Ueba and Fujikawa in 1974.[106,298] Together with the iliac crest it remains the mainstay for extremity reconstruction today. Many variations have been described that allow tailoring of the graft to meet specific needs, including reconstruction of combined bone and soft tissue loss in one setting.

ADVANTAGES

Pedicle vs. Free flap

Vascularized bone grafts allow living bone tissue to be transplanted to an adjacent or remote location and survive by maintenance or restoration of blood flow. Free vascularized bone grafts require microvascular anastomoses to a recipient site artery and vein, whereas pedicle grafts are moved with their blood supply undisturbed to an adjacent area. Pedicle flaps may have orthograde (conventional)[39,40]

or retrograde flow[179,241,331] through a distally based pedicle with satisfactory results.

Biology of Conventional Bone Grafts

Bone graft may be obtained from the patient (autograft), another individual (allograft), or another species (xenograft). Autografts may be nonvascularized or vascularized and may be largely cancellous or corticocancellous in composition. Autografts are superior in general to allograft or xenograft material. For most bone defects less than 6 cm with a well-vascularized bed, adequate soft tissue cover, and absence of infection, a conventional cancellous or corticocancellous bone graft is generally recommended.[20] Cancellous bone has greater inductive capacity than cortical bone and should be used unless mechanical stability is required.

The process of bone graft incorporation is by "creeping substitution," a process of gradual vascular ingrowth, resorption, and replacement of necrotic bone. This process was described by Barth in 1895.[12] Creeping substitution results in rapid revascularization in small cancellous grafts but is slow and incomplete in cortical bone. As much as 40% to 50% of lamellar bone remains necrotic, and the revascularization process that does occur causes significant mechanical weakening, owing to bone resorption at 6 to 12 months.[20,35,259] Allografts, like autografts, must also be replaced by living bone. They are replaced more slowly and less completely and invoke a local and systemic immune response that diminishes stimulus of new bone formation. This effect may be diminished by freezing, freeze drying, irradiating, or decalcifying the bone or eliminated with the use of immunosuppressive drugs.[84,89,119,186,204,244,323] Structural nonvascularized grafts of all types have substantial problem with fatigue fracture, even years after the surgical procedure. Successful grafting requires a well-vascularized bed, adequate immobilization, and protection from excessive stress by rigid internal fixation.[68]

Biology of Vascularized Bone Grafts

Unlike conventional bone grafts, vascularized bone remains alive and dynamic in its new site. Because of its preserved circulation, cell survival is much better than conventional grafts.[9,18] As a result, the process of bone graft incorporation

---

*See references 24, 31, 40, 41, 49, 69, 72, 124, 131, 146, 162, 178, 212, 216, 238, 241, 271, 284, 286, 287, and 331.

by creeping substitution is obviated,[12,20,35] and significant osteopenia is not seen.[47] The result is improved strength, healing, and stress response as compared with nonvascularized bone grafts.* The incidence of stress fracture is lower than in massive structural autografts or allografts.[68,84,96,210,257,310] Furthermore, union is more rapid and bone hypertrophy in response to applied stress may occur with time.[51,76] Bone healing is more likely in difficult circumstances, including scarred or irradiated beds, or in avascular bone. In experimental models, vascularized grafts are superior to otherwise identical nonviable grafts in healing to adjacent bone when direct contact is blocked by muscle[8] or when the adjacent bone is necrotic and without measurable blood flow.[270]

In a study of osteocyte viability, Arata and coworkers reported that osteocyte counts in the cortex of vascularized grafts were 89% of normal controls. There were substantially fewer surviving osteocytes in conventional grafts.[9] Survival of cells results in less remodeling during revascularization. As a result, bone mass is maintained after transfer, as compared with conventional grafts,[47] and the effects of osteopenia are avoided. Vascularized grafts have superior material properties. These include strength, toughness, and elastic modulus two to four times greater than conventional structural grafts.[48]

The ability of vascularized grafts to adapt to applied stress by hypertrophy is a frequently observed phenomenon. This response is an essentially different process from the reactive callus formation of fracture healing[76] and results from an extraperiosteal reaction.[118] Hypertrophy does not invariably occur. For example, it is less likely when the graft is significantly stress-shielded by extensive internal fixation or in the absence of weight bearing.[51] Other important factors include age, extent of bone vascularity, and source of bone graft.[76,118] The fibula is more likely to hypertrophy than iliac crest or rib.

Other Advantages

In addition to superior cell survival, maintained circulation, and mechanical properties, vascularized grafts have other significant advantages over conventional grafts. These include the possibility to restore longitudinal growth by inclusion of growth plate,[26,30,63,291,326] revascularize necrotic bone,[†] improve local blood flow in scarred soft tissue beds,[213,279] and reconstruct composite tissue loss in one procedure by inclusion of skin, muscle, tendon, nerve, and other tissues with the bone graft.

INDICATIONS

Based on the information just reported, it would seem that vascularized autografts would be ideal for grafting under most circumstances. Their use as free tissue transfers is technically demanding, however, and pedicle grafts are often more limited in dimension, pedicle length, and hence indications. Prolonged operative times and extensive dissection increase the risk of complications, and donor site morbidity may be significant. For bone defects under 6 to 8 cm with normal soft tissues, conventional techniques remain the method of choice under many circumstances.

Segmental Bone Loss

Vascularized transfer is indicated, however, in segmental bone defects larger than 6 to 8 cm owing to tumor resection,[‡] traumatic bone loss,[§] osteomyelitis, or infected nonunion.[¶]

Their use in smaller defects is reasonable in cases in which "biologic failure" of bone healing is likely or has already occurred.[189] Examples include persistent nonunion after conventional treatment, poorly vascularized bone and/or its soft tissue bed due to scarring, infection or irradiation, and congenital pseudarthrosis.[4,165,182,203,210,302,309]

Other Indications

Other indications include avascular necrosis of bone, composite tissue loss requiring complex reconstruction, joint arthrodesis in exceptional circumstances, and need for longitudinal growth with physeal transfer.

Avascular Necrosis of Bone

Vascularized grafts have been used to treat osteonecrotic bone in the femoral head, scaphoid, talus, and lunate.[‖] Experimental models of avascular necrosis have demonstrated that vascularized bone or arteriovenous pedicle grafts are able to repair necrotic bone by neovascularization and new bone formation extending from the vascularized graft into the damaged area.[86,110,321] In the clinical setting, symptomatic improvement and direct evidence of revascularization on imaging studies have been reported in the femoral head,[220,221,301] talus,[60,117] as well as the lunate[24,69,171,278] and scaphoid.[93,110,134,145,254,262,331] Nonunions of long bones due to osteoradionecrosis are also optimally treated by vascularized bone grafts.

Complex Tissue Loss

Most vascularized bone grafts can be harvested as composite flaps including vascularized skin, muscle, and other tissues. Examples include osteomuscular or osteocutaneous fibular flaps,[13,143] composite groin flaps including skin and/or muscle,[72,225,233,264] and lateral arm fasciocutaneous flaps including a section of lateral humerus.[131,284] Flow-through fibular flaps with a distal microvascular anastomosis of a second free flap allow coverage of large soft tissue defects with bone reconstruction in a single stage (Fig. 50-1). The unique ability of free tissue transfer to solve complex tissue defect problems with a single-stage

---

*See references 9, 17, 18, 40, 61, 79, 201, 202, 239, 240, 331, and 333.

†See references 85, 86, 117, 149, 158, 171, 220, 241, 256, 270, 296, 301, and 331.

‡See references 1, 22, 65, 80, 94, 150, 158, 177, 188, 199, 216, 284, and 315-317

§See references 22, 52, 70, 79, 96, 106, 118, 158, 194, 196, 211, 310, and 314.

¶See references 22, 96, 102, 122, 125, 180, 187, 216, and 317-319.

‖See references 32, 60, 69, 85, 86, 149, 171, 173, 220, 241, 256, 262, 264, 296, and 331.

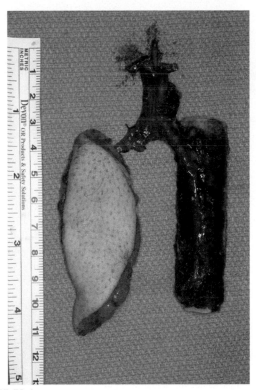

FIGURE 50-1. Osteocutaneous fibula. The fibula may be harvested as a composite flap including skin for coverage or monitoring purposes.

reconstruction makes them highly desirable in these difficult circumstances.

Physeal Arrest

Transfer of vascularized epiphyses may allow continued growth of a limb.[30,63] This is currently practical only for fibular grafts with inclusion of the entire proximal fibula or with digit and vascularized joint transfers. To maintain growth of the proximal fibular physis, the arterial supply of the epiphyseal region must be restored (most commonly by anastomosis of the inferior lateral genicular vessels) and separately identified, with end-to-side anastomosis to the peroneal artery pedicle supplying the fibular shaft.[313] These vessels are the major source of blood supply to the physis, although the anterior tibial and recurrent peroneal vessels also provide some blood flow.[132,285] The procedure is still investigational, but results have been encouraging in experimental animals.[326] Fifty percent of cases from a recent clinical series demonstrated some longitudinal growth.[291]

Osteomyelitis

Infections represent a particularly difficult problem. Application of systemic or local antibiotics and aggressive débridement of necrotic bone and soft tissue must be carried out until the infection is deemed inactive or eradicated. Criteria commonly used to determine inactive sepsis include absence of sinus tracts, negative bacterial cultures, negative C-reactive protein, and a sedimentation rate of less than 15 mm/hr maintained for at least 1 month.[180] When strict criteria for determining quiescence are used, recurrent infection will occur infrequently.

VASCULARIZED GRAFTS FOR UPPER EXTREMITY BONE DEFECTS

The most important sources of vascularized grafts for large upper extremity bone defects are the fibula and the iliac crest. The distal radius is increasingly utilized for carpal nonunion or avascular necrosis, and a number of other donor sites have been used to provide living bone for upper extremity uses, including metacarpal, metatarsal, scapula, rib, pisiform, and vascularized periosteum.

Preoperative Planning

Preoperative planning is vital for successful free tissue transfer. The bony, vascular, and soft tissue anatomy of a particular recipient site must be considered, along with factors related to the bone defect itself. For example, length and location of the bone defect, infection status, soft tissue loss or scarring, and condition of recipient vessels must be determined. The method of bone fixation should be planned in advance. Use of anatomic dissection in the laboratory will enhance familiarity with the regional anatomy.[279]

Recipient Site

If osteomyelitis is present, extensive débridement of all devitalized bone and adequate preliminary soft tissue coverage are prerequisites before vascularized grafting is considered.

Arteriography of the recipient site is frequently to be recommended, particularly in cases where vascular damage is likely.[196,280] Certainly in trauma arteriography is routine, unless both the radial and ulnar arterial pulses are of normal quality at the wrist. In many instances of trauma or postirradiation bone deficiency, the extent of soft tissue injury extends well proximal and distal to the level of bony abnormality.[196,257] Within the reactive zone, a patent vessel may be prone to spasm as well as friability owing to surrounding scar or granulation tissue. This will render any anastomosis potentially flawed. In such situations, planning an anastomosis proximal to the zone of injury is necessary. This may be performed with a sufficiently large flap or long pedicle or at times by the use of vein grafts. Probable need for vein grafting may be determined by preoperative arteriography and by consideration of known factors such as pedicle length and distance of bone from available recipient vessels.

Vein grafting may be done as conventional arterial and venous interposition grafts or by fabrication of a temporary arteriovenous fistula as described by Taylor[279] and by Grenga and Yetman.[91] In the latter circumstance, a reversed saphenous vein graft is anastomosed end-to-side to the recipient artery and end-to-end to the vein. End-to-side arterial anastomoses may have a higher patency rate in free tissue transfer and preserve distal circulation.[83] The shunt is allowed to perfuse while the donor tissue is harvested. Shunts were necessary in 6% of 420 consecutive free tissue transfers in a recent series.[74]

The vascularized graft can be placed in either an orthograde or a retrograde flow position, as dictated by the position of the best vascular anastomosis. Retrograde position has no effect on patency or rate of union.[50] Bony stabilization is performed, followed by vascular anastomosis.

Use of stable internal fixation provides results superior to minimal internal or external fixation.[96] Addition of supplemental cancellous graft at junction sites increases the primary healing rate.

Clavicle

Clavicle bone loss or nonunion can be very difficult to treat effectively. Radiation-induced necrosis of the clavicle has a particularly unfavorable prognosis.[253,306] Partial excision of the clavicle, often advocated in this situation, may result in persisting pain, weakness, sensation of instability, and brachial plexopathy.[2,27,126,258,312,316] Because of the thin soft tissue envelope covering the clavicle, bulky bone and/or soft tissue reconstruction is preferentially avoided. Several methods of surgical reconstruction have been described. In cases involving failed prior plating or infection, conventional nonvascularized iliac tricortical bone graft may not be successful, especially if a significant defect remains in the clavicle. Microvascular fibular transfer combined with autografting has been reported as an appropriate treatment option for difficult nonunions associated with previously irradiated long bones[64]; however, a high failure rate for the clavicular site has been shown.[96,316] Other biologic options include the vascularized transfer of a rib as a composite flap including serratus anterior and/or latissimus dorsi.[57,92] Salvage options such as Dacron graft reconstruction are associated with complications such as stress fracture[66] or erosion of the first rib.[218] A Marlex mesh–enveloped composite graft consisting of a hydroxyapatite prosthesis and autogenous bone has been proposed, although secure fixation of this construct remains a challenge.[250]

Because of its osteogenic capability, vascularized periosteal grafts have considerable potential for the reconstruction of bone defects.[140,265,275] The transfer of free vascularized corticoperiosteal bone flaps seems to be ideally suited for post–radiation-induced fractures or chronic nonunions of the clavicle without substantial bone loss but with poor chances of healing on their own. Successful use of periosteal flaps from the medial femoral condyle has been reported (see Fig. 50-7).[60,75,229] The flap is thin and can be shaped according to the reconstructive requirements without compromising its blood supply. It can be wrapped around the clavicle without visible bulk, thereby avoiding further stress on the previously irradiated overlying skin. It enables clavicular healing at one bone contact site, avoiding the difficulties of interposing, fixing, and healing a bridging vascularized structural graft. Rapid subperiosteal new bone and improved local blood flow both serve to correct many of those changes attributed to radiation necrosis of bone. Although microvascular expertise is necessary, flap exposure and elevation is straightforward. The thoracoacromial trunk artery and vein as well as the descending genicular vessels are constantly present and are of sufficient size for reliable microsurgical anastomoses. Improved healing over other methods has been demonstrated.[59,75]

Humerus

The humerus is difficult to support in the postoperative period. Therefore, if possible, stable internal fixation should be used.[313] Bone fixation of a fibular graft is best performed with plate and screw fixation, with a long compression plate spanning the humerus defect, placing the graft as an inter-

position graft in the defect. Alternatively, compression plating at each end is reasonable. If possible, the fibula should be placed in an intramedullary position if the size of the humerus will allow. If not, end-to-end coaptation should be supplemented with additional cancellous bone graft. In addition to internal fixation, the use of a shoulder spica cast is prudent until bone union has occurred. Vascular anastomoses are straightforward, because the brachial vessels lie adjacent to the bone. End-to-side anastomosis to the brachial artery and end-to-end repair to the cephalic vein or a brachial vena comitans are preferred in most cases.

Forearm

Bone stabilization with rigid internal fixation is relatively easily obtained. In cases of massive bone loss of both forearm bones, the graft may be placed from proximal ulna to distal radius to create a one-bone forearm.[56,208] Alternatively, both bones may be reconstructed with a double-barreled graft or dual fibular grafts. Positioning may be either orthograde or retrograde, depending on the optimal location for vessel approximation. Fixation with dual plating at either end is reasonable (see Fig. 50-10C). Vascular anastomoses to radial or ulnar vessels are easily performed, usually as end-to-side arterial anastomoses. Venae comitantes or superficial (cephalic or basilic) veins are satisfactory for end-to-end anastomosis. A long-arm cast is maintained until radiographic signs of union occur.[313]

Wrist

Vascularized bone grafts have demonstrated clinical promise in the treatment of scaphoid fracture, particularly in nonunions of the proximal pole or associated with avascular necrosis, as well as in the treatment of Kienböck's disease. Grafts used in the wrist are usually pedicle grafts from adjacent radius, pisiform, ulna, or metacarpal. Free microvascular bone grafting has been reported, however.[205] The surgical approach may frequently allow bone graft harvest and recipient site preparation through a single incision. Exposure must not damage the vascular pedicle or its anastomotic connections. In most cases, exposure and protection of the pedicle precede preparation of the recipient site. The method of graft placement and stabilization is carefully planned in advance.

SPECIFIC VASCULARIZED GRAFTS: LONG BONE RECONSTRUCTION

Fibula

 Anatomy

The fibula is the most used vascularized bone graft because its structure and shape are appropriate for diaphyseal locations. A long, straight segment of 26 to 30 cm in length may frequently be harvested and osteosynthesis securely obtained to the recipient bone.

The blood supply to the fibula, as in other long bones, is derived normally from a nutrient artery via radially oriented branches that penetrate the cortex and anastomose with the periosteal vessels.[121,289] The resulting blood flow is centrifugal from medulla to cortex. This arrangement is the norm for the fibula, which has a single nutrient vessel entering its middle third from the peroneal artery. Additional periosteal branches from the peroneal and anterior tibial artery also supply the diaphysis.[81]

The proximal epiphysis is supplied by an arcade of vessels of which the lateral inferior genicular vessels are the most important.[291] This vessel must be anastomosed if physeal growth is desired.[26,62,63,291]

Transfer of a fasciocutaneous skin paddle up to 10 × 20 cm is made possible by a series of fasciocutaneous or myocutaneous perforators from the peroneal artery that typically pierces the soleus muscle adjacent to the lateral intermuscular septum (Fig. 50-2).[143,324] The location of the perforators may be determined in the operating room before skin incision by use of a Doppler ultrasound stethoscope.

Osteomuscular flaps including flexor hallucis longus, portions of soleus, or peroneal muscles may also be raised using the same peroneal artery pedicle.[13,41,42]

The peroneal pedicle has a length of 6 to 8 cm and an arterial diameter of 1.5 to 3.0 mm. Two venae comitantes lie on either side of the artery.[295]

Technique
Usual Free Flap

Two methods of fibular harvest have been described, including the original posterior approach developed by Taylor[281] and the preferred lateral approach of Gilbert, described later with some modifications.[82,313] Exposure must protect the peroneal vessels, which lie between the tibialis posterior and flexor hallucis muscles (see Fig. 50-2).

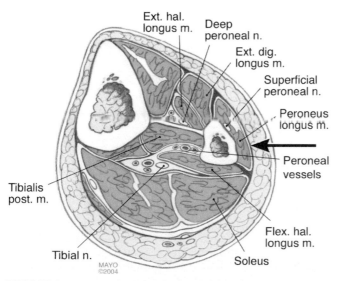

FIGURE 50-2. Harvest of a fibular free bone graft is performed from a lateral approach. The initial dissection is between peroneus longus and soleus. Dissection proceeds anteriorly, sequentially elevating the muscles of the lateral and anterior compartments, interosseous membrane, and tibialis posterior to identify the peroneal vessels. The flexor hallucis longus is the last muscle to be divided. (Copyright 2004, Mayo Foundation.)

The patient is positioned supine with a small sandbag beneath the ipsilateral buttock and another secured to the table near its foot to allow the patient's foot to rest securely with the knee flexed. The entire leg is draped free. Next, a pneumatic tourniquet is inflated. The fibula is measured, and its middle third is identified. An incision is made directly along the fibular longitudinal axis laterally, extending through skin and subcutaneous tissue (Fig. 50-3A). The anterior border of a skin flap is incised at this step. This exposes the broad tendon of the peroneus longus, which is easily identified. A fat stripe posterior to the tendon identifies the interval between the peroneus longus muscle and the soleus. This interval is developed with blunt dissection, beginning in the middle third of the bone (see Fig. 50-3B). The cutaneous vascular perforators supplying the skin may be visualized at this point passing either through the lateral intermuscular septum or, more commonly, through the adjacent anterior centimeter of soleus. As the soleus is reflected posteriorly, one can identify the flexor hallucis muscle belly covering the posterior surface of the bone and obscuring the peroneal vessels from view.

The flexor hallucis longus muscle origin lies well distal to the fibular neck. Proximal to the muscle, the peroneal vessels are identified as they pass deep to the muscle's origin (see Fig. 50-3C). The vessels should be mobilized carefully from the posterior surface of the fibula, to prevent their inadvertent injury when the bone is divided.

Dissection is continued progressively proximally, elevating the soleus tendon of origin from its fibular attachment. Muscular branches of the peroneal vessels to the soleus will be visualized during the dissection and should be ligated and divided unless a composite osteomuscular flap with soleus is desired (see Fig. 50-3D). The soleus is completely detached from the proximal fibula.

Next, the lateral compartment muscles are elevated from the fibula. *Proximally, this must be done subperiosteally to avoid injury to the peroneal nerve.* The nerve must be visualized and protected at this proximal level, lying directly on the bone of the fibular neck and proximal diaphysis. As the muscle is elevated in a distal direction, the superficial branch of the nerve lies further from the bone, and an extraperiosteal dissection plane will better preserve the bone blood supply. This dissection should leave small occasional wisps of muscle rather than a large muscular cuff on the bone surface, because this will form a necrotic barrier to revascularization should the anastomosis fail (see Fig. 50-3E).[251]

The anterior compartment is elevated similarly. Again, care is needed proximally to protect the deep branch of the peroneal nerve (see Fig. 50-3F). The anterior tibial artery will be identified, as will the interosseous membrane at the conclusion of this dissection. Depending on ease of visibility, the interosseous membrane may be divided at this point (see Fig. 50-3G) or the bone divided proximally and distally first. Bone division is carried out with a Gigli saw, protecting neurovascular structures with careful circumferential retraction and blunt passage of the saw cable (see Fig. 50-3H). The middle third of the bone, at a minimum, must be raised to preserve the nutrient artery supply. Harvesting more of the proximal third will improve visualization of the peroneal artery pedicle at the conclusion of the graft elevation. Although the entire proximal fibula may

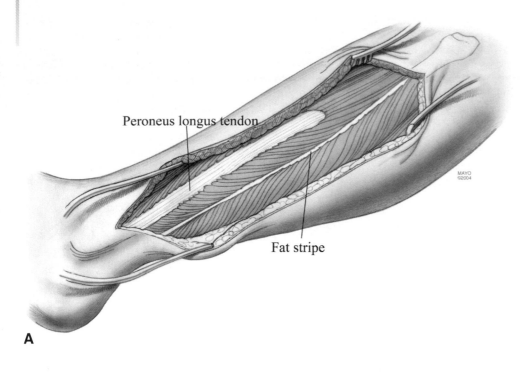

Peroneus longus tendon

Fat stripe

A

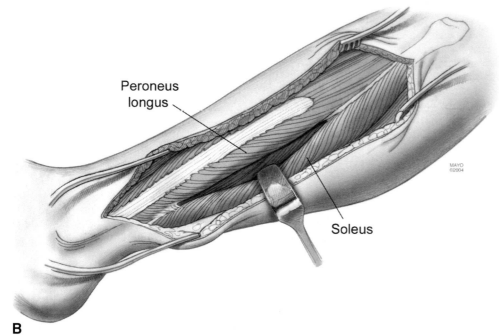

Peroneus
longus

Soleus

B

FIGURE 50-3. Technique of fibula harvest. See description in text. **A,** The fat stripe dorsal (posterior) to the peroneus longus tendon marks the plane of the initial dissection. **B,** Opening the soleus/peroneus longus interval at mid tibia. (Copyright 2004, Mayo Foundation.)

Continued

be harvested if articular surface or physis is required, 7 to 8 cm of distal fibula should be preserved to prevent valgus instability of the ankle (see Fig. 50-3I) . In children, a distal tibiofibular syndesmotic fusion is necessary with an iliac crest interposition graft and screws to prevent ankle instability (Fig. 50-4). Fusion is not necessary in adults.

After the interosseous membrane and bone are divided, the peroneal artery is identified at the distal osteotomy and ligated (see Fig. 50-3J). A long suture tag is left on the proximal stump to facilitate proximal dissection of the vessel. Dissection then proceeds from distal to proximal.

Viewing the fibula from dorsally, the muscle of the tibialis posterior muscle is now exposed after division of the interosseous membrane. The tibialis posterior muscle and posterior fascia must be divided to expose the peroneal vessels (see Fig. 50-3K). The muscle is teased away carefully first, ligating muscular perforators as they are encountered. A tissue plane is identified just anterior to the ligated peroneal vessel. This is the posterior fascia of the tibialis posterior, which is next divided to expose the artery. The dissection must be meticulous to identify and ligate multiple muscular perforators and to protect the underlying vessels.

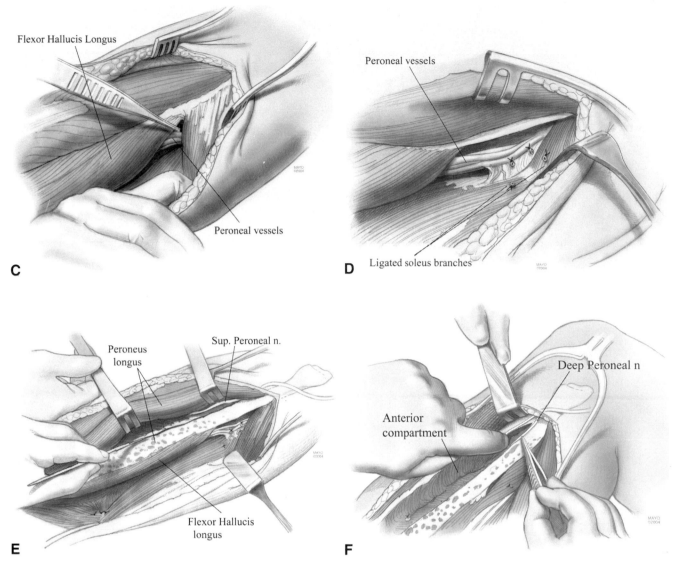

FIGURE 50-3—cont'd. C, Follow the flexor hallucis longus muscle on the posterior surface of the fibula to its proximal origin. The peroneal vessels will then be visualized passing anterior to the muscle. **D,** Ligate any muscular branches to soleus and complete dissection of soleus from fibular neck. **E,** Dissect the lateral compartment muscles from the fibula, beginning subperiosteally proximally until superficial peroneal nerve is identified and protected. Dissection then proceeds extraperiosteally distally. **F,** The deep peroneal nerve is identified, and the anterior compartment muscles are dissected from the fibula in a similar fashion.   *Continued*

At this point, only the vascular pedicle and the flexor hallucis longus muscle belly remain attached to the bone. The flexor hallucis longus tendon may be divided at this point if the muscle is to be included with the fibula as an osteomuscular flap. In most cases, it is not, and the flexor hallucis longus is carefully incised at its fibular origin, protecting the peroneal vessels at all times (see Fig. 50-3L). Additional perforators will frequently require ligation.

Finally, the vessels are dissected as far proximally as possible to their origin from the posterior tibial artery. Separation of the artery and venae comitantes from each other is desirable at this time, passing vessel loops around both veins and the artery. At this point, the sole remaining attachment of the fibula is its peroneal vessel pedicle (see Fig. 50-3M). The tourniquet is then released, and the bone is

allowed to perfuse while careful hemostasis is obtained in the leg. The artery and veins are occluded with microvascular clamps, ligated proximally, and divided to detach the flap. I prefer to use a curved clamp for the artery and straight clamps for the veins, to avoid later confusion. Two suction drains are placed, one between the flexor hallucis longus and soleus and another subcutaneously. The flexor hallucis longus is then loosely repaired to the peroneal muscle with a running absorbable suture. The skin is closed in layers.

Osteocutaneous Flap

The inclusion of skin is made possible by several fasciocutaneous perforators from the peroneal artery that supplies the skin at intervals, particularly along the middle third of the bone. If a cutaneous flap is elevated with bone, the

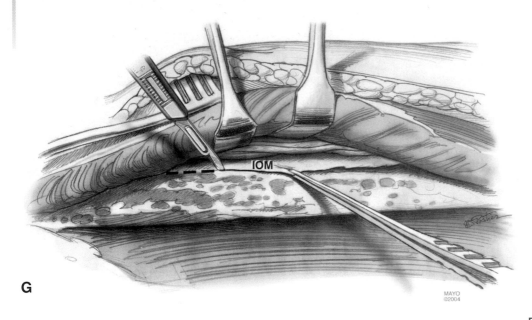

G

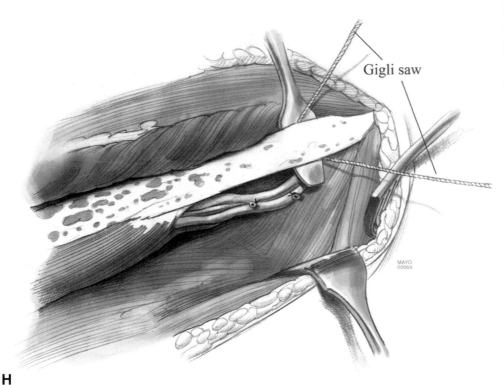

Gigli saw

H

FIGURE 50-3—cont'd. G, The interosseous membrane (IOM) is divided from anteriorly. The tibialis posterior muscle is then visible. **H,** The proximal fibular cut is made, protecting the peroneal vessels and nerve.   *Continued*

locations of the major fasciocutaneous perforators are identified with a Doppler ultrasound stethoscope before tourniquet elevation, because their exact position and number vary considerably between individuals. They may be readily identified midlaterally by an audible pulse using the probe, near the soleus/peroneal junction (lateral intermuscular septum). Alternatively, the exact placement of the skin island can be determined by visualization of the vessels directly after the anterior incision is made.[313] The dissection proceeds exactly as for a conventional fibular graft, except

that the peroneus-soleus interval is left undisturbed in the middle and distal thirds until the peroneal vessels are exposed anteriorly (after fibular osteotomies and division of the tibialis posterior). Isolation of the perforating vessels is performed by division of the posterior skin flap at this point and their mobilization back to the peroneal vessels. To avoid problems with excessively tight skin closure and compartment syndrome, the donor site at the skin paddle area should be closed by a split-thickness skin graft, unless a small "buoy" flap only is taken.

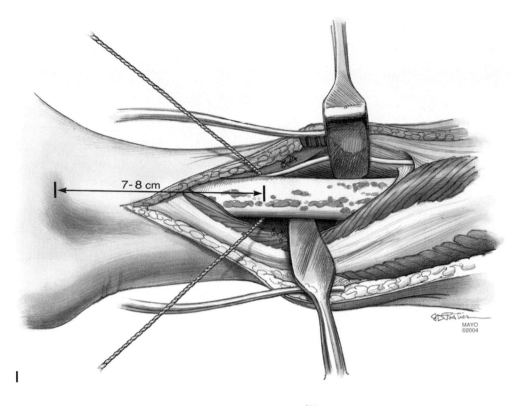

I

FIGURE 50-3—cont'd. I, The distal fibular cut is made, preserving 7 to 8 cm of distal fibula. **J,** The peroneal vessels are visualized and ligated distally, located between the flexor hallucis longus and tibialis posterior.
Continued

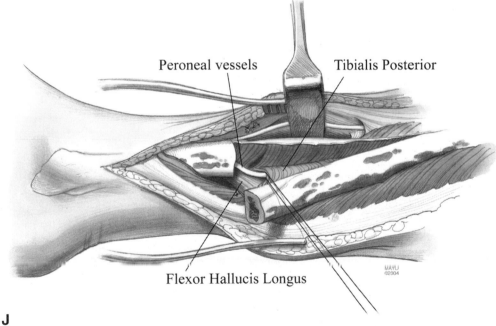

J

Peroneal vessels Tibialis Posterior Flexor Hallucis Longus

Fibula With Physis

Inclusion of the proximal growth plate to restore physeal function is not widely performed, and results have been somewhat unpredictable.[291] Nevertheless, it remains a reasonable procedure when no other options exist. The exposure requires a posterior approach proximally, with a transverse incision at the popliteal fossa, coursing distally along the lateral border of the fibula. The lateral inferior genicular vessels are identified on either side of the lateral head of the gastrocnemius, facilitated by release of the soleus from its proximal origin while carefully protecting the peroneal nerve. The inferior lateral genicular vessels are followed beneath the lateral head of the gastrocnemius to their origin from the popliteal vessels. Once the vessels are isolated the fibular head is released by division of the biceps femoris tendon and iliotibial band attachments, release of the lateral collateral ligament, and tibiofibular joint capsule. The genicular vessels are tagged distally, ligated proximally, and divided. The remainder of the fibular dissection is performed otherwise as described previously. To simplify the

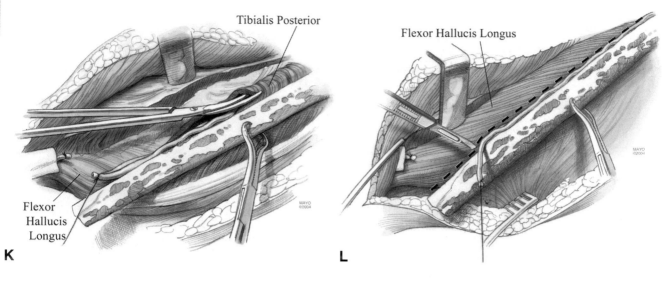

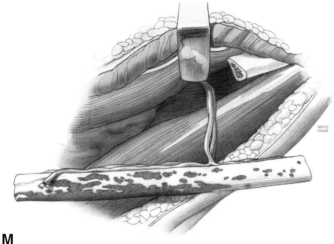

FIGURE 50-3—cont'd. **K,** The tibialis posterior muscle is then divided from distal to proximal, exposing the peroneal vessels. It is necessary to identify and ligate multiple muscular branches. **L,** The flexor hallucis longus muscle is next removed from the fibula. **M,** The fibula is then isolated on its proximal peroneal vessel pedicle.

CRITICAL POINTS: VASCULARIZED FIBULA BONE GRAFT

INDICATIONS

- Segmental bone loss greater than 6 to 8 cm
- Biologic failure to heal
  - Failed conventional treatment
  - Poorly vascularized bone and/or adjacent tissue bed due to scar, infection, irradiation, or congenital pseudarthrosis
- Avascular necrosis of bone
- Composite tissue loss including bone
- Arthrodesis of joints in exceptional circumstances
- Physeal transfer for growth disturbance

PEARLS

- Rigid fixation improves primary union rate.
- Use secondary conventional graft if healing fails to occur after 6 months.

- Harvest more fibula than is likely needed. This provides the possibility of altering the position and final length of the peroneal vascular pedicle to meet recipient site needs, based on normal variations in its position along the length of the fibular shaft.
- Composite osteocutaneous, osteomuscular, or osteomusculocutaneous fibular flaps provide the ability for continual circulation monitoring and providing soft tissue coverage of small to moderate defects.

TECHNICAL POINTS

- Posterior dissection first; identify fat stripe between peroneus longus and soleus muscle in mid leg. Dissection in this plane will protect the flexor hallucis muscle and underlying peroneal pedicle.

CRITICAL POINTS: VASCULARIZED FIBULA BONE GRAFT—cont'd

- Anterior dissection begins subperiosteally proximally, until superficial peroneal nerve is identified and protected. Thereafter, extraperiosteal dissection preserves bone periosteal blood supply.
- The anterior compartment dissection proceeds in an identical fashion, ending with release of the interosseous membrane.
- The fibula is then osteotomized, and the distal peroneal vessels are ligated.
- The tibialis posterior is released from an anterior perspective, exposing the peroneal vessels and ligating multiple muscular branches.

- Release of the flexor hallucis muscle completes the dissection.

PITFALLS

- Children may develop a hindfoot valgus deformity at the donor site unless a distal tibiofibular syndesmotic fusion is performed.
- Previous osteomyelitis cases must have negative cultures, a normal sedimentation rate and C-reactive protein levels before bone transfer to minimize risk of reactivation of infection.

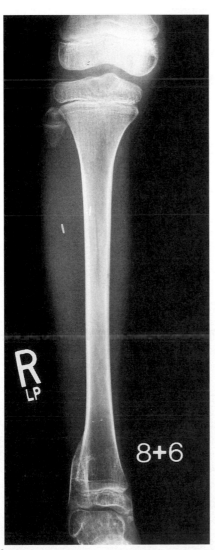

FIGURE 50-4. Fusion of the distal tibiofibular interval prevents the development of valgus instability of the ankle in children.

microsurgical anastomosis, Wood recommends end-to-side suture of the genicular artery and vein to the peroneal vessels on a back table before revascularization of the fibula at the recipient site.[313] Alternatively, they may be sutured to vessels at the site of fibular implantation.

Fibula With Muscle

Although the fibula may be harvested with peroneal muscle, donor site morbidity precludes this. Instead, the lateral portion of soleus and/or the flexor hallucis longus muscle may be used. The flexor hallucis longus provides only enough muscle to cover the distal fibular segment. A larger muscle, sufficient to obliterate dead space or provide coverage, may be preferred. In this instance, use of the lateral portion of the soleus is appropriate.[13] This is easily accomplished by sparing the soleus muscular branch(es) visualized during exposure of the peroneal pedicle, as described earlier. The dissection proceeds unchanged until the end of the elevation, when the soleus is divided longitudinally in its mid substance. The tibialis posterior artery and tibial nerve are carefully protected during this process.

Double-Barrel Flap

Strength can be improved particularly for femoral applications, or two segments can be separated sufficiently to allow simultaneous reconstruction of radius and ulna by use of a "double-barrel" graft.[122] After harvest, the free fibula graft is osteotomized at its midpoint without dividing its vascular pedicle. This produces two vascularized bone grafts that require only one set of anastomoses. This folded fibula provides twice the cross-sectional area of a single fibula transfer when placed in a single bone. This technique has been successfully used in long bone defects of the upper and lower limbs.[198] The proximal strut is vascularized by both a periosteal and an endosteal blood supply, whereas the distal strut is vascularized by a periosteal blood supply alone. This so-called double barrel free vascularized fibular graft has been employed in patients with segmental bone defects of single bones when improved strength is desirable and for adjacent bony defects of the radius and ulna.[70,122]

Iliac Crest

 ## Anatomy

The iliac crest receives dual blood supply from the superficial circumflex iliac artery (SCIA) and the deep circumflex iliac artery (DCIA).[23] Of the two, the DCIA system is most important (Fig. 50-5).[231,282] Musculocutaneous perforators penetrating the abdominal wall 1 cm proximal to the iliac crest provide its nutrition. In the experience of several authors, the skin paddle has been less reliable than a standard groin flap, particularly if slightly rotated in relation to underlying bone.[23,81,214,230,283] Its size, when based on the DCIA, is quite variable, ranging from 7 × 10 to 15 × 30 cm.[282] The entire iliac bone, however, is well supplied by the DCIA via multiple perforating arteries at the points of muscle attachment.[193,201] It remains the pedicle of choice for osteocutaneous flaps, although double-pedicle flaps have been described using both SCIA and DCIA vessels and may be desirable.[143,225]

The DCIA arises from the external iliac artery 1 cm proximal to the inguinal ligament. Several branches supply the internal oblique and iliacus muscles, as well as the lateral femoral circumflex vessels. It courses obliquely cephalad and laterally between extraperitoneal fat in the transversus muscle until it reaches the anterior superior iliac spine. At this level it pierces the transversus muscle to run between it and the internal oblique muscle along the inner lip of the iliac crest adjacent to the iliacus muscle. At its origin, the mean diameters of the artery and vena comitans are 2.78 mm and 3.60 mm, respectively.[114]

Although the entire crest may be harvested, it has a practical limit of 10 cm in length as a vascularized graft because of its curved shape. It is relatively less suited for diaphyseal reconstruction than the fibula, because remodeling for tolerance of weight bearing is prolonged.[257] Furthermore, osteosynthesis is difficult and weak.

Indications

The principal advantages of this graft are its largely cancellous nature and the large amount of soft tissue that may be raised with bone as a combined osteomusculocutaneous flap. In such flaps, a more reliable skin flap may be obtained with inclusion of both superficial and deep circumflex iliac vessels. The advantages of the osteocutaneous flap include the ability to (1) supply vascularized bone to what is frequently a poor recipient bed for a bone graft, (2) reconstruct both soft tissue and bony defects simultaneously, and (3) be used in facilities without capability for microvascular surgery when used as a pedicle flap for the upper extremity.[219] It may also be used for smaller defects. Reports exist of its use for metacarpal tumors and scaphoid nonunion, for example.[100,205]

Technique

Free Flap

The patient is positioned supine with a sandbag beneath the ipsilateral buttock. The patient is draped to the midline anteriorly, costal margin proximally, and as far posteriorly as possible. The leg is draped free to facilitate hip flexion for wound closure. The skin flap is marked, with its axis along the inner margin of the iliac crest, centered at a point 4 to 8 cm posterior to the anterior superior iliac spine.[282] The pubic tubercle, anterior superior iliac spine, femoral pulse, and iliac crest are marked. The skin flap is then incised along its medial margin, extending it medially along the inguinal ligament and obliquely inferiorly along the femoral pulse. Just proximal to the inguinal ligament, the external oblique is incised, exposing the inguinal canal contents. These are secured and retracted medially with an elastic cord. The floor of the canal (internal oblique and transversalis fascia) is incised to visualize the DCIA and accompanying veins. After identifying their origin, they are traced laterally toward the anterior superior iliac spine, ligating multiple small branches as well as the large ascending branch. The lateral femoral cutaneous nerve is identified and spared if it lies below the vessels. It will occasionally pass superficially and must then be divided for later repair. The external and internal oblique and transversus muscle are then sectioned 2 cm medial to the iliac crest insertion to preserve the skin blood supply. At this point, the vessels are not visualized. Finally, the lateral skin incision is made and the tensor fascia femoris and gluteal vessels are dissected extraperiosteally from the outer table of the ilium. The ilium is then osteotomized, and the pedicle is divided to complete the harvest. Closure is important to prevent herniation, first approximating transversalis to iliacus fascia and then internal and external oblique to gluteus and tensor fascia femoris. Skin closure is facilitated by hip flexion.

Vascularized Periosteal Grafts

Periosteal grafts have been demonstrated experimentally to produce predictable new bone formation, provided they have adequate vascularity.[140,275,297] Bone formation after free vascularized transfer of periosteum may be enhanced by enclosing a cancellous bone graft in a periosteal wrap.[223]

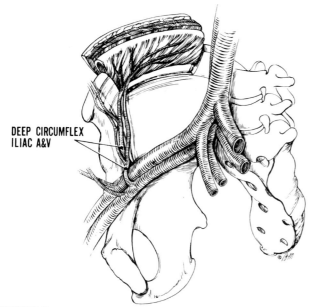

DEEP CIRCUMFLEX ILIAC A&V

FIGURE 50-5. The osteocutaneous groin flap based on the deep circumflex iliac artery and vein.

A variety of donor sites have been identified, including clavicle, fibula, ilium, humerus, tibia and femur, among others.* In the upper extremity, thin corticoperiosteal grafts and small periosteal bone grafts harvested from the supracondylar region of the femur have proven to be of great use, based on either the descending genicular or the medial superior genicular artery and vein (Fig. 50-6A).[60] This graft is elastic and readily conforms to small tubular bones. It has been successfully used for clavicle, humerus, and forearm applications, including pathologic fractures from radiation necrosis and other recalcitrant nonunions.[60,75]

Medial Femoral Condyle Periosteal or Corticoperiosteal Flap

Technique

A free vascularized thin corticoperiosteal bone graft containing a variable amount of vascularized cancellous bone can be obtained from the medial femoral condylar and supracondylar region in a rather straightforward manner.[59,60,103,207,223,229] Based on the descending genicular artery, an 8-cm segment of vascularized distal femoral bone may be harvested from the medial femoral condyle for use in the mandible or smaller defects in other locations.[60,103,159] The surgical approach is made with a longitudinal skin incision overlying the adductor magnus and sartorius in the distal medial thigh. By retracting the vastus medialis anteriorly and the sartorius muscle posteriorly, the descending genicular vessels and superiomedial genicular vessels are visualized in the floor of the vastus compartment. These medial genicular vessels form a robust, arching arcade on the surface of the medial femoral condyle (see Fig. 50-6A). A graft is outlined to include these vessels. Distally and posteriorly, care must be taken to avoid injury of the medial collateral ligament. The superior margin is the reflection of knee joint capsule at the medial patellar facet. Proximally, the change in cortical thickness at the diaphyseal-metaphyseal margin limits elevation. The periosteum, together with fragments of the underlying outer cortex, is elevated with the accompanying vessels, generally no more than 5 × 7 cm in dimension (see Fig. 50-6B). If needed, the flap may include a wedge of cancellous bone for applications such as scaphoid nonunions. Although either a descending or medial superior genicular vascular pedicle will support the graft, the descending genicular is preferred for its larger size and longer length. When dissected proximally to its origin from the superficial femoral vessels in Hunter's canal, a pedicle length of 7 cm may be readily obtained. The corticoperiosteal graft is pliable (Fig. 50-7) and may be wrapped around the clavicle, radius, or ulna and secured with heavy nonabsorbable suture (see Fig. 50-6C). Microvascular anastomoses are performed to adjacent vessels. An end-to-end anastomosis of both vessels to the thoracoacromial trunk vessels is preferred for the clavicle. Vessel patency and a bleeding flap surface confirm a successful transfer. A skin buoy flap can be transferred for continuous monitoring if desired. Postoperatively, a shoulder immobilizer is used for 6 to 8 weeks. Passive range of motion is then initiated.

---

*See references 46, 59, 60, 148, 207, 228, 265, 325, 328, and 332.

CRITICAL POINTS: FREE CORTICOPERIOSTEAL FLAP FROM MEDIAL FEMORAL CONDYLE

INDICATIONS

- Radiation necrosis of the clavicle
- Persistent nonunion of radius and ulna
- Scaphoid nonunion with avascular necrosis

PEARLS

- Vascular supply includes both the descending genicular and medial-superior genicular vessels. Either may be used to support the flap, depending on relative size.

TECHNICAL POINTS

- Make skin incision along inferior border of vastus medialis.
- Elevate vastus medialis from its compartment to identify descending genicular vessels.
- Identify medial superior genicular vessels distally, near the posterior femoral condyle.
- Realize the vessels lying on the periosteum form a semicircular network that can be elevated with fragments of underlying thin metaphyseal cortex as a pliable periosteal flap.
- Alternatively, use a smaller area including cancellous bone for small areas of bone loss.
- Follow the vascular pedicle proximally to its point of origin from the superficial femoral artery and vein in Hunter's canal.
- Dissection remains extra-articular.

PITFALLS

- Avoid injury to medial collateral ligament.
- Patients should expect some mild medial knee pain, persistent for up to several weeks.

POSTOPERATIVE CARE

- Allow full weight bearing and knee motion as comfort permits, generally within 2 to 3 days of surgery.

OTHER VASCULARIZED GRAFTS FOR RECONSTRUCTION OF LONG BONES

Rib

The rib, although used in early reports,[34,101,172] is generally not suitable for upper extremity reconstruction because of its membranous, weak structure and curved shape.[196,200] When based on its anterior internal mammary or supracostal arterial blood supply, only periosteal vessels are supplied.[18,101]

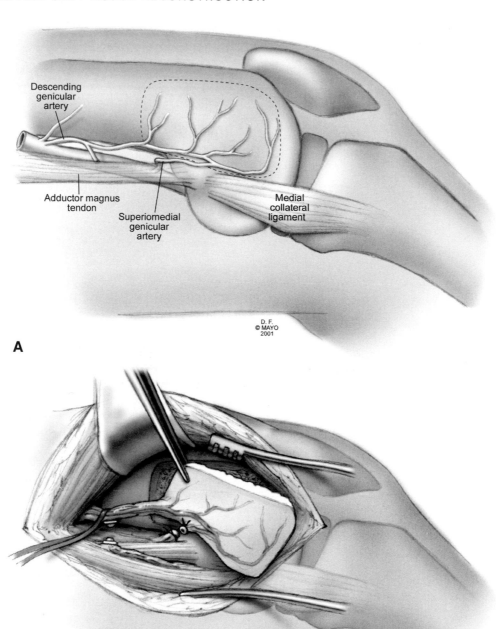

A

B

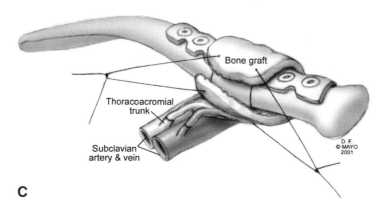

C

FIGURE 50-6. Corticoperiosteal flap (medial femoral condyle). **A,** Anatomy. **B,** Flap elevated from medial femoral condyle. **C,** Flap wrapped around clavicle with vascular connections to thoracoacromial trunk. (Copyright 2001, Mayo Foundation.)

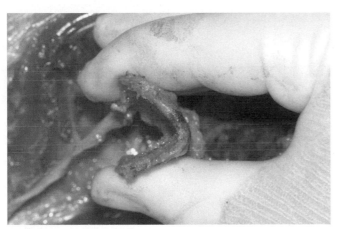

FIGURE 50-7. Corticoperiosteal flap. The flap is sufficiently flexible to wrap around small tubular bones.

The posterior rib graft, which includes its nutrient artery, requires ligation of the dorsal branch of the posterior intercostal artery.[201] Because this vessel supplies the spinal cord, the potential for causing paraplegia exists.[18,102] Furthermore, dissection is difficult and usually requires thoracotomy.

Scapula

Scapular free flaps may be based on the lateral border (lateral scapular osteocutaneous flap)[287] or on the medial ridge of the scapula.[271,286] The lateral flap is based on the circumflex scapular circulation and is usually taken as a composite flap.[189] The dissection requires division of the teres major and minor, resulting in some shoulder impairment. The medial flap, based on the same pedicle, depends on periosteal blood supply for bone nutrition. No donor site morbidity has been reported, although scapular winging from division of the serratus anterior is a likely potential problem.

Humerus

Portions of humerus diaphysis can be taken at the lateral intermuscular septum as part of an osteocutaneous lateral arm flap. In addition, periosteal flaps may be raised from the humerus among other locations, which have been successfully used to reconstruct bone defects.[265]

Manufactured Bone Grafts

Another future possibility is the creation of pedicled vascularized bone grafts in desired shapes. This has been demonstrated in the laboratory by implantation of vascular bundles into bone fragments or demineralized bone matrix.[184,321] When arteriovenous pedicles are enclosed in titanium, hydroxyapatite, or polyethylene chambers, or wrapped with vascularized periosteum in vivo, bone formation and remodeling occurs in the shape of the chamber along with microangiographic evidence of a sprouting vascular network as early as 4 weeks.[184,185,193] Similarly, Khouri has demonstrated the ability to transform muscle into bone of any desired shape using silicone rubber molds containing the recently purified osteoinductive factor osteogenin, when coated with demineralized bone matrix.[138] These findings support the concept of creating a preformed vascularized bone graft to reconstruct segmental bone defects.[184,193] Demonstration of clinical applicability remains to be performed.

Vascularized Bone Allografts

The ability to safely utilize living bone allografts would be an important advance in reconstructive surgery. Expendable vascularized autograft sources are limited, primarily to the fibula and iliac crest for larger defects. These grafts are generally poor structural replacements for missing metaphyseal or diaphyseal bone, particularly in the humerus, femur, and tibia, owing to gross size mismatch. In these locations, load sharing by rigid internal fixation, external fixators, allograft + autograft composites, or a protracted period of non–weight bearing and/or bracing is necessary if risk of stress fracture is to be minimized.[96] An ideal replacement for such large segment bone and joint defects would be a living bone and/or joint allogeneic transplant that exactly matches the dimension and structural property of the missing tissue. The survival of nonautogenous transplants at present relies on modulation of the immune system, using either long-term immunosuppression or induction of tolerance.[119] Long-term use of immunosuppressive drugs causes significant risk of opportunistic infections, malignancy, and organ toxicity.[144,209,227] Alternatively, induction of a state of donor-specific tolerance also carries the potential for significant morbidity and mortality, including causing graft versus host disease.[36,136,142] Given the problems just mentioned, it is not surprising that living musculoskeletal allografts have been seldom used clinically. A 27-cm femoral vascularized diaphyseal graft was performed without immunosuppression recently,[43] and both knee joint and femoral diaphyseal allografts have subsequently been transplanted in 8 patients.[107-109] Postoperative immunosuppression included long-term maintenance with cyclosporine and azathioprine.[109] There were two failures due to infection. Rejection was not monitored, other than a bone biopsy 2 years later. Another single case of a vascularized allogeneic fibula transplanted from mother to child with short-term immunosuppression resulted in nonunion and a secondary autologous bone graft.[9]

At the present time, however, bone and tissue antigenicity require use of immunosuppressive regimens that cannot be justified in patients with nonlethal conditions.[85,86,89] Characterization of the immune response to vascularized bone allografts may subsequently allow more specific modification of the host response and/or graft tissue.

MONITORING

Thrombosis of the vascular pedicle in a vascularized bone graft results in conditions less favorable for vascular invasion and the usual process of bone graft incorporation than a conventional bone graft.[251] Monitoring of graft viability in the immediate postoperative period is therefore desirable. A variety of methods have been to assess viability on an intermittent basis, for the purposes of planning subsequent treatment and anticipating outcome. These include selective angiography,[76,127,146] monitoring of healing and hypertrophy with serial radiographs,[81] bone biopsy or observation of bleeding on subsequent surgery, early[99] bone scans,[25,54,128,155,236,240,276,333] generally in the first postoperative week, as well as use of Doppler ultrasonography[263] or single-photon emission computed tomography.[190]

Intermittent monitoring methods, however, will not detect acute thrombosis. Continuous monitoring is possible with the use of a surface or implantable laser Doppler velocimeter,[99,129,237] thermocouple probe,[169] and measurement of local hydrogen production[245] or use of a skin paddle as a "buoy flap."[324] Detection of thrombosis allows revision of the anastomosis and salvage of a significant number of failing free tissue transfers.

Buoy Flap

By far the most feasible continual monitor is a fasciocutaneous "buoy" flap, which enables direct observation of the transferred tissue.[324] This method is preferred by most authors, allowing immediate return to the operating room if loosening of the dressing, altering limb position, or trial of anticoagulation does not reverse the observed changes in 1 to 2 hours.

Implanted Laser or Ultrasonic Probes

Although measurement of blood flow in an imbedded free flap is difficult, special probes have been used effectively. Karcher and coworkers reported effective monitoring of 11 bone flaps with a laser Doppler endoscopic probe and a screw implant. Postoperative monitoring was possible for 48 hours.[129] In Schuurman and associates' study of free fibular transfer, an occlusion rate of 10%, with 50% successful salvage was seen with use of a laser Doppler probe.[237]

A miniature Doppler ultrasonic probe is also available, designed to be secured to the outflow vein of the flap via a silicone rubber cuff.[139,272] The device was successful in salvaging 20 instances of thrombosis or spasm in 16 of 135 consecutive free flaps.[139]

Arteriography

Arteriography allows assessment of bone viability at a single point in time. Lau and Leung studied five cases of vascularized bone grafts using angiography 6 to 8 weeks after surgery and found the results to be comparable to clinical progress.[146]

Bone Scan

Experimentally, positive bone scans correlate with vessel patency when done before the end of the first week, before the onset of creeping repair in both vascularized and nonvascular autografts (Fig. 50-8).[240] Use of dynamic imaging provides a more accurate, even semi-quantitative linear relationship between scan values and bone blood flow.[197]

Bone scans obtained in the first 1 to 2 weeks after flap transfer have been demonstrably useful in clinical and

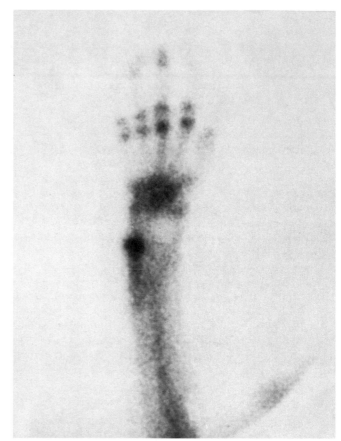

FIGURE 50-8. A bone scan 4 days postoperatively demonstrates excellent uptake in a fibular graft placed in the radius.

experimental studies, correlating well with preserved circulation and clinical outcome.[120,146,333] In these studies, patients with a "hot" postoperative radionuclide were more likely to have a successful clinical outcome than those with negative or equivocal scans. In one series, only one of seven patients with poor scans healed primarily, and two cases (almost 30%) resulted in frank failure, necessitating removal of the transferred bone.[333]

RESULTS OF VASCULARIZED BONE GRAFTING: BONE DEFECTS

Results by Donor Bone

Fibula

After review of 478 vascularized fibular grafts performed for all indications,* the primary union rate was 68%, with ultimate healing after supplemental bone graft in 82%. Healing as well as hypertrophy depends on a number of variables, including patient age, weight-bearing location, type of graft used, method of fixation, as well as the vascular status of the graft. Hypertrophy, when it occurs, is seen by

---

*See references 1, 39, 40, 56, 76, 87, 94, 98, 123, 125, 165, 177, 181, 186, 195, 199, 210, 255, 257, 269, 274, 290, 295, 302, and 309.

an average 13.5 months postoperatively.[51] It occurs primarily in young individuals (age < 20) and is more common in the lower extremity when stresses of weight bearing were not shielded by rigid fixation spanning the fibular graft (Fig. 50-9).[51] Fibulas are more likely to hypertrophy than other grafts.

Harvest of the fibula, although remarkably free from frequent complications, is not totally innocuous. Removal of a vascularized portion of the fibula is associated with a low prevalence of motor weakness and sensory deficits in the foot. The prevalence of pain in the ankle and lower limb increases with time, with some patients having a late onset of the symptoms.[303] Detailed gait and strength analysis demonstrated resolution of initially moderate knee and ankle-foot motion changes when evaluated more than 10 months after harvest.[327] Foot inversion and eversion strength was measurably weaker than normal, the latter inversely proportional to the length of resected fibula and ankle evertor muscle strength.

Iliac Crest

Vascularized iliac crest grafting is subject to higher rates of complications with lower overall success when compared with the fibula.[81,230,232,233,257,319] A summary of 97 flaps in the six reports just cited reveals an average time to union of 7 months, with prolonged protected weight bearing (mean, 18 months). Overall frank failure rate was somewhat higher than that with fibular grafts, with eventual union in 67% (38% requiring secondary bone grafting). Most authors are dissatisfied with the skin flap, noting a frequent tendency for necrosis of a part or all of the soft tissue.[22] Suggested solutions include use of an osteomuscular flap only, utilizing the internal oblique muscle, or the use of a double pedicle of both DCIA and SCIA.[214,230] Revision of the anastomosis is more commonly required than for fibular grafts.[257]

Results by Location

A review of 21 vascularized grafts to the upper extremity included graft placement in the humerus in 11 patients, radius in 5, ulna in 3, and clavicle in 2. Overall, primary bone union occurred in 15 patients (71.4%), and eventual union was achieved in 17 patients (81%). The most favorable results were achieved in cases of forearm bone reconstruction (100% union). Clavicle nonunions and shoulder fusions with vascularized bone carried a worse prognosis.[316] Results for shoulder fusion can be improved with improved stability using allograft proximal humerus/fibula composite grafts with rigid internal fixation. Average time to union for all locations is approximately 6 months, without significant difference based on anatomic location.[96]

Results by Diagnosis

The results of vascularized bone grafting differ significantly by diagnosis. A history of infection had the least favorable results overall. In a large series of 160 vascularized grafts, defects with infection had a primary union rate of 49% and an overall union rate of 77%. Grafts performed for trauma, tumor, and congenital anomalies without infection had primary and ultimate union rates of 69% and 84%, respectively.[96] Similar results may be found in other reports.[310]

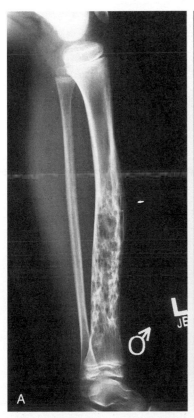
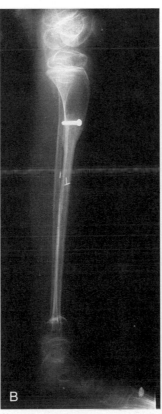
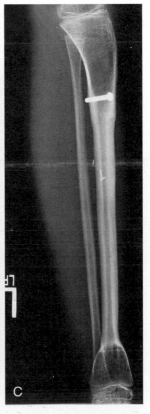

FIGURE 50-9. Resection of an adamantinoma of the tibia in an 8-year-old boy. **A,** Postoperative lateral radiograph. **B,** Successful union was seen 4 months postoperatively. **C,** Hypertrophy of the vascularized fibula graft is obvious in this 23-month postoperative view.

Tumor

Vascularized grafts are useful in limb salvage surgery of aggressive upper extremity tumors, including benign lesions such as giant cell tumor and aneurysmal bone cyst as well as primary bone malignancies (Fig. 50-10).[188,195,199,206] Many patients will receive preoperative and postoperative chemotherapy and/or radiotherapy, with the associated morbidity. Postoperative chemotherapy or radiotherapy probably increases the incidence of stress fracture, but most fractures heal, often without surgery.[1] Han and colleagues reported successful union in 81% of 69 patients.[96] In another review of 26 patients with malignant or locally aggressive bone tumors treated with limb salvage and reconstruction by free vascularized bone grafts, only 4 had complications. In these 4 patients there were three nonunions, two infections, and one stress fracture. The average duration of immobilization was 3.8 months in the upper extremity, and time to union was 5 months.[80]

Infection

The results are less satisfactory for patients who had had the reconstruction for bone loss due to osteomyelitis.[96] Experience with infected pseudarthrosis with segmental osseous defect, treated by débridement and microvascular bone transfer, has demonstrated an increased potential for a number of complications. These include recurrent infection, occasionally leading to amputation,[22,216] and nonunion. It is critical that vascularized bone transfer be delayed until sepsis is inactive. Criteria used for determining inactive sepsis include absence of sinus tracts, negative bacterial cultures, negative C-reactive protein, and a sedimentation rate of less than 15 mm/hr, maintained for at least 1 month after the last clinical evidence of infection.[180] Recurrent infection was seen after vascularized bone grafting in 16% of patients with osteomyelitis in the large Mayo Clinic series.[96]

In the forearm, infected nonunions may not respond to conventional treatment. Dell and Sheppard reported success with the use of vascularized fibular grafts and conversion to a one-bone forearm after failure of as many as six procedures.[56] The fibula was fixed to the ulna proximally and the radius distally with internal fixation, and this was supplemented with an external fixator in three of the four patients. All wounds healed and all bone junctures healed, with one requiring supplemental cancellous grafting.

Trauma

The prognosis is better for traumatic nonunion without infection. Union rates are typically greater than 90%, when patients requiring supplemental grafting are included.*

---

*See references 22, 96, 106, 112, 118, 166, 196, 211, 309, and 310.

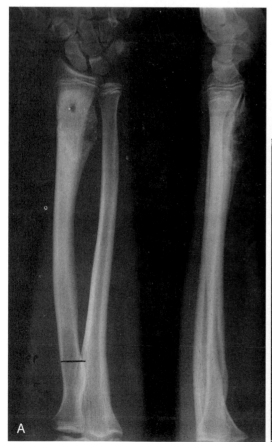
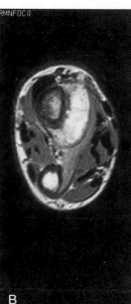
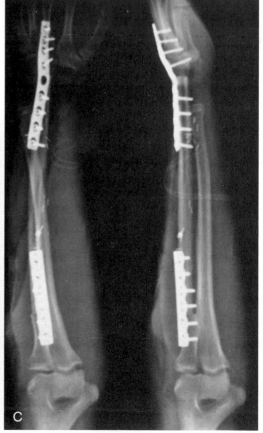

FIGURE 50-10. Osteogenic sarcoma of the distal radius, with diaphyseal medullary extension in a 14-year-old boy. **A,** Preoperative radiographs. **B,** Preoperative MRI demonstrating a large soft tissue extension on the palmar surface of the radius. **C,** Immediate postoperative radiographs. The majority of the radius has been excised and reconstructed with a vascularized free fibular graft, including a wrist arthrodesis distally.

Although some have reported poorer union rates for trauma than for tumor indications,[158] this group had the highest union rate overall in Han's series (primary union 76%, overall 92%).[96] Residual limb shortening and other problems are common, occurring more frequently in patients with scarred and relatively avascular soft tissues surrounding the long bone defects (Fig. 50-11).[158]

Congenital Pseudarthrosis of the Forearm

The use of vascularized grafts for congenital tibial pseudarthrosis has been shown to be demonstrably superior to conventional methods, including bone graft, electrical stimulation, corticoperiosteal graft, or osteotomy of the involved bone.[182,210,302,309] Vascularized grafts have been used successfully in pseudarthrosis of the forearm as well. In the forearm, creation of a one-bone forearm may be reasonable, especially if conventional bone grafting has failed.[203] Wide resection of associated neurofibromatosis is required. With this initial resection and a vascularized graft, good results may be anticipated.[165]

For Epiphyseal Transfer/Growth

The superiority of vascularized growth plate transfer to nonvascularized transfer for physeal replacement has been well documented in experimental models.[26,30,326] Clinically, the ability of near-normal longitudinal growth after digit replantation or toe transfer in children has been well documented.[132] The application of epiphyseal transfers to problems such as radial club hand and physeal arrest of long bones is currently showing substantial promise but remains in the developmental phase.[79] Transfer of the proximal fibula with vascularized proximal physis allowed long-term longitudinal growth in four of eight cases in one report.[291]

COMPLICATIONS

Impaired Vascularity

Vessel thrombosis occurs in approximately 10% of free fibular grafts, as detected with continual laser Doppler flowmetry and confirmed by surgical exploration.[237] If thrombosis occurs, it is likely that the surrounding cuff of necrotic soft tissue may impede neovascularization. Experimentally, the viability of thrombosed vascularized bone grafts is significantly less than conventional nonvascularized grafts as quantified by measurements of bone blood flow, new bone formation, and osteocyte counts.[251] Thus the process of creeping substitution of necrotic bone is likely less extensive in failed vascularized grafts than in conventional grafts.

Delayed Union: Need for Secondary Bone Graft

Secondary bone grafting will be necessary in a substantial number of patients treated with vascularized bone grafts of the long bones. As cited earlier, primary healing occurs in roughly 68% of vascularized fibular grafts, with poorer results in some locations and with a diagnosis of osteomyelitis. Most who do not heal primarily may benefit from a secondary bone graft. Because the mean time to healing is 6 months for fibular grafts and 7 months for iliac

crest grafts, timing of a secondary graft is generally somewhat longer, frequently at or before 12 months after the vascularized graft. A largely cancellous autograft at the ununited junction is usually sufficient. Problems associated with insufficient internal fixation may require revision at that time.

Stress Fracture

Stress fracture of a long graft is not uncommon, particularly in the lower extremity.[279] Minami and coworkers reported an incidence of 12 fractures occurring in 10 of 53 patients (23%).[182] Provided the graft has adequate vascularity, rapid formation of callus at the fracture site and hypertrophy of the bone is observed thereafter, although displacement is common and requires stabilization. Fracture was less common (9%) in the Mayo Clinic series.[96] Of these 12 fractures, 2 occurred in the radius and 1 in the ulna. Stress fractures may occur in the humerus as well, however (see Fig. 50-11B).

The time of fracture occurrence may be significant, because most occur within the first year.[181] Fractures in this time period generally have adequate circulation, as demonstrated by postoperative bone scan,[96] but have had insufficient time to undergo hypertrophy. Late fractures are uncommon and are associated with negative or equivocal bone scans. Most stress fractures occur through the transferred bone, rather than at its junctions

When the fracture occurred in adults, union is often relatively easily obtained. Nondisplaced upper extremity fractures will heal in a cast alone, whereas displaced fractures require internal or external fixation with or without bone grafting.[96,182] A vascularized graft should be protected against fatigue fracture during the first year, allowing a gradual increase in mechanical loading that enhances remodeling and hypertrophy.[51]

Complications Related to Specific Donor Sites

Fibula

Donor site complications are unusual and mostly transient.[189] A review of 132 free fibular grafts from the Mayo Clinic demonstrated donor site problems in 10 patients (8%). These included transient peroneal nerve palsy,[5] flexor hallucis longus contracture,[1] stress fracture of the ipsilateral tibia,[1] and compartment syndrome.[1,96] Closure after harvest of an osteocutaneous fibula should include use of a split-thickness skin graft to minimize the risk of compartment syndrome postoperatively.

In children, valgus deformity of the ankle may occur unless a distal tibiofibular fusion is performed proximal to the physis (see Fig. 50-4).[181] No similar sequelae have been seen at the knee when the fibular head is harvested for articular surface or physis.[291]

Donor site morbidity, studied by Youdas and Wood at two time points postoperatively, manifested as minimal alterations in knee and ankle-foot motion with gait analysis at less then 10 months postoperatively.[327] After 10 months, no significant gait abnormalities were discernable, although impaired strength of ankle inverters and everters persisted, the extent of which was inversely proportional to the length of the graft. Others have reported similar results.[88]

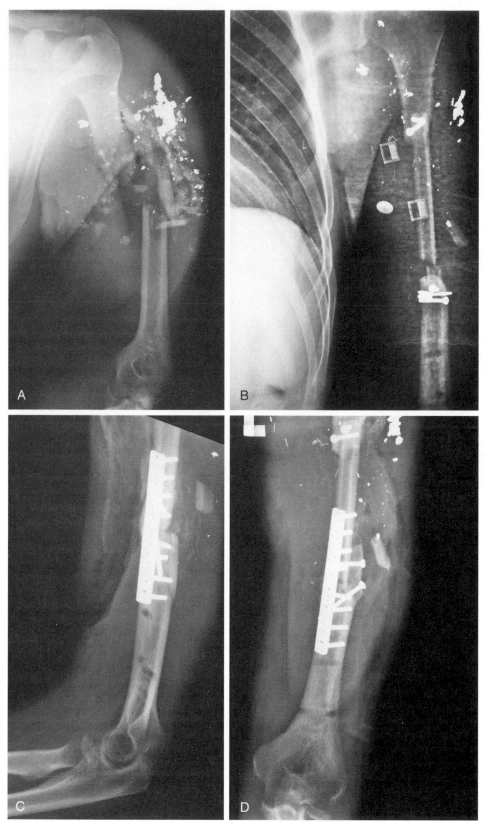

FIGURE 50-11. Gunshot wound in a 23-year-old man. **A,** Fragmentation of the humeral diaphysis before débridement. A large anterior wound was closed with a pedicled latissimus dorsi flap placed as an elbow flexorplasty to reconstruct the missing biceps muscle. **B,** A simultaneous fibular graft reconstructed the bone defect. A stress fracture occurred shortly after removal of a bridging external fixator several months later. **C and D,** Supplemental onlay bone grafting and plate fixation allowed healing of the fibula without further complications.

An extensive review of fibular donor site morbidity by Vail and Urbaniak demonstrated mild weakness in 10% of patients at 3 months postoperatively and a sensory deficit (unspecified) in 5% to 12%. Pain at sites other than the ankle was noted in 9 (3.6%) of the 247 limbs at 3 months and in 8.9% (95% confidence interval, 5.5% to 14.1%), according to the Kaplan-Meier analysis, at 5 years. The prevalence of pain in the ankle also increased with time, from 4 (1.6%) of the 247 limbs at 3 months to 11.5% (95% confidence interval, 7.4% to 17.6%), according to the Kaplan-Meier analysis, at 5 years. Removal of a vascularized portion of the fibula is associated with a low prevalence of motor weakness and sensory deficits in the foot. The prevalence of pain in the ankle and lower limb increases with time, with some patients having a late onset of the symptoms.[303]

Iliac Crest

Complications related to the iliac crest include incisional hernias and partial loss of the cutaneous portion of composite flaps. The surgical approach to the vascular pedicle is through the inguinal canal, raising the risk of an abdominal hernia.[96]

CARPAL VASCULARIZED BONE GRAFTS

Indications

Vascularized bone grafts may be applied to the carpus to aid or accelerate fracture healing, replace bone deficiency, or aid in direct revascularization of ischemic bone. Most commonly, and with increasing frequency, vascularized grafts are applied to treat scaphoid fractures and pseudarthroses and Kienböck's disease.

Sources of Vascularized Grafts for Carpal Pathology

The use of vascularized bone grafts for carpal pathology has been described by others, transposed on a pedicle from the pisiform,[33] metacarpal head,[212] or proximal metaphysis,[235] from the palmar and dorsal radial aspect of the radial metaphysis,* or from the diaphysis of ulna or radius.[93] Free microsurgical transfer is also possible.[205] Many of these grafts require extensive dissection, need an additional surgical incision, and have limited blood supply. Palmar radius grafts, in particular, require dissection in the vicinity of important radiocarpal ligaments and/or have unpredictable nutrient artery locations.[241]

Dorsal Radius

The blood supply to the distal dorsal radius is robust and constant, provided by a series of longitudinal vessels originating from the radial artery or anterior interosseous artery and venae comitantes, which demonstrate consistent spatial relationships to surrounding anatomic landmarks and constant distal anastomotic vascular connections. The possibility of raising vascularized dorsal radius grafts based on branches of the posterior division of the anterior interosseous or radial artery has been recognized by several authors.[113,161,174,331] Recently, the descriptive and applied anatomy of the extraosseous and interosseous vascular supply of the distal radius was described in some detail, including the design of several reverse flow pedicle grafts applicable to the carpus.[241] These grafts are relatively easily harvested through the same operative field used for carpal exposure, based on arteriovenous pedicles whose position relative to anatomic landmarks (extensor retinaculum and dorsal compartments) is constant. Their location allows vascularized bone grafting for Kienböck's disease or scaphoid nonunion with minimal if any additional morbidity. Blood flow is provided by a reverse-flow mechanism in both artery and venae comitantes analogous to the radial forearm flap,[153] with demonstrable preservation of flow possible by inclusion of cutaneous islands whether based on the radial artery or posterior division of the anterior interosseous artery.[21,113,161,243,246,247,331] Experimental studies in the canine distal radius have demonstrated that similar reverse-flow pedicle bone grafts have measurable flow immediately after elevation and marked hyperemia when reevaluated 2 weeks later.[293,294]

Palmar Radius

Palmar radius grafts have been used, based on a pronator quadratus pedicle (palmar metaphyseal arch) or palmar radiocarpal arch.† Flow through the pedicle may be based on the anterior interosseous artery, harvesting the graft from the lateral aspect of the palmar radius, or on the terminal palmar metaphyseal or palmar radiocarpal branches of the radial artery when the bone is harvested from the medial palmar radius (Fig. 50-12B).[95,167,241] Inclusion of the palmar radiocarpal vessels places important palmar radiocarpal ligaments at risk, and the nutrient supply of the more proximal palmar metaphyseal arch within the pronator quadratus muscle is small and highly variable in location.[241] These grafts are further limited by the need for carpal exposure through important radiocarpal ligaments. This limits exposure and may risk radiocarpal instability postoperatively. Nevertheless, excellent clinical results have been reported with this flap.[95,167]

Pisiform

The pisiform receives blood supply from the ulnar artery via its deep volar and dorsal carpal branches.[176] The dorsal carpal branch is the major vessel, with at least two descending branches entering the proximal tip of the bone. This allows elevation of a pedicled pisiform graft that may be used to replace the lunate[33,69,105,322] or, when placed as a decorticated graft with the lunate, to revascularize it.[24]

Second Metacarpal

A small amount of bone may be raised as a vascularized graft from the second metacarpal, based on the first dorsal metacarpal artery.[15,31,137,156,164,235,329,330] The second metacarpal may be harvested entirely for skeletal thumb reconstruction associated with destruction of the index

---

*See references 21, 29, 73, 134, 145, 151, 163, 167, 217, 246, and 247.
†See references 29, 73, 95, 134, 145, 151, 167, 217, and 241.

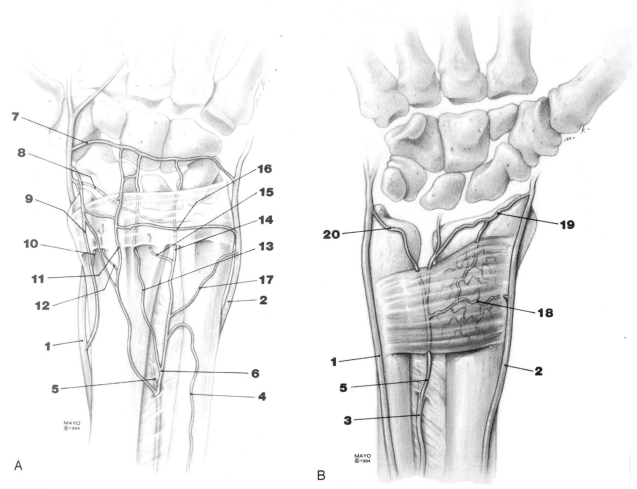

FIGURE 50-12. The vascular anatomy of the distal radius. **A,** Dorsal radius blood supply. Two superficial vessels lie on the surface of the extensor retinaculum (the 1,2 intercompartmental supraretinacular artery [ICSRA] [9] and the 2,3 ICSRA [11]). Two deep vessels lie directly on the radius beneath the tendons of the fourth and fifth extensor compartments (the 4th extensor compartment artery [ECA] [13] and 5th ECA [14]). **B,** The palmar blood supply is provided by two arches connecting the anterior interosseous vessels and the radial artery (palmar carpal arch [19] and palmar metaphyseal arch [18]). 1, radial artery; 2, ulnar artery; 3, anterior interosseous artery; 4, posterior interosseous artery; 5, anterior division of anterior interosseous artery; 6, posterior division of anterior interosseous artery; 7, dorsal intercarpal arch; 8, dorsal radiocarpal arch; 9, 1,2 ICSRA; 10, second compartment branch of 1,2 ICSRA; 11, 2,3 ICSRA; 12, second compartment branch of 2,3 ICSRA; 13, 4th ECA; 14, 5th ECA; 15, fourth compartment branch of 5th ECA; 16, dorsal supraretinacular arch; 17, oblique dorsal artery of the distal ulna; 18, palmar metaphyseal arch; 19, radial portion of palmar radiocarpal arch; 20, ulnar portion of palmar radiocarpal arch. (Copyright 1994, Mayo Foundation.)

finger or partially as an elective procedure for carpal pathology.[171] The arc of rotation allows transposition within the radial side of the hand, for applications in the thumb and carpus.[212] Dorsal proximal metaphyseal grafts have been used successfully for scaphoid nonunions and Kienböck's disease.[156,235,329,330]

INDICATIONS FOR VASCULARIZED GRAFTS IN THE WRIST

Kienböck's Disease

Treatment of Kienböck's disease remains controversial, with a large number of treatment options available, including lunate excision,[133,135] lunate replacement with artificial

replacement,[3,19,67,130,215,304] pisiform,[33,104,105,322] or fascia, unloading procedures such as joint leveling or angular osteotomies of the radius or ulna,* capitate shortening,[5] or intercarpal arthrodesis,[44,111,183,252,305,308] as well as direct lunate revascularization with isolated arteriovenous pedicles[110,277,278,321] or vascularized bone grafts.[24,69,93,171,176] In addition, salvage procedures for advanced changes with arthrosis may be necessary, including proximal row carpectomy or complete wrist arthrodesis.

Experimental studies have demonstrated the ability of vascularized bone grafts to revascularize ischemic bone.[85,110,321] The main function of the procedure appears to be the provision of vessels into avascular bone.[296]

---

*See references 6, 7, 111, 141, 154, 168, 192, 222, 242, 288, 307, and 311.

Vascularized grafts in general have demonstrated satisfactory clinical results in Kienböck's disease, with excellent pain relief and improvement in range of motion and strength. Radiographic progression of lunate and carpal height collapse occurred in 0% to 15% of patients in three studies,[24,171,278] and radiographic and magnetic resonance imaging (MRI) evidence of revascularization are found after surgery.[110,171,278] These types of grafts may be especially useful in cases of ulnar-positive or neutral Kienböck's disease, when joint leveling is contraindicated to avoid ulnar impaction syndrome.[53] The lunate may be expanded with the graft, resulting in improvement of the lunate index and carpal height ratio postoperatively in stage IIIA disease.[171] Their use is questionable with displaced coronal fractures of the lunate, owing to the unreliable healing of such fractures,[171] or in cases with marked carpal collapse, which may progress radiographically with osteoarthritic changes or fragmentation of the lunate.[278] Protection during early healing is necessary, to prevent lunate collapse with revascularization.[10,152]

Scaphoid Nonunion

The scaphoid is the most frequently fractured carpal bone. With prompt appropriate diagnosis and treatment, over 90% will unite. Unfortunately, failure to diagnose acute injury, or surgically treat displaced scaphoid fractures, increases the risk of nonunion substantially.[45,273] The development of scaphoid foreshortening and associated carpal instability with elapsed time contribute to the risk of nonunion.[273] In addition, fractures of the proximal third heal less readily, in part secondary to vascular compromise in the proximal fragment.[115]

Most scaphoid fractures that fail to heal with inlay or wedge conventional grafts probably have impaired vascularity as a contributing factor, as demonstrated by sclerosis of the proximal pole on radiography and MRI and by absence of punctate bleeding at the time of surgery.[38,90,170,191,260] The use of conventional grafts such as the Matti-Russe volar inlay graft may be contraindicated in the presence of an avascular fragment.[90]

Vascularized bone grafts have been proposed as appropriate methods to increase the rate and frequency of healing in fractures with poor prognosis. As early as 1965, Roy-Camille used the palmar tubercle of the scaphoid based on an abductor pollicis brevis muscle pedicle for this problem.[226] In recent years, palmar distal radius grafts,[29,95,134,145,147,151,167,175,235] dorsal radius grafts,* second metacarpal base,[235] free medial femoral condyle,[59] and free iliac grafts[14,77,78,97,205] have demonstrated improved results as compared with conventional grafts in difficult circumstances. These include displaced acute fractures with small proximal fragments or bone deficiency requiring grafting, failed conventional grafts, and nonunion of proximal pole fractures, especially when associated with avascular necrosis.[248,261,270] Alternatively, inlay bone grafting coupled with vascular bundle implantation may be considered.[11,71,110]

---

*See references 28, 55, 157, 175, 234, 261, 262, 268, 292, 299, and 331.

VASCULARIZED GRAFTS FOR THE WRIST: HARVEST OF DORSAL RADIUS GRAFTS

 Anatomy

Four extraosseous vessels contribute nutrient vessels to the distal radius and ulna (see Fig. 50-12A and B). They demonstrate consistent spatial relationships to surrounding anatomic landmarks and supply bone with predictable groups of nutrient arteries. They receive contributions from the radial, ulnar, and anterior and posterior interosseous arteries (see Fig. 50-12). The anterior interosseous artery divides into anterior and posterior divisions proximal to the distal radioulnar joint. Its posterior division together with the radial artery are the primary sources of orthograde blood flow to the distal radius. They also supply nutrition to soft tissues, making possible fabrication of composite pedicle flaps that include the posterior interosseous nerve, skin, and muscle.[243,331]

The four vessels supplying nutrient arteries to the dorsal radius are best described by their relationship to the extensor compartments of the wrist and the extensor retinaculum. Two of the vessels are *superficial* in location, lying on the dorsal surface of the extensor retinaculum between the first and second and the second and third dorsal compartments. At these locations, the retinaculum is adherent to an underlying bony tubercle separating their respective compartments, allowing nutrient vessels to penetrate bone. Because of their location, they have been named the 1,2 and 2,3 intercompartmental supraretinacular arteries (1,2 and 2,3 ICSRA) (see Fig. 50-12A).[241,246,248]

Two *deep* vessels also provide nutrient vessels to the dorsal distal radius. They lie on the surface of the radius in the floor of the fourth and fifth dorsal compartments. They are consequently named the fourth and fifth extensor compartment arteries (4th and 5th ECA).[241]

The 1,2 ICSRA (see Fig. 50-12A; Table 50-1) originates from the radial artery approximately 5 cm proximal to the radiocarpal joint, passing beneath the brachioradialis muscle and tendon to lie on the dorsal surface of the extensor retinaculum. Distally, it enters the anatomical snuffbox to anastomose to the radial artery and/or the radiocarpal arch. This distal origin is the "ascending irrigating branch" described previously.[331] It is the smallest of the four vessels (mean internal diameter of 0.30 mm). Like all of the vessels, it is accompanied by venae comitantes. It provides several small nutrient arteries to the bone (see Table 50-1).

Its position superficial to the retinaculum and directly on the bony tubercle between the first and second extensor compartments makes its dissection and use as a vascularized pedicled graft to the scaphoid fairly straightforward. However, its arc of rotation is short and its nutrient artery branches small in number and caliber. The vessel itself is occasionally absent. These factors may significantly limit its usefulness in other carpal bones and in some patients.

The 2,3 ICSRA (see Fig. 50-12A; see Table 50-1) originates proximally from the anterior interosseous artery or the posterior division of the anterior interosseous artery. It runs

Table 50-1

EXTRAOSSEOUS VESSEL CHARACTERISTICS: DISTAL RADIUS

Artery	Artery Present (%)	Internal Diameter (mm) (mean [range])	Provides Nutrient Arteries to Bone
Posterior division AIA	100	0.71 (0.20-1.18)	No
1,2 ICSRA	94	0.30 (0.14-0.58)	Yes
2nd EC branch of 1,2 ICSRA	56	0.16 (0.14-0.19)	Yes
2,3 ICSRA	100	0.35 (0.14-0.55)	Yes
4th ECA	100	0.38 (0.28-0.72)	Yes
5th ECA	100	0.49 (0.27-0.76)	No
rPCa	100	0.47 (0.19-0.76)	Yes
pMeta	100	0.50 (0.30-0.74)	Yes

AIA, anterior interosseous artery; ICSRA, intercompartmental supraretinacular artery; ECA, extensor compartment artery; rPCa, radial half of palmar carpal arch; pMeta, palmar metaphyseal arch.

From Sheetz KK, Bishop AT, Berger RA: The arterial blood supply of the distal radius and ulna and its potential use in vascularized pedicled bone grafts. J Hand Surg [Am] 20:902-914, 1995.

superficial to the extensor retinaculum directly on the dorsal radial tubercle (Lister's tubercle) to anastomose with the dorsal intercarpal arch, and in some cases the dorsal radiocarpal arch and/or the 4th extensor compartment artery. It has a mean internal diameter of 0.35 mm. The number, location, and size of its nutrient branches are shown in Table 50-1. These nutrient branches often penetrate deep into cancellous bone. One large proximal branch enters the radius in the floor of the 2nd extensor compartment. Like the 1,2 ICSRA, the 2,3 ICSRA is easily based as a retrograde pedicle for a vascularized bone graft because of its position superficial to the retinaculum (see Fig. 50-12A). Because of its midaxial dorsal position, its arc of rotation reaches the entire proximal carpal row. Its nutrient arteries are somewhat larger and more likely to supply cancellous bone than those of the 1,2 ICSRA, particularly if a proximal branch to the floor of the second compartment is included. It is potentially useful for Kienböck's disease or proximal scaphoid nonunion.

The 4th ECA (see Fig. 50-12A; see Table 50-1) lies directly adjacent to the posterior interosseous nerve on the radial aspect of the fourth extensor compartment. In a minority of cases, the vessel may be found within the 3,4 septum for most of its course. Proximally, this artery originates from the posterior division of the anterior interosseous artery or its fifth extensor compartment branch. It anastomoses distal to the radius with the dorsal intercarpal arch, and in most cases to the dorsal radiocarpal arch. Connections to the neighboring 2,3 ICSRA and/or the 5th ECA are common. It has a mean internal diameter of 0.38 mm. The 4th ECA is the source of numerous nutrient vessels to the floor of the fourth compartment that frequently penetrate cancellous bone (see Table 50-1). The vessels entering more distally tend to supply primarily cortical bone, whereas those more proximal are more likely to penetrate cancellous bone.

The 5th ECA (see Fig. 50-12A; see Table 50-1) is generally the largest of all the dorsal vessels supplying nutrient branches (mean 0.49 mm internal diameter). It is located in the radial floor of the fifth extensor compartment, passing mostly through the 4,5 septum in one third of specimens.[241] This vessel is supplied proximally by the posterior division of the anterior interosseous artery and anastomoses distally with the dorsal intercarpal arch. It may also make connections with the 4th ECA, the dorsal radiocarpal arch, the 2,3 ICSRA, and/or the oblique dorsal artery of the distal ulna. Thirty-nine percent of the 5th ECAs in the study of Sheetz and coworkers had a branch that supplied one or two nutrient vessels to the floor of the fourth compartment (fourth extensor compartment branch of 5th ECA).[22] It is perhaps most useful as a large conduit of retrograde flow from the intercarpal arch to other vessels with more consistent nutrient branches. Its large diameter and multiple anastomoses allow creation of a vascular pedicle that can reach almost anywhere in the hand (see Fig. 50-12A).

Distal Anastomoses

A series of arches across the dorsum of the hand and wrist provide anastomoses with these intercompartmental and compartmental arteries. These include the dorsal intercarpal arch (dICa), dorsal radiocarpal arch (dRCA), and dorsal supraretinacular arch (see Fig. 50-12A).

The dICA (see Fig. 50-12A) receives contributions from the radial and ulnar arteries and the 5th ECA and frequently anastomoses with the 2,3 ICSRA, 4th ECA, dorsal radiocarpal arch (67%), and 1,2 ICSRA. The dorsal intercarpal arch does not contribute nutrient arteries to the distal radius or distal ulna except indirectly through arteries with which it connects. It is an important part of several potential grafts because of its anastomotic connections. The arch can be used as a source of retrograde arterial flow, allowing proximal vessel ligation and graft mobilization.

The dRCa (see Fig. 50-12A) receives a contribution from the radial artery and at least two additional sources such as the dorsal intercarpal arch (67%), 4th ECA (59%), 2,3 ICSRA (52%), 1,2 ICSRA (52%), and/or the 5th ECA (23%).[241] It contributes significantly to the dorsal distal radius via small nutrient arteries. These nutrient branches enter bone just proximal to the radiocarpal joint and proceed perpendicularly to supply cancellous bone in the extreme distal end of the metaphysis (Table 50-2). Because of its close proximity to the radius and location on or deep to the superficial joint capsule, it has limited usefulness as a potential source of retrograde arterial flow owing to limited arc of rotation and difficult dissection.

A dorsal supraretinacular arch (see Fig. 50-12A) provides anastomoses between the arteries running parallel to the radial and ulnar diaphyses. It is not a single artery but, rather, an anastomotic network of small vessels connecting the dorsal arteries. Because of its small-caliber vessels, it is not of use in providing retrograde bone graft pedicle blood flow.

1,2 ICSRA Graft

Grafts based on a retrograde 1,2 ICSRA pedicle were originally described by Zaidenberg and coworkers for scaphoid nonunion.[331] The vessel lies superficial to the extensor retinaculum rather than lying on periosteum as originally described and is thus easily visible after retraction of the skin and subcutaneous tissue. This graft is useful for most scaphoid nonunions but cannot be used for other carpal bones owing to its limited arc of rotation. In some individuals, a more proximal branch of the 1,2 ICSRA enters the floor of the second compartment, ending as a large nutrient vessel. A graft centered on this branch results in a pedicle long enough to reach the lunate.[241]

Harvest Technique (Fig. 50-13)

The extremity is elevated for exsanguination and a tourniquet is inflated. Use of an Esmarch bandage before tourniquet elevation will make vessel visualization more difficult. The bone graft donor site and scaphoid are exposed through a gently curvilinear dorsoradial incision paralleling the course of the extensor pollicis longus tendon (see Fig. 50-13A). Branches of the superficial radial nerve are identified and protected. Once the subcutaneous tissues are gently raised from the retinaculum, the 1,2 ICSRA and venae comitantes are visualized on the surface of the extensor retinaculum. They are dissected carefully toward their distal anastomosis with the radial artery and venae comitantes in the floor of the anatomical snuffbox. A vessel loop is placed around the distally based pedicle to protect it during later dissection. Next, the first and second dorsal compartments are opened at the graft elevation site to create a cuff of retinaculum containing the vessels and their nutrient branches (see Fig. 50-13B). The center of the graft should be 1.5 cm proximal to the radiocarpal joint to include the nutrient vessels.

Scaphoid Preparation

Before the graft is elevated, a transverse dorsal-radial capsulotomy is made to expose the nonunion site (see Fig. 50-13C). In most cases, this will be a proximal pole fracture in which a dorsal inlay graft is most appropriate. If this is the case, a 2- to 3-mm bur or small, sharp osteotomes are used

Table 50-2
NUTRIENT ARTERY CHARACTERISTICS

Artery Supplying Nutrient Arteries	No. of Nutrient Arteries (mean [range])	Nutrient Artery Internal Diameter (mm) (mean [range])	Distance from Nutrient Artery Penetration to RC Joint (mm) (mean [range])	% of Nutrient Arteries that Penetrate Cancellous Bone (%)
1,2 ICSRA	3.2 (0-9)	<0.10 (<0.05-0.15)	15 (4-26)	6
2nd EC branch of 1,2 ICSRA	1 (1)	0.16 (0.14-0.19)	21 (17-28)	57
2,3 ICSRA	1.8 (0-5)	0.11 (0.07-0.19)	13 (3-24)	22
2nd EC branch of 2,3 ICSRA	1.4 (1-4)	0.19 (0.09-0.28)	18 (14-32)	48
4th ECA	3.2 (1-6)	0.16 (0.07-0.29)	11 (3-19)	45
4th EC branch of 5th ECA	1.2 (1-2)	0.15 (0.15)	10 (6-12)	43
dRCa	2.6 (0-7)	0.18 (0.14-0.29)	4 (1-12)	79
pMeta	2.0 (0-5)	<0.10 (<0.05-0.20)	12 (10-34)	20
rPCa	6.0 (2-10)	0.15 (0.04-0.33)	6 (1-15)	70

RC, radiocarpal; ICSRA, intercompartmental supraretinacular artery; ECA, extensor compartment artery; dRCa, dorsal radiocarpal arch; pMeta, palmar metaphyseal arch; rPCA, radial half of palmar carpal arch.

From Sheetz KK, Bishop AT, Berger RA: The arterial blood supply of the distal radius and ulna and its potential use in vascularized pedicled bone grafts. J Hand Surg [Am] 20:902-914, 1995.

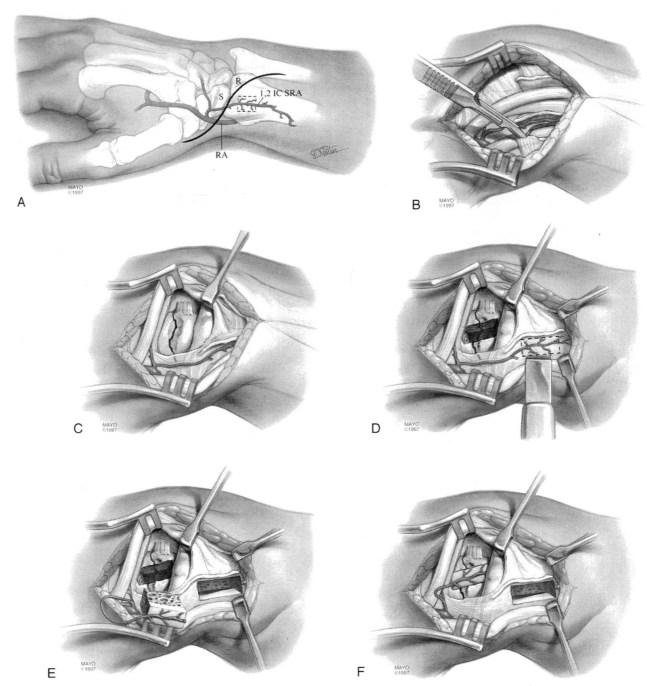

FIGURE 50-13. Treatment of scaphoid nonunions with a 1,2 ICSRA pedicle bone graft. **A,** A curvilinear dorsoradial incision is used for exposure of the scaphoid and the 1,2 ICSRA. **B,** The 1,2 ICSRA is identified on the surface of the extensor retinaculum. The first and second dorsal compartments are opened on either side of the vessels. **C,** The scaphoid nonunion is visualized after the vessel is identified and protected. **D,** A trough for a dorsal inlay graft has been prepared, spanning the nonunion. A distal radius graft including the 1,2 ICSRA is outlined. **E,** The graft is raised and transposed to the nonunion site. **F,** The graft placed as a dorsal inlay. (Copyright 1997, Mayo Foundation.)

Continued

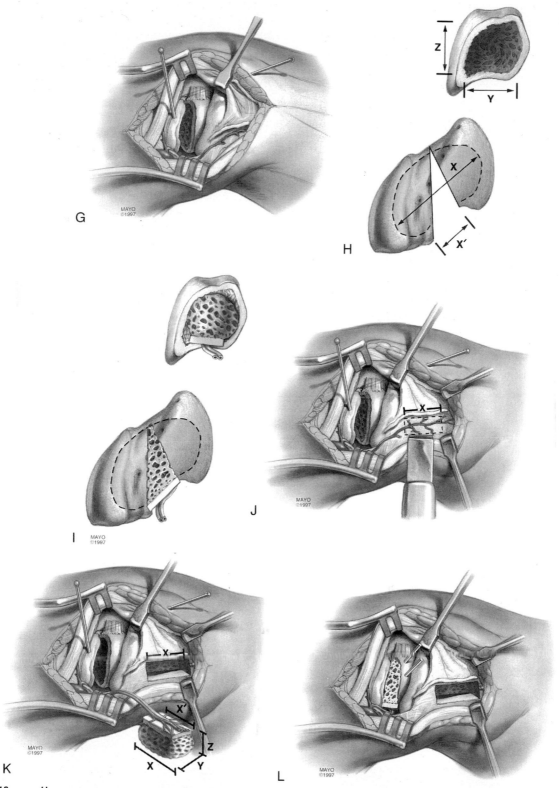

FIGURE 50-13—cont'd. G, Exposure of a scaphoid waist fracture with a humpback deformity requiring a palmar wedge graft. **H,** The dimensions of an ideal wedge graft are determined. **I,** The graft will be placed with the vessels and radial cortex palmarly. **J** and **K,** The dimensions of the scaphoid defect are used to plan the radius pedicle graft dimensions. **L,** The use of supplemental internal fixation is important when using vascularized grafts for scaphoid nonunion. (Copyright 1997, Mayo Foundation.)

to prepare a slot to receive the bone graft, curetting any fibrous tissue from the nonunion site (see Fig. 50-13D). The slot will span the nonunion, unless the proximal pole fragment is very small. If the proximal pole is very small, the graft is shaped to lie within the concavity of the proximal pole fragment and slot into the distal fragment. Alternatively, a wedge graft may be used to expand the scaphoid length through the radial approach (see Fig. 50-13G to L). In some cases, a limited radial styloidectomy may improve exposure but is not generally necessary. For either method, the size and orientation of the bone graft are carefully determined before graft elevation.

Types of Grafts
Dorsal Inlay Graft
Most of the cases in which vascularized grafts have been used have been proximal pole nonunions. In these cases, the use of a dorsal inlay graft is generally appropriate, allowing the graft to bridge the nonunion, facilitating stability and early union.

Preparation of the nonunion site should be performed after pedicle dissection but before graft elevation, as described earlier. Careful inspection of the midcarpal and radiocarpal joint surfaces of the scaphoid is mandatory to prevent articular surface injury during creation of the trough. If the proximal pole fragment is very small, the bone graft is placed within it rather than fitted into a dorsal slot. The graft is removed from the radius, outlining the desired shape using small, sharp osteotomes and protecting the distally based pedicle. The proximal origin of the 1,2 ICSRA may be ligated or cauterized with a bipolar forceps. The graft is then pried from the metaphyseal bone using an osteotome placed

in the proximal cut at the desired depth (approximately 1 cm) (see Fig. 50-13E). Before placement of the graft, my colleagues and I now prefer to stabilize the scaphoid with internal fixation before graft placement. This is generally done with a cannulated scaphoid screw placed antegrade from the proximal pole. Graft placement is facilitated by raising an ulnar-based retinacular flap to include the third dorsal compartment. Retraction of the extensor pollicis longus then allows direct visualization of the scaphoid, scapholunate ligament, and scaphocapitate joint. With the wrist flexed, the guide wire can be easily placed in the mid axis of the scaphoid. Screw placement follows and results in its placement sufficiently palmar so as to not interfere with the bone graft. The graft is then placed and carefully reshaped as needed to allow it to be placed snugly in the slot with sufficient press-fit interference to maintain stability (see Fig. 50-13F).

Interposition (Wedge) Graft (see Fig. 50-13G to L)
Alternatively, when scaphoid foreshortening and angular displacement require its elongation, a vascularized graft may be placed through a dorsoradial approach as a wedge graft. In this circumstance, the scaphoid is again prepared before graft elevation. The maximal dimensions of the palmar cortical defect (X) and internal defect (X') are noted (see Fig. 50-13H). When used as a wedge graft, the vessels are placed palmarly to allow a palmar cortical strut for structural stability (see Fig. 50-13I). A graft sufficiently large to fill the internal scaphoid defect should be raised. Careful graft preparation will allow its use with a volar cortical strut trimmed to the appropriate length and a longer internal cancellous "football-shaped" extension. This allows

---

CRITICAL POINTS: DORSAL DISTAL RADIUS PEDICLE GRAFT FOR NONUNION OF SCAPHOID

INDICATIONS
- Established scaphoid nonunion
  - Proximal third location
  - Avascular proximal pole

PREOPERATIVE EVALUATION
- Computed tomography with reconstructions
- MRI with gadolinium enhancement

PEARLS
- Screw fixation is preferred to enhance stability and chance for healing.
- It is useful to stabilize scaphoid with guide wire before insetting graft.

TECHNICAL POINTS
- Elevate without Esmarch exsanguination before tourniquet elevation.

- Use 1,2 ICSRA pedicle, visible on surface of retinaculum.
- Mobilize distal portion of vessel to radial artery/venae comitantes before capsular exposure.
- Use as dorsal inlay graft in most circumstances. Prepare slot only after carefully identifying scapholunate ligament and radiocarpal and midcarpal articular surfaces of scaphoid.
- Stabilize scaphoid first with guide wire directed from proximal to distal. Guide wire usually lies palmar to location of graft.
- Shape graft to appropriate size. Compress with forceps slightly to allow press-fit.
- Compression from screw placement plus press-fit provides adequate graft stability.

POSTOPERATIVE CARE
- Maintain cast immobilization until early computed tomographic evidence of healing is seen.

the scaphoid internal angles to be corrected while simultaneously filling the central cancellous defect with living bone.

Graft Placement

Once the scaphoid is prepared, a graft of appropriate dimension, including the vessels and cuff of retinaculum between the first and second compartments, is raised. The location of harvest is positioned to include the nutrient vessels, centered a mean 15 mm from the radiocarpal joint margin.[241] In many cases, inspection with loupe magnification will permit visualization of nutrient branches. Graft elevation begins with the ligation of the 1,2 ICSRA and accompanying veins *proximal* to the graft. Next, the vessels are meticulously dissected subperiosteally distal to the graft to separate them from the radial styloid and joint capsule. To improve the arc of rotation, the pedicle may be dissected to its distal radial artery anastomosis. With the vessels mobilized, the graft is carefully separated from the radius with sharp osteotomes. Distally, the pedicle must be retracted first dorsally and then palmarly as the distal osteotomy is created in two stages. The cancellous bone is fragile, requiring attention to detail to prevent its fracture as the graft is levered out from the radius. Once the graft is free on its distal pedicle, the tourniquet may be briefly released to allow demonstration of robust bleeding on the surface of the vascularized bone graft. It may be reinflated once the surgeon is satisfied with the vascularity of the bone. The graft is transposed beneath the radial wrist extensor tendons to reach the nonunion site, where it is gently impacted into position. In the case of the typical dorsal inlay graft, the vessels and cortical bone are positioned to lie on the dorsal surface of the scaphoid. For use as a wedge graft, the cortical bone is positioned palmarly. Wedge graft cortical bone is gently trimmed from the cancellous bone to create a cortical surface of the proper dimension for scaphoid lengthening, while allowing additional cancellous bone to fill any medullary defect in the scaphoid.

Role of Internal Fixation

Supplemental internal fixation is necessary for scaphoid nonunions, even with the use of vascularized grafts. In most cases, a scaphoid screw may be safely placed without jeopardy to the pedicle. Alternatively, one or two Kirschner wires may be used and have been satisfactory in my colleagues and my experience.[262] A meta-analysis of scaphoid nonunion literature has demonstrated that Kirschner wire fixation results in higher rates of pseudarthrosis than when screws are used.[175] My preferred method was discussed previously—placing the screw in an antegrade direction before graft placement.

2,3 ICSRA Graft

The 2,3 ICSRA allows elevation of a vascularized graft from the dorsal tubercle of the distal radius via its distal anastomosis to the dorsal intercarpal arch. Its placement is ideal for the lunate or the proximal scaphoid pole. Because the pedicle is located directly overlying the scapholunate ligament, it must be fully mobilized, generally with graft elevation as well, before a capsulotomy may be performed.

Harvest Technique

Elevation is performed similarly to the 1,2 ICSRA and is likewise technically relatively simple because of its superficial location on the surface of the extensor retinaculum overlying Lister's dorsal radial tubercle. The graft should be centered 13 mm proximal to the radiocarpal joint, in order to include its nutrient vessels. In Kienböck's disease, the graft is oriented to allow the dorsal radial cortex and attached vessels to enter the lunate oriented vertically (ligated proximal vessel placed deeply into lunate), using the underlying graft cortical bone as a strut to help prevent lunate collapse during revascularization (Fig. 50-14F). Dissection through subcutaneous tissues must be gentle to avoid injury to the vessels on the retinacular surface. Once the retinaculum is exposed, the 2,3 ICSRA and its venae comitantes will be visible lying on Lister's tubercle. They are dissected distally with a narrow cuff of perivascular tissue, carefully mobilizing them to the level of the dorsal intercarpal arch. A communicating branch with the dorsal radiocarpal arch will require ligation or bipolar electrocautery. Exposure of the second and third extensor compartment contents is necessary, making two parallel incisions through the retinaculum on either side of Lister's tubercle and the overlying vessels. Retraction of the extensor pollicis longus allows better visualization of the distal course of the 2,3 ICSRA. Once the pedicle is dissected, a bone graft including Lister's tubercle is then raised with an osteotome. Graft elevation should be centered approximately 13 mm proximal to the radiocarpal joint to include the nutrient vessels.[241] The graft and its distal pedicle are retracted distally, allowing capsulotomy for placement of the graft in the carpus. Placement as a dorsal inlay graft for proximal pole union is done as described in the earlier section on the 1,2 ICSRA graft. Graft insetting for core revascularization of the lunate is described in the following section.

5 + 4 ECA Graft

A 4th ECA graft based on retrograde flow from the intercarpal arch may also be useful in Kienböck's disease.[171] Its arc of rotation consistently reaches the lunate, and the nutrient arteries are numerous and large. The 4th ECA vessel is quite small distal to the radiocarpal joint in many patients. As a result, in most cases I now prefer to use the 5th ECA as the source of retrograde blood flow, with antegrade flow to the 4th compartment vessel nutrient branches via their common origin (see Fig. 50-12A). The large diameter of the 5th ECA provides optimal blood flow to the bone graft, and straightening of the "Y" bifurcation creates a very long pedicle twice the length of each vessel.[160] This allows it to reach anywhere in the carpus, while allowing its easy protection from injury during wrist capsulotomy and carpal bone exposure owing to its ulnar location. In nearly every wrist studied by Sheetz and colleagues, the 5th ECA had no nutrient branches to bone.[241]

Harvest Technique (see Fig. 50-14A to F)

Bone graft harvest requires identification of the 5th ECA by opening the fifth dorsal compartment. A dorsal wrist incision is made to expose the extensor retinaculum. A single retinacular flap is created for wrist capsule exposure,

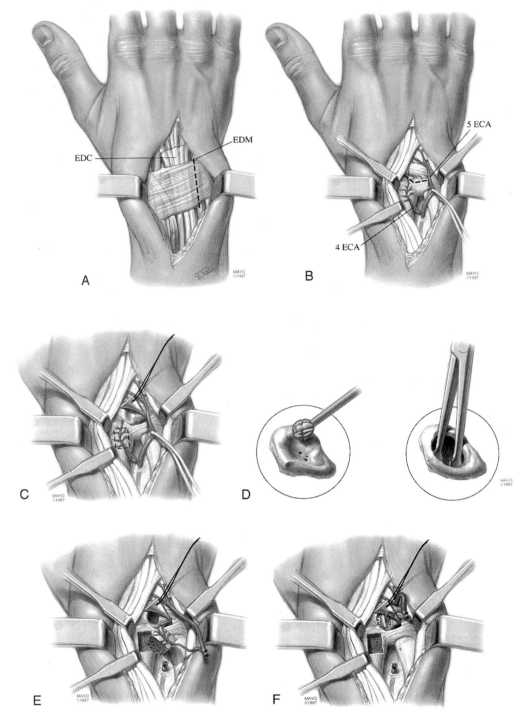

FIGURE 50-14. Vascularized graft for Kienböck's disease using the 5 + 4 ECA pedicle graft. **A,** The 5th ECA is exposed by opening the fifth extensor compartment. **B,** The 5th ECA is traced proximally to its origin from the posterior division of the anterior interosseous artery. The 4th ECA branch origin is identified and traced distally, raising a radially based retinacular flap. **C,** A ligament-sparing capsulotomy exposes the lunate. **D,** Necrotic bone is removed from the lunate, and the remaining bone expanded to normal dimensions. **E,** The graft is elevated, providing retrograde blood flow through the 5th ECA into the 4th ECA. **F,** The graft is inserted vertically into the lunate. (Copyright 1997, Mayo Foundation.)

radially based, with its initial opening directly overlying the fifth compartment (see Fig. 50-14A). The 5th ECA and accompanying veins are easily visualized on the radial aspect of the compartment with retraction of the extensor digiti minimi tendon, lying adjacent to the septum separating the fourth and fifth compartments and occasionally lying within the septum. Its distal anastomotic connections must be meticulously protected. The artery is traced proximally to its origin from the anterior interosseous artery. During this mobilization, the oblique dorsal artery to the distal ulna and the communicating branch with the posterior interosseous artery must be ligated and divided. Proximal to the distal radioulnar joint, the 4th ECA origin should be identified for inclusion with the distally based 5th ECA pedicle (see Fig. 50-14B). A bone graft is then

elevated overlying the 4th ECA, including its nutrient artery branches, which enter the cortex a mean 11 mm proximal to the joint (see Fig. 50-14C). This creates a lengthy pedicle with retrograde flow from the 5th ECA, continuing in an orthograde fashion into the other vessels. A bone graft is then raised based on one or both of these vessels.

Graft Insetting: Lunate

Once the graft is elevated and retracted distal to the lunate on its pedicle, a capsulotomy is performed to expose the joint. My colleagues and I prefer a dorsal ligament-sparing approach (see earlier and Fig. 50-14C).[16] The lunate is inspected; if it is not fragmented, vascularized bone grafting is feasible. Necrotic bone is removed with the aid of direct

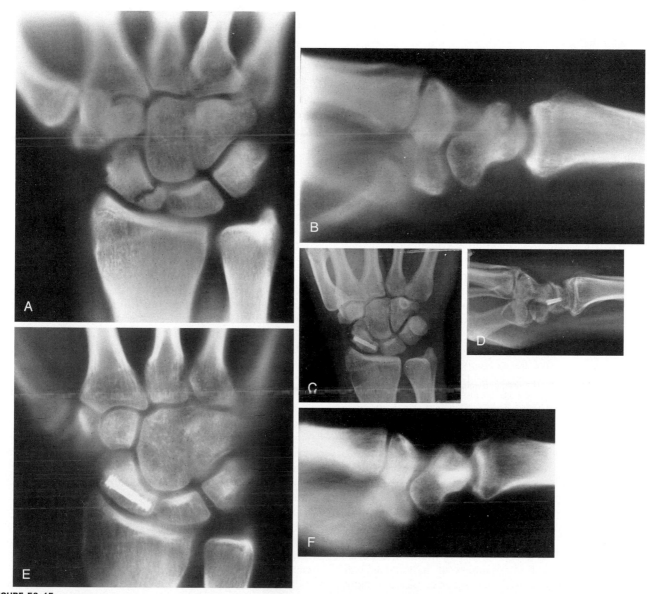

FIGURE 50-15. A 32-year-old man with chronic scaphoid proximal pole nonunion. **A** and **B,** Preoperative anteroposterior and lateral tomograms. A 1,2 ICSRA bone graft was inserted as a dorsal inlay pedicle vascularized graft. **C** and **D,** Postoperative radiographs demonstrate stabilization with a cannulated scaphoid screw. The fracture demonstrated early union at 8 weeks. **E** and **F,** These tomograms at 4 months postoperatively show complete consolidation.

inspection and an image intensifier, leaving a shell of intact cartilage and subchondral bone through a dorsal opening. This opening is placed to avoid injury to the dorsal scapholunate or lunotriquetral ligaments. The lunate may be expanded gently to normal dimensions using a small elevator if it collapsed (see Fig. 50-14D). The bone graft is then placed into the lunate, orienting the pedicle vertically and with the cortical surface on which it lies arranged to serve as a proximal-distal oriented strut to maintain lunate height during revascularization (see Fig. 50-14E and F). No internal fixation is necessary provided the lunate is not fractured and the graft is carefully shaped and impacted into the bone.

Joint Unloading: Kienböck's Disease

Unloading of the lunate is important postoperatively, because lunate collapse most likely results from loss of mechanical integrity due to the cellular processes after restoration of blood supply.[10] This may be accomplished by use of an external fixator,[171] capitate shortening, intercarpal fusion, or temporary pinning of the intercarpal joint. The latter allows motion as early as 3 weeks postoperatively, while maintaining the pins in place for 3 months.[320] External fixation is generally maintained for 6 to 8 weeks postoperatively.

Results

Scaphoid

Vascularized bone grafting has been applied to the scaphoid in an effort to improve results of treatment of nonunion. Roy-Camille used the palmar tubercle of the scaphoid on an abductor pollicis brevis pedicle in 1965.[226] Grafts from the palmar distal radius based on a pronator quadratus pedicle resulted in successful treatment of 13 nonunions in two series.[29,134] Zaidenberg and coworkers reported successful results with a dorsal reverse-flow pedicle graft from the distal radius in 11 cases,[331] using the vessel subsequently described as the 1,2 ICSRA.[241] My colleagues and my initial experience was similar, with successful healing in 15 patients with established scaphoid nonunions (Fig. 50-15).[261,262] Of these, 6 patients had radiographic or MRI suggestion of proximal fragment avascular necrosis and 6 had early radiocarpal joint degenerative changes. Time to union averaged 11.1 weeks (range, 5.5 to 16 weeks), judged by bridging trabeculae on trispiral tomography. Subjectively, 66% were very satisfied with the results of surgery. Three patients, all with preoperative degenerative changes, had additional surgery. Fair and poor results, seen in 5 patients, correlated with degenerative arthritis at follow-up in the majority, whereas only 2 patients with good or excellent results had any arthritic changes. The experience with vascularized bone grafting of the scaphoid has not been uniformly successful, however. Whereas most authors report more than 90% healing,[59,93,97,145,157,167,299,329,331] others demonstrated healing rates from 27% to 80%.[28,77,268] Variations in type and length of internal fixation, numbers of individuals with documented avascular necrosis, and other variables certainly may affect results. One published meta-analysis of scaphoid nonunions has demonstrated that vascularized bone grafts provide better union rates overall in scaphoids with avas-

cular necrosis and a trend to better results than conventional grafts in patients who have failed previous surgery.[175]

Kienböck's Disease

Core revascularization of the lunate using vascularized pisiform grafts or arteriovenous pedicles has been generally successful in relieving symptoms in two recent series.[24,69] In the later study, 26 patients with 28 procedures were followed for an average of 6.7 years (range, 2.5 to 9.3 years) with periodic clinical and radiographic evaluations including a final comprehensive assessment that included trispiral tomography and MRI. Every patient experienced subjective improvement, was pleased with the result, and was able to resume his or her previous job. Pain and grip strength improved significantly, as did wrist motion to a lesser extent. Based on MRI, lunate reconstruction proved successful in 37% of the cases and stabilized the disease process in an additional 23 cases. Overall, 43% good and excellent, 43% fair, and 14% poor results were observed.[24]

The results of nine vascularized grafts obtained from the radial metaphysis in patients with Kienböck's disease, using the reverse-flow pedicles described earlier, were reported by Mazur and associates.[171] These included grafts based on the 2,3 ICSRA in two patients, 4th ICA in four, 5+4 ICA in two, and palmar radiocarpal arch in one. The procedure was used without joint leveling in four patients who had ulnar-neutral or ulnar-positive variance. Three patients with ulnar-negative variance had a concomitant radial shortening. Eight of the nine patients had external fixation for temporary lunate unloading. Follow-up averaged 32 months (range, 7 to 90 months). Grip strength improved 25%, ultimately measuring a mean 86% of the opposite side (range, 60% to 100%). Range of motion was not significantly different from preoperative status. Radiographic measurements demonstrated no change in the modified carpal height ratio, lunate index, or scapholunate angle. Only two patients were without lunate collapse preoperatively, based on carpal height ratio value. Both progressed postoperatively, although absolute numerical change was slight. MRI data demonstrated progressive signs of revascularization with time (Fig. 50-16). Normalization of T2 values was seen first, generally by 18 months, followed by T1 values by 36 months.

CONCLUSION

Vascularized bone grafting is indicated in the upper extremity after segmental bone loss of greater than 6 cm as a result of trauma, infection, or tumor resection. It is also indicated in smaller long bone defects in the presence of radionecrosis, failed prior graft, scarred beds, or need for composite tissue reconstruction. Currently, restoration of growth by inclusion of epiphysis is possible as well. Primary sources of vascularized bone for reconstruction of long bones include the fibula and iliac crest.

In the wrist, vascularized grafts have proven value in scaphoid fracture and nonunion as well as Kienböck's disease. Reverse-flow pedicle grafts from the dorsal distal radius are preferred donor sites, owing to their predictable anatomy, robust blood supply, and location directly adjacent to the scaphoid and lunate.

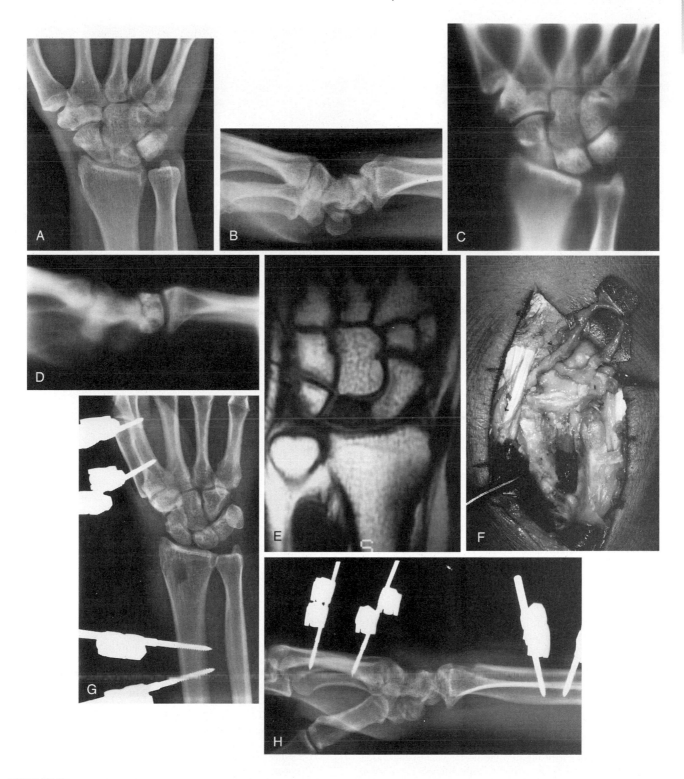

FIGURE 50-16. A 27-year-old woman with Kienböck's disease. **A** and **B,** Preoperative radiographs. **C** and **D,** Tomograms demonstrate the sclerotic changes of Kienböck's disease. **E,** Preoperative MRI demonstrated absence of a lunate signal on T1- and T2-weighted images. **F,** A 2,3 ICSRA pedicle graft raised from the distal radius. **G** and **H,** Immediate postoperative radiographs demonstrating graft placement and temporary lunate unloading with an external fixator.

Continued

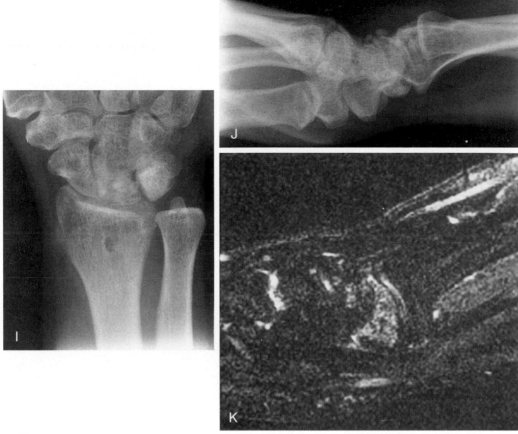

FIGURE 50-16—con t'd. **I** and **J**, Radiographic appearance 8 months postoperatively. **K**, T2-weighted MRI (lateral projection) 8 months postoperatively demonstrating an increase in the lunate signal.

ANNOTATED REFERENCES

24. Bochud RC, Buchler U: Kienböck's disease, early stage 3—height reconstruction and core revascularization of the lunate. J Hand Surg [Br] 19:466-478, 1994.

   Vascularized pedicle grafts were applied to stage IIIA Kienböck's disease in this study. The pisiform, isolated on its vascular pedicle and decorticated, was placed within the lunate to restore normal height and shape. All 26 patients experienced subjective improvement, were pleased with the result, and able to resume working. Grip strength improved significantly. Interestingly, carpal height decreased 4.7% at final follow-up and arthrosis increased in 55% of patients. Overall, 43% good and excellent, 43% fair, and 14% poor results were observed. These findings demonstrate that successful clinical results are the norm when using vascularized bone grafts in patients with Kienböck's disease. Clinical improvement does not always correlate with positive changes in objective radiographic parameters.

51. de Boer HH, Wood MB: Bone changes in the vascularized fibular graft. J Bone Joint Surg Br 71:374-378, 1989.

   The most common problems encountered at the recipient site after vascularized bone grafting include stress fracture and delayed union or nonunion. The authors studied the dynamics of grafts placed across 62 large skeletal defects. Stress fractures occurred in 25% of the cases at an average time of 8 months after surgery. Hypertrophy was more common when the limb was mechanically loaded; it was enhanced where the graft was not bypassed by internal fixation. The length of the graft and the use of additional bone graft material had no influence on the incidence of stress fracture or on hypertrophy. The authors concluded that a vascularized graft should be protected against fatigue fracture during the first year, allowing a gradual increase in mechanical loading to enhance remodeling and hypertrophy.

71. Fernandez DL, Eggli S: Non-union of the scaphoid: Revascularization of the proximal pole with implantation of a vascular bundle and bone-grafting [see comments]. J Bone Joint Surg Am 77:883-893, 1995.

110. Hori Y, Tamai S, Okuda H, et al: Blood vessel transplantation to bone. J Hand Surg [Am] 4:23-33, 1979.

   The authors of these two studies demonstrate in experimental and clinical results that implanted arteriovenous bundles can undergo neoangiogenesis and revascularize adjacent necrotic bone. Such a method represents an alternative to vascularized bone transplantation for Kienböck's disease and scaphoid nonunion.

96. Han CS, Wood MB, Bishop AT, Cooney WP: Vascularized bone transfer. J Bone Joint Surg Am 74:1441-1449, 1992.

   This large series of 160 iliac crest and fibula vascularized bone grafts summarizes the outcomes for skeletal defects resulting from nonunion, tumor resection, traumatic bone loss, osteomyelitis, or congenital anomaly. The information presented provides useful statistics regarding union by location and diagnosis, as well as donor and recipient site complication rates.

107. Hofmann GO, Kirschner MH: Clinical experience in allogeneic vascularized bone and joint allografting. Microsurgery 20:375-383, 2000.

The possible use of living non-autogenous bone to more accurately match the size and shape of a large skeletal defect represents another possible means to improve current results following massive bone loss. Both allogeneic and xenogeneic sources may eventually bear clinical fruit. The potential has been demonstrated in the clinical series of segmental bone and joint vascularized allotransplants reported by Hofmann and colleagues.

138. Khouri RK, Koudsi B, Reddi H: Tissue transformation into bone in vivo: A potential practical application. JAMA 266:1953-1955, 1991.

The ability to engineer new vascularized bone in any desired size or shape holds great promise for future reconstructive problems. A variety of methods have been used. In this study, the authors demonstrate that mesenchymal tissue, such as muscle, into cartilage and bone can be induced to transform by application of osteogenin, an osteoinductive factor, and by demineralized bone matrix in a rat model. Using silicone rubber molds and readily available muscle flaps, the authors demonstrate the potential to create autogenous, well-perfused bone matching the exact shape of the mold. This and similar studies demonstrate the potential of new technology to eventually create skeletal replacement parts.

229. Sakai K, Doi K, Kawai S: Free vascularized thin corticoperiosteal graft [see comment]. Plast Reconstruct Surg 87:290-298, 1991.

This paper describes a thin corticoperiosteal graft harvested from the medial condylar and supracondylar areas of the femur, based on the articular branch of the descending genicular artery and vein, that consists of periosteum with a thin (0.5 to 1.0 mm) layer of outer cortical bone. The technique is clearly described, as well as the results in six patients with fracture nonunion of the upper extremity in which conventional treatment had failed.

241. Sheetz KK, Bishop AT, Berger RA: The arterial blood supply of the distal radius and ulna and its potential use in vascularized pedicled bone grafts. J Hand Surg [Am] 20:902-914, 1995.

My colleagues and I investigated the extraosseous and intraosseous blood supply of the distal radius and ulna and defined potential vascularized pedicled bone grafts for carpal pathology. Several known arteries were described in greater detail, and numerous previously undescribed arteries were found and investigated. Some of these grafts provide a wider arc of rotation, greater ease of harvest, and/or improved vascularity compared with many previously described grafts.

270. Sunagawa T, Bishop AT, Muramatsu K: Role of conventional and vascularized bone grafts in scaphoid nonunion with avascular necrosis: A canine experimental study. J Hand Surg [Am] 25:849-859, 2000.

The effectiveness of vascularized and conventional bone grafts in the treatment of carpal fracture nonunion with avascular necrosis was evaluated in 12 adult dogs. The proximal third of the radiocarpal bone was removed bilaterally and frozen in liquid nitrogen. Its replacement, leaving a 4-mm gap, simulated a scaphoid fracture nonunion with avascular necrosis. A dorsal radius inlay graft was placed across the gap. The graft was nonvascularized, or conventional on one side, and vascularized with a reverse-flow arteriovenous pedicle on the other. After a healing period, quantitative assessment of bone blood flow, fracture healing, and bone remodeling was conducted. Seventy-three percent of the vascularized grafts and none of the conventional grafts healed. At 6 weeks, bone blood flow in the proximal pole was significantly higher on the side of the vascularized graft, as was quantitative histomorphometric evidence of bone remodeling. These experimental data support the clinical value of pedicled reverse-flow vascularized grafts in the treatment of carpal fracture nonunions with avascular necrosis, including proximal pole scaphoid nonunions.

303. Vail TP, Urbaniak JR: Donor-site morbidity with use of vascularized autogenous fibular grafts. J Bonc Joint Surg Am 78:204-211, 1996.

One hundred and ninety-eight consecutive patients (247 vascularized fibular grafts) were studied to determine the prevalence of morbidity at the fibula donor site after the grafts had been obtained. Motor weakness was a transient complaint, resolving by 3 months, but sensory complaints and ankle pain increased over 5 years to 11.8% and 11.5%, respectively. Whereas free vascularized fibular grafts remain ideal for many applications, this morbidity must be weighed against the benefits. The desirability of seeking solutions not requiring an autogenous bone transplant is apparent based on the results reported by these and other similar studies.

331. Zaidenberg C, Siebert JW, Angrigiani C: A new vascularized bone graft for scaphoid nonunion. J Hand Surg [Am] 16:474-478, 1991.

This seminal article describes the application of a new vascularized bone graft from the distal dorsoradial radius to long-standing scaphoid nonunion. The results in 11 patients demonstrated a decreased period of immobilization and a higher union rate than reported results for conventional grafts. Many subsequent papers have further refined the technique and largely affirmed these results.

CHAPTER 51

Vascularized Joint Transfers

Guy Foucher

Finger joints play a critical role in function of the hand. Their function, however, can be absent, disturbed, or destroyed because of congenital conditions, trauma, or disease. Three main levels can be involved: the proximal interphalangeal (PIP) joint, the metacarpophalangeal (MP) joint, or the first carpometacarpal (CMC) joint. In a study by Hume and associates,[105] the useful range of motion for 11 daily activities was found to be 61 degrees for the MP joint, 60 degrees for the PIP joint, and 39 degrees for the distal interphalangeal (DIP) joint. Many methods of joint reconstruction have been developed, but all of them fall short of the ideal requirement, which is a painless, stable, strong, durable joint with full range of motion and, in children, potential for growth. Alternatives for the treatment of damaged joints include amputation, fusion, prostheses, spacers, nonvascularized joint transfer, and vascularized joint transfer (free or island).

Finger amputation is rarely indicated for joint damage except in cases of complex associated lesions involving a single finger. Fusion can afford relief of pain and provide stability, durability, and, usually, good strength, but at the cost of mobility. Arthrodesis must still be thought of as a good operation, at least in adults and in certain joints such as the thumb MP or CMC joint. In other locations fusion may disturb the overall function of the hand, especially with multiple PIP or MP joint involvement.

In patients with massive metacarpal loss involving the MP joint of a central single ray, I have proposed fusion of the base of the remaining proximal phalanx to an adjacent one, usually the long and ring fingers; this is performed by transverse interposition of a bone peg (harvested from the injured metacarpal) in the web, supplemented by a transverse Kirschner wire to form two bars of a ladder.[46] This "scaffold" procedure avoids collapse and allows motion to be transmitted by the neighboring intact MP joint. However, this operation deprives the normal finger of independent motion, and I cannot recommend this operation for the second or fifth rays, where collapse and subsequent clinodactyly could occur. Despite constant improvement, prosthetic implants or spacers[184] are still associated with significant problems relating to stability, durability, and mobility, and they remain contraindicated in young patients except when they may be used with new techniques allowing osteointegration.

Some indications for vascular joint (and epiphysis) transfer in congenital conditions are alluded to, but two new techniques are not discussed in this chapter because they have not been used in hand joint reconstruction (joint homotransplantations[200] with immunosupression) or because results are not yet available (joint tissue engineering). However, both are under experimental study and when available clinically they may make the information in this chapter entirely obsolete.

PREOPERATIVE EVALUATION

The simplest situation for joint reconstruction is in the acute reconstruction where the loss is easily evaluated. One of the most frequent indications is a compound dorsal loss of skin, extensor mechanism, and bone at the PIP or MP joint level. In secondary surgery, a thorough history from the patient and of the trauma is mandatory. Post-traumatic or postoperative infection leads to a delay in the surgical reconstruction for at least a few months. Each anatomic structure of the finger has to be carefully evaluated clinically. The function of the flexor tendon is assessed during mobilization of the neighboring intact joint. Preoperative rehabilitation is sometimes necessary to recover some strength. Then the extensor mechanism and the skin are examined to anticipate problems during joint reconstruction. In some cases a first stage of skin replacement may be necessary, but usually enough skin can be harvested en bloc with the vascularized joint to obviate this need.

One of the main points is to ensure that the vascularity of the finger is good. At least one patent digital artery is necessary to contemplate reconstruction. The finger Allen test is not always possible owing to difficulties with flexion of the damaged joint, and a Doppler examination is favored. An arteriogram is rarely necessary except in very complex trauma. Indeed, in the absence of a patent digital artery any operation except amputation or joint arthrodesis is usually contraindicated. For some vascularized joint transfers two patent arteries are necessary as in homodigital island DIP to PIP transfer. Thorough radiographic examination is also necessary, to confirm destruction of the joint and measure the bony defect. Posteroanterior, lateral, and oblique views should be obtained for this evaluation. Careful examination of the potential donor site is always mandatory, and this allows the patient to be informed concerning any possible sequelae.

Finally a global assessment is conducted to evaluate the patient (hand dominance, bilateral involvement, multilevel injury, associated pathologies [mainly vascular]) as well as his or her desire (functional and cosmetic) and level of compliance. Indeed, compliance is particularly important in complex reconstruction of the hand as with a vascularized joint transfer. Preoperative splinting helps in evaluating the level of cooperation. If the splint is not worn according to the advice of the surgeon and therapist, it is risky to embark on a complex operation, because splinting is always necessary in the postoperative period. I have also found consultation with a psychologist useful in these patients as well, and my colleagues and I have the services of such an individual full time in our unit.

Anatomy

A good knowledge of the anatomy and vascularization of the joints of the hand and foot is mandatory. If one is not familiar with the vascular anatomy of the joints, dissection of injected cadavers' extremities is a useful prelude to embarking on this type of surgery.

Hand Joints

The reader is referred to pertinent textbooks for a discussion of anatomy of the hand. Vascularization of the PIP and DIP joints is provided mainly through the palmar system.[217] The palmar collateral arteries have retrotendinous epiphyseal branches that anastomose to each other, with small "twigs" going to the bone, the volar plate, and ligaments.[2,5,32,182] The dorsal skin is also vascularized through the palmar system and can be harvested along with the extensor mechanism as a compound tissue transfer. At the PIP level two branches of the palmar collateral digital artery run transversely between the distal border of the A2 pulley and the insertion of C1. They then pass under the checkrein ligaments of the volar plate and unite in an arch that is convex distally along the proximal border of the plate.

In an unpublished anatomic study, Bolleker has demonstrated that this arcade runs at a variable distance from the joint space according to the finger (index mean, 8.5 mm; middle finger, 9 mm; ring finger, 7.7 mm; and little finger, 6.7 mm). The distal arch is of a smaller diameter and quite transverse at a mean distance of 4.5 mm from the joint (4.6 for the index, 4.5 for the middle finger, 4.8 for the ring finger, and 4 mm for the little finger).

At the DIP level, the proximal transverse arch is formed by two branches emerging from the palmar collateral digital artery between the distal border of the A4 pulley and the proximal border of the C3 pulley. The convexity of the arch is distal. The distance of the arch from the joint space is variable (index finger, 6 mm; middle finger, 6.5 mm; ring finger, 7.6 mm; little finger, 5.5 mm). This distal arch is more the exception than the rule (noted in 1 of 36 dissections), and the two small transverse branches run at a variable distance from the joint space (1 to 4 mm).

In another work (in which 100 fingers were dissected)[4] it was noted that the radial digital artery of the index and the ulnar digital artery of the little finger did not contribute in 20% and 32% of fingers, respectively, because it was inter-rupted proximal to the PIP joint. This interruption was previously noted in the dissections of Brunelli and Brunelli,[6] who found this anatomy in 10% of index fingers and 15% of little fingers. Finally, it is also of relevance to remember that the dominant artery of each finger (as far the diameter is concerned) is the one closest to the central axis of the hand, which means the ulnar for the index or the radial for the ring finger.[182]

Toe Joints

Although their anatomy is similar, the toe PIP joint is rather small in comparison to the PIP joint of the finger. Mobility in flexion is good, but frequently there is a slight claw deformity that may be reduced by passive flexion of the metatarsophalangeal (MT) joint. In children, only one growth plate is present and it is located at the base of the middle phalanx.

The MT joint is larger but quite similar to the MP joint and possesses some lateral stability but a limited range of flexion in comparison to the range of hyperextension. Two growth plates are present, one on each side of the joint. The extensor and flexor mechanisms are similar to those of the hand. Innervation of the MT joint arises from the terminal branch of the deep peroneal nerve running along the dorsalis pedis artery and from the cutaneous dorsal medial branch of the superficial peroneal nerve.[125]

The vascularization pattern of the second toe has been known for a long time,[87,97,125,137] but only a few studies have been devoted to the vascular pattern of the joints.[125,203,216] A Chinese study[125] demonstrated that the blood supply of the MT joint is mainly dependent on the articular branch of the first metatarsal artery. This constant artery is found in three different patterns (Fig. 51-1): (1) most commonly (60% of cases), the artery branches off the first dorsal metatarsal artery at the distal third of the metatarsal bone (see Fig. 51-1B); (2) in 18% of cases, the articular vessel arises from the origin of the first dorsal metatarsal artery (see Fig. 51-1A); and (3) in the case of a first dorsal metatarsal artery passing beneath the interosseous muscle (12%), the articular vessel branches off close to the joint (see Fig. 51-1C). The authors found additional branches emerging from the first plantar metatarsal artery, but they were inconsistently found and always communicated with the dorsal system. A Japanese study[203,216] and personal unpublished data stressed that vascularization of the PIP and MTP joints of the second toe is provided by both the dorsal and plantar vessels, which do communicate (Fig. 51-2). Furthermore, my colleagues and my study* underlined the role of a fundamental vessel that has been overlookedin the literature—the second plantar metatarsal artery (Fig. 51-3), which is a constant, reliable vessel passing in close contact to the plantar plate of the second MTP joint.

In two other specific transfers (rotatory transfer of the trapezoid-trapeziometacarpal joint for first CMC joint reconstruction and transfer of the distal radioulnar joint for wrist arthroplasty), the anatomy is briefly discussed with the technical description.

---

*See references 46, 47, 53, 54, 56, 58, 60, 62, 67, 69, 71, and 75.

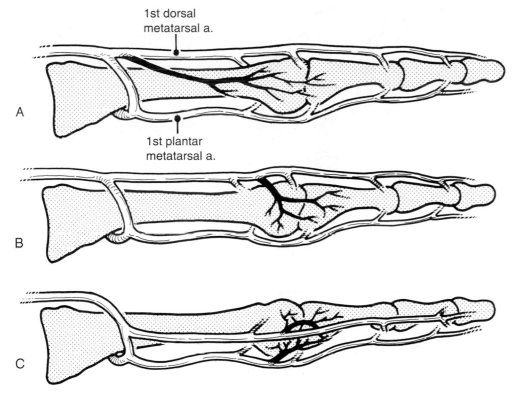

FIGURE 51-1. PIP and metatarsophalangeal joint vascularization patterns according to Kuo and colleagues.[125]

1st dorsal metatarsal a.

1st plantar metatarsal a.

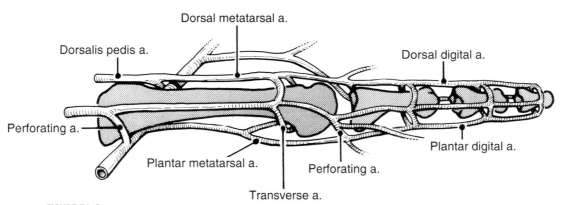

Dorsal metatarsal a.

Dorsalis pedis a.

Dorsal digital a.

Perforating a.

Plantar metatarsal a.

Perforating a.

Plantar digital a.

Transverse a.

FIGURE 51-2. PIP and metatarsophalangeal joint vascularization according to Yoshizu and associates.[216]

BRIEF HISTORY AND BASIC SCIENCE

Surgeons have long sought to provide a biologic joint replacement by using specialized tissues with a similar anatomic configuration (Table 51-1). These attempts fall into three major categories: perichondrial joint grafts, allografts, and autografts (vascularized or nonvascularized half or whole joint transfers).

Several basic problems are common to all biologic reconstructions. Successful transplantation of functioning organs depends on rapid reestablishment of the circulatory perfusion of their tissues if the transplants are to survive and function. Curiously, when bone and cartilage are transplanted, difficulties begin when the process of revascularization is established.[93] Ischemic loss of synovium is responsible for poor production of synovial fluid, which is the sole means of nutrition for the articular cartilage.[114] Moreover, the circulation of synovial fluid depends on movement of the joint, and prolonged immobilization causes trophic changes in articular cartilage.[39,131] The role of denervation in degenerative change in transplanted joints, although poorly documented,[34,118] is probably relatively unimportant.[10]

Nonvascularized joint autografts and allografts have been extensively studied, but sound clinical series providing long-term results concerning ranges of motion, degenerative changes, and/or the percentage of growth in young patients are scarce. Satisfactory joint motion usually occurs after half and whole joint transfers* independently of articular cartilage survival.[8,9,34,36,37,102,118,120,129]

_____

*See references 14, 18, 19, 34, 35, 36, 90, 94, 102, 118, 119, 129, 133, 138, 153, and 155.

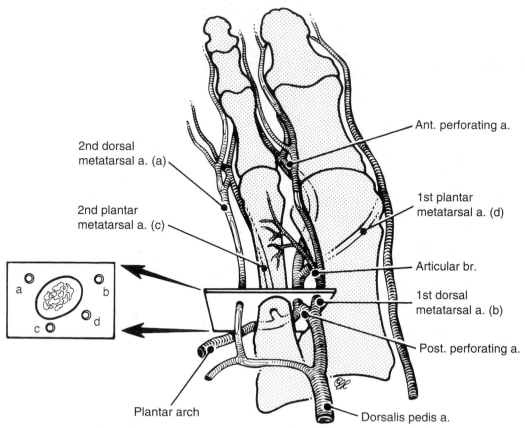

FIGURE 51-3. The vascular pattern of the second web space in the foot, which has been overlooked in the literature. The second plantar and/or dorsal arteries frequently can be used.

In my colleagues and my experience,[54] and throughout the literature,[114] the results of perichondrial autografts have been quite unpredictable. This operation is applicable to only very limited problems in which damage is confined to the articular cartilage in the presence of normal bone structure.

Allografts have been the least successful method experimentally. However, most research with allografts has been concentrated on large weight-bearing joints such as the knee (see Table 51-1). Nonvascularized autografts of half and whole joints have also been studied extensively, experimentally as well as clinically. Experimental, radiologic, and histologic studies have demonstrated degenerative changes in cartilage, with survival of only scattered deep layers and progressive replacement with fibrotic tissue.

Small clinical series have been published on whole joint replacement using a toe or transposition of a normal joint from an otherwise irreparably damaged digit as a free nonvascularized whole joint transfer. Technically, several points have been stressed. The smaller the graft, the sooner revascularization takes place. On the other hand, bone periosteum and joint capsule have to be kept intact. Several authors have demonstrated that limited but satisfactory joint motion usually occurs after half and whole joint transfer independently of articular cartilage survival.

The growth of nonvascularized joint transfers in young patients remains controversial. In experiments, several authors have demonstrated some growth,[36,94,100,163] whereas others have not.[98,99] Clinically, isolated successful cases have

been published.[81,82,94,198,205] Two short but encouraging series[90,207] stressed that the reasons for success or failure of growth were not apparent. Age (the optimum was 6 months) and technique (conservation of periosteum) seem to be important contributing factors.

Taking into account that most problems in transfer of nonvascularized joints arise from delay in bone revascularization, it seemed logical that preservation or reestablishment of nutrient vessels could be the solution. Vascularized grafts are histologically indistinguishable from normal joints with viable subchondral bone. Functionally, only slight to moderate hyperplasia of the synovium with some restricted motion has been demonstrated. Survival of the epiphyseal plate with growth has been demonstrated experimentally and clinically. Vascularized transfers based only on metaphyseal blood supply provide some (but not normal) growth. It seems advisable to use epiphyseal vessels to obtain normal growth. It is necessary to keep in mind that overgrowth may be seen after fractures or in association with inflammatory conditions and that decreased growth may result in patients with chronic disease or prolonged immobilization.

TYPES OF VASCULARIZED JOINT TRANSFER

Post-traumatic reconstruction and congenital conditions are considered separately. Reconstruction may involve the fingers, the CMC joint, or the wrist.

Table 51-1
HISTORY OF JOINT TRANSPLANTATION

Nonvascularized Joint Transfer

Homografts

1908-1925: Lexer[128,129] first performed successful cases of homografts of half and whole joints.

A number of series had high rates of failure.[12,13,102,140,152,173,201]

Small fragments survive better.[13,24,102,132,155,157]

Autografts

1902: Tietze[187] was the first to use a proximal phalanx taken from the big toe.

1913: Goebbel[89] reported the substitution of a finger joint by a toe joint.

Growth

There was experimental demonstration of some growth[36,94,100,163] or absence of growth.[98,99]

Clinically, isolated successful cases have been published[81,82,94,198,205] and two series[90,207] stressing the reasons for success or failure of growth. Age (the optimum was 6 months) and technique (conservation of periosteum) seem to be important contributing factors.

Vascularized Joints

1968: Judet[115,117] experimental demonstration of long-term survival in a dog knee model.

1967: Buncke[10] performed first island, vascularized joint transfer.

1976: Foucher[57] performed first free, compound toe joint transfer.

A number of clinical series have been reported.[43,44,52,54-57,62,63,125,150,172,191-196,216]

Finger Joint Reconstruction

The hand remains the ideal source to provide a similar joint. Two techniques can be used for finger reconstruction: (1) heterodigital transfer from a "banked" finger (another finger sacrificed because of complex injury), either as an island or as a free transfer (from a nonreplantable digit), or (2) a homodigital DIP-to-PIP island joint transfer. The technique is the same whatever joint is transferred (either the MP, PIP or DIP) and whatever the recipient level (PIP or MP), but it becomes more demanding when the donor finger is not sacrificed.

Transfers Between Fingers (Heterodigital Transfers)
Heterodigital Island Transfer
Heterodigital island transfer can be performed acutely or secondarily as a reconstructive procedure.[54,56,69,71] Regional anesthesia by nerve blocks can be used, and no special instruments are necessary except loupe magnification and microsurgical instruments.

First, the recipient site is prepared by skin débridement, the extensor and intrinsic tendons are prepared, and the bone is cut. The volar plate is thinned, with care taken to not violate the flexor sheath. On the donor finger, a dorsal skin flap is outlined so that a circular scar is avoided; two or three dorsal veins are dissected proximally and retracted to harvest enough extensor tendon to allow an overlapping suture. Then one digital artery is dissected free, with as much fat kept around the vessel as possible; the accompanying nerve can be used as a vascularized nerve if needed. This nerve, however, is not necessary for joint preservation, and no subsequent Charcot's change in the transferred joint has been published to my knowledge. Distally, the artery is cut at the level of the future bone section. Then a double osteotomy isolates the joint while keeping the volar plate intact and preserving the vascular bundle. The length of the intercalated segment has to be slightly shorter than the actual recipient defect to avoid a natural tendency toward flexion deformity as a result of increased flexor tendon tension if the transferred joint renders the finger too long.

The compound transfer remains attached solely by its veins and artery and can be transferred to the recipient site, usually through a dorsal subcutaneous route to decrease dorsal scarring. Bone stabilization can be done in many ways, but I favor placing the transferred joint within the medullary canals of the recipient phalanges combined with interosseous wiring or Kirschner wires. This technique will decrease the possibility of making the finger too long. When the fragment is a very small one (e.g., when the DIP joint is used as a donor), a single longitudinal Kirschner wire has been most frequently used to stabilize the transferred joint in extension. The flexor tendon sheath is then reattached to the donor volar plate to decrease the mechanical advantage, and the extensor tendon is secured by overlapping with maximal tension.

At the PIP joint level the donor joint extensor tendon is divided into two slips, one that is secured to the central slip and the other to a lateral band. Finally, the donor finger is treated according to its potential function, either by arthrodesis, shortening, or ray amputation. Mobilization begins usually at 4 to 6 weeks with dynamic extension splinting to avoid attenuation of the extensor suture. Splinting in flexion is postponed until 8 weeks.

The main advantage of this technique is to replace "like by like" but at the price of sacrificing the joint of a neighboring finger. For this reason, the indications for this procedure are rare. However, when a finger has to be amputated in the presence of injury to the other digits, it is mandatory to think about using "spare parts," and a vascularized joint from the amputated finger offers an excellent spare. Such an indication is illustrated by a case in which the patient was referred to us for shortening of a stump with flexion deformity of a PIP joint precluding any prosthetic fitting. Despite the fact that a checkrein ligament release was necessary on this joint, vascular arch preservation was possible and the joint was transferred to a stiff deformed index finger, improving both donor and recipient sites. In case of traumatized fingers, it is necessary preoperatively to confirm the presence of at least one patent artery in the donor and recipient sites. A short proximal phalanx stump after transferring a PIP joint could be particularly sensible to cold when deprived of a patent digital artery.

Free Heterodigital Island Transfer
The technique of free heterodigital island transfer is basically the same as that described earlier except that a microsurgical step is necessary.[20,51,124] The joint is harvested from a nonreplantable finger. Any joint could be used on the condition that one artery and one vein can be found. Arterial

anastomosis is usually performed in situ with a collateral digital artery. The proximal ends of veins of the transferred skin flap are sutured to the distal end of veins in the recipient finger. Compound transfer of the joint with soft tissue may allow reconstruction of nerve loss as well as the arterial flow of the finger via a flow-through anastomosis of the artery.[51,124]

This type of transfer is rarely indicated, as confirmed by the few cases published in the literature. Indeed when a finger cannot be replanted, usually the bone and the vessels are extensively destroyed, precluding the use of such a technique. When technically possible, the range of motion is probably superior to the acute transfer of a toe vascularized joint as proposed by Tsai and coworkers.[195] DIP-to-PIP joint acute free transfer from a nonreplantable finger is demonstrated in Figure 51-4.

Transfers in the Same Finger (Homodigital DIP-to-PIP Transfers)

The technique differs only slightly from that of heterodigital island transfer in that the finger is conserved and precise technique is mandatory.[52,55,56] Four incisions are drawn (Fig. 51-5), the first longitudinally from the DIP joint down to the web to allow dissection of the sacrificed artery and prepare some proximal space to accommodate the folded vessels. Three transverse incisions are used, two to isolate a dorsal skin flap at the DIP joint level and one at the PIP joint level to fit the transfer. To allow the extensor tendon to be cut close to the PIP joint, the dorsal hinged flap of the middle phalanx is gently lifted and two or more dorsal veins are saved for the transfer. Then the DIP joint is harvested by performing two transverse osteotomies 6 to 10 mm apart while avoiding the nail matrix distally and the insertion of the volar plate proximally. Next, the collateral artery is severed at the level of the distal bone cut and the compound island joint flap transferred to the PIP joint level as previously described.

Distally, an arthrodesis is performed along with reinsertion of the flexor profundus to maintain strength (this is particularly relevant for the fifth finger where the superficialis could be defective). A longitudinal Kirschner wire is passed through the arthrodesis site and the transfer with the new PIP joint in full extension. Some flexion is possible at the arthrodesis site, which is usually stabilized by an oblique Kirschner wire. Then the extensor tendon is repaired under maximal tension (to avoid any lack of extension) with one strip sutured to the recipient central band and the other to the best intrinsic tendon. Finally, the vessels are folded and buried in the web before skin closure with some trimming of the long dorsal flap at the middle phalanx level.

The principle of this transfer is derived from the fact that the DIP joint contributes only 15% of the arc of finger joint mobility as compared with 80% for the PIP joint. The finger is simplified to become a two-joint system, but the mobility provided more proximally avoids the finger catching and

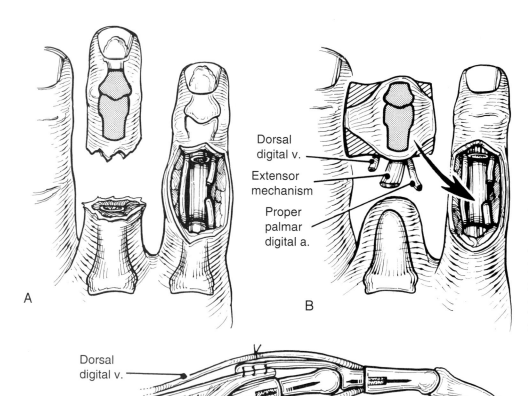

Dorsal digital v.

Extensor mechanism

Proper palmar digital a.

Dorsal digital v.

Proper palmar digital a.

A

B

C

FIGURE 51-4. A, A destroyed PIP joint of the index finger with an intact flexor tendon. The third finger is not suitable for replantation, but the DIP joint is intact. **B,** The third finger DIP joint is harvested as a compound transfer for index finger PIP joint reconstruction. **C,** The proper digital artery of the long finger is sutured to the recipient artery of the index finger.

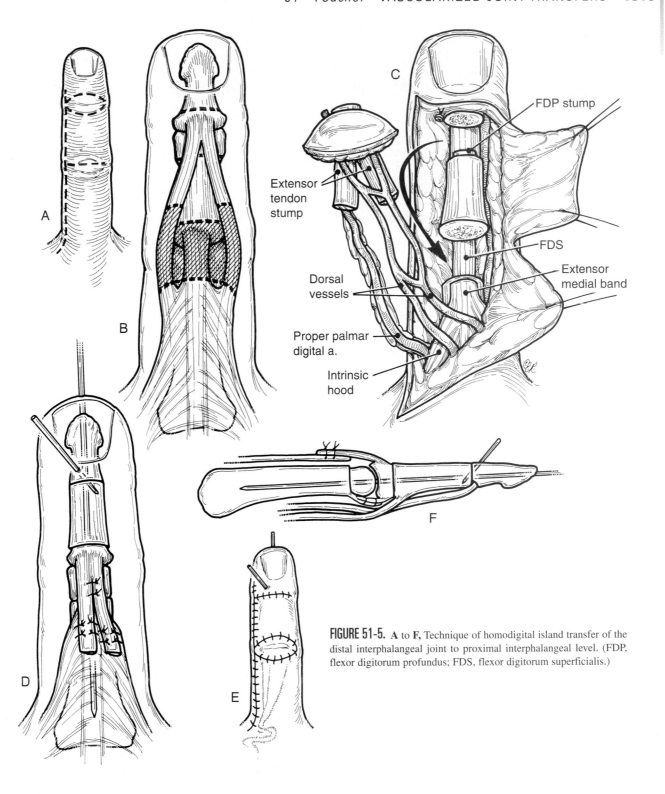

FIGURE 51-5. A to **F**, Technique of homodigital island transfer of the distal interphalangeal joint to proximal interphalangeal level. (FDP, flexor digitorum profundus; FDS, flexor digitorum superficialis.)

interfering with hand function. A functioning flexor tendon and two patent digital arteries are necessary prerequisites. I have transferred some already partially stiff DIP joints, but the range of motion expected after transfer remains more limited and an intact DIP is preferred. The best results are obtained at the fifth finger level where the huge mobility of the MP joint in flexion compensates for the limited motion of the DIP.

Free Vascularized Toe Joint Transfer

Two types of joints are available for free vascularized toe joint transfers: the PIP and the MT joints of the second and/ or third toe. Several transfer techniques have been described in post-traumatic conditions: (1) toe PIP joint transfer for finger MP and PIP joint reconstruction, (2) MTP joint transfer for MP joint reconstruction, (3) double PIP joint transfer[155] for MP joint reconstruction, and (4) the "twisted

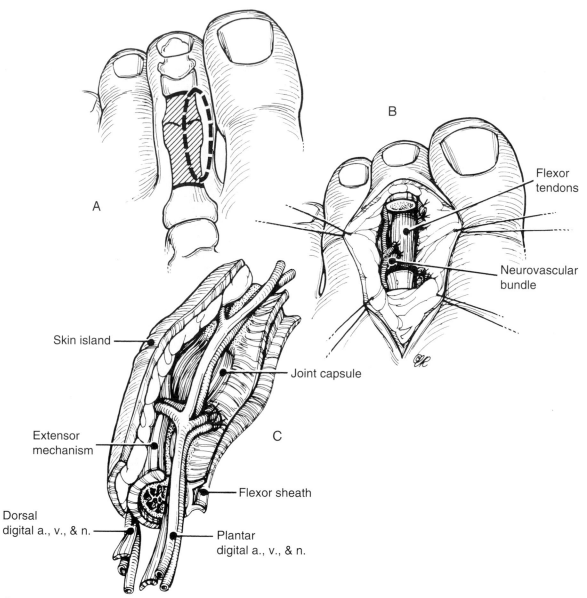

FIGURE 51-6. Technique of second toe PIP joint transfer according to Tsai and coworkers.[195] A small skin island is used as a visible monitor of viability.

toe flap" technique to add a joint in a "wraparound" thumb reconstruction.[47-49,53,58,63,64,107,190] In congenital differences, epiphysis and joint transfer present some special indications.

Toe PIP Joint to Finger PIP Joint

Only a few papers are available on transfer of a toe PIP joint to a finger PIP joint.* The technique as described by Tsai and coworkers[192] is as follows:

Preoperatively, routine radiographs and selective angiograms are performed on the foot and the hand. Under general anesthesia, two surgical teams prepare the donor and recipient sites simultaneously. Through dorsal and plantar incisions, the dorsalis pedis and first dorsal metatarsal arteries are dissected, along with the dorsal veins. A small skin island over the tibial and dorsal aspect of the PIP joint of the second toe is preserved as a visible monitor of the underlying circu-

lation (Fig. 51-6). The tibial-side digital artery is divided distally at the level of the DIP joint, with preservation of the articular and metaphyseal branches. The fibular-side artery is preserved by ligating its articular and metaphyseal branches. The extensor mechanism is then cut proximally and distally, and the joint is isolated by distal disarticulation through the DIP joint and by proximal osteotomy through the first phalanx. The hand is prepped, the involved PIP joint is excised, and a suitable artery is prepared. The joint is transferred and stabilized with an interosseous wire and longitudinal Kirschner wire. The extensor mechanism is then reconstructed, and the arterial repair is done usually by end-to-side anastomosis. At least two veins, including the distal saphenous vein, are sutured.

Among the variations proposed, Yoshizu and associates[216] favored anastomosis of the medial plantar digital artery to a common volar digital artery and Ellis and colleagues[33,122,192] harvested a skin flap from the lateral aspect of the great toe on the same vascular stem to allow good skin cover. This

---

*See references 17, 23, 41, 43, 52, 54, 56, 62, 69, 71, 75, 122, and 191-196.

technique makes preservation of the second toe easier than when harvesting a large skin flap in block with the joint from the second toe (Fig. 51-7).

The indications for this procedure vary according to the surgeon, but the main advantage of this technique is to provide a compound transfer providing bone stock, joint, extensor tendon, and skin as well as potential growth in children, long-term cartilage preservation, and lateral stability. With the exception of children, limited range of motion with some lack of extension (which has to be accepted to provide useful range) has been the rule more than the exception, limiting the indication to multiple joint involvement. In such cases, providing some motion (30 to 40 degrees) with lateral stability at the level of the index finger could be an acceptable indication.

Shibata[174] has published one case of PIP joint transfer in a symphalangism. A small island flap is harvested with the PIP joint of the homolateral second toe, en bloc with the extensor mechanism, perfused by one collateral artery, preserving the contralateral vessel for perfusion of the toe. A longitudinal incision is used at recipient level with preservation of the lateral bands of the extensor, and the symphalangized joint is carefully excised by double osteotomy to allow its transfer to the donor site. Crossed Kirschner wires were used for joint stabilization. In the single case report mobility was 102 degrees at a 4-year follow-up.

Toe MT Joint to Hand MP Joint

With the patient under epidural and brachial plexus block anesthesia, this operation consists of four steps:

1. The joint is exposed at the recipient site through a curved skin incision. The ulnar side of the extensor hood is incised and retracted, and the joint is resected. The radial artery and the cephalic vein are approached through a separate incision. A small branch of the superficial radial nerve

can be dissected at the wrist level to be sutured to the nerve of the transplanted joint.

2. The donor site is prepared by dissection of the distal branches of the great saphenous vein and first dorsal metatarsal artery. The terminal branch of the deep peroneal nerve is also dissected.

3. The graft is turned 180 degrees around its longitudinal axis, that is, in a dorsal-to-volar direction. Bone fixation is done with Kirschner wires, and the vessels are anastomosed: the dorsalis pedis to the radial artery, the great saphenous vein to the cephalic vein, and the deep peroneal nerve to the superficial branch of the radial nerve. Last, the extensor mechanism is sutured and the skin closed.

4. At the donor site, the defect in the toe is filled with either the finger joint or a cancellous bone graft.

Postoperative treatment includes prophylactic antibiotics and low-molecular-weight dextran for several days. The Kirschner wires are removed at 4 weeks, at which time functional exercises are encouraged. The cast on the foot is removed at 4 weeks, and walking is allowed.

One of the major shortcomings in this type of MT joint transfer has been the difficulty in incorporating a skin flap because of the rotation of the transfer. In an effort to solve this problem, Smith and Jones[179] described a technique using an eccentrically placed dorsalis pedis flap (Fig. 51-8). The nondominant lateral digital artery is freed from its attachment to the skin flap. With this maneuver, the flap remains dorsal after rotation of the joint. Alternatively, the skin could be lifted from the fibular aspect of the great toe.

To overcome this technical difficulty, some authors prefer to use the PIP joint of the toe for MP reconstruction.[196] As outlined by Chen and associates,[17] in children, the potential for growth is better with the two epiphyses of the MT joint.

Donor Site Treatment

Different attitudes are proposed in the literature concerning the donor toe. Some authors favor preservation of the donor toe, others sacrificed the toe but preserved the second metatarsal bone, and some prefer a proximal ray resection with reconstruction of the intermetatarsal ligament.[23,56,60] In fact, the length of the harvested bone stock frequently guides the decision. When only a PIP or an MT joint is removed from a toe without skin, a bone graft is frequently the best option, mainly when the bone could be harvested from the recipient finger. Otherwise, the decision to harvest an iliac bone graft,[17,122,175] insert a Silastic block,[148] or maintain the floating toe[192] (isolated or "syndactylized" to the neighboring toe[175]) has to be discussed preoperatively with the patient. When some skin from the same toe is transferred at the same stage, preservation of toe length requires some type of skin cover (e.g., a cross toe flap from the plantar aspect of the third toe). It is relevant to mention that a pseudarthrosis is rarely a painful issue at the donor site, and some authors allow early walking despite bone grafting.[122]

Joint Reconstruction at the Wrist Level

Distal Radioulnar Joint Transfer for Wrist Arthritis

Roux and coworkers[166] have proposed with one illustrated case the transfer of the distal radioulnar joint (DRUJ) as an island pedicle for reconstruction of the radiocarpal joint. In

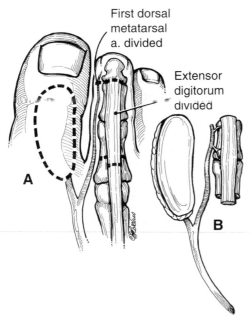

First dorsal metatarsal a. divided

Extensor digitorum divided

A

B

FIGURE 51-7. Technique allowing harvesting on the same vessels. **A,** Drawing of the flap on the long toe. **B,** Composite transfer of the flap of the first toe and the interphalangeal joint of the second toe.

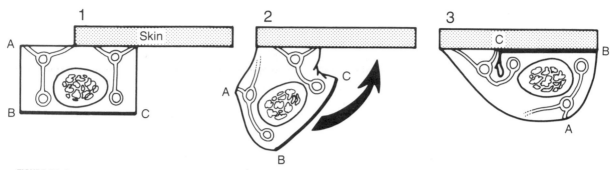

FIGURE 51-8. A skin flap can be harvested with the metatarsophalangeal joint after turning the joint upside down (Smith and Jones).[179]

their anatomic study of 40 cadaver wrists, all joints were vascularized by small branches of the distal posterior perforating branch of the anterior interosseous artery, either directly or through an anastomosis with the posterior interosseous artery. Harvesting the DRUJ was always possible on the anterior interosseous artery and in 38 of the 40 dissections on the posterior interosseous artery. The authors performed the clinical transfer in a 68-year-old patient with stiff and destroyed radiocarpal and ulnocarpal joints as an alternative to arthrodesis, which the patient refused. A dorsal approach was used to dissect the distal perforating branch of the anterior interosseous artery. Through an anterior approach, the pronator quadratus was lifted and an arthrotomy allowed to facilitate the precise bone cut. The vertical cut was at the level of the crest separating the scaphoid and lunate fossae. The transverse one was perpendicular and prolonged at the same level in the distal ulna (Fig. 51-9). The DRUJ was freed from the attached radiocarpal and ulnocarpal ligaments and rotated with the ulnar fragment positioned distally. The cartilage of the radiolunate joint was removed. A proximal row carpectomy with some shortening of the capitate makes room to accommodate the transfer, which was fixed by Kirschner wires. All the stability was provided by preserving the capsule and ligaments of the wrist, which were reinserted. In a personal communication, Roux mentioned that he has performed five such transfers with only one proceeding to arthrodesis, the other patients having some 45 degrees of mobility.

Toe MT Joint to Hand First CMC Joint

The already described technique of MT joint transfer including a skin flap can be used in some congenital thumb hypoplasias (see Chapter 41) and in rare cases of posttraumatic reconstruction of the base of the thumb. In posttraumatic major dorsal skin, bone, and joint loss of the base of the thumb, Macionis[134] has transferred an MT joint with a dorsal skin flap. The transfer was reversed to use the MT joint as a first CMC joint and provide a long metatarsal segment for metacarpal reconstruction (Fig. 51-10). A long arterial and vein pedicle was necessary to allow vascular anastomoses with the recipient radial artery. Good stability and some mobility were obtained.

In thumb hypoplasia two joints have been used, the MT and the PIP joints. Nishijima and colleagues,[148] in a case report used a two-stage operation beginning with a "Z"-plasty for the web, an abductor minimi digiti quinti myocutaneous flap, and a Silastic rod as a first stage for later flexor tendon grafting. The second step was a transfer of the PIP joint of the second toe with a small skin island to monitor the trans-

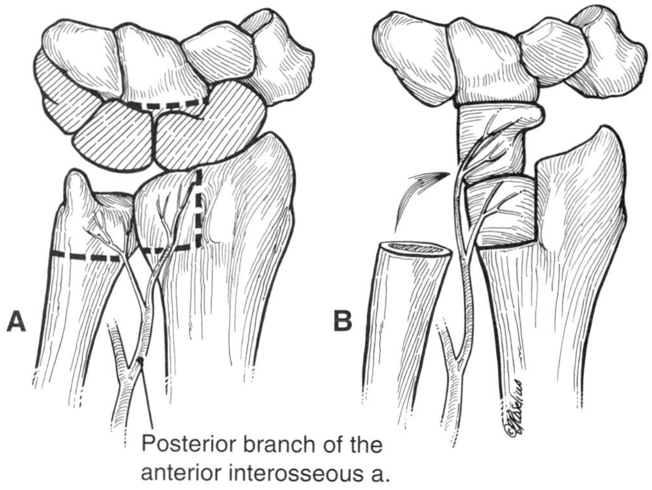

Posterior branch of the anterior interosseous a.

FIGURE 51-9. Reconstruction of the radiocarpal joint by an island rotation transfer of the distal ulnocarpal joint, based on the posterior branch of the anterior interosseous artery. A first row carpectomy allows for interposing the joint.

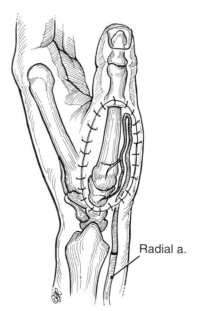

Radial a.

FIGURE 51-10. Reconstruction of a traumatic loss of the base of the thumb by a compound transfer of skin, tendons, bone, and joint. The MT joint is reversed to allow use of the full length of the metatarsal bone.

fer. At the same stage the flexor superficialis of the ring finger was transferred for finger flexion, the flexor of the middle finger rerouted dorsally for IP joint extension (EPL), and the extensor indicis proprius for MP joint extension (EPB).

The few other authors who have performed such reconstruction have used the MT joint to provide some circumduction. Initially proposed by Yamauchi and coworkers,[213,214] the team of Tajima has popularized the technique,[175,185,186] but only two small series are published.[78,186] A short proximal bone segment of the metatarsal is used, and the dorsal aspect of the joint is faced palmarward at the recipient level to allow more flexion than extension. Tendon transfers consist in advancing the abductor pollicis longus to the proximal phalanx and the extensor indicis proprius to the ulnar side of the same phalanx. The MP and IP joints of the thumb are fused and opposition is provided by a flexor superficialis ring finger transfer. In a later publication[175] the same team proposed preventing hyperextension of the MT joint by capsulodesis with variable tendon transfers. The radial artery was absent in three of their four cases, and end-to-side anastomosis was performed with the ulnar artery. The authors consider that if cultural factors are taken into account, the comparison with a small group of pollicizations was favorable in terms of strength, motion, stability, appearance, and donor site sequelae.

Rotational Transfer in Island of the First and Second CMC Joint

Messina[142] published a technical note with one illustrative case of reconstruction of the first CMC joint by an island transfer of the second CMC joint. The radial artery in the first interosseous space gives dorsal branches to the two adjacent CMC joints. The author proposed through a dorsal approach to isolate en bloc the two joints by a transverse osteotomy of the first and second metacarpal bones (Fig. 51-11). To avoid a scissor deformity a transverse Kirschner wire stabilized the two first metacarpals. Proximally, the capsule and ligaments of the scaphotrapezial-trapezoid (STT) joint were disinserted from the distal bone block. Then the bone block was rotated 180 degrees in a horizontal plane and the radial artery was moved to the palmar aspect. The bones were stabilized with Kirschner wires. There are no published results concerning the results of this clinical case, and considering the average mobility of the second CMC joint it is difficult to imagine that it could provide more than a few degrees of motion.

Wrist Reconstruction in Radial Aplasia

Vilkki[199] has proposed a technique for correction of wrist deformity in radial aplasia (or radial club hand—Bayne type IV). At the optimal age of 1 or 2 years the first step of soft tissue distraction is performed. An external fixator is placed on the ulnar side and distraction (0.8 mm per day) is undertaken until alignment of the hand on the distal ulna is obtained (mean distraction 33 mm during an average of 6 weeks). The second step is a vascularized MT joint transfer, harvesting the whole second metatarsal bone (length, 42 to 50 mm) and the dorsal skin, which is filleted. The donor site is prepared to transfer the joint to the radial side of the ulna (Fig. 51-12). The tight radial muscle mass is released and separated into dorsal and palmar components. The first phalanx of the second toe is fixed to the base of the second metacarpal bone, and the second metatarsal bone is fixed to the lateral aspect of the ulna proximal to the epiphysis. Stabilization is provided by Kirschner wires, and the external fixation is maintained for 9 weeks. Microvascular anastomosis can be demanding on the hypoplastic "expanded" radial artery, and an end-to-side anastomosis is recommended by the author. Nine cases followed for a mean of 6 years have confirmed that the pace of growth of the toe allowed maintaining the correction (mean, radial tilt 25 degrees) and providing some mobility (flexion from 60 to 90 degrees and extension from −20 to +20 degrees). Three severe early complications occurred, including two necroses of the transferred tissue and one fracture of the transplanted joint. No impairment in growth of the ulna was encountered (mean length, 67% of normal).

Author's Preferred Methods of Treatment

Indications in Trauma Cases

The potential advantages of vascularized joint transfers are several. Useful range of motion in an acceptable arc and good lateral stability can be obtained, and strong opposition to the thumb in pinch is provided. A 25-year follow-up for Merle and my first case of free vascularized joint transfer[57] has demonstrated clinical durability and persistence of the

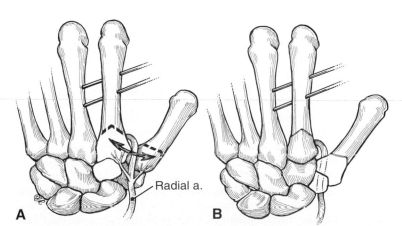

FIGURE 51-11. Reconstruction of the first CMC joint by reversing an island bloc formed by the first and second CMC joints, based on the branches of the radial artery.

Radial a.

A   B

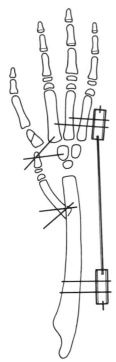

FIGURE 51-12. Technique of Vilkki in radial club hand (Bayne 4) with an MT joint with full length of metatarsal fixed on the radial aspect of the ulna and distally fixed to the base of the second metacarpal bone.

cartilage space, thus corroborating experimental data. Nevertheless, the two main advantages of this technique are the possibility of growth in young patients and the unique possibility of a one-stage reconstruction by a compound transfer that provides not only a joint but also bone stock, extensor mechanism, and skin flap.

However, several disadvantages must be emphasized as well, primarily insofar as vascularized joint transfer from the toes is concerned: (1) the procedure is long, lasting 3.5 hours on average; (2) it must be performed under general anesthesia with hospitalization required (average, 5.3 days); and (3) a danger of failure exists, as in other microsurgical procedures.

Based on my personal series with successive reviews of vascularized joint transfers for PIP joint reconstruction,[54,60,62,69,71,75] it is possible to tell the patient that active range of motion will be a mean of 55 degrees for the heterodigital islands (9 cases with a mean follow-up of 45 months), 57 degrees for the homodigital DIP-to-PIP transfers (11 cases with a mean follow-up of 28 months), 65 to 80 degrees for the free heterodigital transfers (2 cases),35 degrees for toe joint transfers in adult patients (12 cases with a mean lack of extension of 39 degrees), and 64 degrees in the children (5 cases with a mean lack of extension of 25 degrees). The worst results are found with the free toe joint transfer. This is confirmed by a collective review of 89 vascularized toe joints (in 51 adults and 28 children).[196] At MP level the active range of motion was 29.9 degrees when using the MT joint and 35 degrees with the PIP joint, and at the PIP level active range of motion was 26.7 degrees.

Thus, at the PIP joint level, toe vascularized joint transfers fall short of their goal because of restricted range of motion. I think that it is not a good option in adults, but it remains useful, mainly in multiple PIP joint involvement, in young growing patients and in large complex losses (skin, bone, extensor tendon) with a normal flexor tendon. In fingers at the MP joint level indications are similar, but in the case of double reconstruction it seems better to reconstruct the skin cover first. As for the PIP joint, the second and third rays are reconstructed most frequently. These radial fingers are more necessary for lateral stability than for amplitude, contrary to the situation with the ulnar digits. For all the preceding shortcomings I favor the alternative transfer of a finger joint when possible. In multiple digital injuries I carefully assess the possibility of an island or free vascularized finger joint transfer from a nonsalvageable segment.

Transfer of an MP joint when performing a pollicization of a finger stump on a first metacarpal amputation deserves special mention. I have transferred the index MP joint in three such cases, but the average mobility was only 30 degrees.[68] Nevertheless, stability at this level is more relevant than mobility, and careful positioning is of paramount importance owing to lateral mobility of the transferred joint. In one of the cases, the transferred epiphyses had excellent growth. I have performed only one case of hand-to-hand transfer of a proximal phalanx and an MP joint (of the little finger) on an index ray in a metacarpal hand with a moderate range of motion of 45 degrees.[74]

Specific Transfers

PIP Joint Reconstruction

For PIP joint reconstruction, I continue to use the technique that my colleagues and I described originally,[57,58,60,62] that is, use of the second toe. Specific details must be emphasized. I do not use preoperative angiography. The operation is performed with the patient under general anesthesia with careful monitoring of the core temperature. A one-team approach avoids most of the pitfalls inherent in matching the length and size of arteries, veins, nerves, and tendons.

The first step is toe dissection. A cutaneous flap is drawn distally to the DIP joint, and proximally a long tail is taken from the dorsum of the foot. A dorsal approach alone is sufficient for the dissection.[41,44,47,49,50,59,60,63,66] After dissection of the venous arch and the great saphenous vein, the dorsalis pedis artery is dissected just beneath the extensor hallucis longus tendon. The field of dissection then moves to the first web to look for the dorsal metatarsal artery, which is superficial to the intermetatarsal ligament. If the diameter of this artery is not sufficient, I proceed with extensor tendon section and proximal osteotomy of the second metatarsal, which is then lifted with a bone hook. This osteotomy has two advantages: (1) it provides a wide approach to the plantar arterial system of the first and second intermetatarsal space, and (2) it facilitates closure of the donor site (when preservation of the donor toe is not contemplated).

When none of the arteries possesses a suitable diameter, two (or even three) are taken in continuity with the dorsalis pedis artery, and then the toe is divided distally through the DIP joint. A review of the complication rate has demonstrated that there was no failure when the transfer was fed by more than one artery.[42,59] The skin is split on the medial line of the plantar aspect, and two lateral flaps are reflected until the vascular bundle is reached (Fig. 51-13). The flexor sheath is then opened longitudinally and medially to remove the flexor mechanism, with care taken to avoid injuring the retrotendinous vessels and the vascularization of the plantar plate. The first phalanx is osteotomized to the length needed. A bone peg can be harvested from the discarded metatarsal for bone stabilization at either the donor or recipient site (double transfer). Once the compound transfer is pedicled on only its artery (or arteries) and vein, the tourniquet is released. A local topical vasodilator (lidocaine 5%) is applied to the artery, and the foot is wrapped with hot wet sponges.

Preparation of the hand is performed through a classic longitudinal dorsal incision, but extensive excision of scarred tissue is possible because of the large skin flap of the compound transfer. The flexor sheath is cleared out and the remaining volar plate made thinner. The bone ends and the extensor mechanism are prepared. A separate approach (ideally horizontal) is performed in the first intermetacarpal space, with dissection of the radial artery and one superficial vein. The skin is undermined between the two incisions to provide a channel sufficient for the vascular bundle. The length of missing bone and vessels needed is measured, and the dissection of the foot is completed. The phalanges of the toe are usually trimmed to allow intramedullary penetration at the recipient site. Then the vein and artery are divided. When length permits, the dorsalis pedis artery and the proximal plantar arch are harvested so that the latter can be intercalated as a "T"-shaped graft (Fig. 51-14).

The compound joint is then transferred to the recipient finger and the bone secured. I have used different types of osteosynthesis (intramedullary screw, Kirschner wire, bone peg, and wiring), but I have not noted any difference in postoperative motion when comparing methods or techniques of internal fixation. Most frequently, I have used a buried intramedullary pin and an oblique Kirschner wire in adults and a single longitudinal Kirschner wire in young patients, with

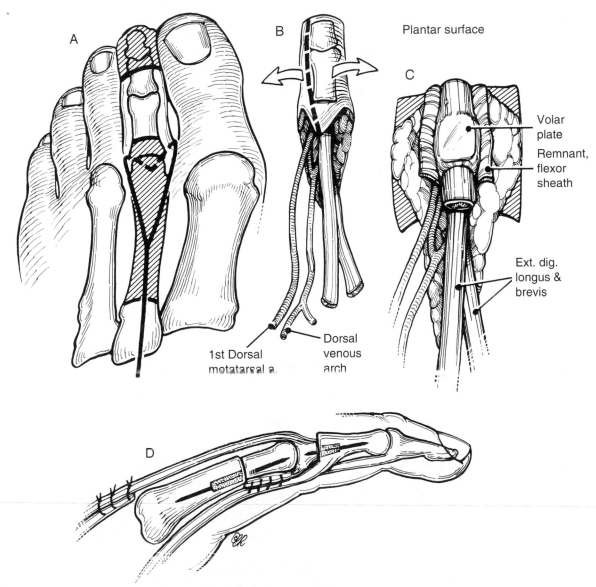

FIGURE 51-13. Author's technique for PIP toe joint compound transfer. **A,** A large flap is harvested. **B,** The plantar skin is split on the midplantar aspect. **C,** Two lateral flaps are reflected and the flexor mechanism removed, with preservation of part of the sheath for later repair. **D,** Intramedullary bone penetration and suture of the recipient's flexor sheath to the rims of the donor site pulleys.   *Continued*

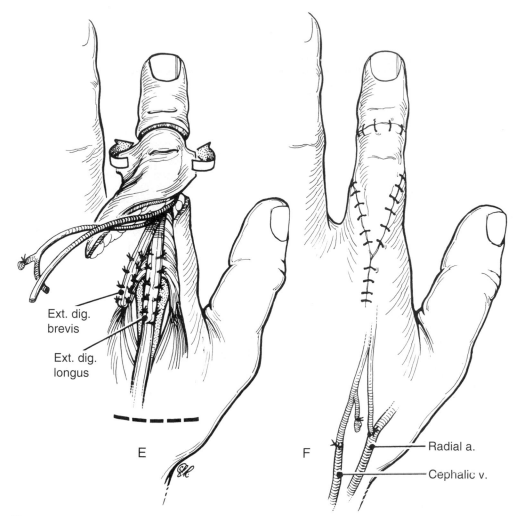

E

Ext. dig. brevis

Ext. dig. longus

F

Radial a.

Cephalic v.

FIGURE 51-13—cont'd. E, Extensor tendon suture. The extensor brevis is sutured to the intrinsic mechanism, and the longus is sutured to the extrinsic extensor tendon. **F,** Vessel anastomoses: end-to-side suture with the radial artery and end-to-end suture with the cephalic vein.

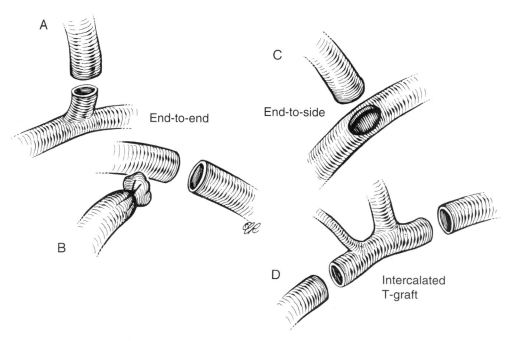

A

End-to-end

B

C

End-to-side

D

Intercalated T-graft

FIGURE 51-14. Four types of arterial suture can be performed. **A,** End-to-end suture with the princeps pollicis artery. **B,** End-to-end suture with the radial artery. **C,** End-to-side suture with the radial artery. **D,** The dorsalis pedis artery in continuity with the plantar arch is intercalated as a "T"-shaped graft (in this case, two feeding arteries have been harvested from the foot).

care taken to avoid any rotation of the intercalated fragment. This also avoids one of the major pitfalls, intercalation of a segment that is too long (it is preferable that it be slightly shorter). The remnant of flexor sheath of the toe is sutured to the rim of the recipient sheath to prevent bowstringing of the flexor tendon. The extensor mechanism is sutured with overlapping and the joint in full extension. The extensor hallucis longus is separated in two bands. One is secured to the central band of the tendon on the dorsum of the first phalanx and the other to the intrinsic tendon. The bundle is then passed through the subcutaneous tunnel while avoiding any twisting, and the skin flap is carefully trimmed, inserted, and sutured. The vessels are then sutured in an end-to-side or end-to-end ("T"-shaped) fashion for the artery and in an end-to-end fashion for the single vein. The tourniquet is then removed and the donor site is closed after hemostasis is obtained. Intermetatarsal ligament reconstruction is performed, and the skin is closed over small drains.

My colleagues and my policy of second-ray amputation is based on problems encountered after donor site grafting (nonunion and delayed walking). On the other hand, a study by a foot surgeon based on 20 cases of second-toe amputation[145] has demonstrated that in a case of amputation of the toe with the metatarsal left in place there was a consistent tendency to hallux valgus deformity. This decreased after ray amputation except when the angle between the first and second metatarsals was greater than 20 degrees. In such cases, reconstruction of the second toe has to be considered. I do try to preserve the second toe when the amount of bone stock transferred is limited.

The last step is assessment of viability of the flap at the recipient site before application of the dressing. Moderate elevation is prescribed postoperatively, and visualization of the skin allows direct monitoring of the transfer. Low-molecular-weight dextran is infused for 5 days with 325 mg of aspirin daily. No antibiotics are given. The patient can be discharged from the hospital on the fifth day. A clinical trial of early mobilization in a dynamic dorsal splint did not correlate with the final range of motion; therefore, I routinely prescribe 4 weeks' immobilization followed by pin removal and active motion with dynamic extension splinting. Nightly passive flexion splinting is delayed until the fifth week.

Other Transfers

Three other techniques are worthy of mention: (1) double transfer for MP or PIP joint reconstruction, (2) adjacent PIP joint reconstruction (hand) by adjacent toe PIP joint transfer, and (3) "twisted two toes" transfer for thumb reconstruction.

Double Transfer of MT and PIP Joints (Same Toe) to Adjacent MP Joints

The MP joint can be reconstructed by using either the PIP or the MTP joint of the toe. When two adjacent MP joints have to be reconstructed, it is possible to harvest both vascularized joints from the second toe (Fig. 51-15). The MT joint is raised on the second plantar metatarsal artery and rotated 180 degrees on its axis. The PIP joint is raised on the first dorsal (or plantar) artery. This technique requires a good extensor mechanism and good skin coverage in the hand. When transferred for index and middle finger reconstruction, it is preferable to put the PIP toe joint in the index finger to provide good lateral stability, because the MT joint is too lax to resist the pressure of the thumb.

Transfer of Adjacent PIP Joints (Second and Third Toe) to Adjacent PIP Joints of the Hand

For reconstruction of an adjacent PIP joint, Tsai and associates[192] have used the PIP joints of the second and third toes with partial syndactylization. To avoid this major cosmetic drawback, I prefer to harvest each joint on a separate pedicle (Fig. 51-16). a first plantar or dorsal metatarsal artery for the PIP joint of the second toe and the second plantar metatarsal artery for the third toe. In such cases, I amputate the second ray and use part of the second metatarsal for reconstruction of the third toe.

CRITICAL POINTS: PIP JOINT TOE TO PIP JOINT FINGER TRANSFER

INDICATIONS

- Mainly children
- Multiple huge compound PIP joint loss in adult

PREOPERATIVE EVALUATION

- Flexor mechanism intact

PEARLS

- Interposed bone/joint segment must not be too long.
- Extensor mechanism is sutured under maximal tension to the central band and intrinsic tendon.

TECHNICAL POINTS

- Core temperature is monitored.
- All the vessels of the first and second space are dissected trying to harvest more than one artery to feed the transfer.
- Distal skin flap is sutured before vessel anastomoses (to have proper vessel length)
- The second toe is preserved when possible or the second ray is amputated.

PITFALL

- Extensor lag is very common.

POSTOPERATIVE CARE

- Immobilization in PIP joint extension for at least 6 weeks (because early mobilization does not improve motion)
- Splint with dynamic extension (allowing flexion) for 2 weeks
- Splint in flexion not earlier than 8 weeks (during the day) with extension splint at night for at least 3 months

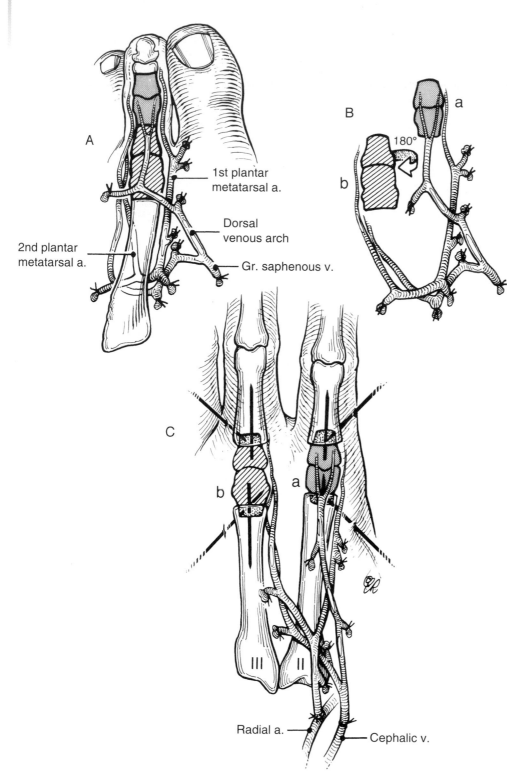

FIGURE 51-15. The metatarsophalangeal joint and PIP joint of the second toe are lifted on separate bundles to facilitate double MP joint reconstruction.

Labels within figure: 1st plantar metatarsal a.; 2nd plantar metatarsal a.; Dorsal venous arch; Gr. saphenous v.; Radial a.; Cephalic v.; 180°

"Twisted Two Toes" Transfer

Finally, a vascularized joint transfer can be incorporated into a wraparound technique for thumb reconstruction in a "twisted two toes" (TTT) technique.[47,49,58,63,64,66,107,123,190] The skin and nail complex based on the first dorsal (and/or plantar) metatarsal artery are taken from the ipsilateral big toe. A piece of vascularized bone longitudinally harvested from the distal phalanx of the great toe is incorporated into the flap. This longitudinal bone-harvesting technique[47,49,61,63] that I use in all "custom-made" thumb reconstructions (including bone)

has several advantages: it avoids bone resorption, provides good fixation for the pulp and nail support, allows curving of the nail to decrease its visual projection ("illusion" technique[49,61]), and does not shorten the great toe.[48] The PIP joint is lifted en bloc with the first and second phalanx on the second plantar (or rarely, the dorsal) metatarsal artery, with the flexor superficialis and the extensor mechanisms being harvested at the same time. Both arteries are taken in continuity with the dorsalis pedis artery, which is used for a "T"-shaped intercalated graft. The joint is buried into the big

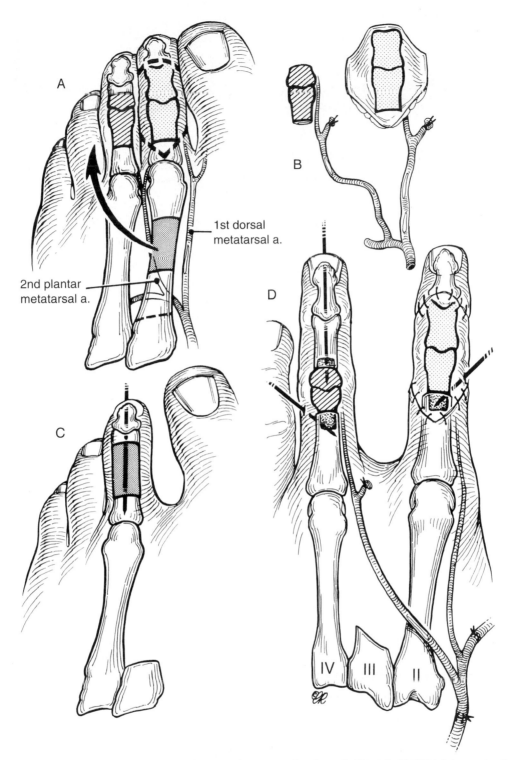

FIGURE 51-16. The PIP joints of the second and third toes are harvested on separate bundles to facilitate double PIP joint reconstruction. **A** and **B,** Double transfer of PIP joints of second and third toes on the first and second metatarsal artery. **C,** Reconstruction of the third toe by a bone graft from the second metatarsal proximally cut. **D,** Reconstruction of the PIP joints of the index and ring fingers (ray transfer of the middle finger) with interposition of the artery at the snuffbox level.

toe flap, and the second phalanx is attached to the longitudinal piece of bone of the great toe by a Kirschner wire (Fig. 51-17). In this way, a two-phalanx "custom-made" thumb is constructed and may then be transferred to the thumb stump in the standard manner. Either a graft or an ulnar-based triangular flap tailored from the stump is used to cover the ulnar side of the filleted big toe skin. At the donor

site, the proximal part of the second metatarsal bone is removed, the intermetatarsal ligament repaired, and the filleted second-toe skin wrapped around the skeleton of the big toe with a "Z"-plasty.

Initially, I have limited this "twisted two toes" technique to amputation of the thumb at the MP joint level, but recently I have also used it for more proximal amputations[49,107] by

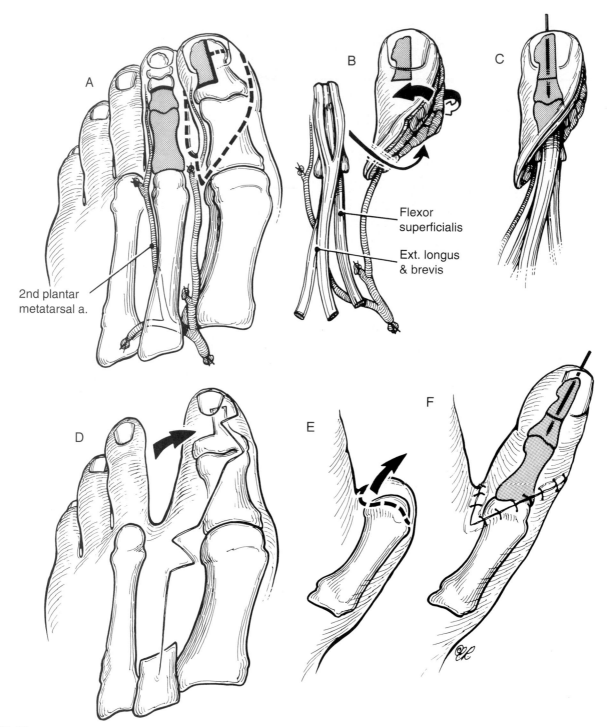

FIGURE 51-17. "Twisted two toes" technique. **A** and **B,** A sheath of skin, the nail complex, and a piece of loose bone are taken from the great toe; the PIP joint with extensor and flexor tendons is harvested from the second toe. **C,** The bones of the first and second toes are joined by a Kirschner wire and the skin wrapped around. **D,** The filleted flap of the second toe covers the great toe defect. **E** and **F,** A lateral flap is elevated from the thumb stump to cover the lateral aspect of the transfer.

including the MT joint of the second ray tilted palmarly about 45 degrees to avoid hyperextension deformity.

In thumb reconstruction, the "twisted two toes" technique is indicated in some amputations located close to the MP joint. It has several advantages over the classic "wraparound"[144] and total second-toe transfer in that it provides (1) a vascularized skeleton (avoiding resorption) with two phalanges (matching the normal thumb), (2) one

joint (plus a proximal hemijoint or an MP joint when necessary) with extensor and flexor mechanisms, (3) firm support for the pulp and nail, and (4) a growth plate in children.

Indications in Congenital Conditions

The indications in congenital conditions are even less frequent than in trauma cases. I have performed one case of

CRITICAL POINTS: "TTT" TRANSFER FOR THUMB RECONSTRUCTION

INDICATIONS

- Amputation at MP joint level or more proximal (with at least one third of proximal metacarpal) with intact fingers (or four-fingered hand)
- Replace wraparound in children because it provides growth

PREOPERATIVE EVALUATION

- Radiographs (no arteriogram)

PEARLS

- Do not make the thumb too long, because mobility is limited.

TECHNICAL POINTS

- Core temperature is monitored.
- The homolateral foot is selected (better nerve on ulnar side).
- The skin envelope with the nail and a piece of vascularized bone (cut longitudinally) is harvested from the great toe based on one artery of the first web space.
- Vascularized joint(s), PIP (and MT) of the second toe, are harvested based on the plantar artery of the second web space (en bloc with extensor and flexor apparatus).

- Simple shifting (not twisting) of the joint in the skin envelope is done.
- A triangular flap (radially based) is lifted on the thumb stump.
- Longitudinal Kirschner wire maintains the joint in extension and gives distal fixation to the fragment from the great toe.
- Suturing of the extensor and flexor tendons is done.
- Distal skin suturing is done before vessel anastomoses (to avoid kinking).
- Arterial and vein sutures are done at the snuff-box level (through a transverse incision).
- The second toe is usually sacrificed with the filleted skin (and nail) used to cover the great toe (which is not shortened).

PITFALL

- Twisting of arteries when inserting the skeleton of the second toe inside the skin envelope of the great toe (mainly if arterial segments are short)

POSTOPERATIVE CARE

- Kirschner wire removed at 5 weeks
- Splinting in flexion (daytime) and in extension (at night)

---

vascularized PIP toe joint transfer in an isolated symphalangism of the ring finger under the pressure of the family, despite the acknowledged absence of a functional problem. The final range of motion at 1 year was 65 degrees. The two other conditions in my experience were some rare cases of symbrachydactyly and thumb hypoplasia. Indeed, one of the major problems in surgery of congenital conditions is the preservation of growth potential, and any lengthening procedure without a growth plate frequently needs to be redone a few years later to keep pace with the growth of the other fingers (or toe transfer). Only a vascularized epiphysis can provide such growth.

Second-Toe MT Joint to the Thumb CMC Joint

Reconstruction of the CMC joint in certain cases of congenital thumb ray hypoplasia can be performed by an MTP joint transfer, which provides bone stock, mobility, stability, and growth plates. MT joint transfer provides an acceptable solution to the occasional case of congenital thumb ray hypoplasia such as type IIIB (in Blauth's classification[1] modified by Manske[135]), where the CMC joint is missing and the thumb is moderately hypoplastic. In such cases, pollicization remains the best option functionally.[7] In Asia and Arabia, preservation of a five-fingered hand is of outstanding importance. Such cultural importance is less frequent in white patients. But if the patients' parents refuse to "sacrifice" the index finger for pollicization, a vascularized MT joint transfer tilted in some extension could be the base of a more complex and

sometimes multi-stage reconstruction. In such cases the amount of bone stock from the first phalanx is limited and in some type IIIB patients bone graft interposition may be necessary. However, it is also possible to switch the donor segment and use the metatarsal, which is longer, to compensate for the absence of metacarpal bone. This transfer improves the cosmetic aspect, allows growth, and provides satisfactory stability and mobility.[78] A skin flap can be transferred at the same time to improve the thenar eminence, thus facilitating the secondary abductor digiti minimi opponensplasty (Huber transfer). Abduction can be reconstructed at this first step depending on the degree of radial hypoplasia.

In fact, reviewing our cases with a long follow-up[78,80] my colleagues and I found that growth of the hypoplastic thumb itself remains unpredictable. The transferred MT joint has a good growth, but the joint has some tendency to adopt a flexed position. I currently do not perform "early" transfer (before 1 year of age to facilitate cortical integration) and I favor performing reconstruction only when the thumb has sufficient growth and is integrated by the child in large grasp. Fine pinch is usually performed between the index and middle finger (explaining the index pronation seen after such reconstruction). Frequently when the reconstruction is delayed, in absence of any use of the thumb, the relatives accept pollicization. Only in some cultural backgrounds (Asian, Arabic families) the refusal is usually definitive. In such cases, early transfer can be performed, because there is no reason to "punish" the infant. The relatives have to be aware that multiple operations are necessary: first webplasty, stabilization of the MP joint when unstable, correction of a pollex abductus, and intrinsic reconstruction. The extrinsic reconstruction (flexor pollicis longus and extensor pollicis) is optional at this setting. Hypoplasia of all the radial aspect of the hand and forearm can present major difficulties in finding enough tendons for transfer. Finally, in such early reconstructions, a secondary distraction lengthening procedure may be necessary if there is insufficient growth.

CRITICAL POINTS: MT TOE JOINT TO FIRST CMC JOINT TRANSFER

INDICATIONS

- Type IIIB (absent first CMC joint) and refusal of pollicization
- Early transfer in families with certain cultural backgrounds
- Late transfer (6 to 10 years) in case of sufficient growth and cortical integration

PREOPERATIVE EVALUATION

- Radiographs confirming type IIIB

PEARLS

- Delayed decision in white patient until integration or exclusion of the thumb in grip

TECHNICAL POINTS

- Core temperature is monitored (no drop of temperature).
- A dorsal flap is harvested from the dorsum of the foot.
- MT joint is harvested on two arteries, including the second plantar metatarsal artery.
- MT joint is placed in extension to allow contact with small finger in opposition.
- Recipient ulnar artery is taken in case of absence of radial artery.
- Tendon transfer is done for abduction of the thumb.
- The second toe can be preserved.

PITFALL

- Risk of insufficient thumb growth (careful follow-up and secondary lengthening)

POSTOPERATIVE CARE

- Immobilization of the thumb for 4 weeks
- Splint with dynamic extension and flexion at 5 weeks
- Second stage (web flap, MP joint stabilization, Huber-Littler transfer) at 3 months

Epiphysis and Joint Transfer in Symbrachydactyly

In symbrachydactyly,[76,79] the thumb is sometimes hypoplastic with a defective proximal phalanx and a short, unstable thumb. I have noted this problem in type IIC patients (with mitten hand) and in type IIIB patients with a monodactylous hand. In some type IIC patients with a mitten hand, the index finger is very hypoplastic (and frequently "floating" owing to absent metacarpal bone) and the first web space is insufficient. If the second ray is sacrificed, a joint and epiphysis could be preserved on its vascular bundle and transferred as an island. Both collateral arteries need to be operatively assessed to select the best for the transfer (but the ulnar one facilitates the transfer to the thumb). After excision of the "anlagen" replacing the proximal phalanx, the vascularized segment of bone, cartilage, joint, and growth plate is interposed and fixed with a small (0.6 mm) Kirschner wire. Such a transfer is quite demanding; growth is present but not normal in my limited experience of four cases, and mobility remains nonmeasurable. However, the main advantages are to obtain stability, provide some growth, and improve the first web.[151]

In symbrachydactyly type IIIB (monodactylous hand with brachymesophalangy of the thumb), there are several alternatives: the thumb could be lengthened by a second toe transfer (the second toe of the opposite foot allowing reconstruction of one finger), a nonvascularized phalanx, or a vascularized free epiphysis transfer from one toe (second or third). An empty pouch with a distal nail invites the interposition of a bone graft, but when using a nonvascularized transfer the growth is limited. Growth is sufficient when using a nonvascularized toe phalanx for finger reconstruction but does not keep the pace of the growth of a vascularized second toe transfer. When a toe transfer is selected for finger reconstruction I favor transfer of a vascularized epiphysis to the hypoplastic thumb.[79,80]

POSTOPERATIVE COMPLICATIONS

Thrombosis of the vessels is a classic complication of microvascular procedures that can be avoided by using multiple arteries to feed the transfer. When thrombosis occurs, however, it has to be diagnosed early by careful monitoring of the skin flap incorporated into the transfer. In case of skin necrosis, mainly in very young patients, the transfer can be saved by moving a remote flap onto the "non"-vascularized joint. Infection, although not mentioned in the literature, should be managed by standard techniques.

Delayed bone healing does not seem to be a problem at the hand level, but it has been mentioned frequently in the foot.[97,122,192,216] Stiffness of the vascularized joint transfer remains a major problem. My colleagues and I have tried to improve joint mobility preoperatively in the foot by splinting at night, but without success. Even when early mobilization was instituted, limitation of both active and passive extension (as noted in total second-toe transfers) was found consistently after toe vascularized joint transfer.* There are several possible reasons for this: (1) preexisting claw deformity of the donor toe, (2) deficient or insufficient tension on

---

*See references 17, 23, 45, 54, 57, 58, 66, 97, 122, 192, and 216.

the extensor mechanism, (3) an overly long intercalated bony segment, (4) bowstringing of flexor tendons increasing the lever arm (as seen in digits with damaged pulleys), and (5) extensor tendon adhesions. As noted previously, only some of these factors can be avoided by surgical technique. Tsai and Hanna have studied the mobility of 50 normal second-toe PIP joints[191] and found that lack of extension correlates with age and ranges from 0 to 20 degrees with a total active motion of 27 to 69 degrees.

In my colleagues and my published series of 25 patients,[62] complications were as follows: two failures (8%), one successful reexploration for arterial thrombosis, one pin tract infection, and one discrete area of skin sloughing resulting in secondary scarring. The other "large" series published by Tsai and Hanna[191] involving 29 patients with an average follow-up of 1.9 years gives a complication rate of 48.4%; no motion was recorded in 28%, and in successful cases the total active motion was 46 degrees. The good news is the absence of radiologic deterioration and the persistence of cartilage growth plates in children[23] as well as few sequelae at the donor site. In a series of five cases of MT joint transfer, numbness of the neighboring toe was noticed in two cases, cold intolerance in one, reduced pushoff in one, tender scar in one, and some deformity of the toe in two.[215] The long plantar incision was responsible for tender scars on the bottom of the foot.

CONCLUSION

Vascularized joint transfer may be indicated for post-traumatic and congenital conditions, at the PIP, MP, and CMC level. The main indication after trauma remains a complex situation in which all the "classic" techniques fall short of achieving the range of motion necessary for daily activities. Here again the aphorism of Bunnell is worth keeping in mind: "When there is nothing, a little is a lot," especially when this "little" is painless and stable in space and time. This technique provides the unique advantage of a compound transfer of skin, bone, joint, tendons, and growth plate. Until vascularized homografts or tissue engineering become clinically available, this is a worthwhile technique in limited complex cases.

ANNOTATED REFERENCES

28. Donski PK, Carwell GR, Sharzer LA: Growth in revascularized bone grafts in young puppies. Plast Reconstr Surg 64:239-243, 1979.

   The authors compared in an experimental study on 12 puppies the growth in transplanted vascularized and nonvascularized ulna epiphyses transfers. They stressed that the growth was better in vascularized epiphyses but less than normal and suggested that there was a metaphyseal vascular contribution.

33. Ellis PR, Hanna D, Tsai TM: Vascularized single toe joint transfer to the hand. J Hand Surg [Am] 16:160-168, 1991.

   The authors describe the technique of harvesting the skin from the lateral aspect of the hallux, based on the first dorsal metatarsal artery. This trick facilitates preservation of the second toe after harvesting the joint. They reviewed 31 single joint transfers. In the 26 performed for traumatic loss, the range of motion was an average 27.2 degrees after a mean follow-up of 22.6 months. Complications were frequent (50% of patients).

87. Gilbert A: Composite tissue transfers from the foot: Anatomic basis and surgical technique. *In* Daniller AL, Strauch B (eds): Symposium on Microsurgery. St. Louis, CV Mosby, 1976, pp 230-242.

   In this classic paper the authors described the vascularization of the toes and demonstrated the possibility that the first dorsal metatarsal artery runs under part of the interosseous muscles but remains superficial at the level of the intermetatarsal ligament.

105. Hume MC, Gellman H, McKellop H, Brumfield RH Jr: Functional range of motion of the joints of the hand. J Hand Surg [Am] 15:240-243, 1990.

   It is of interest to know the "functional" arc of motion of the finger joints during a variety of daily living activities. The functional arc of the MP ranges from 33 to 73 degrees (average, 61 degrees), and for the PIP joint it is 36 to 86 degrees (average, 60 degrees).

176. Singer DI, O'Brien BM, McLeod AM, et al: Long-term follow-up of free vascularized joint transfers to the hand in children. J Hand Surg [Am] 13:776-783, 1988.

   Vascularized joint transfers in four children were reviewed after an average follow-up of 6.6 years. Growth contribution of PIP joint transfer was limited owing to the presence of only one epiphysis (0.4 cm growth). Growth in the two epiphyses of the transferred MT joints was close to normal with good range of motion (even in absence of "upside-down" positioning).

193. Tsai TM, Ogden L, Jaeger SH, Okubo K: Experimental vascularized total joint autografts: A primate study. J Hand Surg [Am] 7:140-146, 1982.

   This study compared autogenous vascularized and nonvascularized joint transfers in the monkeys' hands. The surviving nonvascularized transfers (four of nine) demonstrated necrosis of the hyaline cartilage and degenerative changes. The surviving vascularized joints (seven of nine) had more constant bone union (66% vs. 30%) and preserved cartilage (up to 45 weeks).

199. Vilkki SK: Distraction and microvascular epiphysis transfer for radial club hand. J Hand Surg [Br] 23:445-452, 1998.

   The author provided medium-term results (mean, 6 years) of nine clinical cases of type IV Bayne radial clubhand treated by an original technique. After soft tissue distraction, an MT joint with full length of the metatarsal was transferred onto the radial side of the wrist to correct the deformity and provide mobility. In six cases the correction persisted at follow-up with good preservation of ulna length (67%) and good wrist stability. Mobility was more in flexion (60 to 90 degrees) than in extension (−20 to +20 degrees).

215. Yang XB: The donor foot in free toe or joint transfers. J Hand Surg [Am] 25:382-384, 2000.

   In their series of 84 cases of second toe transfers reviewed after a mean follow-up of 6.5 years to assess the donor foot, 5 had a free MT joint transfer. Eighty-six percent of the 84 patients recovered completely within 6 months. Pain on movement, fatigability, numbness, difficulty in running, and callus formation were seen in 2 cases of joint transfer. Cold intolerance, difficulty in standing on the toes, and tender scar were noticed in 1 case each. Some foot deformity was present in 3 cases.

CHAPTER 52

Toe-to-Hand Transplantation

Fu-Chan Wei

Toe-to-hand transplantation has been intimately related to the development of microsurgical free tissue transplantation, which may be considered one of the most important advances in the history of reconstructive surgery. The first one-stage human toe-to-thumb transfer was performed by Young[1] in 1966 using the second toe, with Cobbett[15] performing a transfer of the great toe to the thumb in 1968. Many clinical reports using various forms of toe transfer followed during the 1970s and 1980s.* Toe transplantation has become a widely accepted option for thumb reconstruction because of its prevalent functional role in opposition.

However, in contrast to thumbs, finger reconstruction using toe transplantation has been somewhat controversial and less acknowledged, owing to either the possibility of functional compensation in the hand after finger amputation or a relative lack of adequate experience among our surgical colleagues. Nonetheless, the absence of fingers is still a clinical problem that limits hand function and causes psychological suffering. Physical impairment and deformity are more severe with mutilating injuries involving multiple digits. When properly indicated, reconstruction with like tissue transferred from the feet is undoubtedly a good alternative to restore function and appearance after finger amputations. In contrast to the results obtained with the use of prostheses or some conventional techniques,[7,29,38,56,67,81,88,89] microsurgical toe transfer is the only procedure that provides functioning digits with acceptable appearance and sensibility.[50,93,107] Reports of the use of toe transplantation for finger reconstruction include multiple digit reconstruction with bilateral toe transplantation,[68,73,84,111,112] combined transplantation of the second and third toes,[86] combined transplantation of the third and fourth toes,[85,114] single transplantation of the third toe,[103,117] and other toe combinations transplanted as one unit.[11,116] Microsurgical restoration of distal digital function with partial toe transfer was first mentioned in 1979 by Buncke and Rose,[6] who used pulp neurosensory free flaps for finger reconstruction. In the past 10 years more attention has been focused on this complex anatomic region and various surgical procedures have been described and refined for distal digit reconstruction, including vascularized nail grafts,[42] toe hemipulp free flaps,[50]

lesser toe wraparound procedures,[41,51,98] and partial transplantation of the lesser toe.[19] It is evident from this brief perspective that the role of microsurgical toe transplantation for reconstruction of the hand has substantially evolved and potential options are still unlimited.

This chapter shall focus mainly on toe-to-finger reconstruction but will cover a few aspects of toe-to-thumb reconstruction (to avoid too much repetition with the later chapter on thumb reconstruction).

GENERAL CONSIDERATIONS

In general, it is acknowledged that not every patient with digital amputation will be a candidate for future microsurgical toe-to-hand transplantation. In selecting suitable patients for this type of reconstruction, the amputation level, number of involved digits, and the patient's needs and motivations must be considered beforehand. For instance, a distal amputation in one digit might be psychologically more important and meaningful for one patient than a metacarpal hand deformity for another, although a higher functional deficit is present in the second patient. The patient's overall general health, medical problems, and associated injuries should be considered as well. Although advanced age is not a contraindication to toe transplantation, functional requirements in the hand are lower and postoperative rehabilitation is more difficult in elderly patients. Furthermore, a higher risk of microvascular complications and less sensory recovery can be expected with advanced age.[17] Occupation, hand dominance, and activity levels are all important factors to keep in mind. Surgical indications may also differ from country to country, depending on the levels of workers' compensation coverage and job opportunities.[46,82]

The location and number of missing digits are important for establishing reconstructive priorities.[101] Radial pulp defects in the index and middle finger and the ulnar aspect of the thumb are more important for fine pinch and handling of small objects.[123] With multiple digit amputation, it is recommended that reconstruction encompass at least two adjacent fingers. The radial digits (index and middle) are more important in patients with occupations that require fine manipulation, whereas the ulnar digits (ring and middle) are more necessary in laborers requiring powerful grasp.[99,107]

---

*See references 69, 70, 83a, 95, 97, 105, 106, 109-111, and 120.

When toe-to-hand transplantation is considered as a reconstructive option, the donor site defect should be extensively discussed with the patient. Although foot function is not restricted for most ambulatory activities with resection of one or two toes, it might be limited to a certain extent for specific activities, such as some sports. Foot cosmesis, on the other hand, should not be overlooked and could be important in some cultures and in young patients. Finally, surgeons must have expertise and familiarity with the various toe transplantation procedures to avoid failures and complications and to offer the patient an optimal result.

Initial Care and Preoperative Evaluation

Digital replantation, including utilization of the distal parts, remains the best option in acute management of traumatic amputations. This is a reliable procedure that must be attempted whenever indicated and possible.[9,25] Toe transplantation for digit reconstruction must be considered from the time of initial injury, however. It should be discussed with the patient and relatives as an option for future reconstruction, when practical, even before replantation. This is particularly true in those patients with multiple digit amputation and when conditions for replantation are not ideal, for example, in severe crushing or avulsion injuries.[83,91] If replantation fails or is not feasible, toe transplantation for reconstruction should be planned during initial care. Bone, tendon, and neurovascular bundle length must be preserved after débridement of all nonviable tissue and adequate soft tissue coverage provided (Fig. 52-1).[59,104,106] The length of all anatomic structures retained in the stump will most likely determine the type of toe transplantation and its functional and aesthetic outcome. Moreover, preservation of stump length will reduce the possibility of requiring nerve or tendon grafts and the use of vein grafts for vascular anastomoses during finger reconstruction, thus avoiding extensive dissection in the donor foot.

Bone and Joint

It is a common mistake to excessively shorten the digital skeleton to achieve primary closure of the wound with local flaps. For skeletal fixation with toe-to-hand transplantation, bone stumps as short as 5.0 mm in length can be used for intraosseous wiring.[121] It is therefore recommended that bone length be preserved to the extent that complete soft tissue coverage is still possible. Every effort should be made to maintain functioning joints or the cartilage surface with the articular capsule. The transferred toe can be harvested through disarticulation and the joint capsule directly repaired with the recipient finger with good functional results, particularly in thumb reconstruction.[80,119] Metacarpal stumps can be augmented to the desired length with a nonvascularized bone block,[2,102] thus avoiding proximal transmetatarsal osteotomies during toe transfer and preserving metatarsal length, which minimizes donor foot morbidity.

Tendons

Preservation of the extensor mechanism in the finger is important for maintenance of balance between the intrinsic and extrinsic systems involved in extension. For distal amputations, the extensor apparatus should be left in situ on the digital stump and the intrinsic insertions over the proximal phalanx preserved. For more proximal amputations at the metacarpophalangeal (MCP) joint level, retention of the extensor hood is advocated for the same reasons.[59,104] Conservative débridement of flexor tendon length is important in distal digit amputations because functional results are better when the insertion of the flexor digitorum superficialis (FDS) is present. For more proximal amputations, the finger flexors must be left in situ, although they might be shortened for future tendon repair in zone III. By preserving the flexor tendons in place, it is possible to maintain the integrity of the pulley system, which is vital for future function, especially the A1 and A2 pulleys.

Vessels

The digital arteries and veins are seldom intact after crushing or avulsion injuries. Every effort should be made to retain the arteries' length in nonreplantable digit amputations because these can be used as recipient vessels for toe transplantation in the future. The ulnar digital artery in particular is larger than its counterpart in the radial digits. The veins are less often a matter of concern inasmuch as a rich venous network on the dorsum of the hand is usually present.

Nerves

For prevention of the potential development of neuromas in amputation stumps, proximal resection of the digital nerves has been advocated.[36] When toe-to-hand transplantation is considered for future reconstruction, the nerves' length must be preserved because recovery of sensation is faster when neurorrhaphies are performed closer to the transferred toe.

Skin

Instead of using local or regional flaps to cover the wound, soft tissue augmentation with a pedicle groin flap is a better alternative. The use of local flaps may increase morbidity, create additional deformity, and decrease functional rehabilitation.[21,39,71] The redundant skin provided by a groin flap may later prove useful for covering the transferred toe (see Fig. 52-1). Additionally, it may be used for protection of the pedicle, creation of an adequate web space, and improvement in scar quality. Besides this, when there is enough skin available on the recipient finger (or hand), it will be possible to minimize the amount of skin included during toe transfer, thus facilitating primary closure of the foot and enhancing donor site appearance as well.[19,106]

Primary Versus Secondary Toe-To-Hand Transplantation

Traditionally, toe-to-hand transplantation has been performed as a second-stage procedure once definitive coverage of the defect is provided. However, it can also be performed primarily (with the wound still open after injury). Recently, comparative results in 144 secondary and 31 primary toe-to-hand transplants showed a survival rate of 96.5% in secondary transplantation and 96.9% with primary transplantation. There was no statistical difference between the two groups in terms of intraoperative anastomotic revision, re-exploration, complications, and secondary procedures.[124]

Primary toe-to-hand transplantation can be performed safely. It reduces hospital stay and helps regain hand function and the patient's body image in a shorter period of

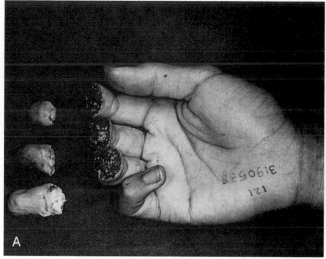

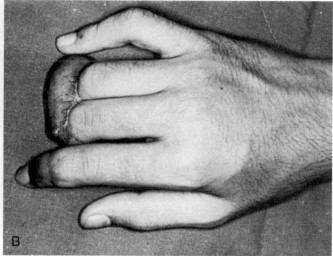

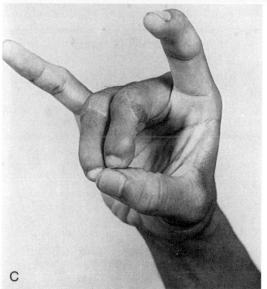

FIGURE 52-1. A, Distal amputation of the index, middle, and ring fingers. **B,** Only the index finger was successfully replanted, and the middle and ringer finger stumps were covered with a pedicled groin flap after débridement and preservation of the fingers' skeleton, tendons, and neurovascular bundle length. **C,** Final result showing pinch function after reconstruction involving bilateral partial second-toe simultaneous transplantation.

time. It is recommended in highly motivated, well-informed patients in good physical condition and when wounds are well demarcated and clean (Fig. 52-2).

RECONSTRUCTIVE OPTIONS

Thumb Amputation

Although the thumb amputated at the interphalangeal (IP) joint level is still able to perform its basic functions, fine manipulation ability and hand appearance are compromised. Therefore, when replantation is not possible, toe transplantation should be always offered as one of the reconstructive options even at a distal level. The thumb can be reconstructed with either the great toe or a lesser toe. Transfer of the great toe can include the entire toe or modified transfers including the great toe wraparound flap, trimmed great toe, twisted toe, and many others. The methods of thumb reconstruction should be individualized with considerations given to the functional and cosmetic needs of the patient as well as donor site morbidity. In general,

thumbs reconstructed with the great toe and its variants have a better functional and aesthetic result than those reconstructed with lesser toes.

Single Finger Amputation

In the same way that replantation of single digit amputations has been a matter of debate for many years,[91] reconstruction of one digit with toe transplantation has not been widely accepted. Because the functional deficit in the hand is minimal when only one finger is missing, some authors believe that sacrificing a toe for finger reconstruction (other than the thumb) is not justified, especially in the nondominant hand.[34,35,38,81] Although this statement may apply to some patients, when suitable, finger reconstruction with like-tissue transplantation from the foot usually offers satisfactory results, particularly in distal finger amputations.[100,108,123]

Reconstruction of Distal Digit Amputation

The distal end of a digit is the part of the hand most frequently injured. It is defined as the end portion of the digit distal to the insertion of the flexor pollicis longus in the

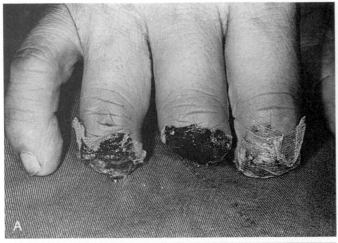

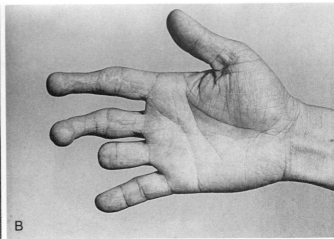

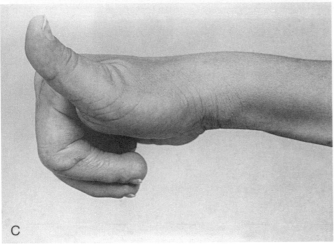

FIGURE 52-2. A, Amputation of the index, middle, and ring fingers 7 days after débridement in a patient who sustained a severe crushing injury. The finger stumps are prepared for primary reconstruction by toe transplantation. **B** and **C,** After using two second toes for index and middle finger reconstruction, full active extension and flexion are possible.

thumb or the FDS in the finger.[19,108] The highest density of innervation in the body surface is contained in the finger pulp; hence it is considered the "end organ of touch."[18,30] Specialized components of the distal digit include a sensate glabrous pulp and stable adherent nail. Glabrous skin characteristics allow resistance to wear and tear and provide a nonslippery surface for grasping. Attachment of the pulp skin to the underlying distal phalanx by a network of septa prevents excessive gliding and shearing of the skin. The fatty tissue arrangement between the septa allows the pulp to conform to the shape of objects in pinch and grasp.[30] The nail plays a major role in tactile sensibility of the pulp and in tip pinch[62,125] and is an important aesthetic component, especially in women and some cultures.[127]

The ideal reconstruction in this part of the finger should maintain digital length with adequate soft tissue padding, provide near-normal sensation, and result in recovery of nail function. Reconstructive options using partial toe transplantation in distal defects include a combination of different portions of the nail, pulp, and distal phalanx from the great or lesser toes. Depending on the defect, vascularized nail grafts,[42,63,73] onychocutaneous flaps,[40,41] wraparound flaps,[51,98] pulp and hemipulp flaps,[16,50,72] and partial lesser toe transplantation[19,100,108] can be selected for reconstruction (Fig. 52-3).

Amputations between the base of the distal phalanx and the middle of the middle phalanx require partial toe transfer with inclusion of the distal IP joint and the flexor and long extensor tendons.[19] Modern jobs and hobbies very often demand the presence of all digits (for instance, using a computer keyboard or playing a musical instrument). When properly indicated, this is probably one of the amputation levels for which the most rewarding results are obtained with toe-to-finger transplantation (see Fig. 52-1).

Reconstruction of Proximal Digit Amputation
Finger amputation between the FDS insertion and the web space (base of the proximal phalanx) presents a more controversial indication for reconstruction with lesser toes, because a shorter finger might result. If the finger amputation has occurred distal to the middle of the proximal phalanx, the second or third total toe (with the proximal interphalangeal [PIP] joint) can still be long enough to achieve adequate function and aesthetic results in some patients (see Fig. 52-2). Because of the length discrepancy with the remaining fingers that may result, more proximal amputations in a single finger might not be suitable for reconstruction with total toe transplantation. Nevertheless, a functional finger with suboptimal but acceptable appearance can still be achieved in highly motivated patients.

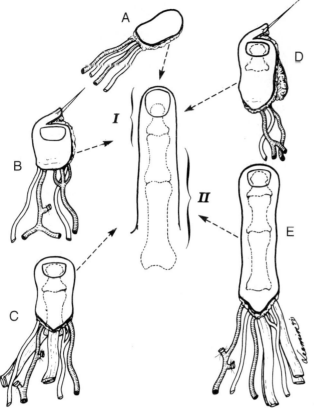

FIGURE 52-3. Single finger amputation levels and reconstructive options with toe-to-finger transplantation. A pulp toe flap (**A**), vascularized nail graft (**B**), partial lesser toe (**C**), or wraparound lesser toe flaps (**D**) may be used for distal finger amputation (I). Total lesser toe transplantation (**E**) is used for proximal finger amputation (II).

Multiple Digit Amputation

Reconstruction of Multiple Distal Digit Amputation

The same principles previously described for single digit distal amputation are used for the reconstruction of two or more fingers with distal amputation. Priority should be given to reconstruction of the index and middle fingers because they play a more important role in global hand function, specifically in fine manipulation.[100,108]

Reconstruction of Multiple Proximal Digit Amputation

In proximal amputation of two or more fingers, the main purpose of reconstruction is to provide improved prehension ability. It is therefore recommended that reconstruction of at least two fingers be considered.[99,101] The advantages of this approach are provision of (1) useful tripod pinch, (2) stronger hook grip, (3) lateral stability, and (4) handling precision (Fig. 52-4). Reconstructive options for adjacent finger amputations include two separate lesser toe transplantations or a combined second and third (or third and fourth) toe transplantation on a single vascular pedicle. In amputations distal to the web space, two separate lesser toes are preferable because transplantation of combined second and third toes will create an objectionable syndactylous appearance.[86,87,102] For finger amputations proximal to the web space, reconstruction with combined second and third toe transplantation is a better choice (Fig. 52-5). An additional consideration when planning tandem second and third toe transplantation for reconstruction of two adjacent digits is the length of the remaining fingers. As a general rule, the remaining fingers have to be shorter than the tip of the normal little finger; otherwise the transplanted unit

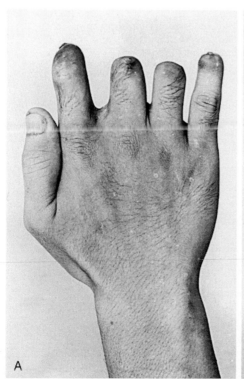

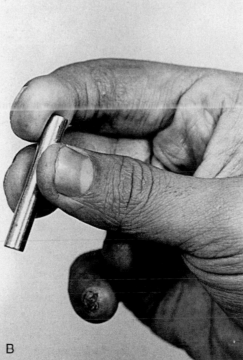

FIGURE 52-4. A and **B,** With multiple digit amputation it is better to aim at reconstructing at least two adjacent fingers to provide useful tripod pinch, stronger hook grip, lateral stability, and handling precision.

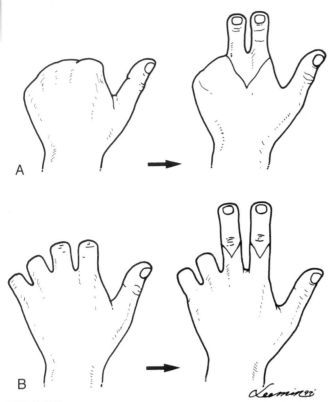

FIGURE 52-5. In digit amputation proximal to the web spaces, combined second- and third-toe transplantation is advocated (**A**), whereas in digit amputation distal to the web spaces, bilateral second-toe transplantation in one stage is selected (**B**).

cannot simulate the pinch point and grasp arch of full-length fingers.[86,87,102]

In cases with an intact articular surface on the metacarpal, the tandem toes can be disarticulated at the metatarsophalangeal joint and the joint capsule and ligaments circularly divided and used for reconstruction of the MCP joint (composite joint reconstruction). If the metacarpal articular surface has been damaged or is absent, transmetatarsal toe transplantation is performed.

A more severe functional deficit and deformity are present when mutilating hand injuries involve all digits at a proximal level with or without thumb amputation, a condition referred to as *metacarpal hand*.[60,96] My colleagues and I have proposed a new classification of metacarpal hands[52,54,107,111,112] and defined specific reconstructive options with toe transplantation (Tables 52-1 and 52-2).

This classification divides the metacarpal hand into two types for reconstructive purposes. In type I, amputation has occurred in all fingers proximal to the middle of the proximal phalanx, and either the thumb is intact or amputated distal to the IP joint (considered the minimum functional length required for precise prehension). In type II, amputation of all fingers is proximal to the middle of the proximal phalanx, with thumb amputation proximal to the IP joint. In type I metacarpal hand it is recommended that at least two adjacent digits be replaced. Depending on the finger amputation level relative to the MCP joint (subtypes IA, IB, and IC), bilateral lesser toes or combined second and third toe transplantation may be used for reconstruction. In type II metacarpal hand, a systematic strategy needs to be followed

Table 52-1
TYPE I METACARPAL HAND

Subtype	Level of Finger Amputation	Recommendations
IA	Distal to the MCP joint	Bilateral second toes for amputations distal to the web space Combined second and third toes for amputations proximal to the web space (transproximal phalanx transfer)
IB	Through the MCP joint with an intact metacarpal articular surface	Combined second and third toes (composite joint transfer)
IC	Through the MCP joint with a damaged metacarpal articular surface or transmetacarpal amputation	Combined second and third toes (transmetatarsal transfer)

Table 52-2
TYPE II METACARPAL HAND

Subtype	Level of Thumb Amputation	Recommendations
IIA	Distal to the metacarpal neck	Whole or trimmed great toe transfer (transproximal phalanx transfer)
IIB	Proximal to the metacarpal neck with adequate thenar muscle function	Preliminary distraction lengthening or interpositional bone graft followed by whole or trimmed great toe transfer *or* Transmetatarsal second-toe transfer
IIC	Any level with inadequate thenar musculature	Thumb reconstruction in a second stage after finger reconstruction *and* Tendon transfer to restore opposition
IID	Any level with a damaged CMC joint	Same as in IIA and IIB but aiming at reconstructing an immobile thumb post

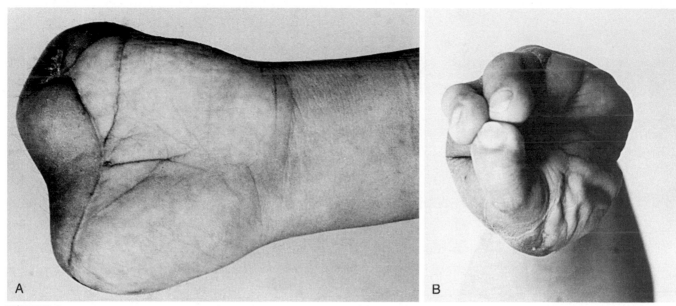

FIGURE 52-6. **A,** Metacarpal hand subtype IIB: amputation of the thumb and all fingers proximal to the MCP joint, with good thenar muscle function. **B,** Tripod pinch after reconstruction of the thumb by trimmed great toe transplantation and reconstruction of the two radial fingers by combined transplantation of the second and third toes from the contralateral foot.

for the selection of donor toes and reconstructive stages. If thenar muscle function is adequate (subtypes IIA and IIB), simultaneous reconstruction of the thumb and two adjacent fingers in one stage is preferable (Fig. 52-6). On the other hand, if thenar muscle function is inadequate (subtype IIC), a staged reconstruction is planned with the fingers reconstructed first and a prosthetic thumb post used temporarily after finger reconstruction to assist in determining the length and position of the transferred toe for thumb reconstruction during the second stage (Fig. 52-7). Even more complex are conditions in which both hands are involved because selection of donor toes should take into account prevention of functional impairment and foot deformity.[107,112]

In bilateral type II metacarpal hand, the dominant hand can be reconstructed with three toes to achieve tripod pinch and the nondominant hand with two toes to provide key or pulp-to-pulp pinch.[52,54] The total five toes can be harvested from the right second and third and the left great, third, and fourth toe sparing the second toe for foot balance. Our experience has revealed good functional recovery of the hands and no significant donor site morbidity in such an approach (Fig. 52-8).

 Anatomy for Toe Dissection

Most surgical procedures involved in partial or total toe(s) transplantation use the arterial pedicle to the great and second toe. Several authors have proposed different classifications of the vascular anatomy in the first metatarsal space.[27,31,48] All of them describe anatomic variations in the origin of the first dorsal metatarsal artery (FDMA) and the relationship between the FDMA and the interosseous

muscle and intermetatarsal ligament. Each of these descriptions has created an image of a complex and highly variable network of vessels in the first-second metatarsal interspace, thus making the vascular anatomy, which is essential in toe harvesting, difficult to understand.

Currently, in most surgical techniques, vascular dissection begins proximally in the dorsum of the foot to identify and follow the course of the dorsalis pedis artery and its continuity as the FDMA.[27,48] In my experience with more than 1200 toe harvests, the FDMA was the dominant artery in approximately 70% of cases, the first plantar metatarsal artery (FPMA) was dominant in 20% of cases, and in the remaining 10% both arteries had the same caliber. In the presence of a plantar-dominant arterial system, dissection of the dorsal aspect in the first metatarsal space need only include one superficial vein and there is no need to deepen the dissection to identify the artery, which might damage the foot and is a waste of time.

It is easier to harvest the great or second toe (or any of the various flaps designed in this anatomic region) by identifying the dominant vascular pattern in the first web space at the beginning of the dissection and proceed with dissection of the artery in a retrograde fashion.[115] Dissection always starts in the dorsal aspect of the first web space, where the junction of the lateral digital artery with the great toe and the medial digital artery with the second toe, which arises from the FDMA, is identified over the intermetatarsal ligament (Fig. 52-9). Further dissection of the pedicle is then carried out 2 to 3 cm from this junction proximally. If a dorsal-dominant system is present, retrograde dissection of the FDMA is facilitated by early ligation of the smaller plantar vessel and the FDMA is isolated proximally. In most cases the artery is superficial to the muscle; however, it may be localized within or deep to the interosseous muscle. If both vessels have a similar caliber, it is preferable to dissect the FDMA because the dissection is much easier and straight-

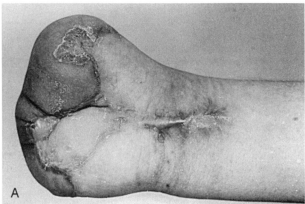

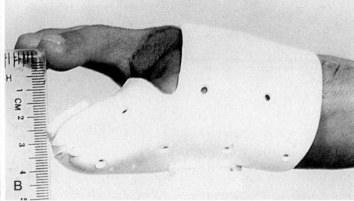

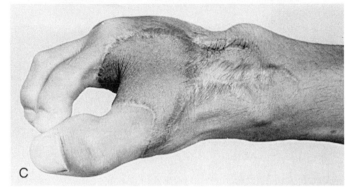

FIGURE 52-7. **A,** Metacarpal hand subtype IIC. **B,** After reconstruction of two adjacent fingers with combined second- and third-toe transplantation, a post is used to enhance pinch function of the transplanted unit and to determine the future position of the toe that will be used for thumb reconstruction. **C,** Eight months after thumb reconstruction by total great toe transplantation, the patient has stable pinch function.

forward.[115] If a plantar-dominant system is noted and the FDMA is either absent or very small, the dissection is continued afterward during the plantar dissection.

The FPMA is usually isolated up to the middle of the metatarsal shaft on the plantar surface. At this point the union between the FPMA and the dorsalis pedis artery is located at the proximal communicating artery (or deep perforator) (Fig. 52-10). If a longer arterial pedicle is required, dissection of the communicating branch in continuity with the dorsalis pedis artery may be too tedious and destructive to the foot. Thus it is advisable to divide the FPMA and use a vein graft for the vascular anastomosis.

Retrograde dissection has proven to be particularly helpful in partial toe transplantation for distal digit reconstruction when only a short pedicle is needed. If this approach is used, proximal dissection of the vascular pedicle is not necessary. Moreover, routine preoperative angiography of the donor foot is not required when this approach is used to harvest any toe or flap based on the arterial system of the first metatarsal space.[115]

SURGICAL TECHNIQUES

Total or Trimmed Transplantation of the Great Toe

Indications
Total transfer of the great toe is selected for thumb reconstruction when the amputation level is at either the proximal phalanx or metacarpal level. It aims to provide a new thumb with a better range of motion and a broader pulp surface for a more powerful pinch. However, it is often too large to

simulate the normal thumb on the opposite side. The great-toe wraparound technique was developed by Morrison[64] using the great toenail, skin envelope, and a conventional bone graft to circumvent the size problem. Although it yields a nice-looking thumb, it does not provide a mobile IP joint. Trimmed transplantation of the great toe[94,95,110] combines the advantages of total transfer and the great-toe wraparound techniques. It is indicated when there is an unacceptable size difference between the thumb on the normal opposite side and the great toe to be harvested, especially when a mobile IP joint is desirable.

Author's Preferred Methods of Treatment: Flap Design and Elevation In Trimmed Transplantation of the Great Toe

The great toe usually looks stouter than the thumb with wider transverse and anteroposterior diameters. The discrepancy involves bony as well as soft tissue elements (Fig. 52-11A). To assess the size discrepancy between the great toe and the normal thumb, the circumference in the great toe and the normal thumb is measured at three points: (1) the nail eponychium, (2) the widest point (corresponding to the IP joint), and (3) the middle of the proximal phalanx. The thumb measurements are transposed to their corre-

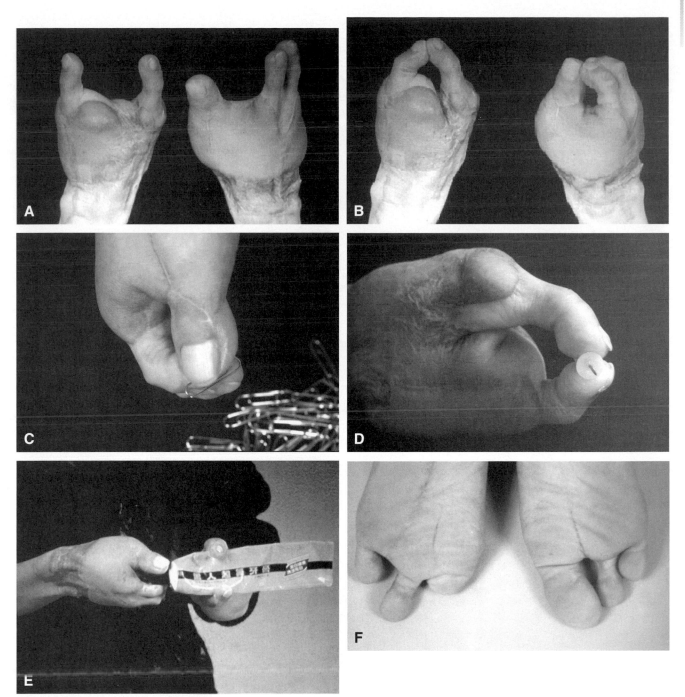

FIGURE 52-8. **A** to **E,** Bilateral metacarpal hand type IIB reconstructed with a total of five toe transplantations to provide tripod pinch for the right dominant hand and pulp-to-pulp pinch for the left nondominant hand. **F,** Both donor feet have no callus formations, which is evidence of good maintenance of the original weight-bearing areas.

sponding points on the great toe. An additional 2 to 3 mm is added to each measurement to allow direct closure without tension. The residual medial skin strip usually measures 0.5 to 0.8 cm in width, which represents the difference between the toe and the thumb circumferences. This should be tapered to a point around the tip of the toe, leaving 2 mm of nail fold to facilitate skin closure. The proximal skin incision is determined by the level of thumb amputation and is usually marked in a circular or "V" shape (see Fig. 52-11B). Although it is possible to trim the nail together

with the underlying nail bed, this is not recommended because the nail fold may become deformed.

The procedure starts with identification of one sizeable vein and the dominant arterial supply in the first web space. The vascular pedicle is dissected in a retrograde fashion to the desired length and diameter. Branches of the deep peroneal nerves are preserved. The extensor tendon is then dissected on the dorsal side, and the neurovascular bundle and the flexor tendon are isolated on the plantar side. Care is taken to place the incision on the plantar aspect lateral to

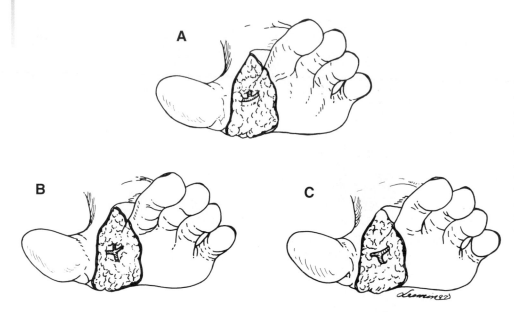

FIGURE 52-9. Retrograde dissection of the first web space in the foot. **A,** In approximately 70% of dissections, the first dorsal metatarsal artery (FDMA) is the largest vessel (dominant) and gives origin to the dorsal proper digital arteries to the great toe and the second toe. **B,** In 10% of cases, the FDMA and the first plantar metatarsal artery (FPMA) have the same caliber. **C,** In 20% of cases the FPMA is the dominant vessel (see the text).

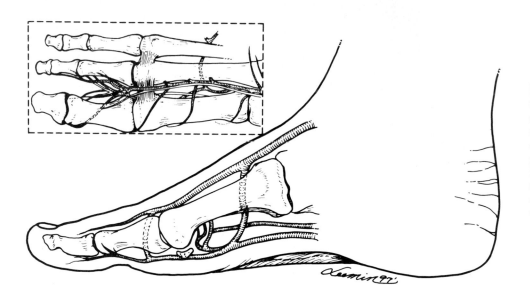

FIGURE 52-10. Anatomic relationships between the first dorsal metatarsal artery over the intermetatarsal ligament and the first plantar metatarsal artery. Communicating branches are present in the web space distally and in the base between the first and second metatarsal bones (also known as the deep perforator or proximal communicating artery).

the head of first metatarsal, to prevent a scar over the weight-bearing area.

Next, the medial skin strip is incised and elevated from distal to proximal. The incision is deepened to the periosteum at the tip of the distal phalanx (see Fig. 52-11C) but remains superficial to the medial collateral ligament on the medial surface of the IP joint. The second incision is then made all the way through the periosteum. The collateral ligament, joint capsule, and periosteum are elevated as a single, thick, and strong composite soft tissue envelope, which my colleagues and I designate a peri-joint flap. This subperiosteal (peri-joint flap) elevation is continued along the hemi circumference, to the middle of the plantar surfaces of both the proximal and distal phalanx (see Fig. 52-11D). A longitudinal osteotomy (see Fig. 52-11E) is then performed with an oscillating saw, while carefully protecting the neurovascular bundle. This removes a 4- to 6-mm width

of the medial joint prominence along with a 2- to 4-mm width of the phalangeal shafts. A smooth contour of the osteotomy edges is obtained using a high-speed bur. The hemi-circumferential composite joint flap is redraped and the redundant portion is trimmed followed by repair under proper tension with interrupted sutures using nonabsorbable material. The repair should be tight enough to maintain joint stability (see Fig. 52-11F). The medial skin incision is also approximated with interrupted sutures (see Fig. 52-11G). Care should be taken to prevent injury to the nail bed or matrix, because this can result in a deformed nail. Finally, the proximal phalanx is osteotomized, preserving at least 1.0 cm of the base of the proximal phalanx and leaving the great toe attached only by its vascular pedicle. After removal of the tourniquet, the transplant is allowed to perfuse for at least 20 minutes before proceeding to transplantation (see Fig. 52-11H). The donor site is closed primarily. The

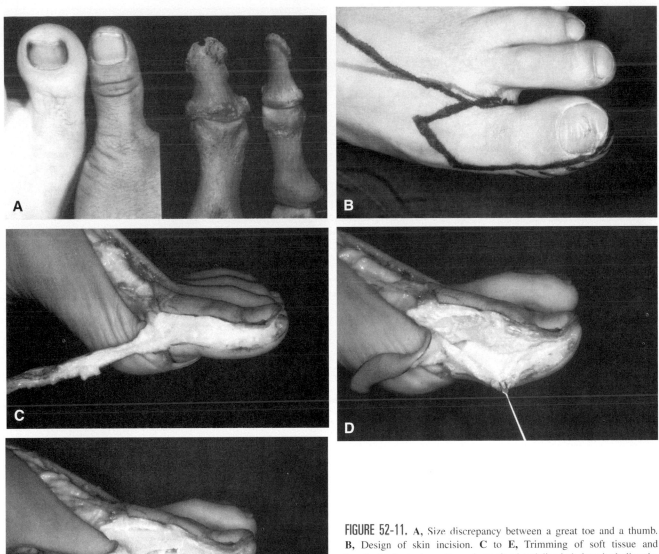

FIGURE 52-11. **A,** Size discrepancy between a great toe and a thumb. **B,** Design of skin incision. **C** to **E,** Trimming of soft tissue and longitudinal osteotomy through proximal and distal phalanx including the IP joint. *Continued*

osteotomy edges are smoothed and the remaining proximal portion of the medial skin flap of the great toe can be utilized to assist tension-free closure, if required.

The amputated stump is prepared through a cross incision creating four flaps (see Fig. 52-11I). These flaps are mobilized to prepare the bone, extensor and flexor tendons, and digital nerves. These flaps also allow smooth closure of skin between the recipient site and transplanted toe for a better appearance of the reconstructed thumb. The recipient artery can either be the common digital artery (our first choice), the princeps pollicis artery, or the radial artery in the anatomical snuff box. The bone, extensor and flexor tendons, recipient artery, vein, and nerves are prepared at the recipient site in the usual manner.

The flap insetting and repair of tendons and neurovascular bundles are as performed as described in other sections of this text. In closing the wound defect, skeletal length preservation and good skin coverage are important. In transplantation of the great toe it is advisable to preserve at least 1.0 cm of the proximal phalanx to maintain foot span for better appearance and to preserve push-off function of the donor foot. Skin grafting of the donor site should be avoided. With adequate planning there should rarely be any problem in tension-free closure of the wound in the foot. No drains are required in the donor site.

Partial or Total Transplantation of the Second Toe

Indications

Although selection of the second toe for thumb reconstruction may be controversial,[3,28,44,95] use of the second toe

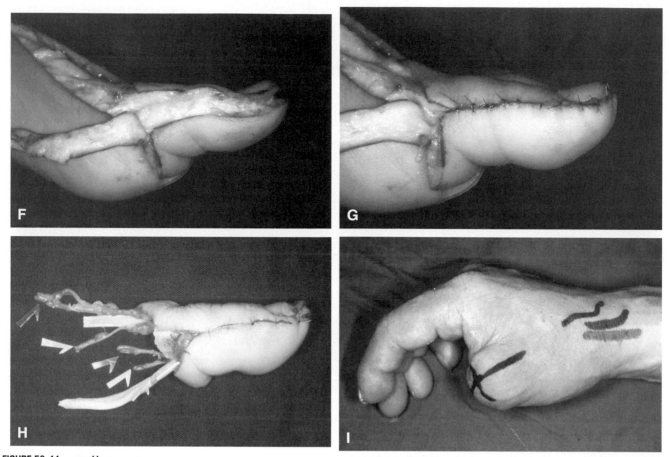

FIGURE 52-11—cont'd. **F** and **G,** Tight closure of the peri-joint flap and skin. **H,** Harvested trimmed great toe. **I,** Preparation of amputation stump through a cross incision creating four flaps.

Continued

in finger reconstruction is well accepted. Partial transplantation of the second toe is used for digit amputations distal to the insertion of the superficial flexor tendon (Fig. 52-12),[19,100,108] whereas total transplantation is used for the reconstruction of more proximal finger amputations (Fig. 52-13).[4,23,40,75]

Flap Design and Elevation

Most surgical techniques designed to harvest the second toe use a combined dorsal and plantar approach.[3,4,28,44,55,75,79] Foucher and Norris[24] suggested harvesting of the second toe alone from a dorsal approach to avoid incision and dissection of the fibrofatty tissue in the plantar surface and allow faster recovery and early walking. In addition, the blood supply to the second toe is theoretically improved because the first and second dorsal metatarsal arteries and the plantar arteries are included in a vascular network. Access to the plantar structures from the dorsal approach is facilitated by removing the second metatarsal bone. For less experienced surgeons, this technique can be more difficult and entail excessive manipulation of the vessels, which might increase the risk of pedicle injury and postoperative vascular complications. Furthermore, resection of the second metatarsal is not necessary in many cases and the plantar skin flap usually included in the transferred toe is often needed to provide glabrous skin on the volar aspect and cover the pedicle in the recipient hand.

Author's Preferred Method of Treatment: Flap Design and Elevation

The length of the second toe to be harvested is determined before surgery and depends on the level of finger amputation and radiographic findings. Two microsurgical teams always work simultaneously to reduce surgical time and intraoperatively assess the exact length of the tendons, nerves, and vascular pedicle in the toe before dividing them. The dorsal and plantar skin flaps are designed in a "V" shape to ensure primary wound closure without tension. The vertex of the "V"-shaped skin incision is marked 5 to 10 mm proximal to the osteotomy site on the dorsal and plantar aspects of the toe, and the two divergent points of the "V" flap are marked at the midpoint of the first and second web space. The incision is extended proximally in a lazy-"S" course for exposure of the vessels and nerves. On the plantar surface this incision is always designed in a vertical direction and the weight-bearing surface avoided.

The skin in the dorsal flap is incised and elevated superficially to protect the dorsal veins. Only one sizable vein, usually in the first metatarsal space, is selected and dissected proximally. The dissection continues distally in the first web space, where the dominant arterial pattern is identified and dissected in a retrograde direction (see Anatomy). All fatty

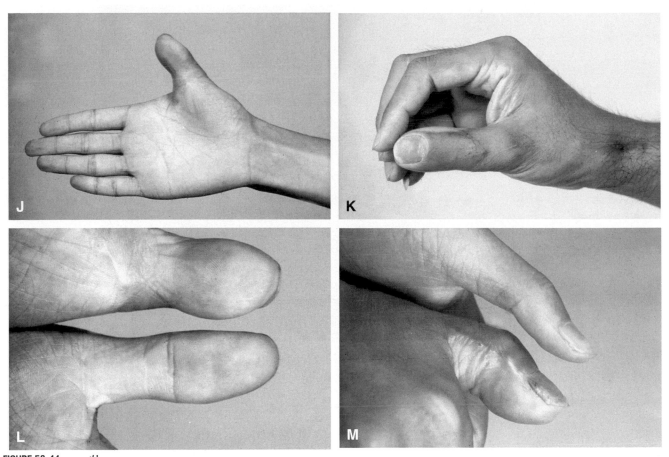

FIGURE 52-11—cont'd. **J** to **M,** Appearance and function of a clinical case. Note preservation of 30 degrees of active range of motion in the trimmed IP joint.

tissue is carefully removed from the nerves and vessels, and the transmetatarsal ligament is then divided. In a dorsal-dominant arterial system, the FDMA is dissected proximally until adequate length is obtained. If a plantar-dominant system is present, dissection on the dorsal surface is necessary only for the vein and the FPMA is isolated afterward. All small veins and arteries in the second metatarsal space are divided. Branches of the superficial peroneal nerve in the first and second metatarsal space are dissected and used together with the proper digital nerves only when sensory recipient nerves are available; otherwise, only the digital nerves are used for sensory recovery of the transplanted toe. The extensor retinaculum is opened and the extensor digitorum longus and brevis tendons are isolated and followed distally.

The skin flap on the plantar aspect is raised to the base of the proximal phalanx with only 2 to 3 mm of subcutaneous tissue left attached to the dermis. All fibrofatty tissue between the plantar skin and neurovascular bundles is discarded to minimize anteroposterior bulkiness and maximize joint motion in the reconstructed finger. The proper digital nerves are identified distally in the web space, close to the proper digital plantar arteries on the medial and lateral aspects. Both plantar nerves are dissected proximally up to their union with the respective common digital nerves, which also contains the proper digital nerves to the great and third toe. When a long proper digital nerve is required, these two nerves are dissected along their course before dividing them. Next, the flexor tendon sheath is approached and vertically opened to expose the short and long flexor tendons.

To facilitate tailoring and insetting of the toe it is advisable to extend the dissection for several millimeters distal to the osteotomy site. This allows skeletonization of the artery and nerves and removal of all fibrofatty tissue, especially that between the skin and the flexor tendon in the plantar aspect.[97] These refinements are more meaningful in partial transplantation of the second toe, which is associated with a higher incidence of vasospasm. Often the vessels need to be tunneled under the skin proximally, and fixation of the partial toe transfer is critical for a good cosmetic and functional result.[19]

Once all the anatomic structures have been isolated and the required length has been determined, the nerves are divided and marked with 6-0 nylon. The flexor tendons are pulled out and cut. In total transplantation of the second toe, the proximal phalanx is cut at the proper level or the metatarsophalangeal joint may be disarticulated and the proximal phalanx shortened to the length needed in the reconstructed finger (see Fig. 52-13). In partial transplantation, the veins, nerves, and tendons are dissected distal to the PIP joint and the middle phalanx is osteotomized in a dorsal-to-plantar direction; otherwise, the distal toe is disarticulated at the PIP joint (see Fig. 52-12). The tourniquet is then released and the toe allowed to reperfuse for at least 20 minutes before dividing the main artery and vein.

The donor site in the foot should be closed primarily without tension. It is not necessary to repair the intermetatarsal ligament, and no drains are used. In unusual cases in which primary closure is difficult, metatarsopha-

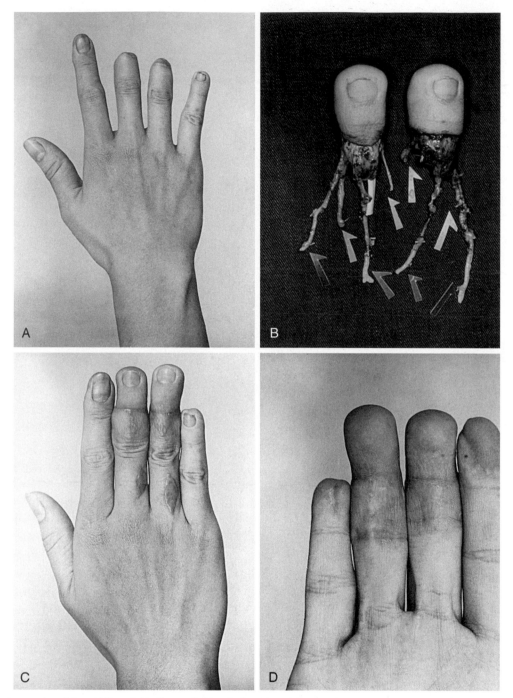

FIGURE 52-12. **A,** Amputation of the middle and ring fingers distal to the insertion of the superficialis flexor tendon. **B,** Bilateral second toes harvested with an osteotomy at the middle of the middle phalanx level. **C** and **D,** Result 3 months after reconstruction.

langeal joint disarticulation or transverse metatarsal amputation is performed. Skin grafting of the donor site should be avoided to prevent foot morbidity and deformity.

Wraparound Flap of the Second Toe

Indications

Despite the fact that great toe wraparound was initially described for thumb reconstruction,[64] this flap can also be used for other injured fingers.[51] Wraparound flaps may be elevated from a lesser toe as well. My colleagues and I

advocated the second-toe wraparound flap for finger reconstruction because the size usually matches the distal digit better, especially the toenail.[98] However, it may also be used for thumb reconstruction (although the nail size may be different), particularly in patients who do not accept or cannot tolerate partial loss of the great toe.

The second-toe wraparound flap is indicated for the reconstruction of a circumferential or dorsal hemi-circumferential loss of skin and nail that is localized distal to the proximal portion of the middle phalanx, with intact skeleton, tendons, and PIP joint (Fig. 52-14).[98] No tendons

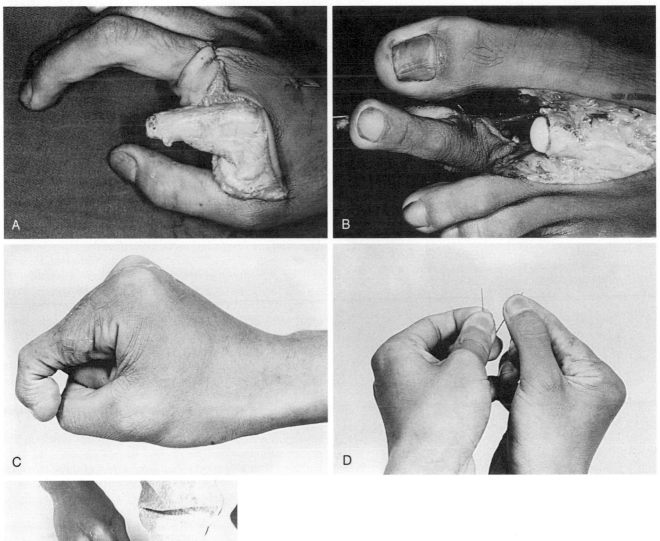

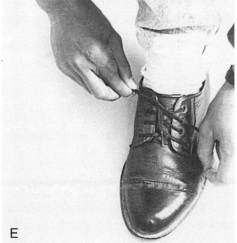

FIGURE 52-13. A, Proximal amputation of the index finger after recipient site preparation. **B,** Disarticulation of the second toe at the PIP joint in preparation for repair with the corresponding joint capsule and ligaments in the recipient finger (composite joint reconstruction). **C,** Ten months after surgery, active range of motion of the PIP joint was 68 degrees. **D and E,** The patient is able to use his finger for daily manual activities and fine manipulation.

are harvested with the second-toe wraparound flap, but the distal phalanx is always included to prevent swiveling, instability, and bone resorption of the reconstructed finger.

Flap Design

The second-toe wraparound flap can be designed on either foot, depending on the nail configuration, size of the defect, previous surgery or injury to the foot, and the patient's preference. The design of the incisions in the hand and foot should avoid scars on the radial aspect of the index and middle fingers or on the ulnar aspect of the thumb,

ring, and little fingers. Proximally, the dorsal and plantar skin incisions are usually outlined in a circular or "V" shape.

The same guidelines described for harvest of the second toe are used to dissect the wraparound flap but with skeletonization of the neurovascular bundle emphasized. The distal phalanx of the second toe is always included and the tendons are cut close to their insertion. The remaining portion of the toe is always disarticulated at the metatarsophalangeal joint to close the wound and provide an aesthetic appearance.

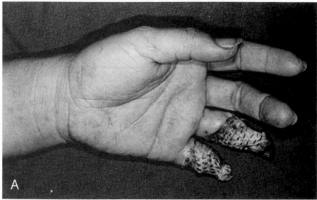

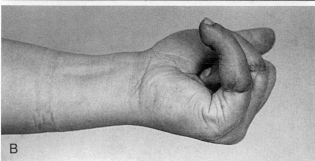

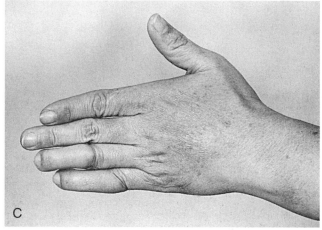

FIGURE 52-14. A, After an avulsion injury of the ring and little finger, circumferential loss of skin and nail with an intact skeleton, tendons, and PIP joint is noted. **B** and **C,** Result 6 months after reconstruction with bilateral second-toe wraparound flaps.

Pulp and Hemipulp Flaps

Indications

Pulp or hemipulp neurosensory free flaps from the great toe or second toe are indicated for large finger pulp defects that cannot be covered with local or regional flaps (Fig. 52-15) or when the use of these flaps may create unacceptable donor site morbidity or restrict global function of an already compromised hand. Although local flaps have many indications for repairing pulp defects, under certain circumstances they may be inconvenient because of limited mobility, size, position, and time of immobilization. In addition, the anatomic features of the toe pulp cannot be imitated by other tissue; specialized skin with rich sensory innervation is unique to the fingers and palm, and, ideally, any defect in these surfaces should be repaired with "like tissue."[5,16,22,37,40,50,72,123]

Pulp flaps are also indicated when sensory recovery is essential for proper hand function and protection. Although pulp free flaps are best indicated for thumb reconstruction, they are also useful for other finger defects in patients with special jobs or hobbies that require critical sensation in all fingers (e.g., an artist or musician).

In cases in which regenerating axons are too far from the injured surface or local sensory neurotization cannot be reliably expected, pulp flaps are an excellent alternative. In addition, they may be used to replace skin grafts or local flaps previously used for pulp reconstruction that result in an unstable or painful scar.[108,123]

Flap Design and Elevation

The great toe is selected more often than the second toe as a donor source of pulp flaps because of the following reasons: (1) the great toe has better superficial sensation than the second toe (two-point discrimination, 7 to 18 mm vs. 10 to 25 mm),[5] (2) more donor tissue can be obtained from the great toe, and (3) it is possible to directly close the donor defect, thus enhancing faster recovery and causing less morbidity.

The flap may be designed on the lateral aspect of the pulp in the great toe or the medial hemipulp in the second toe and be extended to the first web space proximally, depending on the size of the defect in the recipient finger. The deep peroneal nerve supplies these surfaces, and its sensory innervation overlaps with that of the corresponding proper digital nerves; hence, two nerves always need to be included with a hemipulp flap from either of these two toes. The skin incisions are outlined according to a template of the recipient site defect or a drawing of the finger defect on the surgeon's corresponding finger to compare with the patient's toe. Outlining of the incision for dissection of the pedicle follows the course of the proper digital artery to the great or second toe in continuity with the first dorsal and plantar metatarsal arteries in the first web space.

During elevation of the flap, special care should be taken to dissect all superficial veins on the lateral and dorsal surface of the great toe in continuity with one sizable vein. Next, the dominant artery to the great and second toes is localized in the first web space and dissected in a retrograde fashion. All small arterial branches must be skeletonized with the subcutaneous tissue removed and the adventitia layer stripped off (see Fig. 52-15B) to facilitate passage of the vessels in the subcutaneous tissue during insetting of the flap.

When primary closure of the defect is not possible, a split-thickness skin graft (usually from the instep area) is required to close the donor site defect. Because delayed healing in the toe can prolong foot recovery and walking, skin grafting of the donor site should be performed with the utmost care.

First-Web Neurosensory Flap

Indications

The first web space in the foot provides glabrous skin thinner than that of the second or great toe pulp. Its rich sensory innervation makes this flap a good option for resurfacing bigger soft tissue defects in one finger (Fig.

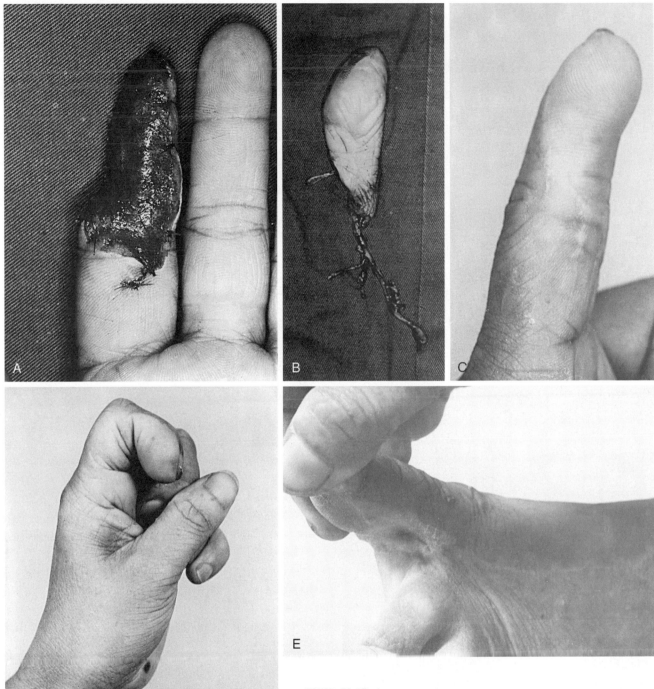

FIGURE 52-15. **A,** Avulsion injury of the index finger involving skin and subcutaneous tissue in the palmar aspect. **B,** Hemipulp free flap from the great toe. **C** and **D,** Final result showing full flexion and extension of the reconstructed finger. **E,** Donor site appearance after primary closure.

52-16) or even in the palm with minimal subcutaneous tissue.[6,21,33,37,43,57,61,78] A flap extending to the tip of the great and second toe can be as wide as 7.3 cm and as long as 14 cm (Fig. 52-17).[78] Adjacent fingers with contiguous defects in the pulp or in the proximal ventral aspect may be reconstructed with one first-web neurosensory flap and a temporary syndactyly, which is divided later.[123]

The first web receives its blood supply from the distal communicating artery that connects the first dorsal and plantar metatarsal arteries. If the design of the flap includes an extension to the lateral aspect of the great toe and/or the medial aspect of the second toe, the respective digital arteries should be included in the pedicle dissection. Innervation of the dorsal aspect is mainly provided by the

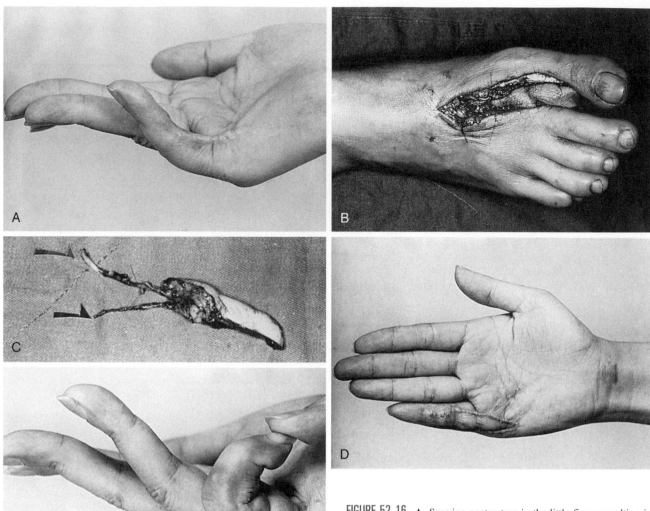

FIGURE 52-16. **A,** Scarring contracture in the little finger resulting in extension limitation and painful flexion. **B** and **C,** Neurosensory free flap from the first web space. **D** and **E,** Although only 3 months has elapsed since reconstruction, full finger extension and flexion are observed.

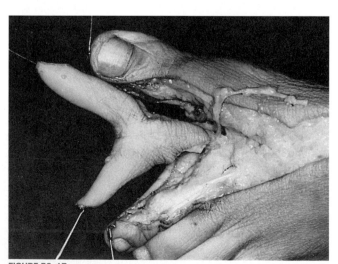

FIGURE 52-17. A large neurosensory skin flap harvested from the first web space can include the lateral aspect of the great toe and the medial aspect of the second toe.

deep peroneal nerve and to a lesser extent by the superficial peroneal nerves. However, when a wider flap with extension to the hemipulp of the great or second toe is designed, the respective common digital nerves in the plantar aspect should be included as well.

Flap Design and Elevation

The flap is outlined according to the size of the defect in the hand. The posterior border of the flap is incised first and the incision extended in a lazy-"S" fashion over the dorsal surface between the first and second metatarsals to the level of the metatarsal head. After isolating one sizable vein draining the flap, the artery is dissected distally over the intermetatarsal ligament. When the FDMA is dominant, retrograde dissection of this artery in continuity with the dorsalis pedis artery is straightforward. The deep peroneal nerve lies beside the artery along its course, under the extensor retinaculum proximally. The rest of the island flap is readily dissected. If the FDMA is very small or absent, elevation of the island flap starts on the plantar aspect of the web space, where the FPMA is localized. From this point the artery is dissected in retrograde fashion until the desired length is obtained, or if the vessel is too short a vein graft can be used for the vascular anastomosis.[115] There is no need to abandon the procedure if the FDMA is not present, as has been proposed.[55] A split-thickness skin graft is used to close the donor site and sutured in place with a tie-over dressing.

Vascularized Nail Graft

Indications

Microvascular nail transplantation is performed to ensure adequate blood inflow to the nail bed.[42,63,77] In contrast to nonvascularized nail grafts, these usually "take" better and provide adequate function and superior aesthetic appearance.[78,126] Vascularized nail grafts may be used for fingertip injuries involving the nail bed or for nail reconstruction after tumor excision. They are also a good option for replacement of nail deformities that are painful or aesthetically unacceptable to the patient (e.g., post-traumatic hook nail deformity). In most instances there is damage or loss of adjacent tissue such as the eponychial fold, pulp, and skeleton (Fig. 52-18).

Technically, it is easier to transfer the whole second or third toe distal to the middle of the middle phalanx instead of trying to use nail segments with small flaps and possibly compromising venous outflow.[41] Whenever a larger amount of soft tissue is included with the transplanted toenail, a variable amount of normal tissue might need to be removed in the recipient finger for proper insetting.[19]

Flap Design and Elevation

The great toe usually matches the thumbnail better and may be trimmed to fit fingernails as well. Still, it is not used frequently because of the secondary deformity created in the donor foot. Although the second toenail is somewhat smaller than a fingernail and has a squared shape, it looks similar to the finger counterparts and the resultant donor defect in the foot is minor.[77] The design of the dorsal skin flap that is included with the toenail should incorporate the small veins on the dorsal surface of the toe. Usually the dorsal skin flap extends from the eponychial fold up to the IP joint in the great toe and to the PIP joint in the second toe. The entire width of the nail, including both lateral eponychial folds, is harvested. The size of the pulp tissue to be harvested is determined by the size of the defect in the finger pulp. However, for inclusion of the dorsal proper digital artery, more than half of the pulp on the medial side of the second toe (or the lateral side of the great toe) must be harvested together with the vascularized nail graft. If all of the distal segment of the finger needs reconstruction, a second-toe wraparound flap is a better option (see earlier). The proper digital nerve is included to restore nail sensation and function.

Dissection of the artery is similar to the technique described previously under Anatomy. It is important to emphasize that the small veins on the dorsal surface of the distal toe should be carefully dissected in continuity with one sizable vein tributary of the saphenous venous system to ensure dependable venous return.

After raising the dorsal flap, the extensor tendons are exposed and divided close to their insertion. Next, the nail is harvested together with all of the distal half of the distal

phalanx by doing a transverse osteotomy in the great toe (Fig. 52-19) or including the entire distal phalanx after distal IP joint disarticulation in the second toe (author's preferred method). In either of these two instances, the periosteum should be left attached to the nail and the skeleton exposed after reflecting the pulp flap from the distal phalanx on the plantar surface. Before doing the osteotomy, the artery, vein, and nerves in the pedicle should be protected from potential injury.

Morrison described technical modifications in which the width of the great toenail is decreased by trimming the lateral edges of the nail matrix.[63] In the great toe, the donor site defect may be closed with a cross-toe skin flap, which is divided 2 weeks later. In second- or third-toe vascularized nail grafts, proximal metatarsophalangeal disarticulation is favored because of the possibility of direct closure and better appearance of the donor site. Nevertheless, if the patient's desire is to preserve the remaining toe, cross-toe skin flaps from the adjacent toe may be used to close the defect. Whenever a cross-toe flap is planned, the risk of complications and potential morbidity should be remembered.

Transplantation of the Third Toe

Indications

Single transplantation of the third toe to the hand is indicated when (1) the second toe is not available or is not suitable for transfer because of previous injury, surgery, or deformity; (2) the second toe is on the same foot from which the great toe was removed (usually for thumb reconstruction in bilateral metacarpal hands) and the second toe is therefore spared for gait; and (3) the third toe provides a better size match for finger reconstruction than the second toe does.[117]

Author's Preferred Method of Treatment: Flap Design and Elevation

Preoperative planning and the operative technique are similar to that for transplantation of the second toe and need not be repeated. The third toe receives its blood supply from the second and third dorsal metatarsal arteries and the second and third plantar metatarsal arteries. Because the majority of patients undergoing transplantation of the third toe have already had or will undergo transplantation of the great or second toe, the second metatarsal pedicle is either not available or must be preserved for subsequent transfer of the great or second toe. Therefore transfer of the third toe is usually based on the third common plantar digital artery (Fig. 52-20).[117] Although this artery might be smaller, it is usually bigger than the second or third dorsal metatarsal arteries. It is simpler and quicker to proceed directly to dissection of the plantar vascular pedicle and, if necessary, to use a vein graft for the vascular anastomosis. In most cases, however, the pedicle is long enough to reach the proper digital artery in the proximal phalanx. The donor site is closed in the same way as described for the second toe.

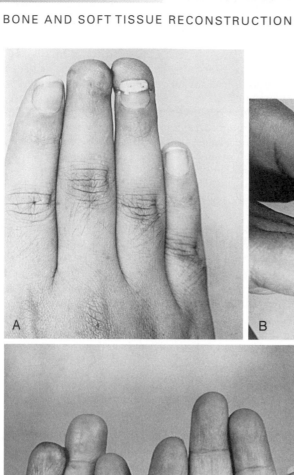

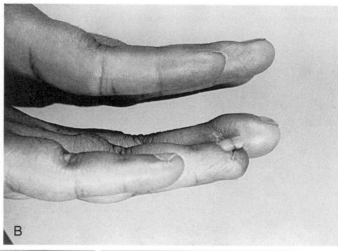

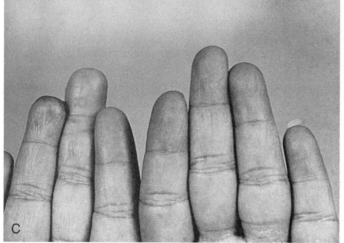

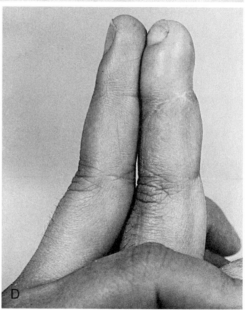

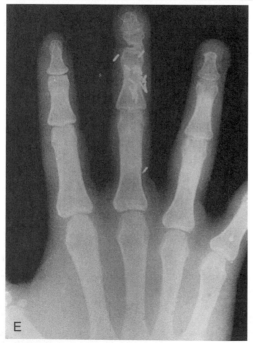

FIGURE 52-18. A, Middle and ring fingertip amputation covered with a pedicled flap. The patient's major complaint was anesthesia and nail absence in the middle finger. **B** to **D,** Result after nail reconstruction of the middle finger with a partial second-toe transplantation, including the whole of the distal phalanx. Comparative views with the other intact digits are presented. **E,** Radiograph showing fixation in the middle phalanx with intraosseous wiring.

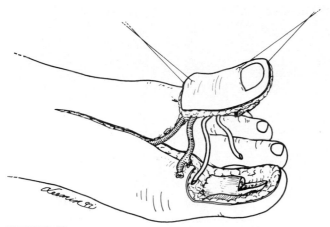

FIGURE 52-19. Vascularized nail transfer from the great toe. The nail bed is harvested through a transverse osteotomy in the distal phalanx.

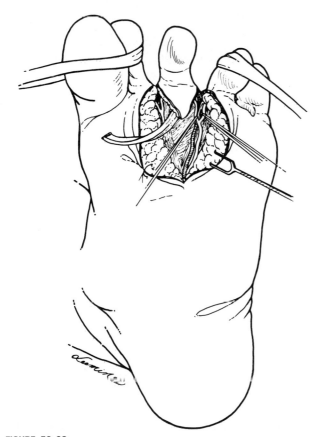

FIGURE 52-20. Dissection of the third toe depicting the third common plantar digital artery and nerve in the plantar surface.

Combined Transplantation of the Second and Third Toes

Indications

Combined transplantation of the second and third toes is indicated for reconstruction of two adjacent fingers after traumatic amputation proximal to the digital webs.[86,102] With this approach, tripod pinch function, hook grip capability, and greater lateral stability are provided.[87,96,99,101,102] When indicated, additional advantages of combined transplantation of the second and third toes over bilateral transplan-

tation of both second toes include the following: (1) only a single set of recipient vessels is required, which might otherwise be difficult to locate in severely injured hands when two different toes are used; (2) less operative time is required; and (3) potential morbidity in the donor site is limited to one foot only, thus allowing earlier postoperative ambulation.

Nevertheless, because of its length limitation, it cannot be expected that a combined transplant accurately simulates the functional capabilities of full-length fingers, particularly in point pinch and arch of grasp (Fig. 52-21). Optimal function is attained when the reconstructed fingers and the remaining fingers are of relatively uniform length, with the distal tip of the normal little finger used as a guide.[102] If the remaining digits extend beyond this point, the tandem transplantation of the second and third toes will be shorter and contribute less to smooth prehension.

The level of digit amputation is used to determine the osteotomy level of the second and third toes. If 5 to 6 mm of length is present in the proximal phalanx of the fingers, the toe osteotomy will also be at the proximal phalanx. The toes are harvested through metatarsophalangeal joint disarticulation (see Fig. 52-21C), and the bases of the proximal phalanges are shortened during toe insetting and the periosteum elevated to the osteotomy level. During subperiosteal dissection and osteotomy of the phalanx, all anatomic structures in the toe must be protected from injury and excessive manipulation of the neurovascular pedicle should be avoided. Active range of motion in the MCP joint of the reconstructed fingers will be similar to that observed in intact MCP joints.[102]

If the cartilage surface in the metacarpal heads and the joint capsule and ligaments are intact, the tandem toes are transplanted together with the respective metatarsophalangeal joint capsule and ligaments for composite joint repair in the hand. In this case, active range of motion of 52 degrees (range, 30 to 80 degrees) can be expected.[80] In addition, when the toes are disarticulated at the metatarsophalangeal joint, the metatarsal heads and metatarsal arch are preserved in the donor foot, which is important for an even weight-bearing surface and prevention of a "scissors deformity" in the donor foot.[102]

In a more proximal transmetacarpal amputation, both toes can be harvested with a transmetatarsal osteotomy. Previously it was suggested that the bony arch be reconstructed with a nonvascularized bone graft after transmetatarsal amputation of both toes.[102] However, this approach is no longer recommended, because no functional difference was revealed in a recent biomechanical gait analysis and from my clinical observations when no bone grafts are used to reconstruct the metatarsal defect.

Author's Preferred Method of Treatment: Flap Design and Elevation

Formerly, radial digital amputations were reconstructed by using combined transplantation of the second and third toes from the contralateral foot, whereas the ipsilateral toes were

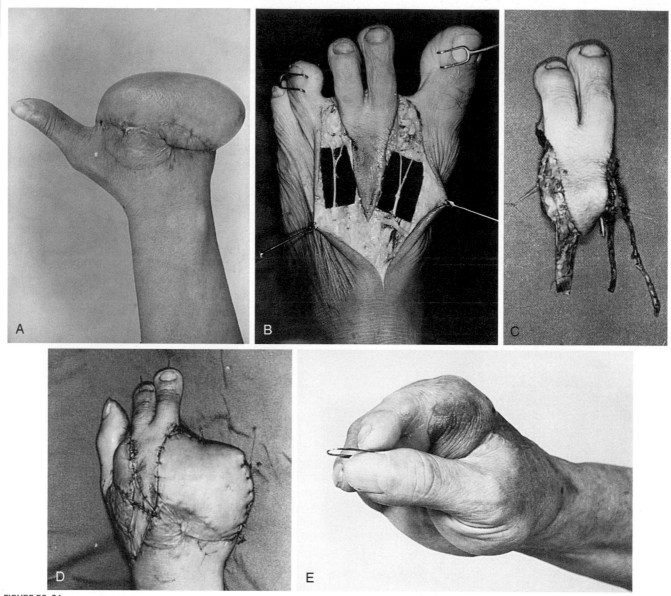

FIGURE 52-21. A, Metacarpal hand subtype IB. **B,** Dissection of branches of the superficial peroneal nerve in the first and third metatarsal spaces. The width of the "V"-shaped dorsal skin flap should not extend beyond the midpoint in the first web and the third web. **C,** Tandem second and third toes disarticulated in the metatarsophalangeal joint. **D,** Immediate result after inset of the transplanted unit for reconstruction of the radial fingers. **E,** Fourteen months after reconstruction, tripod pinch is adequate.

used for the reconstruction of ulnar digital amputations, with the aim of placing the longer second toe in a more acceptable central position.[87,102] Nowadays, when only one second and third toe combination is needed, I always harvest the tandem toes from the left foot because more demand is made of the right foot in daily ambulatory activities. The right foot is selected only when the left foot is not suitable, for example, if the great toe from the same foot has been or shall be used for thumb reconstruction in multiple toe transplantation cases (see Fig. 52-7). Skeletal length in the digits can be adjusted by the level of osteotomy in the proximal phalanges or metacarpals and the toe phalanges or metatarsals.

Skin flaps with a "V" shape are outlined on the dorsal and plantar aspects of the second and third toes. The skin incisions should not extend beyond the midpoint of the first

and third web space in the foot (see Fig. 52-21B). By including narrow skin flaps with the toes it is always possible to close the donor site directly without tension.

Dissection of the flap starts on the dorsal aspect of the foot, with isolation of one donor vein going to the saphenous venous system connecting all draining small veins from the second and third toes. Then the first web space is dissected to identify the dominant vascular pattern to the second toe (see Anatomy). The branches of the superficial peroneal nerve to the second and third toes are dissected free (see Fig. 52-21B). After isolating the vessels and nerves on the dorsal surface, the extensor tendons to the second and third toes are raised and cut. To preserve the vessels communicating between these two toes, it is advisable to avoid excessive manipulation of the soft tissue connections in the second web space, especially when the bone is dissected distal to the metatarsophalangeal joint. Next, the plantar skin flap is raised to the base of the proximal phalanx in both toes, and all fibrofatty tissue under the skin and over the plantar neurovascular bundles is carefully removed. The following three nerves are identified on this surface and included in the surgical unit: (1) the proper digital nerve to the second toe, which is found in the medial aspect of the second toe; (2) the second common digital nerve to the second and third toes, which is located between the two toes; and (3) the proper digital nerve to the third toe, which is in the lateral aspect of the third toe.

Recently my colleagues and I assessed the arterial blood supply in 57 combined transplantations of the second and third toes in 54 consecutive cases.[13] Re-exploration secondary to arterial insufficiency (vasospasm or thrombosis) was required in almost 20% of cases after revascularization using the dominant artery. Our current tendency is therefore to also preserve the second and third common plantar digital arteries and use one of these two vessels for a second arterial anastomosis, especially when arterial perfusion to the third toe is uncertain.

The osteotomy site is exposed in both toes, and all anatomic structures except the main vascular pedicle are divided and dissected a few millimeters distal to the osteotomies. The two phalanges are cut or disarticulated and the tandem toes are allowed to reperfuse for at least 20 minutes before being transplanted. The incisions should always be closed without tension. Skin grafting on the donor site is unacceptable and can lead to severe complications in the foot.

Other Toe Transplantations

Combined transplantation of the third and fourth toes or even triple toe transplantation from the same foot[11] can be used for severe multiple finger amputations, for example, in bilateral metacarpal hands and in patients who are highly motivated or have special jobs. Although the foot deformity may be very conspicuous, no significant functional limitation is usually observed when these combined toes are properly removed.

Recipient Site Preparation

A surgical approach with one team preparing the recipient site and another harvesting the toe provides several advantages: (1) the proper length of all anatomic structures usually included in any flap from the foot is verified before being divided, (2) there is no need for extensive dissection of the foot and hence less morbidity in the donor site may be anticipated, and (3) operative and anesthetic times are considerably reduced, which is reflected in less fatigue for the patient and surgeons. Routinely, the recipient site is prepared under a bloodless field with conventional tourniquet control and the dissection is performed with the aid of loupe magnification.

Skin Incisions
The amputation stump is always cross-incised to create four skin flaps for exposure of the bone, tendons, and distal nerves. The skin flaps are sufficiently undermined and the redundant fatty tissue is properly trimmed off to obtain thin skin flaps with wide mobility over the stump skeleton (see Fig. 52-13A). Flexibility in mobilizing the skin flaps off the underlying structures is very important for shaping the flaps to fit smoothly with the triangular skin flaps of the toe during insetting.[97] The recipient artery may be identified by (1) using a separate incision on the ulnar side of the proximal phalanx or distal palm, especially in distal finger reconstruction, or (2) extending the stump incisions proximally to this area. A separate incision in the snuffbox is usually made if the radial artery is selected. This incision must be connected with the digital stump through a wide subcutaneous tunnel to allow passage of the donor vessels without compression; otherwise it is better to open the skin between the two incisions.

Bone and Joint Preparation
Periosteal dissection should be minimal to expose the fixation site in the recipient bone. The bony surface of the stump is smoothed to provide good contact and stability, which are essential for adequate bone union (Fig. 52-22). Whenever the joint is going to be repaired, the joint capsule and ligaments must be carefully dissected while exposing the cartilage surface.

Tendon and Pulley Preparation
Usually the extensor tendon is located close to the bony stump, and every effort should be made to not detach it (especially in distal finger reconstruction) because extensor mechanism integrity is essential for finger function. The flexor tendons have different locations in distal and proximal finger amputations (see later), and the pulley system must be preserved while exposing the tendon. To achieve a

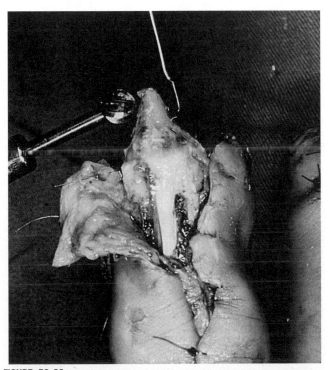

FIGURE 52-22. Recipient site preparation. The distal end of the bone is regularized to attain stability and good bone contact with the transplanted toe.

functional result, it is critical to have good tendon excursion, so all tendon adhesions should be removed at this stage if necessary. Most tendons can be repaired at the mid-palm level, with enough distance left from the tenorrhaphy site to the A1 pulley for smooth excursion. In distal finger reconstruction, the insertion of the FDS must be carefully exposed together with the flexor digitorum profundus (FDP) over the middle phalanx shaft level. It is seldom necessary to repair the flexor tendon at the wrist level. If no flexor tendons are available, the FDS tendon from the adjacent finger may be transferred primarily.

Nerve Preparation

The proper or common digital nerves are close to the edge of the stump in most cases of distal finger amputation, and these are used for neurorrhaphy with the transferred toe. In deciding the proper site for anastomosis in a normal or relatively normal recipient nerve, the appearance of the fascicles under the microscope is a good guide. More proximal recipient nerves in the palm, including the palmar cutaneous branch of the median nerve and dorsal sensory branches of the ulnar nerve, may be selected if the distal nerves have been avulsed. Nerve transfers from the ulnar side of the long or ring finger or sensory branches of the superficial radial nerve on the dorsum of the hand may be used as well.

Vessel (Artery and Vein) Preparation

The proper digital arteries at the proximal phalanx level may be used for anastomosis in distal finger reconstruction. Because of their larger size, the proper digital artery on the ulnar side is selected more often than the proper digital artery on the radial side. Common digital arteries in the palm are a good option for more proximal amputations provided that the arterial arch in the hand was not involved in the initial injury. The recipient arteries should be meticulously dissected and the adventitia layer stripped off to avoid postoperative vasospasm. If these vessels are too small for vascular anastomosis, it is advisable to select a larger artery such as the radial artery in the anatomical snuffbox or the princeps pollicis artery. Vein grafts should be considered if the donor artery is short (e.g., a plantar-dominant system) or the proximal arteries are required for anastomosis, instead of struggling to increase the length of the donor artery in the foot or anastomose the vessels under tension.

One vein is generally dissected on the dorsal aspect of the hand and used as a recipient vessel. More proximal veins can easily be mobilized when these are not found distally.

Toe Fixation Technique

Usually, the following sequence is suggested for insetting the transplanted toe.

Skeletal Fixation

In toe-to-hand transplantation, intraosseous wires, Kirschner wires, and rigid fixation systems have been used for bone fixation.[23,90,92,121] In addition, an intramedullary bone peg may be used in combination with wires.[45] Parallel or coronal and sagittal intraosseous wiring is used frequently. According to the experience of Yim and myself with parallel

intraosseous wiring in 68 toe-to-hand transplants in 47 patients, an overall nonunion rate of 1.5% was observed after a mean follow-up of 30 months.[121] Some of the advantages of this technique include the following: (1) stability is provided for early mobilization, thus preventing tendon adhesions and improving the overall range of motion in the reconstructed digit (Fig. 52-23); (2) any slight angulation and malrotation can be corrected with appropriate splints in the early postoperative period (Fig. 52-24); (3) it is a simple, quick, and inexpensive method; and (4) it can be applied to a stump of phalanx as short as 5.0 mm (see Fig. 52-23D), so the intact proximal joint may be preserved.

For intraosseous wiring, 2.0 mm of healthy bone between the holes and the bony edge in the skeleton stump is enough for bone healing. Two parallel 1.0-mm holes are made through both cortices in the distal part of the bony stump in a dorsal-to-volar direction. After placing the toe in its proper position, the angle and rotation of the toe are determined and two parallel holes are drilled in the phalanx of the toe. Next, 2-0 (28-gauge) stainless steel wires are introduced through the corresponding holes and twisted while the position of the toe is carefully adjusted. The wire ends must be placed away from the gliding extensor tendon to avoid tethering.

For composite joint repair, the volar plate and collateral ligaments of the toe are attached to the corresponding structures on the finger with nonabsorbable sutures.[80,119] The volar plate has to be repaired with proper tension to prevent postoperative hyperextension of the joint. This technique has been used primarily with combined transplantation of the second and third toes.[80,119]

Tendon Repair

After fixing the bone, the extensor tendon is repaired. The tendon is sutured with the PIP and MCP joints in full extension to minimize flexion deformity. The extensor longus tendon of the toe is inserted through two separate longitudinal slits made in the extensor in the finger, and these are sutured with nonabsorbable suture. Next, the long flexor tendon of the toe is sutured to the FDP tendon. Because the insertion of the FDS is intact in distal finger amputations, the FDP is repaired only to provide stability in power pinch. When the FDP is located distal to the FDS insertion, it is directly repaired; however, if the FDP is not present distally, the flexor tendon of the toe can be sutured to the distal portion of the FDS insertion. For proximal finger amputations, only the FDP is repaired, usually in zone III, to prevent entrapment of the anastomotic site by the remaining pulleys during tendon excursion. The tension between both tendons should be adjusted so that the finger forms a natural cascade with the other digits.

After completion of the tendon repair, a single Kirschner wire is inserted through the IP joints to maintain the finger in full extension, which prevents the transferred toe from clawing. To minimize claw deformity it has been proposed that the extensor digitorum longus attachment be released from the capsule of the metatarsophalangeal joint and the extensor digitorum brevis be sutured to the dorsal expansion of the interosseous tendon.[19] In my experience, the best results have been obtained with tight extensor tendon repair and night splint application with the finger in full extension for at least 1 year.[19,97,106]

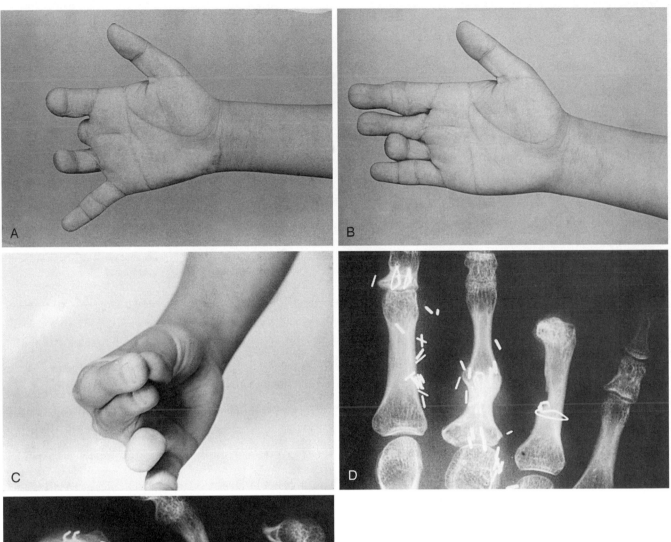

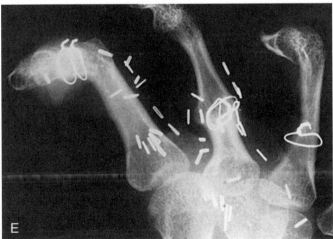

FIGURE 52-23. A, Multiple digit amputation. **B** and **C,** Adequate tripod pinch after index finger reconstruction by partial second-toe transplantation and middle finger reconstruction by total second-toe transplantation. **D** and **E,** Radiographs with the index finger under extension and flexion 8 months after surgery. In the index finger, 3.0 mm of proximal bone in the middle phalanx was used to fix the toe and preserve the proximal joint.

Nerve Repair

The nerves are anastomosed in an end-to-end fashion with 10-0 nylon. Usually only the proper digital nerves are repaired; however, if enough recipient nerves are available, the dccp and superficial peroneal nerves may be individually repaired. When only one digital nerve is available proximally, the different toe nerves can be sutured together with this nerve and priority given to the proper digital nerves.

Skin Closure

The skin is adjusted and temporarily closed after ending the neurorrhaphies and before performing the vascular anastomoses. Hence, swelling and tension during wound closure immediately after reperfusion are minimized. The four skin flaps built in the recipient stump are tailored and interposed with the triangular flaps of the transferred toe to create a smooth surface. Inadequate skin coverage in toe transplan-

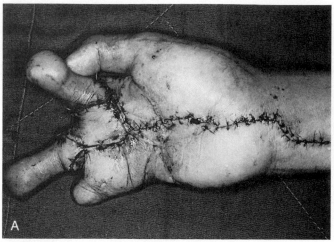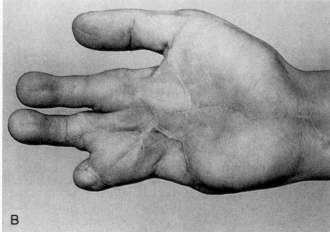

FIGURE 52-24. A, Bilateral second-toe transplantation. Immediately after surgery, significant rotation of both fingers is observed. **B,** Four months after rehabilitation therapy, good alignment of the transferred toes was achieved.

tation is a major cause of complications. Conversely, a "cobra deformity" may result when redundant skin is left at the junction between the transplanted toe and the digit, and excessive fatty tissue is a common cause of bulbous appearance with unpleasant results.[97]

Vascular Anastomoses

The arterial anastomosis is performed first. Once completed, the venous return should be observed for several minutes. Whenever the blood outflow proves to be insufficient, the arterial anastomosis and the entire course of the vessel must be reassessed. If perfusion of the toe is suspect (e.g., into the third toe in combined transplantation of the second and third toes), a second artery can be used for anastomosis.[12]

The remaining wounds in the finger are closed and the vein anastomosis is completed through a separate incision in the dorsum of the hand. If there is some tension in closing the skin, it is advisable to partially close the wound and use skin grafts to cover the remaining raw surface; with adequate preoperative planning, however, tension on the skin during closure is uncommon. Small Silastic drains are used to prevent hematoma accumulation, and contact of the drain with the vascular anastomoses must be avoided.

POSTOPERATIVE MANAGEMENT

The patients are hospitalized on average for 5 days in the microsurgery intensive care unit, where specialized nurses can continue close monitoring of the transplanted toe and the patient's general condition. The proximal portion of the palm and wrist is gently wrapped with the fingers uncovered for continuous observation. The hand and forearm are kept slightly elevated atop a smooth support to reduce edema formation. Bulky dressings are not recommended because of the following reasons: (1) blood clots are retained around the wounds and their removal could induce vasospasm, in addition to presenting a higher risk of infection, and (2) it is not possible to start early postoperative rehabilitation.

An initial bolus of 100 mL of dextran 40 (low molecular weight) is rapidly administered intravenously 10 minutes before completion of the arterial anastomosis, followed by a continuous infusion (25 mL/hr) during the next 4 to 5 days. Aspirin (325 mg/day) is administered for 2 weeks to reduce the risk of platelet aggregation.

Prophylactic antibiotics (cephalosporins) are used in elective cases and in primary toe transplantation. In prolonged surgical cases or potentially contaminated wounds, gentamicin is added initially and the antibiotics subsequently adjusted according to bacterial sensitivity in the event of an infection.

Vascular conditions in the toe are subjectively monitored by direct observation of skin color, turgor, and capillary refill and objectively monitored by measurement of the surface temperature in the toe in comparison to the adjacent normal finger and opposite hand and assessment of artery patency by Doppler ultrasound.

The donor foot is gently covered with nitrofurazone (Furacin)-impregnated gauze over the wound and a light fluff dressing. No splints are used in the donor foot or the recipient hand. Two days later the foot is uncovered and no further dressings are used.

COMPLICATIONS

Vascular Complications

Vasospasm, the most frequent vascular complication, is usually observed in the first 3 postoperative days. It occurs more often in distal digit reconstruction with partial toe transplantation. Precipitating factors should be controlled, including cold temperature in the recovery room, patient anxiety, and excessive manipulation of the hand. Prevention consists of trying to maintain optimal systemic blood pressure, supplying adequate fluid therapy, providing constant analgesia, and lowering the hand below the heart level. If vasospasm occurs, initially some skin sutures may be removed and continuous heating with a heat lamp instituted. Additionally, 2% lidocaine can be intermittently instilled over the partially opened wounds. Sublingual nitroglycerin or nifedipine[67] and regional blocks[66] may help in unrelieved vasospasm; however, if no circulation is restored after observation for a reasonable time (1 hour), prompt re-exploration in the operating room is mandatory.

In some cases an incomplete adventiectomy or a small hematoma may be responsible for local vasospasm. Once the adventitial layer has been completely excised or the hematoma evacuated, the vasospasm may be relieved; instillation of papaverine may be helpful as well. Revision of the vascular anastomosis is indicated if the vasospasm persists or the arterial anastomosis is thrombosed. If preserved, the second or third plantar metatarsal arteries can be used for a second arterial anastomosis in combined second- and third-toe transfer, provided that the arterial insufficiency is secondary to inadequate blood supply.[12]

Venous thrombosis after toe-to-hand transplantation is uncommon and usually related to compression of the vein as a result of inaccurate insetting or hematoma accumulation.

In most instances it is feasible to salvage the transplanted toe after reexploration.[12,121] However, 3.5% of cases[97,124] still end up failing. The possibility of re-exploration and failure must be extensively explained and understood by the patient and relatives before surgery, as in any other microsurgical procedure.

Other Complications

Skin coverage and wound healing problems are probably the most common complications in toe-to-hand transplantation. Very often these are secondary to partial necrosis of the thin skin flaps raised in the toe or in the recipient site, particularly when a groin flap was previously used. When the subjacent tendons and nerves are exposed, immediate action should be taken to provide soft tissue coverage and prevent desiccation of these structures and subsequent sequelae.

SECONDARY PROCEDURES

According to different authors, secondary procedures may be required in up to 20% of cases after toe-to-hand transplantation, and these are required when the function of the transferred toe falls short of expectations.[23,28,32,49,92,122]

In a previous study of 133 toe-to-hand transplantations in our unit, secondary procedures for functional improvement were necessary in 19 (14.3%) transfers after an average time of 8.8 months.[122] The incidence of secondary procedures on tendon, bone, joints, and soft tissue was 9.0%, 1.5%, 2.3%, and 3.8%, respectively. Tenolysis was the secondary procedure most commonly performed (6.8%), followed by arthrodesis (3.0%) and web space deepening (3.0%). In my experience, secondary procedures yield satisfactory results, particularly flexor tendon tenolysis.

Other secondary procedures are sometimes required after toe-to-hand transplantation. These include tendon and nerve grafts, tenorrhaphies, tendon transfer, osteotomies, and capsulotomies.

Small revisions are also used for aesthetic improvement after toe-to-finger reconstruction. Pulp plasties are minor procedures performed under local anesthesia and are used to improve bulbous-appearing reconstructed fingers.[97,118] Scar revisions and "Z"-plasties in the junction between the transplanted toe and the recipient finger are used for correction of soft tissue irregularities that result from inadequate tailoring and adjustment of the skin during toe insetting.[97]

DONOR SITE MORBIDITY AND GAIT ANALYSIS

Foot deformity is more evident after resection of the great toe or combined second and third toe than after removal of the second toe alone. Besides the alteration in appearance, a few complications, including hypertrophic scarring and partial skin necrosis, are observed in the donor foot. Both are usually related to the elevation of very thin flaps to dissect the proximal pedicle in the dorsum of the foot and to excessive tension during wound closure because of inadequate surgical planning.

Recently, biomechanical function of the foot before and after harvesting the second toe and combined second and third toe was evaluated. In 36 patients with removal of the second toe, gait and force plate foot pressure analysis were evaluated during stance and walking. The results showed increased loading on the first toe during stance, with the third toe becoming unloaded with increased loading of the first metatarsal during walking.

Nevertheless, preoperative comparative results were not statistically significant, and it was concluded that transplantation of the second toe is associated with minimal biomechanical foot changes and problems.

Foot kinetics before and 6 months after combined second- and third-toe transfer was also assessed in 17 patients. The analysis revealed no significant change in gait parameters such as walking velocity, cadence, step length and width, duration of stance phase, and the percentage of single and double limb support phases. However, it was found that harvesting of combined second and third toes unloaded the metatarsal region and increased the load on the big toe and, to a lesser extent, the heel, which was adequate compensation for the simultaneous loss of these two toes. Clinically, there were also no significant complaints from these patients.

Therefore, there should not be any hesitation in using this surgical procedure for finger reconstruction in properly selected patients, provided that the precautions related to toe harvesting and postoperative care of the donor site described before are adhered to.

REHABILITATION

Rehabilitation after toe-to-hand transplantation is aimed at improving motor capability and sensory function of the transplanted toe.[47,53]

Motor Rehabilitation

Early controlled motor rehabilitation not only prevents joint stiffness and tendon adhesion but also enhances coordination and dexterity of the reconstructed hand. The rehabilitation program developed in our unit consists of five stages starting from the first postoperative day.[54]

1. *Protective stage* (days 1 to 3). During this stage psychological support is provided to the patient while remaining hospitalized in the microsurgery intensive care unit for observation of toe viability. The importance of this stage revolves around establishing an interaction between the patient and the hand therapist.

2. *Early mobilization stage* (day 4 to week 4). In this stage, rehabilitation is directed at preventing excessive swelling and joint stiffness. During day 4 to week 2, the hand is kept about 1 ft higher than the heart level. On day 4, gentle passive range-of-motion exercises of the joints are commenced by individually moving each joint about 15 degrees. Special care should be taken to not compromise the viability of the transferred toe while performing the exercises. In the second week, the joint distal to the bony union site is moved through a full range of motion while keeping the wrist in neutral position. In the third and fourth weeks, the proximal joints are moved as much as possible, with full range of motion avoided so as not to interfere with bone healing. A light-pressure tubular bandage with the fingertips left exposed is also applied at this time, and the patient is taught gentle massage. A protective splint is provided between exercises. As a general principle, the splint should be placed in a position that prevents stress on the repaired tendons or neurovascular structures.

3. *Active motion stage* (weeks 5 to 6). During this stage, gentle active exercise is added to the passive exercise and the splint is changed to a dynamic one, if necessary. During the sixth week, once the tendons have healed, blocking flexion and extension exercises are initiated. Compression bandages are always used to help reduce edema and minimize scar formation, which are additional aims of this rehabilitation stage. Ultrasound and scar massage are used to produce a softer scar and increase the range of motion.

4. *Activities of daily living training stage* (weeks 7 to 8). Rehabilitation aims at providing tasks that require training to strengthen muscle power and improve the range of joint motion. According to patient capabilities, different manual jobs that simulate daily manual activities are assigned.

5. *Prevocational training stage* (week 8 on). During this stage, vocational activities are designed to further improve muscle strength and hand dexterity and coordination. To prevent a claw deformity, the patient is encouraged to use night-time extension splints for at least 1 year. The patient is encouraged to resume normal activities with the reconstructed hand and sometimes to attend interactive group sessions with other patients who have also received toe-to-hand transplantation. Individual psychological support therapy is indicated only if required.

Sensory Rehabilitation

It is difficult to achieve functional sensory recovery after toe-to-hand transplantation without sensory rehabilitation.[17,53] Sensory re-education is directed at helping the patient interpret the altered sensory impulses reaching the brain from peripheral nerves.[18,113] This does not make axons grow faster or cause receptors to form, but it uses higher cortical functions such as concentration, learning, and memory to maximize the sensory function provided by the regenerated nerves. The program of sensory re-education is divided into early and delayed stages. In the early stage, re-education focuses on facilitating the perception of touch submodalities with correct localization. Training is initiated when the patient can perceive 30-cps vibrations from a tuning fork with the reconstructed fingertip and is continued according to a sequence of sensory recovery observed by Dellon.[18]

Late-phase sensory re-education focuses on size and shape discrimination and object identification. This program is begun following the recovery of touch sensation. It consists of touching several objects with different texture, size, and shape, the nature of which the patient attempts to appreciate with the tip of the transplanted toe instead of the adjacent normal finger surface. It can be implemented as a home rehabilitation program with significant improvement in the final result.[113]

In a study of sensory recovery after toe-to-hand transplantation, my colleagues and I[93] found good relationship between Meissner corpuscle number and two-point discrimination.

Donor Site Rehabilitation

The patient is allowed to walk a few steps on the heel of the donor foot after the second week. It must be emphasized that any contact with the anterior plantar weight-bearing surface should be avoided during this recovery time. The sutures in the donor foot should not be removed earlier than 3 weeks after operation. After 4 weeks the patient is allowed to walk with a normal gait.

CONCLUSION

From 1985 to May 2004, a total of 1734 toe transplantations were performed in 1553 patients at our institution (Table 52-3): 27% (467/1734) of them were used for thumb reconstruction and 73% (1267/1734) for finger reconstructions. The success rate in this series is 97%. From this experience we can conclude that toe-to-hand transplantation is reliable

Table 52-3

TOE TRANSPLANTATIONS AT CHANG GUNG MEMORIAL HOSPITAL, JANUARY 1985-MAY 2004

	No. Patients	No. Toes
Second toe	836	836
Great toe	288	288
Combined second and third toe	178	356
Vascularized joint	66	66
Pulp	93	93
Glabrous	46	46
Third toe	39	39
Fourth toe	4	4
Combined third and fourth toe	3	6
Total	1553	1734

and useful for missing thumbs and finger reconstruction. It provides unique functional and aesthetic results that other reconstructive techniques cannot achieve.

ANNOTATED REFERENCES

104. Wei FC: Tissue preservation in hand injury: The first step to toe-to-hand transplantation. Plast Reconstr Surg 102:2497-2501, 1998.

The traditional management of amputated digital stumps usually involves shortening of bones, tendons, and neurovascular bundles to facilitate wound closure. Contrary to the traditional management, the authors emphasize in this article the preservation of those structures during initial treatment. The base of the phalangeal bone with an intact joint should be maintained. The tendons and neurovascular bundles should not be shortened, and local flaps for stump wound coverage should be avoided.

CHAPTER 53

Thumb Reconstruction

W. P. Andrew Lee and A. Neil Salyapongse

It is in the human hand that we have the consummation of all perfection as an instrument.

SIR CHARLES BELL[12]

The hand without a thumb is at worst nothing but an animated fish-slice, and at best a pair of forceps whose points don't meet properly.

JOHN NAPIER[173]

Despite a long-standing recognition of the uniquely *human* way of using the hand, anthropologists have only recently defined the significance of the structure of the human hand that allows us to forego an arboreal lifestyle in pursuit of activities ranging from computer programmer to auto mechanic to surgeon.[259] Their findings focus in large part on the anatomic features allowing three "grips" that differentiate the human hand and that of other hominids. These grips, the *pad-to-side*, *three-jawed chuck*, and *five-jawed cradle/chuck*, are all possible owing to the structure of the human thumb. As described by Napier, the absence of the thumb, whether due to failure of formation or loss from trauma, significantly impairs hand function. In previous editions of this textbook, Drs. Kleinman and Strickland have provided an excellent summary of the past 125 years of efforts by hand surgeons to preserve and, if necessary, reconstruct thumb function. As they predicted, many of these creative techniques have given way to the demonstrated success of microsurgery, including improved initial thumb salvage via replantation as well as reconstruction using free toe transfer. Unchanged from their writings is the dictum that, for the willing and motivated patient, "reconstruction of an opposable thumb should be attempted whenever possible by using whatever technical pathways are available to the surgeon."

With a few notable exceptions, techniques used when reconstructing the thumb after trauma are not unique to this digit. Skin grafts, local or regional flaps, free tissue transfer, and distraction/lengthening are all discussed at length in their respective chapters. A brief review of the evolution of thumb reconstruction outside of microsurgical techniques is provided to give the reader some perspective on the breadth of procedures that have been developed. After this we place the available procedures within a framework that will help guide the clinician when planning thumb reconstruction. For the details of operative techniques described in other chapters, cross references are provided and any elements of peculiar significance to the thumb are noted. Apart from the advances in microsurgery and refinements in toe transfer techniques, few changes in the procedures used for thumb salvage and reconstruction have taken place. Given this, we will follow the lead of Drs. Kleinman and Strickland by describing procedures unique to thumb reconstruction in detail, with attention to both preoperative planning and postoperative care.

HISTORICAL REVIEW

Although technical advances have changed surgical methods, the general surgical philosophies of thumb reconstruction have remained relatively constant since their inception. In the latter part of the 19th and early 20th centuries, two distinct surgical philosophies evolved: (1) optimizing the function of what remains via local thumb phalangization after partial amputation, essentially a deepening of the first web space as first described by Huguier,[103] and (2) distant pedicle flap attachment with delayed secondary detachment, described in 1897 by Nicoladoni.[174] The principle of phalangization continued to evolve throughout the 20th century as techniques such as the "Z"-plasty, four-flap "Z"-plasty,[18] dorsal rotational flap,[21] and metacarpal lengthening[144] were used to provide additional web span and depth. Nicoladoni's staged great toe-to-thumb transfer and the delayed pedicle finger transfers of Guermonprez[84-86] and Luksch[138] are clearly mirrored in our current microvascular toe-to-thumb and occasional finger-to-thumb transfers.

Also during the late 19th century, the groundwork for the development of the neurovascular island flap was laid.[55,74] In addition to its role in plastic surgery and craniofacial reconstruction,[35] this work would become the basis for the third persistent theme in thumb reconstruction: Gosset's revolutionary concept of transfer of a digit on its own neurovascular pedicle. In introducing this technique, Gosset not only revolutionized contemporary traumatic thumb reconstruction but also pioneered the seminal principles of reconstruction for a congenitally absent thumb. His initial recommendations involved simple lateral displacement of the index ray without bony shortening. Subsequently modified to include metacarpal recession and rotation, intrinsic muscle transfers, and skin flaps specially designed to produce a wide first web space free of scar,[24a,78a] pollicization via nonmicrovascular transfer of the long,[16,73,90,110,140,148] ring,[15,30,33,169,181,211] and little[115,126] fingers remains one of the mainstays of thumb reconstruction.

The fourth pathway to thumb reconstruction was represented by osteoplastic thumb creation.[4,176-178,181,213] Used extensively before World War II, osteoplastic reconstruction was performed in either one or two stages. The first step involved attaching the injured thumb stump to a random tubed pedicle of vascularized skin and subcutaneous tissue from the abdomen or groin; an iliac crest corticocancellous bone graft could be inserted and fixed to the residual thumb either at a second stage (division of the tubed pedicle) or during the primary formation of the pedicle. As recently as 1955, advances in osteoplastic thumb reconstruction were reported with Moberg's introduction of the "island pedicle" transfer of vascularized, sensible cornified skin from an uninjured portion of the hand to restore stereognosis to the tactile portion of the osteoplastic thumb.[164] This technique has been widely practiced and remains a fundamental approach in complex thumb reconstruction after trauma.[35]

GENERAL CONSIDERATIONS

An ideal reconstruction of the thumb would "replace like with like," restoring both function and appearance. Replantation has demonstrated great success in that it restores the actual lost thumb, often yielding excellent functional outcomes.* When replantation fails or is not feasible, the surgeon must re-create the likeness of the thumb. Deconstructing the ideal thumb function into its basic elements will assist the surgeon in choosing a reconstructive technique to provide an optimal outcome. Although authors differ in the specific breakdown of thumb requirements, two broad categories must be addressed. These are sensation and opposition. Sensation may be further divided into freedom from pain and adequate sensibility to interact with or, at least, protect itself from the environment. Opposition, the hallmark of "thumbness," necessitates length, stability/strength, and mobility.† Exactly how important each of these factors becomes will vary depending on the needs of the patient: the jeweler who seeks sensibility and mobility may require different management than the manual laborer who may sacrifice mobility for stability and power.

For a patient to consistently use a reconstructed thumb, it must have painless skin coverage, be durable enough for normal use, and have at least protective, if not normal, sensation.[244] Thus, regardless of the level of amputation and planned thumb length after reconstruction, every attempt should be made to restore at least an acceptable level of sensory cognition after thumb salvage or reconstruction.‡ Procedures should be selected to provide a predictably satisfactory level of tactile perception and stereognosis. Failure to achieve this quality was the most consistent reason for patient thumb disuse after many early reconstructive techniques (despite the fact that other functional requirements may have been met by the procedures). The use of neuro-vascular island pedicle techniques, sensory-innervated cross-finger flaps, and other methods of transferring innervated skin has greatly enhanced the ability to restore sensation when carrying out thumb salvage after trauma or congenital etiology.

First among the components of opposition is length; amputations that deprive the thumb of the distal phalanx or, at most, just proximal to the interphalangeal (IP) joint, may not require reconstruction.[117,191,196,199,206,232,244] Loss at or more proximal to the shaft of the proximal phalanx, however, will usually leave a stump inadequate for pinch and grasp functions.[193,222] In order to oppose the remaining digits, a thumb of sufficient length must be *antiposed* (abducted, slightly extended, and pronated).[166,201,236] Whereas thumb IP flexion does result in slight pronation of the distal phalanx,[95] normal motion at the metacarpophalangeal (MCP) or IP joints is not mandatory. In contrast, active thumb function depends on preserving a full arc of circumduction at the carpometacarpal (CMC) joint.[28,91,166,197] If a substantial range of CMC motion cannot be attained, an essentially sensate prosthesis may be created by arthrodesing the thumb in nearly full abduction-opposition (40 degrees of abduction, 15 degrees of extension, 120 degrees of metacarpal pronation)[117] so that other mobile digits can be flexed to meet it. Thus, strength and mobility, although more closely approximating normal thumb opposition, may be sacrificed to provide a stable, if immobile, post for resistance during pinch and grasp.

Additional considerations when counseling a patient regarding the options for thumb reconstruction include age, sex, occupational demands, hand dominance, and the subjective needs of the patient. Once the patient has expressed interest in a restorative or reconstructive effort, an open and honest dialogue between the patient (or family) and surgeon is necessary before any final decision can be made. Rehabilitation after any reconstructive procedure will be critical to obtaining a successful outcome; the patient must be motivated and should fully understand that his or her effort during therapy will play at least an equal, if not greater, part than the surgery in regaining a functional thumb.

THUMB RECONSTRUCTION AFTER PARTIAL OR COMPLETE TRAUMATIC LOSS

Thumb function after amputation depends primarily on the remaining elements. Consequently, most algorithms for management of thumb reconstruction begin by stratifying the injury by level of loss.§ Division of the thumb into functional levels has varied slightly from one author to the next[95,127]; however, in developing an approach to the reconstructive needs of the thumb, we prefer to stratify thumb defects after the style of Lister.[127]

---

*See references 58, 88, 116, 120, 124, 142, 220, 235, 242, and 247.

†See references 28, 37, 64, 95, 117, 118, 127, 134, 143, 168, 191, 197, 199, 201, 241, and 244.

‡See references 26, 28, 90, 91, 96, 117, 127, 164, 236, and 243.

§See references 9, 23-25, 28, 29, 53, 80, 88, 95, 116, 118-120, 127, 128, 142, 160, 168, 197, 199, 218-220, 229, 232, 235, 239, 241, 242, 244, 255, 256, and 258.

Acceptable length with poor soft tissue coverage: these injuries are typically tip or pulp amputations that leave adequate length and functional thenar musculature and basal joint mobility for opposition. Additional requirements for these injuries focus on sensibility/sensitivity and durability of skin coverage.

Subtotal amputation with questionable remaining length: this group encompasses the widest range of needs, beginning with injuries requiring only soft tissue coverage to those demanding reconstruction analogous to total amputations. Choice of procedure will be chiefly determined by the patient's perceived needs.

Total amputation with preservation of the basal joint: although intrinsic thumb function will be lost to varying degrees, the foremost requirement of amputations at this level is restoration of length. The extent of remaining intrinsic function as well as the chosen reconstructive technique will determine how the new thumb is motored.

Total amputation with loss of the basal joint: again, provision of length is critical, but functional opposition becomes more difficult. Either a substitute for the basal joint must be provided in the reconstruction, or the thumb must be arthrodesed in antiposition.

The following sections present our rationale for this division, including definition of the differing reconstructive needs at each of these levels, and describe in detail the surgical options available.

Acceptable Length with Poor Soft Tissue Coverage

Even complete amputation of the thumb at the level of the IP joint, when treated with appropriate revision amputation, rarely results in significant functional deficit.[77] Therefore, this level has been described as the "compensated amputation zone."[58,143] If the skeletal and soft tissues have suffered damage sufficient to make restoration of a stable, sensate thumb tip unlikely, completion amputation and closure may provide a more immediate and equally functional outcome.[44,60,154,215] In this setting, it is important that closure be carried out by using sound amputation principles, including careful identification and proximal resection of the digital nerves.[44,60,154,215] If these techniques are properly carried out, a good stump in the distal third of the thumb can function well with almost no functional disability.[61,143,191,194,201,205,244]

A broad spectrum of injury exists short of complete amputation or unsalvageable trauma to the distal thumb. Goals of treatment include restoration of skeletal stability, coverage of the thumb with durable, painless skin, and restoration of adequate sensory perception. The specific procedures used to accomplish these goals will vary depending on the amount and depth of tissue loss, and an attempt should be made to salvage all viable tissues consistent with these objectives. Although injuries to the palmar pad of the distal phalanx of the thumb may be managed by the same coverage techniques that are applicable to fingertip injuries, the approach may be somewhat different as one strives to preserve length.*

The choice of reconstructive procedure for soft tissue deficits over the distal thumb depends primarily on the size of the defect. When the loss of skin and subcutaneous tissue from the terminal aspect of the distal phalanx is small (typically less than 1 cm^2) and no exposed bone is present, reasonable treatments include allowing spontaneous healing by secondary intention, free skin grafts,[36,44,225] lateral triangular advancement flaps,[47,78,122,199,246] "V-Y" advancement flaps,[7,59,67,68,76,122,203] and a variety of other techniques.† For these small defects, we prefer conservative, open treatment to allow the wound to heal through secondary intention. The advantage of spontaneous healing resides in more favorable wound contraction, which will result in a minimal defect with nearly normal sensation preserved.[36,117,229] At the time of presentation, patients undergoing conservative treatment should have the wound cleansed and covered with a nonadherent dressing. The initial dressing is removed at 48 hours and daily dressing changes performed thereafter until the wound has completely closed. Patients should be counseled that a few weeks may elapse before the thumb tip has healed.

Loss of greater than 50% of the distal portion of the thumb pad, tendon denuded of sheath and soft tissue coverage, and bone stripped of its periosteum may jeopardize not only the function of the injured thumb but also the preservation of thumb length. Under these circumstances, more complex reconstructive procedures ranging from palmar advancement flaps to cross-finger flaps and neurovascular island or radial sensory-innervated cross-finger flaps may be warranted. Each of these techniques is considered in detail in the following sections.

Palmar Advancement Flap

Originally described by Moberg,[161] the palmar advancement flap provides one of the best reconstructive options for loss of greater than half of the distal thumb pad. It has the advantage of bringing well-innervated palmar thumb skin distally to resurface the pad lesion, thereby restoring nearly normal sensory perception with durable skin and subcutaneous tissue. Resurfacing of the thumb tip is accomplished by advancement of a palmar flap containing the neurovascular structures with or without proximal skin release and interpositional grafting.[76,114,157,161,190,199,205,246] This flap has proven most useful in covering defects ranging from slightly greater than 1 cm to "quarter sized"[114] or as much as 2 cm.[190] The thumb is uniquely suited for this flap in that flexion of the thumb IP joint as much as 45 degrees to provide sufficient advancement of the flap will not result in a long-term flexion deformity.[114,190] In practice, we find that advancement of the flap by more than 1.5 cm is facilitated by a proximal transverse releasing incision,[5,76,205] which can decrease the need for acute IP flexion and increase the amount of tissue that can be mobilized.[76,205] Although the defect created by the releasing incision may be left to heal by secondary intention,[76] coverage with a full-thickness skin graft provides a closed wound and decreases the propensity for wound contraction.

CRITICAL POINTS: PALMAR ADVANCEMENT FLAP

INDICATIONS

- Palmar thumb pad defects greater than 1 cm² but less than 2 cm in length
- Exposed distal phalanx devoid of periosteum

TECHNICAL POINTS

- Perform thorough débridement of the defect.
- Incise skin in midaxial line beginning at wound and extending proximally on the radial and ulnar aspects of the thumb up to the proximal thumb crease.
- Dissect the flap, containing the subcutaneous tissue and both neurovascular bundles from the flexor sheath.
- Test tension on flap by providing distal traction.
- If additional length is necessary, extend incisions/dissection onto the thenar eminence.
- Flex MCP and IP joints of thumb to 30 to 45 degrees.
- Suture distal flap to remaining nail, nail bed, or skin.
- Apply nonadherent dressing and thumb spica splint.

POSTOPERATIVE CARE

- Inspect wound at 7 to 10 days.
- Switch to a thermoplastic thumb spica splint.
- Begin active range-of-motion exercises at 3 weeks.
- If necessary to achieve extension, dynamic splinting may start at 3 weeks.

Palmar Advancement Flap Without Proximal Releasing Incision

This technique is best for terminal distal phalangeal pad defects 1.5 cm or less in length. Under tourniquet control, necrotic and ragged bone is trimmed from the distal phalanx and thorough soft tissue débridement is carried out (Fig. 53-1A). Midaxial incisions are made over the radial and ulnar sides of the thumb and extended proximally from the lesion to the proximal thumb crease. Placement of the incisions across the dorsal apices of the flexion creases facilitates dissection dorsal to the neurovascular bundles. The palmar flap is then carefully dissected from the underlying flexor tendon sheath; the flap should include subcutaneous tissue and both neurovascular bundles (see Fig. 53-1B). The mobility of the flap is tested by distal traction to determine whether any additional soft tissue undermining or releases are necessary. If tension is too great, the midaxial incisions may be extended proximally onto the thenar eminence. The MCP and IP joints of the thumb are flexed 30 to 45 degrees.

The distal edge of the flap is sutured to the remaining nail, nail bed, or terminal skin remnant, and radial and ulnar sutures are used to complete skin closure (see Fig. 53-1C).

Palmar Advancement Flap With a Proximal Releasing Incision

Use of a proximal releasing incision allows the palmar advancement flap to cover defects up to 2.5 cm in length. As in the case of the palmar flap without a releasing incision, appropriate bone and soft tissue débridement should be carried out under tourniquet hemostasis (Fig. 53-2A).

CRITICAL POINTS: PALMAR ADVANCEMENT FLAP WITH PROXIMAL RELEASING INCISION

INDICATION

- As per standard palmar advancement flap, with defects greater than 2 cm and less than 2.5 cm in length

TECHNICAL POINTS

- Perform thorough débridement of the defect.
- Incise skin in midaxial line beginning at wound and extending proximally on the radial and ulnar aspects of the thumb up to the proximal third of the proximal phalanx.
- Connect the midaxial incisions via a transverse palmar incision.
- Identify and mobilize the neurovascular bundles.
- Dissect the flap, containing the subcutaneous tissue and both neurovascular bundles, from the flexor sheath.
- Test tension on flap by providing distal traction.
- If additional length is necessary, extend incisions/dissection onto the thenar eminence.
- Flex MCP and IP joints of thumb to 30 to 45 degrees.
- Suture distal flap to remaining nail, nail bed, or skin.
- Apply a full-thickness skin graft to the proximal thumb flap harvest site.
- Apply nonadherent dressing and thumb spica splint.

POSTOPERATIVE CARE

- Inspect wound at 7 to 10 days.
- Switch to a thermoplastic thumb spica splint.
- Begin active range-of-motion exercises at 3 weeks.
- If necessary to achieve extension, dynamic splinting may start at 3 weeks.

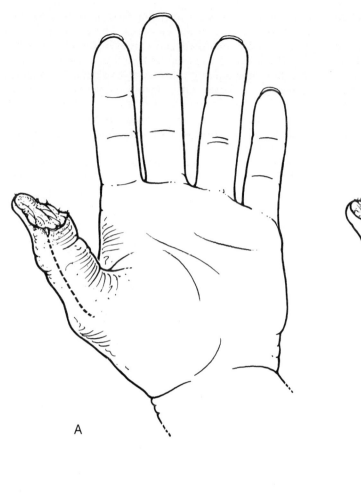

A

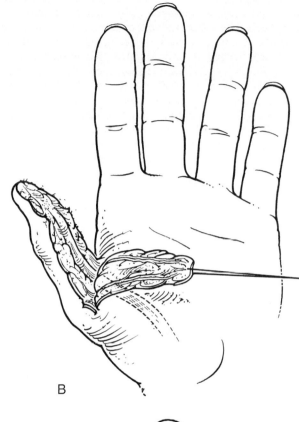

B

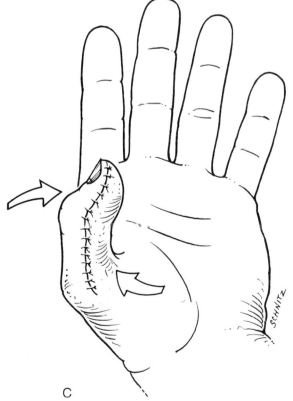

C

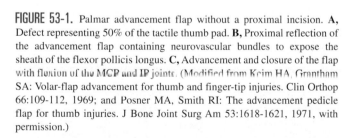

FIGURE 53-1. Palmar advancement flap without a proximal incision. **A,** Defect representing 50% of the tactile thumb pad. **B,** Proximal reflection of the advancement flap containing neurovascular bundles to expose the sheath of the flexor pollicis longus. **C,** Advancement and closure of the flap with flexion of the MCP and IP joints. (Modified from Keim HA, Grantham SA: Volar-flap advancement for thumb and finger-tip injuries. Clin Orthop 66:109-112, 1969; and Posner MA, Smith RI: The advancement pedicle flap for thumb injuries. J Bone Joint Surg Am 53:1618-1621, 1971, with permission.)

Dissection begins at the radial and ulnar edges of the wound via midaxial incisions. How far proximal these midaxial incisions are carried depends on the method chosen to close or cover the wound created by the relaxing incision. If the advancement needed is only slightly greater than can be achieved without a relaxing incision, then options such as ending each incision as a "Z"-plasty over the thenar eminence or creating a "V-Y" advancement flap just proximal to the proximal thumb crease may allow primary closure of all wounds. More often, however, when significant advancement is required, the midaxial incisions should be carried to the level of the proximal third of the proximal phalanx. At

this point, a transverse incision should be used to connect the proximal ends of the incisions. The neurovascular bundles must be identified and carefully mobilized (see Fig. 53-2B). The flap can then be raised in a distal to proximal direction, maintaining a plane of dissection just superficial to the flexor sheath. On reaching the proximal portions of the midaxial incisions, the flap will consist of skin, subcutaneous tissue, and both neurovascular bundles. This "islandized" flap may then be advanced to the thumb tip and sutured into place (see Fig. 53-2C). As when insetting the standard palmar advancement flap, it may be necessary to flex both the IP and MCP joints to relieve tension on the

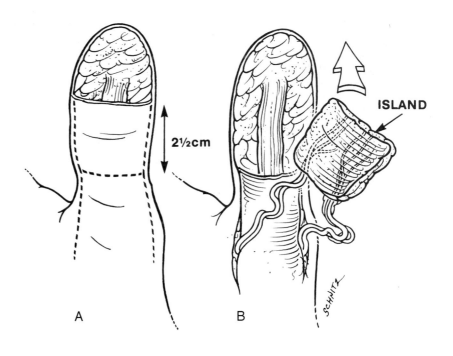

FIGURE 53-2. Palmar advancement flap with a proximal releasing incision. **A,** A 2.5-cm defect of the distal phalangeal thumb pulp and outlines of incisions for the advancement flap. **B,** Elevation of the flap and mobilization of the neurovascular bundles through the proximal incision. **C,** Advancement of the flap to close the defect. **D,** Free skin graft coverage of the proximal donor area. (Modified from Vilain R, Michon J: Plastic Surgery of the Hand and Pulp. New York, Masson, 1979, with permission.)

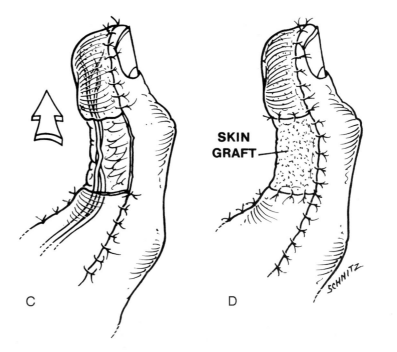

closure. The resulting gap between the proximal end of the flap and the proximal releasing incision is covered with a full-thickness skin graft harvested from the volar wrist, antecubital fossa, or groin (see Fig. 53-2D).

At the conclusion of either palmar advancement flap, a dressing consisting of nonadherent gauze, fluffed cotton gauze, and a thumb spica splint is applied. Care in shaping the thumb spica should be taken to maintain the flexion applied to achieve a tension-free closure. The splint and dressings are removed to allow inspection of the flap and, if used, skin grafts at between 7 and 10 days. Thereafter, a removable orthoplast thumb spica splint is applied to prevent overextension of the thumb. After 3 weeks, the patient begins active range-of-motion exercises and, if necessary to regain full extension, dynamic splinting.

Although the primary use of these flaps occurs in acute situations, they may also be employed for thumb resurfacing at a later period when inadequate coverage exists.[157,161,183,205] Choosing the appropriate wound for reconstruction with these flaps provides the best chance for a successful outcome. The required advancement should not exceed 2.5 cm and should include, if at the upper end of this distance, plans for a proximal releasing incision. Despite the excellent dorsal vascularity of the thumb, it is possible to induce ischemia in the ungual area; therefore, it is advisable to not dissect the pedicle too far.[246] Other risks worth including in preoperative counseling include sloughing of bits of bone or nail during the immediate postoperative period[114] and the possibility of flexion contractures of the IP joints.

Heterodigital Flap Reconstruction

Loss of the entire palmar surface of the thumb distal phalanx presents a wound too great to be covered with a palmar advancement flap. Simple skin grafting may preserve length, but it will not fulfill the priorities of restoring durable, painless skin. Initially developed for coverage of exposed tendon or bone and for loss of a significant amount of skin and subcutaneous tissue from the palmar surface of the fingers,[49,87,237] a cross-finger flap designed from the proximal phalanx of the index finger will often provide excellent coverage of these lesions with satisfactory skin and subcutaneous tissue and adequate recovery of sensation.* This flap, and its innervated variations, substitute a delayed skin flap from an adjacent digit for delayed flaps historically based on cross-arm, thoracic, or abdominal donor sites. The reliability and ease of performance of these flaps has made them the mainstay for larger tissue losses in the distal third of the thumb despite the development of numerous, more elaborate techniques, including transfer of the tip of the fifth finger,[228] free toe pulp transfers,[195,223] a one-stage advancement rotational flap combination,[76,102,111,199] use of "kite or flag flaps" from the index finger,[65,105,165,216,260] a dorsal flap based on the first web space,[146,149] or a flap hinged on the ulnar side of the thumb and rotated distally.[22]

Occasionally, irreparable damage to the digital nerves of the thumb resulting in permanent sensory loss in the palmar tactile pad will accompany soft tissue loss in the distal third of the thumb. The patient with this wound may suffer substantial disability owing to impairment of pinch and grasp function. Under these circumstances, it may be appropriate to use a neurovascular island pedicle transfer as first suggested by Moberg[161] and Littler[132] and extended by others.†

The technique, however, is very demanding and the quality of sensory return has been challenged.[11,170]

Cross-Finger Flap to the Thumb

Under tourniquet hemostasis, acute wounds should be thoroughly débrided and the wound margins excised. Some attempt to convert the lesion into a square or rectangular defect may facilitate flap design and inset, but this should not override the preservation of viable palmar skin, especially along the radial aspect of the thumb, which will represent the most distal aspect of the cross-finger flap. Blotting the wound with a sterile piece of paper will produce a template corresponding in size to the defect. This template may be cut from the paper and traced onto the dorsoradial aspect of the index finger after having adducted the thumb against the side of the index finger to determine the appropriate level for the base of the flap (Fig. 53-3A). Because of the unique rotational motion of the thumb, the base of the flap will originate palmar to the midaxial line of the index finger and extend across the dorsum of the proximal phalanx as far as the defect size requires. A slightly oblique configuration of the donor flap will aid in positioning it against the pad lesion.

Incisions are then made along the proximal, ulnar, and distal borders of the flap through the skin and subcutaneous tissue down to the level of the paratenon. The flap is raised in an ulnar to radial direction in the plane just superficial to the extensor paratenon. As dissection proceeds radially toward the base of the flap, the cutaneous ligaments of Cleland must be cut to increase mobility of the flap. Dorsal veins running in the subcutaneous tissue may be divided with bipolar cautery, but small veins in the radial corner of the flap should be preserved to ensure its viability (see Fig. 53-3B). On completion of dissection, the tourniquet is deflated and hemostasis achieved using bipolar cautery.

A nearly full-thickness skin graft is patterned slightly larger than the donor defect and harvested from either the ipsilateral antecubital fossa or the groin. The graft excess will be applied to the base of the flap as it spans the space between the apposed thumb and index finger. Inset of the flap to the proximal, radial, and distal thumb wound is performed using fine, nonabsorbable sutures. The skin graft is then applied to the donor defect and sutured in place with fine chromic gut suture. The inset of the skin graft is completed by suturing to the ulnar aspect of the thumb defect, thereby creating a closed wound (see Fig. 53-3C and D). The skin graft and flap should be covered with a nonadherent dressing followed by cotton gauze. The gauze overlying the skin graft should be moistened and conformed to the wound. These dressings are held in place by rolled cotton gauze, and the thumb and index are immobilized in a palmar splint extending across the hand and wrist.

Motion is permitted in the ulnar three fingers to prevent stiffness, and a dressing change at 7 days is used to assess the viability of the flap and the "take" of the graft. The flap may be safely divided after 10 to 14 days. Some recommend

---

*See references 9, 36, 50, 56, 99, 100, 117, 149, 150, 189, 191, 192, 199, 201, 202, 217, 228-230, and 246.

†See references 93, 95, 101, 121, 132, 133, 135, 170, 186, 199, 201, 204, 224, 229, and 231.

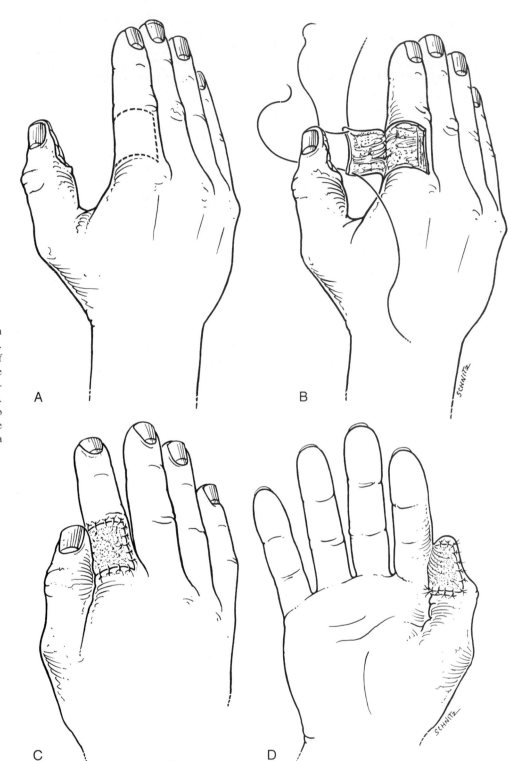

FIGURE 53-3. Cross-finger flap from the index finger to the thumb. **A,** Large defect involving most of the distal pulp of the thumb; outline of the cross-finger flap on the proximal phalanx of the index finger. **B,** Placement of the flap on the thumb defect. **C** and **D,** Position of the thumb and cross-finger flap with a free graft covering the donor defect.

elevation of the wound edges and inset of the flap as well as closure of the index donor site during division of the flap. Although this is possible, the wounds will heal as effectively by secondary intention without the risk of constricting either finger by attempting inset and closure. We advise daily dressing changes to the divided flap wounds until complete closure has occurred. Active and passive range-of-motion exercises are begun immediately after division of the flap.

Satisfactory sensory return has been found in several long-term studies of cross-finger flap performance,[99,183,230] and the technique is reliable and well tolerated by the patient and provides sufficient padding for long-term heavy thumb use (Fig. 53-4). Disadvantages and complications include a sometimes unsightly defect over the dorsum of the index finger, which may be particularly annoying to children and women, and some occasional problems with digital joint stiffness or thumb web contracture.

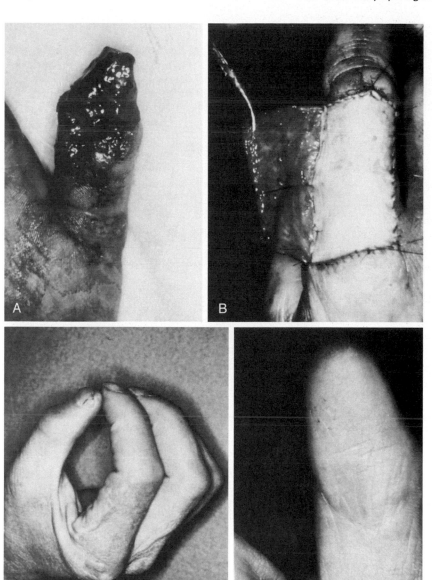

FIGURE 53-4. Cross-finger flap coverage of a large thumb defect. **A,** Large avulsion defect involving the entire palmar aspect of the distal phalanx of the thumb. **B,** Large cross-finger flap designed from the dorsum of the proximal phalanx of the index finger. The donor site has already been covered with a skin graft. **C,** Appearance of the thumb and donor defect at 3 months. **D,** Cosmetic appearance of the thumb pad at 3 months with satisfactory sensation and durable coverage. (From Strickland JW: Restoration of thumb function following partial or total amputation. *In* Hunter JM, Schneider LH, Mackin EJ, Bell JA [eds]: Rehabilitation of the Hand. St. Louis, CV Mosby, 1978, with permission.)

Innervated Cross-Finger Flap

Protective sensation and two-point discrimination after cross-finger flaps return most predictably in patients younger than 20 years old; in patients older than 40, nearly half will fail to regain protective sensation. In an attempt to improve on these outcomes, large cross-finger pedicle flaps that carry a sensory branch of the radial nerve have been described.* With the exception of the axial, bipedicled neurovascular island flap developed by Paneva-Holevich and Holevich,[182] each of these flaps differs from a traditional cross-finger flap primarily in that additional dissection over the first web space is used to facilitate inclusion and transposition of a dorsal sensory branch of the radial nerve.[1,17,72] Walker and colleagues[248] determined that the ultimate sensibility of these flaps is a mixture of the median and radial

nerves, and Hastings[92] has described a "dual innervated cross-finger" or island flap that repairs the dorsal sensory branch of the index radial digital nerve to the ulnar digital nerve of the thumb in an effort to improve cortical recognition of the flap as a thumb. Other variations have also been described,[45,98,160,194,207] and, although rarely required, the procedure has a definite place among the reconstructive options for restoration of thumb sensibility.

Radial-Innervated Cross-Finger Flap

After appropriate débridement under tourniquet hemostasis, a pattern matching the size of the acute defect or the defect to be created to provide sensory restoration to the denervated thumb is created. Markings for the size and location of the cross-finger flap are carried out in a manner identical to the noninnervated cross-finger flap. If necessary, the flap can be extended over the MCP joint for resurfacing of larger defects. Beginning at the midpoint of the proximal

---

*See references 1, 17, 72, 97, 99, 160, 194, 199, 207, and 248.

CRITICAL POINTS: CROSS-FINGER FLAP

INDICATION

- Loss of the entire palmar surface of the thumb distal to the IP joint

TECHNICAL POINTS

- Thoroughly débrided wound.
- Blot wound with sterile paper to form a template.
- Align the thumb with the radial aspect of the index finger to determine the level for the base of the flap.
- Trace the template onto the dorsal index finger.
- Incise the proximal, ulnar, and distal borders of the flap.
- Raise the flap in a plane just superficial to the extensor paratenon.
- On the radial aspect of the flap, divide Cleland's ligaments to increase mobility of the flap.
- Deflate tourniquet and achieve hemostasis before flap inset.

- Inset the flap along the proximal, radial, and distal margins of the wound.
- Harvest a full-thickness skin graft (antecubital fossa or groin) and inset this in the donor site using fine chromic sutures.
- Apply a nonadherent gauze dressing to the flap/graft and apply saline moistened gauze to the skin graft.
- Immobilize the thumb and index via a palmar splint crossing the hand and wrist.

POSTOPERATIVE CARE

- Inspect wound at 7 days.
- Divide the base of the flap at 10 to 14 days.
- Allow divided bridge to heal by secondary intention.
- Begin active range-of-motion exercises immediately after flap division.

---

transverse outline of the flap, an oblique incision extends proximally over the dorsal ulnar border of the first web space to a level several centimeters proximal to the midportion of the thumb web (Fig. 53-5A). A large dorsal sensory branch of the radial nerve may be identified running deep on the muscle fascia in the proximal portion of this incision and traced distally into the proximal margin of the flap. Complete mobilization of the nerve from the proximal edge of the flap to the base of the web space incision is

necessary to prevent undue tension on the nerve after transposition. Small branches of the nerve encountered during mobilization should be divided.

Once the radial sensory branch has been mobilized, the cross-finger flap is incised and elevated as in the case of a standard cross-finger flap. A solitary, but significant difference from the standard flap is that care must be taken when incising the proximal transverse border of the flap to avoid injury to the radial sensory branch as it enters the flap. When

CRITICAL POINTS: RADIAL-INNERVATED CROSS-FINGER FLAP

INDICATIONS

- Similar to cross-finger flap
- Damage to the terminal digital nerve with tissue loss as per the standard cross-finger flap

TECHNICAL POINTS

- Débride, create template, and outline flap as per standard cross-finger flap.
- Incise the skin obliquely, beginning at the midportion of the proximal flap incision and extending along the ulnar border of the first web space.
- Stop incision a few centimeters proximal to the midportion of the thumb web.
- Bluntly dissect a branch of the radial sensory nerve, typically found running deep on the muscle fascia.
- Trace nerve up to the flap.

- Dissect the flap as per the standard cross-finger flap, taking care not to divide the nerve as it enters the flap.
- Incise from the proximal margin of the thumb wound along the radial aspect of the first web space.
- Stop this incision at the proximal end of the incision used to identify the radial sensory nerve branch.
- Deflate the tourniquet and achieve hemostasis.
- Bluntly dissect and elevate the radial sensory nerve branch.
- During inset of the flap, transpose the nerve to the incision created on the ulnar aspect of the thumb.
- Harvest a graft large enough to allow coverage of the harvest site as well as the nerve pedicle at the proximal flap inset.

POSTOPERATIVE CARE

- As per the standard cross-finger flap.

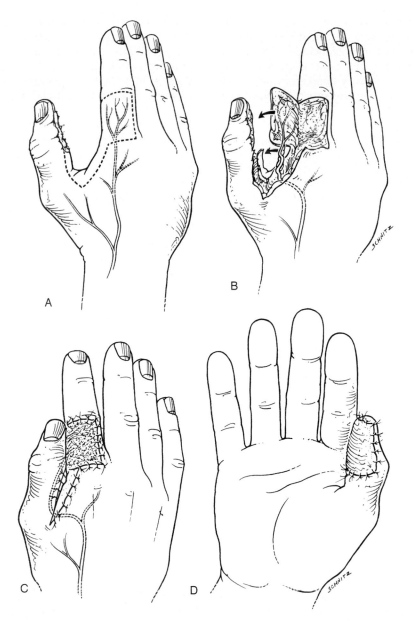

FIGURE 53-5. Radial sensory nerve–innervated cross-finger flap. **A,** Outline of the cross-finger flap with dorsal web incisions connecting to the thumb defect. The incision is made dorsal and proximal to the thumb web to prevent a subsequent scar contracture. The position of the dorsal sensory radial nerve is depicted. **B,** Reflection of the flap after dissection of the nerve branch. **C** and **D,** Position of the thumb and transferred flap with closure of incisions and free graft coverage of the donor defect. (Modified from Gaul JS Jr: Radial innervated cross finger flap from index to provide sensory pulp to injured thumb. J Bone Joint Surg Am 51:1257-1263, 1969, with permission.)

the flap has been mobilized to its base, the thumb is brought along the side of the index finger to check the positioning of the flap into the recipient defect (see Fig. 53-5B).

A connecting incision is made along the ulnar border of the thumb and carried proximally to the previous oblique incision extending from the flap. At the time of flap attachment, the nerve is carefully transposed from the dorsum of the index ray to the ulnar thumb incision after undermining has provided a satisfactory trough in which it can lie without tension. Suturing of the ulnar thumb incision and the connecting dorsal radial index incision will secure the position of the nerve, and the defect over the dorsum of the proximal phalanx is covered with a full-thickness skin graft dissected

from the antecubital fossa or groin. As in the standard cross-finger flap, enough graft is harvested to provide coverage of the exposed pedicle by suturing into the free ulnar edge of the thumb defect (see Fig. 53-5C and D).

A dressing and splint identical to that described for the standard cross-finger flap are applied. Flap monitoring and division are likewise as described earlier. In addition to active and passive motion rehabilitation, a protocol of gradually increasing pressure stimuli is added with the goal of increasing appropriate cortical recognition of the transferred flap. Risks inherent in using the innervated cross-finger flap include those related to damage to the mobilized branch of the radial sensory nerve secondary to undue tension or manipulation. Sensory return may only be protective, and the patient may continue to interpret thumb sensation as being that of the dorsal index finger. Nonetheless, the radial sensory-innervated cross-finger flap is a useful procedure when faced with irreparable sensory damage to the thumb with no other available source for reconstruction (Fig. 53-6).

Dual-Innervated Cross-Finger Flap

Under tourniquet hemostasis, thumb débridement, pattern creation, and flap design are carried out as described for the standard cross-finger flap. An incision is made from the proximal aspect of the flap along the radial aspect of the index metacarpal to the recess between the base of the index metacarpal and extensor pollicis longus. A second incision is then extended distally along the dorsoulnar aspect of the thumb metacarpal to the MCP joint and more distal thumb defect just palmar to the midaxial line (Fig. 53-7A).

Flap elevation is initiated along the distal and ulnar incisions on the index. As the incision is carried down to the level of the peritenon, small veins are divided with bipolar electrocautery. The flap is elevated in a dorsal-to-palmar direction while preserving the peritenon of the extensor mechanism and including all neurovascular structures within the flap. Along the incision coursing proximal over the index metacarpal, flaps are elevated superficial to the neurovascular structures. No attempt is made to separately dissect out the two to four terminal branches of the dorsal sensory radial nerve to the dorsal index. The subcutaneous tissue surrounding the dorsal sensory radial nerve contains veins and, in most instances, the first dorsal intermetacarpal artery; a narrow 0.5- to 1-cm-wide strip of this subcutaneous tissue should be raised down to the level of the investing muscle fascia to incorporate these nerve branches and, if the flap is to be transferred as an island pedicle, the artery and veins (see Fig. 53-7B). If an island flap is planned, the first dorsal intermetacarpal artery should be identified proximally before raising the subcutaneous portion of the flap to ensure that it is contained in the pedicle. Although most often, as stated by Foucher,[65] the artery runs superficial to the fascia, it may run deep to the fascia in 15% or consist of two vessels, one superficial and one deep, in 10%.[92] At the level of the MCP joint, the dorsal branch from the index radial digital nerve (median nerve distribution) is identified and dissected back to its origin. The connecting incision to the thumb is completed, and the ulnar digital nerve amputation stump proximal to the thumb defect is identified.

Transposition of the flap with the dorsal sensory radial nerve branches is accomplished as described earlier, and inset begins radially (see Fig. 53-7C and D). Before completion of the proximal and distal inset, microneurorrhaphy of the palmar ulnar digital nerve of the thumb to the more distal dorsal sensory nerve branch of the transposed flap is accomplished (Fig. 53-8). The connecting incisions are closed, and skin grafts are applied to the donor area.

Postoperative care, flap division, and rehabilitation are identical to that for the radial-innervated cross-finger flap previously described.

Neurovascular Island Pedicle Flap

Although historically developed before the innervated cross-finger flaps, the neurovascular island pedicle flap now plays a smaller role in the armamentarium of the hand surgeon. This stems not only from the increased technical difficulty of the procedure but also from the requirement of sacrificing palmar sensation along the ulnar aspect of another digit. As a result, important preoperative considerations include the selection of a donor digit and determination of the amount of digital skin and subcutaneous tissue to be brought with the pedicle. The main factor in choosing the donor digit is the status of the median nerve; if the median nerve function is intact, the ulnar aspect of the long finger provides a long neurovascular pedicle that can facilitate transposition of the flap. In the absence of median nerve function, an ulnar-innervated digit must be chosen; under these circumstances, the ulnar aspect of the ring finger may serve as a donor. In either setting, the ulnar aspects of the digits do not participate in pinch, making sacrifice of tactile surface an acceptable deficit. In general, the size of the flap should correspond to the deficit created by adequate débridement of the scarred and insensate tissue along the thumb defect; occasionally, it may be reasonable to use an "extended" neurovascular island transfer that consists of almost the entire ulnar palmar half of the donor digit to provide the widest possible areas of sensory restoration.[104,170,204,224,229,240] Thompson[238] emphasized that it is not necessary to apply the flap to the absolute tip of the thumb unless it is required for soft tissue coverage and that the position should favor the ulnar side of the thumb.

Variations on the flap have involved attempts to improve innervation as well as creative use of extended flaps. Several authors[2,3,66,94] have advocated suture of the divided proper digital nerve of the neurovascular island pedicle flap to the distal stump of a previously severed thumb digital nerve to improve sensation. Chen and Noordhoff[38] reported one case in which the entire distal phalanx of the thumb was resurfaced with twin neurovascular island flaps taken from the ulnar and radial sides of the middle and ring fingers.

Before beginning, it is necessary to determine the size of the thumb defect to be resurfaced; this measurement will mandate the size of flap to be used. Because most clinical conditions warrant the use of an extended flap involving the entire length of a donor digit, this technique is described here (Fig. 53-9A).

Under tourniquet hemostasis, the flap is outlined on the ulnar aspect of the donor digit; it extends from well out on the pad of the distal phalanx along the midline of the palmar aspect of the digit and terminates just short of the proximal digital crease. Small darts are created at the IP creases, and the flap extends posteriorly beyond the midlateral line to the dorsal aspect of the digit. A midlateral proximal continuation is then used to connect the digital incision with a series of palmar zigzag incisions. A paper template with the exact size and configuration of the flap is used to outline the recipient area on the palmar aspect of the thumb. A proximal connection into the palm is also provided in this area to facilitate passage of the flap. Under magnification, the dissection begins in the palm, and the neurovascular bundle to the web space is identified. The digital artery to the radial side of the adjacent finger is identified and ligated well away from the arterial bifurcation. The digital nerves to the adjacent sides of the long and ring fingers are carefully teased apart well into the mid palm. The artery and nerve to the ulnar side of the donor finger have now been isolated as far

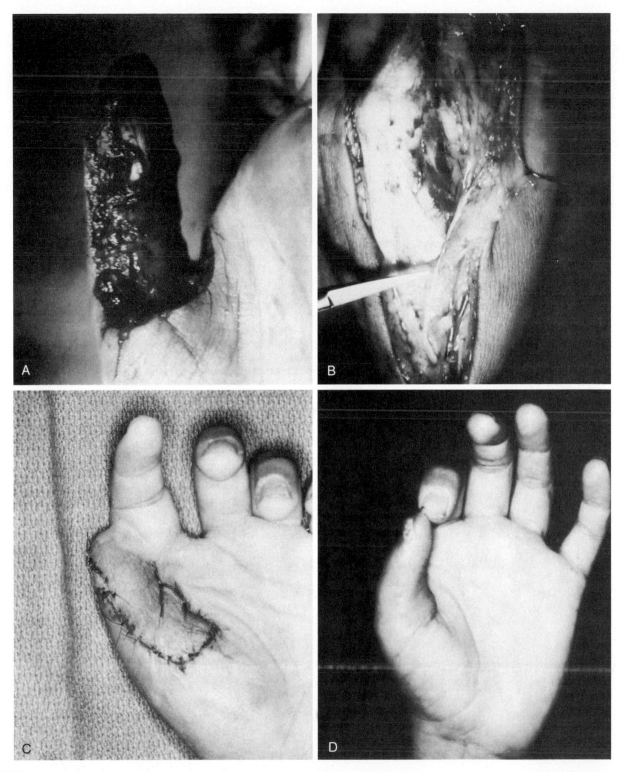

FIGURE 53-6. Large radial sensory nerve–innervated cross-finger flap. **A,** Avulsion of the entire palmar thumb after forceful removal of a circumferential pipe. **B,** Use of a large sensory-innervated cross-finger flap from the index finger and second metacarpal. Scissors indicate the nerve branch within the flap. **C,** Appearance of the flap on the palmar aspect of the thumb at the time of detachment (3 weeks). **D,** Appearance of the thumb with satisfactory motion and sensation at 9 months. (From Strickland JW: Restoration of thumb function following partial or total amputation. *In* Hunter JM, Schneider LH, Mackin E, Callahan AD [eds]: Rehabilitation of the Hand. St. Louis, CV Mosby, 1984, with permission.)

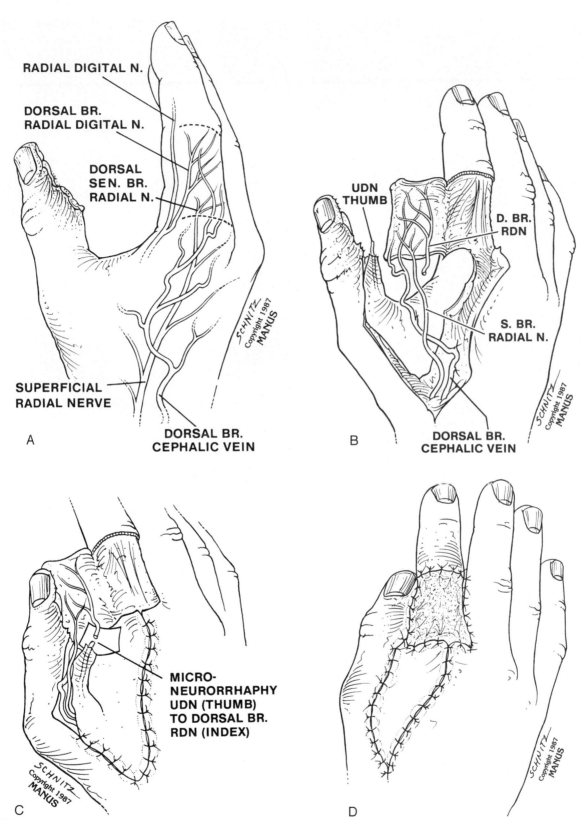

FIGURE 53-7. Dual innervated cross-finger flap. **A,** The dorsal sensory branch of the index radial digital nerve predictably innervates the distal dorsal aspect of the index proximal phalanx. **B,** Elevation of an index-to-thumb cross-finger flap with joining incisions for transposition of the dorsal sensory branch of the radial nerve. **C,** Microneurorrhaphy of the thumb ulnar digital nerve (UDN) to the dorsal branch of the index radial digital nerve (RDN). **D,** Appearance of the flap at closure. (From Hastings H 2nd: Dual innervated index to thumb cross finger or island flap reconstruction. Microsurgery 8:168-172, 1987, with permission.)

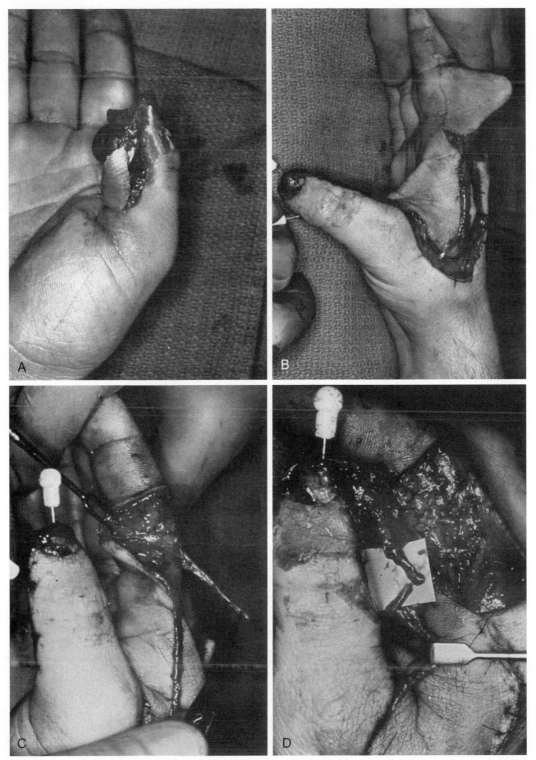

FIGURE 53-8. Use of the dual innervated cross-finger flap. **A,** Crush amputation of the pulp and nail bed of the thumb distal phalanx with a proximal phalangeal fracture. **B,** Dissection of the dorsal sensory radial nerve branches along the surrounding soft tissues to be transposed to the thumb. **C,** The dorsal branch of the index radial digital nerve provides ample pedicle for microneurorrhaphy to the thumb ulnar digital nerve after transposition of the cross-finger flap. **D,** Microneurorrhaphy of the index dorsal branch of the radial digital nerve to the ulnar digital nerve of the thumb. With a short regeneration distance, sensory return is rapid, predictable, and cortically perceived as the thumb. *Continued*

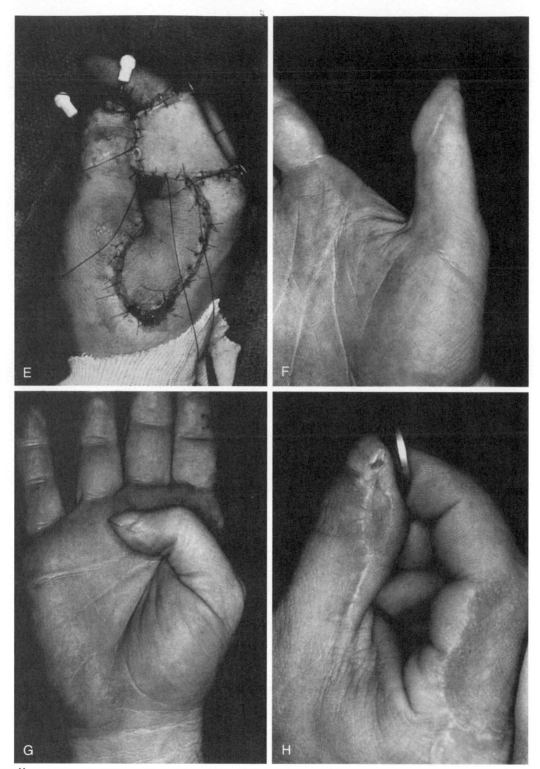

FIGURE 53-8.—cont'd E, A thick split-thickness skin graft is applied to both the donor area and the intervening pedicle between the index finger and thumb. **F** to **H,** Final appearance and function of the resurfaced thumb.

as the base of the finger and are dissected distally into the island flap. Incisions are then made about the entire periphery of the flap, and dissection is performed distally and carefully continued in a proximal direction while incorporating skin, subcutaneous tissue, and the neurovascular bundle, which should be protected by the surrounding soft

tissue. The flap is freed on its neurovascular pedicle to the level of the mid palm. Small vascular branches are cauterized and transected during this dissection.

Skin and scar within the previously outlined recipient site on the thumb are excised, and a bridge between the proximal thumb incision and the proximal end of the palmar incision

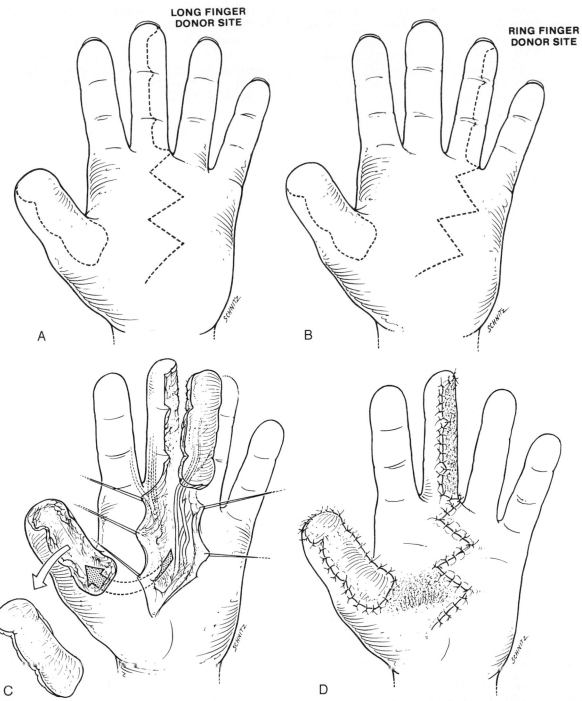

FIGURE 53-9. Neurovascular island transfer from either the long or ring finger to provide sensate coverage of the thumb. **A,** Neurovascular island flap using the ulnar side of the long finger. An extended island flap is designed with an identical defect patterned over the palmar aspect of the thumb. **B,** Use of the ulnar aspect of the ring finger, which is designed and transferred in a similar manner, is depicted. **C,** Mobilization of the island flap on its neurovascular pedicle and preparation of the recipient bed on the thumb. Note the areas of undermining required between the palmar and thumb incisions *(dotted arrow).* **D,** Completed transfer of the neurovascular island flap with a free graft on the donor area of the long finger. Care must be taken to avoid a longitudinal scar along the palmar aspect of the donor finger. (Modified from Reid DAC: Reconstruction of the mutilated hand. *In* Rob C, Smith R, Pulvertaft RG [eds]: Operative Surgery: The Hand, 3rd ed. London, Butterworths, 1977, with permission.)

is carefully undermined in an area just deep to the palmar aponeurosis (see Fig. 53-9B). A suture placed in the distal end of the island pedicle flap is used to gently pull the flap from the palmar wound into the thumb wound, with great care taken to not damage or twist the pedicle (see Fig. 53-9C). It is important to create some redundancy of the pedicle to prevent tension and ensure viability and sensibility of the flap.

The transferred flap is loosely tagged in place in the recipient defect, and the tourniquet is released. Troublesome bleeders are ligated, and the vascularity of the flap can be assessed. Completion of flap suture and repair of the palmar and proximal digital wounds is carried out at this time. A full-thickness skin graft taken from the groin is then sutured into the donor defect (see Fig. 53-9D).

The skin graft is covered with a nonadherent dressing and moist gauze, following which a compressive dressing is applied to the entire hand. The dressing over the distal tip of the thumb should be opened to expose the most distal portion of the flap and allow monitoring of viability. Full dressing change at 7 to 10 days is carried out, and motion is permitted at 3 to 4 weeks.

Potential complications include partial or complete flap necrosis, failure of the graft, or stiffness of the donor finger. Obviously, the loss of sensate skin in the donor finger is considerable; however, when the indications are appropriate, the restoration of good palmar sensory skin to the critical tactile pad of the thumb is functionally justified. Few adults will convert sensory recognition of the transferred flap to that of the thumb.[99,170]

Summary: Reconstruction of Soft Tissue Defects of the Thumb

The primary goal in treating tissue loss of a thumb of adequate length is to provide or improve skin coverage while optimizing the chance for return of satisfactory sensation without pain. Although providing additional length is not necessary at this level, techniques directed at preserving stump length or covering significant palmar soft tissue losses may be useful. The choice of procedure will be dictated primarily by the size of the defect. Defects less than 1 cm^2 and healing by secondary intention will provide adequate coverage with no additional donor wound. For defects less than 2.5 cm in length, the palmar advancement flaps offer excellent coverage with minimal morbidity and no need for sensory cortical reorganization. Larger lesions may require one of the heterodigital flaps. Circumferential soft tissue loss with preservation of the underlying skeletal and tendinous structures often requires reconstruction using

---

CRITICAL POINTS: NEUROVASCULAR ISLAND PEDICLE FLAP

INDICATIONS

- Extensive loss of the palmar thumb pulp
- Loss of terminal digital nerve innervation, particularly of the ulnar thumb

TECHNICAL POINTS

- Choose donor digit based on remaining intact innervation: either ulnar long finger (median intact) or ulnar ring finger (ulnar intact).
- Determine size of defect to be resurfaced and create template.
- Outline template on ulnar aspect of the donor digit, extending from distal palmar pad to just short of the proximal digital crease.
- Center the template such that the donor flap begins at the midpalmar aspect of the digit and extends onto the dorsum of the donor digit.
- Add small darts to the flap design at the IP creases.
- Connect the proximal flap design via an incision along the midlateral aspect of the digit to a series of zigzag incisions on the palm.
- Create the palmar thumb defect to fit the flap design.
- Extend the recipient site via an incision into the palm in a similar fashion to the donor digit extension, leaving a skin bridge of 1 to 2 cm between the donor zigzag incision and the thumb proximal incision.
- Identify the common digital artery/nerve to the donor web space.
- Ligate the proper digital artery to the adjacent (nondonor) finger radial aspect at least 5 to 10 mm away from the bifurcation.

- Tease apart the common digital nerve into the proximal palm, separating the donor ulnar nerve from the adjacent radial sensory branch.
- Dissect the donor artery and nerve to the base of the flap.
- Incise the margins of the flap.
- Raise the flap, including skin, subcutaneous tissue, and the neurovascular bundle.
- Undermine the skin bridge between the two proximal extending incisions just deep to the palmar aponeurosis.
- Place a suture in the distal flap and pass this through the tunnel into the thumb defect wound.
- Gently pull the flap through into the thumb defect.
- Tag the flap in place and release the tourniquet.
- Achieve hemostasis.
- Inset the flap with fine, nonabsorbable sutures.
- Harvest a full-thickness skin graft and inset this into the donor defect using fine chromic sutures.
- Apply a nonadherent dressing and moist gauze; leave the thumb tip of the dressing open to facilitate monitoring of the flap.
- Apply a volar resting splint from fingertip to distal forearm and a gentle compressive dressing.

POSTOPERATIVE CARE

- Inspect the flap/graft at 7 to 10 days.
- Begin active range-of-motion exercises at 3 to 4 weeks.

local and regional flaps for hand coverage (see Chapters 47 and 48). A secondary, but important, consideration will involve the extent of nerve damage. Radial sensory-innervated cross-finger flaps and neurovascular island pedicle flaps are procedures that occasionally may be used for acute thumb injuries with loss of skin, subcutaneous tissue, and one or both digital nerves. Although these procedures result in varying degrees of impairment to their respective donor areas and often involve some difficulties with patient cortical interpretation, they are time-honored methods of improving function in certain instances of devastating palmar thumb loss and are best used as secondary restorative methods.

Subtotal Amputation With Questionable Remaining Length

Amputations of primarily the palmar soft tissues can be managed as described in the preceding section; however, because the tissue loss extends to involve the phalanges the requirement for a thumb of adequate length for opposition begins to fail. Although provision of extra thumb length in the setting of acute injury has been performed,[239a] the surgeon is more commonly presented with a patient who has undergone a completion amputation at the initial presentation and who now seeks advice regarding reconstructive options. Under these circumstances it is imperative that the choice of reconstruction, ranging from none to free toe transfer, be carefully tailored to the patient's needs. Minimal bone loss, up to the level of the thumb IP joint, will be unlikely to significantly impair function. In contrast, loss of length proximal to the midportion of the proximal phalanx decreases hand span, creating difficulty with grasping large objects and problems with dexterous pinch. After amputation at this level, most thumbs retain acceptable CMC rotation and an adequate thumb/index finger cleft. Functional requirements at this level therefore include added length with preservation of sensibility, mobility, and stability and a pain-free status of the thumb.

When unsalvageable amputations occur near the distal portion of the proximal phalanx, satisfactory thumb function can usually be achieved by procedures designed to deepen the first web space and create a widened thumb/index finger interval. These procedures have been called phalangization, and they use methods that deepen the interdigital cleft so that the first metacarpal and remaining proximal phalanx are relatively lengthened.* This may be accomplished by simple scar-lengthening techniques; local, regional, or distal pedicle flaps; or, when necessary, free tissue transfer. The indications for these techniques vary according to residual thumb length, amount of first web contracture, mobility of the first metacarpal, and the condition of the web space skin and muscle.† Apart from their use in thumb reconstruction, these techniques may also prove useful when contracture of the first web space has occurred after thumb reconstruction by another procedure such as free toe transfer.

---

*See references 6, 20, 21, 36, 56, 63, 64, 85, 100, 103, 108, 131, 135, 136, 139, 154-156, 158, 172, 177, 179, 199, and 212.

†See references 4, 20, 21, 63, 103, 135, 136, 139, 158, 172, 212, and 245.

"Z"-Plasty Procedures

"Z"-plasty techniques are designed to lengthen the distance between the apices of the "Z" at the cost of narrowing the distance between the endpoints of the "Z." The simple and the four-flap "Z"-plasty take advantage of both actions to increase the thumb/index finger span and simultaneously deepen the first web space. Prerequisites for effective web space deepening via "Z"-plasty include (1) at least half of the proximal phalanx remains, (2) the skin is minimally scarred, (3) the first metacarpal is mobile, and (4) there is no muscle contracture.[26,100,199,229,260] The following sections discuss the concepts of "Z"-plasty, including proper flap design, mobilization, and repositioning as applied to the first web space.

Simple "Z"-Plasty of the Thumb Web

Under tourniquet hemostasis, the central limb of the planned "Z" is marked on the distal ridge of the first web space, extending from the proximal digital crease of the thumb to approximately 1 cm proximal to the proximal digital crease of the index finger at a point that corresponds with the radial confluence of the proximal and middle palmar creases. Using these landmarks as guidelines decreases the likelihood of extending the flap onto the ulnar thumb or radial index finger. Oblique proximal palmar and distal dorsal limbs oriented at 60-degree angles to the central limb are then designed with their length corresponding to the length of the central limb. Local scar, previous incisions, or possible approaches for other reconstructive procedures may result in a need to reverse the direction of the two oblique limbs (proximal dorsal and distal palmar). Either combination seems to work satisfactorily (Fig. 53-10A), but the combination of proximal palmar and distal dorsal parallels the interthenar crease and affords excellent cosmesis to the closure.

After incising the skin, dissection is carried down to the level of the muscle fascia. The flaps are carefully undermined just superficial to the muscle fascia to avoid vascular compromise. Care should be taken during the dissection to avoid injuring, if present, a distal arterial connection between the indicis radialis and princeps pollicis vessels. Deepening of the web space is facilitated by incision of the fascia over the first dorsal interosseous muscle and partial division of its distal mass (see Fig. 53-10B). Abducting the thumb will tend to begin transposing the flaps; as the span between the thumb and index increases, the distance across the web space, from dorsal to palmar, decreases. This decrease is compensated for by the recession of the first dorsal interosseous muscle. Once the flaps are reversed and sutured in place, the result is an increased web span and deepened web space (see Fig. 53-10C and Fig. 53-11).

Four-Flap "Z"-Plasty of the Thumb Web

Under tourniquet hemostasis, the central limb of the "Z"-plasty is drawn on the distal edge of the thumb web ridge as described for the simple "Z"-plasty (Fig. 53-12A). Proximal palmar and distal dorsal limbs at angles varying from 90 to 120 degrees relative to the central limb are then made with their lengths equaling that of the longitudinal incision. The angles formed by these three limbs are bisected by oblique lines, equal in length to the prior limbs, extending from their apices and yielding four angles ranging from 45 to 60

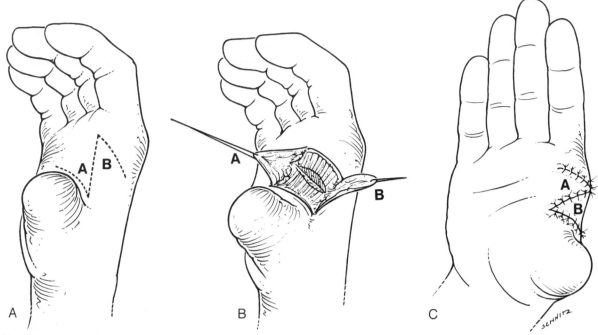

FIGURE 53-10. Simple "Z"-plasty of the thumb web. **A,** Design of the "Z"-plasty. The preferred angles are approximately 60 degrees. **B,** Flaps reflected with partial recession of the web space musculature. **C,** Appearance of the flaps after reversal and suture. Comer sutures are preferred in the tips of the flaps.

CRITICAL POINTS: FOUR-FLAP Z-PLASTY

INDICATIONS

- Amputation near the midportion of the proximal phalanx
- Minimal scarring of the first web skin
- Absence of first web muscle contracture
- Mobile first metacarpal

TECHNICAL POINTS

- Mark the central limb of the planned "Z" on the distal ridge of the first web space, beginning at the proximal digital crease of the thumb and extending to 1 cm proximal to the proximal digital crease of the index.
- Design proximal palmar and distal dorsal limbs at an angle between 90 and 120 degrees relative to the central limb; the combined length of these limbs should equal the length of the central limb.
- Add two more limbs, each equal in length to the proximal and distal limbs and each positioned to bisect the angle between the proximal/distal limbs and the central limb.
- Incise the skin along the markings, and gently undermine the flaps.

- If necessary to provide added depth, incise the musculature to deepen the web space.
- Transpose the flaps such that the common border of the central flaps (the central limb) comes to lie against the proximal and distal incision sites.
- Transpose the proximal palmar and distal dorsal flaps such that their medial edges (previously the bisecting limbs) are joined.
- Inset the flaps with fine, nonabsorbable suture.
- Apply a nonadherent gauze and gentle compressive dressing.

POSTOPERATIVE CARE

- Examine wound at 10 to 14 days.
- Switch to a thermoplastic splint to maintain web space.
- Begin active and passive range-of-motion exercises immediately after the first dressing change.
- Wean the web spacer splint over the course of a few weeks.

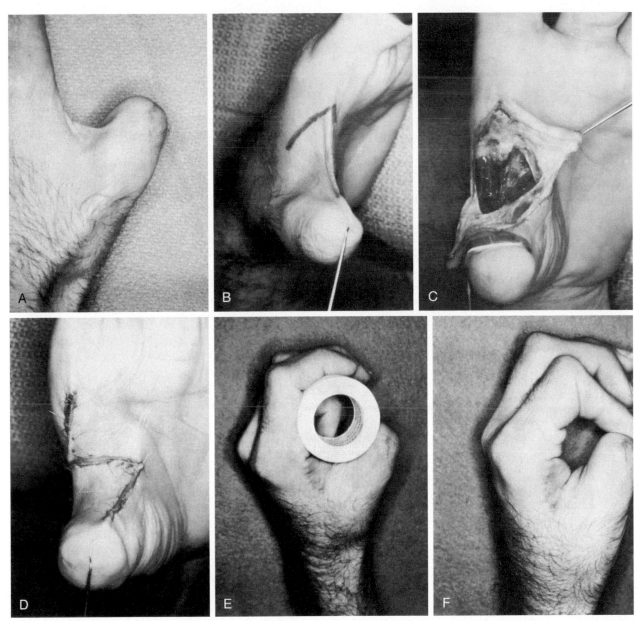

FIGURE 53-11. Simple "Z"-plasty of the thumb web. **A,** Limited thumb-index cleft following amputation through the midproximal phalanx. **B,** Design of the "Z"-plasty. **C,** Reflection of flaps with partial recession of the first web musculature. **D,** Appearance of the "Z"-plasty after reversal and suture of flaps. **E and F,** Effective deepening of the thumb web 3 months postoperatively. (From Strickland JW: Restoration of thumb function following partial or total amputation. *In* Hunter JM, Schneider LH, Mackin E, Callahan AD [eds]: Rehabilitation of the Hand. St. Louis, CV Mosby, 1984, with permission.)

degrees (see Fig. 53-12B and C; Fig. 53-13A). The flaps are reflected on their bases by gentle undermining, and a small recession of the thumb web musculature may be carried out to provide further depth.

The flaps are then transposed so that the common border of the two middle flaps previously formed by the central limb now comes to lie against the proximal and distal incision sites (see Fig. 53-12D and E). The proximal palmar and distal dorsal flaps are rotated to the midline, and their medial edges, previously formed by the oblique bisecting incisions, are joined. The flaps are then sutured in place without tension. Completion of flap transposition should result in a substantial increase in web depth (see Figs. 53-12F and 53-13B).

At the conclusion of the procedure, the wound is dressed with nonadherent gauze and a compressive dressing consisting of adequate gauze to maintain the expanded web space is applied. The wound is examined at an interval ranging from 10 to 14 days, at which time the bulky dressing is exchanged for a static, custom-fitted splint. Therapy consisting of active and passive range of motion begins after this initial dressing change; the patient continues to wear the web spacer splint when not performing range-of-motion exercises. Use of the splint is gradually weaned over the following few weeks based on the individual patient's progress with therapy.

These simple skin mobilization techniques, occasionally combined with short distal muscle recession, can provide

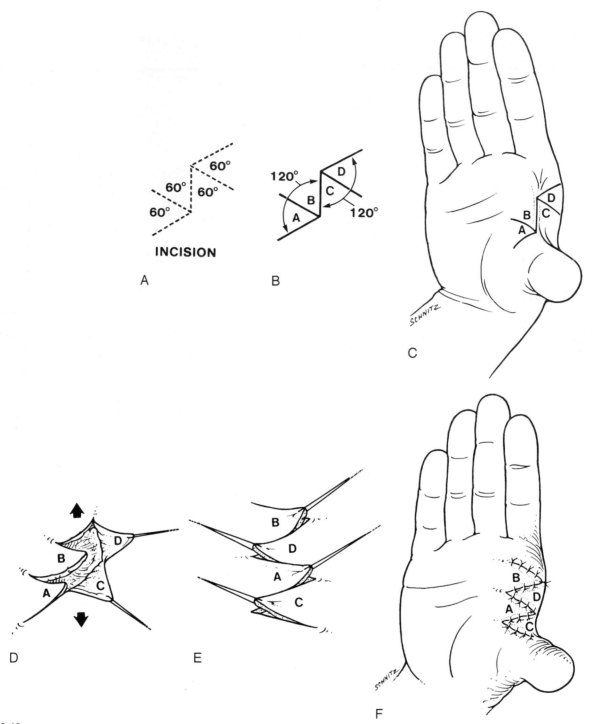

FIGURE 53-12. Four-flap "Z"-plasty of the thumb web. **A** and **B,** Two 120-degree-angle opposing incisions are bisected to form four 60-degree flaps. **C,** Design of the flaps in the first web space. **D,** Incision, elevation, and undermining of the flaps. **E,** Flap position after interposition. **F,** Appearance of the thumb web after interposition of the flaps. (Modified from Broadbent TR, Woolf RM: Thumb reconstruction with contiguous skin-bone pedicle graft. Plast Reconstr Surg 26:494-499, 1960, with permission.)

reliable deepening of the thumb web and relative lengthening of the shortened thumb. When measured, the gain in depth varies from 1.5 to 2 cm, which should result in improved ability to grasp larger objects. The main potential complication with these techniques is necrosis, either partial or complete, of the flaps; the risks can be minimized with careful planning and dissection of the flaps.

Dorsal Rotational Flap

When at least half of the proximal phalanx of the thumb remains but extensive scarring of the first web skin or an adduction contracture of the first metacarpal exists, "Z"-plasty techniques are no longer useful. To phalangize the residual thumb stump, sequential division of all restraining skin, muscle, scar, and capsular adhesions may be necessary.

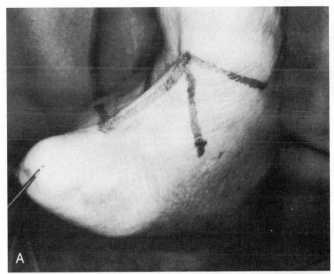

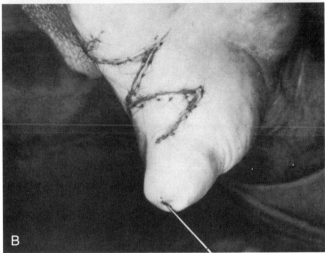

FIGURE 53-13. Four-flap "Z"-plasty of the thumb web. **A,** Design of flaps (see the text and Fig. 53-12). **B,** Appearance of the thumb web immediately after transposition and suture of the flaps.

Such extensive mobilization is likely to result in a significant skin deficit over the first web. Several dorsal rotational flap techniques have proven effective in deepening the first web space and mobilizing and resurfacing the metacarpal phalanx unit.* Advantages of web space coverage by a dorsal rotational flap include both the excellent quality of the skin and the sensory perception that it brings into the web.

Phalangization of the First Metacarpal With Dorsal Rotational Flap Coverage

With the use of tourniquet anesthesia, a continuous linear dorsal and palmar incision is carried through the first web, beginning dorsally at the level of the trapeziometacarpal joint and extending along the ulnar border of the first metacarpal to the first MCP joint, where it passes through the thumb web and continues palmarward into the palm at the base of the thenar eminence (Fig. 53-14).

---

*See references 21, 36, 62, 135, 183, 199, 212, 221, 225, 229, and 246.

Sharp dissection is continued just ulnar to the extensor pollicis longus. With careful technique to protect sensory branches of the radial nerve, the origin of the first dorsal interosseous muscle is stripped from the metacarpal; or, if the muscle has become scarred or fibrotic, it is divided. The radial artery must be identified as it dips between the two heads of the first dorsal interosseous muscle just beyond the trapeziometacarpal joint. By following the artery distally, the princeps pollicis artery can be identified and protected as the border of the adductor pollicis is defined. Both the oblique and transverse heads of the adductor are divided; and by gentle abduction traction on the first metacarpal, a determination can be made about the adequacy of mobilization of the first ray. Stripping of the opponens pollicis muscle may be required to mobilize a severely contracted first metacarpal. In some instances, muscle release will not result in complete mobilization of the first metacarpal and release of the CMC joint capsule or occasionally trapezial excision may be necessary. The capsule of the trapeziometacarpal joint is opened transversely through a palmar incision, and a similar capsulectomy on the dorsal ulnar side of the joint is sometimes used. The mobilized thumb is stabilized in the corrected position by transfixing the first and second metacarpals through their proximal segments with two nonparallel Kirschner wires (see Fig. 53-14D) or with an external fixator (Fig. 53-15). Tourniquet release is carried out at this point, and all brisk bleeding vessels are controlled and the vascularity of the thumb confirmed before re-inflation. Trial rotation of a paper pattern placed over the dorsum of the hand will help determine the proper size and configuration of the flap. The incision is continued from the ulnar aspect of the first web dorsally across the radial aspect of the MCP joint of the index finger and onto the dorsum of the proximal phalanx of that digit. It is then brought proximally over the dorsum of the hand to approximately the base of the fourth metacarpal, although the exact configuration can best be determined by the paper pattern technique just described (see Fig. 53-14B and C). The dorsal flap is dissected free from the peritenon overlying the extensors of the fingers, and although there is minimal interference with the dorsal veins of the hand, a few sizable veins should be ligated distally and brought with the flap (see Fig. 53-14C). Gentle undermining is carried out, and an occasional additional dorsal ulnar skin release may be necessary to bring the flap into proper position to cover the defect. The flap is then sutured in place, and the resulting triangular defect over the dorsal radial aspect of the hand is covered with either a dissected, nearly full-thickness graft from the groin or a split-thickness graft taken with a dermatome (see Fig. 53-14D).

A nonadherent gauze and saline-moistened cotton dressing is used over the graft. Kirschner wires are bent and trimmed, and a compressive dressing is applied to the hand, wrist, and forearm. The flap and grafts are first checked at 7 to 10 days and the sutures removed at 2 weeks. Active and passive therapy for digital mobilization begins at 2 to 3 weeks; during this initial rehabilitation a custom-made first web splint is worn to provide additional maintenance of the web space. The pins are removed at 4 to 6 weeks, after which the patient is gradually weaned from continuous use of the web splint. Continuous monitoring of the status of the web space will be necessary for 1 year, and night splinting

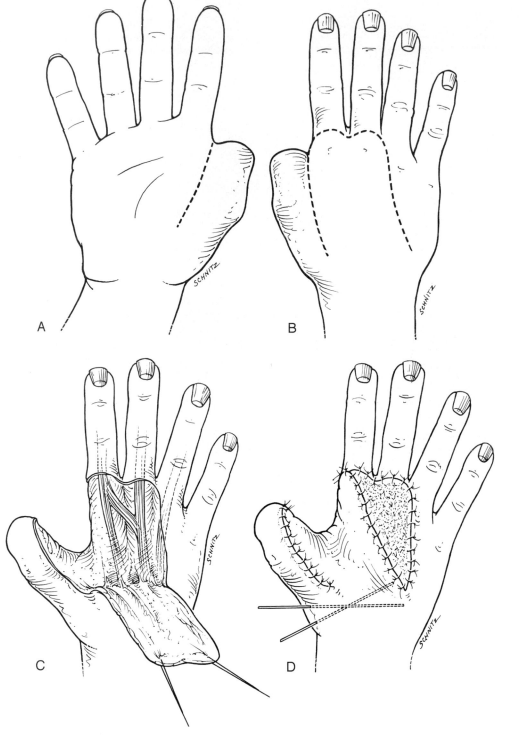

FIGURE 53-14. Release of adduction contracture of the first web space with dorsal rotational flap coverage. **A,** The palmar web–dividing incision is a continuous linear incision from the first web space to the thenar crease paralleling the medial margin of the thenar musculature. **B,** Linear incision over the dorsum of the first web with approximate outline of the dorsal rotational flap. **C,** First web defect after division of restraining skin, soft tissue, and muscle with abduction of the first metacarpal. Elevation of the dorsal rotational flap down to the peritenon overlying the extensor tendons is complete. **D,** Appearance of the first web after coverage with the dorsal rotational flap. Kirschner wires hold the thumb in abduction during healing, and a free skin graft is used to cover the donor defect. (Modified from Brown PW: Adduction-flexion contracture of the thumb: Correction with dorsal rotation flap and release of contracture. Clin Orthop 88:161-168, 1972, with permission.)

with a web spacer may be necessary throughout that time period.

Long-standing severe adduction contracture of the first metacarpal is a crippling deformity, particularly when a portion of the distal thumb has been lost. Surgical release of the deformity is accomplished by meticulous sequential division of all contracting elements and will result in a substantial skin and soft tissue deficit, which may be well covered by the use of a rotation flap from the dorsum of the hand (Fig. 53-16).

Potential complications include hematoma formation, flap loss, graft failure, or recurrent adduction contracture. If the surgical procedure is carefully carried out with attention to technical detail and if proper postoperative care is used, the incidence of these problems should be minimal. Additional reconstructive procedures such as tendon transfers may be necessary to further enhance thumb function; however, restoration of the web space and improvement in thumb posture alone should have a profoundly favorable influence on hand performance (Fig. 53-17).

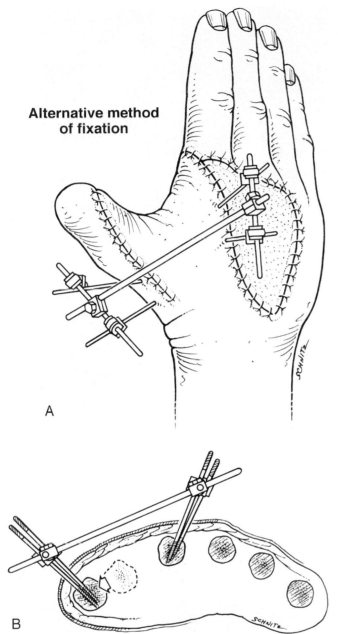

Alternative method of fixation

A

B

FIGURE 53-15. An alternative method of fixation of the first and second metacarpals after first web space deepening. The use of a mini-external fixator is depicted. **A,** Purchase pins in the lateral aspect of the first metacarpal and dorsum of the second metacarpal with a transfixing bar used to stabilize and maintain the web. **B,** Transverse section to depict the position of the fixator pins in the metacarpals.

Regional and Distant Flaps

Just as damage to the first web skin and muscle contractures rendered the simple "Z"-plasty inadequate for thumb phalangization, addition of damage to the skin overlying the dorsum of the hand removes the possibility of deepening the web space with a dorsal rotation flap. In this setting, a remote pedicle source must be sought to provide quality coverage after releasing procedures. A variety of regional and distant flaps have been employed for coverage of defects on the hand, and these flaps may serve equally well for releasing contractures of the first web space and providing greater hand span. Because the locations and techniques

for elevating these flaps are described in detail in other chapters (see Chapter 47), they will be mentioned only briefly here. The distally based radial forearm[56] and posterior interosseous[48,184,261] flaps are both capable of reaching the first web space and providing excellent soft tissue coverage to allow web space deepening and expansion. When trauma to the arm has rendered both of these regional flaps unusable, free tissue transfer either alone, as in the lateral arm flap,[209] or as an adjunct to free toe transfer, may be used to augment the first web space.

Although seldom used owing to the awkwardness of positioning and the inconvenience of even simple activities such as donning a shirt, distant pedicled flaps such as the groin flap, pectoral flap, or cross-arm flap[172,199,227] can be used occasionally in these circumstances to provide excellent resurfacing of the first web space. Unlike the groin and pectoral flaps, the limited size of the cross-arm flap makes it less useful for general hand wound coverage; however, the flap can provide thin, supple skin for web space resurfacing and the contour of the arm is excellent for maintaining the web space while the pedicle is being vascularized.[172] The medial aspect of the arm bears the thinnest skin as well as a thin subcutaneous layer, making it the preferred donor site for the flap. Given its potential, albeit rare, utility in phalangization and web space creation, we will include a description of the cross-arm flap technique.

First Web Space Deepening with Cross-Arm Flap Coverage

Release of the first web space is carried out in a manner identical to that described for the dorsal rotational flap (Fig. 53-18A; see also Fig. 53-14). The abducted position of the thumb is maintained by the use of Kirschner wires crossed between the bases of the first and second metacarpals or by the use of an external fixator. The hand is then brought into place against the opposite arm in such a manner that the ulnar border of the hand can rest against the anterior medial surface of the forearm with the thumb comfortably placed around the inner aspect of the upper arm. Patterns are used to design a proximally based triangular flap that can be used to resurface the dorsal half of the divided web space (see Fig. 53-18B). The flap is meticulously elevated, including skin and subcutaneous tissue, and temporary split-thickness skin coverage is placed on the arm and palmar hand defects. Moist cotton stent dressings over the graft are important, and the position of the arm is maintained by the use of a plaster Velpeau dressing. At 2 to 3 weeks the patient is returned to the operating room and a corresponding triangular flap is designed proximally, which is then dissected out and turned into the palmar defect after the free graft is excised. Defatting of the flap is not usually necessary, and excellent restoration of the web space can be achieved in this manner (see Fig. 53-18C). A bulky dressing to maintain the web space is applied and changed at 7 to 10 days. Suture removal and web space splinting with a custom fit spacer are performed at 2 weeks. Rehabilitation and pin removal occur on the same schedule followed for the dorsal rotational flap. Likewise, monitoring for web space contracture may be necessary for up to 1 year, and night splinting with the web spacer may be necessary.

The cross-arm flap can provide excellent coverage after release of the first web space in patients with amputations

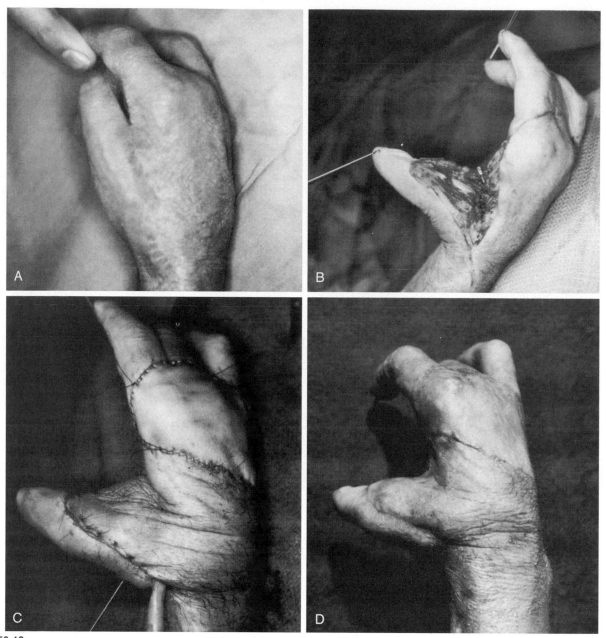

FIGURE 53-16. Phalangization of a severely contracted first metacarpal with a dorsal rotational flap. **A,** Severe, long-standing adduction contracture of the thumb after amputation through the proximal phalanx. **B,** Appearance of the thumb web after release of skin, soft tissue, web space musculature, and the basilar thumb joint. **C,** Coverage of the thumb web with a large dorsal rotational flap. **D,** Appearance of the thumb web at 3 months.

of the thumb through the middle third of the first ray. The procedure restores excellent skin and subcutaneous tissue both palmarly and dorsally without a need to use the frequently compromised dorsal hand skin. It has the disadvantage of a resulting defect on the opposite arm, and although it can in general maintain the hand in a position of function, it does cause obvious limitation of upper limb function during the period of obligatory immobilization. Nonetheless, it has proved to be an effective technique for web space widening and deepening and relative thumb lengthening in certain instances (Fig. 53-19).

Subtotal amputations at or proximal to the midportion of the proximal phalanx are unlikely to achieve adequate length solely through phalangization procedures. At this level, the reconstructive options overlap with techniques used to provide an opposable thumb in the setting of total amputation with preservation of the basal joint.

Total Amputation With Preservation of the Basal Joint

Although not the only possible reconstruction at this level, the reliability of free toe transfer procedures, the availability of microsurgical instrumentation, and the familiarity of most hand surgeons with the techniques have made free toe transfer the optimal choice for these amputations (Fig. 53-20A to D). Either great or second-toe transfer is often an excellent restorative option that can provide the necessary length,

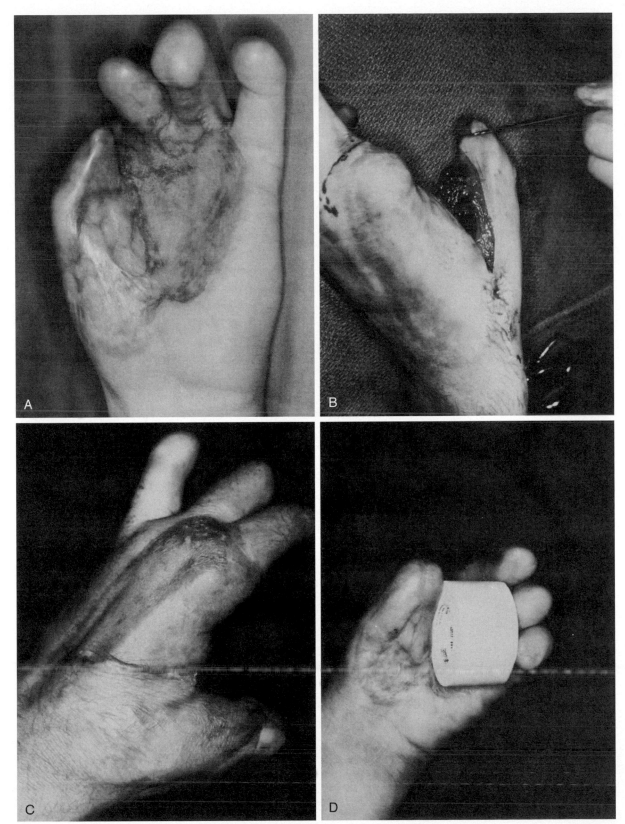

FIGURE 53-17. Phalangization of a damaged metacarpal-phalanx unit. **A,** Tightly contracted thumb metacarpal and proximal phalanx with poor skin coverage after a combination crush-burn injury. **B,** Mobilization of the metacarpal and division of the contracted web with excision of skin and division of the first dorsal interosseous and adductor pollicis muscles. **C,** Improved abduction of the phalangized thumb at 4 months. **D,** Improved grasp and pinch at 4 months. (From Strickland JW: Restoration of thumb function following partial or total amputation. *In* Hunter JM, Schneider LH, Mackin E, Callahan AD [eds]: Rehabilitation of the Hand. St. Louis, CV Mosby, 1984, with permission.)

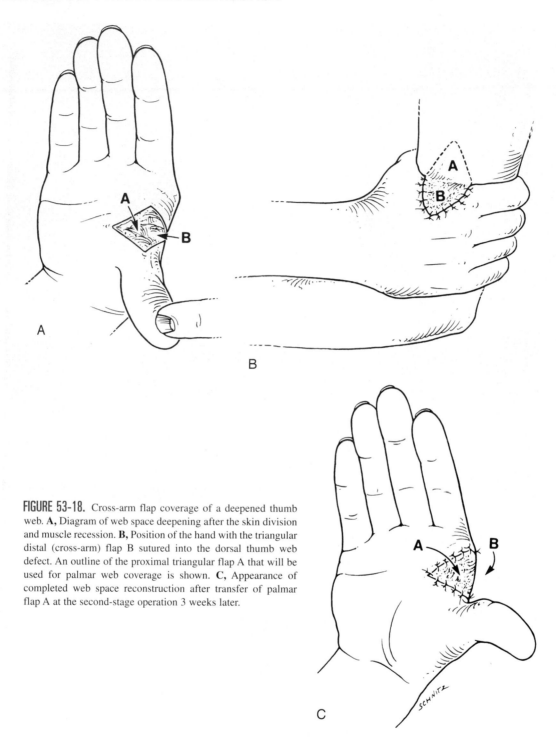

FIGURE 53-18. Cross-arm flap coverage of a deepened thumb web. **A,** Diagram of web space deepening after the skin division and muscle recession. **B,** Position of the hand with the triangular distal (cross-arm) flap B sutured into the dorsal thumb web defect. An outline of the proximal triangular flap A that will be used for palmar web coverage is shown. **C,** Appearance of completed web space reconstruction after transfer of palmar flap A at the second-stage operation 3 weeks later.

mobility, and sensibility for a functional thumb (see Fig. 53-20E and F). Given the evidence of excellent outcomes with free toe transfer (see Chapter 52),[41,69,168,253,254] the majority of patients seeking thumb reconstruction who require additional length will be prime candidates for these procedures. On occasion, there may be many patients who are unwilling to accept the cosmetic alteration of the foot or for whom athletic performance may be compromised after sacrifice of a toe. Alternative methods include metacarpal distraction/lengthening techniques, the use of osteoplastic reconstruction, and pollicization of an injured or partially

amputated digit.[156a] Distraction osteogenesis, as discussed at length elsewhere (see Chapter 54), may be useful when the amputation has spared a substantial amount of the first metacarpal. Under optimal conditions, progressive metacarpal distraction can safely result in 3 to 4 cm of additional length for patients with traumatic thumb amputation. Although distraction can provide additional length, motoring of the digit will depend on the residual function of the intrinsic muscles of the thumb. With increasingly proximal amputations, motor function may need to be provided through tendon transfers.

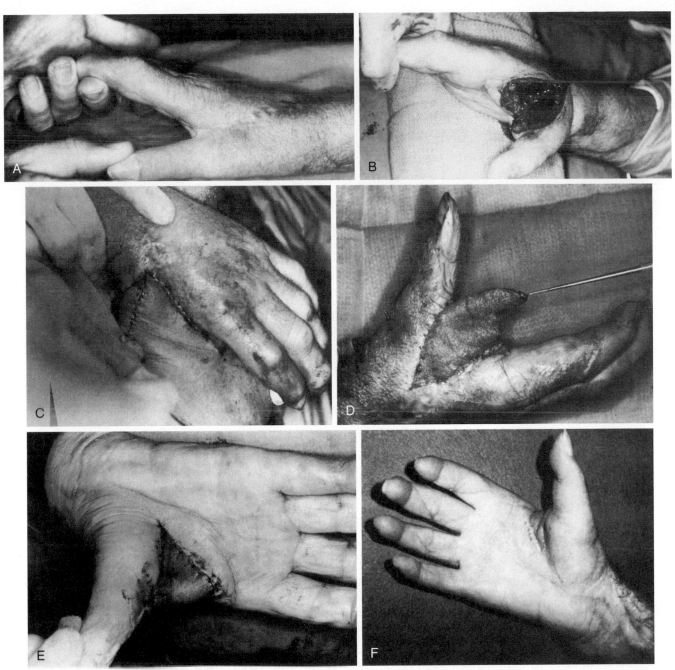

FIGURE 53-19. Clinical application of the cross-arm flap technique. **A,** Tightly contracted first web space with severe injury to the dorsal skin. **B,** Appearance of the thumb web defect after skin, muscle, and scar division. **C,** Appearance of the dorsal first web space coverage with the distal triangular upper arm flap. **D,** At 3 weeks after satisfactory healing of the dorsal flap the proximal triangular flap is transposed into the palmar web defect. **E,** Appearance of palmar web coverage at the time of insetting. **F,** Appearance of the first web space reconstructed with this technique.

Osteoplastic Reconstruction

Osteoplastic reconstruction, or thumb reconstruction by means of a bone graft covered with a pedicled flap, was first attempted by Nicoladoni[174] in 1897. Early reports of successful thumb reconstruction with the use of bone graft and tubed pedicle techniques* made this a preferred method of thumb reconstruction during the first half of the 20th

century; however, results were plagued by the inability to provide adequate sensory perception to the reconstructed thumb and significant resorption of the bone graft inside the pedicle. Moberg[162,163] and Littler[133,135] improved sensation by suggesting that a neurovascular island pedicle transfer be used as part of osteoplastic reconstruction of the thumb, and the use of large, extraperiosteal, tricortical iliac crest grafts may have reduced the extent of bone resorption.[127,167] Although toe-to-thumb free transfer procedures have largely supplanted osteoplastic reconstruction, it may still prove useful when there is good basilar joint motion, the fingers

*See references 4, 9, 11, 14, 54, 81, 83, 141, 174, 175, 185, 187, 188, 205, 208, 233, and 252.

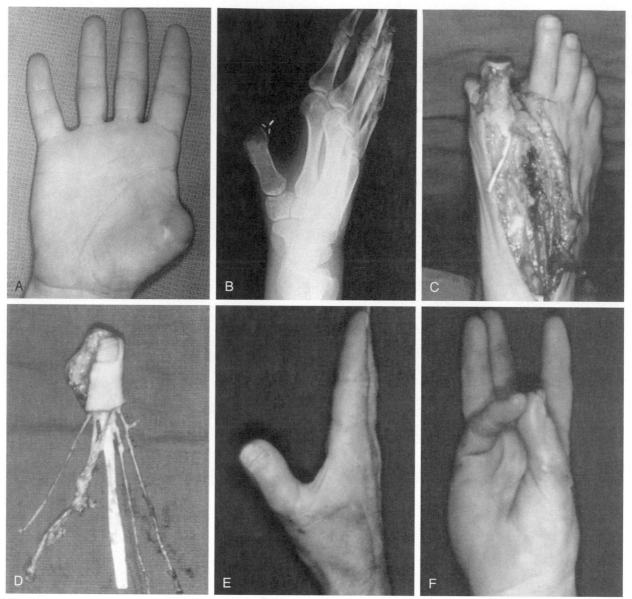

FIGURE 53-20. **A,** Nondominant right hand of a 36-year-old laborer after traumatic crush amputation of the thumb. **B,** Under ideal circumstances, the tissues of the amputation stump can be prepared at the time of initial débridement for ease of identification during later reconstruction (note the vascular clips on the digital arteries and nerves). The remaining musculotendinous units (e.g., extensor and flexor pollicis longus) should be pulled out to physiologic length and sutured securely at the distal end of the stump. This maneuver will prevent myostatic contracture of potential motor units. **C,** Harvest of the great toe for microvascular transplantation to an amputated thumb stump can, under select physiologic and psychological circumstances, provide greatly enhanced hand function after traumatic thumb amputation. **D,** The wraparound great toe flap relies on restoration of bony length, vascular inflow and outflow, increased thumb strength by extensor and flexor pollicis longus tenorrhaphy, and direct neurorrhaphy of the plantar digital nerves to the recipient radial and ulnar digital nerves of the thumb stump. **E** and **F,** Six months after "wraparound" great toe microvascular transplantation, the patient demonstrates excellent thumb opposition and thumb flexion across the palm to the small finger.

are normal or too badly damaged for transfer, and toe transfers or lengthening techniques are not appropriate.[127]

Variations on the osteoplastic theme include the Gillies "cocked-hat" flap, which uses local tissue to cover the bone graft (Fig. 53-21) and composite flaps based on the pedicled radial forearm flap.[13,19,34,46,56,145,257] Biemer and Stock[13] described a one-stage total thumb reconstruction using a composite flap containing skin and subcutaneous tissue, a segment of radial bone, a length of the lateral cutaneous nerve of the forearm, and two veins. The elevated flap is turned 180 degrees, and the radial bone is fixed to the first metacarpal. The digital nerves of the thumb are sutured to

the nerves in the flap, and vein anastomosis is optional. Foucher's technique[70] varies in that it restores sensation by means of a neurovascular island pedicle flap.

Osteoplastic Reconstruction of the Thumb: Two-Stage

Stage I (Fig. 53-22A to D)   A groin flap that includes the superficial circumflex iliac artery is patterned and raised on the same side as the hand whose thumb is to be reconstructed (see Chapter 47). The flap should have a width of 7.5 cm and a minimum length of 12 cm, with its free

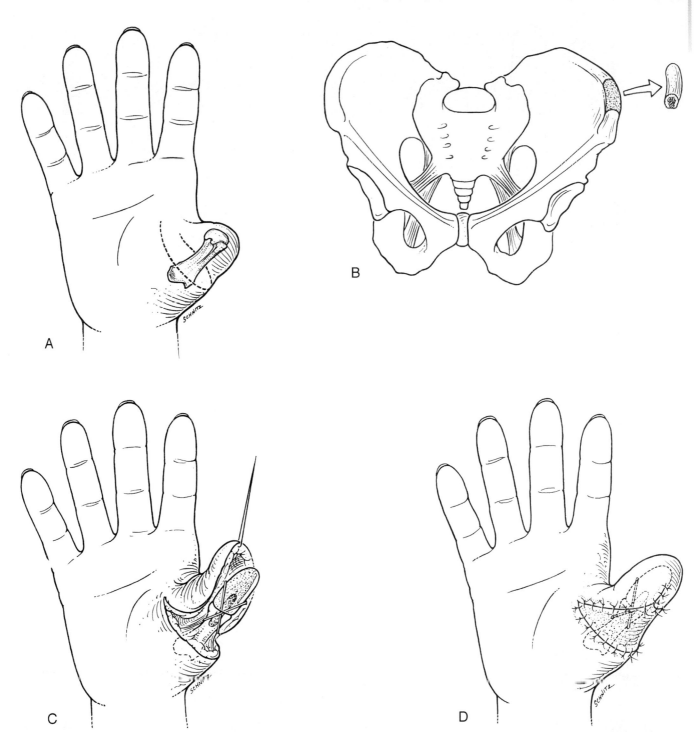

FIGURE 53-21. Gillies' "cocked-hat" flap. **A,** Outline of the incisions around the base of the thenar eminence. **B,** Tricorticocancellous iliac bone graft to elongate the first metacarpal. **C,** The flap is reflected and the graft is held in place with crossed Kirschner wire fixation. The graft may be stemmed for insertion into the metacarpal, or a cortical peg may be used to bridge the graft-metacarpal interval, as shown here. **D,** The flap brought back to cover the bone graft. A free skin graft covers the thumb defect. (Modified from Reid DAC: Reconstruction of the mutilated hand. *In* Rob C, Smith R, Pulvertaft RG [eds]: Operative Surgery: The Hand, 3rd ed. London, Butterworths, 1977, with permission.)

end positioned over the lateral prominence of the underlying iliac crest. A large extraperiosteal tricortical bone graft is then taken from the iliac crest; the graft should be 7 to 8 mm thick, 5 to 6 cm long, and 1.5 cm wide (see Fig. 53-22B).

Under tourniquet hemostasis, adequate débridement of scar, skin, and any necrotic bone from the distal metacarpal is carried out. A cuff of viable skin over the first metacarpal should be reflected to increase the vascular contact area of the flap. A small curet is used to fashion a hole in the medullary canal of the metacarpal, and the bone graft is shaped with a motorized bur to produce a stout cortical stem 2 cm in length. The graft is inserted and secured in the metacarpal so that its flattened raw edge is facing the

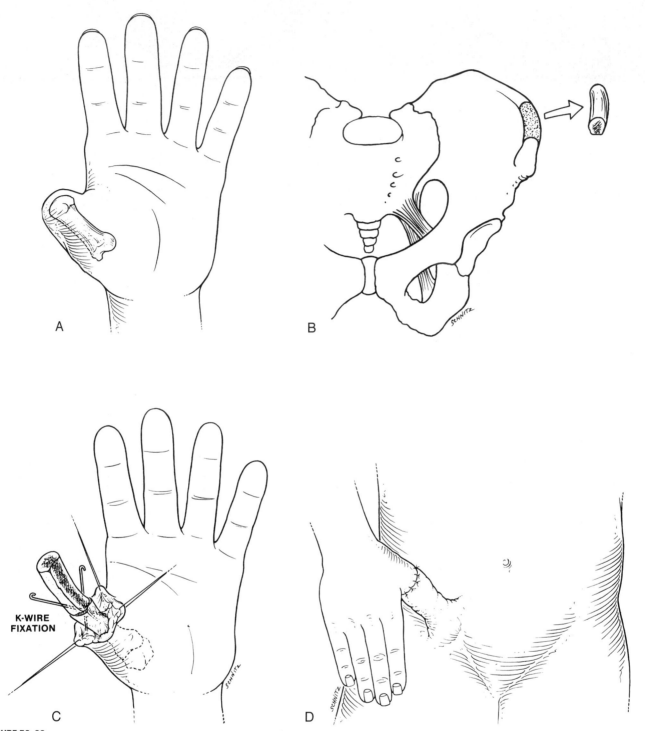

FIGURE 53-22. Osteoplastic reconstruction of the thumb. **A,** Thumb amputation through the metacarpophalangeal joint. **B,** Site of removal of extraperiosteal tricorticocancellous iliac crest bone graft. **C,** Preparation of the recipient site with insertion of the iliac crest graft into the first metacarpal shown here with Kirschner wire fixation. **D,** Bone graft coverage with a tubed groin flap. (Modified from Simonetta C: Reconstruction of the thumb by tube pedicle, bone graft and island flap. *In* Reid DA, Gosset J [eds]: Mutilating Injuries of the Hand. New York, Churchill Livingstone, 1979, with permission.)

index finger in opposition with the first metacarpal (see Fig. 53-22C). Lister has suggested that the fit of the graft peg into the metacarpal should be tight enough to enable lifting of the arm by the graft after insertion; however, fixation is typically secured by longitudinally or obliquely placed pins. The distal tip of the graft is shaped with a rongeur to remove any sharp edges and approximate the length of the IP joint of the normal thumb.

The substantial amount of subcutaneous fat present in most groin flaps necessitates defatting of the distal tip of the flap before inset. After careful removal of an adequate amount of fat, the flap is tubed along most of its length. The donor defect is undermined and closed without excessive tension, and the bone graft is inserted into the tube with the suture line coming to lie palmarly in preparation for insertion of the neurovascular island flap during the second

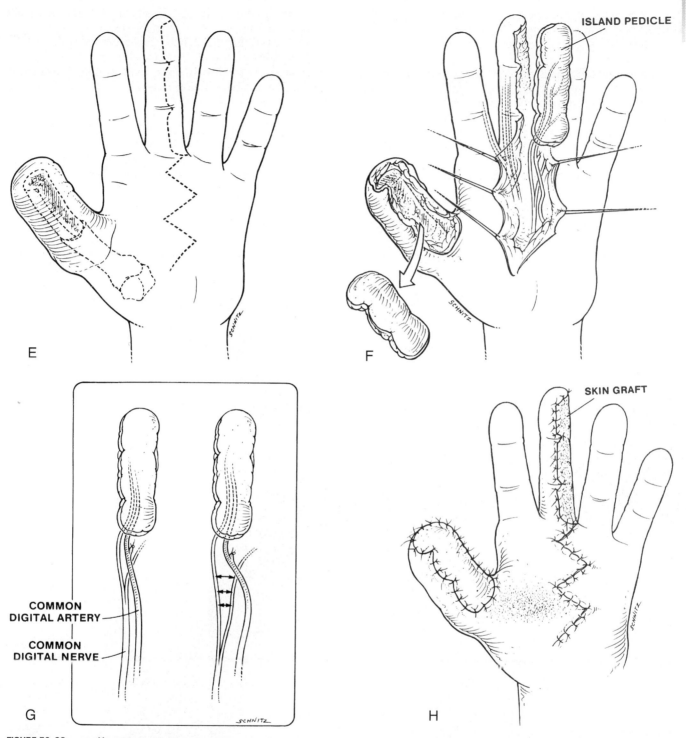

FIGURE 53-22—cont'd. E, Incisions for the use of an extended neurovascular island pedicle flap to provide vascularized and innervated skin on the palmar aspect of the reconstructed thumb. **F,** Transfer of the neurovascular island flap to the palmar thumb defect at the time of flap detachment. **G,** Severance of the digital artery to the opposite web and careful intraneural separation of the common digital nerve in preparation for tension-free transfer of the neurovascular island flap. **H,** Completion of neurovascular island transfer with a free skin graft to the donor defect in the long finger.

stage. The free end of the pedicle is then sutured to the expanded metacarpal skin defect (see Fig. 53-22D). Care is taken to avoid tension, twisting, or "kinking" of the pedicle; and a low-suction drain is placed in the groin wound for 24 to 48 hours. A soft Velpeau-type restraining dressing is used to comfortably immobilize the arm. Throughout the period of neovascularization of the flap, the patient is instructed to move the untethered fingers and wrist through a full range of

motion. The debate over how long to wait before pedicle division and performance of the second stage ranges from just over 8 days (provided an ischemic preconditioning protocol has been followed)[39,40] to 4 weeks.[214] Methods of assessing the readiness of the flap for division include fluorescein[151] testing, laser Doppler flowmetry,[39] and pulse oximetry.[57] Whichever testing modality is used, if question of the length of flap viability remains at 10 to 14 days, partial division of the flap and ligation of the superficial circumflex iliac artery may be performed under local anesthesia.

Stage II (see Fig. 53-22E to H)   At the time of complete tube release, whether at the time of initial assessment or after the partial delay procedure, an extended neurovascular island flap is raised from the ulnar aspect of the long finger and dissected well into the palm as described earlier. When re-creating the defect into which the flap will be placed, the surgeon should extend the defect over the distal aspect of the bone graft and dissect down to the raw bone on the palmar

side of the graft (see Fig. 53-22F and G). Passage, inset, and donor site closure are identical to the standard neurovascular island flap (see Fig. 53-22H).

A plaster-reinforced compressive dressing is used postoperatively for 7 to 10 days, and cast immobilization is continued until bony union is complete at 6 to 8 weeks. Gradually increasing use of the reconstructed thumb is then permitted.

Although rarely necessary, this type of thumb reconstruction is fairly rapid and does not require the use of other digits or toes (Fig. 53-23). Its disadvantages lie in the obligatory insult to the long finger and the tendency to continue

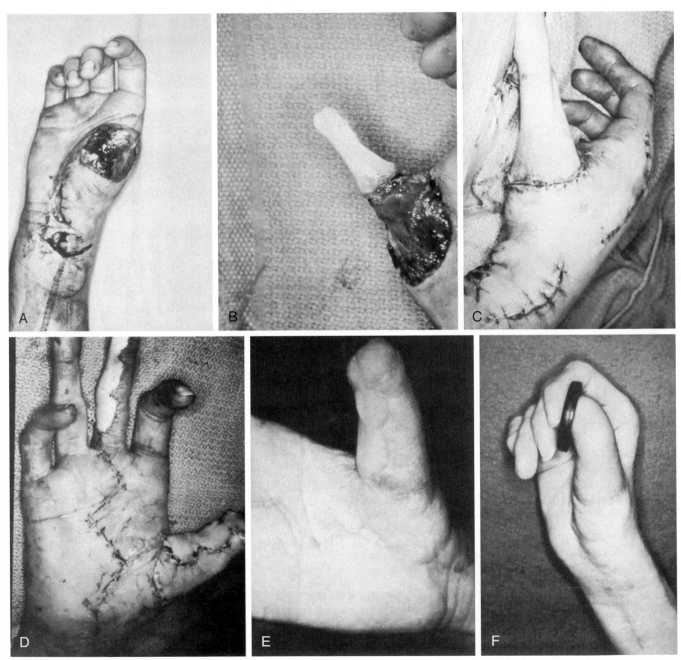

FIGURE 53-23. Osteoplastic reconstruction of an amputated thumb. **A,** Traumatic amputation of the thumb through the first metacarpal. **B,** Bone graft using the preserved proximal phalanx of the amputated thumb. **C,** Application of a thin, tubed upper abdominal pedicle flap. **D,** Transfer of an extended neurovascular island pedicle flap from the ulnar aspect of the long finger at the time of pedicle flap detachment. **E** and **F,** Appearance of the thumb unit at 9 months with satisfactory pinch and grasp functions. (From Strickland JW: Restoration of thumb function following partial or total amputation. *In* Hunter JM, Schneider LH, Mackin EJ, Bell JA [eds]: Rehabilitation of the Hand. St. Louis, CV Mosby, 1978, with permission.)

to perceive the reconstructed thumb unit as the long finger, although this may be a less bothersome phenomenon with the passage of time. The potential complications are numerous and include partial necrosis of the groin flap, loss of blood supply or diminished sensory perception in the neurovascular island flap, failure of the free graft to the long finger, and nonunion or resorption of the bone graft.

Composite Radial Forearm Island Flap

This procedure has the advantage of providing a well-vascularized skin and bone flap and, with the addition of an extended neurovascular island pedicle flap, avoids the staging necessitated by conventional osteoplastic methods. Preoperative requirements are those of the standard radial forearm flap (see Chapter 47), including a patent ulnar artery and palmar arch. The finding of a predominantly radial blood supply or the absence of an ulnar artery would preclude the use of this procedure.

The flap is designed from the palmar and radiodorsal aspect of the forearm, beginning several centimeters proximal to the radial styloid. It should be 7 to 8 cm in length and 6 to 7 cm in width (Fig. 53-24A). After preparation of the distal thumb stump, the flap, including the radial artery and its venae comitantes, is carefully raised. Great care is taken to not damage the cutaneous branches of the radial nerve or the blood supply to the radius just proximal to the styloid process. One or more small branches from the radial artery should be identified entering the pronator quadratus muscle and extending down to the periosteum of the radius. These vessels must be protected, often necessitating leaving a small amount of muscle attached to the radius. A bone flap measuring from 2 to 4 cm is patterned on the lateral side of the radius and designed to include the perforating branches from the radial artery. The bone is osteotomized with either powered or conventional bone instruments, with care being taken to protect the radial artery and perforating vessels. After ligating the radial vessels proximally, the entire flap is mobilized as a composite unit to the level of the anatomical snuff box. The abductor pollicis longus and extensor pollicis brevis tendons are freed proximally by releasing the distal

---

CRITICAL POINTS: COMPOSITE RADIAL FOREARM ISLAND FLAP

INDICATIONS

- Few, given the success of toe-to-thumb microvascular transfer
- Loss of the thumb at the mid to proximal metacarpal level
- Intact remaining digits, making sacrifice for pollicization less desirable
- Patency of the ulnar artery and superficial palmar arch

TECHNICAL POINTS

- Design a flap 7 to 8 cm in length and 6 to 7 cm wide over the volar, radiodorsal aspect of the forearm.
- Débride the distal thumb stump.
- Raise the flap as per a standard distally based, radial forearm flap.
- As dissection approaches the radial styloid, identify a branch of the radial artery coursing to or through the pronator quadratus and the underlying radius periosteum.
- Osteotomize a corticocancellous bone graft 2 to 4 cm long and 1.5 cm wide including the entry point of the feeding vessel from the radial artery.
- Ligate the radial vessels proximally, and elevate the composite flap to the level of the anatomical snuff-box.
- Incise the distal portion of the first dorsal extensor compartment to release the abductor pollicis longus and extensor pollicis brevis tendons
- Pass the composite flap under the abductor pollicis longus/extensor pollicis brevis and

extensor pollicis longus tendons and the overlying skin bridge into the dorsal aspect of the thumb wound.

- Avoid kinking or twisting of the pedicle during passage; if passage is difficult, create connecting incisions in the skin to facilitate passage.
- Orient the cancellous portion of the osseous portion of the flap such that it faces the index finger with the residual thumb metacarpal in opposition.
- Secure the bone portion of the flap to the thumb metacarpal using a small plate or Kirschner wires.
- Harvest a neurovascular island pedicle flap and transpose to the palmar aspect of the composite flap in the standard fashion.
- Release the tourniquet, achieve hemostasis, and inspect the transferred flaps for viability.
- Inset the flaps using fine, nonabsorbable suture.
- Harvest a split-thickness graft and inset this in the radial forearm harvest site.
- Harvest a full-thickness skin graft and inset this in the neurovascular island flap defect.
- Apply nonadherent gauze, a gentle compressive dressing, and a volar resting splint.

POSTOPERATIVE CARE

- Inspect the flaps at 1 week.
- Apply a short-arm/thumb spica cast after the initial dressing change.
- Continue cast immobilization for 6 weeks (possibly longer depending on bone healing).
- On cessation of casting, begin active and passive range-of-motion exercises.

FIGURE 53-24. Composite radial forearm flap. **A,** Incisions to be used for thumb reconstruction entailing a composite radial forearm island flap and neurovascular island flap taken from the ulnar side of the long finger. The radial flap is approximately 7 × 7 cm and is raised from the distal volar lateral forearm. **B,** Elevation of the flap together with a segment of the distal radius with careful preservation of radial artery communications between the skin and bone graft *(inset)*. The artery is ligated proximally, and the flap is tunneled under the first dorsal compartment. The position of the bone graft and the flap is shown. The neurovascular island pedicle flap is raised in preparation for palmar resurfacing of the reconstructed thumb. **C,** Dorsal appearance of the composite radial forearm flap and bone graft in position; a small T-plate is used for fixation. Note the position of the radial artery. **D,** Completion of the thumb reconstruction, with skin grafts used to cover the radial side of the long finger and the volar forearm. (Modified from Foucher G, Van Genechten M, Merle M, Michon J: Single stage thumb reconstruction by a composite forearm island flap. J Hand Surg [Br] 9:245-248, 1984, with permission.)

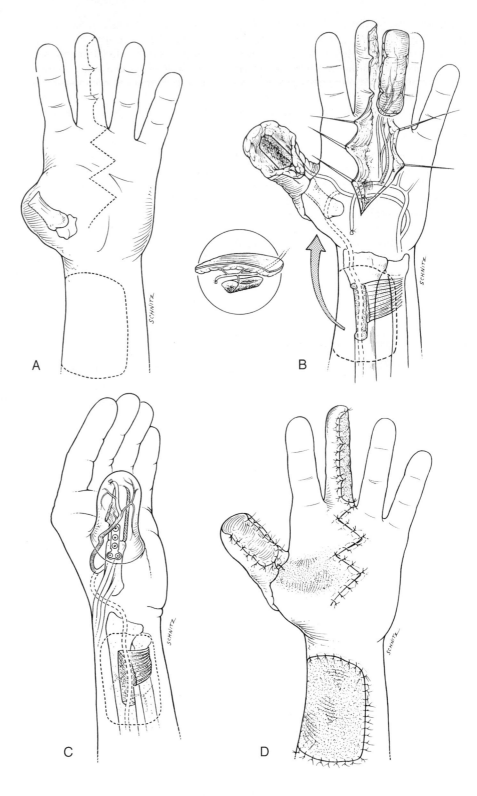

portion of the first dorsal compartment. The composite bone-skin preparation is then passed in a palmar-to-dorsal direction beneath the abductor pollicis longus, extensor pollicis brevis, and extensor pollicis longus. The flap is then passed under the skin bridge of the first web space to the level of the distal thumb wound. Connecting incisions are often used if scar tissue makes this passage difficult. The segment of bone is secured to the metacarpal with its cancellous raw edge facing the index finger and the first

metacarpal in opposition. Fixation is secured by longitudinal or obliquely placed pins or by the use of a small plate. Distal shaping and trimming of the graft ensures a smooth configuration. The forearm skin now provides coverage in a nearly circumferential fashion around the graft and the distal aspect of the remaining metacarpal or proximal phalangeal bone (see Fig. 53-24B).

At this point an extended neurovascular island pedicle flap taken from the ulnar side of either the long or ring finger can be placed on the palmar aspect of the bone graft to provide sensory perception and complete the reconstruction (see Fig. 53-24D). A split-thickness skin graft taken from the opposite anterior thigh is used to close the forearm donor area after adjacent muscle has been mobilized over the defect created by the removal of radial bone. The tourniquet should be released before application of a dressing to ensure sufficiency of the blood supply to both flaps, and exploration of the vascular pedicle must be carried out if any problems exist.

A plaster-reinforced compressive dressing is applied and sufficient portions of both flaps are left exposed to allow for continuous monitoring of their vascularity. A dressing change is carried out at 1 week, and a plaster short-arm/thumb spica cast is applied at 2 weeks and continued for 6 weeks. Additional immobilization may be necessary depending on the appearance of bone healing.

Advantages of the composite radial forearm island flap include elimination of the necessity of staging and the excellent vascularity brought with both flaps that helps minimize the possibility of flap failure. As the bone segment is vascularized, the technique should prevent bone resorption, which is probably the most significant disadvantage of osteoplastic thumb reconstruction.

Disadvantages of the procedure include a considerable cosmetic defect created in the area of forearm flap harvest and the possibility of distal radius fracture. Although no microvascular anastomoses are required, the dissection must be carried out under loupe magnification to ensure that no damage occurs to the radial artery or its venae comitantes and to maintain the vascular supply to the bone graft. When carried out correctly, this procedure would seem to be the most effective means of osteoplastic thumb restoration (Figs. 53-25 and 53-26).

Pollicization of an Injured Digit

Not infrequently, injuries that result in loss of the thumb also cause partial destruction or amputation of adjacent digits, which creates the possibility for transfer of an injured digit or distal metacarpal to the base of the proximal phalanx of the thumb or to the first metacarpal to restore length and sensory perception.* The most common digital injuries associated with thumb loss are partial or complete amputation of the index or index and long fingers. This creates an ideal situation for pollicization of the index or long finger stump to the thumb remnant. This procedure not only adds length to the thumb but also serves to widen and deepen the first web space by providing a ray resection of the second metacarpal.

When both the thumb and index finger have been lost and the long finger has been damaged or partially amputated, transposition of the stump of the long finger may be carried out by techniques almost identical to those described for pollicization of the index stump. Occasionally, satisfactory index function will be preserved with damage or amputation to the long finger, thus making it the best candidate for transposition. Although transfer of an injured ring or small finger[159] may occasionally be indicated, concomitant damage to the index or long fingers makes them much more fre-

---

*See references 27, 35-37, 42, 43, 51, 52, 75, 81, 82, 89, 106, 107, 112, 131, 147, 152, 153, 159, 166, 197-200, 204, 205, 208, 226-228, and 249.

CRITICAL POINTS: FIRST METACARPAL BONE LENGTHENING

INDICATIONS

- Loss of the thumb at the MCP level
- Retention of at least two thirds of the first metacarpal
- Good skin coverage of the thumb stump

TECHNICAL POINTS

- Create a curvilinear incision over the dorsum of the first metacarpal.
- Retract the extensor tendons to expose the bone.
- Mark the planned osteotomy site at the middle of the metacarpal.
- Place the fixation hardware (Kirschner wires or threaded half pins, depending on the distraction mechanism chosen) proximal and distal to the planned osteotomy site.
- If residual proximal phalanx remains, place distal pins into the proximal phalanx to prevent MCP flexion as distraction progresses.
- Create a transverse osteotomy with an oscillating saw.
- Close the incision and apply the distraction apparatus.

POSTOPERATIVE CARE

- Several days after the osteotomy, begin distraction.
- Distract the metacarpal at 1 to 1.5 mm/day.
- Continue distraction for 20 to 35 days until the desired length is achieved.
- In children, immobilize the distracted thumb for 2 to 3 months until complete ossification of the distraction callus occurs.
- In adults (>15 years of age), primary bone grafting of the distraction site with a corticocancellous pelvic graft will speed the healing process.
- Perform web space deepening (see Four-Flap "Z"-Plasty) at the same time as corticocancellous grafting.

quent candidates for transfer, and the techniques described here are limited to these two digits.

Pollicization of an Index Finger Stump

Under tourniquet hemostasis, an incision is designed circumferentially around the base of the index finger, at about the level of the MCP joint, to join as a "V" over the dorsal hand proximal to the midportion of the second metacarpal. An incision originating from the tip of the "V" curves transversely to the ulnar aspect of the first metacarpal. This

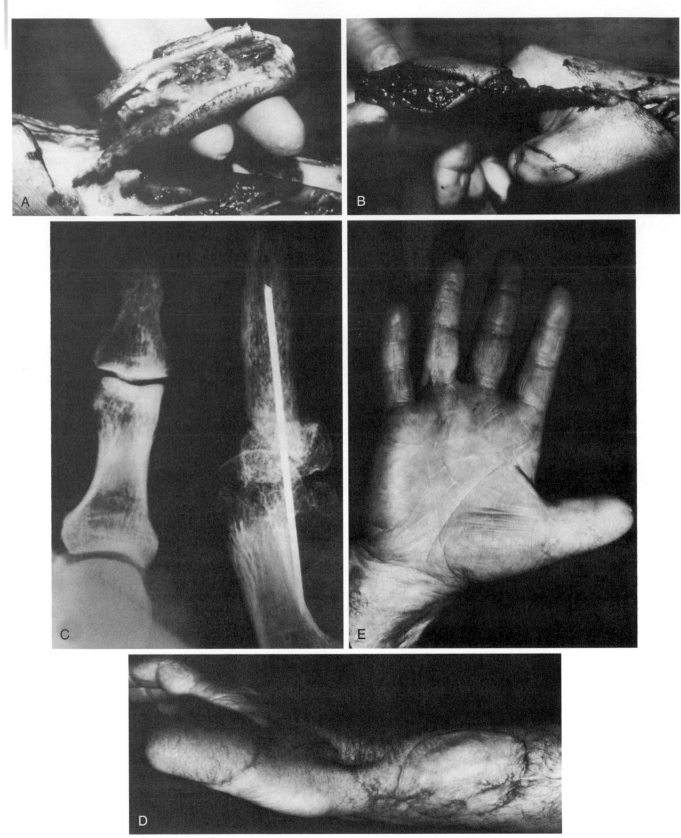

FIGURE 53-25. **A,** Appearance of the composite radial forearm island bone flap on its radial neurovascular pedicle. **B,** The flap after passage onto the back of the hand in preparation for distal passage into the thumb. **C,** Radiographic appearance of the bone graft after it has been added to the base of the proximal phalanx and fixed with a single longitudinal Kirschner wire. **D** and **E,** Appearance of the thumb reconstruction 3 months after the use of a composite radial forearm island bone flap. (Courtesy of Guy Foucher, MD, with permission.)

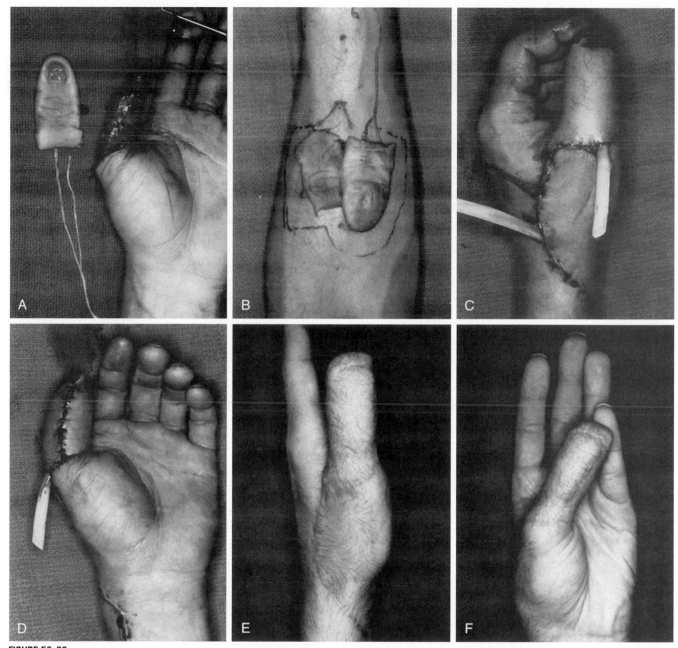

FIGURE 53-26. Coverage of a degloved thumb with a patterned radial artery forearm flap. **A,** This thumb was totally degloved from the MCP joint distally, including skin and digital nerves. **B,** The avulsed skin was used as a pattern for the radial artery forearm flap. Note the oversizing of the skin pattern to ensure adequate coverage. **C and D,** The thumb immediately after completion of radial forearm flap coverage. **E,** Appearance of the thumb at 3 months. **F,** The reconstructed thumb demonstrating pinch to the small finger. Sensation could be enhanced with a dual innervated cross-finger flap or by an extended neurovascular island pedicle flap. (Courtesy of Hill Hastings II, MD, with permission.)

creates a flap that will be used to cover the new first web (Fig. 53-27).

Skin flaps are carefully raised with initial dissection carried out palmarly. Under magnification, the digital nerve to the radial side of the index finger is identified together with the radial digital artery. The flexor tendons are identified, and the neurovascular bundle to the index and long fingers is then delineated. Careful dissection will isolate the digital artery to the radial side of the long finger, which is then clamped and ligated well beyond the bifurcation of the common digital artery. Under magnification, the digital nerves to the adjacent sides of the index and long fingers

are carefully teased apart well back into the palm (see Fig. 53-27B and D).

By alternating dissection from the palm to the dorsum, the second intermetacarpal space is developed beginning in the web and proceeding proximally. The transverse intermetacarpal ligament is divided, and the interossei in the cleft are separated down to the proximal part of the intermetacarpal interval by blunt dissection. Flexor and extensor tendons are left undisturbed.

The index metacarpal is now completely exposed subperiosteally, and an osteotome or reciprocating saw is used to divide it obliquely at its base. The amount of additional

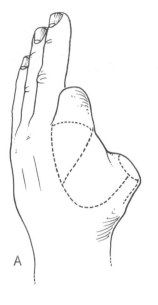

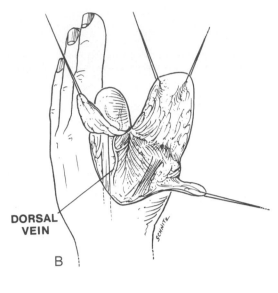

FIGURE 53-27. Pollicization of an index finger stump. **A,** Incisions used for index stump transposition. **B,** Elevation of flaps and mobilization of the second ray. Identification of a dorsal vein is shown. **C,** Diagram depicting the areas of the second metacarpal to be divided and excised *(stripes)* before transfer of the distal metacarpal and proximal phalangeal stump. **D,** The palmar flap with intact neurovascular bundles and flexor tendons following division of the radial digital artery to the long finger. (From Reid DAC: Reconstruction of the mutilated hand. *In* Rob C, Smith R, Pulvertaft RG [eds]: Operative Surgery: The Hand, 3rd ed. London, Butterworths, 1977, with permission.)
Continued

DORSAL VEIN

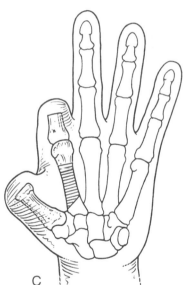

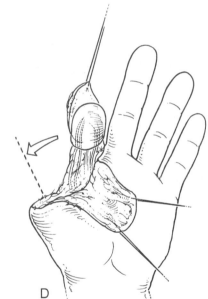

CRITICAL POINTS: POLLICIZATION OF AN INDEX FINGER STUMP

INDICATIONS

- Loss of the thumb at or near the MCP level
- Partial amputation to the index finger

TECHNICAL POINTS

- Incise circumferentially around the palmar base of the index finger near the MCP joint.
- Extend this incision dorsally as a "V" proximal to the midportion of the second metacarpal.
- Incise from the tip of this dorsal "V" transversely toward the ulnar aspect of the thumb metacarpal and distally along the ulnar aspect of the thumb metacarpal.

- Raise the dorsal flaps to the level of the MCP, taking care to leave at least one dorsal vein to the stump intact.
- Identify the radial digital nerve/artery and flexor tendons to the index finger.
- Identify the radial digital artery to the long finger, and ligate it well away from the bifurcation of the common digital artery.
- Tease apart the digital nerves to the ulnar index and radial long finger into the palm.
- Alternate between palmar and dorsal dissection to separate the second intermetacarpal space; sharply divide the transverse intermetacarpal ligament and bluntly separate the interossei.

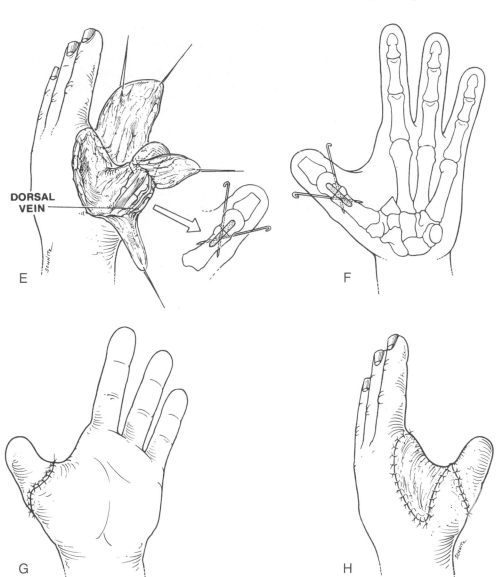

DORSAL VEIN

E

F

G

H

FIGURE 53-27.—cont'd E, Transfer of the index stump to the first metacarpal, again with preservation of a dorsal vein. Fixation by means of a bone peg and crossed Kirschner wires is shown. **F,** First and second metacarpal fixation with proximal deletion of the second metacarpal. **G,** Wound closure on the palmar surface of the transposed index stump. **H,** Use of the palmar flap to create a thumb-long finger cleft.

CRITICAL POINTS: POLLICIZATION OF AN INDEX FINGER STUMP—cont'd

TECHNICAL POINTS—cont'd

- Expose the second metacarpal subperiosteally.
- Obliquely osteotomize the second metacarpal at its base.
- Resect an appropriate amount of metacarpal based on required thumb length (amputations at the MCP level typically require metacarpal just proximal to the neck).
- Remove scarred bone and cartilage from the thumb stump.
- Transfer and fix the index stump to the residual thumb metacarpal; before performing osteosynthesis with a compression plate or crossed Kirschner wires, pronate the transferred index finger to align its palmar surface with the palmar surface of residual thumb.

- Release the tourniquet and achieve hemostasis.
- Transfer the lateral flap into the new web defect.
- Inset flaps with fine, nonabsorbable sutures.
- Dress the area with nonadherent gauze, a compressive dressing, and splint.

POSTOPERATIVE CARE

- Inspect wound at 10 to 14 days.
- Apply a short-arm/thumb spica style cast; maintain cast until bony union occurs.
- After cessation of casting, a thermoplastic web spacer splint should be worn and weaned off over several months.
- Active and passive range-of-motion exercises are begin immediately after removal of the cast.

metacarpal to be removed will depend on the exact level of thumb loss, but this is usually just proximal to the metacarpal neck for amputations at the MCP joint level. The stump to be pollicized should now be quite mobile, attached only by its two neurovascular pedicles and the flexor and extensor tendons.

At this point the thumb stump is prepared by the removal of all scarred bone and cartilage. At the time of transposition, a small bone peg may be fashioned from the removed section of the second metacarpal and used to traverse the

bony juncture (see Fig. 53-27E). The limiting factor in the transfer is the length of the neurovascular pedicles, and great care must be taken to not put these structures under tension. Obliquely placed Kirschner wires or a small compression plate is used to secure fixation of the transferred digit (see Fig. 53-27F). The tourniquet is released to ensure hemostasis and the vascularity of the transferred digital stump. Skin defects are closed by transposing the lateral flap into the cleft created by transposition (see Fig. 53-27G and H and Fig. 53-28).

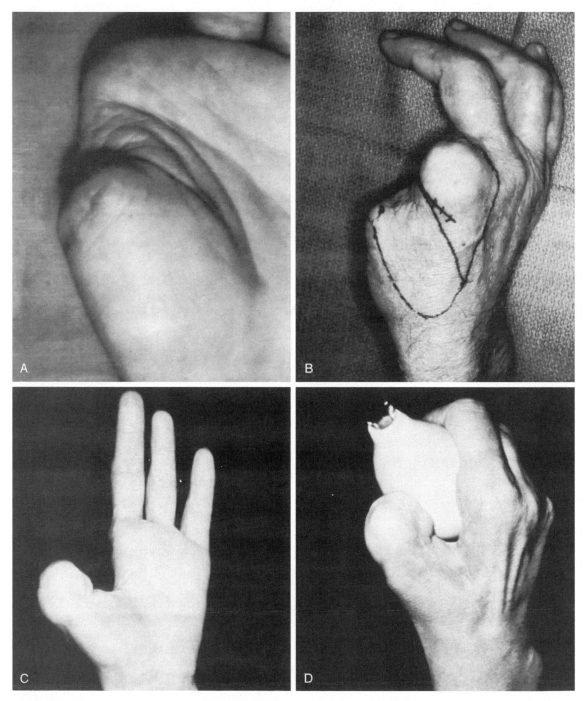

FIGURE 53-28.   Pollicization of a second metacarpal stump. **A,** Old amputations of the thumb and index finger through the MCP joints. **B,** Incisions outlined for pollicization of the index stump to the first metacarpal. **C,** Appearance of the transferred index metacarpal at 6 months. **D,** Restoration of pinch and grasp after transfer. (From Strickland JW: Restoration of thumb function following partial or total amputation. *In* Hunter JM, Schneider LH, Mackin E, Callahan AD [eds]: Rehabilitation of the Hand. St. Louis, CV Mosby, 1984, with permission.)

Postoperatively, the hand is kept in a large plaster-reinforced compressive dressing for 2 weeks and a plaster cast is continued until bony union occurs. A lightweight web space–maintaining splint should then be worn at least intermittently for several additional months (Fig. 53-29).

In the setting of a functional index finger, pollicization of a long finger stump differs slightly from the technique of index transfer. Dorsal incisions are similar, but the palm is approached through an additional zigzag incision (Fig. 53-30A and B). Through the palmar incision, the digital arterial bifurcations are identified and the proper digital arteries to the ulnar side of the index finger and the radial side of the ring finger are exposed and carefully ligated and divided well away from the bifurcations (see Fig. 53-30C). The common digital nerves are carefully separated from each other well back into the palm. Dissection, exposure, and division of the third metacarpal proceed as for the index technique (see Fig. 53-30D). Transfer of the digit differs in that after ensuring that the neurovascular bundles have been mobilized well into the palm, a subcutaneous tunnel is made to the distal aspect of the first metacarpal, which has been cleared of scar tissue and trimmed to strong, well-vascularized bone. The isolated middle finger stump is then

passed through the tunnel, and additional tailoring of the bone ends will be necessary to ensure proper positioning of the pollicized stump. At this point it may be possible to identify the stump of the extensor pollicis longus, free it from its scar tissue, and trim it to good tendon tissue. Tendon repair to the extensor tendon of the transferred long finger stump may then be completed under appropriate tension. Closure of the donor defect is accomplished by approximating the index and ring fingers by suturing their opposing deep transverse metacarpal (intervolar plate) ligaments, and closure of the palmar wound and web space is carried out (see Fig. 53-30E).

These techniques entailing the transfer of stumps of injured index or long fingers to create additional thumb length are perhaps the most practical and efficient of all the thumb reconstructive techniques because they use functionless and sometimes obstructing parts that by virtue of their excellent sensibility can substantially improve function in their new position (Fig. 53-31). Potential complications include partial or complete necrosis of the transferred part, nonunion of the bony juncture, and flap or graft necrosis. With careful planning, precise surgical technique, and appropriate postoperative care, these procedures should have a

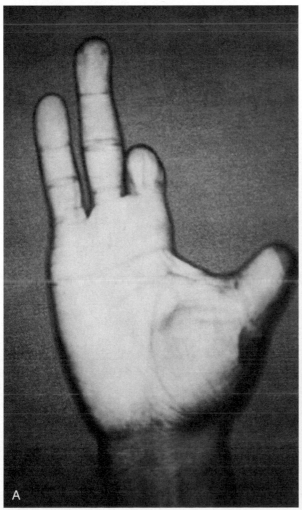
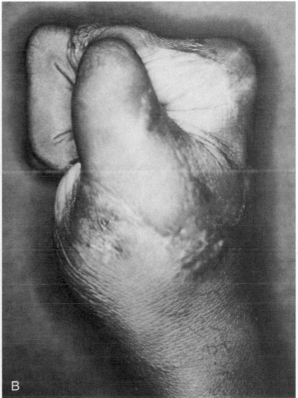

FIGURE 53-29. Palmar (**A**) and dorsal (**B**) views of a hand 6 months after pollicization of the stump of the proximal phalanx and MCP joint of the index finger.

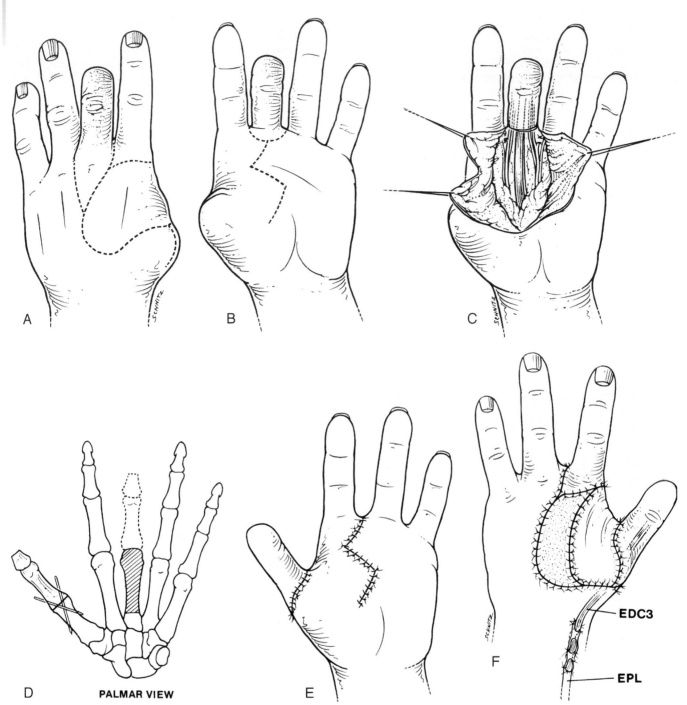

FIGURE 53-30. Pollicization of the stump of the long finger. **A,** Dorsal incision creating a dorsal lateral flap for thumb web coverage. **B,** Palmar incisions. **C,** Palmar dissection showing isolation and ligation of the ulnar digital artery to the index finger and the radial digital artery to the ring finger. **D,** Diagram of bony transfer using phalangeal bone from the long finger stump and ray excision of the third metacarpal *(stripes).* **E,** Closure of the palmar wound after completion of the pollicization. **F,** Dorsal wounds after completion of web space reconstruction using the dorsal flap with free skin graft coverage of the donor defect proximal to the index finger. Suture of the extensor pollicis longus (EPL) to the extensor digitorum communis of the long finger (EDC3) is shown. (Modified from Reid DAC: Reconstruction of the mutilated hand. In Rob C, Smith R, Pulvertaft RG [eds]: Operative Surgery: The Hand, 3rd ed. London, Butterworths, 1977, with permission.)

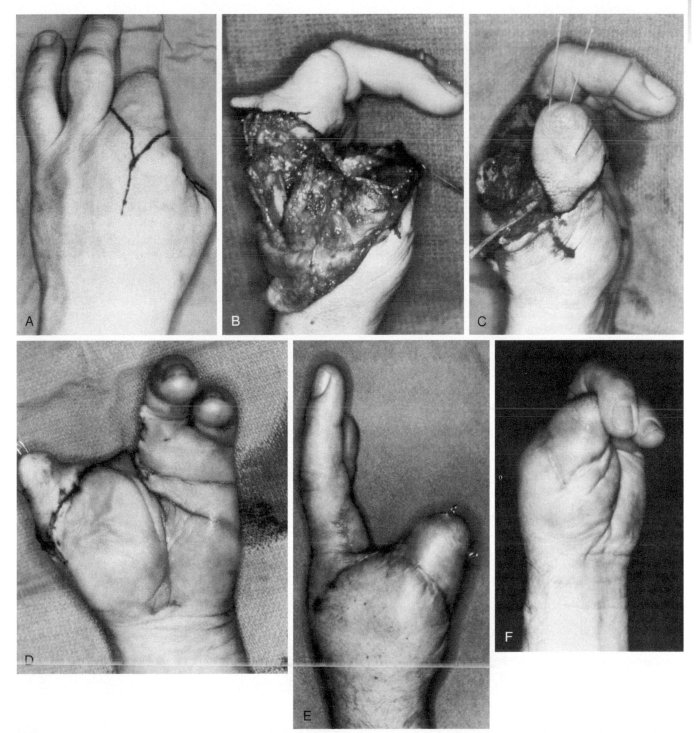

FIGURE 53-31. Transposition of a stump of the long finger after traumatic amputation of the thumb through the MCP joint and the index finger through the distal second metacarpal. **A,** Appearance of the dorsal hand with proposed skin incisions. **B,** Reflection of the dorsal flap, mobilization of the third metacarpal and long finger stump, and preparation of the first metacarpal recipient site. **C,** Appearance of the long finger stump immediately after transference to the thumb position. **D,** Palmar appearance of the transferred digital stump at the time of wound closure. **E,** Appearance of the thumb-ring finger cleft at 3 months. **F,** Restoration of satisfactory pinch between the pollicized long finger stump and the ring finger.

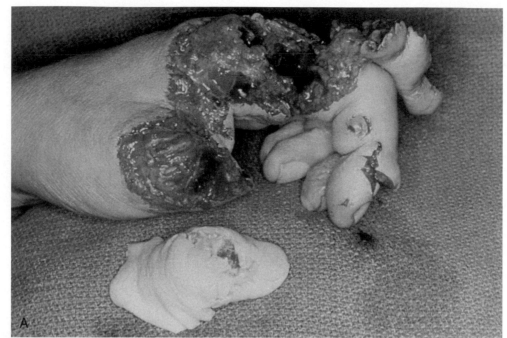

FIGURE 53-32. **A,** Left hand of a 47-year-old laborer mangled by an auger. Because of the nature of this double-level untidy crush amputation, the thumb was not salvageable. The index finger, however, still viable and well innervated in spite of major injury, was used to restore thumb function by primary pollicization at the time of injury. **B,** Appearance 3 weeks after primary pollicization of the index finger. **C,** Loss of index finger flexor tendons required arthrodesis of the IP joint (done here by compression screw fixation).

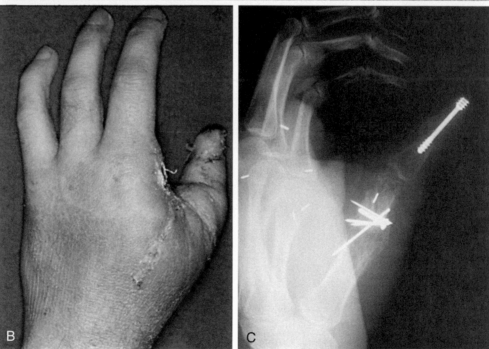

high degree of predictability and patient acceptance despite the fact that the cosmetic appearance of the reconstructed thumb may be somewhat bulbous.[229]

Figure 53-32 illustrates the use of a badly damaged index finger to replace a nonsalvageable thumb.

Total Loss with Destruction of the Basal Joint

Amputations up to, but not including, the basal joint of the thumb may be successfully reconstructed with either free toe transfer or pollicization as described in the previous section. Loss of the basal joint of the thumb, however, leaves the surgeon with the unattractive option of a thumb arthrodesed in opposition (such as might be achieved through an osteoplastic technique), pollicization, or free

transfer of an injured digit from the opposite hand.[10,171] The chief advantage of the pollicization and free digit transfers is that the hyperextended MCP joint may substitute for the lost basal joint of the thumb.

Pollicizations of normal index or ring fingers have emerged as the most popular techniques, and each has its advocates. Littler[129-131,134,136,137] has championed index pollicization on the grounds that it is technically simpler, provides restoration of excellent thumb function and sensation, and is cosmetically pleasing. LeTac[125] and others[30,71,79,123,210] have suggested that the index finger is too long and that its deletion deprives the hand of the most important prehensile digit. They prefer ring finger transfer to the thumb position because there is a minimal sacrifice of normal hand function and excellent cosmetic and functional recovery can be achieved. Regardless of the digit transposed, pollicization as described for congenital thumb deformities (see Chapter 41) may allow restoration not only of the basal joint but also of the motors lost due to injury to the thumb intrinsics.

CONCLUSION

Restoration of a functional thumb after injury remains one of the chief responsibilities of the hand surgeon. Attempts at restoration should begin at the time of injury with adequate débridement and coverage of small injuries and, in the cases of more significant amputation, attempts at replantation. When loss is limited to the soft tissue of the tip, a multitude of local flaps have been successfully used to reconstruct the defect. We have detailed the most commonly used and reliable techniques, although many others have been reported. Intermediate levels of loss may be treated with phalangization, but as more surgeons become facile with microsurgical procedures, free toe transfer becomes the most attractive option. With destruction including the basal joint, pollicization of another digit remains the best method of restoring thumb function. Although the procedure offered to the patient may be governed by these guidelines, the successful reconstruction will be one that provides adequate function for the patient with an acceptable loss from the chosen donor site.

ANNOTATED REFERENCES

24a. Buck-Gramcko D: Pollicization of the index finger: Methods and results in aplasia and hypoplasia of the thumb. J Bone Joint Surg Am 53:1605-1617, 1971.

Because of the thalidomide disaster in Europe, Buck-Gramcko was in a unique position to treat an unusually large number of children with congenital abnormalities. Although Littler was the first to describe modern pollicization techniques (see reference 131), Buck-Gramcko refined the method and provided clear, detailed illustrations of the technique in this classic article.

70. Foucher G, Van Genechten F, Merle M, Michon J: Single stage thumb reconstruction by a composite forearm island flap. J Hand Surg [Br] 9:245-248, 1984.

For subtotal amputations of the thumb, Foucher and colleagues propose a composite flap consisting of the distally based radial forearm fasciocutaneous flap and a segment of bone from the radius vascularized by a branch from the radial artery included in the flap. Benefits include confining the donor site to the injured arm, avoiding microvascular procedures, and avoiding the sacrifice of another digit.

72. Gaul JS: Radial-innervated cross-finger flap from index to provide sensory pulp to injured thumb. J Bone Joint Surg Am 51:1257-1263, 1969.

Although not the first to describe a radial-innervated cross-finger flap, Gaul presents the use of the radial sensory branch to the index finger with a cross-finger flap performed in the standard fashion (as opposed to other, earlier descriptions such as that of Bralliar). His clear, intraoperative photos offer an excellent guide to performance of this flap.

77. Goldner RD, Howson MP, Nunley JA, et al: One hundred eleven thumb amputations: Replantation vs. revision. Microsurgery 11:243-250, 1990.

Given that thumb reconstruction offers at best a second-line therapy to replantation (when possible), it is useful to compare the outcomes of the first-line therapy to that of revision amputation in treating thumb injuries. The authors conducted a rigorous study of hand function after replantation and revision amputation. Their results suggest that revision amputation is as functional as replantation and may offer better lateral pinch strength.

78a. Gosset J: La pollicisation de l'index (technique chirurgicale). J Chir 65:403, 1949.

Perhaps one of the seminal texts in thumb reconstruction, Gosset provided the first description of the transfer of an index finger isolated on its neurovascular pedicle. Although his transfer was employed for traumatic reconstruction post World War II, his techniques have been refined and expanded to provide the procedure now used for congenital pollicization.

93. Henderson HP, Reid DAC: Long term follow up of neurovascular island flaps. Hand 12:113-122, 1980.

Although composed of only 20 patients, this follow-up of the outcome of neurovascular island flaps represents one of the largest published studies and its results continue to be confirmed by other investigators. In particular, only 5 of the 20 patients demonstrated complete sensory reorientation, a finding that corresponds well with recent reports showing limited cortical remapping in adults who have undergone this procedure. Nonetheless, useful sensation did persist in 19 of 20 patients, confirming that the flap works in principle.

134. Littler JW: On making a thumb: One hundred years of surgical effort. J Hand Surg [Am] 1:35-51, 1976.

As evident in the title, Littler's article is significant for detailing the long and innovative history of thumb reconstruction. Although interesting primarily for the historical perspective, the evolution of techniques described helps define our understanding of what constitutes a "thumb."

144. Matev I: Thumb reconstruction through metacarpal bone lengthening. J Hand Surg [Am] 5:482-487, 1980.

Matev reports on his experience with 35 patients treated via metacarpal osteotomy and distraction osteogenesis over a 12-year period. His results show successful lengthening of thumb metacarpals by 3 to 4 cm in a wide age range of patients. He also suggests that patients older than age 25 undergo bone grafting rather than await callus consolidation. Emphasis is placed on web-deepening procedures as adjuncts to successful thumb reconstruction.

156a. Michon J, Merle M, Bouchon Y, Foucher G: Functional comparison between pollicization and toe-to-hand transfer for thumb reconstruction. J Reconstr Microsurg 1:103-110, 1984.

The authors compared reconstruction of thumb amputations of four types: absent thumb with normal remaining digits, absent thumb with partially mutilated other digits, the metacarpal hand, and distal thumb amputation. Their results shed light on the strengths of each technique in various degrees of injury. When applicable, pollicization provides better fine motor control and discriminative sensation; toe-to-hand transfer uniformly provides better strength.

161. Moberg E: Aspects of sensation in reconstructive surgery of the upper limb. J Bone Joint Surg Am 46:817-825, 1964.

Moberg's emphasis on sensibility in the upper limb, ranging from defining useful tactile gnosis to warning against hypersensitivity, continues to offer hand surgeons a measure by which we can judge our outcomes. This article has spurred many of the innervated flap reconstructive techniques described in this chapter.

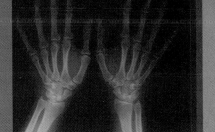

CHAPTER 54

Distraction Lengthening in the Hand and Upper Extremity

William H. Seitz, Jr.

The concept of limb lengthening is not new.[26,91] Application of this concept to develop the procedure of increasing the functional length of a skeletally deficient hand to provide enhanced mechanical advantage, prehension, and grip has gone through an evolution in technique and technology. Since the first reports of digital lengthening by Kessler and colleagues[60] and Matev,[69] their techniques and the techniques that Wagner used in the long bones of the lower extremity have been successfully applied to the hand and upper extremity by many authors.* Refinement of these techniques has included incorporation of more streamlined lengthening devices, use of slower distraction rates, incorporation of toe phalangeal transfers, and, more recently, application of Ilizarov's techniques of callus distraction to create primary new bone formation in the distraction gap.[†]

Distraction provides a mechanism for restoring functional length to a traumatically or congenitally skeletally deficient hand and allows maintenance of a layer of sensate, vascular tissue over the lengthened part throughout the period of construction and/or reconstruction. Alternative methods of reconstruction obviously exist (notably composite vascularized tissue transfers and the use of prosthetic replacement parts).[41,62,65,75,76,98,108,109] However, these techniques are not applicable in all situations and have their own limitations and drawbacks. Distraction lengthening has offered an additional and still-evolving management tool for the treatment of skeletally deficient hands given the proper indications.[15,17,22,32,63,71,88]

APPLICATIONS IN THE UPPER EXTREMITY

Indications

Distraction lengthening can be a viable reconstructive technique in a child or adult with skeletal deficiency caused by trauma or congenital absence. It may also be used for the slow distraction of soft tissue contractures such as those encountered in a burn or in a radial clubhand (radial agenesis).[18,86,111] The technique has application throughout the upper extremity. With traumatic loss of bone from the humerus as seen in severe gunshot wounds, following very short above-elbow amputations (creating a stump too short for prosthetic fitting), or with severe congenital deficiency such as phocomelia, humeral lengthening allows creation of a much more functional limb (Fig. 54-1).[25,37,95,97,106]

In the forearm, traumatic amputation or skeletal deficiency from a segmental loss can be managed by segmental bone transport for purposes of filling a defect gap or for functionally lengthening a short below-elbow segment after amputation (Fig. 54-2). Very short forearms such as those encountered in radial clubhand (Fig. 54-3) or major discrepancies of radial or ulnar length (as in multiple hereditary exostoses) have been managed with callus distraction.*

Distraction techniques have been used about the wrist to stretch soft tissues for correction of radial clubhand deformity in early infancy. Later in life it has been used in conjunction with forearm lengthening and centralization or radialization of the wrist concomitantly.[18,48,63,86,88,111]

In the hand, distraction lengthening can be applied to congenital or post-traumatic partial absence of the digital rays involving either a thumb or multiple digital rays.[†] The primary goal is improvement of length to enhance mechanical advantage, prehension, and grip, which in turn imparts improved use of the extremity and thereby affords functional improvement and, secondarily, cosmesis. However, the technique should not be considered solely for cosmetic purposes, and its use in an isolated short digit such as that found in isolated brachymetacarpia must be carefully evaluated to make sure that there really is significant functional impairment before undertaking this complicated surgical procedure. When a functional defect of the thumb or multiple digits involving the metacarpals and/or phalanges is present, however, the technique of digital lengthening can restore a very functional prehensile unit by distraction of the

---

*See references 20, 24, 27, 28, 36-40, 47, 50, 58, 60, 61, 64, 67, 73, 80, 81, 85, 86, 95, 101, 112, and 118.

[†]See references 1, 3, 4, 8, 16, 18, 19, 22, 24, 25, 30, 31, 33-35, 46, 53-55, 59, 69, 74, 83, 92, 94, 96-98, 100, 103, 106, and 111.

---

*See references 15, 22, 28, 36, 67, 85, 96, 100, 103, 106, and 111.

[†]See references 17, 24, 27, 32, 49, 56, 61, 92, 94, 97, 98, 101, and 118.

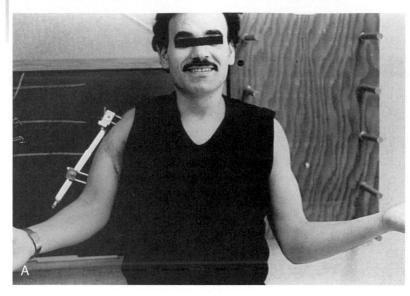

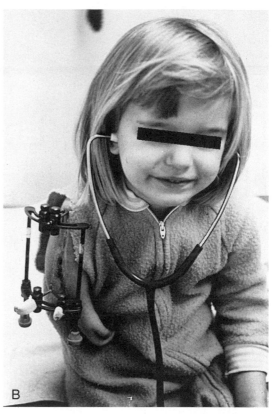

FIGURE 54-1. Distraction about the shoulder and upper arm can be very well managed by applying a half-frame lengthening apparatus in the lateral position. **A,** After segmental traumatic bone loss. **B,** For severe congenital hypoplasia.

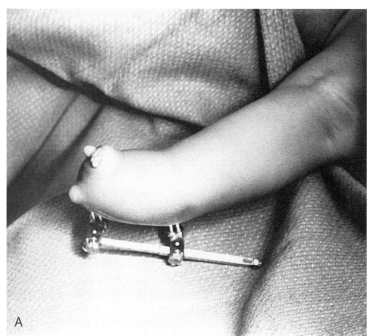

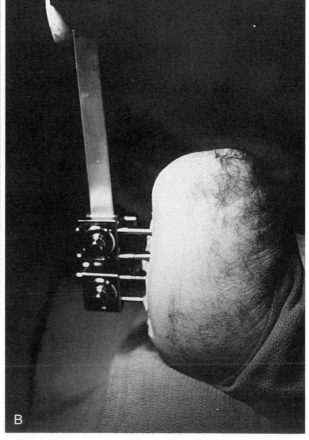

FIGURE 54-2. Lengthening of a short dysfunctional below-elbow amputation stump is well managed by using a miniature half-frame lengthener in a congenital amputee (**A**) or by using a larger half-frame device in an adult after traumatic amputation (**B**).

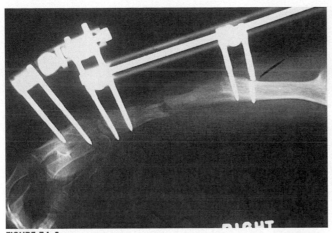

FIGURE 54-3. Functional elongation of a short forearm in a patient with a radial clubhand can be achieved through a half-frame distraction apparatus while hand position is maintained with a neutral set of pins in the hand to stabilize the carpus.

existing skeletal architecture or when following the addition of transplanted bone.[24,38,97,118] Replantation surgery has proved to be quite effective for management of digital loss but may be limited in the presence of abnormal neurologic or vascular development or when multiple digital deficiencies exist for which harvesting multiple toes for microvascular transfer might well leave a more significant functional defect in the foot.[75,76] Such considerations must be carefully weighed by the surgeon (and family) and discussed carefully with the patient during the decision-making process before surgery.

Contraindications and Family Counseling

Aside from situations in which lengthening may be considered solely for cosmesis, other contraindications to this technique do exist. This technique should not be used in noncompliant patients. It is therefore very important for the surgeon to get to know the patient and/or the family before undertaking this surgical procedure. The patient and family must be fully aware of the duration of the procedure, the potential for complications, the necessity of daily monitoring and pin site care, and the need for avoidance of dangerous or injurious activities. They must be aware of the importance of regular careful follow-up appointments and that this is a labor-intensive technique requiring regular evaluation and input from the surgeon, therapist, patient, and family. Trying to accomplish this successfully over a long distance can be difficult unless arrangements are made well in advance for careful regular follow-up.

Problems and complications are not uncommon, and all involved must be aware of this and be ready to deal with them when they occur to prevent the evolution of minor problems into major complications.[78,94]

As noted previously, other relative contraindications include single-digit deficiencies (other than the thumb), for which there may be other more appropriate means of management. Additionally, when considering lengthening of a shortened forearm segment and centralization in radial agenesis, distraction lengthening is contraindicated in the presence of a stiff or ankylosed elbow joint. In such an instance, the wrist itself may be functioning as the elbow joint, and reconstructive techniques could well result in loss of function (e.g., as in eating and hygiene care).

TECHNIQUES OF DISTRACTION LENGTHENING

Two-Stage Lengthening Techniques

Staged lengthening techniques have been used in the long bones by Wagner and others.[20,36,37,112] In the hand, these techniques have been adapted by a number of investigators.[24,27,38-40,61,118] Staged lengthening of the forearm and humerus has been reported by Dick and others.[34,35]

The technique includes an initial osteotomy, application of pins or wires in connection with either a full-frame or half-frame device to establish as much length as possible at the operating table, and performance of one or more daily incremental lengthenings of 1 to 2 mm (Fig. 54-4). Wagner has made the point that the periosteum should be fully divided to ensure no resistance to lengthening.[112] This relatively rapid elongation has been associated with varying degrees of discomfort, and rapid lengthening of the soft tissues has limited their ability to accommodate physiologically. Pain and limitation of soft tissue tolerance have limited the extent of lengthening and use of this technique (Fig. 54-5).

When the limit of lengthening has been achieved, a second operation is performed for the harvest, insertion, and fixation of an intercalary bone graft. Donor sites have included the iliac crest, fibula, and toe phalanges, as well as allograft, depending on the location and size of the bone graft needed (Fig. 54-6).

The form of fixation likewise depends on the size of the bone graft and the extent of lengthening. This has varied from Kirschner wires, to miniature plates and screws in the hand, to larger plates and interfragmentary screws in the forearm and humerus (Fig. 54-7). Additionally, depending on the degree of internal fixation and the age of the individual, tertiary surgical procedures in the form of hardware removal must frequently be performed and the hand or extremity subsequently protected until full healing has been achieved. This duration is frequently longer when an interposed segment of nonvascularized bone is used.

Reported complications with this technique include pain, infection, need for multiple re-operations, graft resorption, hardware failure, soft tissue necrosis, reactive hypertension, angular joint subluxation and contractures, ischemia, and even death.[44,72,105,112,115,121]

Even though staged lengthening is known to have inherent limitations, this technique has provided the foundation for newer concepts in limb lengthening and is still successfully used on occasion.[50,58] Its advantages include a potentially shorter duration of use of the external fixation apparatus and therefore fewer pin complications. As newer techniques of bioabsorbable internal fixation develop, the need for tertiary surgical procedures may also diminish.

One-Stage Lengthening-Distraction Osteogenesis (Callotasis)

The concept of distraction osteogenesis uses the principle of slow distraction through an area of healing fracture callus.

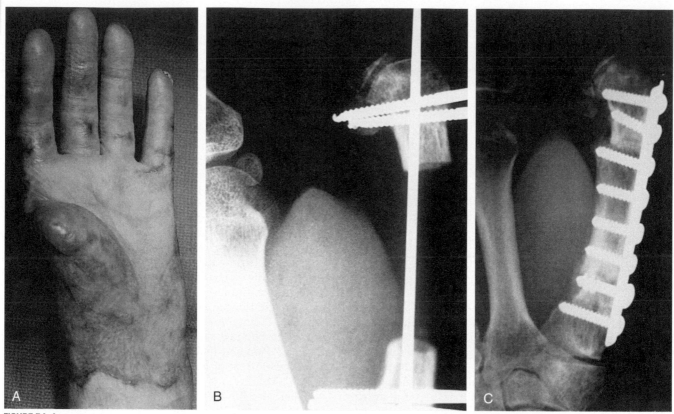

FIGURE 54-4. Staged distraction lengthening for re-creation of a thumb after a burn and amputation of the thumb (**A**) can be achieved by means of distraction across a centrally placed Kirschner wire (**B**) to maintain longitudinal position despite thickened surrounding scar tissue. After length is achieved, a secondary procedure is then done to provide stable internal fixation of a free bone graft (**C**), which may take a significant amount of time to incorporate.

This technique in the long bones has been pioneered by Ilizarov, De Bastiani,[30] Monticelli and Spinelli,[72] and Paley,[77-79,92] and its biology has been elucidated by Aronson, Green, and others.* Application of the principles of callotasis to the upper extremity is recent, but the few reported cases and series have demonstrated the ability to elongate skeletal segments with complete consolidation to normal healthy bone by using a single surgical procedure with fewer complications than with staged lengthening.† The very slow distraction achieved with multiple lengthenings of very small distances throughout each day has two advantages: (1) less discomfort and (2) adaptation of the surrounding soft tissue structures to permit increased degrees of lengthening while maintaining soft tissue viability.

The technique includes preinsertion of fixation pins or wires, local incision at the site of planned bone division, careful elevation and preservation of the periosteum, controlled osteotomy, periosteal repair, wound closure, and device assembly. After the operation, there is a delay period to allow for early healing and preliminary callus formation, followed by a period of slow distraction attained by multiple small lengthenings performed on a daily basis. Circular

frame and hybrid devices have been recommended for correction of angular deformities in the long bones of the upper extremity, but they are complex to apply and cumbersome for the patient to wear and they require "through-and-through" placement of pins that can tether and injure vital soft tissue structures as the lengthening process develops (Fig. 54-8). In the hand, circular frames are extremely cumbersome, whereas half-frame lengtheners with threaded half-pins provide adequate fixation and minimize the bulk of the applied hardware.[92,94,97,98]

Complications of Callotasis

The technique of callotasis is not without its complications.[7,29,52,78,104,110,122] As in any form of external fixation, pin tract infections and stiffness probably represent the largest single group of complications.[87,90] Deep infections can occur but are rare and less common than after secondary bone grafting and internal fixation.[50,92,94,97]

Joint subluxation or angular deviation can occur with callotasis as easily as it can with staged lengthening.[104,115] Adequate control of adjacent joints during the lengthening process can avoid or minimize such complications. Joint contractures should be surgically released before lengthening, and proximal and distal segments should be stabilized as noted in the descriptions and illustration shown later in this chapter.

Adjacent joint stiffness must be carefully watched and minimized with physical therapy and exercises. In lengthening the forearm, both the digital flexors and extensors can

---

*See references 1, 2, 5, 6, 9-14, 16, 18, 19, 21, 22, 25, 28, 34, 35, 42, 43, 45, 51, 53-55, 57, 59, 66, 68, 74, 77-79, 82-84, 99,102, 113, 114, 116, 117, 119, and 120.

†See references 15, 17, 22, 32, 48, 49, 56, 63, 64, 67, 70, 71, 88, 89, 92, 93, 94, 96, 97, 100, 103, 106, 107, and 111.

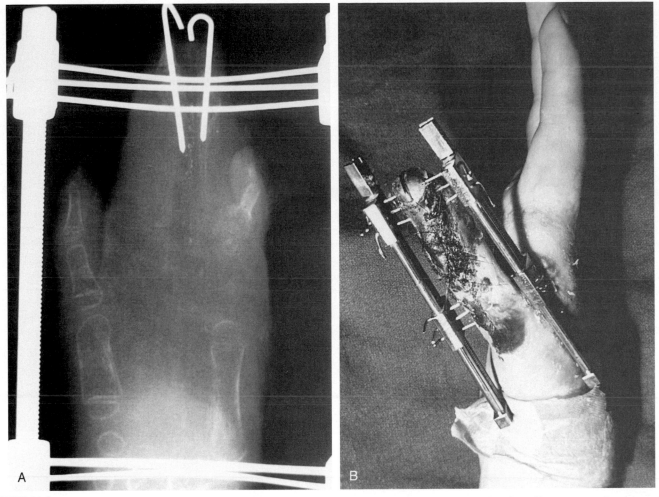

FIGURE 54-5. Rapid lengthening using through-and-through pins can be associated with failure of bone regeneration (**A**) and/or may cause tissue necrosis (**B**), which makes intercalary bone grafting difficult and necessitates flap coverage.

become tight. In the humerus, the elbow may develop a flexion contracture.

Angulation of the lengthened segment can be avoided by lengthening over a central guidewire as described by Wenner.[71,115] Dhalla and coworkers have demonstrated this to be a valuable tool when lengthening very short congenital phalanges when only a single fixation pin can be placed on either side of the osteotomy.[32] This is particularly useful in adult lengthenings (especially lengthenings of the thumb). When forearm lengthening is being performed for radial agenesis, wrist deviation can be avoided by stable fixation of the hand with pins inserted in the metacarpals, thereby avoiding the angular tethering effect of the tight anlage of soft tissue on the radial side of the forearm (Fig. 54-9).

Premature consolidation, or early union of the regenerate bone in the distraction gap, is a complication that limits the overall obtainable length. This complication usually stems from inadequate patient education or noncompliance, which causes a delay in lengthening that allows premature healing.[78,94] In young patients, who have robust healing potential, there is also a tendency to more rapidly consolidate than in an adult.

Failure of consolidation in the distraction gap can be the result of rough handling of the surrounding soft tissues or periosteum and consequent damage to the blood supply at the site of intended neo-osteogenesis. It may also be the result of attempted lengthening through dysvascular bone or an overly rapid lengthening rate. Regenerate bone may also fail to develop as a result of inadequate maintenance of distraction tension because of an unstable fixator, device failure, or pin loosening and/or breakage.[15,78,94]

Fracture of the lengthened segment can occur at a pin site or through the regenerate bone. This complication may be minimized by proper technique of initial insertion of the pins, attentive pin site care during the lengthening and consolidation period, avoidance of trauma, and maintenance of adequate fixation until the regenerate bone is fully consolidated, with additional protection after device removal. Radiographic evidence of consolidation of at least three cortices should be obtained before device removal.[113] This is sometimes difficult to assess, and, recently, ultrasound has been evaluated as a quantifier of bone regeneration.[2] Interestingly, when a fracture does occur, it frequently results in increased bone mass and secondary strength of the bone at the site of fracture. In general, fixation should be maintained for at least *twice* the original duration of lengthening in children and three times that duration in adults. For example, a lengthening of 30 mm (30 days) should be

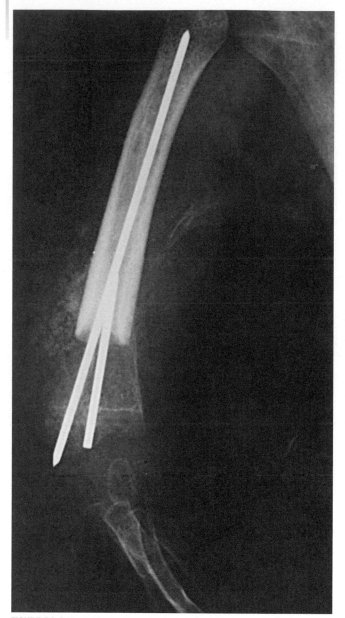

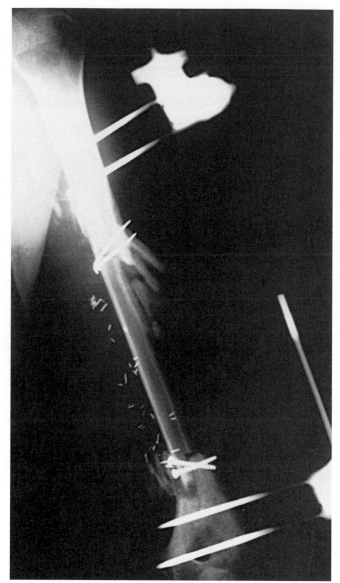

FIGURE 54-7. A vascularized fibula graft (with internal fixation) can speed healing across a large distraction gap after segmental bone loss.

FIGURE 54-6. In a large segmental distraction gap where neo-osteogenesis cannot be achieved, allograft can be used. In this case an adult ulna has been used to bridge an area of distraction in congenital hypoplasia of the humerus.

allowed to consolidate for another 2 months in children and 3 months in adults.

Pain is a much less frequent complaint in patients when the technique of callotasis is used. If pain does occur, it is more frequently seen in adults than in children, especially in lengthenings that are performed after trauma. This may be due to stretching of local nerve structures, the ends of which have been transected and embedded in scar tissue and are now being stretched. When pain occurs in children, it is usually the result of transient local infection or it occurs when the maximum tolerable soft tissue tension has been achieved. This usually signals the end point of lengthening, and as distraction stops, the symptoms usually resolve.[122]

Less commonly than in rapid lengthening, distal soft tissue erosion can occur if there is poor initial coverage (as in lengthening through poorly vascularized scar tissue or inadequately grafted or insensate skin). This problem can be avoided by careful monitoring during the lengthening process and, if needed, by preoperative flap coverage.

Physeal injury can occur but is usually avoidable by means of careful pin placement outside the physeal plates. In very short extremities this can be achieved by lengthening across the joint while controlling the stability of that joint. Careful application of fixation pins can avoid growth arrest, deformity, pain, ligamentous instability, and contractures. Lengthening can be performed through a physeal plate with the formation of exceptionally good regenerate bone, but this should be reserved for children nearing skeletal maturity because it results in physeal closure after lengthening.[33,69]

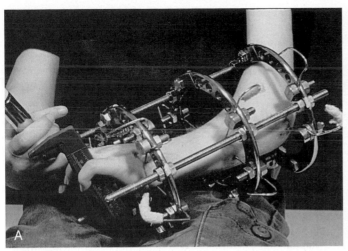 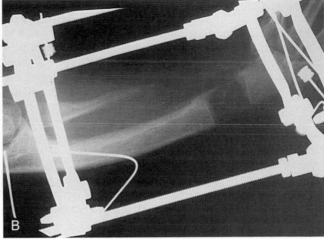

FIGURE 54-8. Circular frame distraction can be used for longitudinal lengthening while correcting angular deformities slowly, but this is a very cumbersome apparatus (**A**) that limits hand use during the lengthening process. The circular frame is quite stable, however, as seen in this case of forearm lengthening in a radial clubhand where the distal set of pins stabilizes the hand over the carpus (**B**). (Courtesy of Melvin P. Rosenwasser, MD, Columbia Presbyterian Medical Center, New York.)

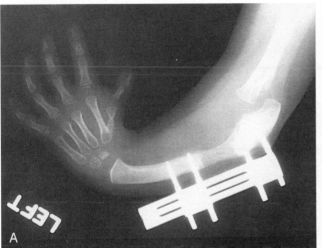 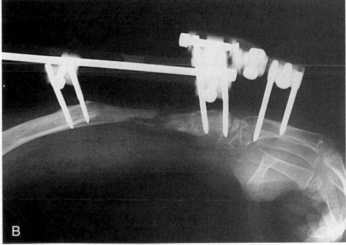

FIGURE 54-9. Loss of hand stability can result during forearm lengthening in a patient with radial agenesis if only the ulna itself is secured and the hand is not stabilized over the forearm. **A,** This patient had recurrent radial deviation despite prior centralization. **B,** Maintenance of appropriate hand position over the forearm can be achieved through a static set of pins in the metacarpals while the forearm is lengthened with a more "streamlined" half-frame device after acute correction of the angular deformity.

Author's Preferred Method of Treatment: Half-Frame Lengthening by the Technique of Callotasis

Callotasis—the distraction of healing fracture callus to create an elongated skeletal segment—has proved to be an effective technique.[1,59,83,94,97] Slow distraction affords relatively little discomfort during the phase of elongation. It is well tolerated by the surrounding soft tissues and allows stretching of these soft tissues to occur simultaneously with the formation of new bone.[57,68,99,120] The price one pays is a period of time during which consolidation of the new bone must occur, and this requires a longer duration of time in the lengthening device itself. Nonetheless, this technique has

distinct advantages over other methods when secondary procedures must be performed for bone grafting and/or additional internal fixation, each of which may be associated with additional complications. To make the procedure of de novo new bone formation through a single-staged procedure an acceptable alternative, it must also have a reasonably low rate of serious complications and devices must be chosen that are "livable" for the patients during the period of fixation. This requires careful attention to surgical detail and the use of streamlined devices.

Pin Placement/Device Orientation

Humerus
Half-pin placement in a monolateral frame configuration for lengthening of the humerus eliminates the cumbersome circular frame and is most easily undertaken through lateral

placement of the pins.[23] This may entail either straight lateral, anterolateral, or posterolateral placement, depending on soft tissue constraints. The anterolateral or lateral position is most convenient when the patient is solely responsible for performing the lengthening task and pin site care (Fig. 54-10).

The half-frame can also be used to lengthen a very short humeral amputation stump to facilitate better prosthetic fitting (Fig. 54-11).

Forearm

Lengthening of the forearm may be undertaken to correct a particularly short, below-elbow amputation stump or to repair a deformity or short forearm (e.g., radial agenesis, multiple hereditary exostoses, Madelung's deformity, or severe discrepancy as a result of physeal growth arrest) (Fig. 54-12).

Circular fixation has been used to provide slow correction of *angular deformity* of a forearm or about a joint, as may occur in multiple hereditary exostosis or Madelung's deformity. This requires extreme attention to detail during the lengthening/angular correction phase. We have found it equally efficacious with much less complexity to perform an angular corrective osteotomy as the actual subperiosteal osteotomy to reestablish appropriate alignment, followed by lengthening along a single axis.[15,22,48,63,70,89,92,93,96]

When possible, pin placement should be along the radial aspect if the radius is the bone being lengthened or along the ulnar aspect if the ulna is the bone to be lengthened. With very proximal stump lengthening, care should be taken to stabilize the elbow joint through a separate set of pins in the humerus (Fig. 54-13). When distal lengthening is being carried out, the hand should be stabilized (especially in a radial clubhand) with a third set of pins to prevent deviation of the carpus (see Fig. 54-9). Radial or ulnar placement also minimizes muscular tethering while allowing the reasonably low-profile device to minimally intrude on function.

Radial Club Hand

Children with severe radial aplasia are good candidates for utilizing the principles of distraction lengthening as long as they have a mobile and stable ulnohumeral joint. Taking away the hyperflexion of the wrist in the face of a stiff elbow or one with synostosis prevents the child from being able to get his or her hand to the mouth. Children with supple elbows with radial agenesis, however, are faced with a hyperflexed and radially deviated wrist and significantly foreshortened forearm. When a good elbow is present, the ability to provide a stable hand centrally situated on a forearm of more normal length can provide a significant functional as well as cosmetic enhancement.[88]

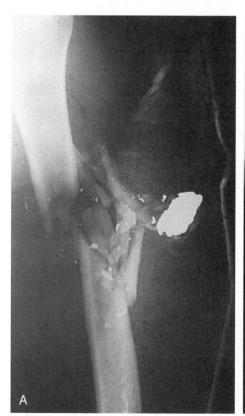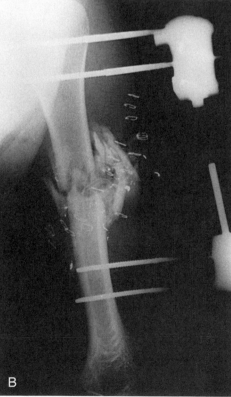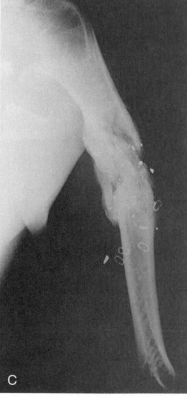

FIGURE 54-10. Humeral distraction. Neo-osteogenesis can be used to restore segmental bone loss after trauma. **A,** A gunshot wound with significant comminution and loss of bone substance has resulted in a 3-inch shortening of the humerus. **B,** After débridement and compression through a half-frame lengthening apparatus, the soft tissues have been repaired and early callus formation is achieved in the first week after injury. Slow distraction is then applied at a rate of 1 mm daily (see the text for details) until anatomic length has been achieved. **C,** After consolidation, a functional humerus of satisfactory length is achieved.

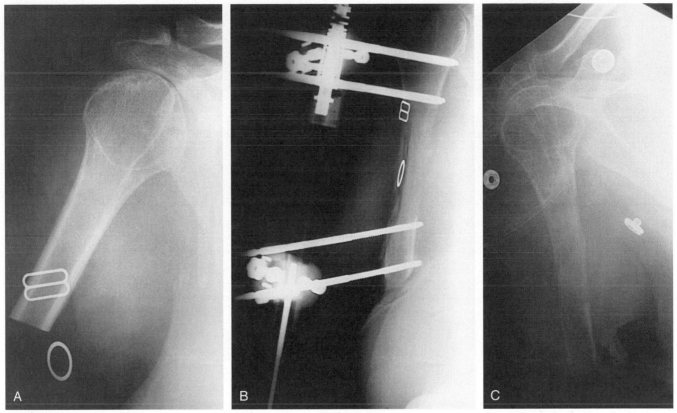

FIGURE 54-11. The very short above-elbow traumatic amputation in this obese patient (**A**) precludes fitting with an above-elbow prosthesis and would require a shoulder disarticular socket. Half-frame lengthening (**B**) was used to achieve satisfactory length to accommodate elbow prosthetic fitting (**C**).

When the child presents for treatment in infancy, a two-staged process of distraction can be instituted. Manual stretching and splinting for the first 6 months of life helps to maintain reasonable flexibility in the otherwise tight radial soft tissues. At 6 months of age, we have found success in using a half-frame lengthening device attached between the proximal ulna and the metacarpals to gradually elongate the soft tissue envelope while extending the carpus distally in a more "radialized" position beyond the distal end of the ulna. Once satisfactory length and alignment have been achieved between the soft tissues and the forearm and the hand is appropriately axially positioned beyond the terminal aspect of the ulna, secondary osteotomy and lengthening can be performed with a second half-frame device, resulting in a "docking" of the distal ulna up against the proximal carpus as length is achieved. After consolidation, both fixators are removed in the operating room and a capsular reefing is performed. At the same time of the device removal, tendon transfers and/or pollicization can be performed if needed. This process has provided good early hand position and finger function with a more normal-length forearm allowing early use for bimanual activities at a very early age (Fig. 54-14).

In all cases, it is important in a child to avoid damage to the physeal plate, unless the child is nearing completion of skeletal maturity, in which case lengthening can be performed through the physeal plate itself.[33,69] This offers a site with very rich osteogenic potential, but after consolidation of the lengthened bone, no further growth can or will occur at this physeal plate.

Metacarpals/Phalanges

In the hand itself, half-pin placement follows a dorsal oblique approach to avoid injury to tendons and the intrinsic musculature. When multiple devices are to be used for lengthening of multiple fingers, an arcuate alignment of pin insertion that follows the natural arch of the hand should be chosen to avoid crowding of the devices one on top of another and preventing satisfactory application and adjustment (Fig. 54-15). Palmar pin placement, or through-and-through pin placement, is not needed, is cumbersome, and will interfere with hand function. We have found that individual finger lengthening with separate devices is preferable because it allows maintenance of individual digital excursion throughout the lengthening and consolidation period and is preferable to using single through-and-through devices to lengthen multiple rays simultaneously. Again, physeal plates should not be injured unless the patient is nearing the point of skeletal maturity. Lengthening across the metacarpophalangeal (MCP) joint has not proved to be problematic. Some degree of joint distraction is frequently seen, but this has been found to aid in the rapid return of functional motion and can avoid the problems of MCP subluxation if the joint capsule is lax proximally and the soft tissues are tight distally (Fig. 54-16).

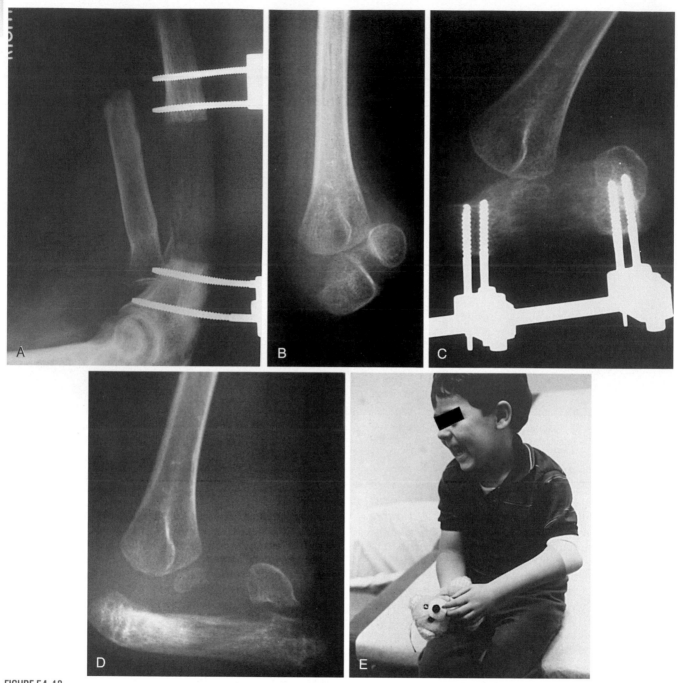

FIGURE 54-12. Forearm callotasis. A short below-elbow stump in an obese patient precluded the use of a below-elbow suction socket. Callotasis lengthening achieved length while spontaneously generating new bone formation (**A**). Similar lengthening can also be achieved in a severe congenital amputation at the elbow (**B** to **D**) to allow functional prosthetic fitting of an otherwise unusable below-elbow prosthesis (**E**).

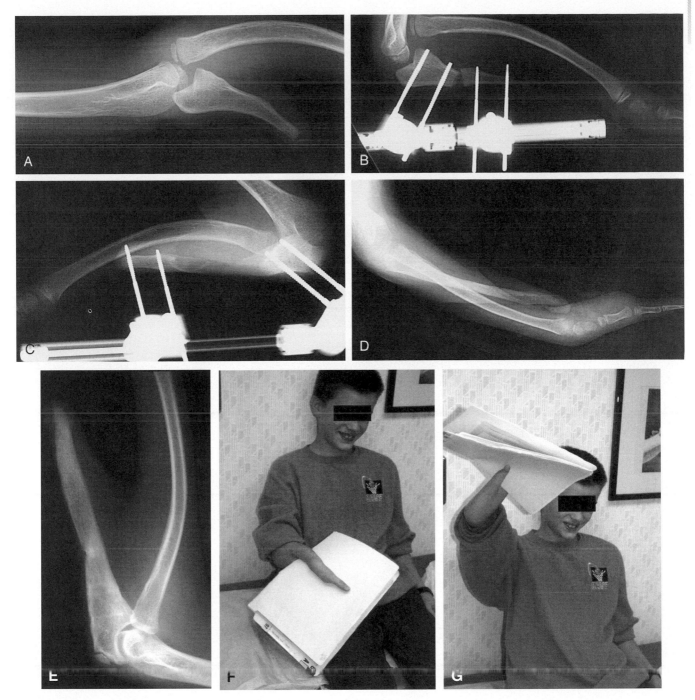

FIGURE 54-13. Special situations in forearm lengthening about the elbow. Forearm lengthening was used to create a useful appendage in this child with severe ulnar agenesis and a single radial digit (**A**). Angular correction and half-frame callotasis lengthening were performed (**B** and **C**) to ultimately create a new digit to be used as a prehensile post as in a Krukenberg procedure (**D** to **G**). *Continued*

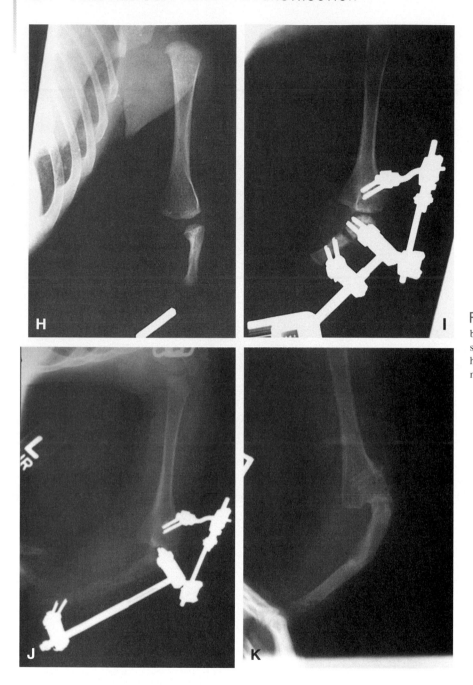

FIGURE 54-13—cont'd. An unstable elbow must be recognized (**H**) and managed by outrigger stabilization with a separate set of pins in the humerus (**I**) for successful lengthening while maintaining stability (**J** and **K**).

Application of distraction to soft tissue contractures, such as in the first web space after severe burns, has also been shown to be an effective use of slow, sustained lengthening techniques with minimal surgical disruption of surrounding skeletal and soft tissue architecture (Fig. 54-17).

Device Choice

The choice of lengthening apparatus should reflect the surgeon's comfort in using that device. Ideally, the device should be relatively simple to apply and adjust, versatile for use in different locations, yet adaptable to a variety of potential anatomic variations. Strength or durability is important for survival of the device throughout the period of length-

ening, and some degree of flexibility or resilience may be important for the promotion of osteogenesis via controlled transmission of subtle vibratory stimuli to the regenerate bone.[11,53,79,82]

We have successfully used multiple monolateral designs, including the small Wagner lengthener (Howmedica, Rutherford, NJ), a monotube spring-loaded lengthening apparatus (Howmedica), the EBI Orthofix small lengthener (with and without custom modification) (EBI, Parsippany, NJ), and the Mini Hoffman lengthener for the fingers (Stryker/Howmedica). All use predrilled, threaded, self-tapping half-pins and are quite secure in their monolateral configuration.

Other available devices include the lengthening apparatus designed by Norman Cowen (Distraction, Inc.,

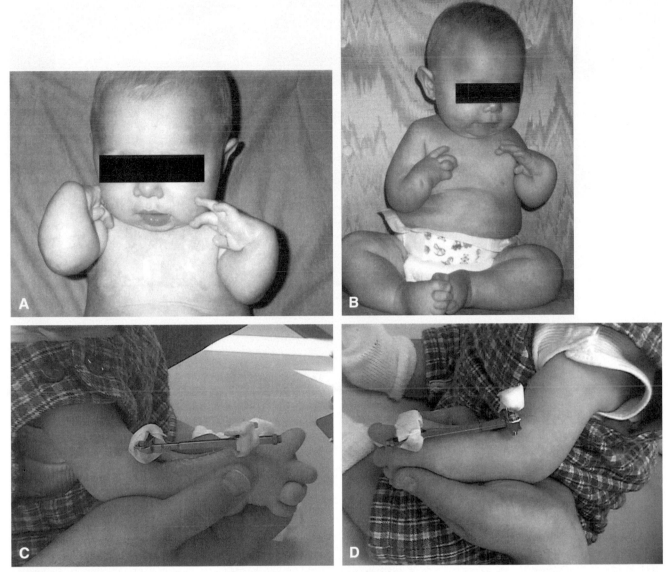

FIGURE 54-14. Three-month-old with bilateral severe radial club hand and foreshortened forearms but with good elbows is seen before treatment. **A** and **B,** Passive soft tissue stretch was performed until 6 months of age. **C** and **D,** Bilateral soft tissue distraction was performed as a first surgical procedure at age 6 months to align the carpus over the end of the ulna. *Continued*

Washington, DC) and the Patel lengthener (George Tiemann & Co., Hauppauge, NY), which have the capabilities of using either Kirschner wires or threaded half-pins. These are variations of Matev's original lengthening apparatus, which was a through-and-through, full double-frame lengthening apparatus using Kirschner wires.

Predrilled, threaded half-pins are preferable in that they achieve secure purchase in the bone through two cortices each. With the use of at least two pins, rotation and angular control are ensured. The problem of blindly skewering important soft tissue structures such as tendons and neurovascular structures that one encounters after passing through bone when through-and-through pin fixation is used is not encountered with half-pin insertion. Smooth pins such as Kirschner wires allow motion at the pin/bone interface and

therefore increase the risk of infection. This is greatly minimized by the tighter pin/bone interface provided by threaded half-pins.

Surgical Technique

Regardless of the location and the specific device chosen to perform the lengthening procedure, the technique requires certain specific technical principles that are constant with each surgical intervention. Surgery itself is performed with either general or very well executed regional block anesthesia to afford complete relaxation and patient comfort. The procedure is performed in the operating room, and an image intensifier is used to verify the proper site of pin placement, osteotomy, and final position of the pins and device.

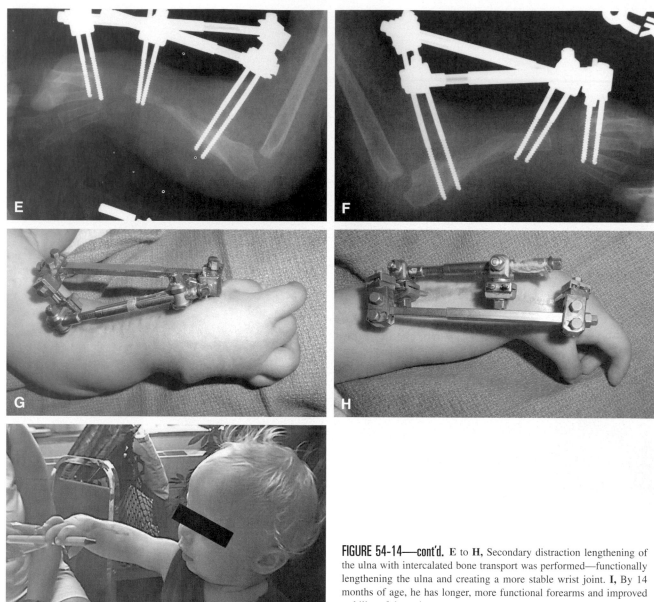

FIGURE 54-14—cont'd. E to **H**, Secondary distraction lengthening of the ulna with intercalated bone transport was performed—functionally lengthening the ulna and creating a more stable wrist joint. **I,** By 14 months of age, he has longer, more functional forearms and improved stability of the wrists.

Skin Incision

A longitudinal incision is made directly overlying the site of pin insertion. After hemostasis is obtained, blunt dissection is used to spread, divide, and protect important soft tissue structures. The length of the incision should be slightly longer than the distance between the two fixator pins to be used. The periosteum is sharply incised with a scalpel and carefully retracted partially to identify the boundaries and contour of the bone. Under direct vision, predrilling is performed through the appropriate drill guide for the device being used. One drill bit is inserted with a power driver and left in place. A second bit is passed, again using the drill guide, through two cortices of the bone and removed. Next, an appropriate-sized, self-tapping, threaded half-pin is inserted into the second drill hole and left in place, at which point the initial drill bit is removed and replaced

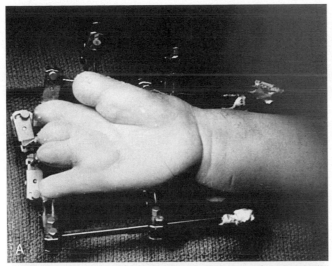

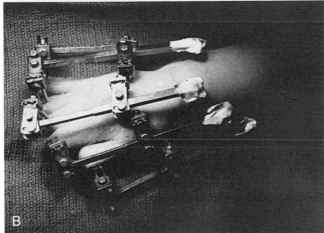

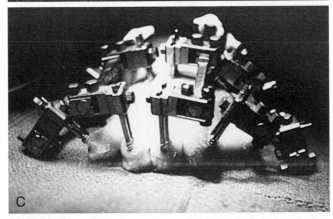

FIGURE 54-15. **A** and **B,** Lengthening of multiple digits can be achieved by using individual half-frames. These should be placed in arcuate fashion dorsally (**C**) to allow palmar tactile stimulation during the period of lengthening.

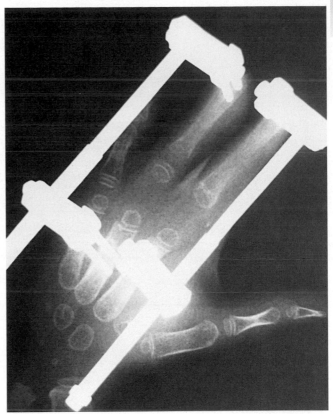

FIGURE 54-16. When very rudimentary phalanges exist, distraction across the MCP joint is possible and effective. Care should be taken to avoid damage to the physeal plate at the base of the phalanx. Distraction across the MCP joints provides enough capsular and ligamentous distraction to maintain flexibility and mobility of the fingers after removal of the device.

with a threaded half-pin of appropriate length and size (Fig. 54-18).

Distal pin placement is performed by using the same technique. In the humerus, 4-mm pins are used; in the forearm, 3-mm pins; and in the metacarpals and phalanges, 2-mm pins. Predrilling is performed with a drill equal to the size of the "core diameter" of the threaded half-pin chosen. The following drill bits are usually required: 4 mm, 3.2 mm, 3 mm, 2.0 to 2.5 mm, 2 mm, and 1.5 mm.

It is helpful to visualize the entire width of the bone to ensure central pin placement (and therefore avoid eccentric drilling or the creation of open section defects). The first of the two drills may be more easily started if an awl is used to create a superficial pilot hole in the cortex. Once the two sets of two pins are inserted, if adjacent joint stabilization is of concern, a third set of pins may be inserted, again in a similar fashion (see Fig. 54-13).

When lengthening is performed in the digits, a single longitudinal incision is made over a span of anywhere from 2 to 6 cm, depending on the bony architecture. This allows pin placement at either end of the incision and central osteotomy of the bone to be lengthened (Fig. 54-19).

Osteotomy

At a central point between the two main sets of pins, the periosteum is again incised and this time elevated circumferentially only at the site where the osteotomy is to be performed. Blunt protective retractors are used to protect the bone and ensure complete circumferential elevation of the periosteum. The osteotomy is then performed with either an

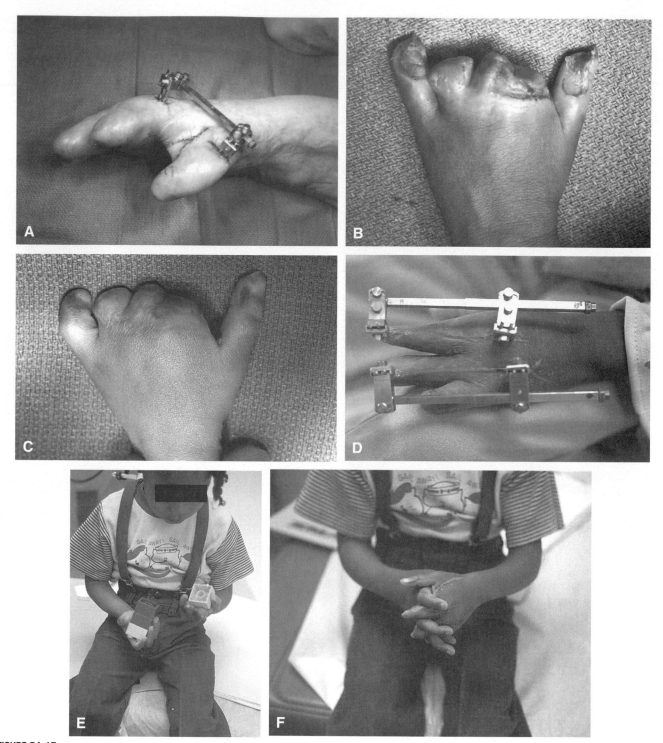

FIGURE 54-17. After burns with severe contractures and loss of digital length, soft tissue distraction can be performed to open up the thumb/index finger web space (**A**). In burns with multiple digital loss (**B**), adequate soft tissue must be achieved (**C**) before lengthening (**D**) to provide a functional outcome (**E** and **F**).

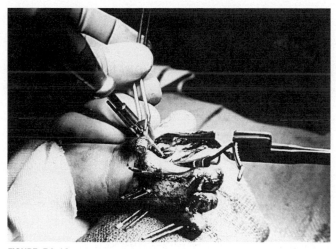

FIGURE 54-18. The surgical procedure for insertion of the lengthening apparatus is essentially the same at any level but requires the most precision in a small hypoplastic hand. Adequate visualization of the bone is essential for central pin placement. Power equipment and a drill guide are used to predrill holes for the threaded half-pins.

osteotome in adults or a blunted scalpel blade in younger children. It is imperative to preserve and protect the periosteum so that it may be closed over the site of osteotomy after completion of that portion of the surgical procedure. The osteotomy itself should *not* be performed with a power oscillating saw or other heat-producing instrument. Additionally, great caution must be taken to avoid periosteal damage and therefore help ensure satisfactory regenerate bone formation (Fig. 54-20).

Ilizarov described a somewhat different technique of cutting the bone, which he called a "corticotomy." This was done by percutaneous insertion of an osteotome and first cutting only the cortex facing the surgeon and then the cortices anterior and posterior to this, with the "far" cortex left intact. He would then fracture this remaining cortex with a rotational movement of the rings. Subsequent studies have shown that this method probably entails greater potential for injury to the blood supply, with no difference in the ability to form new bone when compared with an osteotomy. We therefore prefer to incise the periosteum and do a careful, well controlled osteotomy rather than a corticotomy, especially in the small tubular bones of the hand.

The preferable site of osteotomy is metaphyseal, but it may be diaphyseal as well. Metaphyseal bone generally tends to form new bone faster.[13,107] A diaphyseal osteotomy is usually associated with the slowest regeneration, but in younger children this is not usually an issue. Transepiphyseal osteotomy gives probably the most rapid results in terms of the rate of formation of new bone. However, as mentioned, once this has been performed, no further growth will be obtained from that physeal plate.[33,68]

Closure

At this point, before device assembly and after checking pin position, soft tissue closure is performed. The periosteum is sutured with 6-0 absorbable suture (see Fig. 54-20). Other

major soft tissue structures are allowed to fall back into place in the forearm and upper arm. The subcutaneous tissue is approximated with inverted simple sutures of absorbable material, and then the skin is closed, usually with interrupted simple sutures. Occasionally the skin may be approximated with a running subcuticular suture once the devices are assembled and secured in place. After this is completed, a sterile bulky soft dressing is applied for the first 5 days in children and 7 days in adults (the so-called delay period).

THE LENGTHENING PROCESS

The lengthening process commences from the fifth day after surgery for children and the seventh day for adults. Four daily increments of 0.25 mm each are performed at breakfast, lunch, dinner, and bedtime. This slow distraction through small increments causes gentle disruption and stimulation of the healing fracture callus, which mechanically signals the production of endosteal and periosteal new bone formation. First, fibrovascular tissue develops along with proliferation of sinusoidal blood vessels. This is followed by early bone matrix production by osteoblasts and then progressively more order and gradual maturation of the cortices and intramedullary trabecular bone. Ultimately, normal bone marrow architecture forms once complete consolidation has occurred.[4,8-10] This process continues through the lengthening period, but consolidation is not completed until some time after the lengthening has ceased. In general, the period of consolidation takes an additional two to three times the duration of the lengthening itself. If 30 mm of length is obtained over 30 days, an additional 60 days in children and 90 days in adults will generally be needed before consolidation is complete and the bony architecture stable enough for removal of the lengthening apparatus. In very young children this process is faster than in skeletally mature patients.

A record of each daily lengthening is kept by the patient or parent on a chart by checking off each lengthening, which is then compared with the calibration on the lengthening apparatus itself to confirm that the lengthening is proceeding appropriately.

A number of different lengthening devices are available, and the surgeon should be familiar with the ratio of each turn to the amount of length achieved. For digital lengthening, we have found the mini digital lengthener by Stryker/Howmedica (Fig. 54-21) to be useful for both children and adults. One-half turn of the lengthening screw produces 0.25 mm of length. We find it helpful to mark a blue and a red mark on the head of the turn screw 180 degrees opposite each other; this makes it easier to keep the record by simply alternating colors with each turn. Pin site care is done twice daily at the time the dressing is removed for an additional week. The pin sites are cleaned with a sterile cotton-tipped swab moistened with hydrogen peroxide. This helps remove coagulated and crusted blood from around the pin sites. After this first week of cleaning is complete, transition is made to cleaning in a similar manner with alcohol, still twice daily. This helps dry up the skin around the pin sites. We have found that twice-daily cleaning allows adequate removal of debris from around the pins without overstimu-

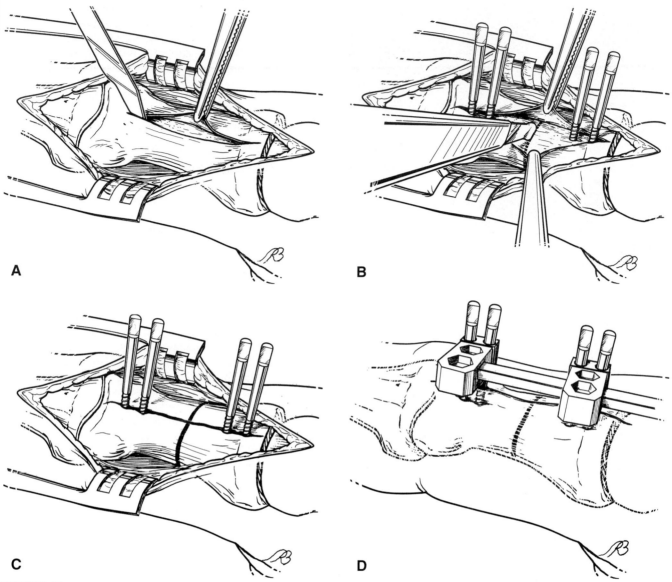

FIGURE 54-19. **A,** Meticulous dissection and preservation of the periosteum is required so that it may be repaired before closure to ensure adequate callus formation. **B,** A gentle osteotomy is performed, taking care to protect the underlying periosteal sleeve. **C,** Fixator pins are applied, taking care to place both pins in a bicortical fashion. **D,** The fixator is assembled with the bone ends in neutral apposition.

lating or irritating the surrounding skin. At this point the patient is permitted to take a daily shower and cleanse the area with fresh running water, but the hand or arm is not to be immersed. After showering, the extremity and pin sites are dried with a clean towel and then cleansed with alcohol as noted.

COMPLICATIONS

Reported complications include pin tract infection, deep infection, soft tissue compromise with distal tip necrosis, premature consolidation preventing adequate lengthening, and inadequate consolidation after lengthening has been completed. Lengthening through tight soft tissue structures

without adequate control of the proximal or distal joints has also resulted in angular deformities or joint subluxation. Fracture has occurred through the regenerate bone if the lengthening apparatus is removed prematurely and through pin sites if there has been infection or loosening of the pins. Pin loosening, bending, and breakage or device failure has resulted in loss of fixation and failure to form regenerate bone, ultimately requiring bone grafting and internal fixation.

Most of these complications, however, can frequently be prevented by avoiding the pitfalls that can occur throughout the treatment process.[78,92,110] Pin site infection can be minimized by careful handling of soft tissues, predrilling of the bone with a sharp drill bit, careful insertion of the pins to provide adequate fixation, and diligent postoperative pin

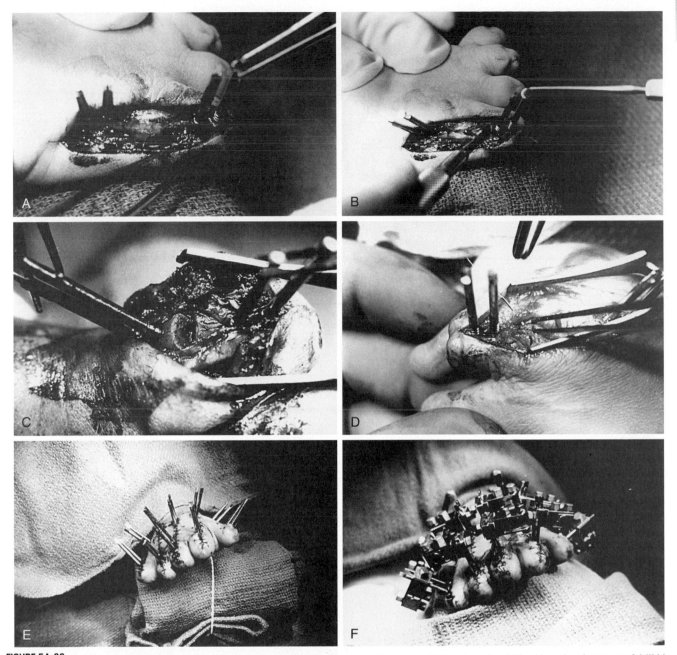

FIGURE 54-20. **A,** The dorsal approach to a hypoplastic finger has been used for central power predrilling through a drill guide and replacement of drill bits with 2.0-mm self-tapping threaded half-pins. **B,** Osteotomy was performed with a curved-tip scalpel blade in this young child (an osteotome is used in older children and adults) after periosteal elevation and protection. **C,** The subperiosteal osteotomy has been completed and both sides of the rudimentary bone to be lengthened are fully mobilized. **D,** Periosteal closure with 6-0 absorbable suture is performed. **E,** Skin closure is achieved with absorbable sutures around the fixator pins. **F,** When multiple digits are to be lengthened, complete closure is achieved before the application of multiple devices in arcuate fashion.

site care. Soft tissue damage at the tip of the lengthened extremity can be minimized by careful observation of the tip to watch for signs of excessive tightness or diminished vascularity, a sign to stop or at least slow down the lengthening process. Also, lengthening should not be done through severely scarred or poorly vascularized skin and subcutaneous tissue. Occasionally, preoperative flap coverage made over the distal tip can avoid such a complication.

Careful education and compliance of the patient and family are important to ensure that the lengthening process begins and continues on a precisely timed schedule. If this can be ensured, premature consolidation can almost always be avoided. Inadequate bone regeneration is usually the result of lengthening through dysvascular bone or bone in which the periosteum has been severely stripped or damaged. Careful, gentle handling of the periosteum

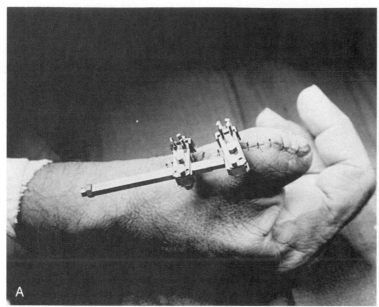
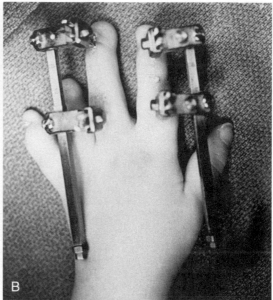

FIGURE 54-21. The Mini Hoffman lengthening device (Howmedica, Rutherford, NJ) is useful in both adult (**A**) and pediatric (**B**) digital lengthening and provides secure fixation during the lengthening process.

with meticulous closure and choice of location for the osteotomy through well-vascularized bone helps avoid this complication.

Patience and careful observation of radiographs to ensure completion of consolidation, cortical continuity on at least three sides, and a confluent appearance of the intramedullary bone help avoid fracture through prematurely unprotected regenerate bone because of early device removal. The device should remain in place under tension until such radiographic evidence has been achieved. Joint luxation or angular deformity can be avoided by securing control of the joint through a third set of pins across that joint. Pins of

adequate size placed in parallel and appropriately spaced for the fixation device can avoid pin bending and breakage. The device used should be of appropriate size and durability to tolerate the forces at the particular level of the extremity. Satisfactory mechanical condition of the device should be checked by the surgeon before clinical use in the operating room. These fundamentally simple steps can greatly reduce the occurrence of complications and contribute to a successful outcome.

The outcome of these procedures has proved in our experience to provide a high level of patient (and parent) satisfaction through enhanced prehensile function (Fig. 54-22).

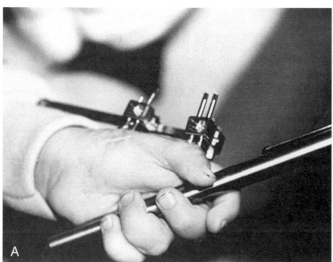
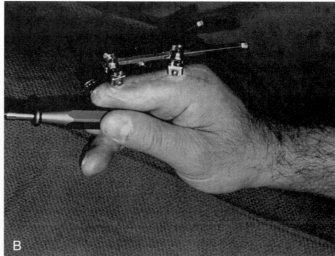

FIGURE 54-22. The lengthening device should be positioned in such a way as to allow the child (**A**) or adult (**B**) to use the hand during the lengthening process. This affords preparation for later functional use of the hand from the outset.

CRITICAL POINTS: DISTRACTION LENGTHENING IN THE HAND AND UPPER EXTREMITY

INDICATIONS

- Functional skeletal deficiency
- Congenital/developmental/traumatic
- Hypoplasia/growth arrest/amputation/segmental bone loss
- Phalanges/metacarpals/radius/ulna/humerus

PREOPERATIVE EVALUATION

- Evaluate the degree of skeletal and soft tissue deficiency.
- Radiographs are usually adequate.
- Evaluate stability/mobility of adjacent joints.
- Consider alternative techniques (microvascular tissue transfer, prosthesis).
- Set realistic goals (function over cosmesis).
- Prepare patient/parents for labor-intensive postoperative course.
- Get to know patient/family (multiple consultations/visits); compliance is mandatory.
- Discuss potential complications and need for auxiliary surgery with patient/family.

Pearls

- Identify noncompliant/unrealistic patient/family.
  - Offer other treatment/suggest second opinion.
- Educate patient/family well.
- Let patient/family talk to others who have "been through it."

Pitfalls

- Noncompliance/inadequate education
- Leads to poor follow-up

TECHNICAL POINTS

- Use dorsal approach.
- Note that multiple rays "fan out" pin insertion: dorsal radial/dorsal central/dorsal ulna.
- Carefully preserve periosteum.
- Use central pin insertion.
- Use two threaded half-pins on either side of osteotomy.
- Perform a careful, gentle osteotomy (no power saw).
- Carefully repair the periosteum.
- Apply stable fixator/lengthener (unilateral half-frame).
- Add static stabilizing pins with outrigger to unstable adjacent joints.
- Use bulky soft compression dressing.

Pitfalls

- Inadequate fixation
- Lengthening through dysvascular bone

- Rough tissue handling (especially periosteum)
- Through-and-through pins leading to traction injury to nerves/vessels
- Unrecognized soft tissue contracture joint instability
- Off-center, poorly drilled pin sites resulting in loose pins and, thus, infection

Pearls

- Release scar contractures.
- Central Kirschner wire can prevent angular deviation (especially thumb).
- Preoperative flap coverage can be used if there is poor skin distally to ensure viable vascular skin.
- Correct angular deformity with closing wedge osteotomy.

POSTOPERATIVE CARE

- Remove dressing after 5 days for child and 7 days for adult.
- Perform pin site care twice daily (use hydrogen peroxide for first week, thereafter alcohol).
- Perform four lengthenings daily of 0.25 mm (at breakfast/lunch/dinner/bed time).
- Keep chart to record lengthenings and pin site care.
- Follow up weekly with radiographs.
- Stop lengthening when desired/maximal length is achieved.
- Consolidation: leave device in place for two to three times the duration of lengthening.
- Remove device when there is good radiographic evidence of healing.
- Apply splint/cast if there is a question of incomplete healing.
- At first sign of pin site infection, begin oral antibiotics.
- Slow the rate of lengthening if pain develops late in lengthening process.

Pitfalls

- Noncompliance/poor follow-up/inadequate pin care
- Delay in treating pin site infection
- Overdistraction leading to pain/skin breakdown
- Premature device removal leading to regenerate fracture

Pearls

- Have patient/family bring chart to weekly visit.
- Emphasize need for compliance daily.
- If pain develops, slow the rate of lengthening to one to two (0.25-0.5 mm) times daily.
- If poor/inadequate bone regeneration is noted on a radiograph, remove fixator earlier and use bone grafting.

ANNOTATED REFERENCES

4. Aronson J: The biology of distraction osteogenesis. *In* Bianchi-Maiocchi A, Aronson J (eds): Operative Principles of Ilizarov: Fracture Treatment, Nonunion, Osteomyelitis, Lengthening, Deformity Correction. Baltimore, Williams & Wilkins, 1991, pp 42-52.

    In this chapter in a landmark text discussing the principles developed by Ilizarov for distraction lengthening, the author details in a stepwise fashion the biology of distraction lengthening through healing fracture callus. The histologic stages of new bone formation related to the development of stress/tension during lengthening are detailed and set a rational foundation for the principles of callus distraction from the point of surgical intervention through device removal.

22. Cattaneo R, Catagni MA, Guerreschi F: Treatment of radial agenesis with the Ilizarov method. Rev Chir Orthop Reparatice Appar Mot 87:443-450, 2001.

    This retrospective review of 15 cases in which an Ilizarov frame was utilized to treat radial agenesis demonstrates the effectiveness of soft tissue distraction as a first stage followed by lengthening. The authors use this technique, although they have elected to perform a compression arthrodesis of the wrist using the same device. Unfortunately a rather subjective evaluation technique is utilized in which the majority of the patients were rated as average, only one was rated as poor, whereas the aesthetic result was good or excellent in 12 of the 15 lengthenings. The importance of this paper is that the long-term results demonstrated stability and maintenance of alignment with reasonable functional hand use over an extended period of time (1 to 16 years).

23. Cattaneo R, Villa A, Catagni MA, Bell D: Lengthening of the humerus using the Ilizarov technique. Description of the method and report of 43 cases. Clin Orthop 250:117-124, 1990.

    In this retrospective review, the authors detail the application of a distraction apparatus for a variety of pathologic states to restore functional length to the humerus. This large series demonstrates the surgical technique of using a circular frame to lengthen the humerus. It provides a foundation for the application of this technique to a variety of conditions. Some of the problems with use of a circular device despite satisfactory outcomes provide a rationale for utilizing more streamline lengthening apparatus.

25. Cowan NJ, Loftus JM Jr: Distraction augmentation manoplasty: Technique for lengthening digits or entire hands. Orthop Rev 7:45-53, June 1978.

    In this classic paper, the authors demonstrate application of distraction lengthening to multiple fingers using free bone transfers to fill the distraction gap. This paper provides a foundation for the use of lengthening techniques for the creation of functional digits but demonstrates the limitations of lengthening of multiple digits with a single full frame and emphasizes the need for subsequent surgery, including division of the artificially created syndactyly when this technique is utilized. It provides a foundation on which newer techniques have been built.

32. Dhalla R, Strecker W, Manske PR: A comparison of two techniques for digital distraction lengthening in skeletally immature patients. J Hand Surg [Am] 26:603-610, 2001.

    In this paper the authors demonstrate utilization of a technique requiring fewer pins to lengthen terminal bones in the hands of skeletally immature children when there is minimal room to implant half pins. They use a central Kirschner wire and single pins on either side of the osteotomy, achieving satisfactory length and outcome; however, this technique was associated with a higher complication rate. It appears to have a valuable role in very short terminal skeletal structures as an alternative to lengthening across a joint.

48. Horii E, Nakamura R, Nakao E, et al: Distraction lengthening of the forearm for congenital and developmental problems. J Hand Surg [Br] 25:15-21, 2000.

    Thirty-five callus distractions of the forearm reviewed by the authors in 23 patients. Eleven patients carry the diagnosis of congenital dysplasia while 12 demonstrated growth disturbances from tumors or infection. The authors noted a correlation between a slower healing rate with older children with congenital hypoplasia while those with developmental problems demonstrated excellent healing and callus formation regardless of age. However, in the second group the authors demonstrate the problems with early device removal resulting in callus deformity. They also demonstrate the effectiveness of two separate shorter lengthenings to both correct length discrepancy and reduce an unstable radial head (which had been chronically dislocated). This paper illustrates the importance of controlling unstable segments during the lengthening process and initiating the process earlier in the face of congenital shortening of the forearm.

49. Houshian S, Ipsen T: Metacarpal and phalangeal lengthening by callus distraction. J Hand Surg [Br] 26:13-26, 2001.

    In this series of 14 patients, individual lengthening of 12 metacarpals with two cases of phalangeal lengthening resulted in satisfactory functional outcome. The authors demonstrate the importance of careful periosteal preservation and repair as a key to successful regenerate bone formation. Pin tract infections were noted in 5 patients; and in those patients with thumb lengthening, "Z"-plasty was needed as an auxiliary surgical procedure. This paper further demonstrates the effectiveness of this technique in both children and adults with both congenital and traumatic skeletal deficiency.

50. Ilizarov GA: The tension-stress effect on the genesis and growth of tissues: I. The influence of stability of fixation and soft-tissue preservation. Clin Orthop 238:249-281, 1989.

    This landmark paper provides a foundation for the use of longitudinal traction through healing fracture callus within an intact periosteal sleeve and provides the basis for generation of newly formed bone when the callus is disrupted very slowly and gradually in multiple lengthenings throughout the day. The author's vast clinical experience is used to demonstrate application of this technique throughout all the long bones of the skeleton.

51. Ilizarov GA: The tension-stress effect on the genesis and growth of tissues: II. The influence of the rate and frequency of distraction. Clin Orthop 239:263-285, 1989.

    In this second part of Ilizarov's landmark paper, the author demonstrates the rationale for multiple daily lengthenings of small increments with a maximum of 1 mm per day. This and the prior paper have been the foundation for application of callus distraction techniques throughout the body and provide the rationale for all subsequent clinical series that seek to use this technique while eliminating the need for intercalated bone graft.

56. Joist A, Neuber M, Frebel T, Joosten U: Callus distraction of the first metacarpal bone for thumb reconstruction after traumatic amputation. Unfallchirurg 103:1073-1078, 2000.

    The authors here demonstrate the effectiveness of callus distraction lengthening of the thumb metacarpal after traumatic amputation in a large series of 34 patients with follow-up in 31. The average length achieved was 78% compared with the uninjured side. This provided functional prehension and use in activity of daily living rated as excellent in 20 patients, good in 9, and unsatisfactory in 2. Complications were noted in 12 patients; 11 of these were limited to infections that responded to oral antibiotics and fracture through incompletely healed callus in one. These very functional results with relatively minor complications provide support for the use of this technique for reconstruction of an amputated thumb as a viable alternative to microvascular toe transplantation.

60. Kessler I, Baruch A, Hecht O: Experience with distraction lengthening of digital rays in congenital anomalies. J Hand Surg 2:394-401, 1977.

Another landmark article provides the foundation for the use of distraction techniques for constructing functional digits in children born with congenitally hypoplastic hands. In this paper, the authors note the relatively poor rate of regenerate bone formation (probably owing to rapid lengthening techniques) and advocated insertion of intercalated bone grafts as a second stage. The through-and-through technique utilizing Kirschner wires in a cumbersome double frame device made central ray lengthening difficult but was particularly useful in the thumb.

63. Launay F, Jouve JL, Guillaume JM, et al: Progressive forearm lengthening in children: 14 cases. Rev Chir Orthop Reparatrice Appar Mot 87:786-795, 2001.

The authors demonstrate the effectiveness of a half unilateral frame lengthening device for forearm distraction in 14 cases. They recommend the effectiveness of closing wedge osteotomy for primary angular correction and use of intramedullary wire to help maintain this correction during the lengthening and healing process. They noted the presence of the rod helped maintain correction, avoid regenerate fracture, and enhance healing but demonstrated a relatively slow healing index of 62 days per centimeter of bone lengthened. It provides rationale for using a unilateral frame even in the face of angular deformity as an alternative to the more cumbersome and complicated circular frame devices.

69. Matev IB: Thumb reconstruction through metacarpal bone lengthening. J Hand Surg 5:482-487, 1980.

This classic review of a pioneer's experience in utilizing distraction lengthening of the thumb again provides a foundation for subsequent studies utilizing distraction to reconstruct traumatically amputated thumbs. Initial use of callus distraction in the periosteal sleeve showed very long waiting periods for bone regeneration that today would be considered an unacceptably long period of containment. It provided the initial rationale for early bone grafting but provides a glimpse of the potential for effective callus distraction, which has later proven to be possible.

70. McCarroll HR. Congenital anomalies: A 25 year overview. J Hand Surg [Am] 25:1007-1037, 2000.

In this comprehensive review paper, the author reviews a quarter century evolution in the understanding and care of congenital hand anomalies. Within this framework, he chronicles the evolution of the use of distraction lengthening in the hand and forearm providing examples of older, more cumbersome devices while acknowledging the evolution of new techniques utilizing more streamlined devices. This paper acknowledges the importance of distraction lengthening in the armamentarium of the surgeon caring for congenital differences.

71. Miyawaki T, Masuzawa G, Hirakawa M, Kurihara K: Bone-lengthening for symbrachydactyly of the hand with the technique of callus distraction. J Bone Joint Surg Am 84:986-991, 2002.

Although only a small series of only four patients, long-term results of metacarpal callus distraction demonstrated improved pinch and grasp function and prehensile use of the hand in everyday activities while maintaining satisfactory sensation for patients with significant loss of function due to symbrachydactyly of the ulnar side of the hand. The results generated stable posts with basilar joint mobility that could be functionally opposed to the thumb and index fingers. The authors utilized a half-frame device and intramedullary Kirschner wires simultaneously lengthening two metacarpals at once.

88. Raimondo RA, Skaggs DL, Rosenwasser MP, Dick HM: Lengthening of pediatric forearm deformities using the Ilizarov technique: Functional and cosmetic results. J Hand Surg [Am] 24:331-338, 1999.

The authors demonstrate the technique and effectiveness of substantially lengthening very shortened forearms achieving between 3.6 and 8.1 cm of increased length with an average healing index between 0.6 and 1.9 months per centimeter lengthened, with total treatment times ranging between 3 and 12 months. Despite a significant complication rate including pin tract infections, finger contractions, nonunion, and a case of finger, wrist, and elbow contractures, the authors note that ultimately good functional results and very satisfying cosmetic results were obtained in the majority of the patients. All patients had previously undergone wrist stabilization, pollicization, and/or tendon transfers to improve prehensile function. Angular correction was achieved gradually through asymmetrical lengthening with the circular Ilizarov device, which as demonstrated was quite cumbersome.

89. Rudolf KD, Preisser P, Partecke BD: Callus distraction in the hand skeleton. Injury 31(Suppl 1):113-120, 2000.

The authors here demonstrate the effectiveness of callus distraction for reconstruction of the thumb and fingers after traumatic amputation and/or skeletal loss in 27 patients in whom 36 digits were lengthened. Of interest is the authors' ability to combine the technique of distraction with other forms of reconstruction such as a wraparound flap to recreate a functional opposable thumb. Complications were noted in nine cases. Only three were pin tract infections, but pin breakage and/or loosening were noted in five (probably related to poor pin insertion techniques or inadequate device control). The need for additional surgical procedures included bone grafting in 3 cases, correction of fixator position in 10, web space deepening in 7, and release of contractures of the carpometacarpal joint in 4. These complications and secondary procedures demonstrate the importance of meticulous attention to surgical detail and choice of a stable device that probably could have avoided a number of the complications and need for secondary surgery. Web space deepening, however, is noted to be an important adjunct even in the face of satisfactory lengthening without complications.

96. Seitz WH Jr, Froimson AI: Callotasis lengthening in the upper extremity. Indications, techniques and pitfalls. J Hand Surg [Am] 16:932-939, 1991.

In this paper, the authors detail strict indications and contraindications and provide a stepwise surgical technique for the successful performance of callus distraction in the hand and upper extremity. Experience obtained through careful review and analysis of complications have demonstrated procedural pitfalls that have led to those complications and that if avoided can help reduce their occurrence.

97. Seitz WH Jr, Froimson AI: Digital lengthening using the callotasis technique. Orthopedics 18:129-138, 1995.

This paper details the effectiveness of the technique of callus distraction in digital reconstruction in both congenital and post-traumatic deformities. Application of surgical techniques in both children and adults is presented. The importance of careful postoperative follow-up and patient selection is emphasized with recommendations for postoperative rehabilitation.

107. Toh S, Narita S, Arai K, Tsubo K: Distraction lengthening by callotasis in the hand. J Bone Joint Surg Br 84:205-210, 2002.

This paper presents the results of distraction lengthening in 26 digits of 18 adult patients all resulting from traumatic amputation. Again, the authors demonstrate effective functional outcome and acknowledge the importance of avoidance of complications (3 months per centimeter healing index without complications, compared with 5 months per centimeter healing index in patients with complications). In all cases, a half-frame device was utilized. Five patients required bone grafting, four of whom demonstrated fracture through incompletely healed callus. The authors note improved rate of healing and neo-osteogenesis when osteotomy was performed in proximal metaphyseal bone as opposed to diaphyseal bone. This paper's importance lies in its recognition of the effectiveness of this technique in adults while reminding the reader that healing is both slower and somewhat less predictable and may have a higher rate of need for secondary bone grafting in this population.

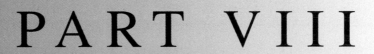

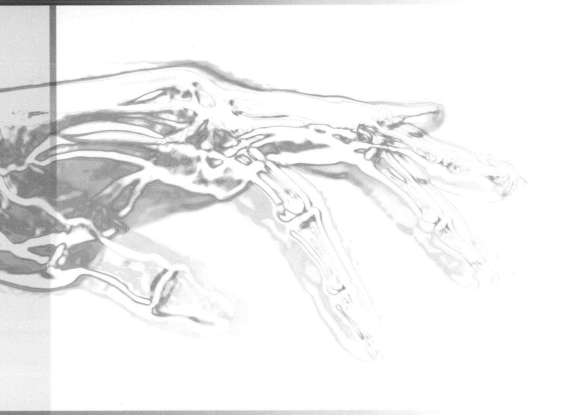

PART VIII

Other Disorders of the Upper Extremity

CHAPTER 55

Amputations

Peter J. L. Jebson and Dean S. Louis

Amputations in the upper extremities may occur as a result of trauma, an elective decision involving congenital deformities,[1] or acquired pathologic conditions such as malignant tumors.[273,275,279,281,283,285,294,299] Amputations may occasionally be self-inflicted because of a psychological disturbance or in an attempt to defraud an insurance company.[6] Functional rehabilitation is the primary consideration after an amputation. Special considerations may occur with malignant tumors. The surgeon's initial responsibility is to know the patient's occupation and avocations and to appreciate the patient's emotional attitude regarding the amputation. This latter facet of the patient's dilemma is the most difficult to assess. Failure to appreciate the patient's attitude and ability to adjust to the injury may compromise an otherwise successful operative procedure. The patient's adjustment may be tempered by the individual's self-concept and concern with body image, as well as cultural background.

As surgeons, we tend to be largely influenced by the experience of our mentors early in our careers and later by our own expanding experience. We hold fast to those methods that prove satisfactory in our hands and quickly seek alternatives to those procedures that do not work well for us. The numerous articles referred to in this chapter attest to the reasoned contributions of many authors who treat seemingly similar amputation situations by widely disparate methods. The multiplicity of techniques for the management of digital tip injuries* is a clear example of the conundrum facing an inexperienced surgeon confronted with such a problem. To some surgeons, the more technically demanding procedures such as cross-finger flaps† and advancement flaps[177,191,193] have great appeal. For others, the simpler procedures of split-thickness grafting,[21,49,103,109,110,117] shortening of bone followed by primary closure,[75,97,137] or healing by secondary intention[76,91,97,98,105,107] have gained preference. There is clearly no best way to handle all situations, and no amount of verbiage should convince any of us otherwise. Rather, we are faced with alternatives based on modifying information relating to the patient. This is particularly true of distal amputations involving the digits. More proximal amputations involving levels at the wrist or more cephalad become less controversial because they are related more to specific prosthetic requirements than to the relative choices of the patient and surgeon.

Simply stated, the goals of amputation surgery in the upper extremity should be (1) preservation of functional length, (2) durable coverage, (3) preservation of useful sensibility, (4) prevention of symptomatic neuromas,[85,270] (5) prevention of adjacent joint contractures, (6) short morbidity, (7) early prosthetic fitting when applicable, and (8) early return of the patient to work and play.

CRITICAL POINTS: GOALS OF AMPUTATION SURGERY

- Preservation of functional length
- Durable coverage
- Preservation of useful sensibility
- Prevention of symptomatic neuromas
- Prevention of adjacent joint contractures
- Short morbidity
- Early prosthetic fitting where applicable
- Early return of patient to work and other activities

The treatment of any amputation in children, whose ultimate roles in life are less well defined, should be approached with a conservative attitude. Late reconstruction is generally preferable to any early radical ablative procedure. Adults with well-defined functional roles may be better served by a more aggressive attitude when it will accelerate their functional rehabilitation.

At times the decision to perform other alternatives of limb salvage versus amputation may be difficult. No reliable injury severity score exists as a guide for treatment decision making after severe upper extremity trauma. Consultation on these difficult cases with a knowledgeable colleague is helpful for all concerned. It will reassure the patient and the family and be helpful should medicolegal matters ensue. If a colleague has reviewed the case, it is also helpful to document this in the patient's medical record.

---

*See references 66, 75-77, 80, 90, 97, 109, 110, 114, 118, 125, 127, 129, 135-138, 144, and 152.

†See references 154, 165, 166, 168-173, 175, 179, 180, 183, 185, 194, and 197.

Although replantation or attempted salvage of a severely traumatized limb at times is an option, it may represent a technical triumph rather than the patient's best interests. The total needs of the patient must be considered. A carefully thought out and meticulously performed amputation should not be considered ablative. It more properly should be considered reconstructive and rehabilitative. Recent literature has emphasized the social and economic consequences of finger amputations.[8,29] The enthusiasm for the successful technical accomplishment of replanting an amputated finger part versus closure and early rehabilitation has been dampened by poor patient outcomes at a greater financial cost, namely, lost wages and the cost of hospitalization and therapy. Cold intolerance is still a problem despite replantation.[45]

CORTICAL REORGANIZATION AFTER AMPUTATION

Investigators have recently focused their attention on the patient's ability to adapt after an amputation, specifically the reorganization of the cerebral cortex motor system.[50,51,60] Several elaborate studies have demonstrated that the functional plasticity of the cerebral cortex occurs independent of the type of amputation (i.e., finger, forearm, or above elbow) and can occur as quickly as 10 days postoperatively.[60] Reorganization of the motor system has been noted in patients more than 20 years after amputation. Differential patterns of corticospinal output can occur, yet not all patients with an amputation have evidence of reorganization. This is an exciting development, but its relevance with respect to rehabilitation after amputation is not well understood at this time.

DIGITAL TIP AMPUTATIONS

An amputation of the fingertip is the most common type of amputation seen in the upper extremity and at the same time provokes the greatest controversy. Although it is generally agreed that the length of the thumb should be maintained by reasonable means, there is less agreement about the wisdom or necessity of maintaining length of the other digits. Multiple ingenious techniques have been developed to advance local skin or transfer skin from an adjacent digit to ensure coverage of an area where bone is exposed. Microvascular reattachment of an amputated fingertip has also been described. No set of rules can be laid down that will serve as a satisfactory guide to the application of each of these techniques. Every surgeon, in consultation with each patient, must choose the type of coverage that appears to be most appropriate for that individual's needs and within the technical abilities of the surgeon. Regardless of choice of treatment, the goals of preserving functional length and restoring adequate sensibility remain constant.

Digital Tip Amputations With Skin or Pulp Loss Only

When the digital tip is amputated, the geometry of the defect dictates the various treatment possibilities. The loss may be transverse or oblique, with more volar skin loss than dorsal skin loss, or the reverse may be true. Some slicing amputations may result in skin loss primarily from the ulnar or radial side of the digit and spare the distal tip.

Primary Closure

Primary closure of a distal tip amputation of pulp may be an option if the location and amount of skin loss permit the placement of sutures without excessive tension. It is difficult to compare the results of primary closure with other methods because the majority of tip amputations lack sufficient mobile dermis for a tension-free primary repair. Primary closure, when possible, was shown in the series of Holm and Zachariae[97] to give results equivalent to conservative healing by secondary intention (88% good results). However, in the series reported by Sturman and Duran,[137] 51% of the patients complained of tenderness and had some disability. Clearly, more studies using comparable patients and level of soft tissue loss are needed to resolve the contradictory conclusions of the available reports.

Nail Horns

The formation of a nail horn can be a very frustrating complication for both the patient and the surgeon after a fingertip injury. Unfortunately, a nail horn may develop despite the surgeon's best efforts to ablate the nail matrix. We routinely caution the patient about the potential development of nail horn formation postoperatively.

We resect the entire nail matrix if the amputation is very proximal, that is, at or through the lunula. An attempt is made to resect the *entire* matrix, both sterile and especially germinal, which means thoroughly scraping the dorsal cortex of distal phalanx with a curet. A common error is to fail to resect the nail-producing tissue that resides on the underneath surface of the proximal nail fold (see Chapter 10).

Split-Thickness Grafting

Split-thickness skin grafting has been a popular method for coverage of the exposed pulp.[21,49,95,113] However, in a follow-up study conducted with a minimum follow-up of 5 years, Holm and Zachariae[97] found that only 56% of the patients who had undergone skin grafting considered their results to be good, compared with 90% of patients treated conservatively with a wound that was permitted to heal by secondary intention. The most important complaints after skin grafting were induration and fissuring of the skin and reduced sensibility in the area of the graft, as well as complaints about the donor site. Cold sensitivity was present in 39% of the patients treated conservatively and in 33% of those who received a split-thickness skin graft. Hypoesthesia was present in 26% of those treated conservatively and in 67% of those who were treated with a skin graft. Primary suturing, when possible, also had the same level of patient satisfaction as simple conservative management (90% good results). The authors concluded that split-thickness skin grafting offered no advantages for fingertip coverage.

Sturman and Duran[137] monitored 235 patients for a minimum of 1 year and reported their late results from these procedures. Seventy percent of the patients who had split-thickness skin grafts reported tenderness in the area of the graft, and in 41% the tenderness was considered to be marked. Cold sensitivity was present in 49% of the patients who had split-thickness skin grafts, including 27 of the 53 who had thumb or index tip amputations. Fifty-nine percent of the latter group avoided the injured digit when the pickup test was used. Thirty-two percent of them noted diminished touch sensibility. The average two-point discrimination measured was 5 mm, markedly worse than the normal 2 mm.

Ridley[126] performed biopsies of split-thickness skin grafts that had been taken from the forearm and placed on the hand and demonstrated that, although there had been some architectural modification of the skin from the forearm to its new location, there were no dermal ridges in the graft and Meissner's corpuscles were absent in the three patients studied at an average follow-up of 4 years. These findings may account for the diminished sensibility observed in sites of split-thickness skin coverage. Some authors[100,132,189] have maintained that there is an improved reinnervation density when hypothenar skin is grafted to cover a digital defect. There is no histologic support for such a contention. Jabaley's work[101] suggests that sensory end organs may be reinnervated after nerve section and repair but that new ones do not form de novo. It is difficult to see, then, how transplanted skin could assume a sensory testing pattern that is like the recipient area rather than like the donor site. These reports are in conflict and point to the need for more studies and a critical skepticism of the information available at this time. The central perception of an applied distal stimulus in an effort to evaluate the return of sensibility to a grafted site may be spurious. In small grafted areas the stimuli may be not only to the grafted site but also to the surrounding tissue, thus giving a nearly normal value for the test.[100]

Bojsen-Moller and coworkers[75] reviewed a series of 134 digital tip injuries in 110 patients who were treated by skin grafting, shortening of the digit, or conservative (nonoperative) treatment. They found that the period of unfitness for work was no longer for those treated conservatively than it was for those treated by other surgical methods. They also observed that conservative treatment was almost always uncomplicated whereas in some of the surgical cases there were complications such as infection or graft failure that prolonged treatment. Tenderness after amputation was the most common late symptom. From their data they concluded that management of amputation by shortening and primary closure was inferior to skin grafting or conservative treatment. There is also ample evidence from the studies of Illingworth,[98] Bossley,[76] Das,[88] and Douglas[91] that conservative management of fingertip injuries in children, when there is no exposed bone, is the preferred method. The studies of Holm and Zachariae[97] and Louis and colleagues[107] reported that appropriate conservative management in adults is as effective as and comparable to that in children (Fig. 55-1). Additional studies have confirmed the success of dressing changes and healing by secondary intention for the management of fingertip injuries.[64,83,121]

Several alternative forms of conservative treatment have been proposed. They all have in common the use of a nonadherent dressing, which is changed periodically until healing is completed. Some authors prefer an occlusive splint over the dressing. However, this is a matter of individual choice inasmuch as the reported results seem equivalent. The skin remaining on the amputated part may be sewn back to the fingertip as a *biologic dressing* after appropriate cleansing and trimming.

Cold intolerance is a consequence of the injury itself and was found in as many as 39% of those treated conservatively, but the incidence was even higher in those treated with other methods.[77,97,107,144] Although early coverage and wound closure may be accomplished by means of a split-thickness skin graft, there is no assurance that the patient's problem will end at this point. In fact, it is more likely that the finger will be cold intolerant, suffer dysesthesias, and have diminished sensibility. As noted later (see Authors' Preferred Method of Treatment), the best option for a tip amputation without exposed bone, regardless of age, is the simplest yet effective technique of healing by secondary intention with dressing changes.•

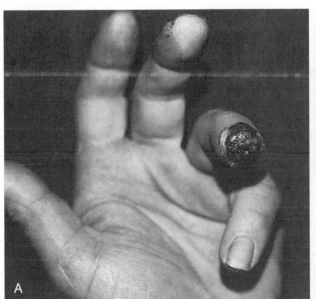
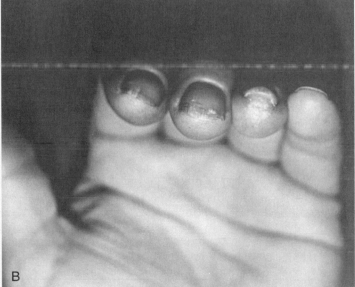

FIGURE 55-1. **A,** Nondominant ring finger in a 53-year-old machinist who lost the fingertip in a transverse fashion just distal to the distal phalanx. **B,** The injury was treated by the open technique (healing by secondary intention) and is seen here 6 weeks post injury. Notice how the tip has recontoured.

Digital Tip Amputations With Exposed Bone

Most of our patients with digital tip amputations and exposed bone are managed in the emergency department. They undergo skeletal shortening and primary closure under digital block anesthesia. The patient is usually seen within 48 to 72 hours for a wound check, and the dressing is changed at that time. Dry dressings may be used if the wound has been closed. Alternatively, wet to dry dressings are applied twice daily if the wound is healing by secondary intention. Patients are taught to perform their own dressing changes.

Oral antibiotics are not routinely prescribed. The use of oral antibiotics is based on surgeon preference and the degree of wound contamination, as well as on individual patient factors. If the patient is a diabetic or immunocompromised or the wound is grossly contaminated, prophylactic antibiotics are appropriate. However, if adequate cleaning and débridement of the wound have been performed, antibiotics are not routinely prescribed.

Supervised occupational therapy is not necessary for most patients, but a program of tip desensitization is initiated once the wound has fully healed, under the supervision of a hand therapist (see p. 1981). If the patient has unacceptable digital swelling, Coban wrapping and range-of-motion exercises are used. This is a home program that the patient personally performs after being instructed on a one-time basis by the therapist. Coban wrapping and range-of-motion exercises are begun within 48 hours, usually after the first dressing change. Tip desensitization is not performed until the wound is fully healed. In our experience, manual laborers may be expected to return to work without restriction by 6 to 8 weeks. However, if the workplace is able to facilitate an early return-to-work program with restrictions, we encourage this.

The development of a hooked nail is avoided by careful attention to wound closure of a fingertip amputation and avoiding the loss of bony support for the nail bed. Closure of a fingertip amputation by pulling the nail bed over the distal phalanx should be avoided. If a satisfactory amount of distal phalanx is absent, the nail bed must be trimmed back to the same level at the end of the bone so that it does not curve over the end of the bone and subsequently lead to the development of a hooked nail. If a hooked nail develops, we recommend revision with shortening of the phalanx and nail bed to a comparable level. Alternatively, a local advancement flap may be used to replace a soft tissue tip. We prefer these simple approaches rather than attempts at free vascularized transfer of toe tips, distal phalanx, and nail.

When no bone is exposed at the time of digital tip amputation, the decision-making process becomes one of whether coverage is to be undertaken (and if so what type) or whether healing should be allowed to proceed by secondary intention. When bone is exposed in the wound, the question then becomes whether length should be preserved (necessitating coverage of the site) or if sacrifice of length is justifiable in the given situation. Because the primary aim is to restore function to the injured individual, many of the wounds with exposed bone may be converted to wounds with no bone exposed by rongeuring followed by closure. Alternatively, if there is no possibility of direct closure, coverage may be accomplished by means of a local rotation flap or by other methods such as a V-Y advancement flap using the Atasoy-Kleinert or Kutler technique as indicated.

Each technique of tip coverage must be evaluated on its own merits and the particular requirements of the individual patient and always compared with nonoperative management using dressing changes and closure by secondary intention. Familiarity with the few good follow-up studies is mandatory if the surgeon's judgment is to be guided by historical experience rather than the technical appeal of some of the procedures mentioned, which unfortunately have a high incidence of complications and questionable value to the patient.

The following section describes various techniques of flap coverage that have been advocated for tip amputation with exposed bone. In the surgical literature it is not unusual to find that the originator of a technique reports results that are far superior to those obtained by others. This certainly appears to be the case with many of the techniques that have been devised for the management of digital tip amputations. We therefore have focused on studies reported by surgeons other than the originators of the specific techniques. In these studies the results suggest that significant complications are associated with most of these more complex forms of treatment.

In reviewing the follow-up studies of Illingworth,[98] Bossley,[76] Holm and Zachariae,[97] Bojsen-Moller and colleagues,[75] and Conolly and Goulston,[85] we have come to the inevitable conclusion that an adult with a fingertip injury in which there is pulp loss has between a 30% and 50% chance of having some cold intolerance and an approximately 30% chance of having some aberration in sensibility, regardless of which wound management technique is used. These features appear to be the consequence of *the injury itself* and not *the treatment*.

Atasoy-Kleinert Volar V-Y Flap

In 1970 Atasoy and associates[148] described a triangular volar V-Y flap advancement (Fig. 55-2) for reconstruction of the distal pad with preservation of length when bone is exposed. They suggested that the procedure was applicable to most fingertip amputations, even those in which bone was not exposed. They believed that it was contraindicated in injuries in which there was an oblique flap with more palmar skin loss than dorsal and in situations in which there was extensive skin loss as a result of the injury.

Digital or metacarpal anesthesia is instituted before preparation of the wound. After surgical preparation of the hand, a Penrose drain is used to exsanguinate the digit, which is wrapped circumferentially in a distal-to-proximal direction and then unwound, leaving the proximal wrapping to be clamped with a hemostat to serve as a tourniquet. A pattern may be made to cover the dimensions of the defect and then transposed proximally to the cut edge of the skin that is to be advanced. The base of the triangle will be the distal cut edge, and an appropriate triangle of skin is made according to the pattern, with the apex of the triangle being at the distal interphalangeal (DIP) flexion crease. The full thickness of the skin only is cut. The digital nerves and blood vessels of the flap are preserved. Separation between the flexor sheath and subcutaneous tissue facilitates advancement of the flap distally. The tourniquet should be let down to ensure that the flap is viable. Warm soaks and local anesthetics may eliminate vasospasm. If the flap shows no vascularity, it should be inset anyway to provide coverage and essentially serve as a biologic dressing. A carefully performed dissection should avoid such a problem. The base of the triangle is carefully

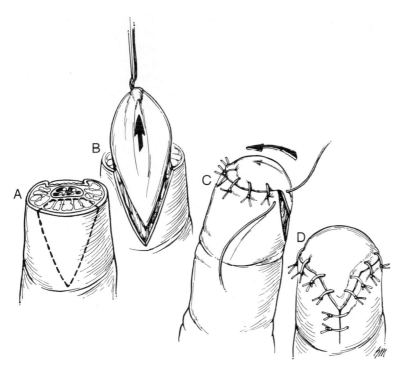

FIGURE 55-2. **A** to **D**, The Atasoy-Kleinert volar V-Y technique is applicable to distal tip injuries with bone exposed and when the distal injury is either transverse or oblique and sloping in a volar distal-to-dorsal proximal direction. In injuries with more volar pad loss, there is usually insufficient skin for this technique to be used.

contoured and sutured to the nail bed or remaining nail, and the resulting "V" incision on the palmar aspect of the digit is closed, thus converting it to a "Y" (see Fig. 55-2). Some slight defatting may be necessary to facilitate tension-free skin closure. Postoperative management consists of sterile dressings over the surgical sites that allow early motion of all adjacent joints and a return to progressively active motion as healing ensues.

In their initial report, Atasoy and associates[148] reported that 56 of 61 patients who were available for follow-up had normal sensibility and normal motion. However, a follow-up study conducted by Frandsen[165] in 1978 found hypoesthesia or dysesthesia in 7 of 10 patients with triangular volar flaps. Four of the 10 patients had subjective complaints of cold intolerance, and 5 of the patients also had difficulty grasping objects. Conolly and Goulston[85] had unsatisfying results in 4 of 7 patients treated by this technique. The results were deemed unsatisfactory because of persistent paresthesias or impaired sensibility. Tupper and Miller[195] reported diminished sensibility in all 16 of their patients tested by two-point discrimination and Von Frey monofilaments. Eight of their patients reported hypersensitivity, particularly cold intolerance. Again, it is believed that such symptomatology is common to all fingertip amputations regardless of the treatment approach.

Kutler Lateral V-Y Flaps

Kutler,[182] in 1944, was apparently the first to describe the use of V-Y advancement flaps for digital tip injuries (Fig. 55-3). His technique used two triangular flaps developed and reflected from lateral positions to cover the tip of the digit.[183] Shepard[190] reported excellent results with a modification of Kutler's technique in 28 traumatic amputations and nine reconstructive procedures, and his article describes the technical details of the procedure very clearly. He suggested

that the Kutler technique is most applicable to oblique palmar and transversely oriented amputations.

Preparation of the digit is similar to that used in the Atasoy technique. The tip of the digit is débrided as necessary. Two triangular flaps are developed from the midlateral aspect of each side of the digit, and the incisions are made just down through the dermis. The subcutaneous tissue is similarly mobilized from the phalanx on a deep plane. Both triangles are advanced to the midline distally and sutured together.

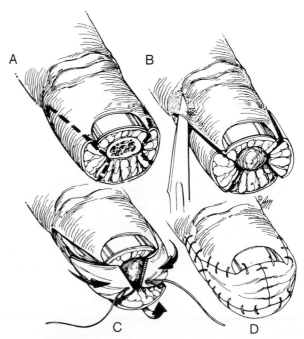

FIGURE 55-3. **A** to **D**, Kutler lateral V-Y technique.

The "V" apex of the triangle is closed in a "Y" fashion, and the surrounding edges and nail bed, or nail, are carefully sutured to the distal edges of the advanced flaps.

Haddad[172] reported on a series of 20 cases treated with this technique and stated that slight skin necrosis occurred at the edges if the flaps were too large; he therefore limited the length of the pedicle in its longest dimension to between ¼ and ⅜ inch. Subjective evaluation in a series of 22 patients was reported by Freiberg and Manktelow,[166] who noted mild hypersensitivity and numbness in 7 of 22 patients. Frandsen[165] reported a follow-up study of 14 patients who underwent Kutler's technique and found subjective complaints of coldness in 8 patients (57%), tenderness on percussion in 10 (71%), difficulty in grasping small objects in 6 (43%), and slight hypoesthesia or dysesthesia in 10 (71%) when objectively measured.

Volar Flap Advancement

Keim and Grantham[178] credited Moberg with the technique of volar flap advancement for coverage of thumb tip amputations. Snow[193] also advocated this technique for fingertip amputations when length is to be maintained. Advancing volar skin on its neurovascular pedicle provides the dermis with sensibility without losing length. Arons[147] has modified this slightly with the addition of a terminal dermal graft for

padding, and sometimes a skin graft may be added at the base of the digit to gain length (see Chapter 47).

Regional anesthesia is obtained, the limb is exsanguinated with an Esmarch bandage, and a pneumatic tourniquet is inflated. The distal tip is appropriately débrided, and mid-axial incisions just dorsal to the flexion crease at each of the interphalangeal (IP) joints are made on both sides of the digit. The flap is completely separated from the underlying flexor tendon sheath, advanced to the distal tip, and sutured to the nail bed and to the adjacent sides of the digit. The tip of the flap may need to be shaped to fit the distal defect (Fig. 55-4). The lateral portions of the skin are then sutured in place.

This method is definitely more appropriate for the thumb than for the fingers. Reported complications are fixed flexion deformity of the DIP joint and necrosis of the entire volar flap. The studies of Caplan and coworkers,[153] Leffert and associates,[217] and Armenta and Lehrman[146] suggest that the blood supply to the flexor tendon apparatus must be compromised for this flap to be used. Although we know of no reports of tendon nutritional difficulties after the use of this technique, it does represent a theoretical disadvantage of this method. This technique is generally thought to be more applicable to the thumb because of its more mobile skin and less likelihood of subsequent flexion contracture. However,

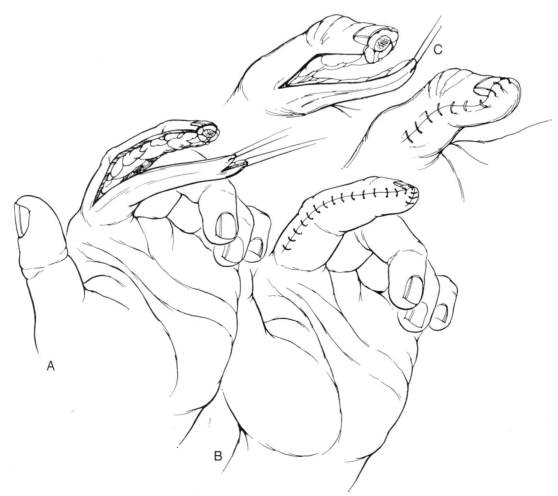

FIGURE 55-4. A to **C,** Volar advancement flap for coverage of a distal index finger amputation with bone exposed. This technique is more applicable to thumb tip injuries in which less than 1 cm of flap advancement is required for coverage. The injudicious use of this technique in a finger can result in significant complications, including necrosis of the entire flap.

in both the thumb and fingers flap advancement is limited to 1 cm.

When the volar skin is lost and the profundus insertion is exposed, a thenar flap is preferred in a young patient who has oblique loss involving the index and long fingers but no preexisting degenerative arthritis of the proximal interphalangeal (PIP) or DIP joints. If the ring or small fingers are involved, a cross-finger flap is preferred. However, use of these flaps is reserved for these particular circumstances, and we have not encountered a case that has not been amenable to healing by secondary intention.

Cross-Finger Pedicle Flap

The cross-finger pedicle flap technique, first described by Gurdin and Pangman[171] in 1950, has found acceptance when other techniques for local flap coverage are not possible and in those situations in which it is deemed advisable to maintain length. Examples of such circumstances are distal amputation of the index finger or thumb and situations in which multiple digits are injured and maintenance of length in the remaining injured tips is considered to be of critical importance.[199] Figure 55-5 illustrates the technique for coverage of an index fingertip when the level of the injury is just distal to the lunula.

The operative procedure is carried out using regional anesthesia, and the limb is exsanguinated to facilitate hemostasis. The flap may be based proximally or distally, depending on the needs of the particular situation. The example shown here, where the adjacent ulnar digit is used and the flap is laterally based, is perhaps the most common application of this technique. A pattern is used to determine the size of the defect to be covered, and this is then placed over the donor area so that the appropriate pedicle can be fashioned for transfer. It is helpful to use a cloth pattern, which can be folded, to simulate the planned pedicle and give an approximation of the amount of joint flexion that will be necessary in the recipient finger. It is important to make a template in this fashion rather than visually estimate the necessary size of the graft. We prefer to cut the template 2 mm larger around its three sides to ensure a tension-free final flap.

Once the template has been made, the donor site is outlined with a marking pen. With careful tissue handling, the flap is reflected, with care being taken to preserve venous drainage at the base of the flap. The dissection is carried down to the plane between the paratenon of the extensor mechanism and the subcutaneous fat. Once the flap is reflected, its vascularity is checked by temporarily deflating the tourniquet. Three of the four available margins of the flap are then sutured in place on the recipient site. The fourth margin is sewn down at the time of flap detachment and closure. A full-thickness skin graft from the ipsilateral antecubital region or groin is used to cover the defect on the extensor surface of the donor digit. In circumstances

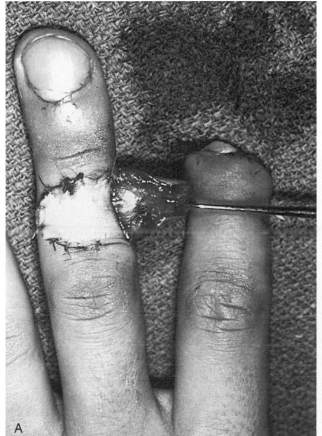
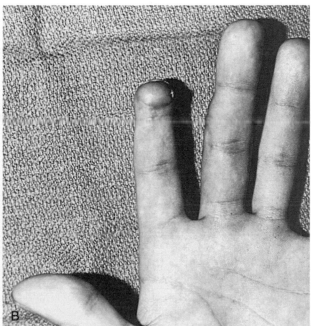

FIGURE 55-5. A, Radially based, dorsal midphalangeal cross-finger flap has been raised with coverage of the donor site by means of a full-thickness skin graft taken from the groin. Care should be taken to not put undue tension on the base of the flap. **B,** Coverage of this fingertip after the use of a cross-finger flap for maintenance of length in the index finger.

in which there is undue tension on the vascular pedicle of the flap, a Kirschner wire transfixing the middle phalanges of the two fingers may be helpful to prevent excessive tension and torsion of the flap. A bulky soft dressing may be reinforced with a plaster splint. At 2 to 3 weeks the pedicle is detached and inset to the recipient site in contour with its margins. The carrier portion of the pedicle flap is reinserted with removal of an appropriate amount of the full-thickness skin that was previously applied for initial coverage.

After detachment of the flap, motion of the digits is encouraged to mobilize all the adjacent joints. Follow-up studies by Sturman and Duran,[137] Kleinert and associates,[180] and Johnson and Iverson[176] have indicated that the return of sensibility to cross-finger flaps as measured by two-point discrimination tests shows excellent reinnervation in the majority of these flaps with progressive improvement occurring with the passage of time. Technique of the cross-finger flap (and other flaps in this section) is also described in detail in Chapter 47.

Thenar Flap

In 1926 Gatewood[168] described the technique of a thenar flap for coverage of digital tip injuries in which there was exposed bone. This was subsequently expanded on by Flatt[161] in 1957 and modified by Smith and Albin[192] with a technique that they describe as a thenar "H-flap." The indications for a thenar flap are quite similar to those for a cross-finger flap, namely, when preservation of length is considered important and other techniques that have less potential for complications are not applicable. The purported advantages are (1) perfect tissue match, (2) abundance of subcutaneous tissues, and (3) inconspicuous donor site.[186] To avoid the potential for joint stiffness with a permanent flexion contracture and/or unsightly scar in the donor area one must keep in mind the three cardinal technical principles outlined by Melone and colleagues[186]: (1) design the flap near the metacarpophalangeal (MP) crease of the thumb and avoid the midpalmar area; (2) fully flex the MP joint with whatever amount of flexion is required in the IP joints of the recipient finger; and (3) detach the pedicle 10 to 14 days postoperatively and begin immediate active range of motion. Figure 55-6 shows the thenar "H-flap" as described by Smith and Albin.[192] This technique is applicable to injuries to the tips of the index and long fingers, but the two ulnar digital tips will not comfortably flex to the thenar eminence; therefore, this technique should not be used for coverage of those digits.

Thenar H-Flap (Smith and Albin)

The area of contact of the injured digital tip with the thenar eminence is outlined with a sterile pen. An H is drawn on the skin approximately 20% wider than the previously outlined area. The transverse limb of the incision is made at the most distal contact point of the fingertip with the thenar eminence (see Fig. 55-6A). Square proximal and distal flaps are elevated, including the subcutaneous tissue. The proximal flap is sutured to the fingertip, and the distal flap is sutured to the proximal margin of the defect on the volar side of the injured finger (see Fig. 55-6B). The proximal flap is then advanced distally and the distal flap advanced proximally to close the donor defect. A soft dressing is applied, and 2 weeks later the flap is detached. The fingertip is closed

with the proximal flap, and the distal flap is advanced into the thenar defect (see Fig. 55-6C). This closes the donor site primarily and avoids the potential problem of an unsightly scar in the thenar eminence. Variations of this flap may be used for radial or ulnar digital loss and would be designed with the base appropriately oriented with regard to the location of the defect.

An alternative technique, as used by Gatewood,[168] Flatt,[161] and others, is to elevate a proximally based flap and suture it to the injured tip in a fashion similar to that just described but to use a full- or split-thickness skin graft for the thenar defect when the flap is divided and inset.

Contraindications to either the cross-finger flap or the thenar flap would be any general condition that might lead to finger stiffness, such as rheumatoid arthritis, Dupuytren's contracture, any connective tissue disease involving the hand, and advanced age with its concomitant degenerative changes. Complications seem to be more prevalent in those patients older than 30 years of age with a greater tendency for the development of joint stiffness. We believe that the risk of this complication is a relative contraindication to the use of the thenar flap in patients older than 30.

In an interesting follow-up study, Porter[120] compared the results of 56 pedicle flaps with 44 free grafts. On the basis of this follow-up study, it was his belief that sensibility was better in cross-finger and thenar flaps and that these flaps gave an excellent cosmetic result. He also concluded that Wolfe's full-thickness grafts were superior to split-thickness skin grafts. He had little use for pectoral flaps because of their bulkiness. In terms of subjective and objective sensibility evaluation, of the five methods evaluated in his study, the results were superior with the thenar and cross-finger flaps.

Distant Flaps

Chest, abdominal, and cross-arm flaps are occasionally useful when the amputation has resulted in major skin loss but with preservation of digital length. Kralova[181] illustrated examples of the use of these methods, which should be used very selectively inasmuch as the donor sites may be unsightly. Joint stiffness may also ensue from prolonged immobilization.

Island Flaps

A number of elegant and ingeniously conceived island flaps have been described for digital reconstruction, including coverage of tip amputations. These flaps are an alternative to the well-established soft tissue procedures such as the cross-finger or thenar flaps. Proposed advantages of island flaps include the avoidance of prolonged digital immobilization in an awkward position, single-stage reconstruction permitting early rehabilitation, introduction of an independent blood supply to provide a good soft tissue bed for nerve grafting or repair, satisfactory restoration of a well-padded sensate digital pulp, the potential for a composite tissue transfer, a wide selection of donor sites, and a greater arc of rotation for mobilization of the flap over longer distances. However, island flaps are more technically demanding and are associated with such complications as flap failure, joint contracture, and cold intolerance. In addition, they have not proved to be more advantageous than simpler methods of achieving coverage of a fingertip amputation, such as skeletal shorten-

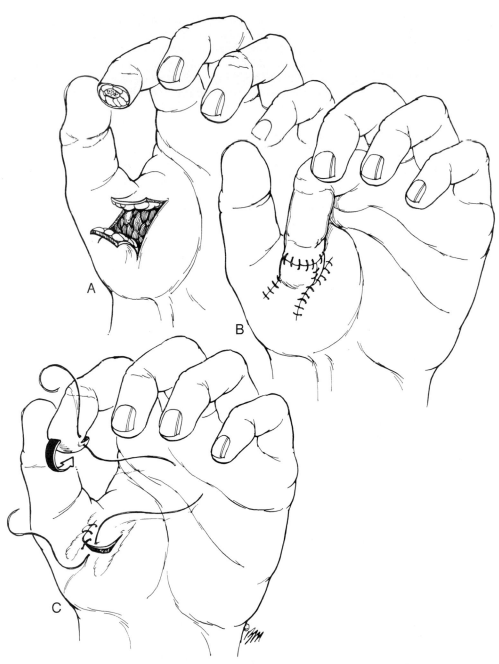

FIGURE 55-6. **A** to **C,** The thenar "H-flap" as described by Smith and Albin.[192] (See text.)

ing and primary closure, healing by secondary intention, or an appropriately indicated and performed local advancement flap. The use of an island flap may be beneficial in select cases, and the reader is referred to a recent review article[163] to become familiar with the indications and surgical techniques (see also Chapter 47).

 Authors' Preferred Method of Digital Tip Amputation

We prefer to treat all digital tip injuries with no exposed bone nonoperatively, with dressing changes as indicated and allowing healing by secondary intention.

In single digit injuries with exposed bone, treatment depends largely on an interview with the patient or with the parents in the case of an injured child. As we have gained more experience, we have performed fewer local and distant flaps in an effort to cover a small portion of exposed bone. A fingertip amputation will not usually heal with adequate soft tissue over protruding bone. Rongeuring a small protruding portion of a phalanx with healing by secondary intention, thus converting a wound with exposed bone to one without exposed bone, is our preferred method.

Most patients and parents (and even house officers) need to be convinced that closure by secondary intention is both rational and the optimal method of treatment. "Before" and "after" photographs of a clinical example to help educate the patient and family regarding the efficacy of this method are invaluable and can make the process of acceptance much easier.

AMPUTATIONS THROUGH THE THUMB

Because of the critical importance of the thumb in pinch, sensibility in the distal skin is vital. From the foregoing discussions it is apparent that split-thickness and full-thickness skin grafts lead to diminished sensibility and frequently to hypoesthesia, dysesthesias, and cold intolerance. For this reason, if the distal tip of the thumb incurs a soft tissue injury and no bone is exposed, we prefer to allow it to heal by secondary intention. Any amputation of the thumb distal to the IP joint is an extremely functional level for almost all patients. Coverage of exposed bone in the distal phalanx by skin that is hypoesthetic, dysesthetic, or tender may lead to functional loss of the tip as the patient bypasses the sensitive area. Specialized techniques such as cross-finger flaps[194] and radially innervated sensory flaps[203] have been used to cover this area where a most critical need for sensibility exists. These and other methods for the management of thumb injuries are discussed in detail elsewhere (see Chapters 47 and 53).

The social and economic consequences of extensive loss of the thumb when replantation was or was not done have been reviewed by Chase[202] and by Hovgaard and coworkers.[204]

AMPUTATIONS FROM DIP TO MP JOINT (EXCLUSIVE OF THE THUMB)

By definition, amputations that occur at levels proximal to the digital skin pad involve bone, and at the distal phalangeal level they involve part of the nail, nail matrix, or nail bed. Nail bed injuries are discussed in Chapter 10. When maintenance of length is considered desirable, one of the local or distal flap techniques described previously in this chapter may be indicated. If sacrifice of bone length will facilitate functional recovery, the tip of the exposed phalanx may be rongeured back beneath the overlying surface, and then skin grafting, healing by secondary intention, or primary suture may be used to gain coverage and closure of the area.

Through the DIP Joint

When an amputation has occurred directly through the IP joint, it is appropriate to shorten the phalanx as necessary to gain primary closure of the defect at the time. Whitaker and colleagues[223] presented experimental and clinical data suggesting that there was less inflammation if the articular surface of the middle phalanx was preserved. However, we believe that the shape and contour of the amputation stump should be made to resemble the normal distal phalangeal tuft. This is accomplished by rongeuring off the volar and lateral condylar prominences. The flexor tendon end should be inspected to ensure that there is no contamination more proximal in the digit. The digital nerves should be dissected and transposed away from the cutaneous scar to an area where the inevitable neuromas will not become symptomatic because of contact. A technique reported by Gorkisch and coworkers[24] may prove useful in this regard (see page 1981). We have no personal experience with this technique, but in light of their excellent results it does have a definite appeal. The flexor and extensor tendons should be inspected and their cleanliness established; they should not be sutured to each other. This will inevitably limit the excursion of both and therefore compromise function of the remaining digits. This may be especially noticeable in the flexor digitorum profundus tendons to the ulnar three digits, where fixation of one will limit mobility of the others.

Authors' Preferred Method of Management For Specific Amputation Levels

DIP Disarticulation

Our preferred method of management for an amputation through the DIP joint is skeletal shortening and primary closure. We routinely denude all articular cartilage from the head of the middle phalanx. Care should be taken to appropriately shape and contour the amputation stump. Identification and resection of the digital nerves to prevent neuroma formation is essential.

Complications of Digital Amputation: The Lumbrical-Plus Finger

Distal release of the flexor digitorum profundus tendon to the index finger may lead to a "lumbrical-plus" habitus.[219] As the independent profundus and its lumbrical move proximally, increasing tension develops in the lumbrical tendon and its contribution to the intrinsic extensor of the PIP joint. As active flexion of the digit is attempted, further proximal migration of the lumbrical may put sufficient tension on this lateral band to cause paradoxical extension of the PIP joint. Sectioning the lumbrical tendon and thereby allowing the superficialis to regain control of the PIP joint may alleviate the problem. It is not necessary to perform this lumbrical sectioning at the time of the amputation unless a lumbrical-plus deformity is identified at that time. In any event, if the deformity does occur, lumbrical tendon sectioning can be performed using local anesthesia on an outpatient basis.

Through the Middle Phalanx

Once amputation has occurred proximal to the DIP joint of the index finger, most patients will transfer pinching and picking up small objects to the tip of the long finger (Fig. 55-7). Therefore, efforts to preserve length by flap coverage for injuries proximal to the DIP joint are not warranted (except in very special circumstances, e.g., multiple amputations in the same hand). Rather, the bone should be shortened sufficiently to allow primary coverage by available skin without tension (Fig. 55-8). As long as an amputation through the middle phalanx is distal to the superficialis insertion, the middle phalangeal segment will be able to participate effectively in grasping activities (Fig. 55-9), although PIP flexion is virtually always quite limited if the middle phalanx stump is short. If amputation has occurred proximal to the insertion of the superficialis, there will be no active flexion control of the remaining portion of the middle phalanx; therefore its preservation becomes more of a cosmetic and less of a functional consideration (Fig. 55-10).

Amputations through the PIP joint should be carried out similarly to those through the DIP joint, with denuding of articular cartilage, shaping of the condyles of the proximal phalanx, and coverage with local skin.

For amputations that have occurred through the middle phalanx and distal to the superficialis insertion, our preferred method of management involves skeletal shortening and primary closure. However, if this involves excessive short-

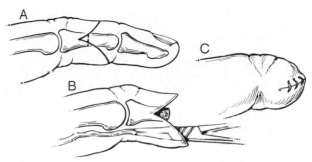

FIGURE 55-8. **A** to **C,** Use of volar and dorsal skin flaps for coverage when a distal amputation in the finger is indicated, that is, distal to the MP joint. Volar flap coverage is considered preferable because of its greater sensibility. This technique is also applicable when primary closure is desired by means of bone shortening. The digital nerve is sectioned after distal traction to allow the inevitable neuroma to form at a location proximal to the cutaneous scar.

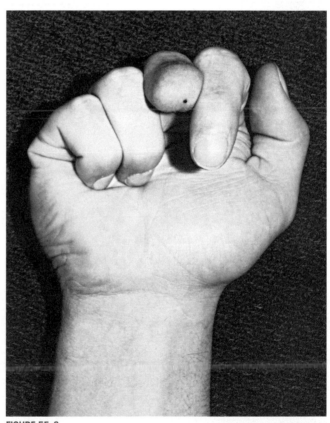

FIGURE 55-9. When amputation through the middle phalanx occurs distal to the insertion of the superficialis, PIP flexion is markedly limited, and the middle segment is capable of participating in the grasping of large objects.

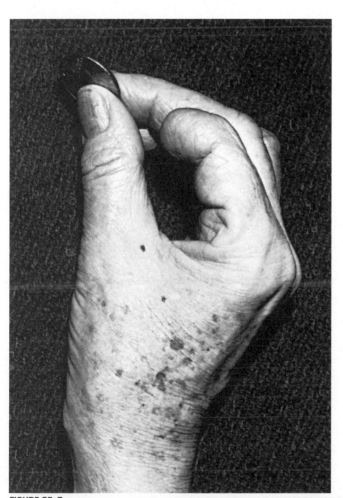

FIGURE 55-7. In a patient with an amputation proximal to the DIP joint of the index finger, pinch will virtually always be transferred to the long fingertip.

ening of the middle phalanx or if a significant portion of the middle phalanx is involved, the use of a flap or an alternative coverage procedure to maintain and preserve length should be considered. If the superficialis tendon has also been injured and is traumatically absent, there is no purpose in preserving length (unless cosmesis is an issue) because PIP joint motion will not occur. Skeletal shortening and primary closure should be performed in such an injury.

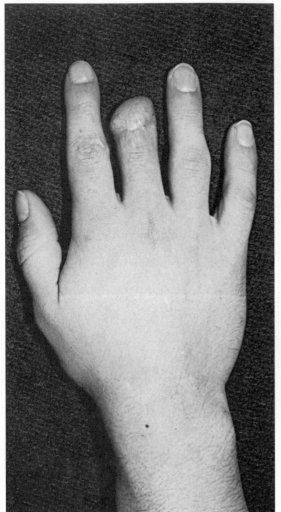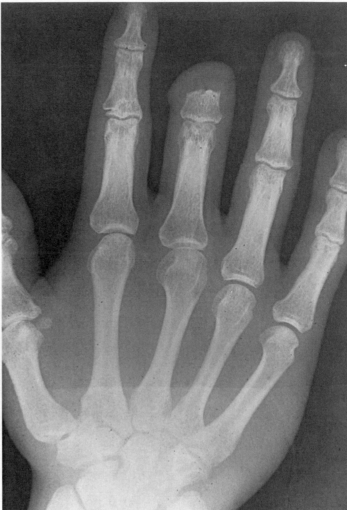

FIGURE 55-10. Note the amputation proximal to the insertion of the superficialis through the middle phalangeal segment. Although no flexion control of the middle phalangeal remnant is possible, the length preservation of such an amputation may be helpful in preventing small objects from falling through the hand.

Through the Proximal Phalanx

If amputation has occurred proximal to the PIP joint (Fig. 55-11A), the remaining proximal segment is under motor control of the intrinsic muscles and the extensor digitorum communis. This will allow active flexion of the proximal phalanx of approximately 45 degrees. Any remaining segment will participate in gripping to that extent and further serve to keep small objects in the palm (see Fig. 55-11B).

However, if the amputation has occurred near or at the MP joint level, especially in the central two rays (namely, the long and ring fingers), functional problems such as dropping small objects through the defect will result (Fig. 55-12) and further consideration of prosthetic replacement or a more proximal ray amputation with closure of the defect as described later should be contemplated.

RAY AMPUTATIONS

Amputation involving the entire metacarpal, as well as the phalanges, or with preservation of the metacarpal base is

---

CRITICAL POINTS: GUIDANCE REGARDING SPECIFIC DIGITAL AMPUTATION LEVELS

- Amputations through the DIP joint are managed by skeletal shortening and primary closure.
- In amputations through the middle phalanx, bone should be shortened to allow primary coverage by available skin without tension. If possible, the amputation level should be distal to the superficialis insertion.
- Amputations through the PIP joint are managed the same as those through the DIP joint.
- If amputation through the proximal phalanx is near the PIP joint, some useful gripping function is preserved. If amputation is near or at the MP, ray amputation is usually the procedure of choice.

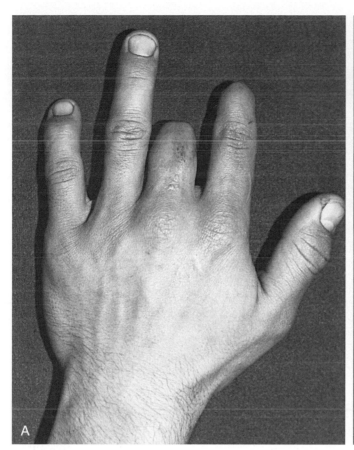 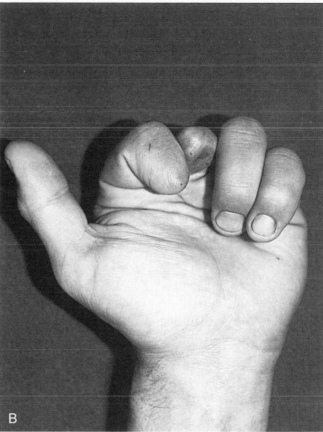

FIGURE 55-11. A, This patient sustained amputations through the distal portion of the middle phalanx of the index finger and through the PIP joint of the long finger. The difference between the functional capacities of these two levels of amputation is clearly demonstrated. **B,** In the long finger, flexion is entirely under control of the intrinsic musculature. The finger is capable of approximately 45 degrees of MP joint flexion, whereas the index finger middle phalangeal segment can fully participate in grasping activities because of the intact flexor digitorum superficialis.

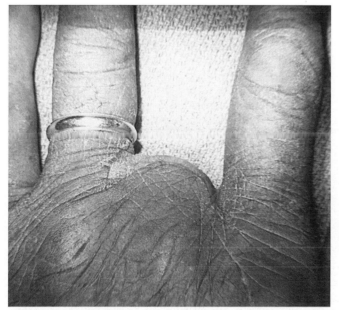

FIGURE 55-12. Preservation of a very short proximal phalangeal remnant, such as that seen here, is of little overall value to the hand because small objects will fall through the defect and be a functional annoyance. Ray amputation with either distal intervolar plate ligament approximation or index ray transposition will not only improve hand function but also result in a more aesthetically pleasing hand.

frequently indicated after trauma, infection, or failed replantation or as part of a tumor resection. It may also be necessary in the reconstruction of a congenitally deficient hand in an attempt to close central defects or to "phalangize" marginal metacarpals by creating a web. Some have argued that ray resection narrows the palm and decreases grip function.[273] However, the narrower palm must be weighed against other impairments related to the gap created by the missing digit, especially for the long and ring fingers. Small objects may fall through this area, especially in the case of an isolated amputation at this level. Amputation of the index finger at the MP joint may lead to problems with the projecting metacarpal head impeding the thumb web or bumping into objects (Fig. 55-13).

Certainly, the loss of any single ray has consequences affecting the ultimate functional strength of the hand. Murray and colleagues[241] demonstrated that power grip, key pinch, and supination strength were diminished by approximately 20% of normal in 26 patients who had index ray amputations but no hypoesthesia after this procedure. Pronation strength in the same group of patients was diminished by 50% of the predicted value. In a long-term functional outcome analysis of 58 patients with an index ray resection and 12 patients with an amputation through the proximal phalanx, Karle and coworkers[238] failed to demonstrate any significant differences in loss of strength when both techniques were

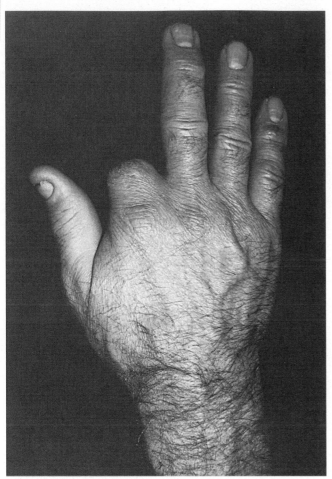

FIGURE 55-13. This proximal phalangeal remnant of the index finger serves only as an impediment to the thumb–long finger web and is a source of painful stimuli when the amputation stump abuts objects that are grasped with the remaining normal digits. A ray amputation in this circumstance is functionally and cosmetically more desirable.

compared. The loss of grip strength after an index ray amputation was 29% to 34% compared with a 21% to 28% loss after an amputation through the proximal phalanx. Patients with an amputation through the proximal phalanx demonstrated a better functional outcome whereas the aesthetic appearance of the hand rated higher after the ray amputation. Comparable clinical assessments of function after ray amputations of the long, ring, and small fingers are not available, but it would seem to be a reasonable assumption that their contribution to the overall strength of the hand would likewise be of significance. Peimer and associates[243] demonstrated in a retrospective series of patients who underwent a primary or reconstructive single ray resection that unsettled compensation/litigation issues are associated with statistically significant differences in grip strength, key pinch, oppositional pinch, and Minnesota Rate of Manipulation Test results. While such patients had poorer results, their study documented a high rate of satisfaction overall with respect to the appearance and function of the hand. Primary ray resection reduced the total costs associated with the injury and subsequent disability.

Ray amputation is most frequently undertaken as an elective procedure consequent to disability resulting from a pre-vious injury to a digit that renders it either functionally impaired or useless. It may also be undertaken in the treatment of tumors or infections. In special circumstances, it may be part of a reconstructive program where phalangization of the metacarpals is facilitated by removing one or more rays toward this end. Ray amputation at the time of initial trauma may occasionally be indicated.[243,248] However, in multiple injuries, the principle of saving all viable tissue should, of course, be followed. Metacarpal bone, which might at first appear to be destined for later ablation, may serve as a good source of bone graft for subsequent reconstruction. The principles of spare-parts surgery espoused by Chase[252,253] should be kept in mind under these acute traumatic circumstances.

Index Ray Amputation

In a review of 41 patients with index trans-metacarpal amputation, Murray and colleagues[241] found hyperesthesia interfering with function in 37.5% of the patients; in 10% it was disabling. Their conclusion was that excessive mobilization of the radial digital nerve to the index finger was responsible for this; and in 9 of the patients who underwent subsequent exploration, the symptoms were not relieved. Fisher and Goldner[231] reported a similar problem in 5 patients. It is of interest that this complication usually appears 6 to 8 weeks after surgery, and although it may initially be relieved by a subsequent procedure, the symptoms may recur at approximately the same time interval. Of 34 patients who had elective ray amputations in the series of Murray and associates, 21 complained of pain in the preexisting stump before their trans-metacarpal amputation. Only 3 of these patients experienced complete relief of their symptoms after the procedure. This information is important in terms of advising the patient preoperatively about the possibility of persistent postoperative symptoms.

Murray and associates[241] found no difference in pinch strength in patients who had no transfer performed to augment the second dorsal interosseous tendon when compared with those who had such a transfer. Transfer of the first dorsal interosseous to the insertion of the second dorsal interosseous has been suggested, but according to these data it appears to be unnecessary. In 11 of 28 cases in which the second dorsal interosseous was augmented by transfer of either the first dorsal interosseous or one of the long flexors of the index finger, there was an intrinsic-plus deformity evident on clinical examination. From these data it would appear that procedures designed to augment the second dorsal interosseous not only are unnecessary but may lead to significant complications as well.

The cosmetic appearance of an index ray amputation is highly acceptable (Fig. 55-14). Garcia-Moral and colleagues[232] found no statistical difference between normal hands and a hand with index ray resection except for a 14% loss of grip strength. The loss of an index finger alone does not represent a major impairment to the usual activities of daily living.

We have encountered patients who developed carpal tunnel syndrome after a ray amputation as a result of proximal migration of the transected flexor tendons into the carpal canal. This occurred with one index and one long finger ray amputation. In one case, triggering occurred when the proximal migration of the long finger lumbrical hung on the distal edge of the transverse carpal ligament.

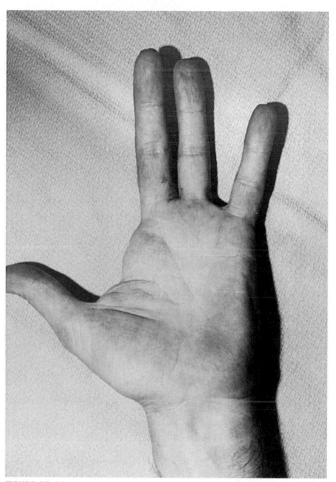

FIGURE 55-14. The cosmetic appearance of an index ray amputation is quite acceptable. Aside from some loss of grip strength, there is little functional impairment.

Authors' Preferred Method of Index Ray Amputation

Regional anesthesia is preferred for this procedure. Depending on the reason for the amputation, the limb may be exsanguinated with an Esmarch (Martin) bandage. If an infection or a tumor is the reason for amputation, exsanguination by compression is not appropriate and the limb may be exsanguinated by prolonged limb elevation or manual compression of the brachial artery. Circumferential skin incisions are made on the index finger at the mid-proximal phalangeal level when possible. This is continuous with a dorsal incision that overlies the index metacarpal (Fig. 55-15A). The skin is intentionally left long distally so that it can be trimmed to the proper length when the procedure is completed. It should be noted that this technical point is especially important when performing ray amputations of the middle two rays because if not enough skin remains, a web contracture will result. The longitudinal dorsal incision overlying the index metacarpal is carried down through subcutaneous tissue. Dorsal veins are ligated as necessary. The extensor digitorum communis and extensor indicis proprius tendons are transected at the level of the

second metacarpal base. The distal stumps of the tendons are then reflected distally, and a longitudinal periosteal incision is made along the index metacarpal. This is carried down to the metacarpal base distal to the proximal metaphysis, where the bone is transected distal to the extensor carpi radialis insertion (see Fig. 55-15B). The metacarpal is elevated subperiosteally from its soft tissue bed. Dissection is then carried around the distal circular portion of the incision. The tendon of the first dorsal interosseous is identified and sectioned. The lumbrical to the radial side of the index finger is likewise tenotomized at its insertion into the hood.

By proceeding around the volar side of the digit one can identify the neurovascular bundles. The vessels are appropriately ligated at this time. The nerves are dissected out distally into the middle phalangeal segment if possible, and a ligature is placed about each nerve proximal to the point where it is to be transected. This will facilitate translocation of the nerve later in the operation. The flexor tendons are identified, transected, and allowed to retract into the palm. The tendon of the first palmar interosseous is transected.

Dissection now reveals the remaining attachments between the volar plate, deep intervolar plate (deep transverse metacarpal) ligament, preosseous bands of the palmar fascia, and proximal portion of the flexor tendon sheath. These attachments are divided sharply, and the amputation specimen is removed at this point. The digital nerves that have intentionally been transected distally in the finger are carefully dissected proximally, with their connections with the palmar skin left undisturbed (see Fig. 55-15C). The ligatures that were previously placed around the nerves distally are transposed proximally into the interosseous space between the first and second dorsal interossei to provide protection from external trauma (see Fig. 55-15D). The periosteal sleeve is closed after hemostasis is obtained. Interrupted sutures are used for the skin, and a soft dressing is applied. Early motion is encouraged.

Long Finger Ray Amputation

Two techniques of ray amputation of the long fingers are useful. They differ in that the technique of Carroll[226] involves transposition of the base of the index metacarpal to the base of the long finger metacarpal (Fig. 55-16) and thereby closes the space that would exist between the index and ring fingers. The alternative technique is to preserve the deep intervolar plate ligaments between the ring and index fingers and suture them together (Fig. 55-17), thus closing the potential space in this fashion. The advantage of Carroll's technique is that it gives immediate closure of the space that remains when the long finger ray is removed. The disadvantage is that protection must be provided by means of a cast for several weeks with the MP joints of the index and ring fingers included and flexed to 45 degrees. Radiographic assessment may necessitate further immobilization until the osteotomy has healed, and delayed bone healing or nonunion can occur (see Fig. 55-18). Thus there is the potential for greater morbidity with this technique. In his series of 43 patients, Carroll[226] reported only one nonunion. Carroll[226] also reported his results in 20 cases in which the entire index metacarpal was transposed to the base of the capitate and an arthrodesis was performed between the base of the index metacarpal

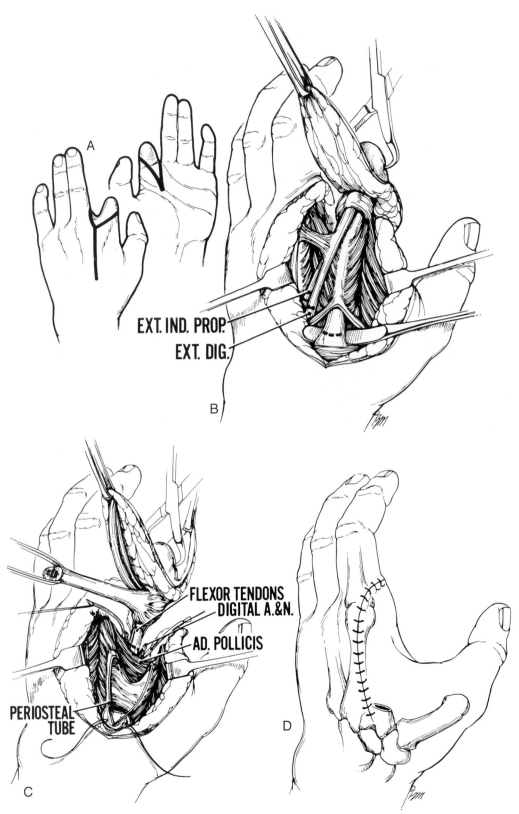

FIGURE 55-15. **A** to **D,** Technique of index ray amputation. The index metacarpal is transected at its metaphyseal flare. Special care should be taken to transpose the digital nerves into the interosseous space to prevent the formation of a symptomatic neuroma. Excessive dissection of the digital nerves, especially the radial digital nerve to the index finger, should be avoided to prevent potential hyperesthesia in the newly created web.

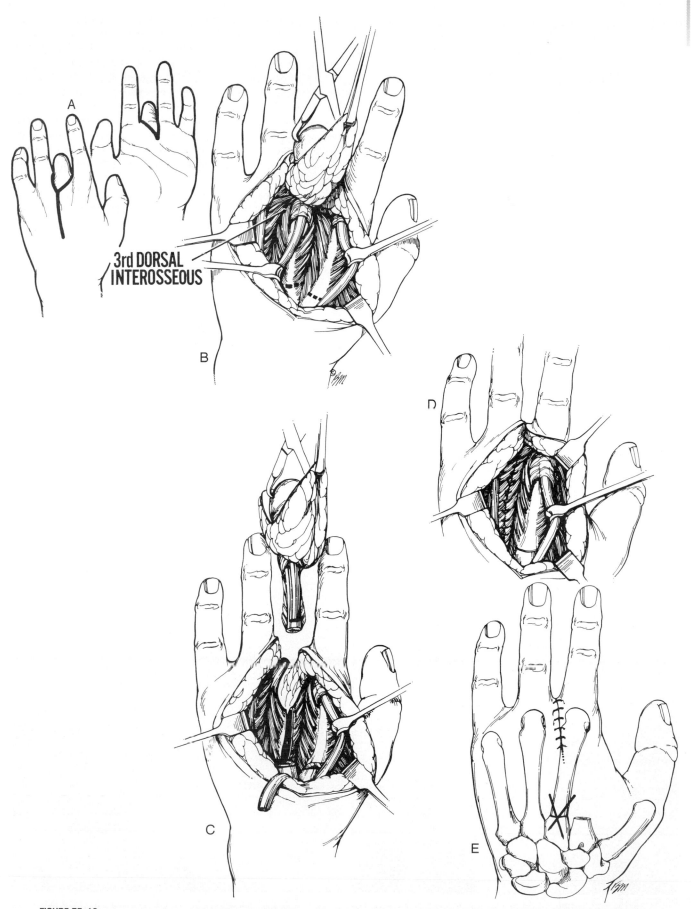

3rd DORSAL INTEROSSEOUS

FIGURE 55-16. **A** to **E,** Technique of transposition of the index metacarpal to the base of the long finger metacarpal as described by Carroll.[226]

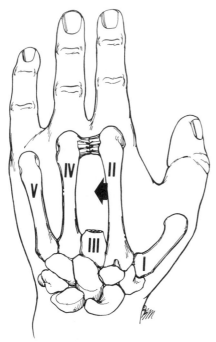

FIGURE 55-17. Alternative technique for long finger ray amputation with distal suture of the deep intervolar plate ligaments to close the space between the index and long fingers.

and capitate after the transposition. He noted no difference in the two techniques but preferred osteotomy at the base of the index metacarpal and osteosynthesis of this transposed metacarpal shaft to the base of the third metacarpal. Figure 55-18 illustrates an example of transposition as advocated by Carroll; however, it also demonstrates a nonunion at the base of the transposed index ray. The osteotomy site in the long finger metacarpal was made too far distally. If ray transposition of the index finger is done, it is important to perform the osteotomy at the metacarpal base. In our experience a more distal osteotomy has a higher incidence of nonunion.

Chase[11] proposed a similar technique but used an intramedullary bone graft as well as transfixation wires. In addition, rigid fixation with plates and screws may be used.[234] The alternative technique does not involve an osteotomy, but it depends on accurate approximation of the adjacent soft tissues to obtain closure of the web. Moreover, it may be helpful to transfix the metacarpals with a transverse pin to ensure correct rotational alignment. Colen and colleagues[228] have also reported excellent results with the use of digital ray transfer for central digital loss. These authors believed that the transfer improved their ability to close the central gap. They demonstrated preservation of an excellent range of motion, 50% of grip strength, and 83% of pinch strength. Posner[246] has also advocated this technique.

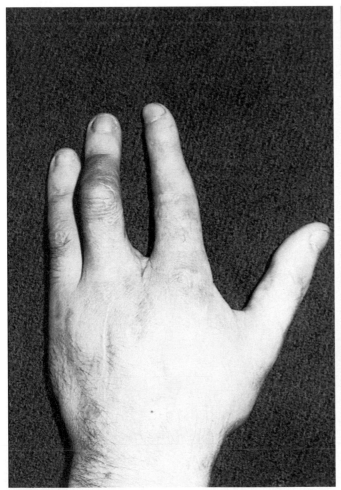

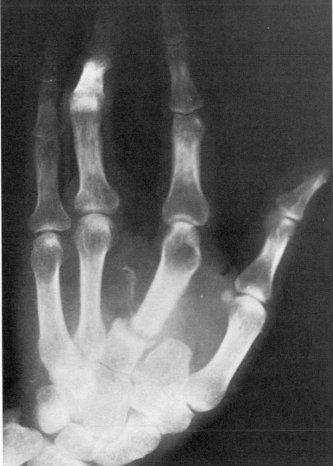

FIGURE 55-18. Transposition of the index ray to the base of the long finger metacarpal. In this situation the osteotomy was made too far distally at the diaphysis, resulting in a nonunion.

Peze and Iselin[244] reported their technique for closing the central gap that is present when the long finger ray is amputated. They created a distally based wedge in the capitate with its apex proximally. When the wedge was closed, the central defect was eliminated as the index and ring fingers were brought together. Their clinical results looked excellent.

Long Finger Ray Amputation With Transposition of the Index Finger (Carroll[226])

After satisfactory regional or general anesthesia is obtained, the limb is exsanguinated and a tourniquet is applied. A dorsal incision is made that extends along the shaft of the long finger ray dorsally (see Fig. 55-16A). The distal ends of the incision are carried out over the proximal phalangeal skin to preserve sufficient skin for closure of the commissure between the index and ring fingers. The extensor digitorum communis tendon to the long finger is divided proximally after the initial exposure has been made. The long finger metacarpal is osteotomized at its base distal to the extensor carpi radialis brevis insertion (see Fig. 55-16B) after subperiosteal dissection has been carried out and the intrinsic muscles reflected. The second dorsal interosseous, the lumbrical, and the third dorsal interosseous tendons are divided. Volar dissection is carried out in a fashion similar to the procedure for the index finger, and the blood vessels are ligated and the digital nerves transected as far distally as possible. The flexor tendons are divided and allowed to retract proximally. The deep intervolar plate ligaments are transected. Next, the preosseous bands of the palmar fascia are dissected out and the ray is removed (see Fig. 55-16C).

After removal of the ray, the base of the index metacarpal is exposed subperiosteally and an osteotomy is performed at its metaphyseal flare (see Fig. 55-16D). The index metacarpal is then transposed to the base of the long finger ray, and after correct rotation has been accurately aligned, the base is transfixed with two crossed Kirschner wires or a longitudinal wire (see Fig. 55-16E). More demanding step-cut osteotomies have been described by some authors,[246] which we do not use.

A mini-fragment plate can be used as an alternative method of fixation. Hanel and Lederman[234] have reported a technique of index ray transposition using a 2.7-mm plate with excellent results in 10 patients. The deep intervolar plate ligaments are approximated distally, and the digital nerves should be transposed into the muscular interosseous space to protect the inevitable neuroma from external trauma in a more superficial position. At times it may be helpful to use a transverse interosseous Kirschner wire from the index to the long finger metacarpal to ensure correct rotational alignment.

A drain may be used, depending on the indication for the amputation. After hemostasis is obtained, the dorsal fascia and skin are closed. The commissure is fashioned to reflect a dorsal-volar slope of the web skin between the index and ring fingers. External immobilization for 6 to 8 weeks is usually required to ensure healing of the osteotomy. The MP joints of the index and ring fingers must be included in the cast (preferably in at least 45 degrees of flexion), but the PIP joints should be left free for active motion. When rigid plate fixation is used, cast immobilization may not be necessary and early mobilization of the MP joints is permitted.[234]

Long Finger Ray Amputation Without Transposition

When osteotomy and transposition are not desired, the deep intervolar plate ligaments are sutured distally to one another (see Fig. 55-17) and stabilization is carried out by means of a transverse intermetacarpal Kirschner wire during the period of healing. Postoperative management is essentially the same, although with this limited soft tissue procedure it is not necessary to immobilize the hand for more than 4 weeks. Modifications of this technique have been described by Steichen and Idler[249] and more recently by Lyall and Elliott.[239]

Ring Finger Ray Amputation

Preoperative preparation and the skin incisions are the same as those used in the other ray resections. As with the third ray, two procedures are available for management of ray resection of the ring finger. Anatomically, although almost no mobility in the carpometacarpal joints of the index and long finger rays exists, there is 15 to 30 degrees of mobility between the bases of the fourth and fifth metacarpals and the hamate, with which they share a common articulation. It is therefore possible for the base of the fifth metacarpal to slide radially if the entire metacarpal shaft of the fourth metacarpal is excised. This possibility is enhanced by the anatomic fact that no tendinous attachments to the base of the fourth metacarpal exist as they do in the remaining metacarpals in the hand.

Ring Finger Ray Amputation Without Transposition

A racquet-shaped incision is created distally over the proximal phalanx or its remnant (see Fig. 55-26A). A proximal longitudinal incision is made over the fourth metacarpal, continuous with the racquet incision. The incision is carried down through subcutaneous tissue, beginning dorsally. The dorsal veins are preserved when possible. The extensor digitorum communis tendon to the ring finger ray is transected proximally and the tendon is reflected distally. An incision is made through the periosteum down to the metacarpal shaft. Subperiosteal dissection is carried out, and the base of the metacarpal is identified at its articulation with the hamate. The dorsal carpometacarpal ligaments are incised; subsequently, by detaching the articulation and palmar flexing the metacarpal, the volar carpometacarpal ligaments may be divided. Care must be taken to avoid damage to the ulnar nerve and artery, which lie immediately volar to the fourth carpometacarpal joint. The metacarpal base is elevated, and further dissection frees the metacarpal from its underlying bed. The lumbrical and second volar and fourth dorsal interosseous tendons must be transected. Dissection is then carried out around the volar aspect of the amputation site, the digital vessels are identified and ligated, and the digital nerves are transected at their most distal portion. The flexor tendons are divided sharply after incision of the palmar fascia. The deep intervolar plate ligaments are identified and appropriately transected close to the volar plate with careful preservation of the digital nerves. The palmar fascial attachments are incised, and the ray is removed.

The deep intervolar plate ligaments are approximated with nonabsorbable suture (Fig. 55-20), and the digital nerves are transposed dorsally into the interosseous space. The periosteal tube is closed, and wound closure is carried out in routine fashion. A transverse interosseous Kirschner wire may be used to stabilize the two metacarpals if the surgeon's judgment so dictates. Again, care must be taken to prevent rotational malalignment. The cosmetic appearance of the hand is usually quite satisfactory (see Fig. 55-19).

A bulky dressing is applied at this point, and early motion of the remaining digits is encouraged. All dressings are removed by the third week. If a pin has been used for transfixion, it is removed at that time. Return to full function is usually accomplished by the sixth to eighth week. With time, the bases of the fifth and third metacarpals come to partially approximate one another (Fig. 55-21).

Rowland and associates[247] described a technique that includes excision of the carpometacarpal ligaments between the fifth metacarpal and hamate and repositioning of the fifth metacarpal next to the third metacarpal after excision of the fourth metacarpal. Their results in four patients showed satisfactory hand function.

Plasschaert and Hage[245] used a flap of adjacent skin to preserve the web between the center digits as an alternative to the previously described techniques (Figs. 55-22 to 55-25). This alternative provides a cosmetically and functionally excellent web for central ray amputations.

Ring Finger Ray Amputation With Transposition of the Fifth Metacarpal

The fifth metacarpal may be transected at its base and transposed to the base of the fourth metacarpal as an alternative means of closing the space between the small and long finger rays. The technique is similar to that for index transposition to the long finger as previously described. A racquet incision is made around the proximal phalangeal remnant of the ring finger (Fig. 55-26A). Dorsal prolongation of this incision is made between the fourth and fifth metacarpals. With appropriate attention to venous drainage, the extensor digitorum communis tendon to the ring finger is transected proximally. Care must be taken to preserve the extensor communis slip to the fifth finger, which may be small and mistaken for a junctura tendinum. The fourth metacarpal is exposed subperiosteally, and a transverse osteotomy is made through the metaphyseal flare with an oscillating saw. The metacarpal is freed distally, and the lumbrical and second volar and fourth dorsal interosseous tendons are divided. The volar extent of the dissection is carried out by identifying the neurovascular bundles, ligating the digital vessels, and transecting the digital nerves at the most distal level possible. The palmar fascia, flexor sheath, and flexor tendons are divided; the deep intervolar plate ligaments are identified and transected; and the

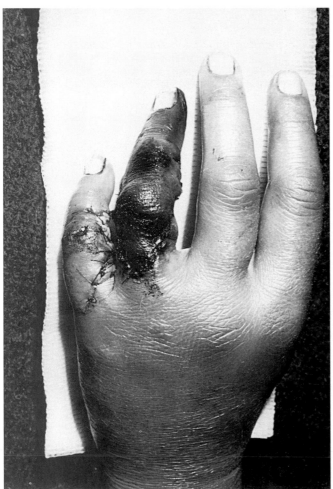
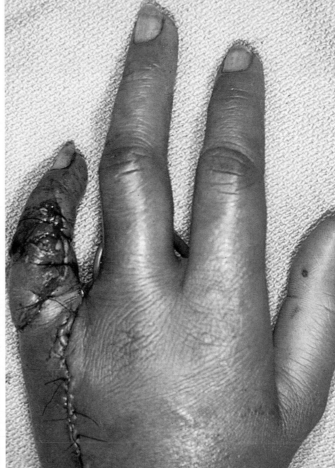

FIGURE 55-19. A gangrenous ring finger after a crushing injury necessitated ray amputation of the ring finger. Closure of the web was performed by excising the entire fourth metacarpal, including the base.

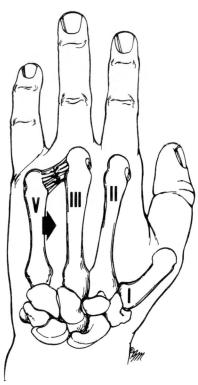

FIGURE 55-20. Suture of the deep intervolar plate ligaments (with subsequent migration of the fifth metacarpal base radially across the hamate) is a satisfactory procedure for accomplishing a ring finger ray amputation.

specimen is removed. Dissection is then carried out in sub-periosteal fashion to allow an osteotomy through the base of the fifth metacarpal just distal to its metaphyseal flare. The fifth metacarpal origin of the fourth dorsal interosseous is stripped to mobilize the fifth metacarpal shaft for transposition. The subperiosteal tube of the fourth metacarpal is then closed.

The fifth metacarpal, now freed from its basilar attachment, is transposed to the base of the fourth metacarpal and transfixed there by two crossed Kirschner wires or a longitudinal wire after rotational alignment has been secured (see Fig. 55-26B). The deep intervolar plate ligaments are approximated at this point with a nonabsorbable suture, and if deemed advisable by the surgeon, a transverse Kirschner wire may be inserted distally between the two metacarpals. The wounds are closed in routine fashion, with care being taken to fashion the interdigital commissure appropriately. Dry sterile dressings are applied after the tourniquet has been deflated and hemostasis obtained. Attempts to lengthen the transposed ray by making the osteotomy of the fourth metacarpal distal to that of the little finger should be avoided. Such attempts will create a tension tenodesis and limit digital motion.

Postoperative management is similar to that described for the other ray amputations. A plaster cast should be used for 6 to 8 weeks postoperatively. If a Kirschner wire is used distally, it is left percutaneously. The pin is not incorporated in the cast because as the swelling recedes, a wire incorporated in the plaster will wiggle and set in motion an inflammatory reaction at its site of cutaneous entry. This may necessitate wire removal earlier than desired.

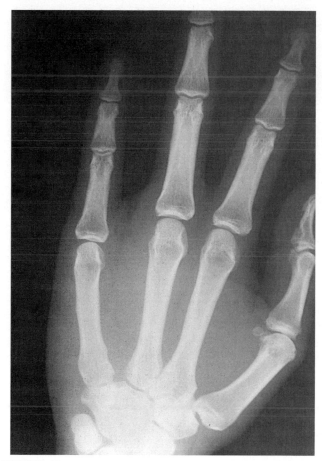

FIGURE 55-21. Radial migration of the base of the fifth metacarpal. Suture of the deep intervolar plate ligaments partially closes the commissure between the long and small fingers.

DeBoer and Robinson[229] added an intercarpal osteotomy and fusion of the capitate and hamate to close the space. We have no experience with this technique, but it does appear to have its own unique complications.

Authors' Preferred Method of Long and Ring Finger Ray Amputation

Both of us prefer ray resection without transposition because of the potential complications (particularly nonunion) and the need for prolonged immobilization postoperatively after a transposition.

Authors' Preferred Method of Fifth Ray Amputation

Amputation of the fifth ray requires preservation of the metacarpal base because of the insertions of the flexor carpi

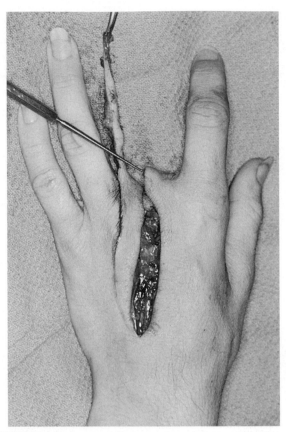

FIGURE 55-22. The web-preserving incision as described by Plasschaert and Hage[245] has been an effective modification to preserve the commissure.

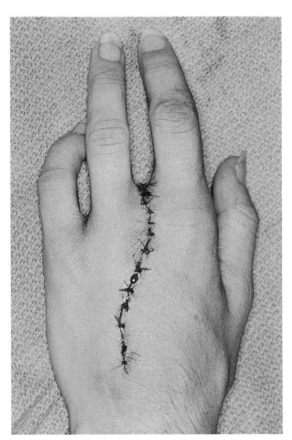

FIGURE 55-23. After closure of the wound shown in Figure 55-22 with appropriate skin resection, the commissure is preserved and the interdigital space is narrowed.

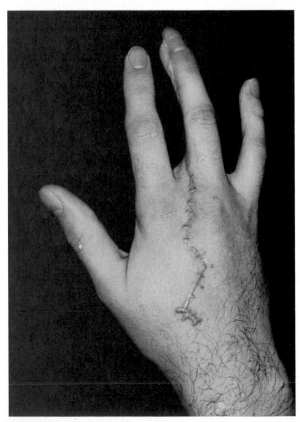

FIGURE 55-24. Early postsurgical photograph shows preservation of the web after a long finger ray resection.

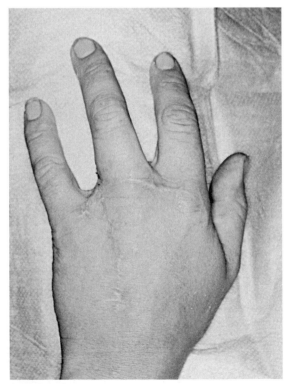

FIGURE 55-25. Preservation of the commissure between the small and long fingers after ring finger ray amputation with closure of the intervolar ligaments.

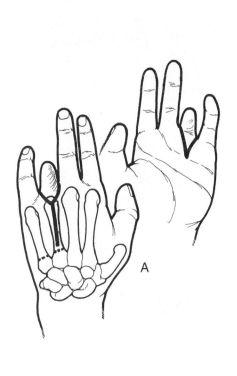

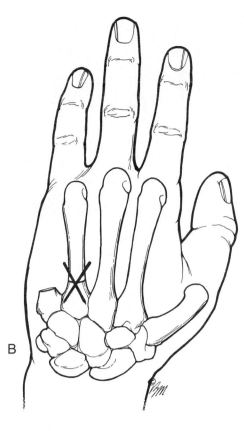

FIGURE 55-26. A and **B,** This alternative technique for ring finger ray amputation may be performed with or without bone grafting and trans-metacarpal pin or plate and screw fixation. However, the morbidity associated with healing of the osteotomy usually does not warrant this procedure.

ulnaris and extensor carpi ulnaris tendons at this level. The procedure (Fig. 55-27) is accomplished by means of an incision curved around the proximal phalanx, if that remnant is present, with care taken to identify the dorsal sensory branches of the ulnar nerve as the incision is carried proximally over the fifth metacarpal shaft. The extensor digiti minimi and extensor digitorum communis tendons to the small finger are transected proximally and reflected distally. Subperiosteal dissection is carried out around the base of the metacarpal, and the bone is osteotomized at its metaphyseal flare with an oscillating saw. The metacarpal is reflected distally. The conjoint tendon of the abductor digiti minimi and flexor digiti minimi is divided distally, and the third volar interosseous and lumbrical tendons are transected. The digital vessels are ligated, and the digital nerves are ligated distally in the wound, to be transposed later into the interosseous space to protect them from direct trauma. The deep intervolar plate ligament between the ring and small fingers is divided. The flexor tendons are divided, the remaining attachments of the palmar fascia to the digit are released, and the ray is removed (Fig. 55-28). The hypothenar muscles are used to cover the gap but are not sutured directly into the fourth dorsal interosseous muscle. This provides adequate padding for the ulnar side of the hand. It is not advisable to reattach the hypothenar muscles to the tendon of the fourth dorsal interosseous because this is unnecessary and possibly undesirable. After approximation of the muscle bellies, the cutaneous wound is closed in routine fashion after appropriate hemostasis has been obtained. A bulky dressing is used for postoperative care, and the patient is encouraged to move all fingers actively. The cosmetic appearance of a fifth ray amputation is usually excellent (Fig. 55-29).

CRITICAL POINTS: RAY AMPUTATIONS

- Most frequently undertaken as an elective procedure based on severe functional disability from a previous injury.
- Usually the primary treatment of choice for total ring avulsion injury.
- In ray amputations, skin should be left long distally to ensure enough skin for optimal commissure closure; otherwise, a web contracture can result.
- Authors prefer resections without transposition to avert complications such as nonunion and the need for prolonged postoperative immobilization.
- Amputation of the fifth ray requires preservation of the metacarpal base.

MULTIPLE DIGIT AMPUTATIONS

The principles governing the management of elective or traumatic amputations when they involve a single digit, whether it involves a finger or thumb, are relatively straightforward and generally agreed on by most hand surgeons. Modification of the procedures previously described is generally based on the needs of the individual patient. Amputations that involve multiple digits simultaneously are usually the result of acute trauma, most frequently of a mechanical nature. However, thermal and cold injuries, as well as vascular disturbances,

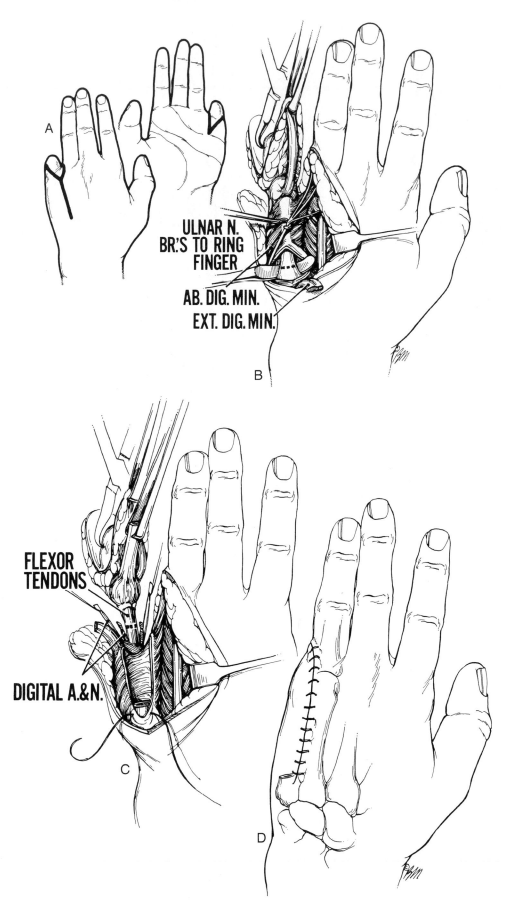

ULNAR N.
BR.'S TO RING
FINGER

AB. DIG. MIN.
EXT. DIG. MIN.

FLEXOR
TENDONS

DIGITAL A.&N.

FIGURE 55-27. A to **D,** Ray amputation of the small finger is accomplished by transection of the metacarpal at its base, with the hypothenar muscles preserved to serve as an ulnar pad for the hand.

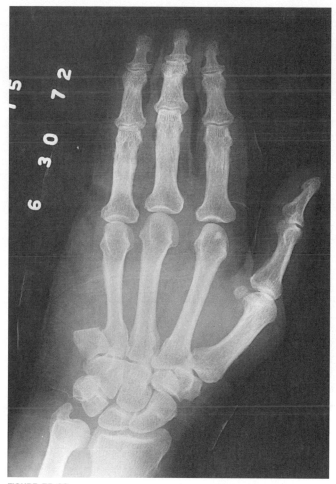

FIGURE 55-28. Appropriate level for bone resection of the small finger metacarpal in which the tendinous insertions of the flexor and extensor carpi ulnaris muscles are preserved.

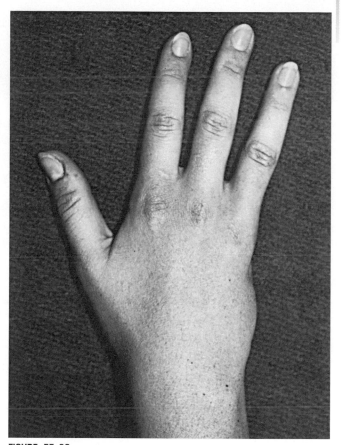

FIGURE 55-29. The appearance of the small finger ray amputation is cosmetically quite acceptable.

may result in the necessity for multiple digit amputations. The basic principle in such situations is to save all viable tissue by whatever means appropriate and to preserve the tissue for possible reconstruction at a later date.[253,254]

Figure 55-30 shows the dominant right hand of a 17-year-old boy who sustained an injury in a mechanical corn picker. Preservation of the remnants of the index and small finger proximal phalanges was extremely important to the boy's subsequent function, not only for writing (see Fig. 55-30) but also for grasping activities. This example clearly demonstrates the principle of preserving length when feasible and salvage of all possible tissue for later reconstruction.

Later reconstruction may involve shifting or ablation of parts. The 43-year-old woman in Figure 55-31 sustained a punch press injury to her nondominant hand. The press spared her thumb metacarpal and a remnant of the proximal phalanx, and she had a proximal phalangeal amputation level of the four remaining digits. A distant inframammary flap was used to cover the denuded end of her thumb, as well as the exposed phalanges. Subsequently, it was possible to remove the index metacarpal and shift dorsal skin into the thumb/long finger web, thereby "phalangizing" the thumb. This allowed the patient good pinch and grasp in this area. Preservation of length in this circumstance was

extremely important for subsequent restoration of function.

Rose and Buncke[264] have used selective finger translocation after multiple digit amputations. They have taken the least severely damaged digits and placed them where they will be most functionally useful. This is a natural extension of microsurgical technique.

Figure 55-32 demonstrates another severe injury involving multiple digits. In this situation a punch press was responsible for creating the central defects in both hands. The bony elements of the proximal portion of the ring finger on the right hand were gone, as well as one of the neurovascular bundles. However, the flap was viable. It was filleted and used to close the defect, again salvaging all possible usable parts.

Occasionally, later revision will be required to functionally improve the situation, as seen in Figure 55-33. The

CRITICAL POINTS: MULTIPLE DIGIT AMPUTATIONS

- In initial repair the goals are to preserve length when feasible and to save all viable tissue for possible late reconstruction.

- In some cases later revision will be required to improve function.

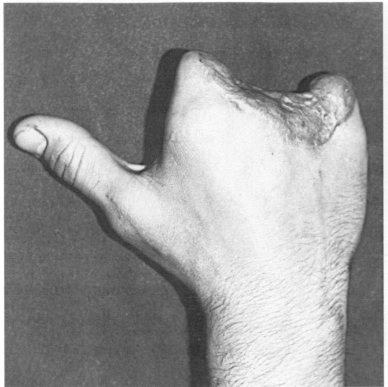
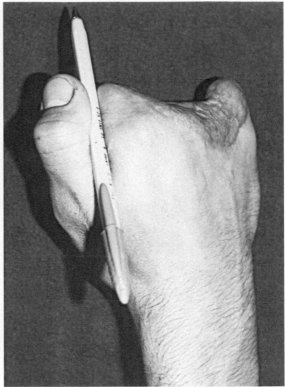

FIGURE 55-30. In multiple digit amputations, preservation of all possible length is important. In this situation the proximal phalangeal remnant of the index finger was important for pinching and especially for writing.

metacarpals that were preserved at the time of the original closure projected into the web and created functional difficulties for the patient. Therefore, the bases were preserved and the remaining distal portions of the metacarpals were removed, much to the satisfaction of the patient. Reconstruction after traumatic amputation at the level of the distal metacarpals creates ample opportunity for the exercise of surgical ingenuity. It is extremely important, however, that all possible tissue be saved initially to allow for such later reconstruction.

AMPUTATIONS THROUGH THE CARPUS

Amputations through the carpus or more distally through the bases of the metacarpals do not have the possibilities for the same functional restoration (see Fig. 55-31). Intrinsic musculature is absent, and although coverage may be possible with local or distant skin, the capability of pinching and grasping is absent.[46] This may initially create a dilemma for both the patient and surgeon. More proximal amputation and fitting with a conventional prosthesis are certainly considerations, especially in terms of early functional rehabilitation of the patient. However, at the time of the initial traumatic event, the injured patient may be incapable of making this decision. It is therefore preferable to save what is salvageable and allow time for the patient to come to a decision after having an opportunity to functionally evaluate the alternatives.

Figure 55-34 illustrates an amputation that runs obliquely from the thumb metacarpal proximally through the carpus

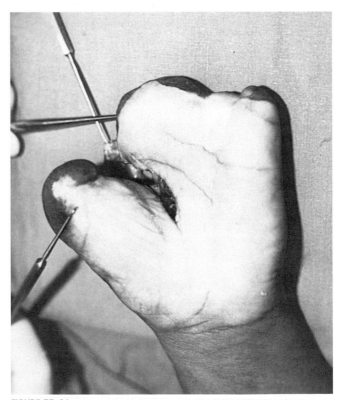

FIGURE 55-31. Preservation of all length in the proximal phalanges and in the thumb metacarpal facilitates later index ray resection and "phalangization" of the thumb by means of a dorsal transposition flap. This illustrates the potential for subsequent reconstruction once initial coverage and preservation of length have been maintained by skin flap coverage.

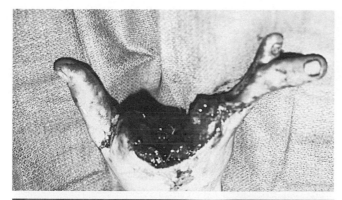

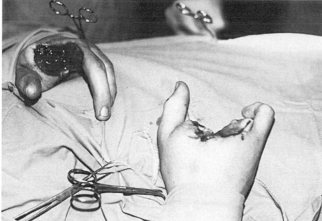

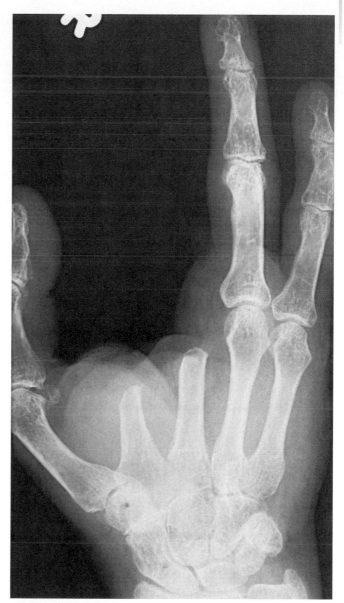

FIGURE 55-32. Preserved viable skin from the filleted ring finger was used for subsequent coverage of the cutaneous defect incurred by this severe punch press injury.

FIGURE 55-33. Preservation of the second and third metacarpal remnants was accomplished at the time of the initial procedure in this individual. However, because the remnants projected into the web, they were subsequently removed with preservation of the metacarpal bases and the tendon insertions.

on the ulnar side. Certainly, there is no possibility of pinch or grasp. The skin is sensitive, however, and this woman preferred to keep the stump as it was because she considered it preferable to a more proximal amputation level and prosthetic device. A cosmetic hand was fashioned for her, which she wore for social occasions. At home she used the stump with the remaining wrist flexion and extension to hold objects against her body and accomplish other tasks. The presence of wrist mobility does impart some function to a stump of this sort, and it should not be ignored. With modern prosthetic techniques, it is possible to fashion a prosthesis that can incorporate the preserved wrist joint and allow for a terminal device without the necessity of attachments proximal to the elbow.[323,329] Preservation of the radiocarpal joint eliminates the necessity for a wrist unit incorporated into the prosthesis and is therefore extremely useful.

WRIST DISARTICULATION

According to Tooms,[56] a survey of surgeons in this country indicated a preference for long below-elbow amputation over wrist disarticulation. There was a time when this was perhaps an appropriate accommodation to the capabilities of prosthetic fabrication; however, current technology and biomaterial fabrication techniques have made the application of functional prosthetic devices possible for practically

any level of amputation in the upper extremity, including wrist disarticulation. The advantage of preserving the distal radioulnar joint (DRUJ) is that full pronation and supination are possible, assuming the joint is uninjured, and this in itself improves the capability of the amputee. Preserving the radial styloid flare improves prosthetic suspension. Therefore, when possible, the DRUJ should be preserved, even though prosthetic fitting may be more challenging than for below-elbow amputees. Conventional wrist units are not used because of excessive length and myoelectric fitting is also difficult. When the amputation is an elective procedure, preoperative consultation with the surgeon's own local prosthetist regarding the preferred level may be worthwhile.

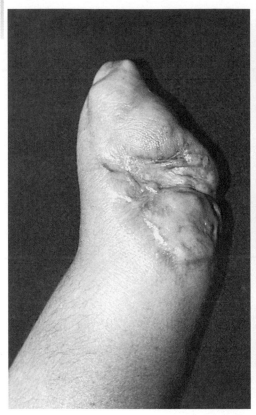

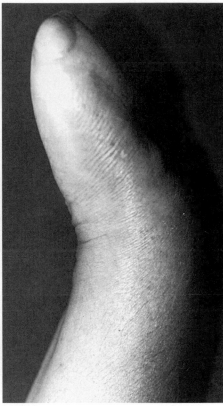

FIGURE 55-34. When given the option, this woman considered her trans-metacarpal amputation with preservation of wrist motion preferable to a more proximal amputation level and prosthetic fitting.

 ## Authors' Preferred Method of Wrist Disarticulation

The patient is positioned on the operating table in a supine position, and a tourniquet is used when possible. More distal amputations may be done under intravenous regional or axillary block anesthesia. When the circumstance involves a tumor or infection, exsanguination of the limb by means of an Esmarch (Martin) wrap is contraindicated. Some surgeons prefer to use general anesthesia or an interscalene block in patients with an infection in the limb distally because of the potential problems of lymphatic spread with the use of axillary block anesthesia. If a tourniquet is to be used but it is not desirable to exsanguinate the limb, the limb may be drained by limb elevation or manual compression of the brachial artery. At the completion of all amputations, the tourniquet is released and hemostasis obtained before final wound closure.

When the amputation level has been defined by the acute traumatic situation, management of the remaining tissue follows basic surgical principles. All blood vessels should be ligated and care taken to allow the transected tendons to retract proximally. The nerves should be managed in such a way as to encourage the inevitable neuroma to form at a site that will not come into contact with the prosthetic wall or become entrapped in the healing wound. Two methods have been used for this. One is to put gentle longitudinal traction on the nerve and transect it so that it can retract to a more proximal level. Because of difficulties encountered with this technique, we prefer to make a more proximal (longitudinal) incision between the pronator teres and brachioradialis just

distal to the elbow flexion crease and doubly ligate the median, ulnar, and superficial radial nerves at this point. This causes a neuroma-in-continuity to form at this site and be buried beneath the proximal muscles, where it is less likely to be a symptomatic problem.[270] We have not found it necessary to ligate the antebrachial cutaneous nerves in the proximal forearm. In an acute situation, skin coverage will depend entirely on the level of transection and what remains for closure. In elective cases, the procedure is carried out as follows.

A long palmar flap and short dorsal flap are fashioned at a level sufficiently distal to the radioulnar joint to allow the volar flap to be reflected dorsally for final closure (Fig. 55-35). It is preferable to take excess skin at this point, which can be fashioned at the conclusion of the procedure to give an appropriate contour (Fig. 55-36). Flaps are reflected in a proximal direction and all veins are ligated. The superficial branch of the radial nerve and the dorsal sensory branch of the ulnar nerve will be identified during this portion of the procedure. If they are to be proximally ligated as indicated earlier, they may be transected without fear of consequences. In some individuals, the lateral antebrachial cutaneous nerve may be quite prominent on the radial side, and if so, it may be ligated proximal to the wound margin. The medial antebrachial cutaneous nerve is handled in a similar fashion when it is identified. Next, it is most important to identify the radial and ulnar vessels and to doubly ligate them proximal to the wrist. After transection of the vessels, the median nerve is transected. The flexor and extensor tendons are pulled distally and transected. Electrocautery may be used to obtain hemostasis of both the anterior and posterior interosseous vessels. A transverse dorsal

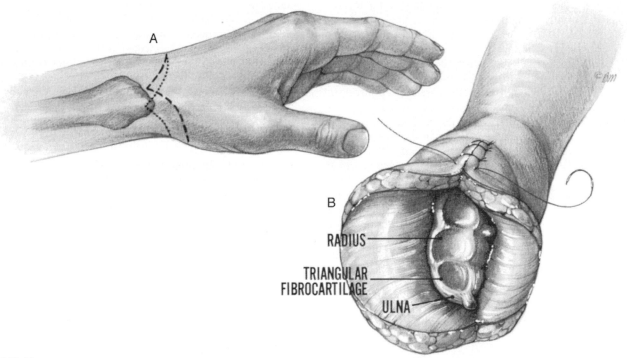

FIGURE 55-35. **A** and **B,** Disarticulation of the wrist has the advantage of preserving pronation and supination. With modern prosthetic techniques, this is a very functional level of amputation. Care must be taken in the course of the operation to preserve the distal radioulnar joint ligaments and the triangular fibrocartilage complex to maintain distal radioulnar joint stability.

incision of the dorsal radiocarpal joint gives visual access to the radiocarpal joint. Circumferential dissection may then be carried out to divide all the radiocarpal capsular and ligamentous attachments, which allows the amputated part to be removed. It is important to preserve the radioulnar ligaments, capsule, and triangular fibrocartilage complex and avoid damage to the distal radioulnar joint. The prominent styloid processes must be rounded off. After removal of the amputated specimen, the skin flaps are fashioned to eliminate redundancy. The subcutaneous tissue and skin layers are closed. A soft dressing is applied with compression in a distal-to-proximal direction. A proximal incision is made, as previously noted, to gain access to the median, ulnar, and radial nerves for proximal ligation.

FOREARM AMPUTATIONS

Below-Elbow Amputation

In general, amputations below the elbow should preserve the maximum length possible,[2,54-57] thereby preserving maximum pronation and supination. This technique of fashioning flaps is illustrated in Figure 55-37.

In elective amputations below the elbow, the flaps are fashioned distal to the intended level of bone amputation.[54,56,57] With more proximal levels of amputation and muscle transection, the skin flaps will shift proximally as the muscles are divided, but they can easily be retracted and closed appropriately. In general, anterior and posterior flaps of equal dimension are created and reflected proximally. Ligation of the superficial veins and proximal ligation of cutaneous nerves are carried out at this point. The dorsal and volar

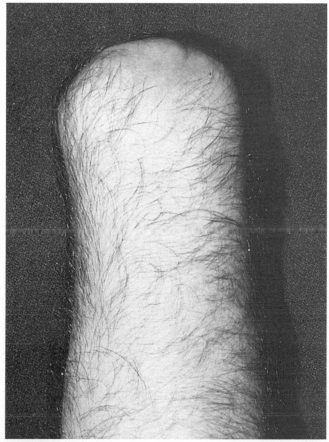

FIGURE 55-36. Satisfactory stump closure for a wrist disarticulation level. Preservation of the distal radioulnar joint is important because it preserves pronation and supination.

antebrachial fascia is incised, and, depending on the level of amputation, either the tendons or muscle bellies are divided after the radial and ulnar vessels are ligated. For all long below-elbow amputations and certainly for those more proximally, we prefer to ligate the nerves doubly through a separate incision, if necessary, to bury them underneath the muscle bulk proximally.[270] The muscle bellies are incised just distal to the planned level of bony resection. The anterior and posterior interosseous vessels should be ligated or coagulated with electrocautery. An incision in the periosteum is then carried out sharply and circumferentially. The bone is transected at the desired level at this time, and the specimen is removed. The bone ends are smoothed with a rasp. Bone wax may be used to cover the exposed ends. We prefer not to use wax because we have encountered patients who later presented with the material extruding from their amputation stumps. Wound closure is accomplished after hemostasis has been obtained by the usual means after release of the tourniquet. The skin flaps can then be carefully fashioned; the subcutaneous tissue and skin are closed in separate layers. A drain is sometimes helpful, depending on the surgeon's judgment. The stump is dressed and wrapped circumferentially with an elastic bandage applied more firmly distally than proximally to prevent stump edema. If a drain is used, it is removed after 24 hours. Immediate active motion of the elbow and shoulder are encouraged to prevent joint contractures. The patient is instructed in stump wrapping during the early postoperative period. When stump shrinkage has subsided, early prosthetic fitting is undertaken.

Short Below-Elbow Amputation

The technique for amputation of the proximal forearm is quite similar to that used for amputation in the middle and distal thirds. It is, however, important to note that when a very proximal amputation is carried out (i.e., proximal to the bicipital tuberosity), it may be advisable to reattach the biceps tendon proximally to the ulna if necessary to facilitate prosthetic fitting at this level. When elbow flexion is present, approximately 5 cm of ulnar bone length is sufficient to allow below-elbow prosthetic fitting. The biceps tendon should be attached to the ulna at a position approximating its resting length. Too distal an attachment may result in a flexion contracture. Jones and Blair[269] have demonstrated a unique salvage of a below-elbow stump as an alternate to an above-elbow amputation level by means of a free latissimus dorsi flap.

Krukenberg's Procedure

In 1917 Krukenberg described an imaginative operative procedure that converts a forearm stump into radial and ulnar rays. The two opposing rays created by this procedure provide a pincer-like grasp that is motored by the pronator teres muscle. The indications for this operative procedure have been the subject of many debates in the literature.[317,318] One generally agreed-upon candidate for this operation is a bilateral upper extremity amputee who is also blind. A relative indication may also exist in a sighted bilateral upper extremity amputee. Performance of the procedure on the dominant side eliminates the necessity for visual contact for all "manual" activities because of the proprioception and stereognosis present in the created stump. This may also allow for effective maneuvering in the dark and at night. Performance of this procedure does not preclude the use of a standard prosthesis and thus gives the individual the option of prosthetic use.

Swanson and Swanson[318] advocated the use of this procedure in selected juvenile amputees. Nathan and Trung[313] described modified skin incisions that, when possible, allow for primary closure without the use of skin grafts. The use of other than local skin for coverage will, of course, depend on the reason for the amputation. Descriptions of the operative procedure by Swanson and Swanson[318] and by Nathan and Trung[313] are recommended. Gu and colleagues[308] have further modified the procedure by removing all the forearm musculature except the pronator teres, the flexor carpi ulnaris, the brachioradialis, and the supinator. They also keep the length of the forearm trunk at 12 to 15 cm, which allows for better flap closure. Garst,[307] in a large series of 35 operations, also selectively removed portions of the flexor and extensor muscle mass with the aim of debulking the stump. He did not believe

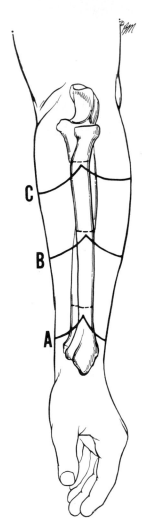

FIGURE 55-37. Three levels of amputation. More distal amputations preserve forearm rotation. The more proximal level has no rotation but does preserve elbow flexion and still allows the use of a below-elbow prosthesis.

that its application should be limited to blind double amputees. His experience in developing countries, where expensive prostheses are not available, expanded the indications for use of the procedure. This procedure is not recommended as a primary procedure at the time of an amputation but rather as a secondary procedure after appropriate counseling because of cosmetic concerns. Less than 10 cm of residual limb length from the tip of the olecranon and an elbow flexion contracture greater than 70 degrees are relative contraindications to this procedure.

ELBOW DISARTICULATION

Elbow disarticulation has the advantage over an above-elbow amputation of allowing transmission of humeral rotation to the prosthesis distally because a snug fit at the flare of the humeral condyles can be achieved (Fig. 55-38). Because of this feature, some surgeons and prosthetists prefer this highly acceptable level of amputation over a more proximal amputation level.

Skin flaps are fashioned according to the circumstances of the amputation. Typical anterior and posterior flaps of relatively equal dimension can be carried out in elective circumstances, but practically any flap designed will adequately serve for coverage at this level. After the flaps have been designed, they are reflected proximally over the humeral condyles. Anterior exposure initially is preferred, with the brachial artery and accompanying veins proximal to the elbow identified and doubly ligated. The medial brachial and antebrachial cutaneous nerves are identified and ligated proximally. The median nerve is identified just medial to the brachial artery and should be transected or ligated sufficiently proximal to allow it to retract under cover of the biceps muscle. The ulnar nerve is identified behind the medial epicondyle or more proximally; it is either allowed to retract or ligated proximally under cover of the triceps muscle. The biceps tendon is transected and allowed to retract proximally. The brachialis muscle is removed from its attachment to the coronoid process. The flexor-pronator origin is reflected distally from the medial humeral condyle. The joint is entered anteriorly. The lateral antebrachial cutaneous nerve is ligated proximally and permitted to retract beneath the biceps and brachialis muscles. The radial nerve is identified beneath the cover of the brachioradialis and is either ligated or allowed to retract proximally between the brachialis and brachioradialis. The extensor musculature is then divided in a circumferential fashion, and the radiohumeral and ulnohumeral joint capsules are divided posteriorly to complete the amputation. If the patient is very thin, it may be advisable to cover the end of the humerus with a reflected flap of brachialis, biceps, or triceps. Again, a drain may be used if deemed necessary. A simple two-layer closure may also be used if the patient has sufficient subcutaneous fat. By design, the resulting stump of an elbow disarticulation is somewhat more bulbous than an above-elbow amputation at a more proximal level. This characteristic allows rotation of the humerus to be transmitted to the prosthesis. If a drain is used, it is removed after 24 hours. Immediate amputation stump management involving edema management, wrappings, and early prosthetic fitting is essential.

ABOVE-ELBOW AMPUTATIONS

Amputations above the elbow should also maintain all possible length.[54,56,57] In traumatic amputations, additional bone resection to allow primary closure should be avoided if at all possible. Even split-thickness skin grafting to maintain length is preferable to more radical proximal bony excision. This is especially true in circumstances in which the level is close to the axillary fold. Amputations of the humerus at this level or more proximally are essentially treated as shoulder disarticulations, and virtually all shoulder motion is lost, particularly abduction-adduction maneuvers. Prosthetic fitting for amputations above the elbow requires the use of a suspension system, which is accomplished by means of one of a variety of harness devices.[3,47,320,325,328]

CRITICAL POINTS: CARPUS AND UPPER LIMB AMPUTATIONS AND DISARTICULATIONS

- The surgeon should make optimal use of modern prosthetic techniques; devices can be fabricated for practically any level of amputation.
- Both below-elbow and above-elbow amputations should maintain all possible limb length.

Skin flaps of equal dimension should be designed (Fig. 55-39) with appropriate length so that the suture line will lie over the end of the stump. In traumatic situations it is acceptable to fashion a flap with available skin, which may place the suture line in a medial-lateral or more anteroposterior position. After the skin flaps have been reflected proximally, the brachial artery and vein are identified and doubly ligated proximal to the level of planned bony resection. The radial, median, and ulnar nerves are either proximally ligated or pulled distally, transected, and allowed to retract under the proximal musculature. The flexor and extensor muscle masses are transected just distal to the level of intended bone resection. Usually, muscle division between 1 to 2 cm distal to the level of intended bone resection will allow retraction to the level of the bone end. The periosteum is divided and the bone is then transected. At this point the tourniquet, if one was used, should be released and hemostasis obtained by vessel ligation or electrocautery. The anterior and posterior fascia over the flexor and extensor muscle masses may be sutured to each other to cover the end of the stump. Alternatively, closure may be accomplished in two layers by using the subcutaneous tissue and skin to fashion the end of the stump. We prefer to close the anterior and posterior fascia over the stump. However, because of the bulk, it may be necessary at times to trim some of the muscle fibers to contour the final stump.

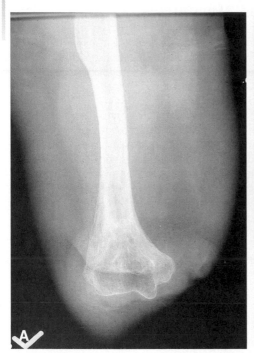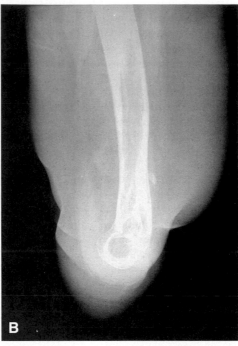

FIGURE 55-38. Anteroposterior (**A**) and lateral (**B**) radiographs depicting a post-traumatic elbow disarticulation.

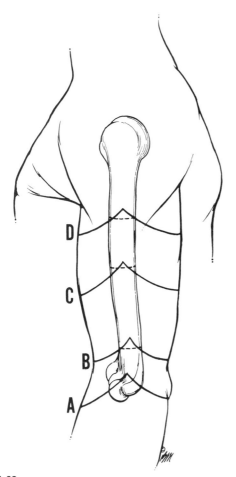

FIGURE 55-39. Four levels of amputation, including elbow disarticulation and proximal humeral amputation.

Amputation of the Arm at the Level of the Pectoralis Major

From a prosthetic point of view, amputations at this level will function as a shoulder disarticulation because independent motion of the proximal humerus will not be available. The prosthetic component must grasp the shoulder girdle to have a satisfactory fit. However, preserving the proximal portion of the humerus does apply contour to the shoulder, and no matter how small the remaining proximal portion is, it will be of some aid in gaining better purchase for the prosthesis.

The incision begins anteriorly at the coracoid process and continues distally and posteriorly over the anterior edge, the insertion, and subsequently the posterior margin of the deltoid muscle (Fig. 55-40A). After incision of the skin and subcutaneous tissue, this flap is reflected in a proximal direction. The cephalic vein is identified in the deltopectoral groove and ligated proximally. The pectoralis major tendon is sectioned at its insertion on the humerus (see Fig. 55-40B). The deltoid tendon is transected distally, and the muscle is reflected in a proximal direction (see Fig. 55-40C). Care should be taken at this point to not injure the axillary nerve, which may be seen on the undersurface of the deltoid muscle. The pectoralis minor and coracobrachialis may now be clearly visualized; and in the interval between them the neurovascular structures are identified. The axillary artery and vein are doubly ligated and transected. The nerves are pulled distally, transected, and allowed to retract proximally. The conjoint tendon of the teres major and latissimus dorsi muscles is severed at its insertion on the bicipital groove. The tendons of the biceps and triceps are transected just distal to the intended level of bone resection and allowed to retract. The humerus is transected just proximal to the insertion of the pectoralis major. The end of the bone is smoothed with a rasp. The triceps and coracobrachialis may be sutured as a myofascial flap over the exposed end of the humerus. The deltoid is then reflected distally and the wound is closed in a layered fashion. As an alternative, the deltoid muscle and the lateral skin flap may be reflected downward to cover the end of the humerus and the wound subsequently closed in two layers through subcutaneous tissue and skin (see Fig. 55-40D).

Shoulder Disarticulation

The initial exposure for a disarticulation of the shoulder is identical to that used for an amputation through the proximal humerus (Fig. 55-41A). After the axillary vessels have been ligated, the thoracoacromial artery is identified just at the medial border of the pectoralis minor tendon, where it arises from the second portion of the axillary artery. The acromial branch may be seen lying on the pectoralis minor tendon and coursing toward the acromion. This vessel should be ligated and allowed to retract (see Fig. 55-41B). The median, ulnar, musculocutaneous, and radial nerves are identified in the interval between the short head of the biceps and the coracobrachialis; they are retracted distally, sharply transected, and allowed to retract beneath the pectoralis minor. The tendons of the coracobrachialis and the short head of the biceps may be sectioned at their conjoint origin from the coracoid process. Exposure of the latissimus dorsi and teres

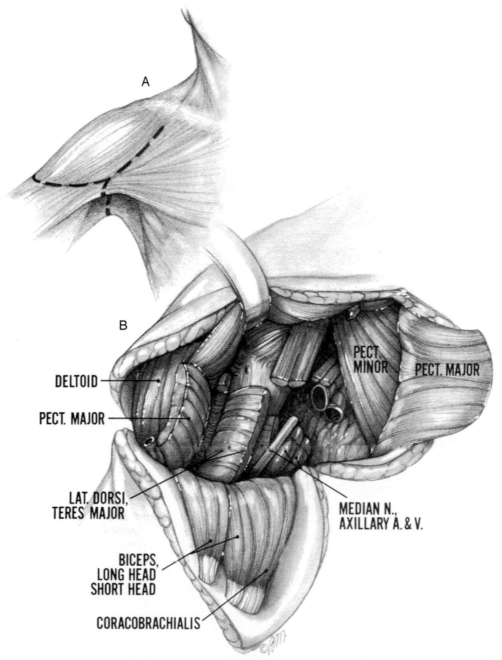

FIGURE 55-40. **A** to **D,** Amputation through the proximal humerus above the level of the pectoralis major preserves the contour of the shoulder but is functionally equivalent to a shoulder disarticulation. The muscular sling (shown in **C**) for coverage of the end of the humerus is optional but is an alternative way of covering the end of the bone.   *Continued*

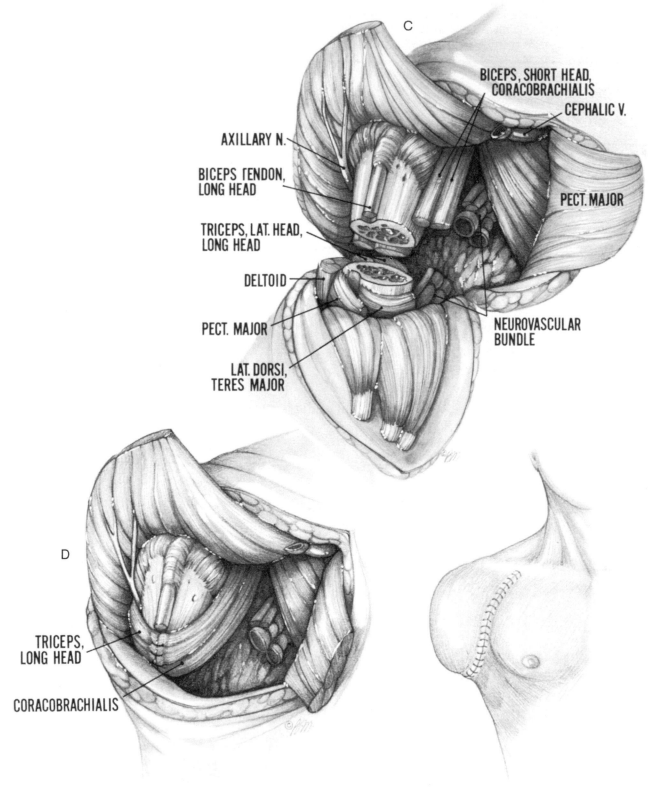

FIGURE 55-40—cont'd.

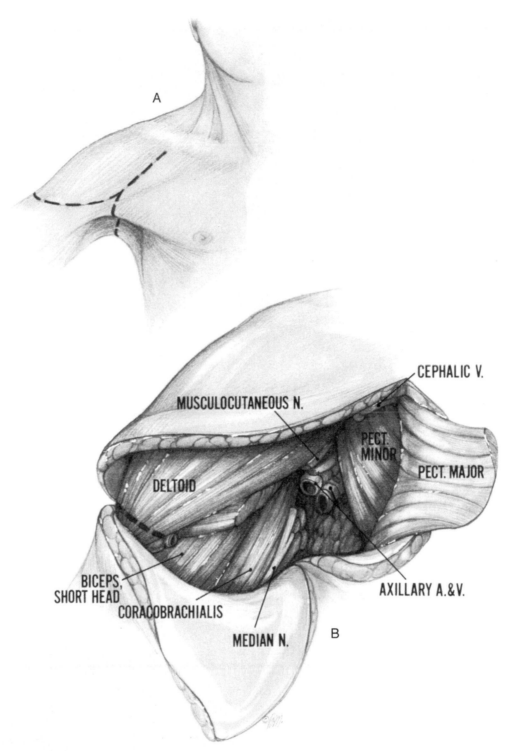

FIGURE 55-41. **A** and **B,** Shoulder disarticulation. The transaxillary approach with an extension over the deltoid and with proximal exposure along the deltopectoral groove gives excellent access to the shoulder joint, with sequential division of all muscle groups. *Continued*

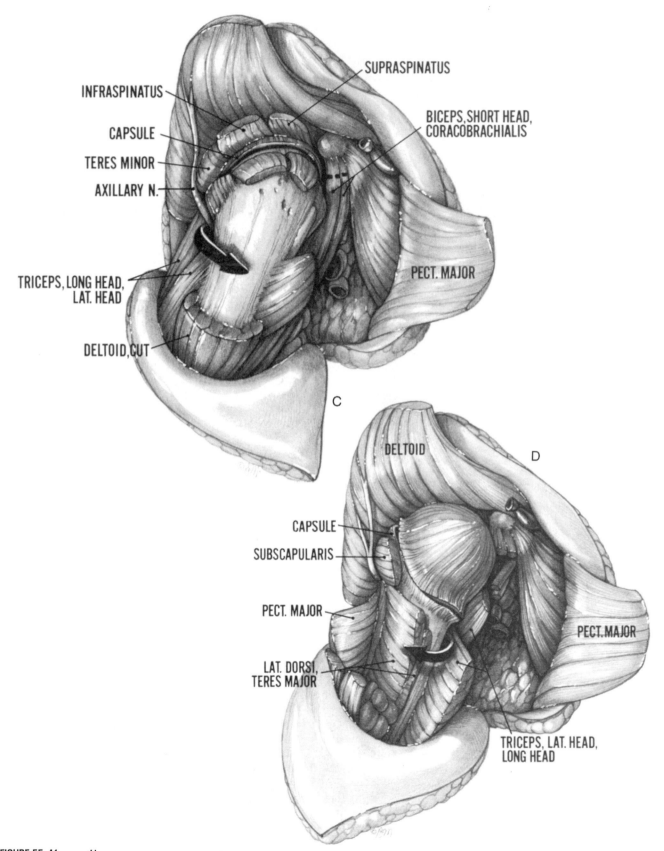

FIGURE 55-41—cont'd. C, After division of the pectoralis major and deltoid, the muscles attached to the coracoid arc divided; and with the arm internally rotated, the rotator cuff is severed. **D,** After the anterior musculature and the triceps are divided, the limb is externally rotated to give access to the glenohumeral joint capsule.

Continued

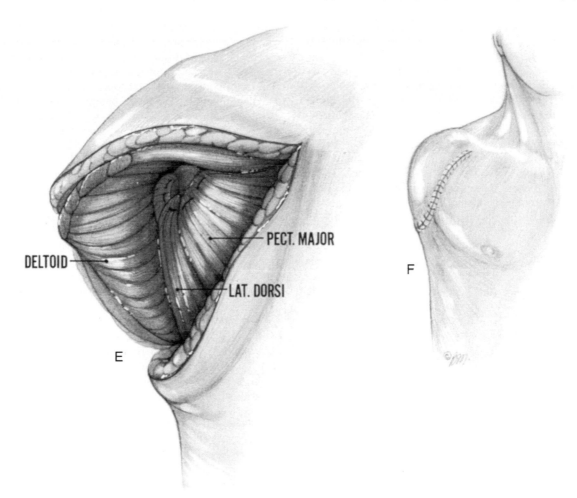

FIGURE 55-41—cont'd. **E** and **F,** The pectoralis major and latissimus dorsi muscles may be approximated over the empty glenoid. If the acromion is unduly prominent, it may be appropriately shaped.

major tendons is now possible, and these tendons are sectioned near their insertions. With further external rotation, the subscapularis tendon may be identified and should be sectioned, along with the anterior aspect of the joint capsule. With distal traction and internal rotation, the short external rotator muscles may be identified at this point; they likewise should be sectioned at their insertions on the greater tuberosity (see Fig. 55-41C). With subsequent section of the long head of the biceps, the triceps insertion, and the remaining capsule of the shoulder joint, disarticulation of the limb will be completed (see Fig. 55-41D). The deltoid muscle flap and its overlying skin are reflected to meet the inferior margin of the incision. This flap is then trimmed as necessary to provide contour and eliminate redundant tissue after the disarticulation. Alternatively, the ends of the latissimus dorsi and pectoralis major may be sewn together at the level of the glenoid (see Fig. 55-41E). If the acromion process is unduly prominent, it may be rounded off to a more acceptable appearance. The wounds are closed in routine fashion, and drains are used if indicated.

FOREQUARTER AMPUTATION

Forequarter amputation is a procedure that fortunately is infrequently performed. Its principal application is in the palliative or curative management of advanced malignant tumors involving the shoulder girdle or proximal humerus.[278,289,293] In addition to removal of the arm and distal upper extremity, the entire bony pectoral girdle, including the clavicle and scapula, is removed. This is an extremely disfiguring operation and is usually resorted to only as a palliative measure or in unusual cases of severe limb trauma. Before consideration of such an extensive procedure, thorough assessment of the extent of the tumor by means of computed tomography and magnetic resonance imaging of the affected area and the lungs should be performed. A study by Merimsky and colleagues verified that a forequarter amputation, when performed for palliative purposes, resulted in an improved quality of life and performance status in severely ill patients with an advanced malignancy involving the proximal upper extremity.[293]

Anterior Approach (Berger)

Two techniques have gained acceptance, the first being the anterior approach described by Berger.[277] For this procedure the patient is positioned on the operating table in a lateral position after general anesthesia has been induced. Maintenance of position is aided by an inflatable patient support. The limb is draped free, and the surgical field should be prepped from the opposite nipple line both anteriorly and posteriorly and up onto the neck. The first incision begins anteriorly just lateral to the sternocleidomastoid muscle. It is extended laterally over the clavicle and posteriorly over the acromioclavicular joint and then carried posteromedially along the vertebral border of the scapula to its inferior angle. A second incision is made laterally through the axilla, along the border of the latissimus dorsi, and then carried superiorly just medial to the deltopectoral groove, back to join the original incision (Fig. 55-42A). The incisions are deepened circumferentially down to the myofascial layers throughout the extent of the dissection. The nerves in the supraclavicular region are identified in the anterior portion of the incision, sectioned, and retracted cephalad. The platysma is sectioned. The medial third of the clavicle is exposed circumferentially by careful subperiosteal dissection. The external jugular vein may be encountered and should be retracted or ligated. The clavicle is carefully osteotomized just lateral to the sternocleidomastoid by means of a Gigli saw (see Fig. 55-42B). Further distal subperiosteal dissection of the clavicle is carried out to the extent of the acromioclavicular joint; and after dividing the conoid and trapezoid ligaments, the clavicle is removed by disarticulation of the acromioclavicular joint. The subclavius muscle is divided medially. The pectoralis major tendon is sectioned and the muscle retracted medially. The clavicular origin of the pectoralis major may be reflected distally or sectioned, depending on its bulk, to facilitate further exposure. The deltoid is retracted laterally. The tendons of the pectoralis minor, coracobrachialis, and short head of the biceps are divided at their insertions on the coracoid process of the scapula to further facilitate exposure of the neurovascular bundle. The subclavian artery and vein are doubly ligated and allowed to retract. The transverse cervical artery and vein and the suprascapular artery and vein are ligated as they cross laterally from the thyrocervical trunk (see Fig. 55-42C). Branches of the brachial plexus are identified, ligated proximally, and allowed to retract.

The posterior portion of the incision is then entered superiorly to allow sequential sectioning of the trapezius throughout its attachment to the scapula. The levator scapulae and both rhomboids are sectioned at their attachments to the scapula. With distal and lateral traction on the limb, the omohyoid is seen and sectioned. The fibers of the serratus anterior are then sectioned throughout their muscular and tendinous attachments to the scapula. The only muscle remaining at this point is the latissimus dorsi, which connects the shoulder girdle to the thorax. The muscle may be detached from the limb and the amputation completed by sectioning its tendinous attachment. Before this final move it is advisable to look for any remaining vascular attachments to prevent additional blood loss.

Posterior Approach (Littlewood)

The posterior approach to forequarter amputation, as advocated by Littlewood[291] in 1922, has continued to remain popular with some surgeons.[294-296] The presumed advantage of this technique is that the vessels are approached from their posterior aspect at the termination of the procedure without having to dissect through all the anterior structures, including the clavicle, before gaining vascular control. In addition, the easiest part of the forequarter amputation is

done initially, so release of the limb is very nearly complete when the anterior portion of the procedure is begun.

The patient is positioned in a lateral position with the limb that is to be amputated facing upward. An inflatable patient support may be used to assist in maintenance of the patient's position. The prep begins from the nipple line anteriorly and posteriorly to the opposite side of the chest, and the appropriate sterile field is created. The incision that is used has three components (Fig. 55-43A). The anterior part begins at the medial third of the clavicle and continues over the acromion. It is carried dorsally over the posterior aspect of the deltoid and then inferiorly to parallel the axillary border of the scapula. At the inferior angle of the scapula the incision is directed transversely toward the spine. This creates a large medially based skin flap, which allows exposure of the vertebral border of the scapula. The descending anterior limb is the second part of the exposure and is connected with the anterior portion of the preceding incision. The incision is carried down through the deltopectoral groove anteriorly. The third component of the exposure goes through the axillary fold inferiorly and connects the two previous limbs of the incision. The posterior portion of the wound is developed first and is carried down through subcutaneous tissue to elevate a large flap, which is reflected posteriorly toward the midline. Through this incision the posterior structures are identified and sectioned. The trapezius is identified, detached from the spine and the lateral portions of the acromion and the clavicle, and reflected in a superior direction. The levator scapulae, rhomboids, and attachment of the latissimus dorsi to the inferior angle of the scapula are transected (see Fig. 55-43B). The transverse cervical artery and suprascapular vessels are identified and doubly ligated. With traction on the limb, the omohyoid muscle is identified and likewise released from its attachment to the superior aspect of the scapula. The limb is then freed from its posterior attachments to rotate into an anterior position, where the neurovascular structures can be identified. The subclavian artery and vein are doubly ligated and transected. The components of the brachial plexus are individually identified, sharply transected, and allowed to retract medially. The anterior limb of the incision is then developed and carried down through subcutaneous tissue to expose the superior aspect of the clavicle. The nerves in the supraclavicular region are identified and transected after traction has been applied to allow them to retract beneath the proximal skin flap. The platysma is divided. Subperiosteal dissection of the clavicle is carried out, and the clavicle is divided just lateral to the attachment of the sternocleidomastoid muscle. The clavicle is then reflected laterally and the subclavius muscle divided. The attachments of the pectoralis major are released from the clavicle, and the tendons of the pectoralis major and latissimus dorsi are transected. The tendinous attachments to the coracoid process, namely, the short head of the biceps, pectoralis minor, and coracobrachialis, are likewise divided. At this point the remaining structure to be divided is the serratus anterior, which is easily approached through either portion of the incision. After severing this muscle, the limb is freed. After maintenance of hemostasis, the skin margins are approximated and an appropriate dressing is applied.

The long-term prognosis of this type of procedure is not good with respect to survival and prosthetic use. One recent

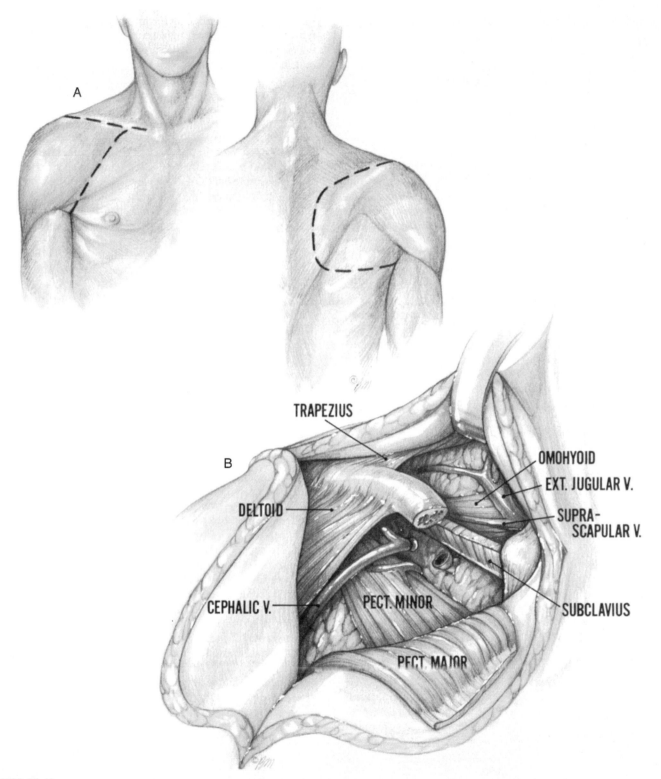

FIGURE 55-42. A, The classic forequarter amputation as originally described by Berger. The anterior part of the incision begins lateral to the sternocleidomastoid with a descending limb that goes along the deltopectoral groove and down through the axilla. The posterior limb then follows the vertebral border of the scapula to meet with the original anterior incision over the neck. **B,** The anterior part of the exposure is undertaken first to gain vascular control. Care must be taken when removing the clavicle from its bed.   *Continued*

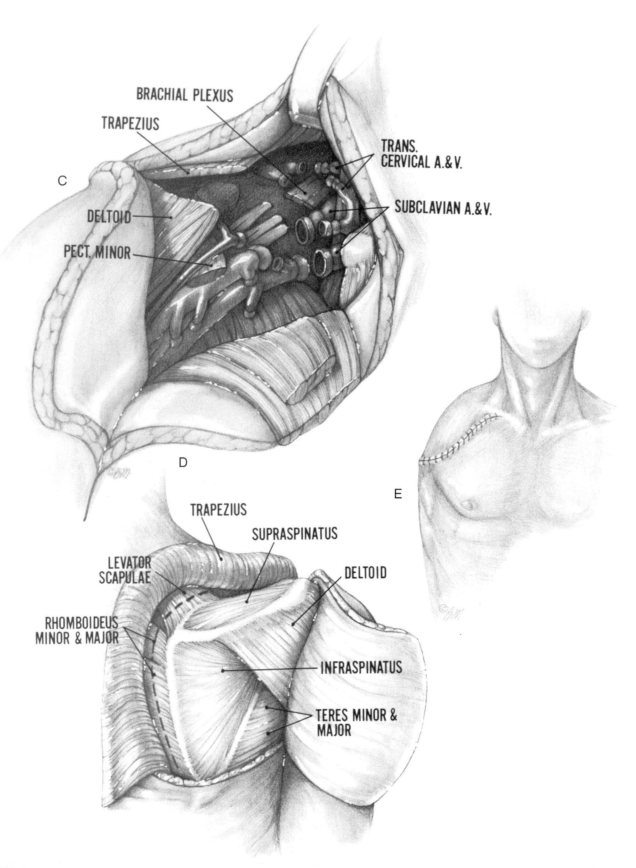

FIGURE 55-42—cont'd. C, After the clavicle has been removed, dissection is carried out to sever the anterior attachments of the shoulder girdle to the chest wall. **D** and **E,** The posterior attachments of the scapula to the chest wall are released sequentially after the anterior dissection has been completed.

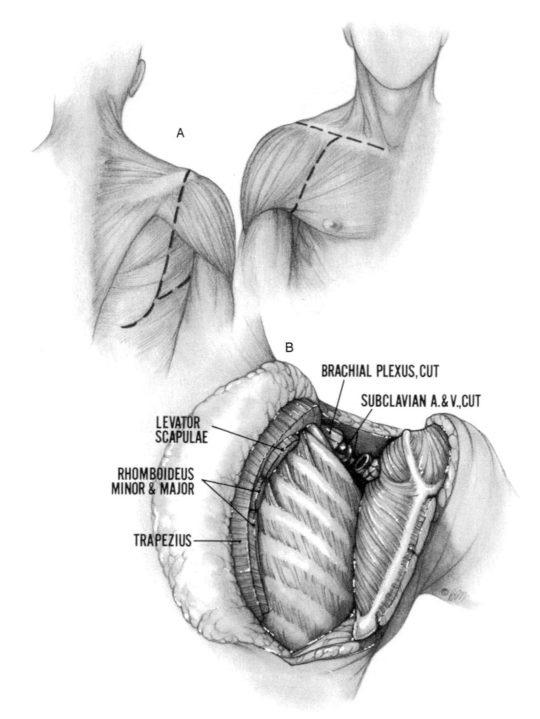

FIGURE 55-43. **A** and **B,** The posterior approach to forequarter amputation was described by Littlewood[291] and differs from the anterior exposure in that the neurovascular structures are managed after the posterior exposure has been made.

study reported a 23% 5-year survival rate that is directly related to the preoperative diagnosis, namely, an upper extremity malignancy.

Radical Forequarter Amputation

Roth and coworkers[301] described a radical forequarter amputation that includes the chest wall. This is used for extensive tumors that involve the shoulder girdle, chest wall, or axilla or for axillary metastases associated with recurrent breast

carcinoma. It is unlikely that most hand surgeons would be involved in this type of procedure. It is mentioned only for completeness.

Tikhor-Linberg Procedure (Resection of the Shoulder Girdle With Preservation of the Arm)

There are few good alternatives to a forequarter amputation when the amputation is indicated; however, for well-localized tumors of limited extent and for other special circum-

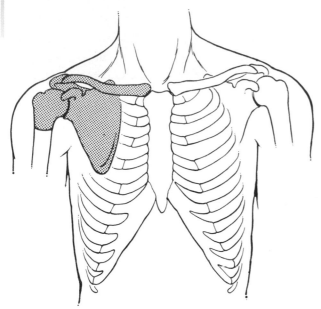

FIGURE 55-44. The Tikhor-Linberg[298] resection of the shoulder girdle is rarely indicated, but it does offer an alternative to interscapulothoracic, or forequarter, amputation in carefully selected individuals. The procedure involves excision of the clavicle, scapula, proximal humerus, and adjacent soft tissue attachments while preserving the distal upper extremity and its neurovascular components.

stances, the Tikhor-Linberg[303] resection (Fig. 55-44) may preserve distal function and obviate the need for the more severely mutilating aspects of a forequarter amputation. Pack and Crampton[298] reported their experience with four patients who underwent this procedure, and in all cases the results seem to have been preferable to forequarter amputation. It should be noted that during the same time interval they performed 102 forequarter amputations, perhaps indicating the relatively limited application of this procedure.

The operative approach is begun with an incision identical to that seen in the anterior approach to a forequarter amputation (see Fig. 55-42A). The incision may be modified, depending on the nature of the tumor or other condition and the presence or absence of cutaneous involvement. The anterior limb of the incision starts at the medial end of the clavicle and proceeds laterally over the tip of the acromion. The inferior aspect of the incision extends from the clavicular portion distally along the deltopectoral groove and then across through the axilla. The posterior portion continues up along the vertebral border of the scapula superiorly and connects with the anterior portion of the incision. The clavicle is exposed subperiosteally and transected lateral to the attachment of the sternocleidomastoid muscle. It is subperiosteally resected from its bed. The pectoralis major is transected at its insertion and reflected in a medial direction. The pectoralis minor, the short head of the biceps, and the coracobrachialis are transected at the coracoid process. The deltoid is reflected from its anterior attachments and from the scapula laterally and posteriorly. The long head of the biceps is resected anteriorly, and the long and short heads of the triceps are resected posteriorly. The humerus is transected at the appropriate level, depending on the individual case. The

posterior portion of the procedure is quite similar to that involving forequarter amputation. The trapezius is elevated from its attachment to the scapula and clavicle. With careful dissection over the superior part of the incision, the transverse cervical and the suprascapular arteries are divided at this point. The levator scapulae, rhomboids, and omohyoid are transected from their scapular attachments. The serratus anterior is divided from its attachment to the chest wall. The inferior angle of the scapula is separated from its attachment to the latissimus dorsi. By lateral traction, any remaining soft tissue attachments between the neurovascular bundle and the specimen may be removed at this time to free the specimen.

Varying amounts of overlying skin may be taken, depending on the nature of the problem to be dealt with. In addition, it may be possible to perform some reattachment of the remaining arm musculature proximally, either to the rib cage or to the soft tissue attachments about the hemithorax. Closure of the wound over a deep drain is accomplished in two layers.

EARLY POSTSURGICAL PROSTHETIC FITTING

Early prosthetic fitting of the upper extremity amputee has many advocates.[322,323,331,334,340] Burkhalter and coworkers[322] reported their results with immediate and early postsurgical prosthetic fitting in 96 upper extremity amputees, including nine individuals with shoulder disarticulation. In contrast to patients with lower extremity amputations, in whom vascular insufficiency and problems with wound healing are a major concern, most upper extremity amputees have excellent vascularity in the amputation stumps and are much less prone to wound breakdown and other attendant problems with wound healing. The major advantage of the application of modified upper extremity prostheses in the early postsurgical period is the early performance of bimanual activities. In addition, early prosthetic fitting allows for patient education in prosthetic use during the wound-healing phase and thus shortens the period of morbidity and hastens functional rehabilitation. Details of the technique are available in the excellent article by Burkhalter and coworkers.[322] Reports regarding continued prosthetic use are varied. Pinzur and associates[337] reported a high usage rate when an aggressive protocol was used after amputation. Jones and Davidson,[333] on the other hand, found only a 37% usage rate of 8 hours per day in a series of 27 patients monitored over a 9-year period in Australia. Wright and colleagues[342] reported a 94% usage rate for below-elbow amputees. More proximal amputees in all reported series have a much lower usage rate.

PAIN PROBLEMS AFTER AMPUTATION

Despite the surgeon's efforts to prevent amputation stump symptoms by careful tissue management, some patients will have stumps that are dysesthetic. This is a problem that occurs most frequently with distal digital injuries. It may also occur with more proximal amputations when a neuroma is superficially located or in continuity with the scar. Surgical translocation of the neuroma will usually improve symptoms. In the digits, however, dysesthesias may occur even though there is no clinical evidence of a discrete neuroma. As emphasized by Wilson and Carter-Wilson,[61] an early aggressive approach to this potential problem may prevent long-term impairment of function.

Gross and Watson[347] have suggested that excision of the remaining remnant of distal phalanx when it is extremely short (less than 17 mm) is effective in relieving pain and restoring function. They demonstrated this in a series of 21 patients who had dysfunctional fingertips after the preservation of short distal phalangeal segments.

Suzuki and associates[356] reported the pathologic findings in the cervical cord of a patient who underwent amputation at the shoulder 38 years previously. Not surprisingly, anterior horn cells, spinal ganglion cells, and large myelinated fibers of both the anterior and posterior roots were reduced in number. Schady and colleagues[354] demonstrated intact somatosensory function in eight patients who had proximal nerve stimulation at an average duration of 13 months after amputation. This microneurography resulted in precise distal localization of the parts previously amputated. The localization was quite precise. They concluded that the somatosensory system is capable of processing information long after peripheral sensory fields have been eliminated.

Desensitization Modalities

Desensitization has been recognized as an effective way of managing these perplexing situations. The physiologic basis for the dysesthesias and their response to desensitization techniques are not entirely understood at this time. The work of Sica and associates[52] demonstrated that the amplitude of the cortical evoked response of the contralateral somatic sensory cortex was diminished in patients with partial limb amputations. Interestingly, they found an increased amplitude of the evoked response in the proper area corresponding to the uninjured limb on the same side as the partial amputation. It would appear that the cerebral cortex makes adaptations when its peripheral afferents are interrupted. Exactly how this information relates to dysesthesias after amputation is unclear. Empirically it would seem that desensitization techniques are effective because of this adaptability of the central nervous system to repetitive stimuli.

Several techniques of desensitization have been suggested, but in general these are related to either early return to functional activities as advocated by Fisher and Boswick[346] or intensive supervised programs of progressive resensitization to textures and objects as outlined by Barber[344] and others.

It is not uncommon to encounter patients who for a variety of reasons (financial, transportation, personal) do not have access to a hand therapist. In such patients we review a home program with them with an actual demonstration of how to perform desensitization to the fingertip. The patient is provided with an instructional handout we have developed that illustrates how to rub and tap the fingertip against various different smooth and rough surfaces such as sandpaper and cloth. We ask the patients to spend 10 minutes, four times a day on the program for a minimum of 6 weeks. We emphasize the importance of being compliant and also the functional consequences/limitations of the hypersensitive finger.

Phantom Limb Pain

Phantom limb pain remains another persistent and poorly understood problem that is extremely difficult to treat. Jensen and colleagues[351] performed a prospective study of 58 patients who were to undergo an amputation. Most of these were for occlusive vascular disease involving the lower extremities. They demonstrated a correlation between the presence of preamputation limb pain and postamputation phantom limb pain. A gradual diminution in phantom limb pain from 72% at 8 days postoperatively to 59% at 2 years was demonstrated. There is good evidence that phantom limb pain after lower extremity amputation can be prevented or diminished by perioperative epidural anesthesia or postoperative intraneural anesthesia applied to the transected nerves.[343,344,352] However, similar data involving upper extremity amputees are not available at this time.

Phantom Limb Sensation

After an amputation some patients may develop the phenomenon of phantom limb *sensation* in which they feel that the amputated part(s) is still present. The mechanism for this bothersome phenomenon is not well understood, but it is of considerably less concern than phantom limb pain. Fortunately, phantom limb sensation does not require any specific treatment except reassurance because in most patients it resolves gradually over time.

Painful Neuromas

Finally, it appears that surgeons' efforts should be directed at those peripheral factors that they may be able to control, particularly with regard to neuroma formation. In this regard, Gorkisch and colleagues[24] described a new technique of centrocentral nerve coaptation, which in their experience limited symptomatic neuroma formation. They reported success in 29 of 30 patients treated by this method, which involves the juncture of two proximal nerve stumps, for example, the proper digital stumps of the index finger. They make a more proximal transection of the fascicles, thus creating an interposed graft. The new central ends then regrow toward each other through this newly created graft. The exact mechanism by which this frustrates the process of neuroma formation is

---

CRITICAL POINTS: POSTAMPUTATION PAIN PROBLEMS

- Dysesthetic amputation stumps occur even with careful tissue management, especially with distal digital injuries.
- Desensitization programs may improve outcomes in digital amputations.
- Phantom limb pain remains poorly understood and difficult to treat.
- Amputation neuromas should be identified, but treatment is difficult.

unclear, but they have made the same observation in an experimental animal model that served as the basis for their clinical work. Corroboration by other studies is needed.

Yuksel and colleagues[359] demonstrated that epineural grafts were significantly more effective in preventing neuroma pain when compared with a ligature or epineural flap. Another study demonstrated the effectiveness of preserving the digital nerves via a neurovascular island flap that is used to cover the proximal amputation stump, or, in the case of a ray resection, is de-epithelialized and buried between the adjacent metacarpals.[355] Clearly, the innovative surgical techniques confirm that there is no consensus on how to effectively manage the amputated finger with a painful neuroma.

Psychological Aspect of Hand Amputations

There is an expanding literature regarding investigations on the psychological impact of hand injuries. Grunert and colleagues[362-367] have had a unique experience in this regard inasmuch as a psychologist is an actual part of their hand evaluation team. They have shown that the severity of the initial exposure and visualization of the traumatic event can lead to frightening flashbacks and a post-traumatic stress disorder. They strongly suggest psychological consultation within the first 3 days after injury. They have found the use of various psychometric tests to be helpful in not only predicting outcomes but also successfully returning the injured patient to gainful employment.

It is clear that preinjury attitudes, motivation, and desire have a strong influence on how an individual will deal with a traumatic event.[360,361] It is also becoming evident that these same factors may influence an individual's response when there has been no amputation.[368]

ANNOTATED REFERENCES

88. Das SK, Brown HG: Management of lost fingertips in children. Hand 10:16-27, 1978.

    This article is important because of the controversy regarding the management of fingertip injuries in children. The authors reviewed their series of 60 children who underwent split-thickness skin grafting, local flap coverage, or a conservative (nonoperative) approach. They, and others subsequently, demonstrated that local wound care is the preferred approach for children with a fingertip injury distal to the insertion of the terminal tendon.

148. Atasoy E, Ioakimidis E, Kasdan ML, et al: Reconstruction of the amputated fingertip with a triangular volar flap. J Bone Joint Surg Am 52:921-926, 1970.

    This classic article is the original description of the volar V-Y advancement flap for closure of dorsal oblique or transverse fingertip amputations. The authors reviewed the indications and summarized their results in 56 patients with a fingertip injury. The reported advantages of this technique are its simplicity, minimum amount of scarring, excellent cosmetic result, and preservation of normal sensation.

161. Flatt AE: The thenar flap. J Bone Joint Surg Br 39:80-85, 1957.

    In 1955, Flatt wrote a paper about hand injuries and the use of the thenar flap. Controversy ensued because of his statement that he was "yet to have an ungrateful patient" with

the use of the technique. The follow-up to that paper was this publication that provided technical details and postoperative instructions to avoid the possible causes of "imperfect results." The surgeon who wishes to incorporate the thenar flap into his or her armamentarium of soft tissue coverage of fingertip injuries should review this paper.

171. Gurdin M, Pangman WJ: The repair of surface defects of fingers by trans-digital flaps. Plast Reconstr Surg 5:368-371, 1950.

    This is the original description of the indications and technical details of the trans-digital (now known as the cross-finger) flap. The technique was advocated as a simple, yet effective method to repair a soft tissue defect of the finger with exposed bone or tendon.

180. Kleinert HE, McAlister CG, McDonald CJ, Kutz JE: A critical evaluation of cross finger flaps. J Trauma 14:756-766, 1974.

    This is a follow-up article to a previous analysis of cross-finger flaps in the hand. The original article resulted in controversy regarding the several aspects of the technique, specifically (1) the criticism that the technique should not be used in the thumb and little finger; (2) that it was contraindicated in patients older than 40; and (3) that there was reported sensory re-innervation potential of these pedicle flaps. Kleinert and his colleagues demonstrated that the age of the patient and the digit involved are not contraindications to the use of a cross-finger flap. Their study was the first to document functional sensory re-innervation of the flap in a high percentage of cases.

183. Kutler W: A new method for fingertip amputation. JAMA 133:29-30, 1947.

    Kutler was apparently the first to suggest lateral V-Y advancement flaps based on the terminal branches of the proper digital arteries. Although this article was written nearly 60 years ago, the technique remains in use today and is useful for fingertip injuries with an intact nail matrix and exposed distal phalanx.

186. Melone CP, Beasley RW, Carstens JH: The thenar flap: An analysis of its use in 150 cases. J Hand Surg [Am] 7:291-297, 1982.

    Melone and his colleagues described what they called the "three cardinal technical principles" of thenar flaps: (1) flap design near the metacarpophalangeal (MP) joint crease and avoidance of the midpalmar area; (2) full flexion of the MP joint and, when feasible, the interphalangeal joints of the recipient finger; and (3) flap detachment at 10 to 14 days postoperatively with immediate active range of motion exercises. In their large series of 150 cases, donor site problems were "infrequent" and joint contractures developed in only six (4%) patients.

189. Schenck RR, Cheema TA: Hypothenar skin grafts for fingertip reconstruction. J Hand Surg [Am] 9:750-753, 1984.

    The subjective and objective results of full-thickness skin grafting from the ipsilateral hypothenar region were reviewed in 20 patients with 25 fingertip injuries. The donor site was selected because it is convenient and reliable. All of the patients could differentiate between coarse and smooth texture, none complained of hypersensitivity, and all reported that the donor site was cosmetically acceptable. The technique is an alternative to a local flap and is particularly useful in those injuries involving palmar and lateral pulp loss in which a local advancement flap is not feasible.

190. Shepard GH: The use of lateral V-Y advancement flaps for fingertip reconstruction. J Hand Surg [Am] 8:254-259, 1983.

    Shepard had a particular interest in fingertip injuries, and during the 1980s he presented and published several excellent reports regarding these very common injuries. This 1983 article contains the most precise details of the V-Y flap to be found in the literature.

243. Peimer CA, Wheeler DR, Barrett A, Goldschmidt PG: Hand function following single ray amputation. J Hand Surg [Am] 24:1245-1248, 1999.

The authors assessed and contrasted the results of primary and secondary/reconstructive ray amputation. They demonstrated that primary ray resection is associated with less total cost with respect to the injury itself and subsequent disability. The majority of patients returned to their preinjury occupation and were subjectively satisfied with the appearance and function of the hand. A very curious finding was the significant differences in grip strength, key pinch, oppositional pinch, and rate of manipulation test results in those patients who had unsettled litigation/compensation issues. These differences could not be explained on a physical/anatomic basis, implicating secondary gain issues.

249. Steichen JB, Idler RS: Results of central ray resection without bony transposition. J Hand Surg [Am] 11:466-474, 1986.

The authors reviewed their experience with central ray resection without bony transposition, which at that time was controversial because of the criticisms of inadequate closure of the defect and the resultant angulation and rotation of the adjacent digits. In their retrospective review of 13 patients, all but one patient was satisfied with the aesthetic and functional outcome. No late scissoring or malrotation occurred.

293. Merimsky O, Kollender Y, Inbar M, et al: Is forequarter amputation justified for palliation of intractable cancer symptoms? Oncology 60:55-59, 2001.

The authors attempted to demonstrate, in a difficult group of patients, that a palliative forequarter amputation, while considered disfiguring, improves the quality of life and performance status of severely ill patients with an advanced malignancy of the shoulder girdle or proximal humerus.

307. Garst RJ: The Krukenberg hand. J Bone Joint Surg Br 73:385-388, 1991.

Classically, the Krukenberg amputation was said to be indicated in bilateral blind amputees. This author said that is "too restrictive." This study evaluated the Krukenberg cineplasty operation in forearm amputees, the majority of whom had a post-traumatic amputation and were *not* blind. Thirty-five Krukenberg procedures were performed over 36 years by a surgeon in a developing country where the cost of prosthetic devices made their use prohibitive. All of the patients had a good pincer grip, could use their stumps bimanually, and were employed and self supporting.

336. Pillet J: Esthetic hand prosthesis. J Hand Surg [Am] 8:778-781, 1983.

Any hand surgeon who wishes to view the remarkable color photographs of Dr. Jean Pillet's aesthetic hand prostheses is encouraged to review this important article. Pillet elegantly demonstrated the superb technology available even 20 years ago for cosmetic replacement in upper extremity amputations.

363. Grunert BK, Devine CA, Matloub HS, et al: Flashbacks following traumatic hand injury: Prognostic indicators. J Hand Surg [Am] 13:125-127, 1988.

This group of investigators has raised our awareness of the various psychological symptoms that many patients experience after a hand injury. It is essential that any surgeon involved in the care of such patients understand that psychological evaluation, when indicated, and appropriate management are just as important as a well performed surgery. Failure to recognize the psychological impact can compromise the rehabilitation process of such patients.

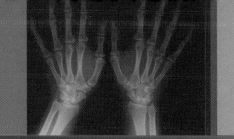

CHAPTER 56

Compartment Syndrome

Ayan Gulgonen

ompartment syndrome is used to describe the group of clinical signs and symptoms associated with elevated interstitial tissue pressure within a rigid, limited space called a compartment. In the previous editions of this textbook, "Fasciotomy: The Treatment of Compartment Syndrome"[145] and "Management of Established Volkmann's Contracture"[179] were discussed in different chapters. Although these two clinical entities are treated in different ways, both of them constitute a spectrum of disease that stems from pathologically elevated tissue pressure. Furthermore, the treatment strategy for this spectrum of disease is somewhat complex and the success of the initial treatment very much determines the long-term prognosis. Therefore, in this edition these two topics are combined and extended to cover the whole spectrum of the disease under a "unified concept."[111]

HISTORY AND DEFINITION

Clinical awareness of the sequela of the compartment syndromes dates to the end of the 19th century when Richard von Volkmann published a few case reports in 1869.[182] These initial reports consisted of a description of the deformities, which were subsequently known as Volkmann's ischemic contractures. He later reorganized his data and attempted to analyze the causative factors leading to the contractures. In his classic article published in 1881, he described the relation between the contracture and the ischemic conditions that resulted from trauma, fractures, bandaging, and edema.[183] Bernays (1900),[11] Edington (1903),[45] and Rowland (1905),[146] described the histologic characteristics of the disease and emphasized that increased interstitial fibrosis was present in the muscle in all stages of the disease. Hildebrand[74] was the first to note nerve contusion and scarring and defined this as a poor prognostic factor.

Until 1910, only the pathology and the clinical picture of contracture were clearly described. The authors in these early reports also proposed treatment alternatives. In 1906, Bardenheuer suggested that surgical decompression (fasciotomy) of the forearm fascia might be a method of treatment.[8] Early diagnosis and prevention of the disease was still not possible owing to the lack of understanding of the mechanisms leading to contracture. In 1910, Rowland pointed out that circumferential dressings caused congestion and edema.[147] Murphy (1914) agreed with this and proposed that "internal tension" played the leading role in the pathogenesis of the disease.[122] These two authors proposed the "internal pressure theory" as the etiology of contracture.

In the following years, vascular causes were scrutinized. In 1922, Brooks investigated the arterial and venous obstruction models on animals.[20] He concluded that only the venous occlusion model was reliably reproduced in animal models and produced a similar picture of Volkmann's ischemic contracture in animals. Later, Jepson (1926) agreed with Brooks and further defined fasciotomy in dogs to relieve the increased pressure and perhaps prevent sequela.[86] During World War II, Griffiths[67] and Foisie[50] put forward the "arterial theory" of Volkmann's ischemic contracture and tried to explain the occurrence of the disease based solely on arterial spasm.

Bywaters and Beall[28] described a deadly form of the disease, "crush syndrome," and reported massively swollen limbs, myonecrosis, renal failure, and often death in patients crushed during the aerial bombardment of London during World War II. Interestingly, they did not know at the time that this clinical entity was connected to compartment syndrome or, as it was known at the time, Volkmann's ischemic contracture.

Within the following decades, various operative techniques were described. Benjamin (1957)[10] recommended a transverse division of the fascia of the antecubital fossa followed by a longitudinal division of the deep forearm fascia. Seddon (1956) proposed the excision of the infarct.[168] Eaton and Green[42] described the surgical anatomy in more detail and proposed secondary wound closure with split-thickness skin grafts and relaxing incisions. Whitesides and coworkers included carpal tunnel release with the standard forearm fasciotomy.[188]

From the pathophysiologic standpoint, the relationship between the compartment syndrome, Volkmann's ischemic contracture, and crush syndrome was not firmly established until 1970s. It is now understood that in all these clinical entities the primary pathologic event is increased compartment pressure within a confined space, producing similar circulatory and functional loss wherever the process is located and whatever the initiating cause.[14,58,72,104,111,121,190] The duration and the severity of this pathologically increased pressure determine the progression of the disease to Volkmann's ischemic contracture or to crush syndrome. This "unified concept" is the synthesis of the accumulated experience of all the just-mentioned authors in this field (Fig. 56-1).

The terms *compartment syndrome, acute compartment syndrome,* and *compartmental syndrome* denote the same pathophysiology regardless of the cause. Subacute compartment syndrome has been defined in patients who do not develop typical signs and symptoms of the acute syndrome but rather progressive flexion contracture of the fingers and who later develop the typical chronic sequelae.[41,44] Recurrent and chronic compartment syndromes represent the painful clinical picture seen usually in the lower extremity that is induced by exercise.[3,38,99,136] This condition, however, does not show the typical severe signs of acute compartment syndrome and resolves with rest; the increased compartment pressure is transient but may also progress to acute compartment syndrome. A more descriptive term for this clinical entity may be *chronic exertional compartment syndrome.*[8,73] Finally, crush syndrome is an acute compartment syndrome associated with rhabdomyolysis, myoglobinemia, and acute renal failure.

ACUTE COMPARTMENT SYNDROME

Pathophysiology

There are various theories accounting for increased tissue pressure in compartment syndrome. Rowland described the arteriovenous (AV) gradient theory that has been supported by Matsen.[112] To this, the "ischemia-reperfusion" theory for cellular injury may be added. Whereas Matsen's AV gradient theory explains the physical injury in a more clinically relevant way, understanding the pathophysiology of the

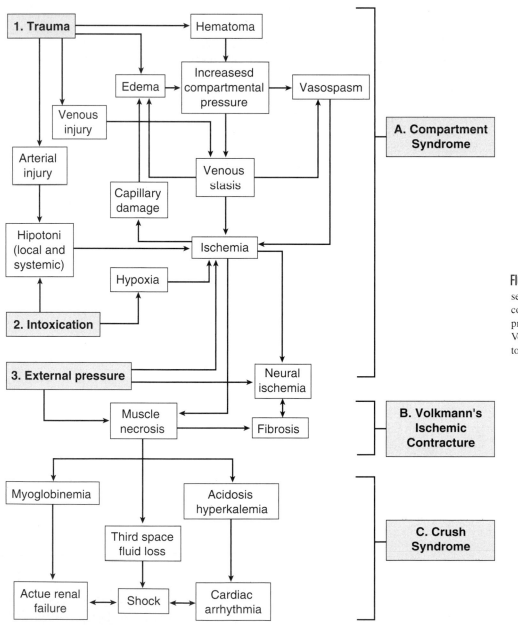

FIGURE 56-1. The duration and the severity of pathologically increased compartment pressure determine the progression of the disease to Volkmann's ischemic contracture or to crush syndrome.

ischemia-reperfusion injury may result in opportunities for better therapeutic interventions.

The relationship between local blood flow (LBF) and the AV gradient can be expressed by the following equation:

$$LBF = (Pa - Pv)/R$$

The local blood flow in a compartment equals the local arterial pressure (Pa) minus the local venous pressure (Pv) divided by the local vascular resistance. Matsen and Rorabeck[115] stated that if the AV gradient is significantly reduced, the role of local vascular resistance becomes relatively less and, for clarity, can be ignored. Because veins are collapsible, the pressure inside them cannot be less than the local tissue pressure; hence, when tissue pressure rises, the pressure on the local veins must also rise and the local AV gradient decreases.[112] When this occurs, local blood flow is reduced to the point where it no longer meets the metabolic needs of the muscles and nerves. The AV gradient theory clarifies why in the presence of increased tissue pressure or a reduction in local arterial pressure (such as that seen in hypotension, hemorrhage, peripheral vascular disease, arterial occlusion, and limb elevation above the heart) the circulatory effect of any given increase in tissue pressure is exaggerated by lowering the local AV gradient. With lowering of the local AV gradient, oxygen perfusion of the muscles and nerves decreases, function ceases, and muscle ischemia progresses to death of the muscle and its subsequent replacement by dense fibrous tissue, which in turn causes a "strangulation neuropathy."[26,132,167] While this theory allows us to understand the basic role of physics leading to reduced oxygen perfusion in a closed compartment, more complex events occur at the cellular level.

Regardless of the cause, ischemia results in the depletion of intracellular energy stores. Derangements in oxidative or glycolytic energy production and the resulting depletion of adenosine triphosphate cause profound disturbances in myocyte ion hemostasis with cytosolic Ca^{2+} overload. Once a critical level of free Ca^{2+} accumulates in the myocyte, neutral proteases, phospholipases, and other degenerative enzymes are activated, resulting in myofibril and membrane phospholipid damage, respectively. The net result of these events is myocyte lysis with release of toxic intracellular chemicals into the extracellular microenvironment. Local accumulation of these products may cause microvascular damage, producing capillary leak and rising intracompartmental pressure.[96,184] Neutrophil activation and adherence to the damaged vascular wall further increase the capillary leak and the compartment pressure.[9,32,171,172] Experimental trials have suggested that inactivation of white blood cells by antiadhesion antibodies[137] or after induction of leukopenia with chemotherapeutic agents[148] can alleviate the development of postischemic compartment syndrome. Also, interference with eicosanoid metabolism,[29] calcium influx,[128] platelet activation,[124] and nitric oxide synthesis[123] appear to diminish the effects of ischemia-reperfusion injury. Finally, it has been shown that pretreatment with mannitol, catalase, and other oxygen free-radical scavengers before the onset of reperfusion can diminish the ischemia-reperfusion injury.[9,170,184] These experimental observations have obvious implications relevant to the clinical setting.

Etiology

Injuries that are known to be associated with compartment syndrome have been listed by Matsen,[112] and Rowland has modified this list (Table 56-1).[145] Each injury has its own special ramifications for treatment, but one factor that they all share is a high incidence of compartment syndrome. When these injuries are encountered, the physician should be aware that the patient must be monitored closely for tissue ischemia.

Table 56-1
INJURIES KNOWN TO CAUSE COMPARTMENT SYNDROME

Decreased Compartment Volume
Tight casts, dressings, or air splints

Tourniquet

Lying on limb

Entrapment under collapsed weights

Closure of facial defects

Application of excessive traction to fractured limbs

Limb lengthenings

Thermal injuries, burn eschar

Increased Compartment Content
Bleeding

Major vascular injury
    Coagulation defect
    Bleeding disorder
    Traumatized vascular hamartoma
    Anticoagulant therapy
    Postoperative status
    Increased capillary permeability
    Reperfusion after ischemia
    Arterial bypass grafting
    Embolectomy
    Ergotamine ingestion
    Cardiac catheterization
    Trauma
    Fracture
    Contusion
    Wringer injuries
    Intensive use of muscles
    Exercise
    Seizures
    Eclampsia
    Tetany
    Thermal burns
    Electrical burns
    Intra-arterial drug injection
    Cold
    Orthopedic surgery
        Revascularizations and replantations
        Reduction and internal fixation of fractures
    Snakebite
    Increased capillary pressure
    Intensive use of muscles
    Venous obstruction
        Venous ligation
    Diminished serum osmolarity: nephrotic syndrome
    Infiltrated infusion

Continued

Table 56-1

INJURIES KNOWN TO CAUSE COMPARTMENT SYNDROME—cont'd

Increased Compartment Content—cont'd
 Pressure transfusion
 Metastasis to skeletal muscle
 Leaky dialysis cannula
 Muscle hypertrophy
 Infection
 Capillary leak syndrome
 Acute rhabdomyolysis
 Tendon avulsion
 High-pressure injections
 Duchenne's muscular dystrophy

Displaced supracondylar humerus fractures, most common in children between 3 and 13 years of age, are a classic cause of Volkmann ischemic contracture.[23] The anteriorly displaced humerus can damage the brachial artery, vein, and median nerve with its sharp edge, as well as causing these structures to get stuck between the bone and fascia. Furthermore, compartmental pressure can increase through bleeding, thus increasing edema, which impairs venous return and, hence, if not properly treated, leads to ischemia.[131] A direct injury to the main artery and/or vein at or above the elbow, if not immediately treated, can also result in ischemia in the forearm flexor compartment because of insufficient circulation and venous stasis.[180] In these cases the deep forearm compartment and proximal muscles are primarily affected (Fig. 56-2).[198]

The most common causes of Volkmann's contractures seen in developing countries are bandages or casts that are too tight or badly applied, not only for supracondylar fractures but also for forearm bone fractures, by unqualified practitioners (including some simple injuries that would have healed in time without treatment). In such cases, circulatory problems and necrosis are seen at the pressure area itself, leaving the proximal area of the forearm intact (Fig. 56-3).

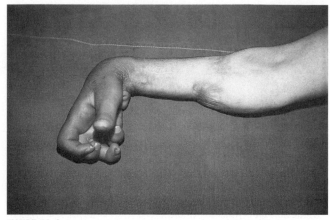

FIGURE 56-3. A Volkmann ischemic contracture deformity seen as a late case caused by tight casting of the distal forearm after fractures of the radius and ulna 2 years previously (Holden II, severe type).

In earthquakes causing mass casualties, prolonged direct pressure of collapsed buildings on crushed extremities can result in acute compartment syndrome cases (Fig. 56-4). The characteristic of earthquake injuries is that they affect large muscle groups, especially in the lower extremities. Hundreds of immediate fasciotomies need to be done (Fig. 56-5). There may be large numbers of very severe cases of muscle crush resulting in ischemic necroses, contractures, and amputations, as well as myoglobinemia and acute tubular necrosis leading to crush syndrome and death in cases where intensive care and dialysis services are not available. Following first aid, rapid transport to main hospitals with intensive care and dialysis services can be life saving. In the months after mass casualties, there will still be a need to treat the complications and resultant deformities in numerous patients.[68]

Individuals exposed to high doses of barbiturates, and others who are unconscious and in coma lose all protective reflexes and can rest on a hand or arm for long periods. Their extremities are exposed to continued pressure, which can cause acute compression neuropathies as well as interference with the circulation, thus increasing compartmental

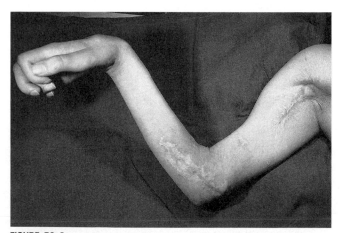

FIGURE 56-2. A case of Volkmann's ischemic contracture involving the whole upper extremity (Holden I, severe type) developed after 6 months as a sequela of brachial artery injury in the upper arm, which was originally treated within the first 10 hours after injury.

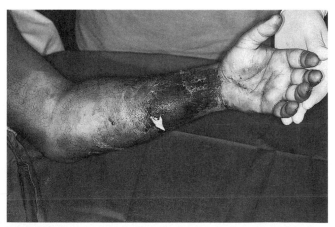

FIGURE 56-4. An earthquake victim whose forearm was exposed to prolonged direct pressure up to 10 hours under a collapsed wall, developed an acute compartment syndrome.

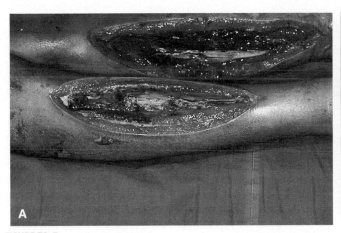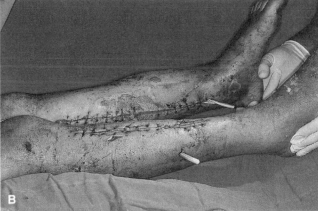

FIGURE 56-5. **A,** Fasciotomy incisions in a patient brought in the day after evacuation from a collapsed building. Fasciotomies were performed as emergency treatment for acutely developing compartment syndromes in the lower extremities. **B,** Secondary wound closure 36 hours after the immediate fasciotomies after débridement of necrotic muscle.

pressure and leading to muscle necrosis.[25] Hypovolemia resulting from intoxication increases the ischemic effect. The literature further indicates that causes such as intra-arterial barbiturate or intravenous hypertonic solution injections,[169] snake bites[100,145] (see later), hemophiliac bleeding,[108] and birth trauma[31,95] can cause increased intracompartmental pressure. Thermal and electrical burns combined with crush injury can cause compartment syndrome by producing intramuscular edema; moreover, burned skin loses elasticity and hinders tissue expansion, acting like a too-tight dressing.[110] The lower extremity muscle ischemia variously known as the tibialis anterior syndrome,[91] march gangrene,[12] or anterior crural ischemia results from overwork of the muscles[89] and is seldom encountered in the upper extremity.[87]

Diagnosis

The diagnosis of compartment syndrome is primarily a clinical one based on symptoms and signs of muscle and nerve ischemia.[120] The most important symptom is pain. Persistent, increasing pain (usually out of proportion to that expected from the existing injury), not decreased by immobilization, and increase in pain despite elevation of the limb are the most typical findings. Normally, elevation decreases edema and pain, owing to a decrease in local hydrostatic pressures; but in compartment syndromes (because intercompartmental pressure and stasis remain unaffected) the AV gradient decreases with elevation and the vicious cycle leading to ischemia continues—hence the pain.[105] In children, profound anxiety, in the presence of an increasing analgesic requirement, has been found to be a reliable indicator of a compartment syndrome.[103] Sensory problems, paresthesias, and paralysis are other important findings that indicate nerve ischemia. The nonmyelinated type C sensory fibers carrying fine touch and mediating symptoms such as paresthesias are the tissues most sensitive to hypoxia; sensory disturbances are usually the first clinical symptom of compartment syndromes. In addition, the passive muscle stretch test[145] and a sense of stony numbness during palpation of the proximal forearm are typical findings. However, distal circulation may be unhindered in spite of increased pressure in the deep forearm compartment, and the distal

radial artery may continue to pulsate. Because compartment syndrome occurs at tissue pressures (30 to 40 mm Hg) well below systolic arterial pressure (120 mm Hg in average), the distal pulses are rarely obliterated by compartmental swelling, yet there may not be adequate circulation in the muscles and nerves.[13,46,76,107] Due to patent return of flow in the superficial veins, the color of the fingers may be unaffected.[113,161] A palpable distal pulse and positive Doppler flowmeter measures of the blood flow do not rule out the possibility of an early acute compartmental syndrome. Arteriography is only of importance in evaluating whether an artery has been injured or blocked.

In cases of head injury with loss of consciousness or intoxication, the clinical signs are limited. Similarly, a patient with an associated brachial plexus injury may present with no distal pain. The fact that regional anesthesia of long duration (in replantation or flap operations) can also relieve pain and thus conceal a compartmental syndrome must also be taken into account.[119] Intracompartmental pressure monitoring is necessary whenever the diagnosis is in question.

Various methods of measuring compartment pressure exist. Whitesides and colleagues[187] described an infusion technique that measures the pressure necessary to overcome tissue pressure while injecting a minute quantity of saline into a closed compartment (Fig. 56-6). Other procedures include Matsen's continuous infusion and monitoring technique (Fig. 56-7),[114] the wick-catheter technique, which measures the free transmission of interstitial fluid pressure,[121] and Weiner's catheter technique with fiberoptic transducer tips.[186] There are also commercially available monitors in sterile disposable packets (e.g., the Stryker STIC device) specifically designed for tissue pressure measurements.[145] A simple setup for measuring compartment pressure involves the use of an arterial pressure monitoring device hooked up to a needle that is inserted in the compartment in question. Generally, fasciotomy is recommended in cases in which the compartmental pressure rises above 30 to 45 mm Hg and does not decrease.[179] However, subfascial pressure measurements reflect muscular circulation in an indirect way, paying no attention to simultaneous decreases in arterial pressure or the AV gradient, so

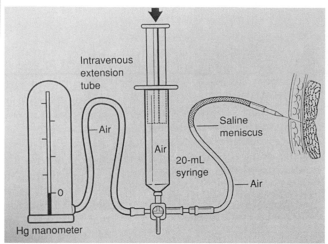

FIGURE 56-6. Whitesides' method of measuring tissue pressures. The three-way stopcock is open to the 20-mL syringe and to both extension tubes. The pressure within the closed compartment is overcome by injecting a minute quantity of saline. When the shape of the meniscus changes from a convex to a flat configuration, the pressure is read on the manometer. This is the compartment pressure. The meniscus must be level with the site of the needle tip to have an accurate reading. (From Whitesides TE, Heckman MM: Acute compartment syndrome: Update on diagnosis and treatment. J Am Acad Orthop Surg 4:209-218, 1996. Copyright 1996, American Academy of Orthopaedic Surgeons.)

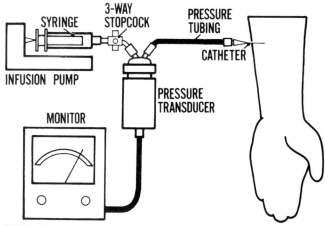

FIGURE 56-7. The advantage of Matsen's technique is that a muscle compartment can be monitored continuously for as long as 3 days.

their clinical value requires attention to technique and interpretation.[105] Radioisotope clearance using xenon-133 is valid as a direct method of muscle circulation measurement,[97] but there are practical difficulties in its clinical application. Steinberg and Gelberman have developed a device consisting of a low-friction piston probe and a flat-bed recorder to quantify the tissue hardness.[175] While the diagnosis of compartment syndrome remains primarily a clinical one, documentation of compartment pressures is advisable if the equipment is available.

The duration of compression is obviously an important factor in estimating the seriousness of a compartment syndrome. In clinical situations, it is difficult to know the time course of intramuscular pressure from the patient's

initial injury to the first measurement of intracompartmental pressure.[72] Therefore, the level of interstitial tissue pressure alone must not be taken as an absolute factor in determining the diagnosis of a compartment syndrome, but it must be integrated with all the other clinical data.[140]

Nerves are particularly sensitive to ischemia. Experimental studies show that at 30 mm Hg of diastolic blood pressure, disturbances of nerve conduction start to develop, whereas beyond 50 mm Hg nerve conduction stops completely.[72] After 8 hours of total ischemia, irreversible changes in the nerve can be expected.[189]

Direct nerve stimulation can be useful in differentiating nerve dysfunction secondary to compartment syndrome from a more proximal nerve, spinal cord, or head injury. Two 25-gauge needles are placed 1 cm apart near the motor nerve as it enters the muscle compartment in question. A battery-powered nerve stimulator is sufficient to evoke a muscle response if the muscle is viable.[145] Somatosensory evoked potential monitoring of nerve dysfunction with actual or impending compartmental hypertension has shown a high degree of accuracy in experiments.[139] Computed tomography and magnetic resonance imaging are of no value in diagnosing impending or acute compartment syndrome and are only of value for delineating the areas of edema and the degree of muscle death resulting from compartment syndrome.[102,103] Laboratory findings such as an increase in creatine phosphokinase levels or myoglobulin in blood and urine are of no practical value in an emergency situation.[104] In short, the clinical picture, with pain (increasing with elevation and positive stretch test) and stony numbness to palpation, paresthesia, and paralysis, ought to be given precedence; and when a patient is examined in the light of this possibility, there is little chance that a compartment syndrome will be missed (Table 56-2).[129] Medicolegally, however, the measurement of intracompartmental pressure with one of the just-described techniques should be advocated in clinical instances when the findings are equivocal.

When circulation in the muscles and nerves stops owing to increased compartmental pressure, an irreversible condition arises unless this pressure is relieved within 6 to 8 hours; the muscle fibers can be lost irreversibly if a delay ensues. This critical time period may be shorter if the injury has a crush component along with the ischemic injury. Therefore, only early diagnosis and treatment can prevent Volkmann's contractures. It can be seen that, however, the clinical findings can be masked, which may result in irreversible muscle ischemia and necrosis.[129]

Treatment

Acute Stage

Early treatment involves first the removal of external pressure if this exists. Any tight cast or bandage should be completely removed. If the fracture or dislocation has not been reduced accurately, as is often the case in supracondylar fractures, a further attempt at reduction is indicated.

The treatment of acute compartment syndrome is immediate fasciotomy.[43,164] Emergency fasciotomy and decompression can be done without a tourniquet to avoid making the ischemia worse and to permit intraoperative nerve conduction studies.[108] When dealing with mass casualties in

Table 56-2
DIFFERENTIAL DIAGNOSIS OF COMPARTMENT SYNDROME, ARTERIAL INJURY, AND NERVE INJURY

Sign or Symptom	Compartment Syndrome	Arterial Injury	Nerve Injury	Obtunded Patient
Pain with passive stretch	+	±	–	±
Paresthesia or anesthesia	+	+	+	?
Paresis, paralysis	+	+	+	?
Pulses	+	–	+	±
Palpation	+	±	–	+
Hand position	+	–	–	+
Increased pressure in compartment	+	–	–	+

Adapted from Mubarek SJ: Treatment of acute compartment syndromes. *In* Willy C, Sterk J, Gerngrob H, et al (eds): Das Kompartment-Syndrom. Berlin, Springer-Verlag, 1998, p 128.

overstrained facilities it is obvious that there is no need of tourniquets. However, for elective cases it is usually preferred to start the operation using an inflatable tourniquet and to observe the revascularization of the muscles and nerves in the reactive hyperemic period after its release.[68]

Instead of a straight longitudinal incision, it is preferable to enter the anterior forearm through a long sinuous skin incision (Fig. 56-8). This starts distally between the thenar and hypothenar mounds (Fig. 56-8A), releasing the carpal tunnel, and then continues parallel to the wrist crease (Fig. 56-8B) and along the ulnar border of the distal forearm (Fig. 56-8C) (avoiding the palmar cutaneous branch of the median nerve and, if necessary, providing an approach to Guyon's tunnel for release of the ulnar nerve). In the mid forearm it crosses over to the radial side (so as to be able to create a flap to expose and cover the median nerve) and then curves back toward the ulnar border as it approaches the flexor carpi ulnaris and the ulnar nerve at the elbow. The apex of the flap is just radial to the medial epicondyle on the ulnar side of the elbow flexion crease (Fig. 56-8D and E). This flap prevents linear contracture across the antecubital fossa and provides a cover for the brachial artery and median nerve when the wound is left open. During the procedure, damage to the cutaneous nerves is avoided and as many longitudinal veins as possible are retained. Through extensive fasciotomy incisions, decompression of the superficial and deep compartments is achieved. After compartment release, if the muscle bellies still appear pale, tense, and avascular, epimysiotomy of individual muscle bellies should be carried out.[41]

If there is a direct injury to a main artery and/or vein at or above the elbow, these interruptions of the main trunks

should be treated at the same stage with fasciotomy. The incision can be extended cephalad by following the course of the brachial artery (see Fig. 56-8E). If the radial pulse is not palpated, the anterior elbow region and lacertus fibrosus are systematically opened to expose the brachial artery and vein and to decompress them. Sometimes arterial blood flow recovers immediately; in other circumstances a thrombectomy or even a repair with a vein graft may be necessary. Arterial vascular exploration, as well as fasciotomy, is an important part of the emergency treatment in these cases.[140]

Secondary revascularization gains importance in cases that arrive in the early mid term, that is, in the first 6 to 12 hours after injury. In ischemic conditions due to arterial lesions or emboli, late fasciotomies combined with delayed revascularization may bring about limited regeneration in mildly ischemic regions.[41,57,145] During the same operation, early release of the median nerve can be done with resection of all irreversibly damaged necrotic tissues to diminish the risk of infection (Fig. 56-9).[68]

If there is no circulatory problem of the involved extremity, late fasciotomy will usually not help and, owing to the potential for problems with soft tissue coverage and secondary infection, is contraindicated.[49,189] Prophylactic fasciotomies, however, are almost always required after any repair of a ruptured axillary or brachial artery and in replantations and transplantations, even if there are no signs of an obvious compartment syndrome.[7,33,166] Prophylactic fasciotomies of all compartments involved are the most reliable interventions to prevent the development of compartment syndrome in these cases (Fig. 56-10).[75]

If the injury causing compartment syndrome is proximal to the forearm compartments (e.g., injuries of the main

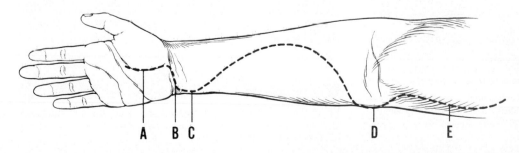

FIGURE 56-8. The author's preferred skin incision for performing a volar forearm fasciotomy (see the text for reference points A to E).

A   B   C   D   E

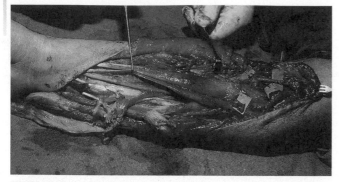

FIGURE 56-9. Repair of the brachial artery at the elbow 12 hours after injury. Below the arterial repair, the separated ends of the ulnar nerve are seen that will be repaired at this stage. The already necrotic parts of the muscles are to be excised meticulously.

vessels, upper arm total or subtotal amputations, a comatose patient sleeping on the arm, or supracondylar fractures of humerus), the deep flexor compartment that contains the flexor digitorum profundus, flexor pollicis longus, and pronator quadratus, as well as the palmar interossei, is mostly affected. If the etiology is a direct trauma (such as in too-tight casts or crush injury to the forearm), necrosis of the muscles nearer to the surface can also arise together with

soft tissue damage, as well as increased pressure in the deep flexor and extensor compartments. In severe cases, the extent and severity of the ischemia expand, even requiring the release of the extensor and intrinsic compartments (Fig. 56-11).

When there is increased pressure and edema in the intrinsic compartments of the hand, incisions are made in the dorsal, thenar, and hypothenar regions for emergency fasciotomy procedures (Fig. 56-12A). Each compartment consisting of a palmar aponeurosis and vertical septa is decompressed individually with incisions from dorsal or palmar regions.[87] Decompression of the finger can be carried out with midaxial lateral incisions along the most dorsal portion of the joint flexor creases (see Fig. 56-12B).[145]

Acute fasciotomies performed promptly and correctly help muscles to regain their normal color and enable them to respond to direct stimulation. If the fasciotomies are done during the first 3 to 4 hours, healing is ensured with no lasting morbidity. After 4 to 5 hours, if irreversible necrosis is already present in the compartment, this localized area can clearly be identified during fasciotomy by its dirty pale color as soon as the circulation and color have returned to normal in other areas after release of the tourniquet (Fig. 56-13). At this early operation, in addition to fasciotomy, meticulously performed resection of any necrotic region is necessary to prevent otherwise inevitable late contracture. Pale color, no return of circulation in the reactive hyperemic phase, and no response to stimulation are pathognomonic for irreversible damage of the muscles.[68]

There are also cases in which there are direct injuries to nerves in addition to compartment syndrome. The median or ulnar nerve can be crushed between displaced segments of a supracondylar fracture or any displaced fragment can press on a nerve (Figs. 56-14 and 56-15). A direct crush can also cause nerve ruptures. In any acute compartment syndrome due to trauma, after relieving the pressure of the compartment, one must look for a direct injury to vessels and nerves inside and/or outside of the compartment; if these exist, repair should be done at this first operation (see Fig. 56-9).

Immediate or early closure of the skin to protect the open tissues from dryness, infection, and necrosis is important. This is best done by leaving the fascia open and apposing

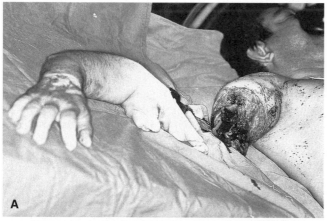

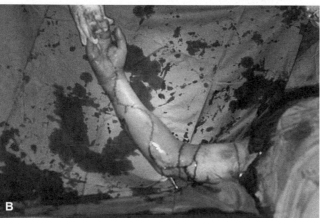

FIGURE 56-10. **A** and **B,** An upper arm amputation below the shoulder was done within 3 hours after the accident. Together with replantation, prophylactic fasciotomies of all forearm compartments were performed with primary skin closure.

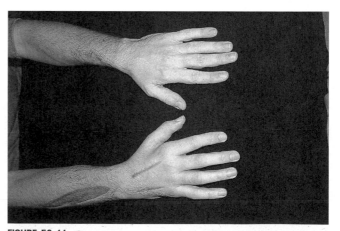

FIGURE 56-11. The left arm of a patient seen 6 months after emergency fasciotomies of the extensor and intrinsic compartments. Moderate atrophy of the intrinsic muscles still exists.

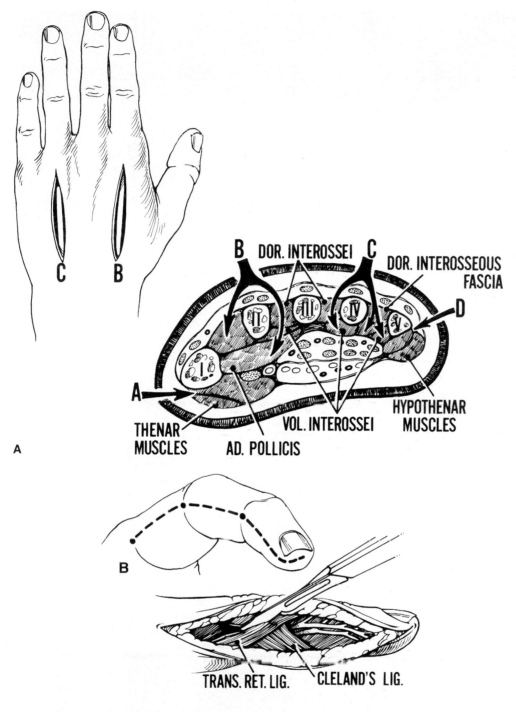

A

B

FIGURE 56-12. A, Both dorsal and volar interosseous compartments and the adductor compartment to the thumb can be released through two longitudinal incisions over the second and third metacarpals (B and C). The thenar and hypothenar compartments are opened through separate incisions (A and D). **B,** Correct placement of a midaxial incision in the finger. A flexion contracture of the finger may occur if the incision is placed too far volarward.

the skin with loose stitches. After prophylactic fasciotomies, or in mild cases, this is usually possible (see Fig. 56-5). If the edematous muscles herniate through the incision and the skin margins stay wide open, split-thickness skin grafts are the simplest and most commonly used method for at least temporary wound coverage.[18] This can be done at the same stage after emergency fasciotomy (Fig. 56-16). Because immediate closure of soft tissues after fasciotomies in mass casualty situations is not always possible (and usually not advisable), secondary closures are performed after 72 hours (at the latest within 3 to 5 days). In severe cases, when there are tissue defects with large necrotic areas of muscle and superficial infection develops, early secondary application

of myocutaneous free flaps with their rich vascularity can salvage an extremity (Fig. 56-17).[33] In our experience, failure to perform early or secondary closure of fasciotomies in the wake of the earthquakes resulted in numerous complications such as infection, necrosis, and, thus, amputation.[68]

Hyperbaric oxygen may be useful in helping the revitalization of the involved muscles, but only in borderline cases and only after fasciotomies have been performed. Sympathetic blocks appear to be ineffective because maximal local vasodilation is already present.[41,43] Medical treatment is mainly adjuvant with antispasmodics, vasodilators, corticosteroids, and antibiotics.[108] However within recent years, oxygen-radical scavengers and mannitol have gained

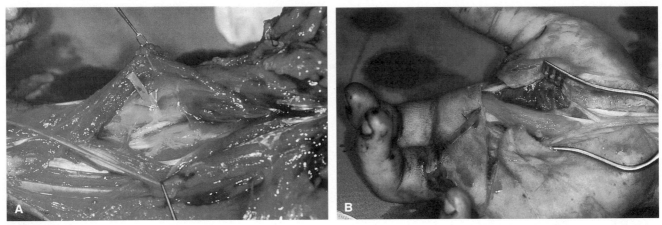

FIGURE 56-13. A, Dirty pale color of part of the deep flexor and pronator muscles around the median nerve immediately after the release of tourniquet in reactive hyperemic phase indicates irreversible necrosis. **B,** Lumbrical of the index finger with its pale color and insensitivity to stimulation is an indication that it will become necrotic and fibrotic and therefore is to be resected at this stage.

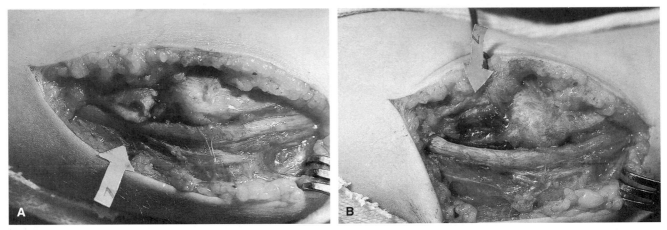

FIGURE 56-14. A, Ulnarly displaced proximal segment of humerus compressing the ulnar nerve before it enters the cubital tunnel after a supracondylar fracture. **B,** Release of the nerve after resection of the compressing bone.

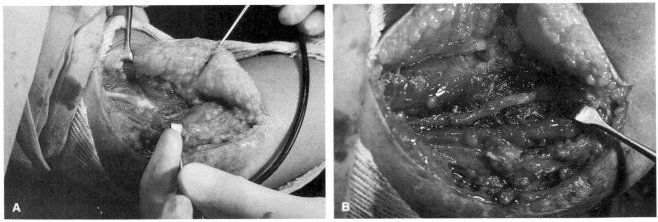

FIGURE 56-15. A, Median nerve found embedded between the slightly anteriorly displaced humerus and the distal fragment 6 weeks after a supracondylar fracture in a child who had "prolonged pain syndrome" in addition to a mild ischemic contracture. **B,** Decompression and external neurolysis of the median nerve out of the entrapment of fresh callus.

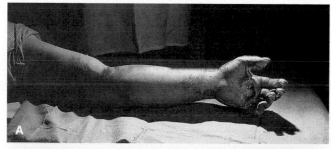

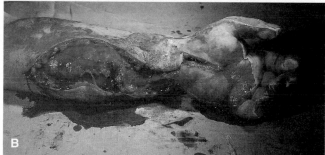

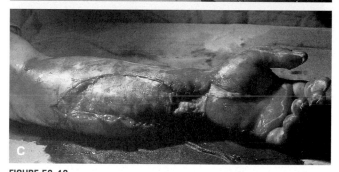

FIGURE 56-16. **A,** Compartment syndrome developing after a crush of the forearm under a hot press. **B,** Immediate fasciotomies with herniation of edematous muscles. **C,** Same-stage soft tissue coverage with split-thickness skin graft, leaving the fasciotomies open.

interest as complementary agents to reduce the swelling and edema, and hence the compartment pressure, in compartment syndromes.[139,170] This effect is attributable to mannitol's oxygen-radical scavenger effect (reducing ischemia-reperfusion injury) and its hyperosmolar capabilities (reducing tissue edema).[127] After fasciotomy, proper splint-ing with elevation of the extremity above the heart is recommended to promote venous drainage and reduce swelling.

Secondary Stage

Within a matter of days, and often despite emergency treatment (fasciotomies are seldom performed within the first 4 hours), Volkmann's contracture becomes established.

The major limiting factor in treatment at this early secondary stage is the condition of the skin. Edema with purulent blisters, loss of epidermis, and contused areas imply that any surgical procedure would lead to secondary infection.[66] Improvement in the condition of the skin and soft tissues may take 4 to 6 weeks. The extent and location of muscle necrosis and subsequent fibrosis and nerve involvement vary according to the type and site of the compression.

In general, in local crush injuries that are limited to a specific region, only the muscles in the affected region become ischemic and necrotic, and the more proximal muscle mass remains intact. Even in very severe compression with loss of all directly affected flexor and extensor muscles, as well as the distal intrinsics, this viable proximal muscle can be available for secondary reconstruction. In contrast, if the injury to the vessels and stasis in the veins is located proximal to the fascial compartment, the proximal muscle portions turn ischemic whereas the distal portions may remain intact because of circulation through surface collateral veins. However, in very severe cases, almost all the flexor mass as well as the extensor and/or intrinsic muscles are fibrotic. These are the cases that will usually require functional free muscle transfers.

During the interval before surgery, physical therapy with active-passive stretching, careful electrical stimulation, and dynamic splinting are continued. Because limitation of muscle excursion by fibrosis gradually leads to loss of joint motion and subsequent joint, ligament, and capsule contracture, this early conservative therapy is a very important part of the overall treatment. It is preferable to start reconstructive efforts 3 to 4 months after the acute injury, when soft tissue coverage is optimal and scar tissue formation in the muscle is complete but the yellow, friable tissue can still easily be scooped up with scalpel and curet (Fig. 56-18).

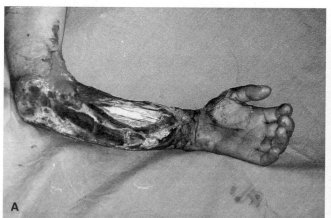

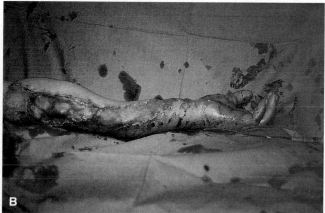

FIGURE 56-17. **A,** Severe necrosis of the soft tissues and muscles from a crushing injury. **B,** Extremity salvaged with free vascularized myocutaneous latissimus dorsi transfer combined with skin grafts.

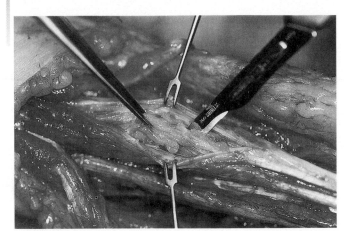

FIGURE 56-18. Resection of the yellow friable necrotic tissue after epimysiotomies of the individual muscle fascia.

This timing is early enough to save nerves before irreversible entrapment takes place and late enough for the maturation of muscle fibrosis before it gets stony hard. However, in patients with severe neuralgia (the "prolonged pain syndrome"),[79] as well as in cases with soft tissue coverage problems (see Fig. 56-17), earlier operative

intervention with neurolysis, necrotic tissue excision, and reconstruction of soft tissue coverage may be necessary.

THE ESTABLISHED CONTRACTURE

Classification

A number of classifications are reported for different kinds of ischemic contractures.[77,79,167,178,197] In most of the classifications, a high percentage of patients who had to be classified in the same group may clinically show a great variety in the manifestation of contracture. Holden's classification,[77] which divides cases into two main types based on the etiology (as contractures distal to or at the site of the injury), can be combined with a modified Tsuge's classification[178] for each group separately as either mild, moderate, or severe (Fig. 56-19). This will provide a more or less systematic approach to treatment that can be adapted to each case according to (1) the severity of the contracture of the joints and of the muscles, (2) the degree of nerve and vessel damage, (3) the condition of soft tissue coverage, (4) the function of the remaining muscles and nerves, and (5) the availability of other functioning muscles for reconstruction.

In Holden I types the injury to the vessels and stasis in the veins are located proximal to the fascial compartment.

In Holden I, mild type, the degeneration of the muscles is located in the deep flexor compartment, mainly as limited

CRITICAL POINTS: COMPARTMENT SYNDROME

ETIOLOGY

- Vascular injury
  - Supracondylar fracture
  - Vascular trauma
  - Amputation
- Crush injury
- External compression

DIAGNOSIS

- Clinical
  - Pain, paresthesias in distal hand
  - Hard, stony feel to forearm
- Objective
  - Compartment pressure measurement
  - Pressure should be less than 30 to 40 mm Hg

MANAGEMENT

- Fasciotomy
- Release all involved compartments
- Management of vascular/nerve injury
- Secondary closure versus split-thickness skin grafting

PITFALLS

- Failure to diagnose
- Failure to adequately release compartments

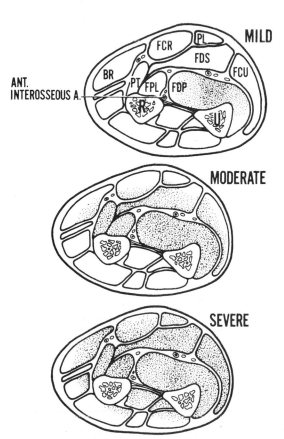

FIGURE 56-19. The extent of muscle involvement in Tsuge's classification of Volkmann's ischemic contracture, which details Holden II type contractures.

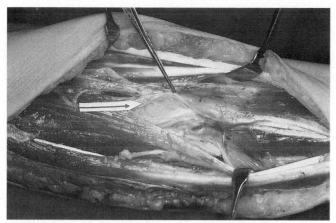

FIGURE 56-20. Limited infarction of the muscle bellies of some of the deep flexors in a Holden I, mild type of established contracture.

infarction of the profundus muscles (Fig. 56-20). The clinical picture is characterized by flexion contracture of long and ring fingers and occasionally of the little and index fingers. The flexor pollicis longus and pronator teres may also be partially affected, with contracture of the thumb and some supination restriction of the forearm. The superficial flexors are not involved. There are usually light sensory disturbances in the area of median nerve sensibility. A cordlike induration is palpable on the flexor side of the forearm. A tenodesis effect can be demonstrated (i.e., the contracted finger can be extended by flexing the wrist). There is no paralysis of the extrinsic or intrinsic muscles and no fixed joint contractures.

In Holden I, moderate type, also known as the "classic or typical type," the moderate muscular degeneration is in the deep flexor compartment, affecting the flexor digitorum profundus, flexor pollicis longus, and pronator teres, but there may also be partial involvement of the wrist flexors and the flexor digitorum superficialis (Fig. 56-21).

The wrist is held in a flexed position, and the fingers show an "intrinsic-minus" deformity. There are sensory disturbances in the area of the median and sometimes the ulnar nerves. There are also borderline cases with rather diffuse degeneration in the flexor compartments and severe nerve involvement overlapping to the "severe type."

Holden I, severe type results in muscular degeneration of all flexors and pronators and partial or total involvement of the extensors, and occasionally the intrinsics, with severe degrees of contracture (see Fig. 56-2). The median nerve is always involved, with the ulnar nerve usually severely involved as well. Soft tissue coverage may be tight but stays more or less intact since there was no direct trauma. The forearm muscle mass has a firm "woody" consistency.

The deformation of the hand and fingers is usually in an intrinsic-minus position, characterized by hyperextension at the metacarpophalangeal (MCP) joints and flexion at the interphalangeal (IP) joints. Although extrinsic and intrinsic contractures are associated and may occur simultaneously, the resultant concomitant clawhand is produced by contracture of the more powerful extrinsic finger flexors and extensors.[14] If this severe type is the result of a maltreated supracondylar humeral fracture in childhood, there is a remarkable length discrepancy between the forearms. Long-standing cases with secondary fixed joint contractures and failed reconstructive efforts, considered primarily moderate in type, can also be included in this category.

Holden II type is caused by direct trauma (e.g., externally applied localized pressure, tight dressings, entrapment under heavy objects, local crush injuries, forearm fractures, or thermal injuries) with ischemia developing at the site of the injury. These cases can also be classified in three types as either mild, moderate, or severe.

In Holden II, mild type, the muscle injury is in the limited area of direct trauma, with the muscles being partially fibrotic, and the extent of necrosis is usually unrelated to the anatomic limitations of the forearm compartments (Fig. 56-22). Other soft tissues and nerves may also be directly traumatized but without interruption or entrapment of the nerves. The proximal portion of the forearm is protected and is thus clinically normal. Depending on the site and expansion of the localized contracture, the fingers may be in an intrinsic-minus position, usually with a tenodesis effect without fixed contractures.

In Holden II, moderate type, the soft tissues at the site of injury are usually scarred or contracted. In this area of localized trauma, all the superficial and deep flexors from the surface inward are involved (in circumferential injuries the extensors may be involved as well), with potential involvement of both the median and ulnar nerve. These localized nerve lesions, whether due to entrapment in the scarred muscles or direct injury, can cause neuralgias, paresthesias, and sometimes dystrophic changes at the fingertips (Fig. 56-23). Paralysis of distal muscle may be present as well, clinically presenting as an intrinsic-minus deformity. Again the proximal part of the forearm remains intact.

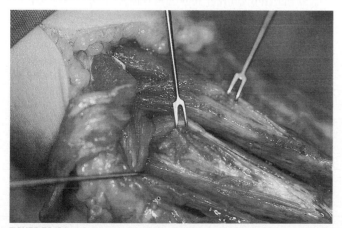

FIGURE 56-21. Diffuse partial infarct of the muscle bellies of the proximal flexor muscles.

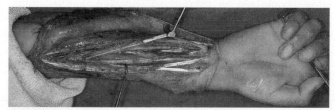

FIGURE 56-22. Ischemic necrosis of the distal bellies of superficial flexors in a Holden II, mild type after tight casting.

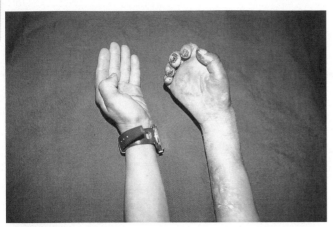

FIGURE 56-23. Trophic changes in the fingertips of an ischemic contracture case with severe nerve involvement. Pressure areas of tight casting can be seen in the forearm. Typical intrinsic-minus posture developed at 3 months owing to muscle and nerve fibrosis.

Holden II, severe types are usually neglected or improperly treated cases beginning in childhood but may also follow severe localized crush injury or entrapment under collapsed weights in mass casualties. From the site of injury to distally, the whole extremity is usually atrophic and severely contracted with neural involvement (see Fig. 56-3). The fingers show a fixed intrinsic-minus deformity. In more distal injuries with overwhelming intrinsic contracture, an intrinsic-plus deformity may develop with adduction of the thumb and MCP flexion and IP extension contractures of the fingers. In injuries occurring in childhood, there are differences in forearm length.

Operative Treatment

The usual operative treatment, preferably starting 3 months after the acute injury, is performed through the same incisions described for emergency fasciotomies (see Fig. 56-8).

Holden I, Mild Type

Tenolysis and tendon lengthening with "Z"-plasties, after having removed the concomitant areas of the deep flexors, will usually be sufficient to bring the fingers and the wrist into a neutral position, correcting the tenodesis effect.

The wrist flexors and flexor pollicis longus can also be lengthened if necessary. A disadvantage of this technique is the additional weakening produced in the already impaired muscles; therefore, this technique is performed as the sole procedure only in mild or limited cases with healthy superficial flexors; otherwise it is combined with tendon transfers. In any ischemic contracture, exploration of the median nerve should not be overlooked. Because muscle-sliding procedures do not enable release of one muscle more than the other, these are usually not performed in mild cases.

Holden I, Moderate ("Classic") Type

Different methods of treatment are described for this type of contracture. In cases in which the extent of muscle degeneration is moderate, leaving enough intact contractile elements for active flexion even in the deep flexor compartment, a muscle slide technique is performed with release

applied as a whole, as was described by Page in 1923[130] and Scaglietti (who added neurolysis as a systematic step) in 1936.[163] This method is still in use today,[105] and Tsuge has described the operation in detail.[179]

Muscle Slide Technique

The tourniquet is applied as high on the arm as possible. The classic fasciotomy incision is made. The subcutaneous tissue is separated to the ulnar and radial sides along the incision, and the skin flaps are retracted. The subcutaneous veins are spared whenever possible, and only when unavoidable are they ligated and divided. Effort is made to protect the medial cutaneous nerves of the forearm by gently retracting them to the side.

The fascia is excised, beginning in the antecubital fossa. After confirming the muscle origins of the medial epicondyle, the ulnar nerve, median nerve, and brachial artery and vein are identified. The ulnar nerve is first dissected along the supracondylar ridge, dissecting distally behind the medial epicondyle to the tendinous arch between the humeral and ulnar heads of the flexor carpi ulnaris. When releasing the nerve, care is given to minimize damage to the concomitant vessels; the nerve is gently retracted with a Penrose drain to prevent secondary injury. After identifying the median nerve proximal to the elbow, the nerve is traced distally to the proximal border of the pronator teres, which is freed from surrounding tissue. At this point, part of the aponeurosis is separated from the biceps. Next, a periosteal elevator is inserted between the brachialis and the common flexor-pronator origin from the medial epicondyle. The elevator's end is brought out between the humeral and ulnar heads of the flexor carpi ulnaris on the anterior side of the joint. When inserting the elevator, attention is paid to avoid injury to the ulnar nerve (Fig. 56-24).

The origin of the flexors is dissected, detaching the muscle subperiosteally using a scalpel. The origins of the pronator teres, flexor carpi radialis, and palmaris longus are also released. The deeper muscles are next released: the humeral head of the flexor carpi ulnaris and the origins of the flexor digitorum superficialis.

Next, the ulnar head of the flexor carpi ulnaris is detached subperiosteally by inserting a periosteal elevator along the posterior border of the ulna, where the bone can be directly palpated subcutaneously. The extent of detachment needed depends on the degree of flexion contracture. It is generally necessary to release the entire proximal portion of the muscle from the central part of the ulna, occasionally extending the release to the middle and distal third. Particular care is taken not to harm the ulnar nerve when carrying out release procedures of the humeral origin on the medial side of the olecranon (see Fig. 56-24).

The flexors are detached from the ulna medially and anteriorly beginning with the flexor carpi ulnaris and all attachments of the flexor digitorum profundus down to the interosseous crista (the bony ridge from which the interosseous membrane arises). Dissection of the periosteum is carried to the interosseous membrane and then continued along the radial side. At the same time, detachment is carried out on the proximal side from the ulnar tuberosity until the oblique cord is exposed. Finally, by bringing together the detached muscles from the proximal and ulnar sides at the interosseous space on the proximal

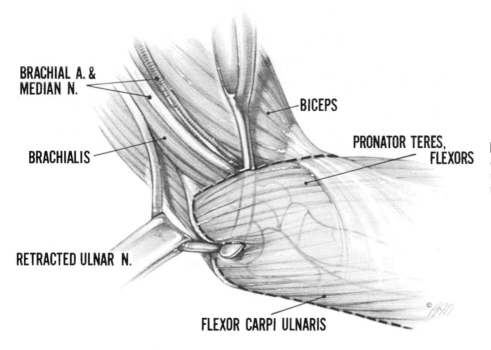

BRACHIAL A. & MEDIAN N.

BICEPS

BRACHIALIS

PRONATOR TERES, FLEXORS

RETRACTED ULNAR N.

FLEXOR CARPI ULNARIS

FIGURE 56-24. The muscle-sliding operation of the flexor muscles. Both the median and ulnar nerves are identified and protected (see text).

side, the contracture should be nearly completely released. It is essential that the detachment of the muscle-tendon unit be conducted close to the bone (Fig. 56-25).

It is helpful to occasionally flex and extend the fingers during the detachment procedure to determine the site causing contracture and whether the amount of release is sufficient. When the muscle has been detached at the interosseous space on the proximal side, the fibrous band will rupture with a crackling sound when the fingers are extended, and the state of improvement in finger extension can be readily appreciated. Detachment of the muscle at the interosseous space is performed with great care so that the common interosseous artery and vein that pass through this space are not injured. Care is also taken to avoid injuring the

interosseous artery, vein, and nerves when detaching the flexors from the interosseous membrane.

In moderate types, it may be necessary to detach the flexor pollicis longus from the radius as well. It is advisable to use magnification when performing detachment of such fine structures. The extent of the dissection is shown in Figure 56-26. By pulling the brachioradialis toward the radial side, the radius, to which the pronator teres is attached, is exposed. The insertion of the pronator teres is dissected and separated from the radius. Care is taken so as not to injure the sensory branch of the radial nerve when exposing the flexor pollicis longus muscle belly on the deep side of the pronator teres. The flexor pollicis longus muscle is then detached subperiosteally from the radius. This is

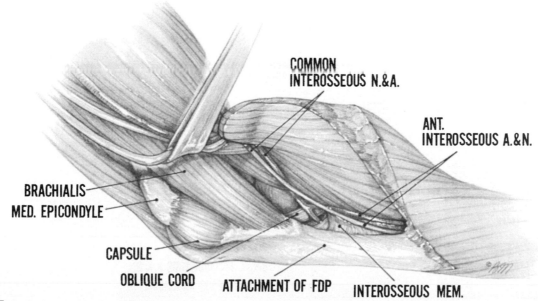

COMMON INTEROSSEOUS N. & A.

ANT. INTEROSSEOUS A. & N.

BRACHIALIS
MED. EPICONDYLE

CAPSULE

OBLIQUE CORD   ATTACHMENT OF FDP   INTEROSSEOUS MEM.

FIGURE 56-25. Muscle slide operation. The extent of detachment depends on the degree of flexion contracture, but generally it is necessary to release the entire proximal portion from the ulna, occasionally extending this into the middle and distal thirds.

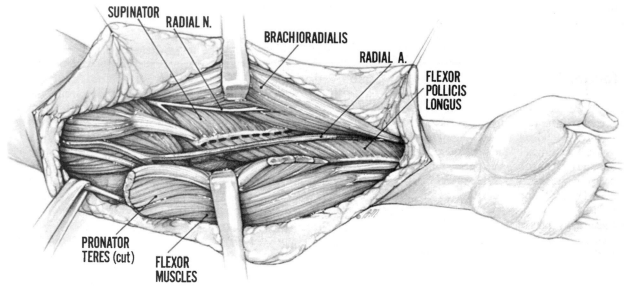

FIGURE 56-26. For the moderate type of contracture, it is necessary to also detach the radial flexor muscles from the radius (see text).

accomplished by using a periosteal elevator beginning distally and working proximally, proceeding along the border of the supinator to the proximal interosseous space. Attention is paid to avoid injury to the vessels that run through this space. When the detachment along the radial side and that on the ulnar side come together, the entire flexor mass can be shifted distally the distance deemed necessary. It is possible to shift the flexors 3 to 4 cm in this case (Fig. 56-27). The procedure is concluded by releasing the nerves that pass through the indurated muscles. When the degree of muscle fibrosis is severe, a greater degree of release and thus of distal muscle slide is required to correct the contracture. However, because muscle power is reduced proportionately in relation to the amount of the slide, it is probably better to close the wound leaving some degree of contracture. Proper aftercare includes the postoperative use of dynamic splinting.

Proper application of these procedures should bring about satisfactory results. The surgeon need not be too con-

cerned about recurrence of contracture so long as enough contractile element for active flexion remains in the deep compartment and technically adequate and atraumatic muscle detachment is accomplished. However, in borderline cases with rather diffuse degeneration in the deep flexor compartment, a "slide" releases mostly noncontractile, fibrous and fatty tissue rather than functional muscles; therefore, tendon transpositions are preferred.

If the superficial flexors remain intact despite complete scarring of the flexor pollicis longus and flexor digitorum profundus, they can be transposed to the distal tendons of these deeper muscles. The wrist flexors, which usually remain partially intact, can also be transposed to the finger flexors. Transposition of the extensor muscles becomes an option when there is insufficient muscle tissue in the flexor compartment. According to the individual situation, a wrist extensor can be used for finger flexion and the extensor indicis proprius, extensor digiti minimi, or brachioradialis for the flexor pollicis longus (Fig. 56-28). The hand is

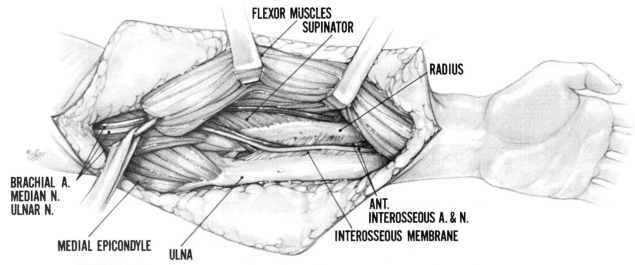

FIGURE 56-27. All of the flexor muscles have been detached, and the muscle slide operation has been completed.

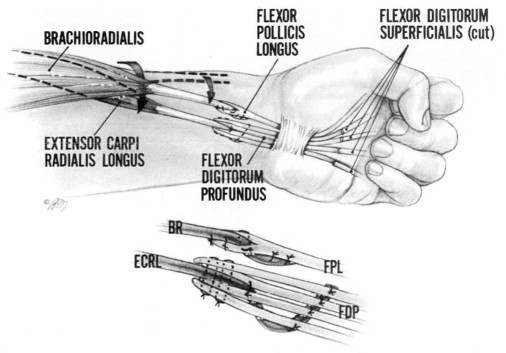

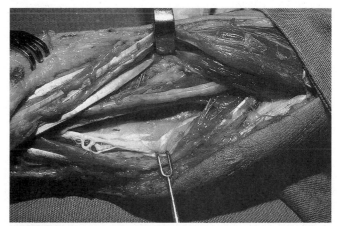

FIGURE 56-28. The author's preferred transfers are brachioradialis to flexor pollicis longus and extensor carpi radialis to flexor digitorum profundus. Details of the tendon junctures are shown.

immobilized for 3 weeks in a palmar plaster splint with the wrist in 10 degrees of extension and the fingers in flexion. Voluntary movement and physical therapy are begun when the cast is removed, and dynamic splinting is started 5 or 6 weeks after surgery. Tendon transpositions are usually performed at the same operation as excision of the necrotic muscle, extensive pronator slide, and neurolysis of the nerves. In most of the typical cases of Volkmann's contracture, satisfactory functional results can be expected.

If the initial fasciotomy incisions were carried out ignoring described hand surgery principles, these initial incisions can still be used for secondary intervention, but the contracted scars are corrected on closure with "Z"-plasties or tissue transfers as necessary.

In the treatment of all ischemic contractures, exploration and neurolysis of the involved nerves with excision of the entire mass of scarred tissue are as important as tendon operations.[66] In any Volkmann's contracture case, the nerves are almost always affected to some extent. Besides muscle ischemia, the median nerve itself is usually damaged if embedded in the ischemic zone (Fig. 56-29). External neurolysis of both the median and ulnar nerves must be performed throughout the forearm, and epineurectomy and interfascicular nerve dissection under the microscope may also be necessary.

In Holden I, moderate or severe types, the necrotic and scarred areas in the nerves are usually seen in areas of classic nerve compression.[126] For the median nerve these are under the arch of the flexor digitorum superficialis, between the two heads of the pronator teres, between the superficial and deep flexors, and in the carpal tunnel. The ulnar nerve may be affected between the two heads of the flexor carpi ulnaris muscle, but is sometimes spared. The radial nerve is rarely affected. In established contractures, while performing total excision of scar tissue and neurolysis, the

FIGURE 56-29. Release of the median nerve that was embedded in ischemic muscles of the deep flexors.

usually thickened epineurium is resected (Fig. 56-30) and interfascicular neurolysis is added when needed. After release of the tourniquet, return of circulation in individual nerve fascicles is checked under the microscope. If return of circulation is established after tourniquet release, which is usual in moderate types, the nerve procedure is considered sufficient (Fig. 56-31). The operation can then continue with other procedures such as muscle slides, tendon transpositions, or tendon lengthenings. The patient is kept under clinical and electrodiagnostic observation throughout functional recovery.

Holden I, Severe Type
Besides muscular degeneration of all deep flexors and pronators, there is partial or total involvement of the superficial flexors, extensors, and occasionally the intrinsics with severe degrees of nerve ischemia. If the circulation in the

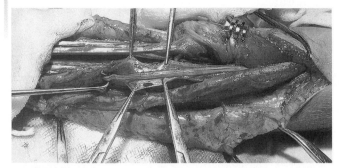

FIGURE 56-30. Epineurectomy of the thickened epineurium with internal neurolysis of the median nerve.

nerve does not return after external and internal neurolysis and there is visible scarring (Fig. 56-32A), the individual nerve fascicle groups should be examined under high magnification and the scarred parts of the nerve should be resected proximally and distally until normal nerve tissue is seen. The defects created are then spanned by nerve grafts (see Fig. 56-32B).

In contractures with a total sensory deficit and severe functional loss, a section of the median nerve, mostly between the two fibrotic heads of the pronator teres, may also be completely fibrotic (Fig. 56-33) or the caliber of the nerve is reduced to less than one half of normal. In these cases long nerve grafts are needed to restore at least protective sensation to the hand and fingers (Fig. 56-34).

If there is not enough healthy muscle for tendon transfer, especially in cases where there is extensive scarring of all the flexor and extensor muscles below the elbow, functioning muscle transfers are indicated.[80,109] These have provided new opportunities for treatment in severe cases of Volkmann's contracture.[33,47] Usually, the latissimus dorsi and gracilis muscles are used.[48,98] Because the extra skin is usually not needed in Holden I, severe types, the gracilis muscle—whose skin island is not reliable in the distal third—is usually preferred, because of less donor site morbidity and the reliability of the major neurovascular pedicle (see Chapter 49). In cases where soft tissue reconstruction is also needed, the voluminous latissimus dorsi muscle with its larger and dependable skin island is usually preferred (see Fig. 56-17).[47]

The arterial pedicle is anastomosed to branches of the radial, ulnar, or anterior interosseous arteries. Lengthening the vascular pedicle with a vein graft and directly anastomosing it to the brachial artery, so as to perfuse it at high

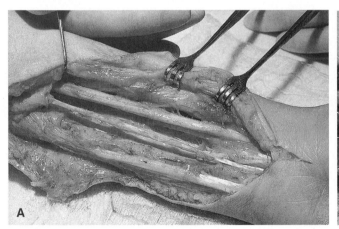
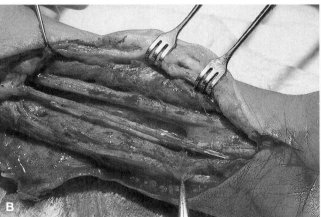

FIGURE 56-31. **A,** The external neurolysis of the median nerve after resection of the ischemic muscles. The tourniquet is still up. **B,** Return of circulation immediately after tourniquet release. Petechial bleedings and homogeneous circulation along the epineurium can be seen; there the procedure is sufficient.

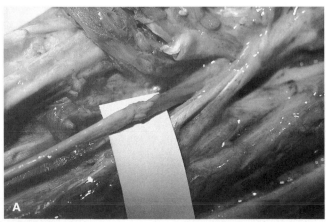
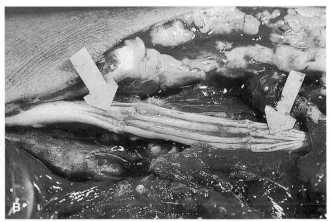

FIGURE 56-32. **A,** Median nerve prepared under the fibrotic pronator teres turns out to be fibrotic. Starting point of fibrosis in individual fascicule groups can clearly be differentiated under the operating microscope. **B,** After resection of fibrotic fascicules, each fascicle group is replaced with separate sural nerve grafts enabling topographic adaptation at both healthy ends with 10-0 sutures.

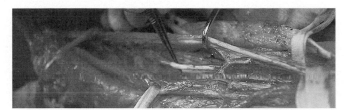

FIGURE 56-33. Complete fibrosis of a 5-cm long portion of the median nerve is seen after excision of fibrotic muscles in mid forearm.

pressure, has proved to be a safe approach.[48] Previous preparation of the vessels is important to limit the ischemic period of the transferred muscle. Marking sutures are placed in the muscle before dividing its origin and insertion to ensure correct resting tension after transfer. Veins and nerves are connected after tourniquet release. The motor nerve of the muscle is sutured to the anterior interosseus nerve, which is normally spared in Volkmann's ischemic contractures. Healthy fascicles on the cut surface should be identified under the microscope, and an exact apposition of suitable fascicles with 10-0 sutures is performed. It is better to suture the donor nerve to the motor branch of the muscle at the point where it enters the muscle; this shortens the reinnervation period that starts after 4 to 6 months. During this time, physical therapy with careful electrical stimulation is important. Functioning muscle transfers can be combined with long nerve grafts to the median and/or ulnar nerve as necessary. Because the nerve grafts are covered with vascular tissue, there is a dramatic increase in sensory recovery. Muscle strength usually reaches one third of the healthy hand. The final outcome of hand function depends strongly on the severity of contracture preoperatively, the interval between development of contracture and reconstruction, the method of treatment, and prompt participation in a hand rehabilitation program.[79]

In Holden I types, the most significant hand impairment is not caused by intrinsic contractures but rather by secondary problems due to sequelae of ischemic extrinsic muscles in the forearm. The treatment of the extrinsic finger contractures with tendon and nerve surgery, if there is no so-called intrinsic Volkmann's, can also correct the intrinsic-minus deformity. Otherwise, existing intrinsic contractures or intrinsic-plus deformity developing after the treatment of extrinsic contracture should be addressed in a second stage.[14]

Arm-length discrepancies seen in long-term follow-up of Volkmann contractures due to poorly treated supracondylar fractures in childhood may be disturbing for patients. If hand function is satisfactory, bone-lengthening operations (which may lead to recurrence of the contracture) are usually not advised.

In management of Holden II types, the incisions should be adapted according to the existing scars and contracture of the soft tissues. The carpal tunnel is usually opened, but the proximal incision at the forearm need not be elongated to the elbow.

In Holden II, mild types with limited local necrosis and scar tissue formation at the site of injury, the contractures are corrected by passively flexing and extending the fingers after complete resection of scar tissue and exploration of the nerves. Because the proximal parts of the muscles are healthy, individual tendon lengthening of the involved superficial or deep flexors, as well as the wrist flexors, with "Z"-plasties at different levels is usually sufficient for complete reconstruction. Tendon transpositions and additional soft tissue coverage are rarely required in these mild types.

Holden II, moderate types, which are the most common, are caused by localized injuries starting from the skin inward toward the bone. In the end, all these tissues are scarred and contracted with a typical intrinsic minus deformity of the wrist and fingers (Fig. 56-35). Paresthesias and neuralgias are usually present. The tissues proximal to the injury are undisturbed, so there is almost no indication for free functional muscle transpositions. By proper planning of the skin incisions, the primarily damaged area and existing soft tissue contractures can occasionally be corrected with "Z"-plasties, but skin grafts or flaps are usually required for coverage. Because the nerves in areas of localized muscle necrosis are also affected and may need grafting, and soft tissue cover is often poor, a pedicled flap or free tissue transfer may be needed.

In these Holden II, moderate types, following forearm fascial incision, carpal tunnel release, and muscle belly

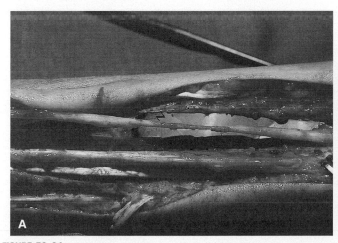

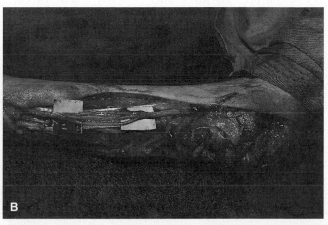

FIGURE 56-34. A, Due to compression between the fibrotic deep and superficial flexors, the caliber of the median nerve is reduced to a thin segment. **B,** Resection of the fibrotic segment and bridging the gap with sural nerve grafts is combined with a proximal muscle slide of flexor origins.

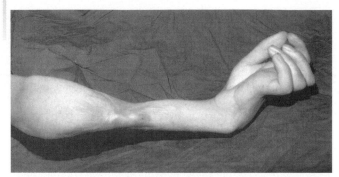

FIGURE 56-35. Holden II type flexion contracture due to severe localized injury from the skin inward to the bone. Note typical intrinsic-minus appearance of the finger.

epimysiotomy, meticulous resection of all scarred muscles is performed and the entrapped nerves are released. The usually thickened epineurium is resected, followed by interfascicular neurolysis if necessary. The circulation of nerves is evaluated after tourniquet release in the reactive hyperemia phase. Proximal muscle slides are not usually performed because detachment of these healthy muscles will potentially diminish their functional capacity. Instead, if only the distal half or distal two thirds of the forearm is involved, tendon lengthening or grafting at the musculotendinous junctions is performed. Transpositions of the wrist flexors to the deep finger flexors or to the flexor pollicis longus can be combined with opponensplasty, using one of the remaining superficial flexors. Wrist extensors can also be utilized (Fig. 56-36). In circumferential injuries, tenolysis of extensor muscles may also be required.

In Holden II, severe types, severe wrist flexion contracture is usually seen with contracture of the intrinsic muscles. In late cases with inadequate initial management, the whole extremity from the site of injury distally may be severely atrophic with tight and stiff soft tissues and fixed joint contractures with fibrous ankylosis (Fig. 56-37).

Victims of mass casualties with delay in treatment due to the situation may develop this type of deformity despite emergency treatment, which is seldom sufficient. In cases in which there are no healthy forearm muscles, free functioning myocutaneous transfers, combined with long nerve grafts to provide protective sensation, can solve the motor, sensory, and soft tissue problems to some extent (Fig. 56-38).

In the nonfunctional and severely deformed extremity, simple contracture release may be useful to facilitate extremity hygiene in the palm, wrist crease, or antecubital fossa and to facilitate dressing and positioning of the extremity.[14] Even in the most severe cases, the significance of reconstruction of protective sensation is to be emphasized.[17]

In late cases with severe fixed contractures of the wrist, proximal row or total carpectomy or arthrodesis of the wrist can be performed.[66] If the proximal joint surface of the capitate and the cartilage of the distal radius are not damaged, some correction and useful movement of the wrist can be achieved by proximal row carpectomy. In typical Volkmann's contracture of the forearm, there is usually a flexed wrist, hyperextended MCP joints, lack of IP joint extension of the fingers, and an adduction contracture of the thumb.[177] In cases of intrinsic Volkmann's contracture, which can also be seen in combination with ischemic contracture of the forearm muscles, the typical deformity of the hand gives an intrinsic-plus position of the fingers, with flexed MCP and extended IP joints and an adducted thumb with a hyperextended IP joint (Fig. 56-39).[21] The usual procedures to correct intrinsic paralysis in the hand (e.g., tendon transpositions for lumbrical reconstruction or opponensplasty) are usually useless or impossible in cases with extrinsic muscle contracture, because there are usually ischemic contractures of the intrinsic muscles of the hand itself.

In cases of intrinsic Volkmann's contracture, the main functional handicap is the inability to open the hand for

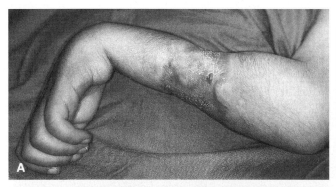

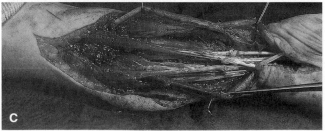

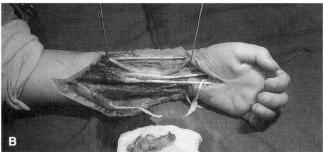

FIGURE 56-36. **A,** Holden II, moderate type deformity caused by tight bandaging with soft tissue damage in the pressure area and nerve involvement with thenar atrophy. **B,** Excision of localized fibrosis and neurolysis of the median and ulnar nerves. **C,** Tendon transfers of flexor carpi ulnaris to the flexor digitorum profundus and the middle finger flexor digitorum superficialis to the flexor pollicis longus.

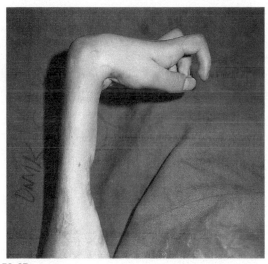

FIGURE 56-37. Fixed wrist contracture at 90 degrees with atrophic distal forearm in a late case of Holden II, severe type contracture.

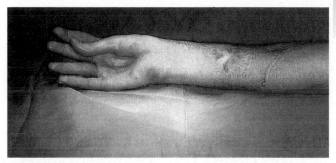

FIGURE 56-39. Typical intrinsic plus contracture of the finger and the thumb in a case of Volkmann's contracture.

grasping even medium-sized objects.[23] It is therefore necessary to resect the whole first dorsal interosseous and most of the adductor pollicis muscles that are fibrotic to release the adduction contracture of the first web space and to perform soft tissue reconstruction by local flap transposition from the dorsum of the hand or with a free or

pedicled flap. These procedures are generally combined with arthrodesis of the thumb MCP joint and intrinsic muscle release of the fingers. In mild cases of finger intrinsic contractures, Littler's release operation (excision of the oblique and lateral bands) will suffice. In severe cases, releasing all the adhesions through small longitudinal incisions over the metacarpal heads, with release of all the interosseous and abductor digiti minimi tendons, accessory collateral ligaments, and arthrolysis of the MCP joints is

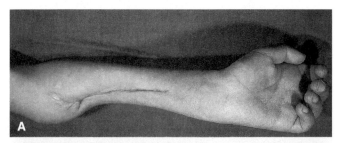

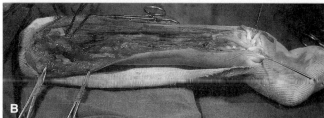

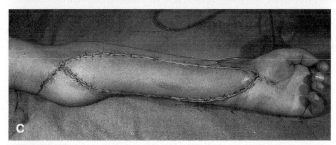

FIGURE 56-38. **A,** Holden II, severe type ischemic contractures with soft tissue deficit. **B,** Appearance after excision of all fibrotic tissues. **C,** Free functioning myocutaneous transfer of the latissimus dorsi, using the interosseous nerve as the motor branch, with a large skin island for soft tissue coverage.

CRITICAL POINTS: MANAGEMENT OF VOLKMANN'S ISCHEMIC CONTRACTURE

MILD CONTRACTURE

- Skin release, "Z"-plasty lengthening of tendons

MODERATE CONTRACTURE

- Resection of scarred muscles
- "Z"-plasty tendon lengthening
  In Holden I type—muscle slide
  In Holden II type—tendon transfers according to individual situation
- Exploration and release of both the median and ulnar nerves
- Possible soft tissue coverage

SEVERE CONTRACTURE

- Innervated free muscle transfer for function and coverage
- Reconstruction of protective sensation (neurolysis or nerve grafting)
- In Holden II type (carpectomies or arthrodesis of the wrist, correcture of intrinsic contractures)

PEARLS

- Proper early management prevents development.
- Avoid sliding muscle with some function too distally in Holden II type.
- Do not forget possible need for coverage after surgery on tendons and nerves.

preferred. Hyperextension deformity usually does not develop, owing to the existing soft tissue tightness and contractures.[30]

In cases with severe wrist flexion contracture combined with contracture of the intrinsic muscles, there is also fixed radial deviation of the metacarpals with ulnar deviation of the fingers (as in rheumatoid arthritis). Dorsoulnar wedge resection osteotomies at the base of the second and third metacarpals, performed at the same time as proximal row carpectomy or arthrodesis of the wrist, may correct radiopalmar deviation of the metacarpals as well as the wrist flexion deformity.

The Management of Snake (Pit Viper) Bites

Spencer Rowland and William C. Pederson

Approximately 98% of venomous snakebites are inflicted by pit vipers,[133,135] with the remaining 2% inflicted by coral snakes, captive snakes, and foreign venomous snakes.[134] Approximately two thirds of poisonous snakebites occur on the hands and upper extremities.[138] Because of the high incidence of upper extremity and hand involvement,[39] it is natural for physicians who treat hand and upper extremity injuries to have more than an inquisitive interest in the subject. This section is by no means meant to be a treatise on the subject because the material is voluminous and controversial. Those physicians taking on responsibility for the total treatment of a snake-envenomated patient must be familiar with the physiologic problems that can arise and must be capable of handling them medically. Surgical management of the patient may be relatively straightforward, but the problems that can arise when treating pit viper bites may require experience in hematologic, cardiovascular, renal, respiratory, neurologic, and electrolyte management.

CHARACTERISTICS OF PIT VIPERS

Rattlesnakes, cottonmouths (water moccasins), copperheads, pigmy rattlesnakes, and massasaugas are the pit viper snakes (Crotalidae).[152] They are characterized by heat-sensitive pits located between the eyes and the nostril (Fig. 56-40). With these heat-sensitive pits they can make a direct hit on a warm-blooded animal that they cannot see.[150] Pit vipers can be further identified by eyes that have vertical elliptical pupils ("cat's eye") and a single row of subcaudal scutes or scales.[40,134] The genus *Crotalus* is further characterized by horny segments on the tail known as rattles.[92]

ENVENOMATION

Envenomation is a term implying that sufficient venom has been introduced into the body to cause either local signs at the site of the bite and/or systemic signs.

The venom apparatus of the Crotalidae consists of a gland, a duct, and one or more fangs on each side of the head.[191] The venom consists of 5 to 15 enzymes, 3 to 12 nonenzymatic proteins and peptides, and at least 6 other unidentified substances.[155,191] The venom contains hemotoxin, neurotoxin, venotoxin, cardiotoxin, and necrotizing factors.[150] The venom almost instantly alters blood vessel

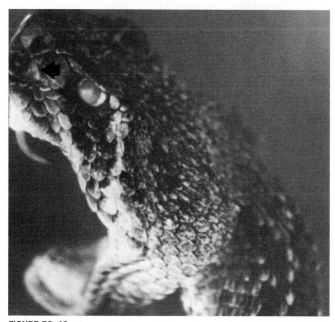

FIGURE 56-40. The heat-sensitive pit, which enables the pit viper to strike warm-blooded animals it cannot see, is seen as an indentation between the nostril and the eye *(arrow).*

permeability, which leads to loss of plasma into the tissue and breakdown of blood cells.[150,153,155,160] This results in immediate tissue edema and ecchymosis and is probably responsible for the cardinal signs of local envenomation. These signs consist of severe burning pain, rapid swelling, ecchymosis, and local necrosis and sloughing about the fang marks (Fig. 56-41). These local cardinal signs usually occur within 10 minutes of envenomation,[156] and it is unusual to have an onset longer than 20 minutes after the bite. If symptoms and signs do not occur within 4 hours, it is almost certain that envenomation has not taken place.

Systemic signs that may occur after the local signs are secondary to toxic effects on the cardiovascular, hematologic, nervous, and respiratory systems. Bleeding, coagulation, and prothrombin times may be altered, which may result in hematuria, epistaxis, and other bleeding problems. The hematocrit blood level may fall rapidly, along with the platelet count[101] and fibrinogen levels.[22,71,181]

A rapid fall in blood pressure and a decrease in circulating blood volume may occur along with pulmonary

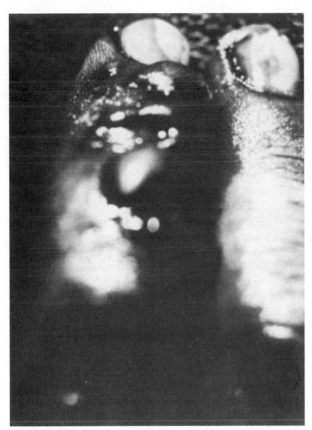

FIGURE 56-41. Blood blisters are characteristic of local envenomation after pit viper bites. The fang mark's entrance into the skin can be seen only by removing the blisters.

edema.[151] Death, although rare, is associated with destruction of red blood cells and the intimal lining of blood vessels, particularly those of the pulmonary system.[191]

Systemic signs of envenomation include weakness, sweating, faintness, nausea, and vomiting. Paresthesias and numbness about the scalp, face, lips, fingers, and toes may occur.[156] Perioral and periorbital muscular fasciculations[19,69,70] may be expected.

Envenomation from the Mojave rattlesnake differs from envenomation by other pit vipers in that the initial symptoms may be myotoxic and neurologic and frequently associated with severe hypotension.[85] The characteristic tissue signs seen with the other North American Crotalidae bites are frequently minimal or absent, as is fibrinogenolysis and thrombocytopenia. Severe rhabdomyolysis- and myoglobinuria-associated kidney failure has been reported along with severe hypocalcemic tetany, all of which should be treated with appropriate antivenom treatment and support therapy.

TREATMENT

First Aid

Prompt transfer to a medical facility is the most appropriate first-aid measure.

No time should be lost in reaching an appropriate medical facility after a snakebite, but the following measures may be helpful if they can be done immediately after the bite has occurred.

1. The patient should be kept emotionally and physically quiet. Studies on experimental animals show that the median lethal dose (LD_{50}) of venom can be decreased by decreasing physical activity.[185,191]
2. Kill the snake if practical, but do not lose time in attempting to retrieve the snake. Identification of the snake by the treating physician may aid in treatment. If the snake is retrieved, handle the snake with a stick. Decapitated pit viper head reactions may sometimes persist for up to an hour.[94,191]
3. A small rubber tourniquet should be loosely applied immediately proximal to the bite in such a fashion that it occludes lymphatic and intracellular drainage only. It should not be tight enough to block the arterial or venous circulation. The tourniquet should be moved proximally as the swelling advances (Fig. 56-42)
4. Incision and suction are contraindicated unless done by an experienced person or if one cannot reach a medical

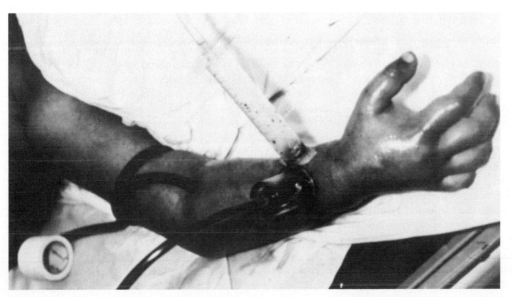

FIGURE 56-42. The tourniquet should not be tight enough to block arterial or venous circulation and should only retard lymphatic and intracellular edema. Cup suction is safer than mouth suction, which may infect the wound and can also envenomate the individual giving first aid if a mucosal lesion exists.

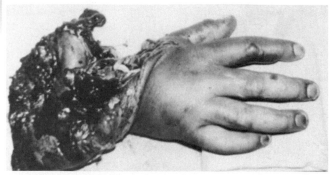

FIGURE 56-43. Prolonged icing of a hand may cause added tissue damage by potentiating the necrotic effect of the venom locally. Application of ice was used in the treatment of this child, who was bitten on the index finger by a rattlesnake. Amputation was required because of frostbite, not as a result of snakebite. (Courtesy of W.S. Lorimar, Sr., MD.)

facility within 1 hour and symptoms and signs of envenomation are present (localized burning pain, rapid swelling associated with ecchymosis). This is established by making an incision ¼ inch linear and ¼ inch deep in each fang mark and starting cup suction (see Fig. 56-42).[81-84] Mouth suction could be dangerous if the person applying the suction has a mucosal cut. Suction of snakebite wounds, one of the oldest forms of treatment, has been recorded as early as 200 BC.[93] McCollough and Gennaro[116] demonstrated by radioisotope studies that 50% of tagged crotalid venom injected subcutaneously into dogs could be removed by suction if instituted within 3 minutes of injection. The benefit from suction decreases 30 minutes after the bite and is probably of little value after 1 hour.[59,116,118,159] Little or no venom can be recovered from the advancing edema.[159]

5. The envenomated part should be immobilized and kept at heart level if possible.
6. Ice and/or cooling of the wound or extremity should not be used in any form (Fig. 56-43).[6,142,143,156]

HOSPITAL TREATMENT

Once the patient has reached the hospital, the following steps have been suggested by Wingert and Wainschel[191]:

1. Identify the snake. Approximately 20% of all bites in the United States are nonpoisonous.[156,157]
2. Evaluate the symptoms and signs. Antivenom administration is not indicated for snake-bitten patients without local or systemic manifestations of envenomation,[174] but the snakebite victim should be hospitalized for observation. (We recommend 23 hours.) Did envenomation of the patient occur? Russell[154] reported three patients bitten by the same pit viper. The last patient required no treatment because no envenomation had occurred, a so-called dry bite.[173] Presumably, the snake had injected all of its venom into the first and second patients. If envenomation did occur within the last 60 minutes, we believe that in the emergency department a lymphatic tourniquet should be placed above the progressive swelling, incisions made in the bites, and suction started.

3. Tests that should be done immediately after pit viper envenomation are a complete blood cell count (CBC); urinalysis; platelet count; prothrombin time (PT); partial thromboplastin time (PTT); bleeding time; determinations of blood glucose concentration, blood urea nitrogen level, and electrolyte levels; and type and cross-match.[156,157] Other frequently ordered tests are red blood cell indices, sedimentation rate, clotting and clot retraction times, arterial blood gas measurements, serum protein levels, and fibrinogen titers. Electrocardiography is performed on all patients with moderate to severe envenomation, and renal function tests are often useful.[155,156,193]
4. Measure and record the circumference of the injured extremity. Marking the skin in ink at the sites selected for measurement will ensure accurate serial comparisons and should document proximal migration of the edema. These measurements should be repeated every 15 to 20 minutes[156,191,193] inasmuch as they serve as an index of progression of the poisoning and a guide for antivenom administration.

Grading the Severity of Envenomation

All bites should be immediately graded for severity of envenomation. Various grading methods have been used to determine this factor.[27,59,117,191] One such method based on local and systemic reactions has been recommended by the Committee on Trauma of the American College of Surgeons.[4,6]

Patients in whom pain, swelling, ecchymosis, systemic symptoms, or abnormal laboratory findings develop within 30 minutes to 1 hour of the bite are appropriate candidates for antivenom therapy. Antivenom is most effective when given within 4 hours of the snakebite.

No Envenomation. No local or systemic signs are present. Clean the wound and give antibiotics and tetanus toxoid if indicated. Do not apply ice. Order a CBC, bleeding time, PT, PTT, platelet count, and urinalysis for blood cells.

The patient should be admitted as a medical emergency and carefully observed until there is clear evidence that envenomation has not occurred or is minimal.

If there is the slightest suggestion of envenomation, the patient should have a repeat of the aforementioned blood tests before discharge from the hospital. We have seen a patient who was discharged from a hospital emergency department after having "minimal swelling" of the ankle after a snakebite. Fifteen hours later she was seen with minimal swelling and pain but with a PTT greater than 200 seconds, a PT greater than 50 seconds, and a platelet count of 50/mm^3—a potentially life-threatening situation.

Minimal Envenomation. Local symptoms and signs (swelling, pain, or ecchymosis) are present, as well as a few systemic symptoms and signs (signs such as hypotension, vomiting, sweating, ptosis, paralysis, and muscle fasciculations and symptoms such as nausea, dizziness, perioral paresthesia, and weakness). Laboratory abnormalities are minimal.

Moderate Envenomation. Swelling that progresses beyond the area of the bite is a feature of moderate envenomation. Some systemic features are present, such as vomiting, sweating, weakness, dizziness, perioral paresthesia, ptosis, paralysis, and muscle fasciculations. Laboratory findings are abnormal and consist of abnormal clotting factors, a fall in hematocrit and platelets, and so on.

Severe Envenomation. In severe envenomation, local symptoms and signs are marked and systemic symptoms and signs are severe. Significant abnormalities are noted in laboratory results.

Intravenous Lines

Start two separate intravenous infusions, one line for the support of blood pressure and one line for administering antivenom.[191]

Antivenom

Administer an adequate amount of antivenom intravenously (see the appropriate brochure accompanying the antivenom for guidelines). Almost all authorities agree that antivenom is the single most important therapeutic measure and recommend its use as the initial treatment of all serious envenomations.*

Gennaro and McCollough[59] have shown that radiolabeled antivenom accumulates at the site of the bite faster after intravenous administration than after intramuscular or subcutaneous injection. Antivenom should never be injected into a finger or toe[156] and not locally.[191] Antivenom is most effective when given within 4 hours of the bite. It is of questionable value if given after 24 hours, but it should still be tried.[156] We believe that skin testing and the administration of snake antivenom should be done in an intensive care unit because of the possibility of an anaphylactic reaction to components of the antisera.

Antivenom (Crotalidae) Polyvalent (ACP)

There are two types of antivenom available in the United States for the treatment of snakebites. Antivenom (Crotalidae) Polyvalent (ACP) has been available from Wyeth Laboratories since 1954. It is produced by exposing horses to the venom of the Eastern diamondback, Western diamondback, and tropical rattlesnakes as well as the fer-de-lance. This antivenom is composed of neutralizing IgG immunoglobulins with a molecular weight of approximately 150,000 daltons.[35] Because of the similarities in venom between snake species, this antivenom is considered to be effective for the treatment of envenomation by all species of rattlesnake found in North and South America.[125] Although it has been proven to provide therapeutic benefit in animals, there have been no randomized, prospective studies in humans.[35] Nonetheless, its therapeutic benefits are accepted in the management of snakebite. This is despite the fact that acute allergic reactions to the horse serum component of this antivenom have been reported in up to 20% of treated patients.[125] Most of the reported allergic reactions have been limited to urticaria, however, and are generally well managed with intravenous antihistamines (diphenhydramine or H_2-blocking agents).[125] Patients can also develop late serum sickness reactions to ACP, which have been reported in the 18% to 86% range in retrospective studies.[65]

In a study involving 26 patients who received ACP,[88] immediate hypersensitivity occurred in 6 patients (23%). Cutaneous manifestations occurred in 3 of these patients, whereas the other 3 had anaphylaxis. Twenty patients were available for follow-up; and of these, serum sickness developed in 10. The authors concluded that skin testing was not reliable in predicting immediate anaphylaxis or delayed serum sickness; however, in their series, treatment of antivenom allergic reactions was "uniformly effective with no mortality, minimal morbidity, and no chronic sequelae."[88] Weigert and Wainschel,[191] after performing skin tests on 211 patients envenomated by pit vipers, demonstrated a false-positive rate of 50% and a false-negative rate of 8%.

The first vial of antivenom must be given very slowly and with extreme caution, with resuscitation equipment and drugs (diphenhydramine [Benadryl], epinephrine) immediately available. Forks[51] suggests that if a patient has a reaction to horse serum, treatment with the antivenom should be temporarily discontinued and diphenhydramine given intravenously. Horse serum proteins may cause degranulation of mast cells with release of histamines. Urticaria and pruritus result from this reaction and are best treated with intravenous antihistamines.[51] The antivenom may then be restarted and increased or decreased as tolerated by the patient.[51]

Serum sickness (pruritus, skin wheals, lethargy, fever, and lymphadenopathy) may occur 1 to 3 weeks after the administration of the antivenom.

It has been reported that some degree of serum sickness will occur in patients who receive over 70 mL (7 vials) of the antivenom[191]; however, most authors believe that the risk of serum sickness is less serious than are the complications of pit viper envenomation.†

The following dosage based on the degree of envenomation was suggested by the American College of Surgeons Committee on Trauma in February 1981[4]:

Minimal: 0 to 4 vials
Moderate: 5 to 9 vials, especially in children and the elderly
Severe: 10 to 15 vials

Antivenom should be administered only intravenously[51] and the directions accompanying Wyeth's antivenom followed. If symptoms progress, the original dose should be repeated at 2-hour intervals until no further increase in edema, pain, paresthesia, or muscular fasciculation occurs.[51] There is no maximal dosage of antivenom. Children should be given one and one-half to two times the initial adult dose.[51]

Crotalidae Polyvalent Immune Fab (Ovine) (CroFab; FabAV)

CroFab is a sheep-derived antivenom that was approved for use in the United States by the FDA in October 2000 and is marketed by Savage Laboratories. It consists of purified Fab immunoglobulin fragments obtained from sheep immunized with venom of the Western diamondback, Eastern diamondback, and Mojave rattlesnakes and the cottonmouth or water moccasin.[162] It has a molecular weight of approximately

---

*See references 15, 53, 116, 117, 141, 156, 157, 176, 194, and 195.
†See references 15, 53, 116, 117, 141, 156-158, 191, 194, and 195.

50,000 daltons and is purified to remove the majority of sheep proteins as well as the more immunogenic Fc fragments.[35] In animal models of snakebite, this antivenom has been found to be up to 5.2 times more potent than ACP against a number of different crotaline snake venoms.[35] This antivenom was subject to prospective, controlled clinical trials before its approval by the U.S. Food and Drug Administration.[34-36]

Early clinical trials noted several allergic reactions to this serum, including anaphylaxis, angioedema, urticaria, and delayed serum sickness.[34] The case of anaphylaxis was related to a too-rapid infusion of the antisera, which resolved with appropriate systemic management and did not recur with a secondary slower infusion of the antivenom.[78] In these early trials, however, there was an issue concerning the purification of the antisera that resulted in an excess of Fc fragments that was thought to have led to these increased reactions. Later clinical experience after governmental approval of the antivenom has shown a decrease in hypersensitivity reactions; however, mild symptoms of possible late serum sickness were noted.[149] It is generally believed that this newer antivenom has a lower incidence of acute and delayed allergic side effects.[218]

The suggested initial dosage of CroFab is 4 to 6 vials given intravenously to achieve "initial control" of the symptoms of envenomation. If initial control is not achieved within 1 hour, an additional 4 to 6 vials should be given intravenously.[162] The manufacturer suggests dilution of the initial dose in 250 mL of saline that is administered over 60 minutes. The infusion should proceed slowly over the first 10 minutes at a rate of 25 to 50 mL/hr to observe for allergic reactions. If no reaction is observed, the rate can be increased to the 250 mL/hr rate.[162] Because the half-life of the Fab fragment is short, further treatment with an additional 2-vial dose every 6 hours for up to 18 hours may be necessary, depending on the status of the patient.

Due to this shorter half-life, some problems with recurrence of symptoms after initial treatment have been seen with CroFab. Patients have been noted to have a recurrence of swelling and coagulopathy after initial management when antivenom treatment was not continued after the initial dosage.[16,149] The clinical significance of late asymptomatic elevation of clotting abnormalities has been questioned in the literature, however.[196] Despite this, most authorities agree that treatment of significant envenomations with CroFab should continue until coagulation parameters stabilize.[16,196]

Blood and Blood Products

The coagulopathies encountered in pit viper envenomation usually improve with the administration of antivenom; however, when indicated, platelets, fresh frozen plasma, and blood may be needed.[51] Coagulopathy problems are best handled by a hematologist. Ten to 20 U of fresh-frozen plasma has been suggested by Forks[51] in the presence of prolonged PT and PTT. Clotting studies should be repeated at 2-hour intervals until the results are normal. Blood products should only be used for clearly defined indications.[24]

Antibiotics

A broad-spectrum antibiotic should be administered to cover aerobic coliforms and histotoxic anaerobic organisms. Gentamicin in combination with chloramphenicol has been recommended by one author.[90] At least one case of a patient developing necrotizing fasciitis due to *Aeromonas hydrophila* infection after snakebite has been reported.[5]

Tetanus Prophylaxis

Appropriate antitetanus prophylaxis should be given. Parrish[134] presented a patient who recovered from severe envenomation only to die of tetanus 2 days later because he had never received immunization against tetanus.

Systemic Corticosteroids

Corticosteroids, although advocated by some authors,[61,62] have been shown to be of no benefit in preventing tissue damage.[1,37,165,192]

Ice and Cooling

Ice should not be used.[142] Investigators have shown that cooling potentiates the necrotic effect locally.[2,116,159,192-195] Cryotherapy, once recommended to prevent dissemination of the venom, has been a significant factor leading to the amputation of extremities (see Fig. 56-42).[60,116,142,194]

Surgical Management

There is a great deal of disagreement regarding the role of surgical treatment in the management of snakebites. As previously mentioned, if an incision is made to the depth of each fang mark and suction applied within the first 30 minutes of pit viper snakebite, a great deal of venom can be removed.[81-84] Glass[61-63] recommended surgical exploration of all snakebites to determine the extent of the envenomation, débride the wound, and perform a fasciotomy if needed. Watt[185] recommends that a dermotomy of finger bites be done routinely. Garfin and associates,[52-54,56] to the contrary, have stated that the incidence and degree of necrosis in edematous limbs after pit viper bites are not altered by fasciotomy. Russell[156,157] has treated more than 650 cases of snake venom poisoning and has never had to do a fasciotomy. He states that "the use of fasciotomy usually reflects an insufficient dosage of antivenom, or no antivenom, during the first 12 hours following the bite."

Garfin and Mubarak[55] have pointed out that because of the severe pain and acute swelling that occur after snakebites, it is difficult to differentiate the acutely swollen limb from a true compartment syndrome. For this reason, they and others[55,56,144] recommend intracompartment pressure monitoring to help make the correct diagnosis. If the diagnosis of compartment syndrome is made, fasciotomy is carried out without delay after coagulation studies are done.

There have been a few reported cases of snakebite-induced compartment syndromes that have "resolved" after treatment with antivenom.[64,106] In one case no compartment pressures were measured before scheduling for surgery, which was cancelled after clinical improvement with antivenom treatment. In the other case, the patient received antivenom and hyperbaric oxygen treatment for a compartment syndrome in the thenar muscles. From the perspective of a hand surgeon, late hand function was not assessed adequately. In our opinion, these reports remain in the anecdotal sphere, and we believe that fasciotomy should be performed after snakebite if elevated intracompartmental pressures are documented.

Authors' Preferred Method of Treatment

Pit viper bites differ from other compartment syndromes in that the venom is injected directly into the skin and subcutaneous tissue with resultant immediate tissue edema, ecchymosis, and rapid swelling (Fig. 56-44). The venom may or may not be injected into a closed compartment, but it usually is. The severe swelling of the skin and soft tissues outside a compartment can be of such a degree that the circulation will be impaired (Fig. 56-45). This is particularly true of the digits of the hand (Figs. 56-46 and 56-47). When we first see a snakebite victim in whom the tissues of the envenomated extremity have the appearance of impaired blood supply and/or compartment syndrome, the patient is prepared for surgery regardless of whether antivenom was or is being administered, but only after blood coagulation studies have been done. As shown in Figure 56-48, skin and subcutaneous swelling can be so great as to cause impairment of the blood supply and subsequent tissue loss. If this condition exists, a fasciotomy of the underlying compartment as described earlier is done at the same time, without measuring compartment pressures (Fig. 56-49). In almost all instances, if the swelling is severe enough to necessitate a dermotomy, the fascia has been penetrated and intracompartment swelling is present. Failure to release skin that is too tight and compromises local blood flow can lead to

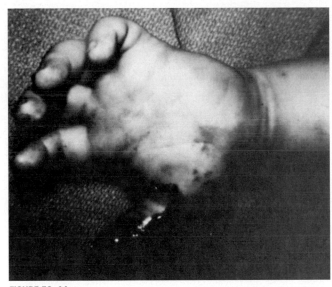

FIGURE 56-44. This child was bitten on the thumb. Note the bloody blister and spreading of the fingers secondary to rapid swelling.

significant tissue loss in the hand, which may necessitate later coverage (Fig. 56-50). Local tissue necrosis at the site of the fang marks is débrided, but no other débridement is done at this time.

If after a snakebite no clinical evidence of impending tissue loss secondary to severe swelling exists and there is no clinical evidence of a compartment syndrome, no surgery is performed. As emphasized previously,[53,55,56] the pain and degree of swelling after a pit viper bite can make the clinical diagnosis of compartment syndrome a difficult one and may necessitate continuous intracompartment pressure monitoring. The guidelines for decompression of the soft tissues outside a compartment are nebulous and based on past experience; however, the question of whether a closed compartment should be opened should be settled by measuring compartment pressure.

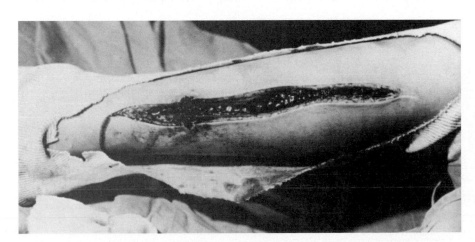

FIGURE 56-45. The necessity for dermotomy is well demonstrated in this patient; bleeding from the skin or subcutaneous tissues is minimal after the initial incision.

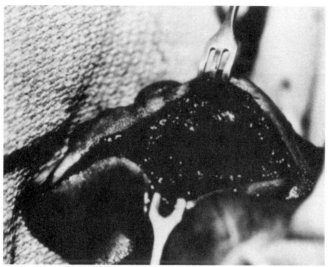

FIGURE 56-46. Dermotomy and decompression of the entire finger are indicated when this degree of swelling and suggillation (ecchymosis) is present.

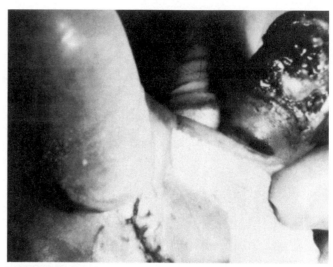

FIGURE 56-48. Dermotomy and fascial release were not done on this thumb despite severe swelling secondary to snakebite. Tissue loss occurred.

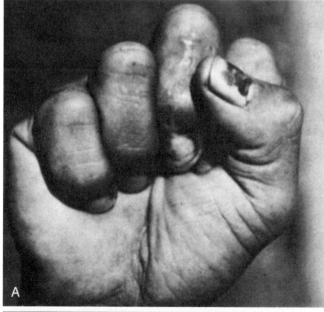

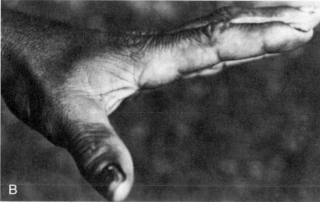

FIGURE 56-47. Active flexion (**A**) and extension (**B**) of the index finger after decompression of the finger and volar compartment of the forearm for snakebite.

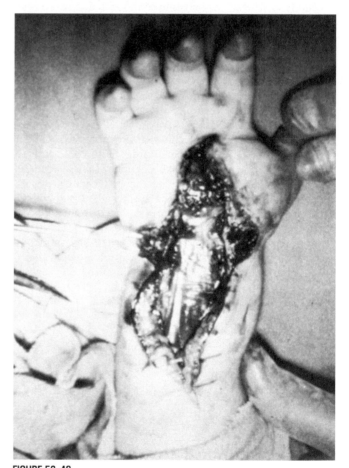

FIGURE 56-49. Fasciotomy relieved the acute swelling in the volar forearm compartment of this child with a snakebite. There was no loss of muscle tissue or function.

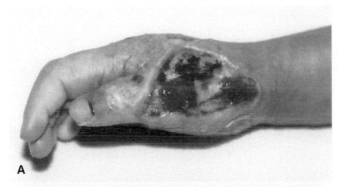

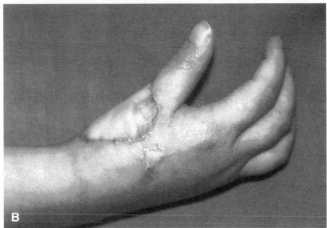

FIGURE 56-50. **A,** Hand of a child who suffered a rattlesnake bite 2 weeks previously on the dorsal thumb. Surgery was delayed due to severe hypersensitivity reaction to ACP antivenom with necessity for care in an intensive care unit for 10 days. **B,** Hand after débridement of wound and coverage with pedicled radial forearm flap.

ANNOTATED REFERENCES

16. Boyer LV, Selfert SA, Cain JS: Recurrence phenomena after immunoglobulin therapy for snake envenomations: II. Guidelines for clinical management with crotaline Fab antivenom. Ann Emerg Med 37:196-201, 2001.

   This paper discusses the proper dosing and length of therapy with the newer snake antivenom (Fab). These authors noted a recurrence of swelling and coagulopathy after treatment with the recommended original dosing. Because of this they have suggested a modified protocol to attempt to avoid these problems.

65. Gold BS, Dart RC, Barish RA: Bites of venomous snakes. N Engl J Med 347:347-356, 2002.

   This article presents a contemporary overview of the management of snakebites. It discusses the use and complications of both the standard antivenom (ACP) and the newer Fab antivenom.

79. Hovius SE, Ultee J: Volkmann's ischemic contracture: Prevention and treatment. Hand Clin 16:647-657, 2000.

   This is a current review of the management of Volkmann's ischemic contracture. The author's emphasis, however, is on prevention. They give guidelines for management and monitoring of high-risk patients as well as indications for surgery to prevent the development of muscle contracture.

111. Matsen FA III: Compartmental syndrome: A unified concept. Clin Orthop 113:8-14, 1975.

   This is one of the classic articles on the pathophysiology, diagnosis, and management of compartment syndromes. Dr. Matsen was one of the first authors to present a "unified concept" to help with the understanding of the etiology and progression of increased compartmental pressure to a compartment syndrome. This article should be read by all with further interest in this area.

178. Tsuge K: Treatment of established Volkmann's contracture. J Bone Joint Surg Am 57:925-929, 1975.

   This is another classic article dealing with the late management of Volkmann's contracture. Although not dealing with more current techniques (i.e., free innervated muscle transfer), it does cover nonmicrosurgical techniques as discussed in the text.

174a. Spiller HA, Bosse GM: Prospective study of morbidity associated with snakebite envenomation. J Toxicol Clin Toxicol 41:125-130, 2003.

   This recent article is one of the few that really discusses the morbidity and "outcomes" related to snakebite in the United States. The authors studied 81 patients who had documented envenomation and treatment. They found that patients with hand bites had "reduced function" for a mean of 14 days, with a mean loss from work of 14 days as well.

189. Whitesides TE, Heckman MM: Acute compartment syndrome: Update on diagnosis and treatment. J Am Acad Orthop Surg 4:209-218, 1996.

   The lead author of this paper is one of the pioneers in the measurement of compartment pressures for the diagnosis of compartment syndrome. This paper discusses the diagnosis and evaluation of patients with suspected compartment syndrome. The parameter for ischemia in this paper is 10 to 20 mm Hg below diastolic blood pressure, and the authors advocate fasciotomy if the pressure rises above 20 mm below the patient's diastolic pressure.

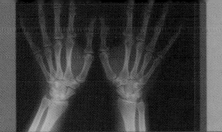

CHAPTER 57

Complex Regional Pain Syndrome

L. Andrew Koman, Gary G. Poehling, Beth P. Smith, and Thomas L. Smith

After trauma, abnormally intense and inappropriately prolonged pain that is not a reflection of actual or impending tissue damage may delay or prevent recovery and has a strong negative impact on health-related quality of life. The classification of abnormal, post-traumatic pain is complicated and encompassed in the term *complex regional pain syndrome* (CRPS). The term *reflex sympathetic dystrophy* (RSD), a descriptor of post-traumatic pain, is established in the lay, medical, and legal literature despite the absence of defined pathophysiology and/or consistent clinical symptoms and signs. RSD is a condition considered to be present in a subset of patients contained within the broader category of CRPS. In spite of the introduction of the name CRPS, much of the contemporary literature used RSD, algodystrophy, and other descriptors.[4] Therefore, the term RSD is used in this text wherever it was originally used by the cited authors. The term *causalgia*, or intractable pain after a partial nerve injury combined with an unrepaired vascular insult, has been expanded to include any abnormal post-traumatic nerve injury. Because pathognomonic criteria are lacking for RSD, a taxonomic system based on consistent definitions and objective quantifications of clinical findings is desirable. Therefore, the concept of CRPS is proposed to replace the current myriad of empirical descriptions (Table 57-1). The purpose of this chapter is to present diagnostic criteria that define clinical subtypes of CRPS and

Table 57-1
SYNONYMS FOR COMPLEX REGIONAL PAIN SYNDROME

Acute atrophy of bone	Post-traumatic pain syndrome
Algodystrophy	Post-traumatic sympathetic dystrophy
Algoneurodystrophy	Post-traumatic vasomotor abnormality
Causalgia state/syndrome	Post-traumatic vasomotor instability
Chronic traumatic edema	Reflex nervous dystrophy
Major causalgia	Reflex neurovascular dystrophy
Major traumatic dystrophy	Reflex sympathetic dystrophy
Mimo-causalgia	Shoulder-hand syndrome
Minor causalgia	Shoulder-hand-finger syndrome
Minor traumatic dystrophy	Sudeck's atrophy
Neurodystrophy	Sympathalgia
Neurovascular dystrophy	Sympathetic algodystrophy
Osteoneurodystrophy	Sympathetic mediated pain
Pain dysfunction syndrome	Sympathetic neurovascular dystrophy
Painful post-traumatic osteoporosis	Sympathetic overdrive syndrome
Peripheral trophoneurosis	Transient osteoporosis
Postinfarctional sclerodactyly	Traumatic angiospasm

to provide treatment approaches based on physiologic criteria. Chronic unilateral CRPS that is sympathetically independent demonstrates decreased perfusion of the affected limb, symmetrical sympathetic innervation and norepinephrine synthesis, but decreased norepinephrine release on the affected side.[121]

PREOPERATIVE EVALUATION AND DIAGNOSIS

Clinical Definitions

CRPS is initiated by extremity trauma, compounded by post-traumatic events (e.g., tight casts), influenced by external influences, exacerbated by preexisting physiologic makeup, and affected by congenital and/or genetic factors.[67,71,172,175,178] Because pathognomonic physiologic or metabolic markers are absent, *the diagnosis of CRPS is clinical.* The existing taxonomy of RSD may be confusing and may imply inappropriate physiology. Therefore, the name CRPS has been proposed to define the clinical subtypes of extremity pain formerly classified as RSD.[1,274] Three types of CRPS have been proposed: type 1, "classic" RSD without identifiable peripheral nerve injury; type 2, RSD associated with a peripheral nerve injury or causalgia; and type 3, other entities producing extremity pain such as myofascial syndrome (Table 57-2).[1,154,274] Although the existence of type 3 CRPS is controversial,[274] its acceptance expands the concept to include all extremity pain dysfunction under a CRPS designation. In this chapter, RSD will be subdivided into CRPS type 1 and type 2; CRPS type 3 will not be discussed. As of July 2001, RSD was the most common descriptor, followed by algodystrophy, transient osteoporosis, and CRPS.[4] Since then, the frequency of use of the name CRPS has increased and the importance of consistent diagnostic criteria and reproducible nomenclature has been emphasized.[289]

The diagnosis of CRPS is contingent on regional pain combined with autonomic dysfunction, atrophy, and functional impairment (Fig. 57-1). CRPS may include sympathetically maintained pain (SMP) or sympathetically independent pain (SIP).[274] This classification represents a significant departure from recent recommendations,[1,6,172,178,254] recognizes the dynamic nature of dystrophic responses, and stresses the value of reliable and consistent clinical

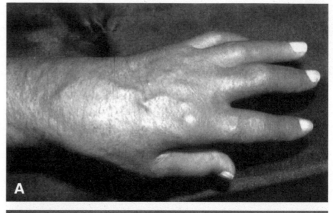

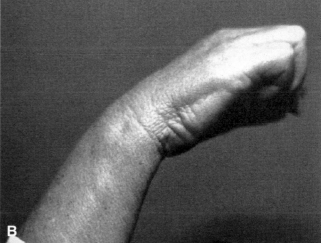

FIGURE 57-1. A, Hand of patient with CRPS and swelling and autonomic dysfunction. **B,** Hand and forearm of patient with CRPS with trophic changes and arthrofibrosis.

definitions.[274] The diagnosis of SMP is based on pain relief with sympatholytic medications or sympathetic blocks[35,249,250]; however, SMP may become SIP over time.[35] In the absence of anatomic, physiologic, or metabolic marker(s) that are pathognomonic for CRPS, the diagnosis must be based on clinical criteria. Early recognition along with prompt treatment of CRPS is the single most important predictor of functional recovery and pain relief. Objective and reproducible methods to assess pain, quantify trophic change, define autonomic dysfunction, and measure functional impairment are important to provide consistent treatment regimens and assess outcome reliably.[176] The availability of objective physiologic and clinical data provides a method to assess empirical protocols, evaluate random treatment selections, and eliminate patients with inappropriate diagnoses.[256] The natural history of CRPS after distal radius fracture suggests that permanent impairment is frequent in spite of prompt recognition and treatment.[14,15,30] Follow-up of patients frequently demonstrates a persistent impairment of their affected extremities; however, significant disability using guidelines from the American Medical Association does not always coexist with impairment[111]; work cessation for over 1 year is not infrequent (30%), changes in occupation are common, and psychological disorders are often coincident.[111,112]

Table 57-2
CLASSIFICATION OF COMPLEX REGIONAL PAIN SYNDROME

Type 1	Reflex sympathetic dystrophy (pain, functional impairment, autonomic dysfunction, dystrophic changes without clinical peripheral nerve lesion/injury)
Type 2	Causalgia (pain, functional impairment, autonomic dysfunction, dystrophic changes with a diagnosable peripheral nerve injury)
Type 3*	Other pain dysfunction problems (e.g., myofascial pain)

*Not discussed in this chapter.

Neuropathic Versus Nociceptive Pain

Neuropathic pain is defined as pain initiated or caused by a primary lesion(s) or dysfunction of the peripheral or central nervous system.

Nociceptive pain results from damage to tissues due to thermal, mechanical, chemical, or other irritants. Unfortunately, these distinctions are often combined and confusing in the literature dealing with CRPS. Neuropathic pain may be associated with CRPS type 1, or neuropathic pain may be considered as a distinct entity depending on the source (Table 57-3).

Demographics

Eighty percent of patients with RSD diagnosed within 1 year of injury will improve significantly,[178,281] and it is reported that 50% of patients with untreated symptoms lasting more than 1 year will have profound residual impairment.[293] RSD can develop in children and adolescents,* but the majority of RSD patients are between 30 and 55 years of age, with the median age being 45. The incidence of cigarette smoking is higher in RSD patients, and cigarette smoking is statistically linked to RSD.[8] Women are affected three times more frequently than men,[203] except following wartime casualties.[155] Data suggesting a possible familial and/or genetic predisposition to RSD have been presented but have not been confirmed.[126] In Olmstead County, the incidence of CRPS was 5.5/per 100,000 person-risk years and the female:male ratio was 4:1.[259] A predisposition to CRPS type 1 has been suggested on the involved side of hemiplegic patients.[110,127] Structural nociceptive injury (e.g., injury to the superficial radial nerve during an operation) that initiates or potentiates dystrophic pain is diagnosed in fewer than 50%.[172,178] Fracture of the distal radius and ulna is the most *common* injury producing RSD, which in turn may complicate the postinjury recovery in 20% to 39% of patients.[15,30,99] The natural history of CRPS after distal radius fractures may vary from other entities with finger stiffness or "poor function" at 3 months past injury correlating with residual RSD at 10 years.[103] Furthermore, CRPS is more likely to occur after distal radius fracture in the presence of tight casts[102] or the presence of a nociceptive event such as compression of median nerve, overdistraction, instability of distal radioulnar joint, or ulnar fracture.[141,264] Carpal tunnel surgical release complicated by postoperative dystrophic pain is commonly encountered in referral centers.[178]

Common nerve injuries occurring during operative procedures that may precipitate CRPS include (1) injury to the palmar cutaneous branch of the median nerve during carpal tunnel surgery, (2) damage to the superficial branch of the radial nerve during surgical approaches to the first and second dorsal compartments for tenosynovitis, and (3) trauma to the dorsal branch of the ulnar nerve during a surgical approach to the distal ulna.[169,173] In association with simultaneous median nerve decompression at the wrist and partial palmar fasciectomy for Dupuytren's contracture, CRPS may produce devastating consequences.[231,312]

Table 57-3
DEFINITIONS

Pain	An unpleasant perception associated with actual or potential cellular damage
Analgesia	Absence of pain in response to an insult that should produce pain
Neuropathic pain	Pain initiated or produced by a primary lesion(s) or dysfunction of the peripheral or central nervous system
Nociception	Response to an unpleasant (noxious) stimulus that produces pain in humans under normal circumstances, owing to thermal, mechanical chemical, or other irritants of non-neural tissues
Allodynia	Pain in a specific dermatomal or autonomous distribution associated with light touch to the skin; a stimulus that is not normally painful
Hyperalgesia	Increased sensitivity to stimulation (includes allodynia and hyperesthesia)
Hyperesthesia	Increased sensitivity to simulation (pain on response to a mild non-noxious stimulus)
Sympathetic pain	Pain in the presence of and/or associated with overaction of the sympathetic fibers; by definition, the pain is relieved by sympatholytic interventions
Hypoesthesia	Decreased sensitivity to stimulation
Hyperpathia	Abnormally painful reaction to a stimulus
Dysesthesia	An unpleasant abnormal sensation
Paresthesia	An abnormal sensation

From Gracely R, Price D, Roberts W, Bennett G: Quantitative sensory testing in patients with complex regional pain syndrome (CRPS) I and II. *In* Janig W, Stanton-Hicks M (eds): Reflex Sympathetic Dystrophy: A Reappraisal, Vol. 6, Progress in Pain Research and Management. Seattle, 1996, pp 151-170.

Psychological Issues

CRPS is not a psychogenic condition. Extensive reviews of the existing literature do not support a psychological causation,[39,54,60,132,204,236,292,303] and no personality disorder related to RSD has been verified.[21,60,140] However, chronic pain is known to play a role in psychological well-being, with 50% of 283 consecutive patients admitted to pain centers, regardless of etiology, fulfilling the criteria for personality disorders.[68,105] Dependent, passive-aggressive, and histrionic personality disorders are common in those with chronic pain and are seen in patients with CRPS.[132] Behavioral responses reducing extremity use exacerbate edema and atrophy.[60]

Psychological Problems Mimicking CRPS

The differential diagnosis of CRPS includes psychological conditions including conversion disorders and clenched fist syndromes.[79,125,159,199,280,284] The patient with SHAFT (sad, hostile, anxious, frustrating, and tenacious) syndrome is

---

*See references 23, 27, 74, 107, 120, 192, 267, 273, 274, 296, 306, and 307.

difficult to discern from a patient with CRPS without active suspicion. A history of multiple operations, absence of consistent clinical findings, multiple treating physicians, a myriad of medications, psychiatric treatment, absence from work, disproportionate self-characterization and verbalization of symptoms, crying from pain, and family history of disability are common factors.[159] Misdiagnosis associated with abnormal postures is documented.[280] Dysfunctional postures are defined, such as holding an upper extremity in a fixed posture, and associated with a lack of objective findings (e.g., trophic changes, edema, osteopenia, radiographic and/or fixed contractures).[280]

Symptoms and Signs

Pain associated with CRPS is seen in a variety of clinical manifestations (Table 57-3). The pain may be described as burning, throbbing, pressing, cutting, searing, shooting, and/or aching. *Hyperalgesia,* the perception of pain greater than would be expected, may be primary, affecting the area of injury, or secondary, affecting nontraumatized surrounding areas or the entire limb. The zone of primary pain may aid in the localization of a *nociceptive* focus; however, diagnoses of the etiologic trigger event may not be possible until successful sympatholytic management of the secondary hyperalgesia is complete. *Allodynia,* or perception of pain initiated by normally innocuous stimuli, is a characteristic of sympathetically maintained CRPS. *Hyperpathia,* or pain produced by painful stimuli that appears with a delay, outlasts the initiating stimulus, and spreads beyond the normal neural distribution is encountered frequently. It is important to differentiate *spontaneous pain* from stimulus-evoked pain.[82]

Quantifying subjective complaints of pain by the use of standardized and/or validated instruments or questionnaires allows an objective analysis of symptoms.[174] Useful instruments include the Visual Analog Scale (VAS),[63,147,184] the Rand Corporation Short Form 36 (SF 36),[278,299] the McGill Pain Questionnaire,[63,175] and/or self-administered questionnaires designed to assess upper extremity symptoms/function.[7,190,191] A self-administered questionnaire for the assessment of severity of symptoms and functional status in carpal tunnel syndrome is applicable in dystrophic states after carpal tunnel surgery or secondary to injuries of the median nerve at the wrist and allows the examiner to follow graphically the patient's health-related quality of life (Fig. 57-2).[176,190] Cold intolerance, or pain on exposure to cold, may be analyzed by the McCabe Cold Sensitivity Severity Scale.[217]

The importance of standardized physiology testing and instruments is supported by the lack of reproducibility using isolated clinical evaluation by published criteria.[289] The recent introduction of scoring systems modified from Gibbons and Wilson[115] to improve classification and severity is promising.[82,313]

Trophic changes—stiffness; edema; osteopenia; atrophy of hair, nails, and/or skin; and/or hypertrophy of skin (or hyperkeratosis)—may be present in patients with CRPS (see Fig. 57-1). Changes in skin, hair, and/or nails are seen within 10 days of onset in 30% of extremities with CRPS type 1 (RSD).[22] Osteopenia is common, involves both cortical and cancellous (trabecular) bone, and requires significant demineralization for visualization on plain radiographs (Fig. 57-3).[30] Objective analysis of demineralization requires dual-photon absorptiometry or quantitative scintigraphy.[13,30] Stiffness and atrophy of joints, muscles, and

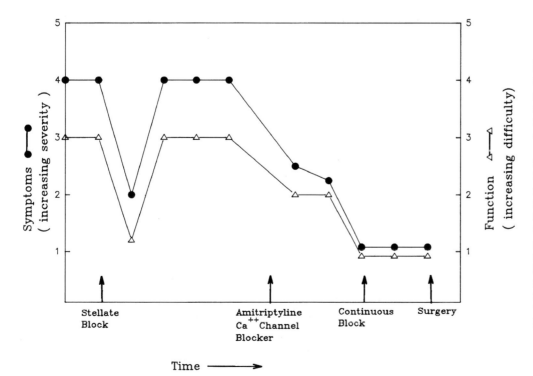

FIGURE 57-2. Symptoms and function in a dystrophic patient after carpal tunnel surgery may be monitored objectively with appropriate instruments.[190] The self-administered carpal tunnel questionnaire contains 11 questions regarding hand/wrist symptoms and 8 questions regarding hand/wrist function; symptoms are rated numerically from none (1) to severe (5), and function is rated from no difficulty (1) to cannot do at all (5). A numerical score that reflects symptoms and function can be monitored over time, and the effects of intervention can be analyzed objectively. (From Koman LA [ed]: Bowman Gray Orthopaedic Manual. Winston-Salem, NC, Orthopaedic Press, 1996.)

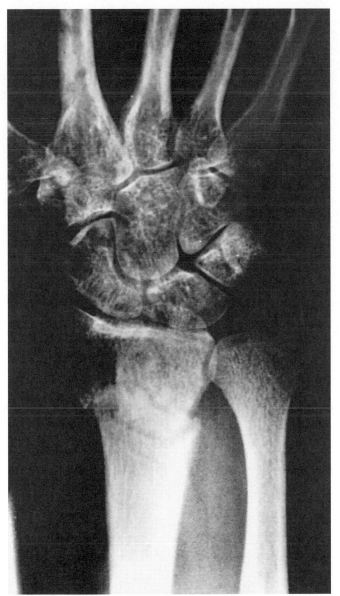

FIGURE 57-3. Plain radiographs of a patient with type 1 complex regional pain syndrome after fracture of the distal ends of the radius and ulna. The fracture line is visible. There is diffuse osteopenia in addition to juxtacortical demineralization and subchondral erosions and cysts. (From Koman LA [ed]: Bowman Gray Orthopaedic Manual. Winston-Salem, NC, Orthopaedic Press, 1996.)

tendons may be apparent during endurance testing.[172,178] "Fixed" dystonic posturing has been described.[29]

Autonomic Function

The *autonomic nervous system* controls microvascular perfusion and sweat gland activity. Abnormalities of autonomic and/or vasomotor control are seen during the course of CRPS in most patients, and loss of thermoregulatory control is common.[58] Affected extremities (hands) may be either *"hot"* or *"cold,"* and significant differences in digital temperature occur between affected and unaffected extremities in 80% of patients.[20,22] Abnormalities in thermoregulation/

vasomotion usually occur[171,241] and may vary depending on the progression of clinical stages.[183,268] Autonomic control may be evaluated by an assessment of total digital blood flow, which comprises both thermoregulatory and nutritional components, and by an analysis of sudomotor activity-sweating and piloerection. A medical history will reveal symptoms of autonomic dysfunction in 80% of patients.[58] Symptoms include abnormal sweating (excessive sweating or anhidrosis), vasomotor alterations, and heat and/or cold sensitivity (intolerance). Vasomotor changes may be described as a redness or a bluish discoloration of the extremity either at rest or, more commonly, with the limb dependent. Evidence of autonomic dysfunction can be detected in 98% or more of patients by using sophisticated technology during the painful stages of CRPS.[174,183,241] Digital perfusion and its components can be analyzed by digital temperature measurements, laser Doppler fluxmetry, plethysmography, and vital capillaroscopy. Sweating may be analyzed by resting sweat output, the quantitative sudomotor axon reflex test (QSART),[203] changes in galvanic skin response,[160,200,201] or asymmetry of somatosensory evoked potentials in the affected and the contralateral extremity.[51]

Sympathetic nervous system function, as reflected in laser Doppler fingertip blood flow and vasoconstriction response to deep inspiration varies by stage. Stage 1 patients exhibit increased blood flow but an unchanged vasoconstriction response, whereas stage 2 patients demonstrate decreased blood flow and stronger vasoconstriction.[149]

Functional impairment may be analyzed by using standardized assessments of hand function, such as the Moberg pickup test.[227] In addition, quantitative evaluation of extremity function before, during, and after stress with computerized equipment may detect subtle functional changes reflecting stiffness or atrophy.[172,176] Thus, the use of standardized tests and various computerized systems can document functional impairment that may be difficult to quantify by traditional methods.[172,176]

Physical Examination

The clinical characteristics of CRPS are related to altered extremity physiology. The magnitude of symptoms and signs is a reflection of the initiating event, postinjury response, inherent adaptability, interventional modalities, and time. Classic dystrophic progression from acute (less than 3 months) to dystrophic (3 to 6 months) to chronic (greater than 6 months) occurs infrequently because of individual variability and the effects of partial treatment. Patients with CRPS who are evaluated for a painful, hot, swollen, and stiff hand are easily recognizable; however, the precipitating nociceptive trigger (e.g., contusion of the superficial radial nerve) may not be identified until the SMP is managed and the dystrophic manifestations are treated. Once allodynia and hyperpathia are alleviated, a careful examination may delineate an underlying disorder that may be amenable to treatment.[177] Partially treated or variants of CRPS may be subtly manifested and can be overlooked as "poor results" or "noncompliant patients." In the postoperative or post-traumatic period, unusual swelling, stiffness, pain, and restlessness may represent a dystrophic response.

The physical examination should include a neurologic assessment and evaluation of the cervical and thoracic spine. The presence of cervical disease (either discogenic or degenerative) may exacerbate CRPS—a form of "double crush syndrome." Cervical spine and shoulder range of motion should be recorded, and the brachial plexus should be evaluated. The arm should be assessed to rule out evidence of vascular or neurologic compression within the thoracic outlet. An adhesive capsulitis, or "shoulder-hand syndrome," is a frequent sequela that may be overlooked unless the shoulder is examined. Hypersensitivity, vascular adequacy, edema, sensibility, joint range of motion, motor function, grip, pinch, fibrosis, sweating, and vasomotor tone must be evaluated. Grip is frequently abnormal and should be assessed carefully.[112]

Mechanical Nociceptive Focus

The identification of nociceptive foci, which include peripheral nerve lesions and mechanical derangements, is important. Evaluation before and after sympatholytic intervention may delineate "trigger events" that might have initiated and/or propagated dystrophic symptoms.[177] Nociceptor input may be associated with SMP or SIP.[132] However, early diagnosis and prompt surgical correction of SMP associated with peripheral nerve injury is an effective management approach.[158]

Authors' Perspective

The manifestation of CRPS is quite variable, and a classic swollen painful hand is not always present. Commonly, the patient's condition is thought to be a "poor" result after surgery or minor trauma. Examination reveals subtle, yet retrospectively more obvious, symptoms and signs of a dystrophic process. The time course of CRPS may vary considerably, with mild symptoms preventing recovery without pathognomonic findings. Individual variability is tremendous. Many patients with undiagnosed CRPS recover spontaneously; others "smolder" in the early stage of dystrophy for prolonged periods of time. Occasionally, within a short time period patients progress rapidly from painful, hot, and swollen *to* painful, cold, and stiff, *to* stiff and painless. CRPS can affect a single digit, an isolated peripheral nerve distribution, or an entire limb. *Early diagnosis is aided by a high index of suspicion and the recognition that dystrophy can occur after any traumatic event.*

Diagnostic Testing

Pain Threshold Evaluation

The use of specific standardized evaluations and/or tests provides reproducible and objective information with regard to pain-pressure thresholds.[63,124]

Rubber-tipped algometers,[40] dolorimetry,[12] monofilaments,[172,176] computer-controlled stimuli,[195] or evaluations of thermal pain threshold[124,245] may be used to provide a quantitative measure of hyperpathia and/or allodynia. For example, pain perception from a 2.83 Von Frey monofilament (normally not painful) in a specified area or dermatomal distribution defines the extent of allodynia. Success or failure of treatment can be assessed by repeated evaluations. Decreased pain from the same-size or larger monofilament documents improvement; persistent pain from the same-size or a smaller-diameter monofilament suggests ineffective management. Monofilaments provide the most practical method to assess and monitor allodynia and hyperesthesia. Von Frey monofilaments are available in pocket kits, are inexpensive, and provide useful bedside sensibility and pain threshold data.

Radiography

Regional osteopenia can be seen on plain radiographs in approximately 80% of extremities affected by CRPS.[14,15,113,181] Significantly decreased mineralization is necessary for changes to be visualized on standard anteroposterior and lateral radiographs (see Fig. 57-3).[11] Classic Sudeck's atrophy includes diffuse osteopenia with juxtacortical demineralization and subchondral erosions or cysts. Genant and associates have described five radiographic patterns of resorption: irregular resorption of trabecular bone in the metaphysis creating a patchy appearance, subperiosteal bone resorption, intracortical bone resorption, endosteal bone resorption, and surface erosions in subchondral and juxtachondral bone.[113] Although osteopenia is more easily visualized in metaphyseal areas, recent data confirm that the densities of cortical and cancellous bone are affected equally in patients with CRPS.[13,30]

Bone Scan (Scintigraphy)

Three-phase technetium-99m bone scanning (TPBS) is performed commonly[25] and has assumed a significant role in the diagnosis of RSD.[64,179,180,206,241,276,314] With TPBS, the first or "dynamic" phase lasts 2 to 3 minutes and provides an assessment of digital perfusion; the second phase, "blood pool image" or "tissue phase," allows an assessment of total perfusion over a 3- to 5-minute period; and the third phase, a standard bone scan, evaluates radiotracer uptake in bony structures (Fig. 57-4).[310] In patients with CRPS, the use of a forearm or arm tourniquet or blood pressure cuff may affect radiotracer accumulation in the hands and/or in digits during phases I and II.[70] Traditionally, scans have been considered "positive" if there is asymmetrical flow in phases I, II, and/or III.[181] However, more recent reports suggest that the diagnostic yield of phase III alone equals the diagnostic yield of the three-phase scan (Fig. 57-5).[206,304] Mackinnon and Holder have stated that a "strictly interpreted" phase III scan with "diffuse increased tracer uptake in the delayed image is diagnostic for RSD."[144] Although a positive third-phase scan provides specific corroboration of the clinical diagnosis of CRPS, the sensitivity of scintigraphy is insufficient to provide stand-alone criteria and should be used to corroborate clinical suspicion. In the majority of studies, a "positive" scan has a high specificity but poor sensitivity.[64,175,181,241,304] Quantitative scintigraphy provides useful physiologic data, allows quantitative assessment of regional bone loss associated with complex regional pain,[30,69] and adds useful diagnostic information.[176] However, bone scan data do not correlate with symptoms, do not provide prognostic information, and are unable to aid in the prediction of which interventional approaches might be successful.[170,241]

In the majority of patients, abnormal bone turnover reflected in the TPBS is diffuse throughout the hand and wrist (see Fig. 57-5). The segmental distribution of RSD isolated to a digit, a single ray, or multiple rays can be evaluated by a bone scan to delineate the affected areas.[166]

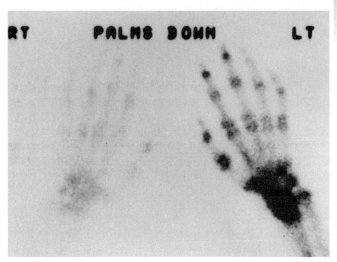

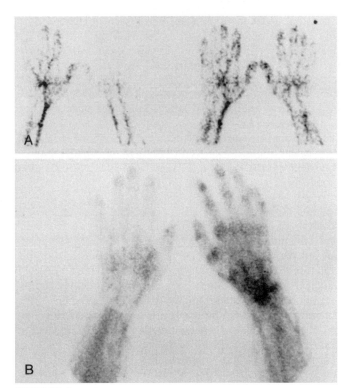

FIGURE 57-4. Three-phase bone scans. Phase I (**A**), a "dynamic phase," evaluates vascular perfusion by visual or quantitative analysis or radiotracer uptake after an intravenous injection. Each image represents a 3- to 5-second interval and allows an assessment of flow dynamics. Phase II (**B**), a "blood pool" image, documents total tissue uptake of tracer during the first 3 to 5 minutes after injection. Phase III is a conventional bone scan (see Fig. 57-5). (From Koman LA [ed]: Bowman Gray Orthopaedic Manual. Winston-Salem, NC, Orthopaedic Press, 1996.)

FIGURE 57-5. An abnormal (phase III) bone scan demonstrating increased periarticular uptake throughout the hand. This is a scan of the patient whose radiograph is seen in Figure 57-3. Notice the increased radiolucency at the fracture site. (From Koman LA [ed]: Bowman Gray Orthopaedic Manual. Winston-Salem, NC, Orthopaedic Press, 1996.)

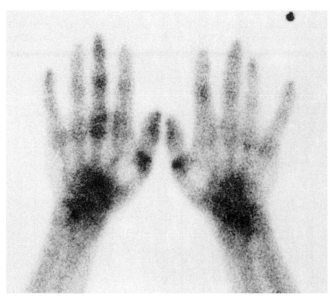

FIGURE 57-6. Segmental periarticular uptake confined to a digit in a bone scan of a patient with complex regional pain syndrome isolated to the long finger. (From Koman LA [ed]: Bowman Gray Orthopaedic Manual. Winston-Salem, NC, Orthopaedic Press, 1996.)

Although TPBS is used frequently, there is no evidence to support (1) diagnostic accuracy in variant or partially treated CRPS or late-stage CRPS,[143] (2) prognostic data that predict outcome,[174] or (3) value in determining management decisions.[143,170,172,177,241]

At this time, a "positive" third-phase bone scan is not a prerequisite for the diagnosis of CRPS or SMP.[185] Bone scans do not correlate with traditional staging criteria for RSD, are not part of the diagnosis of SMP or CRPS,[185,274,275] do not predict recovery, and will not predict the potential for response to treatment.[169,173,241,304] However, the presence of a positive third-phase bone scan provides objective support for the clinical diagnosis of CRPS.

Evaluation of Autonomic Control

Autonomic function controls sweating and microvascular perfusion. Evaluation of sympathetic control or, more specifically, sympathetic dysfunction associated with characteristic pain provides objective and sensitive methods to corroborate clinical suspicion of CRPS.

Regulation of Microvascular Flow

Under normal conditions, total digital blood flow is composed of 80% to 95% thermoregulatory flow and 5% to 20% nutritional flow; the distribution of nutritional versus thermoregulatory flow is governed by complex factors that control arteriovenous shunting.* Abnormal autonomic control of microvascular perfusion in patients with CRPS is reflected, in part, by ischemia secondary to inappropriate arteriovenous shunting and decreased nutritional flow.[150,174,183,215,237] The importance of nutritional flow in the pathogenesis of CRPS is supported by the segmental distribution of trophic events, the rapidity of action of successful sympatholytic interventions, and the similarity of pain patterns in patients with contrasting clinical findings. Abnormal arteriovenous shunting in bone has been documented in patients with CRPS.[69,215] Nutritional deprivation may exist

---

*See references 90, 91, 93, 94, 96, 173, 175, 232, and 241.

in both a "warm, swollen" hand with high total flow and a "cold, stiff" hand with low total flow. The common underlying finding in both clinical situations is the nutritional deprivation (Fig. 57-7). Pain relief in CRPS is not dependent on peripheral vasodilatation (thermoregulatory flow) after spinal cord stimulation,[162] suggesting the importance of nutritional flow. In addition, there is growing evidence that physiologic subgrouping, in contradistinction to staging based on timing, is important. For example, "warm" CRPS responds differently to intervention than "cold" CRPS.[238]

Total digital flow—composed of thermoregulatory and nutritional components—may be analyzed by digital temperature measurements, laser Doppler fluxmetry, and vital capillaroscopy.[24,90-96,149,150,174,237,241] *The use of a stressor to physiologic homeostasis—thermal, emotional, or ischemic—is necessary to obtain reproducible information, to evaluate dynamic response patterns over time, and to maximize sensitivity* (Fig. 57-8).[57,89,171,174,184] A technique that combines a stressor with measurement technique is isolated cold stress testing. In this procedure, total digital blood flow and microvascular perfusion may be evaluated by monitoring digital temperature and laser Doppler fluxmetry before, during, and after controlled stress.[175,240,241] The heterogeneity of digital microvascular perfusion may be analyzed by laser Doppler techniques and is reflected in average pulp temperature readings.[298] Nutritional flow may be measured directly by vital capillaroscopy (Fig. 57-9).[92,95,174] Analysis of temperature, laser Doppler fluxmetry, microvascular perfusion, and nutritional flow permits an objective determination of autonomic/vasomotor stability, as well as physiologic staging of autonomic-sympathetic performance, defines the adequacy of nutritional flow, and provides an assessment of the effects of interventions.[174,176,178,183,200,202] For example, the effectiveness of sympathetic blockade may be assessed by analysis of digital temperature measurements and microvascular perfusion during stress (Fig. 57-10). Laser Doppler perfusion imaging (LDPI) provides an assessment of perfusion over a 12 × 12-cm area and may be used to assess the effects of a sympathetic block on skin blood flow.[270]

Sudomotor Function

Analysis of sudomotor activity may be achieved by cumulative unstimulated resting sweat output,[200-203] QSART,[200-203] galvanic skin response,[178] combined temperature and peripheral autonomic surface potential (PASP) reflex response,[167] and analysis of sympathetic skin response (SSR) evoked by activation of sympathetic unmyelinated efferent fibers.[51,89,262] These techniques can be used to obtain quantitative measurements of sweat function, which then can be contrasted to contralateral or ipsilateral areas and/or normal controls. When combined with microvascular perfusion indices of temperature and/or laser Doppler fluxmetry, these data supplement the clinical examination, document autonomic dysfunction, and provide objective evidence of the effect(s) of intervention.[174,178,200-203]

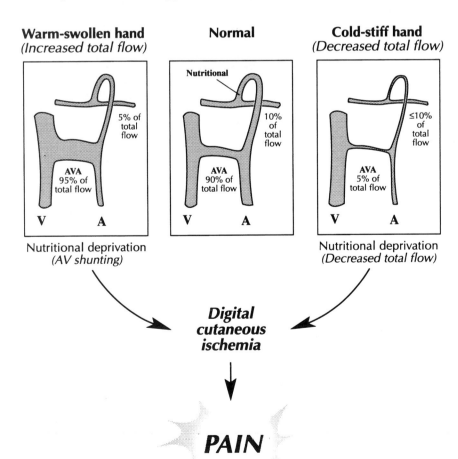

FIGURE 57-7. In a warm, swollen hand with increased total digital blood flow and in a cold stiff hand with decreased digital flow, abnormal arteriovenous (AV) control through arteriovenous anastomosis (AVA) may produce or contribute to abnormally decreased nutritional blood flow and pain. (From Koman LA [ed]: Bowman Gray Orthopaedic Manual. Winston-Salem, NC, Orthopaedic Press, 1996.)

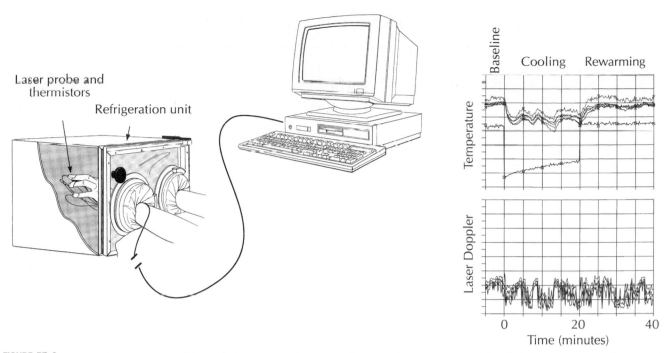

FIGURE 57-8. Digital microvascular physiology can be evaluated by using an isolated cold stress test combining digital temperature and laser Doppler fluxmetry measurements. Digital temperatures are monitored with thermistors attached to each digit of both extremities. Microvascular cutaneous perfusion is assessed with a laser Doppler probe attached to one digit of each extremity. Digital temperature and laser Doppler fluxmetry measurements are sampled by using custom computer software, and the results of the test are plotted for analysis. (From Koman LA [ed]: Bowman Gray Orthopaedic Manual. Winston-Salem, NC, Orthopaedic Press, 1996.)

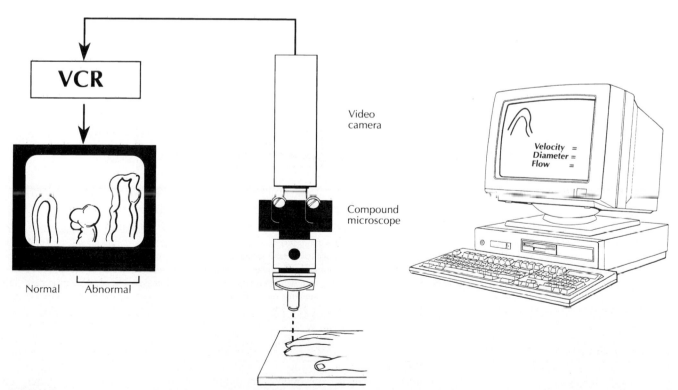

FIGURE 57-9. Nutritional capillaries may be visualized directly through a compound microscope, which provides visualization of cell motion within the capillaries and permits the identification of normal and/or abnormal capillary morphology. Videotape analysis facilitates quantitation of the diameter of the capillaries and velocity of flow within the ascending and descending capillary loop. Abnormal morphology diagnostic of collagen vascular disease can be observed. (From Koman LA [ed]: Bowman Gray Orthopaedic Manual. Winston-Salem, NC, Orthopaedic Press, 1996.)

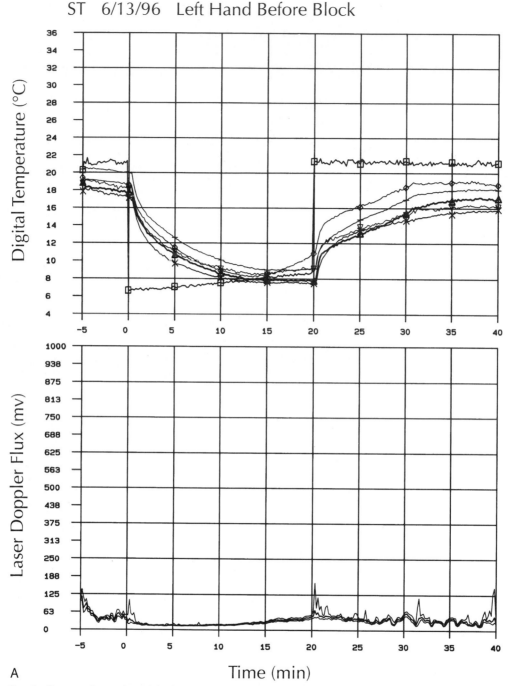

ST   6/13/96   Left Hand Before Block

A

Time (min)

FIGURE 57-10. Laser Doppler fluxmetry in a patient with clinical reflex sympathetic dystrophy before (**A**) and after (**B**) sympathetic blockade. Temperature of all five fingers of the left hand and the environmental temperature *(indicated by squares)* are plotted in the upper portion of the graphs. Laser Doppler measurements were monitored with a probe placed on the left ring finger. Baseline temperatures and laser Doppler measurements were taken for 5 minutes. For the cooling phase, the hands were inserted into the refrigeration unit for 5 minutes. After cooling, the hands were removed from the unit and allowed to rewarm at room temperature. After the sympathetic block, digital temperatures were increased markedly during all phases of the testing procedure. The amplitude of laser Doppler flux was increased after the block, thus confirming modulation of sympathetic input (chemical sympathectomy). (From Koman LA [ed]: Bowman Gray Orthopaedic Manual. Winston-Salem, NC, Orthopaedic Press, 1996.) *Continued*

Diagnostic Sympathetic Blockade

CRPS may be sympathetically maintained (SMP) or sympathetically independent (SIP). Relief after sympatholytic interventions defines SMP. Pain relief after parenteral, oral, or topical pharmacologic preparations or after neural blockade confirms the influence of the sympathetic nervous system and supports receptor-mediated abnormalities.[247,]

[249,275] Pain relief after an intravenous injection of phentolamine (a mixed α_1- and α_2-adrenergic blocking agent) is considered presumptive evidence of SMP,[249] or it may be considered diagnostic for SMP.[247] Phentolamine testing is compromised unless the drug is administered in conjunction with placebo injections. Intravenous phentolamine may produce profound transient side effects, including headache

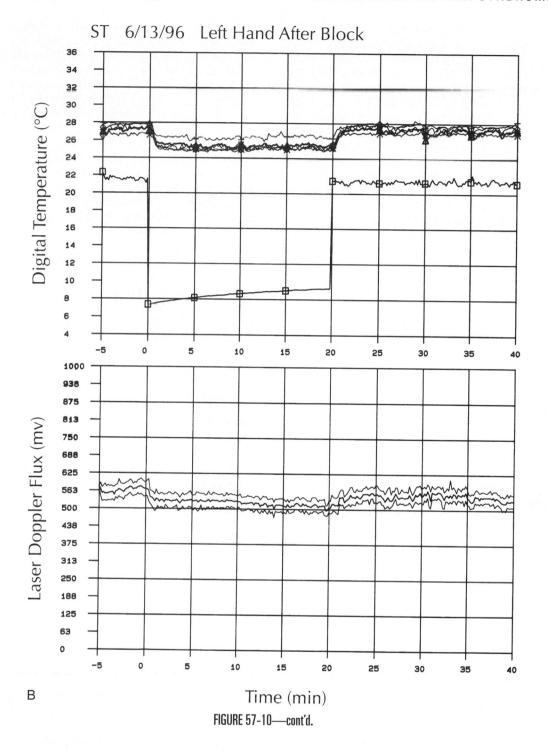

ST   6/13/96   Left Hand After Block

B

Time (min)

FIGURE 57-10—cont'd.

and hypotension. However, such administration negates the concerns over inadequate needle placement (e.g., stellate block) or dose delivery (e.g., somatic nerve block) that are associated with pharmacologic blockades and the need to verify sympatholysis.[274,310] Unlike other pharmacologic end-organ blockers (e.g., bretylium, guanethidine, reserpine), phentolamine has no therapeutic indications and is used only as a diagnostic modality. Recent data indicate that adequate sympathetic blockade does not consistently correlate with the extent of pain relief and that the duration and density of the block may alter clinical response.[287]

Regional Blockade

Sympathetically maintained pain may be diagnosed by nerve blocks of the stellate ganglion, epidural space, brachial plexus, or peripheral nerves.[178] Diagnostic blocks are usually obtained with short-acting or intermediate-acting local anesthetics (e.g., lidocaine). A stellate ganglion block is the most common diagnostic test performed in patients with CRPS. Stellate ganglion blocks may be achieved by injections at the transverse process of C6 (Chassaignac's tubercle) or by a medial approach at C7 (see Chapter 2).[274] Injection of the stellate ganglion or sympathetic trunk adequate to obtain sympatholysis is dependent on variations in patient anatomy, the presence or absence of scarring in or around the sympathetic chain, drug diffusion characteristics, and the ability and skill of the administrator. Therefore, adequate interpretation of results requires verification of sympatholysis. This can be accomplished by indirect signs such as Horner's syndrome, nasal congestion, and/or facial anhidrosis or by direct evidence of sympathetic nerve block such as an increase in temperature (≥3°C), venous engorgement of the hand veins, dry skin, changes in skin color, and characteristic laser Doppler changes (see Fig. 21-11).[175,211,274] Indirect "signs" of blockade are mediated by preganglionic fibers and can occur without sympathetic blockade. Therefore, it is imperative to have objective evidence of blockade before dismissing patients or declaring patients as having SIP. Effective stellate ganglion blocks—even when administered by experienced anesthesiologists—occur in only 70% to 75% of cases.[274] Therefore, objective determination of the adequacy/effectiveness of autonomic blockade is important.[211] Furthermore, a patient who does not respond favorably to peripheral sympathetic blockade may have symptomatic relief with a continuous sympathetic block or from epidural blockade.[53]

Thermography

Thermographic techniques provide a large quantity of temperature data, allow comparison of both upper extremities, and permit rapid repeated measurements over time.[83,98] However, peer-reviewed data do not support the use of thermography as a superior alternative to other conventional diagnostic modalities.[16] Recent data suggest that higher temperatures indicated by thermography do not correlate with skin surface flow in RSD,[215] and the use of temperature alone cannot distinguish RSD from "chronic upper limb pain."[57] Thermographic data must be interpreted strictly to be effective. Misleading color-coded asymmetry patterns may be created by inappropriate sensitivity settings; that is, settings should exceed 0.5°C to 1.0°C per color band.[266] Repeated measurements over time from the same subject(s) are reproducible, are consistent, reflect skin blood flow, and correlate with symptoms in a variety of painful pathologic entities.[266] The use of a stressor strengthens thermographic data, which is a reflection of total skin blood flow,[131,175] and significantly improves the predictive and diagnostic value of telethermography.[131]

Endurance Testing

Objective evaluation of extremity function can be accomplished by using standardized tests and computerized analysis systems. These evaluations document overall functional capacity, verify gross and fine motor skills, and quantitate strength and endurance. Repeating these measures over time provides a sensitive and reproducible methodology that is capable of delineating subtle functional deficits, documenting the effects of intervention (management), and defining the magnitude of permanent impairment.[172,176,178]

Authors' Approach to Diagnosis

Because successful treatment of CRPS is influenced positively by the rapidity of diagnosis and treatment, early clinical recognition of this syndrome is crucial. A dystrophic process should be considered in all patients experiencing pain that is out of proportion to the traumatic or surgical insult and that is inappropriately influencing function or outcome. High-risk groups for CRPS include patients with peripheral nerve injury, distal radius and ulna fractures, or crushing trauma; however, CRPS may affect any person with an injury. In the postoperative period, painful and excessive swelling combined with vasoconstriction or vasodilatation suggests CRPS. The diagnosis of CRPS is clinical, and symptoms must include pain, trophic change, autonomic dysfunction, and functional deficit. If the diagnosis is suspected, instruments to quantitate pain (e.g., McGill Pain Questionnaire and VAS),[222] overall symptoms, and function (e.g., self-administered carpal tunnel questionnaire)[190] are administered. Objective measures of hyperpathia/allodynia are preferred, if possible, and responses to measured stimuli such as monofilaments are quantifiable. Edema is estimated or measured by volumetric analysis. Function is assessed by questionnaires and/or verified by standardized methods (e.g., grip, pinch, Moberg pickup test, computerized instrumentation). The use of standard instruments, appropriate questionnaires, and reproducible objective tests assists in confirming the diagnosis and aids in monitoring the efficacy of interventions.

Physiologic staging of autonomic function is determined by an analysis of temperature and laser Doppler fluxmetry before, during, and after a cold stress. Nutritional capillary perfusion is assessed by vital capillaroscopy. Temperature and laser Doppler fluxmetry data provide reproducible and sensitive information that provides an estimate of physiologic function, documents pathophysiology, and guides treatment decisions. Although not used routinely, TPBS (bone scan) provides confirmative information when combined with clinical prerequisites. Intravenous phentolamine, stellate ganglion blocks, epidural injections, or somatic nerve blocks are used to verify the presence of SMP and predict the efficacy of oral sympatholytic drugs. After the use of oral or parenteral sympatholytic medications, the location of any identifiable nociceptive foci is identified.

HISTORICAL REVIEW

- Ambrose Paré, 16th century: burning pain after phlebotomy of Charles IX
- Percivall Pott, 1771: pain after nerve injury
- Silas Weir Mitchell, 1864: description of causalgia
- Leriche, 1916: post-traumatic "burning" pain
- Sudek, 1900: bone demineralization
- Evan, 1947, and Bonica, 1973: term *reflex sympathetic dystrophy*
- Complex regional pain syndrome, 1991

Silas Weir Mitchell published the first descriptions of dystrophic pain after peripheral nerve trauma.[225,226] The term *causalgia* (Gk., "burning pain") was used to describe symptoms after partial disruption of the median nerve and transection of the brachial artery.[225,226] Since Mitchell's description, pain after trauma or injury has received a great deal of attention. Post-traumatic persistent burning pain, abnormal vasoconstriction/vasodilatation, and diminished function were attributed to the sympathetic nervous system by Leriche in 1916.[188,189] The importance of distinguishing

SMP from SIP was emphasized by Roberts in the 1980s[254] and that importance has been reemphasized in the 1990s.[1]

Regional demineralization *(inflammatory bone atrophy)* accompanying post-traumatic pain was described by Sudek in 1900.[282] The term *reflex sympathetic dystrophy* was introduced by Evans[88] in 1947 and was expanded to include secondary peripheral and central neurovascular events by Bonica[36-38] in 1973. The term *reflex sympathetic dystrophy* is firmly entrenched in medical, lay, and legal documents and is used synonymously with a large variety of descriptors (see Table 57-1). It is believed by many to be inappropriately broad[1,6,76,153,154,274] because it implies—without significant documentation—that the sympathetic nervous system is causally related to the entire process.[38,154,235] RSD has been characterized as a disease of "medical understanding" in the absence of a discrete pathophysiologic disorder.[234] Recent emphasis has been placed on clarifying these taxonomic difficulties. Dobyns proposed that abnormal function related to pain should be grouped broadly under the term *pain dysfunction syndrome.*[5,76] Subsequent investigators have stressed the importance of differentiating SMP from SIP and have defined the former as a better descriptor of RSD.[1,172] However, recent reports regard the concept of SMP as questionable because of the lack of proper placebo controls and the failure to include chronic "neuropathic" subjects.[244,294,295] To avoid undocumented emphasis on the sympathetic nervous system and to prioritize clinical characteristics, CRPS has been proposed as an inclusive category that includes subgroups based on clinical and/or pathophysiologic manifestations of dystrophic pain.[153,154] Under the CRPS system, disorders previously considered to be RSD and causalgia are classified as CRPS type 1 and type 2, respectively (see Table 57-2). These disorders can be differentiated further into SMP or SIP depending on the response to sympathetic interventions.[35,153,154]

PHYSIOLOGY OF PAIN

Normally, pain is perceived only in the presence of actual or impending cellular tissue damage; in the absence of continued trauma, persistent pain is pathologic. Painful peripheral nociceptive experiences that include cellular damage produce secondary inflammation by activating and sensitizing polymodal low-threshold mechanoreceptors and nociceptor afferent neurons, which produce, in theory, ectopic chemosensitivity to α-adrenergic agonists.[55,72,77] This information is relayed via the process of *transduction* through small myelinated (Aδ), large myelinated (Aβ), and small unmyelinated (C) afferent fibers to the dorsal horn of the spinal cord, where *sensitization* of wide dynamic range (WDR) neurons contributes to central nociceptive discharge (Fig. 57-11A).[45,77,212,236,239] Within the dorsal horn, excitatory amino acids serve as the principal neurotransmitters. Transmitters include *N*-glutamate, aspartate, α-amino-3-hydroxy-5-methyl-4-isoxazopropionic acid (AMPA), *N*-methyl-D-aspartate (NMDA), and substance P. Of these, the NMDA receptor-transmitter interaction produces long-lasting potentials, is refractory to stimulation, and is theorized to play an important role in CRPS types 1 and 2.[151] Nociceptive input is modulated via descending pathways, and both peripheral and central factors are required for the

perception of pain (see Fig. 57-11B).[43,44] Pain intensity is determined by the magnitude and extent of the initiating/ongoing event, afferent input, efferent modulation, and central nervous system (CNS) interpretation. The conscious appreciation of nociceptive (painful) experiences is dependent on a complex interplay of afferent and efferent information modulated and balanced by physiologic adaptations. Vasomotor disturbances may result from a variety of mechanisms, including antidromic vasodilation, vasoparalytic dilatation, normal somatosensory reflexes, and denervation supersensitivity.[77] Responses to nociceptive stimuli may vary significantly among individuals. The presence of nociceptive-induced inappropriate transmitter-receptor activity can affect peripheral microcirculatory control and thereby result in impaired nutritive flow[174,175,182,237,258] and may sensitize CNS pathways.[77]

Perception of Pain

By definition, CRPS does not exist in the absence of pain. Peripheral injury stimulates endogenous inflammatory mediators via nociceptive pathways. Repetitive trauma/injury may alter protective responses by producing earlier activation through sensitization. In addition to providing central input, local nociceptors initiate the direct release of peptides and neurotransmitters, control the inflammatory process, and promote tissue repair. Pain requires cognitive recognition.

Pain Mediators/Receptor Control

A variety of non-neurogenic and neurogenic mediators participate in the transmission of information interpreted as pain. Non-neurogenic mediators include bradykinin, serotonin, histamine, acetylcholine, prostaglandins E_1 and E_2, and leukotrienes. Neurogenic mediators—biologically active peptides produced by primary afferent neurons—potentiate or inhibit nociceptive information. These mediators include substance P, vasoactive intestinal peptide, calcitonin gene-related peptide, gastrin-releasing peptide, dynorphin, enkephalin, galanin, somatostatin, cholecystokinin, γ-aminobutyric acid, dopamine, and glycine.[169]

The role of α-adrenergic receptors and local blood flow in sympathetically maintained complex regional pain states is well documented,[44,46,72,86,108,145,247,248,251] and relief of pain after intravenous phentolamine—a mixed α_1 and α_2 antagonist—is considered pathognomonic for SMP (CRPS type 1).[249,250] Abnormal regulation of adrenoreceptor function and/or modulation in neural and vascular structures is the major common control pathway supporting the concept that RSD (SMP) is a *receptor disease.*[104,247,248] Presynaptic and postsynaptic receptors are involved and affect nociceptive foci, blood flow, nutritional perfusion, and peripheral nerve excitability.* The pathologic mechanisms involved in the compromise of extremity blood flow and neural control include (1) abnormal neurotransmitter release secondary to nociceptive foci, (2) abnormal receptor distribution, and/or (3) alterations in receptor sensitivity (e.g., up- or down-regulation).

---

*See references 24, 62, 84, 174, 183, 237, 239, 247, and 258.

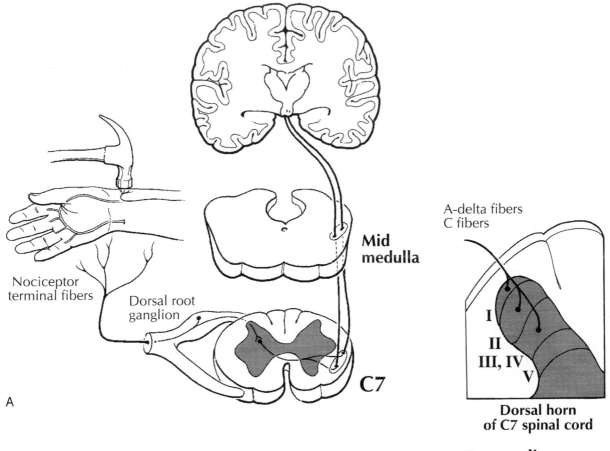

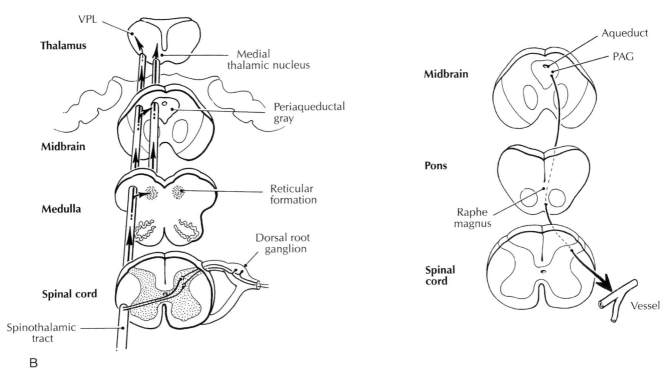

FIGURE 57-11. A, Abnormal central nervous system modulation of afferent sensory stimuli may contribute to the development of a dystrophic response after an injury that produces a peripheral nociceptive focus or "trigger." **B,** Ascending and descending pathways in the spinal cord and brain. PAG, periaqueductal gray matter; VPL, ventral posterolateral nucleus. (From Koman LA [ed]: Bowman Gray Orthopaedic Manual. Winston-Salem, NC, Orthopaedic Press, 1996.)

Gate Theory of Pain

The "gate theory" is an appropriate aid in the conceptualization of pain. The theory assumes that a finite amount of information can be received at the spinal cord or cortical level. The "gate" is the dorsal horn of the spinal cord. Thus, painful information displaced or modified by less noxious input cannot be processed through the gate. Although as yet unproven, certain general principles relating to pain processing can be conceptualized by using this theorem.[223]

Acute Versus Chronic Pain

Acute pain is initiated during tissue injury or destruction, and the presence of acute pain may be beneficial or harmful. Beneficial effects include physiologic responses for the maintenance of blood pressure, cardiac output, intravascular volume, and appropriate homeostasis. Acute pain warns the host of danger, prevents inappropriate motion of an injured extremity, and may diminish additional harm from repetitive injury. Persistence of pain beyond the need for protective action is unpleasant and may induce hypertension, tachycardia, coagulopathy, hyperglycemia, anxiety, fear, and chronic pain. Chronic pain that occurs in the absence of ongoing tissue destruction or that provides an inappropriate reflection of intensity, magnitude, and/or duration of tissue damage/compromise is pathologic. Although the pathophysiology of chronic pain is incompletely understood, the following processes can contribute to its establishment: persistent mechanical irritation of peripheral neural structures, incomplete regeneration of peripheral nerves, abnormal neurotransmitter activity, nutritional deprivation secondary to abnormal arteriovenous shunting, and/or central imprinting.

After trauma or surgery, a transient period of dystrophic extremity function is normal. It is abnormal for hyperpathia (increased pain), allodynia (painful responses to normally nonpainful stimuli), vasomotor disturbances, and functional deficiencies to persist. If untreated, these conditions may progress to permanent compromise of the extremity. Posttraumatic alterations in extremity physiology follow a variable time course. Therefore, the abnormal prolongation of these otherwise normal responses is pathologic, and, over time, irreversible changes in anatomic structures or physiologic processes may occur (Fig. 57-12). *CRPS may therefore be considered an abnormally severe and/or prolonged manifestation of a normal postinjury response.* Abnormally prolonged dystrophic events may damage or compromise the arteriovenous shunt mechanism,[174,183] produce arthrofibrosis,[174] cause excessive osteopenia,[30] alter neuroreceptor function,[247,248] and/or result in central pain imprinting.[176]

TREATMENT

Principles

The efficacy of pharmacologic and therapeutic modalities cannot be predicted reliably by existing classifications or diagnostic categories. Therefore, a treatment approach that relies on pathophysiologic findings and functional considerations has distinct clinical advantages and provides information that allows the use of medications in a specific and consistent fashion. Patients with CRPS may have SMP or SIP. In general, patients with the latter have a poorer prognosis, do not respond as well to sympatholytic modalities, and may be more likely to progress to chronic pain and disability. The diagnosis of sympathetically independent CRPS should be reserved for patients with CRPS (1) that was but is no longer relieved by sympatholytic intervention and/or (2) that has the clinical symptoms and signs of CRPS—pain, atrophy, autonomic dysfunction, and functional impairment—but is not relieved by sympatholytic

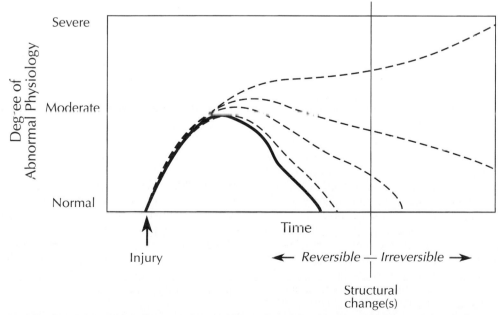

FIGURE 57-12. Abnormal physiologic events after trauma are "normal"; the majority of patients *(solid line)* recover spontaneously from the trauma. An abnormal prolongation of the intensity of these events and dystrophic pain of varying magnitude and duration *(broken lines)* is pathologic. Irreversible changes may occur and convert sympathetically maintained pain to sympathetically independent pain. (From Koman LA [ed]: Bowman Gray Orthopaedic Manual. Winston-Salem, NC, Orthopaedic Press, 1996.)

intervention. Identification and localization of a nociceptive focus provide significant etiologic information. The correction of a nociceptive abnormality by surgical intervention may improve recovery and diminish the need for prolonged use of medication.[158] After a favorable response to oral sympatholytics, it may be possible to identify a specific cutaneous nerve injury, correct this underlying mechanical nerve problem, facilitate recovery, and improve functional outcome. By definition, patients with CRPS type 2 (causalgia) have an identifiable or documented peripheral nerve injury. Surgical interventions that correct nerve damage or protect the nerve may decrease the nociceptive focus, lessen symptoms, and enhance function.[158] Similarly, patients with CRPS type 1 (classic RSD) may have a non-neural or mechanical nociceptive focus, which if corrected will facilitate recovery of the extremity.[176]

The choice of intervention may be influenced by physiologic staging, which, in turn, facilitates the selection of appropriate pharmacologic agents. The goal should be to correct the pathophysiologic manifestations of CRPS. Before treatment selection, clinical or laboratory testing should determine (1) the extent of sympathetic tone (increased, normal, or decreased); (2) the presence or absence of edema; (3) the amount of total digital flow (as elevated, normal, or decreased); and (4) the status of nutritional flow (decreased or normal).

If sympathetic tone is increased (based on clinical judgment or objective testing), sympatholytic medications aimed at correction of neural or vascular adrenergic tone should be used. On occasion, the only manifestation of abnormal tone may be inappropriate arteriovenous shunting with decreased nutritional flow. Edema should be managed with physical modalities or specific pharmacologic management. Estimates of total blood flow and the components of flow may also guide treatment decisions. In summary, *treatment of CRPS is complex and may involve simultaneous and/or sequential use of a myriad of modalities.*

Therapy and Adaptive Modalities

Multidisciplinary Approach to Management

Although CRPS can be managed effectively by a single physician, a multidisciplinary team approach is often advisable to optimize outcome. Professional input from the surgeon, primary care practitioner, psychologist, hand therapist, case worker, and/or psychiatrist is often beneficial. The inclusion of a rehabilitation specialist, case worker, and/or workers' compensation coordinator may be of benefit. The lead member is determined by the circumstances of the pain process. For example, in the acute phase of CRPS type 2 after a distal radius fracture and median nerve injury, care is often best coordinated by a hand surgeon. Under other circumstances, a primary care physician, anesthesiologist, or psychologist might be the most appropriate to coordinate care (e.g., in a patient with CRPS type 1 with persistent symptoms after more than a year of active treatment). Pain clinics are a valuable resource, should be incorporated into management plans, and should not be used as a "dumping ground." Continued involvement of the initial treating physician throughout the process optimizes management. After the dystrophic process is quieted, one or more mechanical foci may be evident that will not be apparent to an isolated practitioner. A physician who understands the injury process and is knowledgeable in the diagnosis and management of upper extremity disorders should be involved in the ongoing management of the patient.

Authors' Preferred Method— A Multidisciplinary Approach

Our management protocol involves the use of anesthesiologists, a pain control clinic, psychologists, case workers, and therapists. In acute active phases of the dystrophic process, the diagnostic testing and treatment decisions are coordinated through our offices in concert with a hand therapist and the case manager. Direct referrals for specific evaluations and/or treatments are made as needed. If blocks are required, referral is made to an anesthesia-directed pain clinic, where resuscitative equipment and skilled personnel are available. The choice of intervention is discussed with the physician administering the block(s), and follow-up is coordinated in both offices. In more chronic cases, patients are referred for primary management or consultation, depending on the circumstances.

Hand Therapy

The use of physical therapy in the management of CRPS is well supported.[133,172,302] Therapeutic regimens should address the entire limb. Restricted shoulder motion from secondary adhesive capsulitis is often insidious in onset and debilitating over time. Maintenance (or restoration) of shoulder motion is necessary to optimize recovery,[80] and it may have a profoundly positive impact on health-related quality of life. If present, limited elbow motion may be debilitating. Joints in close proximity to the area of trauma and the small joints of the hand and wrist are most frequently involved with arthrofibrosis and secondary restricted range of motion. Prevention of arthrofibrosis is important because, once established, it is difficult to manage. Although physical therapy modalities alone may provide dramatic improvement,[302] many patients require concomitant pharmacologic intervention and adaptive therapies[172,176] and/or surgery.[133,158] *The mainstay of therapy should include active and passive range of motion, including stress-loading activities, transcutaneous electrical nerve stimulation (TENS) desensitization techniques, and/or sensory re-education.*

Adaptive Modalities

Adaptive therapeutic modalities include TENS, contrast baths, continuous passive motion, intermittent positive pressure with pneumatic pumps, and hydrotherapy.[2,110,198,221,252] TENS units are theorized to decrease pain by blocking input and have been shown to increase extremity blood flow.[252]

Pharmacologic Interventions

On the basis of empirical, theoretic, and documented modes of action, a variety of oral, topical, and parenteral pharmacologic interventions are used to treat CRPS. Theoretic mechanisms of drugs that control pain associated with dystrophic or causalgic responses include membrane stabilization (e.g., anticonvulsants, local anesthetics), competitive inhibition of neurotransmitters (e.g., bretylium, guanethidine), receptor blockade (e.g., terazosin), blockade of end-organ effects of sympathetic stimulation (e.g., nifedipine), desensitization of central pain-signaling neurons (e.g., α_1- and α_2-blocking agents), and blockade of sympathetic-somatic coupling (e.g., guanethidine). Some of these drugs may exhibit more than one mode of action (e.g., guanethidine). Few of the drugs used in the management of CRPS are listed for "pain management" in the accompanying package insert approved by the U.S. Food and Drug Administration (FDA). Rather, their usage is based on largely empirical data and an assessment of risk/benefit. *Before using the drugs discussed in this chapter, each practitioner should be familiar with the pharmacology, side effects, potential complications, indications, and contraindications for each* (see accompanying tables).

Oral and Topical Medications

Antidepressants

Antidepressants are frequently used in the management of chronic pain. Originally they were used empirically to relieve post-traumatic depression; however, they also provide analgesia and modulate sympathetic hyperactivity in the peripheral and central nervous system.[61,97,207,228,288,301] Antidepressants used in CPRS include tricyclic antidepressants, tetracyclic antidepressants, atypical antidepressants, and selective serotonin reuptake inhibitors.

Tricyclic antidepressants, which have been used since the early 1960s, are the most common agents used in the management of CRPS. A decrease in SMP is based on interference with postganglionic reuptake of amines, down-regulation and desensitization of presynaptic α_2 and serotonergic receptors, and reduction of the synthesis and release of norepinephrine.[279,288] Variation in the biogenic amines of each of these antidepressants produces differential receptor affinity and accounts for the differences in clinical response. Therefore, one antidepressant may prove efficacious in one patient and not in another. The most commonly used tricyclic antidepressants include imipramine, amitriptyline, doxepin, desipramine, nortriptyline, and protriptyline (Table 57-4).[61,85]

Drug selection should be individualized to account for potential side effects, drug interactions, comorbid conditions, previous response to the drug, and patient age. The most common side effects of tricyclic antidepressants are anticholinergic, cardiovascular, and CNS effects (see Table 57-4). Long-term treatment with these drugs is tolerated, and abrupt discontinuation should be avoided because of the potential untoward side-effects. Chronic treatment requires physician monitoring.

The *tetracyclic antidepressant* maprotiline (Ludiomil) is pharmacologically similar to imipramine and blocks the reuptake of norepinephrine more than that of serotonin. The anticholinergic properties of this drug are significant and may complicate its use (see Table 57-4).

Trazodone (Desyrel), an *atypical antidepressant*, can be used to treat CRPS. Mechanisms include preferential blocking of the reuptake of serotonin and binding to adrenergic (α_1 and α_2) receptors.[139] Once-per-day dosing is possible; however, the effects of α-adrenergic blockade are often difficult to tolerate and include tremor, hypertension, bradycardia, dizziness, and sedation.

The use of *selective serotonin reuptake inhibitors*, or second-generation antidepressants, has increased in prevalence significantly over the past decade. These drugs include fluvoxamine (Luvox), paroxetine (Paxil), fluoxetine (Prozac), and sertraline (Zoloft) (Table 57-5).[224,291] Selective serotonin reuptake inhibitors bind preferentially to the presynaptic serotonin carrier in the CNS and thereby inhibit serotonin reuptake. Side effects, which may be significant, tend to diminish after 1 to 2 weeks. Even though the efficacy of selective serotonin reuptake inhibitors used in treating chronic pain is not well defined, these agents are used frequently for that purpose. Selective serotonin reuptake inhibitors are commonly used in conjunction with low-dose tricyclic antidepressants; the use of both drugs has a synergistic effect in many patients. Tricyclic antidepressants exhibit greater sympatholytic effect and should be used before or in addition to a serotonin reuptake inhibitor.

Anticonvulsants

Anticonvulsants were first used to treat hyperpathic pain and later to treat CRPS.[48,220] Although their mechanism of action is unknown, it is postulated that these compounds stabilize excitable nerve membranes, limit neuronal hyperexcitability, and inhibit trans-synaptic neuronal impulses in the CNS.[42,139,156,207,279] Anticonvulsants are often used in combination with other medications (e.g., tricyclic antidepressants). Phenytoin (Dilantin), carbamazepine (Tegretol), valproic acid (Depakene), and gabapentin (Neurontin) are the most commonly used anticonvulsants in the management of CRPS (Table 57-6).

Membrane-Stabilizing Agents

The oral use of local anesthetics provides a new approach to the management of CRPS.[139,228,286,300] Local anesthetics selectively depress neuronal activity within the spinal cord, decrease C fiber polysynaptic conduction, reduce α motor neuron reflexes, and diminish noxious thermal and chemical reflexes.[61] However, the exact mechanism by which local anesthetics reduce pain is unclear. The development of oral membrane-stabilizing agents was based on the observation that lidocaine, when used intravenously, provided relief from chronic pain.[139,300] Tocainide (Tonocard) and mexiletine (Mexitil) are available as oral medications (Table 57-7). Unfortunately, the side effects of tocainide are common (40% to 80% of patients experience side effects) and include serious idiosyncratic reactions such as interstitial pneumonitis, psychosis, encephalopathy, neutropenia, lupus-like syndrome, agranulocytosis, anemia, hepatitis, and convulsions. Mexiletine is less commonly associated with severe complications, but known drug reactions associated with its use include lupus-like syndrome, abnormal liver function, blood dyscrasias, and impotence.[139] Therefore, the use of these drugs in patients with CRPS is limited to very severe and/or refractory cases.

Adrenergic Compounds

The role of α-adrenergic receptors and transmitters is well documented in CRPS with SMP (Table 57-8).[10,61] Adrenergic agents useful in the management and/or diagnosis of SMP and variant forms of CRPS include α_1 antag-

Table 57-4
ANTIDEPRESSANTS

Drug	Mechanism of Action		Dosage (Range)	Common Side Effects				
	Action	Efficacy		Anticholinergic Effects	Orthostatic Seizures	Conduction Hypotension	Abnormalities	Sedation
Tricyclic Antidepressants								
Imipramines (Tofranil, SK-pramines)	Blocks reuptake of amines Serotonin Norepinephrine	++++ ++	50-75 mg (50-300 mg)	+++	+++	++++	++++	++
Amitriptyline	Blocks reuptake of amines Serotonin Norepinephrine	++++ ++	25-75 mg (50-300 mg)	++++	+++	+++	++++	++++
Doxepin (Sinequan, Adapin)	Blocks reuptake of amines Serotonin Norepinephrine	+++ ++	50-75 mg (50-300 mg)	+++	+++	++	++	++++
Desipramines (Norpramin, Pertofrane)	Blocks reuptake of amines Serotonin Norepinephrine	+++ ++	50-75 mg (50-300 mg)	+++	++	+++	+++	++
Nortriptyline (Aventyl, Pamelor)	Blocks reuptake of amines Serotonin Norepinephrine	+++ +++	25-50 mg (50-150 mg)	+++	++	+	+++	+++
Protriptyline (Vivactil)	Blocks reuptake of amines Serotonin Norepinephrine	+++ ++++	10-20 mg (15-60 mg)	+++	++	++	++++	+
Tetracyclic Antidepressants								
Maprotiline (Ludiomil)	Blocks reuptake of amines Serotonin Norepinephrine	+ ++	50-75 mg (50-225 mg)	+++	++++	++	+++	+++
Atypical Antidepressants								
Trazodone (Desyrel)	Blocks reuptake of amines Serotonin Norepinephrine	+++ ±	50-150 mg (50-600 mg)	+	++	+++	+	+++

++++, Marked; +++, moderate; ++, minimal; +, none.

From Koman LA (ed): Bowman Gray Orthopaedic Manual. Winston-Salem, NC, Orthopaedic Press, 1996.

Table 57-5
SELECTIVE SEROTONIN REUPTAKE INHIBITORS

	Fluvoxamine (Luvox)	Fluoxetine (Prozac)	Paroxetine (Paxil)	Sertraline (Zoloft)
Blocks Presynaptic Serotonin Reuptake	Moderate serotonin affinity	Minimal serotonin affinity	Pronounced serotonin affinity	Moderate serotonin affinity
Dosage	Start at 50/mg/day, increase to 100-300 mg/day	20-80 mg/day	Initially 20 mg/day Average, 50-100 mg/day (titrate to effect)	Initially 50 mg/day Average, 50-100 mg/day (titrate to effect)
Common Side Effects	Headaches, nausea, sleep disorders	CNS: headache, sleep disorders, agitation GI: nausea Other: chills, weight loss	CNS: asthenia, sleep disorders GI: nausea Other: male sexual dysfunction	CNS: agitation, sleep disorders, headache GI: nausea Other: male sexual dysfunction

From Koman LA (ed): Bowman Gray Orthopaedic Manual. Winston-Salem, NC, Orthopaedic Press, 1996.

Table 57-6
ANTICONVULSANTS

	Phenytoin (Dilantin)	Carbamazepine (Tegretol)	Valproic Acid/Valproate (Depakene)	Gabapentin (Neurontin)
Starting Dose (Maximum Dose, mg)	100 mg tid (up to 400 mg/day)	100 mg bid (1200 mg/day)	250 mg qid (3000 mg/day)	600-800 mg tid (2400 mg/day)
Mechanism of Action	Membrane stabilization	Blocks sodium influx across cell membranes	Stimulates GABA production	Unknown; assumed to be GABA related
Side Effects				
Gastrointestinal	Nausea, vomiting, constipation, hepatitis, liver damage	Nausea, vomiting, jaundice (hepatocellular, cholestatic)	Nausea, vomiting	Anorexia, flatulence
Hematologic	Thrombocytopenia, leukopenia, megaloblastic anemia	Aplastic anemia, agranulocytosis, thrombocytopenia	Thrombocytopenia, anemias, clotting disorders	Purpura
CNS	Nystagmus, ataxia, dizziness, convulsion	Dizziness, drowsiness, ataxia	Sedation, tremor, hallucinations, headache	Somnolence, dizziness, ataxia
Other	Rashes	Rashes, epidermal neurolysis, congestive heart failure	Hepatic failure, dysmenorrhea, pancreatitis	Fatigue, hypertension
Contraindications	Liver disease, pregnancy	Bone marrow depression, simultaneous monoamine oxidase inhibitors	Liver disease, pregnancy	Care must be taken in patients with renal disease

GABA, γ-Aminobutyric acid.

From Koman LA (ed): Bowman Gray Orthopaedic Manual. Winston-Salem, NC, Orthopaedic Press, 1996.

Table 57-7

COMPARATIVE CHARACTERISTICS OF INTRAVENOUS AND ORAL LOCAL ANESTHETIC AGENTS USED FOR CHRONIC PAIN: MEMBRANE-STABILIZING AGENTS

	Lidocaine	Mexiletine (Mexitil)	Tocainide (Tonocard)
Dosage	3 mg/kg (range, 2-6 mg/kg). Test dose over 20-30 min	10 mg/kg/day	20 mg/kg/day
Side Effects			
Cardiovascular	Bradycardia, hypotension	Palpitations, chest pain, syncope	Hypotension, ventricular arrhythmias
CNS	Dizziness, nervousness, apprehension, euphoria	Dizziness, tremor, headache	Dizziness Uncommon: encephalopathy and psychosis
Other		Nausea, vomiting	Blood dyscrasias, pulmonary fibrosis, nausea, rashes
Contraindications		Cardiogenic shock: second-or third-degree atrioventricular block (if no pacemaker)	Second- or third-degree atrioventricular block in absence of pacemaker; heart failure

From Koman LA (ed): Bowman Gray Orthopaedic Manual. Winston-Salem, NC, Orthopaedic Press, 1996.

onists, α_2 antagonists, combined α_1 and α_2 antagonists, and α_2 agonists (see Table 57-8).[10,18,66,168,247,249]

Phentolamine (Regitine), first introduced as a diagnostic test for RSD, produces nonselective, competitive α-adrenergic blockade by affecting postsynaptic α_1 receptors and presynaptic α_2 receptors.[10,139,249,250] Theoretically, the resulting chemical sympathectomy produces peripheral vasodilation, increases nutritional blood flow, and decreases non–microvascular-mediated adrenergic sensitization. Decreased pain or pain relief after intravenous phentolamine

(25 to 30 mg) is pathognomonic for adrenergically driven SMP.[249] Patients with a positive response to intravenous phentolamine are likely to respond to other forms of sympatholytic intervention. The use of phentolamine as a definitive test for CRPS is hindered by the presence of false-negative tests and the absence of placebo controls.[244]

Nonselective adrenergic oral medications include phenoxybenzamine (Dibenzyline), which is a nonselective and irreversible postsynaptic α_1 antagonist and a presynaptic α_2 antagonist. Unfortunately, the drug is poorly tolerated

Table 57-8

ADRENERGIC AGENTS

	Phentolamine (Regitine)	Phenoxybenzamine (Dibenzyline)	Prazosin (Minipress)	Terazosin (Hytrin)	Clonidine (Catapres)
Administration and Dosage	IV infusion; 25-30 mg/ 100 mL saline in 20 min	PO: 5-120 mg/day	PO: 1 mg once at bedtime up to tid	PO: 1 mg qid	Topical, intrathecal, or PO: 1 mg/hr patch weekly 1 mg PO tid initially
Action/Mechanism	Postsynaptic α_1 antagonist Presynaptic α_2 antagonist	Postsynaptic α_1- antagonist Presynaptic α_2- antagonist $\alpha_1 > \alpha_2$	Postsynaptic α_1 antagonist	Postsynaptic α_1 antagonist	Presynaptic α_2 antagonist
Side Effects	Hypotension, cardiac arrhythmias, weakness, nausea, dysrhythmias	Orthostatic hypotension	Orthostatic hypotension	Orthostatic hypotension	Dry mouth, drowsiness

From Koman LA (ed): Bowman Gray Orthopaedic Manual. Winston-Salem, NC, Orthopaedic Press, 1996.

by many patients; however, the pain relief it provides may be dramatic.[114] Prazosin (Minipress) and terazosin (Hytrin) block postsynaptic α_1 receptors selectively without affecting presynaptic α_2 receptors and may diminish symptoms such as allodynia and vasospasm.[277]

α_2-Adrenergic agonists may also be effective. Clonidine (Catapres), a selective presynaptic α_2 agonist in the CNS, is used clinically in three divided doses or as a continuous transcutaneous patch. In patients with edema and hyperalgesia, dramatic improvement may result from α_2 agonist stimulation.[18,66,168,279]

Calcium Channel Blockers

Calcium channel blockers have been demonstrated to improve symptoms in selected patients with CRPS (Table 57-9).[156,246,255,300] Although their mechanism of action in the treatment of CRPS is unclear, calcium channel blockers decrease sympathetic tone by preventing calcium release after stimulation of adrenergic receptors. Nifedipine (Adalat, Procardia) and amlodipine (Norvasc) are the most commonly used. By inhibiting extracellular calcium passage through L-channel(s) in the vascular smooth muscle membrane, the effects of adrenergic agents are blocked and vasoconstriction is diminished. Use of these drugs often results in significant diminution of pain, which may correlate with increased nutritional perfusion and diminution of abnormal arteriovenous shunting.[174,249,250,300]

Corticosteroids

High success rates have been reported with the use of corticosteroids in the management of CRPS.[50,116,179-181] The exact mechanism of action of these agents in dystrophic pain has not been elucidated, although they are believed to stabilize membranes.[139] A high starting dose (e.g., 60 mg of prednisone) rapidly tapered over a period of 5 to 10 days is commonly used.[180,181,263] Long-term use of low doses (2 to 5 mg) is also advocated.[50,116,117,128,180,181] The use of corticosteroids remains controversial because of their potential side effects, complications, and variable benefits. Side effects include adrenohypophyseal suppression, hirsutism, and abnormal fat deposition. Complications include avascular necrosis of osseous structures (i.e., the femoral head). Corticosteroids have also been infused regionally in a Hannington-Kiff protocol as an intravenous bolus distal to a proximal tourniquet.[135,137]

Neuromuscular Blocking Agents

Botulinum A and B toxins have been utilized in the management of acute and chronic pain. These agents are injected into muscle or skin with reported relief of muscle spasm, dystonia, and skin hypersensitivity through incompletely delineated mechanisms that include inhibition of substance P and decreased muscle overactivity.[9]

Others

Free Radical Scavengers

Dimethyl sulfoxide (50%) (DMSO) showed favorable results in a randomized controlled trial in "warm" CRPS type I and N-acetylcysteine (NAC) in "cold" CRPS. Both groups—DMSO and NAC—were more effective if patients were treated early.[238] In addition, DMSO is cost effective compared with NAC.[290] DMSO is not FDA approved in humans.

Authors' Approach to Oral Medications

Drug selection should be based on physiologic staging and should address symptoms or specific lesions. In patients with SMP, an estimate of total flow, nutritional flow, edema, and symptoms may guide the decision process. Combination drug treatment is used frequently, often in conjunction with hand therapy (i.e., stress loading), adaptive therapy, and TENS stimulation. Various combinations of drugs may be used; two drugs from separate classes are often more effective than two drugs from one class. For example, patients with sympathetically maintained pain, high total blood flow, and nutritional shunting without edema may be given amitriptyline and phenytoin in combination with a stress-loading program. If treatment is successful, total flow will be decreased by minimizing arteriovenous shunting, nutritional flow will increase, and pain will be relieved.

In patients with pain associated with a cold, stiff, atrophic hand, evaluations usually indicate compromised nutritional flow.[241,258] The use of a calcium channel blocker combined with a serotonin reuptake inhibitor should increase nutritional flow and thereby relieve symptoms. Transcutaneous nerve stimulators may also increase nutritional flow by inhibiting smaller nociceptive fibers.[198,221,252] Hyperalgesia with significant edema is managed initially by transdermal clonidine in conjunction with a tricyclic antidepressant and/or a serotonin reuptake inhibitor. Corticosteroids are

Table 57-9
CALCIUM CHANNEL BLOCKERS/CORTICOSTEROID

	Nifedipine (Adalat, Procardia)	Amlodipine (Norvasc)	Corticosteroid
Dosage	10-30 mg PO tid or 30-90 mg qid sustained	2.5-5 mg/day	10 mg/day PO
Mechanism of Action	Blockade of calcium channel on vascular smooth muscle cell	Blockade of calcium channel on vascular smooth muscle cell	Decreases inflammation, unknown
Common Side Effects	Headaches, peripheral edema, postural hypotension	Headaches, postural hypotension	Multiple, including edema, circulatory problems, paresis, dermatologic, cataracts

From Koman LA (ed): Bowman Gray Orthopaedic Manual. Winston-Salem, NC, Orthopaedic Press, 1996.

seldom used because of fear of avascular necrosis. Patients should be monitored carefully by objective data when possible. In the absence of clinical improvement, oral medications should be altered or augmented by parenteral interventions. Other additional oral and topical medications used to treat CRPS include capsaicin,[49,100] ketanserin,[65,134] calcitonin,[119,233] transdermal nitroglycerin,[148] and prostaglandin E$_1$ ointment.[214] Ketanserin, a selective S$_2$ serotonergic antagonist, has been documented to provide relief of RSD pain in a double-blind, placebo-controlled crossover study.[134]

Parenteral Medications

Intravenous Regional Infusion

Infusion of drugs into an isolated extremity for analgesia was described by Bier in 1908; intravenous drug infusion for dystrophic pain was used first in the 1970s by Hannington-Kiff.[135] The latter's protocol, with or without minor modifications, is used by most anesthesiologists and pain specialists to deliver intravenous drugs. In CRPS the most common pharmacologic agents used with this technique are reserpine, guanethidine, bretylium tosylate, and corticosteroids (Table 57-10).* A randomized, double-blind comparison of intravenous guanethidine, reserpine, and normal

---

*See references 26, 65, 78, 87, 101, 108, 118, 122, 135-137, 145, 152, 196, 197, 218, 219, and 243.

saline demonstrated significant and equal improvement with all three at 30 minutes and no differences in outcome at 24 hours.[34] Tourniquet-induced analgesia may be involved in the short-term pain relief observed after the Hannington-Kiff protocol.[34] Guanethidine and reserpine are no longer available commercially in the United States and, in general, are not indicated clinically in the management of CRPS type 1 or 2. The use of intravenous corticosteroids in the management of CRPS is not supported by any controlled clinical trials. Bretylium tosylate (Bretylol) is the only drug approved and labeled (as of August 2002) by the FDA as an intravenous competitive blocking agent. Bretylium produces a transient release of norepinephrine from postganglionic sympathetic nerve endings, thereby preventing release of norepinephrine. It is well tolerated and appears to be effective in selected patients.[106,138,145] Bretylium or corticosteroids may be used in conjunction with regional anesthesia for surgical procedures in patients requiring reconstructive procedures or to facilitate mobilization of stiff joints by manipulation under anesthesia.[80] In rare cases, lasting relief may be obtained after a single intravenous infusion of a sympatholytic drug or corticosteroid; however, in many cases, sequential blocks (three to five) are required. Intravenous regional droperidol, an α-adrenergic antagonist, has been evaluated in a double-blind, placebo-controlled crossover study.[165] Effectiveness of intravenous ketorolac and lidocaine is reported.[283] Intravenous regional phenoxybenzamine "appeared" to produce long-term relief in five patients.[210]

Table 57-10
PARENTERAL MEDICATIONS

	Methods of Administration and Usual Dosage	Mechanism of Action	Major Short-Term Disadvantage or Side Effects	Contraindications
Bretylium	IV regional: 100-200 mg	Norepinephrine-blocking agent; depletion of terminal vesicle of norepinephrine		
Clonidine	Continuous epidural: 10-40 mg/hr	Diminishes regional sympathetic outflow by direct action at the spinal cord	Hypotension, transient sedation	Advanced renal insufficiency, atrioventricular block greater than first degree, concurrent use of α agonists or α antagonists
Cortisone	IV regional: 100 mg	See Table 57-9	See Table 57-9	See Table 57-9
Guanethidine	IV regional: up to 30 mg; usually must be repeated; no longer available in the United States	Norepinephrine neuron blocking agent; stabilization of postsynaptic membrane	Orthostatic hypotension	Tricyclic antidepressants
Phentolamine	IV injection: 5-15 mg	α-Adrenergic blocker	Hypotension	Coronary artery disease
Reserpine	IV injection: no longer available in the United States	Norepinephrine inhibitor	Orthostatic hypotension	Depression

From Koman LA (ed): Bowman Gray Orthopaedic Manual. Winston-Salem, NC, Orthopaedic Press, 1996.

Diagnostic Intravenous Infusion

Intravenous infusions are used for diagnostic purposes; there are no current treatment programs that use such infusions. Intravenous phentolamine is used to determine the presence of α-adrenergically mediated sympathetic pain,[10] and intravenous lidocaine may be used to assess the potential efficacy of oral membrane-stabilizing agents.[61]

Epidural Agents

Epidural corticosteroids and clonidine have been used and may provide relief in selected patients.[75,86,251]

Intra-arterial Medications

Intra-arterial injection of reserpine and guanethidine has led to subjective improvement,[52,101,118] but there have been no published placebo-controlled or blinded trials or documented treatment protocols using intra-arterial drugs in the management of CRPS.

Percutaneous Neural or Ganglionic Blockade

Neural blockade of the stellate ganglion, brachial plexus, or spinal cord/nerve roots is effective in relieving CRPS in a large percentage of cases (see Diagnostic Sympathetic Blockade on page 2024). A series of blocks performed at 3- to 14-day intervals is often necessary to achieve adequate sustained relief.

Continuous Autonomic Blockade

The use of prolonged and/or continuous sympathetic blockade for the management of chronic pain is well established.[28,142,194] Sympathetic blockade may be achieved by continuous infusion of local anesthetic over the area of the stellate ganglion or paravertebral ganglia, along the brachial plexus, or within the epidural space. Specific blocks include "anterior scalene," "axillary," or "brachial" (Fig. 57-13). Epidural blocks have been used successfully in the lower extremity[59] and provide an alternative method to effect sym-

pathetic blockade in the upper extremity.[53] Blocks should be performed by experienced physicians and in the presence of resuscitation equipment and ventilatory support. Epidural blocks may be effective in patients who demonstrate no improvement after peripheral sympathetic blockade,[53] and brachial plexus blocks may provide relief in patients unresponsive to stellate ganglion blocks.[81] Complications include complete or temporary motor and sensory blockade, which may compromise respiration,[305] as well as bleeding and nerve irritation. However, with proper patient selection, sustained improvement can be observed in 50% to 70% of patients.[41,194]

Biofeedback/Acupuncture

Self-hypnosis and/or biofeedback may be useful in the management of properly selected patients.[3,23,32,33,109,130,239] Acupuncture (using electrodes and/or transdermal needles) has also been advocated for the management of CRPS.[23,47,186,187,216] These techniques should be used judiciously.

Authors' Preferred Methods of Treatment: Parenteral Medications

The administration of intravenous medications via variations of the Hannington-Kiff technique should be guided by highly controlled protocols based on documented and progressive improvement with sympatholytic blockade. We do not refer patients for reserpine, guanethidine, or corticosteroid intravenous infusion; instead, in selected patients bretylium blocks, which are administered every other week for 6 to 8 weeks, are effective. Patients are seen between blocks and examined for a nociceptive focus, symptoms

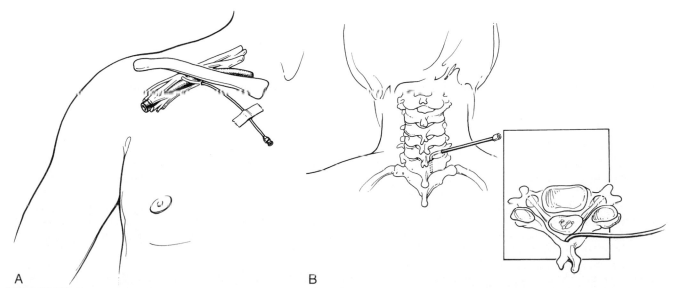

FIGURE 57-13. Placement of (**A**) continuous blockade with a brachial plexus catheter and (**B**) continuous cervical epidural blockade. In both cases a small Silastic catheter is introduced percutaneously and continuous blocking agents or other medications are injected via a pump mechanism. (From Koman LA, Poehling GG: Reflex sympathetic dystrophy. *In* Gelberman RH [ed]: Operative Nerve Repair and Reconstruction. Philadelphia, JB Lippincott, 1990, pp 1497-1524.)

and function are quantified, and physiologic testing is performed. We prefer continuous autonomic blocks (e.g., epidural) for 3 to 7 days and verify the effectiveness of the block by stress testing after 24 to 36 hours of blockade. It is important to monitor the patient closely by objective criteria, and courses of "blocks" should be based on the attainment of prospective goals within a predetermined time frame.

Intravenous bretylium should be considered if regional blockade is necessary for other indications. In general, we have found continuous autonomic blockade to be more effective than a series of regional infusions. Continuous autonomic blockade is efficacious in selected patients; it may attenuate the dystrophic process, thereby allowing the identification of a nociceptive focus. Furthermore, its use for 3 to 5 days may alleviate symptoms, may allow the patient to return to a satisfactory functional level, or may prevent recurrence or exacerbation of pain after surgical intervention. Biofeedback is used in conjunction with psychological support in selected patients who demonstrate appropriate psychological profiles established by objective testing (e.g., Minnesota Multiphasic Personality Inventory [MMPI]).

Surgical and Ablative Therapies

Sympathectomy
Chemical
Chemical sympathectomy effected by the injection of phenol or other agents along the sympathetic trunk provides clinical efficacy in selected patients. For this procedure, 4% to 7% phenol is injected into the nerve or ganglia with computed tomography used for localization. This allows a reversible axonotmesis with recovery in 3 to 6 months. Theoretically, this effects pain relief without complete transection of the nerves and diminishes the possibility of delayed hypersensitivity from receptor up-regulation. Peripheral sympathectomy that increased perfusion after arterectomy, which includes the resection of sympathetic fibers on peripheral blood vessels, was first described by Leriche.[189,190] Although resection of major blood vessels is not recommended in CRPS, the role of sympathectomy continues to be evaluated and has been reported anecdotally.

Surgical
Surgical sympathectomy has been reserved for patients with refractory CRPS because results are variable. Short-term effectiveness is common, and success after sympathectomy has been reported after failure of other treatment modalities. Successful surgical sympathectomy requires complete sympathetic denervation of the appropriate limb fibers from the stellate ganglion to T2 and T3.[46] Thorascopic ganglionectomy is currently being used with satisfactory success rates.[265] The effects of proximal sympathectomy on distal sympathetic tone (as reflected by increased blood flow) last from 6 to 24 weeks. The etiology of loss of efficacy is postulated to be secondary to up-regulation of distal receptors, which may produce supersensitivity to circulating or endogenous catecholamines and prompt recurrence of symptoms. However, in some patients the pain relief after sympathectomy is sufficient to break the dystrophic cycle, and improvement persists. Patients occasionally experience an increase in pain and symptoms after sympathectomy.

Therefore, temporary (3- to 6-month) chemical sympathectomy of the autonomic sympathetic nervous system may be preferable to transection of neural structures. When this technique is used, nerve regeneration will occur and receptor up-regulation either does not occur or is diminished. Radiofrequency ablation of the cervicothoracic ganglion has also been recommended.[308,309] Recently, the use of intrathecal or epidural administration of drugs such as clonidine has been advanced.[251]

Summary
Critical analysis of the peer-reviewed literature to assess the effects of both chemical and surgical sympathectomy for neuropathic pain concluded that this clinical practice "is based on poor quality evidence, uncontrolled studies, and personal experience. Furthermore, complications of the procedure may be significant..."[208] and "denervation supersensitivity of blood vessels and intense vasomotion may be associated with recurrence of pain...."[22] These findings are in agreement with observations by the authors.

Implantable Devices
Peripheral Nerve Implants
Implantable electrical stimulators have been placed on painful peripheral nerves[123] throughout the nervous system.[17,19,146,182,193,229,253,297,311] These include stimulators for gray matter, the dorsal column, the spinal cord, and peripheral nerves. Current devices allow placement of multiple electrodes on peripheral nerves and of long-lasting implantable pulse generators and use of remote programming.

Implantable Spinal Cord Stimulation
The role of implanted spinal-cord stimulation (SCS) for CRPS and successful pain relief has been reported in 50% of patients otherwise unresponsive to treatment.[164,269] SCS in selected patients relieves pain without improving function[161] and is more effective and less expensive than standard treatment.[163]

Central Nervous System Ablative Techniques
CRPS has been treated with bilateral anterior cingulotomy with only short-term palliation.[260]

Management of the Neural Dystrophic Focus
If a nociceptive (dystrophic) focus, or trigger area, is identifiable, direct treatment of the abnormality may provide significant relief.[158] Nociceptive foci, identifiable in fewer than 50% of patients, may be mechanical or neural. If diagnosed, the underlying focus should be managed by conventional procedures after maximal pharmacologic control is achieved. If symptoms persist, surgical correction of the defect/deformity may be helpful. The most recognized neural problems contributing to a dystrophy include neuroma, neuroma-in-continuity, and secondary compression neuropathies.

Diagnosis and Management of Neural Problems
Neuromas develop in 30% to 40% of significant nerve injuries and may precipitate a dystrophic response, complicate clinical management, and interfere with health-related quality of life. A partial nerve injury, when complicated

by a neuroma-in-continuity, is characterized by allodynia, hyperpathia, and vasomotor abnormalities; sudomotor changes are common and cold sensitivity may be significant.[56] Compression neuropathies are frequently seen in patients with CRPS[129,173] and may either be the precipitating causal event or occur secondarily. Most frequently, the median nerve is involved within the carpal canal; involvement at the elbow is less frequent. The ulnar nerve at the cubital tunnel or within the wrist may also be involved. The posterior interosseous branch of the radial nerve may be compressed above or within the supinator (radial tunnel syndrome).

Physical examination after sympatholytic intervention may be required to verify the clinical suspicion of neuroma, neuroma-in-continuity, or compression neuropathy. Local anesthesia of the suspected nerve proximal to the suspected injury may be helpful and provides confirmation of clinical suspicion.

Principles of Management

Surgery on neural structures compromised by neuromas, neuroma-in-continuity, or compression is indicated if symptoms persist after nonoperative modalities, including sympatholytic medications. An acute dystrophic flare of a quiescent dystrophy is possible in the postoperative period. Surgical choices include neurolysis, neurorrhaphy, neural relocation, environmental modification, and/or a combination of these procedures.[205,230,262]

If a neural insult is identified and is correctable surgically, the nerve is explored via an extensile incision. All adhesions are released and the nerve is evaluated under magnification, with an operating microscope if necessary. The appropriate treatment option depends on clinical findings, the location and type of nerve (i.e., motor, sensory, or mixed), preoperative nerve function, the location of the injury, the quality of the neural bed and its environment, and the general needs and condition of the patient. With a complete nerve transection or a neuroma-in-continuity, the following general principles apply:

- Avoid tension on the repair site(s) by performing nerve grafts from the sural nerve or, for small nerves, a branch of the medial or lateral antebrachial cutaneous nerves.
- Manage adhesions between the skin and nerve by a "Z"-plasty, local flaps, or distant flaps.
- If excessive scarring or adhesions develop, modify the neural bed by the use of autologous fat, rotational muscle flaps, pedicled muscle or fascial flaps, free muscle transfer, or autologous or allograft venous wraps.[123,157,173,213,271,272]
- Minimize internal neurolysis.
- Include sympatholytic intervention (e.g., continuous autonomic blockade), pharmacologic palliation, physical therapy, and early active and passive range of motion in postoperative care.
- Establish hemostasis to prevent hematoma formation.
- Avoid constrictive postoperative dressings.

In the treatment of compression neuropathy, the dystrophic response is managed by sympatholytic medications and/or autonomic blockade and the nerve is evaluated clinically. If symptoms are sufficient to justify intervention, location of the compression neuropathy is confirmed by

peripheral nerve conduction velocities or interstitial pressure measurements[99] (see also Chapter 56). Complete release of the involved nerve is important. If there is damage to the neural bed or the neural bed is compromised, modification of the neural environment is appropriate.[176,242] The patient may be treated postoperatively with appropriate sympatholytic oral medications and/or continuous autonomic blockade to minimize postoperative pain and prevent dystrophic flare.

Surgical Technique for the Management of Injury to the Superficial Branch of the Radial Nerve Complicated by CRPS

The superficial radial nerve may be injured by trauma or during surgical release of the first or second dorsal compartment of the wrist. Options for treatment include proximal transection of the nerve in normal tissue beneath the brachioradialis muscle or exploration with neurolysis and/or repair.

The nerve should be approached through an extensile incision incorporating the previous scar if necessary. The nerve may be adherent to the tendons, the tendon sheath, or overlying skin; regional fat necrosis is common.[261] To facilitate dissection, the nerve should be identified proximally and distally in an unoperated or uninjured area while working toward the area of injury. While working from normal to abnormal tissue, the nerve is isolated to expose existing lesions. A decision is then made regarding management of the injury. If repair is selected, microscopic dissection and repair of injured fascicles is performed end-to-end or with a nerve graft. If the nerve is to be transected, it may be resected to a level of surrounding normal tissue or relocated to an unscarred area (Fig. 57-14). Either a sural nerve or a forearm nerve is harvested from a separate incision to accomplish nerve grafting. Based on experience with six patients with injured superficial radial nerves and CRPS, our preference is to use the sural nerve to avoid a potential nociceptive focus in the same extremity. During preoperative assessment, donor nerves may be blocked proximally so that the patient appreciates the degree of potential numbness in the donor nerve field that will be experienced after the surgery. The sural nerve is harvested through a separate lateral incision in the leg. The grafting is then completed with 8-0 or 9-0 nonabsorbable suture under the operating microscope.

Excessive scar-related attachment of the nerve to underlying tendon structures or to overlying skin requires environmental modification. Although this may be achieved by a variety of means, we prefer covering the nerve with a section of the adjacent cephalic vein or harvesting a separate vein from the leg or arm. Alternatives include glutaraldehyde-preserved umbilical vein grafts,[213] local or free fat grafts, and a free muscle transfer.[157] After repair, the tourniquet is deflated, bleeding is controlled, and a drain is placed. Subcutaneous tissue is closed with absorbable suture, and the skin is approximated with nonabsorbable suture and/or staples. If chromic suture is chosen, it should not be allowed to come into contact with neural tissues because it may induce nociceptive nerve pain. A drain is placed to prevent hematoma formation. Postoperative reactivation of the dys-

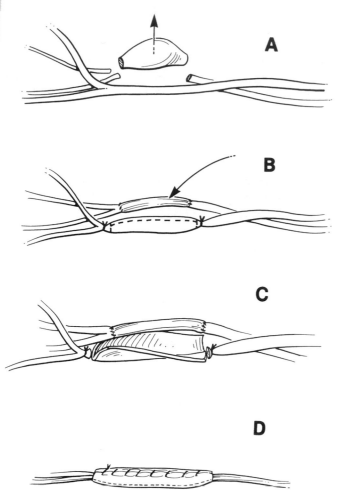

FIGURE 57-14. Authors' preferred treatment of a neuroma of the superficial branch of the radial nerve. **A,** Resection of the neuroma. **B,** Repair with a sural nerve graft and ligation of the cephalic vein. **C,** Longitudinal split in the resected segment of vein. **D,** Cephalic vein wrapped loosely around the nerve repair. (From Koman LA [ed]: Bowman Gray Orthopaedic Manual. Winston-Salem, NC, Orthopaedic Press, 1996.)

trophic process is a major concern, but this may be minimized by continuous autonomic blockade for 3 to 5 days after surgery.

Revision of Carpal Tunnel Surgery

Persistent mechanical pain associated with dystrophic symptoms after release of the transverse carpal ligament or neurolysis of the median nerve is a difficult problem. The nociceptive focus may result from internal or external scarring, neuroma-in-continuity, and/or transection of a nerve branch (e.g., the palmar cutaneous branch of the median nerve). When SMP is associated with a demonstrable peripheral nerve lesion, surgical intervention/correction of the underlying lesion may provide significant palliation.[158] If external adhesions or mechanical problems contribute to the nociceptive focus, environmental modification may be necessary.

CRITICAL POINTS: MANAGEMENT OF PAINFUL MEDIAN NERVE WITH CRPS

INDICATIONS

- Quiescent or stable sympathetically maintained CRPS with mechanical pain
- Previous neurolysis with scar and decreased nerve mobility

PREOPERATIVE EVALUATION

- Demonstrate painful nerve gliding.
- Evaluate peripheral nerve conduction velocities.
- Note a positive response to sympatholytic intervention.

PEARLS

- Careful, unless pain is relieved with splinting and sympatholytic treatments.
- Preoperatively, place continuous autonomic blockade.

TECHNICAL POINTS

- Perform extensile neurolysis.
- Excise synovitis.
- Mobilize nerve.
- Cover nerve with fat, muscle flap, vein, or free tissue transfer.

PITFALLS

- Failure to confirm ability to control postoperative pain with oral or parenteral drugs or continuous field or nerve blocks
- Iatrogenic nerve injury
- Failure to mobilize nerve
- Failure to provide good soft tissue between skin and nerve and nerve and tendons

POSTOPERATIVE CARE

- Begin early range-of-motion exercises of fingers and wrist.
- Maintain vigorous pain management for 1 to 7 days with parenteral and/or oral agents.
- Note that continuous blocks are very helpful.
- Allow unrestricted motion when comfortable.

Authors' Preferred Method of Treatment: Revision of Carpal Tunnel Surgery

The nerve is approached through an extensile excision and identified proximally and distally in "normal" tissue. The nerve is then traced distally to the "take off" of the palmar

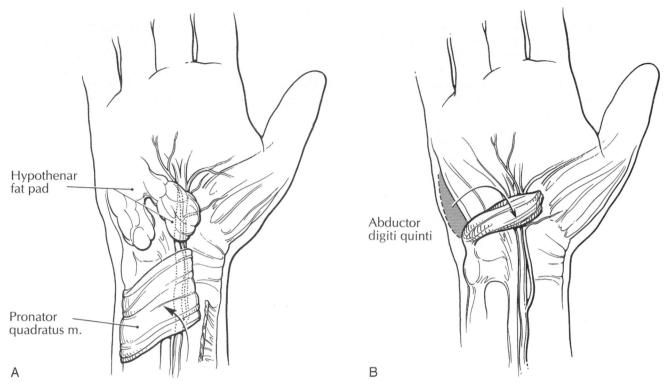

FIGURE 57-15. Options for modifying the environment surrounding an injured median nerve at the wrist include transposition of (**A**) pedicled hypothenar fat, the pronator quadratus muscle, or (**B**) the abductor digiti quinti muscle. (From Koman LA [ed]: Bowman Gray Orthopaedic Manual. Winston-Salem, NC, Orthopaedic Press, 1996.)

cutaneous branch, which is dissected separately and protected unless already damaged. Dissection in a distal-to-proximal direction is performed while avoiding injury to the branches. The entire nerve from the distal portion of the forearm in normal tissue to the terminal proper and common digital nerves and motor branch(es) should be identified. The superficial palmar arch should be identified and protected. Internal neurolysis should be avoided, if possible. If a *neuroma* or *neuroma-in-continuity* is encountered, it may be dissected under the operating microscope and either repaired, grafted, or resected to a better position. All the sensory branches and the recurrent motor branch(es) are identified.

If there is significant scarring between the nerve and the surrounding subcutaneous tissue, tendons, skin, or synovium, the neural environment should be modified. Options include placing a local or distal autologous flap, using local pedicle muscle flaps (e.g., abductor digiti quinti, palmaris brevis, and pronator quadratus), using forearm fascia, transferring distal free tissue (i.e., fascia, omentum, muscle), or wrapping the scarred nerve with an autologous or allograft vein, usually the saphenous vein (Fig. 57-15). If venous wrapping is selected, either autogenous saphenous vein or allograft umbilical vein (BioVascular) may be wrapped directly around the median nerve with a space left through which the palmar cutaneous branch can exit (Fig. 57-16).[157,213,257] The palmar cutaneous branch, if scarred or injured, may be wrapped separately with a small vein from the forearm, or a piece of the umbilical vein may be placed around the vein and nerve in sandwich fashion. If autologous vein is used, it can be wrapped around the nerve in a "barber pole" fashion.

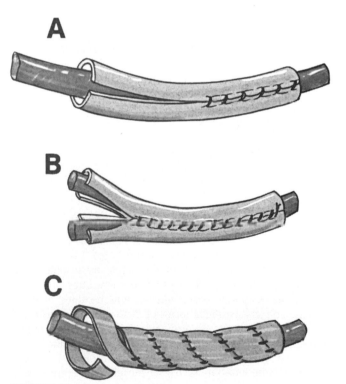

FIGURE 57-16. Alternative methods of covering a nerve with an autologous vein. **A,** The vein is split and then repaired. **B,** If the vein is large enough, branches may be managed by a second longitudinal slit in the nerve, which is then closed to form two sleeves. **C,** For a larger nerve the vein may be "wrapped" in barber-pole fashion. (From Koman LA [ed]: Bowman Gray Orthopaedic Manual. Winston-Salem, NC, Orthopaedic Press, 1996.)

The saphenous vein is seldom large enough to fold around the median nerve itself but will wrap easily around the branches. The graft should be sutured proximally and distally with a 5-0 or 6-0 nonreactive suture. *Chromic suture should be avoided because chemicals released from the suture can create a nociceptive neural focus.*

Injury to the palmar cutaneous branch of the median nerve is common. If this branch is injured, the branch may be resected and moved to an unscarred area or repaired by using end-to-end anastomoses or an interposition nerve graft. For grafting, we prefer, when possible, to use a short branch of the medial or lateral antebrachial cutaneous nerve. This graft may be harvested through a separate oblique incision in the forearm. Nerve repair is accomplished under the operating microscope with 9-0 to 10-0 nonabsorbable suture on 75- to 130-μm needles.

Before completion of the procedure, the tourniquet is released, bleeding is controlled, and a suction drain is placed. Postoperatively, the limb is protected from pain and dystrophic flare by the use of continuous autonomic blockade. Motion of the affected extremity is initiated in a controlled active program or by using continuous passive motion over the 3- to 5-day period of hospitalization for the continuous blockade.

Management of Mechanical Nociceptive Foci

Mechanical nociceptive foci are encountered frequently and include internal derangement of the wrist, cartilage flaps in the carpometacarpal area, injury to the triangular fibrocartilage complex, and injury to the distal radioulnar joint. Once the dystrophy is quieted, the diagnosis can be verified, and, if clinically indicated, surgical correction is performed.

Secondary Joint Deformities—Late Stage Treatment

Surgical correction of secondary joint deformities from arthrofibrosis may be necessary after CRPS. Fixed contractures of the metacarpophalangeal (MCP) joints in extension and the proximal interphalangeal (PIP) joints in flexion or extension are common. In addition, the shoulder, elbow, and wrist may have restricted motion.

Early management of CRPS will diminish the development of contractures; manipulation under sympatholytic block has been advocated to prevent such contractures. However, disuse and segmental ischemia may produce arthrofibrosis in spite of active intervention. Surgery on contracted joints should not be initiated until maximal nonoperative improvement has been achieved. In general, the waiting period should be a minimum of 3 to 6 months after successful elimination of the active dystrophic pain. This policy is in contradistinction to early intervention of identifiable peripheral nerve injuries, which should be dealt with as soon as it is safe in terms of dystrophic symptoms.[158]

When nonoperative improvement has reached a plateau and symptoms warrant intervention, release of the MCP and/or PIP joints can be achieved. Indications for surgery are joint pain without diffuse dystrophic symptoms and arthrofibrosis that interferes with functioning. Persistence of MCP and PIP joint contractures is devastating because it prevents adequate hand function and interferes with health-related quality of life. If necessary, all four MCP joints and all four PIP joints can be released in a single operation. It is important for the patient and physician to understand that this is a salvage procedure and that improvement in gross hand function, reduction in pain, and improved quality of activity is both the long-term and the short-term goal; restoration of full flexion and/or extension is not a reasonable goal or expectation. Surgery is performed to allow the hand to achieve improved function, to facilitate MCP joint motion, and to make active grasp and release less cumbersome and painful. The range of motion achieved intraoperatively rarely persists postoperatively.

Authors' Preferred Method of Treatment: MCP and PIP Contractures

After placement of an epidural or brachial plexus catheter, adequate surgical anesthesia is obtained. The MCP and PIP joints are approached through oblique dorsal incisions. The extent of adhesions in the extensor mechanism and the degree of arthrofibrosis are identified. Major findings in the MCP joint in the presence of an extension deformity include contracture and thickening of the collateral ligaments, adhesions of the volar plate and metacarpal neck, dorsal capsular tightness, and intrinsic muscle contracture. PIP joint motion is limited by contracture of the extensor mechanism, as well as by collateral ligaments and volar plate adherence. Tendon-splitting incisions are avoided by approaching the MCP joints from the radial side and moving the extensor tendon ulnarly. The joint capsule is opened and the collateral ligament identified. Often, erosions are present beneath the collateral ligament; the collateral ligament is invariably hypertrophied and contracted. The true and accessory collateral ligaments are released from the metacarpal head on the radial and ulnar sides; a small elevator is used to mobilize the volar plate without detaching it from the phalanx. Rarely is it necessary to transect the volar plate. After release of the collateral ligaments and freeing the volar plate, the MCP joints should move from neutral to greater than 90 degrees of flexion without subluxation (see Fig. 57-17).

If necessary, the PIP joint is approached through a dorsal incision. Tendon splitting is avoided with the extensor mechanism retracted after releasing both transverse retinacular ligaments. The lateral band and central slip may be moved radially or ulnarly to allow ready access to the joint. The joint is dissected, collateral ligaments are released, and the volar plate is freed (Fig. 57-17).

After sequential release of the MCP and PIP joints, the intrinsics are tested. If an intrinsic contracture exists, an intrinsic release is performed. Once these procedures are completed, all these joints should move through a satisfactory range of motion greater than or equal to 170 degrees, and the joints should be stable. If stability is in question, the MCP joint is pinned in full flexion and the PIP joint in 35 to 45 degrees of flexion. Continuous passive motion or an active and passive range-of-motion program is used postoperatively.

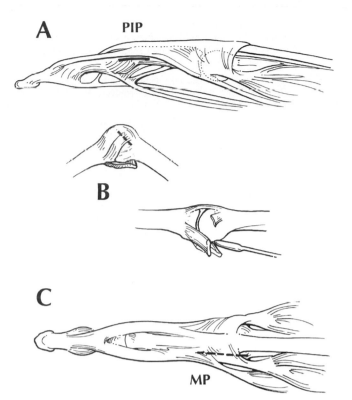

A PIP

B

C

MP

FIGURE 57-17. Release of the MCP and PIP joints. **A,** Through an oblique dorsal incision, the PIP joint is exposed by elevating the extensor mechanism after release of the transverse retinacular ligament. **B,** The capsule is then incised and the collateral ligament released. Dorsal adhesions may require lysis. **C,** The MCP joint (MP) is approached by incising a portion of the sagittal bone, reflecting the extensor tendon ulnarly, and incising the capsule. Collateral ligaments are then released. (From Koman LA [ed]: Bowman Gray Orthopaedic Manual. Winston-Salem, NC, Orthopaedic Press, 1996.)

The results of MCP joint release are gratifying, and usually 80% to 90% of the intraoperative range of motion is maintained. However, release of the PIP joint is less satisfactory. Although patients report significant symptomatic relief and improved health-related quality of life, joint range of motion averages approximately 50% of that observed intraoperatively.

Amputation

Amputation is reported in CRPS. Indications for amputation are recurrent infection, massive edema, or to improve function; however, patients are rarely symptom free,[73] prosthesis use is rare,[73] recurrence of CRPS is frequent,[73] and a psychosocial dysfunction persists.[285]

If necessary, amputation of limbs with CRPS requires perioperative sympatholytic treatment with oral medications and sympathetic block. Immediate prosthetic fitting is advisable and psychological support helpful.

Postoperative Management and Expectations

Natural History

The natural history of treated and untreated CRPS is variable. In general, early treatment portends a better outcome, but this is not always true. Therefore, it is wise to inform the patient that residual pain and stiffness may occur. In many patients, if not most, RSD is not a progressive condition.[313] Spread of CRPS symptoms to other body areas, while reported, is rare. Most patients who develop additional areas with CRPS sustain causal insults that trigger the dystrophic response.[209]

Moderate to severe CRPS after distal fracture of the radius may be more recalcitrant; however, only 3.5% to 7% of patients who initially had features of CRPS after distal fracture of the radius showed significant symptoms at 1 to 2 years.[31] In contrast, 26% of 55 patients with CRPS after distal fracture of the radius followed for 10 years continued to demonstrate symptoms and signs of CRPS, with "poor finger function" at 3 months correlating with symptoms at 10 years.[103] In 28 patients with debilitating CRPS after distal fracture of the radius referred for management by orthopedic surgeons, multimodal management including surgery improved function but did not eliminate residual disability.

Postoperative management is dependent on the type of procedure. However, sympatholytic intervention using parenteral or oral agents is important and exacerbation is rare. Patients should expect prolonged rehabilitation, continued use of oral non-narcotic agents for 3 to 6 months, and residual disability. For example, surgical release of intrinsic muscles or MCP or PIP joints will decrease "stiffness" but will not restore full range of motion (50% improvement is average).

CONCLUSION

The pathophysiologic entity known as CRPS includes classic RSD and causalgia. The diagnosis is based on the clinical finding of pain combined with autonomic dysfunction, trophic changes, and functional impairment, which may be supported by a variety of objective instruments and tests. Sympathetically maintained pain is encountered frequently but is not a prerequisite for diagnosis. Early diagnosis and prompt intervention correlate with maximal recovery. Treatment is multifaceted and, if possible, based on physiologic criteria and objective determination of effectiveness. Surgical correction of underlying mechanical/neural foci is appropriate in selected patients.

It is crucial that patients understand that symptoms, signs, and morbidity are common after nonoperative or operative management. This is especially true after fractures of the distal radius and CRPS. Stiffness at 3 weeks frequently portends long-term problems. In addition, long-term use of sympatholytic drugs may be required.

The surgical management of chronic deformity in the absence of pain is possible; however, re-exacerbation of a dystrophic response is possible. Therefore, perioperative pain control with continuous epidural or peripheral catheters is prudent for 3 to 5 days. Alternatively, continuous field block catheters may be utilized. Although recurrent CRPS is infrequent, rarely are salvage procedures—repeat neurolysis of a nerve, resection of a neuroma, release of contractures—100% successful. Improvement of 50% or more is common; complete recovery is rare.

ANNOTATED REFERENCES

61. Czop C, Smith TL, Rauck R, Koman LA: The pharmacologic approach to the painful hand. Hand Clin 12:633-642, 1996.

    A review of the pharmacologic options useful in the management of RSD and CRPS. It includes the indications, contraindications, and dosage of oral, intravenous, intra-arterial, and intramuscular medications.

73. Dielissen PW, Claassen ATPM, Veldman PHJM, Goris RA: Amputation for reflex sympathetic dystrophy. J Bone Joint Surg Br 77:270-273, 1995.

    Management of 28 patients who underwent 34 amputations in 31 limbs is detailed. The major indication was infection and was frequent; however, RSD was recurrent and only 2 used prostheses.

142. Hobelmann CF Jr, Dellon AL: Use of prolonged sympathetic blockade as an adjunct to surgery in the patient with sympathetic maintained pain. Microsurgery 10:151-153, 1989.

    This article presents the results of surgery after RSD and the use of prolonged sympathetic blocks to aid perioperative recovery and prevent re-exacerbation.

145. Hord AH, Rooks MD, Stephens BO, et al: Intravenous regional bretylium and lidocaine for treatment of reflex sympathetic dystrophy: A randomized, double-blind study. Anesth Analg 74:818-821, 1992.

    An important trial that demonstrates the effectiveness of bretylium in RSD.

157. Jones NF: Treatment of chronic pain by "wrapping" intact nerves with pedicle and free flaps. Hand Clin 12:765-772, 1996.

    This article highlights the role of environmental modification of painful nerves serving as a nociceptive focus in RSD.

158. Jupiter JB, Seiler JG 3rd, Zienowicz R: Sympathetic maintained pain (causalgia) associated with a demonstrable peripheral-nerve lesion. J Bone Joint Surg Am 76:1376-1384, 1994.

    This landmark article demonstrates the importance of surgical management of injured nerves in managing RSD. In this small series, active nerve repair or intervention and perioperative continuous block eliminated or improved RSD.

185. Lee GW, Weeks PM: The role of bone scintigraphy in diagnosing reflex sympathetic dystrophy. J Hand Surg [Am] 20:458-463, 1995.

    A review of the literature that evaluates the role of bone scans in diagnosis. Nineteen studies in the English literature are reviewed critically with the conclusion that "three phase bone scintigraphy should not be used as a major diagnostic criteria in diagnosing reflex sympathetic dystrophy."

199. Louis DS, Lamp MK, Greene TL: The upper extremity and psychiatric illness. J Hand Surg [Am] 10:687-693, 1985.

    Classic article on psychiatric problems that may masquerade as CRPS in the hand.

240. Pollock FE Jr, Koman LA, Smith BP, et al: Measurement of hand microvascular blood flow with isolated cold stress testing and laser Doppler fluxmetry. J Hand Surg Am 18:143-150, 1993.

    The importance of physiologic staging of RSD in CRPS is detailed in this article. RSD does not follow specific time courses. Proper treatment depends on the aberrant physiology.

280. Stutts JT, Kasdan ML, Hickey SE, Bruner A: Reflex sympathetic dystrophy: Misdiagnosis in patients with dysfunctional postures of the upper extremity. J Hand Surg [Am] 25:1152-1156, 2000.

    Classic description of postures mimicking in 43 patients with CRPS or RSD.

293. Veldman PHJM, Reynen HM, Arntz IE, Goris RJA: Signs and symptoms of reflex sympathetic dystrophy: Prospective study of 829 patients. Lancet 342:1012-1016, 1993.

    This article details the demographics of RSD.

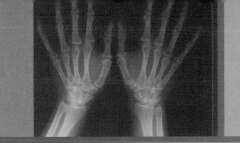

CHAPTER 58

Factitious Disorders

Dean S. Louis and Morton L. Kasdan

On occasion a patient will present with symptoms or physical findings that do not follow the usual injury or disease paradigms. The symptoms may be out of proportion to the physical findings, or the physical findings may not make sense based on the historical record. When such circumstances occur, it behooves the examining physician to consider the possibility that the patient's agenda may be something other than wellness.[3,7,11,13]

A variety of terms have been used to describe these presentations. These include *malingering, factitious disease,* and *conversion reactions.*[24,25] These are only a few of the various and often confusing designations that apply to some of the conditions that the hand and upper extremity surgeon may have to recognize. The complexities of the psychiatric diagnoses are not pertinent here but are referenced elsewhere.[2,14]

The majority of the diagnoses that we have seen fit into one of the major categories just listed. There are some recognizable patterns of clinical presentation that should instantly alert the evaluating physician. It is important to recognize current psychiatric thought in this area. LoPiccolo and colleagues[14] have summarized this as follows, "While malingering[10] represents a *conscious* intent to deceive for the purpose of obtaining an easily identifiable goal (secondary gain), it should not be confused with factitious disorders. Factitious disorder is also defined as an *intentional* production of symptoms, but differs from malingering in that it is always considered pathological, and in that its goal is an internal rather than an external incentive, i.e. to assume the sick role."[4,17] Previous thought had denied attribution to personal motivation and referred to unconscious mechanisms to explain the observed behavior. Both malingering[10] and factitious disorders may be detected by either situational behavior or secondary (videotaped) surveillance. The former would occur when an individual was observed in the work place, social environment, or inpatient facility where he or she is seen by the staff to be performing contrary to any self-described limitations. Secondary surveillance usually involves direct videotaping from a concealed location of the individual performing a task or tasks that the person says he or she cannot do because of a specific condition (e.g., lifting a heavy trash can or other object when incapacitating low back pain is the major complaint). Although malingering and factitious disorders are "first cousins," they have a major difference. A malingerer is *feigning* illness, whereas a person with a factitious disorder is *causing* illness.

RECOGNIZABLE FACTITIOUS DISORDERS

Factitious Lymphedema

Patients who present with factitious lymphedema[8,15,16,19,22] usually have a history of the mysterious appearance of painless swelling of the limb and a denial of any knowledge of the cause of the problem. The site of the edema is at a defined point anywhere from the shoulder distally (Fig. 58-1).

Once this pattern of factitial illness is recognized (also of diagnostic significance) treatment may be effective. Patient hospitalization with controlled elevation will result in a rapid decrease in the edema. If it persists with constant elevation, then late night rounds may reveal a tourniquet somewhere about the limb. An alternate outpatient technique is the application of a shoulder spica cast. Psychiatric and/or psychological consideration should be sought. There is no indication for surgical intervention.

Factitious Ulceration

Patients with factitious ulceration usually present with a history of trivial trauma, subsequently developing lesions that will not heal (Fig. 58-2). The easiest way to confirm that

---

Editor's note (DPG): Some readers may think it inappropriate to have a chapter on factitious disorders in a book on operative surgery. Everyone would agree that the patients described in this brief chapter are clearly those in whom we should want to avoid operative intervention, but an accurate diagnosis in such patients is not always clearly apparent and virtually never easy to prove. It is precisely because these patients do constitute a pitfall for the unsuspecting hand surgeon that the editors deemed it necessary to include the chapter.

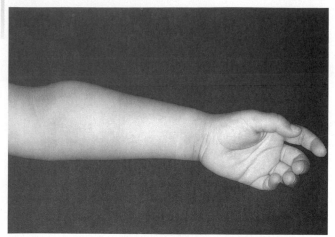

FIGURE 58-1. This 37-year-old woman presented with a history of mysterious swelling of her left hand. There is an obvious area of tourniquet compression just distal to the elbow flexion crease. This was the initial presentation of a long-involved and convoluted series of events that ended with severe flexion contracture of all fingers.

the lesion is factitious is to cover the area with a cast so that the patient cannot manipulate the wound.[18] Healing under such circumstances helps to confirm the diagnosis.

Dysfunctional Postures

There are a host of nonfunctional hand postures that patients assume.[6,16] These have some common characteristics and usually present as a claimed inability to use the hand (Figs. 58-3 to 58-5). In the classic position of the clenched fist[21] the ulnar three digits are held in a flexed position while the thumb and index fingers are fully mobile and functional.

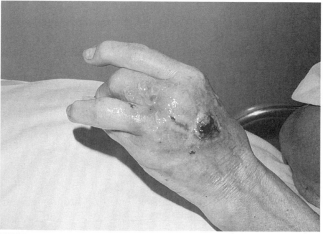

FIGURE 58-2. This patient was seen in consultation in an inpatient psychiatric ward. She held her hand in a dysfunctional posture. She had had a minor traumatic injury to the dorsum of her hand and refused to return to an abusive home situation. The wound would not heal. The wound was painted with fluroscein dye and covered with a dressing. The next morning an ultraviolet light was focused on the opposite hand, revealing marked fluorescence, indicating wound manipulation by the patient. (From Phelps DB, Buchler U, Boswick JA: The diagnosis of factitious ulcer of the hand: A case report. J Hand Surg [Am] 2:105-108, 1977.)

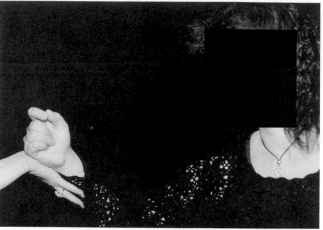

FIGURE 58-3. This patient stated that she was injured in 1994 when she slipped on something and threw her right arm up, causing her right forearm to strike a door handle. She claimed that her entire right upper extremity was numb and she was unable to use the hand. She held it in the fixed position as shown. She had been diagnosed with reflex sympathetic dystrophy. She would not actively move her digits but had a full range of motion with gentle passive manipulation. There were no trophic changes on clinical examination nor diminished mineralization of the bones on radiography. Surveillance documented full use of the extremity. Old medical records indicated the patient had similar episodes in the past and had claimed disability against two other employers.

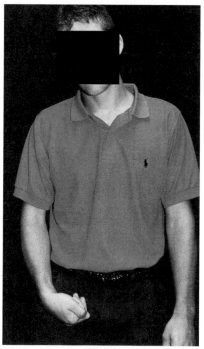

FIGURE 58-4. When first seen in June of 1995, this 23-year-old man claimed that he had been injured in 1994 when a heavy object struck the dorsum of his right hand. At the time of his evaluation, he held his right upper extremity in the fixed posture and claimed he was unable to use the right upper extremity for anything. He had been diagnosed with reflex sympathetic dystrophy and had undergone multiple blocks and insertion of a dorsal column stimulator. Bilateral radiographs documented symmetrical and normal mineralization of the bones. Video surveillance clearly indicated full active and strenuous use of the entire upper extremity was present. The grand jury returned a true bill of indictment for felony fraud. He pleaded guilty to a lesser charge of making a false sworn statement.

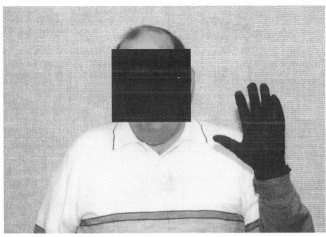

FIGURE 58-5. When first seen in 1989 this 53-year-old man claimed he did not have good use of his left hand. He was a diabetic and was noted to have a diffuse neuropathy. The patient had a full range of active motion but would immediately return his hand to the stiff, extended position. The significance of the black glove he wore to each visit was not clear. He was drawing disability benefits.

There are many variations on this theme, including, but not limited to, the adducted thumb, extension of the digits, and combinations of all of these.

We are aware of a case in which the examining physician was sued for performing a vigorous passive examination that the patient claimed hurt her and worsened her condition. The message here is that it may be prudent for the physician to merely observe and record active motion (or lack thereof) when the patient says he or she cannot move from a certain position.

DIFFERENTIAL DIAGNOSIS OF FACTITIOUS DISORDERS

There are many clinical presentations that may be factitious,[1] but the ones illustrated here are the most common patterns observed in two disparate practices over a 30-year period. The assumption inherent in this chapter is that all recognized medical conditions have been excluded and that the evaluating physician is now trying to figure out what is really going on. A recognition of the entities mentioned will make them a part of "recognized medical conditions."

MISTAKEN DIAGNOSIS

Factitious illness is probably one of the most frequently underdiagnosed, misdiagnosed, and mistreated conditions seen in medical practice. It is also one of the most difficult to prove. Perhaps the person whose diagnosis is not apparent to the initial evaluating physician will ultimately be diagnosed correctly. What is a problem is the misdiagnosis or incorrect labeling of factitious illness. The most frequent misdiagnosis is that of complex regional pain syndrome (CRPS) or reflex sympathetic dystrophy (RSD).[23] This misdiagnosis may occur at multiple levels from primary care physicians to advanced surgical specialties. The unfortunate

scenario is that once misdiagnosed, these patients frequently are treated inappropriately. The proliferation of practitioners who make a living off the symptom of pain is increasing. Unfortunately the misdiagnosis of CRPS or RSD may have devastating effects. A patient who indeed has a factitious condition may accept the fact that he or she has a real disease and accept treatment for it. When the diagnosis of CRPS or RSD is made, the usual treatment is one or more stellate ganglion blocks. Unfortunately the nonspecific criteria frequently used under these circumstances to establish a diagnosis often lead to misdiagnosis and overtreatment.

Consider the patient under these circumstances. If the diagnosis of factitial disease is correct and the patient is trying to manipulate a circumstance, then it is likely that the patient would accept a specific diagnosis and submit to treatment, confirming that the patient is ill. This results in the nocebo effect[5,9,12,20]—the expectation of illness, in some ways the opposite of the placebo effect. If an individual wishes to be ill for whatever reason, and this is then sanctified by a specific diagnosis, such as CRPS or RSD, and receives treatment for it, his or her path to wellness may be forever impeded, especially if litigation is involved.

MANAGEMENT OF PATIENTS WITH FACTITIOUS DISORDERS

There are neither easy solutions nor uniformly applicable paradigms for dealing with these difficult patients. Most of the patients with factitious disorders have secondary gain as a major confounder, and most are seeking benefits from one insurance source or another. It is the hand surgeon's responsibility to recognize these patterns of factitious disease and refer or suggest referral for psychiatric evaluation.

ANNOTATED REFERENCES

4. Bellamy R: Compensation neurosis. Clin Orthop 336:94-106, 1997.

   Bellamy presents a thorough discussion of the implications that workers' compensation has on patients' wellness. He emphasizes the benefits of illness behavior on the part of claimants and how the system fosters this.

5. Benson H: The nocebo effect: History and physiology. Preventive Med 26:612-615, 1997.

   The nocebo effect is a belief that something adverse is going to happen or that the diagnosis given means that the person given the diagnosis is not going to do well. It is in many ways the opposite of the well-known placebo effect. This is an excellent review of centuries of antecedents of these mind-body conflicts.

6. Dobyns JH: Pain dysfunction syndrome. *In* Gelberman R (ed). Operative Nerve Repair. Philadelphia, JB Lippincott, 1991, pp 1489-1494.

   One of the most knowledgeable hand surgeons in the realm of pain dysfunction syndromes is Jim Dobyns, who in this chapter covers this broad topic and compares and contrasts the findings in distinct categories. He clearly explains the dichotomy between reflex sympathetic dystrophy (complex regional pain syndromes) and other presentations of dysfunction.

8. Grunert BK, Sanger JR, Matloub HS, Yousif NJ: Classification system for factitious syndromes in the hand with implications for treatment. J Hand Surg [Am] 16:1027-1030, 1991.

This pivotal study evaluated 29 patients with factitious disorders. It used the Minnesota Multiphasic Personality Disorder (MMPI) to assess trends and revealed that there were two personality profiles: those that were angry and hostile and those that were dependent. The results with the latter group regarding return to work were far better than those with the former. A complete evaluation by a psychological professional was recommended.

9. Hahn RA: The nocebo phenomenon: Concept, evidence, and implications for public health. Preventive Med 26:607-611, 1997.

The author describes patients' expectations and how they influence behavior, differentiating two forms. The first is one in which the patient is expecting to die from the surgery and does die, not because of the operation but because of the expectation. The second form of the problem is that which involves a patient whose general attitude is negative and all of these expectations are fulfilled even though the patient's problem would not be expected to result as it did.

12. Kasdan ML, Lewis K, Bruner A, Johnson AL: The nocebo effect: Do no harm. J Southern Orthop Assn 8:108-113, 1999.

This brief report from a hand surgeon's perspective details how giving a patient a label, or "diagnosis," especially when it is suspicious and not based on sound criteria, can lead to the patient's acceptance of the "illness role." The failure of the physician involved to understand the nature of the patient's complaints, and the misapplication of the term *reflex sympathetic dystrophy* as well as the application of invasive and questionable surgical procedures, only led to profound dysfunction.

13. Lazare A: Conversion symptoms. N Engl J Med 305:745-748, 1981.

This is one of the clearest explanations of conversion symptoms that we have read. It discusses in detail the diagnosis of conversion symptoms and the associated loss of sensory and motor function that defy medical explanation. The rationale for this behavior is presented in detail.

14. LoPiccolo CJ, Goodkin K, Baldewicz TT: Current issues in the diagnosis and management of malingering. Ann Med 31:166-174, 1999.

This is a definitive article regarding the intentional reporting of symptoms where no disease exists. The conscious intent to deceive where a known objective (i.e., financial gain) is anticipated (malingering) must be considered when the history and physical findings do not make sense. This article also reviews the American Psychiatric Association's classifications of malingering and factitious disorders.

15. Louis DS, Lamp MK, Greene TL: The upper extremity and psychiatric illness. J Hand Surg [Am] 10:687-693, 1985.

This paper reviews a large series of patients (33) who presented with a variety of recognizable problems consistent with factitious illness. The follow-up averaged 4½ years. At the time this was written, self-causation was suspected but not established as it is now.

18. Phelps DB, Buchler U, Boswick JA: The diagnosis of factitious ulcer of the hand: A case report. J Hand Surg [Am] 2:105-108, 1977.

Suspecting a nonhealing ulcer to be factitious, the authors painted the wound with a tetracycline solution and later demonstrated wound manipulation by fluorescence of the fingers of the uninvolved hand.

19. Reading G: Secretan's syndrome: Hard edema of the dorsum of the hand. Plast Reconstr Surg 65:182-187, 1980.

This report of five patients details the relationship of workers' compensation to persistent edema of the hand, ulceration, and failure of wounds to heal. It brings into question the previous concept of "Secretan's syndrome" and hand edema of the dorsum of the hand as a distinct pathologic entity.

20. Schweiger A, Parducci A: Nocebo: The psychologic induction of pain. Pav J Biol Sci 16:140-145, 1981.

A group of healthy college students were evaluated who responded to suggestions that they would develop headaches after the application of an electrical current that was simulated but never happened. This was compared with the other group who were exposed to another challenge where headache was only listed as one of the side effects. This study suggests the susceptibility of people to anticipated or perceived outcomes even when the provocative events do not occur.

21. Simmons BP, Vasile RG: The clenched fist syndrome. J Hand Surg [Am] 5:420-427, 1980.

As one of the earliest papers explaining the dysfunctional positioning of the hand in the fisted position, this article emphasized the use of psychotherapeutic help and biofeedback. The futility of various treatment measures is explained as well as the positive effect of psychotherapy when it was followed.

22. Smith RJ: Factitious lymphedema of the hand. J Bone Joint Surg Am 57:89-94, 1975.

Smith's classic article involves 22 cases of factitious lymphedema with some outstanding pictures of the problem and a clear delineation of the personal characteristics of the patients with the problem. This is a must-read reference.

23. Stutts JT, Kasdan ML, Hickey SE, Bruner A: Reflex sympathetic dystrophy misdiagnosis in patients with dysfunctional postures of the upper extremity. J Hand Surg [Am] 25:1152-1156, 2000.

Sixty-three percent of patients in this study who presented with a dysfunctional posture of the hand were previously diagnosed as having reflex sympathetic dystrophy (RSD). After careful review, not one of these patients fulfilled stringent criteria for RSD. The paper emphasizes the frequency of this misdiagnosis and the consequences of inappropriate treatment.

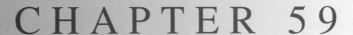

CHAPTER 59

Rheumatoid Arthritis and Other Connective Tissue Diseases

Paul Feldon, Andrew L. Terrono, Edward A. Nalebuff, and Lewis H. Millender

Reconstructive hand surgery has been established as an effective component in the overall management program of a patient with rheumatoid arthritis. Approximately 25% of all arthritis surgery is now performed on the hand.[1] However, it should be understood that hand reconstruction does not restore normal function to rheumatoid hands. Pain may be alleviated, severe deformity prevented or corrected, and appearance and function improved; but motion and dexterity will be limited, and weakness will remain a significant disability.[2-13] Because of the difficulty in consistently restoring or improving function, careful judgment must be used when recommending reconstructive surgery.

The purpose of this chapter is to describe the surgical techniques used to correct rheumatoid hand deformities. However, an understanding of these techniques is only one requirement—the surgeon must also appreciate the natural history of the disease and deformities. In addition, the surgeon must understand the functional needs and limitations of each patient to make appropriate judgments regarding the indications for surgical treatment.[14] By working closely with the rheumatologist, orthopedic surgeon, and physical, occupational, and hand therapists, the hand surgeon will have a better understanding of the overall treatment program and thereby provide the best care possible for these patients.[15,16]

SURGICAL CONSIDERATIONS IN THE ARTHRITIC PATIENT

The care of a hand affected by rheumatoid arthritis differs in many respects from that of a hand affected by trauma. In a rheumatoid patient, an ongoing process of joint and tendon destruction can persist for many years. Involvement of one joint affects adjacent joints. Involvement of adjacent joints or recurrent disease can nullify the effects of previous surgery. The manifestations of the disease vary for each patient. Cooperation between the rheumatologist and the surgeon is essential to provide appropriate surgical recommendations for each individual. The surgeon must understand both the pathophysiology and the natural history of the disease.[17-25]

Rheumatoid arthritis is a systemic condition affecting synovial tissue. All deformities, joint destruction, and pathologic anatomy that occur in patients with rheumatoid arthritis are the result of the way in which the diseased and hypertrophied synovial tissue alters its surroundings. Rheumatoid synovium destroys articular cartilage by a poorly understood enzymatic reaction, invades subchondral bone, and stretches the soft tissues that support the involved joint. It also surrounds and invades the flexor and extensor tendons. The result is disruption of the normal architecture of the hand and wrist, and loss of the normal delicate balance of flexor and extensor forces across adjacent joints of the hand-wrist unit.

Nearly all the surgical procedures performed on the rheumatoid hand and wrist fall into one of five groups: synovectomy, tenosynovectomy, tendon surgery, arthroplasty, and arthrodesis.[1]

Judgment regarding the type and timing of surgical procedures for reconstructing the rheumatoid hand and wrist requires experience. An individual treatment plan must be formulated for each patient based on the status of the hand and the patient's needs, as well as the expertise and experience of the surgeon. The presence of deformity is not, in and of itself, an indication for surgery, because many patients maintain good function in spite of significant deformity. We believe that reconstructive rheumatoid hand surgery is not for the occasional hand surgeon.[26-30]

The surgeon treating a rheumatoid hand must work within the framework of the patient's medical, social, and economic problems. This requires coordination and interaction with the other professionals involved with the patient's care. Good rapport with the patient is essential, because the reconstructive program usually spans many months, and often years.

The patient's disease pattern affects the surgical approach in rheumatoid reconstruction. In general, synovectomy is indicated for patients with mild disease controlled by drugs who experience persistent synovitis in one or two joints. However, synovectomies are contraindicated in patients with rapidly progressive joint disease. In these patients, frequent observation is required so that reconstructive surgery can be performed before the development of severe deformities. Early tenosynovectomy may be required in patients with rapidly progressive disease to prevent tendon rupture. With the advent of anti–tumor necrosis factor (TNF) therapy, communication between the rheumatologist and the hand surgeon is especially important in the patient with aggressive disease. Before embarking on surgical treatment, the optimal medical regimen should be established.

Better results are possible when reconstruction is performed before severe fixed contractures occur and before significant subluxation or dislocation occurs. After the capsule and supporting ligamentous structures have stretched, the lack of adequate soft tissue support makes the maintenance of joint alignment and function more difficult. Caution must be used when considering reconstructive surgery in patients with mild deformities who are basically healthy and active but who are frustrated because of their general loss of function. They want to pursue their avocations or sports activities but may not have the strength or endurance to do so. Hand surgery cannot restore full function in these patients and may weaken the hand even further; therefore, it is not indicated, because it would not produce the desired or expected end result. Such patients need to understand their disease and modify their activities. A hand therapist can be helpful in this situation.

Hand surgery also can lead to disappointing results in patients who have significant destruction of multiple joints but who have minimal pain and who function relatively well in spite of their disease. Many of these patients are older and place fewer demands on their hands. Unless surgery can provide either significant pain relief or a dramatic change in function, the patient's expectations of reconstructive surgery may not be fulfilled.

Patients' expectations should match the surgeon's goals and anticipated results. They must know that some deformity, especially at the metacarpophalangeal (MCP) joints, is likely to recur after surgery. Nonetheless, Vahvanen and Viljakka[31] reported a high rate of patient satisfaction after reconstructive surgery for rheumatoid disease. There is no substitute for in-depth preoperative discussion between the surgeon and the patient.

MEDICAL CONSIDERATIONS IN THE RHEUMATOID PATIENT

Certain factors should be considered in rheumatoid patients scheduled for hand surgery. A careful preoperative evaluation will alert the surgeon to these factors, and appropriate consultation can be obtained before surgery if needed. Discovering an unexpected condition on the day of surgery that might alter or delay the reconstruction is always disrupting and frustrating.[32]

Cervical spine involvement may be subtle. It is worthwhile to identify instability of the cervical spine preoper-atively so that appropriate measures can be taken to protect the neck during surgery if general anesthesia is required. Cervical spine stability should be evaluated clinically as well as radiographically, because there may not be a close correlation between neurologic deficit and radiographic findings. A history of numbness or paresthesias with cervical motion must be heeded.

Temporomandibular joint involvement may compromise intubation during general anesthesia. The anesthesiologist should be aware of such involvement so that adequate plans can be made for nasotracheal or fiberoptic intubation if these become necessary.

Pulmonary involvement can occur from the disease itself (pulmonary rheumatoid nodules or interstitial fibrosis) or as the consequence of antirheumatic therapy with gold, penicillamine, or methotrexate.

Felty's syndrome (splenomegaly and neutropenia), although rare, can cause a profound decrease in white blood cell count and thereby increase the susceptibility to infection.

Drug therapy must be taken into account when planning surgery. Systemic corticosteroids and penicillamine can delay wound healing. Methotrexate can affect liver function, which may affect the choice of anesthesia. There have been conflicting reports on infection rates in patients on methotrexate who undergo surgery for rheumatoid arthritis.[33-35] We have not noticed an increased incidence in reconstructive hand surgery.

Gold, penicillamine, and methotrexate can suppress platelet counts. Aspirin affects platelet function for several days, and discontinuing aspirin before extensive surgery may be prudent. Nonsteroidal anti-inflammatory medication affects platelet aggregation only for several hours. These drugs are withheld preoperatively for a period equal to five times the dose interval schedule. For example, drugs given four times daily are withheld for 2 days before surgery. Those given once daily are withheld for 5 days. These medications can be restarted within 48 hours after surgery. In general, we also withhold anti-TNF medications in a similar fashion to methotrexate.

Every effort should be made to minimize the use of narcotics after surgery. It is easy for patients with chronic pain to become dependent on oral narcotic analgesics, although this is rare in the rheumatoid population. The use of patient-controlled analgesia, whereby small amounts of medication are delivered intravenously by pump on demand, has been effective in controlling pain and in decreasing the total amount of pain medication used in the postoperative period.

STAGING HAND SURGERY

One of the difficult tasks in rheumatoid surgery is the formulation of a plan for the systematic reconstruction of the hand. Although there are no hard-and-fast rules, some general principles can be outlined. The priorities for hand surgery in rheumatoid patients are (1) alleviation of pain, (2) improvement of function, (3) retardation of progression of the disease, and (4) improvement of appearance. Appropriate decisions are made more easily if each of these priorities is considered for each patient. Relief of pain is the foremost goal. The indications for surgery to relieve pain are clear and predictable; fusions and arthroplasties accomplish this.

Pain may be the most important factor in determining a rheumatoid patient's ability to work. Many patients with severe deformities can work because they are able to adapt to their functional limitations. In contrast, patients with much less deformity but with significant pain are less able to continue gainful employment.[36] A painful wrist or thumb usually takes precedence over dislocated MCP joints of the fingers. Acute carpal tunnel syndrome or proliferative dorsal tenosynovitis with a single tendon rupture is allocated high priority to prevent permanent loss of median nerve function or more tendon ruptures.

Loss of function is not synonymous with deformity, and careful evaluation and discussion are needed before any surgery to improve function is undertaken. Patients with adequate function, in spite of deformity, may not benefit from surgery.

Undetected carpal tunnel syndrome often can be aggravated by any surgical procedure in the hand. Therefore, carpal tunnel release should be considered before, or in conjunction with, other surgical procedures on the volar aspect of the wrist.

Each joint must be evaluated both individually (Table 59-1) and as part of the whole hand. We usually correct MCP joint deformities before treating proximal interphalangeal (PIP) joint deformities.[37-39] An exception to this is the severe boutonnière deformity, which should be corrected before or at the same time as the MCP joint, because a severe flexion deformity at the PIP joint compromises the result of the MCP joint surgery. Conversely, an extension deformity of the PIP joint concentrates the flexion at the MCP joint and enhances the MCP motion. Therefore, extension deformities at the PIP joint can be corrected at a later time.

PIP joint deformity is often the result of a primary MCP joint deformity. Treating the MCP joints first may simplify treatment of the PIP joints. Just restoring MCP joint alignment and motion can provide a significant improvement in hand function, even with imperfect PIP joint function. The converse is not necessarily true; reasonable PIP joint motion does little to improve hand function if the MCP joints remain fixed in flexion (Fig. 59-1).[40]

If extensor tendon reconstruction is required in addition to MCP joint surgery, we reconstruct the MCP joints before the extensor tendons are treated. This facilitates postoperative rehabilitation, because active MCP joint flexion is necessary for restoring MCP joint motion after arthroplasty, but MCP extension can be provided with a dynamic splint.

Extensor tendon reconstruction can be done at a second stage without compromising the previous MCP joint surgery.[40]

Most patients have bilateral hand problems that require surgical treatment. When similar problems are present bilaterally, we discuss the situation with the patient and allow him or her to help us decide on which hand to operate first. However, when only one hand is severely disabled, it takes precedence over the other hand. This staging allows the patient to have one hand for daily needs while the other hand is being rehabilitated after surgery. During the rehabilitation period, the nonoperated hand must perform additional work, and this alone may induce a flare of synovitis.

It is better to do preventive surgery such as synovectomy, dorsal tenosynovectomy, and even median nerve decompression before considering reconstructive surgery. As emphasized by Souter,[41] it is best to begin a reconstructive program with surgical procedures that are predictable in their outcome and effect and to progress in stages to those procedures that are less predictable. Thus, such procedures as wrist stabilization and distal ulnar excision can be performed first, followed by thumb MCP joint fusion, distal interphalangeal (DIP) fusion in the fingers, and MCP joint arthroplasty.

It may be prudent to operate on the less involved hand first, especially in an apprehensive patient. This approach can prevent progressive deformity, provide a better overall result, and allow the patient to assess the potential of further reconstruction. The effect of proximal joint function on the wrist and hand must be considered in preoperative planning. Shoulder and/or elbow reconstruction, if indicated, should be done before hand reconstruction so that rehabilitation of the hand after surgery is not impeded by more proximal problems. Proximal and distal joints must be evaluated before any surgery, because they can affect what type of surgery is performed. If elbow flexion is limited, for example, the ability of the hand to get to the mouth may be compromised if the wrist is corrected into a more extended position. Therefore, the wrist should be fused in a neutral or slightly flexed position, or the elbow flexion should be increased.

Occasionally, it is necessary to consider hand deformities and upper extremity limitations in view of lower extremity problems. If a painful or deformed hand prevents the use of ambulatory aids such as crutches or walkers, it may be necessary to perform upper extremity surgery before lower extremity surgery. In general, patients with a rheumatoid wrist problem require fusion to allow the use of ambulatory aids.

Hospital stays should be coordinated so that the total number of admissions (and anesthetics) is reduced. Frequently, hand surgery and foot surgery can be performed simultaneously by two teams. When the patient is ready to ambulate after lower extremity surgery, modified walking aids such as platform crutches or walkers are used. The patient's therapy and rehabilitation programs also must be coordinated among the therapists caring for the upper and the lower extremities.

In this chapter, we include our philosophy of the management of difficult rheumatoid hand problems. We summarize the pathology of the deformities and our indications for surgery, as well as the results that can be expected from the procedures. A large reference list has been included, and

Table 59-1
STAGES OF RHEUMATOID JOINT INVOLVEMENT

Stage	Description
1	Synovitis without deformity
2	Synovitis with passively correctable deformity
3	Fixed deformity without joint changes
4	Articular destruction

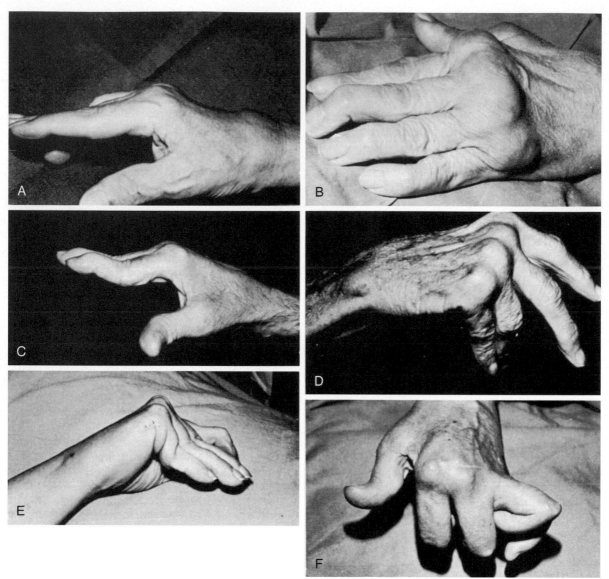

FIGURE 59-1. Examples of stages of rheumatoid hand deformities. **A,** Stage 1: Early MCP joint synovitis without deformity. Note early dorsal tenosynovitis. **B,** Stage 2: Moderate MCP joint synovitis without dislocation of the MCP joints and without marked bony destruction. **C,** Stage 2: Early MCP joint subluxation with swan neck deformity. Both of these deformities are correctable passively, and there is no cartilage or bone destruction. The patient is a candidate for intrinsic release, synovectomy, and extensor tendon relocation. **D,** Stage 3: Classic example of MCP joint dislocation without PIP joint involvement. Note absence of wrist joint subluxation and minimal subluxation of the distal ulna. Extensor tendon function is intact. **E,** Stage 3: Fixed dislocation of the MCP joints with secondary swan neck deformity. Note mallet deformity of the DIP joint in the index finger. **F,** Stage 4: Severe hand deformity with fixed dislocation of the MCP joints and fixed flexion contractures of the PIP joints. The patient has had previous synovectomy. Salvage surgery includes PIP joint arthrodeses and MCP joint arthroplasties. (From Millender LH, Nalebuff EA: Evaluation and treatment of early rheumatoid hand involvement. Orthop Clin North Am 6:697-708, 1975, with permission.)

readers are encouraged to refer to the original articles by many authors in this field to enhance their understanding of the principles and procedures described here.

OTHER CONNECTIVE TISSUE DISEASES (RHEUMATOID VARIANTS)

Psoriatic arthritis, systemic lupus erythematosus, and scleroderma are three uncommon arthritic diseases that superficially resemble rheumatoid arthritis. These diseases frequently involve the hand and wrist and thus are sig-

nificant to the hand surgeon. Each of these diseases has distinct features affecting the type of deformities seen and the treatments needed to adequately care for these patients. The specifics of the surgical techniques are discussed in the corresponding section on rheumatoid arthritis.

Psoriatic Arthritis

Psoriatic arthritis is a rheumatoid variant that is classified as one of the seronegative spondyloarthropathies, along with Reiter's syndrome, ankylosing spondylitis, and the arthritis of inflammatory bowel disease. The classic finding in psoriasis is a scaly, erythematous rash.[42] Approximately 5% of patients with psoriasis have some type of inflammatory arthritis. The skin lesions precede the arthritis changes in most cases, but 15% to 20% of patients develop the skin lesions after the onset of the arthritis.[43] This rash may be extensive or localized to small patches on the scalp, face, or extremities. Direct skin involvement can occur on the hand and complicates surgical treatment, because of the enhanced risk of infection. Cultures of *Staphylococcus aureus* have been found in psoriatic skin.[44] The psoriatic rash improves with ultraviolet light, which is one of the main treatments for this condition. Because the skin condition often improves during the summer, this should be taken into account when scheduling elective surgery on a hand with a significant psoriatic rash. The diagnosis of psoriasis can also be made by characteristic changes in the nails.[45,46] It has been stated that 80% of patients with psoriasis have nail changes, but this finding is present in only 15% with arthritic involvement. Psoriasis of the nails alone without overt evidence of cutaneous disease is infrequent. The most common nail finding is pitting and represents involvement of the proximal matrix. Other nail findings include leukonychia and crumbling of the nails.[45]

The pattern of joint involvement in psoriatic arthritis varies widely: 95% of such patients have peripheral joint involvement; 25% have a polyarthritis similar to rheumatoid arthritis; and 5% have classic DIP joint disease with erosion of the terminal phalanges, DIP joint destruction, nail pitting, and onycholysis. Osteolysis is common, with destruction of bone and ultimate widening of the joint spaces. Bone proliferates along the margins of the bone on the distal side of the joint. The proximal bone tapers and, when associated with the distal bone changes, leads to a "pencil in cup"[47] appearance. Osteolysis most commonly affects the DIP joints[42] but can involve all the finger joints, resulting in digital shortening. In its full-blown stage, these patients have arthritis mutilans. Because of collapse of the digits, the condition has been called "opera glass hand."[48] The collapse of the fingers can also occur in rheumatoid patients but is more frequently seen in those with psoriatic arthritis. Although osteolysis is the most frequent radiographic finding in the psoriatic hand, spontaneous ankylosis can also occur. In digits with spontaneous or surgical fusion, the digital length is maintained.[48] It is common for the distal joints to fuse spontaneously, but this can also occur at the PIP level. Most patients with hand involvement have combinations of osteolytic and fused joints. In our experience, ankylosis of the digital MCP joints does not occur. Inflammation of the periosteum, tendons, and tendon insertions may be a factor in the fusiform swelling of digits in this disease, so-called sausage swelling or psoriatic dactylitis, with significant soft tissue swelling around the joints. The radiographs readily show the periarticular soft tissue enlargement that explains the clinical appearance. Fusiform swelling of the digits is best treated by medical means.

Psoriatic arthritis causes hand deformities similar to those seen in rheumatoid arthritis, with several typical differences, including psoriatic skin lesions.[42] There is a much lower incidence of tenosynovitis and tendon ruptures than noted in rheumatoid arthritis.[43,49] Therefore, tenosynovectomy and other tendon surgery are uncommon in psoriatic arthritis. The subcutaneous nodules associated with rheuma-

toid arthritis are not found in this condition. Unlike rheumatoid disease, which tends to be symmetrical, these patients usually have asymmetrical involvement of the hands. This asymmetry is also present within the hand, with apparently unaffected digits adjacent to involved fingers that are short or demonstrate significant deformity.

Although individual patients may have both osteolysis and ankylosis, one of these characteristics is usually more prominent than the other, making it possible to categorize patients into different groups, which helps determine treatment choices. We now use a modification of the Moll and Wright classification,[50] based directly on the radiographic and clinical changes seen in these hands. In psoriatic arthritis there can be (1) spontaneous fusions that maintain digital length, (2) osteolysis with bone loss, or (3) joint stiffness with rheumatoid arthritis–like deformities. It is important to stress that the extent of bone loss can vary from mild to extensive. Spontaneous ankylosis can also involve single or multiple joints.[51]

Digital Deformity

The most common deformities seen in the psoriatic hand are flexion deformities of the PIP joints without the corresponding distal joint hyperextension characteristic of the boutonnière deformity.[49,52] As a consequence of the flexed PIP joint, the MCP joints are often hyperextended and ultimately become stiff. Severe fixed flexion deformities are best treated by fusion rather than by arthroplasty. Swan neck deformities, which are common in rheumatoid arthritis, occur occasionally in psoriatic arthritis but often result from a distal joint mallet deformity rather than originating at the PIP level.

In contrast to rheumatoid arthritis, patients with psoriatic arthritis tend to have MCP joint extension contractures rather than flexion contractures. Postoperative motion after MCP arthroplasty may be limited compared with that usually obtained in rheumatoid patients. If arthroplasties are done, more bone should be resected to allow adequate space for the implant. In our experience with MCP arthroplasties, we have found that the risk of infection is higher in this group.[44] Fixed flexion deformities of the MCP joints appear in patients with stiff or extended PIP joints. These patients have difficulty grasping large objects because of the limited MCP extension frequently associated with a contracted thumb web space.

The DIP joints are involved frequently but rarely need treatment, because they tend to fuse spontaneously. Arthritis mutilans, which results in severe loss of bone stock with collapse and shortening of the digit, is not uncommon and must be treated early and aggressively by joint fusions using bone grafts to restore digital length (Fig. 59-2).[52,53]

Thumb Deformity

Each of the three thumb joints can be involved in psoriatic arthritis. As noted in rheumatoid arthritis, the most common deformity includes MCP joint flexion and interphalangeal (IP) joint hyperextension. Hyperextension deformities of the MCP joint are rare in this group. The patients do develop stiffness at the carpometacarpal (CMC) joint level, which greatly reduces thumb function. Surgical procedures should include MCP and/or IP fusions. It is advisable to pronate the thumb as part of the fusion to improve the thumb index

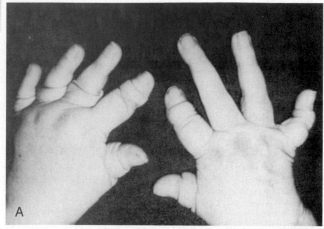

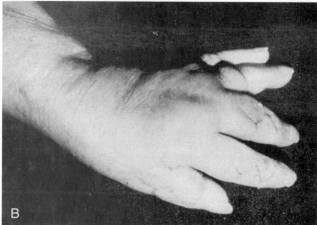

FIGURE 59-2. A, Arthritis mutilans with typical "opera glass" hand deformities. **B,** Fusions of the IP joints of the index and middle fingers and of the IP and MCP joints of the thumb using iliac crest bone grafts to restore pinch function.

pinch. At the basal joint, to restore or to maintain thumb motion, we prefer a resection arthroplasty with a ligament suspension,[54] as is used in osteoarthritis.[51]

Wrist Deformity

Wrist involvement is common in psoriatic arthritis.[49] Presently, we limit wrist surgery in psoriatic arthritis to fusion and excision of the distal ulna.[55] Spontaneous intercarpal fusion can alleviate the need for additional wrist surgery if the alignment is good and the motion is not painful. We continue to use Steinmann pin fixation techniques to achieve a total wrist fusion. Intramedullary fixation in the third metacarpal is necessary when there is considerable carpal bone loss. The intermedullary technique can be used when the patient has intact or fused carpal bones.[55,56] We do not recommend wrist arthroplasty for patients with psoriatic arthritis.

Systemic Lupus Erythematosus

Systemic lupus erythematosus (SLE) is a multisystem disease with common joint and hand involvement.[47] It may involve many major organs of the body, such as the heart, lungs, and kidneys.[57] Pericarditis is the most common heart problem, with pleuritis affecting pulmonary function. It has been reported that 50% of lupus patients have clinical manifestations of renal disease. Skin lesions occur in 85% of these patients, with a typical erythematous blush in the butterfly area on cheeks and across the bridge of the nose often noted after sun exposure. Another common rash is an erythematous maculopapular eruption that may also occur after sun exposure on the fingers and palm.[57]

Patients with SLE are often initially diagnosed as having rheumatoid arthritis or "nonspecific" arthritis.[57] In children, the most common initial diagnosis is rheumatic fever. At present, the generally accepted way to diagnose SLE is based on the American Rheumatism Association Preliminary Criteria. A patient needs to have 4 of 14 criteria, either simultaneously or serially, to make the diagnosis of SLE. Some of these criteria are LE cells, arthritis, Raynaud's disease, facial erythema, pleuritis, pericarditis, or uremia.[57]

Lupus patients are predominantly young women, with a female-to-male ratio of 9 to 1.[57] This condition is more common in black women than in white women, with an average age at onset between 15 and 25 years.[57] Hand involvement can include symmetrical joint swelling, tenderness, pain with motion, and morning stiffness. Raynaud's disease is common.[58] Joint deformities are the most predominant hand manifestations of SLE.[59,60] Although the deformities may appear similar to those seen in rheumatoid arthritis, ligamentous and volar plate laxity, as well as tendon subluxation leading to joint imbalance, are the hallmark of this disease rather than joint destruction.[61,62] The joint deformities occur without the erosive destruction of the articular cartilage seen in other forms of arthritis. The wrist, digits, and thumb are the most frequent sites of involvement, and the ankles, elbows, and shoulders are least often affected.[61,62] The joint deformities occur without the erosive destruction of the articular cartilage seen in other forms of arthritis. The wrist, digits, and thumb are the most frequent sites of involvement, and the ankles, elbows, and shoulders are least often affected.[61,62] Radiographs show deformity, but with normal-appearing joint spaces (Fig. 59-3). Tenosynovitis can occur and may be present without joint involvement.

Patients with SLE are best managed with a team approach. These patients may have serious medical problems that take priority over the hand and wrist deformities. A rheumatologist or internist should carry out the medical treatment of this condition. Patients without major organ involvement are usually treated symptomatically with nonsteroidal anti-inflammatory drugs.[57] In more serious cases, corticosteroids are indicated. With regard to specific wrist and hand involvement, a cooperative effort between a hand therapist and surgeon is ideal.

The initial treatment of passively correctable deformities, which are the hallmark of SLE, is best carried out by exercises and splinting. We do not believe that the common deformities of SLE will be permanently corrected by these methods, but it is possible to maintain function for an extended period of time and, thereby, delay surgery. Patients can be taught to stretch tight ulnar intrinsics that are secondary to digital ulnar deviation at the MCP joint level. Wrist splints are helpful to maintain wrist alignment. Resting splints at night are useful to keep the fingers in proper alignment at the MCP joint level. For the passively

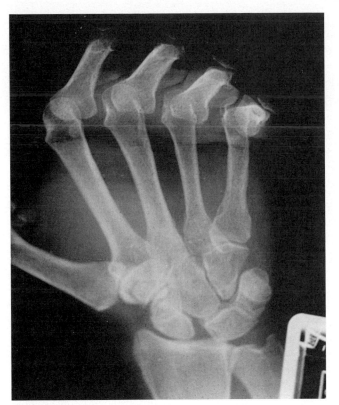

FIGURE 59-3. Lupus causes deformities similar to those seen in rheumatoid arthritis but without joint destruction. Note the ulnar deviation and volar subluxation of the MCP joints, the secondary radial deviation of the metacarpals, and the scapholunate dissociation in the absence of joint space narrowing, periarticular erosions, and cyst formation.

correctable swan neck deformities of the fingers, the patient can wear Silver Ring splints that resemble jewelry and are well accepted by patients. Commercially available Lamb Wire Foam splints are useful for early boutonnière deformities. The risk of "conservative" nonoperative treatment may be progression to fixed deformities that alter the treatment options for the surgeon. Therefore, it is the surgeon's role to determine when it is appropriate to modify the course of the disease by surgical intervention.

Wrist Deformity

Deformities can often be corrected passively, but attempts to reconstruct the deformities by soft tissue procedures are associated with a frustratingly high recurrence rate. Thus, arthroplasties and/or fusions may be necessary, even though the joints have been preserved and look uninvolved on radiographs. Surgery in lupus patients should be performed before fixed deformities occur. With regard to the wrist, the most useful surgical procedures are limited and total wrist fusions. For complete wrist dislocations, total wrist fusion is the procedure of choice.[55] Longitudinal Steinmann pin fixation is our preferred technique to obtain total wrist fusion.[55,63,64] For ulnar translocation of the carpus, realign the wrist with either radiolunate or radiocarpal fusions, thus maintaining midcarpal motion.[55] In our opinion, there is no place for flexible implants in the lupus wrist. We have no experience with total wrist replacement in SLE and doubt the wisdom of its use in a situation in which stability

and soft tissue balance are so critical to success. The lax ligaments characteristic of lupus do not provide the essential support to prevent recurrent deformity. Realignment of the wrist reduces the risk of secondary finger deformities. However, most of the deformities at the MCP joint level are primary as a result of soft tissue changes at the local level.

A common wrist problem is dorsal subluxation of the ulna. In addition to being unsightly, causing pain, and restricting wrist rotation, it can cause attrition extensor tendon ruptures.[62,65] Dorsal wrist tenosynovitis is uncommon in SLE. When tendon ruptures do occur, they are generally the result of attrition. A Darrach procedure is useful in lupus. Stabilization of the remaining ulna with a portion of the extensor carpi ulnaris (ECU) tendon or the ulnar carpal ligaments should be performed to prevent dorsal migration.[66,67] It is important to bevel the dorsal lip of the resected ulna to minimize subsequent attrition tendon ruptures over a sharp bone edge.

Digital Deformity

The characteristic finger deformity at the MCP joint is ulnar deviation and volar subluxation.[60,62] These patients demonstrate excellent finger flexion with a loss of active extension while maintaining passive extension. With time, they gradually lose passive extension. The sequence of pathologic findings is as follows: Subluxation of the extensor tendon ulnar to the metacarpal head occurs; and as this support is diminished, the proximal phalanx subluxes volarly. The joint capsule becomes thinned, and a defect in the dorsal capsule occurs. With increasing ulnar deviation, the ulnar intrinsic muscle shortens, with subsequent hyperextension deformity at the PIP level. At first, the deformity is passively correctable, but gradually this mobility is lost. In spite of the MCP deformity becoming fixed, the articular cartilage is preserved.

In a previous review of this subject, we noted that soft tissue realignment of the extensor tendons did not maintain correction in 21 of 30 digits.[62] In each of these fingers, the deformity recurred and often became fixed. Swanson arthroplasties were performed either for fixed MCP joint deformities or in those digits in which soft tissue corrections had failed. We concluded that arthroplasty with a silicone implant was indicated, even though the metacarpal head was intact, with normal-appearing articular cartilage.[62] Zancolli reported success in maintaining MCP joint alignment in rheumatoid arthritis by attaching the extensor tendon to the proximal phalanx, which minimized recurrent tendon subluxation.[68] Wood and associates, using the same technique, corrected recurrent extensor tendon subluxation in a large group of patients that included two with SLE.[69]

 Authors' Preferred Method of Treatment

During the past 5 years, we have attempted to restore MCP alignment and function by soft tissue surgery, including extensor tendon relocation and tenodesis. In patients with full passive correction, we approach the joint dorsally. A central defect in the joint capsule is repaired, and the extensor tendon is relocated on to the dorsum of the joint directly to the bone, as described by Wood and associates.[69] As part of the soft tissue rebalancing, the contracted ulnar sagittal fibers are released and the radial sagittal fibers are reefed to try to rebalance the support of the extensor tendon directly over the joint. The aim is to restore full MCP extension when direct traction is applied to the extensor tendon.

Although we have completely released the ulnar intrinsic in many patients, there have been late complications. In a few fingers, we noted late radial deviation with tightness of the radial intrinsic. For this reason, we now believe that a complete ulnar intrinsic release is not without risk and prefer, instead, to step-cut and lengthen the ulnar intrinsic. We believe that intrinsic transfers that are useful in correcting severe ulnar deviation in rheumatoid arthritis are particularly dangerous in SLE. All the soft tissue surgery that we perform is designed to restore alignment and balance to the joint. It may be foolhardy to think that restoration of local anatomy can withstand the tissue changes in SLE. However, we believe that the deformities can be corrected and the need for joint replacement thereby delayed or avoided. These same soft tissue repairs are indicated in patients with fixed MCP joint deformities requiring prosthetic replacements.

Prolonged postoperative splinting is required after MCP surgery whether or not implants are used. The joints are held in good alignment for 6 weeks before motion is initiated. Once MCP motion is begun, the fingers are splinted together as a unit to maintain alignment and concentrate flexion at the MCP level. Dynamic splinting is also used to support extension and maintain digital alignment during the early healing stage.[70]

Occasionally, we have treated SLE patients who also demonstrate excessive finger MCP joint hyperextension. In this situation, a "lasso procedure" described by Zancolli for ulnar nerve palsy is combined with the dorsal soft tissue balancing.[71,72] In this procedure, one slip of the sublimis tendon is passed around the A1 pulley to restrain MCP joint hyperextension.

PIP Joint Deformity

Finger IP joints can have hyperextension, flexion, or lateral deformities that occur as a result of stretching of the supporting tendons, collateral ligaments, and volar plate mechanism. With mild and early deformities, soft tissue procedures useful in rheumatoid arthritis can be carried out.[38,64] Unfortunately, these deformities often become severe and fixed, making arthrodesis the treatment of choice. Restoration of IP alignment, even by fusion, is essential if long-term MCP joint corrections are to be maintained.[70]

Thumb Deformity

The thumb is commonly involved in SLE. It is often the first place where hand deformities occur.[61,62] A frequent primary manifestation is lateral subluxation of the distal joint. However, the distal joint deformity can be a secondary response to primary deformity at the MCP level. With MCP joint hyperextension, the distal joint rapidly assumes a flexed position, whereas the reverse occurs with MCP

flexion deformities.[73,74] The treatment of choice is surgical fusion, which restores thumb stability and function. In addition, the correction of the IP joint deformity lessens the chance of reciprocal deformity at the more proximal MCP joint.[73,74]

The thumb MCP joint can also be the primary site of deformity. Subluxation of the extensor tendons is common in SLE, and the thumb is no exception. As extensor pollicis longus (EPL) support diminishes, the MCP joint assumes a flexed position.[73,74] Lateral instability may also occur in long-standing cases as a result of laxity of the collateral ligaments. Initially, passive correction is possible, but later the deformity becomes fixed. As a response to the severe flexion, the metacarpal assumes an abducted position and the distal joint hyperextends, producing the typical type I thumb deformity.[73,74]

Authors' Preferred Method of Treatment

If passive MCP joint extension is possible, there are two surgical approaches that we have found useful: EPL rerouting[73,74] and MCP joint arthrodesis. EPL rerouting is preferred if the distal joint of CMC joint requires fusion to provide stability. This procedure restores active MCP extension while maintaining mobility, thereby relieving some strain on the CMC joint. However, certain modifications are in order. These include reefing the collateral ligaments for lateral support and postoperative splinting for 6 weeks. Temporary Kirschner wire fixation is important to maintain the corrected position. Joints in SLE patients ordinarily do not get stiff after immobilization. The typical range of postoperative flexion is about 40 degrees and is usually achieved even with 6 weeks of immobilization.

When the flexed MCP joint cannot be passively corrected or is hyperextended, or if the CMC and IP joints are good, arthrodesis is the procedure of choice. The joint should be fixed in 15 to 20 degrees of flexion. Arthroplasty of the MCP joint with a flexible implant might be considered, but our experience with this approach in SLE patients has not been as successful as in those with rheumatoid arthritis. SLE patients tend to regain excessive motion and fracture the prosthesis, with recurrent deformity. If both the MCP and IP joints are fused, it is imperative to maintain motion at the thumb CMC joint.

Primary subluxation or dislocation of the thumb CMC joint also occurs in lupus. If the MCP and IP joints are well aligned and stable, fusion of the CMC joint can be performed, resulting in a general improvement in thumb alignment and function.[61,62] It is important to stabilize the CMC joint with the metacarpal in a slightly abducted position. However, excessive metacarpal abduction must be avoided, because it may lead to excessive MCP joint flexion and dislocation, with a further reduction of thumb function. A prosthetic replacement is not indicated.[61]

An alternative to CMC fusion is soft tissue stabilization, which is essential if the MCP and IP joints are fused. Realignment of the metacarpal with the flexor carpi radialis

(FCR) tendon is effective for maintaining stability with[54] or without[75] a resection arthroplasty. Temporary Kirschner wire fixation can be used.

Scleroderma

Scleroderma (systemic sclerosis) is a generalized disease with involvement of the skin, gastrointestinal tract, kidneys, lungs, and heart and often the hands. It is more frequent in females than males. Although the etiology of this condition is unknown, it is thought to be a disorder of the small blood vessels and connective tissue that leads to fibrosis. The fibrosis of the skin affects primarily the face and hands, altering the patient's appearance and leading to severe finger deformities, with subsequent loss of hand function. The facial involvement contracts the skin around the mouth, thereby reducing the patient's ability to open the mouth. Scleroderma patients tend to look alike.

A common early manifestation is Raynaud's phenomenon, with intermittent vasospasm and reduced digital circulation. During these episodes, the fingers become white and then turn blue and finally reddish. The reduced digital circulation can lead to skin ulcers, gangrene of the fingertips, and ultimately digital amputations. The acronym CREST has been used to describe the common features of systemic sclerosis: calcinosis, Raynaud's phenomenon, esophageal dysfunction, sclerodactyly, and telangiectasia. The term *overlap syndrome* is used for those scleroderma patients with associated findings characteristic of lupus, dermatomyositis, or rheumatoid arthritis.

There are two forms of systemic sclerosis: a type with limited and localized skin involvement and a more common diffuse type. Patients with the diffuse type more frequently develop finger joint contractures and digital deformities. Subcutaneous or intracutaneous calcinosis can occur within a single digit, causing painful hard areas at the fingertips, or it may be widespread within the hand and arm. The skin can break down over these areas and discharge a white toothpaste-like or chalky material. The term *sclerodactyly* is used to describe the appearance of the fingers, which become slender with thin, shiny, and sclerotic skin.

Digital Deformity

The deformity patterns seen in scleroderma are diverse, but certain combinations are common. The most frequent deformity is the progressive development of PIP flexion contractures (Fig. 59-4). These patients gradually lose the ability to actively extend the PIP joints and then develop flexion contractures that become severe and fixed. The extensor mechanism over the joints thins and ultimately ruptures. The skin blanches and ultimately breaks down, exposing the underlying tendon or the open joint. The danger of joint infection or osteomyelitis is real. Therefore, keeping areas of skin breakdown clean before surgical correction is critical. As patients develop increasing flexion of the PIP joint, they compensate by hyperextending at the MCP joint level. Initially, the MCP joints maintain active flexion, but with time, the collateral ligaments, joint capsule, and overlying skin contract, severely limiting MCP joint flexion.

The development of PIP joint hyperextension is also encountered in scleroderma but is infrequent. This deformity is secondary to the development of MCP joint subluxation in flexion, similar to patients with rheumatoid arthritis. The prominent metacarpal head can erode the overlying skin.

The skin and muscles of the first web space often shorten, and a first web space contracture develops. This reduces thumb mobility and diminishes the ability to grasp large objects between the thumb and index finger.

Surgery on the scleroderma patient's hand is usually performed to improve function and to relieve pain. It is unlikely that splinting and exercises can stop the progression of deformity. Scleroderma poses distinct problems for the hand surgeon. The deformities encountered are similar to those seen in rheumatoid arthritis. However, the altered circulation and skin changes associated with this disease adversely affect the surgical options and treatment. Wound healing is compromised, and surgical exposure is limited because of tight skin and poor circulation, complicating surgical options.

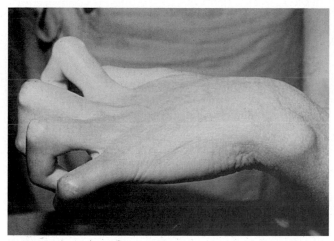

FIGURE 59-4. Scleroderma typically causes severe PIP joint contractures, which result in compensatory hyperextension of the MCP joints.

Authors' Preferred Method of Treatment

Increasing deformity with functional loss, the development of skin breakdown, and extruding calcific material are common indications for surgical consultation. The most common indications for surgery are vascular insufficiency with digital ulceration, calcinosis, and finger and thumb deformities.

Ulceration. Ulceration at the tips of fingers is the result of poor circulation and may be extremely painful. The ulceration is often slow to heal. Skin breakdown at the PIP or MCP level results from a combination of decreased circulation and pressure from underlying bone prominence secondary to joint deformity. These open wounds can progress to deep infections, but with splinting and good wound care they often heal. They require frequent dressing changes, occasional débridement, and protective splinting. Range-of-motion exercises should be curtailed to protect the underlying joint, because the risk of joint sepsis or osteomyelitis is real. At the fingertips, the underlying phalangeal tufts can resorb, and if gangrene ultimately develops, autoamputation can occur or surgical amputation will be needed. These ulcerations are best treated with local topical antibiotics such as silver sulfadiazine. Wound cultures usually reveal *S. aureus*, and appropriate antibiotics are used if an infection is present. Resection of a bony prominence or joint fusion may be the only way to heal open wounds over the MCP or PIP joints. However, with patience, many open areas spontaneously heal and therefore should initially be treated conservatively.[76]

Calcinosis. Calcinosis can be intracutaneous or subcutaneous. According to Jones and associates, its frequency is 15% in the diffuse type of scleroderma and 44% in the limited cutaneous variety.[77] Calcium deposits can occur within a single digit or be widespread throughout the hand. They cause symptoms when they are close to the surface and cause local skin breakdown. The deposits are quite firm and produce tender areas in the finger pulps that interfere with the patient's ability to pick up objects. They can spontaneously extrude calcific material. The calcific material can be removed surgically in the distal pulp. In areas with digital nerves in close proximity, only a limited removal is carried out. Usually a curet is used rather than a scalpel. This is a particularly common approach in the thumb. Irrigation with saline solution is also used to safely remove as much material as possible. Occasionally, after removing the calcium deposit, the fingertips are left open to allow spontaneous healing rather than using sutures through compromised skin. In most cases, a partial removal or debulking may be enough to relieve the patient's symptoms.[77] Isolated calcific masses in the forearm can be surgically excised without risk of circulatory or nerve problems.

Deformity of Digital Joints. Surgery at the DIP joints is usually either amputation or fusion. Amputation may be required if the patient develops gangrene, osteomyelitis of the distal phalanx, or a septic DIP joint. This surgery is best done under regional anesthesia with tourniquet release before closure to check for adequate circulation. The skin flaps are closed loosely to avoid any compromise of the skin. However, any surgery at the distal level is risky because of diminished circulation. Therefore, the surgeon must proceed cautiously because of the possibility of postoperative gangrene and subsequent amputation.

The PIP Joint. At the PIP joint level, the most common deformity is fixed flexion. There is frequently skin blanching or breakdown, with exposure of the extensor mechanism. In late cases, there may be a complete slough of the extensor mechanism, with exposure into the PIP joints. Hand function decreases as the fixed flexion deformity increases. To improve grasp, patients compensate with MCP joint hyperextension, which itself becomes fixed unless an attempt is made to maintain this motion. The circulation at the PIP level is better than in the distal part of the finger.

Thus, it is possible to operate with less risk at the PIP joint, even with infected or exposed joints.

In our opinion, fusion is the procedure of choice for the common fixed PIP joint flexion contracture. The bone resection as part of the fusion procedure, combined with skin resection, makes it possible to achieve primary healing. The overall functional result of a PIP joint fusion is determined in large part by the range of motion of the MCP joints. With good MCP function, the PIP joints can be fused in less flexion. If MCP motion is reduced, it should be regained surgically by either capsulotomy or arthroplasty before proceeding with PIP joint fusions. With severe flexion contractures, there may be an intraoperative circulatory problem as the digit is straightened. In that situation, it may be necessary to either accept less correction than usual[77] or perform a digital sympathectomy to improve the circulation and preserve the correction. Sympathectomy is usually not performed at the same setting.

Some surgeons have reported their use of Swanson flexible implant arthroplasties at the PIP joint level. However, the ultimate gain in motion in reported cases has been small.[78] In addition, the amount of bone resection required for implant insertion can lead to considerable digital shortening. We do not recommend this approach.

The MCP Joint. At the MCP level, the circulation approaches normal levels. The area is warm to palpation, and therefore the surgeon has the ability to carry out more extensive surgery with normal wound healing. However, tight skin poses a significant problem when one tries to achieve additional flexion. Although it is possible to insert flexible implant prostheses at this level, the risks are increased over resection arthroplasty, which can also restore satisfactory motion. However, with shortened dorsal skin and fixed MCP hyperextension, the situation changes. Faced with this dilemma, the surgeon can safely approach the metacarpal heads via a palmar approach and carry out a wide resection of the metacarpal heads to restore flexion. When faced with fixed MCP hyperextension and severe fixed flexion of the PIP joints, it is imperative that the MCP flexion be restored by resecting the metacarpal heads through a volar incision before correcting the PIP flexion contractures by fusion. We have noted considerable remodeling of the metacarpal heads after resection, which makes this technique a viable alternative to implant surgery in these patients. In patients with MCP flexion deformities, a standard dorsal approach is used.

First Web Contracture. Another area treated surgically in scleroderma is the tight first web space between the thumb and index finger. Opening the web space and releasing the tight deeper structure may require release of the tight adductor attachment to the thumb and the addition of a skin graft. Selected fusions of the IP or MCP joint of the thumb are also helpful when deformities of the thumb reduce the ability to achieve an adequate thumb-index pinch. In some patients, resection of the trapezium may be required to restore thumb metacarpal abduction.

Vascular Insufficiency

Surgical approaches to improve digital circulation have focused on attempts to decrease the sympathetic innervation of the digital vessels. Flatt,[79] Wilgis,[80] and Jones[81-83] each described various techniques to strip the adventitia of the common digital arteries in the palm. Each of these techniques has resulted in temporary improvement in digital blood flow, with increases in skin temperature and improvement in the healing of fingertip ulcers. Jones[81] investigated digital circulation in scleroderma patients by several methods, including digital plethysmography, cold stress testing, and intra-arterial digital subtraction angiography. Cold stress testing involves measurement of digital temperature, pulse volume readings, or laser Doppler flow values of the digits before and during exposure of the hands to a cold environment and during subsequent rewarming.[81] At surgery, he inspects the entire superficial palmar arch, looking for segmental occlusions to determine the need for interposition vein grafts. He also inspects for constrictive fibrous tissue around the small vessels that can be excised. He calls this surgical approach "decompressive arteriolysis." Unfortunately, patients undergoing these various techniques often continue to have pain and develop recurrent ulceration within 2 years. However, it is an exciting new approach in the management of diminished distal circulation in these patients.[81,82]

RHEUMATOID NODULOSIS

Subcutaneous nodules are common in rheumatoid arthritis and are seen occasionally in patients with SLE. These nodules occur frequently in the olecranon areas (Fig. 59-5B) and on the extensor surfaces of the forearms. They can be tender and a source of discomfort to the patient if they are large. They can occur on the dorsal aspects of the hand (see Fig. 59-5A), where they are unsightly, or on the palmar surfaces of the digits, where they may interfere with hand function because of pressure sensitivity or compression of digital nerves. They may cause erosion of the overlying skin and can form a draining sinus from necrosis of the central core of the nodule. Nodules that form in the subcutaneous areas on the volar surfaces of the digits can interfere with function, because pressure during grip or pinch causes discomfort.

Symptomatic nodules can be resected. Meticulous hemostasis should be obtained, particularly in the region of the olecranon. The use of a drain (brought through normal skin) usually prevents or minimizes the formation of postoperative hematoma or seroma. On the palmar surfaces of the digits, care must be taken to protect underlying structures, particularly the neurovascular bundles, and to maintain sufficient skin to allow primary closure. If the wound cannot be closed, skin grafts should be used.

Rheumatoid nodulosis has been described as a separate clinical entity (rheumatoid variant) and is characterized by multiple subcutaneous nodules, usually on the hands, and is associated with intermittent polyarthralgias, absent or minimal joint involvement, subchondral cystic radiolucencies, and a positive rheumatoid factor. Involvement of the hands by prominent subcutaneous nodules, often in clusters, can be extensive. When unsightly, resection of multiple nodules can dramatically improve the appearance of the hand. There is some tendency for these nodules to recur after excision.[84,85]

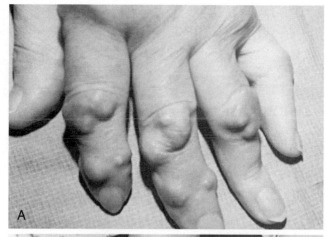

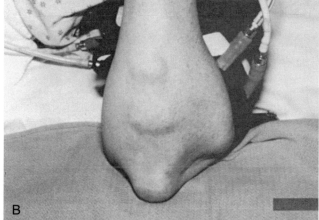

FIGURE 59-5. **A,** Rheumatoid nodulosis on the dorsal aspects of the fingers. **B,** Rheumatoid nodules on the posterior aspect of the forearm and in the olecranon region can cause considerable discomfort. Resection of these nodules is done through longitudinal incisions.

RHEUMATOID ARTHRITIS

Tenosynovitis

Rheumatoid arthritis is a disease of the synovium. The synovium-lined sheaths that surround many of the tendons about the hand and wrist can be affected by proliferative synovitis in the same way as are the synovium-lined joint spaces. Tendon sheath involvement is common and may occur months before the symptoms of intra-articular disease are noted.[86-89]

The three common sites of tendon sheath involvement are the dorsal aspect of the wrist, the volar aspect of the wrist, and the volar aspect of the digits (Fig. 59-6). Rheumatoid tenosynovitis can cause pain, dysfunction of tendons, and, ultimately, tendon rupture after invasion of the tendons by the proliferating synovium. Recent analysis by transmission and scanning electronic microscopy has demonstrated intracellular collagen, dysplastic fibrils, and reduced collagen fibril diameter in involved tendons.[90] Treatment can relieve pain and, if instituted before secondary changes in the surrounding structures and before tendon ruptures have occurred, can prevent both deformity and loss of function. For this reason, dorsal, volar, and digital tenosynovectomy are often the first surgical procedures indicated in rheuma-

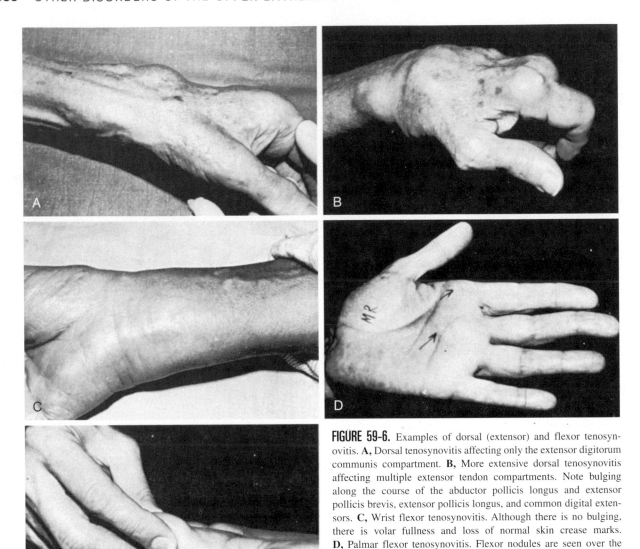

FIGURE 59-6. Examples of dorsal (extensor) and flexor tenosynovitis. **A,** Dorsal tenosynovitis affecting only the extensor digitorum communis compartment. **B,** More extensive dorsal tenosynovitis affecting multiple extensor tendon compartments. Note bulging along the course of the abductor pollicis longus and extensor pollicis brevis, extensor pollicis longus, and common digital extensors. **C,** Wrist flexor tenosynovitis. Although there is no bulging, there is volar fullness and loss of normal skin crease marks. **D,** Palmar flexor tenosynovitis. Flexor nodules are seen over the volar surfaces of the MCP joints in the index and long fingers. **E,** Digital flexor tenosynovitis presenting as volar fullness over the proximal phalanx. (From Millender LH, Nalebuff EA: Evaluation and treatment of early rheumatoid hand involvement. Orthop Clin North Am 6:697-708, 1975, with permission.)

toid patients.[89-94] Fifty to 70 percent of patients with tenosynovitis have been found to have infiltration of the tendon by proliferative tenosynovium at the time of prophylactic tenosynovectomy.[95-97]

Anatomy of the Tendons and Tendon Sheath

On the dorsal aspect of the wrist, the deep fascia thickens to form a band approximately 3 cm in width. This dorsal retinaculum functions as a pulley for the extensor tendons that run in compartments directly beneath it. Six separate compartments are formed by vertical septa, which run from the volar surface of the retinaculum to the dorsal surface of the radius and ulna. These compartments are referred to numerically. The first (most radial) compartment contains the abductor pollicis longus (APL) and extensor pollicis brevis (EPB) tendons; the second contains the extensor carpi radialis longus and brevis (ECRL and ECRB); the third, the extensor pollicis longus (EPL); the fourth, the extensor digitorum communis (EDC) and extensor indicis proprius (EIP); the fifth, the extensor digiti quinti (EDQ); and the sixth, the extensor carpi ulnaris (ECU). Each of the tendons within these compartments is surrounded by tenosynovium, which begins just proximal to the proximal edge of the retinaculum and continues distally to the level of the metacarpal bases. The tendons distal to this area are covered by paratenon rather than by tenosynovium.

On the volar aspect of the wrist, the flexor tendons of the fingers and thumb and the median nerve pass into the hand under the transverse carpal ligament (flexor retinaculum). This thick ligament extends across the volar aspect of the carpus attached to four "pillars"—the trapezium and the scaphoid on the radial side of the wrist, and the hamate hook and pisiform on the ulnar side—to form the roof of the carpal canal. Just before the finger flexors enter the carpal canal, a common sheath of tenosynovium surrounds them. The flexor pollicis longus (FPL) tendon runs in a separate tendon sheath.

The tendon sheaths of the index, middle, and ring fingers extend from mid palm to the DIP joints. The sheaths of the thumb and small finger continue proximally into the carpal tunnel. The flexor tendons within the digits are enclosed in a snug fibro-osseous canal that is lined by synovium.

Dorsal (Extensor) Tenosynovitis in the Wrist

Dorsal tenosynovitis is characterized by swelling on the dorsal aspect of the wrist. This may be subtle or massive. It may involve one tendon, a combination of tendons, or all the tendons in the dorsal compartments. Because the dorsal skin of the wrist and hand is thin and is displaced easily as tenosynovium proliferates, dorsal tenosynovitis usually is obvious and may be the first sign of rheumatoid arthritis. Isolated dorsal tenosynovitis is painless. Because of this, patients tend to ignore the swelling, and tendon rupture is frequently the first manifestation of the condition. When patients with dorsal tenosynovitis complain of pain, one must look for involvement of the radiocarpal or radioulnar joints.

Although early in the disease the synovial tissue remains thin and distends the sheath with fluid, as the disease progresses this tissue thickens and develops a more solid appearance, similar to that found within joints affected by advanced rheumatoid arthritis. Small fibrinoid "rice bodies" occasionally fill the tendon sheaths. The hypertrophic synovium adheres to the tendon surfaces and may eventually invade the tendon substance, resulting in weakening and, not infrequently, rupture of the tendon. Occasionally, rheumatoid nodules are found within the tendon substance.

Spontaneous or drug-induced remission of early dorsal tenosynovitis may occur. Rest and/or local injection of a steroid solution also may result in remission. However, if the proliferative synovitis progresses, remission becomes unlikely. The dorsal tenosynovitis becomes unsightly, and the risk of tendon rupture increases. For this reason, early dorsal tenosynovectomy is recommended (i.e., if there is no improvement after 4 to 6 months of appropriate medical management). Although the appearance of the tendons within the compartments affected by tenosynovitis may be poor (as evidenced by fraying), tendon rupture rarely occurs after dorsal tenosynovectomy is performed.[91-103]

Authors' Preferred Method of Treatment: Dorsal Tenosynovectomy (Fig. 59-7)

A straight (preferred) or gently curved longitudinal incision is made over the dorsal aspect of the wrist just to the ulnar side of the midline. Full-thickness skin flaps, including the subcutaneous tissue, are reflected to expose the underlying extensor retinaculum and deep fascia. The superficial branches of the ulnar and radial nerves remain in the sub-

cutaneous tissue of the flaps and thus are protected. Longitudinal veins are preserved if possible, but transverse communicating veins are divided. A longitudinal incision is made through the deep fascia and the extensor retinaculum, entering into the sixth extensor compartment. Transverse incisions are made above and below the retinaculum, allowing it to be reflected as a flap. The retinaculum is incised over the sixth compartment as a single, radially based flap. As each extensor compartment is opened, its vertical septum is divided. Care is taken to protect the EDQ and EPL tendons, which are contained tightly in their separate compartments. The EPL is at risk, because it changes direction distal to Lister's tubercle and crosses the tendons contained in the second dorsal compartment. The first dorsal compartment is not opened unless it is involved significantly. Hypertrophic synovium is removed from each extensor tendon sheath in a systematic manner. A limited dorsal tenosynovectomy can be done through a single compartment incision (e.g., the fourth) if indicated. The synovium is dissected from the extensor tendons with small scissors or with a rongeur. As much of the diseased synovium is removed as possible, although it is sometimes necessary to leave material that is densely adherent to the extensor tendon surface. Frayed areas of the tendons are repaired with interrupted sutures of fine material. If an area of tendon appears so attenuated or frayed that tendon rupture appears imminent, the tendon at risk can be sutured to an adjacent extensor tendon above and below the area of damage, or the frayed and attenuated areas can be imbricated. If extensive tendon infiltration is found, similar infiltration may be present in other areas or on the contralateral side, and early surgery in these areas should be considered to prevent rupture. A description of the pathologic findings recorded in the operative note is invaluable for future reference.

After a complete tenosynovectomy has been performed, the wrist joint is evaluated. If synovitis is present, the joint is opened and a wrist synovectomy is performed using a small, curved rongeur. The dorsal aspects of the ulna and radius are examined, and any bony spicules, which might cause attrition ruptures, are removed with a rongeur. The distal ulna is resected if it is dislocated and prominent dorsally. This is discussed in greater detail in the section on the distal radioulnar joint (DRUJ).

The dorsal retinaculum is passed deep to the extensor tendons and sutured in place to provide a smooth gliding surface beneath the tendons. If bowstringing is anticipated as a potential problem (e.g., in a patient with good wrist extension), half of the retinaculum may be retained over the tendons (Fig. 59-8). Studies on the function of the extensor retinaculum suggest that at least a portion of the retinaculum should be retained over the extensor tendons if at all possible.[104] The ECU tendon may be stabilized in a dorsal position by a narrow segment of the retinaculum.

The tourniquet may be released and bleeding controlled before final closure. If the tourniquet is released and bleeding is minimal, no drain is necessary. However, a small Penrose or suction drain will prevent hematoma formation if the tourniquet is not released. The hand and wrist are immobilized in a bulky conforming dressing and volar plaster splint. The wrist is held in neutral and the MCP joints in extension. The IP joints are left free. The drain is removed 24 to 36 hours after surgery. Dorsal tenosynovectomy can

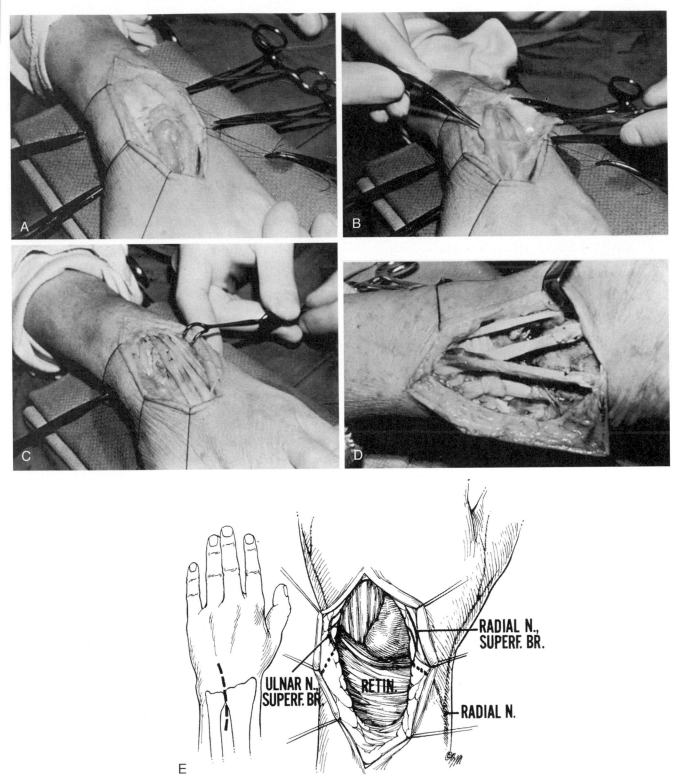

FIGURE 59-7. Surgical technique of dorsal tenosynovectomy. **A,** A straight dorsal incision has been made. The extensor retinaculum and the bulging dorsal tenosynovitis are seen. **B,** The retinaculum has been incised in the midline and reflected radially and ulnarward. Tenosynovitis is seen surrounding the extensor tendons. **C,** Dorsal tenosynovectomy and retinacular relocation completed. The dorsal retinaculum has been placed deep to the extensor tendons. **D,** Capsular closure is completed and tendon transfer is performed. Note extensor carpi ulnaris relocation using a portion of the dorsal retinaculum. **E,** Exposure for dorsal tenosynovectomy. We prefer a straight rather than a slightly curved incision *(as shown)*. Note superficial branches of radial and ulnar nerves protected in skin flaps. (**A** to **C** from Millender LH, Nalebuff EA: Preventative surgery: Tenosynovectomy and synovectomy. Orthop Clin North Am 6:765-792, 1975, with permission.)

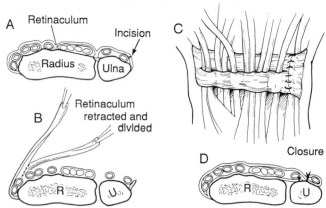

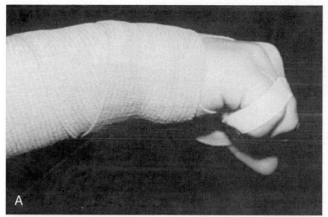

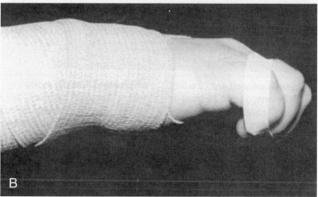

FIGURE 59-8. Dorsal tenosynovectomy is done by elevating a radially based flap of extensor retinaculum as shown in **A** to **C**. If the extensor carpi ulnaris (ECU) tendon has subluxated volarward, a sling of retinaculum is used to relocate and maintain the ECU dorsal to the axis of wrist flexion, as shown in **D. A,** An incision is made over the sixth compartment. **B,** The flap of retinaculum is elevated, dividing the vertical septa between compartments. The flap can be divided transversely to form two separate flaps. **C,** One flap is placed beneath the extensor tendons and one is placed over the tendons. **D,** ECU subluxation is corrected with a sling formed by incising the retinaculum at its ulnarmost insertion, passing this flap under and around the ECU tendon, and suturing the flap to itself on the dorsal aspect of the wrist to contain the tendon. (From Williamson SC, Feldon P: Extensor tendon ruptures in rheumatoid arthritis. Hand Clin 11:449-459, 1995, with permission.)

FIGURE 59-9. Postoperative MCP joint exercises can be done with the PIP and DIP joints taped in flexion. This maximizes extensor tendon excursion as the MCP joint moves from flexion (**A**) to extension (**B**).

be performed in conjunction with other procedures such as thumb fusion, volar synovectomy, or finger tenosynovectomy.

Postoperative Management. Hand motion is started 24 to 48 hours after surgery. Active extension and flexion exercises are emphasized. Motion usually returns rapidly, but in a patient with a low pain threshold, formal hand therapy may be required. The MCP joint should be splinted in extension to prevent extensor lag until active extension is possible. The wrist is supported with a volar splint for 2 weeks after the procedure.

When patients have difficulty regaining active MCP joint extension, taping the fingers with the PIP and DIP joints in flexion during active extension exercise is helpful in improving joint motion. All the extensor power is concentrated at the MCP joint level, and extensor tendon excursion is increased over the areas of surgery (Fig. 59-9).

Complications. Complications after dorsal tenosynovectomy are infrequent. The most serious complication is skin necrosis or skin slough. When this occurs, the extensor tendons are exposed and are at risk for rupture or scarring. Hematoma formation under the thin dorsal flaps of rheumatoid patients (especially those on corticosteroids) is the most frequent cause for delayed skin healing. Special care must be taken to prevent hematoma formation. The skin is closed without tension. A drain should be used routinely. The proximal and distal ends of the wound can be left open if necessary to avoid hematoma formation. A layered closure to cover the tendons with subcutaneous tissue can sometimes be done. Occasionally, it is useful to put the

extensor retinaculum over the tendons to protect them if a skin breakdown occurs. Sutures should not be removed prematurely. If skin slough occurs, the wound can be treated by débridement and skin coverage. The MCP joints are splinted in extension until the wound has healed by secondary intention in 2 to 3 weeks

Occasionally, postoperative adhesions may result either in an extensor lag of the MCP joints or in loss of active finger flexion. Hand therapy is adjusted to emphasize flexion or extension as necessary. If pain or flexor weakness prevents flexion, passive flexion exercises and dynamic flexion splints are added. If a significant extensor lag develops, a dynamic dorsal extension splint is used. Loss of motion after dorsal tenosynovectomy occurs more often in those patients whose tendons are found to be in poor condition at the time of surgery, those with multiple joint involvement, and those with low pain tolerance.

Tenolysis after dorsal tenosynovectomy is rarely necessary. However, if significant impairment of function persists after 6 months of therapy, tenolysis should be considered.

Flexor Tenosynovitis in the Wrist

Whereas swelling on the dorsal aspect of the wrist often is prominent because of the thin skin in the area, hypertrophic synovitis on the volar aspect of the wrist may not be obvious. However, proliferative synovitis of the flexor tendon sheaths occurs commonly and affects the anatomic struc-

CRITICAL POINTS: DORSAL TENOSYNOVECTOMY

INDICATIONS

- Persistent dorsal tenosynovitis after 4 to 6 months of appropriate medical management
- Extensor tendon rupture

PEARL

- Tape IP joints in flexion for postoperative exercise if patient has difficulty regaining active MCP extension.

TECHNICAL POINTS

- Use straight midline incision.
- Use transverse incisions distal and proximal to retinaculum.
- Use longitudinal incision volar to sixth compartment.
- Elevate radially based retinacular flap by dividing septa between compartments.
- If tenosynovitis is limited to a single compartment, use longitudinal incision for limited tenosynovectomy.
- Remove tenosynovium from each tendon.
- Repair frayed tendon/suture tendon at risk for rupture to adjacent tendon.
- Remove tenosynovium infiltrating tendon substance and repair.
- Perform synovectomy of wrist joint if necessary.
- Perform distal ulnar resection if necessary.
- Transpose retinaculum beneath tendons; split transversely and transpose half/reattach half left dorsal to preserve function.
- Stabilize ECU in dorsal position with retinacular flap if necessary.
- Close skin over drain.

POSTOPERATIVE CARE

- Splint with wrist in neutral and MCP joints in extension.
- Leave IP joints free and start finger motion within 24 hours.
- Use wrist splint for 2 weeks after patient is able to maintain active MCP extension.

tures in the area.[105-107] Compression of the median nerve may occur, resulting in the symptoms of carpal tunnel syndrome.[108-111] Restriction of the free-gliding motion of the flexor tendons results in impaired active and passive motion of the fingers.[112,113]

As in extensor compartment tenosynovitis, flexor tenosynovitis eventually destroys the outer surfaces of the tendons. The tendons become adherent to one another, and, as synovial tissue invades the tendon substance, tendon ruptures may occur. There may occasionally be complete destruction of the flexor tendons within the confines of the carpal canal.[114]

Although rheumatoid flexor tenosynovitis may respond temporarily to local corticosteroid injection, we believe that early surgical decompression of the carpal canal combined with flexor tenosynovectomy is indicated to prevent permanent damage to the median nerve. Flexor tenosynovectomy with decompression of the nerve prevents permanent pain, numbness, thenar muscle loss, and spontaneous rupture, as well as preserving independent tendon gliding function.

Authors' Preferred Method of Treatment: Flexor Tenosynovectomy (Fig. 59-10)

An incision is made in the mid palm, parallel to the thenar crease, and is extended proximally, curving ulnarward at the wrist. The incision is extended above the wrist 4 to 5 cm in a zigzag manner. Care is taken to protect the palmar cutaneous branch of the median nerve at the level of the wrist flexion crease. The deep fascia at the level of the wrist is divided to expose the median nerve. The palmar fascia is incised and separated from the superficial surface of the transverse carpal ligament. The transverse carpal ligament is divided to open the carpal canal.

The median nerve is freed from adherent synovial tissue. The motor branch of the median nerve is identified and traced into the thenar musculature. If compression of this branch by the fascia of the thenar muscles has occurred, the fascia is divided. The hypertrophic tenosynovium surrounding the flexor tendons is excised, and areas of tendon fraying are repaired as described for the extensor tendons. Occasionally, unsuspected ruptures of the deep flexor tendons may be discovered at this time. Therefore, it is critical that the function of the flexor tendons be known before surgery. If the flexor tendons are functioning by pulling through scar tissue, complete removal of all diseased tissue is not done. Careful dissection is required when performing an extensive flexor tenosynovectomy, and thought must be given to the consequences of separating each of the deep flexor tendons out of the mass of tenosynovium binding them together. It may be more prudent to separate the superficial flexor tendons and leave the deep flexor tendons in situ (i.e., not separate the flexor digitorum profundus into its four component tendons but merely separate them en masse from their scarred bed).

After tenosynovectomy is performed, the floor of the carpal canal is inspected and palpated. Any exposed bony spicules, particularly over the volar surface of the scaphoid bone, are removed with a rongeur, because these can result in tendon rupture by attrition. Exposed bony surfaces are covered by mobilizing and suturing local soft tissue.[115] Ertel and colleagues [4,116,116a] described a volar rotation

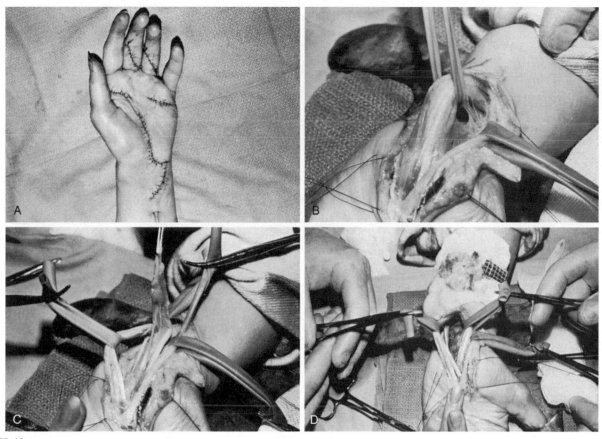

FIGURE 59-10. Surgical technique of wrist flexor tenosynovectomy. **A,** Incisions for wrist, palm, and digital flexor tenosynovectomy. The tube seen emerging from the skin proximal to the incisions is a small Penrose drain, which we prefer over suction catheters for postoperative drainage. A Penrose drain is seen proximal to the skin incision. Either a Penrose or a suction drain should be used routinely after tenosynovectomy. **B,** Flexor tendons exposed at the wrist and elevated into the wound. The median nerve is retracted with a Penrose drain. **C,** Flexor tenosynovium excised from the flexor tendons. **D,** Flexor tenosynovectomy completed. The median nerve is retracted to the radial side of the wound. (**A** to **F** from Millender LH, Nalebuff EA: Preventative surgery: Tenosynovectomy and synovectomy. Orthop Clin North Am 6:765-792, 1975, with permission.) *Continued*

CRITICAL POINTS: VOLAR TENOSYNOVECTOMY

INDICATIONS

- Symptoms and/or signs of median nerve compression
- Persistent tenosynovitis after injection/medical management
- Flexor tendon rupture

PEARLS

- If multiple flexor profundus tendon ruptures are found at time of surgery, do not perform tenosynovectomy, but leave flexor digitorum profundus mass intact.
- If "catching" is found when testing for tendon excursion after tenosynovectomy, check for flexor tendon nodules in digits and/or palm.

TECHNICAL POINTS

- Make an incision from mid palm (parallel to thenar crease) to 4 to 5 cm proximal to wrist flexion crease.

- Protect palmar cutaneous nerve.
- Expose and protect median nerve in forearm.
- Divide volar fascia and transverse carpal ligament longitudinally under direct vision.
- Perform tenosynovectomy.
- Inspect floor of carpal canal and débride scaphoid osteophyte and cover with soft tissue rotation flap if present.
- Check for free tendon excursion.

POSTOPERATIVE CARE

- Splint wrist in neutral.
- Start immediate active finger motion.

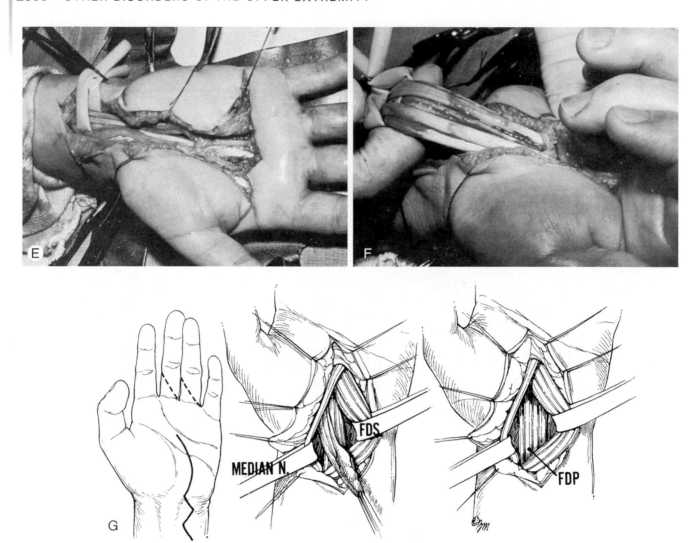

FIGURE 59-10—cont'd. E, If there is extensive palmar disease, a palmar flap may be raised to provide additional exposure. **F,** After completion of flexor tenosynovectomy, nearly full tendon excursion is demonstrated. **G,** Drawing of the technique. FDS, flexor digitorum sublimis; FDP, flexor digitorum profundus. (**A** to **F** from Millender LH, Nalebuff EA: Preventative surgery: Tenosynovectomy and synovectomy. Orthop Clin North Am 6:765-792, 1975, with permission.)

flap to close the defect if primary closure is not possible (Fig. 59-11).

Traction is applied to the flexor tendons to check finger motion. Smooth motion of the fingers and thumb should be present. "Catching" signals the presence of tendon nodules in the palm or digits. If smooth motion of the tendons is not present, the involved tendon must be explored as far distally as necessary to remove the nodules. After removal of the nodules, the defect in the tendon is repaired with interrupted fine sutures.

Flexor Tenosynovitis in the Digits

As described previously, the fibro-osseous canal is lined by synovium. This canal is not distensible, and even mild synovial hypertrophy can affect finger function significantly. Discrete rheumatoid nodules can form in one or both flexor tendons within the sheath. Such nodules may occur at different levels. The size of these nodules and their relationship to the annular pulleys determine the degree of finger dysfunction.[117-120]

Four clinical patterns of rheumatoid "trigger finger" have been described, based on the size and location of the nodules.[102,121] Small, localized areas of disease cause catching of the tendons during flexion.[122] This is type I triggering, which resembles the triggering that occurs in non-rheumatoid stenosing tenosynovitis. In type II digital tenosynovitis, flexor tendon nodules are present in the distal palm, which causes the finger to lock as it is flexed. In type III triggering, a nodule in the flexor profundus tendon in the region of the A2 pulley over the proximal phalanx causes the finger to lock in extension. Type IV flexor tenosynovitis is manifested by generalized tenosynovitis within the fibro-osseous canal. There is palpable swelling on the volar aspect of the digit and limitation of motion. Usually, active motion is more restricted than passive motion. This loss of finger motion may result in stiffness of the IP joints as the periarticular soft tissue structures contract. As the IP joints become stiff, the diagnosis becomes more difficult, because one cannot tell whether the lack of finger motion is because of joint stiffness or restricted excursion of the flexor

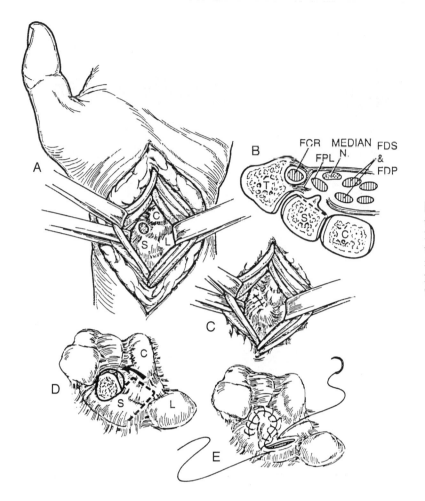

FIGURE 59-11. A scaphoid osteophyte can erode through the volar wrist capsule (**A**), resulting in the "Mannerfelt lesion," an attrition rupture of the flexor pollicis longus tendon. **B,** During a volar tenosynovectomy, the osteophyte is resected and the defect in the capsule closed either primarily (**C**) or with local rotation flaps of the wrist capsule (**D** and **E**).

tendons. Prolonged flexor tenosynovitis within the fibro-osseous canal ultimately can result in tendon rupture. Flexor tenosynovectomy and excision of flexor tendon nodules are indicated regardless of the type of tenosynovitis and/or triggering present.[92,117,121-123]

Authors' Preferred Method of Treatment: Digital Tenosynovectomy (Fig. 59-12)

We explore the flexor tendon sheaths of rheumatoid patients with digital tenosynovitis through zigzag incisions on the volar aspect of the digits. Such incisions can be extended proximally or distally to provide additional exposure if necessary. If multiple fingers are involved, a single transverse incision across the distal palm can be used to expose the proximal portions of the flexor tendon sheaths. The diseased tenosynovium surrounding the tendon is excised. However, the annular pulleys are preserved to prevent bowstringing of the flexor tendons. The pulleys may be narrowed if necessary, but as much pulley as possible is preserved.

Nodules within the flexor tendons are excised and the defects closed with fine sutures. After complete tenosynovectomy and nodule excision have been performed, traction is applied to the flexor tendons to confirm smooth

gliding. Occasionally, another nodule is present at a different level within the fibro-osseous canal and is revealed only after the obvious nodule is excised and flexor tendon excursion is tested. If passive flexion of the finger is greater than the flexion obtained by traction applied to the tendon, additional tenosynovectomy is necessary. The objective of flexor tenosynovectomy is to make active and passive finger flexion equal. Gentle manipulation of stiff joints can be performed to restore passive joint motion at this time. Ferlic and Clayton[117] recommended excising one slip of the flexor digitorum superficialis (FDS) tendon to decompress the fibro-osseous canal. We do not use this method routinely but prefer it to resecting excessive amounts of annular pulley to allow free excursion of the tendons. The entire FDS tendon may be excised if it is severely diseased and prevents complete "pull-through" of the flexor digitorum profundus (FDP) tendon.

Postoperatively, finger motion is started early, usually the day after surgery. The patient is taught to stabilize each joint of the operated finger in sequence to exercise the superficial and deep flexor tendons independently and thereby avoid adhesions between these two tendons.

Tendon Ruptures

Tendon ruptures in the hand are common in rheumatoid arthritis. The cause and location of these ruptures vary. Attrition ruptures occur as the tendon moves across bone roughened or eroded by chronic synovitis. Attrition ruptures of the extensor tendons occur most frequently either at the

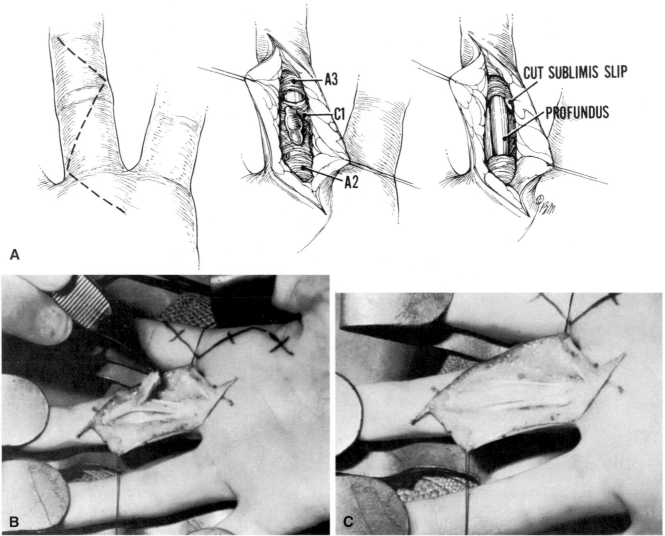

FIGURE 59-12. Digital flexor tenosynovectomy. **A,** The tendon sheath is approached through an extensile zigzag incision. Note the annular pulleys; and synovium usually bulges through the thin cruciate pulleys. As much annular pulley as possible is preserved when tenosynovectomy is performed. One half of the superficialis tendon can be excised to allow free excursion of the remaining tendons without compromising annular pulley function. **B,** Tenosynovium is excised from the flexor digitorum profundus. Both slips of flexor digitorum superficialis can be seen. **C,** The flexor digitorum profundus and flexor digitorum superficialis are seen at the completion of flexor tenosynovectomy. (**B** and **C** from Millender LH, Nalebuff EA: Preventative surgery: Tenosynovectomy and synovectomy. Orthop Clin North Am 6:765-792, 1975, with permission.)

distal end of the ulna or at Lister's tubercle, which acts as a bony pulley for the EPL tendon. Attrition ruptures of the flexor tendons occur on the volar aspect of the wrist where they contact the scaphoid. Tendon ruptures also may be caused by direct tendon invasion of rheumatoid tenosynovium, which erodes and weakens the tendon, or by ischemic necrosis from diminished blood supply caused by pressure from proliferative synovium under the dorsal retinaculum, transverse carpal ligament, or flexor tendon pulleys.[4,114-116,124-133]

The treatment options for rheumatoid patients with tendon ruptures are fusions of various joints and tendon transfers. Smith[134] pointed out the significant differences between tendon transfers done in rheumatoid and non-rheumatoid patients. In the rheumatoid patient, (1) the joints to be moved by the transfer may be stiff or unstable; (2) the bed through which the transfer passes may be scarred or irregular, compromising tendon excursion; (3) the tendons to be

transferred may have been weakened by ischemia or by tenosynovial invasion; and (4) if the wrist, MCP, and/or PIP joints are stiff or deformed, the tenodesis effect of wrist motion or the complementary motion of the MCP and PIP joints cannot be relied on to enhance the performance of the transferred tendons. These factors must be considered carefully when planning tendon transfers to reconstruct rheumatoid tendon ruptures.

Diagnosis

Extensor Tendon Ruptures

Although the correct diagnosis of tendon rupture usually is not difficult, it requires both an observant patient and an informed physician. The sine qua non of tendon rupture is the sudden loss of finger extension or flexion. Tendon ruptures usually are painless and commonly follow trivial hand use or activity. Rheumatoid patients who become accustomed to frequent variations and limitations of hand function are likely to delay medical attention unless the functional loss after a tendon rupture is obvious to them or is quite significant. Isolated ruptures of the EDQ or EPL may cause only limited functional loss and, therefore, may go unrecognized or be overshadowed by more significant deformities.[130]

The factors leading to a single tendon rupture, unless corrected, are often responsible for subsequent ruptures with more significant functional loss. Frequently, after a rupture of the extensor tendon of the small finger, the ring finger extensor ruptures, followed by the long finger extensor, and so on (Fig. 59-13). This occurs as the remaining intact tendons shift ulnarward and become abraded over the roughened edges of the distal ulna. Thus, the usual progression of extensor tendon ruptures is in a radial direction, affecting the index finger last. In our experience, multiple extensor tendon ruptures (especially those that occur in rapid sequence) are the result of attrition as the tendons wear against a bony spicule on the ulnar aspect of the wrists, as described by Vaughan-Jackson.[132]

Although the sudden loss of extension of the ring, small, and middle fingers is most likely the result of multiple extensor tendon ruptures, three other conditions occur in rheumatoid arthritis that can mimic tendon rupture and should be excluded before surgery to restore extensor power to the fingers is performed. The most common of these is MCP joint dislocation, which results in a flexed and ulnar-deviated position of the finger. The lack of passive MCP joint extension and the presence of palpable and/or visible extensor tendons on the dorsal aspect of the hand make the differential diagnosis between MCP joint dislocation and extensor tendon rupture straightforward. The second condition to be excluded is displacement of the extensor tendons into the valleys between the metacarpal heads. When this

occurs, extensor force is lost, as the tendons now lie volar to the axes of motion of the MCP joints. In this condition, the posture of the fingers is similar to that which occurs in cases of multiple extensor tendon ruptures. Differentiation between extensor tendon rupture and displacement of the tendons between the metacarpal heads sometimes can be made if the patient is able to maintain MCP joint extension actively after the joints are extended passively. This is not always the case, however; and occasionally it is necessary to explore the tendons at the level of the wrist at the time of MCP arthroplasty to verify their continuity. The treatment for subluxation of the extensor tendons is relocation over the MCP joints with or without MCP joint arthroplasty.

The least common but most difficult condition to diagnose among those simulating multiple extensor tendon rupture is paralysis of the common extensor muscle secondary to posterior interosseous nerve compression as the result of elbow synovitis.[135-140] Several subtle differences allow tendon rupture to be differentiated from muscle paralysis. Patients with posterior interosseous nerve compression usually demonstrate some radial deviation of the wrist because of paralysis of the ECU muscle, in addition to the absence of active finger extension. Soft tissue fullness about the elbow signals proliferative synovitis of the radiohumeral and ulnohumeral joints, which can result in compression of the posterior interosseous nerve. In posterior interosseous nerve compression, the extensors of the middle and ring fingers may be weaker than those of the index and small fingers.[134] Thus there is a greater extensor lag of the middle and ring fingers than of the index and small fingers. In contrast, in rheumatoid attrition ruptures, the ring and small finger extensors are involved first. The best diagnostic test is the presence or absence of MCP joint extension as the wrist is flexed. A positive "tenodesis effect" is found in the paralytic condition, because the extensor tendons are in

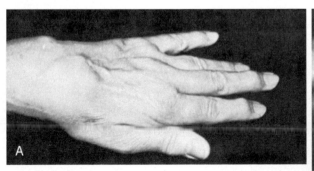
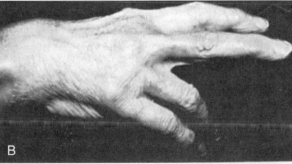
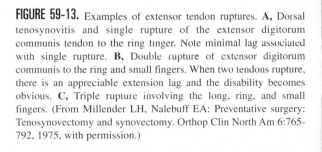
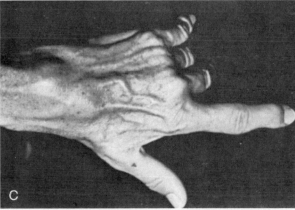

FIGURE 59-13. Examples of extensor tendon ruptures. **A,** Dorsal tenosynovitis and single rupture of the extensor digitorum communis tendon to the ring finger. Note minimal lag associated with single rupture. **B,** Double rupture of extensor digitorum communis to the ring and small fingers. When two tendons rupture, there is an appreciable extension lag and the disability becomes obvious. **C,** Triple rupture involving the long, ring, and small fingers. (From Millender LH, Nalebuff EA: Preventative surgery: Tenosynovectomy and synovectomy. Orthop Clin North Am 6:765-792, 1975, with permission.)

continuity. With tendon rupture, flexion of the wrist usually has no effect on finger extension, because the extensor tendons are not in continuity. In addition, patients with multiple extensor tendon ruptures usually have dorsal tenosynovitis or a prominent distal ulna, which predisposes to extensor tendon rupture, whereas patients with posterior interosseous nerve compression may have no such findings about the wrist.

Flexor Tendon Ruptures

Flexor tenosynovitis is not uncommon in rheumatoid arthritis. Although carpal tunnel syndrome is the most common manifestation of flexor tenosynovitis at the wrist, weakness, loss of dexterity of the hand, local or radiating pain, and/or discomfort with hand use can occur. Tendon gliding becomes restricted, and progressive loss of active finger flexion ensues. A discrepancy between active and passive finger flexion is characteristic of rheumatoid flexor tenosynovitis. Triggering, locking, loss of the normal finger cascade, and loss of active flexion may occur, particularly with tenosynovitis in the palm or in the fibro-osseous canals. Joint stiffness makes concomitant flexor tenosynovitis more difficult to detect. Flexor tendon ruptures occur but are much less common than extensor tendon ruptures.

Ertel and coworkers[4,116] found that the presence of inflammatory flexor tenosynovitis adversely affects the outcome of reconstructive surgery. That is, there is less restoration of function after a tendon transfer done for a rupture caused by inflammatory synovitis than after one done for an attrition rupture.

The most common flexor tendon to rupture is the FPL. Patients with this rupture lose active flexion of the IP joint of the thumb. It occurs when the tendon is eroded by a volar osteophyte on the scaphoid that penetrates the volar wrist capsule and is known as the "Mannerfelt lesion."[115] The diagnosis of FPL rupture is not difficult unless there is a fixed hyperextension deformity or stiffness of the IP joint.

An isolated rupture of the FDP tendon results in the inability to flex the DIP joint actively. A condition that mimics FDP tendon ruptures and, in fact, is a precursor to such ruptures is a rheumatoid nodule in the tendon within the fibro-osseous canal of the finger. The nodule restricts profundus excursion, and there is loss of active flexion of the DIP joint. This condition is discussed on page 2067.

Rupture of both the superficial and deep flexor tendons causes such obvious functional loss that the diagnosis is straightforward. The patient lacks active PIP and DIP joint motion and can flex the finger only at the MCP joint. Of course, passive motion of the finger must be present to conclude that both tendons are ruptured.

After a flexor tendon rupture is recognized, the site of rupture must be determined. Flexor tendon ruptures can occur at the wrist, in the palm, and within the finger. Palpation for fullness (or lack thereof) within the finger can be useful in this regard. Ultimately, surgical exploration is often necessary to determine the exact site of rupture.

Treatment of Extensor Tendon Ruptures (Table 59-2)
Rupture of the EPL

Rupture of the EPL is common in rheumatoid arthritis (Fig. 59-14).[66,96,129,130,141,142] The functional loss varies, depending on the functional capacity of the EPB and on the status of

Table 59-2
TREATMENT OPTIONS FOR EXTENSOR TENDON RUPTURES

Type of Rupture	Treatment
Ruptures—all	Dorsal tenosynovectomy Remove bone spikes Retinacular relocation to cover bone Ulnar head resection as needed
Single rupture	Primary repair Adjacent suture Intercalated graft
Double rupture Usually EDC of ring and small finger, EDQ	As for single rupture plus: EIP transfer
Triple rupture	As for double rupture plus: FDS$_{mid}$ through interosseous muscle or around side Wrist extensor especially if wrist fusion EPL if MCP fusion
Quadruple rupture	As for triple rupture plus: another FDS

EDC, extensor digitorum communis; EDQ, extensor digiti quinti; EIP, extensor indicis proprius; FDS, flexor digitorum sublimis; EPL, extensor pollicis longus.

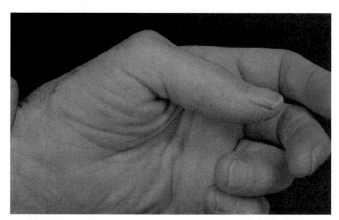

FIGURE 59-14. Extensor pollicis longus tendon rupture. Note that the major deformity is loss of MCP joint extension. The IP joint can be extended by intact intrinsic tendons, as seen in this patient.

the thumb joints. Although spontaneous rupture of the EPL may cause a "droop" or incomplete extension of the IP joint of the thumb, more commonly the patient maintains the ability to extend this joint in spite of the rupture. IP joint extension is a shared function of the EPL and the intrinsic muscles of the thumb. The intrinsics alone can extend this joint to neutral; the EPL is necessary for IP joint hyperextension. The patient with an EPL rupture loses extension of the MCP joint, because the EPB is not strong enough to extend this joint by itself. Occasionally, no deformity occurs at either the MCP or IP joint level, and the diagnosis is often missed unless a specific test for tendon function is done by asking the patient to extend the thumb with the palm resting on a flat surface while the examiner palpates the tendon of the EPL at the wrist level.

If the tendon is ruptured and the functional loss and/or deformity is significant, EPL function should be restored. The options available include end-to-end repair, tendon graft, or tendon transfer.[143] Although a tendon rupture occasionally can be repaired by end-to-end technique, this is an exception and should not be expected. In general, tendon grafts through areas of rheumatoid tissue tend to become adherent. However, a graft used to repair an EPL rupture can function satisfactorily. The power and long excursion of the thumb flexor overcome the adhesions that form on the dorsum. The proximal motor must not be scarred or contracted for this to be effective, and, for this reason, we prefer tendon transfers for the treatment of EPL rupture. The two most commonly used tendons for transfer are the EIP and extensor carpi radialis longus.[134] We prefer to use the EIP for several reasons: (1) it can be taken from the index finger at the MCP joint level without interfering with the index finger function; (2) in our experience, the patient does not lose independent extension of the index finger as a result of this transfer;[144,145] and (3) we do not like to weaken radial wrist extension, which is very important in maintaining proper wrist alignment.[95,129,130]

Authors' Preferred Method of Treatment

The EIP tendon is identified at the level of the MCP joint; it is usually the most ulnar of the two tendons.[146] It is withdrawn at the wrist through a second transverse incision and passed subcutaneously to the thumb. In the past, we did an end-to-end or weaving connection of the transferred tendon with the distal stump of the EPL. This was always tedious, and the adjustment of proper tension was difficult once the tendon was sutured. Now we pass the tendon directly to the MCP joint level and weave it into the extensor

mechanism. A temporary suture is used to judge tension. With the correct tension, the thumb remains in extension when the wrist is flexed. With the wrist extended, passive flexion of the thumb to the small finger pulp should be possible. Weaving of the tendon through the extensor mechanism results in a strong connection and allows us to start motion with confidence after 4 to 5 weeks of immobilization. The result of a properly performed tendon transfer to restore EPL function is usually excellent. If necessary, a dorsal tenosynovectomy and excision of a prominent, dorsally displaced distal ulna are performed at the same time as the EIP transfer.

Rupture of the Finger Extensors (see Table 59-2)

Single Tendon Ruptures. Although single tendon ruptures can involve any finger, the small finger is affected most often. The patient demonstrates incomplete extension of the finger at the MCP joint level. The amount of extensor lag depends on whether both the EDQ and the EDC tendons are ruptured. With an isolated EDQ rupture, MCP joint extension may lag only 30 to 40 degrees. The contribution of the EDC to extension of the small finger is tested by holding the index, middle, and ring finger MCP joints in flexion and asking the patient to extend the small finger. An increased extensor lag demonstrates loss of the contribution to extension provided by the EDC. Because of the danger of additional ruptures that complicate treatment, patients with a single tendon rupture are advised to undergo early surgical reconstruction. The surgical treatment of an isolated rupture of any one finger extensor is relatively easy, and the functional result is usually excellent (Fig. 59-15).[95,129,130,147,148]

Operative Technique. An end-to-end repair of a ruptured extensor tendon is feasible occasionally. Nalebuff uses this technique whenever possible and feels that the results are superior to adjacent tendon suture. In this technique, the MCP joints are extended to allow direct end-to-end repair of the ruptured tendons. The adjacent intact tendons look too long and the fingers are out of sequence when the direct repair is completed. This should be expected. The posture of the hand improves 7 to 10 days

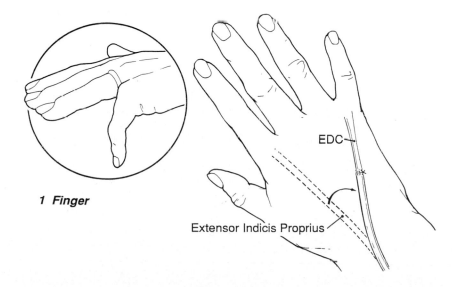

1 Finger

EDC

Extensor Indicis Proprius

FIGURE 59-15. The extensor indicis proprius tendon is transected over the MCP joint and transferred to the extensor digiti quinti (EDC) (small) tendon stump. (From Williamson SC, Feldon P: Extensor tendon ruptures in rheumatoid arthritis. Hand Clin 11:449-459, 1995, with permission.)

after surgery as the proximal end of the repaired tendon stretches out. The wrist is splinted in extension to allow the MCP joints to flex slightly

If direct repair is not possible, we prefer to suture the distal tendon stump to an adjacent extensor tendon. Dorsal tenosynovectomy and removal of any bony spicules from the distal end of the ulna (or ulnar head resection) should be done at the same time to eliminate the cause of rupture. The dorsal retinaculum should be transferred deep to the extensor tendons to provide a bed for gliding if bone is exposed. This is done before the tendons are reconstructed. Partial transfer of the retinaculum is described in the section on tenosynovectomy. Adjacent tendon suture is particularly easy for an isolated rupture of the middle or ring finger. For example, the distal end of the EDC tendon to the small finger or the EDQ is woven through the EDC of the ring finger and sutured. Similarly, the distal end of the ring finger EDC can be transferred to the long finger EDC. If there has not been major loss of tendon substance, an end-to-end repair can be done. Nonabsorbable suture material is used, and tension is determined by restoring the appropriate extensor stance (in sequence) to the fingers. The tension must be sufficiently tight so that when the wrist is flexed moderately, the fingers are maintained in complete extension and, when the wrist is extended moderately, the MCP joints flex only 20 to 30 degrees.

The use of intravenous regional anesthesia simplifies the task of judging proper tension. After the tendon suture has been completed, the tourniquet can be released. When voluntary muscle control is regained, the patient is asked to extend the fingers. If there is a lag in extension, the tendon tension can be corrected at this time. Skin closure is done under local infiltration anesthesia if this technique is used.[95,147] If the tourniquet is not released, a drain is used to prevent a subcutaneous hematoma.

Multiple Ruptures of the Extensor Tendons. As additional tendons rupture, the surgical treatment becomes more complicated. With double ruptures of the long and ring finger extensors, it is still possible to use the adjacent suture technique; the stump of the ring finger tendon is attached to the small finger tendon, and the stump of the long finger tendon is attached to the index finger tendon. If the EDC to the small finger is not present, the ring finger tendon stump can be sutured to the EDQ.

Options and Techniques for Extensor Tendon Reconstruction

Ring and Small Finger Ruptures. Double ruptures more frequently involve the ring and small fingers (Fig. 59-16). Although the adjacent suture technique can be done in some of these patients by connecting both distal tendon stumps to the long finger tendon, there may be difficulty with the small finger. The distal tendon stump of this finger may be so short that it cannot reach the ring finger tendon without excessive abduction of the small finger. In this situation, a different method is required, and we use the EIP as a tendon transfer. It is not necessary to divide the tendon as far distally as when it is used for a thumb tendon rupture. Other tendon transfers, such as the ECU, have been advocated to restore extension in this situation. However, this wrist extensor is very important in maintaining wrist alignment and power, and we believe that it is best left in its normal position. In addition, it does not have the same excursion as the finger extensors, and its use results in lack of either full flexion or extension of the small finger. We have occasionally used the ECRB tendon as a transfer, with satisfactory but not excellent results.

When the extensor tendons of the ring and small fingers rupture (the so-called double rupture), MCP joint extension can be restored with two tendon transfers: the EIP to the small finger and the distal stump of the ring finger to the intact common extensor tendon of the long finger.

Rupture of More Than Three Extensor Tendons. As additional extensor tendons rupture, restoring finger extension becomes more difficult. With three or four extensor tendons gone, the adjacent suture technique combined with EIP transfer is no longer sufficient to restore extensor power. In addition, independent and dexterous use of the index finger for pinch and pick-up functions may be lost if the EIP

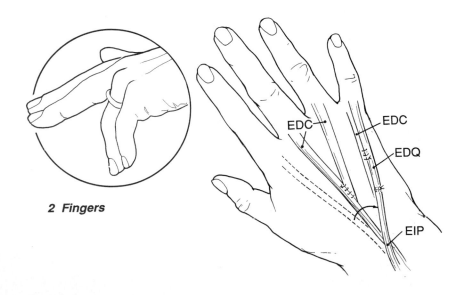

2 Fingers

EDC — EDC — EDQ — EIP

FIGURE 59-16. The extensor digitorum communis (EDC) (ring) tendon stump is sutured side to side to the EDC (long) tendon, and the extensor indicis proprius (EIP) tendon is transferred to the EDC (small) and/or extensor digiti quinti (EDQ) tendon stumps. (From Williamson SC, Feldon P: Extensor tendon ruptures in rheumatoid arthritis. Hand Clin 11:449-459, 1995, with permission.)

is used for transfer. A donor tendon for transfer that has a strong motor, is expendable, and has the necessary length to reach the distal tendon stump just proximal to the MCP joints is needed. The superficial flexor tendons meet these criteria.[148] The FDS transfer was advocated first by Boyes[149] for radial nerve palsy. He showed that patients learned to use a former finger flexor as an extensor. In his technique, the transferred tendon was brought through a wide opening in the interosseous membrane to provide a direct route to the site of connection. We prefer this routing of the tendon transfer through the interosseous membrane in patients who have no scarring in the region of the distal forearm and/or wrist. This more direct route of the sublimis tendon provides optimal function of the transfer. A window large enough to allow the muscle belly of the superficialis, rather than just the tendon alone, to be passed into and through the membrane should be made in the interosseous membrane. This helps preserve maximal excursion of the tendon after transfer. (See Chapter 31 for details of the Boyes transfer through the interosseous membrane.)

We modified the Boyes technique in patients with scarring in the dorsal wrist area either from previous surgical procedures or from long-standing tendon ruptures. In these patients, we use the long finger FDS instead of the ring finger sublimis tendon as a motor to avoid a decrease in grasp power, and we route the tendon subcutaneously around the radial aspect of the forearm rather than going through

the interosseous membrane and the area of scarring. This direction of pull was chosen to eliminate the risk of pulling the fingers into increased ulnar deviation. The technique for the modified transfer is described later (Fig. 59-17).

The transfer is performed through three incisions. A small transverse incision is made in the distal palmar crease, and the tendon is divided after applying proximal traction. This provides enough length to reach the MCP joints. A second incision is made on the volar aspect of the forearm. This should be placed ulnar to the midline so that the final transfer passes deep to the skin incision and thus minimizes tendon adherence. The third incision is made on the dorsal aspect of the hand where the transfer is attached to the extensor mechanism of the ring and small fingers. Usually, we suture the middle finger tendon to the adjacent index finger tendon. Care must be taken to route the transferred tendon deep to the superficial radial nerve. Otherwise, symptomatic compression of the nerve may occur from the tendon passing over the nerve.

With quadruple tendon ruptures, two superficial flexor tendon transfers are used: one to restore extension of the index and middle fingers, the other to restore ring and small finger extension (Fig. 59-18). Again, the judgment of tension is critical. The transfer should be tight enough to have a tenodesis effect, as described previously. There is a tendency for the transfer to stretch postoperatively because of the strong flexor pull.

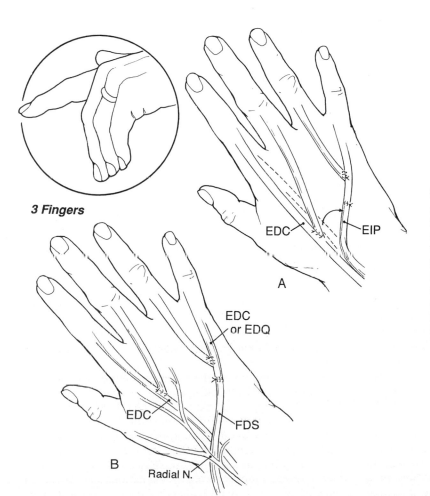

3 Fingers

FIGURE 59-17. **A,** The EDC (long) tendon stump is sutured side to side to the EDC (index) tendon, and the EIP tendon is transferred to the EDC (ring) and EDC (small) tendon stumps. **B,** If the EIP tendon cannot be used for transfer, the FDS (ring) tendon is transferred to the EDC (small) and EDC (ring) tendon stumps. Note that the FDS is passed *beneath* the superficial radial nerve. The EDC (long) is sutured side to side to the EIP or EDC (index) tendon stump. EDQ, extensor digiti quinti. (From Williamson SC, Feldon P: Extensor tendon ruptures in rheumatoid arthritis. Hand Clin 11:449-459, 1995, with permission.)

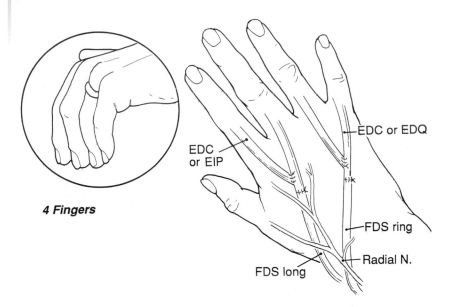

4 Fingers

FIGURE 59-18. The donor FDS (ring) tendon is passed around the radial aspect of the forearm and transferred to the EDC (small) and EDC (ring) tendon stumps. The FDS (long) is transferred to the EDC (index) and EDC (long) tendon stumps. EDQ, extensor digiti quinti; EIP, extensor indicis proprius. (From Williamson SC, Feldon P: Extensor tendon ruptures in rheumatoid arthritis. Hand Clin 11:449-459, 1995, with permission.)

We have used the FDS transfer in patients who have had previous wrist fusion. These patients are able to achieve satisfactory extension of the fingers without the benefit of any tenodesis effect.

In patients with multiple tendon ruptures and advanced disease of the thumb MCP joint, this joint can be fused and the EPL used as a tendon transfer to the finger extensors.

We have found that primary intercalary or "bridge" grafts can be useful, particularly for triple tendon ruptures. The palmaris longus tendon or, if the wrist is fused, one of the wrist extensors can be used for the graft.[150] The dorsal wrist incision is extended proximally, and the proximal stumps of the ruptured extensor tendons are located and dissected free from scar and adherent soft tissue. The tendon in the best condition is selected for the motor. The bridge graft is inserted between the proximal and distal tendon ends using an interweaving technique. The graft should be put in tightly, as the muscle will gradually stretch postoperatively. Bora and associates[151] reported excellent results (MCP joint motion, 10 to 75 degrees) in a long-term follow-up study using the palmaris longus as a "loop" tendon graft to bridge the extensor tendon defect after multiple tendon ruptures (Fig. 59-19). The considerations and alternatives for extensor tendon transfers have been summarized by Smith.[134]

Tendon Transfers in Patients With Fused Wrists. In patients with fused wrists, the wrist motors can be used to restore finger extension. As noted before, the excursion of these muscles is limited. However, they are valueless with the wrist fused and can be used to extend the fingers without diminishing the power of finger flexion that results when a FDS transfer is used. We have used both wrist extensors and flexors to restore finger extension in this situation. The wrist extensors may be of sufficient length for transfer if they are dissected from their insertions on the bases of the metacarpals and the wrist unit is shortened slightly when the radiocarpal joint is prepared for fusion. The wrist flexors frequently are not long enough to reach the ruptured tendon ends, and a supplementary tendon graft is needed. In performing a wrist fusion that is to be followed later by a second-stage tendon transfer for multiple extensor tendon rupture, one or more silicone-rubber rods can be inserted at the time of the wrist fusion. This makes the second-stage tendon graft procedure easier and minimizes the risk of postoperative adhesions.

Multiple Ruptures With MCP Joint Disease. The not infrequent situation of multiple extensor tendon ruptures with associated MCP joint disease warrants attention. We do not try to restore finger extension by tendon transfer before restoring joint motion. Unless the MCP joints can be extended passively, any transfer will become adherent. Thus, a staged reconstruction usually is necessary. Initially, an MCP arthroplasty is done. Postoperatively, dynamic splinting substitutes for the absent extensor tendons. At the second stage, appropriate transfers are done to provide active extensor power. With experience, it is possible to combine the MCP joint arthroplasty with a tendon transfer in a single operative procedure. The arthroplasty is done in the routine fashion, after which an FDS tendon is brought around the forearm and sutured to the extensor mechanism at the arthroplasty site. The postoperative management of patients with combined arthroplasty and tendon transfers is geared toward protecting the tendon transfer. Therefore, active motion is delayed for 3 weeks. Restoration of complete active motion is not expected in these cases. The results of a combined procedure fall short when compared with an arthroplasty in the presence of normal tendons or with a tendon transfer in the presence of minimally involved joints.

Treatment of Flexor Tendon Ruptures
Rupture of the FPL
The most common flexor tendon to rupture in rheumatoid arthritis is the FPL. It is usually secondary to attrition at the level of the carpal scaphoid bone and has been referred to as the Mannerfelt lesion.[115,131] The functional loss is variable. If the patient has a good IP joint, the loss is apparent. If the MCP joint has significant involvement or is fused, the loss of any IP joint motion results in substantial functional loss. Either terminal joint stability or restoration of active motion must be provided. Even if the IP joint is fused to provide

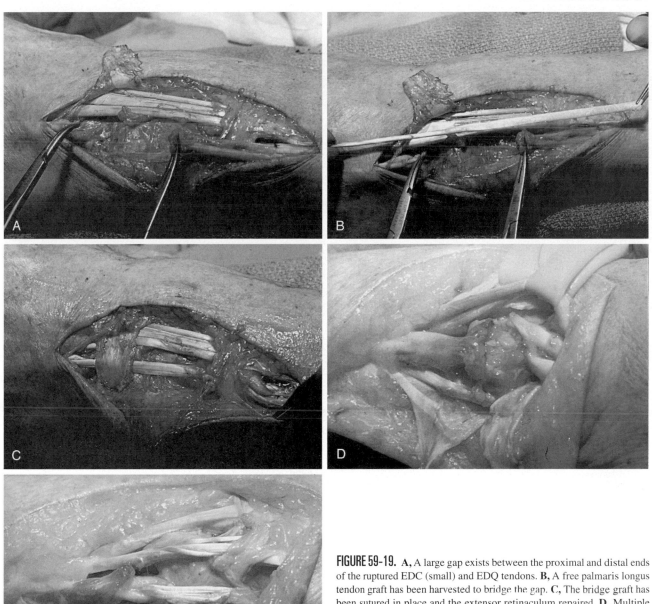

FIGURE 59-19. **A,** A large gap exists between the proximal and distal ends of the ruptured EDC (small) and EDQ tendons. **B,** A free palmaris longus tendon graft has been harvested to bridge the gap. **C,** The bridge graft has been sutured in place and the extensor retinaculum repaired. **D,** Multiple tendon ruptures can also be reconstructed using bridge grafts (**E**).

stable pinch, the volar aspect of the wrist must still be explored. The bony spicule that has disrupted the FPL will affect the tendons of the index finger next and must be removed. One of our patients was found to have ruptures of both the superficial and deep flexor tendons of the index and middle fingers, in addition to the thumb flexor.

Operative Technique (Fig. 59-20).   The volar aspect of the palm and wrist is exposed through a curved incision along the thenar crease and is extended proximally in a zigzag manner. The bony spicule on the ulnar aspect of the scaphoid bone, which protrudes into the radial side of the carpal canal, is removed, and the exposed bone is covered by

mobilizing adjacent soft tissues.[4,116] Attention then is directed toward restoration of tendon function. The surgical choices include the use of a bridge graft, a standard tendon graft, or a tendon transfer. If both tendon ends can be identified at the wrist level, we prefer to insert a short bridge graft.[112] The palmaris longus is suitable for this, but if it is not present, a slip of the FCR or one of the multiple slips of the APL can be used. If the distal tendon stump cannot be brought into the wrist incision, we either use a full-length tendon graft or transfer a superficial flexor tendon. We prefer to use the superficial flexor of the long finger as the motor, because it is longer and avoids compromise of the grip function of the ring and small fingers. The superficial

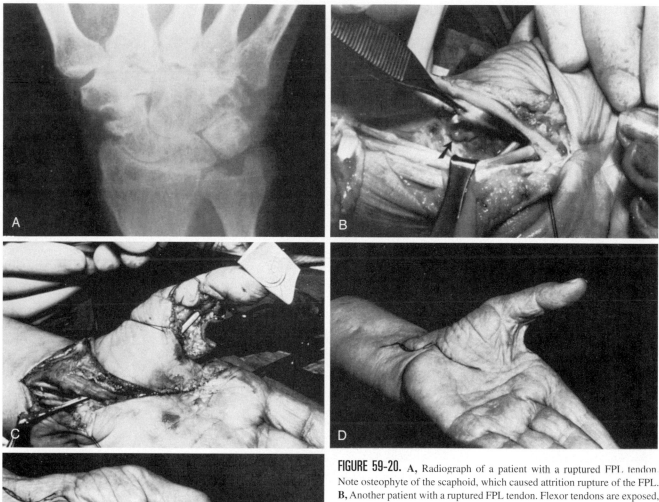

FIGURE 59-20. A, Radiograph of a patient with a ruptured FPL tendon. Note osteophyte of the scaphoid, which caused attrition rupture of the FPL. **B,** Another patient with a ruptured FPL tendon. Flexor tendons are exposed, and the ruptured FPL is held with forceps. Synovium from the scaphotrapezial joint can be seen *(arrow)*. A sharp spur on the scaphoid can be palpated adjacent to this capsular tear. Note the ruptured proximal tendon and intact finger flexors. **C,** Flexor tendon graft attached by pull-out wire before proximal repair. **D** and **E,** Range of motion of the IP joint of the thumb 4 months postoperatively. (From Nalebuff EA: Reconstructive surgery and rehabilitation of the hand. *In* Kelly WN, Harris ED, Ruddy S, Sledge CS [eds]: Textbook of Rheumatology, 2nd ed. Philadelphia, WB Saunders, 1985, pp 1818-1826, with permission.)

flexor is detached in the distal palm and sutured to the volar aspect of the distal phalanx of the thumb with a pull-out suture. A soft rubber catheter or a tendon passer is used to bring the tendon through the sheath and pulley mechanism. The stump of the flexor pollicis longus is elevated, and the underlying cortex is roughened before final attachment of the graft or transfer. A carpal tunnel release and flexor tendon tenosynovectomy usually are performed at the same time. The thumb and wrist are immobilized in moderate flexion for 3 weeks, after which active motion is started.

Rupture of the FDP

Rupture of one or more of the deep flexor tendons is not uncommon. If a patient with these ruptures can maintain superficial flexor function (both in range of motion and in strength), the functional loss is minimal. The treatment should match the degree of functional loss. If the distal

tendon stump becomes adherent, the patient may lose active flexion but may maintain enough stability of the DIP joint to preclude the need for surgical stabilization.

The most important factor determining the type of treatment is the level of tendon rupture. Flexor tendon ruptures can occur within the finger, at the palm, or at the wrist level. The palm is the easiest level at which function can be restored. Ruptures in the palm may be less obvious if the ruptured tendon adheres to the adjacent deep flexors. This obscures the diagnosis, as DIP joint flexion is possible with the finger extended, and the flexor mass pulls on the distal tendon end through scar tissue, but not when the finger is flexed actively or passively at the PIP joint. This situation can be confused with a flexor tendon nodule that blocks active excursion of the profundus tendon. Clues to the proper diagnosis include the lack of a palpable nodule and an alteration of the resting finger posture, with the finger assuming a more extended position than the adjacent fingers.

Flexor tendon ruptures at the palm and wrist levels are best treated by suture of the distal tendon ends to the adjacent intact tendon, although small bridge grafts can be used at the wrist level. Adjacent tendon suturing cannot be done if the rupture occurs within the fibro-osseous canal. In this case, surgery is performed only to remove diseased synovium from the intact superficial flexor, which is now vital to the function of the finger. Caution should be used in considering staged flexor tendon reconstruction of the FDP through an intact FDS. The results with this technique have not been good.[4,116] If the DIP joint hyperextends, we prefer to stabilize the DIP joint rather than consider a flexor tendon graft through an intact FDS tendon.

Rupture of the FDS

Loss of FDS function alone causes no obvious functional loss. In fact, as described previously in the section on tenosynovitis, we occasionally resect half of the FDS to restore proper function of the deep flexor tendon. The diagnosis of FDS rupture can be made only by careful examination. The treatment should not jeopardize existing tendon function. However, suture to adjacent tendons within the palm or the wrist is feasible. A tenosynovectomy should be done to protect the FDP tendons.

Rupture of Both Superficial and Deep Finger Flexor Tendons

The loss of both flexor tendons of a finger results in obvious and significant functional loss: the finger "sticks out" from the other fingers and thereby "gets in the way." Restoration of active finger flexion is a goal that is not always possible to achieve. For this reason, it is far better to be aware of early nodular tenosynovitis and to perform a prophylactic tenosynovectomy before tendon rupture occurs. If the ruptures have occurred at the wrist, function can be restored by suture to adjacent tendons or by a bridge graft of the FDP tendon with the suture lines placed proximal and distal to the carpal tunnel area. It is not necessary to reconstruct FDS tendon ruptures at the wrist. Therefore, an intact portion of a ruptured FDS tendon can be used for bridge grafts to reconstruct ruptured FDP tendons.

If the rupture is in the palm, adjacent suture to an FDP tendon or the transfer of an FDS to the distal profundus stump can be done.

Within the fibro-osseous canal, the same problem encountered in tendon laceration at this level exists, except that the situation is worse. The disease is not localized, and the dissection needed for exposure leaves a very poor bed for tendon grafting. In addition, the adjacent joints may have restricted and/or painful motion. In our experience, free flexor tendon grafts have not produced good results in patients with rheumatoid arthritis. Occasionally, if no other alternative is available, we perform a staged flexor tendon reconstruction using a silicone-rubber tendon rod, particularly in younger patients who have minimal joint involvement. The technique is essentially the same as those described for post-traumatic flexor tendon reconstruction.

Finally, because of advanced age, poor status of the IP joints, or generalized disease, the wisest choice for some patients in whom both flexor tendons have ruptured within

the finger is to fuse both the PIP and DIP joints in a functional position. In this way, satisfactory function can be restored and pain diminished. Suturing the proximal flexor tendon stumps to the base of the proximal phalanx may augment MCP flexor strength if there is free excursion of the flexor tendon proximal to the rupture. Of course, this is a last resort, but it should be considered as a method of handling this complicated problem in selected patients.

THE WRIST

The wrist is the "keystone" of the hand. A painful, unstable, and deformed wrist impairs hand function regardless of the status of the fingers.[6,8] In addition, wrist deformity is a major cause of finger deformity, and unless wrist alignment is preserved or restored, maintaining correction of finger deformities is difficult if not impossible.[152,153] An understanding of the pathophysiology of rheumatoid wrist disease is necessary to appreciate the effects of wrist involvement on hand function and finger deformity.[22,154-158]

Natural History of Rheumatoid Wrist Involvement

Rheumatoid synovitis follows predictable patterns. In the wrist, the ulnar styloid, the ulnar head, and the midportion of the scaphoid frequently are the earliest to be involved by rheumatoid synovitis. Progressive synovial proliferation in these areas leads to the various patterns of wrist deformity.

In the ulnar compartment, synovitis stretches the ulnar carpal ligamentous complex and results in changes that Backdahl called the "caput ulna syndrome."[159] This syndrome is the result of destruction of the ligamentous complex, including the triangular fibrocartilage complex, which allows dorsal dislocation of the distal ulna, supination of the carpus on the hand, and volar subluxation of the ECU.[160-162] The caput ulna syndrome (seen in up to one third of rheumatoid patients undergoing hand surgery) can result in significant disability. Patients with this syndrome complain of weakness and pain that are aggravated by forearm rotation. Examination of the wrist reveals prominence of the distal ulna, instability of the DRUJ, limited wrist dorsiflexion, and supination of the carpus on the forearm. As the ECU tendon subluxates volarward, normal function of this tendon is diminished, allowing the wrist to deviate radially and setting the stage for attrition ruptures of the ulnar extensor tendons.[163]

Radiocarpal involvement by proliferative synovitis begins beneath the radioscaphocapitate, or "sling," ligament in the region of the deep volar radiocarpal ligament.[107,164] Destruction of these ligaments eventually results in rotatory instability of the scaphoid. In this condition, the scaphoid assumes a volar-flexed position. There is secondary loss of carpal height and radial rotation of the carpus and metacarpals on the radius. The combination of rotatory subluxation of the scaphoid, volar subluxation of the ulnar carpus, and dorsal subluxation of the distal ulna produces relative supination of the wrist in relation to the distal forearm. This common pattern of wrist collapse results in imbalance of the extensor tendons, radial shift of the metacarpals,

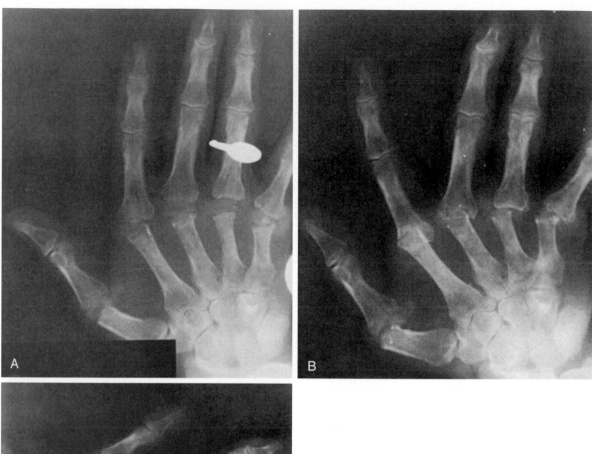

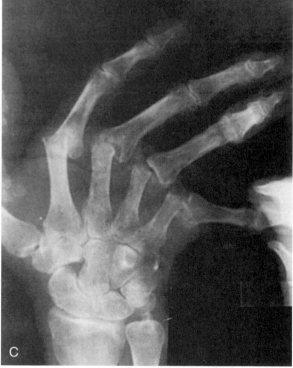

FIGURE 59-21. A, Radiograph taken 4 weeks after implant arthroplasties of the MCP joints. There is an early collapse deformity of the wrist with vertical rotation of the scaphoid, scapholunate dissociation, and dorsal rotation of the lunate. Note the radial deviation of the metacarpals associated with the wrist collapse, and note the reciprocal ulnar deviation of the MCP joints. **B,** Two years after MCP arthroplasty, increased wrist deformity with ulnar translocation of the carpus and severe recurrent deformity of the MCP joints with fracture of the implants have occurred. **C,** The wrist deformity can be corrected passively. Note that the scapholunate dissociation is corrected as the wrist is held in the neutral position.

and ulnar deviation of the fingers.[165,166] This deformity is thought to be one of the important factors initiating ulnar deviation of the MCP joints, as well as recurrence of ulnar deviation after MCP joint arthroplasty (Fig. 59-21).[153,167,168]

The untreated, end-stage rheumatoid wrist is dislocated volarward with complete destruction of the carpal bones and complete dissociation of the radioulnar joint. Early surgical treatment can prevent this severe pattern of destruction.

Operative Treatment for Rheumatoid Radiocarpal and Radioulnar Joint Deformities

Surgical procedures for the radiocarpal and radioulnar joint are either preventive or reconstructive. Preventive procedures include radioulnar joint and radiocarpal joint synovectomy, balancing of wrist extensors, and tenosynovectomy. Reconstructive surgery includes distal ulnar excision, reconstruction of the ulnocarpal ligamentous complex, radiocarpal joint arthroplasty, partial wrist fusion, and total wrist arthrodesis.[55,160,163,165,169-187]

Synovectomy of the Radiocarpal and Radioulnar Joint

Indications. The indications for wrist joint synovectomy have never been clearly established. There are no studies that demonstrate conclusively that synovectomy changes the natural course of rheumatoid disease. In addition, because the wrist is a multiarticulated complex joint, total synovectomy is impossible. The indications for wrist synovectomy vary among hand surgeons. Lipscomb[188] and others have recommended a several-month trial period of conservative therapy before synovectomy. Flatt and Ellison[189] advocated early synovectomy because of the rapid joint destruction that can occur when active synovitis does not respond to medical therapy. Hindley and Stanley[190] found relative sparing of the midcarpal joint and suggested that early synovectomy may prevent progression. Ishikawa and coworkers[191] found that synovectomy can provide significant pain relief, even in advanced disease. Synovectomy in some cases can thus be an alternative to wrist fusion.

We use wrist synovectomy in the small group of patients with persistent, painful wrist synovitis and minimal to moderate radiographic involvement. Shapiro and colleagues,[192] Thirupathi and associates,[193] Allieu and coworkers,[194] and Brumfield and colleagues,[195] in separate long-term follow-up reviews of wrist synovectomy, found consistent and dramatic relief of pain and varying loss of wrist motion after wrist synovectomy. Alnot and Fauroux found that the progression after early synovectomy was slow.[196] Of importance, Shapiro found that grip strength was maintained, not weakened, after synovectomy.

Operative Technique: Dorsal Approach for Synovectomy (Fig. 59-22). The wrist is exposed as described for dorsal tenosynovectomy using a straight, longitudinal incision. Flatt and Swanson have recommended entering the sixth extensor compartment and reflecting the entire extensor retinaculum as a radially based flap, releasing each of the dorsal extensor compartments except the first.[6,197,198] Alternatively, the retinaculum may be opened over the fourth dorsal compartment and reflected as radially and ulnarly based flaps. The terminal branch of the posterior interosseous nerve can be found consistently on the floor of the fourth dorsal compartment, deep to the extensor tendons.

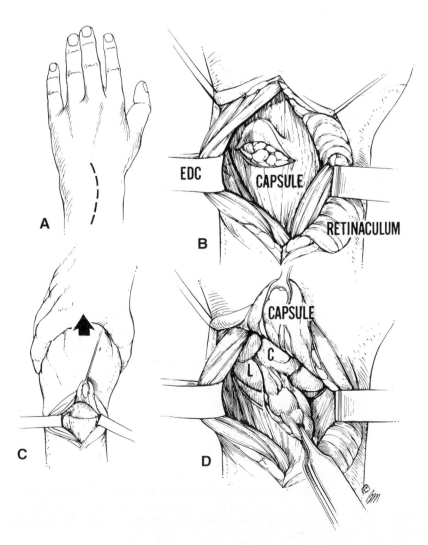

FIGURE 59-22. Technique for wrist joint synovectomy. **A,** The extensor tendons are exposed. We now prefer a straight incision rather than a slightly curved one as shown. A dorsal tenosynovectomy is performed. **B,** Extensor tendons are retracted and wrist capsule is exposed. **C,** Transverse capsular incision exposes the underlying synovium. **D,** Proximal and distal carpal rows are exposed, and synovectomy is performed with a rongeur. Capsular flaps are preserved for closure. EDC, extensor digitorum communis.

This is an articular branch that innervates the wrist joint. It can be resected to partially denervate the wrist joint for pain relief.[199-201]

A transverse or "U"-shaped incision is made in the wrist capsule, and a distally based flap is elevated to expose the wrist and intercarpal joints. The distally based capsular flap allows the wrist capsule to be reefed easily to stabilize the wrist joint by limiting flexion. Synovium usually is seen bulging from the proximal and distal carpal rows. Traction applied to the hand distracts the joints and allows the synovectomy to be performed with a small rongeur. A small, blunt periosteal elevator can be used to provide better exposure within the joint. Periarticular erosions are curetted. If the triangular fibrocartilage is intact, synovium is removed from the area between the triquetrum and the fibrocartilage.

The DRUJ is exposed through a longitudinal incision proximal to the triangular fibrocartilage. The forearm is rotated to provide exposure as the synovectomy is performed. Bony spurs are removed from the distal ulna, and, again, periarticular erosions are curetted.

After the synovectomy has been completed, the capsular incisions are closed with interrupted nonabsorbable sutures. Closure is performed with the forearm in supination to minimize the tendency for the ulna to subluxate and to allow a tighter closure of the DRUJ capsule. Tendon rebalancing, dorsal tenosynovectomy, and relocation of the dorsal retinaculum are performed if necessary. The tourniquet may be released at this point and hemostasis obtained. A Penrose or suction drain is placed in the subcutaneous area before skin closure.

A bulky compression dressing is applied. The wrist is splinted in neutral, and the forearm is held in full supination with a sugar tong splint. The drain is removed in 24 hours. Forearm supination is maintained for approximately 3 weeks. At that time, the splints are removed and both forearm and wrist range-of-motion exercises are started.

The length of postoperative splinting depends on the degree of wrist ligament laxity present preoperatively and the degree of ligament disruption found at the time of surgery. The greater the laxity, the longer the wrist is splinted postoperatively. Splinting for 4 to 6 weeks may be necessary to allow enough capsular healing to provide stability. We have found that the optimal range of motion after surgery is 30 to 40 degrees of flexion and the same range of extension.

Adolfsson and Nylander[202] performed a limited series of arthroscopic dorsal wrist synovectomies with good short-term results. Although we have only a small series using this technique, our early results are encouraging. We have found little morbidity and a more rapid recovery after this procedure compared with open wrist synovectomy.

Operative Technique: Volar Wrist Synovectomy. A volar wrist synovectomy can be done when a flexor tenosynovectomy is indicated. Both Straub and Ranawat[185] and Taleisnik[107] advocated volar wrist synovectomy in conjunction with wrist flexor tenosynovectomy to prevent destruction of the deep volar ligaments and secondary rotatory subluxation of the scaphoid.

When present, volar wrist synovitis is manifested by bulging of the volar capsule. The skin incision described for volar tenosynovectomy is used. A transverse incision is made over the bulging volar wrist capsule. Traction is applied to the hand, and synovium is removed from the volar portion of the wrist with a rongeur. The volar capsule is closed with interrupted nonabsorbable sutures. The postoperative management is the same as that described for dorsal tenosynovectomy.

Distal Ulnar Excision and Reconstruction of the DRUJ Complex

Involvement of the DRUJ is a common cause of disability in the rheumatoid wrist. For this reason, distal ulnar excision and reconstruction of the triangular fibrocartilage and the DRUJ are performed frequently in wrists affected by rheumatoid arthritis.

Distal ulnar excision was described first by Smith-Peterson and coworkers for rheumatoid arthritis.[29] It remains our procedure of choice because it is reliable and allows adequate exposure to perform a DRUJ synovectomy and to reconstruct the triangular fibrocartilage complex. Swanson described distal ulnar excision and replacement with a silicone-rubber implant.[161,197,203] We no longer use this implant because of problems with bone resorption beneath the implant collar, fracture of the implant stem, dislocation of the implant, and particulate synovitis. The importance of soft tissue reconstruction to correct supination of the carpus and subluxation of the distal ulna has been emphasized by many authors.[159,161,162,181,182,204-211] Total loss of the triangular fibrocartilage ligamentous complex complicates the correction of the supination of the carpus on the distal forearm and the dorsal subluxation of the ulna.

Distal ulnar excision for symptoms of the caput ulna syndrome usually is performed in conjunction with dorsal tenosynovectomy and tendon transfer for ruptured extensor tendons or in conjunction with wrist joint synovectomy or wrist joint reconstruction.

Other surgical techniques are available to reconstruct the DRUJ destroyed by the rheumatoid process. There has been renewed interest in fusion of the distal ulna to the sigmoid notch of the radius with resection of a segment of ulna to allow rotation of the forearm (the Sauvé-Kapandji procedure)[166,212,213] following reports by Taleisnik[214,215] and by Hales and Burkhalter.[216] Taleisnik[166] believes that the Sauvé-Kapandji procedure is indicated for younger patients with painful DRUJ dysfunction because it provides stable fixation of the ulnar head, preserves ulnocarpal support, restores forearm rotation, and results in a better cosmetic appearance than does distal ulnar resection. He prefers the Sauvé-Kapandji procedure to distal ulnar resection in patients with impending ulnar translocation not severe enough to warrant radiolunate fusion. In our experience, the Sauvé-Kapandji procedure does not prevent or correct ulnar translocation in the rheumatoid patient.

We prefer radiocarpal fusion for patients with established or impending ulnar translocation of the carpus. A segmental ostectomy of the ulna similar to that done in the Sauvé-Kapandji procedure occasionally can be used to restore partial forearm rotation in patients with juvenile rheumatoid arthritis who have had spontaneous fusion of the DRUJ. Bowers[217] described hemiresection of the DRUJ with preservation of the ulnar styloid process and interposition of soft tissue between the distal ulna and radius. This procedure preserves the ligaments that arise from the styloid process and support the ulnar side of the carpus. Watson and colleagues[218] have yet another approach to reconstructing the DRUJ destroyed by rheumatoid arthritis. They use a resection arthroplasty of the joint that preserves the entire length of the ulna, including the styloid process and the attachments of the triangular fibrocartilage and the joint capsule. This allows rotation throughout the range of forearm motion without contact of the ulna with the radius. All these procedures have specific advantages and should be considered as alternatives to the standard procedure of distal ulnar resection in selected patients.

Operative Technique: Distal Ulnar Excision and Reconstruction of the DRUJ. The surgical principles of distal ulnar excision are important and include the following: (1) limited resection of the distal ulna (2 cm or less) to minimize instability of the remaining ulna, (2) synovectomy of the DRUJ, (3) correction of carpal supination by suturing the remnant of the triangular fibrocartilage complex to the dorsoulnar corner of the radius, and (4) reconstruction of the dorsal capsule and extensor retinaculum with relocation of the ECU from volar to dorsal.

The wrist joint is approached through the dorsal longitudinal wrist incision described previously. The extensor retinaculum is opened. It is usually thin and/or adherent over the capsule of the distal ulna, which makes separation of these two layers difficult. Identification of the volarly subluxed ECU also may be difficult. The tendon usually can be palpated on the ulnar aspect of the wrist. Often, tenosynovium is noted bulging in the region of the sixth dorsal compartment. Occasionally, the entire sheath of the sixth compartment is destroyed and the tendon is frayed or ruptured. If the ECU has subluxated volarward, it is released and replaced dorsal to the axis of wrist flexion. It can be held

in place with a sling of tissue fashioned from the extensor retinaculum.

A longitudinal capsular incision is made over the distal ulna. The capsule and triangular fibrocartilage are reflected from the ulna and preserved. The periosteum of the ulna is elevated, and small bone retractors are placed around the distal ulna. The distal ulna can be sectioned with a bone cutter, an osteotome, or a power saw. A towel clip is used to apply traction to the bone fragment when the soft tissue attachments are divided. Approximately 2 cm of bone is resected. If excessive bone is removed, stability of the distal ulna may become a problem.

After the bone is removed, a complete synovectomy of the DRUJ is performed. Although the triangular fibrocartilage has often been destroyed, if it is present it should be protected during the synovectomy.

Reconstruction of the soft tissue support for both the DRUJ and the radiocarpal joint is important to correct carpal supination and to stabilize the distal ulna. If the triangular fibrocartilage and the radioulnar ligamentous complex are present, they are sutured tightly to the dorsal and ulnar aspect of the radius.

Various methods have been used to stabilize the distal ulna after resection of the ulnar head. Blatt and Ashworth[219] incised the volar capsule to form a distally based flap. The flap is brought dorsally and fixed to the ulna to reconstitute the ligament (Fig. 59-23).

Linscheid and Dobyns used a different method.[207] A Kirschner wire is used to hold the carpus to the radius in the corrected position. A distally based strip of the ECU tendon is detached, woven through the ulnar collateral ligament and any remnants of the triangular fibrocartilage, and sutured to the radius (Fig. 59-24). The dorsal radioulnar capsule is

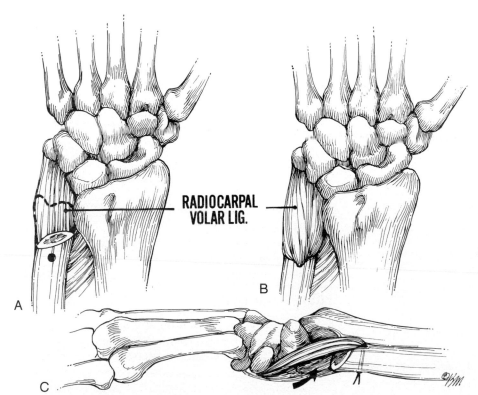

RADIOCARPAL VOLAR LIG.

A   B   C

FIGURE 59-23. Stabilization of the distal ulna using a flap of volar capsule. **A,** After distal ulnar excision and synovectomy are completed, a distally based flap of volar capsule is reflected. **B,** The free proximal end is brought dorsalward and sutured to the dorsal cortex of the ulna through drill holes. The flap acts as a volar restraining ligament to prevent dorsal subluxation of the distal ulna. **C,** Volar flap sutured over the dorsal cortex of the distal ulna.

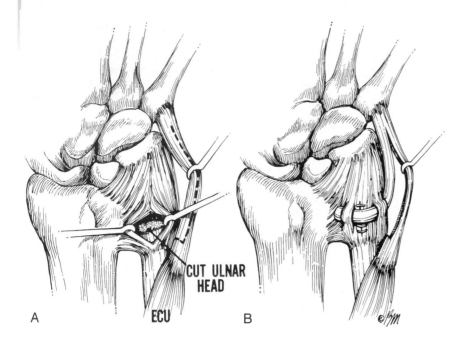

CUT ULNAR
HEAD

A   ECU   B

FIGURE 59-24. Reconstruction of the DRUJ after synovectomy and distal ulnar excision. **A,** The dorsal capsule of the DRUJ is opened longitudinally, a synovectomy is performed, and the distal ulna is excised. (The slip of tendon to be stripped from the extensor carpi ulnaris [ECU] is shown by the *dotted line.*) **B,** A strip of ECU is mobilized, passed through the ulnar aspect of the joint capsule, across the dorsal aspect of the joint, and sutured to the dorsal capsule over the radius to correct the supination deformity. The radioulnar joint capsule is imbricated to correct the dorsal subluxation of the distal ulna. The dorsal retinaculum can be used to further reinforce the radioulnar joint capsule. The dorsal edge of the distal ulna should be beveled and smoothed to avoid postoperative attrition ruptures.

closed tightly, imbricating the tissues when necessary. This is facilitated by supinating the wrist to relocate the ulna. After this, the extensor retinaculum is relocated deep to the tendons. The position of the ECU tendon is corrected if necessary (see later).

Another method[66,67,126,220] uses a distally based slip of ECU tendon. The tendon slip is passed through the distal end of the ulna, through a hole made in the dorsal cortex of the ulna, and then is sutured back onto itself (Fig. 59-25).

Breen and Jupiter[221] used a distally based slip of the flexor carpi ulnaris (FCU) and a proximally based slip of the ECU to stabilize the distal ulna after ulnar head resection.

Ruby and colleagues[222] described transferring the origin of the pronator quadratus to the dorsal aspect of the ulna, placing the muscle belly between the radius and the ulna to stabilize the distal ulna after resection of the ulnar head. Their long-term results were satisfactory, but their study did not include rheumatoid patients.

A Penrose or suction drain may be placed if the tourniquet is not released. A bulky hand dressing is applied with the wrist and fingers splinted in extension and the forearm in supination. The dressing is changed in 24 hours, at which time the drain is removed. Finger motion is begun immediately. When the fingers are not being exercised, they are

CRITICAL POINTS: DISTAL ULNAR RESECTION

INDICATIONS

- Painful synovitis
- Painful/limited DRUJ range of motion
- Extensor tendon attrition rupture

PEARLS

- Use sugar tong splint postoperatively if necessary to control pain.
- Click and/or crepitus are not uncommon for several weeks after surgery but usually resolve spontaneously after several months.

TECHNICAL POINTS

- Use a dorsal longitudinal incision.
- Release and relocate ECU tendon if subluxated volarward.
- Use limited resection of distal ulna (2 cm or less) through longitudinal capsulotomy.

- Perform synovectomy.
- Bevel dorsal edge of ulna to minimize risk of postoperative tendon rupture.
- Taper end of ulna to smooth "bullet" shape.
- Correct carpal supination by suturing remnant of triangular fibrocartilage complex/volar capsule to dorsal edge of radius.
- Stabilize ulna with tendon slip/pronator quadratus if necessary.
- Reconstruct dorsal capsule to stabilize and pad distal ulnar stump.
- Close skin over drain.

POSTOPERATIVE CARE

- Apply a short-arm splint for 2 to 3 weeks.
- Allow gentle forearm rotation as tolerated and increase forearm motion exercise after 3 weeks.

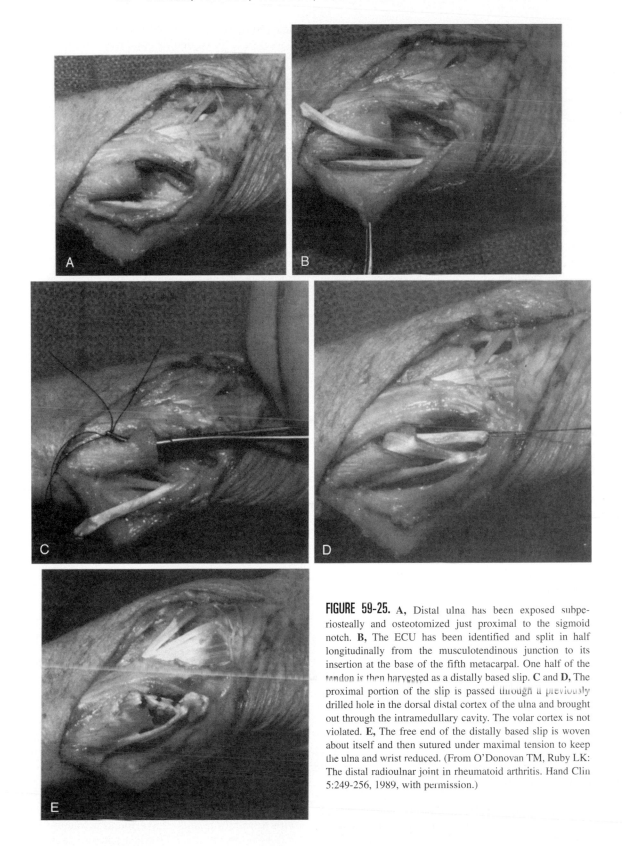

FIGURE 59-25. **A,** Distal ulna has been exposed subperiosteally and osteotomized just proximal to the sigmoid notch. **B,** The ECU has been identified and split in half longitudinally from the musculotendinous junction to its insertion at the base of the fifth metacarpal. One half of the tendon is then harvested as a distally based slip. **C** and **D,** The proximal portion of the slip is passed through a previously drilled hole in the dorsal distal cortex of the ulna and brought out through the intramedullary cavity. The volar cortex is not violated. **E,** The free end of the distally based slip is woven about itself and then sutured under maximal tension to keep the ulna and wrist reduced. (From O'Donovan TM, Ruby LK: The distal radioulnar joint in rheumatoid arthritis. Hand Clin 5:249-256, 1989, with permission.)

splinted in extension until the patient is able to extend them actively.

If the preoperative deformity or instability was minimal and if a satisfactory ligamentous reconstruction and tight capsular closure were possible at surgery, short-arm splints provide adequate immobilization postoperatively. Occasion-ally, a sugar tong splint to limit forearm motion is useful for pain relief in the first few days after surgery. Gentle forearm motion is allowed gradually as the postoperative pain and swelling decrease. However, if the soft tissue closure was suboptimal, the forearm should be maintained in supination with a long-arm splint or cast for 2 to 3 weeks to allow soft tissue healing before forearm motion exercises are started. It is not uncommon to have mild crepitus or a click during forearm rotation for the first few weeks after motion is started. This usually diminishes gradually and resolves entirely after several months.

Ulnar Head Excision—Complications. The most frequent complication after distal ulnar excision is painful forearm rotation. This often responds to prolonged splinting and a gentle motion exercise program under the direction of a therapist. No surgery is indicated for 3 to 4 months, unless a definite cause for the symptoms is evident. If the symptoms do not remit after several months and there is instability of the distal ulna on examination, a soft tissue stabilization procedure using the ECU to reinforce the DRUJ joint capsule can be considered.

We have had several extensor tendon ruptures after distal ulnar resection in rheumatoid patients. These occurred from attrition by the sharp edge of the distal ulnar shaft. We now bevel the dorsal edge of the distal ulna at the osteotomy site and use local tissues to provide a soft tissue layer over the distal end of the ulna after ulnar head resection.

Tendon Transfers to Restore Wrist Balance

A frequent wrist imbalance in rheumatoid arthritis is supination and ulnar translocation of the carpus on the radius. As stated previously, this deformity is associated with the caput ulna syndrome and rotatory instability of the carpus. In the caput ulna syndrome with volar subluxation or dislocation of the ECU tendon, there is unopposed radial deviation of the carpus from the pull of the radial wrist extensors. This is exacerbated if there is a concomitant intercarpal dissociation with collapse deformity of the scaphoid.

Clayton advocated correcting wrist imbalance by transferring the ECRL to the ECU in patients who cannot actively ulnarly deviate the wrist.[170,171,223,224] We have used this transfer in patients with radial deviation of the wrist that is correctable passively. The procedure should be considered in conjunction with wrist joint synovectomy, dorsal tenosynovectomy, and distal ulnar excision. However, our indications for this procedure are limited, because most of our patients already have advanced wrist involvement with fixed deformity. In these advanced cases, correction requires major reconstructive surgery (wrist fusion).

Hastings and Evans advocated balancing the wrist by repositioning the ECU into its normal dorsal position.[225] Preoperatively, to evaluate if the relocated ECU will function, place the forearm in supination and evaluate wrist extension. If the ECU functions as an extensor in this position, it will function appropriately in the relocated position. If not, an ECRL transfer is indicated.

Operative Technique: ECRL Transfer. After dorsal tenosynovectomy, distal ulnar excision, and ligamentous reconstruction are performed, the ECRL is divided at the base of the second metacarpal. This can be done through either a separate small incision or the primary surgical incision. The tendon is rerouted dorsal to the finger extensors and sutured into the repositioned ECU tendon. At the completion of the transfer, the wrist should maintain a neutral position in the coronal plane (radial and ulnar deviation). The wrist is splinted in the corrected position for 4 weeks before beginning exercises.

ECU Tendon

Operative Technique: Repositioning. During any surgical procedure on the dorsal aspect of the wrist, the ECU tendon should be released from its volarly subluxated position and repositioned in its normal dorsal position. If the extensor retinaculum has been reflected radially, a strip of this retinaculum can be split and looped around the ECU to hold the tendon dorsal to the axis of wrist flexion. Alternatively, when the retinaculum has been reflected radially and ulnarward, the ulnar portion can be placed deep to the ECU and used as a sling to hold the tendon in the corrected position. If there is a tendency for the tendon to subluxate, it can be sutured to the capsule over the dorsal aspect of the carpus.

Reconstruction of the Radiocarpal Joint

The indications for reconstruction of the radiocarpal joint by either arthrodesis or arthroplasty include deformity and instability that interfere with function, persistent pain unresponsive to conservative therapy, and progressive destruction of the joint seen on radiographic examination.

Historically, arthrodesis has been the reconstructive procedure of choice for the rheumatoid wrist.[185,226-232] In 1965, Clayton advocated the use of an autogenous bone graft and a Steinmann pin for fixation.[170] In 1971, Mannerfelt and Malmsten described the use of a Rush rod, which was introduced into the third metacarpal and driven across the radius, obviating the need for external fixation.[179] In 1973, we reported a modification of the techniques described by Clayton and Mannerfelt in 60 patients who underwent wrist fusion.[180] All of our patients had relief of pain and improved hand function. Although wrist fusion diminishes pain, wrist motion is lost, which is in itself a disability, especially in patients with stiffness of the opposite wrist (Fig. 59-26).

Total wrist arthroplasties have been used with inconsistent results.[173,233-235] In the mid 1970s, Swanson developed the silicone-rubber wrist arthroplasty for reconstruction of the rheumatoid wrist.[197,236,237] Since that time it has been the implant used most frequently for wrist arthroplasty. In 1980, we reported our early results in 35 Silastic wrist implant arthroplasties.[175] At that time, we concluded that the procedure was preferable to wrist fusion in most patients. In the first edition of this book, we stated that "in patients with persistent pain, relatively good alignment, functional wrist extensors and adequate bone stock, we prefer silicone implant wrist arthroplasty."

In 1986, we reviewed the long-term follow-up (average 5 years) of 71 patients who had undergone wrist arthroplasty with Silastic implants.[238] We found a fracture rate of 20% and a failure rate of 25% when fractures and revisions for pain and recurrent deformity were combined. Fatti and associates[239] reviewed 53 silicone-rubber implant arthroplasties and found 90% good results in patients followed less than 2.5 years. However, the percentage of good results dropped to 60% in those patients followed for more than 2.5 years. Stanley and Tolat reviewed 50 silicone-rubber

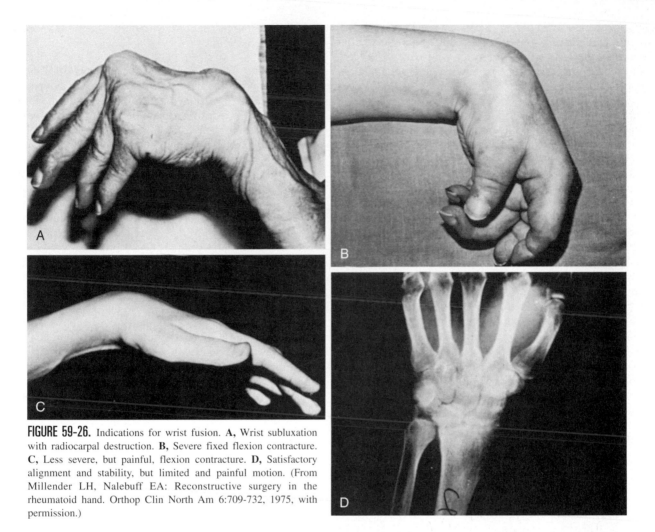

FIGURE 59-26. Indications for wrist fusion. **A,** Wrist subluxation with radiocarpal destruction. **B,** Severe fixed flexion contracture. **C,** Less severe, but painful, flexion contracture. **D,** Satisfactory alignment and stability, but limited and painful motion. (From Millender LH, Nalebuff EA: Reconstructive surgery in the rheumatoid hand. Orthop Clin North Am 6:709-732, 1975, with permission.)

implant arthroplasties with an average 8-year (range, 6 to 11.8 years) follow-up. There were 66% excellent and good results at the latest follow-up. The fracture rate was 22%, and the reoperation rate was 14%.[240] Although silicone synovitis has been noted after the use of some silicone-rubber implants in the hand and wrist,[177,241] this condition has not occurred in our series of wrist arthroplasties. The use of metal grommets may decrease the fracture rate.

Based on these reports, we have narrowed our indications for Silastic implant wrist arthroplasty. We now limit this procedure to those patients who will have low demand on the wrist after surgery in addition to the previously described criteria of functional wrist range of motion, wrist extensors in good condition, minimal wrist deformity, and good bone stock. We believe strongly that bilateral wrist arthroplasties are contraindicated. Those patients who do undergo wrist arthroplasty and require crutches as an ambulatory aid should use only forearm or platform crutches. Patients with arthroplasties should use wrist splints for any activity that will place stress on the wrist. (The operative technique of Silastic wrist arthroplasty is described elsewhere in this text.)

Choice of Operation for the Rheumatoid Wrist
Because of the increased number of surgical options now available for the reconstruction of joints affected by rheuma-

toid arthritis, preoperative clinical evaluation must be done carefully. After this, a considered recommendation for treatment can be made. Patient education, nonoperative treatment (including splinting and the judicious use of steroid injections), and hand therapy with modification of wrist use patterns are all important.

Distal ulnar excision alone may be indicated in a patient whose symptoms are limited to the radioulnar joint and whose radiocarpal joint is stable and functional, even when the radiocarpal joint shows significant destruction on radiographs.[242,243] Distal ulnar excision combined with radiocarpal synovectomy can be performed when there is mild to moderate loss of articular cartilage from the radiocarpal joint or early erosive changes within the carpus.

We have found (as have others[192,193]) that synovectomy alone can slow or even prevent progression in some cases. When soft tissue procedures or limited bony procedures are not appropriate, the decision to perform a total wrist arthrodesis or an implant arthroplasty must be made.[244] We have had no experience with total wrist arthroplasty using a metal-plastic prosthesis. Others have obtained reasonable results with newer implant designs.[97,245]

In summary, our indications for wrist arthroplasty with a Silastic wrist implant have decreased; we favor limited wrist fusions in patients with early collapse patterns of the wrist and in those with destruction limited to the radiocarpal joints. We advise wrist fusion in patients who require radio-carpal reconstruction but who are likely to place high demand on the wrist after surgery or who have significant wrist deformity or instability, poor wrist extensor function, or poor bone stock.

Partial Wrist Fusion

Partial wrist fusion has applications in rheumatoid as well as non-rheumatoid wrist disease.[55,165,178,187,246-248] Limited wrist fusion is useful in those rheumatoid patients whose disease has destroyed the radiocarpal joints but has left the mid-carpal joints relatively unaffected. Taleisnik demonstrated the paucity of ligaments in the midcarpal region of the wrist.[249] Because the synovium is concentrated in areas with abundant ligaments, the midcarpal area is the last to become involved and frequently is preserved even when the radio-carpal joint is not.

The earliest wrist changes in the rheumatoid patient occur as the volar ligaments stabilizing the proximal row are lost, resulting in vertical rotation of the scaphoid, dorsi-flexion or volarflexion of the lunate, and/or ulnar translo-cation of the lunate. These changes can be arrested in their early stages before progressive collapse and joint destruc-tion occur by fusion of the scaphoid and lunate to the radius. Of course, a destroyed radiocarpal joint can be salvaged by this fusion as well.[55,178] Limited arthrodesis of the involved joints combined with a synovectomy of the less involved joints may relieve pain yet preserve 25% to 50% of wrist motion (Fig. 59-27).

Operative Technique: Partial Wrist Arthrodesis. The wrist is exposed as described previously for synovectomy. The proximal and midcarpal rows are identified, and a synovectomy is performed using a small rongeur. Articular cartilage is removed from the joints selected for limited fusion. Cancellous bone is exposed by removing or "fish-scaling" the subchondral plate. The contours of the individ-ual carpal bones are preserved to allow apposition of the prepared surfaces. It is important to preserve the overall dimensions of the carpus; that is, the carpal bones should not be "collapsed" onto one another after the cartilage and subchondral are removed. Rather, the resulting space should be filled with bone graft. When a proximal row fusion is performed, we usually fuse the radius, scaphoid, and lunate bones. If the articular surface of the scaphoid is preserved, the fusion may be limited to the radiolunate articulation alone, as reported by Chamay and colleagues[246] and Linscheid and Dobyns.[178] If a midcarpal fusion is necessary, we include all the joints surrounding the capitate.

Autogenous bone graft is used to supplement the fusion site. Cancellous bone is packed between the individual bones to be fused. The distal ulna can be used as bone graft if a distal ulnar excision has been performed. Alternatively, bone may be harvested from the distal radius either by

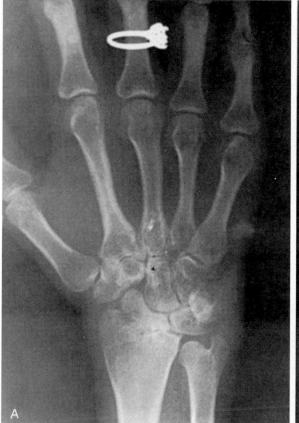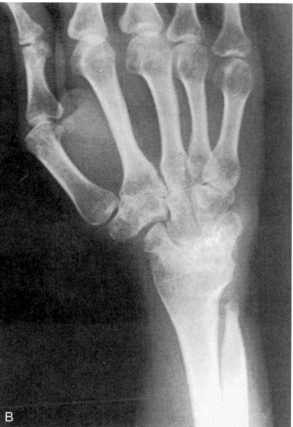

FIGURE 59-27. Partial wrist fusion. **A,** Isolated destruction of the radiocarpal joint and ulnar translocation of the carpus with preservation of the midcarpal joints. **B,** Correction of wrist alignment with preservation of some wrist motion by partial wrist fusion (radius-scaphoid-lunate).

removing Lister's tubercle or by making a small window in the dorsal cortex of the distal radius.[250] We prefer internal fixation with multiple 0.045-inch smooth Kirschner wires for the midcarpal joints and small cannulated screws (Acutrak, Herbert-Whipple, or ASIF) for the radiocarpal joints. These may be cut beneath the skin or left protruding through the skin. The Shapiro stapling device can be used to augment internal fixation.[251]

Postoperatively, the wrist is immobilized in a short-arm cast for 4 to 6 weeks, at which time the Kirschner wires are removed. Short-arm cast immobilization for an additional 3 to 4 weeks is necessary until there is evidence of solid fusion on radiographs. We expect to retain 25% to 50% of normal wrist motion after limited wrist arthrodesis.

Taleisnik[252,253] has described partial wrist fusion combined with carpal bone implant arthroplasty in selected rheumatoid patients with radiocarpal destruction or ulnar translocation and an unsatisfactory midcarpal articular surface of either the capitate or the scaphoid. If the articular surface of the head of the capitate has been eroded, he excises the proximal pole of the capitate and replaces it with either a Silastic condylar implant or a soft tissue spacer, such as a rolled-up length of tendon graft ("anchovy"). If the articular surface of the scaphoid is unsatisfactory, but the capitolunate articulation has been preserved, he fuses the lunate to the radius and replaces the scaphoid with a Silastic implant. In both procedures, the radiocarpal joint is stabilized and midcarpal motion is maintained.[163]

Operative Technique: Wrist Arthrodesis (Fig. 59-28). The wrist is exposed through a dorsal longitudinal incision similar to that for the wrist procedures described previously. A dorsal tenosynovectomy and associated procedures are performed. The radiocarpal joint is exposed by elevating a distally based flap of wrist capsule. The distal ulna is exposed and excised as described previously. The radioulnar capsule and triangular fibrocartilage are preserved for closure later. With traction and moderate flexion, a synovectomy of the radiocarpal joint is performed. The radial collateral ligament is released from the radial styloid, avoiding the APL and EPB tendons located in the first dorsal compartment. The cartilage and sclerotic bone are removed from the distal radius and proximal carpal row with a rongeur to provide proper alignment. The amount of bone resected is determined by the degree of deformity and subluxation.

In the standard procedure, the medullary canal of the radius is perforated with a pointed awl to provide a channel for the Steinmann pin to be used for internal fixation. The largest pin that will fit the medullary canal of the radius is selected. The pin is tapped through the carpus to exit between the second and third or between the third and fourth metacarpals, depending on the alignment between the carpus and radius. The pin should exit between the MCP joints. After this, the pin is tapped with a mallet retrograde into the previously prepared channel in the radius and countersunk approximately 2 cm proximal to the level of the MCP joints. Cutting the pointed end of the pin with a sterile bolt cutter minimizes the risk of penetrating the cortex as the pin is advanced by tapping it with a mallet. Power should not be used to insert the pin into the radius because of the increased chance of cortex penetration or fracture. Bone chips from

the resected segment of the ulna are packed into the radiocarpal joint before the carpus is impacted against the radius. One or two small staples or an obliquely placed Kirschner wire may be used to provide additional fixation of the radiocarpal joint if necessary. The Kirschner wire generally has to be removed later; the staples can remain in permanently.

If there is severe loss of carpal bone stock, the Steinmann pin is introduced into the third metacarpal to provide stability. If the MCP joints are dislocated and MCP joint arthroplasties are indicated, the rod can be drilled through the distal end of the metacarpal and countersunk proximally and an MCP joint arthroplasty can be performed subsequently. If MCP joint arthroplasty is not indicated, the Steinmann pin is introduced into the third metacarpal through a hole in the cortex made just proximal to the collateral ligament. This avoids passing the pin through the interosseous muscles and through the MCP joint. Leaving the rod buried in the metacarpal has not caused problems.

This method requires that the wrist be fused in a neutral position, that is, the metacarpal is aligned with the radius. We have found that this is an excellent wrist position for most rheumatoid patients and have used this method for patients requiring bilateral wrist fusions. The position of the wrist can be varied only 5 to 10 degrees by adjusting the direction of the pin as it is driven into the radius. The position of the wrist cannot be altered after the rod has been inserted. The single rod, albeit large in diameter, does not provide secure rotatory stability of the carpus to the distal radius.

Two-Pin Modification of Feldon. Feldon uses a modification of the technique described earlier for wrist fusions in both rheumatoid and non-rheumatoid patients. The wrist is prepared as described previously. Instead of using a single large Steinmann pin, two relatively thin Steinmann pins ($3/32$- to $7/64$-inch diameter) are inserted through the second and third web spaces between the metacarpal bones, across the carpus, and into the medullary canal of the radius. This results in a "stacked-pin" effect in the radius that provides rotational stability as well as anteroposterior and lateral stability, without the need for supplementary internal fixation (Fig. 59-29). The pins are thin enough to be bent after insertion into the radius, allowing final correction and adjustment of the wrist position. Thus, if slightly more dorsiflexion is desired after the rods are in place, the wrist is gently manipulated into the correct position. The use of thinner pins minimizes the potential for compression of the intrinsic muscles of the hand (interossei) by a large rod. Care must be taken to insert the pins through the dorsal portion of the web space to avoid potential damage to the neurovascular structures in the palm. It is sometimes helpful to make a small window in the dorsal cortex of the distal radius. This allows the pins to be guided into the medullary canal of the radius under direct vision. The pins may lie dorsal to the capitate bone because of the configuration of the wrist: this is not of concern (see Fig. 59-29B). Additional cancellous bone graft may be harvested from the distal radius as well. The pins are cut short beneath the skin in the web spaces and are removed after solid bony union has occurred, usually between 4 and 6 months postoperatively, or if they become symptomatic. However, the pins have been left in situ for many years without adverse effect.

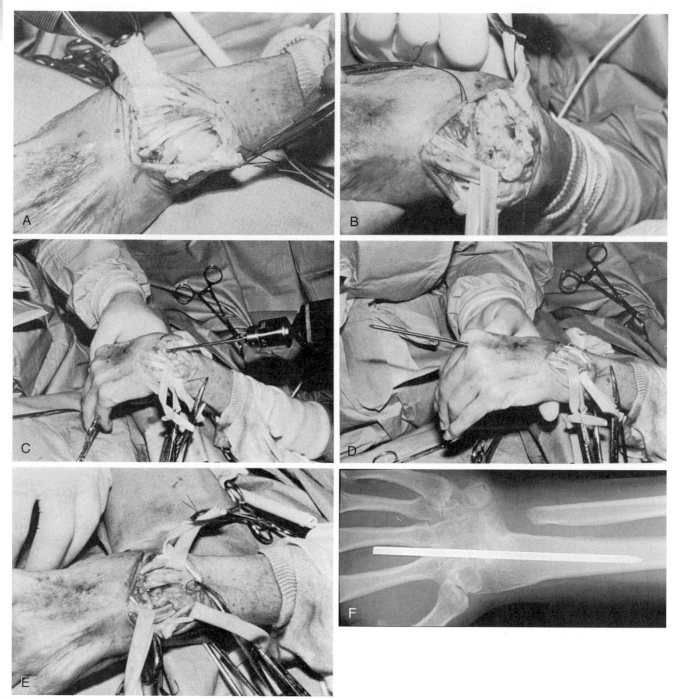

FIGURE 59-28. Technique for wrist arthrodesis. **A,** Slightly curved dorsal incision with the extensor retinaculum reflected and dorsal tenosynovectomy performed. **B,** Cartilage and sclerotic bone excised and cancellous bone exposed. Note the medullary canal of radius perforated to test the size of the Steinmann pin. **C,** A Steinmann pin introduced into the carpus exits between the second and third metacarpals. **D,** The Steinmann pin is driven into the radius and countersunk between the second and third metacarpals. **E,** The capsule is closed and the extensor retinaculum transposed or reconstructed. **F,** The postoperative radiographic appearance. (**A** to **E** from Millender LH, Nalebuff EA: Reconstructive surgery in the rheumatoid hand. Orthop Clin North Am 6:709-732, 1975, with permission.)

The pins are removed under local anesthesia by making a vertical incision in the web space and grasping the pin end with a 10- to 12-inch "diamond-jaw" needle holder.

Solid union has been obtained in more than 30 patients over the past several years. This technique has been used in rheumatoid patients even when carpal bone stock has been minimal. The advantages of this method include ease of hardware insertion and removal, the ability to adjust the position of the wrist at the time of surgery in both the anteroposterior and the lateral planes, and stable fixation even with suboptimal bone stock.

Tourniquet release, drainage, and closure are performed as described previously. A bulky dressing and a sugar tong or long-arm splint are used until the first dressing change. After this, only a short-arm cast or splint is necessary if the internal fixation is stable and the soft tissue reconstruction

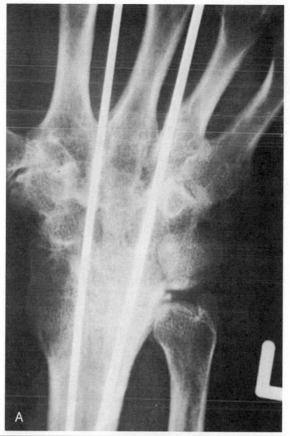

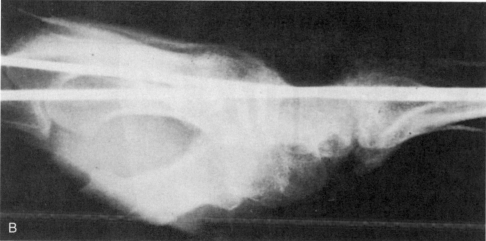

FIGURE 59-29. Wrist fusion using dual intermetacarpal-intramedullary Steinmann pins for internal fixation. **A,** Solid fusion was obtained with the wrist in slight ulnar deviation. **B,** The wrist is in slight dorsiflexion. The pins are positioned on the dorsal aspect of the wrist to minimize the risk of damage to the soft tissue structures in the palm and to facilitate placement of the pins in the medullary canal of the radius. Note that the Steinmann pins may lie dorsal to the fused carpus.

of the DRUJ will allow early forearm rotation. The forearm is held in supination for 2 to 3 weeks if this joint must be protected. Short-arm cast or splint immobilization facilitates early motion of the elbow and shoulder, as well as the forearm, and is much easier for patients to tolerate. The patient may walk with platform crutches 7 to 10 days after wrist fusion.

When the single Steinmann pin technique is used, the pin is not removed unless it causes discomfort or migrates. Rarely, the pin migrates distally enough to penetrate the skin. Should this occur, the pin is removed and supplementary external fixation is used if appropriate. Reintroduction of a pin that has come through the skin should be avoided because of the risk of infection.

Combined Wrist Arthrodesis and MCP Joint Arthroplasty (Fig. 59-30)

It is not unusual for a patient with severe rheumatoid arthritis to require both wrist fusion and reconstruction of the MCP joints. Ordinarily, this would necessitate two separate surgical procedures. However, we have performed both procedures during one operation.[254] This combined procedure is indicated in patients with painful wrists (but without significant wrist deformity) who are appropriate candidates for MCP joint arthroplasty. The single, definite contraindication for this combined procedure is a severely deformed or dislocated wrist that would require extensive exposure to correct the radiocarpal alignment.

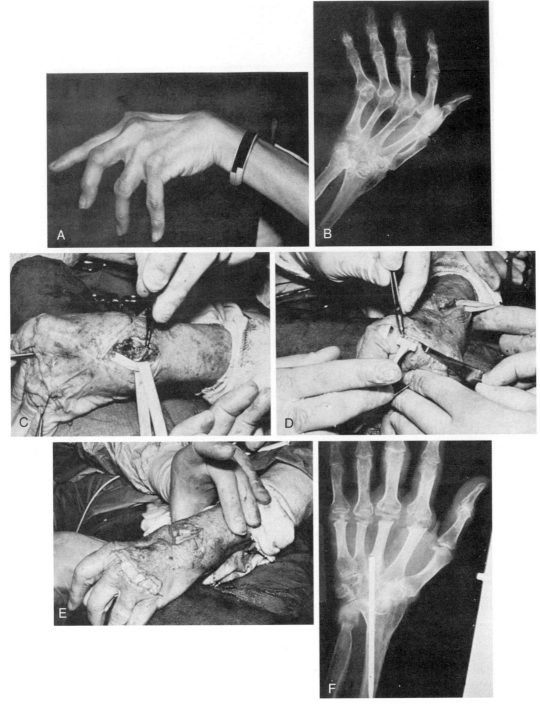

FIGURE 59-30. Wrist fusion combined with MCP joint arthroplasty. **A,** A patient presented with a painful wrist and dislocated MCP joints. **B,** Radiograph demonstrates the destroyed wrist joint and dislocated MCP joints. **C,** Minimal dorsal tenosynovectomy is performed, the distal ulna is excised, and the distal radius and carpus are crushed with a rongeur to form a fusion mass. The metacarpal heads have been resected, and the Steinmann pin has been introduced. **D,** After the Steinmann pin has been countersunk and a bone plug packed into the metacarpal to prevent distal migration of the Steinmann pin, the implants are introduced. **E,** Completed procedure before closure. **F,** Radiographic appearance. Note how far the Steinmann pin has been countersunk in the third metacarpal.

A less extensive exposure, without dislocation of the radiocarpal joint, is used to prepare the wrist for fusion. This allows the MCP joint arthroplasty to be performed with minimal risk of excessive postoperative edema and its attendant risk of skin slough and other complications. The procedure is a modification of the technique for wrist arthrodesis described earlier.

Operative Technique. A dorsal-ulnar skin incision is made, exposing the EDQ and, if necessary, the EDC. The distal ulna is excised, and a limited dorsal tenosynovectomy is performed. An arthrotomy of the radiocarpal joint is made either through the radioulnar joint capsule or through a separate dorsal radiocarpal capsular incision. Through these incisions, synovectomy, débridement, and preparation of the joint for fusion can be accomplished with a small rongeur. We have found that by removing the cartilage and sclerotic subchondral bone and by softening the distal radius and carpus to form a fusion mass of cancellous bone, solid arthrodesis can be obtained.

Preparation is facilitated by applying traction to the hand to distract the joints. If there is moderate flexion or deviation of the radiocarpal joint, alignment can be restored through the limited capsular incision by removing more of the radial styloid and/or carpus with a rongeur. After adequate preparation, the medullary canal of the third metacarpal can be aligned with the radius. After preparation of the wrist, the MCP joint arthroplasties are performed using a transverse incision over the metacarpal heads. Before introducing the MCP joint implant, a large, smooth Steinmann pin is introduced into the third metacarpal through the distal end and tapped through the carpus into the radiocarpal joint. The pin is introduced into the medullary canal of the radius under direct vision. Intraoperative radiographs are obtained to confirm appropriate pin position. After the pin has been tapped into the radius, radiocarpal stability is evaluated. The distal end of the pin is cut and countersunk 3 to 3.5 cm into the metacarpal bone to allow room for the MCP joint implant. Care must be taken not to countersink too far, or adequate purchase on the metacarpal will be lost. After the pin is countersunk, cancellous bone is tamped into the medullary canal before introducing the implant. This ensures that the rod will not back out. The MCP joint arthroplasties are completed in the usual manner. Routine closure over drains and immobilization in a bulky dressing with a volar plaster splint complete the procedure.

Postoperative management for combined wrist fusion and MCP arthroplasty is the same as for MCP joint arthroplasty alone. A volar wrist splint is used for 4 to 6 weeks. This splint may be combined with the dynamic splint used for the postoperative management of MCP joint arthroplasties, or the dynamic splint can be fabricated over a plaster volar wrist splint.

Complications of Wrist Fusion

Complications after wrist fusion were reviewed by Clendenin and Green.[255] The most frequent complication in their series was pseudarthrosis. In our experience, pseudarthrosis occurs infrequently in the rheumatoid patient, usually is asymptomatic, and rarely requires further treatment. Ryu and associates[256] described producing a fibrous nonunion intentionally in rheumatoid patients. Other complications occurred rarely but included deep wound infection, superficial skin necrosis, transient median nerve or superficial radial nerve compression, fracture of the healed fusion, and pin migration.

THE MCP JOINTS

The MCP joint is the key joint for function of the fingers. Rheumatoid destruction of this joint results in severe deformity and functional loss. MCP joints are condylar, allowing motion in two separate planes. Because of this anatomic configuration, their inherent stability is less than that of the IP joints, and, therefore, they are more vulnerable to the deforming forces present in rheumatoid arthritis.

The causes of deformity of MCP joints have been the subject of much debate. There are multiple factors leading to the classic ulnar drift and volar dislocation seen in rheumatoid patients. An understanding of the various factors leading to these deformities is important for the surgeon dealing with these problems.[17,51,123,257-269a]

Etiology of Rheumatoid MCP Joint Deformities

The deforming forces begin as proliferative synovitis stretches the capsule and ligamentous structures. In the MCP joints, this proliferation occurs in the recess between the metacarpal head and collateral ligament attachment, resulting in fraying and fragmentation of the collateral ligaments. Flatt believes that loosening of the ligaments markedly decreases the stability of the joint and is one of the early factors leading to progressive deformity.[259] The normal MCP joint is stable in full flexion, with little lateral motion possible in this position. However, in the rheumatoid patient, the flexed MCP joint often can be deviated 45 degrees.

The following factors affect the altered MCP joint, ultimately resulting in volar subluxation or dislocation and ulnar deviation: wrist deformity, flexor and extensor tendon forces, intrinsic muscle imbalance, and the forces of gravity and pinch. Wilson and Carlblom[123] described the interaction of these forces in detail.

Shapiro[167,168] showed that wrist collapse leads to radial deviation of the metacarpals and, subsequently, to an increased tendency for ulnar deviation of the MCP joints affected by the rheumatoid process. This is an expansion of the intercalary collapse theory of Landsmeer. Pahle and Raunio,[153] Hastings and Evans,[225] and others have confirmed these observations.[266,268,270]

The extrinsic extensor and flexor tendons also affect ulnar drift.[271] In the rheumatoid hand, the extensor tendons often are shifted or even dislocated ulnarward. Selective stretching of the radial-side transverse lamina (sagittal band) fibers by synovial proliferation and the normal ulnar shift of the extensor tendons during MCP flexion as the fourth and fifth metacarpal bones descend (which may be increased in rheumatoid arthritis by laxity of the fourth and fifth CMC joints) contribute to this ulnar subluxation.

Flexor tendon forces also contribute to MCP joint deformity.[272] Flatt demonstrated that during pinch there are palmar and ulnar forces in the index and long fingers and a palmar force at the MCP joint levels in all four fingers.[6] Stretching of the collateral ligaments of the MCP joints, which support the flexor tendon sheath, allows a volar and ulnar shift of the A2 pulley mechanism, which can increase the tendency toward MCP joint deformity significantly. The anatomic configuration of the joint and the forces of the intrinsic mechanism contribute to the ulnar deviation tendency.

Indications for Operative Treatment of the MCP Joint

Operative procedures for the MCP joint are either preventive or reconstructive. The only potentially prophylactic procedure is synovectomy (Fig. 59-31). Reconstructive procedures

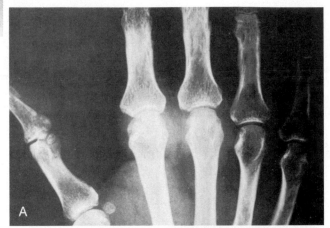

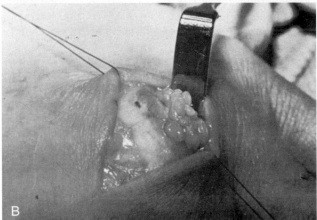

FIGURE 59-31. Indications for MCP joint synovectomy. **A,** Radiograph shows minimal cartilage loss, no bony destruction, and no deformity. **B,** Note proliferative synovium bulging dorsally and stretching the extensor mechanism.

include soft tissue surgical reconstruction and various types of arthroplasties.

Synovectomy

The indications for either synovectomy alone or synovectomy with soft tissue reconstruction are difficult to define, because no study has shown definitively that these procedures affect the natural course of the disease. Although synovectomy is considered by some to arrest the local disease or to slow progression of the disease and allow erosive lesions to heal, recurrence is always possible. Recurrent synovitis may occur as early as several months or as late as many years following the procedure. It is impossible to predetermine those patients that are likely to develop recurrence. In addition, 30% to 50% of patients with rheumatoid arthritis will have spontaneous remission, making it difficult to evaluate the effectiveness of any preventive surgery.[273-278] Because of the inconclusive results after synovectomy, most rheumatologists and surgeons today take a conservative attitude toward synovectomy of the MCP joints.

Synovectomy is indicated for the infrequent patient with persistent MCP joint synovitis, minimal radiographic changes, and minimal, if any, evidence of deformity. Intermittent, painful synovitis (which is infrequent) is an additional indication for synovectomy. Before considering synovectomy, the patient must have had an adequate trial of conservative therapy, which includes systemic medication, splinting, and up to three local intra-articular corticosteroid injections.[279] Chemical synovectomy in digital joints using thiotepa has been reported to give favorable results, but this technique needs further investigation.[280]

We consider a 6- to 9-month period of conservative therapy necessary before performing synovectomy. Within this period, some patients being considered for the procedure will have a medical remission, and unnecessary surgery will be avoided. Others undergoing conservative therapy will show rapid joint destruction, and these patients would not have good results from synovectomy. The third group of patients on conservative therapy will continue to have persistent localized synovitis with minimal, if any, deformity and minimal radiographic changes. These patients, we anticipate, will benefit on a long-term basis from synovectomy.

Combined Synovectomy and Soft Tissue Reconstruction

Our indications for combined synovectomy and soft tissue reconstruction to correct deformity are limited, because the persistence of multiple deforming forces and the progression of the disease frequently result in recurrence. Synovectomy with soft tissue reconstruction is considered in a patient who is a candidate for synovectomy but who also has early volar subluxation and ulnar drift. If the disease appears to be progressing slowly and the patient is young, soft tissue reconstruction may slow recurrence of the deformity. Occasionally, a patient presents with the inability to extend the MCP joint actively because of complete dislocation of the extensor tendons but the ability to maintain active extension if the MCP joints are extended passively. Extensor tendon relocation with synovectomy is indicated for this patient.

We believe that, in view of both the high incidence of recurrence and the alternative of MCP arthroplasty, which has proved to be an effective, predictable, and long-lasting procedure, soft tissue surgery alone is indicated infrequently.[37,197,219,281-288a]

Contraindications to MCP Joint Surgery

There is a group of patients for whom surgery should not be suggested. Although these patients have definite subluxation, ulnar drift, advanced radiographic changes, and a weakened grip, they are usually pain free and have good hand function. Although MCP joint deformity is present, surgery will not increase their function and would probably weaken their grip. These patients are best treated with night splints and observation every 3 to 4 months. If they maintain satisfactory function, observation should be continued. If they show progressive deformity and dysfunction, they will become candidates for operative treatment.

Operative Techniques for the MCP Joint
MCP Joint Synovectomy (Fig. 59-32)
MCP joint synovectomy on multiple joints is performed through a transverse incision centered over the dorsal aspect of the joints. Synovectomy for a single joint may be performed through a longitudinal incision located just ulnar to the joint. The longitudinal incision also is used when

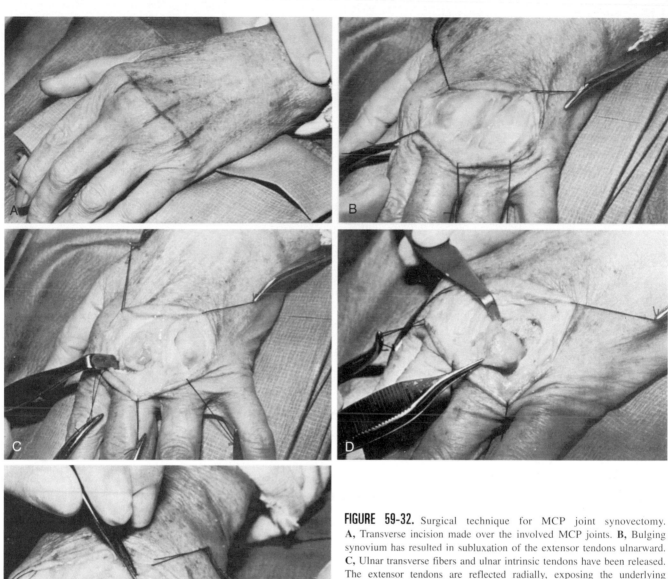

FIGURE 59-32. Surgical technique for MCP joint synovectomy. **A,** Transverse incision made over the involved MCP joints. **B,** Bulging synovium has resulted in subluxation of the extensor tendons ulnarward. **C,** Ulnar transverse fibers and ulnar intrinsic tendons have been released. The extensor tendons are reflected radially, exposing the underlying synovium within the MCP joint. **D,** MCP joint synovectomy is performed. **E,** At completion of the MCP joint synovectomy, articular cartilage of the metacarpal head is demonstrated. (From Millender LH, Nalebuff EA: Preventative surgery: Tenosynectomy and synovectomy. Orthop Clin North Am 6:765-792, 1975, with permission.)

multiple procedures are being performed in one finger, thereby decreasing the risk of excessive swelling. The initial skin incision must not be too deep to avoid damage to the extensor tendons that lie immediately beneath the skin. The dorsal veins and nerves are located within fat pads in the interdigital spaces. These structures must be protected, because injury to them may result in painful neuromas or dysesthesias and/or increase the risk of postoperative swelling, with resultant adherence of the extensor mechanism.[283]

The extensor mechanism is exposed, and the areolar tissue overlying the sagittal bands is separated so that the degree of extensor tendon subluxation to the ulnar side of the joint can be determined. In early cases, there is minimal subluxation of the tendon and no significant intrinsic tight-

ness. We prefer to expose the joint by making an incision through the ulnar-side sagittal band, volar to and parallel with the extensor tendon. Others enter the joint from the radial side. Swanson described splitting the extensor mechanism in the mid-dorsal line to avoid damaging either the radial or the ulnar intrinsics. Intrinsic release is performed at this stage, if necessary (see later).

The extensor mechanism is separated from the underlying capsule with small, blunt-tipped scissors. This dissection is often difficult, because the capsule has been thinned and disrupted by proliferating synovium that has herniated dorsally or because the capsule is scarred and adherent to the extensor mechanism. The transverse orientation of the fibers of the sagittal bands serves as a guide to the plane between the capsule and the extensor mechanism. The extensor mechanism is retracted radially, and the joint capsule is incised transversely. Bulging synovium is excised by sharp dissection or with a small rongeur. Traction applied to the finger allows easier access to the volar pouch. Synovectomy of the recess between the collateral ligament and metacarpal neck is performed with a small pituitary rongeur or a curet. Cystic areas of the metacarpal head are curetted.

After completing the synovectomy, the extensor mechanism is repositioned. If the mechanism subluxates ulnarward, it must be secured as described on page 2095. No attempt is made to close the dorsal capsule. The wound is closed over a Penrose or suction drain placed in the subcutaneous area, and a bulky conforming dressing is applied. Active motion is begun 1 to 2 days postoperatively, and a program of dynamic splinting similar to that after MCP joint arthroplasty is used for 4 weeks.

Intrinsic Release (Fig. 59-33)

Intrinsic release usually is performed in conjunction with MCP joint synovectomy or MCP joint arthroplasty, but it may be performed as an independent procedure in one or more fingers.[289,290] Either a transverse or a longitudinal incision may be used. After the dorsal neurovascular structures have been mobilized and the extensor mechanism has been identified, areolar tissue is freed from the entire ulnar side of the extensor mechanism. The sagittal, transverse, and oblique fibers of the intrinsic mechanism are identified. A longitudinal incision is made in the sagittal band adjacent to the extensor tendon. A curved hemostat is passed beneath the transverse fibers and oblique fibers to exit around the thickened portion of the oblique fibers. These structures are divided, and a section of the oblique fibers may be excised. If a release of the bony attachment is required to obtain adequate position of the MCP joint, the proximal portion of the tendon is grasped with a clamp and, using scissors, the tendon attachment into the proximal phalanx is sectioned.

In the small finger, the abductor digiti quinti is a strong, ulnar-deforming muscle that must be released. A blunt retractor is used to hold the skin and subcutaneous tissue out of the way. The dorsal branch of the digital nerve of the small finger is protected. The fascial sheath is incised to expose the hypothenar muscles. The abductor digiti quinti is separated from the flexor digiti quinti and is selectively sectioned at its musculotendinous junction. The ulnar neurovascular bundle lies just volar to these muscles and must be protected. Flatt emphasized the importance of releasing

only the abductor digiti quinti without sacrificing the flexor digiti quinti. He showed that releasing the flexor digiti quinti results in limited MCP joint flexion and increased weakness.[6]

Harris and Riordan[290] described an alternative method of releasing tight intrinsics. After the intrinsic mechanism is exposed, a triangular portion of the oblique fibers is excised. With this method, the transverse fibers, which act as a yoke to flex the MCP joints, are left intact.

Flatt[291] described a modified intrinsic release that he uses for early subluxation of the MCP joint or for persistent flexion contracture. He releases that portion of the transverse fibers that aids flexion of the MCP joint. If tightness persists after this release, the bony attachment of the intrinsic tendon is released as well.

Crossed Intrinsic Transfer

Straub[11,292] introduced the crossed intrinsic transfer as an additional method to restore finger alignment and prevent recurrent ulnar drift. In principle, the intrinsics are released from the ulnar sides of the index, long, and ring fingers and transferred to the radial aspect of the adjacent fingers to provide additional radial stability. Although we do not use this procedure frequently, Oster and colleagues[285] found that it can provide effective long-term correction of ulnar drift. In a subsequent follow-up study, El-Gammal and Blair[293] found a decrease in active range of motion of the MCP joint after 5 years.

Crossed intrinsic transfer is performed in conjunction with MCP joint synovectomy and soft tissue reconstruction. The intrinsic tendons of the index, long, and ring fingers are exposed as described previously. In Straub's method, the tendon is released from the extensor mechanism over the midportion of the proximal phalanx and dissected proximal to its musculotendinous junction. The bony attachment is released from the base of the proximal phalanx to allow free excursion of the muscle-tendon unit. Each tendon is transferred to the radial intrinsic mechanism of the adjacent finger. The tendon is woven into the lateral band and sutured.

Flatt and associates[294] believe that the intrinsic transfer performed as described here may cause a swan neck deformity. Flatt sutures the intrinsic tendon to the radial collateral ligament of the adjacent finger rather than weaving the tendon into the lateral band of the adjacent finger.[6,294]

In Flatt's method, the intrinsic tendons are exposed and released as described earlier. The extensor expansion is opened on the radial side to expose the collateral ligament. The intrinsic tendon is sutured to the radial collateral ligament at its phalangeal attachment using several interrupted 4-0 sutures. The tension at which the attachment is made is correct if complete finger alignment is restored at the completion of the repair. The finger is splinted for 3 weeks before beginning exercises. A dynamic splint is applied then and is used for an additional 3 weeks.

Extensor Tendon Relocation

Realignment of an ulnarly dislocated extensor tendon is necessary to correct deformity, restore extension, and prevent recurrent dislocation. The degree of extensor tendon subluxation varies from minimal to complete dislocation with the tendon fixed within the intermetacarpal valley.

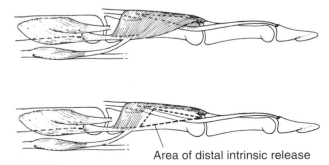

Area of distal intrinsic release

FIGURE 59-33. Technique for ulnar intrinsic release. The ulnar intrinsic tendon is exposed, and a triangular section of the extensor hood including the lateral band is resected.

Several different operative techniques have been described to centralize the extensor tendon.[72,295,296]

Longitudinal incisions are used when only one or two fingers are to be done. If all four fingers are to be done, adequate exposure can be obtained through a transverse incision. The subluxated extensor tendon is identified, and the sagittal fibers along its ulnar side are incised. A hemostat is placed beneath the transverse and oblique fibers of the intrinsic tendon on the ulnar side, and an intrinsic release is performed. The extensor tendon is dissected free and relocated over the dorsal aspect of the MCP joint. The tendon may be maintained in the relocated position by one of three methods. The simplest but least effective method is to reef the stretched radial sagittal fibers. After the tendon has been relocated, the lax fibers are imbricated with an absorbable 4-0 suture. We use this procedure when there is no tendency for the tendon to resubluxate. However, if there is a tendency for radial deviation of the wrist, which increases the tendency for ulnar subluxation of the tendon, more secure fixation of the tendon must be obtained.

An effective method is that described by Harrison.[297] A 4-cm slip of extensor tendon, 5 mm wide, is detached proximally and freed distally to the distal portion of the MCP joint. This is passed through a hole drilled into the dorsal cortex at the base of the proximal phalanx. Zancolli[72] described a method for rebalancing and stabilizing the extensor mechanism by attaching the extensor tendon to the proximal phalanx through drill holes.

We prefer a modification of the Harrison procedure that does not require a hole drilled into the bone (Fig. 59-34A and B). We have found that attachment of the tendon slip described earlier to the thick capsule at the base of the proximal phalanx is satisfactory. After the tendon slip has been prepared, a transverse incision is made through the capsule on the dorsal aspect of the proximal phalanx. The tendon slip is passed from outside to inside, then out through the capsule and extensor mechanism on the radial side, and finally sutured back to the extensor tendon. This maintains the extensor mechanism in the centralized position. The fingers should be moved through their full range of motion passively after the procedure has been completed to be sure that the tendon stays centralized and does not subluxate either to the ulnar side or to the radial side of the MCP joint. Flexion of the MCP joint should not be restricted significantly after the tendon has been centralized.

We also have had good results with direct attachment of the extensor tendon to the proximal phalanx. The attachment is made by either suturing the tendon to the joint capsule just proximal to the base of the proximal phalanx or attaching the tendon directly to the dorsal aspect of the proximal phalanx with a suture passed through drill holes in the proximal phalanx or a small bone anchor (see Fig. 59-34C).

Postoperative Management for Soft Tissue Procedures

At the completion of the surgical procedure, a bulky conforming dressing is used to immobilize the hand with the MCP joints in extension and in correct alignment. The drain placed in the subcutaneous area is removed on the first postoperative day, and the hand is re-splinted. Exercises, supervised by a hand therapist, are begun within the first 3 to 4 days. The fingers are protected during the exercises

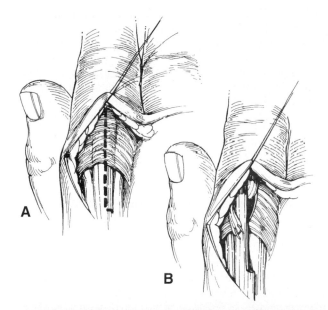

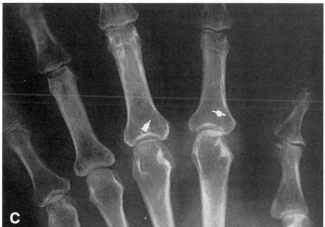

FIGURE 59-34. **A,** A strip of extensor tendon is split from the ulnar side of the extensor tendon and passed through the underlying joint capsule, and through the radial portion of the extensor mechanism before being sutured to itself. **B,** The tendon strip is sutured to itself, centralizing the extensor tendon by attaching it to the underlying joint capsule. **C,** Ulnarly subluxated extensor tendons of the index and long fingers have been relocated by using small bone suture anchors to attach the extensor tendons directly to the proximal phalanges, just distal to the MCP joint.

and are splinted in extension between exercise periods. Exercises are performed three or four times a day. On the fifth to seventh postoperative day, a dynamic splint is fabricated to maintain finger alignment and MCP joint extension but also to allow active flexion. This splint is worn during the day, and a plaster "resting" splint is used at night. Both splints are used for 4 to 6 weeks after surgery. Long-term splinting and carefully supervised therapy are important in preventing the recurrence of deformity.

MCP Joint Arthroplasty in Rheumatoid Arthritis

In the late 1950s and early 1960s, Vainio, Riordan, and Fowler described techniques to correct the deformities of arthritic MCP joints.[321,332] These procedures included joint resection and the interposition of soft tissues between the metacarpal and proximal phalanx. Despite improved digital alignment and moderate motion from these resection arthroplasties, the results were unpredictable and recurrent deformities were common.[305]

Swanson, in the mid 1960s, devised a flexible hinge implant to improve the reliability of the resection/interposition arthroplasty. The silicone rubber implant was designed to function as an internal splint that would maintain alignment and stimulate a capsular response termed *encapsulation*.[327] The flexible stem of the implant was allowed to glide in the medullary canal.[333] The combination of the implant and scar tissue provides joint stability and alignment, while allowing a reasonable arc of motion. Swanson called his implant a "load-distributing flexible hinge." The Swanson silicone implant is composed of a high-molecular-weight, cross-linked silicone elastomer. In 1975, an improved silicone elastomer with a fourfold increase in tear propagation strength was made available for use. The most recent modifications have further increased the fatigue-crack growth resistance and have been used since 1986.[298]

The result was a resection arthroplasty with a painless and functional arc of motion and which was much more reliable and predictable than a resection arthroplasty alone.

Flexible hinge arthroplasty has remained the most accepted and widely performed technique for treatment of severely involved MCP joints in rheumatoid arthritis. However, strict attention to technical detail is necessary for this operation to succeed.[311,312,325] Recently, new implant designs have sought to replicate the anatomy of the MCP joint to preserve function and improve on the limitations of silicone arthroplasty.

Indications

The goals for implant arthroplasty of the MCP joint are pain relief, correction of deformity, and improvement in function and appearance. Implant arthroplasty should fulfill the criteria outlined by Flatt and Fischer in 1969[306]: restoration of functional range of motion, adequate stability, and resistance to lateral and rotational forces. Linscheid suggested the addition of biologic compatibility, adequate material

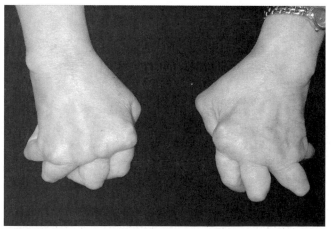

FIGURE 59-35. This patient has rheumatoid arthritis with severe hand involvement. The MCP joints are dislocated, flexed, and ulnar deviated. The PIP joints are also involved. This patient was treated with selected PIP joint fusions for fixed flexion deformities and in a second stage, MCP arthroplasty.

properties and the opportunity for adequate soft tissue reconstruction.[310]

The typical patient with rheumatoid arthritis has a combination of MCP joint ulnar deviation and volar subluxation deformity, pain from synovitis, deformities at other joints, and grasp weakness. MCP joint arthroplasty can improve the patient's function by correcting deformity as well as relieving pain and improving appearance. Combined and/or staged procedures may be necessary (Fig. 59-35).

Initially, MCP joint reconstruction surgery was advocated only for patients with severe deformity and limited function. This standard has been modified with increased confidence in the outcomes of arthroplasty. Current trends favor surgery in less deformed hands for the following reasons: (1) Less bone is resected in the patient with mild deformity compared with the patient with severe deformity. (2) Soft tissues such as the capsule and collateral ligaments are better preserved, which ultimately facilitates soft tissue reconstruction. Nevertheless, silicone MCP joint arthroplasty is not indicated for mild deformities. Likewise, radiographic deformity alone is not a sufficient indication for MCP joint reconstruction. Realistic goals and expectations by both the patient and surgeon are necessary ingredients for a successful outcome in MCP joint surgery.

Contraindications

Active infection is a contraindication to MCP arthroplasty. A previous MCP joint infection is a relative contraindication to implant surgery. The surgeon should give consideration to the duration of the infection and pathogens involved. Bone loss and soft tissue problems after an adequately treated infection may preclude arthroplasty.

Other general contraindications include inadequate skin coverage, compromised neurovascular status, insufficient bone stock, and an irreparable musculotendinous system.[326]

Patients with severe progressive rheumatoid arthritis (arthritis mutilans) may have inadequate bone to support or receive the implant. Typically, the phalanges and metacarpals of patients with juvenile rheumatoid arthritis have very small intramedullary canals that may make it impossible to insert even the smallest implant. In such cases, simple resection arthroplasty should be considered to realign the digits.[330,331] Extensor tendon dysfunction must be considered but it is not a contraindication to MCP joint arthroplasty. MCP joint arthroplasty and extensor tendon reconstruction can be done as either a combined procedure or in stages.[313]

Patients with multiple deformities from rheumatoid arthritis may require a staged reconstruction.[313] Wrist deformity and or pain must be considered when planning MCP joint surgery. A fixed radial deviation deformity of the wrist will lead to recurrent ulnar deviation of the fingers after arthroplasty (Fig. 59-36).[324] If there is significant wrist pain, hand function will still be limited even after successful MCP joint reconstruction. Therefore, the wrist problem should be addressed before or in combination with MCP joint reconstruction.

Arthroplasty Options

Many implants have been used over the past 30 years in attempt to achieve pain-free, well functioning MCP joints. These can be categorized into one of three design-types: metal hinged prostheses (Flatt), flexible implant (Swanson),

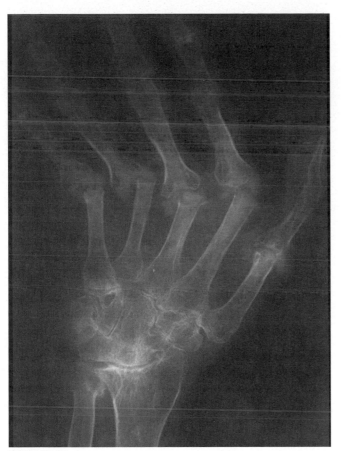

FIGURE 59-36. This patient had failed MCP arthroplasties with fractured implants secondary to a fixed radial deviation deformity of the wrist. This is treated by correction of the wrist deformity and subsequent revision MCP arthroplasties. When performing revision MCP arthroplasty, the procedure is identical to the initial technique and there are no shortcuts.

and third-generation prostheses. The first hinged prostheses used for MCP arthroplasty were simple metal uni-axis hinges. Evolution of this type resulted in multi-axis hinges with combinations of metal, ceramic and polymer components. Despite early promising results, recurrent deformity, dislocation, and loosening plagued these designs in the longer term.

Flexible silicone implants have been the most extensively used and studied and currently remain the implant of choice. These implants have a class 2 designation from the U.S. Food and Drug Administration (FDA). Despite their limitations, they are relatively easy to implant, can be revised without undue difficulty, and are reasonable in cost.

The group of third-generation prostheses includes surface replacement prostheses and hybrids of hinged and flexible prostheses. The most recently studied with long-term follow-up is the pyrolytic carbon MCP implant.[303] These FDA class 3 implants have an articulating, unconstrained design with a hemispherical head and grooved, offset stems, re-creating the bony anatomy. The material is made up of an isotropic carbon coating over a graphite substrate with similar wear properties to ceramic. These designs were developed to provide greater strength and durability. Flexible implants may not be adequate for younger patients with higher grip strength and longer life expectancy. Patients with less advanced rheumatoid disease, post-traumatic

arthritis, and primary osteoarthritis will benefit most from restoration of anatomy with a surface replacement arthroplasty. Functional ligaments and muscles surrounding the joint are critical in providing joint stability and the ultimate success of this type of arthroplasty.[299]

Surgical Technique
Flexible Implant Arthroplasty
There are three major design choices in flexible implant arthroplasty: the original Swanson design (Wright Medical), the Avanta (Avanta Orthopaedics), and the Neuflex (Depuy) implants. We have the greatest experience with the Swanson implant, although the surgical technique for each of the designs is essentially identical.

A single longitudinal incision may be used when the surgery is confined to a single digit.

When two or more arthroplasties are done simultaneously, a single transverse skin incision is made over the affected MCP joints. With multiple joint implantations, the surgery is started on the index finger and proceeds sequentially to the small finger. In patients with rheumatoid arthritis, the skin is often thin and care should be taken to avoid damage to the underlying veins, superficial nerves and extensor tendons. The skin is retracted with sutures, and the extensor mechanism of each digit is exposed by blunt dissection. It is usually necessary to divide the junctura between the index and middle fingers and separate the conjoint tendon going to the ring and small fingers.

Attenuation of the radial sagittal band fibers and ulnar translocation of the extensor tendons is common. The tendons and extensor mechanism are elevated from the underlying joint capsule after the ulnar side of the extensor tendon is identified and freed. Release of the shortened ulnar sagittal band often is required to mobilize the extensor tendon. We prefer to approach the joint from the ulnar side to release these fibers (Fig. 59-37). A longitudinal incision is made between the volar edge of the extensor tendon and the sagittal fibers. Adherences between the extensor tendon and the underlying joint capsule are freed, and the extensor tendon is retracted to the radial side to expose the MCP joint capsule.

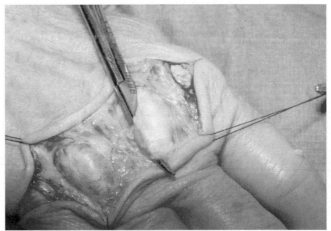

FIGURE 59-37. A transverse incision is used to expose the MCP joints. The superficial nerves and veins that run between the metacarpal heads are preserved. The ulnar sagittal band is identified with a hemostat and then released with a transverse incision parallel to the extensor tendon.

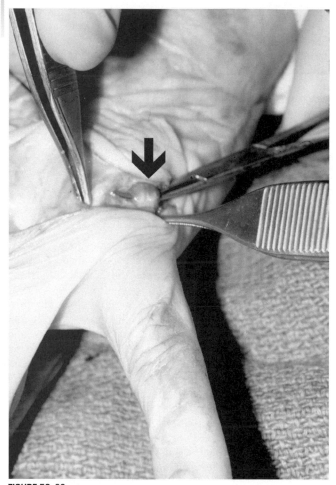

FIGURE 59-38. The ulnar intrinsic is identified in the hemostat and released to correct the significant ulnar deviation of the MCP joint.

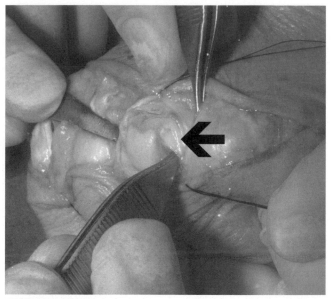

FIGURE 59-39. The capsule has been incised and the MCP joint flexed. The collateral ligament can then be identified and released if needed from the metacarpal neck *(arrow)*.

Before the metacarpal head is resected the configuration of the base of the proximal phalanx should be checked. If there is dorsal erosion, the base of the proximal phalanx is squared by resecting bone from the volar portion of the base of the phalanx (Fig. 59-40). In this case, less of the metacarpal head will be resected. If the proximal phalanx is

The ulnar intrinsic tendon is identified and released in most cases (Fig. 59-38). Passing a right-angled retractor around the tendon will help isolate the tendon and will protect the neurovascular bundle volar to it. It is tagged with a suture if a crossed intrinsic transfer or lengthening is planned. Release of the ulnar intrinsic will help correct ulnar deviation of the finger. If the intrinsic is not contributing to the deformity at the MCP (or the PIP) joint, we do not divide it.

A longitudinal midline incision is made through the joint capsule, and exposed synovium is removed. The collateral ligaments usually need to be released to correct the deformity and/or allow access to the joint. However, if there is minimal deformity and the collateral ligaments are competent, release of the ligaments may not be necessary.

A knife blade is placed in the collateral ligament sulcus at the metacarpal neck and swung dorsalward along the neck to detach the collateral ligament origin while preserving its distal attachment to the proximal phalanx. Flexion of the joint facilitates this (Fig. 59-39). Preserving the radial collateral ligament is especially important for reconstructing the joint. Reattachment of this ligament allows correction of the ulnar deviation deformity and provides resistance to the lateral forces generated during pinch.

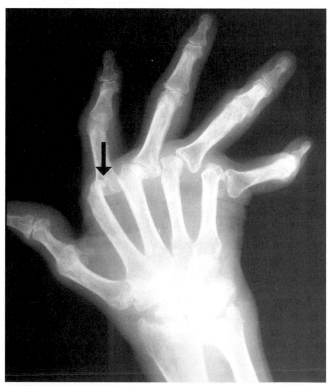

FIGURE 59-40. This preoperative radiograph demonstrates dorsal erosion of the proximal phalanx of the index finger *(arrow)*. This should be recognized preoperatively to avoid perforation of the proximal phalanx and/or excessive bone resection of the metacarpal.

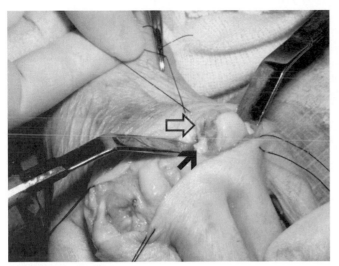

FIGURE 59-41. After the collateral is released *(closed arrow)* the periosteum is stripped proximally *(open arrow)* to provide tissue for collateral ligament repair when needed.

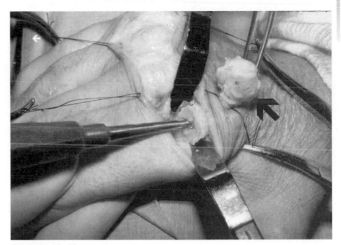

FIGURE 59-42. The metacarpal head has been removed *(arrow)* perpendicular to the metacarpal, and the medullary canal is perforated with an awl.

not checked first, too large a space for the implant may result after bone has been resected from both sides of the joint to provide flush surfaces for the barrel of the implant to rest against.

The metacarpal head now can be resected. The periosteum is incised transversely at the proposed resection site on the dorsal aspect of the metacarpal neck. The periosteum is left intact proximally to provide tissue for reattachment of the collateral ligament and capsule (Fig. 59-41). With the use of an oscillating saw oriented perpendicular to the shaft, the metacarpal head is resected level with the origin of the collateral ligaments. This is best done with the joint flexed and a flat elevator placed on the volar surface of the metacarpal for support. The synovectomy now can be completed and the amount of space available for the implant checked by applying distal traction to the finger. If there is not enough space to accommodate the implant, more of the metacarpal head is resected. It is better to err on the side of too little initial bone resection than too much resection.

Flexion of the joint exposes the base of the proximal phalanx. The base is brought dorsal to the metacarpal. Resection or release of the volar plate may be necessary to allow adequate exposure and alignment of the proximal phalanx. This may also gain additional space for the implant after bone resection. Care is taken to avoid injury to the flexor tendons while releasing the volar plate. A limited flexor tenosynovectomy can be performed at this time if needed, and flexor tendon excursion can be checked.

The base of the proximal phalanx should be completely exposed. An oscillating saw or rongeur is used to provide a flush base to the proximal phalanx. Usually only the joint margins or, if necessary, a thin portion of the subchondral bone need be removed.

After bone removal is completed, a pointed awl is introduced into the medullary canals of the proximal phalanx and metacarpal (Fig. 59-42). The phalanx is prepared first since it usually determines the size of the implant to be used. This will prevent over-reaming of the metacarpal. The exception to this is in the fourth (ring) metacarpal. The canal of this metacarpal is usually narrower than that of the ring finger

proximal phalanx and is prepared first to avoid over-reaming the proximal phalanx. The Swanson reamers are used to shape a rectangular opening in the proximal phalanx, which helps resist rotation of the implant stem. Power burs with a blunt leading tip can be helpful when the diaphysis is constricted. For the index and long fingers, the rectangular opening should be angled so that it is slightly more dorsal on the radial side and volar on the ulnar side. This will supinate the fingers slightly, facilitating opposition to the thumb and thereby chuck pinch. In the other fingers, the rectangular opening will be parallel to the volar surface of the proximal phalanx. Preparation of the metacarpal is similar with the rectangular opening parallel to the volar surface of the bone.

At this point, it is essential to confirm that there is sufficient space for implant insertion. A 1-cm space is ideal and will usually allow placement of the implant without buckling (Fig. 59-43). If the space is too small, insertion of

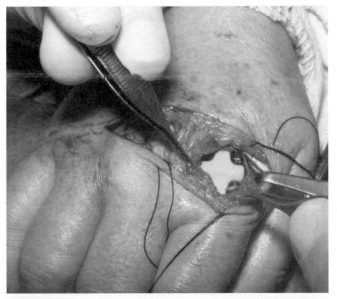

FIGURE 59-43. Trial implant is in place, and an adequate space for the implant is demonstrated.

the implant will be difficult and subluxation may then occur, resulting in limited joint motion and/or recurrent deformity. The space can be increased by several methods: release or resection of the ulnar intrinsic and capsule, release or resection of the volar plate, and resection of additional bone.

The joint is now ready for implant insertion and soft tissue reconstruction. A 2-0 absorbable suture is woven into the radial collateral ligament at the base of the proximal phalanx for the index and middle fingers. Traction applied to the suture after placement will deviate the proximal phalanx radialward if the suture has been properly placed (Fig. 59-44). The collateral ligament need not be repaired for the ring and small fingers unless this is necessary to correct finger alignment. The radial collateral ligament of the index and middle fingers usually is sutured to the periosteal sleeve on the dorsal and radial aspect of the metacarpal. The ligament can be reattached through drill holes on the dorsal/radial edge of the metacarpal if there is not adequate periosteum. The suture is not tied until after the implant is in place.

The implant is inserted using smooth forceps to minimize injury to the implant surface. Glove powder should not contact the implant because it will adhere to the implant and can lead to a particulate synovitis. Implant insertion is done with the metacarpal and the proximal phalanx positioned at right angles to one another. Usually the metacarpal stem is inserted first. The central portion of the implant is held with a smooth instrument while the phalanx stem is inserted. The joint is extended to seat the implant. Check to be sure that both stems of the implant are in their respective medullary canals. If the implant buckles with the joint extended or dislocates with the joint flexed, there is not enough space and either a soft tissue release or additional bone resection must be done. The finger is held in extension and slight radial deviation while the collateral ligament suture is tied with sufficient tension to maintain the joint in 10 to 15 degrees of radial deviation. Redundant capsule is trimmed, and the capsule is closed to cover the implant. Capsular closure helps to protect against implant dislocation and speeds the encapsulization process. If doing multiple implants, the most radial finger is done first and the more ulnar digits aligned to it.

Extensor Tendon Centralization

Laxity of the radial sagittal fibers and ulnar displacement of extensor tendon after implant insertion typically requires reinforcement of the radial side. If there is mild subluxation, placement of several 4-0 absorbable mattress sutures will shorten the radial sagittal fibers and bring the extensor tendon into a centralized position. If the tendon is dislocated or does not stay centralized during passive MCP joint flexion, a more formal centralization procedure will be necessary. These are described on page 2095. Once all implants are in place, the previously divided tendon junctura are repaired, if possible (Fig. 59-45). At the conclusion of the procedure, the fingers should align in a slight radial deviation. Passive MCP joint flexion of 70 to 80 degrees should

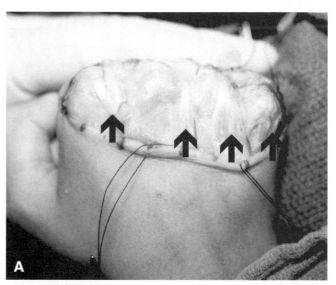

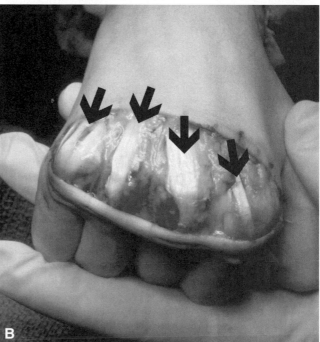

FIGURE 59-45. This is an example of an extensor tenodesis. **A,** The extensor tendons are ulnarly subluxed *(arrows)*. **B,** A tenodesis of the tendon to the proximal phalanx has been performed. With full MCP flexion the extensor tendons remain centralized *(arrows)*.

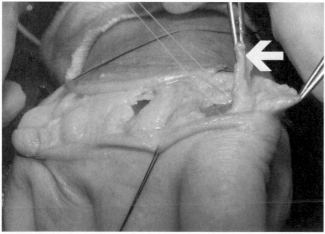

FIGURE 59-44. The radial collateral ligament is held in forceps *(arrow)* and prepared for repair in slight overcorrection.

be possible without capsular suture failure or extensor subluxation. The skin edges are closed with 5-0 nylon sutures. In most cases, with careful attention to hemostasis, we close the skin with the tourniquet still inflated. A drain placed in the subcutaneous space helps prevent postoperative hematoma formation. A well-padded hand dressing is applied with the MCP joints supported as follows: the position of immobilization of the MCP joints is determined by their preoperative position. If the major problem was ulnar deviation or subluxation without fixed flexion, the fingers are placed in a functional position with the MCP joints slightly flexed. If the patient had severe MCP joint flexion deformity preoperatively with weak or absent extension, the MCP joints are splinted in extension. Each finger is maintained in slight radial deviation with tape supporting the ulnar side of the proximal phalanx to protect against ulnar deviation. The wrist is supported in slight extension and neutral deviation by a plaster splint that also supports the MCP joints in the desired position. The PIP joints usually are left free.

Technical Points

An alternative approach to the exposure of the joint is through the stretched radial sagittal fibers. This method requires shortening of the radial sagittal fibers once the implant is in place.

Release of the ulnar intrinsic tendon should be considered based on the amount of deformity present and the finger involved. Specifically, the ulnar intrinsic provides a supination force for the index finger and is helpful in pinch. Therefore, it can be left intact when the deformity is mild and correctable without release.[326] The final decision for release of the ulnar intrinsic can be made after resecting the metacarpal head in patients with mild deformity. If the MCP joint deformity cannot be completely corrected, the intrinsic should be released.

Intrinsic release may also correct a concomitant swan neck deformity by decreasing the extensor force to the PIP joint. However, intrinsic division reduces the patient's ability to spread the fingers in a normal fashion after the arthroplasty. Lengthening of the intrinsic tendon is an alternative to complete division. This should diminish the deforming force while preserving some ulnar intrinsic function. Keeping the intrinsics intact also should be considered in patients with significant laxity, such as in systemic lupus. Complete ulnar intrinsic release in such patients may result in a radial deviation deformity after reconstruction.[314]

Inadequate bone resection and/or soft tissue release can result in not enough space for placement of the implant. This can cause implant fracture and/or limited motion. Implant dislocation can occur if too much bone is resected or if there is inadequate soft tissue release. Sharp bone edges must be smoothed to prevent implant injury.

Perforation of the dorsal or volar aspect of the proximal phalanx can occur during preparation for the distal stem. Typically, an unrecognized proximal phalanx base deformity leads to perforation. This is usually not a problem if the stem is redirected distal to the perforation.

Rehabilitation

Most of our MCP joint reconstructions now are done on an outpatient basis. We recommend the dressing be changed and the drain removed in 1 to 2 days. A static splint to maintain the MCP in the corrected position (nearly full extension and slight radial deviation) is applied and supplemented with soft tape to keep the fingers in proper alignment.

We have learned that a single postoperative protocol does not work for all patients who have had MCP arthroplasties done. A splinting and exercise program for each patient is specifically designed around his or her preoperative deformity and the condition of the soft tissues at surgery.

The initial Swanson protocol used a dynamic splint with slings under the proximal segments of the fingers to maintain MCP joint extension and slight radial deviation. We found that this method often resulted in limited flexion of the ring and small fingers, and we modified it by leaving the slings off of these fingers (Fig. 59-46). Now we use low-profile custom volar splints to support the MCP joints in nearly full extension for 6 weeks. A lip on the ulnar side controls radial deviation. Usually the PIP joints are left free and motion of these joints is encouraged. The splint is removed for range-of-motion exercises several times daily. If the PIP joints are supple, splinting them in extension during the MCP joint exercises will facilitate gaining MCP joint flexion. In patients with relatively mild preoperative deformity (mostly ulnar deviation with minimal loss of extension), Nalebuff prefers placing the MCP joints in the flexed position (intrinsic plus) at the time of surgery and

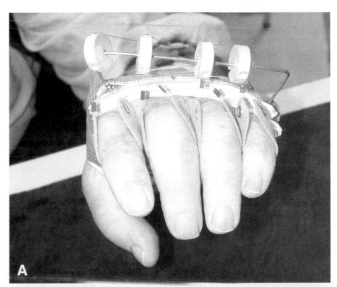

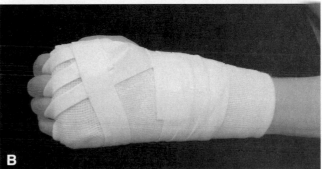

FIGURE 59-46. A, A low-profile dynamic extensor splint can be used to support the MCP joints in extension while allowing active flexion. **B,** A short-arm cast extended distally to support the MCP joints in extension is an alternative to dynamic splinting in selected patients. Note use of tape to maintain MCP joint alignment.

allowing active extension out of the splint. Careful postoperative monitoring is necessary to be sure that the reconstructed joints are responding as desired. The protocol is changed as necessary to accommodate the patient's progress.

In patients who have difficulty in returning for frequent follow-up because of distance or other constraints, we have used a short-arm cast extended distally to support the MCP joints in about 30 degrees of extension for 4 to 6 weeks after suture removal, as described by Simmons.[317] We use dynamic extension splinting for patients with a significant extensor lag at the MCP joints postoperatively or who had moderate preoperative MCP joint flexion deformities. In patients with severe preoperative flexion deformities, casting in extension for 4 to 6 weeks can be used.[317] Gradual mobilization is started after the cast is removed, and a period of dynamic splinting may be helpful after the cast is discontinued.

In general, continuous passive motion usually is not indicated, because it has not been shown to increase the postoperative range of motion.[320] However, it can be of some use in selected patients. We use a static splint to maintain the corrected position at night for 3 months.

The need to customize postoperative splinting and therapy for each patient, taking into account the nature of their disease (e.g., rheumatoid, psoriatic, lupus) and the severity of the deformity before arthroplasty as well as the condition of the soft tissues and flexor and extensor tendons cannot be emphasized enough. Careful planning and close follow-up will maximize hand function after MCP joint arthroplasty.

Complications

The complications associated with MCP joint arthroplasty include recurrent ulnar deviation, extensor lag, limited MCP joint flexion, implant fracture, infection, and silicone-induced particulate synovitis.[301,318] Most patients have some recurrent ulnar deviation and loss of MCP joint extension over time. In one of the largest studies to date, Bieber and colleagues reported on 210 Swanson-design MCP implants.[300] These patients were followed for an average of 5.3 years. At the initial postoperative evaluation, ulnar drift improved from the preoperative average of 25 degrees to less than 5 degrees. The preoperative average extension deficit decreased from 56 to 10 degrees, whereas the average range of motion increased from 17 to 51 degrees. At long-term postoperative evaluation, the average ulnar drift had increased to 12 degrees, the average extension deficit had increased to 22 degrees, and the average range of motion had decreased to 39 degrees. In the longest follow-up period to date, Kirshenbaum and coworkers reported on a series of 144 arthroplasties at an average of 8.5 years from surgery.[309] These authors found an average recurrence of 7 degrees of ulnar deviation. They found that mean extension had improved to a range of 7 degrees to 19 degrees and that mean flexion ranged from 56 degrees to 66 degrees. At the time of the last follow-up, the motion of the MCP joints had not deteriorated significantly. However, range of motion alone is not the only determinant of success or failure of MCP arthroplasty in any given patient.

Reported fracture rates for all designs of MCP silicone implants range from 1% to 26%. When earlier (less tear-resistant) designs are excluded, the incidence of implant fracture varied from 0.9% to 10%.[298] In 1972, Swanson reported a fracture rate for his implant of 1.9% at follow up, ranging from 2 to 5 years.[328] He noted that most implant fractures occurred in the first 6 months after surgery and appeared to correlate to inadequate release of the joint deformity. The studies of Bieber and associates and Kirschenbaum and coworkers found fracture rates for the Swanson design of 0% and 10%, respectively.[300,309] Fracture of the implant does not necessarily lead to recurrent ulnar drift or require revision.[311] Encapsulation of the implant tends to maintain a functional joint even with implant fracture. However, with a significant increase in ulnar deviation or shortening of a finger, implant failure should be suspected and may be confirmed with radiographs of the hand. Bass and coworkers were able to correlate implant fracture and recurrent ulnar drift with the Sutter design implant in patients who underwent MCP arthroplasty.[298]

Titanium grommets can be used to protect the stems of the implant against the bone edges and may decrease implant fracture rates. Schmidt and associates evaluated the effect of grommet use in 151 Silastic MCP arthroplasties.[323] There were no significant differences in the clinical outcomes with respect to swelling, correction of ulnar deviation, range of active movement, and grip strength. However, the use of grommets slightly reduced reactive osteolysis, protected the spacers from breakage, and slightly reduced the amount of pain with only a few additional complications in the mid-term 3.9-year follow-up. The favorable bone response and better bone preservation at the metaphysis with use of grommets, as described by Swanson, was not seen. As such, the main advantage seems to be prevention of implant fracture. The insertion and fitting of the grommets, however, adds to the complexity of the procedure. We limit their use to cases with previous implant fracture or when the resected bone edges are particularly sharp.

Infections around the implants are rare. Deep infection rates, requiring implant excision, have varied from 1.6% to 9%.[298,312] Removal of the implant with a short period of antibiotic coverage usually controls the problem. We do not attempt to reinsert an implant after an infection of the MCP joint has been brought under control. By removing the implant, the operation is converted to a "resection" arthroplasty. The range of motion is reduced, but pain is eliminated and digital alignment can be maintained by splinting for 6 weeks.

Outcomes

In patients with rheumatoid arthritis, the ability to correlate clinical and radiographic parameters to subjective patient interpretation of outcome is difficult, if not impossible. Patient satisfaction and radiographic parameters have not shown significant correlations.[298] The results of MCP joint arthroplasty are as varied as the patients undergoing the procedure. In the largest meta-analysis to date, Chung and colleagues reviewed all published series of the Swanson MCP joint arthroplasty used for treatment of rheumatoid deformity.[302] Based on these authors' findings, use of the Swanson implant has been shown to effectively correct ulnar drift deformity and improve the aesthetic appearance of the rheumatoid hand. Several major research design deficiencies hindered analysis, including unclear overall design, lack of uniform outcome measurements, confounding patient characteristics and clinical factors, and varying follow-up intervals.

One of the most important considerations in MCP joint arthroplasty is the restoration of function. The literature indicates that the expected active range of motion is 40 to 50 degrees (with passive motion typically greater) after uncomplicated arthroplasty. After implant arthroplasty, the functional arc is usually shifted to greater extension, which is usually advantageous for hand function.[302] The postoperative range of motion is influenced by many factors, including the type of arthritis, the condition of adjacent joints, the controlling tendons, and the tissue elasticity of the patient. Hume and colleagues reported that a functional arc between 33 to 73 degrees is necessary for most activities of daily living.[308] Seventy-three percent of MCP joint arthroplasties met this goal in study by Gellman and associates in 1997.[307] This may be misleading because of concomitant deformities of the fingers. It is important to understand that the range of motion alone may not be the ultimate determinant of the outcome of MCP joint implant arthroplasty. Despite good MCP joint motion, hand function may be compromised if finger stiffness or poor position limits grasp or pinch. Several studies report conflicting data. Blair and colleagues examined simulated activities of daily living and did not find significant changes in postoperative function.[301] Conversely, Opitz and Linscheid and Rothwell and associates, in prospective studies, showed improvement in standardized hand function tests.[315,322] In the final analysis, patient satisfaction may be most related to pain relief and improved appearance at moderate-term follow-up (Fig. 59-47).[329]

Quantitative assessment of hand function related to activities of daily living may be a more meaningful outcome measurement than recording range of motion, correction of deformity, strength, and radiographic changes. In 1997, Rothwell and coworkers reported on hand function after Silastic MCP arthroplasties using the Baltimore Quantitative Test of Upper Extremity Function.[322] The results demonstrated that MCP arthroplasty significantly improved hand function within 6 weeks and benefits were maintained up to 4 years. Most improvement occurred in functions requiring pinch, span, or hook grip. The authors attributed this to correction of ulnar drift, stabilizing the fingers for pinch grip, and the change in arc of MCP joint motion, restoring ability to open the hand for grasp. The gains in hand function should continue provided there is not further deterioration in thumb or wrist function. The patients in whom scores declined between 1 year and 3 to 4 years also showed significant deterioration of the shoulder or elbow, which affect ultimate hand function.

In our practice it is common for patients with bilateral hand deformities to request MCP joint arthroplasties in the second hand. To us, this is the best test of patient satisfaction with the operation.

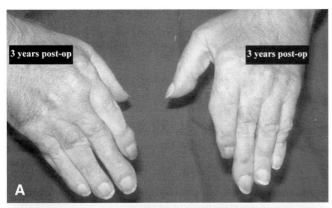
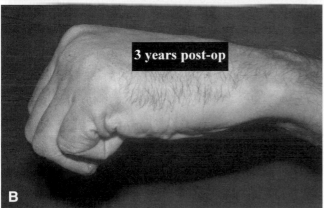

FIGURE 59-47. Appearance at 3-year follow-up after MCP arthroplasty. **A,** Active extension is good with alignment maintained. **B,** Good flexion is preserved.

CRITICAL POINTS: MCP JOINT ARTHROPLASTY

INDICATIONS

- Painful and/or deformed MCP joints from arthritis (rheumatoid, osteoarthritis, post-traumatic)

PEARLS

- Correct wrist deformity before MCP arthroplasty.
- Reconstruct radial collateral ligament with slight overcorrection of deformity.
- Begin supervised hand therapy postoperatively.

TECHNICAL POINTS

- Use a longitudinal incision for a single implant and a transverse one for multiple implants.
- Preserve longitudinal veins and sensory nerve branches.
- Divide ulnar sagittal band.
- Release ulnar intrinsic (if necessary).
- Reflect extensor tendon radialward; preserve joint capsule.
- Divide collateral ligaments at metacarpal neck; preserve radial collateral ligament insertion on proximal phalanx.

Continued

THE PIP JOINTS

PIP Joint Synovectomy

Although synovectomy is performed infrequently at the wrist and MCP joints for the reasons discussed previously, the indications for synovectomy of the PIP joint are broader. Progressive PIP joint synovitis that stretches the extensor mechanism will result in a boutonnière deformity that is difficult to reconstruct. The results of PIP joint arthroplasty are less reliable than those of MCP joint arthroplasty, and PIP joint fusions are more disabling. For these reasons, preservation of PIP joint function is important. In addition, the PIP joint is more stable than the MCP joint and recurrent deformity after synovectomy is less common than after MCP joint synovectomy. PIP joint synovectomy has relatively little morbidity. It can be performed on a single joint on an outpatient basis or in conjunction with other procedures such as tenosynovectomy, MCP synovectomy, or MCP arthroplasty.[142,273,335-341]

Operative Technique (Fig. 59-48). The joint is exposed through a slightly curved incision on the dorsal aspect of the finger. A sharply curved flap is avoided to prevent edema within the flap postoperatively. The extensor mechanism is exposed, preserving the longitudinal dorsal veins. The joint is exposed through a longitudinal incision splitting the central slip or through an incision between the lateral band and the central tendon. The location of the capsulotomy is determined by the site of bulging synovium. Hypertrophic

synovium is removed by sharp dissection or with a small rongeur. Gentle distal traction of the finger and flexion of the joint facilitate the synovectomy.

Occasionally, the synovium bulges laterally. In this case, incising the transverse retinacular ligament and reflecting the lateral band dorsally expose the synovium bulging through the accessory collateral ligament. A longitudinal incision volar to the collateral ligament allows the synovectomy to be performed without injuring the ligament and facilitates the removal of synovium from the volar pouch.

The extensor mechanism is repaired with an absorbable 4-0 suture. A conforming hand dressing is applied with the PIP joint positioned in extension.

Postoperatively, early motion is begun to preserve PIP joint function. Active flexion and extension are started 1 to 2 days after surgery. The joint is splinted in extension, except during exercise periods, for 2 weeks.

FINGER DEFORMITIES

Two finger deformities commonly occur in rheumatoid arthritis: the so-called swan neck and boutonnière deformities. The former is characterized by PIP joint hyperextension with DIP joint flexion, and the latter is the reverse deformity. Neither the swan neck nor the boutonnière deformity is unique to rheumatoid arthritis. Rather, they represent the end result of muscle and tendon imbalance caused by rheumatoid disease. Thus, we occasionally see patients who have both deformities in adjacent fingers of the same hand. Many factors cause these deformities and contribute to the degree of functional loss they produce.[336,342-344] This explains the variety of operations recommended to correct these deformities and the diversity of opinion regarding treatment.[189,345-351]

Swan Neck Deformity

Although all swan neck deformities have a superficial resemblance to one another, they vary considerably. Careful determination of the type of deformity present is essential for the selection of proper treatment. The significant functional loss associated with this deformity is related directly to the loss of motion at the PIP joint. This may range from no loss to partial loss to almost complete loss of flexion. Patients with almost complete loss of PIP joint flexion can be subdivided further into those with and those without preservation of joint space by radiographic examination. We classify these deformities into one of four types, depending on the PIP joint mobility and the condition of the joint surfaces. This classification serves as the basis for our treatment of fingers with swan neck deformities (Tables 59-3 to 59-5).[38,39,344,352-354]

Type I: PIP Joints Flexible in All Positions

Some rheumatoid patients with swan neck deformities demonstrate hyperextension of the PIP joint with DIP joint flexion yet maintain the ability to flex the PIP joint completely. The deformity may originate at either the DIP or the PIP joint. At the DIP joint it starts with stretching or rupture of the terminal extensor tendon attachment, resulting in the

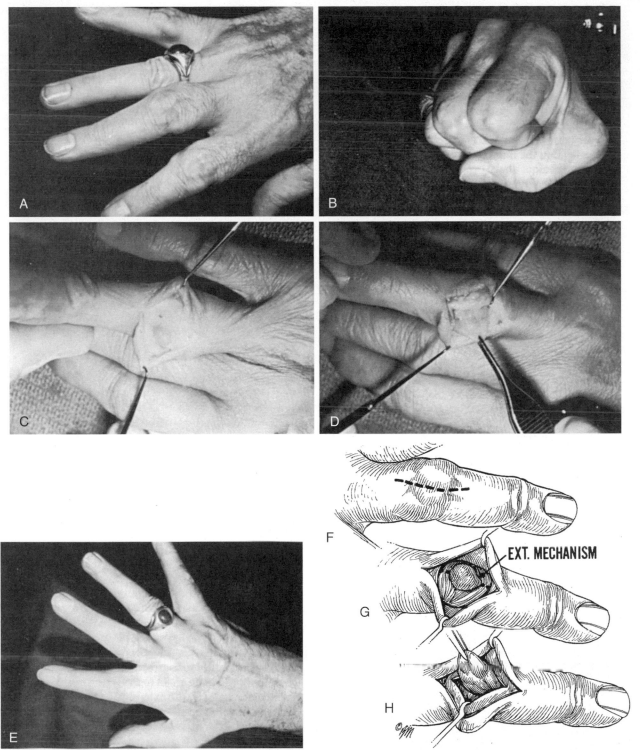

FIGURE 59-48. Technique for PIP joint synovectomy. **A** and **B,** A patient presented with PIP joint synovitis in several fingers. **C,** The extensor mechanism is exposed, demonstrating proliferative synovium bulging between the lateral bands and central slip. **D,** A longitudinal incision through the stretched extensor mechanism exposes the synovium, which is excised sharply. **E,** Postoperative photograph demonstrates full extension. **F** to **H,** Drawing of PIP joint synovectomy technique.

so-called mallet deformity. Extensor mechanism imbalance secondary to DIP joint flexion and associated with laxity of the volar plate of the PIP joint allows the PIP joint to assume a posture of hyperextension. In patients with early deformity, this progression can be observed. However, in patients who present with established deformity, the sequence of

events described can be inferred if the DIP joint deformity is more severe than the PIP joint hyperextension.

In other patients, the deformity may originate at the PIP joint as synovitis stretches out the volar capsule or if rupture of the superficial flexor tendon removes the force restraining PIP joint hyperextension. In these cases, DIP joint flexion is

Table 59-3

CLASSIFICATION SYSTEM OF THE FINGER SWAN NECK DEFORMITY

Type	Characteristics
I	Full range of motion No intrinsic tightness No functional limitations
II	Intrinsic tightness Limited PIP motion with an extended MCP joint with ulnar deviation corrected
III	Stiff PIP in all positions of MCP joint Radiograph good
IV	Severe arthritic changes

secondary. Swan neck deformity originating at the DIP or PIP joint is classified as type I if full passive motion of the PIP joint is maintained. These patients have only a small functional loss related to the limitation of DIP joint extension. They usually do not have associated MCP joint disease.

Treatment of patients with type I swan neck deformity is directed at preventing or limiting the PIP joint hyperextension, restoring DIP joint extension, or both. The use of a silver ring splint can be helpful in correcting PIP hyperextension while allowing motion (Fig. 59-49).[355] Several surgical procedures can be considered. These include DIP joint fusion, dermadesis (volar to the PIP joint), flexor tenodesis of the PIP joint, and retinacular ligament reconstruction.

Table 59-4

TREATMENT OPTIONS FOR SWAN NECK DEFORMITY IN FINGERS

Type	MCP Joint	PIP Joint	DIP Joint
I		Splint Dermodesis FDS sling Littler ORL reconstruction	Fusion
II	Intrinsic release	As for type I	Fusion
III	As for type II MCP joint reconstruction as needed	As for type II PIP joint manipulation Skin release Lateral band mobilization *Check flexor tendons*	Fusion
IV	As for type III	As for type III arthroplasty Fusion	Fusion

FDS, flexor digitorum sublimis; ORL, oblique retinacular ligament.

Table 59-5

SOFT TISSUE PROCEDURES FOR RHEUMATOID FINGER SWAN NECK DEFORMITY

Technique	Indications	Contraindications	Complications
Intrinsic release Manipulation PIP joint	Positive intrinsic tightness test Stiff joint with acceptable articular surfaces	Excessive force required	Injury to extensor mechanism Boutonnière deformity Loss of motion in postoperative period
Skin release	Blanching of skin with full PIP joint flexion		
Sublimis tenodesis Littler oblique retinacular ligamenti reconstruction	PIP hyperextension that interferes with flexion; may be combined with any of the others	Mild PIP deformity with severe mallet deformity (treat with DIP fusion)	Flexion contracture
Lateral band mobilization	Stiff joint with acceptable articular surfaces, not amenable to manipulation	Bone loss, instability, painful degeneration	Boutonnière deformity Loss of motion in postoperative period
Flexor tendon exploration and tenolysis	Active motion limited		

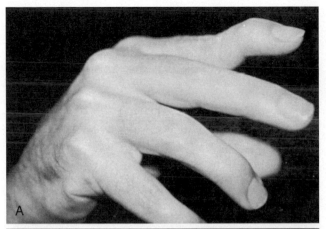

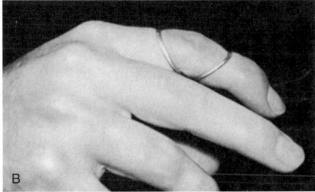

FIGURE 59-49. A mild, supple swan neck deformity (**A**) can be corrected with the Silver Ring splint (**B**).

Distal Joint (DIP) Fusion

Although correction of the flexion deformity of the DIP joint to restore balance to the finger could be obtained by reattaching the extensor mechanism to restore active control of the joint, the reconstructed tendon is subject to the same rheumatoid changes that led to the deformity in the first place. In addition, secondary arthritic changes within the joint may make attempts to restore motion unwise. An alternative treatment is to fuse the DIP joint.[356] We prefer this approach, particularly when the mallet deformity is primary.

We use a dorsal curved skin incision or the "Y" incision described by Swanson.[357] The extensor mechanism is divided transversely. The joint is flexed, and the collateral ligaments are divided to improve exposure. The articular cartilage is removed, and the bone ends are shaped to provide good bony contact. A longitudinal Kirschner wire is used for internal fixation. To be certain that the wire is introduced into the medullary canal of the middle phalanx, we predrill a small hole in the middle phalanx into the canal. Then we pass a slightly larger wire distally through the distal phalanx. This wire should emerge from the pulp just volar to the nail bed. The wire is then passed retrograde across the joint into the predrilled hole in the middle phalanx. Care should be taken not to drill the Kirschner wire too far proximally to avoid damage to the PIP joint. The minimum pin size that should be used is 0.045 inch. The DIP joint is fixed in neutral position (full extension), which is our preferred position in the correction of the swan neck deformity (Fig. 59-50). The Kirschner wire can be either cut off just below the skin or left exposed. If the wire is left exposed, removal after fusion is easy and the risk of pin tract infection is minimized. However, the finger cannot be immersed in water and the protruding pin must be covered to prevent injury to the patient and others. Burying the pin under the skin allows washing of the hand but increases the risk of skin irritation, skin breakdown, and subsequent infection. Usually, we use only one longitudinal Kirschner wire for DIP joint fusion. However, if necessary, an obliquely placed wire is added to control rotation. To facilitate fusion, we commonly add bone grafts to the fusion site. These grafts are essential for patients with extensive erosive changes and significant loss of bony substance.[48] The metacarpal heads removed for implant arthroplasty provide a good source of local bone graft material. External support with a small aluminum splint is advisable for the first 4 to 6 weeks after fusion.

If the pin has been buried, it can be removed in the office after the fusion is solidly healed. Local anesthetic can be injected directly into the skin and subcutaneous tissue overlying the pin, or a digital block can be given. A stab wound is made over the pin, and the pin is extracted with a needle holder. Occasionally, the pin may migrate proximally so that it is completely or almost completely buried in bone. This requires more extensive dissection to locate and remove the pin and should therefore be done in the operating room under optimal conditions that allow removal of some bone from the distal phalanx to expose the end of the pin.

A Herbert screw, Herbert-Whipple screw, or Acutrak small joint fusion system also can be used for internal fixation of DIP joint fusions.[358] These provide rigid internal fixation of the fusion and do not need to be removed after the fusion heals. Intramedullary placement ensures the preferred straight position of the joint. Relatively rigid fixation provided by the screw device precludes the need for prolonged postoperative splinting; 2 to 3 weeks is sufficient.

These screw systems have several disadvantages, however. If the screw is inserted incorrectly, the screw threads can damage the germinal matrix of the nail, resulting in nail plate deformity. The distal phalanx must be large enough to accept the trailing threads of the screw. Fixation can be lost if the leading screw threads extend beyond the isthmus of the middle phalanx and toggle in the soft bone of the metaphysis. We have used these screws more frequently recently and are pleased with the results when attention is paid to the technical details of inserting them (Fig. 59-51).

Operative Technique: Screw DIP Joint Fusion. Before beginning this procedure, check the lateral radiograph of the finger to be sure that the width of the distal phalanx medullary canal is sufficient to accept the screw. The DIP joint is exposed and the joint surfaces are prepared as described previously. The medullary canal of the middle phalanx is located with a 0.035-inch Kirschner wire. The canal is prepared with either a larger Kirschner wire or the appropriate drill/reamer, depending on the type of screw system selected. A 0.035-inch Kirschner wire is inserted through the base of the distal phalanx and into the medullary canal. The wire is driven distally to exit on the tip of the finger just below the hyponychium. A transverse stab wound is made where the Kirschner wire exits. The wire is withdrawn, and the appropriate drill/tap is inserted through the stab wound, into the tuft of the distal phalanx, and advanced

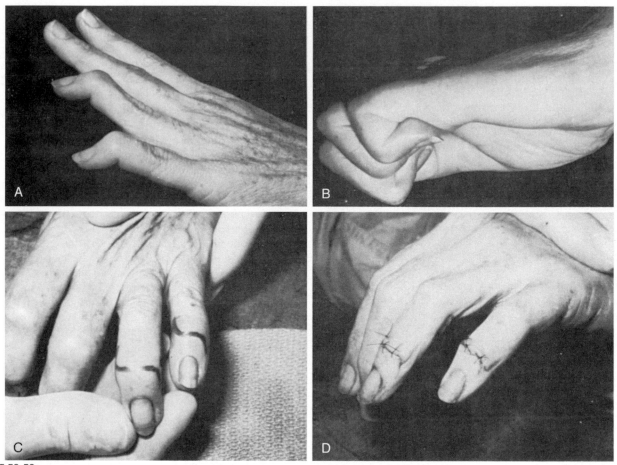

FIGURE 59-50. Type I swan neck deformity with primary defect at the distal joint. **A,** Note mallet deformity of the distal joint with secondary PIP joint hyperextension. **B,** The patient demonstrates full flexion of PIP joints. **C,** One of the incisions used for distal joint fusion. **D,** Improvement in finger posture after distal joint fusion in extension.

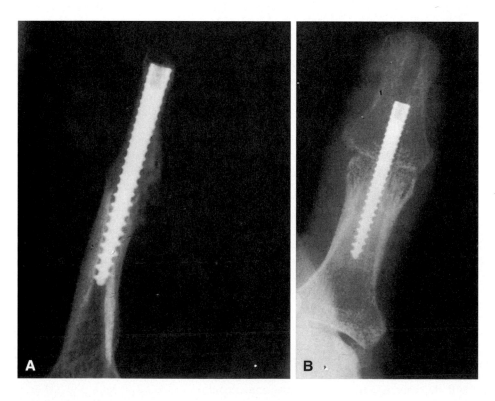

FIGURE 59-51. Self-compressing screws provide excellent internal fixation for small joint fusions in rheumatoid patients. The Acutrak small joint fusion system has been used to fuse the DIP joint of a finger (**A**) and the IP joint of a thumb (**B**).

Continued

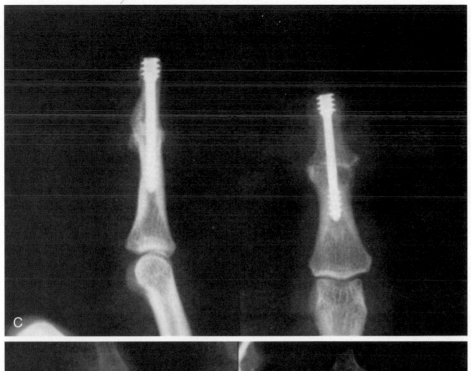

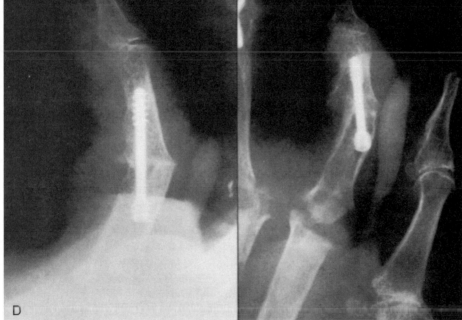

FIGURE 59-51—cont'd. C and **D,** Herbert screws can be used for both DIP and PIP joints in the fingers and for the thumb IP joint. The leading threads of a screw used to stabilize the DIP joint fusion should extend only into the isthmus of the middle phalanx to avoid loss of fixation from toggle of the screw in the softer bone of the metaphysis. MCP joint arthroplasties do not preclude the use of the Herbert screw for PIP joint fusions in the rheumatoid patient.

proximally until it emerges at the base of the phalanx. The appropriate length screw is inserted and advanced until it emerges at the base of the distal phalanx. The screw tip is aligned with the hole in the middle phalanx under direct vision and then advanced with the fusion surfaces held tightly together. The trailing threads of the screw are recessed into the tuft. If too long a screw is used, there may be a sudden loss of fixation as the leading thread passes through the isthmus into the softer and wider portion of the phalanx. Rotatory stability can be augmented by inserting a 0.028- or 0.035-inch Kirschner wire parallel to the screw. Intraoperative radiographs are obtained to confirm proper placement and length of the screw.

Dermadesis

Dermadesis[39] is an operative approach that is used occasionally in patients with type I swan neck deformities. This procedure attempts to prevent PIP joint hyperextension by creating a skin shortage volarly. An elliptical wedge of skin (4 to 5 mm at its widest point) is removed from the volar aspect of the PIP joint. Care is taken to preserve the venous network just under the skin and not to open or disturb the underlying flexor tendon sheath. The skin is closed with the PIP joint in flexion. This technique is helpful only in mild cases and usually fails unless it is done in conjunction with other procedures, such as DIP joint fusion. When PIP joint hyperextension is primary, we prefer to use a stronger checkrein against hyperextension. Our procedure of choice is flexor tendon tenodesis, using one slip of the FDS.

Flexor Tendon Tenodesis ("Sublimis Sling")

Patients with PIP joint hyperextension maintain full passive motion but, as the hyperextension increases, begin to develop difficulty in initiating active flexion. These patients require restoration of strong volar support to the joint. We prefer to use an FDS tendon tenodesis to prevent PIP joint hyperextension. We have found a method of tenodesis similar to that described by Curtis,[359] using one slip of FDS, to be useful in correcting rheumatoid swan neck deformities.

A volar zigzag incision is made over the PIP joint, and the flexor tendon sheath is exposed. The thin portions of the sheath on either side of the A3 pulley are excised, preserving the pulley. The flexor tendons are exposed, and care is taken to avoid injury to the vincula passing between the FDS and the FDP tendons. One slip of the FDS is divided approximately 1.5 cm proximal to the joint. This portion is separated from its corresponding slip but is left attached distally. With the joint in 20 to 30 degrees of flexion, the detached slip is fixed proximally to act as a checkrein against extension. The proximal attachment can be made directly into the bone using a pull-out wire or can be made at the thickened margin of the flexor tendon sheath (distal edge of the A2 pulley) (Fig. 59-52).

In the standard method of attaching the tendon into bone, we drill a small hole perpendicular to the shaft of the proximal phalanx. A pull-out wire is used to bring the tendon into the hole and is tied over a button on the dorsum of the finger. A rubber cushion is fabricated from a Penrose drain or a piece of Esmarch bandage and is placed between the skin and button. The attachment to bone is stronger but is technically more difficult than the attachment to the margin of the fibrous sheath.

An easier technique is to use a small bone anchor with a 2-0 or 4-0 suture to attach the tendon directly to the bone. To attach the tendon slip to the sheath, a transverse slit is made in the distal portion of the A2 pulley; the detached tendon slip is then passed through this and sutured back onto itself. In both methods, the goal is to create a slight flexion

contracture of the PIP joint. For greater purchase, the tendon slip can be attached through or adjacent to the A1 pulley in the distal palm. Postoperatively, the joint is splinted in 30 degrees of flexion. We start flexion at 3 weeks to maintain PIP joint function but block hyperextension for at least 6 weeks.

Nalebuff has modified this technique. He divides the FDS tendon more proximally using a distal palm incision. The FDS slip is then passed around the A1 pulley to prevent PIP joint hyperextension. This technique is simpler and faster and avoids incision in the digit.

Retinacular Ligament Reconstruction

Littler devised a clever technique to prevent hyperextension while restoring DIP joint extension by reconstructing an oblique retinacular ligament using the ulnar lateral band.[85,360] In this procedure, the ulnar lateral band is freed from the extensor mechanism proximally but left attached distally. It is passed volar to Cleland's fibers to bring it volar to the axis of PIP joint motion. The band is sutured to the fibrous tendon sheath under enough tension to restore DIP joint extension and prevent PIP hyperextension. In theory, this approach should solve both the DIP and PIP joint problems simultaneously. However, in a rheumatoid patient who has a primary mallet deformity with destruction of the terminal tendon, no amount of tension applied to the relocated lateral band will restore DIP joint extension. Thus, the net result of this procedure is restriction of PIP joint hyperextension. In rheumatoid arthritis, it is an alternative to dermadesis or flexor tenodesis.

Type II: PIP Joint Flexion Limited in Certain Positions

Some rheumatoid patients with swan neck deformities have restriction of finger flexion only in certain positions. The deformity may appear similar to the type I deformity. However, on examination, PIP joint flexion is influenced by the position of the MCP joint. With the MCP joint extended or radially deviated, passive PIP joint flexion is limited. If the MCP joint is allowed to flex or deviate ulnarward, PIP joint flexion is increased. In these cases, the swan neck deformity is secondary to MCP joint involvement.

As the MCP joints deviate and subluxate and the intrinsics become tight, a secondary swan neck deformity develops as the result of muscular imbalance. Initially this is supple in most positions and becomes stiff only when the MCP joint is in extension and the intrinsics are tightened further. Ultimately, however, the PIP joint becomes stiff regardless of the position of the MCP joint.

In these patients it is not sufficient to restrict PIP joint hyperextension. The intrinsic tightness must be relieved. Any MCP joint disorder that initiates or aggravates the muscular imbalance of the finger (i.e., subluxation or deviation) also must be corrected. This is accomplished by intrinsic release in patients with minimally involved MCP joints and by combined MCP joint arthroplasty and intrinsic release in the others.

Intrinsic Release

Intrinsic muscle release is performed through a dorsoulnar longitudinal incision over the proximal phalanx, as described on page 2098. After this release, PIP joint flexion with the MCP joint extended or radially deviated should be

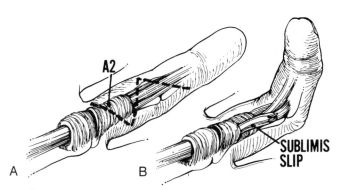

FIGURE 59-52. One technique for superficialis tenodesis to correct swan neck deformity. **A,** Zigzag incision used to expose the flexor tendon sheath. The incision should be extended far enough proximally to expose the A2 pulley. A tenosynovectomy is performed if necessary. **B,** A slip of flexor digitorum superficialis (sublimis) is sectioned proximally, passed through a slit in the A2 pulley, and sutured back on itself.

improved. Intrinsic release can be combined with DIP joint fusion or volar dermadesis to correct the PIP joint hyperextension and restore balance.

In patients with associated MCP joint disease, MCP joint alignment is corrected by implant arthroplasty. Although MCP joint arthroplasty (Swanson) with resection of the metacarpal heads does lengthen the intrinsic tendon, we prefer to resect the ulnar intrinsic tendon as well, to reduce the risk of recurrent intrinsic tightness and ulnar drift of the fingers.

Type III: Limited PIP Joint Flexion in All Positions

In patients with the type I and II deformities described earlier there is only slight to moderate functional loss in spite of the finger deformity. However, patients with marked reduction of PIP joint motion in any position (type III) have significant loss of hand function, because the ability to grasp objects is greatly reduced. Although it might seem logical to assume that patients with stiff swan neck deformities have advanced intra-articular changes that require either fusion to bring the finger into a functional position or arthroplasty to restore active motion, radiographic examination often reveals well-preserved joint spaces. In these cases, the structures that restrict passive motion include the extensor mechanism, the collateral ligaments, and the skin. The first step in the surgical reconstruction of the stiff swan neck deformity is the restoration of passive PIP joint motion. The procedures we use to restore passive motion include joint manipulation, skin release, and lateral band mobilization. Correction of the deformity is delayed until passive motion is restored.

PIP Joint Manipulation

In patients with stiff swan neck deformities, the soft tissues have contracted about the joint. However, with the patient under anesthesia, it is sometimes possible to obtain 80 to 90 degrees of PIP joint flexion by gentle manipulation. PIP joint manipulation is rarely performed alone; it is usually done in conjunction with intrinsic release, MCP arthroplasty, or flexor tenosynovectomy. If the joint is splinted in the flexed position, the tight soft tissues will stretch. After several weeks, the passive motion obtained by manipulation and splinting can be maintained as active motion, provided the flexor tendons have not become adherent. When done in conjunction with MCP arthroplasty, temporary Kirschner wire fixation is used to hold the PIP joint in flexion. This concentrates the postoperative exercises on MCP joint motion. After 10 days, the pins are removed and therapy is directed toward increasing PIP joint motion, using an extension block splint to prevent full extension of the joints. As stated previously, this method has restored 80 to 90 degrees of PIP joint flexion in joints that had been stiff.

When PIP joint manipulation is performed in conjunction with flexor tenosynovectomy, the joints are not pinned but are splinted in the flexed position postoperatively. Usually, after 24 to 48 hours of splinting, therapy can be initiated using extension block splints. Therapy includes active PIP range of motion exercises, with careful splinting in flexion between exercise periods. Initially, exercises are done for 5 minutes, four to six times daily, and increased as pain and endurance allow. Splinting is continued for 2 to 4 weeks, depending on the range of motion obtained. If an extensor

lag of the PIP joint develops, extension splinting may be necessary.

Skin Release

The dorsal skin may limit the amount of passive flexion that can be achieved by manipulation. At some point during the manipulation of long-standing fixed deformities into flexion, the dorsal skin blanches. If this is not relieved, skin necrosis occurs directly over the joint.

Dorsal skin tension can be minimized with an oblique incision just distal to the PIP joint, which allows the skin edges to spread. The defect created is the result of skin contracture (not loss) and closes gradually in 2 to 3 weeks. Although initially we used skin grafts to cover these defects, satisfactory healing by secondary intention has convinced us that grafts are not needed. In fact, leaving this portion of the wound open allows drainage and reduces postoperative swelling and pain. It is important that the skin release be distal to the joint so that the extensor mechanism overlying the joint is covered (Fig. 59-53).

Certain precautions must be observed when joint manipulation is performed. Minimal force should be used to bring the PIP joint into flexion. The soft tissues should stretch, not rupture. Fracture of osteopenic bone must be avoided. Therefore, if manipulation is difficult, we proceed to soft tissue release. The procedure we use most often is lateral band mobilization.

Lateral Band Mobilization (Fig. 59-54)

In established swan neck deformities, the lateral bands are displaced dorsally. Their normal volar shift is lost, and the finger is stiff. We have found that freeing the lateral bands from the central slip using two parallel longitudinal incisions in the extensor mechanism allows the joint to be manipulated gently into full flexion without releasing the collateral ligaments or lengthening the central slip. Full passive flexion often can be achieved by this method. When the procedure is performed under local anesthesia, the shifting of the lateral bands volarward on flexion and their relocation dorsally on extension can be observed during active motion.

When we first used this procedure for stiff swan neck deformities in 1962, our greatest problem was loss of motion after skin closure. Once the skin was sutured, the passive and active motion achieved by the lateral band mobilization was lost. If the skin was allowed to heal before active motion was started, the amount of flexion obtained in the operating room was seldom maintained. We now use a curved dorsal incision with a short oblique limb across the middle segment. The proximal portion of the incision is closed with the finger held in flexion. The distal third of the incision usually is left open. The finger is splinted in flexion for 3 to 5 days to stretch the contracted collateral ligaments. Occasionally, however, it is necessary to release these ligaments, as well as to step-cut lengthen the central slip. A dorsal extension block splint is used to prevent full extension of the PIP joints.[242,355]

Flexor Tenosynovitis Associated With PIP Joint Stiffness

The flexor tendons also must be considered and assessed if optimal results are to be obtained from the procedures described earlier. Flexor tendon tenosynovitis and secondary

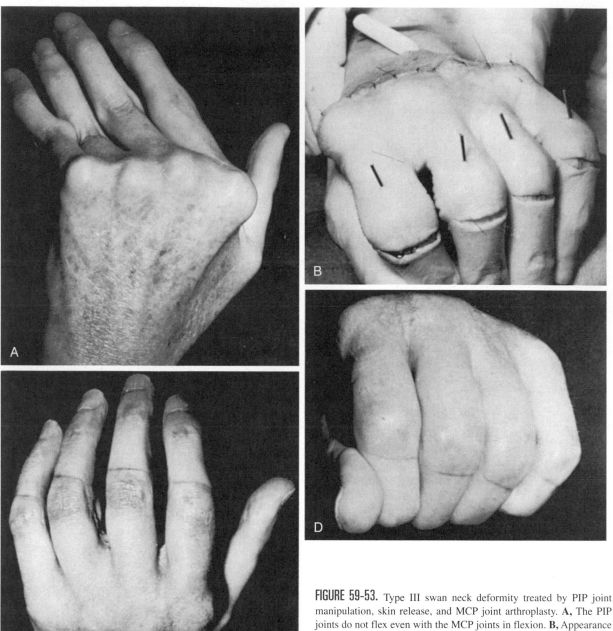

FIGURE 59-53. Type III swan neck deformity treated by PIP joint manipulation, skin release, and MCP joint arthroplasty. **A,** The PIP joints do not flex even with the MCP joints in flexion. **B,** Appearance at surgery after MCP arthroplasty, PIP manipulation with Kirschner wire fixation, and skin release. **C,** Postoperative extension shows improved finger posture. **D,** Range of flexion achieved postoperatively.

flexor tendon adherence are integral etiologic factors of the stiff PIP joint and must be understood to provide adequate treatment. Flexor tenosynovitis that limits active PIP joint flexion can result in stiff PIP joints. Conversely, stiff PIP joints can result in adherence of the flexor tendons. In either case, flexor tenosynovectomy or tenolysis must be a consideration in any treatment aimed at the restoration of PIP joint motion.

Adhesions or rupture of the flexors will obviate any passive motion gained by procedures directed at the extensor mechanism or the soft tissues surrounding the joint.

However, the preoperative assessment of flexor tendon function is limited if stiff joints are present. For this reason, we now determine the status of the flexor tendons in the operating room. If intravenous regional or local anesthesia has been used for either manipulation or lateral band mobilization, the tourniquet is released and the patient is asked to flex the fingers after muscle control has returned. If active motion is not nearly equal to passive motion, anesthesia is reinstituted and the flexor tendons are explored. Adhesions of the tendons are released, and rheumatoid nodules within the tendon are removed. If regional block

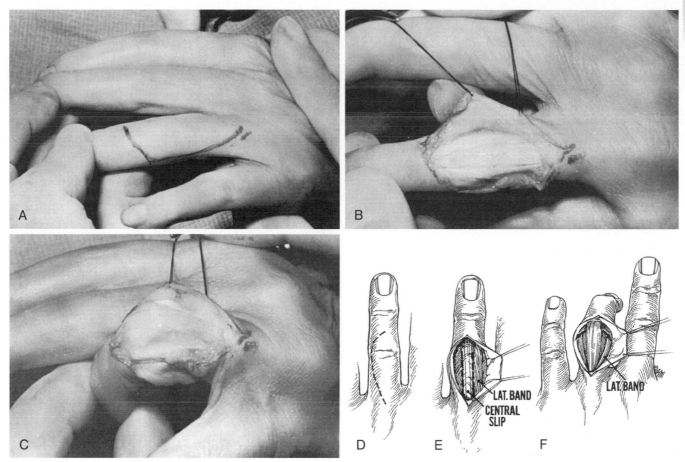

FIGURE 59-54. Type III swan neck deformity treated by lateral band mobilization. **A,** Incision used to expose the extensor mechanism over the PIP joint. **B,** Parallel incisions separate the lateral bands from the central slip. **C,** Flexion obtained after manipulation of the PIP joint. Note volar shift of the lateral bands. **D to F,** Drawing of the technique for lateral band mobilization.

anesthesia has been used, the flexor tendons are exposed in the palm and traction is applied to test flexor tendon excursion. Occasionally, an extensive flexor tenosynovectomy is required to improve flexor tendon excursion. Postoperatively, supervised splinting and active exercises are important in maintaining the motion gained at the time of surgery (see page 2111).

Type IV: Stiff PIP Joints With Poor Radiographic Appearance

Patients with stiff PIP joints and radiographic evidence of advanced intra-articular changes require some type of salvage procedure, either fusion or arthroplasty. The factors that must be considered in deciding between these procedures include the fingers involved, the status of adjacent joints, the status of supporting ligamentous structures, and the status of the flexor tendons. We tend to prefer fusion in the index finger, where lateral stability is particularly important. The status of adjacent joints is also important. If the MCP joints require arthroplasty, we favor fusion at the PIP joint level, although arthroplasty at both levels can be performed with good results in our experience. Although Adamson and colleagues[361] reported less than optimal results with PIP arthroplasty in inflammatory arthritis, their study combined the results in both boutonnière and swan neck deformities. We believe that arthroplasty plays a limited role in the treatment of the flexion boutonnière

deformity, in which the extensor tendon is often compromised. In the swan neck deformity, PIP arthroplasty works well as long as the hyperextension is corrected; a sublimis tenodesis can be performed at the same time if necessary.

Poor lateral ligamentous support and/or associated flexor tendon ruptures also are relative indications for fusion.[362]

PIP Joint Fusion for Swan Neck Deformity

We use a longitudinal skin incision. The extensor mechanism is split in the midline, and the collateral ligaments are detached from the proximal phalanx. The joint is flexed to expose the articular surfaces, which are prepared for fusion by removing the articular cartilage and softening the subchondral bone. At the PIP joint level, we routinely use two crossed Kirschner wires for internal fixation. If the bone stock is adequate and the width of the medullary canal allows, a Herbert screw can be used for internal fixation (see Fig. 59-51). Precise technique is needed to obtain the desired angle of fusion using this method. The position of fusion selected depends on the finger involved and the sex of the patient. In general, the index finger PIP joint is fused in less flexion than that of the middle finger. The degree of flexion is greater in the ring and small fingers to facilitate grip. The amount of flexion chosen ranges from 25 to 45 degrees. In female patients, in whom cosmesis is often more important than strong grasp, less flexion than the so-called functional position is used. The patient's requirements must be discussed and determined preoperatively. It is helpful to have a small sterile goniometer on the instrument table, as it is sometimes difficult to judge the angle of flexion of the PIP joint accurately by eye. Usually the joint is flexed more than is anticipated. Measurement of the angle of flexion after the first pin is inserted allows easy correction before insertion of the final pins.

PIP Joint Arthroplasty

PIP arthroplasty can relieve pain and restore functional motion in joints affected by rheumatoid, degenerative, and post-traumatic arthritis. Arthroplasty techniques include fibrous interposition,[364,365] volar plate advancement,[366] perichondral reconstruction,[367] hinge implants (metallic, metalloplastic, or plastic),[368-374] and semi-constrained prostheses.[375] In this section we address implant arthroplasty.

The PIP silicone arthroplasty was originally used in 1966[370-373] in conjunction with the silicone implants for the MCP joint in rheumatoid arthritis. Over the years the indications have changed and now we find the procedure most useful with degenerative arthritis and certain cases of traumatic arthritis.[376]

Swanson's single-piece polymeric silicone spacer has been the implant arthroplasty of choice for several decades. Use of the flexible silicone spacer was designed to facilitate the development of a fibrous capsule that would provide for a pain-free and functional PIP joint.[371,377] The dorsal hinge design as well as intramedullary stem pistoning was thought to increase "in-plane" functional motion; however, only modest improvements in flexion arcs were reported.[373,374,378,379] Other silicone implants include those made by Avanta and Depuy (Fig. 59-55). Although the material properties are essentially the same, the design features are slightly different. Both Avanta and Depuy PIP implants have a more

volar hinge, which may allow improved flexion arcs without volar impingement.

Although silicone implant arthroplasty has been used with clinical success, complications including hinge failure, angular deformities, bony erosion, and particulate synovitis occur.[363,373,378,379] Failure to replicate normal PIP motion may be a primary contributing factor to hinge joint implant failures. Recently, surface replacement arthroplasties (SRA) of the PIP joint have been developed to improve joint biomechanics.[375] SRA implants are designed to mimic the physiologic articulation of the PIP joints to restore normal motion based on a virtual axis rather than a fixed axis.[377] Minimal bony resection, collateral ligament preservation, and implant design may also improve "out-of-plane" stability with the theoretical advantage when considering arthroplasties of the PIP joints on the radial side of the hand,[375] particularly the index finger, which must be able to resist forces generated during pinch. Current SRA designs include the metal-polyethylene prosthesis (Avanta Orthopaedics, San Diego, CA) and the pyrocarbon prosthesis (Ascension Orthopedics, Austin, TX) (Fig. 59-56).

Indications. Arthroplasty of the PIP joint is primarily used in patients who have persistent pain that has been refractory to several months of intensive nonoperative therapy, including nonsteroidal anti-inflammatory drugs, occasional cortisone injections, temporary splinting, and carefully prescribed hand therapy focusing on activity modification (not range of motion). If PIP motion is greater than 70 degrees, or if the patient can touch the finger to the palm, we recommend PIP arthroplasty cautiously, unless pain is an overriding factor.

The best candidate for PIP joint arthroplasty is the patient with a painful PIP joint from degenerative or post-traumatic arthritis in one of the ulnar three digits who has nearly full extension and limited (20 to 40 degrees) of flexion. When there is good bone stock, minimal deformity, and a preserved extensor and flexor mechanism, the prognosis for eliminating pain and improving motion is good.

We usually do not recommend PIP arthroplasty in painless conditions, especially if there is good MCP and DIP joint motion. However, there are occasional patients with a

A. *Swanson Silicone Finger Implant*
(Wright - Medical Technology)

B. *PIP Soft-Skeletal Implant*
(Avanta Orthopaedics)

C. *Neuflex PIP Joint Implant*
(DePuy Orthopaedics)
DORSAL
SCHNITZ
15° bend
VOLAR

FIGURE 59-55. Silicone PIP implants. **A,** Swanson silicone finger implants (Wright-Medical Technology, Arlington, TN). **B,** PIP soft-skeletal implant (Avanta Orthopaedics, San Diego, CA). **C,** Neuflex PIP joint implant (Depuy Orthopaedics, Warsaw, IN). (From Kobayashi K, Terrono AL: Proximal interphalangeal joint arthroplasty of the hand. J Hand Surgery 3(4): 219-226, 2003. © 2003 by the American Society for Surgery of the Hand.)

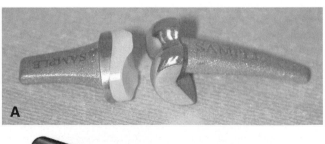
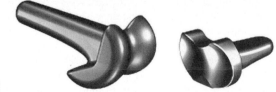

FIGURE 59-56. Surface replacement implants. **A,** SR PIP Implant System (Avanta Orthopaedics, San Diego, CA). **B,** Ascension PIP PyroCarbon Total Joint (Ascension Orthopedics, Austin, TX).

single long, ring, or small finger that is stiff in an extended position who are candidates for the procedure, even though the amount of flexion gained may be less than optimal. Silicone rubber implants usually will not stand up to the repeated stress of pinch and, therefore, are not recommended for the index finger.

PIP joint arthroplasty is often unsuccessful in patients with severe rheumatoid involvement, and particularly in patients with advanced boutonnière deformities. The results in swan neck deformities are much better.[376] Combining PIP joint arthroplasty with MCP joint arthroplasty either as a combined procedure or in two stages is generally not successful. We recommend PIP joint fusions combined with MCP joint arthroplasty for combined involvement. However, in the unusual case of an isolated painful digit with little deformity, preserved bone stock, and functional extensor and flexor mechanisms, PIP arthroplasty may be appropriate.

Contraindications. The worst results after PIP joint arthroplasty have been in patients who have had PIP joint infections or who have had previous failed attempts at tenolysis. The surgery usually fails because of recurrent scar formation. Massive bone loss, severe deformity, and repeated surgery including initial extensive open reductions are relative contraindications for the procedure, and arthrodesis should be considered in these cases.

We are cautious in recommending PIP arthroplasty in digits with significant fixed flexion contractions in the range of 50 degrees or more. In these cases, one must remove excessive bone to insert the implant, and extensive reconstruction of the extensor mechanism with prolonged postoperative splinting is required. Results after these procedures are generally not good. When surgery is indicated in these situations, it may preferable to consider arthrodesis in a more functional position.

In general, we recommend PIP arthrodesis for the index finger because flexion is not as crucial, strong pinch is necessary, and lateral deviation after PIP arthroplasty occurs (Fig. 59-57).[363,373] Volar plate arthroplasty may be a reasonable option for the radial digits given the lateral stability that has been documented after these procedures.[4] However,

we would not absolutely exclude implant arthroplasty in the index PIP joint in certain cases.

Surgical Approaches. PIP arthroplasty can be done through either a dorsal or volar approach. The original dorsal approach has some specific indications and advantages. It is useful if there is a significant flexion contracture that must be corrected and/or if reconstruction or tenolysis of the extensor mechanism is needed. With this approach, the extensor mechanism must be carefully handled, reattached, and then protected during the rehabilitation phase.

The volar approach spares the extensor mechanism, and for that reason is now our preferred approach in patients with degenerative arthritis. It is simple and provides excellent exposure without interfering with the extensor mechanism. Swan neck deformities can be corrected by repairing or reconstructing the volar plate. If flexor tendon adhesions are an additional issue, a volar approach allows easy access for tenolysis (Fig. 59-58). However, the approach puts the digital nerves and vessels at risk and requires strict attention to the orientation of the joint to ensure that the bone cuts are made appropriately and that the implant is inserted corrected. To date, the volar approach cannot be used with surface replacement arthroplasties.

Dorsal Approach. A dorsal slightly curved incision is made to expose the extensor apparatus of the PIP joint. A midline incision is made through the extensor mechanism, protecting the central slip insertion. If length adjustments are necessary to address boutonnière deformities, a distally based flap can be created. Alternatively, an incision can be made between the central slip and one of the lateral bands. The collateral ligaments can be released to allow adequate exposure of the joint surfaces (Fig. 59-59). The surfaces are prepared for arthroplasty with careful attention to preserve the collateral ligament integrity. The head of the proximal phalanx is resected. Preparing the middle phalanx can be the most difficult part of the procedure depending on the amount of deformity at the base. When there are erosions

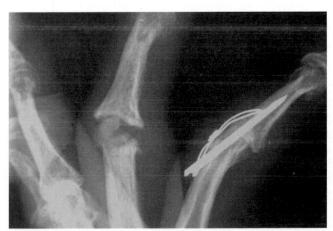

FIGURE 59-57. Status post index finger arthrodesis and middle finger PIP arthroplasty. (From Kobayashi K, Terrono AL: Proximal interphalangeal joint arthroplasty of the hand. J Hand Surgery 3(4): 219-226, 2003. © 2003 by the American Society for Surgery of the Hand.)

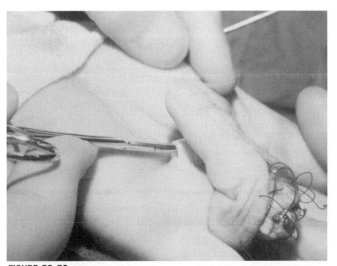

FIGURE 59-58. Flexor tendons can be assessed for adhesions utilizing a small incision located at the proximal border of the A1 pulley. (From Kobayashi K, Terrono AL: Proximal interphalangeal joint arthroplasty of the hand. J Hand Surgery 3(4): 219-226, 2003. © 2003 by the American Society for Surgery of the Hand.)

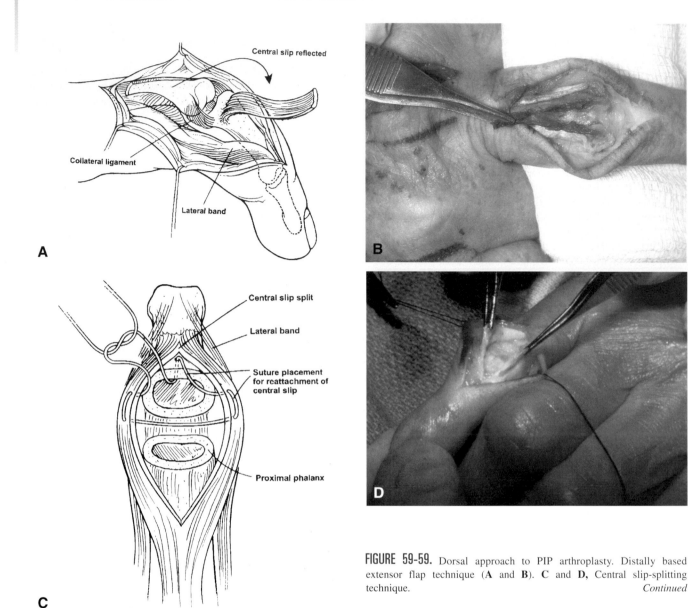

Central slip reflected

Collateral ligament

Lateral band

A

Central slip split

Lateral band

Suture placement for reattachment of central slip

Proximal phalanx

C

B

D

FIGURE 59-59. Dorsal approach to PIP arthroplasty. Distally based extensor flap technique (**A** and **B**). **C** and **D**, Central slip-splitting technique. *Continued*

with large lateral ridges on the sides of the middle phalanx these ridges must be removed to prepare a flat surface for the implant to seat. To do so, the assistant lifts the base and supports the phalanx while the surgeon carefully detaches the collateral ligament from the ridges but is careful not to completely detach the entire ligament from the middle phalanx. A sharp rongeur is used to remove the ridge. The medullary canals of the proximal and middle phalanges are opened with an awl and reamed to fit the selected size implant using the broaches supplied with each of the implant instrument sets. Occasionally, a high speed bur with a blunt leading tip is used to shape the canal. Trial components are used to assess motion and stability. It is sometimes necessary to repair the collateral ligaments to bone if there is laxity. The implant is inserted with the joint hyperflexed. The implant should be stable in the extended position. If the implant dislocates, buckles, or cannot be inserted, the space for the implant usually is too small and more bone must be resected. The extensor mechanism is repaired using either interrupted mattress sutures or a running suture. We prefer

monofilament absorbable suture for this, but nonabsorbable sutures may be used.

Volar Approach. A generous volar zigzag incision is used, centered over the PIP joint. The neurovascular structures are mobilized and protected. A 2- to 3-cm flap of volar pulley including the A3 pulley and a small portion of A2 and A4 are raised. This exposes the volar plate that is detached from its membranous proximal origin and the accessory collateral ligaments, but it is left widely attached to the base of the middle phalanx for later reconstruction. Penrose drains can be placed to retract each flexor tendon on either side of the joint. The joint is then carefully dislocated by hyperextension ("shotgun"), and the joint surfaces are prepared as described for the dorsal approach (Fig. 59-60). Care must be taken to protect the central slip attachment as well as to orient the bone cuts and insert the implant properly.

The flexor tendon must be assessed if full active flexion was not present preoperatively. A trigger finger incision can

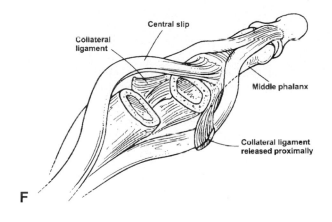

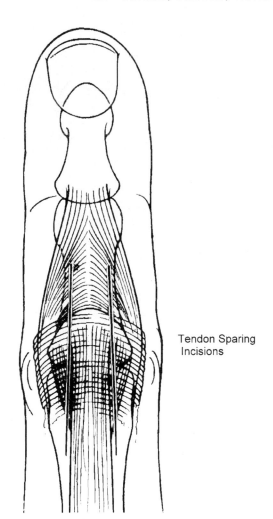

Tendon Sparing
Incisions

FIGURE 59-59—cont'd. E and **F,** Central tendon-sparing technique. (From Kobayashi K, Terrono AL: Proximal interphalangeal joint arthroplasty of the hand. J Hand Surgery 3(4): 219-226, 2003. © 2003 by the American Society for Surgery of the Hand.)

E

be used, and traction can be placed on the tendons to ensure full flexion. Alternatively, if local or intravenous regional anesthesia has been used, the tourniquet can be deflated and active flexion checked.

Closure is done by reattaching the volar plate to soft tissue or bone if necessary. If reattaching to bone, two to three drill holes are made in the base of the proximal phalanx. Alternatively, a miniature suture anchor can be used. The flexor sheath can be used to reinforce the volar plate by placing it deep to the tendons, but it is usually placed in its anatomic position or excised.

The tourniquet is deflated, and meticulous hemostasis is obtained because a postoperative hematoma or excessive swelling can jeopardize the early exercise program. A bulky dressing is applied with a volar splint holding the digits in extension.

Rehabilitation. Early motion is started, usually on the day of or after the procedure, regardless of the approach used. This may be modified if the extensor mechanism has been reconstructed. The dressing is changed 1 to 3 days after surgery. Rehabilitation protocols for dorsal approaches focus on maintaining the integrity of the extensor apparatus and the prevention of adhesions. Early protected active PIP

flexion and independent DIP flexion will minimize adhesions of the extensor apparatus. Usually the PIP joint is maintained in neutral position (full extension) in between exercise periods and at night. A light dynamic extension splint can be started after the sutures are removed. If a significant extension deformity was present preoperatively, the patient is instructed to tape the finger in maximum flexion during the day, releasing the tape hourly for extension exercises.

If the volar approach was used, active flexion and extension can be started immediately, usually with an extension block splint to maintain the PIP joint in 15 to 20 degrees of flexion for the first 2 weeks to protect the volar plate and prevent a hyperextension deformity.

Supervised hand therapy is usually used, and the protocol is customized for each patient based on the preoperative deformity, the condition of the soft tissues, and the type of approach used. This is continued for 4 to 6 weeks. Night and/or resting splints are used for protection after dynamic splinting is stopped.

Outcomes. Large series of Swanson silicone PIP arthroplasties demonstrate an average range of motion of 45 to 60 degrees with approximately 70% of patients getting greater

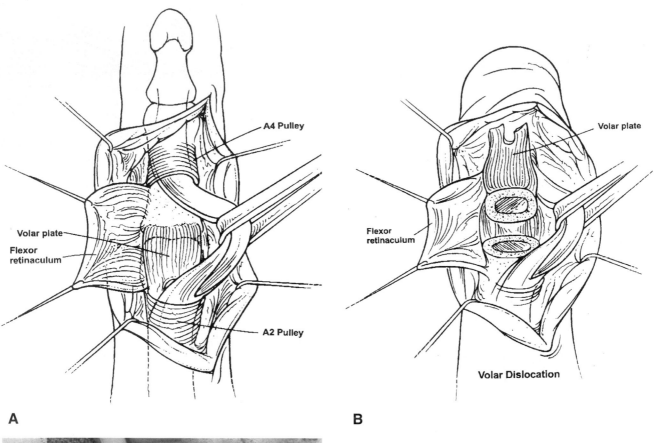

A

B

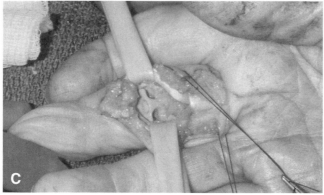

C

FIGURE 59-60. Volar approach to PIP arthroplasty. **A,** Incision centered over volar PIP joint exposes the volar plate that is detached from the proximal phalanx. **B,** Flexor tendons are retracted with Penrose drain, permitting dislocation and preparation of the joint surfaces. **C,** Trial implant inserted to assess stability, appropriate size, and motion. (From Kobayashi K, Terrono AL: Proximal interphalangeal joint arthroplasty of the hand. J Hand Surgery 3(4): 219-226, 2003. © 2003 by the American Society for Surgery of the Hand.)

than 40 degrees.[373,378] Better results are obtained in patients with degenerative and post-traumatic arthritis. Our results for silicone PIP implant arthroplasty are similar to those reported in the literature, with excellent pain relief, good motion, and stability.[12] No fractures, dislocations, or infections have occurred. In our series, patients with post-traumatic arthritis demonstrated an average range of motion of 48 degrees without deterioration or pain at an average follow-up of 7 years (Fig. 59-61).[61] Iselin and coworkers reported on 238 Swanson implants of the PIP joint between 1970 and 1990 noting an average range of motion of −20 degrees of extension to 80 degrees of flexion (long, ring, and little fingers).[381] These authors concluded that results obtained at 12 months were likely to remain at 12 years.

The incidence of infection and dislocation in a large series is approximately 0.4%.[373,378] The implant fracture rate is about 6%,[373,378] with an overall revision rate of 10%.[373]

Reports of bone resorption vary from 1.2%[373] to 35%[363] and may vary with the length of follow-up and person evaluating the radiographs. Foliart reviewed all the literature (70 articles, 15,556 small joint implants) pertaining to complications associated with silicone finger implants and reported very low complication rates.[380] Implant fracture and bone changes occurred in 2% and 4%, respectively. Particulate synovitis and particle-wear lymphadenopathy was less than 1%.[380]

Very little information is available for semi-constrained surface replacement PIP arthroplasty. In 1997, Linscheid and colleagues reported on 66 SRA proximal interphalangeal prostheses utilizing a chromium cobalt proximal component and an ultra-high-molecular-weight polyethylene distal component.[375] The average follow-up was 4.5 years. Eighty percent of fingers suffered from traumatic and degenerative arthritis. The average arc of motion was 47

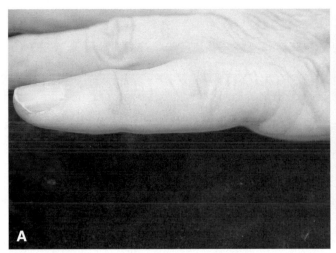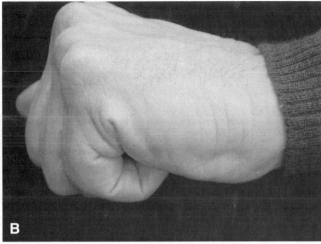

FIGURE 59-61. Fifteen-year follow-up of left small finger PIP arthroplasty demonstrating excellent extension (**A**) and flexion (**B**), which is possible with proper patient selection, precise surgical technique, and supervised rehabilitation. (From Kobayashi K, Terrono AL: Proximal interphalangeal joint arthroplasty of the hand. J Hand Surgery 3(4): 219-226, 2003. © 2003 by the American Society for Surgery of the Hand.)

degrees. Approximately 95% of patients had excellent pain relief. Poor results were associated with previous extensive injury or static deformities. Only one implant demonstrated evidence of component loosening on radiography. "Out-of-plane" deformity was noted in approximately 6% of implants. In 2001, Johnstone reported his experience with 20 SRA PIP implants (CoCr/polyethylene) primarily used for osteoarthritis and post-traumatic pain.[382] Average follow-up was 14.6 months (range, 2 to 34 months). All patients noted pain reduction, with 90% reporting excellent pain relief. No patient lost movement, and 70% of patients demonstrated an average arc of motion of 73 degrees. Poor results were associated with high levels of early postoperative pain and compliance with hand therapy.

CRITICAL POINTS: PIP JOINT ARTHROPLASTY

INDICATIONS

- Persistent PIP joint pain
- Swan neck deformity with joint destruction

CONTRAINDICATIONS

- Infection
- Bone loss
- Unstable joint
- Severe flexion deformity

PEARLS

- Do not overbroach; you will lose stability provided by implant.
- Splint DIP in extension postoperatively to concentrate motion at PIP joint.

TECHNICAL POINTS

- Use volar approach if extensor tendon is normal.
- Use dorsal approach if extensor tendon requires reconstruction (i.e., boutonnière/swan neck deformity).
- Volar zigzag incision centered on PIP joint.
- Mobilize and protect neurovascular bundles.
- Open A3 pulley and retract flexor tendons.
- Detach volar plate proximally.

- Detach collateral ligaments from proximal phalanx (if necessary).
- Perform synovectomy/débridement.
- Resect condyle of proximal phalanx perpendicular to long axis.
- Square off base of middle phalanx.
- Broach middle phalanx first, slightly dorsal to center.
- Rectangular broach provides stability and rotational alignment.
- Broach proximal phalanx.
- Insert trial implant; it should fit flush against bone and extend just beyond medial/lateral cortices.
- Implant should not buckle or dislocate.
- Check flexor tendon excursion (separate incision in palm if necessary).
- Pre-place suture in volar plate.
- Insert implant and then repair volar plate if necessary.

POSTOPERATIVE CARE

- Splint for 3 to 5 days and then start active flexion/extension.
- Use extension block splint, which includes adjacent digit(s), for 4 to 6 weeks.
- Buddy strap for 3 months.

PIP Arthroplasty in Rheumatoid Arthritis

We often perform Swanson implant arthroplasties of the PIP joint for the stiff swan neck deformity if the adjacent joints, soft tissues, and tendons are in good condition. We prefer arthroplasty, particularly in the ring and small fingers, when restoration of grasp is important.

Our standard technique uses the dorsal approach. We do not use the volar approach in rheumatoid swan neck deformities because the lateral band must often be released through a dorsal approach anyway.[383] In the dorsal approach, the extensor mechanism is exposed, split longitudinally in the midline, and reflected to either side of the PIP joint. This allows the tension on the extensor mechanism to be adjusted with a pursestring suture during closure. Nalebuff has modified this approach to avoid damaging the extensor mechanism when this structure is in good condition. The same curved dorsal skin incision is used but is made slightly longer. An incision in the extensor mechanism is made within the lateral bands. Placing the incision within the substance of the lateral band facilitates closure and maintains the integrity of the transverse retinacular ligament. The subtotal extent of the entire extensor apparatus is moved to one side to expose the PIP joint capsule. The fatty areolar tissue lying between the dorsal periosteum of the phalanges and the extensor tendon is preserved to facilitate tendon gliding postoperatively. The collateral ligaments are divided at their origins on the proximal phalanx and preserved for reattachment after insertion of the implant. The distal end of the proximal phalanx is removed, and the medullary canal is prepared to accept the stem of the implant. A sufficient amount of bone is removed to relax tension on the contracted extensor mechanism when the implant is inserted, to avoid having to lengthen the central slip. The base of the middle phalanx is débrided if necessary, and the articular cartilage and subchondral bone are perforated. The medullary canal is prepared to accept the distal stem of the implant. Closure of the extensor mechanism after insertion of the prosthesis must not be so tight as to prevent full passive flexion of the PIP joint. The central slip may need to be shortened if there is insufficient extension of the PIP joint when tested either by the tenodesis effect during passive wrist motion or by proximal traction on the extensor mechanism proximal to the PIP joint. Skin closure is done with the joint in slight flexion. If necessary, the distal portion of the wound is left open to avoid excessive skin tension. Frequently, a palmar incision is made and the flexor tendon excursion checked; a tenolysis is performed if needed. Postoperatively, the fingers are splinted in 20 to 30 degrees of flexion and active and gentle passive range-of-motion exercises are begun within several days after operation.

Boutonnière Deformity

Boutonnière deformity occurs frequently in patients with rheumatoid arthritis. Like the swan neck deformity, it is not specific to this disease and represents an alteration in muscle and tendon balance.[384-387] The deformity has three components: flexion of the PIP joint, hyperextension of the DIP joint, and hyperextension of the MCP joint. Whereas the swan neck deformity in the rheumatoid patient may originate at any of the finger joints, the boutonnière deformity

Table 59-6

TREATMENT OPTIONS FOR FINGER BOUTONNIÈRE DEFORMITY

Stage	PIP Joint	DIP Joint
I—Mild	Dynamic splinting Injection vs. synovectomy	Extensor tenotomy
II—Moderate	Correct any wrist flexion first Extensor reconstruction	Extensor tenotomy
III—Severe	Fusion (standard) Arthroplasty	Extensor tenotomy

begins with flexion of the PIP joint. The changes in the adjacent joints are secondary.

Synovial proliferation within the PIP joints stretches the extensor mechanism. As a result, the central slip is unable to maintain full extension of the joint. The lateral bands displace volarward and become fixed in this position. Shortening of the oblique retinacular ligaments results in hyperextension and limited active flexion of the DIP joint. As the flexion deformity of the PIP joint increases, the patient compensates by hyperextending the MCP joint. When seen early, the deformities are correctable passively. Later, with fibrosis and contracture of the capsular tissues, the deformity becomes fixed. Functional loss as a result of the boutonnière deformity may remain minimal until the late stages. For this reason, the treatment of early boutonnière deformity should be simple and involve minimal risk. Salvage surgery (fusion or arthroplasty) should be performed only for the severe fixed deformities. Our operative approach to the rheumatoid boutonnière deformity depends on the degree of severity. We classify boutonnière deformities as mild, moderate, or severe on the basis of the degree of flexion of the PIP joint, the presence of passive correctability of this joint, and the status of the PIP joint surfaces.[388] This classification helps direct the treatment (Table 59-6).

Stage I: Mild Boutonnière Deformity

In the early stages of the boutonnière deformity, there is only a slight lag (10 to 15 degrees) in PIP joint extension. There may be active synovitis of the joint. The DIP joint may or may not be slightly hyperextended. The MCP joint usually is normal during this early stage. The extensor lag of the PIP joint can be corrected passively. However, when this is done, there is limited flexion of the DIP joint. Flexion of the DIP joint improves as the PIP joint is flexed. The patient's functional loss is related as much to the lack of full DIP joint flexion as to the lack of PIP extension, but functional impairment is minimal at this stage. Any operative treatment of this mild boutonnière deformity should not jeopardize existing function. We treat the mild boutonnière deformity by extensor tenotomy to improve DIP joint flexion.[26] Dynamic splinting to extend the PIP joint is used postoperatively to restore the balance of the finger. This method does not risk loss of PIP joint flexion. If active PIP joint synovitis is present, we consider either local corticosteroid injection or synovectomy in our treatment plan.

Extensor Tenotomy (Fig. 59-62)

We use a longitudinal incision over the dorsal aspect of the middle phalanx. The extensor mechanism can be divided either obliquely or transversely to allow the DIP joint to flex. We prefer an oblique tenotomy, which allows the tendon to be sutured in the lengthened position and provides more tendon surface area for healing. Postoperatively, there may be a slight "droop" of the DIP joint but a significant mallet deformity usually does not develop. This procedure is based on the concept that the oblique retinacular ligament acts to extend the DIP joint. However, the dorsal support provided by the extensor mechanism and joint capsule most likely plays a role in maintaining the normal posture of the joint.

We perform extensor tenotomy under local anesthesia; this allows the alteration of finger stance as well as finger function to be observed at the time of surgery. Occasionally, a significant extensor lag of the DIP joint occurs after the tenotomy. A brief period of postoperative external splinting of this joint usually corrects the problem. If the deformity is not corrected, or if it progresses, the DIP joint can be fused in extension. In most patients, we do not splint the DIP joint postoperatively but encourage active DIP joint flexion with the PIP joint supported by a dynamic, reverse knuckle-bender splint. This is important in restoring proper balance between the two joints.

Stage II: Moderate Boutonnière Deformity

The functional loss of the finger becomes more significant as the flexion deformity of the PIP joint reaches 30 to 40 degrees. Patients usually compensate for this by hyperextending the MCP joint. Although there are significant difficulties involved in reconstruction of a fixed moderate boutonnière deformity, we have found that satisfactory correction of the deformity with preservation of active PIP joint flexion can be achieved. All the procedures described to correct the established boutonnière deformity attempt to restore the extensor power to the PIP joint using local tissue. We do this by shortening the central slip and bringing the lateral bands dorsally. We believe that it is important to combine this procedure with extensor tendon tenotomy at the DIP joint. Unless this is done, there is a risk of restoring PIP extension but markedly limiting DIP flexion. We recommend extensor mechanism reconstruction in patients with moderate progressive deformity if several criteria are met: good dorsal skin, relatively smooth joint surfaces, intact and functioning flexor tendons, and, of course, passive correctability of the PIP joint. Flexion deformity at the wrist should be corrected before attempting to restore PIP joint extension. We prefer to reconstruct the PIP joint extensor mechanism before, or at the same time as, MCP joint arthroplasty, because any residual flexion deformity at the PIP

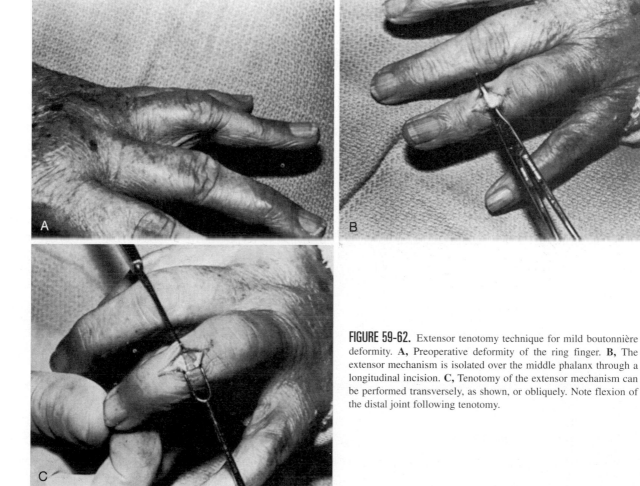

FIGURE 59-62. Extensor tenotomy technique for mild boutonnière deformity. **A,** Preoperative deformity of the ring finger. **B,** The extensor mechanism is isolated over the middle phalanx through a longitudinal incision. **C,** Tenotomy of the extensor mechanism can be performed transversely, as shown, or obliquely. Note flexion of the distal joint following tenotomy.

joint has an adverse effect on achieving MCP joint flexion after MCP joint arthroplasty.

Reconstruction of the Extensor Mechanism
(Figs. 59-63 and 59-64)

A dorsal longitudinal curved incision is made over the PIP joint. A laterally based skin and subcutaneous flap is elevated to expose the extensor mechanism. This places the skin incision away from the site of the extensor tendon repair. The central slip is divided distally, leaving a cuff of tendon attached to the base of the middle phalanx. The central slip is separated from the lateral bands proximally. Inspection of the undersurface of the central slip shows the changes that have occurred from gradual stretching. Approximately ¼ inch (6 mm) of the central slip is excised. The remaining portion is reattached to the cuff of the central slip insertion (which was left intact at the base of the middle phalanx) with nonabsorbable sutures. Two longitudinal relaxing incisions are made just volar to the lateral bands. These divide the transverse retinacular ligaments and allow the lateral bands to be brought dorsally. The lateral bands are sutured either to the central slip or to each other. The posture of the finger should be corrected now. However, there is usually increased resistance to passive DIP joint flexion, or even hyperextension of this joint. The extensor

mechanism overlying the middle phalanx is divided obliquely through the distal portion of the incision, allowing the DIP joint to flex. This procedure allows all of the extensor mechanism force to be concentrated at the PIP joint level.

Adjustment of the tension of the central slip is very important. It should be possible to flex the PIP joint passively 70 or 80 degrees after the central slip has been reattached. The strong flexors act to increase the range of flexion after postoperative splinting has been discontinued.

A Kirschner wire is placed across the PIP joint to maintain full extension during the early postoperative period. The DIP joint is left free, and active motion of this joint is allowed. After 3 to 4 weeks, the Kirschner wire is removed and the joint is protected with a reverse knuckle-bender splint during the day and a padded aluminum splint at night for several weeks.

The postoperative program may be modified according to the finger involved and the amount of PIP joint flexion possible after the Kirschner wire is removed. If several fingers are reconstructed simultaneously, we remove the Kirschner wire from the small finger first. In this finger we accept less correction of PIP joint extension to ensure maximal flexion. The reverse is true for the index finger, in which a loss of some flexion is less significant. If necessary, reconstruction of the moderate boutonnière deformity can

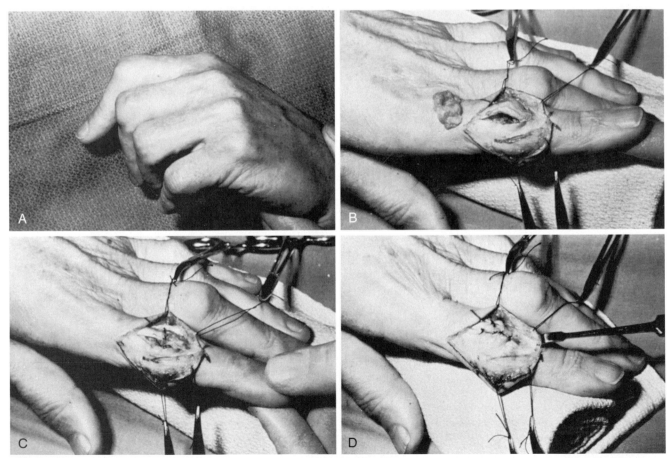

FIGURE 59-63. Technique of extensor mechanism reconstruction for boutonnière deformity. **A,** The patient has a moderate boutonnière deformity of the index finger. **B,** The extensor mechanism is lax after synovectomy. **C,** The central slip has been shortened. Note the relaxing incision volar to the lateral band. **D,** The lateral bands sutured in dorsal position. Note extensor tenotomy over the middle phalanx (at the extreme distal end of the incision).

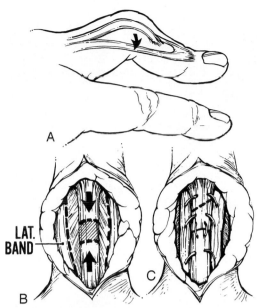

FIGURE 59-64. Extensor mechanism reconstruction for boutonnière deformity. **A,** The arrow shows the fixed volar position of the lateral band. **B,** Lateral bands mobilized. The portion of the central slip to be excised is shaded. **C,** The central slip is sutured in shortened position, and the lateral bands are brought dorsalward and sutured to the central slip.

be performed on all four fingers at the same time. In most patients, however, the criteria necessary for this operation are present in only one or two fingers. Limiting the reconstruction to these fingers simplifies the operation as well as the postoperative splinting and exercise program.

Stage III: Severe Boutonnière Deformity

In time, the boutonnière deformity progresses to the point where the PIP joint can no longer be extended passively. No attempt should be made to restore extensor mechanism function unless the joint can be extended passively without excessive force. In this case, restoration of passive motion by dynamic splinting or serial plaster casting is attempted. Occasionally, soft tissue release (dividing the transverse retinacular ligaments and the accessory collateral ligaments) is necessary to restore passive extension. This is combined with extensor mechanism reconstruction. This extensive surgery is not indicated often.

In severe deformities with poor joint surfaces, the alternative treatment is fusion or arthroplasty. Fusion is the standard method used to correct severe fixed flexion deformities in the rheumatoid patient. It is used in patients whose finger extension is so restricted that they are unable to grasp moderate-sized to large objects.

The position of PIP fusion is chosen to achieve a "functional" position of the involved finger. In the index or middle finger, loss of full flexion is not critical. In patients with severe bilateral boutonnière deformities, we have performed multiple fusions on one hand, leaving the deformities on the other side untreated to maintain the ability to grasp small objects on one side. However, the loss of PIP joint flexion after fusion is compensated, in part, by the gain in MCP joint flexion.

PIP Joint Fusion

Technically, it is easier to perform PIP joint fusion to correct a fixed flexion deformity than to correct a swan neck deformity because of the surplus skin on the dorsal aspect of the finger and the compression of the bone ends that occurs as the joint is straightened. We use either a longitudinal curved incision or, occasionally, a transverse incision over the PIP joint. The extensor mechanism often is nonexistent. The collateral ligaments are divided at their origins on the proximal phalanx. With the finger in maximal flexion, the distal end of the proximal phalanx is removed with an osteotome. The proximal phalanx cut is at a slight angle, directed volarly. The articular cartilage is removed from the base of the middle phalanx, and the subchondral bone is softened with a rongeur. As the finger is straightened, the bone ends are compressed. Bone grafts usually are not needed because of the excellent bone contact.

The position of fusion that we choose varies with the finger involved. We prefer 25 degrees of flexion for the index finger and gradually increase the flexion to 45 degrees for the small finger. As mentioned previously, confirmation of the desired angle of fusion with a sterile goniometer is suggested. A Kirschner wire is passed longitudinally across the joint (Fig. 59-65) and is supplemented by an obliquely placed wire. These can be cut off flush to the bone and left in place permanently or left protruding through the skin to facilitate removal after fusion has occurred. A Herbert screw may be used as described previously for internal fixation (see Fig. 59-51).[358] External splints are used for the first 4 to 6 weeks until the fusion has started to consolidate. If the MCP joints were fixed in hyperextension preoperatively, they are brought into flexion by manipulation, soft tissue release, or arthroplasty.

PIP Joint Arthroplasty

PIP joint arthroplasty using a silicone implant is an alternative method for treating the fixed rheumatoid boutonnière deformity. Because the goal of this procedure is to maintain motion, the extensor mechanism must be reconstructed as part of the procedure. This is done by reattaching the central slip to the base of the middle phalanx. Relocation of the lateral bands dorsally is often required as well, to direct all the extensor force to the PIP joint. Swanson[197,286,287] has shown impressive results with this technique, and we now use it in selected cases.

This approach is particularly appropriate in patients whose deformity involves the ring and small fingers and whose MCP joints are flexible, because preservation of PIP motion in these fingers enhances the ability to grasp. However, we believe that it is not indicated in a severely flexed PIP joint because of the necessity of resecting excessive bone to provide enough space for the implant. PIP joint arthroplasty is discussed in more detail elsewhere in this text.

THUMB DEFORMITIES

Pathophysiology

Rheumatoid thumb deformities represent some of the more difficult problems of rheumatoid reconstructive surgery, especially for the surgeon who is unaccustomed to dealing

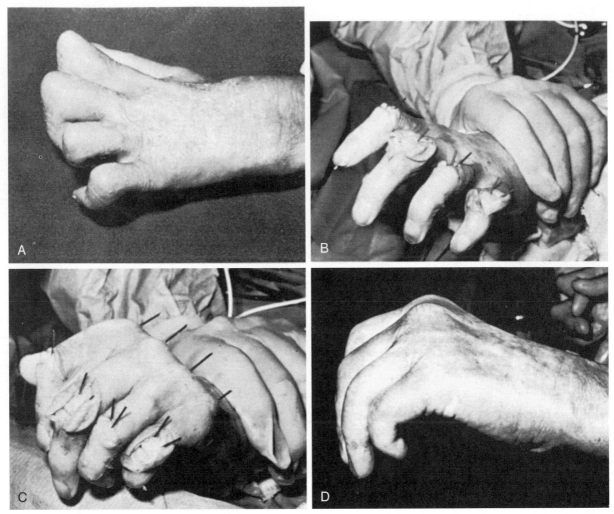

FIGURE 59-65. Severe boutonnière deformities treated by PIP fusions. **A,** Severe fixed flexion contractures of the PIP joints with the MCP joints fixed in extension. **B,** Degree of flexion for fusion increases from the index to small finger. **C,** MCP joints manipulated into flexion and held with Kirschner wires. **D,** Postoperatively, the finger position is improved, and grasp of moderate-sized objects is possible. (From Nalebuff EA, Millender LH: Surgical treatment of the boutonniere deformity in rheumatoid arthritis. Orthop Clin North Am 6:753-763, 1985, with permission.)

with the rheumatoid hand. To evaluate the rheumatoid thumb deformity and to plan appropriate treatment, a clear understanding of the pathophysiology and natural history of these deformities and their resultant clinical disabilities is necessary.

The original classification of thumb deformities suggested by Nalebuff included four groups. This classification was revised to include a fifth and a sixth group. Type I deformity (boutonnière deformity) is the most common, and type III (swan neck deformity) is the second most common. Type IV deformity is seen occasionally, and type II and type V are more rare. Type VI is joint destruction and collapse associated with arthritis mutilans (Table 59-7). Ratliff[389] described an additional deformity: IP and/or MCP joint destruction with instability but without the characteristics of any of the other types.[390-399] Surgical treatment must be individualized for each patient and each joint and includes synovectomy, tenodesis, tendon transfer, arthrodesis, and arthroplasty.

Type I Thumb Deformity (Boutonnière Deformity)

Type I deformity is characterized by MCP joint flexion and distal joint hyperextension. It is usually initiated by proliferative MCP joint synovitis, which bulges dorsally and results in attenuation of the EPB tendon insertion, stretching of the extensor hood, and displacement of the EPL tendon ulnarward and volarly. The collateral ligaments are stretched, and intra-articular joint destruction occurs to varying degrees. This loss of dorsal support results in subluxation of the proximal phalanx on the metacarpal and concomitant hyperextension of the IP joint from the altered pull of both intrinsic muscles and the EPL. The first metacarpal becomes radially abducted to compensate for the MCP flexion. The hyperextension of the IP joint and the flexion of the MCP joint are accentuated when pinch forces are applied to the thumb and, with time, may become fixed. This particular deformity can be described as an "extrinsic-minus" deformity. Rupture of the EPL at the wrist level can therefore result in a similar deformity.

Table 59-7
RHEUMATOID THUMB DEFORMITIES

Type	CMC Joint	MCP Joint	IP Joint
I (boutonnière)	Not involved	Flexed	Hyperextended
I Early	Not involved	Passively correctable	Passively correctable
I Moderate	Not involved	Fixed contracture	Passively correctable
I Severe	Not involved	Fixed contracture	Fixed contracture
II (uncommon)	CMC flexed and adducted	Flexed	Hyperextended
III (swan-neck)	CMC subluxed, flexed, and adducted	Hyperextended	Flexed
III Early	Minimal deformity	Passively correctable	
III Moderate	CMC subluxed	Passively correctable	
III Severe	CMC dislocated	Fixed contracture	
IV (gamekeeper's)	CMC not subluxed, flexed, and adducted	First degree, radially deviated, ulnar collateral ligament unstable	Not involved
V	May or may not be involved	First degree, hyperextended, volar plate unstable	Not involved
VI (arthritis mutilans)	Bone loss at any level	Bone loss at any level	Bone loss at any level

Distal joint hyperextension can be the primary disturbance, with MCP joint flexion being secondary, although this is less common. This may be a result of attenuation of the volar plate of the IP joint, owing to synovitis or a rupture of the FPL tendon that usually occurs in the carpal tunnel. In these patients, IP hyperextension is greater than MCP flexion. Metacarpal radial abduction is usually not a significant component because the MCP flexion is less. Thus, when faced with a patient with a type I deformity, it is necessary to evaluate the MCP and IP joints as well as the individual flexor and extensor tendons that control them.

In the early stage, both MCP and IP joint deformities are correctable passively (Fig. 59-66); however, in time, fixed deformities develop, first of the MCP joint alone and later of both the MCP and the IP joints.

Indications for Operative Treatment (Table 59-8)
There are three clinical stages in the development of type I deformity. Each requires a different type of surgical treatment. In the early stages, there is MCP joint subluxation with IP joint hyperextension, but both joints are correctable passively. Surgical treatment at this stage includes synovectomy of the MCP joint and reconstruction of the extensor mechanism. The original reconstruction of the extensor mechanism as described by Nalebuff is an EPL rerouting procedure in which the long extensor tendon is rerouted through the dorsal capsule of the joint to provide additional extensor force at this level.[73] When this procedure is done, the intrinsic muscles of the thumb act as extensor forces for the distal joint. Synovectomy alone has not been shown to significantly alter the natural history of the disease, and synovitis recurs in 6% to 13% of patients after MCP joint synovectomy.[338,399a,399b,410] EPL rerouting corrects the MCP joint deformity and helps prevent further collapse of the IP joint, but a review of this procedure by Terrono and Millender[400,401] revealed a high late recurrence rate.

However, this procedure does improve function over that period of time.[400]

In the second stage, a fixed MCP joint is present with or without intra-articular joint destruction. The IP joint deformity is correctable passively. Most patients are seen at this stage. Arthrodesis is recommended for the MCP joint if it is totally destroyed and the two adjacent joints are involved minimally. However, if destructive changes are likely to develop at one of the adjacent (CMC or IP) joints, MCP joint arthroplasty or MCP arthroplasty combined with EPL rerouting must be considered. Correction of the deformity at the second stage helps prevent the third stage from developing.

The third and most difficult stage is that of both a fixed MCP joint flexion deformity and a fixed IP joint hyperextension deformity. Treatment is dependent on the status of each of the two joints. If the IP joint is not destroyed and can be released by a dorsal capsulotomy, some degree of IP joint motion can be preserved. However, the deformity usually recurs after IP joint release.[401]

If the deformity is too severe, IP joint arthrodesis is indicated. MCP joint surgery depends on the severity of the deformity, the status of the articular surfaces, and the surgery indicated for the IP joint. If the IP joint has been fused, we try to preserve MCP joint motion either with synovectomy and EPL rerouting or with silicone implant arthroplasty.[402] However, in severely deformed or destroyed joints, combined MCP and IP joint fusions are sometimes indicated. Although Ratliff[389] stated that he had never found an indication for arthrodesis of both these joints, others believe that this is indicated occasionally. If the MCP joint is only moderately stiff and has a salvageable joint surface, intrinsic muscle and ligamentous release with reconstruction of the extensor mechanism is indicated.

Our most common procedure for third-stage deformity is IP joint fusion and MCP joint arthroplasty.[8,400-403] We use the

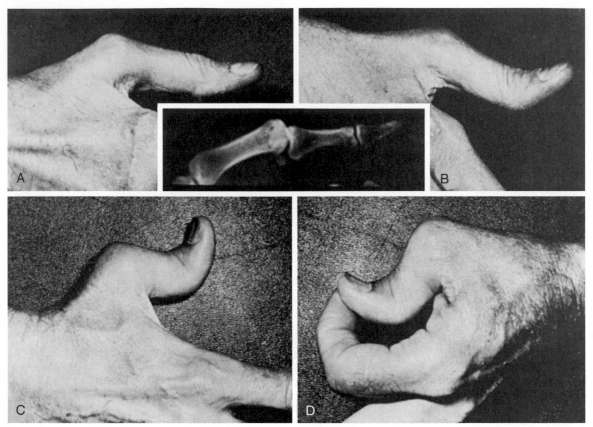

FIGURE 59-66. Type I thumb deformity. **A,** Synovitis of the MCP joint stretches the extensor mechanism, resulting in MCP joint extension lag. Initially, the IP joint is not involved. **B,** MCP joint subluxation with IP joint hyperextension. As the disease progresses, there is MCP joint involvement with cartilage loss and early subluxation. **C,** Advanced type I deformity with fixed MCP and IP joint deformity. **D,** Pinch aggravates the collapse deformity.

Table 59-8
TREATMENT OPTIONS FOR TYPE I THUMB DEFORMITY (BOUTONNIÈRE DEFORMITY)

Stage	MCP Joint	IP Joint
Early	Synovectomy EPL rerouting	Synovectomy Restore FPL function Flexor tenodesis
Moderate	Fusion Arthroplasty	Joint release
Advanced	Arthroplasty	Fusion Joint release

EPL, extensor pollicis longus; FPL, flexor pollicis longus.

hinged Swanson implant designed for the great toe because of its greater strength. The collateral ligaments are tightened during closure, and the MCP joint is splinted for 4 to 6 weeks after surgery to increase stability of the joint.

Type III Thumb Deformity (Swan Neck Deformity)

The second most common thumb deformity is type III, or swan neck, deformity. It is characterized by MCP joint hyperextension, IP joint flexion, and metacarpal adduction.[73] This deformity results from disease at the level of the CMC joint.[347] Synovitis and erosion of the articular surfaces and capsular distention allow dorsal and radial subluxation of the CMC joint as the thumb is used for grasp. Repeated use may result in complete dislocation of this joint. As the joint subluxates, abduction forces are reduced and adduction contracture of the metacarpal develops (Fig. 59-67).

Swanson believes that painful abduction associated with an element of adductor muscle spasm may lead to this deformity.[287] Clayton described contracted adductor muscles preventing abduction of the thumb metacarpal.[404a] Vainio postulated that the adduction contracture developed as a result of joint ankylosis and fibrosis.[278,288] Kessler found that neither the adductor muscle nor the first dorsal interosseous muscle was ever contracted, but he did find contracture and shortening of the fascia overlying these muscles.[100] Our experience confirms Kessler's findings.

Hyperextension of the MCP joint develops secondary to the metacarpal adduction contracture, if the volar plate is lax. As the patient attempts to open the first web space to grasp, the fixed CMC joint deformity prevents metacarpal abduction and extension. The extension forces are transmitted to the MCP joint, resulting in the hyperextension of this joint. These patients can grasp moderate-sized objects only by hyperextending the MCP joint.

Indications for Operative Treatment (Table 59-9)
Patients with type III deformities also are seen in three general stages. In the first stage, a painful CMC joint, weak pinch, and various degrees of radiographic CMC joint

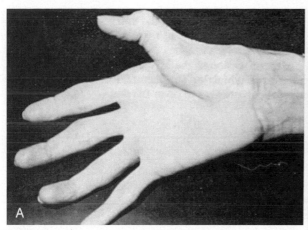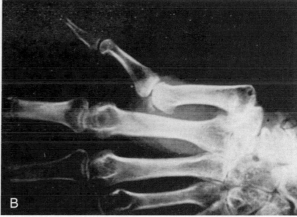

FIGURE 59-67. Type III thumb deformity. **A,** Clinical appearance with carpometacarpal joint subluxation, thumb metacarpal adduction, and secondary MCP joint hyperextension. **B,** Radiograph demonstrates carpometacarpal joint destruction with erosion of the trapezium and metacarpal subluxation.

Table 59-9

TREATMENT OPTIONS FOR TYPE III DEFORMITY (SWAN NECK DEFORMITY)

Stage	CMC Joint	MCP Joint
Early	Resection arthroplasty, LRTI	None
Moderate	Resection arthroplasty, LRTI	Fusion Volar restraint
Advanced	Resection arthroplasty, LRTI Release contracture	Fusion

LRTI, ligament reconstruction tendon interposition arthroplasty.

destruction are seen. At this stage, there is minimal subluxation, minimal deformity, and no secondary MCP joint involvement. Surgical treatment is indicated only for persistent CMC joint pain after proper conservative therapy has failed. Conservative therapy consists of an adequate trial of systemic medications, 2 to 4 months of splinting, and occasional corticosteroid injections. The recommended surgical treatment is hemiarthroplasty. We no longer use implant arthroplasty at the thumb base but instead use a resection arthroplasty with ligament reconstruction and tendon interposition.[54]

Patients in the second stage show varying degrees of CMC joint deformity and mild, passively correctable MCP joint hyperextension (Fig. 59-68). Unless pain is significant, these patients function quite well, except for weakness of pinch. Our recommended treatment for the CMC joint with mild MCP joint deformity is resection arthroplasty and ligament reconstruction,[54] combined with volar tenodesis or sesamoidesis[405] of the MCP joint. We perform MCP joint fusion for advanced deformity or joint destruction.

Advanced type III deformity includes complete CMC joint dislocation with a fixed adduction contracture and a fixed hyperextension deformity of the MCP joint. These patients have significant disability as a result of the contracted first web space, which prevents grasp of moderate-sized objects. The zigzag collapse deformity precludes

adequate pinch. CMC resection arthroplasty with ligament reconstruction and MCP joint fusion is helpful in restoring function to these patients. MCP arthroplasty is not performed for hyperextension deformity of the thumb. We have found, as did Kessler, that nearly complete correction of the metacarpal deformity can be obtained by resecting the base of the metacarpal and, if necessary, releasing the deep CMC ligament. We have found that it is necessary to release the fascia over the first dorsal interosseous muscle only occasionally, and we have never found it necessary to release the adductor muscle. "Z"-plasty of the skin of the first web space is necessary infrequently, because tight skin in rheumatoid patients stretches after bony and other tissue releases have been performed.[282,406,407]

In a patient with SLE, a CMC joint fusion should be done because of increased ligamentous laxity. Shapiro staples[251] are useful for internal fixation in these fusions.

Type IV Thumb Deformity (Gamekeeper's Deformity)

Type IV deformity is characterized by a radial deviation deformity of the MCP joint with secondary adduction of the thumb metacarpal. This occurs as synovitis of the MCP joint stretches the ulnar collateral ligament, resulting in lateral instability of this joint. Secondarily, an adduction contracture of the thumb develops. In some cases, shortening and contracture of the adductor fascia similar to that seen in type III deformity may occur. The important aspect of type IV deformity is that there is no primary CMC joint disease; therefore, treatment is directed toward the MCP joint.

Indications for Operative Treatment (Table 59-10)

For early deformity, MCP joint synovectomy and collateral ligament reconstruction are performed, with release of the adductor fascia if these structures are tight. In advanced cases, either MCP joint arthrodesis or arthroplasty is performed. If fusion is done, it should be accompanied by correction of the adduction contracture. After the MCP joint is stabilized, the thenar muscles function to abduct and oppose the entire thumb ray more effectively and to prevent further adduction of the thumb metacarpal.

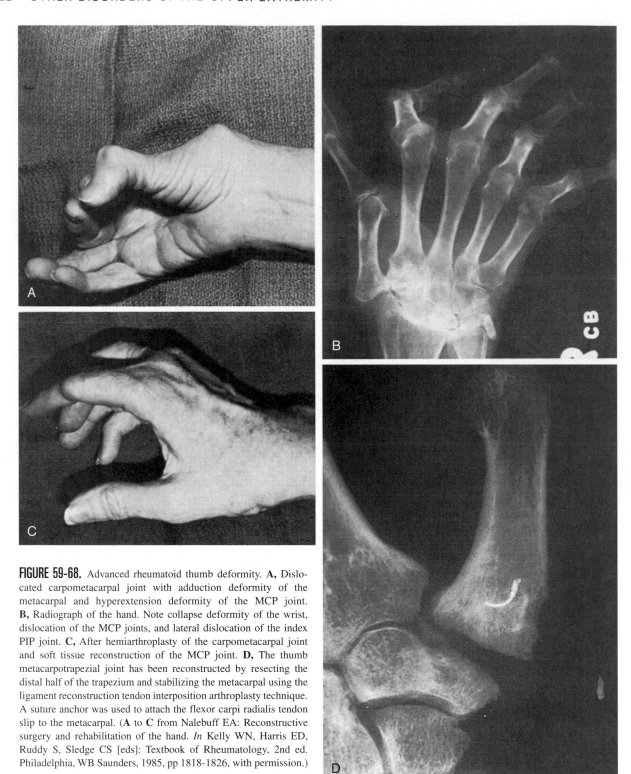

FIGURE 59-68. Advanced rheumatoid thumb deformity. **A,** Dislocated carpometacarpal joint with adduction deformity of the metacarpal and hyperextension deformity of the MCP joint. **B,** Radiograph of the hand. Note collapse deformity of the wrist, dislocation of the MCP joints, and lateral dislocation of the index PIP joint. **C,** After hemiarthroplasty of the carpometacarpal joint and soft tissue reconstruction of the MCP joint. **D,** The thumb metacarpotrapezial joint has been reconstructed by resecting the distal half of the trapezium and stabilizing the metacarpal using the ligament reconstruction tendon interposition arthroplasty technique. A suture anchor was used to attach the flexor carpi radialis tendon slip to the metacarpal. (**A** to **C** from Nalebuff EA: Reconstructive surgery and rehabilitation of the hand. *In* Kelly WN, Harris ED, Ruddy S, Sledge CS [eds]: Textbook of Rheumatology, 2nd ed. Philadelphia, WB Saunders, 1985, pp 1818-1826, with permission.)

Type II Thumb Deformity

Type II deformity, which is seen rarely, is a combination of type I and III deformities. It consists of MCP joint flexion with IP joint hyperextension and an associated subluxation or dislocation of the CMC joint. The treatment of this deformity is similar to that for types I and III deformities.

Type V Thumb Deformity

Type V thumb deformity results from stretching of the MCP joint volar plate. The MCP joint hyperextends, with secondary flexion of the IP joint as tension on the flexor tendon increases. In contrast to the type III deformity, the first metacarpal does not assume an adducted position.

Table 59-10

TREATMENT OPTIONS FOR TYPE IV THUMB (GAMEKEEPER'S)

Stage	MCP Joint
Early	Synovectomy Reconstruction of collateral ligament
Moderate	As for early (rare) Fusion Adductor fascia release
Advanced	Fusion Adductor fascia release

Surgical treatment of the type V thumb deformity is simple; the MCP joint is stabilized in flexion by volar capsulodesis, sesamoidesis, or fusion.

Thumb Deformities Secondary to Joint Destruction

Ratliff described an additional deformity that we see frequently.[389] This is the result of both destruction and instability of the IP joint and/or the MCP joint. Although any type of deformity may develop, lateral deformities are seen frequently at the MCP joint and lateral and hyperextension deformities are seen at the IP joint. These deformities often are the result of the bone destruction and resorption associated with arthritis mutilans. In advanced cases, they cause severe loss of hand function and disability.[48]

Indications for Operative Treatment: Severe Joint Destruction and Arthritis Mutilans

Arthrodesis is the usual procedure of choice for these joints. In patients with arthritis mutilans, arthrodesis should be performed early, before marked bony resorption has occurred. When arthritis mutilans has resulted in marked bone loss, bone grafts will be required to restore or maintain length and to allow fusion to occur.[48,408] Although we have no experience with Harrison-Nicolle "pegs," they may be an alternative in these situations. The pegs are polypropylene implants that are used as internal splints to stabilize the joint, thereby allowing a bony or fibrous ankylosis to develop around the joint and peg.[295,297]

Operative Techniques for Thumb Reconstruction

Surgery is based on which joint is involved. The classification of deformity by type improves the surgeon's understanding of the problem but is not important in the overall treatment.

IP Joint

The surgical techniques used for reconstruction of the IP joint are synovectomy, extensor tendon release (for fixed hyperextension deformities), and arthrodesis of the IP joint.

Synovectomy. Synovectomy of the IP joint may be performed through a dorsal curved or longitudinal incision. Swanson described a "Y" incision centered over the IP joint,

which we have found useful.[357] Another incision that we have used is a longitudinal zigzag incision centered over the IP joint. This protects the terminal branches of the dorsal sensory nerve. After the skin flaps are elevated, the proliferative synovium can be removed from either side of the joint with a small rongeur. A small portion of the extensor mechanism can be detached from the base of the distal phalanx, which, combined with traction on the phalanx, allows easier access to the joint.

Flatt noted that occasionally the major portion of the diseased synovium lies in the volar pouch.[6] In these cases, the synovium may be removed through a midaxial incision on one side of the joint, dividing the accessory collateral ligament. Lipscomb[338] recommended approaching the joint from the side (the ulnar side in all fingers except the small finger) and releasing the collateral ligament to completely dislocate the joint. The collateral ligament is repaired after a complete synovectomy is performed. The joint is protected with a Kirschner wire for 10 to 12 days before beginning motion. We have had no experience with either of these procedures.

After IP joint synovectomy, the joint is splinted in extension for a few days before beginning exercises. The joint should be splinted between exercise periods for 2 weeks to prevent an extensor lag from developing.

IP Joint Release. This procedure is performed in conjunction with MCP joint fusion or arthroplasty in the moderately severe type I deformity. The skin incision used is critical, as the dorsal skin is contracted and thereby limits the amount of flexion that can be obtained. Our usual approach uses a lateral incision on either side of the joint. A tenolysis of the extensor mechanism is performed. The dorsal capsule is incised by sliding the blade volar to the extensor mechanism and then rotating it 90 degrees. The dorsal portion of the collateral ligament is released through each incision, and the joint is manipulated into flexion. Usually the joint can be held in 25 to 30 degrees of flexion without placing the dorsal skin under undue tension.

Alternatively, a "Z"-plasty can be used. A longitudinal incision is made over the midportion of the joint. This provides excellent exposure. The release is performed as described earlier. After the Kirschner wire has been inserted, the incision is converted into a "Z"-plasty. There is rarely sufficient skin to close the incision completely, and a portion of the wound is left open. This epithelializes within 10 to 12 days, after which time the Kirschner wire is removed and exercises are started. For several days after the wire is removed, the joint is protected with a plaster or aluminum splint. Occasionally, an extensor lag develops. In these cases, the joint should be splinted in extension to allow the extensor mechanism to contract. Ten to 25 degrees of active joint flexion after these procedures can be expected; a large range of flexion is never obtained, and the deformity often recurs.[401]

IP Joint Arthrodesis. This is described on page 2107.

MCP Joint

Operative procedures for the rheumatoid MCP joint include synovectomy, synovectomy with extensor mechanism reconstruction, volar release in conjunction with reconstruction of the extensor mechanism for fixed flexion deformities, arthroplasty, and arthrodesis.[297,338,409-411]

Synovectomy. A slightly curved, longitudinal incision, 3 to 4 cm in length, is made over the MCP joint. Radial and ulnar flaps are reflected to expose the extensor mechanism. The sensory branches of the radial nerve must be protected. The joint is exposed by a longitudinal incision between the EPL and EPB tendons, which are reflected ulnarward and radially, respectively. The synovium bulges dorsally, often having ruptured through the joint capsule. A synovectomy is performed with a small rongeur.

Traction applied to the joint gives additional exposure. Synovium should be removed carefully from the recesses on either side of the collateral ligament attachment to the metacarpal head. Synovitis in this area causes the early bony erosions, which are seen radiographically. A small curet is helpful in entering the tight space between the ligament and the metacarpal head. After synovectomy is completed, the extensor mechanism is closed and tightened. The joint is splinted in extension to prevent a flexion deformity. Splinting is continued for 12 to 14 days before beginning exercises. In the thumb, MCP joint stability is more important than motion; therefore, we allow time for adequate soft tissue healing before motion is started.

MP Joint Synovectomy With Extensor Mechanism Reconstruction (Fig. 59-69). These procedures are indicated for early type I deformity in which the joint is preserved and subluxation is correctable passively. Nalebuff,[397] Inglis and coworkers,[412] and Harrison[392] described separate surgical procedures.

In each of the methods, the extensor mechanism is exposed as described for synovectomy. The EPL and EPB tendons are identified. The EPB usually is attenuated, and the EPL often is displaced ulnarly and volarly.

To perform the EPL rerouting described by Nalebuff, the interval between the EPL and the EPB is identified. The EPL is transected over the proximal one third of the proximal phalanx and freed proximally. The attenuated EPB tendon is dissected from the base of the proximal phalanx and detached from the extensor hood. The joint is approached through a transverse incision in the thin portion of the capsule, leaving the thickened portion of the capsule attached to the base of the proximal phalanx. A transverse incision is made in this thicker capsule distal to the joint, through which the EPL tendon will be passed. A complete synovectomy of the joint is performed. The EPL is passed through the hole in the capsule and pulled back over itself. With the joint held in full extension, the tendon is sutured tightly to itself. The EPB is pulled distally and sutured into the side of the EPLs. Nalebuff modified his technique for EPL rerouting. He now transects the EPL tendon more proximally and sutures the EPB tendon to the EPL stump to improve IP joint extension.

The dorsal expansions of the intrinsic tendons on each side of the joint are checked to be sure that they are in their proper position, because they are now the sole extensors of the terminal phalanx. If there is any tendency for these tendons to subluxate volarly, the transverse fibers between the intrinsic tendons over the dorsal aspect of the midportion of the proximal phalanx can be tightened to ensure their direct action on the stump of the EPL tendon. An oblique Kirschner wire is used to hold the MCP joint in extension. The thumb is splinted with the IP joint in extension.

IP joint flexion and extension exercises are started in a few days. The IP joint is protected in extension when not being exercised to prevent an extensor lag. The Kirschner wire across the MCP joint is removed in 4 weeks. However, the MCP joint is splinted in extension for an additional 1 to 2 weeks to allow complete soft tissue healing. All splinting is discontinued 6 weeks after surgery.

Harrison's[297] procedure for reconstructing the MCP joint is similar to the rerouting procedure described earlier, except that a portion of the EPL is tenodesed to the base of the proximal phalanx by passing the split tendon through a hole in the base of the proximal phalanx and suturing it back to itself. The MCP joint is held with a Kirschner wire. The postoperative management is essentially the same as described earlier.

Inglis and coworkers[412] split the extensor mechanism longitudinally between the EPL and EPB tendons to expose the joint and perform a synovectomy. The abductor pollicis brevis and the adductor pollicis are detached from the

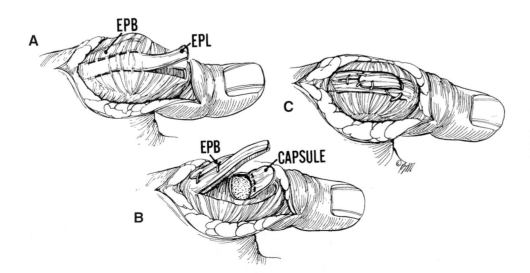

FIGURE 59-69. Extensor pollicis longus rerouting for early type I deformity. **A,** In the standard method of EPL rerouting, the EPL tendon is transected between the MCP and IP joints and elevated proximally. **B,** In Nalebuff's modified technique, the EPL is transected more proximally and the distal stump is sutured to the EPB tendon. **C,** The proximal stump is passed through the MCP joint capsule and sutured back onto itself in both methods.

extensor hood. These two structures are retracted proximally and laterally. After synovectomy is performed, the EPB is sutured tightly to the base of the proximal phalanx through a drill hole. The abductor pollicis brevis and adductor pollicis tendons are brought dorsally and attached to the side of the EPL tendon. These three tendons—the abductor pollicis brevis, adductor pollicis, and EPL—now function together as the extensor mechanism.

MCP Joint Ligamentous Reconstruction for Type IV Deformity. The skin incision described earlier is used. The interval between the EPL and EPB tendons is opened, and the EPL and dorsal expansion of the adductor pollicis are reflected ulnarward. The stretched ulnar collateral ligament is identified. This ligament is detached from the proximal phalanx or metacarpal, whichever end is more attenuated. A synovectomy of the joint is performed. The attenuated portion of the collateral ligament is excised. The end of the collateral ligament is attached to bone using a pull-out suture or suture anchor. The adductor tendon is detached from the base of the proximal phalanx and advanced distally.

The postoperative management is similar to that for the EPL rerouting procedure.

Procedures for Fixed MCP Joint Contractures. The procedures performed for fixed MCP joint contractures are soft tissue release with extensor reconstruction (in mild to moderate cases) and arthroplasty or arthrodesis (for severe MCP joint contractures with extensive cartilage loss). If the deformity is in the range of 25 to 35 degrees and the joint cartilage is involved minimally, soft tissue release may be preferable to arthroplasty or arthrodesis. Flatt[6] described a procedure that we use in these circumstances.

MCP Joint Soft Tissue Release With Extensor Reconstruction. The joint is exposed dorsally. The edges of the extensor mechanism are exposed, and the two winged intrinsic tendons are detached from the EPL distal to the MCP joint. This releases the intrinsic tendon from the IP joint, thereby correcting some of the IP joint extension contracture. IP joint extension is now provided solely by the EPL. If necessary, a dorsal capsulotomy of the IP joint is done to allow additional IP joint flexion. The extensor mechanism is freed proximally, releasing the bony attachments to the base of the proximal phalanx on the radial and ulnar sides. This should allow the MCP joint to extend. If it cannot be extended, division of the accessory collateral ligament is necessary. Synovectomy is done through the standard dorsal capsular incision. The EPB is reattached to the proximal phalanx—either to the capsule or to bone. The two winged intrinsic tendons are reattached to the soft tissues around the neck of the metacarpal to provide abduction and adduction of the entire thumb ray.

A Kirschner wire is used to stabilize the MCP joint. The postoperative treatment is similar to that described for the extensor mechanism reconstruction of the MCP joint on page 2130.

Arthrodesis. The problems with and techniques for arthrodesis of rheumatoid joints differ from those in other clinical conditions and deserve special consideration. In some respects, arthrodesis in these joints is easier than in osteoarthritis or post-traumatic arthritic joints. Exposure is easier because of the laxity of the rheumatoid joint capsule and ligaments, cartilage removal is easier, and, unless there is bony resorption or significant deformity, preparation of subchondral bone and positioning of the bone surfaces before fixation are not difficult. Because of these factors, arthrodesis of rheumatoid joints can be done rapidly, allowing joint fusions to be performed in addition to other major procedures during the allowable period of tourniquet inflation. However, other factors can make arthrodesis of these joints technically difficult. These include marked joint deformity, bone loss, and soft bone that does not afford firm internal fixation.

Arthrodesis of IP and MCP Joints Without Severe Deformity or Bone Loss. Both joints are exposed dorsally, using approaches similar to those for synovectomy. The extensor mechanism and collateral ligaments are divided over the IP joint, allowing it to be dislocated by hyperflexion. Releasing the collateral ligaments from the metacarpal allows adequate exposure of the MCP joint. Cartilage is removed from all surfaces with a rongeur, and soft cancellous bone is exposed over a broad surface. Proximal convex and distal concave surfaces are formed. The surfaces are apposed and checked for firm, stable contact. If MCP joint arthroplasty or other arthroplasty has been performed immediately beforehand, the previously resected bone is morselized and packed into the fusion site before Kirschner wire insertion. Generally, we fuse the IP joint in full extension or in very slight flexion. If necessary, we also rotate the IP joint into slight pronation. A 0.045- or 0.062-inch Kirschner wire is passed distally through the medullary canal of the distal phalanx to exit at the tip, just volar to the nail plate. The exit position of the wire on the fingertip is important. Placement too dorsal will damage the nail bed, and placement too volar will be uncomfortable postoperatively. With the joint held in the selected position, the wire is drilled proximally into the medullary canal of the proximal phalanx using a power drill. The size of the wire is determined by the softness of the bone and the size of the medullary canal.

After the wire is passed, the bone ends are impacted and stability is checked. If stable, one Kirschner wire is sufficient. If not, an oblique wire is added. The end of the wire is cut and buried deep to the pulp. If the pulp is thin or the wire is cut improperly, wire protrusion and pin tract infection make early wire removal necessary and increase the possibility of nonunion. A plaster splint is applied after surgery. If the IP joint alone is fused, an aluminum splint is used to protect the joint for approximately 4 weeks after the sutures are removed.

Several techniques for MCP fusion are available. The MCP joint is approached and prepared essentially as described earlier. In one technique, the joint is transfixed with two crossed Kirschner wires. Although these can be passed retrograde, they are inserted most easily directly across the joint from dorsal and ulnarward on the metacarpal to dorsal and radial on the proximal phalanx, and vice versa. The wires should be directed so that they do not exit on the volar surface of the thumb, thereby putting the flexor tendon and/or digital nerves at risk. Dual parallel Herbert screws or Acutrak screws can be used for internal fixation of MCP joint fusions. Alternatively, a tension band technique can be used.[412a] It provides a more stable construct than Kirschner wires, with earlier function and minimal immobilization. However, the tension band technique is more demanding (Fig. 59-70). Inglis and coworkers[412] recommended fusing the MCP joint in 15 degrees of flexion, 15 degrees of abduction, and 15 degrees of internal rotation. We generally agree with this; however, this position is not sacred. If the CMC joint is unstable, the MCP joint should be fused in more flexion, up to 25 degrees. It is advisable to measure the position of fusion accurately with a sterile goniometer before the final internal fixation devices are inserted. Intraoperative radiographs also are helpful in confirming the appropriate alignment for fusion.

If, after obtaining stable fixation, the position varies from that described earlier and is considered suboptimal, the joint can be bent into a better position if only one small-diameter Kirschner wire has been inserted. The second wire is inserted after the position is corrected.

Arthrodesis in Arthritis Mutilans. Loss of bone stock is the major factor that makes fusion in rheumatoid patients difficult. The amount of loss ranges from thinned cortices and absent medullary cancellous bone to severe bone resorption with shortening, as seen in arthritis mutilans.[48,405] Joint exposure may be difficult because of deformity and/or subluxation, and the soft, thin bone may not hold Kirschner wires well. In general, the technique is similar to that used for fusing any rheumatoid joint. However, certain points should be emphasized. Excellent exposure is mandatory. If "pencil-in-cup" deformities are present at the IP or MCP joints, the bones are exposed by excising the capsule from the rim of the bone and the volar plate from the undersurface of the phalanx and by cutting the cartilaginous and cortical rim transversely to obtain a flat surface.

After this has been accomplished, the joints can be apposed. However, adequate bone stock must be present. If bone stock is insufficient, cancellous bone from other areas (e.g., resected metacarpal heads) is helpful to fill the gap and increase stability. If the metacarpal heads from arthroplasty are devoid of cancellous bone, the cortical bone is crushed and used to fill the cavity. Wires are inserted as described earlier. A second longitudinal or crossed Kirschner wire may be needed for the IP joint.

Bone grafts are important in cases of arthritis mutilans. Shortening is accepted if the joints have fused spontaneously. However, iliac bone blocks often are needed to restore length and to obtain fusion (Fig. 59-71).[48] The joints are exposed and prepared as described earlier. A bone block from the iliac crest is fashioned, wedged into place, and fixed with longitudinal Kirschner wires. Cancellous bone is packed into the remaining space. These fusions are technically difficult and require 4 to 5 months of immobilization postoperatively.

Arthrodesis Using Internal Splints. An alternative to formal arthrodesis in cases of arthritis mutilans or severe bone loss is the use of the Harrison peg.[261,295] In some cases of arthritis mutilans, we have used small Swanson MCP implants in MCP and IP joints. After these are inserted, Kirschner wires are passed across the joint. External immobilization is used for 10 to 12 weeks. This procedure results in fibrous ankylosis but allows some restoration of length with stability of the joint.

Trapeziometacarpal Joint Arthroplasty

Currently, we rarely perform an implant arthroplasty, either partial or total,[8,152,406,407,413] at the thumb CMC joint. More commonly, we resect part of the trapezium and thumb metacarpal to correct the deformity and perform a ligament reconstruction and tendon interposition as described by Burton and Pellegrini.[54,414] MCP joint hyperextension or instability must be corrected at the same time.

A zigzag incision extending from the proximal one third of the metacarpal along the first extensor compartment is used. The sensory branches of the radial nerve have ramified at this level and must be preserved within the dorsal and volar flaps. Injury to these nerves can cause painful neuromas and dysesthesias along the course of the radial nerve. The radial artery is identified as it passes deep to the APL and EPB tendons and is dissected free and retracted. Small branches of the artery that enter the trapeziometacarpal joint are electrocoagulated.

After the radial artery is retracted, the CMC joint capsule is incised longitudinally and released from the base of the metacarpal. Care is taken to preserve the capsule for later closure. The metacarpal base and trapezium are exposed. Enough of each is excised to create an adequate space and to correct the deformity. If necessary, the scaphotrapezial joint is identified and the dissection is extended to this joint. It is easier and safer to remove the trapezium piecemeal with a rongeur than to attempt to remove it in one piece. When the volar surface of the trapezium is removed, care is taken to avoid removing the volar capsule with the bone and to

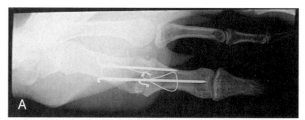

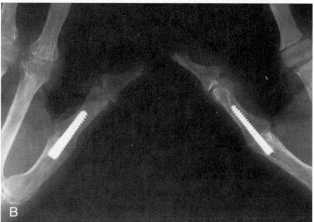

FIGURE 59-70. **A,** Thumb MCP joint fusion using the tension band technique. **B,** The left thumb MCP joint was fused using a standard Acutrak screw, and the right thumb MCP joint was fused using a Mini-Acutrak screw. Both fusions healed solidly in 6 weeks.

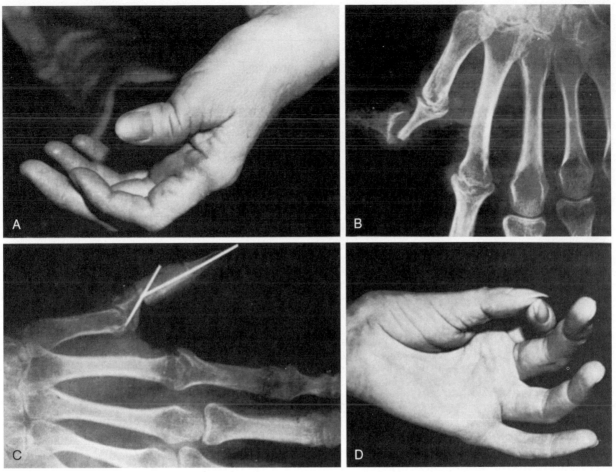

FIGURE 59-71. Unstable distal joint of the thumb fused with a bone graft. **A,** The clinical appearance of the thumb with collapse of the IP joint. **B,** Radiograph shows significant absorption of the distal end of the proximal phalanx. **C,** Postoperative radiograph shows use of bone graft to restore length and facilitate joint fusion. **D,** Note the stable pulp pinch between the lengthened thumb and index finger. The distal joint is fused in slight flexion. **E** and **F,** Drawing of the IP joint fusion technique using a bone graft in patients with severe bone loss. Obtaining internal fixation purchase can be difficult because of the bone loss. Multiple Kirschner wires are used to obtain a stable construct. (**A** to **D** from Nalebuff EA: Reconstructive surgery and rehabilitation of the hand. *In* Kelly WN, Harris ED, Ruddy S, Sledge CS [eds]: Textbook of Rheumatology, 2nd ed. Philadelphia, WB Saunders, 1985, pp 1818-1826.)

avoid damaging the FCR tendon, which passes through a groove in the trapezium.

In the loose, subluxated joint, the metacarpal can be dislocated completely and the entire surface of the metacarpal base visualized. The beveled volar and ulnar surface, which has eroded the dorsal radial facet of the trapezium, can be seen. In stiff, contracted thumbs, resection of the base of the metacarpal is more difficult. After the capsular release, the deep volar CMC ligament may have to be divided to allow adequate exposure. In addition, partial metacarpal resection may have to be performed before the base can be dislocated into the wound. In each case, enough soft tissue release and bony resection should be done to expose the metacarpal base completely.

In our experience, a formal adductor release is rarely necessary. However, if this is indicated, the fascia over the first dorsal interosseous muscle is incised. The distal limb of the incision can be extended and the skin retracted to allow release of this fascia.

The procedure is now performed as described by Burton and Pellegrini.[54,414] The APL should be advanced to ensure adequate postoperative abduction power.

Postoperatively, the thumb is splinted for 4 weeks before Kirschner wire removal (if used), after which splinting is continued for 2 to 4 weeks. Exercises are begun at 4 to 5 weeks, and splinting is discontinued after 8 weeks.

Other thumb surgery, such as MCP joint arthrodesis or IP joint arthrodesis, can be performed at the same time, if indicated. Hyperextension of the MCP joint (as seen in type III deformity) must be corrected at the time of trapeziometacarpal joint arthroplasty. If there is more than 20 to 30 degrees of hyperextension of the MCP joint, a volar capsulodesis or sesamoidesis is indicated. If there is excessive instability or MCP joint destruction, MCP arthrodesis should be performed.

ANNOTATED REFERENCES

288a. Aptekar RG, Duff IF: Metacarpophalangeal joint surgery in rheumatoid arthritis. Long-term results. Clin Orthop 83:123-127, 1972.

A retrospective review was performed on 16 patients with rheumatoid arthritis who had finger MCP joint synovectomy.

This involved 25 hands and 88 joints. Some patients had advanced disease with other procedures also being performed, including tendon realignment and arthroplasty. However, there was a long follow-up of 7.1 years (range, 5 to 9 years). In 36% of the joints the synovitis recurred. However, patients did get the benefit of pain relief and improvement in deformity and appearance. Synovectomy was suggested to be performed before radiographic changes.

151. Bora FW, Osterman AL, Thomas VJ, et al: The treatment of ruptures of multiple extensor tendons at the wrist level by a free tendon graft in the rheumatoid patient. J Hand Surg [Am] 12:1038-1040, 1987.

The results were reported of the treatment of multiple finger extensor tendons ruptures at wrist level in the patient with rheumatoid arthritis by free tendon grafts. Twenty-three patients averaged 65 degrees of active motion at the MCP joints when seen at an average follow-up of 43 months. This is an excellent option for the patient with multiple tendon ruptures.

195. Brumfield R Jr, Kuschner SH, Gellman H, et al: Results of dorsal wrist synovectomies in the rheumatoid hand. J Hand Surg [Am] 15:733-735, 1990.

Dorsal wrist tenosynovectomy was performed on 78 patients with rheumatoid arthritis from 1962 to 1982. This was done in 102 wrists and included intra-articular synovectomies and Darrach resection. Follow-up after surgery averaged 11 years (range, 3 to 20 years). Synovitis recurred in 16 wrists and radiographic evidence of progressive intra-articular destruction was seen in 45 wrists. Wrist synovectomy can decrease pain (pain was diminished in all but 17 wrists) and thereby maintain function. Motion does decrease an average of 13 degrees. However, revision surgery was necessary in 28 wrists.

246. Chamay A, Della Santa D, Vilaseca A: Radiolunate arthrodesis, factor of stability for the rheumatoid wrist. Ann Chir Main 2:5-17, 1983.

Surgical radiolunate arthrodesis appears to be an appropriate procedure to stabilize ulnar translation of the carpus, to correct radial deviation of the wrist and consequently ulnar drift of the fingers, and to restore neutral orientation of the lunate when collapse occurs. The surgical procedure and complications are described.

15. Clayton ML: Historical perspectives on surgery of the rheumatoid hand. Hand Clin 5:111-114, 1989.

The history of rheumatoid hand surgery is reviewed with its multiple contributors.

62. Dray G, Millender LH, Nalebuff EA, Philips C: The surgical treatment of hand deformities in systemic lupus erythematosus. J Hand Surg [Am] 6:339-345, 1981.

Ten patients with systemic lupus erythematosus and with hand deformities were studied. Wrist involvement included distal ulnar subluxation in 14 wrists (with 4 requiring excision) and various degrees of carpal instability in 12 wrists (usually asymptomatic). MCP joint subluxation treated by soft tissue procedures for passively correctable deformities in 30 joints had a failure rate of 70%. MCP joint arthroplasties performed in 33 joints gave fair results in 16 joints with fixed deformities and good results in 17 joints with passively correctable deformities. Thumb deformities always involved all three joints, and maintenance of CMC joint stability was the key to thumb stability. CMC joint stabilization with ligamentous reconstruction gave good results in three of four thumbs. Four CMC joint fusions and two CMC joint implant arthroplasties gave good results. Each was accompanied by appropriate procedures on the MCP joint or IP joint. The treatment of the hand involved with lupus is complex, with many interacting factors. However, unless the disease process can be modified, the failure rate of any soft tissue procedure in the long term is likely to be high. Results of the soft tissue reconstruction of the passively correctable MCP joint may be improved with an extensor tenodesis and prolonged immobilization.

116a. Ertel AN, Millender LH, Nalebuff EA, et al: Flexor tendon ruptures in patients with rheumatoid arthritis. J Hand Surg [Am] 13:860-866, 1988.

One hundred fifteen flexor tendon ruptures were reviewed in 43 hands with rheumatoid arthritis, one hand with psoriatic arthritis, and one hand with lupus erythematosus. Ninety-one tendons were ruptured at the wrist, 4 ruptures occurred at the palm, and 20 ruptures occurred within the digits. At the wrist level, 61 ruptures were caused by attrition on a bone spur and 30 were caused by direct invasion of the tendon by tenosynovium. All ruptures distal to the wrist were caused by invasion of the tendon by tenosynovium. Patients whose ruptures were caused by attrition regained better motion than those whose ruptures were caused by invasion by tenosynovitis; however, motion overall was poor. Patients with isolated ruptures in the palm or at the wrist had the best functional results. Those patients with multiple ruptures within the carpal canal had a worse prognosis. Ruptures of both tendons within the fibro-osseous canal had the worst prognosis. The severity of the patient's disease and the degree of articular involvement had a great effect on the outcome of surgery. Prevention of tendon ruptures by early tenosynovectomy and removal of bone spurs was suggested to be the cornerstone of treatment.

384. Ferlic DC: Boutonnière deformities in rheumatoid arthritis. Hand Clin 5:215-222, 1989.

In patients with rheumatoid arthritis the PIP joints are often involved with a boutonnière deformity. The pathology of the deformity begins with a synovitis of the joint, followed by elongation al the central slip, subluxation of the later bands, and contracture of the retinacular ligaments. Treatment in the early stages can include synovectomy and tendon reconstruction. In the later stages, when the joint is fixed or there is articular surface damage, a joint replacement or arthrodesis is necessary.

190. Hindley CJ, Stanley JK: The rheumatoid wrist: Patterns of disease progression. J Hand Surg [Br] 16:275-279, 1991.

Fifty wrists in 28 patients were followed in a retrospective radiographic review for a mean period of 9.56 years. Patterns of disease and the rates of change in the severity of the disease were determined, with particular reference to the changing relationship in time between involvement of the wrist and hand. In the wrist, there was relative sparing of the midcarpal joint, with a significant correlation between a high incidence of triquetrolunate disease and changes in the ulnar styloid. Wrist disease was found to "protect" the hand for the first 5 years but not after this time. On the basis of these results, earlier surgical intervention is proposed, with the intention of shifting the emphasis of surgery from salvage to preventative or reconstructive procedures.

178. Linscheid RL, Dobyns JH: Radiolunate arthrodesis. J Hand Surg [Am] 10:821-829, 1985.

It was noted that spontaneous radiolunate arthrodesis resulted in painless, satisfactory wrist function. A radiolunate arthrodesis was performed to stabilize the wrist in patients with rheumatoid arthritis and ulna translocation with a maintained midcarpal joint. Twenty-two radiolunate arthrodeses were performed, 16 by a corticocancellous slotted graft, and 6 by a modified Lauenstein procedure in 17 rheumatoid and 5 traumatic cases. Nineteen wrists were available for follow-up at an average of 28 months. Average range of motion was 25 degrees of extension, 30 degrees of flexion, 5 degrees of radial deviation, and 15 degrees of ulnar deviation. Subjective evaluation was good in 14 wrists, fair in 3, and poor in 2. Relief of pain was generally satisfactory, and preoperative grip strength was slightly improved. Progressive degeneration of the midcarpal joint tends to be minimal. Carpal ulnar translation, midcarpal angulation, and radial angulation are corrected. Loss of carpal height is partially corrected in most instances. Radiolunate arthrodesis is a good procedure to stabilize the wrist in the appropriate patient with rheumatoid arthritis.

95. Millender LH, Nalebuff EA, Albin R, et al: Dorsal tenosynovectomy and tendon transfer in the rheumatoid hand. J Bone Joint Surg Am 56:601-610, 1974.

Seventy-three patients with rheumatoid arthritis had tenosynovectomy for tenosynovitis of the finger extensors. In addition, 41 had treatment of extensor tendon ruptures. Dorsal tenosynovectomy prevented subsequent tendon ruptures. However, there were two ruptures caused by a problem with the distal ulnar excision. The indications for tenosynovectomy were presented. These include persistent tenosynovitis despite adequate medical treatment, extensor tendon rupture, and recurrent tenosynovitis. Tendon rupture is an urgent problem because more ruptures may follow. We agree with these suggestions and emphasize the importance of contouring the distal ulna by removing any sharp edges and stabilizing it when needed.

40. Miller-Breslow A, Millender LH, Feldon PG: Treatment considerations in the complicated rheumatoid hand. Hand Clin 5:279-289, 1989.

The rheumatoid patient with complex involvement or multiple deformities of the hand and wrist can be a challenge to the hand surgeon. A systematic and orderly approach is used to formulate and execute a treatment plan that is realistic and that can result in modest, but significant improvement in overall hand function. The evaluation and treatment philosophy that is described can simplify a complicated and seemingly overwhelming situation.

284. Nalebuff EA: Factors influencing the results of implant surgery in the rheumatoid hand. J Hand Surg [Br] 15:395-403, 1990.

A review of the factors influencing the result of implant arthroplasty in the rheumatoid hand is presented.

51. Nalebuff EA: Surgery of systemic lupus erythematosus arthritis of the hand. Hand Clin 12:591-602, 1996.

SLE is one of a group of three uncommon arthritic diseases, including psoriatic arthritis and scleroderma, that superficially resemble rheumatoid arthritis. These diseases frequently involve the hand and wrist. SLE has certain specific characteristics that separate it from the other two conditions. The distinctive features of SLE as well as the treatment indicated to adequately care for these patients are outlined.

269a. Nalebuff EA: Surgery of psoriatic arthritis of the hand. Hand Clin 12:603-614, 1996.

Psoriatic arthritis is an uncommon form of arthritis that poses specific problems. Although there are similarities between this form of arthritis and the more common rheumatoid or degenerative arthritis, this particular entity is unique, and one should be aware of the differences to advise or carry out the appropriate treatment. The distinctive features of psoriatic arthritis and the treatment indicated to adequately care for these patients are outlined.

220. O'Donovan TM, Ruby LK: The distal radioulnar joint in rheumatoid arthritis. Hand Clin 5:249-256, 1989.

Rheumatoid arthritis commonly affects the DRUJ. This can result in pain, instability, or tendon rupture. The goals of surgical reconstruction of the DRUJ are to relieve pain, stabilize the joint, and prevent tendon rupture. A review of the many described procedures and the authors' experience with excision of the distal ulna and soft tissue reconstruction with a distally based slip of extensor carpi ulnaris tendon are presented.

168. Shapiro JS: A new factor in the etiology of ulnar drift. Clin Orthop 68:32-43, 1970.

A retrospective review of a series of 100 rheumatoid hands with serial roentgenograms and clinical material from 20 hands is performed. The author presents these data to show that radial rotation of the wrist and subsequent radial deviation of the metacarpals is the major factor in the development of ulnar drift of the finger MCP joints. Whereas there are many other factors that are involved in the cause of ulnar drift (see article by Smith and Kaplan[266]), this is an important factor and must always be addressed before attempting to correct the ulnar drift.

266. Smith RJ, Kaplan EB: Rheumatoid deformities at the metacarpophalangeal joints of the fingers: A correlative study of anatomy and pathology. J Bone Joint Surg Am 49:31-37, 1967.

A detailed presentation of the normal and abnormal anatomy and the pathology involved in the finger MCP joints of patients with rheumatoid arthritis. The causes of the ulnar deviation of the finger MCP joints are outlined. However, radial rotation of the wrist is not mentioned (see Shapiro[168]). This is a "must-read" for the surgeon involved in the treatment of MCP joint problems in rheumatoid arthritis.

399. Stein AB, Terrono AL: The rheumatoid thumb. Hand Clin 12:541-550, 1996.

The thumb frequently is involved in rheumatoid arthritis and often is a source of significant functional loss, pain, and deformity. The goals of surgery are pain relief, improvement of function, enhancement of appearance, and slowing the progression of disease and can be reached. Specific surgical interventions should be based on the nature and stage of deformity as well as the status of tendons, ligaments, and adjacent joints. Treatment options, in isolation or in combination, include synovectomy, arthrodesis, arthroplasty, and tendon repair or transfer. Although most thumb deformities can be classified as one of six common types, other patterns of deformity also are seen. It therefore is imperative not to operate on pattern recognition alone but to examine each patient carefully and individualize treatment.

193. Thirupathi RG, Ferlic DC, Clayton ML: Dorsal wrist synovectomy in rheumatoid arthritis—a long-term study. J Hand Surg [Am] 8:848-856, 1983.

Dorsal wrist synovectomy, tenosynovectomy of the extensor tendons, excision of the distal ulna, ulnar-side stabilization of the wrist, and placement of the extensor retinaculum underneath the extensor tendons was found to be an effective procedure in wrists with rheumatoid arthritis. Twenty-seven patients who had surgery on 38 wrists were followed for 7.4 years (range, 5 to 14 years). There were 25 women and two men with an average age of 54 years. Over 95% had excellent pain relief. There was significant reduction of wrist motion, but the arc of motion was within a functional range. Subsequent tendon rupture was minimal and even tendons found to be thinned out at the time of surgery remained intact. The carpal height was maintained in 70% of the wrists. Carpal translocation occurred in 44% of the wrists. Subsequently, three patients had a wrist arthrodesis and five had an arthroplasty. Carpal collapse and translocation could not be predicted by preoperative radiographs. Progressive carpal collapse was associated with increasing ulnar deviation of fingers. Progression of carpal collapse and ulnar translocation occurred in a linear fashion with the years of follow-up. These procedures are important for the delay in progression of rheumatoid wrist disease as well as in pain relief.

414a. Williamson SC, Feldon P: Extensor tendon ruptures in rheumatoid arthritis. Hand Clin 11:449-459, 1995.

The best treatment for extensor tendon rupture is prevention, either by medical management or surgical tenosynovectomy before tendon ruptures occur. Once a rupture has occurred, tendon transfer or free tendon grafting can provide acceptable restoration of extensor function. Communication with the rheumatologist is necessary to provide timely treatment for chronic dorsal tenosynovitis (and impending tendon rupture) or for single finger extension loss before the disease progresses to multiple finger extension loss. Consideration always must be given to associated joint involvement when planning surgical treatment.

123. Wilson RL, Carlblom ER: The rheumatoid metacarpophalangeal joint. Hand Clin 5:223-237, 1989.

Reconstruction of the MCP joint affected by rheumatoid disease can pose a challenge to the surgeon and therapist. The multiple initiating and aggravating factors must be taken into consideration during the planning phase before they can be addressed surgically. The results after surgery at the MCP joint are dependent on a number of factors. The most important of these is the general activity of the rheumatoid disease and the patient's response to medical treatment. The individual who requires corticosteroids and antimetabolites may observe a general worsening of his disease state, which will be uninfluenced by surgery at the MCP joints. Patients demonstrating vasculitis may have problems with wound healing and mobilization after MCP joint surgery. The surgeon's ability to rebalance the MCP joint is directly related to the quality of the periarticular soft tissues needed for the reconstructive procedure. The ability of an individual to cooperate in a postoperative program and to apply the principles of joint protection is absolutely necessary. The eventual joint motion is related to tendon function in the hand.

69. Wood VE, Ichtertz DR, Yahiku H: Soft tissue metacarpophalangeal reconstruction for treatment of rheumatoid hand deformity. J Hand Surg [Am] 14:163-174, 1989.

The long-term results of soft tissue MCP reconstruction without articular resection were reviewed in 16 hands of 12 patients with painful ulnar deviation-subluxation deformity. The indications and surgical technique are described. No splinting was used beyond 3 weeks. Patients had either lupus or rheumatoid arthritis. The mean age at operation was 66 years, with mean disease duration of 15.9 years before operation. At follow-up (mean, 81 months), complete pain relief occurred in 88% of patients and 56 degrees and 64 degrees of mean active MCP and PIP range of motion was present, respectively. Ulnar drift was corrected to 6 degrees on the average. The first semi-objective grading scale for MCP reconstruction was introduced. There were 82% good or excellent results. This is a good treatment for an MCP joint with ulnar deviation without volar subluxation that is passively correctable.

CHAPTER 60

Tenosynovitis

Scott W. Wolfe

Painful conditions affecting the tendons of the wrist and hand are perhaps the most common reason for a visit to a hand surgeon. Strictly defined, tenosynovitis refers to inflammation of the synovial lining of a tendon sheath and is abundantly demonstrated by the diffuse, invasive synovitis associated with rheumatoid arthritis (RA). Such *proliferative* tenosynovitis is relatively uncommon, is erosive, is not restricted to the retinacular thickenings of the tendon sheath, and may lead to tendon rupture. Other inflammatory-type causes include deposition diseases such as amyloidosis; crystalline tendinopathy such as calcific tenosynovitis or gout; and septic tenosynovitis, including bacterial, mycobacterial, and viral agents.

A far more common condition is *tendon entrapment*[141] or *stenosing tendovaginitis,*[29] caused by narrowing or stenosis of the tendon's retinacular sheath in such conditions as trigger finger or de Quervain's disease. Because there is a paucity of inflammatory tissue associated with tendon entrapment, the term *tenosynovitis* is misleading and inaccurate from an etiologic perspective. Tendon entrapment occurs about the narrow fibro-osseous canals that provide fulcrums for acute angulation of digital and wrist tendons. The nearly constant motion of a tendon through such a narrow passageway can cause hypertrophy and fibrosis of the retinacular sheath,[59,176] resulting in an impediment to gliding, edema, and, ultimately, catching or locking of the swollen flexor tendon[88] on either side of the sheath. Rarely, these conditions may be initiated by direct trauma. Tendon entrapment is initially characterized by intense local pain, swelling, redness, and, occasionally, crepitus. Over time, the affected retinacular sheath responds by thickening (up to three times normal diameter[64,102] and with fibrocartilaginous metaplasia.[176] Gross pathologic examination rarely demonstrates hypertrophied synovium but rather thickening, nodularity, and attritional changes within the tendon, accompanied by gross thickening of the overlying sheath. The conditions respond well in the early phase to conservative measures such as ice, splinting, rest, and corticosteroid injection and rarely recur after surgical release of the offending retinacular sheath.

PROLIFERATIVE TENOSYNOVITIS

Rheumatoid Arthritis

It has been estimated that tenosynovitis of the hand and wrist will develop in 64% to 95% of patients with RA.[25,109] This differs from other systemic polyarthropathies, such as psoriatic arthritis, in which proliferative synovitis is distinctly uncommon.[18] The process may begin within the synovial lining of the tendon sheath, or it may invade the tendon from involvement of a contiguous joint. Rheumatoid tenosynovitis produces relatively painless bulky swelling along the entire extent of the synovial sheath and is most noticeable at the retinacular boundaries.[150] Because of the thin, expansile dorsal skin of the hand, the disease may be quite prominent dorsally, producing noticeable swelling from the distal retinaculum to the metacarpal bases. The process can be easily differentiated from common wrist tumors such as ganglia or lipomas by the mobility of the mass with the extensor tendons and the tendency of the mass to bunch or "tuck" at the retinacular edge with digital extension.[25] The tenosynovitis of RA is most common on the ulnar border of the wrist over the distal radioulnar joint and most frequently involves the fourth, fifth, and sixth dorsal compartments.

On the flexor surface, the earliest signs of significant flexor tenosynovitis may be painful paresthesias caused by median nerve entrapment beneath the unyielding transverse carpal ligament.[149,150] One study[23] showed that flexor tendon involvement characterized by palmar nodularity along the flexor tendons, crepitus, and frank triggering will develop in 38% of patients with RA. Fusiform swelling of one or more digital flexor sheaths may cause a significant impediment to flexion, pain, and stiffness mimicking rheumatoid arthropathy of the interphalangeal (IP) joints. Rarely, a finger may trigger in RA from entrapment of the profundus tendon by synovitis at the superficialis decussation (Camper's chiasm). Helal described the cardinal sign of this syndrome as an inability to flex the distal IP joint when the proximal IP (PIP) joint was held passively by the examiner in full flexion.[84]

I would like to thank **Dr. Avrum Froimson** for his superb and comprehensive chapter "Tenosynovitis" that appeared in three previous editions of this book and constituted the framework from which this chapter was written.

Gross findings at surgery for RA include abundant red, "angry"-appearing synovium with tenacious attachment to the epitenon and, frequently, infiltrative invasion of the tendon substance. Fibrinoid deposits, or "rice bodies," are usually present amid the masses of swollen tissue. Often the underlying joint capsule is distended by proliferative joint synovitis. The synovial fluid is cloudy and contains abundant white cells, usually a mixture of lymphocytes and polymorphonuclear cells. Histologic findings within the synovium include hypertrophy and hyperplasia of the synovial cells, infiltration with lymphocytes and plasma cells (often containing characteristic eosinophilic aggregates of gamma-globulin known as Russell bodies), and a fibrinous exudate.[27]

Certainly the most pivotal complication of rheumatoid tenosynovial invasion is tendon rupture,[200] which is far more common among the extensor tendons than the flexors.[22] Although the redundancy of both flexor and extensor tendons gives rheumatoid patients the ability to compensate for a single tendon loss in most cases, the event may herald impending rupture of several more. Tendon rupture has been attributed to fibrinoid degeneration of the collagen fibrils,[101] granulomatous replacement of tendon,[109] synovial invasion,[58] and microvascular compromise.[9] The tendency of tendons to rupture at the distal edge of the extensor retinaculum, that is, in the so-called watershed zone of vascular supply,[25] lends credence to the latter theory. Other factors involved in tendon rupture include angulation around a subluxated joint, such as the distal ulna, or abrasion against an irregular bony spicule, such as Lister's tubercle or a malrotated scaphoid.[58,196,212]

Prevention of tendon rupture is the mainstay of treatment for rheumatoid tenosynovitis. Medical management includes aspirin or nonsteroidal anti-inflammatory agents; remittive agents such as hydroxychloroquine (Plaquenil), gold, and penicillamine; chemotherapeutic agents such as methotrexate; and for resistant cases, oral steroids.[5] Rest, ice, splinting, and alterations in medical management should be instituted for approximately 6 months. On occasion, the physician may choose to administer a corticosteroid injection for an acute episode of flexor tenosynovitis, but repeated injections should be avoided because of the risk of accelerating tendon rupture. It is difficult, if not impossible, to predict tendon rupture[25,150]; and if appropriate medical management has failed to control symptoms, surgical tenosynovectomy is indicated.

For a more detailed discussion of rheumatoid tenosynovitis and operative treatment, the reader is referred to Chapter 59.

Crystalline Tendinopathy

Gout

Precipitation of crystalline material within the confines of an enclosed space (joint or tenosynovial space) incites an acute, fulminant inflammatory reaction marked by intense swelling, erythema, and pain. Gout is a disorder of urate metabolism in which the overproduction of uric acid causes hyperuricemia and hyperuricosuria. Monosodium urate is the final common product of purine metabolism, and urate supersaturation is necessary for precipitation to occur.[17] Both hyperuricemia and gout are more common in men, and although hyperuricemia is necessary for gout, it alone is insufficient to cause gout.[17,46,174] Heritable enzymatic defects[17] and racial factors are probably responsible for a predisposition to urate deposition, and a very high incidence has been noted in men from the South Pacific islands of Java and New Zealand.[46,71] A longitudinal study of 1337 healthy medical students demonstrated a cumulative lifetime incidence of 8% and identified significant risk factors as obesity, hypertension, and weight gain at an early age.[175] Gout may also be the initial sign of renal disease secondary to a reduction in uric acid clearance.[209]

A low solubility of monosodium urate is responsible for its crystallization and deposition in peripheral sites, including subcutaneous, intra-articular, and tenosynovial locations. Attempted phagocytosis by peripheral leukocytes releases lysosomal enzymes that produce an intense inflammatory synovitis. If left unchecked, the disease results in the formation of gouty *tophi*, which are large lobulated subcutaneous deposits of monosodium urate crystals commonly seen in the pinna of the ear and the great toe.[199] Deposition in the hand occurs relatively late in the disease and is uncommon with good medical management.[140] Radiographic manifestations of gouty arthritis may precede symptoms in up to 25% of patients and may precede deposition of gouty tophi in up to 42%.[15] Medical control of the disease is the mainstay of treatment and consists of maintenance uricosuric agents such as probenecid and sulfinpyrazone, xanthine oxidase inhibition by allopurinol, nonsteroidal anti-inflammatory agents, intra-articular corticosteroid preparations, and microtubule inhibitors such as colchicine for acute attacks.

Gouty tenosynovitis in the hand can be present without visible tophi or previous involvement of the upper extremity.[73] Often called "the great imitator," gout may masquerade as septic arthritis, RA, or neoplasm, and the diagnosis is often delayed by weeks or months. Initial signs of flexor tendon involvement include marked pain, erythema, acute swelling, and warmth suggestive of acute suppurative tenosynovitis.[1,73,140] Gouty flexor tenosynovitis within the carpal tunnel can compromise the median nerve and result in acute carpal tunnel syndrome.[73,93,140] In unsuspected cases, an intense exudative inflammatory reaction can occur after carpal tunnel release and mimic infection, but this responds well to anti-inflammatory and uricosuric agents.[73] Gout can rarely coexist with RA,[7,169,227] but it is perhaps more frequently misdiagnosed as RA because of its proliferative synovitis[1] and because 10% to 20% of patients with RA have elevated uric acid levels.[199]

Because hyperuricemia exists in 5% to 7% of adult males, a diagnosis of gout should not be based on laboratory values alone. Joint or tenosynovial aspiration, Gram stain, and examination under polarized light is 85% sensitive for the diagnosis of gout and may be helpful in differentiating acute gouty tenosynovitis from RA or infection.[17] Suspected pathologic material must be transported to the laboratory in ethanol rather than formalin to prevent degradation of the monosodium urate crystals.[1,7] Compensated polarized light microscopy will demonstrate negatively birefringent (urate) crystals within granuloma with histologic features otherwise typical of RA.[7]

Other sites of tenosynovial involvement in the hand include the extensor tendons at the dorsal retinaculum,[140] a localized painful mass in the mid palm,[162] and tophi over the dorsal aspect of the IP or MP joints.[38,199] Neglected cases can proceed to intratendinous infiltration,[1] flexion contractures,[199] tendon rupture,[140] and skin ulceration in extreme cases. Acute attacks are generally well handled by the administration of

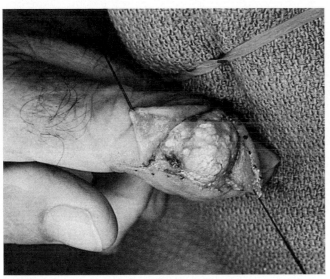

FIGURE 60-1. Excision of gouty tophus involving extensor tendons and the DIP joint. Meticulous skin flap handling is necessary to avoid skin slough and wound breakdown.

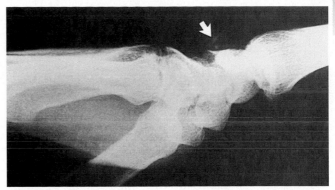

FIGURE 60-2. A small calcific deposit within the extensor carpi ulnaris tendon sheath *(arrow)* explained the extreme pain and loss of motion experienced by this 28-year-old businessman.

colchicine and anti-inflammatory agents,[199] and perioperative medication is recommended to reduce postoperative flares.[140]

Indications for operative management include restoration of joint and tendon mobility, decompression of the median nerve, control of skin breakdown and infection, and removal of painful or disfiguring tophi (Fig. 60-1).[199] Surgical synovectomy, removal of intratendinous deposits, and occasional tendon transfer for rupture may be performed in resistant cases. When excising gouty tophi, care is taken to not undermine involved and compromised skin. Skin grafts are rarely necessary for coverage. Curettage is useful for bony involvement, and extensive stripping of periosteum is avoided.[111] No attempt should be made to completely eradicate a tophus if excision would damage vital neurovascular structures or impair function. Bulky compression dressings are recommended to reduce dead space. Recurrence is rare after subtotal excision of gouty tophi and good medical management.[199]

Calcific Tendonitis

An acute, intensely painful synovitis can accompany the release of calcium salts into the intrasynovial space in joints or tenosynovial sheaths; this can resemble an infectious process.[35,131,142,158,186,225] The disease is not unlike the deposition of calcium about major joints in the body, including the calcific bursitis affecting the hip, knee, shoulder, and elbow. Hypercalcemia is neither necessary nor sufficient to produce ectopic calcifications, and elevated laboratory values and systemic signs are characteristically lacking.

Typically, a patient seeks medical attention for a painful, red, swollen digit or wrist and marked decrease in motion.[35] Delay in diagnosis for up to 2 weeks has been attributed to a relative unfamiliarity with the diagnosis.[142] Redness may occasionally extend proximally and may mimic cellulitis.[158] Differentiation from septic tenosynovitis can be made by a striking lack of systemic findings.[131] Standard radiographs may be dramatic and reveal a large deposit of fluffy calcium, or they may be entirely normal. Specialized views or oblique radiographs may be necessary to demonstrate a surprisingly small soft tissue calcium deposit (Fig. 60-2).[131,158]

The etiology of calcific tendonitis of the hand and wrist is unknown. It has been proposed that intratendinous necrosis from microtrauma caused by everyday use is necessary for calcium deposition to occur.[158] A history of significant trauma preceding the incident is decidedly uncommon. The disease is more commonly reported in women than men, with a female-to-male ratio of 5:1.[225] Calcific tendonitis in children is decidedly uncommon but is identical in its presentation, making the potential for misdiagnosis high.[137] Carroll and colleagues documented the largest reported series of calcific tendonitis in the hand (n = 100) in patients with an average age of 45 (range, 30 to 60).[35] The most frequent site was the flexor carpi ulnaris tendon, a relatively short tendon (5 cm) whose muscle belly is densely anchored to the investing antebrachial fascia by numerous areolar attachments. The tendon travels in a short synovial sheath before enveloping its sesamoid bone, the pisiform, and is continuous with the tendons of origin of the abductor and opponens digiti minimi.

Small asymptomatic intratendinous nodules can occur, as seen frequently in other locations such as the patellar tendon.[131] It is likely that intratendinous calcific deposits remain asymptomatic until a tear in the paratenon or tendon substance liberates the caustic material into the tenosynovial space, where it incites an acute inflammatory reaction. Histologic studies of the crystalline material demonstrate hydroxyapatite in the majority of cases.[225] The material may spread diffusely through the tenosynovial space and cause extensive pain and swelling, followed by gradual macrophage resorption. Free crystals injected into a joint have been demonstrated to precipitate a prostaglandin-mediated acute inflammatory response that includes vasodilatation, increased vascular permeability, and neutrophil ingress.[204] As in other types of inflammatory synovitis, carpal tunnel syndrome has been reported to result from acute calcific tenosynovitis in the flexor tendons.[148,158]

Once the diagnosis has been made, treatment is usually symptomatic only. Splinting and a short course of nonsteroidal anti-inflammatory agents will generally reduce the inflammatory phase within 24 to 48 hours. If the deposit can be localized by radiographs, an attempt at needle aspiration, with or without an injection of lidocaine (Xylocaine) and corticosteroids, may be justified and will give prompt relief of the symptoms.[131,158,186,225] In general, however, these patients respond so well to anti-inflammatory agents that it is not usually necessary to subject them to an injection in an already exquisitely tender site. Follow-up radiographs will usually show complete disappearance of small deposits in 2 to 4 weeks. Resistant or chronic cases with large calcific deposits may require surgical excision, but this is an exception. Incision of the affected tendon will allow extrusion of the material, which resembles "toothpaste."[35]

Other Crystalline Tenosynovitides
Pseudogout
Rarely, calcium pyrophosphate deposition disease (CPPD or pseudogout) can cause an acute fulminant inflammatory tenosynovitis within the carpal tunnel with resultant acute compressive neuropathy of the median nerve.[40,108] Radiographs may reveal fluffy soft tissue calcifications within the carpal tunnel and often reveal calcifications within the triangular fibrocartilage complex. Pathologic examination reveals rhomboid-shaped crystals with faintly positive birefringence under polarized light.

Hydroxyapatite Deposition
Hydroxyapatite deposition has also been reported to cause an acute carpal tunnel syndrome that is recalcitrant to anti-inflammatory agents and rest.[210] Both conditions are best treated by early decompression and excision of the crystalline material.

Deposition Disease

Normal protein products of metabolism that are either under-excreted or poorly metabolized may accumulate and be deposited in the bones, joints, and soft tissues.

Amyloid Deposition
Amyloidosis is a condition resulting from the deposition of a low-molecular-weight serum protein, β_2-microglobulin, in the bones and soft tissues. Excess protein accumulation can result from a rare primary enzymatic defect (Meretoja's syndrome)[168] but more commonly occurs in patients with renal failure who are undergoing peritoneal dialysis[44] or hemodialysis.[13,107,144,188] The protein is not filtered by standard dialysis membranes,[173] and the severity of the disease is proportional to the age of initiation of hemodialysis and the duration of treatment.[98,107]

Hand involvement in amyloidosis is usually characterized by cystic lesions in the carpal bones and destructive arthropathy involving the wrist and IP joints.[4,13,144] In patients with amyloidosis, tenosynovitis is common. Thick, plaque-like accumulations along the flexor tendons within the carpal tunnel have been demonstrated to cause median nerve compression in up to 15% to 20% of patients undergoing hemodialysis.[44,144,188] There is no apparent relationship between carpal tunnel syndrome and the side of arteriovenous fistulas in hemodialysis patients. Infiltrative amyloid tenosynovitis in the palm and digits can cause trigger fingers, flexion contractures, and tendon rupture.[107] Clinical signs of acute inflammatory tenosynovitis are lacking; characteristically, the digit or wrist is chronically swollen along the course of the affected tendons, without significant pain, warmth, or erythema. In a patient undergoing renal dialysis, radial-sided digital paresthesias and decreased digital

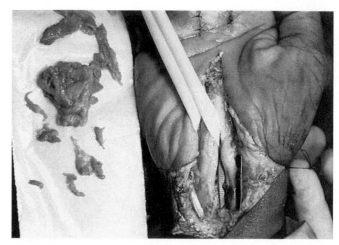

FIGURE 60-3. The more extended operative exposure required for amyloid-induced carpal tunnel syndrome. Note the extensive hypertrophied synovium excised from around the flexor tendons.

motion are strongly suggestive of amyloid tenosynovitis within the carpal canal.

Treatment of amyloid tenosynovitis is surgical, which is highly effective in relieving symptoms of median nerve entrapment and stenosing tenosynovitis. Complete tenosynovectomy through an extended carpal tunnel incision that zigzags across the palmar wrist crease is recommended (Fig. 60-3). Trigger fingers should be approached through standard incisions in the mid palm, and complete tenosynovectomy and division of the A1 pulley should be performed. Digital tenosynovitis may be excised through Bruner incisions, with retention of all other annular pulleys. Recurrence after carpal tunnel release and complete tenosynovectomy is uncommon.

Ochronosis
Alkaptonuria is an extremely rare autosomal recessive defect of tryptophan metabolism caused by a deficiency in the enzyme homogentisic acid oxidase.[34,95] As a result, unmetabolized homogentisic acid is excreted in the urine and deposited in the joints and soft tissues (ochronosis). The protein deposits have a characteristic dark pigmentation that causes darkened urine and deep staining of collagenous tissues.[125] Joint deposition, or accumulation in the intervertebral disk, can lead to severe destructive arthropathy.[125,136] The protein may be deposited within tendons[127] and has been demonstrated to cause stenosing tenosynovitis. Seradge reported a case involving multiple digits of both hands that was unresponsive to corticosteroid injection. Surgical release of the A1 pulley was successful at eliminating the symptoms.[184]

Septic Tenosynovitis

Acute suppurative flexor tenosynovitis is covered in Chapter 3.

Chronic Tenosynovitis

Certain indolent infections can be manifested as subacute tenosynovitis and must be included in the differential diagnosis. These include tuberculosis,[31,116] atypical *Mycobacterium* infection,[45,89,94,106,124,195,216,228] gonococcal tenosynovitis,[12,14,154,178] and fungal infections.[76,82,184,226] These chronic infections are discussed in detail in Chapter 4.

Sarcoid

On occasion, sarcoidosis can be manifested as digital flexor tenosynovitis and must be included in the differential diagnosis of isolated, inflammatory tenosynovitis.[77,135,192] Sarcoidosis is a systemic, immune-mediated granulomatous disease that primarily affects the lungs, spleen, and lymph nodes but may manifest as bone, joint, or tenosynovial involvement in approximately 25% of cases. Radiographs of affected hands typically reveal well-defined cystic granulomatous lesions in the phalanges. The causative agent that triggers sarcoidosis has not been identified. Its progression is variable; it spontaneously regresses in some but progresses to a chronic fibrotic state in others.[60] The disease is more common in women than men and affects blacks 10 times more frequently than whites in the United States. Sarcoidosis may precipitate secondary gout because of an overproduction of purines in the proliferative granulomas. Treatment includes surgical tenosynovectomy and systemic corticosteroids.[135]

Tendon Entrapment

Tendon entrapment (formerly known as *stenosing tenosynovitis*) refers to the mechanical impingement of a tendon in the hand or wrist caused by narrowing of its retinacular sheath. *Tendovaginitis* (Latin = "tendon sheath" and Greek = "inflammation") may be a more precise term than *tenosynovitis* to describe the inflamed and thickened retinacular sheath that characterizes these conditions. Unfortunately, tenosynovitis is generally very broadly defined and has been used to describe a heterogeneous collection of vague aching conditions of the upper extremity.[141,183] Burman[29] tried to clarify the definition as follows: "Tendovaginitis is not tenosynovitis. Before there is stenosing tendovaginitis, there must be nonstenosing tendovaginitis. It takes time to make a sheath stenotic. The latter is reversible, the former is not."

Histologic Findings

The most common types of tendon entrapment are de Quervain's disease and trigger digits, although the process has been reported to affect each of the tendons of the hand and wrist. Tenosynovitis has been cited as the common denominator of a number of affectations of the upper extremity, including carpal tunnel syndrome.[120,172] In patients without a known history of RA or inflammatory disease, however, several studies have failed to detect acute or chronic inflammatory cells in tenosynovial biopsy samples taken from patients undergoing carpal tunnel release.[65,103,120,151,180] Similarly, in Fahey and Bollinger's pathologic analysis of synovium from adults and children who underwent trigger release, synovial proliferation was uncommon (one case), and pathologic findings of degeneration, vascular proliferation, and cartilage formation were limited to the retinacular sheath.[59] Similar histologic analysis of tissue removed during tenolysis for de Quervain's disease or stenosis of the flexor

carpi radialis tendon documented perisynovial fibrous tissue and endothelial proliferation with a paucity of inflammatory tissue.[62,102,115] The lack of pronounced inflammatory findings within the tenosynovium and the demonstration of fibrotic thickening in the retinacular ligament prompted Garsten, in 1951, to coin the term *peritendinitis stenosans* and suggest that the conditions may be related more to intrinsic anatomic and degenerative changes than to occupational factors.[68]

Causative Factors

Although the etiology of tendon entrapment is disputed, certain epidemiologic factors are apparent. These conditions tend to cluster among certain patients, with coexistence of carpal tunnel syndrome, trigger digits, de Quervain's disease, epicondylitis, and subacromial bursitis implicating a more systemic and undefined rheumatic process or predisposition.[64,69,75,115,120,153,158,194,214] Each condition is far more common in women than men,[81,145,153,157,159,167,194,215] and the peak incidence of trigger digits averaged 55 to 60 years of age in several series.[59,97,105,120,206,214] The age distribution of trigger digits has not changed appreciably in more recent series despite an increase in the use of computer keyboards and other "repetitive" tasks.[145,153,157,167,176] Anatomic factors have been proposed to explain the pronounced difference in prevalence among men and women.[28] Degenerative factors may have an etiologic role in the development of flexor tendon entrapment of the digits, as evidenced by the increased incidence of these disorders in the dominant hand.[120,153,157,176] Several studies point to a relationship between activities that require exertion of pressure in the palm while performing forceful grip or repetitive digital flexion, such as arc welding, use of heavy shears, or constant hand-held tool work.[29,59,72,121] Forceful use is unlikely to be the sole etiologic factor, however, as evidenced by the strikingly low incidence in males and an age distribution that peaks in the sixth decade. Trezies and colleagues demonstrated no significant difference between the occupational distribution of patients with trigger digits and that of the general population.[206] Other anatomic and intrinsic factors undoubtedly contribute to a predisposition for the development of tendon entrapment of the hand and wrist.[115,214]

Trigger Digits

Tendon entrapment of the fingers and thumb is one of the most common causes of hand pain and disability. The condition causes painful catching or popping of the involved flexor tendon as the patient flexes and extends the digit. On occasion, the digit will lock in flexion and require passive manipulation of the digit into full extension. Over time, guarding and reluctance on the part of the patient to fully range the digit can lead to secondary contractures at the PIP joint.

Pathology

Twenty-two extrinsic tendons cross the wrist and provide a unique combination of power and dexterity in the hand. Each tendon passes through a series of tight fibro-osseous canals designed to optimize the balance between motion and force production by maintaining the tendon in close apposition to the joint(s) it controls. Division or rupture of a critical retinacular ligament, or *pulley*, will allow the tendon to drift away from the joint's center of rotation and consequently increase the moment arm for force production but effectively lengthen the tendon and limit excursion of the joint.

The phenomenon of tendon entrapment is due to mechanical impingement of the digital flexor tendons as they pass through a narrowed retinacular pulley at the level of the metacarpal head.[120,153,157,176] Proximal phalangeal flexion, particularly with power grip, causes high angular loads at the distal edge of the first annular (A1) pulley. Hueston and Wilson[87] suggested that "bunching" of the interwoven tendon fibers occurs, akin to the effect of pulling a multifilament strand through the eye of a needle, and causes the reactive intratendinous swelling often noted at surgery.[59,105,120,214] The most remarkable pathologic changes are seen in the pulley itself, which demonstrates gross hypertrophy, described by Bunnell as a "whitish, cicatricial collar-like thickening."[28] Microscopic examination demonstrates degeneration, cyst formation, fiber splitting, and lymphocytic or plasma cell infiltration.[59] Recent ultrastructural studies comparing normal and trigger A1 pulleys have demonstrated the presence of chondrocytes in the normal innermost, or *friction,* layer of the normal A1 pulley and chondrocyte proliferation and the presence of type III collagen in the pathologic pulleys.[176] These authors proposed that the A1 pulley and the corresponding surface of the flexor tendon undergo fibrocartilaginous metaplasia under the influence of repetitive, compressive loads.

Demographics

The most common form of trigger finger is the primary type, found in otherwise healthy middle-aged women with a frequency two to six times that seen in men.[59,64,105,120,128,153,157,167,214] Primary trigger finger and thumb occur with approximately the same frequency as de Quervain's disease,[113] and involvement of several fingers is not unusual. In patients with multiple trigger digits, the most commonly affected digit is the thumb, followed by the ring, long, little, and index fingers.[59,120,141,214] Secondary trigger finger can be seen in patients with diabetes, gout, renal disease, RA, and other rheumatic diseases and is associated with a worse prognosis after conservative or surgical management.[39,75,105,191] The lifetime incidence of trigger digits in nondiabetic adults over the age of 30 has been reported to be 2.2%[191] and to be up to 10% in patients with insulin-dependent diabetes mellitus.[191]

Although the flexor tendon sheath is constricted at the metacarpophalangeal (MP) joint, the patient or examining physician often localizes the phenomenon incorrectly to the PIP joint. A locked trigger digit can lead to an incorrect diagnosis of dislocation, Dupuytren's disease, and even focal dystonia or hysteria.[113] Trigger digits can be confused with so-called true locking of the MP joint (see Chapter 9). Except for rare instances of locking caused by a tumor of the tendon or sheath,[110,155,163] a loose body in the MP joint,[26] anomalies of the sesamoids,[185] or entrapment of intrinsic tendon on an irregularity of the metacarpal head,[96,161] the diagnosis should be straightforward and can be confirmed with a simple lidocaine injection into the flexor sheath to unlock the digit. On occasion, de Quervain's disease[59,211,220] and tendon entrapment of the extensor pollicis longus[133] have been demonstrated to cause triggering of the thumb and may lead to an

error in diagnosis. Rarely, localized enlargement of the flexor digitorum profundus can trigger at a stenotic A3 pulley and lead to persistence of symptoms after routine surgical incision of the A1 pulley.[165] Up to 22% of trigger digits in patients with RA may be due to profundus entrapment by synovitis at the superficialis decussation.[84]

Classification

Attempts have been made to classify triggering, but in one such report by Newport and colleagues,[153] no correlation was found between their grading scheme and outcome after injection therapy. I believe that some type of simple classification is useful if for no other purpose than to provide the clinician with a way to record notes in the patient's chart for retrospective review. Several authors have used a scheme such as the following[56,79,147,157] (as modified by Green DP, personal communication, 1997):

Grade I (pretriggering)—Pain; history of catching, but not demonstrable on physical examination; tenderness over the A1 pulley

Grade II (active)—Demonstrable catching, but the patient can actively extend the digit

Grade III (passive)—Demonstrable catching requiring passive extension (grade IIIA) or inability to actively flex (grade IIIB)

Grade IV (contracture)—Demonstrable catching, with a fixed flexion contracture of the PIP joint

Treatment

Nonoperative

Most primary trigger digits in adults can be successfully treated nonsurgically with the use of splinting and cortisone injection. Early series recommended surgical treatment as straightforward and highly effective[28,59,113] and regarded prolonged conservative treatment as "unreliable and expensive."[59] Subsequent follow-up series documented 7% to 9% poor results from surgical treatment, with complications including reflex sympathetic dystrophy, infection, stiffness, and nerve injury.[114] More recent series continue to document infrequent but serious complications, including nerve transection, infection, incisional pain, flexion deformity, flexor tendon bowstringing, and recurrence.[21,36,75,83,153,205] The small but significant risk of complication from open trigger release warrants an attempt at splinting and/or corticosteroid injection.

The popularity of corticosteroid injection has waxed and waned over the past several decades. Among primary trigger fingers and thumbs, corticosteroid injection has a highly satisfactory rate of success, particularly among nondiabetic patients with single digit involvement, a discrete palpable nodule, and a short duration of symptoms (Table 60-1). The only reported complication is a single case of flexor pollicis longus (FPL) rupture that occurred in a 62-year-old patient while opening a file drawer 4 years after two corticosteroid injections for trigger thumb.[203] No other complications of this technique have been reported. A transient rise in blood and urine glucose levels is common in diabetics,[75] and these patients should be advised that this is likely to occur.

Technique of Corticosteroid Injection. There are many different techniques for injecting trigger fingers, but this is my preferred method. A 3-mL syringe is loaded with

Table 60-1
OUTCOMES OF STEROID INJECTION FOR TRIGGER DIGITS

Author(s)	Year	Cortisone Preparation	Findings	No. Digits	Notes
Kolind-Sorensen[105]	1970	Hydrocortisone	67% success overall: 78% in "primary" trigger digits	106	Only 50% success in trigger digits secondary to rheumatoid arthritis, diabetes
Lapidus[114]	1972	Methylprednisolone	"Uniformly good results"	41	Follow-up unspecified
Rhoades et al.[167]	1984	Methylprednisolone	72% resolution overall: 93% resolution if < 4 months	53	Favorable prognosis: single digit, short duration
Marks and Gunther[128]	1989	Triamcinolone acetonide	Single injection: 84% Two injections: 91%	108	Average 44-month follow-up; better outcomes in female patients
Newport et al.[153]	1990	Betamethasone sodium phosphate	One to three injections: 77%	338	Favorable prognosis: single digit, < 6 months' duration; trigger grade had no effect on outcome.
Griggs et al.[75]	1995	Betamethasone sodium phosphate	50% success in diabetics: 72% NIDDM 44% IDDM	121	Incidence of multiple trigger digits and failure of injection statistically increased in IDDM population.
Stahl et al.[191]	1997	Methylprednisolone	Diabetics: 49% Nondiabetics: 76%	60 60	Diabetics: higher incidence diffuse type, multiple digits; 7% complication rate in diabetics
Freiberg et al.[64]	1989	Triamcinolone acetonide	79% resolution overall: 93% "nodular" 48% "diffuse"	101	Improved prognosis: nodular vs. diffuse type; shorter duration of symptoms
Murphy et al.[145]	1995	Betamethasone sodium phosphate	64% resolution steroid group 20% placebo response	24	Sheath distention alone unsuccessful.

IDDM, insulin-dependent diabetes mellitus; NIDDM, non–insulin-dependent diabetes mellitus.

0.9-mL plain lidocaine (no epinephrine) and 0.1 mL sodium bicarbonate. Sodium bicarbonate, in a 1:10 mixture, will neutralize the acidity of lidocaine and effectively reduce the pain of injection. (Marcaine should not be used when mixing with bicarbonate, because precipitation may occur.) One milliliter of soluble corticosteroid solution is added to the mixture; I prefer betamethasone sodium phosphate acetate, but other preparations such as dexamethasone or triamcinolone hexacetonide are equally satisfactory. A 27-gauge needle is applied to the syringe. The hand is prepped with a povidone iodine or alcohol solution and the digits slightly hyperextended. The metacarpal head is palpated and the skin sprayed with ethyl chloride solution for 10 seconds as a local refrigerant/anesthetic. The needle is introduced directly into the flexor tendon over the metacarpal head (Fig. 60-4). Needle placement can be confirmed if necessary by disengaging the syringe from the needle and asking the patient to bend the digit gently; needle motion confirms proper placement. The syringe is replaced and light pressure applied to the plunger while simultaneously withdrawing the needle slowly. When the needle tip emerges from the tendon substance, dramatic relief of resistance is felt, and a fluid wave may be palpated throughout the tendon sheath proximal and distal to the injection site. Generally, no more than 1 to 2 mL of the solution can be injected. The needle is withdrawn and slight digital pressure applied for 30 seconds. As an alternative to midline injection, Carlson and Curtis prefer a midaxial injection site at the level of the midproximal phalanx as a simple and relatively painless access to the flexor sheath.[33]

Splinting. For those who decline injection, some consideration should be given to splinting the involved digit. To test the efficacy of simple splinting for trigger digits, Patel and Bassini compared the outcomes of splinting the MP joint in 15 degrees of flexion with a single injection of betamethasone.[157] At 1-year follow-up, 66% of all digits splinted were symptom free versus 84% of the injected digits. The authors concluded that splinting is an efficacious alternative for patients who are reluctant to consider corticosteroid injection. Rodgers and associates demonstrated 55% resolution of early trigger digits among 31 workers using distal interphalangeal (DIP) joint splinting in full extension for 6 weeks.[170] They proposed that limitation of profundus gliding, decreased differential gliding of the flexor tendons within the sheath, decreased overall use of the digit, or a combination of these factors were responsible for symptom resolution in this manual laborer population.

Surgical Treatment

Pertinent Anatomy. The nine digital flexor tendons pass through the carpal tunnel beneath the median nerve and are tethered to the metacarpals and phalanges by a series of retinacular pulleys. The flexor digitorum profundus and superficialis tendons enter a narrow fibro-osseous tunnel

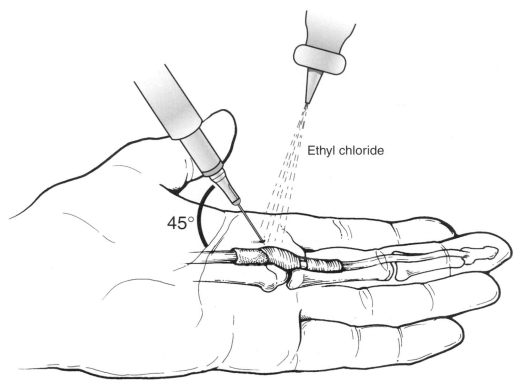

Ethyl chloride

45°

FIGURE 60-4. Author's preferred technique of trigger finger injection (see text).

formed by a groove in the palmar surface of the metacarpal neck and the annular ligament.[43,113] Doyle and Blythe[52,53] demonstrated that the flexor sheath in the finger is a double-walled, hollow, synovial-lined, connective tissue tube that encloses the flexor tendons. A visceral component of the sheath covers each of the enclosed tendons, and a surrounding parietal layer creates a closed, fluid-filled system. These authors identified four annular and three cruciform pulleys (Fig. 60-5). The annular pulleys are thick and rigid. The second pulley (A2), attached to the proximal phalanx, and

the fourth pulley (A4) are the most important functionally. It has been shown experimentally that section of only the first annular pulley (A1), as is done in surgical release of trigger finger or thumb, produces no loss of flexor function. However, division of both the A1 and A2 pulleys causes significant postoperative bowstringing and limitation of active flexion.

The flexor pollicis longus passes through a narrow tunnel formed by the grooved palmar surface of the first metacarpal neck and the transverse fibers of the annular ligament of the

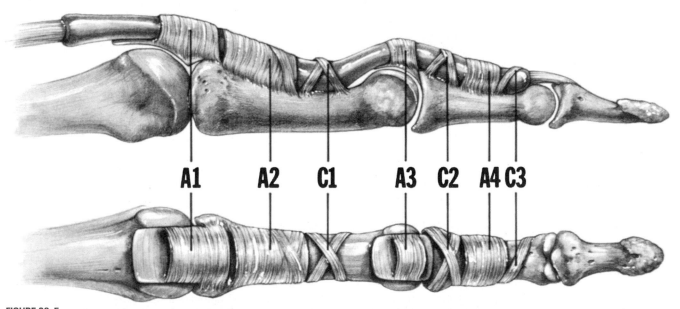

A1   A2   C1   A3   C2   A4 C3

FIGURE 60-5. Doyle and Blythe have identified four annular and three cruciform pulleys in the fingers. (Adapted from Doyle JR, Blythe W: The finger flexor tendon sheath and pulleys: Anatomy and reconstruction. *In:* AAOS Symposium on Tendon Surgery in the Hand. St. Louis, CV Mosby, 1975, pp 81-87, with permission.)

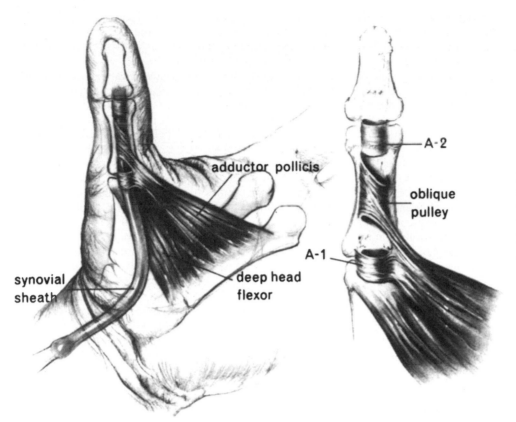

FIGURE 60-6. The flexor pollicis longus passes beneath a similar system of pulleys. Note the important *oblique* pulley just distal to the first annular pulley. (Adapted from Doyle JR, Blythe W: Anatomy of the flexor tendon sheath and pulleys of the thumb. J Hand Surg [Am] 2:149-151, 1977, with permission.)

flexor sheath (Fig. 60-6). The thumb is enclosed in a similar double-layered synovial sheath, and its pulley system consists of two annular and one oblique pulleys.[53] The first annular pulley is 7 to 9 mm wide and located palmar to the MP joint. Embedded on either side of the capsule of the MP joint is a sesamoid bone into which a tendon of one head of the flexor pollicis brevis is inserted. It is at this narrowest point in the sheath of the flexor pollicis that constriction develops. Overlying the proximal phalanx is a second pulley that has been variably described as oblique[53] or transverse[16] but is critically important to prevent bowstringing of the flexor pollicis. The pulley is 9 to 11 mm wide and is continuous with a slip of the tendon of insertion of the adductor pollicis and courses in a ulnar proximal to radial distal direction. These fibers must be preserved during trigger thumb release. The second annular pulley overlies the volar plate of the IP joint, just proximal to the insertion of the flexor pollicis longus on the distal phalanx.

Topographic Anatomy and Skin Incisions.   A study of the relationship of surface anatomy to deep structures in the palm shows that the proximal edge of the first annular pulley almost exactly coincides with the distal palmar crease in the fourth and fifth rays, the proximal palmar crease in the index finger, and halfway between the two creases in the middle finger (Fig. 60-7). A recent anatomic study of 256 cadaveric digits demonstrated that the palmar-digital skin crease lies midway between the proximal edge of the A1 pulley and the PIP flexion crease, thus allowing the examiner to precisely identify the A1 pulley's leading edge based on the distance between the palmar-digital crease and the PIP flexion

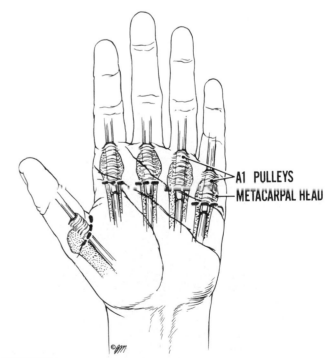

FIGURE 60-7. Incisions for release of trigger fingers and thumb. The index finger is released through an incision in the proximal palmar crease, the ring and little fingers through an incision in the distal crease, and the middle finger through an incision midway between the two palmar creases. The thumb flexor is approached through its TMP crease. In each instance the resultant scar will lie proximal to the metacarpal head prominence.

crease.[219] The proximal edge of the flexor pollicis longus sheath annulus is directly deep to the MP flexion crease of the thumb.[122] The transverse A1 pulley of the thumb is 7 to 9 mm in length and directly overlies the volar plate.

Short transverse incisions placed within the appropriate crease—or for the middle finger release, halfway between the two creases—thus provide excellent exposure of the A1 pulley to be divided. This site also positions the healed incision away from the underlying bony prominence of the metacarpal head, thereby lessening direct pressure on a tender scar in grasping spherical or cylindrical objects.[115] Longitudinal incisions are favored by several authors inasmuch as the extensile approach allows rapid and safe visualization of a longer segment of the flexor tendon, including both the A1 and A2 pulleys.[21,193] It is important to avoid crossing the palmar or digital creases with a longitudinal incision, or a painful contracture may develop. In either approach, the digital nerves and arteries that closely parallel each flexor sheath in the fingers must be protected. In particular, the radial digital nerve of the thumb is vulnerable as it lies quite close to the deep layer of dermis at the flexion crease and will be lacerated if the initial incision is carried too deeply.[36,205] The same nerve can also be injured by blind scissors dissection more proximally, where it crosses the thumb flexor sheath diagonally (Fig. 60-8).

Operative Technique of Open Trigger Digit Release. A padded pneumatic forearm tourniquet is applied, and 5 mL of lidocaine anesthetic is used to infiltrate the skin overlying the A1 pulley and percutaneously fill the flexor tendon sheath. A 1- to 1.5-cm transverse, oblique, or longitudinal incision is made over the involved metacarpal head. In the

thumb, the flexor pollicis tendon is approached through a 1.5-cm transverse incision in the MP flexion crease. Immediately after the skin has been incised, blunt dissection is used to spread the subcutaneous tissues and the palmar fascia to expose the flexor sheath. The digital nerves and vessels are retracted with small right-angle retractors and are not subjected to extensive dissection. The proximal edge of the thickened flexor sheath (proximal side of the A1 pulley) is identified, and a scalpel blade is used to divide the entire A1 pulley under direct vision (Fig. 60-9). Care is taken to not violate the proximal edge of the A2 pulley so as to prevent the potential for bowstringing and loss of digital flexion. Although it has been demonstrated that up to 25% of either end of the A2 pulley can be divided without detrimental mechanical effect on digital flexion,[139] anatomic studies have demonstrated apparent continuity between the first and second annular pulleys in up to 40% to 60% of digits.[118,201] Close inspection will usually identify an oblique cruciate pulley (the C0 pulley) at the proximal border of A2 and serve as a marker for the distal boundary of pulley release.[219] After release, the patient is asked to actively move the digit to confirm complete relief of the triggering. Meticulous hemostasis is obtained via electrocautery, and the wound is closed with two or three monofilament sutures.

A small hand dressing is applied, with all digits left free, and motion is encouraged on the day of surgery. The patient is counseled to use the hand for light activities, and supervised hand therapy is usually necessary only for patients with preoperative fixed flexion contractures. Sutures may be removed 10 to 14 days postoperatively. Most patients can resume full hand use within 3 to 4 weeks of surgery.

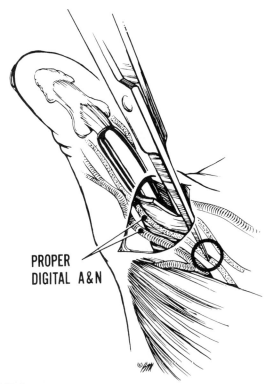

PROPER DIGITAL A & N

FIGURE 60-8. The digital nerves are vulnerable to injury if the skin incision is deepened too quickly or if scissors are inserted too far proximally without visualizing the nerves (*circle*).

CRITICAL POINTS: OPEN TRIGGER FINGER RELEASE

- Make an oblique or longitudinal incision distal to the MP flexion crease centered over MP joint.
- Do not cross flexion creases with longitudinal incision.
- Spread down to flexor sheath; retract neurovascular bundles.
- Sharply divide A1 pulley fibers to expose flexor tendons.
- Preserve A2 pulley in fingers; preserve oblique fibers in thumb.
- Confirm complete release by active flexion.
- Use a small conforming bandage and advise immediate motion. Perform early therapy for fixed flexion contractures.

Percutaneous Trigger Finger Release. Open surgical release of trigger digits is not without complication; in fact, some authors report a dissatisfaction rate as high as 15% to 26%.[21,205] With current demands for increased practice productivity and decreased costs for patient management, a simple office procedure that would provide safe and effi-

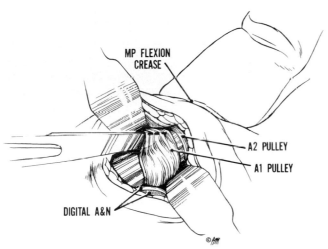

MP FLEXION
CREASE

A2 PULLEY

A1 PULLEY

DIGITAL A&N

FIGURE 60-9. A No. 11 knife blade is used to divide the first annular pulley to relieve triggering in the finger.

cacious treatment for resistant trigger digits would be attractive. Percutaneous trigger release has been reported by several authors to be a safe alternative to traditional open methods using a variety of instruments[56,122,126,202] (Table 60-2). Reported results have been encouraging, with success rates of 74% to 94% at medium-term follow-up and no complications. Incomplete relief of triggering has been reported in a higher percent of patients with grade 4 trigger digits and fixed flexion contractures[79] and among those on hemodialysis.[147] All authors agree that practice on cadaveric hands is recommended before attempting the procedure in patients.

This procedure is done in the office.[56,160] The palm and affected digit are prepped with antiseptic solution and the digit exposed with a fenestrated drape. The MP joints are hyperextended over a rolled towel to displace the neurovascular structures dorsally. The A1 pulley is palpated directly over the metacarpal head. Ethyl chloride is sprayed by an

Table 60-2
PERCUTANEOUS TRIGGER FINGER RELEASE

Author(s)	Year	No. Digits	Findings Instrument	Findings Success Rate	Follow-up (mo)	Notes
Lorthioir[122]	1958	52	Custom "tenotome"	100%		Longitudinal tendon scoring well tolerated
Tanaka et al.[202]	1990	210	4-mm scalpel blade	74%	24	29% poor results in fingers; best results: thumbs
Eastwood et al.[56]	1992	35	21-gauge needle	94%	13	1 repeat release; discouraged for thumbs
Lyu[126]	1992	63	Custom hook device	88%	11	11% conversion to open release; no complications
Stothard and Kumar[197]	1994	18	18-gauge needle	94%		One recurrence; several patients with temporary flexion contractures; superficial tendon scoring
Pope and Wolfe[160]	1995	25 (cadaveric)	19-gauge needle	90%	N/A	Superficial scoring of tendon; not recommended for thumb or index: proximity of digital nerves
	1995	13	19-gauge needle	100%	N/A	5/13 pulleys incompletely divided distally; active trigger necessary to confirm release
Bain et al.[10]	1995 (cadaveric)		14-gauge angiocatheter	68% digits 58% thumb	N/A	Five missed releases; not recommended for thumb or little finger
Nagoshi et al.[147]	1997	67	18-gauge needle	78% idiopathic 62% hemodialysis	9	Active triggering necessary at time of release; higher grades and digits locked in extension do less well with percutaneous method
Cihantimur et al.[42]	1998	34	16-gauge angiocatheter	100%	12	No complications
Dunn and Pess[55]	1999 (cadaveric)	52	Custom push knife	98%	N/A	No nerve or vessel injury; complete release
		26	19-gauge needle	38%		Superficial scoring of tendons
Bain and Wallwork[11]	1999	31	14-gauge angiocatheter	97%	2	Active triggering at time of release; not recommended for locked digits, tenosynovitis
Ha et al.[79]	2001	185	Custom hooked blade	94%	12	No complications; effective for locked digits

assistant as a topical anesthetic, and the skin and flexor tendon sheath are infiltrated with 1 to 2 mL of 1% lidocaine solution using a 27-gauge needle. A 19-gauge needle is placed percutaneously through the annulus, and placement within the flexor tendon is confirmed by asking the patient to slightly flex the digit (Fig. 60-10). The needle is then withdrawn slowly and rotated to align the bevel of the needle along the longitudinal axis of the tendon. A sweeping motion is used to score and section the A1 pulley proximal and distal to the site. Disappearance of a grating sensation indicates complete sectioning of the annulus. The needle is withdrawn, and the patient asked to flex and extend the digit several times. On occasion, a second needle stick is necessary to complete the release. An adhesive bandage is applied, and the patient is instructed to use the hand for activities as tolerated. Patients should be advised to expect a mild to moderate degree of discomfort for several days; ice and anti-inflammatory agents are helpful in the immediate 48 to 72 hours postoperatively.

CRITICAL POINTS: PERCUTANEOUS TRIGGER FINGER RELEASE

- Indicated for recalcitrant digits that have failed one or two corticosteroid injections
- Actively triggering digits may be candidates for percutaneous release.
- The 19-gauge needle using technique of Eastwood[56]:
  - Do not use for thumb and index finger because of proximity of crossing nerves.
  - Hyperextend digit over rolled towel at MP joint to retract nerves.
  - Insert needle into tendon; confirm placement by active tendon motion.
  - Rotate needle to align bevel with tendon; sweep back and forth with tip.
  - One or two needle placements may be necessary to complete division of pulley.
  - Confirm complete release by active flexion of digit

 ## Author's Preferred Method of Treatment

All patients with trigger digits are offered one to two trials of corticosteroid injection. Patients with trigger digits secondary to RA or diabetes are counseled about the reduced success rate with this form of treatment and are not generally offered a second attempt at injection. Resistant primary trigger digits that actively trigger at the time of the office visit may be considered for percutaneous release; active triggering is necessary at the time of release to confirm complete

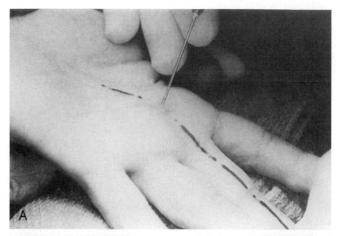

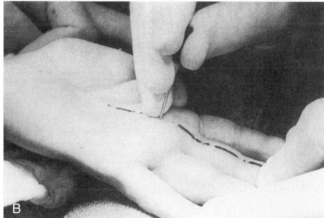

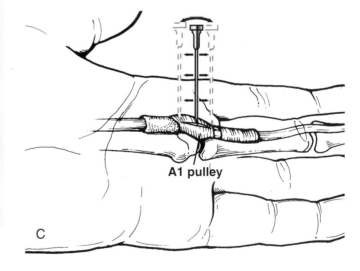

FIGURE 60-10. A, Percutaneous release of a long finger A1 pulley. The MP joint is hyperextended and a 19-gauge needle inserted just distal to the palmar crease. The bevel of the needle is oriented longitudinally with the tendon. The skin markings indicate the path of the flexor tendons. **B,** The needle is stabilized and the pulley is released in a proximal-to-distal direction. Elimination of a grating sensation as the pulley is cut indicates completion of the release. **C,** A proximal-to-distal sweeping motion of the needle is used to lyse the annular pulley. (**A** and **B** from Pope DF, Wolfe SW: Safety and efficacy of percutaneous trigger finger release. J Hand Surg [Am] 20:280-283, 1995, with permission.)

sectioning of the annulus. The technique is not used in the index finger and thumb or for digits with PIP joint contractures. Open release is performed through a 1-cm longitudinal or oblique incision placed in the skin lines and directly over the A1 pulley. The thumb is released through a 1.5-cm transverse incision at the level of the MP flexion crease.

Complications

There have been no reported nerve or vascular complications with steroid injection or percutaneous trigger finger release. If the trigger finger has been locked in flexion for a while before surgery, the patient may require hand therapy and dynamic splinting to overcome a PIP joint flexion contracture.

Digital nerve injury is an infrequent but serious complication of trigger release by the open method.[36,205] Prompt exploration and repair or reconstruction are indicated. A more frequent complication is incisional tenderness at the operative site.[21] Rarely, recurrence has been reported, requiring reoperation.[205,207] Inadvertent sectioning of all or a portion of the A2 pulley can cause bowstringing with resultant loss of full finger flexion.[83] Littler cautioned against "excessive sectioning" of the flexor sheath of the index finger and recommended an incision along the radial border of the A1 pulley to prevent lateral bowstringing of the index flexor tendons on flexion of the digit (Fig. 60-11).[30,222] If the bowstringing does not resolve, pulley reconstruction may be required (see Chapter 7).

Congenital Trigger Thumb

When a child is seen with a thumb locked in flexion, a variety of diagnoses must be entertained, including congenital clasped thumb, absent or aberrant extensor tendons, arthrogryposis, or spasticity (see Chapter 43). The most common etiology of abnormal thumb posturing in flexion or extension is termed *congenital trigger thumb,* although the digit is rarely seen to trigger or catch as occurs in the adult equivalent.[47,92,224] Pathologic specimens document more frequent thickening and synovial proliferative changes in the tendon itself rather than in the annular sheath, as opposed to adult specimens, which show characteristic thickening and degeneration within the sheath.[59,214] A frequent pathologic finding at surgery is nodular thickening in the tendon, referred to as "Notta's node" after the individual who reportedly first described the trigger phenomenon in 1850 (Fig. 60-12).[214]

Although the condition is rare, the true incidence of trigger thumbs is unknown; among all children seen at a major pediatric hospital, the condition was diagnosed in 0.05%.[70] Whether the condition is truly congenital or acquired is of some controversy because the condition is rarely diagnosed at birth.[47,49,143] Some authors contend that the condition is overlooked until at least 6 months of age because of characteristic flexion posturing of the thumb in newborns.[63,218] Among 70 congenital trigger digits treated by De Smet and colleagues, only 3 digits were reported by the parents as present at birth and only 9 before the age of 6 months.[47] In two prospective series involving a total of 5765 newborns, no trigger thumbs were demonstrated in the nursery, and the authors contend that the condition is acquired rather than congenital.[171,187] Within a cohort of 78 children treated surgically for trigger thumb, none presented before age 3 months.[171] The condition has a bilateral incidence of 25% to 33%,[49,59,70,224] and no association with specific congenital anomalies has been demonstrated.[70,224] Trigger thumbs have been reported among monozygotic twins,[59] and two series have reported a hereditary predisposition.[63,218]

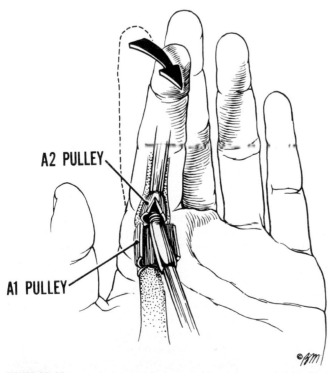

A2 PULLEY

A1 PULLEY

FIGURE 60-11. Incising the second annular pulley can cause bowstringing or ulnar deviation of the finger and should be avoided.

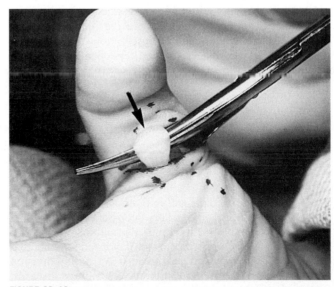

FIGURE 60-12. Inspection of the flexor pollicis longus after release of the first annular pulley reveals the characteristic "Notta's node" *(arrow)* seen in congenital trigger thumbs.

Treatment

Early authors found conservative measures such as observation and splinting to be "uniformly unsuccessful"[59,92] and perhaps causative of deleterious MP hyperextension deformities or fixed IP contractures. A later study of 26 trigger thumbs diagnosed in early infancy by Dinham and Meggitt documented a 31% rate of spontaneous resolution.[49] In children aged 6 to 30 months at diagnosis, however, the same authors cited a recovery rate of only 12% after a 6-month observation period. Ger and coworkers reported no spontaneous resolution among 19 trigger thumbs diagnosed in children younger than 6 months of age and monitored for an average of 44 months.[70] Similarly, Wood and Sicilia found no spontaneous resolution among 37 digits monitored an average of 9 months.[224] Splinting is difficult to maintain, particularly among infants and toddlers. It is unlikely that a 6-month period of observation before surgery will result in any permanent deficit or flexion contracture,[63,224] but surgical treatment will be necessary in virtually all congenital trigger thumbs regardless of age at diagnosis. It is recommended that surgical release be performed before the age of 4 to prevent permanent contracture of the IP joint.

Surgical Technique. A small transverse[70] incision is made over the palpable nodule at the MP flexion crease. Blunt dissection is performed to identify both digital nerves, which lie very superficial at this level. Right-angle retractors are used to retract the neurovascular bundles, and the transverse retinacular pulley is divided to expose the flexor tendon and associated nodule. The oblique fibers of the retinacular pulley system are carefully preserved.[16,53] No attempt is made to excise or reduce the tendon nodule. The flexor tendon should be lifted out of the wound with a blunt instrument to ensure unrestricted range of thumb motion.

Outcomes of surgical release for congenital trigger thumb have been excellent, with no reports of recurrence and few complications.[70,224] McAdams and associates performed a long-term study of 21 patients at an average of 15 years and demonstrated minor deficits in IP extension in 23% of their patients but no functional deficit. Longitudinal incisions in a third of their patients resulted in unsatisfactory scarring and contracture. The authors underscored the importance of a transverse incision and careful preservation of the oblique pulley fibers to prevent changes in tendon mechanics and flexion contracture.[129]

Trigger Digits in Childhood

Rarely, other digits can present with triggering in childhood.[32,59,224] Surgical treatment by release of the A1 pulley is not universally successful, as it is with childhood trigger thumbs, suggesting a different etiology of the condition. In a series of 16 children with 18 trigger digits, Cardon and colleagues demonstrated resolution in triggering in only 10 after A1 pulley division alone. In 6 others, abnormalities of the flexor digitorum superficialis decussation necessitated excision of one or both of its slips.[32] The authors recommend use of an extensile approach to the flexor tendons, so that additional surgery can be performed if A1 pulley division does not resolve triggering. Children with storage diseases, such as Hurler's syndrome, can acquire trigger digits and carpal tunnel syndrome due to abnormal collections of the mucopolysaccharide within and around the flexor tendons.

Surgical decompression has been demonstrated to be successful in improving hand function.[32,208] Seiler and Kerwin reported trigger finger in an adolescent secondary to a painless calcific nodule in the substance of the flexor profundus tendon.[182]

De Quervain's Disease

There are six separate compartments under the dorsal carpal ligament, each lined with a separate synovial sheath membrane (Fig. 60-13). The first of these, which is over the styloid process of the radius, contains the abductor pollicis longus and extensor pollicis brevis tendons. These tendons pass through an unyielding osteoligamentous tunnel formed by a shallow groove in the radial styloid process and a tough overlying roof composed of the transverse fibers of the dorsal ligament attached by vertical septa to bone. This fibrous tunnel is about 2 cm long, whereas the synovial sheath extends from each musculotendinous junction proximally to the tendon insertions well beyond the tunnel itself.

Tendon entrapment of the first dorsal compartment of the wrist is a common cause of wrist and hand pain and disability. Fritz de Quervain has been credited with the description, in 1895, of a specific entity involving the abductor pollicis longus and extensor pollicis brevis sheaths at the radial styloid process.[115,120,159] A similar entity had been reported in the 1893 edition of *Gray's Anatomy* and named "washerwoman's sprain."[121,158] The process is attributed to activities requiring frequent abduction of the thumb and simultaneous ulnar deviation at the wrist. Tension on the tendons of the first dorsal compartment, if sustained and repeated, is said to produce friction at the rigid retinacular sheath, with subsequent swelling and/or narrowing of the fibro-osseous canal.[102,159] Acute angulation of the tendons at the retinaculum occurs with wrist extension, and increased angulation of the tendons in women was suggested by Bunnell to help explain their markedly increased prevalence of the disease.[28] Aberrant tendons and variations in anatomy of the tendons and their sheaths have been thought by several authors to contribute to the process and help explain the poor response to conservative treatment in certain individuals.[29,81,117,121,138]

The diagnosis is usually made without difficulty after eliciting a complaint of several weeks or months of pain localized to the radial side of the wrist and aggravated by movement of the thumb. The average age in most series is in the fifth and sixth decades, and the syndrome may be up to six times more common in women.[81,159,194,215,220] The disease is also frequently diagnosed in a much younger cohort of recent postpartum and lactating females.[8,208] Findings of local tenderness and swelling 1 to 2 cm proximal to the radial styloid and knifelike pain when the thumb is clasped in the palm and the wrist forced into ulnar deviation (Finklestein's test) are diagnostic of the disease.[61,159] Pseudo-triggering of the thumb has been reported in several series[41,59,220] and may be related to the presence of a separate fibro-osseous tunnel for the extensor pollicis brevis tendon.[211]

De Quervain's disease must be differentiated from the less commonly recognized painful condition of intersection syndrome, in which pain, swelling, and, in severe cases, crepitus is found 4 cm proximal to the wrist. De Quervain's disease should also be differentiated by radiograph and physical

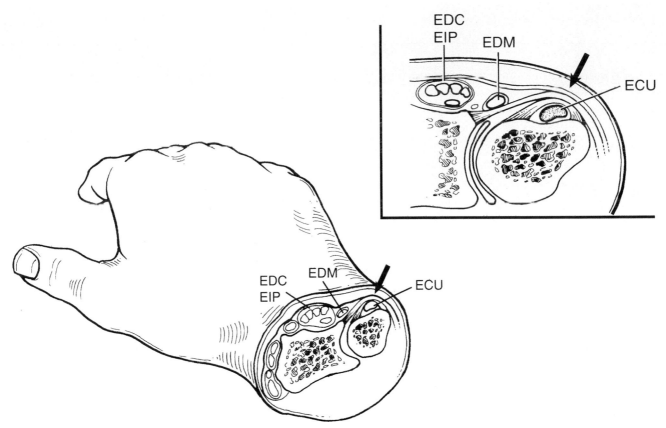

FIGURE 60-13. The six separate synovium-lined retinacular compartments on the dorsum of the wrist. Note the contribution of the extensor carpi ulnaris tendon sheath to the triangular fibrocartilage complex *(arrow)*.

examination from arthritis of the thumb carpometacarpal and/or scaphotrapezial-trapezoid joints, although these lesions may coexist because of their similar demographics.[6,134] Radiographic study also excludes scaphoid fracture and arthrosis involving the radiocarpal or intercarpal joints. Technetium bone scanning may show increased uptake in the distal radius deep to the first dorsal compartment, but it is more likely to be negative. Occasionally, radiographs show localized osteopenia or spurring at the radial styloid[29,194] (Fig. 60-14).

Treatment
Nonoperative
In acute cases, some success has been reported after immobilization in a cast with the wrist gently extended and the thumb widely abducted,[115,121,194] but, in my experience, symptoms tend to recur shortly after removal of the cast when the inciting activity is resumed. In a prospective study, splint immobilization alone led to a 70% failure rate among 37 wrists and was shown to provide no additional benefit when combined with corticosteroid injection of the first dorsal compartment sheath.[215]

As with trigger digits, corticosteroid injection was initially discouraged as ineffective[59] but later hailed as a successful form of treatment for de Quervain's disease.[114,115,120] Success with corticosteroid injection has been reported in 50% to 80% of patients after one to two injections[81,158,215] and is particularly effective in relatively acute cases.[115] A lower rate of success among diabetics has been suggested.[215]

In de Quervain's disease of pregnancy and lactation, non-operative treatment is highly effective, and the condition tends to resolve after cessation of lactation.[8,166,179,181] In a comparative study of splinting and corticosteroid injection, Avci and coworkers demonstrated complete resolution of pain and disappearance of Finklestein's test after methyl-prednisolone injection in nine patients, whereas all patients in the splinted group continued to report pain during the treatment period. Eight of the nine patients in the latter group experienced complete resolution 2 to 6 weeks after cessation of lactation.[8]

Technique of Injection. The radial styloid area is prepped with antiseptic solution. A number of corticosteroid preparations are available and differ predominantly in their solubility and thus their duration of action.[130] Some data suggest that the less soluble preparations may contribute to a higher incidence of local complications, including depigmentation, subcutaneous atrophy, and fat necrosis (Fig. 60-15).[152] Therefore, in this very superficial location I prefer a water-soluble preparation of 1 mL dexamethasone mixed with 0.5 mL of 1% plain lidocaine (no epinephrine). The anesthetic effect of lidocaine allows confirmation of correct needle placement and diagnosis by immediate, temporary relief of discomfort.

The first dorsal compartment tendons can easily be palpated as the patient abducts and extends the thumb. While ethyl chloride is sprayed as a local refrigerant, the examiner's gloved index finger and thumb bracket the tendons at a level

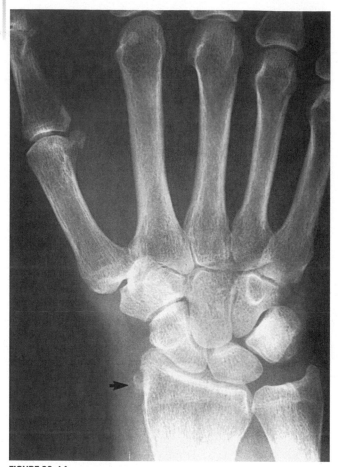

FIGURE 60-14. Anteroposterior radiographs of the wrist in a patient with de Quervain's disease occasionally reveal localized osteopenia or a small spur (*arrow*).

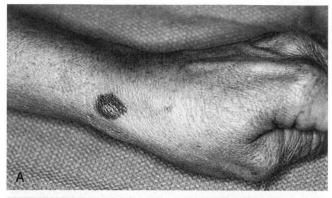

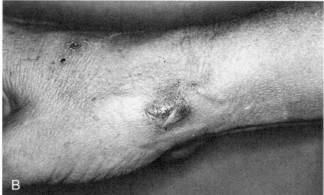

FIGURE 60-15. Local complications from the use of local corticosteroid injections for the treatment of de Quervain's disease. Although successfully relieved of pain, both patients had localized capillary fragility and recurrent transient hemangioma-like lesions at the site of injection.

1 cm proximal to the radial styloid, which serves to steady the patient's wrist and localize the injection site. A 27-gauge needle is introduced into the tendon sheath, and resistance may be felt as the injection is attempted. The needle is slowly backed out of the tendon while pressure is maintained on the plunger, and a fluid wave should be palpable proximal and distal to the injection site as the abductor pollicis longus sheath fills. A portion of the solution should be redirected slightly dorsal (ulnar) to the first site in an attempt to infiltrate a possible separate extensor pollicis brevis sheath.[117] In a study in which radiopaque dye was mixed with a corticosteroid and injected into the first dorsal compartment, 13 of 19 wrists failed to demonstrate dye filling the extensor pollicis brevis subsheath, suggesting that it is technically more difficult to successfully administer the medication to the extensor pollicis brevis compartment.[229] Should the injection fail to relieve symptoms, a second injection may be performed 4 to 6 weeks after the first; however, repeated injections are not indicated and may be detrimental to local tissues.

Surgical Treatment

Pertinent Anatomy. Although early anatomic textbooks showed one long thumb abductor tendon accompanying one extensor brevis tendon passing through a single first dorsal compartment as the normal anatomy, numerous modern anatomic and surgical studies have shown that this is not usually the case.[6,29,61,115,121,159,194] In most reports, fewer than 20% of cases showed the so-called normal anatomy.[91,121,138,198]

In fact, the first dorsal compartment of the wrist is probably the site of the most numerous variations in tendon structure and organization in the upper limb. Failure to recognize these variations can cause persistence or recurrence of pain because of incomplete surgical release of the tendon sheath.[6,19,123]

The extensor pollicis brevis is a phylogenetically young structure found only in humans and gorillas as a separate muscle distinct from the thumb abductor.[102] The muscle is always thinner than the abductor and is absent in 5% to 7% of people.[194] The larger abductor pollicis longus usually has two and sometimes three or more tendinous slips inserting variously into the base of the first metacarpal, trapezium, volar carpal ligament, opponens pollicis, or abductor pollicis brevis.[121,194,198]

In 24% to 34% of specimens in anatomic studies, the first compartment was found to be subdivided by a longitudinal ridge and septum into two distinct osteofibrous tunnels, the ulnar one for the extensor pollicis brevis and the radial containing one or more slips of the abductor pollicis longus.[102,115,117] A third deep tunnel containing an anomalous tendon has also been reported.[121] The reported incidence of separate compartments at surgery is higher than that seen in anatomic specimens in several series,[81,120,177,198,215,221] which raises the possibility that septation of the extensor pollicis brevis increases the probability that nonsurgical treatment will fail. Harvey and associates reported success with one or two corticosteroid injections in 80% of patients and found separate compartments for the abductor pollicis longus and extensor pollicis brevis in 10 of 11 wrists that failed injection and required surgical release.[81] As noted in various published reports of operative findings, either one or both subdivisions of the first dorsal compartment may be stenotic.[121] The recently described *extensor pollicis brevis entrapment test* was reported to be 81% sensitive in its ability to discriminate the presence of a septated extensor pollicis brevis compartment in those patients who had failed corticosteroid treatment and required surgery. The test is a two-part test in which the patient is asked to forcibly (1) extend the MP joint or (2) abduct the CMC joint against resistance from the examiner.[3] Pain during the MP joint portion of the test is said to be a positive predictor of a separate compartment for the extensor pollicis brevis tendon.

The anatomic relationship of the radial artery and nerve to this compartment must be understood to prevent complicating injury to these structures during surgical release of the tendons (Fig. 60-16). The radial artery passes diagonally across the anatomical snuff-box from the volar aspect of the wrist to the dorsum of the web space deep to the thumb abductor and both extensors. It is separated from the first compartment sheath by enough areolar tissue that it need not be exposed during the dissection if the surgeon does not perforate the floor of the sheath distal to the radial styloid. However, two or three terminal divisions of the radial sensory nerve lie immediately superficial to the first dorsal compartment and must be identified and protected during the surgical procedure.[2,164]

The procedure is usually performed with only local infiltration anesthesia. A pneumatic tourniquet around the forearm[90] is well tolerated for the short duration of the proce-dure, and a bloodless surgical field is essential for the identification of radial sensory branches, as well as the anatomic variations discussed earlier.

A 2-cm transverse skin incision is made over the first dorsal compartment about 1 cm proximal to the tip of the radial styloid process (Fig. 60-17). Care is taken to identify and gently retract the one to three radial sensory branches that cross the compartment obliquely by using gentle, blunt longitudinal dissection as soon as the deepest dermal layer of skin has been incised. A common technical error is to transversely incise the subcutaneous fat with the skin knife, which may injure a superficial nerve branch. The exposed annular ligament covering the compartment is sharply incised with a scalpel.

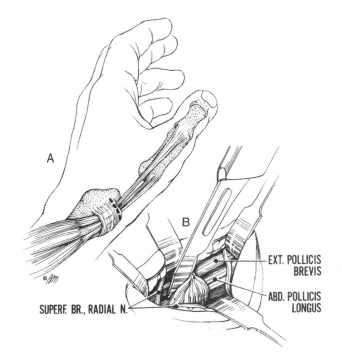

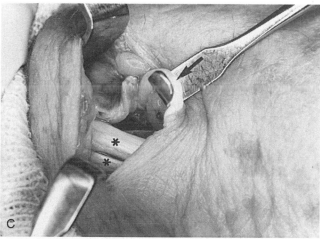

FIGURE 60-17. Tenovaginotomy for de Quervain's disease. **A,** The first dorsal compartment is approached by a short transverse skin incision. **B,** The annular ligament is incised with a scalpel from the snuff-box to the musculotendinous junctions. **C,** Surgical demonstration of a separate compartment for the extensor pollicis brevis (EPB) *(arrow)* after release of the abductor pollicis longus (APL) *(asterisks).*

FIGURE 60-16. Anatomic relationships of the first dorsal compartment.

CRITICAL POINTS: DE QUERVAIN'S RELEASE

- Positive response to diagnostic injection should precede decision for surgery.
- Use a transverse incision; protect numerous superficial sensory nerves.
- Incise sheath on dorsal margin to prevent tendon subluxation.
- Inspect for separate extensor pollicis brevis tendon and excise septa.
- Ask patient to voluntarily move thumb to confirm release.

Complete excision of the entire sheath should be avoided because this has occasionally been associated with painful palmar subluxation of the tendons postoperatively.[2,29,217] Burton and Littler recommended incising the sheath on its most dorsal margin and leaving a flap of palmar sheath to prevent subluxation.[30,222] Although the particular site of sheath incision is disputed,[132] all authors agree that a thorough exploration for separate compartments must be performed, with complete division of all intervening septa and identification of each tendon slip. Unusually thick septa can be excised entirely. If the tenosynovial tissue is thick and opaque, surgical debulking is performed. The tendons are lifted by hook or blunt retractors out of the tunnel to ensure complete decompression from their musculotendinous junctions to a point at least 1 cm distal to the retinacular sheath. The tendons are replaced and the patient moves the thumb to demonstrate free and independent movement of the long abductor and short extensor. It is imperative that the separate tendon of the extensor pollicis brevis be specifically identified by demonstrating passive extension of the thumb MP joint with gentle retraction on the tendon.

Hemostasis is established with cautery after tourniquet release, and the skin is closed with a single intradermal monofilament pull-out suture and adhesive bandages. A soft bulky dressing is applied and thumb motion is encouraged in the immediate postoperative period. If it is thought that the released tendons are unstable after release, a palmar thumb spica splint may be applied with the wrist in 20 degrees of extension for 10 to 14 days, although this is rarely necessary. Thereafter, the patient may begin to resume use of the thumb and wrist as tolerated. Supervised hand therapy is rarely necessary. Localized soreness may persist for 4 to 6 weeks postoperatively and generally responds to wound massage and light use of the hand. It is advised to avoid heavy mechanical activities for the initial 4 to 6 weeks.

Complications

Not infrequently, extravasation of injected corticosteroids into the superficial tissues can cause subcutaneous atrophy, fat necrosis, and/or depigmentation.[6,74,130,152,177] Darker-skinned individuals are particularly prone to this occurrence, and all patients should be counseled before injection about the 5% to 10% risk of this complication. In my experience, these have usually resolved within a year, but persistent symptoms can be severe enough to warrant transposition of healthy skin or fat grafts to the area.

The most serious complication of this operation follows iatrogenic injury to a superficial sensory branch of the radial nerve with the subsequent formation of a painful neuroma.[2,6,119] Overly vigorous retraction of a radial nerve branch without apparent injury may cause a painful neuroma-in-continuity. Injuries to this vulnerable nerve can result in excruciating, disabling symptoms that dwarf the initial symptoms in severity.[222] Management of an inadvertently lacerated radial sensory nerve is a controversial subject. Some authors advise resection of the lacerated nerve to put the resultant neuroma well above the operative scar, where it will be less exposed to repeated contusion.[6] However, not entirely happy with the persistent pain of those who have undergone proximal transposition of painful forearm neuromas, I agree with those who advocate immediate nerve reapproximation by appropriate microsurgical techniques to reduce the likelihood of neuroma formation and minimize hypoesthesia in the thumb and index finger.[119] (For a more detailed discussion of this complication, the reader is referred to Chapter 30.)

Incomplete relief of pain after release of the first dorsal compartment, especially among working women, is not uncommon.[6] Associated diagnoses, including painful carpometacarpophalangeal joint arthritis or instability, are common and may be confirmed with a diagnostic lidocaine injection to the suspected area. If documentation of specific identification and release of both the EPB and APL tendons in the operative report is lacking, some consideration should be given to re-exploration for an unreleased separate compartment.[102] A preoperative lidocaine challenge can be helpful in this instance as well. Hypertrophic or painful longitudinal scars may be modified by "Z"-plasty. For the rare patient with painful palmar or dorsal subluxation of the tendons after release, pulley reconstruction with a slip of extensor retinaculum,[217] a distally based slip of the brachioradialis,[132] or a strip of the second dorsal compartment retinaculum[99] has been described.

OTHER STENOTIC CONDITIONS OF TENDONS AT THE WRIST

 Anatomy

The second compartment contains the two radial wrist extensors, the extensor carpi radialis longus and brevis, respectively. The third compartment contains the extensor pollicis longus tendon, which angulates acutely around Lister's tubercle en route to the distal phalanx of the thumb. Four slips of the extensor digitorum communis tendon and the single extensor indicis proprius tendon compose the fourth compartment. The fifth and sixth compartments each contain a single tendon: the extensor digiti minimi and the extensor carpi ulnaris tendons. The floor of the extensor carpi ulnaris tendon sheath is quite thick and forms an important structural component of the triangular fibrocartilage complex that aids in stabilization of the distal radioulnar joint.[100,189] Although each of the dorsal extensor compartments may be involved in tendon entrapment, the most commonly involved are the first and sixth compartments.

Intersection Syndrome

Pain and swelling about the muscle bellies of the abductor pollicis longus and extensor pollicis brevis are characteristic of intersection syndrome. This area, which lies about 4 cm proximal to the wrist joint, may show increased swelling of a normally prominent area (Fig. 60-18) and, in severe cases, redness and crepitus.[222] Although previously thought to be the result of friction between the muscle bellies of the abductor pollicis longus and the extensor pollicis brevis and the radial wrist extensor tendons,[24,51,86,223] Grundberg and Reagan demonstrated the basic pathology to be tendon entrapment of the second dorsal compartment.[78]

The syndrome, like other stenotic conditions about the hand and wrist, has been associated with activities requiring frequent or repetitive motions of the wrist.[24,29,156] It is frequently seen among athletes, particularly in sports such as rowing and weightlifting.[222] Initial nonoperative treatment consists of modification of activities, a thermoplastic molded wrist splint in 15 degrees of extension, and, in some patients, steroid injection into the second dorsal compartment. The majority of patients thus treated improve and remain permanently asymptomatic.

For those with persistent pain, Grundberg and Reagan suggested a longitudinal incision to approach the radial wrist extensors beginning at the wrist and extending proximal to the swollen area.[78] After incising the deep fascia, release of the second dorsal compartment demonstrates the area of pathology (Fig. 60-19). The tendons are elevated and inspected, and no attempt is made to close the retinaculum. The wrist is splinted in neutral to slight extension for 10 days postoperatively, and patients are advised to use the hand and wrist as tolerated thereafter. Although bowstringing of the extensor tendons is a theoretic problem after incising the dorsal retinaculum, Grundberg and Reagan did not report this in their series of 13 cases.

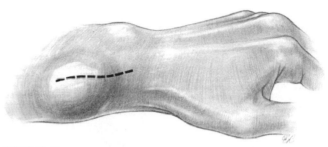

FIGURE 60-18. A patient with intersection syndrome manifests swelling in the area where the abductor pollicis longus and extensor pollicis brevis cross the common radial wrist extensors. The dotted line indicates the location of the surgical incision. (Adapted from Grundberg AB, Reagan DS: Pathologic anatomy of the forearm: Intersection syndrome. J Hand Surg [Am] 10:299-302, 1985, with permission.)

Extensor Pollicis Longus

Tendon entrapment of the extensor pollicis longus occurs rarely but requires early diagnosis and urgent operative treatment to prevent tendon rupture, a complication that is seldom seen in de Quervain's disease, trigger finger, or trigger thumb. The condition is recognized by pain, swelling, tenderness, and often crepitus on the dorsum of the distal radius at Lister's tubercle, around which the long thumb extensor tendon veers toward its insertion on the thumb. Passive or active flexion of the thumb IP joint is associated with pain at the level of Lister's tubercle, and triggering has been reported.[112,133] The tendon has a separate synovial sheath-lined tunnel beneath the extensor retinaculum that may be compromised by blunt trauma[112] or Colles' fracture.[57] Rupture of the tendon has been reported and occurs most commonly in initially undisplaced fractures.[37,50] Its tendency to rupture under these circumstances may be secondary to local ischemia produced by increased pressure within a relatively unyielding fibro-osseous canal. Microvascular studies have demonstrated a watershed zone in proximity to Lister's tubercle, wherein the tendon is entirely dependent on synovial fluid for its nutrition,[57] and may be vulnerable to ischemic rupture after local trauma.[112] The condition may also be caused by degenerative or inflammatory conditions of the wrist.[222]

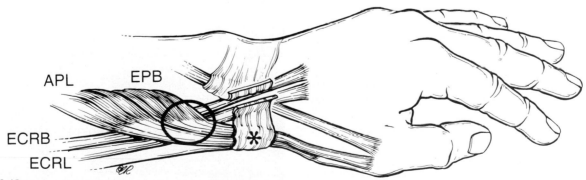

FIGURE 60-19. The *circled area* shows where the extensor pollicis brevis and abductor pollicis longus cross the common radial wrist extensors. The location of the first dorsal compartment where de Quervain's disease occurs is indicated with an asterisk. The second dorsal compartment has been released in the manner recommended for treatment of intersection syndrome.

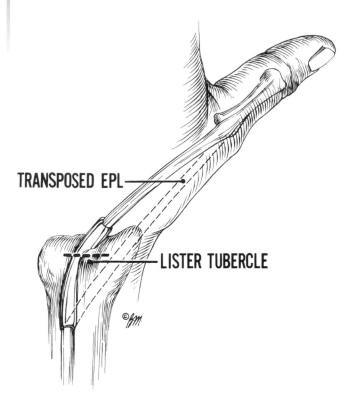

FIGURE 60-20. The extensor pollicis longus (EPL) tendon is rerouted superficially radial to Lister's tubercle (*dotted lines*) to relieve tenosynovitis.

Operative treatment is recommended to prevent attritional rupture of the tendon. The tendon is exposed through a 2-cm dorsal incision centered over Lister's tubercle. Care is taken to avoid injury to small branches of the radial sensory nerve. The third dorsal compartment is identified and incised completely, and the tendon is elevated from its bed and transposed radial to the tubercle. Any osteophytes within the tunnel may be débrided and the tunnel closed to prevent a return to the groove (Fig. 63-20). The skin is closed with a single subcuticular suture, and postoperative splinting is not necessary. Unrestricted use of the hand and wrist is permitted as tolerated.

Fourth and Fifth Extensor Compartments

Although common among patients with RA, primary symptomatic stenosis of the fourth and fifth extensor compartments is extremely rare.[54,85] The condition most commonly affects the extensor digitorum communis tendons to the index and small digits because these tendons angulate more acutely at the distal edge of the retinacular sheath.[29] Isolated extensor indicis proprius tenosynovitis has been reported and is attributed to presence of the distal extensor indicis proprius muscle belly within the retinacular sheath.[190] The process may be initiated after Colles' fracture[54] and has also been thought to be due to increased demands on the extensor tendons secondary to loss of wrist flexion.[29] Clinical findings demonstrate tenderness and swelling over the affected compartment. With the wrist flexed, pain may be elicited at the involved retinacular sheath by attempted MP extension against resistance.[54,190] Pathologic findings show marked

thickening of the tendon sheath, tight stenosis, and sparse inflammatory tissue.[85] Duplicate tendons or anomalous muscle bellies should be suspected in a patient who does not respond to the usual conservative modalities of rest, ice, anti-inflammatory medications, or corticosteroid injection.[85,222]

Extensor Carpi Ulnaris

Reactive tenosynovitis of the extensor carpi ulnaris tendon is not uncommon[66,146] and must be included in the differential diagnosis of ulnar-sided wrist pain. The condition is usually initiated by a twisting injury, followed within 24 to 48 hours by increasing pain and swelling.[68,104] Nocturnal pain is frequent and occasionally severe enough to interfere with sleep. Dysesthesias along the course of the overlying dorsal sensory branch of the ulnar nerve are frequent findings.[48] Because the floor of the extensor carpi ulnaris tendon sheath is an important stabilizer of the triangular fibrocartilage complex,[100,189] the process may be difficult to differentiate from traumatic disruption of this complex.

Pain is generally poorly localized by the patient and frequently felt to be deep within the joint. Pain is increased with all motions of the wrist, and extension/ulnar deviation against applied resistance is indicative of the process. Crepitus may be palpable within the swollen extensor carpi ulnaris sheath (Fig. 60-21).[48,68] The condition may coexist with tendon entrapment of other wrist compartments, triangular fibrocartilage complex tears, distal radioulnar degenerative disease, and carpal tunnel syndrome.[104] Instability of the tendon must be differentiated from tendon entrapment and can be elicited by palpating the tendon while the patient actively rotates the extended wrist from full supination to pronation. The tendon may subluxate, occasionally with an audible snap, as the supinated wrist is brought from extension into ulnar deviation and flexion.[222]

Transient but complete relief of discomfort with lidocaine filling of the extensor carpi ulnaris sheath confirms the diagnosis and differentiates the process from an intra-articular injury. Conservative treatment with ice, extension splinting or casting, and anti-inflammatory agents generally

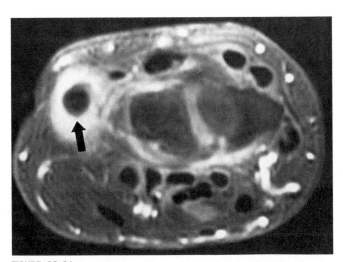

FIGURE 60-21. Magnetic resonance image of the wrist demonstrating abundant tenosynovial thickening and a halo of edema surrounding the extensor carpi ulnaris (ECU) tendon (*arrow*).

provides relief of symptoms.[66,68,80,104] Corticosteroid injection is helpful when splinting and anti-inflammatory medications have failed.[146] On occasion, recalcitrant cases require surgical release of the stenotic retinacular sheath. Among operative cases, splitting or fraying of the extensor carpi ulnaris tendon is frequently observed.

Surgical Treatment

Operative treatment involves complete incision of the fibro-osseous canal of the sixth dorsal compartment through a 3-cm curvilinear incision over the distal radioulnar joint that parallels the course of the underlying ulnar sensory nerve. Care must be taken to identify and protect subcutaneous nerve branches with vessel loops throughout the procedure. Controversy exists about whether retinacular repair is necessary to prevent postoperative instabilty,[48,80] but no reports of instability after release without retinacular repair have been reported.[29,48,68,146] In an effort to resolve this question, Kip and Peimer reported on 17 patients after complete division of the fibro-osseous tunnel with no attempt to repair or reconstruct the retinaculum and found no symptoms or signs of instability.[104]

Flexor Carpi Radialis Tendonitis

The sharp angulation of the flexor carpi radialis tendon across the ridge of the trapezium and the tight fibrous canal through which it runs on its course to the base of the index metacarpal make this tendon prone to stenotic tendovaginitis. The multiplicity of other diagnoses in the immediate vicinity of the tendon, including ganglion cysts, basal joint degenerative disease, scaphoid fractures and nonunions, and de Quervain's disease, may lead to misdiagnosis and prolong the treatment of this condition.

 ## Anatomy

On the flexor surface, the radial and ulnar wrist flexors span the carpal tunnel, and each enters a short tenosynovial sheath where it crosses the wrist joint. The musculotendinous junction of the flexor carpi radialis tendon is located approximately 8 cm proximal to the wrist crease, and the tendon is surrounded by a thin paratenon. The tendon becomes invested by the antebrachial fascia as it approaches the wrist crease and is completely lined by a true synovial sheath from the level of the trapezial crest to the metacarpal insertion distally.[20] Bishop and colleagues[20] demonstrated that the tendon is nearly encircled by the tubercle of the trapezium, which constitutes between 61% and 80% of the wall of the tunnel. Within this tunnel, these authors found the tendon to occupy 90% of the available cross-sectional area. The authors propose that the tendon's narrow fibrous sheath and the rigid anchoring of the tendon to the wall of the trapezium make it vulnerable to both primary stenotic tendovaginitis and secondary injury in association with traumatic or degenerative lesions of the carpus.

Pain is most pronounced at the palmar wrist crease over the scaphoid tubercle. Increased pain with resisted wrist flexion and radial deviation is pathognomonic of the process.[62] Localized swelling may be evident, and a ganglion may overlie the tendon. A successful lidocaine injection in the offending sheath confirms the diagnosis.

The condition typically affects persons in their fifth decade and is more often diagnosed in women. The process does not appear to have a predilection for the dominant hand.[67,213] Most cases develop insidiously, and a history of repetitive flexion/extension of the wrist or blunt trauma is rarely elicited. Fitton and coworkers[62] reported trapezial degenerative disease in 29 of 30 patients and proposed that the neighboring degenerative process was responsible for attrition and fraying of the flexor carpi radialis within the overlying tendon sheath.

Treatment

Nonoperative Treatment

As for other stenotic conditions of the wrist tendons, treatment is nonoperative initially, with a period of splinting, ice, and anti-inflammatory agents. Corticosteroid injection may provide temporary or lasting relief in cases not associated with neighboring degenerative disease or bone spurs. Nonoperative treatment in secondary cases, however, should not be prolonged inasmuch as tendon fraying and rupture have been reported in several cases.[62,213]

Operative Technique

Exposure of the tendon is performed through a 3-cm longitudinal incision over the flexor carpi radialis tendon that extends proximally from the wrist crease. Care must be taken to avoid injury to the nearby palmar cutaneous branch of the median nerve, as well as the thenar branches of the radial sensory nerve. Limited elevation of the thenar muscles can be performed for exposure. The sheath is opened proximal to the fibrous tunnel and dissection carried distally to a point just beyond the trapezial tubercle. The tendon should be elevated and inspected, with frayed or degenerated fibers excised. If the trapezial groove has rough, sharp edges or osteophytes, limited débridement with a small rongeur should probably be done. No attempt is made to approximate the sheath, and the wound is closed with a subcuticular suture. A conforming dressing is applied, and gradually increasing activity is resumed within 7 to 10 days of surgery.

ANNOTATED REFERENCES

20. Bishop AT, Gabel G, Carmichael SW: Flexor carpi radialis tendinitis: I. Operative anatomy. J. Bone Joint Surg Am 76:1009-1014, 1994.

   The authors call our attention to an uncommon cause of radiovolar wrist pain in this two-part anatomic and clinical study. This seminal study details an effective diagnostic and treatment regimen for a largely overlooked tendinopathy.

31. Bush DC, Schneider LH: Tuberculosis of the hand and wrist. J Hand Surg [Am] 9:391-398, 1984.

   This important report of 11 cases of tuberculous tenosynovitis and arthritis details the often striking similarities of TB and rheumatoid arthritic involvement of the hand and wrist. Delay and misdiagnosis are common, and the authors recommend vigilance for this dangerous "mimic" when faced with localized and painless synovitis of the wrist.

35. Carroll RE, Sinton W: Acute calcium deposits in the hand. JAMA 130:422-426, 1955.

By compiling records of 100 patients treated for this exquisitely painful and often misdiagnosed condition, the authors remind us to maintain a high level of suspicion in order to correctly diagnose and expeditiously treat these patients. The flexor carpi ulnaris tendon was the most common location, and specialized radiographs are helpful to confirm the diagnosis.

53. Doyle JR, Blythe W: Anatomy of the flexor tendon sheath and pulleys of the thumb. J Hand Surg [Am] 2:149-151, 1977.

This simple and elegant study detailed the anatomic arrangement and mechanical importance of the oblique and transverse components of the pulley system of the thumb flexor sheath. Division of either transverse component had minimal effect on MP or IP joint flexion, whereas division of the oblique band resulted in significant loss of IP joint flexion. The oblique fibers, which run from ulnoproximal to radiodistal, should be preserved during trigger thumb release and flexor tendon repair.

56. Eastwood DM, Gupta KJ, Johnson DP: Percutaneous release of the trigger finger: An office procedure. J Hand Surg [Am] 17:114-117, 1992.

The authors present a quick, cost-effective and simple technique to safely divide the A1 pulley in an office setting. The technique requires no special instruments and is easily replicated. Subsequent studies have confirmed the authors' caution about use of this technique in the thumb.

59. Fahey JJ, Bollinger JA: Trigger-finger in adults and children. J Bone Joint Surg 36:1200-1218, 1954.

This comprehensive treatise on trigger digits provides the reader with a clear understanding of the pathogenesis, etiology, operative findings, and outcomes of treatment for tendon entrapment in children and adults.

61. Finklestein H: Stenosing tendovaginitis at the radial styloid process. J Bone Joint Surg Am 12:509-540, 1930.

This landmark paper was the first comprehensive American study of this common phenomenon, described over thirty years earlier in Europe. At the time of publication, stenosing tendovaginitis of the wrist was commonly misdiagnosed as inflammatory arthritis, neuritis, or even tuberculous osteomyelitis. Finkelstein described the pathognomonic signs as well as the diagnostic test that bears his name in this clinical, anatomic, and histopathologic analysis. He successfully replicated the syndrome in a rabbit model by chemical, thermal, and traumatic injury to the first dorsal compartment sheath, and conclusively demonstrated the pathologic alterations in the retinacular sheath that are the hallmark of this condition.

78. Grundberg AB, Reagan DS: Pathologic anatomy of the forearm: Intersection syndrome. J Hand Surg [Am] 10:299-302, 1985.

Intersection syndrome had heretofore been mistakenly attributed to friction between the muscle bellies of the abductor pollicis longus and extensor carpi tendons. Drs. Grundberg and Reagan definitively demonstrated pathology confined to the second dorsal retinacular compartment and reported improvement in 13 patients with this rare form of tendon entrapment.

87. Hueston JT, Wilson WF: The aetiology of trigger finger. Hand 4:257-260, 1972.

The authors propose that the spiral arrangement of tendon fibrils within the flexor tendons allows bunching and nodule formation on either side of the stenotic A1 pulley, akin to drawing a multifilament thread through the narrow eye of a needle.

104. Kip PC, Peimer CA: Release of the sixth dorsal compartment. J Hand Surg [Am] 19:599-601, 1994.

Effective methods of conservative and surgical treatment are outlined in this review of 22 patients with a relatively uncommon tendon entrapment of the wrist. The authors demonstrated that reconstruction of the released compartment was not necessary and instability did not develop postoperatively.

141. Moore JS: Flexor tendon entrapment of the digits (trigger finger and trigger thumb). J Occup Environ Med 42:526-545, 2002.

The author presents a well-organized compendium of the literature on this topic and proposes that the term *stenosing tenosynovitis* be discarded in favor of flexor tendon entrapment to more appropriately describe this "uncomplicated and non-controversial" disorder. A balanced review of the literature in support of and against an occupational cause of the condition is provided.

153. Newport ML, Lane LB, Stuchin SA: Treatment of trigger finger by steroid injection. J Hand Surg [Am] 15:748-750, 1990.

The authors present a large series of trigger digits treated with a uniform technique of corticosteroid injection with long-term follow-up and helped to establish corticosteroid injection as the first-line treatment for trigger fingers.

171. Rodgers WB, Waters PM: Incidence of trigger digits in newborns. J Hand Surg [Am] 19:364-368, 1994.

Despite incidence estimates of congenital trigger thumb ranging from 0.5% to 2%, no study had previously examined newborns in a prospective fashion. Rodgers and Waters challenge the commonly held belief that trigger digits in children represent congenital anomalies by finding no trigger digits in a population of 1046 newborns. The authors propose that the condition is acquired and present additional data on 89 trigger thumb surgeries to further support their argument.

176. Sampson SP, Badalamente MA, Hurst LC, Seidman J: Pathobiology of the human A1 pulley in trigger finger. J Hand Surg [Am] 16:714-721, 1991.

This elegant microscopic and immunohistochemical study provided compelling evidence to eliminate the term *tenosynovitis* when describing tendon entrapment of the digits. The authors demonstrated chondrocytic proliferation and fibrocartilage metaplasia in the "friction layer" of the annular pulley, supporting stenosis of the annular pulley as the primary cause of noninflammatory trigger digits.

208. Van Heest AE, House J, Krivit W, Walker K: Surgical treatment of carpal tunnel syndrome and trigger digits in children with mucopolysaccharide storage disorders. J Hand Surg [Am] 23:236-243, 1998.

Because of a high incidence of median nerve entrapment and trigger digits in children with mucopolysaccharide storage disease, these authors recommend routine screening with electrodiagnostic testing. Improvements in survival secondary to bone marrow transplant make prompt recognition and treatment of carpal tunnel syndrome and trigger digits a priority in management of this disease.

CHAPTER 61

The Burned Hand

Günter Germann and Katrin Philipp

Hands are involved in more than 80% of all severe burns. Although each hand represents less than 3% of the total body surface, the American Burn Association categorizes burns to the hand as major injuries.[72a] Even small burns of the hand may result in severely limited function. When burns of the hand occur as part of a major thermal injury, treatment of the hands receives high priority because a patient's ability to perform useful work after recovery is to a great degree determined by the residual hand function. The functional importance of the hand cannot be overemphasized, because severe hand burns may leave individuals unable to work or even care for themselves. The hand plays a crucial role in the individual's evaluation of the environment ("get a grip on a problem"), in communication with others by sending and receiving emotional signals, and in sexuality, and a person's hands are frequently a mirror image of his or her mental state.[110]

Burns to the hand frequently have devastating consequences not only for the functional outcome but also for the aesthetic appearance. Whereas burned areas at the trunk or the lower extremity can be easily hidden under clothing, burned hands are easily visible. The social and professional re-integration of the patient may be delayed owing to the psychological stigma that is caused by the visible mutilation. For these reasons, burned hands deserve great care and excellent conservative and surgical treatment techniques to achieve not only the best function but also the best possible aesthetic result. The statement of Guy Foucher that "hand surgery is also aesthetic surgery" has never been truer than in the treatment of burned hands. The functional importance of the hand gives it a top priority in modern treatment concepts. Early initiation of physical therapy, splinting, passive exercises, topical treatment, and early excision and grafting where indicated are the most important treatment principles. A multidisciplinary team approach including hand surgeons, physical and occupational therapists, and psychologists should be involved from the day of admission to ensure the best quality of care.

EPIDEMIOLOGY

It is estimated that about 1% of the population in Western countries will have a burn injury each year, of which approximately one fourth will require medical care.[8a] This makes thermal injury the most frequently reported accident. The workplace, however, accounts for fewer than one third of burn unit admissions and fire-related deaths. The upper extremity is the most common anatomic area, being involved in up to 89% of burns.[8a,38a] The two main reasons are the protective reflex with which patients try to guard their faces and the fact that the hand, in most instances, is exposed without any form of protection. The dorsum of the hand is predominantly involved in flame or explosion injuries, whereas injuries to the palm are more frequently found in chemical lesions, friction burns, or high-voltage injuries. Thermal energy may be transmitted directly by contact with a hot object or liquid. More commonly, energy is transmitted indirectly, such as when escaping gas from an oven ignites.

 ## Anatomy

The skin and soft tissues of the hand demonstrate some unique properties. The dorsal skin is thin, is very flexible, and lies on a rather thin subcutaneous layer of fatty tissue. This structure provides little mechanical protection but allows maximum tendon excursion and joint mobility without the necessity of excess skin. The wrinkles over the metacarpophalangeal (MCP) joints and proximal (PIP) and distal interphalangeal (DIP) joints deepen with finger extension and stretch with flexion. Similar movements are facilitated by longitudinal creases in the web space. The dorsal skin contains large superficial veins, hair follicles, and sebaceous glands but no sweat glands. The skin is especially thin over the PIP joints where the extensor tendons are at risk. Rupture of the central slip and PIP joint exposure is one of the most frequently encountered complications after deep dorsal burns. The underlying cause for many postburn functional disturbances is the disruption of the coordinated interplay of extrinsic and intrinsic muscles, tendons, and joints.

The palmar skin shows similarities with the plantar skin of the weight-bearing area of the foot. The thick subcutaneous fatty layer demonstrates a honeycomb-like structure that is shock absorbing and provides grip stability by numerous fibrous septa that connect the skin with deep fascia. Thick epidermal layers are found in the areas of greatest mechanical stress. In the finger, Cleland's (dorsal to the neurovascular bundle) and Grayson's ligaments (palmar to the neurovascular bundle) provide stability.

PATHOPHYSIOLOGY

These anatomic properties facilitate direct thermal effects not seen elsewhere in the body.[95] Besides the blood vessels, tendons and joints are also situated very closely beneath the skin surface over the dorsum of the fingers, making these structures extremely susceptible to the effects of thermal energy. The cylindrical form of the fingers with their ligaments limit swelling and volume change in the finger after thermal injury, causing dermal compartment syndromes in circumferential deep dermal burns.[95]

The severity of a thermal injury depends on the amount of transferred energy, which is correlated to the duration of exposure and the temperature of the heat source. Longer exposures to lower temperatures have the same pathophysiologic consequences as short exposures to high temperatures. The character of the skin at the site of injury also determines the depth of the injury. The palmar skin, for example, withstands greater thermal energy than the dorsal skin. The heat leads to coagulation of blood vessels, denaturation of proteins, and an increase in capillary permeability ("capillary leak"). This phenomenon divides the burn wound into a zone of necrosis, a zone of stasis, and a zone of impaired circulation.[43] Insufficient primary treatment, that is, no escharotomy if indicated or insufficient fluid replacement, may convert the zone of stasis into a zone of necrosis ("after burn") (Fig. 61-1).

Intravascular fluid shifts into the interstitial space and causes a protein-rich edema. Burns of more than 20% body surface area lead to a generalized edema, where swelling of the skin is also encountered in nonburned areas. Edema causes several pathologic effects by creating intercellular pressure and decreased circulation. In the intrinsic musculature of the hand this may lead to a compartment syndrome requiring fasciotomy. Intracellular edema is caused by disruption of the sodium pump, resulting in the entry of sodium and water into the cell.[68] In the hand, persistent interstitial edema that has not resolved after 72 hours may lead to subcutaneous fibrosis with subsequent stiffness of the joints.

Blisters are the cutaneous equivalent of intercellular edema accumulation. The blister fluid is rich in proteins and inflammatory cytokines, leukotrienes, and prostaglandins, besides multiple growth factors such as angiogenic factors[82] and platelet-derived growth factor (PDGF), interleukin (IL-6 and IL-8), and transforming growth factor (TGF) alpha.[83] Fluid losses through blistering may be considerable in major burns because the capability of the epidermis to limit loss of water vapor is out of balance, but fluid loss does not play a role in isolated hand burns. Blisters are found in partial-thickness and superficial dermal burns and are less frequent in deep dermal burns (see later description of determination of depth of burns).

MANAGEMENT OF ACUTE HAND BURNS

Treatment Goals

Any burn injury to the hand, even if considered minimal in extent, can still be catastrophic if the burn is severe enough to result in deformities that render the individual unable to perform personal daily functions. One of the major basic principles of management of injuries to the skin and subcutaneous tissue of the hand is to achieve a healed wound as rapidly as possible. Equally important is to avoid complications that may extend the magnitude of the injury.[38a] The basic considerations in treating a burned hand can be divided into treatment goals and treatment principles.

Treatment should always aim at these goals, taking into consideration that the individual circumstances of the patient may lead to a shift in priorities.[36] To achieve these goals it is recommended to follow the basic treatment principles listed in the accompanying box (Fig. 61-2).

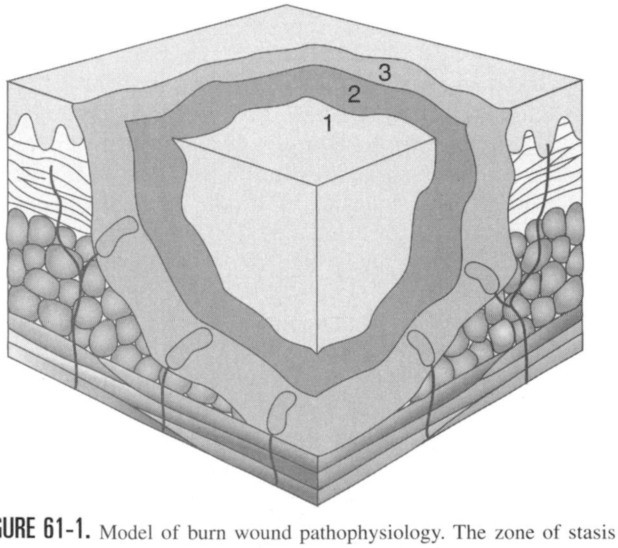

FIGURE 61-1. Model of burn wound pathophysiology. The zone of stasis may convert to a zone of necrosis if no sufficient fluid resuscitation is administered.

BASIC TREATMENT PRINCIPLES OF HAND BURNS

- Evaluation of size and depth of the burn
- Escharotomy if indicated
- Application of proper wound care and dressings
- Decision about conservative or operative treatment
- Initiation of early hand therapy and splinting
- Surgical management: removal of eschar, transplantation of skin grafts, flap coverage if necessary
- Early postoperative physical therapy
- Functional rehabilitation
- Secondary and tertiary corrections if necessary

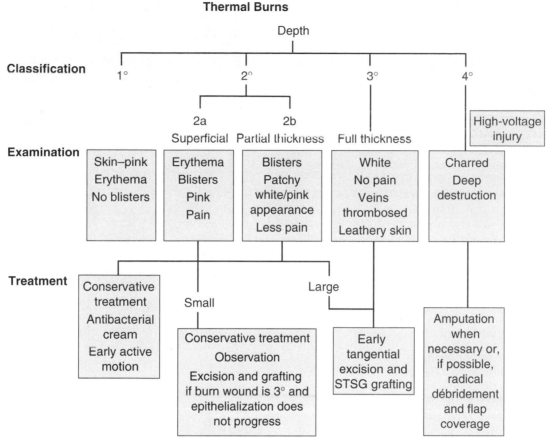

FIGURE 61-2. Decision algorithm for the treatment of cutaneous burns. STSG, split-thickness skin graft. (Redrawn from Germann G, Sherman R, Levin SL: Decision Making in Reconstructive Surgery: Upper Extremity. Berlin, Springer, 1999.)

Initial Evaluation

A careful and comprehensive history of the injury is of great diagnostic value and prognostic importance and may give important information for the necessary treatment decision making. After the history, a thorough physical examination should define the extent and likely depth of the burn, the presence and severity of associated injuries, and the general health of the patient. Physical diagnosis of the depth of burn is initially difficult even with years of experience, but knowledge of the mechanism and circumstances can be of initial assistance to give an indication of the amount of thermal energy conveyed to the tissue.[102]

All injuries should be documented carefully to create a solid foundation for further decisions and to provide a baseline for follow-up and outcome evaluations during the treatment course. Photographic documentation is recommended. The status of perfusion, capillary refill, skin color, and so on has to be documented to facilitate decisions about escharotomies, compartment release, or acute eschar excision.

Classification of Burns

The etiology of the burns can be considered a most useful predictive factor with regard to healing prognosis. Scalds usually result in a mixed depth pattern of injury, frequently involving the palms. Especially in younger patients, scald burns demonstrate a high capacity for spontaneous healing.

A more aggressive approach is indicated in the elderly with thinner skin. Flame burns are the most serious types of burns, except high-voltage injuries. They are usually deep partial-thickness or full-thickness burns, frequently requiring surgical treatment.[36]

Treatment of burns is dictated by the severity of the injury. The severity is determined by the level of thermal energy transmitted to the tissue. Burn wounds have been classified in many ways, although the most common is an anatomic classification of the depth of the wound.

Superficial, first-degree burns are characterized by an erythematous epidermis without blistering and are moderately painful. First-degree burns are those in which cell damage occurs without cell death. These injuries require only symptomatic care, principally directed at relieving pain, usually achieved by the application of cooling lotions and pain relievers. They will heal without scarring, usually in 2 to 3 days, with good return of function.

Superficial partial-thickness, second-degree burns destroy the epidermis and some elements of the basal epidermal regenerating layers of the dermis. They are considered to be the most painful type in the immediate post-trauma period because sensitive nerve endings are not damaged. They have the potential to self-heal by virtue of regeneration from the living epidermal elements remaining in the dermis (sweat or sebaceous glands and hair follicles). Regeneration, however, may be quite prolonged, depending on the depth of injury. In second-degree injuries, the resulting scar formation is directly dependent on the depth of injury and the quality of the regenerated skin is inversely proportional to the depth of injury: the deeper the burn, the poorer the quality of the regenerated skin (Fig. 61-3).

Deep partial-thickness, second-degree burns appear as a moist mottled surface that may be pale or erythematous depending on the depth of the burn. These wounds typically blanch with pressure and refill on release. Nerve endings are still present in the vital layers. The skin still bleeds after a needle prick (Fig. 61-4).

Full-thickness, third-degree burns are characterized by the death of all germinal epidermal elements. The wound extends below the level of the dermis. They show a leathery, unyielding appearance of the skin, which is pale to brown. Since nerve endings are destroyed, pain may not be significant. Because all the dermal appendages, as well as the overlying epidermis, are destroyed, these wounds cannot heal by epithelial regeneration and are not self-healing.

A *fourth-degree injury* involves necrosis of deeper structures such as tendons and bone and is usually only found in contact burns or high voltage injuries (Fig. 61-5).[102]

Determination of Burn Depth

Clinical assessment is of primary importance in the evaluation of the burn depth. The evaluation is based on clinical appearance, the testing of residual sensibility, the pinprick test for bleeding, and evaluation of the capillary refill. These findings are correlated with the classification of the burn. Modern devices such as laser Doppler, high-resolution ultrasound, or spectrometric analyses are interesting adjunctive techniques but have not excelled the clinical assessment.[119]

Control of Edema

Initial delivery of first aid in cases of hand burns includes the immediate cooling of the wound by rinsing with cold tap

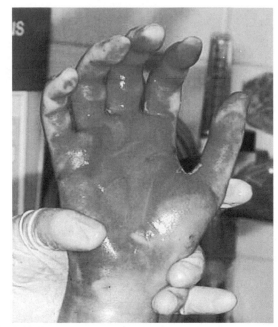

FIGURE 61-4. Deep partial-thickness (second-degree) burn of the palm. The burn will heal spontaneously owing to the healing capacity of the palmar skin.

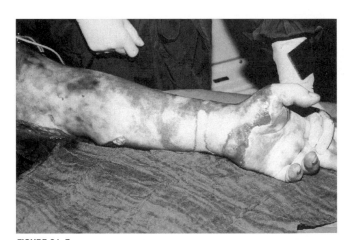

FIGURE 61-5. Deep partial-thickness and full-thickness (third degree) burn of the forearm. This burn will require excision and grafting.

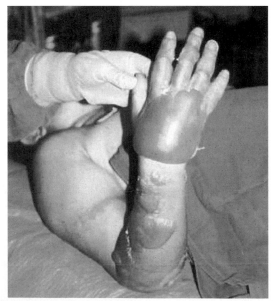

FIGURE 61-3. Superficial thickness (second-degree) burn with blister formation.

water within the first 30 minutes of a burn injury.[91] Cold packs or crushed ice may cause additional harm by decreasing the tissue temperature too much. There is good evidence that the immediate application of cold to a burn wound will reduce subsequent edema formation and may reduce the actual depth of injury by reducing the zone of stasis. A positive side effect is the reduction of pain by cooling the burn wound. Another major defense against edema in early management of acute hand burns is proper positioning of the hand. The strict elevation of the burned hand above the level of the patient's heart is recommended. This elevation must be maintained continuously during the early postburn period.[72a]

Escharotomy

The most important principle in the initial management of the burned upper extremity is maintenance of perfusion, which is ensured by adequate fluid resuscitation to maintain the circulating volume and removal of any mechanical obstruction to flow in the extremity. The tourniquet effect of an unyielding circumferential burn eschar may worsen the situation of postburn edema, and the potential for circulatory insufficiency is great, especially in deep partial-thickness or full-thickness circumferential burns. The initial therapy for constricting burn injuries of the upper extremity should therefore be directed toward releasing the subdermal tissue pressure and maintenance of the circulation.[86,122]

Escharotomy for tight, constricting burns was first described by Fabry of Hilden in 1607. Escharotomy has been commonly indicated in the treatment of circumferential full-thickness burn injuries, with its use increasing over the past three decade.[89a]

Indications for escharotomies include pain, resistance to passive straightening of the fingers, and disappearance of capillary refill in the nail beds. The forearm and hand feel tense to palpation. Doppler measurement of digital or superficial palmar arch pulses may also help but by the time radial or ulnar pulses disappear, tissue ischemia is well advanced.[102] The measurement of subcutaneous pressure with wick catheters has been recommended.[1] Escharotomy is indicated when pressure values of more than 30 mm Hg are found in two separate readings. However, the clinical experience of the surgeon usually obviates the need for pressure management.

The surgeon should carefully plan escharotomy incisions with the aim of releasing areas of circulatory embarrassment and restoring adequate flow, while avoiding injuries to underlying structures, such as nerves or vessels. Escharotomies can be performed either with the use of unipolar cautery or by scalpel. A radial full-thickness incision to decompress the hand and arm is the first step, because there is no risk of any injury to one of the peripheral cutaneous nerves except the superficial branch of the radial nerve. The length of the incision depends on the size of the constricting eschar. The maximum length of the incision extends on the axis from the tip of the acromion, to the lateral edge of the antecubital flexion crease, up to the radial aspect of the distal flexion crease of the wrist.[98,100] If necessary, a medial ulnar escharotomy can be added. The incision line is drawn from the axilla to the medial aspect of the antecubital flexion crease to the ulnar aspect of the distal flexion crease of the wrist (Fig. 61-6A).

In case of tight circumferential burn eschar of the fingers, digital escharotomies should be performed. The ulnar incision can be lengthened along the hypothenar eminence to the midlateral line of the ulnar border of the little finger. The radial escharotomy incision line can be extended along the radial aspect of the thenar eminence and the midlateral aspect of the thumb. The index, long, and ring fingers can be decompressed with similar midlateral incisions on the ulnar aspect of each finger. If the blood supply is not restored adequately by these incisions, the other side of each digit can be released in a similar fashion, thereby performing bilateral digital escharotomies. Decompression (fasciotomy) of the dorsal interossei should be performed with associated edema of the hand and diminished flexion. Small vertical escharotomy incisions are performed on the dorsum of the hand between the metacarpals.[100] Salisbury and coworkers were able to show in a random selection trial that there was an almost threefold increase in the number of fingers that could be salvaged by extended digital escharotomy[96] (see Fig. 61-6A to C).

Spinner and colleagues have pointed out the importance of intrinsic muscle decompression to overcome ischemic contracture of the hands. It is therefore vitally important in deep burns to the upper extremity to detect and prevent any possible loss of fingers or the thumb due to a secondary vascular compromise. If there is significant subfascial edema, an escharotomy can be combined with a fasciotomy for diagnostic and therapeutic purposes.[96,122] The early signs of ischemic necrosis of the intrinsic muscles are hyperextension of the fingers in the MCP joint with flexion of the IP joints.

Splinting

Without appropriate early splinting and positioning, a typical intrinsic-minus posture develops in the severely burned hand owing in great part to swelling of the hand. The injured hand takes the characteristic position of wrist flexion, hyperextension of the MCP joints, and flexion of the PIP and DIP joints. The thumb usually adducts toward the palm with the IP joint hyperextended.[38a] In a short time, edema, inflammation, and immobility are replaced by scarring and fibrosis, resulting in deformities not correctable without surgical intervention. Scar contractures across the dorsum of the hand further accentuate extension of the MCP joints, leading to the so-called claw deformity that is typical of the neglected burn of the hand.

The anti-claw position is essential to prevent permanent contracture deformities. To maintain this position, the hand should be immediately splinted in the so-called position of advantage (or "intrinsic-plus" position; Fig. 61-7). In the position of advantage, the MCP joints are fully flexed and the IP joints are essentially fully extended. The first web space is maximally abducted. In this position the ligaments of the digital joints have the best pre-tension to prevent shrinking of the ligaments. With the burned hand in this position, the dorsal skin is stretched somewhat tight across the metacarpals and there is little room for excessive edema formation. The so-called "position of function" with all digital joints slightly flexed should be avoided at all times because this will inevitably lead to contractures. The elbow should be kept in an extended position, because flexion contractures are the most frequent deformities. The shoulder is best positioned in abduction to prevent axillary contractures.

Hand splints should be applied on the day of injury. Customized splints from thermoplastic material are most effective and can be adjusted to any clinical situation. Whether one chooses to initiate early motion or maintain the hand relatively immobilized for a longer period of time depends principally on the condition of the skin over the PIP joints. Here the skin is very thin, and deep burns over this area frequently lead to disruption of the central extensor mechanism over the PIP joint and the development of a boutonnière deformity. If the burn over the PIP joint is fairly

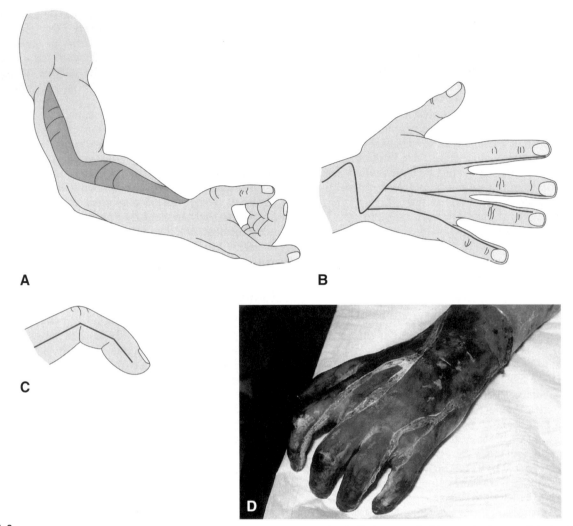

FIGURE 61-6. **A,** Schematic illustration of escharotomy incisions in the upper extremity. **B,** Escharotomy incisions at the dorsum of the hand. **C,** Clinical situation after escharotomy of the dorsum of the hand. **D,** Escharotomy incisions in the digits.

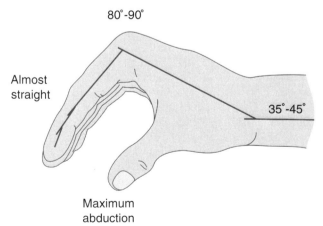

FIGURE 61-7. Ideal splinting position for the hand.

superficial, then early active flexion and extension exercises of these joints can be initiated. However, if the skin over the PIP joint appears to be more deeply burned, it is best to maintain the joints splinted in near full extension. The use of Kirschner wires has been advocated to maintain the PIP joints in extension in deep dorsal burns, but we have seen more problems (such as pin tract infections and joint stiffness) than detectable benefits, so that this technique is used only rarely (Fig. 61-8).

Local Wound Care

Care of the burn wound depends on the depth of the injury, the injury pattern, and the general condition of the patient. The decision-making process is illustrated in Figure 61-2. Basic wound care includes débridement, daily cleansing, prevention of infection by topical agents, and wound dressings.

In the partial-thickness burn, spontaneous healing can be expected within 7 to 14 days, depending on the size of deeper areas. The burn wound should be débrided of all contaminants.[102] Areas of loose skin are removed. The treatment of blisters remains somewhat controversial. Small blisters of less than 1 cm in diameter can be left intact, and the wound allowed to heal spontaneously. It has been proposed that larger blisters should be left intact as a biologic dressing to protect against infection.[37] However, the fluid of burn blisters is rich in prostaglandins and other proinflammatory cytokines such as interleukin-6 (IL-6) and IL-8 that may

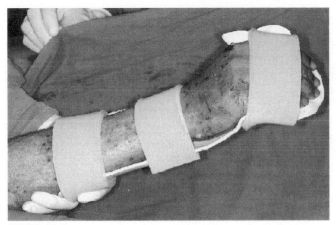

FIGURE 61-8. Custom-made thermoplastic splint in "intrinsic-plus" position.

propagate the burn wound injury, increasing the zone of necrosis.[83,94] The current recommendation for larger blisters is aspiration of the fluid, removal by incision, or débridement of the blisters.[102] Dressings can then be applied directly to the burn wound.

The principle of moist wound healing is used in spontaneously healing wounds. The burn wound should also be cleansed daily either in a hydrotherapy tank or under filtered tap water. This is followed by the application of an antibacterial cream. The cutaneous immune response of the individual against bacteria is neutralized during the edema phase of the burn wound. Administration of antibacterial agents during this period can prevent sequelae such as streptococcal cellulitis or erysipelas of the burned hand.

In superficial thermal injury, agents such as water-soluble bacitracin can be used as an alternative to spontaneous wound healing. A deeper partial-thickness burn wound should be dressed with a topical antibiotic agent with more penetrating capabilities such as silver sulfadiazine (Silvadene). Unless the thermal injuries to the hand are associated with large surface areas, systemic antibiotics are not indicated. Petrolatum (Vaseline) gauze strips and elastic netting are usually used to provide a custom-fit dressing with the opportunity for maximal movement of the extremity. The fingertips should remain visible to allow observation of their color and vascularity. Siliconized gauze can be applied as an alternative.

As the superficially burned areas begin to epithelialize, care must be taken to avoid shear of the new epithelium with dressing changes or exercise. Bland ointments or creams such as Vitamin A & D ointment are helpful to prevent dehydration of the new epithelium. These new epithelial surfaces will require some maturation before recovery of function by the sebaceous and sweat glands.

In recent years more simple and less time-consuming techniques have been introduced. The simplest treatment for superficial partial-thickness burns is a large surgical glove filled with silver sulfadiazine cream. The patient slips the hand into the glove, which is fixed with bandages at the wrist level. Some patients feel uncomfortable in the rather tight-fitting gloves, but for many patients this technique provides a simple, inexpensive solution that is also applicable in developing countries. Harrison and Parkhouse

described the use of silicone oil in a glove for the same purpose.[36] For those patients who cannot tolerate the glove, the large Gore-Tex glove provides a useful alternative (Fig. 61-9). The glove can be left on for several days, and daily dressing changes are easy and almost painless in both techniques.

The Biobrane glove provides an excellent alternative to the techniques just described (Fig. 61-10A to C). The biohybrid membrane of knitted nylon, silicone mesh, and peptides from porcine proteins is perfectly fitted to the hand and then sealed. It is semi-permeable, and small amounts of wound fluid can evaporate through the membrane. Larger fluid collections have to be evacuated through small puncture holes. The glove remains on the wound until the surface is epithelialized and then peels off automatically. Since the glove is transparent, changes in the wound can be observed through the membrane. Dressing changes are not necessary and therefore the high cost of the glove is equalized over time, especially because only limited nursing care is required. The major disadvantage of this method is that the initial wound assessment has to be correct, because only superficial thickness wounds heal spontaneously under the glove. However, our experience has shown that in cases in which patches of deeper burns are detected, the glove can be removed to treat deeper burns with surgical techniques. Similar techniques can be used with polyurethane films such as Opsite or Omiderm or with polyacrylic mesh (Surfasoft).[62] Whereas many authors claim that film dressings tend to lead to superior results in superficial burns, gauze dressings seem to have the same effect, provided that the moist environment of the wound is maintained.

Excision and Grafting

Deep dermal and full-thickness burns of the hand are best treated by early excision and grafting. It is usually accepted that the burn wound is not infected and is suitable for primary surgical treatment within the first 5 days. If this initial ideal period of time is missed, surgery is considered best after a delay of 3 weeks because of the increased risk of graft loss due to infection and excessive bleeding from the inflamed bed of the eschar.[36]

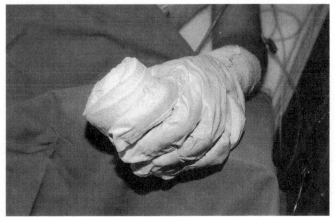

FIGURE 61-9. Gore-Tex glove filled with silver sulfadiazine for conservative treatment of superficial partial-thickness (second-degree) burn.

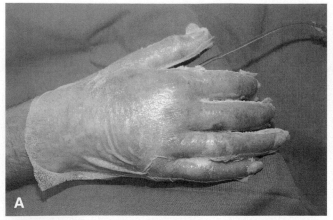

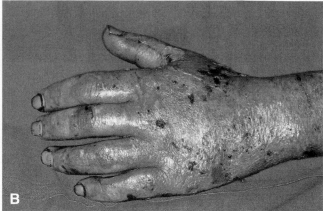

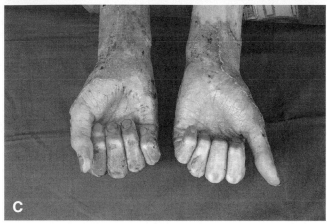

FIGURE 61-10. **A,** Biobrane glove fitted to a superficially burned hand. **B** and **C,** Excellent cosmetic and functional result after spontaneous healing.

Tangential excision is the preferred surgical procedure in hand burns. It involves shaving of the burned skin in thin layers until brisk capillary bleeding is encountered. A typical instrument used in the hand is the Goulian knife, which consists of a single-edged razor blade with a guard. Thin layers of devitalized tissue can be removed until healthy tissue is encountered. It is very important not to leave residual devitalized tissue because this might prevent adequate take of skin grafts, promote wound infection, and delay the process of recovery. Reddish areas of fat are considered to represent the zone of stasis and should be excised. No matter how deep the burn is, one must attempt to preserve the paratenon of the extensor tendons and the fine layer of areolar tissue above the joint capsules to facilitate the acceptance of the skin graft. After excision of the eschar, sponges soaked with epinephrine are then applied to reduce bleeding. The most crucial area is the dorsal skin above the PIP and MCP joints. Failure of the skin graft in these areas almost inevitably leads to exposure of the joint with the consequences of joint infection, cartilage erosion, and joint stiffness.

Débridement can also be performed under tourniquet control. This makes the assessment of the wound a little more difficult and requires more surgical experience but may reduce blood loss. Our procedure includes wrapping of the hand with epinephrine-soaked sponges and tight elastic bandages before releasing the tourniquet and leaving them in place for approximately 20 minutes. Whereas most capillary bleeding usually has stopped at this point, further hemostasis still has to be meticulous.

After bleeding is controlled, skin grafts are transplanted. Resurfacing the wound with split-thickness grafting is considered the gold standard in most cases.[65] There is an ongoing debate whether the grafts should be meshed or unmeshed. Many authors claim that sheet grafts (unmeshed) provide superior aesthetic appearance when compared with meshed grafts. They are thought to produce less scar tissue than meshed grafts and usually provide a more functional result (Fig. 61-11). Meshed grafts have the advantage of facilitating drainage of wound fluid, blood, and bacteria through the mesh. They usually have a higher overall success rate in critical wound beds with some remaining bleeding or in patches of questionable viability.[69] The main disadvantage is the high rate of scar contracture, which frequently leads to major functional disturbances. The mesh-graft expansion ratio used in the burned hand should not exceed 1.5:1 (Fig. 61-12). There are studies, however, that show that there is no significant difference in aesthetics and function between both types after 12 months. In patients with major burns to the rest of the body, skin grafts may be in short supply and mesh grafts may have to be selected for coverage. Our recommendation for the choice of graft depends on the availability of skin graft donor sites and the general condition of the patient. If sufficient donor sites are present, sheet grafts are the first choice, which are harvested as split-thickness grafts. In patients with limited graft availability, meshed grafts are the only alternative. In rare patients with isolated hand burns, the skin grafts can be harvested a little thicker. This results in more supple skin with less contractures and better functional results.

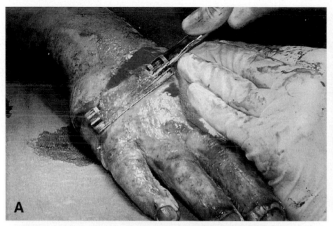

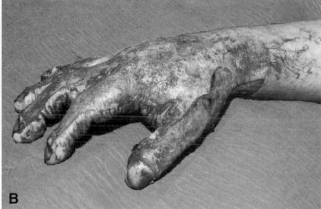

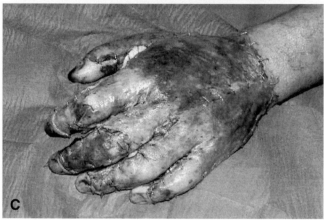

FIGURE 61-11. **A,** Tangential excision of deep partial-thickness burn of the dorsum of the hand. **B,** Result after tangential excision, **C,** Sheet graft transplantation to the excised areas.

Full-thickness skin grafts are not indicated in acute burns. Their success depends too much on a perfect wound bed, perfect hemostasis, and a perfect tie-over dressing. With their significant risk for graft loss, full-thickness grafts are usually reserved for secondary corrections.

The graft is fixed either with single interrupted stitches or a running stitch (4-0 or 5-0). Care should be taken to create smooth transitions between the grafts and the edges of the remaining skin. The wound is dressed with petrolatum or siliconized gauze. Cotton balls are placed over the gauze for a tie-over bolster dressing when necessary. Experimental data suggest that skin grafting is most effective when pressures of 30 mm Hg are exerted evenly over the wound. Clinical experience has shown that a conventional tie-over

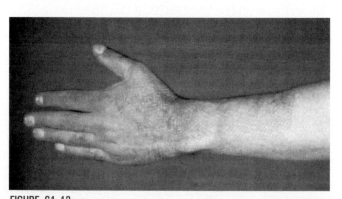

FIGURE 61-12. Cosmetic result of meshed skin graft transplantation to the hand.

bolster reaches this goal. A rather new technique to enhance skin grafting is application of vacuum pressure to the wound. This has shown to yield very good results in skin grafting of chronic wounds, but it is very difficult to apply this technique to a burned hand. Early results with vacuum gloves have been reported, but larger series are still lacking.

In full-thickness burns of the upper extremity and large surface area involvement of the entire body, epifascial excision may be indicated. The skin envelope may be reconstructed with meshed skin grafts in these cases, but this will most likely result in severe postburn contractures. Artificial dermal equivalents such as Integra can be employed under these circumstances. This results in a more pliable skin envelope with less need for corrective surgeries later (Fig. 61-13).

Dressings are left in place for 5 days. The skin graft can be assessed by then, and decisions for further wound care can be made. If the wound begins to smell, dressing changes can be done earlier to avoid graft loss through infection. If the wound is found to be clean, no particular treatment is indicated. Only petrolatum or any similar basic cream is administered to keep the graft moist and supple. If traces of infection such as suppuration or colored crusts are found, all debris should be removed carefully and the wound rinsed with antiseptic ointments such as chlorhexidine (Bactigras) or polyhexanid (Lavasept). All skin graft areas that appear nonvital should be removed. The wound is then redressed with gauze and antiseptic creams such as mafenide acetate (Sulfamylon) or silver sulfadiazine.[36,62] Dressing changes are performed daily until the wound does not show any signs

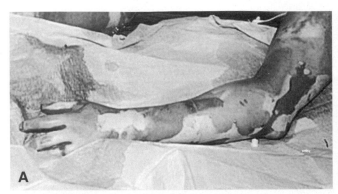

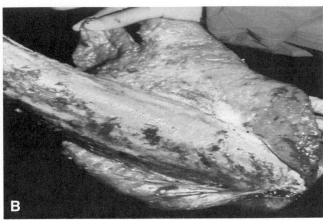

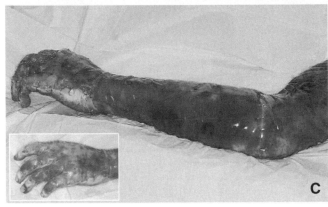

FIGURE 61-13. **A,** Deep full-thickness burn of the left upper extremity. **B,** Epifascial excision of severe full-thickness burn of the left upper extremity. **C,** Application of Integra to the extremity.

of infection. With this technique, many "endangered" grafts may be salvaged.

Special emphasis should be given to postoperative splinting and physical therapy. Splints are an integral part of the postoperative treatment plan. After grafting, the hand is immobilized for 5 days until graft success is assured. Passive physical therapy is then initiated to prevent and reduce stiffness of the joints. Minor graft loss has to be accepted when joint mobility can be maintained. Even in situations in which it is not guaranteed that the graft will "take" over the PIP joints, mobility of the remaining joints has priority. Active range-of-motion exercises are initiated as soon as the patient is awake and conscious.

In rare cases, tangential excision does not suffice. In full-thickness injuries the skin damage may reach down to the paratenon and tendons, and the metacarpal bones or joints may be exposed. In these cases, primary flap coverage is indicated. The choice of flaps depends on donor site availability and the ideal tissue for the particular situation. In younger females and children, a conventional groin flap may be the first choice. The donor site can easily be hidden, the skin is supple, and shoulder immobilized for a groin flap is usually well tolerated. A drawback of this flap is that four to five procedures are required to achieve a definitive result. However, in patients with thick subcutaneous fatty layers, the flap may be too thick, yielding aesthetically nonsatisfying results.

In most situations, in which the general condition of the patient allows more sophisticated procedures, the flaps can be tailored to the individual needs of the patient—free flaps, pedicled forearm flaps, or intrinsic hand flaps. Fascial flaps have proven to be very helpful in coverage of dorsal hand defects, where cutaneous flaps are a better choice than thick

flaps.[24] They provide stable but supple tissue, all secondary reconstructive procedures can be performed under these flaps, and the aesthetic results after grafting with split-thickness skin grafts are pleasing. Temporoparietal fascia, serratus fascia, or anterolateral thigh fascia flaps are most frequently used. They seldom require secondary debulking (Fig. 61-14).

In situations in which large flaps are required, the latissimus dorsi, the anterolateral thigh flap, or a cutaneous flap from the subscapular system would be ideal choices. These flaps are rarely indicated in flame burns but more frequently employed in chemical burns, contact burns, or high-voltage injuries (see later). Secondary surgery is frequently necessary. All principles of physical therapy also apply to a flap-covered hand. After 5 days, flap healing is usually secured and passive exercises can be initiated.

Skin grafting is rarely necessary in palmar burns owing to the enormous capacity of spontaneous healing from skin appendages. This is the reason why thick split-thickness skin grafts are seldom required. Flap coverage may be more common in deep palmar burns. In our hands fascial flaps offer the best solution for this problem. The stability of the tissue is sufficient, and these types of flaps show little tissue shearing that would diminish the quality of the grip. Deep sensation is reported to return within 12 to 15 months.

In children, Pensler and associates[87] found no significant difference in the number of operative procedures with either full-thickness or split-thickness grafts. They claim that the split-thickness skin grafts have less tendency toward hyperpigmentation, leading to superior cosmetic results, are more expeditious to harvest, and preserve donor sites for future reconstruction. In contrast, Pham and associates[88] consider full-thickness skin grafts as a first choice for deep palm burn injuries in children.

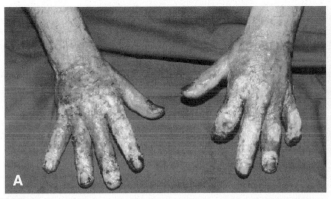 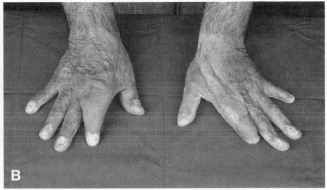

FIGURE 61-14. **A,** Deep contact burn of both hands with exposed PIP joints after failed skin grafts. **B,** Result after free serratus fascia flaps to both hands with skin grafts.

COMPLICATIONS

Complications in isolated hand burns are rare and can usually be avoided by proper treatment. They are more frequent in major burns in which the immune response of the patient is severely suppressed and the patient remains in a catabolic state for a considerable period of time. Three types of complication can jeopardize the treatment result: secondary infection, graft loss, and early hypergranulation.

Secondary Infection

Secondary infection can be a major problem in hand burn injuries. Two areas of the hand are extremely susceptible to secondary infection.[95] The thin skin overlying the dorsum of the PIP joints makes the tendons likely to be injured or result in an open joint. Decreased blood supply may also increase the susceptibility to infection with secondary joint involvement (Fig. 61-15). The nail bed is the other area that is particularly susceptible to injuries. Despite its high vascularity, the nail bed is readily exposed to thermal injury and secondary trauma and infection.

Infected areas are treated with local application of antibacterial creams or ointments (see earlier). Systemic antibiotic therapy is indicated only when clinical signs of cellulitis or ascending lymphangitis are seen. The hand is cleansed and rinsed daily, before antibacterial agents are applied.

Graft Loss

The loss of skin grafts can have several underlying causes.

CAUSES OF SKIN GRAFT LOSS

■ Insufficient débridement with residual layers of nonvital tissue
■ Bleeding of the wound bed with hematoma under the graft
■ Not perfectly fitting tie-over dressing
■ Secondary infection of the wound bed

In case of graft loss or nonvital grafts, the wound must be débrided surgically. All nonvital skin should be removed, the wound bed must be débrided until healthy bleeding is encountered, meticulous hemostasis is mandatory, and regrafting can be performed in the same session. If the wound is seriously infected, the viability of the deeper layers is questionable, or the wound is bleeding too much (owing to the inflammation), it is recommended to prepare the wound for several days with local care and perform early secondary regrafting to avoid additional graft loss.

Early Hypergranulation

Early hypergranulation occurs between nonepithelialized areas of mesh grafts or the borderlines of sheet grafts. It is rarely encountered in large surface area burns, because the immune response of these patients is usually severely impaired. Surgical removal of these hypergranulations is not recommended because it will cause profuse bleeding. Dressing the wound with a corticosteroid-containing gauze (Corticotulle) has proven to be extremely useful. Several days of treatment usually suffice for wound epithelialization. Early treatment with pressure gloves and silicone membranes is mandatory in these patients.

POSTBURN DEFORMITIES

Even if in the initial phase of acute hand burn injury all treatment measures have been executed properly, and despite increasing sophistication in the overall management, postburn deformities still occur and are the most common cause of skin contracture in the hand[53] (Table 61-1). Postburn scarring and contractures affect the function as well as the aesthetic appearance of the hand and remain the most frustrating late complication of a hand burn. If contractures or scarring affect the dominant hand, as they do on most occasions, the vocation and thereby the economic status of the patient suffers. Proper management of these deformities is thus highly desirable. A classification of postburn deformities has been proposed by Achauer[1]:

A. Claw deformity
   1. Complete
   2. Incomplete

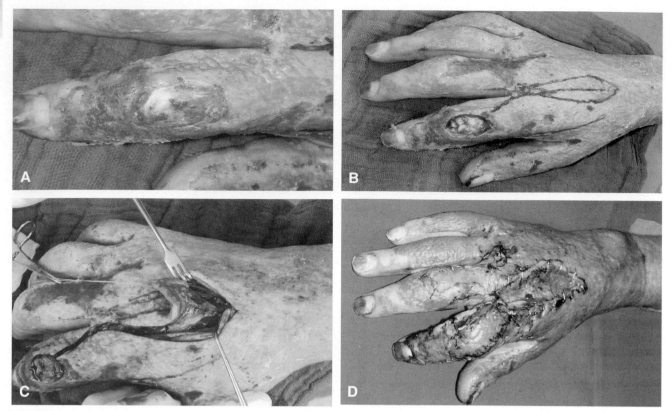

FIGURE 61-15. **A,** Typical exposure of PIP joint after deep partial-thickness (second-degree) burn and graft loss. **B,** Design of a reversed DMCA flap based on the second dorsal metacarpal artery. **C,** Flap raised on its pedicle. The pivot point is in the web space. **D,** Flap after 5 days. Flap perfusion is excellent. Skin graft is used for reconstruction of the donor site.

Table 61-1
POSTBURN HAND DEFORMITIES

First web adduction contractures

Web space contractures

Dorsal skin contractures

Digital flexion contracture

Boutonnière deformity

Dorsal skin deficiency

Digital loss secondary to ischemia

Median and ulnar nerve compression syndrome

B. Palmar contracture
C. Web space deformity
  1. Web space contracture
  2. Adduction contracture
  3. Syndactylism
D. Hypertrophic scar and contracture bands
E. Amputation deformity
F. Nail bed deformity
G. Elbow
  1. Flexion contracture
  2. Deep burn with extensive tissue loss
  3. Heterotopic ossification
H. Axilla

Scars can also be assessed with scoring systems such as the Vancouver Scar Scale,[6] which allow some classification of the inhomogeneous clinical pictures.

Prevention

It is well accepted that the best therapy for burn wound contractures is prevention. Prasad and colleagues[89] suggest that comprehensive treatment efforts have led to a significant reduction in development of burn scar contracture. It appears that factors such as improved management of burn wounds, liberal use of positioning, improved splinting, early maintenance of range of motion, and exercise programs have contributed to this success. The decrease of required reconstructive surgery procedures over time is also reflected accordingly in other articles in the literature. Dobbs and Curreri[22] reported a serious contracture rate of 27% in 681 adult burn patients. Pegg and associates[85] reported on 411 patients having a 7.8% incidence of development of burn scar contracture, and Kraemer and coworkers[51] noted only a 3.7% rate of reconstruction procedures for burn scar release in a population of 839 adults and children with burn injury. These data suggest that improved treatment protocols and consequent splinting for prolonged periods of time are reducing the need for reconstructive readmissions.

Treatment

Usually postburn deformities go along with the tissue deficit. Contractures can be caused by the spontaneous healing of deeper burns, that is, the burn wound itself, or more frequently by the inevitable contracture of transplanted split-thickness skin grafts. This phenomenon occurs more extensively in the acute burn situation, and is less pronounced in elective situations. The clinical impression that secondary split-thickness grafts contract more in burn wound corrections than in other post-trauma situations is shared by many authors, but scientific evidence is lacking. Release of contractures may be performed by various patterns of "Z"-plasties but frequently require skin grafting or flap coverage. Full-thickness skin grafts play an important role in those secondary corrections because they are more similar to normal skin in texture, color, and resilience than split-thickness grafts. However, full-thickness grafts "take" less readily than split-thickness grafts and they may be of limited availability in larger burns.[75] The latter problem, in some situations, may be solved by pre-expansion of the donor sites.[7] Full-thickness grafts have less tendency for contraction, because there is an inverse relationship between thickness of the dermis and graft contraction.[42,46]

Before surgically addressing the problem, a thorough analysis is mandatory. Several questions have to be answered:

1. What is the nature of the contracture or the limiting scarring?
2. Are there any underlying joint problems (e.g., contracture of the ligaments or capsule, cartilage destruction)?
3. Will soft tissue procedures be sufficient?

4. Which type of coverage is adequate after contracture release?
5. From which donor site do I harvest skin grafts or flaps?

Only after these questions have been answered, can a surgical plan be designed. While the most disturbing functional problems are usually addressed primarily, the patient often perceives aesthetic deformities to be more urgent. Decision-making algorithms are illustrated in Figures 61-16 and 61-17.

Nail Bed Deformities

Dorsal scarring over the DIP joint leads to distortion of the eponychial fold, retraction of the eponychium, and proximal nail exposure. In cases of only skin tightness without severe retraction of the nail fold, skin release and skin grafting may be sufficient.

When reconstruction of the nail fold is required or skin grafts are not appropriate, proximally based lateral skin flaps are recommended. The donor site of these narrow flaps can usually be closed primarily, and the resulting tip deformity evens out over time.[1]

Claw Deformities

Claw deformities may be difficult to correct. They usually consist of hyperextended MCP joints and flexion contractures of the PIP joints. In contrast to Achauer's classifi-

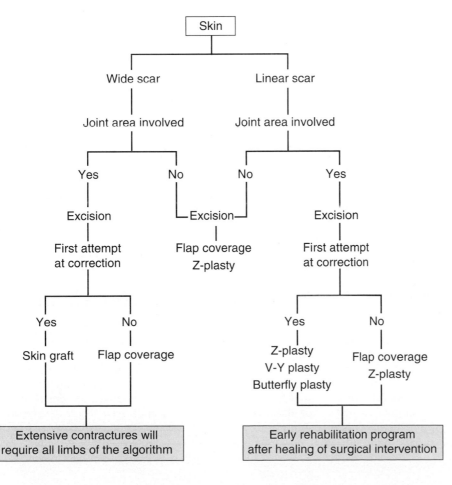

FIGURE 61-16. Decision-making algorithm for skin contractures. (Redrawn from Germann G, Sherman R, Levin SL: Decision Making in Reconstructive Surgery: Upper Extremity. Berlin, Springer, 1999.)

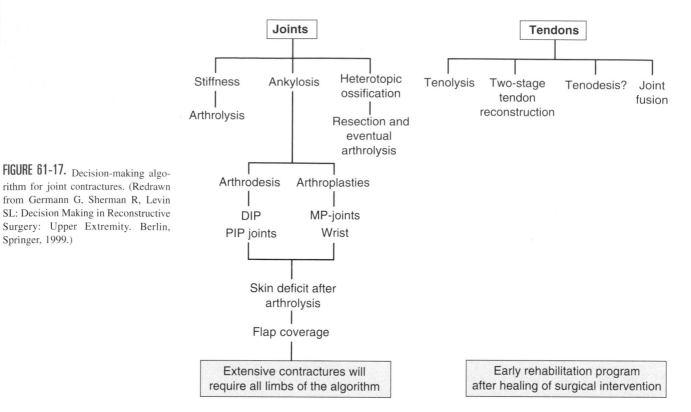

FIGURE 61-17. Decision-making algorithm for joint contractures. (Redrawn from Germann G, Sherman R, Levin SL: Decision Making in Reconstructive Surgery: Upper Extremity. Berlin, Springer, 1999.)

cation, we prefer to divide claw deformities into two categories: (1) those with long-standing fixed deformities with ligament contracture (which will require joint release and coverage) and (2) cutaneous deformities, where simple release of the skin contracture solves the joint position problem.

The first group requires arthrolysis, either from the dorsum or in rare cases from the palmar aspect of the joint. Both approaches to the joint can usually be performed from a dorsal skin incision. These situations usually require some sort of flap coverage because the extensive dissection eliminates all tissue layers where the skin graft is likely to be successful. The same holds true for situations in which the extensor tendon apparatus is exposed and stable soft tissue coverage is required. As mentioned earlier, the choice of flaps depends on the individual profile of the patient and ranges from regional flaps such as the radial forearm flap to distant flaps (groin flap) and microvascular flaps (Fig. 61-18).

Full-thickness skin grafts are preferred when skin grafts will suffice for skin reconstruction. Only in cases of limited availability and/or when other important areas may require the use of full-thickness skin grafts (i.e., the eyelids or lips) are split-thickness grafts used. Temporary fixation with Kirschner wires is indicated only in joints where, after release of cutaneous and ligamentous contractures, there is still an "elastic" resistance found and the patient cannot mobilize sufficient strength to overcome this resistance.

The same holds true for the PIP joint in claw deformities. In most cases there is a relative palmar tissue deficit that requires either full-thickness skin grafting or flap coverage after release. However, local intrinsic hand flaps are usually limited in these hands, so that distant flaps or free tissue

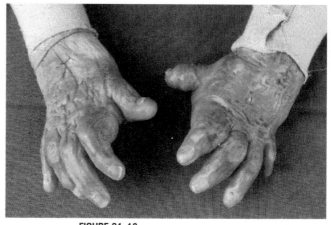

FIGURE 61-18. Bilateral claw deformity.

transfers are frequently indicated because the problem is usually encountered in more than one digit.

Web Space Syndactyly/Interdigital Contractures

There are two mechanisms in burn injuries of the hand that cause interdigital fusion syndactyly. Adjacent burned digits may be allowed to fuse together by the healing process, and granulation or contractures of the digital skin allow distal migration of the web. Contracture of the second, third, and fourth web spaces usually occurs along the dorsal margin of the web. Numerous methods have been developed to improve this surgically, consisting of local flaps and grafts. They usually consist of variations of the "Z"-plasty as 3, 4, or 5 flap ("V-M") plasty. Most important in correcting these deformities is to reconstruct the natural slope of the web space—from dorsal proximally to palmar distally. This re-creates the natural appearance of the web and the natural motion pattern of the dorsal skin creases (Fig. 61-19).

In cases in which any type of "Z"-plasty will not provide sufficient skin, patches of full-thickness skin grafts are used. To achieve a reasonable success rate, the wound bed must be dry, all cavities of the wound surface should be filled with petrolatum gauze, and a tie-over bolster is meticulously applied. Mancoll and associates[70] reported the long-term follow-up of various techniques used to surgically correct interdigital contractures. Although all techniques using skin grafts or local flaps showed a high recurrence rate, "Z"-plasties alone had the lowest recurrence rate. With all techniques, care should be taken during these procedures to avoid damage to the neurovascular bundles in the web space (Fig. 61-20).

Contractures of the Thumb

Contractures of the first web space are usually the result not only of hypertrophic scarring or skin shortage in the web but also contracture of the adductor muscle, fascia, and possibly the basal joint capsule. First web space contractures limit the movement of the thumb at the trapeziometacarpal joint, thus affecting both grasp and pinch.[10a] This can be treated with release of all structures involved and soft tissue reconstruc-

tion with skin grafts or any type of suitable flap. Our experience has shown that in most cases at least the adductor muscle is involved so that division of the adductor is an integral part of the contracture release.

Contractures of the first web space can be released with a variety of techniques, including "Z"-plasties, four-flap "Z"-plasties, local rotation flaps, and full-thickness or split-thickness skin grafts. Distant or free microvascular flaps are infrequently required.[84a] The technique of simple 60-degree "Z"-plasty gives the greatest increase in length and depth of the web space. Woolf and Broadbent have described a four-flap "Z"-plasty with a 90-degree flap on each end of the central incision, with each of these flaps divided into two 45-degree flaps. This technique provides a smoother contour than the standard "Z"-plasty. In addition, rotation flaps have been described by many other authors.

Although the most common contracture of the thumb is adduction deformity, other anatomic deformities are also seen. Less frequently, the thumb metacarpal may be contracted in opposition and extension owing to bands of dorsal hypertrophic scar between the distal radius and the first metacarpal or, conversely, in flexion owing to volar scarring producing flexion of the IP or MCP joint.[104] Correction of these contractures requires surgical release, sometimes combined with wider burn scar excision, followed by appropriate soft tissue coverage,[53] and temporary fusion in selected cases (Fig. 61-21).

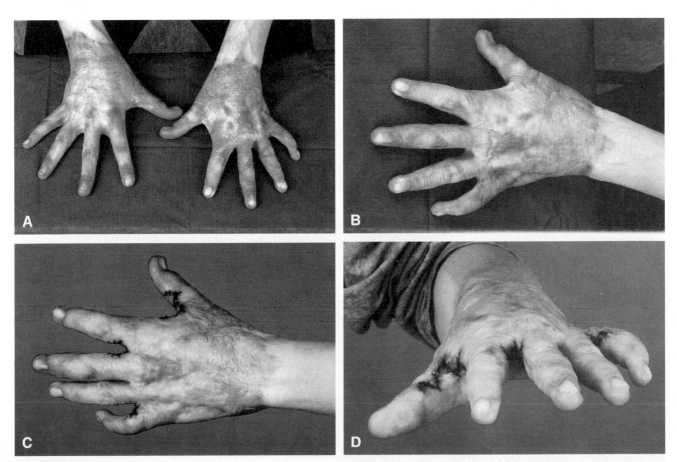

FIGURE 61-19. **A** and **B,** Web space contracture of the first, second, and fourth web spaces of the left hand. **C** and **D,** Result after release of web space contractures by multiple "Z"-plasties.

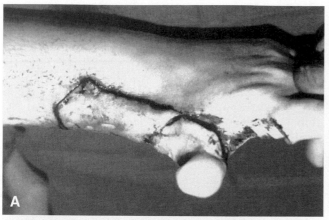

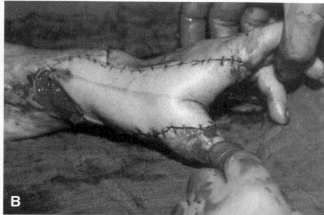

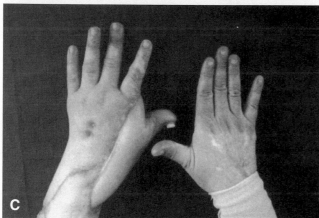

FIGURE 61-20. **A,** Severe contracture of the first web space. **B,** After release of the contracture a posterior interosseous flap is rotated into the resulting defect. **C,** Long-term result.

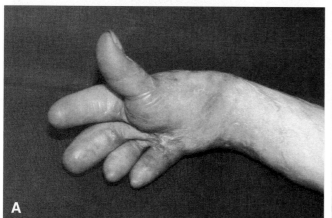

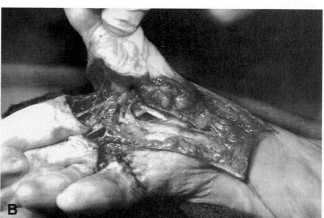

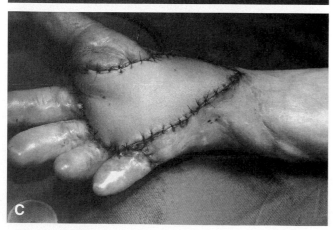

FIGURE 61-21. **A,** Severe adduction contracture of the palm in a 10-year-old child. **B,** Resulting defect after contracture release. **C,** Reconstruction with free parascapular free flap.

Digital Flexion Contracture

Release of flexion contracture of the digits and palm is one of the most commonly performed procedures in burn injuries. The skin of the palmar surface of the hand is specialized because of its unique functional requirements. It is hairless, thick, sturdy, and relatively inelastic and is designed to withstand the heavy demands of daily work. It is the best tactile organ with optimal sensitivity and is rich in sweat glands to provide moisture essential for a sure grasp and touch. The fundamental principle of reconstruction is to replace the lost tissue with similar tissue. Because of the unique similarities with palmar skin, plantar skin is an excellent donor area for skin grafting for the palmar aspect of the digits and hand. Le Worthy first reported split-thickness plantar skin grafting.[56] Webster[121] and Zoltie and colleagues[127] used full-thickness plantar skin grafts from the plantar instep area, and Tanabe and colleagues[108] have described the use of a plantar dermal graft for reconstruction of palmar skin defects of the digits and hand. The similarities between palmar and plantar skin have been described by many authors.[56,80,121,127] Histologically, both have a thick epidermal layer with a well-defined stratum lucidum and a solid stratum corneum. The connective tissue of the dermis in both is less elastic and more compact than dermis elsewhere, providing stability against pressure and shearing forces. Both are hairless and lack sebaceous glands and melanocytes. They have numerous pacinian corpuscles for optimal sensibility and abundant sweat glands to provide moisture. The sweat glands produce multicentric epithelial budding and promote rapid and good quality healing of the plantar area after split-thickness graft harvest. Hyperpigmentation, scarring, and recurrence of contracture are the most common problems encountered with traditional skin grafts to the palm. Skin grafts from the plantar area of the foot provide better results because they have sparse pigment cells and tend to contract less, owing to the less elastic and more compact connective tissue in the dermis.[12] Good cosmetic and functional results are obtained at both donor and recipient sites.[12,108]

Postburn flexion contractures of the fingers functionally impair the digits and restrict the functional capability of the entire hand. They have been classified by Kurtzman and Stern[53]:

Type I: Skin only; MCP in passive flexion; PIP can be fully extended

Type II: Palmar capsular structures; MCP in passive flexion; no passive extension of PIP possible

Type III: Soft tissue, joint structures; fixed PIP regardless of MCP position

The skin shortage between the palmar digital and distal IP skin creases limits the extension of the PIP joint. This deformity can be corrected by releasing the contracted structures and replacing the palmar skin deficiency.[2] When possible, we attempt to achieve release with modified "Z"-plasties, but we prefer full-thickness skin grafts if "Z"-plasty is not sufficient.

Type II deformities frequently require release of the volar plate and division of the checkreins to free the joint. Flap coverage can be indicated in these cases, if the joint capsule or flexor tendons are exposed.

Type III deformities are fixed with joint irregularities and frequent cartilage destruction. These patients are often best served by joint fusion, despite available complex soft tissue reconstruction procedures.

Boutonnière Deformity

The postburn boutonnière deformity is a multifaceted problem, and the damaged central slip of the extensor apparatus is only one facet of it. Deep dermal and full-thickness burns of the dorsum of the PIP joint are a potential cause for the development of boutonnière deformity. Deep dorsal burns damage the central slip of the extensor apparatus over the PIP joint initially or during the healing phase. When this occurs, the lateral bands slide below the axis of rotation of the PIP joint. As a result, the lateral bands become PIP joint flexors rather than extensors, and the PIP joint is flexed up to 90 degrees and is unable to actively extend. The absence of the central slip creates a loss of restraint for the extensor mechanism that allows this system to move proximally. This results in excessive pull on the DIP joint through the lateral bands and subsequent hyperextension at the DIP joint.

Such postburn boutonnière deformities are a challenge to the surgeon and call for a comprehensive approach. The surgical management is extremely difficult, and the results of the various operations are unpredictable. First, it is necessary to eliminate the related contractures of other hand joints and restore passive movement of the PIP joint by preparatory operations; and distraction devices may be necessary for successful tendon plasty.[30] There are a variety of tendon plasty techniques described in the literature. Transposing the lateral bands to the dorsum of the finger and suturing them together has been proposed or, alternatively, the creation of a "figure-of-eight" tendoplasty.[96] Other authors have proposed simple transection of the lateral bands to correct the deformity.[8] A more commonly used technique is to pull a tendon graft through a hole in the base of the middle phalanx to connect it with the lateral bands or with the central slip over the proximal phalanx.[55] Although methods vary, the results are frequently unsatisfactory. Consequently, PIP joint fusion or finger amputation is common and many authors believe that arthrodesis is more effective than tendoplasty.[32,103] By shortening of the finger with fusion, often no additional coverage is necessary and healing time is frequently shorter than with tendon reconstruction.

Contractures of the Dorsum of the Hand

The initial thermal injury of the hand is usually limited to the skin alone, and the underlying tendons and joints are usually spared. Therefore, dorsal contracture is the most common problem encountered after hand burns. This deformity, usually occurring after skin grafting, may be due to unsatisfactory skin coverage, partial graft loss due to wound infection, or inadequate therapy and splinting in the antideformity position.[13] This results in dorsal skin contracture, MCP joint hyperextension, and limitation of finger flexion.[13]

Correction consists of complete excision of the contracted tissues and mobilization of all adjacent joints. Full-thickness skin grafts are the first choice for reconstruction. Resurfacing the dorsum of the hand with full-thickness skin grafts requires a considerable amount of skin, however, which frequently may not be available. Thick split-thickness skin grafts may be a reasonable alternative. A simple solution is to utilize the Crane principle.[77] Subcutaneous tissue can be carried on a skin flap placed temporarily over a wound defect. The skin flap, along with a thin layer of subcutaneous tissue, is later returned to the donor site, leaving a layer of subcutaneous tissue suitable for skin grafting over the original defect.

In any case where there are questions about the quality of the wound bed and the graft "take" rate, flaps should be considered. Besides skin flaps, fascial flaps have proven to be excellently suited to the dorsal hand, because they provide thin, stable, and supple coverage that only requires split-thickness skin grafting. To avoid any graft loss, hemostasis of the fascial flap should be meticulous. If oozing persists, secondary grafting should be considered. This can be done as a secondary bedside procedure 2 to 3 days postoperatively, with the skin graft being harvested at the time of flap transfer (Fig. 61-22).

Amputation Deformity

Patients presenting with significant burns to the hand with digital involvement are always at risk for vascular compromise of the digits. Early escharotomy to preserve the intrinsic muscles of the hand and improve circulation of the digits is crucial. In spite of these procedures, some patients face partial or total amputation of the digits. Such losses both distort the aesthetic appearance of the hand and severely affect its function.

Salisbury[98] points out that it might be inappropriate to concentrate multiple surgical efforts on one finger, if a patient has other extensive problems. Amputation can rapidly relieve the problems of "hooking" or chronic pain in these cases. The overall goal is to do only the operations necessary to rehabilitate the patient.

Reconstruction of the digits is frequently centered on restoration of a three-point grip, involving the thumb and predominantly the index and middle fingers. The thumb represents approximately 40% of hand function, which is why its reconstruction is a primary concern in rehabilitation of the burned hand with multiple digital losses. Any recon-structive procedure is surgically more difficult than in other post-traumatic situations.

Thumb Reconstruction

In thumb reconstruction, the adequacy of soft tissue coverage must be assessed first. If soft tissue coverage is not adequate, flap coverage of the area of the first metacarpal and web space should be undertaken as a first stage. Adequate length, mobility, stability, and sensation as well as aesthetics are the goals of functional thumb reconstruction.[63]

With thumb loss distal to the IP joint, function remains good. Frequently, simple deepening of the web space using "Z"-plasties gives sufficient additional relative length for the thumb. When the proximal phalanx becomes foreshortened, function progressively diminishes. In these deformities, pollicization or transfer of partial digits is very useful and should be considered when the thumb does not have sufficient length to oppose the remaining digits. Littler[64] addressed the issue of thumb reconstruction in patients with multiple digital amputations by performing first-to-second metacarpal transfer using a vascularized osteocutaneous transfer. In such instances, two functionless digits are combined to make a functional thumb. This procedure both lengthens the thumb and creates a newly developed first web space, which allows for pinch.[72a] Although Littler's patients were not burn victims, other plastic surgeons have applied this approach to thumb reconstruction in case of burn injuries of the hand with digital amputation.[117]

Toe-to-thumb transfer is an alternative technique for thumb reconstruction,[41,112] especially in cases in which no digits are available for pollicization. In a severely burned patient with large total body surface area burns, most toes and fingers will be damaged, so pollicization is the more likely solution.

In some cases, for example in electrical injuries, with complete loss of the thumb, toe-to-thumb transfer is a better choice. Frequently, soft tissue shortage is encountered, so that primary coverage procedures such as a groin flap or free tissue transfer are necessary to provide a sufficient soft tissue envelope for the transplanted toe. Technical difficulties in microsurgical procedures of the burned hand include dissection in heavily scarred tissues, shortage of large-

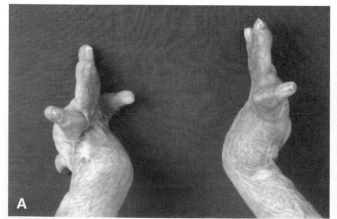
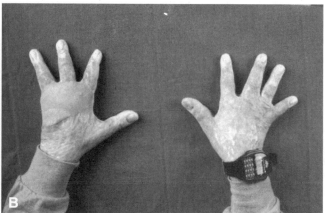

FIGURE 61-22. A, Severe bilateral contraction of the dorsum of the hand. **B,** Long-term result after release and reconstruction of the right hand with full-thickness skin grafts on the left hand with a conventional groin flap.

caliber cutaneous veins, and tight surrounding tissues with the risk of compression to the vascular pedicle after toe transfer.

Modified toe transfers such as en bloc transfers of the second and third toe to facilitate a three-point grip or additional transfers to the fourth or fifth ray may be indicated in severe cases to provide grip in the dominant hand. Whenever possible, local finger transpositions or partial finger transpositions should be employed to use any available intrinsic "spare parts."

Elbow Contractures

Elbow contractures are divided according to the structures involved into intra-articular and extra-articular types, involving skin, musculotendinous units, and the joint capsule. Most contractures are extra-articular flexion contractures. Correction can usually be achieved with all the measures described earlier (see Fig. 61-16). Contraction bands are usually released with any type of suitable "Z"-plasty. Thick split-thickness skin grafts can be used to resurface the volar aspect of the elbow if no vital structures are exposed. The combination of artificial dermis equivalents such as Integra, Alloderm, or Dermacell with split-thickness skin grafts has also yielded favorable results.[20] In deeper defects after release, flap coverage may be indicated. The spectrum of flaps ranges from local and regional flaps to sophisticated free flaps, depending on flap availability and the local situation. The following are the flaps most commonly used:

• Antegrade radial forearm flap
• Posterior interosseous transposition flap
• Recurrent collateral radial artery flap
• Inner upper arm fasciocutaneous flap
• Scapula free flap
• Parascapular free flap
• Anterolateral thigh free flap
• Fascial free flaps (temporoparietal, serratus anterior fascia)

Physical therapy is initiated as soon as graft take is guaranteed or secure healing of the flap is confirmed (Fig. 61-23).

Heterotopic Ossification

In severely burned patients the incidence of heterotopic bone formation is estimated to be in the range of 2%.[23] The incidence is higher in massive full-thickness burns and in elbows that have to be immobilized for a prolonged period. Radiographs are recommended before any contracture release of the elbow to rule out heterotopic ossification. Bone formation is usually found posteriorly and medially and occasionally leads to ulnar nerve entrapment. There are several reports about reduction of bone formation after hip surgery by nonsteroidal anti-inflammatory drugs, but data are sparse in the burn literature and prophylactic use is not applicable. The same holds true for protocols using bisphosphonates.[23,93]

Early excision is indicated only when severe impairment of active motion is caused by the newly formed bone. Otherwise it is recommended to wait until the bone has matured, usually after 12 to 18 months. Maturity can be confirmed by serial radiographs. The surgical approach is through a posteromedial incision. Care has to be taken not to injure the ulnar nerve and to avoid resection of the stabilizing medial collateral ligament complex. An arthrotomy should be part of the procedure to release any intra-articular adhesions. Physical therapy is of utmost importance and should be initiated after 2 days if the wound allows. Continuous passive motion postoperatively has also proven to be useful in our practice in these cases.

Axillary Contractures

Axillary contractures are divided into three groups[54,109]:

Type I patterns involve either the posterior (IA) or, in the majority of cases, the anterior axillary fold (IB).
Type II involve both axillary folds with an island of intact skin in the axillary dome.
Type III involve all structures in the axilla including the skin of the dome.

Contraction bands in both axillary folds are usually addressed by variations of "Z"-plasties if sufficient local tissue is available. In type II patterns, sequential operations are recommended, because the vascularization of the flaps

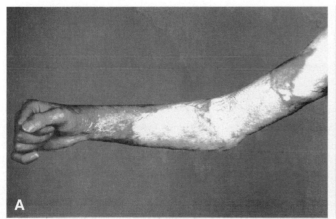
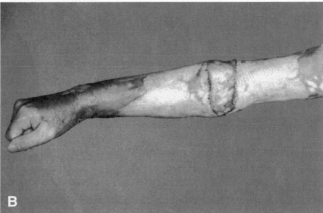

FIGURE 61-23. **A,** Elbow contracture. **B,** Release of elbow contracture by flap transfer.

may be jeopardized by a bilateral approach. Release should be performed to the underlying fascia of the latissimus or the pectoralis muscle to prevent early recurrence.

In type III patterns skin grafting is correlated with an extremely high incidence of recurrence. In this frequently uneven area, the results of skin grafting can be poor and secondary healing further promotes re-contraction. The same holds true for transplantation of dermis equivalents. Flap reconstruction has proven to be very helpful in these cases. Regional flaps such as the pedicled scapular fasciocutaneous, parascapular, or latissimus dorsi flaps are preferred when available. In severe cases in which no regional options exist, one should not hesitate to choose the option of a microsurgical free flap. The spectrum of flaps is identical to those listed earlier for elbow release, with the exception of the fascial flaps (Fig. 61-24).

Reconstructive Tools

"Z"-plasties and their modifications as well as most regional or microvascular flaps are described elsewhere (see Chapters 47 and 48). However, some flaps have proven to be very useful and are discussed here.

Commonly Used Flaps

A number of distant pedicle flaps are available for hand coverage. The choice of flap depends on the type of soft tissue coverage required, along with the experience of the surgeon involved. The entire armamentarium of flaps can be used in burn reconstruction. The spectrum ranges from simple distant flaps such as the random abdominal wall flap to regional pedicle flaps such as the groin flap or the tensor fascia lata flap. The cross-arm flap has also been utilized for acute coverage of burned hands[9] but has been generally abandoned owing to its unsightly donor site. Some of the more commonly employed flaps are described next.

The Random Abdominal Wall Flap

The random abdominal wall flap has the advantage of simplicity, in that no knowledge of specific vascular anatomy is necessary to perform the procedure. The flap is suitable for coverage of the entire hand and fingers. A disadvantage is that the covered hand is inaccessible for inspection. If the patient becomes febrile, operative exploration and takedown of the flap may be necessary to rule out infection. A second disadvantage is that the transplanted skin and subcutaneous tissue retains the characteristics of the fat cells in

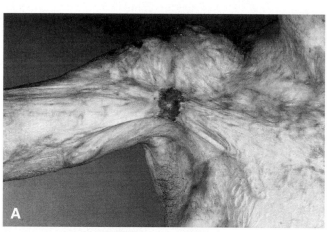

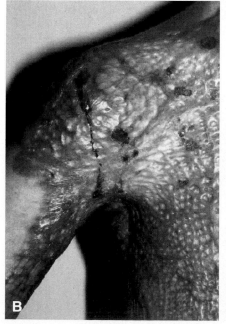

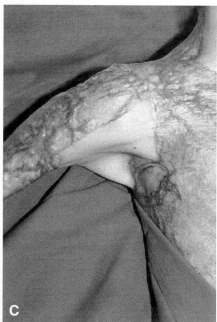

FIGURE 61-24. **A** and **B,** Axillary contracture type II—anteroposterior view. **C,** Contracture release with anterolateral thigh free flap. Note perfect contour with almost free range of motion.

abdominal skin: increase in body weight will result in a thickening of the transposed abdominal flap on the hand that mirrors increased abdominal girth. Finally, the immobility of the hand while in the abdominal tissue pocket results in joint stiffness at the hand, elbow, and shoulder and the donor site is highly unaesthetic.

The Groin Flap

One of the most important distant flaps is the groin flap.[26] Since the pedicled groin flap was first described by McGregor and Jackson in 1972[74] and the free groin flap was first applied clinically by Daniel and Taylor in 1973,[18] the free groin flap has become a well-accepted and widely used method for reconstruction of many types of defects.[16,60,71] The groin flap is a particularly useful flap in burn reconstruction because the groin is usually spared even in large body surface area burns. Use of the groin flap for acute coverage of burned hands has been well described.[34]

The superficial circumflex iliac artery (SCIA) runs parallel to and 2 to 3 cm inferior to the inguinal ligament.[105] This flap can reliably include skin 5 cm inferior and superior to the artery and approximately 5 cm beyond the anterior superior iliac spine. The presence and course of the superficial circumflex iliac artery should be confirmed by Doppler examination before elevation of the flap because this vessel is absent in a small percentage of patients. In such cases, a flap may be developed based on the adjacent superficial epigastric artery. (For further description of this flap see Chapter 47.)

The specific advantages of the free groin flap are large size of the flap, direct closure of donor defect in most cases, a scar situated in a usually hidden area, and reliability of the blood supply.[35] The blood supply to the flap consists of the superficial epigastric artery and/or the superficial circumflex iliac artery and their branches. These two arteries constitute a subcutaneous vascular network to give the flap adequate blood supply. This method, compared with the pedicled groin flap, is more convenient for the patient, the hospitalization time is shorter, and overall costs are lower. The free groin flap has subsequently been used less frequently as other donor sites have emerged, and problems exist with frequent anatomic variations in the groin flap's blood supply, a limited length and inconsistent caliber of the vascular pedicle, as well as excessive bulk in obese patients.[28]

The Tensor Fascia Lata Flap

The tensor fascia lata flap is based on the tensor fascia lata muscle and can be considered a second line of defense in burned hand reconstruction. A fasciocutaneous territory three to four times larger than the muscle can reliably be elevated for a total flap size of up to 15 × 14 cm.[72,105] The anterior aspect of the flap is defined as a line running from the anterior superior iliac spine to the lateral tibial condyle. The distal margin is a point approximately 8 cm superior to the knee. The posterior border runs along a line drawn from the greater trochanter to the head of the fibula. The vascular pedicle, located 6 to 10 cm below the anterior superior iliac spine, is the axis of rotation, allowing coverage of defects of the groin, sacrum, lower abdomen, or hand.[72,73] The use of the tensor fascia lata flap as a pedicled flap for hand coverage allows some shoulder and elbow motion before division of the pedicle. A disadvantage of this flap in burn

patients is the need to place operative incisions on the lateral thigh, normally a prime donor site for split-thickness autografts. Kimura[47] describes experience with a microdissected, thin, free tensor fascia lata perforator flap for reconstruction of hand skin defects. The perforators were anastomosed to the superficial radial artery or to the superficial palmar arch and both comitant veins. These procedures are not to be considered standard procedures and require above-average microsurgical skill with an increased risk of failure in the burned hand.

The Forearm Flaps

Forearm flaps are distally based on either the ulnar or radial artery and provide thin, tailored flap coverage and allow the upper extremity to be properly elevated during the initial phase of healing. Forearm flaps may be raised either as fascial flaps alone on the ulnar or radial artery or as a fasciocutaneous skin. Fascia alone provides a supple layer of subcutaneous tissue that is readily grafted with split skin. The forearm skin is relatively thin and provides acceptable cover for the dorsum of the hand, although it leaves a more obvious donor defect. Nevertheless, with the reversed flow forearm flaps, the donor defects are placed proximally over muscle bellies rather than over the tendons close to the wrist, and donor morbidity in general is low. Very large flaps can be raised if necessary. It is essential to ensure the presence and viability of the palmar arch before embarking on one of these flaps. Generally, the venae comitantes provide adequate venous drainage, and it has not been found necessary to anastomose additional superficial veins.[31,36]

ELECTRICAL INJURY

Epidemiology

Injuries through electric current are infrequently seen, comprising less than 3% of all admissions to specialized burn units in industrialized countries. Two thirds of all injuries are low-voltage injuries. The victims of major electrical trauma are characteristically young, previously healthy men and adolescents. The upper extremity is involved in between 75% and 88% of all electrical injuries.[8a] The patient profiles reflect the risk of occupational exposure: one third of all electrical injuries occur through contact with power lines, and one third are sustained in construction work.[58] Amputation rates range between 40% and 70%,[40] with mortality ranges in the 8% to 14% range. Hospital stay is significantly prolonged.[58] Five years after trauma, more than 50% of the patients still suffer from neurologic problems. In cases of occupational accidents, permanent disability has been noted in 85% of all patients with a high-voltage injury.[113]

Properties of Electricity and Pathophysiology

The history of electrical injuries started with the invention of the electric incandescent lamp by Thomas Alva Edison in 1879 and the death of a theater carpenter in Lyon, France in the same year, who was killed by an alternating current of 250 volts.[45] To understand the pattern of injuries it is helpful to consider the physical properties of electric current. The quantity of charge in a wire is expressed in amperes; one unit is defined as a flow of 6.2×10^{18} electrons per second. The potential difference between two points in a conductor characterizes the electromotive force and is defined in volts. Resistance describes the opposition of electron flow and is caused by collisions of current-carrying charged particles. Resistance is directly proportional to the length of the conductor and inversely proportional to its cross-sectional area and depends on the material of the conductor. The unit of resistance is the ohm. Today, distribution of electrical energy is mainly through alternating current. The motion of the electric charge is periodically reversed. The frequency of this change per cycle is defined as frequency in hertz. Voltage used in households and most industrial fields range, depending on the country, from 110 to 380 volts, for example, for stoves and ovens. Cross-country power lines carry 38,000 volts, most train power lines carry 15,000 volts with 16 hertz. Direct current is used only in specialized applications, such as subway train nets.

The three units of current are related by Ohm's law. It states that resistance equals the ratio of electromotive force and current in amperes:

$$R = V/I$$

Another important equation is Joule's law, which describes the heat production in an electric circuit. The heat in Celsius can be calculated as:

$$H = 0.24I^2 \times R \times t \text{ (duration in seconds)}$$

The extent of tissue damage is determined by current, voltage, duration of contact, tissue resistance, and pathway of flow through the body. Alternating current is more dangerous than direct current with respect to cardiac function. One to 2 milliamperes cause a tingling sensation, and muscular contraction is seen between 8 and 12 mA. More than 20 mA may exceed the "let go threshold" owing to tetanic muscular contractions caused by the alternating current, which can be strong enough to cause joint dislocations and even fractures. One hundred milliamperes can lead to ventricular fibrillation when flowing from hand to foot, with the same current passing through the brain causing immediate unconsciousness.

There are three current theories about the mechanism through which tissue damage is inflicted.

First, tissue resistance is a decisive factor in the extent of damage. The skin demonstrates values between 5,000 and 50,000 ohms/cm^2. The glabrous skin of the palm and feet may have a resistance of 2 million ohms, which can be 1000-fold reduced in the presence of moisture. Where skin resistance is low, the direct cutaneous effect is also low, but a high-energy current flows through the deeper tissues. When the skin resistance is high, low-energy current flows through deeper tissues but the skin manifestation of the burn is significant. The amount of heat generated by the flow of current is also proportional to the resistance of the tissue, which is again determined by the conducting properties and the cross-sectional area. The largest current densities (amps/cm^2) are passed through nerves and arteries, followed by muscle, skin, and bone. Muscle with the largest cross-sectional area passes the largest portion of electricity, although the resistance is relatively low. Areas with small cross-sectional areas such as the elbow or wrist demonstrate a high resistance, which leads (according to Joule's law) to extraproportional generation of heat. These areas are called "choke points."[111] This hypothesis is supported by experimental data from Hunt and colleagues,[40] who showed in rats that the individual conducting properties of tissues are less significant than the resistance related to the cross-sectional area.

The second theory is that current inflicts pores or defects in the cell membrane, leading to severe cell damage and death ("electroporation"). Lee and Kolodney[58] demonstrated that nonthermal electrical forces cause defects in the cell membrane, preferentially in the largest cell populations such as neurons or myocytes. The lesions can be found scattered throughout the muscle ("skipping lesions"). This would explain a portion of the myolysis and persistent neurologic deficits seen in electrical injuries.[19,124]

The third theory is based on a progressive constant release of arachidonic acid metabolites such as thromboxane from disrupted cells. Robson and associates[94] postulated that this will disturb the prostaglandin E_2/prostaglandin $E_{2\alpha}$ balance.

An ongoing discussion circles around this question: Is there progressive tissue damage or is the extent of damage determined primarily at the moment of trauma? Experimental data by Zelt and coworkers[125] speak in favor of a definitive extent of damage at the time of the injury, suggesting that in the clinical situation surgeons may be unable to determine the true extent of the damage.

Many surgeons strongly oppose these data based on their clinical experience. They frequently encounter progressive damage (i.e., ongoing muscle necrosis with serial débridements where healthy muscle had been seen 2 days before). Damage to vascular intima and media may lead to delayed occlusion with progressive damage, supported by local ischemia induced by release of thromboxane metabolites.[94a] The truth most likely lies in between, but it is agreed among burn surgeons that assessment of tissue damage in high-voltage injuries always poses a challenge, even for experienced surgeons.

Mechanism and Classification

Although, as described earlier, many factors determine the extent of tissue damage in electrical injuries, they have been divided for clinical purposes into low-voltage (<1000 V) and high-voltage (>1000 V) injuries.

Arcing occurs between objects of opposite charge and does not require direct contact. It is estimated that approximately 10,000 V can bridge a distance of 1 cm. Although voltage drops immediately after skin contact, temperatures from 3000° to 5000°C are developed for milliseconds, which are enough to inflict severe cutaneous destruction. Direct contact with high-tension lines frequently exceeds the "let go threshold" and the victim suffers continuous flow of current through the body. Flash burns are principally flame burns with ignition of the clothing and follow the same pathophysiologic principles as nonelectrical thermal injuries.

CLASSIFICATION OF ELECTRICAL INJURIES

LOW VOLTAGE

Flash

Direct contact

Cutaneous burn

Muscle contractures

Cardiac involvement

    Arrhythmias, ventricular and atrial fibrillation
    ST-segment/T-wave changes

HIGH VOLTAGE

Flash

Arcing

Direct contact

    Cutaneous burn
    Muscle contractures, fractures, dislocations
    Tissue destruction
        Muscle, nerve, vessels, bone, tendons
    Cardiac involvement
        Arrhythmias, elevated isoenzymes
        Ventricular and atrial fibrillation
        Electrocardiographic changes

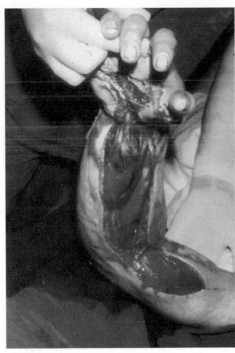

FIGURE 61-25. Clinical situation after high-voltage injury with current flow through the upper extremity.

Clinical Manifestations

High-voltage injuries are often life threatening owing to the combination of deep tissue destruction and large surface cutaneous burns. The clinical manifestations are related to exposure to the current, the pathway through the body, and the patient's premorbid medical status. The majority of injuries involve the hands. Contact burns are localized, deep, depressed, sometimes blistered, and frequently charred, with surrounding redness and swelling. Arcing occurs across flexor surfaces and typically involves the distal forearm, the antecubital fossa, and the axilla.[8a] High-tension injuries are devastating injuries, usually associated with an entrance wound and one or more exit wounds at the points where the current enters and exits the body.[38a] High-tension injuries have a high incidence of compartment syndrome. The main source of damage by the electrical current in the tissues is the conversion of the electrical energy into heat.[25] The heat generated by the electrical injury causes coagulation necrosis of the tissues involved. As explained earlier, the muscles with the largest cross-sectional areas suffer the greatest energy load. The rich vascular network also conveys thermal energy. It is therefore assumed today that bony necrosis is not caused by the poor conducting properties of the bone with a high resistance but by the extremely heated muscle environment. Similarly, intravascular thrombosis can be quite extensive and can lead to occlusion of major vessels. The extent of cutaneous damage is correlated to the skin resistance (see earlier). The upper extremity frequently presents in a fixed flexion contracture position that indicates severe muscle contraction and necrosis and most frequently the presence of a compartment syndrome. The loss of intra-

cellular proteins such as myoglobin due to rhabdomyolysis into the circulation is responsible for myoglobinuria, which may obstruct the renal collection system, potentially leading to renal failure (Fig. 61-25).

Because peripheral nerves are very sensitive to electrical forces, even minor electrical trauma may cause temporary nerve dysfunction. Symptoms of anesthesia, paresthesia, or dysesthesia may occur. Other clinically significant features of electrical injury include refractory cardiac arrhythmias, spinal fractures due to tetanic muscular contraction, other fractures and dislocations, serum electrolyte derangements, and blast trauma.[8a] These coexisting injuries must be diagnosed, assessed, and managed.

Management

Patient evaluation and resuscitation should proceed simultaneously. Stabilization of vital parameters and monitoring should include urinary catheters, central venous access, and invasive hemodynamic monitoring if indicated. Fluid requirements are significantly higher than in pure cutaneous burns, and care has to be taken not to underestimate the amount of fluid necessary to maintain appropriate urinary output, which should be at least 2 mL/kg/hr. In severe muscle destruction, the clinical picture of a "crush syndrome" is seen. Our experience has shown that two and a half to three times as much crystalloid is required in high-voltage injuries compared with similar surface flame burns. Some authors have recommended alkalinization of the urine to improve clearance of hemoglobin and myoglobin from renal tubuli,[3,66] whereas others have used high-volume lactated Ringer's resuscitation alone.[67] Levels of creatine kinase indicate the extent of muscle destruction but are not clearly correlated.

Low or normal levels, however, indicate only little or no dead muscle tissue.

Once the patient's condition is stabilized, a detailed history is essential, followed by a thorough physical examination for skeletal, neurologic, and intra-abdominal injuries. If there is concern about cardiac injury as indicated by electrocardiographic abnormalities on admission, continuous cardiac monitoring, daily 12-lead electrocardiograms, and cardiac isoenzyme analyses are performed to assess direct myocardial damage. Tetanus prophylaxis and antibiotics protecting against clostridial infection should be given.

Surgical Management

Once the patient's condition is stabilized, management is directed toward preservation of function, prevention of infection, ablation of clearly necrotic parts, and resurfacing of defects, especially those over vital structures such as arteries, nerves, tendons, and bone.[8a] Tissue decompression techniques are central to the successful initial treatment of electrical injuries to the upper extremity.[19] Standard escharotomies as described earlier should be combined with fasciotomies. Both escharotomies and fasciotomies should decompress the digits, carpal tunnel, and Guyon's canal. All compartments should be addressed both dorsally and volarly, and the muscle compartments in the hand should be adequately decompressed within 6 to 8 hours.[19] It has to be emphasized that sometimes division of the epimysium is also necessary, but the need for this is based on clinical assessment at the time of surgery. Measurements of intracompartmental pressures may be a useful adjunct, but clinical symptoms such as swelling, pain on passive motion, and firmness are usually sufficient. Skin burns should be incorporated into incision lines. Whereas escharotomies can be performed at the bedside, fasciotomies should be executed in the operating room and have to be considered emergency measures that can be the difference between the need for amputation versus limb salvage. Temporary coverage is recommended until conditions for definitive coverage are reached.

Radical débridement of nonviable tissue should be performed as soon as the patient's condition is stabilized. Regardless of the initial technique, a second-look operation to re-inspect tissues and to débride additional necrotic tissue should be undertaken every 48 hours, until only viable tissue remains.[19] After each débridement, allografts or topical antimicrobial agents are applied to the wounds. Splints are essential between surgeries to reduce pain, maintain position of function, prevent tendon rupture, and protect vascular perfusion.

Assessment of tissue viability can be performed by:

- Clinical evaluation (muscle color, contractile response)
- Scintigraphy with technetium-pyrophosphate
- Magnetic resonance imaging (MRI) with contrast medium enhancement
- Sequential histologic sections
- Perfusion with nitroblue-tetrazolium

Most surgeons rely on their clinical experience, which can be misleading, but clinical evaluation of tissue viability has not been surpassed by imaging techniques, of which scintigraphy is probably the most useful method. Whereas muscle is generously débrided, tendons and nerves are resected if they are clearly necrotic. If viability is questionable, early flap coverage may salvage the structures. If major vessels are occluded, vein graft reconstruction can be performed if well vascularized tissue coverage is provided.[115a] Excision and grafting of damaged arteries, especially at the wrist level, has been described with salvage of involved extremities.[123] Whether more aggressive early surgical reconstruction may prove to be beneficial in long-term patient outcome remains controversial.[19]

Once viability of the remaining tissue is established, skin grafts, local skin or fasciocutaneous flaps, or microvascular free flaps may be used to close the wound and salvage the injured extremity. The method of resurfacing is dependent on the tissue exposed, with split-skin grafts suitable for muscle and local, pedicled, and free flaps used for the coverage of nerves, patent arteries, tendons, and bone. Chick and coworkers[14] have reported promising results with radical débridement and free flap coverage within 3 days of injury based on their experience with trauma to other extremities. Many authors have also applied microvascular techniques for the salvage of limb and function in severe electrical injuries[33,44,101] (Fig. 61-26).

On occasion, tissue destruction in a limb is so extensive that limb salvage would jeopardize the patient's life. In these cases patient survival and functional outcome are best optimized by proximal limb amputation early in the treatment course ("life over limb"), although the threshold for the decision to amputate has moved somewhat higher in recent years. Today, use of microvascular free tissue transfer techniques has added much to limb salvage,[19] although somewhat higher complications rates have been reported in this group of patients.[7a] All reconstructive techniques described earlier and in other sections of this volume can be applied. The selection depends on the size of the defect, the availability of flaps, and the condition of the patient.

Complications

Early complications include vascular occlusion, wound infection caused by residual avascular tissue, systemic sepsis, multiorgan failure, and failure of reconstructive procedures with the consequence of limb amputation. Late sequelae include cataract formation, peripheral neuropathies, pulmonary dysfunction, cerebral hemorrhage, and muscle fibrosis.[19]

Rehabilitation

In view of the devastating nature of these injuries, rehabilitation is an essential part of the treatment regimen. Despite all efforts, many patients are left with permanent disabilities and are not able to return to their original occupation. Besides all conservative measures such as splinting, continuous passive motion, lymph drainage, compression therapy, prosthetic fitting, and intensive physical therapy, operative procedures such as tendon transfers to restore muscle function, transfer of innervated muscles, or toe transfer for missing thumbs are also an integral part of the rehabilitation program.

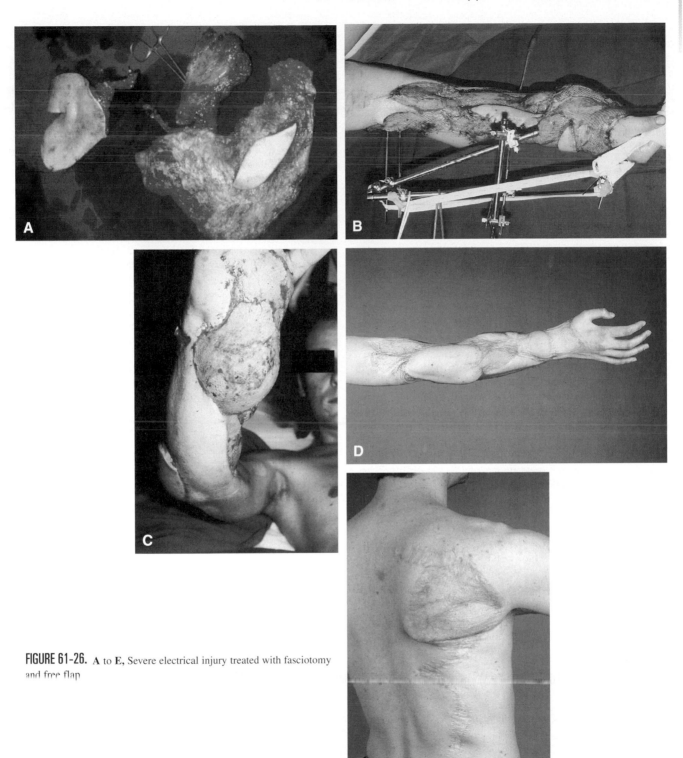

FIGURE 61-26. **A** to **E,** Severe electrical injury treated with fasciotomy and free flap.

CHEMICAL BURNS

Chemical burns are unique injuries that need specialized knowledge and management principles to obtain satisfying outcomes. Literature about therapy for chemical burns is relatively rare. However, chemical burns in our times are common problems, especially for hand surgeons. Various chemicals are widespread in common household and indus-

trial use. Products containing chemicals capable of causing a cutaneous injury number more than 25,000.[17] More than 60% of admissions to the hospital from chemical injuries are work related.[92] The upper extremity is one of the most affected parts of the body, specifically the digits. This implies an average total body surface area involvement of 19.5%. Long hospitalizations with poor wound healing is the rule.[10]

Similar to thermal burns, the damage of chemical burns of the hand is usually limited to the skin. The major difference, however, is that some chemical agents may continue to be active at the site and continue to destroy tissues. Ongoing tissue destruction will occur for as long as the chemical remains active and in contact with the skin. The level of injury depends on the area exposed to the chemicals, the nature and the concentration of the noxious agent, the volume of substance contacting the skin, local characteristics of the skin, and the duration of contact to the chemical[10,92] (Table 61-2). Duration of contact of the noxious agent with the skin is the major determinant of the chemical injury.[92] Most chemical injuries are the result of contact of the individual to either acid or alkaline agents.[10]

Acid burns are classically described as hydroscopic, gaining access through the protective stratum corneum. Cellular dehydration occurs as well as destruction of cell membranes and liquefaction necrosis. The reactions are progressive unless lavage or neutralization therapy is employed to chemically bind, inactivate, or remove the offending agent. Tissue damage depth is limited by the buffering capacity for acids contained in the damaged tissue.

Alkali burns are clinically more latent than acid burns. Alkaline albuminates combine with tissue elements to form fatty soaps. These hydroscopic reactions may continue for days with extensive destruction of tissue.[10] This tissue injury is commonly known as liquefaction necrosis. It allows for a deeper injury in comparison with acid burns due to a continued basic wound milieu produced by the alkaline injury. Because damaged tissue has a limited capacity to buffer alkalis, there is further penetration of the lipophilic alkali, which results in deeper injury.

Management

Chemical burns of the upper extremity do not present any special management problems that have not already been discussed under thermal or electrical injuries. The same careful attention must be given to elevation, immobilization, tetanus immunization status, and monitoring of pulses (Fig. 61-27).

There is no question about the first step in treatment, which is to stop the burning process. Immediately after contact with either acid or alkali, the removal of the patient from the offending chemical agent should be performed and all affected clothing should be removed. The initial goal in the treatment of chemical injuries is immediate dilution, or, better, neutralization of the chemical agent. Lavage that is not thorough enhances absorption of the agent. Water is the appropriate emergent treatment for most chemical contact spills. A water lavage of 1 to 2 hours is recommended for acid burns and longer for alkali burns.[21] Water lavage facilitates dilution of the chemical agent away from the victim, thereby decreasing the chemical load to the skin. In addition, water lavage decreases the rate of the chemical reaction and tissue metabolism and contributes to a restoration of normal skin pH.[92] Both animal studies and human experience confirm the essential fact that copious and continuous water irrigation immediately after chemical exposure is critical to limiting the injury process.[92] A delay of only 15 minutes after contact with a chemical agent may allow the epidermis to be destroyed.

Once the agent has been clearly established, neutralizing substances can be added.[38a] Skin pH measurements using litmus paper give a rough guide to neutralization of the surface skin but does not provide an accurate estimate of the pH of the deeper tissues, where the damage may be ongoing. Pain may also be a useful guide but is not completely reliable because some of the chemicals, such as phenols, demyelinate nerves, making the wound anesthetic.[92]

After adequate removal of the chemical from the injured part, the damaged skin must be protected from infection. Nonviable tissue, blisters, and bullae should be débrided, because they may contain residual concentrations of the chemical agent. Topical antibacterial agents should be applied. Partial-thickness chemical burns are generally managed conservatively with dressing changes. Patients with deep partial-thickness burns of the hands should be hospi-

Table 61-2
COMMON CHEMICAL AGENTS AND THEIR TISSUE DAMAGE CHARACTERISTICS

Agent	Commercial Use	Damage Characteristics	Treatment
Phenol	Cleaning agents, cosmetics, plastics	Protein denaturization, rapid absorption	Water irrigation, cover with oil, no alcohol
Phosphorus (white)		Highly fat soluble	Water irrigation, excision
Lyes	Cement, oven cleaners	Liquefaction necrosis, fulminant initial response, saponify fats, dehydrate other cells	Water irrigation
Hydrofluoric acid	Rust removers	Painful, deep ulcerations below tough coagulum	Local infiltration of calcium gluconates
Hydrochloric acidl	Pool cleaners	Shallow ulcers form with coagulated eschar and base	Water irrigation, magnesium oxide, soaps
Muriatic acid	Toilet bowl cleaners	Hard eschar with indolent ulcer	Water irrigation
Sodium hypochloride	Bleach	Coagulation of proteins	Water irrigation

Adapted from Bentivegna PE, Deane LM: Chemical burns of the upper extremity. Hand Clin 6:253–259, 1990; and Reilly DA, Garner WL: Management of chemical injuries to the upper extremity. Hand Clin 16:215-224, 2000.

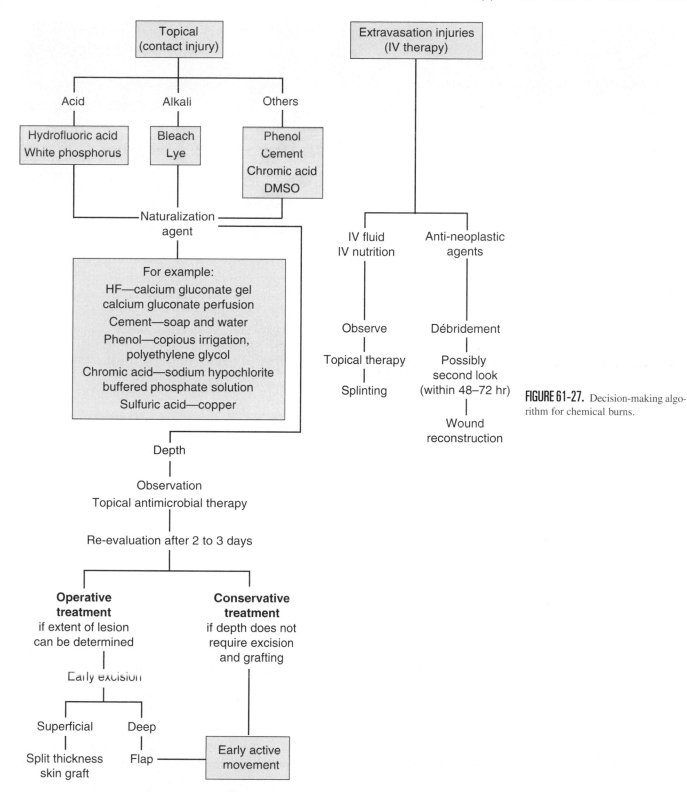

FIGURE 61-27. Decision-making algorithm for chemical burns.

talized and the injured skin should be excised and grafted early in a fashion similar to that outlined for thermal injuries.[10] Deeper injuries may require local or even microvascular flap coverage (Fig. 61-28).

Persistent chemical contact beneath the nail bed can be difficult to treat owing to water's inability to penetrate through the overlying nail. Partial or even complete removal of the nail may be necessary to obtain adequate water irrigation.

Similar to thermal injuries, the fascial compartments of the upper extremity are at risk to develop edema formation. Because the magnitude of a chemical injury may often be underdiagnosed in the early hours post compartment syndromes may be missed in their initial stages unless careful surveillance of the neurovascular status is carried out. Consequently, surgical release of the fascial compartments is performed in a standard fashion and treated as with open burn areas.[92]

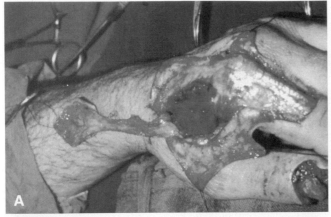

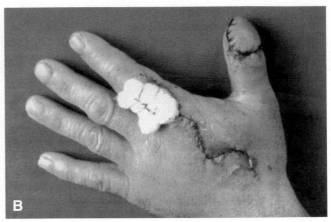

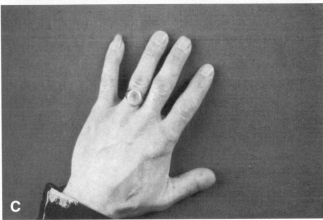

FIGURE 61-28. **A,** Hydrofluoric acid burn of the tip of the thumb with loss of the nail. The area is débrided and a "kite flap" (first DMCA flap) has been raised. The artery is clearly visible in the pedicle, which includes the fascia of the interosseous muscle. **B,** The flap has securely healed in. A full-thickness skin graft is applied to the donor site. **C,** Result is aesthetic appealing.

Treatment of Burns Caused by Specific Chemical Agents

Specific exceptions to the rule of copious water dilution for chemical injuries deserve mention.

Phenol

Phenol was historically used as an antiseptic. Its use was limited by the appearance of cutaneous irritation and systemic symptoms (phenol marasmus). Today, phenol has wide use in industrial substances such as cleaning agents, cosmetics, plastics, and explosives. Phenol is not water soluble, and specific therapy is required. Phenol should be removed from the skin with glycerol or polyethylene glycol.

Hydrofluoric Acid

Hydrofluoric acid is a common industrial chemical. It penetrates the skin, especially areas not protected by the stratum corneum such as the nail bed, and causes severe pain. Treatment consists of immediate water lavage followed by specific fluoride binding therapies. Traditionally, magnesium sulfate solutions have been used with limited success. More recent therapies include 10% calcium gluconate subdermal injections.

Cement

Cement burns are traditionally considered alkali burns because the lime (calcium oxide) component of cement has a pH as high as 12.9. There is usually no initial pain, so the injury remains unrecognized and untreated for hours. The final result usually presents itself as a full-thickness injury that is very slow to heal.

White Phosphorus

Phosphorus is highly fat soluble. Absorption of this chemical is enhanced by oils used topically and should be avoided. Therapy consists of water lavage followed by identification and excision of remaining particles. A dilute solution of copper sulfate (0.05% to 1%) is helpful in identifying phosphorus particles.

FROSTBITE INJURIES

Frostbite is an injury that results from exposure to temperatures that are low enough to cause crystal formation in the exposed tissue. There is risk for tissue exposed to temperatures below −2°C.[11] Frostbite can develop after exposure to these low temperatures for more than 1 hour[49] and usually occurs when protection from the environment is insufficient.[118] The severity of frostbite depends on numerous factors besides the ambient temperature, such as wind velocity ("wind chill factor"), altitude, duration of exposure, wetness of the tissue, the patient's vascular status, and previous exposure to cold injury.[11]

A variety of classification systems have been developed to describe frostbite injuries. Traditionally, cold injuries have been classified into four degrees[50]:

First degree (superficial skin): Erythema, edema, and hyperemia develop in the injured areas; blisters and tissue loss do not occur.

Second degree (full-thickness skin): Erythema, vesicle formation, and superficial skin sloughs occur; no deeper necrosis develops.

Third degree (full-thickness skin and subcutaneous tissue): Local edema and grayish blue discoloration occur and are followed by skin loss down to the subcutaneous level.

Fourth degree: Deep cyanosis without development of vesiculation or local edema is observed. There is necrosis of subcutis or deeper tissues down to muscle, tendon, and bone.

Currently, a more clinically useful classification system considers frostbite injuries as superficial or deep.[114] This classification system is useful because it has prognostic implications and defines frostbite through its fluctuating clinical course. Superficial frostbite results in minimal, if any, tissue loss. In contrast, deep frostbite injuries result in significant tissue loss.[106]

Outdoor winter activities such as skiing, cross-country skiing, or other sporting activities[81] and mountaineering make cold injury a continuous clinical problem. Inadequate clothing, prolonged exposure due to alcohol abuse,[11] psychiatric disorders, or accidents[52] may lead to these injuries. The fingers, toes, nose, and ears are most commonly involved.

Pathophysiology

In the cold-exposed areas blood becomes viscous and circulation in the capillaries slows. Vessel damage leads to fluid extravasation and blistering. Thrombosis may occur in the terminal arterioles. Although cellular dehydration and enzymatic damage undoubtedly contribute to the necrosis of frozen tissue, peripheral circulatory failure may play the major role in determining the extent of eventual tissue loss.[107] Venules clot with thrombi within the first 10 minutes after rewarming. Within 1 hour, most of the capillaries are thrombosed and blood flow is short-circuited through arteriovenous communications. Thus, whereas blood may continue to flow through the larger arterioles and venules, the tissues are not nourished.[107] Two different theories concerning the pathogenesis of frostbite are discussed:

1. Cold injury directly damages the tissue cells.[76]
2. Cold produces injury to the endothelial lining of small blood vessels with a consequent increase in capillary permeability, loss of fluid from the circulation, and intravascular cellular aggregation in the injured area. The clumping of the red blood cells causes occlusion of small blood vessels with resulting tissue ischemia and necrosis.[120]

Diagnosis

Both history and physical examination are important in assessing the depth and degree of frostbite injury. The severity is both proportional to temperature and duration of exposure and depends on the amount of heat lost from tissues.[106]

Various imaging techniques have been tried to more accurately predict the extent and severity of frostbite injury.

Plain radiographs are of no value in determining the ultimate level of demarcation.[106] Technetium-99m (^{99m}Tc) bone scanning has become the standard imaging study employed within the first several days to assess tissue perfusion and viability.[5,29] It allows for evaluation of the microcirculation of both soft tissue and bone.[106] Cauchy and coworkers found a strong correlation between positive uptake and eventual healing.[13a] They showed that ^{99m}Tc bone scanning in the first few days after frostbite injury indicates the level of amputation in severe frostbite in more than 84% of cases.

Barker and coworkers[5] compared MRI and magnetic resonance angiography (MRA) to bone scanning for the evaluation of frostbite injuries.[5] Both MRI and MRA directly image occluded vessels and surrounding tissues. Both define the extent of tissue ischemia well before clinical signs of necrosis. T2-weighted images show increased signal intensity in muscles after disruption of cell membranes as well as increased content of extracellular water, an indicator of cell death. The major disadvantage of MRI and MRA is their high cost compared with bone scans and their frequently limited availability.

Treatment

Management of acute frostbite is carried out in accordance with the guidelines popularized by Mills[78] (Table 61-3).

Early treatment includes a thorough assessment of the patient's general condition and stabilization of other disorders in a routine system of priorities. The restoration of normal body temperature through provision of a warm environment and oral or intravenous administration of warm liquids is the first priority. Immediate local treatment consists of rewarming of the frozen extremity in warm water (40° to 44°C).[38] This emergency treatment is widely accepted as the single most important step in the salvage of tissue and limb function, followed by elevation and splinting of the extremity.[95] Tetanus prophylaxis is given and analgesia as indicated, while some consider antibiotic prophylaxis important for the first few days.[11,106] Local treatment concepts for the affected areas vary. Some reports consider

Table 61-3
MANAGEMENT OF ACUTE FROSTBITE

Restore core body heat

Rapid rewarming of the frozen extremity in a 40° to 44°C water bath

Sedation and/or analgesia

Triple-phase technetium-Tc99m bone scan

Tetanus prophylaxis

Open dressing

Oral ibuprofen

Antibiotics for confirmed infections

Physical therapy

Amputation or surgical débridement only after clear demarcation

Modified from Mills WJ Jr: Frostbite: A method of management including rapid thawing. Northwest Med 65:119–125, 1966.

early débridement of all blisters to be adequate,[11] whereas other authors favor débridement of only the ruptured blisters.[79]

Hydrotherapy is the only adjuvant intervention (daily treatment for 30 to 45 minutes at 40°C) that reliably improves vascularization of the affected tissues after cold injury.[38] Heparinization has been used to prevent intravascular thrombosis, but the results have been inconclusive.[76] Pentoxifylline shows some beneficial effects in animal models[90] but has not become a generally accepted therapeutic agent. Inhibitors of prostaglandin synthesis and inhibitors of free radicals such as superoxide dismutase may be promising agents for the future.[11,48]

Surgical management is conservative. The principle of early excision and grafting is not applied to frostbite injuries, because determination of the extent of tissue damage is extremely difficult and a high capacity for spontaneous healing under the eschar is frequently observed. During the first 9 to 15 days, seriously frostbitten skin forms a black, hard, leathery eschar.[106] Over time, the eschar separates, frequently revealing relatively healthy underlying skin. Some wounds will not heal and instead proceed to complete mummification within 3 to 6 weeks.[84] Once mummification of the involved extremity has taken place, reconstructive or ablative options are to be considered. Primary amputation of an affected digital part is often the most expeditious and least morbid method of restoring function to the remaining digit or hand.[114]

When more extensive upper extremity frostbite injuries are encountered, skin grafts, local rotation flaps, and staged pedicle grafts have been the mainstay of reconstructive techniques. With the advent of microsurgical tissue transfer, the surgical options for extremity reconstruction including restoration of grip function have been significantly broadened. While the functional results have improved by virtue of thin tissue transfer, aesthetic restoration still remains a challenge.[114]

REHABILITATION

As in all hand surgery, planned rehabilitation with intensive physiotherapy and occupational therapy is an essential prerequisite for the best possible results. In general terms, active movement is encouraged as early as possible after thermal injury. Immediately after contracture release, splinting is of the utmost importance. The joints can be immobilized in ideal positions (Fig. 61-29), or dynamic splints can be applied to encourage active motion after surgical corrections (Fig. 61-30).

The first few months after a burn are characterized by a period of scar hypertrophy. Scars become thick, red, and tight, and they limit the range of motion. The patient needs to overcome this tightness with active range-of-motion exercises of all joints every day. An important adjunct to scar management are custom-fitted elastic pressure garments. Linares and coworkers have provided interesting details about the history of pressure treatment.[61] The first full description dates back to Petz in 1790. The first reference was written by Johnson in 1678, who referred to the work of Ambroise Paré from the 16th century. Nason observed in 1942 that ischemia produced by pressure stops

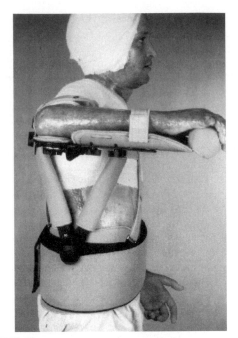

FIGURE 61-29. Adjustable splint after release of axillary contracture.

the formation of hypertophic scarring with ideal pressure ranges between 15 and 40 mm Hg.

Pressure therapy should be initiated as early as 2 weeks after grafting. The pressure garments should be worn 23 hours a day for the initial period of approximately 6 months in burns with prolonged healing time or burns that have required skin grafting.[102] Subsequent pressure garment use is individualized depending on scar quality and response. The exact mechanism by which pressure garments alter scar formation is not yet clear.[84a] However, they improve the quality of scars in both texture and color in the long term (Fig. 61-31). Special spacers may be placed in the web spaces to minimize the problem of compromised web spaces by burn scar contractures.[1]

Silicone sheets have proven to be useful on the dorsum of fingers and web spaces, if placed under the pressure garment gloves. Coban wrapping is useful in controlling edema. Hand therapy continues until function returns to normal or treatment is no longer demonstrating improvement. A maintenance hand therapy program should then be continued.[102]

CRITICAL POINTS: MANAGEMENT OF HAND BURNS

- Avoid any additional injury or an increase in the depth of the burn ("Do no harm").
- Achieve early wound closure.
- Maintain active and passive range of motion.
- Prevent infection or loss of soft tissue coverage.
- Achieve early functional rehabilitation.

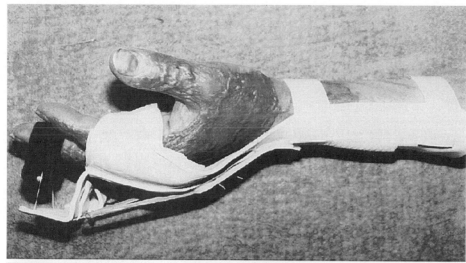

FIGURE 61-30. Active dynamic extension splint after release of extensor tendons.

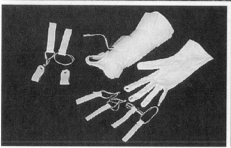

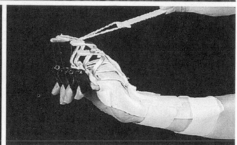

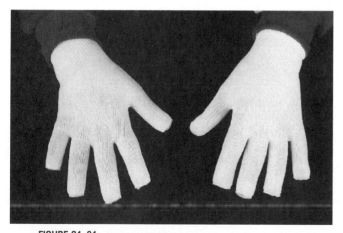

FIGURE 61-31. Custom-fitted pressure gloves after skin graft.

ANNOTATED REFERENCES

3. Arturson G, Hedlund A: Primary treatment of 50 patients with high-tension electrical injuries: I. Fluid resuscitation. Scand J Plast Reconstr Surg 18:111-118, 1984.

   This paper retrospectively investigates the outcome and complication rates of patients with high-tension electrical injuries with special regard to the fluid resuscitation and early internal organ involvement. The paper is of importance owing to the high number of patients and the principal value of the conclusions.

6. Baryza MJ, Baryza GA: The Vancouver Scar Scale: An administration tool and its interrater reliability. J Burn Care Rehabil 16:535-538, 1995.

   The authors describe a pocket-sized tool to aid in scoring burn scars based on the Vancouver Scar Scale. This tool makes the Burn Scar Index a viable measure for clinical practice and research.

10. Bentivegna PE, Deane LM: Chemical burns of the upper extremity. Hand Clin 6:253-259, 1990.

    This paper gives an excellent overview on chemical burn injuries, with special emphasis on specific emergency therapies. It also includes a comprehensive summary of common agents and their toxicity tissue action. Because many of the agents are still in use, reading of this article is recommended.

12. Bunyan AR, Mathur BS: Medium thickness plantar skin graft for the management of digital and palmar flexion contractures. Burns 26:575-580, 2000.

    The technique of plantar skin grafts with reference to take of graft, quality of skin, comparability with digital skin, healing of donor area, and recurrence are discussed in this paper and compared with other techniques and studies. The high number of patients presented in this study makes the results worthwhile.

14. Chick L, Lister GD, Sowder L: Early free flap coverage of electrical and thermal burns. Plast Reconstr Surg 89:1013-1021, 1992.

    This paper is one of the first reports about the controversially discussed concept of early post-traumatic excision and coverage of high-tension electrical burns with free flaps.

18. Daniel R, Taylor G: Distant transfer of an island flap by microvascular anastomoses. Plast Reconstr Surg 52:111-122, 1973.

    Historical paper reporting the first cutaneous free flap.

19. Danielson JR, Capelli-Schellpfeffer M, Lee RC: Upper extremity electrical injury. Hand Clin 16:225-234, 2000.

Excellent review about electrical injuries of the upper extremity. This article gives a good overview about pathophysiology, clinical manifestations, medical management, surgical therapeutic options, and rehabilitation protocols after high-voltage injuries.

23. Evans EB: Heterotopic bone formation in thermal burns. Clin Orthop 263:94-101, 1991.

This paper presents a tutorial review about heterotopic bone formation, which is a rare complication in burned patients. However, knowing about occurrence may help in detecting heterotopic ossification in patients.

26. Giessler GA, Erdmann D, Germann G: Soft tissue coverage in devastating hand injuries. Hand Clin 19:63-71, 2003.

This paper points out the importance of reconstructive algorithms for mutilating hand injuries. It describes the reconstructive ladder that helps in decision making about soft tissue coverage and functional reconstruction.

33. Grotting J, Walkinshaw M: The early use of free flaps in burns. Ann Plast Surg 15:127-131, 1985.

The authors describe case studies on patients with full-thickness burns of the upper extremity in which they considered free flaps as ideal solution for initial wound closure.

39. Herruzo-Cabrera R, Garcia-Torres V, Rey-Calero J, Vizcaino-Alcaide MJ: Evaluation of the penetration strength, bactericidal efficacy, and spectrum of action of several antimicrobial creams against isolated microorganisms in a burn centre. Burns 18:39-44, 1992.

This paper gives a comprehensive comparison on the penetration capacity, bactericidal efficacy, and spectrum of action of eight antimicrobial creams against microorganisms isolated from burn patients.

54. Kurtzman LC, Stern PJ: Upper extremity burn contractures. Hand Clin 6:261-279, 1990.

This article discusses the reconstructive options for axillary, antecubital, wrist, MCP joint, and interdigital web contractures with special emphasis on the techniques and advantages of local flap reconstruction.

62. Lionelli GT, Lawrence WT: Wound dressings. Surg Clin North Am 83:617-638, 2003.

There are currently hundreds of dressings on the market to aid in wound management. This article provides a framework to assist in dressing assessment and selection. Properties of the various dressings are described and compared.

92. Reilly DA, Garner WL: Management of chemical injuries to the upper extremity. Hand Clin 16:215-224, 2000.

This article reviews management of chemical burn injuries of the upper extremity and provides a critical pathway based on the principles of pathophysiology.

98. Salisbury RE: Reconstruction of the burned hand. Clin Plast Surg 27:65-69, 2000.

This article documents problems, pitfalls, and complications of the reconstruction and rehabilitation of the burned hand. A milestone review.

102. Smith MA, Munster AM, Spence RJ: Burns of the hand and the upper limb—a review. Burns 24:493-505, 1998.

This paper outlines the reconstructive principles and a problem-oriented approach to the most common reconstructive problems of thermal injury to the hand and upper limb.

106. Su CW, Lohman R, Gottlieb LJ: Frostbite of the upper extremity. Hand Clin 16:235-247, 2000.

This is an excellent review about frostbite of the upper extremity. It gives a good overview about the pathophysiologic mechanisms, the clinical and radiographic evaluation, the medical management, the surgical therapeutic options, and the late sequelae.

CHAPTER 62

Skin Tumors

Kevin C. Chung

A vast array of tumors may occur in the hand. These range from ordinary skin cancers, typical of those found elsewhere on the body, to several tumors preferentially or exclusively occurring in the hand. Management of hand tumors requires hand surgeons to perform as surgical oncologists and reconstructive surgeons—two roles that are often at odds with one another in their surgical goals. While the surgical oncologist aims to totally eradicate the malignant tumor, sometimes at the expense of functional and aesthetic considerations, the reconstructive surgeon toils to restore the upper extremity to normalcy. An optimal outcome for these patients can only be achieved by strict adherence to oncologic principles, even when following these principles makes the subsequent reconstruction more challenging.

Many types of tumors can grow on the skin. These range from the common basal cell carcinoma that has low metastatic potential to melanoma, which can appear insidiously and metastasize to various other organs. In addition, many tumors are rather unusual (e.g., the sweat gland tumors), whereas others, such as squamous cell carcinoma, are increasing in incidence in the white population because of elevated exposure to ultraviolet radiation.[120] Recent data estimate that there are 1.2 million cases of nonmelanoma skin cancers (basal and squamous cell cancers) in the United States, at an annual cost of treatment exceeding $500 million.[85] Because of the prevalence of skin malignancy, hand surgeons will need to play an integral role in treating skin disorders of the upper extremity. Hand surgeons have a unique understanding of the functional goals of the upper limb and can be instrumental in working with dermatologists in the ablation and reconstruction of many of these disorders. Because the upper extremity is often exposed, many of the skin tumors can be noticed at the beginning stages of their growth. Even the more serious malignancies can be cured when treated early in their evolution. The goal of this chapter is to present tumors arising from the skin of the upper extremity and to provide current treatment recommendations. Tumors that grow under the skin, such as giant cell tumors, ganglion cysts, and glomus tumors, are covered in Chapter 63 on soft

CRITICAL POINTS: STRATEGIES IN TREATING MALIGNANT SKIN LESIONS

INDICATION

- Biopsy confirmation: perform excisional biopsy if defect can be closed primarily. If defect cannot be closed primarily, perform excisional biopsy, incorporating some normal skin at the excision margin.

PREOPERATIVE EVALUATION

- Complete physical examination to look for other suspicious skin lesions and palpate for enlarged epitrochlear and axillary nodes.
- For melanoma, obtain chest radiograph and liver function tests to evaluate for possible distant metastasis. Work with dermatologists and tumor oncologists for comprehensive care of the patient, preferably through a melanoma clinic.

PEARLS

- Develop a working relation with a dermatopathologist to ensure correct diagnosis and adequate clearance of surgical margins.
- Do not ignore other reconstructive options. Skin graft is an excellent option for ease of tumor surveillance, particularly if the tumor is highly invasive and requires monitoring.

POSTOPERATIVE CARE

- Work with a dermatologist to follow the patients on a semi-annual or annual basis.

I wish to acknowledge the comprehensive work of **Earl J. Fleegler, MD,** in the prior editions of this text, which laid the foundation for this chapter. I also appreciated the help of Steven C. Haase, MD, and Sandra V. Kotsis, MPH, in the preparation of this chapter.

tissue tumors of the hand. Whereas the content of this chapter will be comprehensive in addressing most skin tumors, greater emphasis will be placed on the more common varieties, including nonmelanoma and melanoma skin cancers, by illuminating recent treatment recommendations from the National Institutes of Health Consensus Panel and other national and international organizations.

GENERAL PRINCIPLES

Approach to the patient with a skin neoplasm should begin with a detailed history of the lesion, including duration and changes in size or color. One should also consider risk factors for skin cancer, collecting information on history of extensive sun exposure, childhood sunburns, exposure to chemicals, and ionizing radiation. Pathology reports from previous biopsies or excisions should be obtained and reviewed, along with the operative notes, if available (see Critical Points).

Ideally, all physicians should carry out complete inspection of the skin as a part of their physical examination.[44] This requires communicating the reasons and importance for such an examination to the patient. Adequate lighting is necessary. The patient must be completely undressed but covered adequately to prevent embarrassment, because the examination completely evaluates skin from the scalp to the plantar surfaces of the feet. Use of a magnifying lens and even Wood's light is helpful to evaluate certain melanocytic lesions.[60]

Physical examination in patients with skin tumors should include a full hand examination, along with palpation of the regional lymph nodes. Lesion size should be carefully documented in the medical record. If benign lesions are to be followed clinically, photographic documentation of the appearance may help detect changes over time. Photographs are also recommended in the patient with multiple or subtle lesions, which can be marked to help with identification. Radiographs are not essential for most skin lesions unless involvement of underlying joint or bone cannot be ruled out on physical examination. Radiologic evaluation is indicated, however, for very large skin tumors and for those fixed to underlying structures.

Some practitioners may wish to save time and expense by not submitting tissue from benign-appearing lesions to pathology for evaluation. I believe that every skin lesion should be sent for pathologic analysis, no matter how innocuous it appears, because clinical diagnosis may not be perfectly accurate. Any misdiagnosis of a malignant lesion, no matter how infrequent, may have deleterious effects to an individual patient. Large lesions should have orientation stitches placed in one or two areas to help the pathologist interpret the margins in relation to the surrounding anatomy. These guidelines will ensure that a malignancy is never overlooked and that a positive margin can be adequately localized for re-excision.

Small tumors are often easily removed via excisional biopsy by removing an ellipse of tissue that can be closed primarily. It is advisable to design the orientation of the elliptical excision parallel to the long axis of the extremity. This makes subsequent re-excision of the scar easier, if required, and will cause less disruption of the axial lymphatic drainage. Larger tumors, especially those in which malignancy is suspected, are best managed by performing an incisional biopsy first, which can often be performed under local anesthesia. A full-thickness sample of the lesion should be taken from one of the peripheral edges, where it meets normal tissue. This will help the pathologist identify the malignant tissues in the context of the surrounding normal skin. In tumors with ulcerative central lesions, a biopsy from the center of the tumor will often contain excessive necrotic debris and may contain very few malignant cells. The incisions made for the biopsy should not extend beyond what would be excised in any future resection. An accurate tissue diagnosis might significantly change the surgical plan by determining what the margins of excision should be.

If an incisional biopsy of a large lesion returns as a benign diagnosis, the decision to delay or avoid further operation must not be made without careful consideration. It is always possible to miss a malignancy arising in one part of a large, otherwise benign lesion. This sort of "sampling error" must be addressed in the management plan of large "benign" lesions. Often, one can be conservative and perform an initial excision of the tumor with 1- to 2-mm margins. If the pathology examination of the specimen reveals a malignancy or other locally aggressive lesion, the wound can then be re-excised with a more generous margin to conform to current treatment recommendations.

When excision of a neoplastic lesion is undertaken, the margin of excision should be carefully planned and marked preoperatively. In the operating room, special consideration should be given to use of the tourniquet. Typically, the arm is not exsanguinated before tourniquet inflation. It is theorized that tumor cell aggregates may form just distal to the tourniquet, where the flow of blood has been halted. A great deal more has been written about the horizontal or radial margins of resection than about the vertical or deep margins of tumor excision. Conceptually, the radial margin for an individual lesion should incorporate enough surrounding normal-appearing skin to excise the vast majority of subclinical tumor extension that characterizes many skin malignancies. This margin will vary depending on the tumor type, size, and depth of invasion. Some of the more common skin cancers have standardized recommendations for horizontal excision margins, because many clinical trials have been performed to establish guidelines for these margins. But the behavior of less common tumors cannot be so easily anticipated because much of the data available are from case reports or very small series.

The vertical (deep) margin is not often discussed but is no less important. This becomes a critical issue in the distal upper extremity, where very little subcutaneous tissue is interposed between the dermis and the deeper structures. In general, the excision specimen should contain both the epidermis and the dermis. For large tumors, or tumors believed to have an extended vertical component (i.e., nodular melanoma), the resection should include the subcutaneous layer up to (but not including) the next anatomic layer, which may be muscle fascia in the forearm or paratenon in the hand. Resections to this depth will successfully remove the overwhelming majority of skin cancers.

If deeper invasion is suspected in a large tumor, or if a tumor appears to be fixed to deeper structures, appropriate preoperative imaging, including magnetic resonance imaging, should be used to assess the depth of invasion. A skin tumor that invades tendon, joint, or bone must be viewed as a high-risk tumor, and amputation or partial amputation should be considered.

A detailed review of reconstruction of large defects in the hand and forearm is beyond the scope of this chapter. However, a couple of key points should be emphasized regarding the closure of defects after tumor extirpation. If there is any doubt about the margins of the resection, extensive undermining and complicated flap closures should be avoided so that residual tumor cells do not spread throughout the undermined tissues and flap donor sites.

Most large tumor excisions, even radical excisions down to fascia or paratenon, can be closed with a skin graft, unless tendons or bones are exposed after deep resection. Using separate, sterile surgical teams and setup to harvest the skin graft will avoid contamination of the donor site with tumor cells. Although skin grafts on the hand are not always as durable as more complicated flaps, they allow the wound to heal with minimal dissection and make detection of recurrence much easier.

If more durable coverage is required, or deeper structures are exposed that will not heal with skin grafting alone, a variety of local, distant, and free flaps are available. Before proceeding with flap closure, however, complete tumor removal should be confirmed. In some cases, frozen section pathology may be reliable. If the margins are in question, the wound can simply be covered with allograft skin for several days until the final pathology results from the permanent sections are available. Allograft skin will prevent desiccation and infection of the defect while encouraging growth of granulation tissue in the wound. These principles can be applied to nearly every skin tumor found in the upper extremity. In the following sections, many of these tumors and tumor-like conditions are discussed in greater detail.

Concept of Surgical Margin

The issue of surgical margin is important in the operative extirpation of skin tumors; however, it is a concept that is not well understood by surgeons.[1] Because skin tumors, particularly melanoma and squamous cell carcinoma (SCC) and, to a lesser extent, basal cell carcinoma, often extend beyond the visible margin of the tumor, a sufficient surgical margin of resection will ensure that the tumor is completely excised. The wider the margin of resection, the higher the chance of completely extirpating the tumor. Over the trunk and the thighs, wider surgical margins can be closed easily with large flaps or skin grafts. However, in more privileged areas, such as the hand and the head/neck regions, wide excision may compromise the functional and aesthetic appearance, which makes reconstruction much more complex. The issue of surgical margin has been intensely studied in malignant skin tumors and the recommendation is to derive the narrowest surgical margins and still provide a high rate of cure.

Once the tumor is excised, pathologists undertake histologic sections of the specimen to determine whether the "margin is clear." What is often not understood by surgeons is that the pathologists only sample the margins; and a "clear margin" report by pathologists, although reassuring to the surgeon and the patient, only means that the representative sections are free of tumor. These representative sections are only a sampling of the entire specimen, depending on how the pathologist chooses the sampling sections. Because this is a sampling technique, not all margins are examined and tumor skip areas may misrepresent the margins as well. To study the whole specimen comprehensively would require thousands of serial sections.[1] Frederick E. Mohs, in 1936, described a method of fixing skin cancer in situ with serial excision and examination of the tissues to obtain clear margins.[71] This Mohs' procedure, usually performed by dermatologists, is reserved for important aesthetic and functional areas, such as the face (e.g., around the eyes, nose, and ears) and perhaps the fingers. This is an expensive and time-intensive procedure and should not be prescribed for small tumors that can easily be excised. However, it can be quite effective for larger SCC of the fingers when the surgical margin is uncertain and also for recurrent SCC when local tumor control is more difficult.

 Anatomy

Having a fundamental knowledge of the structures of the skin is essential in understanding the development of various types of skin tumors and their behavioral patterns (Fig. 62-1). The dermis lies between the outer aspect of the skin, the epidermis, and the subcutaneous fat. In the dermis, we find skin appendages, including hair follicles and sebaceous glands in the extensor skin surface and eccrine sweat glands in the palmar skin. Masses arising from sebaceous glands are limited to the extensor surface of the hand, whereas the uncommon sweat gland tumors may arise from the palmar skin. Superficial papillary dermis projects into the overlying epidermal ridges. The deeper, reticular dermis lies over the subcutaneous fat and includes the termination of sensory nerve end organs, blood vessels, and lymphatics. Lymph node drainage areas include the epitrochlear nodes in the vicinity of the medial epicondyle of the humerus and more proximally along the cephalic venous drainage in the deltopectoral and axillary areas.[53] Some skin tumors that can metastasize to regional nodes include SCC, melanoma, sweat gland carcinomas, and Merkel's cell carcinoma.

BENIGN TUMORS OF THE SKIN

Pseudotumors

Sebaceous Cyst
These lesions can have an appearance similar to epidermoid inclusion cysts but have a distinct etiology. Arising from obstructed apocrine glands in the skin, these cysts contain sebum rather than keratin (trapped keratinocytes from a puncture wound result in an epidermal inclusion cyst) and usually have a more obvious pore communicating with the surface of the skin. This central pore needs to be excised with the cyst to prevent recurrence. These lesions occasionally appear on the dorsum of the hand and should be excised

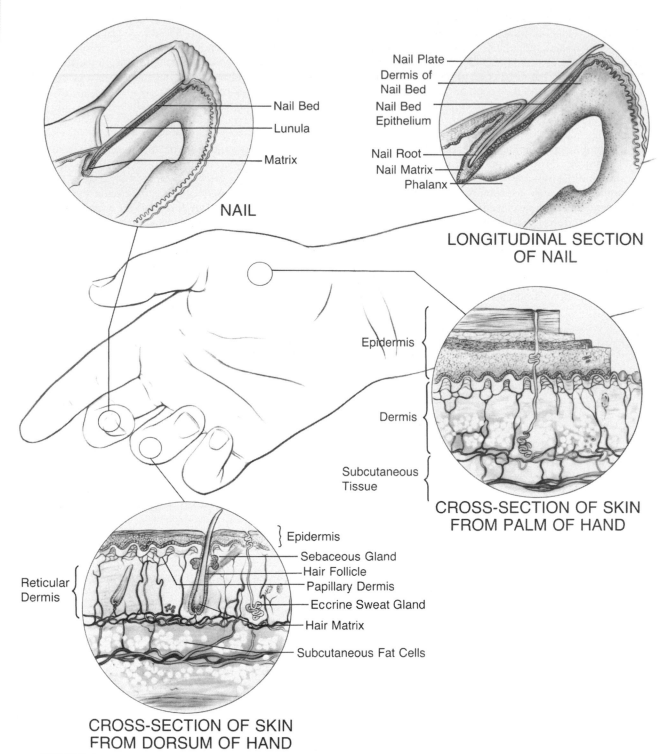

FIGURE 62-1. Histologic anatomy of the skin, showing the differences between thick palmar skin and thin skin of the dorsum of the hand.

when they become problematic. The palmar surface has no sebaceous glands, and these "tumors" are not found there.

Cutaneous Horn

A cutaneous horn (cornu cutaneum) is a protrusion of keratotic material from the skin resembling the horn of an animal. It is often conical and found on sun-exposed areas. Cutaneous horns (Fig. 62-2) can annoy the patient not only

because of their unsightly appearance but also by interfering with hand function and catching on clothing or gloves. Much like systemic "anemia," this is a clinical finding that has multiple possible underlying causes. Benign causes of cutaneous horn include verruca vulgaris, seborrheic keratosis, pyogenic granuloma, fibroma, epidermal nevus, discoid lupus erythematosus, and epidermal inclusion cyst, to name just a few. Malignant or premalignant lesions associated with horns

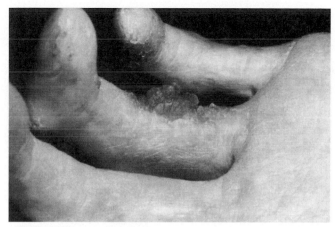

FIGURE 62-2. A cutaneous horn arising from an area of irradiated skin.

include actinic keratosis, basal cell carcinoma, Bowen's disease, Kaposi's sarcoma, and SCC, among others. So-called giant cutaneous horns are often associated with SCC.[10]

Because of the risk of underlying malignancy, excisional biopsy of smaller lesions is indicated. For larger lesions, a diagnostic punch biopsy may help guide therapy, keeping in mind the potential problem of sampling error. Decisions about therapy will be steered by the underlying pathologic diagnosis.

Benign Tumors

Verruca Vulgaris

Common warts, or verruca vulgaris, are caused by infection with human papillomavirus (HPV). Since it was first isolated in 1949, many different subtypes of this small DNA virus have been identified.[107] Types 1 to 4, 7, and 10 are known to cause lesions of keratinized epithelium, whereas other types are implicated in mucosal lesions.[4,129]

Warts are most commonly found at sites of trauma and may involve any portion of the hand. Habitual nail biting may result in periungual lesions.[98] The common wart (verruca vulgaris) is readily identifiable by its rough, raised surface (Fig. 62-3). Plane or flat warts (verruca plana, HPV types 3 and 10) have a slightly different appearance. These small flesh-colored papules tend to occur on the dorsum of the hand in sun-exposed areas.[67]

The natural history of verruca is spontaneous resolution within 1 to 2 years. Clearance of warts may be limited by a person's viral load, immune status, and duration of infection. Lesions that are persistent, interfere with function, or are cosmetically unacceptable should be treated. Excision may also be required to exclude malignancy in cases in which the diagnosis is in question.[67]

First-line treatment for common warts is usually a topical agent, many of which are available without a prescription. Patients should be instructed to pare down the lesions before applying the topical therapy. The most common formulation contains salicylic acid, which is both keratolytic and a local irritant. It works best in preparations that form an occlusive coat, such as collodion.[67] Cure rates of 70% to 80% can be achieved with minimal side effects.[19] Other topical remedies contain glutaraldehyde and occasionally formaldehyde,

but the latter has more side effects, including hypersensitivity and excessively dry, cracked skin, and is used infrequently.

Cryotherapy is increasingly available to both dermatologists and primary care physicians. It is used as a first-line therapy for facial and genital lesions, but it is considered a second-line therapy for lesions of the hand, where it is less well tolerated.[67] Multiple treatments may be required, but cure rates approach 60% to 80%.[14] Residual hyperpigmentation and hypopigmentation have been reported in dark-skinned patients.

Many other therapies have been proposed for treatment of warts. Immunomodulatory agents may have a role in treating immunosuppressed patients, who often develop widespread, recalcitrant HPV infections. Carbon dioxide lasers, pulsed-dye lasers, and photodynamic therapy have shown some promise, but further clinical trials are required to establish their usefulness.[67]

Pyogenic Granuloma

Pyogenic granuloma (granuloma telangiectaticum) usually presents as a solitary reddish nodular tumor of the skin or mucosa (Fig. 62-4). Although the exact etiology is unknown, many believe it is caused by trauma and subsequent infection. In any case, the end result is a chronic vascular lesion that eventually becomes inflamed and generates localized granulation tissue.[122] Spontaneous resolution is unusual.

Many different treatments for this lesion have been described, including excision, curettage, radiation therapy, cauterization, pulsed-dye laser, or silver nitrate.[48,83,84] All of these methods have some incidence of recurrence. Careful excision under magnification, including a margin of normal tissue, has proved to be most effective in some studies.[124] In our experience, excision of the lesion with a 1-mm margin has been curative with no recurrence.

In the subungual location, pyogenic granulomas may be the result of a nail plate puncture wound, whether traumatic or iatrogenic. Repeated silver nitrate applications to the lesion have resulted in resolution; however, nail growth abnormalities may occur and be long standing.

Keratoacanthoma

This rapidly growing skin tumor closely resembles squamous cell carcinoma and therefore deserves careful attention. It usually occurs on sun-exposed, hair-bearing skin, beginning as a small red papule and enlarging rapidly over 1 to 2 months to become a firm, rounded tumor as large as 2.0 cm in diameter (Fig. 62-5). Some authors believe this tumor arises from the epithelium of hair follicles.[101] Typically, a dome shape or a crater with a core of keratinous material develops. At this stage it is considered a mature lesion. The natural history of this lesion is spontaneous regression, which occurs after a latent phase of variable duration. However, in modern practice, most of these lesions are excised before this occurs. It has been noted that some of these masses may be present for a year or more. The final or "involutional" stage is said to leave a prominent scar.[101]

Several characteristics may help differentiate this lesion from SCC. The central keratin plug seen in keratoacanthomas typically occupies the majority of the lesion, whereas large SCCs contain central necrosis. Keratoacanthomas

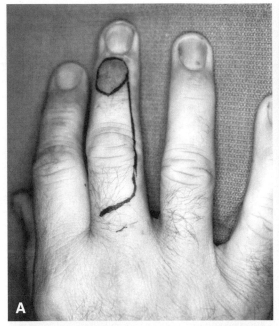

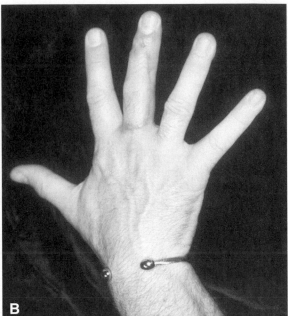

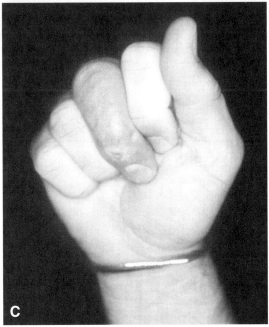

FIGURE 62-3. A 35-year-old man developed verruca vulgaris over the dorsum of his right middle finger. The wart was refractory to all medical therapy and was referred for excision. **A,** The mass was excised and a rotational-advancement flap was designed to cover the defect. **B** and **C,** There was no recurrence of the wart, and he had full range of motion of the digits.

grow very rapidly into an obvious skin tumor, whereas SCCs typically have a more insidious onset.

Etiologic factors associated with the development of keratoacanthoma are numerous. These include, but are not limited to, sun exposure in fair-skinned individuals and genetic inheritance.[42,95,101] Keratoacanthoma may develop in the sites of previous radiation therapy, scar formation, chemical exposure, and in a setting of immunosuppression. HPV and smoking may be involved either directly or as cofactors in the development of keratoacanthoma.[42,101]

This lesion should be excised for accurate diagnosis. Accurate determination of the pathology can only occur when the entire lesion is presented to an experienced pathologist for evaluation. It is sometimes difficult to differentiate a keratoacanthoma from an SCC.

Distal Digital Keratoacanthoma

This rare, destructive variant of keratoacanthoma involves the distal subungual tissue or the proximal nail fold. It differs from true keratoacanthoma in several respects, including its occurrence in non–hair-bearing skin, the lack of a surrounding epithelial collar, less associated inflammation, and a tendency toward deeper invasion. It is a painful tumor that usually arises in the nail bed, causing separation of the nail plate from the bed (distal nail bed tumors) or paronychia-like lesions (proximal nail bed tumors). Like true keratoacanthoma, this variant exhibits very rapid growth, which helps distinguish it from other lesions.[9]

In the subungual location, this rapid growth can result in early bone destruction. Ironically, these tumors can be even more destructive to bone than classic SCCs arising at this

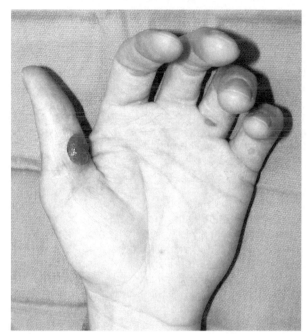

FIGURE 62-4. A 20-year-old man developed pyogenic granuloma over the volar thumb after a cut. Note the red, fleshy appearance of the mass. The tumor was excised with a 1-mm margin with no recurrence.

site. Radiographs will typically show a punched-out area of bone destruction without accompanying sclerosis or periosteal reaction, findings that are common in SCC-associated bony changes.[9]

Because of its tendency toward bony invasion, some favor classifying this neoplasm as a low-grade carcinoma. However, cases of spontaneous regression have been reported, as in true keratoacanthomas.[8,41,82] First-line treatment for this lesion should consist of local excision and curettage, as long as incisional biopsy has conclusively ruled out SCC. In cases in which the diagnosis is unclear, bony destruction is extensive, or the lesion is recurrent, amputation or partial amputation of the digit is warranted.[68] Mohs' micrographic surgery offers a theoretical advantage in getting clear margins at the time of excision but has not been widely used for this tumor.

Other therapies, such as topical 5-fluorouracil, methotrexate, and etretinate, have been tried with anecdotal success.[8,37,118]

Dermatofibroma (Histiocytoma)

These are fibrous tissue tumors that involve the dermis. Pathologic evaluation reveals these tumors to be composed of fibroblasts, collagen, and histiocytes. They are usually solitary, firm, dome-shaped masses that exhibit varying degrees of coloring, including red, brown, or darker colors.[42] In fair-skinned patients, they may be pink or flesh colored. They develop in young adults and are found more commonly in women than men. Etiology may be related to minor, insignificant trauma.

The differential diagnosis of these lesions includes everything from sarcomas to melanoma. Excisional biopsy is warranted and is often the only treatment required, so long as the margins are negative.[42]

Lentigines

These benign pigmented macules result from increased activity of epidermal melanocytes. Although similar in appearance to freckles (ephelides), lentigines are persistent and do not fade in the absence of sun exposure. There are two major types: simple lentigo and solar lentigo. Simple lentigines often appear during childhood, affecting both sun-exposed and non–sun-exposed sites. They are brown or brownish-black macules, usually less than 5 mm in diameter, and generally few in number.[100]

Solar lentigines, also called actinic or senile lentigines, are limited to sun-exposed areas and are quite common on the extensor forearms and dorsum of the hands. Their incidence increases with age, as expected. These lesions may closely resemble melanoma, especially lentigo maligna, and a biopsy may be indicated to establish the nature of the lesion (Fig. 62-6).[100]

Seborrheic Keratosis

These benign neoplasms of keratinocytes are extremely common in middle-aged and older adults. They have a widespread distribution and increase in number and size with age. They begin as a flat area of hyperpigmentation, but thicken as they progress and eventually take on a characteristic, waxy, "stuck-on" appearance (Fig. 62-7). These

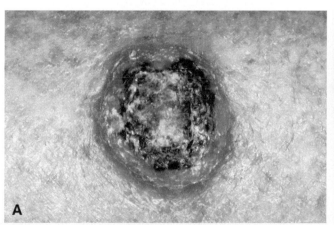

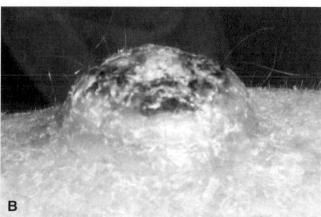

FIGURE 62-5. **A** and **B,** A 2-cm keratoacanthoma that developed over a 2-month period. Note the keratin plug at the center of the tumor. The rapid growth and lack of central necrosis of this large tumor points toward keratoacanthoma instead of squamous cell carcinoma.

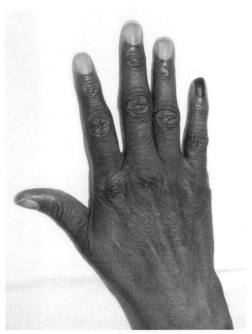

FIGURE 62-6. A 50-year-old African American woman presented with a 4-month history of nail discoloration of the little finger. Fortunately, biopsy showed lentigines and no further treatment was necessary.

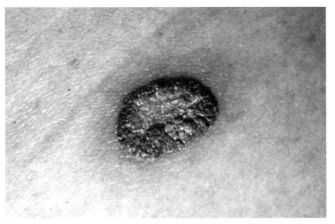

FIGURE 62-7. Seborrheic keratosis with the classic "stuck-on" appearance.

lesions can mimic melanoma and may require biopsy to rule out a malignancy.[100]

If malignancy is not suspected, these benign lesions can be removed by any number of means. Curettage, laser treatment, and cryotherapy have all been used with success. Excision of clearly benign lesions is probably unnecessary.

Melanocytic Nevi

A melanocytic nevus (mole) is a benign proliferation of a type of melanocyte called a nevus cell. Unlike the melanocytes that reside in the basal layer of the epidermis, nevus cells do not have dendritic processes (except nevus cells found in blue nevi) and are clustered rather than evenly dispersed. Both of these cell types can produce the pigment melanin. Melanocytic nevi may be acquired or congenital and common or atypical.

Common Acquired Nevi

Common acquired nevi have a distinct time course. They begin to appear after 6 months of life and increase in size and number during childhood and adolescence. After reaching a peak in young adulthood, these lesions slowly regress with advancing age. Along the way, the nevus will typically become more raised and less pigmented. Each stage in this cycle is marked by a different histologic appearance as the nests of nevus cells migrate from the dermal-epidermal junction into the dermis. Junctional nevi are flat, well-circumscribed pigmented lesions with uniform color, rarely exceeding 6 mm in diameter.[36] These nevi are in the earliest phase of development, when the nevus cell nests are located at the dermal-epidermal junction. Junctional nevi may evolve into compound nevi when their growth extends vertically, such that nevus cells are found both at the dermal-epidermal junction and in the dermis.[36] These lesions are usually raised, uniformly pigmented, and well circumscribed. When the nests of nevus cells move completely into the dermis, it is termed an *intradermal nevus*. These lesions are raised and retain their overlying skin markings. Pigmentation generally fades, however, because the dermal nevus cells often lose their ability to produce melanin.

Acral nevi are located on the palmar and plantar surfaces. They are usually of the junctional or compound type but may have linear streaks of hyperpigmentation. Biopsy is probably indicated in mottled or large (> 7 mm) lesions, especially in older patients.

Longitudinal melanonychia is a descriptive term that refers to tan, brown, or black streaking of the nail caused by increased melanin deposition in the nail plate. Acral nevi involving the nail matrix can present this way. However, in dark-skinned patients, where longitudinal melanonychia is common, it is usually due to increased melanin production by normal nail matrix melanocytes. Dark nail streaks appearing in older patients, streaks that are changing over time, or those that lead to nail dystrophy or extension beyond the nail folds should always be sampled to rule out acral-lentiginous melanoma.

When nevi do not develop normally, they can become atypical and eventually cancerous. Important clinical signs of atypical nevi can be easily recalled by the "*ABCD*" mnemonic: (1) *A*symmetry, (2) *B*order irregularities, (3) *C*olor variation, and (4) *D*iameter over 6 mm. More detailed descriptions of the premalignant and malignant tumors arising from nevi are presented later in this chapter.

A large case-control study has shown a twofold increase in melanoma risk in persons with increased numbers of common acquired nevi.[113] However, most acquired nevi remain benign throughout a person's lifetime. In fact, more than 50% of cutaneous melanomas arise de novo and are not associated with an existing nevus.[113] Therefore, any new, pigmented lesion arising in a patient, especially in a middle-aged or older patient, should be examined very carefully.

Congenital Nevi

Nevi present at birth deserve special consideration. Congenital pigmented nevi are generally larger than acquired nevi and are classified by size into three categories: small (<1.5 cm), medium (1.5 cm to <20 cm), and large or giant

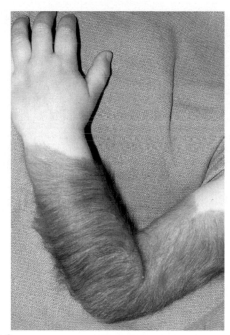

FIGURE 62-8. A 4-year-old girl with giant hairy nevus. The risk of malignant transformation is estimated to be 0% to 9%.[119] After full excision of this giant nevus, complex reconstruction was required. Consultation with the parents is crucial to provide a balanced discussion on the risk and benefits of excision of giant congenital nevus. This patient underwent complete excision of the nevus and expanded abdominal pedicle flap coverage.

(>20 cm) (Fig. 62-8).[59] Giant congenital nevi may be surrounded by multiple smaller "satellite" nevi.

Congenital nevi enlarge in proportion to the child's growth, and they often change from flat, evenly pigmented lesions to raised, mottled ones. Their surface may become nodular or verrucous in texture, with an increased density of coarse terminal hairs.

The risk of developing cutaneous melanoma in giant congenital nevi is not well established. Our recent systematic overview on the malignant potential of large congenital nevi estimated the incidence of melanoma to range from 0% to 9%.[119] These incidence rates reflect crude incidence, assuming that the melanoma risk in these patients remains constant through a lifetime. However, approximately half of the malignancies that have occurred in giant nevi developed in the first 3 years of life, 60% by childhood, and 70% by puberty.[11] The incidence of malignant degeneration in medium-sized congenital nevi is also controversial but is probably about 1%.[96]

The greatest risk of melanoma is found in patients with congenital nevi of the scalp or a posterior axial location, particularly those patients with "satellite" nevi. These patients also comprise those at highest risk for an associated disorder, neurocutaneous melanosis. This proliferation of melanocytes in the central nervous system may cause neurologic symptoms, usually presenting around the second year of life.[50] Magnetic resonance imaging with gadolinium can make this diagnosis. Symptomatic cases have a poor prognosis; the prognosis for asymptomatic cases is unknown.

Small congenital nevi are easily excised; very small lesions are often followed clinically without excision. Large or giant congenital nevi should be excised because of the increased incidence of malignant degeneration, but simple excision of these lesions is often not possible. The ultimate postexcision defect and the complexity of reconstruction must be balanced with the estimated risk of developing melanoma during the child's lifetime.[119] Serial excisions of the lesion, removing no more at each operation than that which can be primarily closed and allowing the surrounding skin to stretch out between procedures, is a common option. When this is combined with tissue expansion and/or local flaps, excision can often be expedited.

Blue Nevi

This variety of benign nevus contains dermal melanocytes that actively produce melanin, unlike the typical intradermal nevus described earlier. These melanocytes have dendritic processes, which also differentiates them from common acquired nevi. Dermal melanin preferentially scatters the shorter wavelengths of light, giving these nevi a blue color; this phenomenon is known as the Tyndall effect.[52] The common blue nevus often arises in adolescence or early adulthood. It usually presents as a solitary lesion, 1 to 10 mm in diameter, and is often found on the dorsal surface of the hands or feet. The presence of multiple blue nevi is associated with some rare syndromes, such as the Carney complex (multiple blue nevi, cardiac myxomas, and endocrine overactivity).[52] A separate entity, the cellular blue nevus, tends to be larger (>1 cm) and more elevated. These are not commonly found on the extremities.

Careful observation, as for any benign nevus, is indicated. Malignant degeneration has been reported within cellular blue nevi, especially those of the scalp, but not within common blue nevi.

Acquired Digital Fibrokeratoma (Acral Fibrokeratoma)

These benign tumors of fibrous tissue usually occur on the acral surfaces (hands and feet) but have been found elsewhere. They have a characteristic appearance: a flesh-colored, hornlike projection with a raised collar of skin at the base. They involve the epidermis, which becomes hyperkeratotic, and the dermis, which demonstrates increased fibrosis. Large, stellate fibroblasts are seen in many of these lesions on histopathologic examination.[97]

These tumors can mimic fibromas, eccrine poromas, and pyogenic granulomas. The Koenen tumor described in the literature is probably a variant of acquired digital fibrokeratoma. Excision is the treatment of choice for this lesion, although recurrence after excision is frequent.

Premalignant Tumors

Keratoses

Sun exposure, especially in fair-skinned individuals, produces cutaneous damage that causes skin atrophy and telangiectasia. These are premalignant lesions that, if allowed to progress, may become SCCs. The same list of etiologic agents described under keratoacanthoma applies here. They are capable of producing lesions that will evolve into SCC or basal cell carcinoma.[12,43,60,95]

Treatment of these actinic keratoses requires excision or destruction by another means such as 5-fluorouracil cream.[95] Prevention is still the best approach and requires protection from sun exposure.

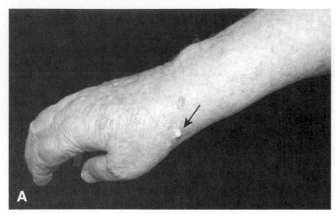
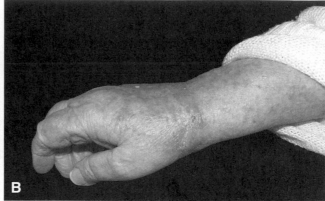

FIGURE 62-9. **A,** Actinic keratosis in a 70-year-old woman. Note the hyperkeratotic scaly lesion *(arrow).* There is a risk of malignant transformation of actinic keratosis into squamous cell carcinoma, although this risk is not well quantified. **B,** The tumor was excised with a 1-mm margin and closed with a rhomboid flap.

Arsenical keratoses are often widespread, especially involving the palmar surfaces of the hand and the plantar surfaces of the feet. They are also keratotic lesions. Changes in these marked by enlargement or ulceration require biopsy and appropriate treatment based on their pathology.[65,95]

Actinic Keratosis

Actinic keratosis represents the third most common reason for consulting a dermatologist, after acne and dermatitis.[39] It presents as a hyperkeratotic lesion with densely adherent scales attached to a pink base (Fig. 62-9). Actinic keratoses are scaly lesions, typically 2 to 6 mm in diameter, and can be skin color, pink, or brown.[3] This lesion is often tender to palpation. Microscopically, it is composed of abnormal proliferations of epidermal keratinocytes; the dysplastic keratinocytes are confined to the lower one third of the epidermis.

These lesions are directly linked to long-term sun damage. As such, they are most common in fair-skinned persons with a history of significant sun exposure. Some of these lesions progress to SCC, whereas some resolve spontaneously. Estimates of the conversion rate to invasive cancer range from 0.1% to 10%[33,69]; the process is believed to take several years to occur.

Cryotherapy or electrodesiccation with curettage have been the traditional mainstays of therapy for individual lesions. In patients with severe sun-damaged skin and multiple areas of actinic keratosis, therapy should treat the entire area that is at risk. Modalities that can address wider areas include topical 5-fluorouracil, dermabrasion, and cutaneous peels (i.e., trichloroacetic acid peel). Oral and topical retinoids may be of some benefit but are not effective monotherapy.[56]

Photodynamic therapy is a newer modality that has shown excellent early results. This modality involves the use of a photosensitizer (usually a porphyrin derivative), applied topically or systemically, which is activated by visible light. Cure rates are similar to that reported for cryotherapy and 5-fluorouracil therapy.[56]

Bowen's Disease

Bowen's disease is the eponym given to intraepidermal SCC, also known as SCC in situ. Although technically confined to the epidermis, these lesions may extend deeply into hair follicles and sebaceous glands. The neoplastic cell is the keratinocyte, and these tumors have some potential for evolution into invasive SCC (about 3% in most studies).[58,85] After this progression occurs, metastasis is not uncommon (one third of cases).[58]

Clinically, these lesions present as erythematous, slow-growing plaques with irregular borders and crusty or scaly surfaces (Fig. 62-10).[66] These may present in any location on the hand, but occurrence on the palmar surface is rare. In 10% to 20% of cases, multiple lesions are present.[27,34,62,92,109] Subungual Bowen's disease is uncommon and is more likely to be a pigmented variant.[90] Obviously, this makes the diagnosis of these lesions very difficult to make before biopsy.

The cause of Bowen's disease appears to be linked to chronic sun damage, given the distribution of lesions on sun-exposed areas.[61,92,99] Accordingly, Bowen's disease is rare in dark-skinned persons, but they may develop this tumor on nonexposed areas.[73] Additional risk factors including arsenic exposure, immunosuppression, ionizing radiation, and chronic dermatoses have been associated with the development of this tumor.[31,40,102,127,128]

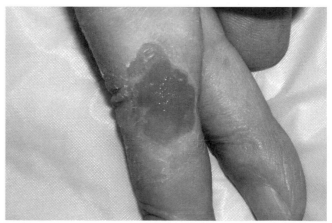

FIGURE 62-10. Bowen's disease in a 40-year-old patient. Note the erythematous, plaquelike appearance of this carcinoma in situ. The mass was excised with a 1-mm margin, and the wound was covered with a skin graft.

Because of the small but real risk of developing invasive cancer, treatment of these lesions is almost always indicated. Thin, slowly progressing lesions in patients at high risk for healing difficulties may be managed by observation alone. Modern treatment of Bowen's disease varies considerably, and controlled studies are scarce. Topical 5-fluorouracil has been very effective in some small studies,[45,89,106,108,111,121] but it can be very irritating and is not always well tolerated. Cryotherapy has been used successfully, with recurrence rates under 10% at 12 months.[28,76] Recurrence appears to be slightly higher with electrodesiccation and curettage (as high as 20%),[108,109] perhaps because this method does not reliably ablate the deeper foci of tumor (i.e., within the pilosebaceous unit). Radiotherapy, while delivering excellent cure rates, appears to result in an unacceptably high incidence of delayed healing.[28] Photodynamic therapy has shown initial clearance rates of 90% to 100% with recurrence rates of 0% to 11% after 12 months.[76,114] Simple excision has been reported to have a recurrence rate between 4.9% and 19% within 5 years.[51,109] Some lesions at difficult sites (particularly the subungual area) might benefit from ablative laser therapy or Mohs' micrographic surgery. Reports utilizing these techniques contain very small numbers of cases.[74]

In summary, there is no single optimal treatment modality for Bowen's disease; several therapies have very similar results. Until randomized controlled studies are available, the choice of therapy should be individualized, considering the morbidity, availability, and cost of each option.

Atypical Nevus (Atypical Mole)

Nevi are said to be atypical if they have any of the characteristics described in the "*ABCD*" mnemonic discussed earlier. Because this is a clinical description, the term *atypical nevus* is preferred over the term *dysplastic nevus,* which was previously used to describe these lesions. Atypical nevi are believed to be potential precursors of melanoma; the presence of just one atypical nevus doubles a person's risk for melanoma. When 10 or more clinically atypical nevi are present, a patient's risk for melanoma is increased 12-fold.

It is not uncommon for patients to have multiple nevi; some fair-skinned patients may have dozens or hundreds of these lesions. When patients present with multiple suspicious lesions, it is often helpful to involve a dermatologist in their care. A competent dermatologist can help the surgeon determine which, if any, of the nevi are clinically atypical. After surgical treatment, the dermatologist can then follow the patient's multiple nevi on a regular basis to help detect changes in nevi that might require further evaluation.

Atypical nevi should be excised with a 1- to 2-mm margin of surrounding skin. The skin excision needs to be full thickness to accurately determine depth of invasion, should melanoma be discovered. Histopathologic evaluation of these lesions should describe the level of melanocytic atypia (none, mild, moderate, or severe) and comment on the margins of the excision. If margins are found to be involved, and atypia is present, conservative re-excision of the nevus is recommended.

Atypical Junctional Melanocytic Hyperplasia

As the name suggests, this term refers to abnormal proliferation of junctional melanocytes. This is a descriptive finding reported by pathologists and not necessarily a distinct clinical entity. Although often seen in association with atypical nevi and melanoma-in-situ, this finding is also associated with 6.2% of clinically benign intradermal nevi.[81] In the latter context, it is a completely benign lesion and re-excision of what was otherwise a benign nevus is not indicated. To summarize, biopsy reports containing the term *atypical junctional melanocytic hyperplasia* should be interpreted carefully. Discussion with the pathologist interpreting the histologic specimen is extremely helpful to gauge the perceived behavior of each individual case. Benign intradermal nevi need no further treatment, whereas melanoma-in-situ will often require a wider excision to be confident of negative margins (see later).

MALIGNANT SKIN TUMORS

Melanoma

Types of Melanomas

Melanoma-in-situ is an early form of melanoma with tumor confined to the epithelial layer (Fig. 62-11). Several clinical pathology terms have been used to identify this favorable tumor type, including *lentigo maligna, atypical melanocytic proliferation,* and *pagetoid melanocytic proliferation.* Lentigo maligna is a type of melanoma-in-situ sometimes referred to as Hutchinson's freckle. This lesion, which often appears on the face of elderly patients, is associated with long-term sun exposure and develops in the same areas affected by actinic keratoses. In the upper extremity, lentigo maligna most commonly appears over the extensor forearm. Beginning as a tan, flat macule, this lesion has a prolonged radial growth phase that may last 1 or 2 decades (Fig. 62-12A). The appearance of papules may signify the onset of a vertical growth

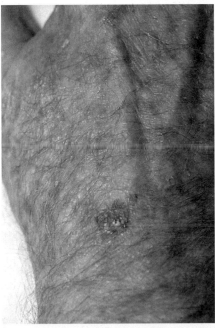

FIGURE 62-11. A 40-year-old man presented with biopsy-proven melanoma-in-situ over the dorsum of the hand. Note the discolored, irregular borders of this 1-cm lesion. This melanoma was excised with a 5-mm margin and the wound was closed with a rhomboid flap, after the margins were cleared.

phase, invasion of the dermis, and development of invasive melanoma or so-called lentigo maligna melanoma (4% to 10% of all melanomas). Because the clinically uninvolved surrounding skin will often contain scattered atypical melanocytes, histologic determination of clear margins may be problematic. It is advisable to excise the lesion with a 5-mm margin and cover the wound with a temporary homograft. The tumor can be re-excised if atypical cells are still detected at the margins. Once a tumor-free margin is established, the wound can be closed definitively with skin graft or flap.

Because this type of tumor is confined to the epithelial layer and has no potential for metastasis, the goal is to completely excise the lesion with a histologically proven clear margin.[93] The long-term survival approaches 99% once the tumor is excised. Although it is customary to use these different descriptive terms for melanoma-in-situ, current convention prefers referring to these lesions simply as melanoma-in-situ.

Superficial spreading melanoma is the most common type of melanoma and represents 70% of melanomas overall (see Fig. 62-12B). This is the variant of melanoma most likely to arise within or contiguous with a melanocytic nevus, and its distribution coincides with areas of greatest nevus density. It begins as a pigmented plaque and has a radial growth phase (months to years) before vertical growth begins. Metastatic spread is correlated with vertical invasion and rarely occurs during the earlier radial growth phase.

Nodular melanoma (15% of all melanomas) has little or no radial growth phase and therefore has increased early metastatic potential (see Fig. 62-12C). It is fast growing and usually arises de novo. Its pigmentation is usually a uniform dark blue-black color, but it may be gray or pink (amelanotic melanoma).

Acral lentiginous melanoma (2% to 8% of all melanomas) is a variant found on palmar and plantar surfaces, the nail apparatus, and mucous membranes. It does not seem to be associated with sun exposure, and it is the most common type of melanoma in populations where melanoma is usually uncommon (African-Americans, Asians, and Hispanics). It is a slow-growing melanoma that has a long radial growth phase before vertical growth begins. Diagnosis is often delayed simply because it is located in areas not routinely examined.

Subungual melanoma usually affects the thumb or great toe and typically arises in the nail matrix (Fig. 62-13). Early lesions may present as longitudinal melanonychia or may be mistaken for subungual hematomas. Because the nail bed is adherent to the underlying bone, the histopathologic fea-

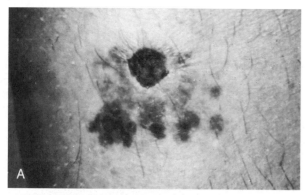

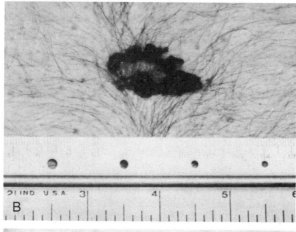

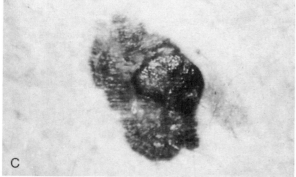

FIGURE 62-12. Types of melanomas (see text). **A,** Lentigo maligna. **B,** Superficial spreading melanoma. **C,** Superficial spreading melanoma with nodule.

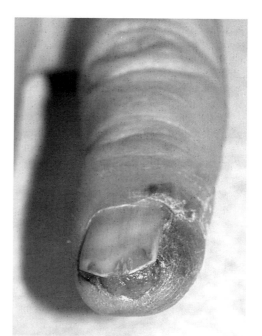

FIGURE 62-13. A 50-year-old man presented with discoloration of the index fingernail bed that was present for over 1 year. Note the involvement of the pulp of the finger and extension of the tumor to the eponychial fold. Biopsy of the tumor showed subungual melanoma, undetermined Breslow's thickness. Ray amputation was performed and sentinel node biopsy contained melanoma. Metastatic work-up showed no other involved organs (stage 2 disease). He is currently on experimental chemotherapy protocol.

tures of subungual melanoma tumor type cannot be assessed reliably using the Breslow's level system.[80] A diagnosis requires a high index of suspicion. For pigmented nail lesions that have persisted for over 2 months, a formal biopsy is necessary. The nail is elevated, and a partial thickness biopsy of the pigmented lesion is performed. The nail is replaced over the biopsy site.

An unusual melanoma subtype is desmoplastic melanoma. This type of melanoma mainly occurs in the head and neck region, but the hand is occasionally involved by this melanoma variant.[21] Histologically, it is similar to lentigo maligna melanoma, but a distinguishing feature is the fibroblastic reaction in the dermis and neural invasion. Although the mean thickness at presentation is 4.3 mm in published series of desmoplastic melanoma, the survival is much more favorable for this thick tumor (5-year survival of 63% compared with 48% for other types of melanoma of comparable thickness).

Treatment

The optimal management of melanoma patients demands a multidisciplinary melanoma clinic. Because of the rapid advancement of many treatment regimens and multiple specialties involved in the care of this disease, a melanoma clinic was formed at the University of Michigan. This clinic has representatives from several disciplines, including surgical oncologists, dermatologists, plastic surgeons, and other ancillary personnel to ensure that appropriate surgical, immunologic, and future surveillance issues are addressed.

For many years, the surgical margin for melanoma has been based on the traditional 5-cm margin. However, skin grafting or flap reconstruction is often required to cover the resulting large excision defects. Two multicenter randomized controlled trials by Veronesi and colleagues[116,117] and Balch and associates[7] have set the stage for narrower resection margins that attained the same survival rates as the traditional wider resection margin. The NIH Consensus Panel[79] and the evidence-based guidelines from the United Kingdom[93] in recent publications further defined the surgical margins for different tumor depths. The following is the recommendation from the recent United Kingdom Consensus Panel, based on the best available evidence in the literature, published concurrently in both the *British Journal of Dermatology*[93] and the *British Journal of Plastic Surgery*.[78]

Breslow's classification, based on tumor thickness, is commonly used to assist in determining excision margins (Fig. 16-14). For in-situ lesions, a 2- to 5-mm clinical margin is adequate and 5-year survival rate ranges from 95% to 100%. For Breslow thickness of less than 1 mm, a 1-cm margin is recommended and 5-year survival ranges from 95% to 100%. For thickness of 1 to 2 mm, a 1- to 2-cm margin is recommended and 5-year survival ranges from 80% to 96%. For thickness of 2 to 4 mm, a 2- to 3-cm margin is recommended, with 60% to 75% 5-year survival. For thickness of greater than 4 mm, a 3-cm margin is recommended and 5-year survival is about 50%.

These recommended margins apply to the peripheral margin. Obviously it is difficult to attain a 1-cm deep margin in the upper extremity, particularly over the dorsal hand. For in-situ lesions, excision of the tumor with some subcutaneous fat is sufficient to eradicate the tumor. For deeper melanomas, one should excise the lesion to the level of the paratenon over the dorsal hand or include the forearm fascia.

More extensive resection, including removal of the tendon structures, may be necessary if the initial deep margin still contains melanoma cells (Fig. 62-15)

A controversial area in the field of melanoma relates to the management of nodal territories. When the regional lymph nodes are enlarged because of tumor invasion, lymph node dissection will afford regional control and potentially prevent metastatic spread of the tumor cells. However, if the draining regional lymph nodes are not palpable, the need for lymph node dissection is less clear. The traditional approach is to perform elective lymph node dissection (ELND) in the axilla for any intermediate-thickness (0.76 to 4.0 mm) melanoma of the upper extremity. ELND provides staging information that will be helpful in prescribing adjuvant treatment. Theoretically, ELND may be curative by interrupting the spread of metastatic tumor cells from the lymph nodes to the rest of the body.[55]

For thin melanomas (<0.76 mm), ELND would provide no therapeutic advantage because regional or systemic metastasis is quite unlikely. The 5-year survival rate associated with this early melanoma approaches 98% with excision of primary tumor alone.[55] On the other hand, for patients with thick melanomas (>4 mm), 62% will have regional nodal metastasis and 72% will have distant diseases.[55] In this situation, ELND is not a curative procedure but serves as a palliative procedure to gain regional tumor control. In most thick melanomas, lymph node dissection for regional control is performed only when nodal metastasis is palpable.

Controversy for ELND revolves around intermediate-thickness melanomas (0.76 to 4.0 mm). Because ELND in the axilla removes most of the lymphatic channels, lymphedema can develop and may be rather disabling. The benefit of ELND needs to be tangible and should outweigh the cost and morbidity of prolonged survival. However, several randomized controlled trials have failed to show a survival advantage for ELND in intermediate-thickness melanomas.[5,6,20,102,114,115] But multivariate analysis from these trials did define the following factors adversely affecting survival: tumor ulceration, trunk site, thicker tumors, and increasing age.[55] Among all the body regions, upper-extremity melanoma has a better prognosis.

The issue with ELND has abated somewhat with a new technique—sentinel node biopsy—in detecting nodal metastasis. The sentinel lymph node is the first node draining a tumor, and this node may represent the metastatic involvement of the lymph node basin.[112] A blue dye or radiocolloid or combination of both is injected around the melanoma site 10 to 15 minutes before lymph node mapping. The sentinel lymph node is identified by the blue stain and/or radiocolloid gamma probe. This sentinel node is excised, and the primary melanoma is widely excised. If the lymph node is positive, ELND is performed for potential cure. If the sentinel node is negative for malignancy, no ELND is performed and the patient is followed per protocol of the melanoma clinic. Many publications have documented the effectiveness of the sentinel node biopsy approach.[46,77,110,112] The morbidity of sentinel node biopsy is much less than formal axillary node dissection, and formal node dissection can be targeted to specific groups of patients with positive sentinel nodes.

Sentinel node biopsy is quite applicable to subungual melanoma, in which the Breslow's depth is often difficult to assess and the staging is quite uncertain for this type of

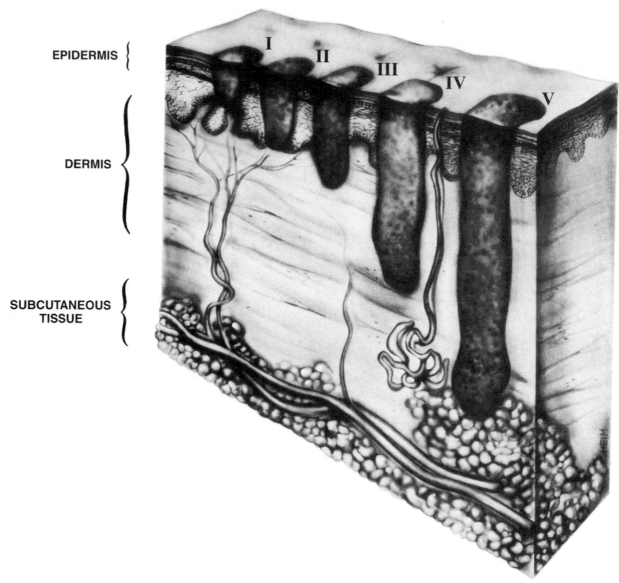

EPIDERMIS

DERMIS

SUBCUTANEOUS
TISSUE

FIGURE 62-14. Clark's classification of melanoma according to level of invasion. This classification system has been replaced by Breslow's classification system based on tumor thickness.

tumor. Because diagnosis of subungual melanoma is often delayed, this type of tumor has a rather poor prognosis, with 5-year survival of 74% for stage I (local) disease and 40% for stage 2 (nodal) disease.[80] Mapping the axillary nodes using the less invasive sentinel node biopsy for subungual melanoma has the advantage of determining the stage of the disease so that appropriate treatment can be prescribed. The local disease for subungual melanoma is controlled with an amputation of the involved digit. Amputation is performed at one joint proximal to the joint closest to the subungual melanoma. For example, if the tumor is limited to the nail matrix, the amputation will be performed at the proximal interphalangeal joint level. For tumors extending to the middle phalanx, the amputation should be performed at the level of the metacarpophalangeal joint. Functional consideration should also come into play when considering the level of the amputation. If the level of amputation results in a digit that hinders hand function, a ray amputation is the prudent approach.

Squamous Cell Carcinoma

Nonmelanoma skin cancer is the most common malignancy in the United States. Estimates from 2001 indicate that there are over 1.3 million cases in this country, consisting of 80% basal cell and 20% SCC.[63] SCCs are the most frequent malignant tumors one encounters on the hand. Despite the prevalence of nonmelanoma skin cancers, the mortality resulting from these skin cancers is still rather modest, with 2300 estimated deaths per year.[43] While basal cell carcinoma is mainly locally invasive and has low metastatic potential, SCC has a much higher risk of metastasis, particularly in immunocompromised populations, such as renal and heart transplant patients (Fig. 62-16).[3,26,30,57,94,115] The risk in transplant recipients is 65 times that of age-matched control subjects

Radiation is also a risk factor for developing SCC, particularly in patients receiving radiation for cutaneous conditions, such as acne, dermatitis, and hemangioma in the 1940s and 1950s. In addition, health care workers and personnel

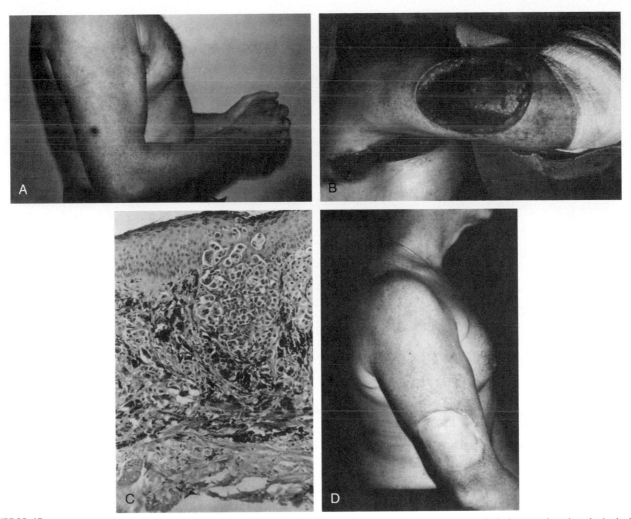

FIGURE 62-15. This 43-year-old man had a biopsy-proven level III to IV (Breslow 1.74 mm) melanoma. **A,** Because the lesion was thought to be in the high-risk group, which raised the question of metastasis to the regional nodes, the patient, after evaluation, was treated with a wide re-excision of the biopsy site (**B**) and regional lymphadenectomy. Recent advances dictate that the axillary lymph nodes will be mapped using the sentinel node technique to avoid potential morbidity with negative elective lymph node dissection. **C,** The histologic appearance of the tumor. **D,** Three years postoperatively the patient was free of any evidence of melanoma.

from certain industries who were exposed to chronic doses of radiation are particularly susceptible.[3] But the most common risk factor for developing SCC is still ultraviolet radiation.[38,87] This tumor may occur in a patient who has inherited abnormalities such as xeroderma pigmentosum.[13,94,95,122]

SCC ranges from slow-growing wartlike lesions under or near the fingernail to large ulcerated or exophytic tumors. One must keep in mind that these tumors have the capacity not only to extend locally but also to metastasize, especially by lymphatics or even hematogenously. Evaluation of the patient, therefore, must include not only a careful history and physical examination but also an evaluation of regional lymphatic drainage. Preexisting lesions of solar (actinic) keratoses, or the multiple keratoses seen with arsenic exposure, may be present for a variable amount of time before the obvious malignancy. In the evolution of these tumors, one occasionally sees an in-situ SCC or Bowen's disease presenting as an erythematous, scaly, perhaps ulcerated area. Assessment of these lesions is frequently made easier by using magnification.[47]

Invasive SCC occurs on sun-exposed regions of the body, most commonly on the head and neck area and the arms.[87]

The dorsum of the hand and forearm are commonly involved areas in the upper extremity. Presentation is varied and can appear as papules or plaques, skin-colored or pink, and smooth or hyperkeratotic.[3] It is often itchy and bleeds easily when traumatized. Invasive SCC appears to arise from actinic keratosis, which is carcinoma-in-situ with tumor confined to the epidermis.

Treatment

For invasive SCCs that are less than 2 cm in diameter, an initial 4-mm surgical margin around the clinical border of the tumor should suffice; for tumors greater than 2 cm, a 6-mm margin is recommended.[16] Cure rate with these margins have been reported at 95%. Of course, the margins need to be identified with sutures so that re-excision can be targeted toward positive margins after histologic examination.

The depth of resection should include some subcutaneous fat, because 30% of the SCC invades the subcutaneous fat to some extent.[16] The wound can be closed primarily, or a rotational flap can be used to cover the defect. For large wounds that cannot be closed without a more involved flap procedure, the wound can initially be covered with a homograft

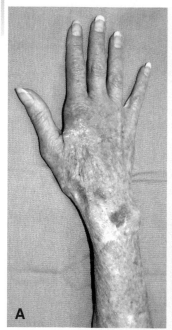
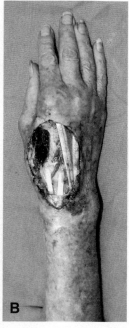
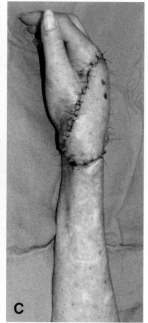

FIGURE 62-16. **A,** A 35-year-old renal transplant female patient presented with margin-positive invasive squamous cell carcinoma of her right hand despite two prior excisions. Note the long incision scar over the index metacarpal. **B,** The prior biopsy scar was excised with a 2-cm margin, with excision of the extensor pollicis longus tendon, periosteum of the index metacarpal, and a 5-mm thickness of the interosseous muscles. **C,** The excised specimen contained residual tumor cells, but the margins were cleared. The defect was covered with a lateral arm free flap, and the extensor indicis proprius tendon transfer was used to reconstruct the extensor pollicis longus tendon.

until the margins are cleared by the pathologists. Skin grafts, local flaps, or free flaps are good reconstructive options, whereas distant pedicle flaps are not recommended for the theoretical problem of seeding a distant site by occult tumor cells. It is reported that 2% to 5% of SCCs metastasize to the axillary nodes.[86] Because of the low incidence of lymph node metastasis, ELND is not performed unless the axillary nodes are enlarged. In this case, node biopsy is followed by formal axillary node dissection if the axillary nodes are involved with the cancer. Five-year survival drops markedly to between 30% and 40% with axillary node metastasis.[94]

Basal Cell Carcinoma

Basal cell carcinomas are malignant neoplasms of the basal epithelium. They are the most common form of skin cancer, affecting 800,000 Americans each year.[70] In the hand, basal cell carcinoma is less frequently seen than SCC. These are usually slow-growing tumors that may present as areas of skin atrophy, pink to reddish discoloration, telangiectatic changes, and, ultimately, ulceration with an elevated, occasionally "pearly" border (Fig. 62-17). There are many variations of this tumor, some of which grow in a very irregular fashion and have a scarlike quality to their advancing edge. These tumors are more frequently seen in sun-exposed areas in patients who have fair skin and hair. Certain basal cell carcinomas are seen in a congenital inheritance pattern, such as with the basal cell nevus syndrome, or in association with the inherited disease xeroderma pigmentosum.[49,91] Although these lesions can be diagnosed early, if neglected they may invade deeper structures and produce significant tissue destruction. Although they rarely metastasize, they do invade tissues locally.

The etiology of basal cell carcinoma is most commonly related to sun exposure. Therefore, avoidance of ultraviolet radiation is an excellent preventive measure. However, once these tumors develop, the patient must be followed carefully, because multiple basal cell carcinomas are frequent

and, in certain types with poorly defined borders, recurrence is not unusual. Among these more-difficult-to-treat lesions is the "superficial spreading type of basal cell carcinoma," which frequently has nests of malignant cells separated from the parent tumor margin.[95]

Several distinct clinical variants of basal cell carcinoma have been described. Nodular basal cell carcinoma is the most common form. These lesions begin as pearly white papules and slowly extend radially, often remaining flat. The central portion typically ulcerates and builds up a scaly crust. It is not unusual for the central ulceration to heal with scarring, giving patients a false sense of "improvement" in the lesion. As time goes on, the lesion continues to grow and the ulceration returns. For this reason, these tumors often present as "nonhealing ulcers."

Other variants are less common. Pigmented basal cell carcinoma can be confused with melanoma, but it usually retains the pearly border and can be identified on close inspection. Cystic basal cell carcinoma behaves much like the nodular variant, but it presents as a smooth, round, cystic mass. Sclerosing or morpheaform basal cell carcinoma is the most troubling variant, because it tends to extend well beyond the visible borders of the lesion, making margins hard to clear surgically. It may appear plaquelike and resemble scleroderma, with very indistinct edges that blend into normal skin. Superficial basal cell carcinoma is the least aggressive variant. It tends to present as a scaly plaque that looks much like eczema. However, careful inspection will often reveal diminutive but characteristic pearly white borders.

Treatment

Treatment can be carried out by a variety of modalities. Excision offers the opportunity to resect the tumor with a margin of uninvolved surrounding barrier tissue, followed by immediate histologic evaluation to confirm the tumor-free tissue. Reconstruction by either direct closure (in small lesions) or skin grafts or flaps is then possible on either an immediate or a delayed basis. Small tumors of the nodular

Excision of these lesions should incorporate about a 4-mm margin of "normal" skin, and the depth of excision should be at the mid-subcutaneous level. A large prospective study has shown that a 4-mm margin will completely excise 95% of basal cell carcinomas under 2 cm in diameter.[125]

Larger lesions (>2 cm) and morpheaform variants will require a much wider excision to ensure clear margins. In these cases, Mohs' micrographic surgery is recommended. This allows for accurate clearance of all margins without removing excess healthy tissue.

Lymphangiosarcoma (Stewart-Treves Syndrome)

This is an uncommon but highly malignant tumor that occurs in postmastectomy patients (Fig. 62-18). Fifty percent of patients die within 19 months of diagnosis,[64,126] and only 9% of patients survive longer than 5 years.[126] Three cases were presented recently, which outlined the recognition of this unusual malignancy of the upper extremity soft tissue.[22] The typical patient who developed this disease had chronic lymphedema for over 10 years and had mastectomy with axillary lymph node dissection followed by radiation to the chest wall. This tumor develops quickly and may appear as a simple bruise. It can present as multiple purplish papules on the skin.

The treatment should be rather aggressive after biopsy confirmation of this malignancy. Amputation of the involved limb should be the preferred option to save the patient's life. Consultation with medical oncologists is useful, because newer adjuvant therapies show promise.

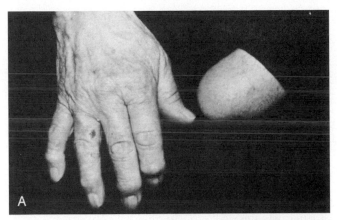

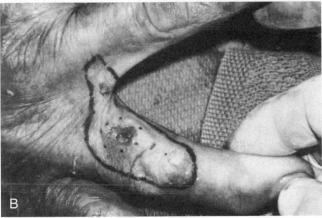

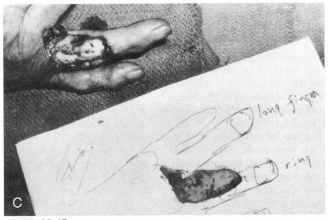

FIGURE 62-17. A, An 82-year-old patient with a previous traumatic amputation of the left hand and an elevated, ulcerated basal cell carcinoma of the right ring finger. **B** and **C,** Excisional biopsy was done in this patient because adjacent premalignant skin changes, as well as the primary lesion, required treatment. Histologic evaluation of the margins of resection is necessary. Note the important use of the drawing to orient the specimen for more precise evaluation of the margins. Incisional biopsy, especially when needed to determine the type of treatment and to limit tumor seeding, is an appropriate alternative.

or superficial type respond well to electrodesiccation and curettage, with low recurrence rates. This approach, however, fails to preserve any tissue for pathologic diagnosis. We generally recommend excision for this malignant tumor. This ensures an accurate diagnosis of the tumor type and variant, as well as an evaluation of both the peripheral and deep margins of excision.

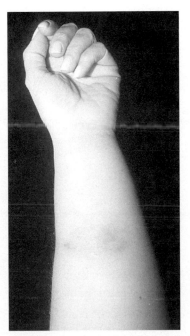

FIGURE 62-18. A 50-year-old woman developed lymphangiosarcoma 25 years after mastectomy and radiation to the chest wall. Note the seemingly innocuous discoloration of the lymphedematous forearm.

Merkel Cell Carcinoma

There is another group of tumors that one occasionally encounters that can produce great difficulty in recognition, treatment, and cure. Merkels cell carcinoma is located in the basal layer of the epidermis, and this cell-neurite complex is considered to be a pressure receptor. Dellon has pointed out that the Merkel cell/neurite complex "is the receptor part of the slowly-adapting fiber/receptor system."[32] Tumors composed of these cells are unusual and are considered malignant. Varying patterns of the tumor cells occur.[93] Merkel cell carcinoma may occur on the extremities. It is described as a "rapidly growing, painless, firm, nontender, bluish-red, intracutaneous nodule 0.5 to 5 cm in diameter."[95]

Treatment recommended in the literature is wide surgical excision with regional lymphadenectomy. Postoperative radiation and chemotherapy should be considered.[25,103] The literature points out that there is a high incidence of distant metastases, as well as a high incidence of recurrence of the tumor and metastases to regional lymph nodes.[54]

SWEAT GLAND TUMORS

Although rare, one of the messages to take away from this discussion is that we must heed patients' inquiries with regard to lumps developing in and about the skin. Just as occurs with more deeply placed tumors, we cannot tell what these lesions are until the patient is evaluated and the mass sampled. This is emphasized by the next group of lesions, which arise from some of the adnexa or appendages of the skin.

Eccrine sweat gland tumors may be encountered in both benign (Fig. 62-19) and malignant varieties. They must be differentiated from other lesions, but this can cause significant difficulty for the pathologist. Differential diagnosis includes giant cell tumors, basal cell carcinoma, SCC, metastatic malignant tumors (e.g., from breast, salivary gland, and lung), and melanoma. The malignant varieties vary widely in their behavior.[17,123] This group of tumors, especially, exhibits a tendency toward local recurrence of benign lesions and may change from benign to malignant varieties over time.[24,29]

Eccrine Poroma

This benign tumor is thought to originate from that part of the sweat gland within the epidermis.[18] It usually presents as an asymptomatic, solitary, soft, raised, or nodular tumor in middle-aged or older patients. Most often seen on the sole of the foot, several have been described in the hand, usually in the palm. Malignant change may be heralded by bleeding, itching, and pain.[88] Treatment in Buckley and colleagues' review is excision with a barrier or margin of surrounding normal tissue. As with all tumors, especially sweat gland

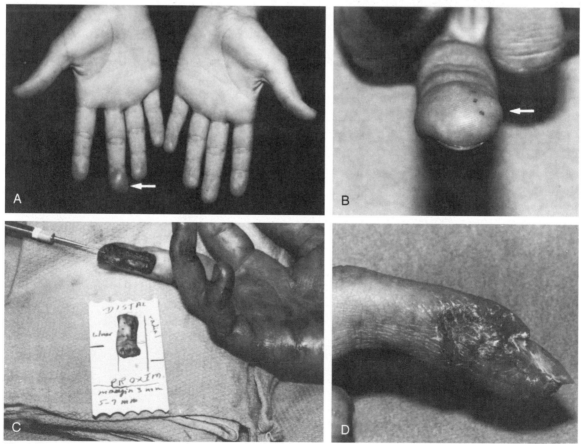

FIGURE 62-19. A, A mass arising from the pulp area in the right middle finger (*arrow*) of a 10-year-old girl. **B,** Recurrence of the tumor was noted approximately 2 years postoperatively. **C,** After biopsy of presumed recurrent giant cell tumor, the diagnosis of benign sweat gland tumor was made. The biopsy showed involved margins, and re-excision included the surrounding skin and underlying collateral ligament. **D,** Early postoperative appearance showing split-thickness skin graft.

tumors, long-term follow-up is recommended.[18] A malignant variant has been described, but it is quite rare.

Chondroid Syringoma

Chondroid syringoma, even in its benign form, can grow quite large. It is seen more commonly in men than in women. The malignant variety not only can recur but also may metastasize.[95]

Eccrine Spiradenoma

Eccrine spiradenoma represents a sweat gland tumor that may involve the upper extremity. This may be noted as a single mass or multiple nodules.

When a nodule enlarges rapidly, one must be more concerned about the possibility of its being a malignancy. These are known for their tendency to locally recur and to spread widely.[95]

Malignant Sweat Gland Tumors

Malignant sweat gland carcinomas that may occur in the upper extremity include clear cell carcinoma, which commonly produces metastatic disease, as well as aggressive digital papillary adenocarcinoma and eccrine adenocarcinoma.[24,29]

Aggressive digital papillary adenocarcinoma specifically involves the digits. The patients are often older. Pain and/or tenderness may be present with this lesion, especially when it ulcerates. Because of this lesion's tendency to grow deeply, local recurrence is not unusual, as is the case with many of the sweat gland tumors. These tumors may metastasize to regional lymph nodes as well as by blood-borne routes to bone, skin, lung, brain, and kidney.[75] The tumors usually have a palmar location, because this is the most concentrated area for sweat glands. In understanding the nature of these lesions, one must realize that local recurrence is common.[35] Metastatic disease is certainly a great concern with these tumors, although some of them may grow to a large size before that occurs.[105]

Following careful evaluation of the patient, including examination of regional nodes and investigation for metastatic involvement, treatment requires tumor excision with good tumor free margins of normal tissue for barriers. The optional margins are not well established by the sparse literature available on these tumors. Some authors have recommended prophylactic regional lymph node dissection. It is still not possible to answer the question as to the efficacy of radiotherapy or chemotherapy for these tumors.[2,75,123] These can be extremely aggressive tumors, even though they may follow a long indolent course.[105]

ANNOTATED REFERENCES

15. Breslow A: Thickness, cross-sectional areas and depth of invasion in the prognosis of cutaneous melanoma. Ann Surg 172:902-908, 1970.

Following Clark's paper, Breslow measured the depth of invasion of melanomas using micrometers and determined that the depth of invasion predicts patient survival. Subsequent randomized controlled trials have shown that the depth of invasion has the greatest prognostic factor, regardless of the type of melanoma.

16. Brodland DG, Zitelli JA: Surgical margins for excision of primary cutaneous squamous cell carcinoma. J Am Acad Dermatol 27:241-248, 1992.

This is a prospective study of 141 primary invasive squamous cell carcinomas. The margins were evaluated serially using Mohs' technique. This is the first study to apply scientific data to establish a clear guideline for excision margin in squamous cell carcinoma. The authors found that 4-mm margins were adequate for most squamous cell carcinoma. Margins of 6 mm were recommended for tumor size of 2 cm or larger, histologic grade 2 or higher, invasion of the subcutaneous tissue, and location in high-risk areas, such as the scalp, ears, eyelids, nose, and lips.

23. Clark WH Jr, Wihm MC: The histogenesis and biologic behavior of primary human malignant melanomas of the skin. Cancer Res 29:705-727, 1969.

This is a classic article that first hypothesized that the level of melanoma invasion has great prognostic significance. The depth of invasion is based on the histologic layers of the skin, which are difficult to quantify because the thickness of the layers varies with each individual. Nevertheless, this seminal paper ushers a new direction in the treatment of melanoma.

42. Fleegler EJ: Tumors involving the skin of the upper extremity. Hand Clin 3:197-212, 1987.

Dr. Earl Fleegler, an authority on malignancies of the skin, has presented a clear and succinct discussion of various skin tumors of the upper extremity. He used case examples to illustrate the management of these conditions, and this article is a quick reference for a surgeon confronted with skin tumors of the upper extremity.

72. Mohs FE: Chemosurgery: Microscopically controlled surgery for skin cancer—past, present and future. J Dermatol Surg Oncol 4:41-54, 1978.

This review article recounted the evolution of Mohs' technique in microscopically controlled excision of skin cancers. This technique is used for excision of melanoma, basal cell carcinoma, and squamous cell carcinoma, particularly when one needs to minimize the amount of tissue resected from privileged areas. Although this technique is used mainly over the face to conserve the amount of tissue resected, its application in the upper extremity is less well defined. It may have a role in clearing recurrent skin cancers of the hand or in removing residual cancer cells after the initial unsuccessful excision attempt.

77. Morton DL: Lymphatic mapping and sentinel lymphadenectomy for melanoma: Past, present, and future. Ann Surg Oncol 8:22-28, 2001.

This article presents the evolution of the concept of sentinel node biopsy. This mode of mapping the draining lymphatic system challenges the traditional method of elective lymph node dissection for melanoma, which adds additional morbidity to a large subset of patients who have no metastasis to the lymph nodes. The sentinel biopsy has become the accepted method in staging intermediate-thickness melanoma (1.0 to 4.0 mm) and is associated with much less morbidity.

79. NIH Consensus Development Panel on Early Melanoma: Diagnosis and treatment of early melanoma. JAMA 268:1314-1319, 1992.

In January 1992, the National Institutes of Health convened an expert panel from various specialties to derive a consensus statement on the diagnosis, treatment, and future direction in melanoma research. This publication helps define the state of melanoma care from leading experts.

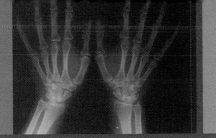

CHAPTER 63

Bone and Soft Tissue Tumors

Edward A. Athanasian

The purpose of this chapter is to present the most recent knowledge regarding specific benign and malignant bone and soft tissue tumors that may be seen in the hand. Tumors occurring in the hand and forearm often have unique growth patterns and potential for metastasis that may be different from those seen elsewhere in the body. Tumors in the hand are relatively uncommon, and most surgeons encounter them infrequently. Knowledge regarding treatment and care of hand lesions is often based on case reports, small case series, retrospective reviews, and a few large general case series. Data from controlled trials are limited but have advanced the use of chemotherapy and radiation therapy and the treatment of soft tissue sarcoma. At times the available information is both contradictory and controversial. It is important for the treating surgeon to understand thoroughly the specific characteristics of the tumor being treated, as well as the systemic treatment of the disease. Of greater importance, however, is knowledge and practice of the principles and guidelines for the treatment of patients with tumors. The reader is strongly encouraged to understand and review the principles of staging, biopsy, resection, and amputation before treating all tumors, particularly those that are malignant. In no other aspect of hand surgery are the implications for uninformed decisions, judgments, or actions more serious than in the treatment of malignant bone or soft tissue sarcomas. Conversely, treatment based on up-to-date knowledge and a thorough understanding of the principles of local and systemic cancer care maximizes the potential to save the patient's life. Only after this concern has been addressed can one focus on the task of salvaging or reconstructing a useful hand or limb. Regular review of treatment principles before treating patients for malignant tumors is imperative and helps to ensure appropriate treatment.

DIAGNOSIS AND MANAGEMENT OF MUSCULOSKELETAL TUMORS

Neoplasms are usually classified in two categories: benign and malignant; in musculoskeletal tissues, malignancies may also be subdivided into low grade and high grade. Cellular growth in benign neoplasms usually proceeds at a much slower rate than in malignant tumors. Benign lesions may be expansile and sometimes encapsulated. Distant spread usually does not occur, and local recurrence is less common in benign than in malignant lesions.

Malignant neoplasia is characterized by a rapid growth rate, atypical cellularity, and poor cell differentiation. Local growth is aggressive and infiltrative; there are only "pseudo-capsules" through which the tumor extends with satellite lesions. Such tumors are likely to spread as blood-borne metastases, and local recurrence rates are high after excision unless a wide margin of normal tissue is included in the resection. Low-grade malignancies grow more slowly and infiltrate early but are less likely to metastasize than to recur locally. *Neither all generic categories nor isolated case illustrations are consistent with these classifications.*

Many benign tumors of the hand or forearm require no treatment, can be diagnosed clinically, and are asymptomatic. However, if a lesion increases in size or becomes symptomatic, or if the physical or radiographic appearance suggests an aggressive process, appropriate staging studies, including obtaining tissue for diagnosis, must be done.[†] Unfortunately, lumps and growths that look innocent may not necessarily be so; every tumor ought to be considered a potential impediment to function, if not to survival. Surgeons need to be familiar with the range of possible diagnoses. A physician is not justified in advising a patient that a mass ought to be "left alone" until the proper diagnosis is established by all appropriate means. Any tumor with an unclear diagnosis on the basis of nonsurgical evaluation should be sampled. If the biopsy proves the tumor to be benign, no further surgery may be necessary. If a malignant or an aggressive nonmalignant lesion is identified, further management is required.

Tumors that are symptomatic or continue to grow need to be diagnosed and staged. The clinical and family history, physical characteristics of the tumor, and data from labora-

*I would like to acknowledge the excellent work of earlier authors who wrote and revised portions of this chapter in previous editions: Alexander C. Angeledes, Gordon B. McFarland, Jr., Waldo E. Floyd III, Richard J. Smith, Clayton A. Peimer, Harold M. Dick, and Owen J. Moy. The principles of aggressive and malignant tumor management as described in great detail by these authors have changed relatively little. I have attempted to enlarge the focus of the chapter and update patient management principles, which have changed as the effect of adjuvants has become better understood.

†See references 34, 56, 82, 112, 119, 156, 157, 162, 164, 348, 494, and 495.

tory and imaging studies provide at least the basis of a clinical impression. If the precise diagnosis is unclear after a complete work-up, a carefully planned biopsy is required to avoid hazards of misdiagnosis and its complications.

CLASSIFICATION AND STAGING OF TUMORS

Managing tumors of the hand and upper extremity does not differ significantly from managing tumors in other parts of the musculoskeletal system. Correct treatment must always take into consideration the size and location of the growth, the histologic grade and clinical behavior, and the potential for metastases.[112,156,157,162,163,348,471,494,495] A thorough understanding of general principles and guidelines is essential for accurate assessment and staging of tumors.

Histologic Grade and Surgical Staging

The histologic grade (G) of a neoplasm is determined by the malignant characteristics of tissue obtained with a biopsy. The accepted classification is as follows:

G0: Benign
G1: Low grade: few cells, much stroma, little necrosis, mature cells, fewer than five mitoses per high-power field
G2: High grade: many cells, little stroma, much necrosis, immature cells, more than 10 mitoses per high-power field

Benign tumors can be classified into three stages[162]:

Latent, stage I tumors usually do not require treatment; they may heal spontaneously and/or remain unchanged.
Active, stage II benign neoplasms grow within a limited zone and are contained by natural barriers; if surgery is required, these tumors are most often controlled by intralesional or marginal excision.
Locally aggressive, stage III benign tumors may both grow and spread beyond natural barriers; excision requires a wide surgical margin or en bloc resection for local cure.

To avoid confusion and differences of opinion about malignant bone tumors, it has become important to establish specific grading criteria for tumors. A classification scheme based on a modified staging system for bone sarcomas was established by the American College of Surgeons Joint Committee on Cancer and End Results Reporting in 1977. It was proposed by W. F. Enneking at the University of Florida and accepted by the Musculoskeletal Tumor Society (MSTS) in 1979 (Tables 63-1 and 63-2). Although this staging system was developed for bone sarcomas, it has also been used to describe and stage soft tissue sarcomas, particularly in the orthopedic surgery community. A comparison of the MSTS system and the fourth and fifth editions of the American Joint Committee on Cancer (AJCC) system has found the AJCC system to be more predictive of systemic relapse.[577] The AJCC staging system incorporates grade, size, depth, and the presence or absence of metastasis to determine the final stage of the lesion. This system should be used preferentially for staging of soft tissue sarcomas (Table 63-3).

The pathologist and surgeon must agree on a surgical grade (G1, G2) of malignancy based primarily on the histologic features of the tumor and also on its gross pathologic appearance, the clinical setting, and the radiologic appear-

Table 63-1
SURGICAL STAGES

Stage	Grade	Site
IA	Low (G$_1$)	Intracompartmental (T$_1$)
IB	Low (G$_1$)	Extracompartmental (T$_2$)
IIA	High (G$_2$)	Intracompartmental (T$_1$)
IIB	High (G$_2$)	Extracompartmental (T$_2$)
III	Any (G) Regional or distant metastasis (M)	Any (T) Regional or distant metastasis (M)

Adapted from Enneking WF: Staging of musculoskeletal neoplasms. *In* Uhthoff HK, Stahl E (eds): Current Concepts of Diagnosis and Treatment of Bone and Soft Tissue Tumors. New York, Springer-Verlag, 1984, pp 1-21.

ance. The histologic grade is determined only after a representative biopsy and careful scrutiny by an experienced musculoskeletal pathologist. The clinical and radiologic status are also important parameters for determining the final tissue diagnosis and surgical grade.

There are two grades of malignant tumors: G1, low-grade malignancy, with low likelihood of metastasis and frequent local recurrence, and G2, high-grade malignancy, with frequent blood-borne metastases. The so-called low-grade malignant tumors can also metastasize but typically are less likely to do so early in their course. The assignment of a grade to a particular tumor is neither easy nor exact, because grading criteria are not quantifiable. Cellular morphology, anaplasia, necrosis, mitoses, and tissue of origin may also be influenced by clinical behavior. Tumors that are known to be exceptionally dangerous (e.g., synovial and epithelioid sarcoma) are most properly classified into a higher grade than their histology would indicate. Two other criteria are important: T, which represents the size and site of the tumor; and M, which designates the presence of detectable metastases.

Location (Site)

Regardless of size, if the tumor is limited to a single anatomic compartment, it will usually be resectable. At the same time, it will be possible to preserve the extremity, as is the case when highly malignant tumors involve the distal phalanges and other acral parts. The basis of defining a *compartment* is the recognition that certain natural anatomic barriers exist that will temporarily contain and delay the spread of a pathologic process, such as infection and neoplasia. For example, an intraosseous tumor contained by the cortices and intramedullary canal of a tubular bone would be considered intracompartmental. However, if this tumor perforates into the surrounding soft tissues, it would then be considered extracompartmental, as it has already crossed a natural barrier. Computed tomography (CT) and magnetic resonance imaging (MRI) enable us to estimate the size and location of a tumor, permitting more accurate preoperative planning than was previously possible.

This concept also applies to soft tissue compartments, but not quite so neatly as with bone tumors. Tumors that involve a flexor tendon in the digit have, in theory, violated the

Table 63-2
SURGICAL PROCEDURES FOR EXTREMITY SARCOMAS

	Surgical Method			
Margin	Limb Salvage	Amputation	**Planes of Dissection**	**Microscopic Appearance**
Intralesional	Debulking, piecemeal excision/curettage	Translesional amputation	Within tumor (palliative)	Tumor at all margins
Marginal	Marginal en bloc excision	Marginal amputation	Within tumor "reactive zone"	Reactive tissue (± microextensions of tumor)
Wide	Wide en bloc excision	Wide through-bone amputation	Through normal tissue but within compartment	Normal tissue (± "skip lesions")
Radical	En bloc resection of entire compartment	Extra-articular disarticulation	Normal tissue: Extracompartmental	Normal tissue

Adapted from Enneking WF: Staging of musculoskeletal neoplasms. *In* Uhthoff HK, Stahl E (eds): Current Concepts of Diagnosis and Treatment of Bone and Soft Tissue Tumors. New York, Springer-Verlag, 1984, pp 1-21.

Table 63-3
AJCC STAGING SYSTEM FOR SOFT TISSUE SARCOMAS

Stage I	
IA	Low grade, small (<5 cm), superficial or deep to fascia
IB	Low grade, large (>5 cm), superficial to fascia
Stage II	
IIA	Low grade, large, deep to fascia
IIB	High grade, small, superficial or deep to fascia
IIC	High grade, large, superficial to fascia
Stage III	High grade, large (>5 cm), deep to fascia
Stage IV	Any metastasis to lymph nodes or distant sites

entire compartment of extrinsic muscle. Tumors may have a propensity to spread proximally along the tendon to the muscle, much as a hematoma may track proximally after a flexor tendon rupture, following the natural barriers of tendon sheath and muscle fascia.

Metastases

The third criterion for malignant tumor classification identifies the patients in whom the tumor has already metastasized to other sites. The final system therefore has three stages, with stage III including all patients with distant metastases, regardless of the other parameters (see Table 63-1). Lymph node involvement is always an important finding, because primary musculoskeletal neoplasms do not commonly spread to regional nodes. Because fewer than 5% of patients with such sarcomas develop lymph node metastases, the differential diagnosis of extremity tumors with possible nodal metastases must always be expanded to include carcinomas and melanomas. Metastases to lymph nodes are significantly more prevalent with rhabdomyosarcoma, epithelioid sarcoma, clear cell sarcoma, and angiosarcoma.

Once the appropriate staging studies are completed, the surgeon will know the anatomic characteristics (the T) of the lesion and whether metastases (the M) are absent or present. A differential diagnosis can then be formulated and the biopsy planned.

EVALUATION PROTOCOL

There are no precise physical characteristics that clearly distinguish aggressive and malignant tumors from benign and reactive lesions. The only definitive test is histologic evaluation of biopsy material. However, because hand tumors may produce such significant dysfunction, and inadequate or unnecessarily aggressive surgery also presents risks, biopsy must be the final step in obtaining a diagnosis. All nonsurgical studies should be completed before surgical biopsy (Fig. 63-1).

Laboratory Studies

Laboratory studies include determination of levels of serum calcium, phosphorus, blood urea nitrogen, and creatinine to evaluate the possibility of metabolic bone disease. The serum alkaline phosphatase and lactase dehydrogenase levels are elevated in some malignancies. A serum immunoelectrophoresis assists in determining if multiple myeloma is present. The hematologic profile and the erythrocyte sedimentation rate are abnormal in the presence of many neoplastic and infectious processes. A urinalysis may detect an occult renal cell carcinoma. Antinuclear antibodies and rheumatoid factor may be positive in patients who have upper extremity swelling secondary to rheumatoid disease.

Diagnostic Imaging

A variety of diagnostic imaging techniques permit analysis and localization of the size and extent of the lesion and its impingement on normal anatomy. Although imaging does not typically offer a specific diagnosis, it provides important clues in the evaluation, analysis, and work-up of a specific patient.

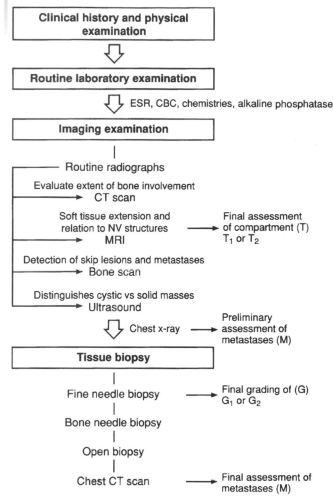

FIGURE 63-1. Suggested evaluation protocol for suspected musculoskeletal neoplasms. NV, neurovascular.

Plain Radiographs

Plain radiographs afford the best possible resolution and detail of bone and adjacent soft tissues. The anatomic region in question should be fully visualized on all radiographs, and this is achieved by taking an adequate number of views. Plain radiographs are the standard for predicting the presence and location of bony involvement. They may also be the most specific radiologic test for bone tumors.

Computed Tomography

Although conventional radiographs offer significant spatial information, the higher resolution of CT produces images that are useful specifically in localizing small tumors within a bone and in identifying soft tissue extension or calcification within such growths. Because of its ability to discriminate varying densities, a CT scan allows visual separation between the medullary canal, cortex, and surrounding soft tissues, often providing critical information concerning anatomic location (T) for tumor staging. Plain chest radiographs are always obtained before performing a biopsy of a suspected malignancy; chest CT scans are useful for staging histologically defined malignant tumors but are not routinely used for prebiopsy screening studies.

Scintigraphy

Radionuclide "bone scan" imaging can be very helpful in detecting primary and metastatic tumors. However, the phenomenon of increased radiopharmaceutical pooling (increased uptake) in a particular bone or soft tissue area is not at all specific or diagnostic. The technique has two time-variable phases. Within minutes after injection, conditions associated with an increased vascularity show abnormally high uptake (trauma, infection, and neoplasia). Later, the isotopes are actively concentrated; in the skeleton, pooling occurs in woven (new) bone, so that any process that forms immature bone would be associated with increased uptake on films done 2 or 3 hours after injection. Radioisotope scans are probably most helpful to demonstrate lesions that may not have been suspected clinically or in anatomic sites not seen on initial images that focused only on the symptomatic region. These findings may be important in patient management, and they have the potential to alter biopsy or therapeutic plans significantly.

Magnetic Resonance Imaging

MRI is a technique that depends on sophisticated computers to produce excellent delineation of soft tissue contrast as well as images in axial, coronal, and sagittal views. For MRI studies, electromagnets generate strong fields that cause cellular nuclei to "wobble" or "vibrate" at specific frequencies. A number of technical factors affect the MRI signal, including echo time (TE), pulse or repetition time (TR), longitudinal or spin-lattice relaxation (T1), and spin-spin relaxation (T2).

The majority of soft tissue tumors have a low signal intensity (i.e., appear darker) on T1-weighted scans and a high signal intensity (i.e., appear brighter or whiter) on T2-weighted studies. Specific problems such as hematoma, lipoma (or liposarcoma), hemangioma, or conditions that involve hemorrhage into an existing tumor zone are known to have a high signal intensity on T1-weighted scans. Obviously, the potential value of MRI is diminished in a region recently subjected to biopsy, trauma, or other surgery.

MRI is a superior imaging technique for the assessment of the soft tissue extent of disease and is particularly beneficial in the evaluation of soft tissue sarcoma. The extent of intramedullary bone involvement can also be readily determined. This facilitates preoperative planning of bone transection level during resection and may aid in the identification of skip metastases that otherwise might not be identified. High-resolution CT offers the benefit of more accurate assessment of cortical bone involvement and may be the preferred technique for evaluating lesions involving the cortex of a given bone. CT is particularly beneficial in identifying occult osteoid osteomas.

Sonography

Sonograms produce images from a differential pattern of transmitted and received echoes. Compared with CT and MRI, sonography produces less detail with respect to precise anatomic relationships and tumor margins. Echo patterns of solid masses are nonspecific, but fluid-filled lesions can be easily differentiated from solid tumors. Sonograms are extremely inexpensive in comparison to the cost of CT and MRI and may be more useful than either for distinguishing reactive and cystic processes.

Biopsy

The biopsy is the last stage of diagnostic management. Biopsy surgery should be planned as carefully as the definitive operation.[348,494] The exact technique used is influenced by history, location, and size of the mass, as well as the experience of the surgeon and the pathologist.

Needle Biopsy

Needle biopsy has an extremely limited role in the diagnosis of lesions in the hand and upper extremity. It can be useful in confirming the histology of a recurrent or metastatic lesion. Needle biopsy produces only a small and often fragmented tissue sample that may be impossible to diagnose or grade accurately. Even if the core biopsy seems clearly diagnosable, the tissue volume may not be representative of the tumor, leading to the possibility of overgrading or undermanagement.

Open Biopsy

Open surgical biopsy is a complex procedure, but one that plays a critical role in determining treatment outcome for aggressive and malignant tumors.[348,494,495] During the biopsy, the patient and surgeon must be prepared for the unexpected. Institutions or clinicians that are not prepared or able to complete all diagnostic studies and also provide definitive surgical and medical-adjunctive management are best advised to refer patients *before* the biopsy is performed.

Hand surgery is most safely and efficiently performed in a bloodless field. The use of a pneumatic tourniquet is acceptable during both open biopsy and surgical treatment of tumors and neoplasms. Limb exsanguination before biopsy is contraindicated before tourniquet inflation because of the risk of seeding or dislodging tumor cells. An entirely satisfactory field is achievable by elevating the arm for 3 to 4 minutes before inflating the tourniquet. Likewise, the use of intravenous anesthesia (Bier block technique), a method that also requires pretourniquet exsanguination, is not appropriate for tumor biopsy or treatment of aggressive bone or soft tissue neoplasms.

A frozen section is necessary at the time the biopsy is performed to determine whether an adequate specimen has been sampled, so that permanent light microscopic and special microscopic evaluations can be carried out subsequently. It is rare to find a pathologist who can consistently provide accurate histologic analysis of a frozen specimen dependable enough to begin treatment.[348,495,547] The definitive treatment plan should be decided on only after the results of all permanent sections, electron microscopic studies, and special tissue techniques are complete and reported. All biopsy specimens should be cultured, and all cultures should be sampled. Although plain chest radiographs are taken before biopsy, chest CT is performed to stage a diagnosed lesion. If the tumor is aggressive or malignant, the biopsy tract itself will be contaminated with tumor cells and must later be excised en bloc with the subsequent resection or amputation specimen. Preferred biopsy incisions are therefore longitudinal and are carefully placed to permit their complete excision without having to extend a dissection margin simply to accommodate a badly placed incision. As a simple rule, the biopsy should be placed in line with or immediately parallel to the incision that may be required for later attempted limb salvage (Fig. 63-2). Transverse and Bruner-type incisions are specifically to be avoided.

Incisional Biopsy

Incisional biopsy is frequently the most appropriate technique for diagnosis of bone and soft tissue masses. It requires excision of an adequate tissue sample that is minimally manipulated. Frozen sections are important to determine specimen sample adequacy. The biopsy incision is located to afford the most direct route to the tumor, thereby ensuring that the fewest tissue planes are disturbed or contaminated.

Correct surgical technique for biopsy is different from all typical surgical dissections. Biopsy involves a direct approach via a longitudinal incision through muscle and other tissues that overlie the mass. Biopsy technique does not include spreading or extensive and vigorous retraction, which has the potential to contaminate a widened area. However, adequate visualization during biopsy, as in any operation, is critical. Because the biopsy tract is cell-contaminated, an approach through a muscle sacrifices only one plane, whereas spreading techniques (i.e., moving muscles aside) contaminate not only the muscle that is retracted but also all surrounding structures. Perfect postsurgical hemostasis is essential to avoid hematoma, which can lead to cellular spread beyond the primary site and biopsy tract. Once the wound is dry and hemostasis is secure after tourniquet release, the wound is closed, not drained. Other than taking steps to avoid pathologic fracture, post-biopsy surgical care is routine while the surgeon awaits the definitive histologic findings.

Excisional Biopsy

Excisional biopsy involves complete removal of a lesion through the reactive zone. An example would be excision of a giant cell tumor of tendon sheath or lipoma. It is a technique that should be reserved for very small lesions (a diameter less than 1 to 2 cm) to avoid compromising subsequent surgical procedures. Extensive contamination of the operative field occurs with this type of biopsy. If this is done for a large tumor, the extent of contamination may increase

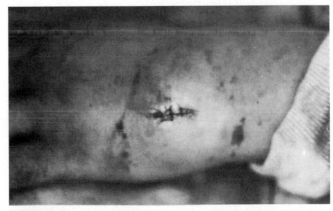

FIGURE 63-2. An open incisional biopsy was performed for a rapidly growing hand lesion. The biopsy site is contaminated with tumor cells; the incision is oriented longitudinally and will be excised as part of the definitive procedure performed later. Frozen section at biopsy verified adequacy of the specimen sample.

the need for soft tissue coverage and increase the risk of both positive margins at definitive resection and subsequent local recurrence. Extensive contamination may preclude subsequent limb salvage and may commit the patient to amputation specifically as a result of the biopsy.

Primary Wide Excision. This type of biopsy requires excision of the tumor with a wide margin or cuff of surrounding normal, nonreactive, healthy tissue. This is an excellent oncologic procedure but requires sacrifice of an extensive amount of normal tissue. Primary wide excision is usually best reserved for very small lesions where the suspicion of malignancy is high and the risks of soft tissue contamination with other forms of biopsy are excessive, as might occur in the carpal tunnel. The decision of when to perform this type of biopsy is usually best made with the assistance of or by a musculoskeletal oncologist.

DEFINITIVE TREATMENT

General Plan of Tumor Excision

Benign Tumors

Nonaggressive, benign neoplasms are usually removed simply by marginal or intralesional operations such as curettage. If there is a question about the adequacy of resection or of the tissue margins, and the diagnosis is already confirmed, a frozen section may be of great assistance for intraoperative sampling of the margins.

Malignant Tumors

In the management of malignancies of the upper limb, preservation of function is secondary to eradication of the disease process.[499] The hand surgeon who undertakes management of a neoplasm must have a thorough understanding of the tumor's biologic behavior, its patterns of local and metastatic spread, and its response to radiotherapy and chemotherapy. Radiation and chemotherapy may allow the surgeon to use less radical tumor margins so that amputation may be avoided and function may be maintained.[112,156,157, 322,420,496,520,521] However, the risk of unnecessary sacrifice of tissue must be balanced against the need for adequate resection, because local recurrence of sarcoma sometimes carries a grave prognosis. One of the major problems in assessing outcome has been the lack of a common procedural language regarding surgical methods; however, uniform use of the Enneking terminology as recommended by the MSTS provides such a means of communication (see Table 63-2).[162]

Treatment should not begin until a neoplasm has been diagnosed definitively and the results of all preoperative studies, including biopsy, are verified. The assumption that a problem can be "handled" by a relatively simple extirpation in the absence of complete diagnostic data is neither justified nor defensible. The risks associated with soft tissue extension from a tumor-contaminated field are too great. Because most tumors are benign, cystic, and nonproblematic, the outcome of those few that are aggressive or truly malignant may be disastrous if we become too casual or complacent. When a malignant tumor or aggressive nonmalignant lesion is identified, carefully planned treatment is required not only to preserve a maximal degree of hand function but also to save the patient's life. Function is secondary to survival.[112,192,348,499,500]

The hand surgeon who seeks to treat a specific neoplasm must have not only a general understanding of the concepts and principles of tumor management but also a detailed knowledge of the tumor's biology, histologic and clinical behavior, tendency to spread locally and widely, and potential response to adjunctive measures. All these considerations may bear significantly on proposed surgical margins and long-term function.[112,156,157,232,322,420,496,520,521] An inade-

---

CRITICAL POINTS: OPEN BIOPSY OF FOREARM AND HAND TUMORS

INDICATION

- Lesions that cannot be diagnosed as benign on clinical and radiographic grounds

TECHNICAL POINTS

- Review case with pathologist before biopsy and confirm pathologist availability.
- Draw limb salvage incision or amputation flaps at the time of biopsy.
- Place longitudinal biopsy incision mark in line with limb salvage incision.
- Confirm biopsy incision will not compromise subsequent amputation flaps.
- Elevate arm only for exsanguination without using Esmarch bandage.
- Inflate tourniquet to ensure bloodless field.
- Dissect through one anatomic plane or muscle to limit contamination field.
- Avoid extensive flaps or retraction to limit contamination.
- Incise directly into tumor to remove a wedge for frozen section and permanent analysis.
- Culture all biopsy specimens.
- Confirm the presence of adequate lesional tissue on frozen section.
- In most cases defer definitive treatment of malignant lesions until permanent analysis confirms diagnosis.
- Obtain perfect hemostasis before closure.
- If a drain is used it should exit the patient immediately in line with the incision to limit contamination.
- Place sutures close to wound edges to avoid additional skin contamination.
- Apply bulky compressive dressing to avoid hematoma.

POSTOPERATIVE CARE

- Limit use of limb until definitive treatment.

quate resection that permits a local recurrence may condemn the patient to a far worse prognosis than would otherwise occur.[29,82,119,165,168,328,464,494]

According to MSTS criteria, compartmental resection and radical excision cannot yet be applied to the hand.[119,142] Most hand tumors occur in spaces rather than in compartments; and although metacarpal excisions may remove a compartment for a stage IA or IIA bone tumor, extirpation of the entire flexor surface or above-elbow amputation would be required to remove the compartment if the neoplasm arose on a digital flexor. Presently there are no data to support a conclusion that the MSTS definitions should be applied uniformly to all parts of an acral compartment. Because the flexor tenosynovium is continuous in the thumb and little finger, but not in the index, middle, and ring fingers, there may be differences in management that can be prudently used with such variations in location. A soft tissue tumor that develops along the dorsum of the wrist requires surgical extirpation of the extensors of several fingers and/or the thumb but not necessarily of the entire muscle compartment proximally or distally. Functional restoration can be achieved via tendon grafts, transfers, or free muscle flaps. True radical excision may be impractical if function of any kind is to be salvaged in lesions of the hand and forearm, and it may be that a 1- to 2-cm margin of normal tissue, especially with tumors that are sensitive to adjuncts, will be safe and allow secondary reconstruction.[114,142,156,287,344,416,427,500,502] The extent of surgical resection for aggressive tumors is dependent on the histologic diagnosis, location, and size. Remote tissues, except when provided by microvascular transfer,[232,547,559,561] should be avoided because of the risk of transferring malignant cells via tissue or flap pedicles.

Principles of Excision for Specific Sites

Distal Phalanx

Malignant soft tissue tumors in the distal phalanx typically involve skin and bone (Fig. 63-3).[92] Safe removal may require excision at the distal interphalangeal (DIP) joint; occasionally, a lesser segment may need to be excised when the lesion, such as a nail bed carcinoma, is more superficial and slow growing. A small portion of dorsal or palmar skin might be used as a local flap to cover the middle phalanx after DIP joint disarticulation. In such an instance, the distal phalanx and DIP joint are sacrificed if the lesion involves or threatens enough tissue, while retaining the tissues at a safe distance from the tumor site. Indeed, if the tumor involves both the dorsal and the palmar surfaces of soft tissue as well as bone, a more proximal transosseous amputation through the middle phalanx is required. In every case, the proximal end of the excision margin should be sampled and inspected by frozen section at operation and later by permanent-technique histology to ensure the safety of the level of removal.

Malignant distal phalangeal lesions require removal with an appropriate cuff of contiguous soft tissue. Lower-grade bone tumors may be managed by distal phalangeal amputation including a soft tissue cuff 1 to 2 cm proximal to the intraosseous tumor, a level that requires transosseous resections through the middle phalanx. It is unlikely that such lesions can be safely removed by DIP disarticulation alone. Cases that present with pathologic fractures or extracompartmental extension usually require removal of the finger at

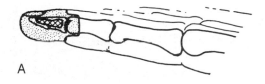

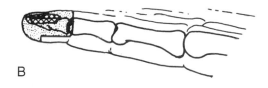

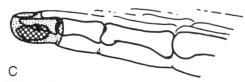

FIGURE 63-3. Malignant lesions of the terminal segment of the finger generally require amputation at or proximal to the DIP joint. **A,** Intraosseous distal phalangeal tumors are amputated at or proximal to the joint, with combined dorsal and volar flap closure. **B,** Dorsal lesions are treated by appropriate tumor excision and volar flap closure. **C,** After removal of a palmar tumor, dorsal flap closure may be possible.

or proximal to the proximal interphalangeal (PIP) level, or even ray resection.

Middle Phalanx

Malignant and aggressive soft tissue tumors in the middle phalanx and those proximal to the region of the DIP joint require amputation at the metacarpophalangeal (MP) joint or metacarpal level or ray resection (Fig. 63-4). In this instance, MP joint disarticulation should allow at least a 2- to 3-cm margin of normal tissue. However, functional and aesthetic considerations strongly recommend ray resection (Fig. 63-5). In theory, bone tumors involving the proximal and middle phalanges may be excised and replaced with bone graft if the lesion is not aggressive and if it has not extended into the soft tissues. However, ray resection is actually a far more practical, functional alternative if both the proximal and middle phalanges are involved. For malignant tumors that have spread beyond bone owing to fracture or slow, progressive extension, ray amputation is clearly indicated. MP joint disarticulation is rarely a safe, practical, functional, or aesthetic choice for treating tumors at these levels.

First Metacarpal

Intracompartmental first metacarpal malignancies may be treated by osseous excision and autogenous or allograft replacement (Fig. 63-6). After removal, biopsy specimens

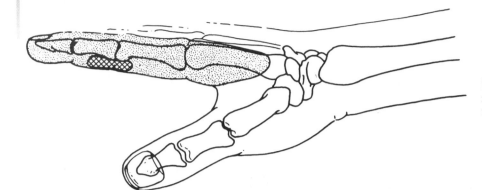

FIGURE 63-4. Tumors of the soft tissue at the middle phalangeal and PIP joint level are best treated by ray resection.

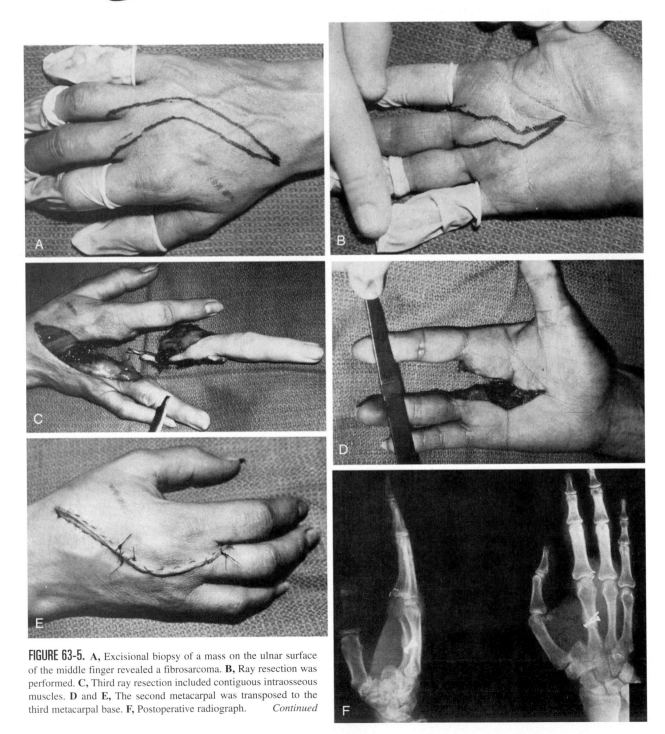

FIGURE 63-5. A, Excisional biopsy of a mass on the ulnar surface of the middle finger revealed a fibrosarcoma. **B,** Ray resection was performed. **C,** Third ray resection included contiguous intraosseous muscles. **D** and **E,** The second metacarpal was transposed to the third metacarpal base. **F,** Postoperative radiograph. *Continued*

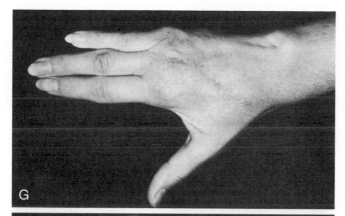

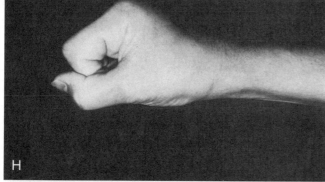

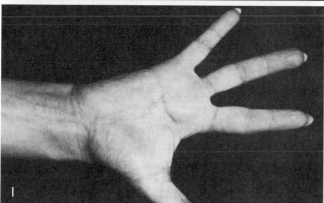

FIGURE 63-5.—cont'd **G** to **I,** Appearance after rehabilitation. Function and aesthetic appearance were retained.

are taken from the soft tissue bed surrounding the excised bone, and the metacarpal is also carefully studied to exclude breakthrough. Replacement by metatarsal or metacarpal allograft, or fibula or iliac autograft, may be considered in appropriate circumstances.[328] Autografting should be done using a second, separate surgical setup and clean gowns and gloves to avoid cross-contamination of the bone donor site. Osteoarticular allografts may be unstable, and arthrodesis may be required at the trapeziometacarpal articulation.

If a bone tumor has broken into soft tissue, a more radical resection is required, including the entire first ray and possibly portions of the web and second metacarpal, to gain a safe margin. If part of the second metacarpal is resected, the "floating index" thereby produced can be considered for direct pollicization if sacrifice of the entire second ray is not required.

Finger Metacarpals

Aggressive and malignant bone tumors of the second through fifth metacarpals generally require en bloc bone excision. A more important treatment decision may be whether removal of one metacarpal alone is possible or whether removal of an entire ray, or pair of rays, is best. Ray excision is usually best for lesions of the second and fifth metacarpals (Fig. 63-7). With the additional consideration of ray transposition, the principles governing removal of the third and fourth rays are no different from those governing the second and fifth. If bone graft has been used for reconstruction, carpometacarpal arthrodesis and MP ligament reconstruction or silicone arthroplasty may be practical. Whatever level is chosen for reconstruction, it is essential that an adequate, safe margin of normal tissue first be excised en bloc with the tumor.

Aggressive tumors of the second through fifth metacarpals that have invaded soft tissue or sustained pathologic fractures often require excision not only of the involved ray but also of the contiguous ray or rays radial and ulnar to the involved digit. A malignant tumor of the second metacarpal that extends into the soft tissues may necessitate removal of the second and third rays or of the first through third rays,

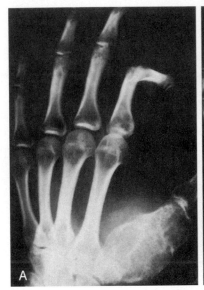
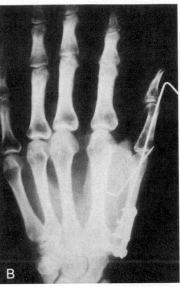

FIGURE 63-6. **A,** Recurrent tumor in the first metacarpal after excision of an enchondroma proved to be a low-grade chondrosarcoma. **B,** The first metacarpal and distal trapezium were removed with contiguous soft tissues and replaced by an allograft, MP reconstruction, and carpometacarpal joint arthrodesis.

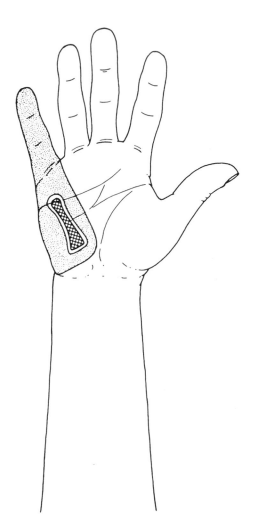

FIGURE 63-7. Malignant tumors of the fifth metacarpal can be treated by ray excision.

while preserving soft tissue of the middle finger as a filet flap to resurface the radial side of the hand. A similar technique can be used on tumors of the ulnar side of the hand. If the second, third, and fourth rays must be removed, the best strategy is usually to osteotomize and supinate the fifth metacarpal to promote effective oppositional pinch and grasp to the thumb. If a tumor of the fourth metacarpal requires removal of the third through fifth rays, the radial aspect of the middle finger or a filet of that digit on its radial neurovascular pedicle can be used to close the ulnar side of the hand. Tumors of the fifth metacarpal may require excision of the fourth and fifth rays. Skin coverage may be possible by using a filet flap from the ring finger.

If a malignant tumor has broken into the mid palm and extends across the metacarpals, removal of all digital rays may be needed to gain an adequate soft tissue margin. Retention of a sensate and relatively mobile thumb may be considerably more aesthetic and functionally satisfactory than a forearm- or wrist-level amputation.[501] However, if a tumor extends proximally from the metacarpals, a more proximal level of hand, wrist, or forearm amputation is required for safe tumor management.

Soft tissue tumors in the palm or on the dorsum of the hand, as well as metacarpal tumors, usually require at least a partial hand amputation. If treated by only local or limited excision, the chance of recurrence and metastasis may be enhanced; below-elbow amputation is necessary to treat these larger tumors. It is unusual for an aggressive soft tissue tumor to be adequately removed by a truly local en bloc excision. At a minimum, aggressive soft tissue tumors, like bone tumors, require ray resection or removal of multiple rays (Figs. 63-8 to 63-10). Central palmar lesions usually require sacrifice of three rays; those on the border are more likely than those in the center to be salvageable by removing only two rays. In the presence of proximal, broader, and larger lesions, all four digits or the entire hand may have to be sacrificed to save the patient.

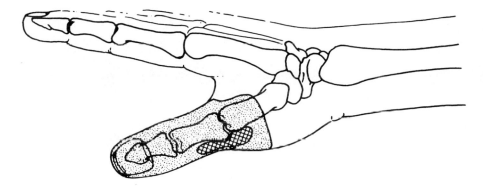

FIGURE 63-8. Malignant soft tissue tumors adjacent to the thumb MP joint require amputation through the metacarpal. More aggressive and extensive tumors may require removal of the entire ray, possibly contiguous with the second metacarpal.

Wrist and Distal Forearm

Malignancies of the proximal palmar hand and volar wrist should not be treated with wide local excision in most cases. A dissection that attempts to "salvage" the median nerve or one or two flexors in the middle of an expanding tumor or reactive zone is likely only to spread the disease. Correct surgical and medical principles of tumor removal and care should be followed (Figs. 63-11 to 63-13).

Tumors that arise on the dorsum may allow preservation of the hand if staging studies show that the lesion has not penetrated into the palm and the excision margin verifies a safe plane of normal tissue. Isolated intraosseous carpal lesions that have not invaded soft tissue are rare but may be excised locally. The carpal bones are intra-articular, so the onset of symptoms is usually associated with synovitis and joint invasion; therefore, below-elbow amputation or complete en bloc excision of the entire radiocarpal articulation and carpus is likely to be necessary.

Growths on the volar aspect of the distal forearm generally require above- or below-elbow amputation, because it is not easy to excise a tumor adequately and still preserve function in and distal to this region after removal of all flexor muscles and tendons, the median and ulnar nerves, and vessels. If a tumor arises in a location that does not specifically involve the ulnar nerve and artery, it may be possible to save a portion of the hand and wrist along with the neurovascular bundle and to consider later reconstruction after longitudinal hemiamputation. Treatment of tumors arising on the radial side of the distal forearm varies according to lesion size and exact location (Fig. 63-14). In many situations, as is true of lesions on the volar side, amputation is probably preferable when all criteria are considered. Tumors on the extreme ulnar side of the wrist may be handled in a way that mirrors those on the radial aspect, although lesions in the extreme end of the ulna may be amenable to wide excision of the distal ulna (Fig. 63-15).

Intracompartmental lesions within the distal radius or ulna can be treated by wide excision of the bone and arthrodesis or autograft replacement.[347,502] In such a situation, transosseous excision must include biopsy of the medullary canal from the retained segment or segments. When tumors have invaded tissues or crossed compartments extensively, above- or below-elbow amputation is required.

Wherever a tumor is located, treatment must be individualized to achieve the goal of functional restoration without risking local recurrence and later distant spread. Because we lack control over the site and origin of the neoplasm, the surgeon's responsibility is confined to intelligent management and treatment, adhering to the proper principles of care.

BENIGN SOFT TISSUE LESIONS

Ganglions and Mucous Cysts

Clinical Characteristics

Ganglion cysts are the most common soft tissue tumors of the hand. These mucin-filled cysts are usually attached to the adjacent underlying joint capsule, tendon, or tendon sheath. Ganglions are most prevalent in women[152] and generally occur (70%) between the second and fourth decades of life. They are not rare in children[339,341,466,554] and have been reported from the first to the eighth decades. Ganglions usually occur singly and in very specific locations; however, they have been reported to arise from almost every joint of the hand and wrist (Table 63-4). The less common ganglions are often associated with other conditions of the hand (e.g., bossing of the second and third carpometacarpal joints, de Quervain's disease, and Heberden's nodes of the distal interphalangeal [DIP] joint). Ganglion cysts have also been reported to cause clinically symptomatic pressure on the median and ulnar nerves of the hand.[68,180,210,337,367,485] Because of their high incidence and prevalence, ganglion cysts should be readily recognized by most hand surgeons. Other conditions that cause diffuse swelling over the dorsum of the wrist, such as extensor tenosynovitis, lipomas, and other hand tumors, must also be considered in the differential diagnosis. The history, physical examination, techniques of transillumination, and aspiration should allow a conclusive diagnosis in most instances.

Patients usually seek medical attention due to cosmetic appearance of the mass, pain, weakness, and concern of potential malignancy. A specific antecedent traumatic event is present in at least 10% of cases, and repeated minor trauma may be an etiologic factor in their development. There is no obvious correlation with patient occupation. Malignant degeneration has never been reported; however, malignant soft tissue tumors are frequently misdiagnosed as ganglion cysts. Ganglions may appear quite suddenly or develop over several months. They may subside with rest, enlarge with activity, and rupture or disappear spontaneously. Although recurrences are rare with proper excision,[18,100,104,185,261] over 50% may recur if incompletely excised.

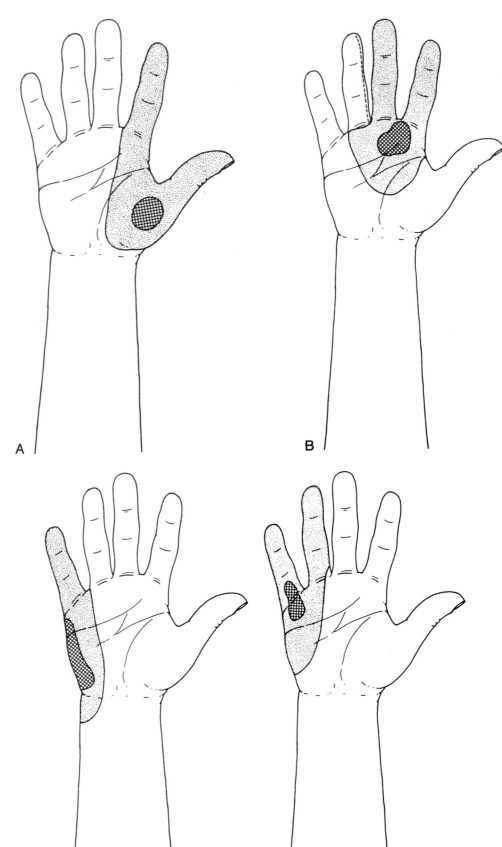

FIGURE 63-9. **A,** Tumors located between the first and second metacarpals may require amputation of both rays for adequate local control. **B,** Tumors between the second and third metacarpals require removal of both rays. **C,** Lesions of the ulnar border of the hand can be treated by fifth ray resection and local flap or skin graft closure. **D,** Large and more aggressive lesions or those extending more radially may need removal of both the fourth and fifth rays.

Radiographs of the involved region are often unremarkable, although intraosseous cysts are occasionally present at the wrist. Osteoarthritic changes are commonly seen with cysts at the DIP or carpometacarpal joints. Communication between the wrist joint and cyst has been demonstrated with arthrograms[16,43,531] but not with cystograms. A one-way valvular mechanism[263] has therefore been postulated to connect the wrist joint to the cyst.

Anatomy

The microscopic description of ganglions is well known. The main cyst may be single or multiloculated and appears smooth, white, and translucent. The wall is made up of compressed collagen fibers and is sparsely lined with

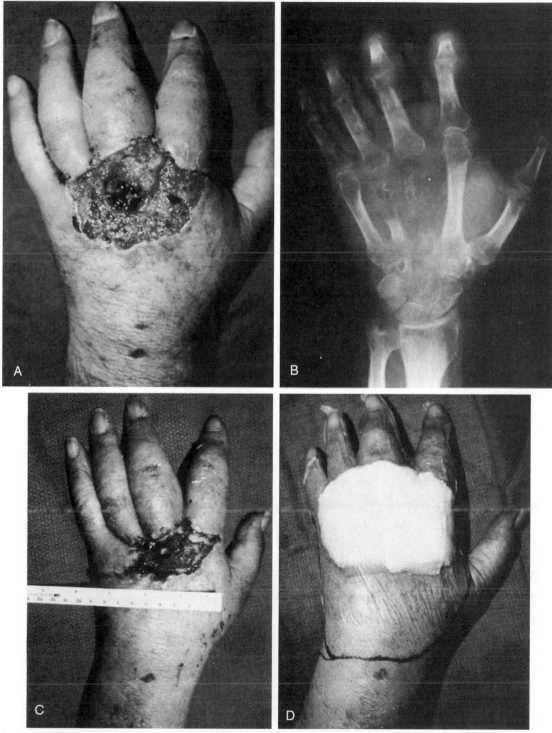

FIGURE 63-10. **A** and **B,** This neglected squamous cell carcinoma progressed to invade and destroy the third and fourth metacarpals (**C**). **D,** The tumor was removed by partial hand amputation.

Continued

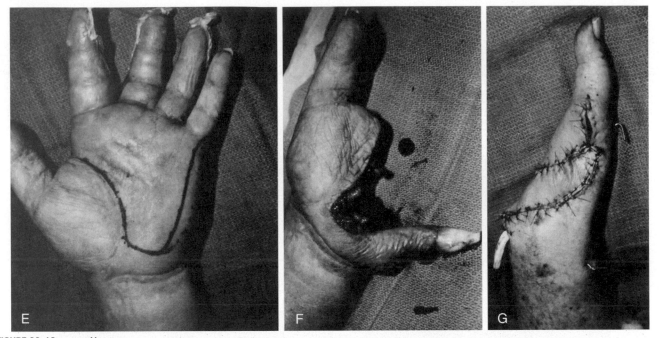

FIGURE 63-10.—cont'd E to **G,** The ulnar skin was retained to resurface the border of the thumb. Axillary node dissection was negative.

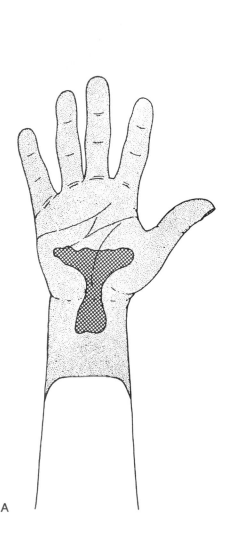

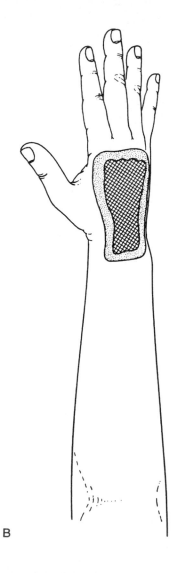

FIGURE 63-11. A, Tumors on the proximal volar palm often involve the flexor tendons and median and ulnar nerves; forearm- or wrist-level amputation is usually required. **B,** Lesions on the dorsum of the hand may not necessarily invade vital neurovascular structures and can be adequately resected en bloc, followed by secondary reconstruction.

A

B

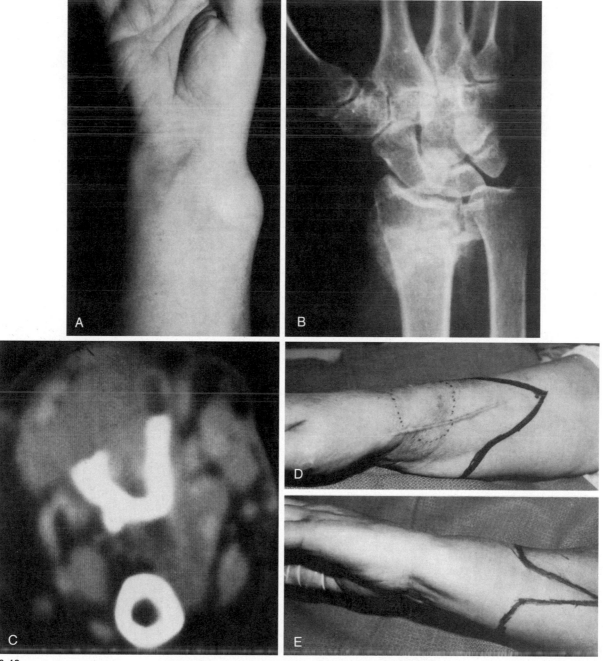

FIGURE 63-12. **A** and **B,** A soft tissue mass of the volar forearm was discovered after treatment and healing of a now apparently pathologic fracture of the distal radius. **C,** CT demonstrates bone invasion. Biopsy revealed fibrosarcoma. **D** and **E,** The tumor was treated by below-elbow amputation with flaps designed to excise the overly generous biopsy incision *(dotted lines).*

flattened cells without evidence of an epithelial or synovial lining. Electron microscopic studies have further confirmed these findings.[331,440]

The capsular attachment of the main cyst reveals mucin-filled "clefts," which have been shown by serial sections to intercommunicate[18] via a tortuous continuous duct connecting the main cyst with the adjacent underlying joint. The stroma surrounding the intracapsular ducts may show tightly packed collagen fibers or sparsely cellular areas with broken collagen fibers and mucin-filled intercellular and extra-cellular lakes. No inflammatory reaction or mitotic activity has been noted.

The contents of the cyst are characterized by a highly viscous, clear, sticky, jelly-like mucin made up of glucosamine, albumin, globulin, and high concentrations of hyaluronic acid. In some cases the mucin may be blood tinged. The contents of the cyst are decidedly more viscous than normal joint fluid.

Pathogenesis

The etiology and pathogenesis of ganglions remain obscure, and a review of the literature reflects the confusion that exists.[163,178,504] Since Hippocrates offered the first recorded description of "knots of" tissue containing "mucoid flesh,"

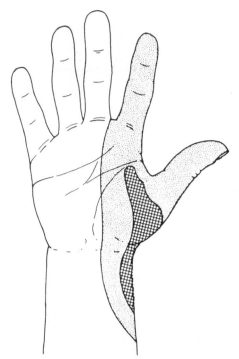

FIGURE 63-13. Aggressive tumors of the radial side of the distal forearm may require amputation of the thumb and index rays as well as the contiguous radial wrist, at a minimum.

numerous speculative theories with little scientific basis have abounded. This became especially true when 18th and 19th century anatomists offered the following hypotheses: (1) synovial herniation (Eller, 1746) or rupture through the tendon sheath; (2) synovial dermoid or rest caused by "arthrogenesis blastoma cell nests" or embryonic periarticu-

lar tissue (Hoeftman, 1876); (3) new growths from synovial membranes (Henle, 1847); and (4) modifications of bursae or degenerative cysts (Vogt, 1881).

Until recently, the most widely accepted theory, initially postulated by Ledderhose (1893) and popularized by Carp and Stout,[87] was that of mucoid degeneration. The fibrillation of collagen fibers, accumulation of intercellular and extracellular mucin, and decreased collagen fibers and stroma cells supported this theory. Mucoid degeneration does not, however, explain why the degenerative process is self-limiting and solitary and usually occurs in adolescents and young adults and why the fluid recurs following aspiration or incomplete excision.

Nonoperative Treatment

Nonsurgical methods of treatment are usually considered initially due to the limited associated morbidity and possibility of success. Nonsurgical treatment has included digital pressure, injections of hyaluronidase or sclerosing solutions,[340] subcutaneous tenotome dissection, and cross-fixation with a heavy suture.[203] Historical folk medicine has mentioned rupture with a mallet or Bible, methods that need not be considered except for their historical interest. Observation has been advocated in the pediatric population owing to the high likelihood of spontaneous resolution.[554]

Aspiration of the ganglion, puncture of the cyst wall, and instillation of lidocaine (Xylocaine) and betamethasone (Celestone) into the capsule or tendon sheath attachments reduces the mass and may alleviate symptoms for varying periods of time.[20,32,54,67] Aspiration may provide long-term relief and has been reported to be effective in 20% to 30% of patients with wrist ganglia.[61] Injection and aspiration of volar wrist ganglions must be approached with caution due to the proximity of the radial artery. Marked subcutaneous atrophy and skin depigmentation may be seen after injection

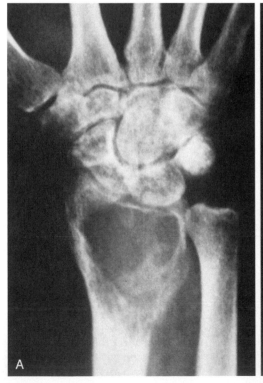

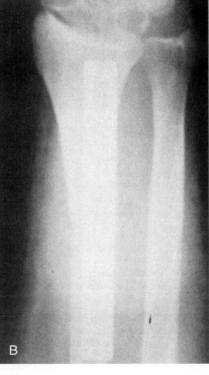

FIGURE 63-14. A, Angiosarcoma of the right distal radius. **B,** Surgical management by en bloc radius excision and allograft replacement.

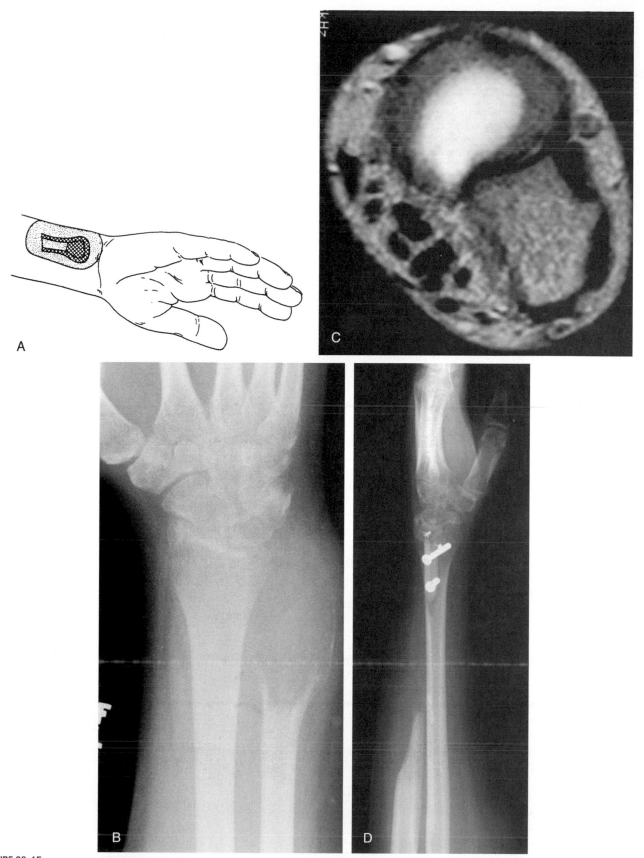

FIGURE 63-15. **A,** Intraosseous tumors of the distal ulna can be managed by en bloc excision. No bone reconstruction is needed in most cases. Tumors with soft tissue extension (**B** and **C**) may require excision of the ulnar cortex of the radius en bloc with the ulna, as was required with this malignant fibrous histiocytoma (**D**). A portion of the remaining ulna was used to augment the radius and support the lunate facet.

Table 63-4
GANGLIONS OF THE HAND AND WRIST

Dorsal wrist ganglion

Volar wrist ganglion

Volar retinacular ganglion (flexor tendon sheath ganglion)

Mucous cyst (ganglion of distal interphalangeal joint)

Other ganglions
  Carpometacarpal boss
  Proximal interphalangeal joint
  Extensor tendon

Miscellaneous locations
  First extensor compartment (dorsal retinacular ganglion)
  Carpal tunnel
  Ulnar canal
  Intraosseous ganglion

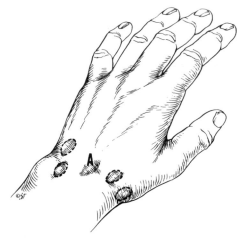

FIGURE 63-16. A few of the many possible locations of dorsal wrist ganglions. The most common site (A) is directly over the scapholunate ligament. The others *(dotted circles)* are connected to the scapholunate ligament through an elongated pedicle.

with triamcinolone (Kenalog), which should be used with great caution or simply avoided.

The most effective nonsurgical treatment is patient reassurance. An explanation of the condition and assurance of its nonmalignant nature are often the only treatment sought or required. Surgery is best reserved for patients with persistently symptomatic ganglions.

Operative Treatment

Open procedures are most commonly done for excision of ganglion cysts. Treatment principles include attempts to minimize scar formation and loss of range of motion. Data regarding arthroscopic approach to both dorsal and volar carpal ganglion cysts have been published.[245,338,398,490] The technique appears to be effective in small case series with local recurrence risk comparable or better than the historic risk of recurrence after open procedures. No comparative or outcome studies have been reported comparing the relative risks and benefits of open versus arthroscopic treatment. It is possible that arthroscopic excision may become the preferred technique if superior outcome is ultimately determined.

Author's Preferred Method of Treatment

Dorsal Wrist Ganglion

Clinical Characteristics. The prototype of all ganglions of the hand is the dorsal wrist ganglion, which accounts for 60% to 70% of all hand and wrist ganglions. The main cyst is usually directly over the scapholunate ligament (Fig. 63-16) and is easily seen and diagnosed. The cyst may occur anywhere else between the extensor tendons, however, and can be connected to the ligament through a long pedicle (see Fig. 63-16). Failure to identify this pedicle and excise its scapholunate ligament attachment increases the likelihood

of recurrence. Careful preoperative palpation of the cyst with digital compression often reveals the extent of the cyst and the direction of the pedicle. Transillumination or aspiration confirms the diagnosis preoperatively. Although ganglions have been reported from other carpal joints, these are rare, and attachments to the scapholunate joint must be ruled out before a dissection is considered complete. A review of the patient's preoperative radiographs to rule out an interosseous component is wise.

Operative Technique. Most dorsal ganglions may be approached through a transverse incision over the proximal carpal row, but a modified incision or second transverse incision may be necessary for ganglions not directly over the scapholunate ligament (Fig. 63-17). The diagnosis of ganglion cyst should be made before commitment to a transverse incision because this type of incision is not readily incorporated into a limb-sparing incision in the event

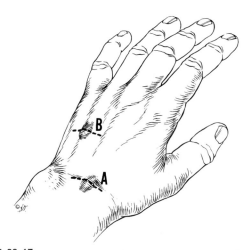

FIGURE 63-17. Transverse incision over the scapholunate ligament (A) used to expose the typical dorsal ganglion. Additional incision (B) to expose a more distant cyst. The main cyst and pedicle are mobilized, passed under the extensor tendons, and delivered through incision A.

of a subsequent diagnosis of a malignant soft tissue tumor. Typically, a dorsal ganglion appears between the extensor pollicis longus and extensor digitorum communis tendons, which are retracted radially and ulnarly, respectively (Fig. 63-18). The main cyst and its pedicle are mobilized down to the underlying joint capsule. With the wrist in volar flexion, the joint capsule is opened along the border of the radius and proximal pole of the scaphoid (Fig. 63-19). The capsule is elevated and retracted distally to expose the capsular attachments to the scapholunate ligament (Fig. 63-20). Smaller

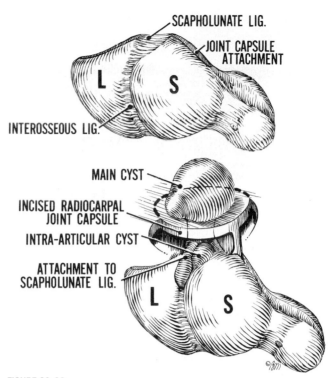

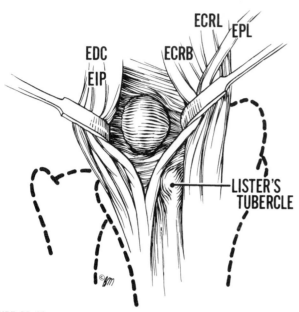

FIGURE 63-18. The dorsal ganglion exposed and mobilized between the extensor pollicis longus (EPL), extensor carpi radialis longus (ECRL), and extensor carpi radialis brevis (ECRB) radially and the extensor digitorum communis (EDC) and extensor indicis proprius (EIP) ulnarly.

FIGURE 63-20. Schematic representation of the cyst in situ. Attachments to the scapholunate ligament are visualized before final excision (*dotted line*).

intra-articular cysts are often seen attached to the scapholunate ligament. The capsular incision is then continued around the ganglion, but all capsular attachments to the ligament are left intact (Fig. 63-21). The capsular incision is extended more laterally if any capsular ducts, which can be identified by small amounts of mucin drainage, are encountered during the dissection. The ganglion and its capsular attachments are then tangentially excised off the scapholunate ligament (Fig. 63-22). A small mucin-filled duct is invariably seen piercing the transverse fibers of the scapholunate ligament. This duct appears to connect the underlying scapholunate joint with the main cyst. Synovial and capsular

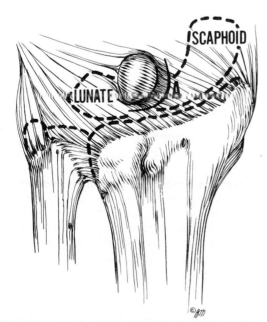

FIGURE 63-19. The initial incision through the joint capsule (A) to expose the scapholunate ligament attachments and intracapsular cysts.

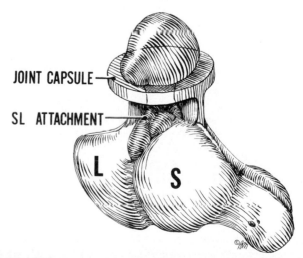

FIGURE 63-21. The ganglion and scapholunate (SL) attachments are isolated from the remaining, uninvolved joint capsule (not shown).

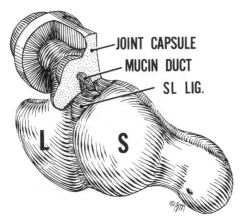

FIGURE 63-22. Tangential excision of the ganglion and attachments off the fibers of the scapholunate (SL) ligament. A minute mucin duct piercing the fibers of the scapholunate ligament is invariably cut during this dissection.

attachments along the distal margin of the scapholunate ligament are also excised to give an unobstructed view of the head and neck of the capitate (Fig. 63-23). If the ganglion ruptures and its anatomic features are lost during the dissection, the dissection should continue until all attachments to the scapholunate ligament have been excised. The excised portion of the joint capsule usually measures approximately 1.0 × 1.5 cm. It is neither necessary nor desirable to cut into the scapholunate ligament, nor is it necessary to curet the scapholunate joint.

The tourniquet is released and hemostasis obtained, and then under tourniquet control the wound is closed and a dressing applied. Attempts to close the joint capsule either primarily or with fibrous flaps are contraindicated. Subcuticular closure with a monofilament, nonabsorbable, pullout suture may minimize scar formation. Splinting the wrist in slight flexion may reduce postoperative flexion loss.

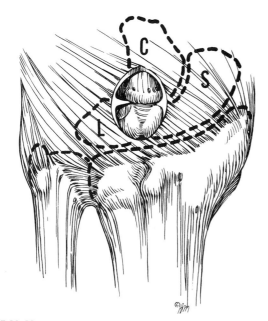

FIGURE 63-23. Completed excision of all attachments to the scapholunate (SL) ligament and the immediate vicinity. Synovial tissue between the ligament and head of the capitate (C) has also been excised. Note that the scapholunate ligaments remain intact.

Postoperative Care. A bulky dressing extending from the proximal forearm to the MP joints is applied and the hand elevated. Early finger motion is encouraged. The dressing and sutures are removed between 7 and 10 days postoperatively. Wrist motion should be initiated and encouraged, especially volar flexion. Hand therapy is continued until a full range of motion has been obtained.

Complications. Early recurrences, the most common complication of ganglion surgery, are usually due to inadequate and incomplete excisions and should rarely occur. Ganglions appearing at the same site years after excision may in fact be new ganglions. Stiffness of the wrist can be avoided by early motion, physical therapy if necessary, and splinting of the wrist in slight flexion in the immediate postoperative period. It is imperative to stress early volar flexion. To avoid keloid or hypertrophic scars, longitudinal incisions across the wrist joint should be avoided. Awareness and respect for the sensory branches of the radial and ulnar nerves prevent neuroma formation, which often defies effective treatment. I have not seen avascular necrosis of either the lunate or scaphoid or scapholunate dissociation after the surgical technique just described.[18,152,556] Ganglions and sprains of the intercarpal ligaments can occur concomitantly after trauma to the wrist and must be distinguished preoperatively. Identification of concomitant wrist pathology may be facilitated with arthroscopic treatment.

Occult Dorsal Carpal Ganglion

Unlike protruding dorsal ganglions, smaller, occult dorsal ganglions are easily overlooked and can often only be palpated with the involved wrist in marked volar flexion. Comparison with the opposite normal wrist is helpful. An occult ganglion may be the cause of unexplained wrist pain and is disproportionately tender. Its intimate relationship to the overlying posterior interosseous nerve has been suggested as the etiology of the exquisite pain and tenderness associated with occult dorsal ganglions.[136] Differentiation of a painful occult dorsal ganglion from sprains of the scapholunate ligament and other intercarpal ligaments with early carpal instability may be difficult, especially after dorsiflexion injuries of the wrist. The presence of a ganglion does not exclude other causes of wrist pain. Dorsal ganglions do occasionally occur in association with an underlying scapholunate diastasis, and they may be blamed for the carpal instability after their excision.[118,152,222] Dorsal prominence of the proximal pole of the scaphoid secondary to intercarpal instability may be confused with a painful occult ganglion and must be diagnosed with appropriate radiographic studies[43,325,531] to avoid a delay in proper treatment. Excising the ganglion alone might not alleviate all the patient's preoperative pain. Excision of the posterior interosseous nerve at the level of the radiocarpal joint may help alleviate pain and add to the patient's postoperative comfort. If other causes of wrist pain and tenderness, especially directly over the scapholunate ligament, can be excluded, an occult dorsal ganglion is best initially treated conservatively with immobilization and steroid injections directly into the dorsal capsule, which may also aid in diagnosis.[474]

In cases in which further diagnostic studies are necessary, some authors have found the use of MRI, CT, and ultrasonography helpful.[179,216,408,409,447,563] The cost-effectiveness of these studies must be kept in mind.

Chronic tenosynovitis of the extensor tendons may be confused with a dorsal wrist ganglion but is easily distinguished by the diffuse nature of the swelling and the puckering seen with digital extension, the so-called tuck sign.

Recurrent Dorsal Ganglion

A recurrent dorsal ganglion can be treated like a primary ganglion, but excision may be more complicated because of scarring. Previous skin incisions should be excised and longitudinal scars may be converted with a "Z"-plasty. Tendons and nerves are identified and delicately cleaned of scar tissue before dissecting the ganglion itself. Excision can then proceed as described earlier.

Dorsal Wrist Syndrome and Impingement

A dorsal ganglion, whether occult or not, is often evidence of a periscaphoid ligamentous injury and frequently associated with a dorsal wrist syndrome.[474,556] Any repetitive or acute trauma to the periscaphoid tissues can lead to a ganglion. In many instances the patient has experienced an acute hyperextension injury. Watson and associates[556] reported a 62% occurrence of ganglions in patients in whom dorsal wrist syndrome was diagnosed. Steroid injections into the capsule at the area of maximal tenderness may be effective for pain relief. When conservative treatment fails, surgery should include excision of the ganglion, thickened soft tissues, bone spurs, and the posterior interosseous nerve. Careful excision of a dorsal ganglion will not lead to carpal instability. The underlying periscaphoid trauma may go on to more advanced instability patterns, however. Soft tissue thickening over the scapholunate area, with or without a ganglion, often leads to impingement against the dorsal radial lip.[556] Excision of this thickened capsule with the posterior interosseous nerve usually relieves pain.

Volar Wrist Ganglion

Clinical Characteristics. The second most common ganglion of the hand and wrist is the volar wrist ganglion (18% to 20%). Most volar ganglions occur either directly over the distal edge of the radius or slightly more distally over the scaphoid tubercle. The former arises from the capsular and ligamentous fibers of the radiocarpal joint and occurs under the volar wrist crease between the flexor carpi radialis and abductor pollicis longus tendons (Fig. 63-24). The main cyst may be intertwined with the bifurcating branches of the radial artery, thus making delicate dissection imperative. The other type of volar ganglion arises from the capsule of the scaphotrapezial joint.

Although volar ganglions may appear clinically small, they can be surprisingly extensive at surgery. Multiloculated cysts extending under the thenar muscles, along the flexor carpi radialis tendon, into the carpal canal, and under the first extensor compartment adjacent to the dorsal branch of the radial artery as far dorsally as the first web space may be encountered. These extensions can often be appreciated preoperatively by careful palpation and digital compression of the ganglion.

It is important to assess the patency of the radial and ulnar arteries. Allen's test should be routinely performed and

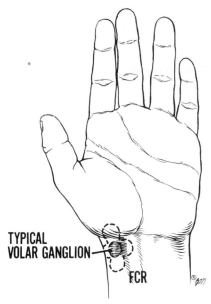

FIGURE 63-24. Typical location of a volar wrist ganglion. Possible subcutaneous extensions *(dotted lines)* are often palpable. FCR, flexor carpi radialis.

ulnar artery occlusion excluded. The surgeon must be aware of the importance of preserving the radial artery, particularly in those patients with a radial dominant circulation.

Operative Technique. Although the surgical technique of excision of a volar ganglion is similar to that for a dorsal ganglion, the exposure and precise identification of the capsular attachments of the volar ganglion are more difficult. The incision must be planned to allow for extension into the carpal tunnel or base of the thenar muscles (Fig. 63-25). Most difficulties are accentuated by a small transverse incision that does not allow adequate mobilization of adjacent structures.

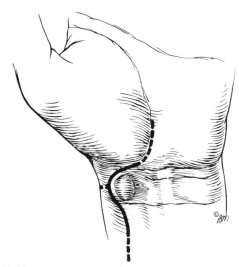

FIGURE 63-25. The usual incision to expose a volar wrist ganglion. Extensions proximally, distally, and even radially are possible *(dotted lines)*. Care must be taken to avoid injury to the palmar cutaneous branch of the median nerve if the incision is extended.

With the skin flaps retracted, the forearm fascia is incised longitudinally and the dome of the cyst identified and mobilized. Particular care is taken to identify and protect the radial artery, which is often intimately attached to the wall of the ganglion and may even be completely encircled by the ganglion (Fig. 63-26). Magnification is helpful.

The pedicle is traced to the volar joint capsule (usually the scaphotrapezial or radiocarpal ligament). The joint is opened and explored and the capsular attachments are excised (approximately 3 × 4 mm). Once the ganglion is excised, the surrounding tissues can be digitally compressed to rule out further mucin-filled pockets. If unidentified extensions are present, they must be excised. Hemostasis, wound lavage, and a simple skin closure (preferably subcuticular) complete the operation. Again, capsular closure is unnecessary and only delays early mobilization.

Postoperative Care. A bulky bandage and elevation of the hand ensure early postoperative comfort. Follow-up care is similar to that for dorsal ganglions, and motion of the wrist should begin within the first 2 weeks after surgery.

Complications. The complications are similar to those of dorsal ganglions. Unexpected branches of the radial sensory or lateral antebrachial cutaneous nerves may be injured and lead to troublesome neuromas. Extensions of the routine incision into the carpal canal must avoid injury to the palmar cutaneous branch of the median nerve. Injuries to the radial artery can be microscopically repaired. Some authors[327] recommend leaving a portion of the cyst wall attached to the artery to avoid arterial injury. Stiffness of the wrist is less common than with dorsal ganglions, but it can occur if early motion is not encouraged. Unpleasant scars are not an uncommon problem on the volar aspect of the wrist and often defy "plastic" revisions. Curved incisions appear to provide more consistently attractive scars, especially near the volar wrist creases (see Fig. 63-25).

Volar Retinacular (Flexor Tendon Sheath) Ganglion

Clinical Characteristics. The third most common ganglion (10% to 12%) of the hand is the volar retinacular ganglion, which arises from the proximal annular ligament (A1 pulley) of the flexor tendon sheath. This ganglion is invariably a small (3 to 8 mm), firm, tender mass palpable under the MP flexion crease (Fig. 63-27). The cyst is attached to the tendon sheath and does not move with the tendon. Needle rupture,[69] followed by a steroid injection and digital massage to disperse the cyst contents, can often delay

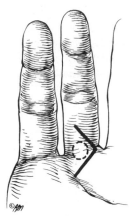

FIGURE 63-27. Volar retinacular ganglion palpable over the proximal tendon sheath and an incision for easy exposure.

or obviate the need for surgery. Several attempts at conservative treatment are recommended before surgery, with the patient's understanding that recurrences may happen. The proximity of the digital nerves must be appreciated.

Operative Technique. The ganglion is approached through an oblique incision over the mass (see Fig. 63-27). Transverse incisions are more popular but often do not allow adequate exposure without undue skin traction and are not easily incorporated into an extensile incision. The incision must also allow identification and mobilization of the radial and ulnar neurovascular bundles. The ganglion can then be traced to the tendon sheath and excised with a small portion of the sheath (Fig. 63-28).

The synovial side of the specimen usually reveals a defect in its smooth, white homogeneous surface suggestive of a communication between the tendon space and cyst.

After skin closure, a simple dressing is applied and early motion allowed.

Complications. Complications and recurrences are rare, although injuries to the digital nerves have been reported.

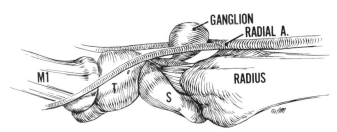

FIGURE 63-26. The usual relationship of the ganglion to the radial artery and volar joint capsule. S, scaphoid; T, trapezium; M1, first metacarpal.

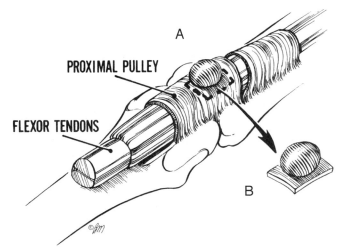

FIGURE 63-28. A, Volar retinacular ganglion in situ on the proximal annular ligament (A1 pulley) of the flexor tendon sheath. **B,** Excised specimen with a surrounding margin of tendon sheath.

Mucous Cyst

Clinical Characteristics. A mucous cyst is a ganglion of the DIP joint and usually occurs between the fifth and seventh decades.[13,19,113] The earliest clinical sign may be longitudinal grooving of the nail, without a visible mass, caused by pressure on the nail matrix (Fig. 63-29). Usually, however, the patient is seen after the cyst has enlarged and attenuated the overlying skin. The cyst (3 to 5 mm) usually lies to one side of the extensor tendon and between the dorsal distal joint crease and eponychium. The patient often has Heberden's nodes and radiographic evidence of osteoarthritic changes in the joint. The cyst and osteophytes should both be treated to ensure a satisfactory result.[154]

Operative Technique. The cyst has historically been approached through an "L"-shaped or curved incision (Fig. 63-30A), and any attenuated or involved skin that cannot be easily separated from the cyst wall is elliptically excised (see Fig. 63-30B). The cyst is mobilized, traced to the joint capsule, and excised with the joint capsule (Fig. 63-31A). From a practical point of view, however, all soft tissue between the retracted extensor tendon and adjacent collateral ligament is excised and the DIP joint left exposed (see Fig. 63-31B). Care is taken to not disturb the insertion of the extensor tendon or nail matrix. With the joint extended and the tendon dorsally retracted, the opposite side is explored and occult cysts or hypertrophied synovial tissue is excised.

Osteophytes can be excised with a rongeur or a fine power bur (Fig. 63-32). Skin closure may require rotation and advancement of the dorsal skin flap[294] or a full-thickness skin graft.

An alternative and my current preferred approach is to make a transverse incision centered over the DIP joint. The base of the mucous cyst is identified and excised while leaving the distal and superficial portion of the cyst intact. Osteophytes and joint capsule are excised and the skin closed. The remaining portion of the cyst will involute over the course of several weeks and skin complications seen with marginal excision are avoided. I have used this technique since its report by Gingrass and colleagues and have not needed to perform any skin coverage.[210] Patients must be educated preoperatively to expect slow resolution of the cyst. My personal experience has confirmed that published in the report.

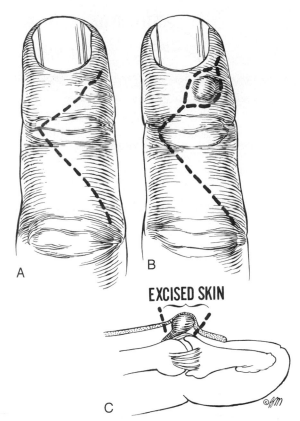

FIGURE 63-30. **A,** The cyst without skin involvement and the overlying incision. **B,** Schematic representation of the extent of the elliptical incision when the skin is attenuated. A skin graft or local rotation flap is usually necessary to close the defect.

Postoperative Care. If a skin graft was used, the distal joint is supported with a cast or splint for 2 weeks. Earlier motion is permitted if a local rotation flap was used. Motion and therapy can then be undertaken until full painless motion has been achieved.

Complications. Recurrences may be due to inadequate excision of the capsular attachments of the ganglion and failure to recognize extensions of the ganglion under the

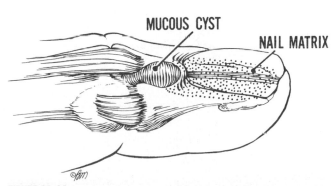

FIGURE 63-29. An early mucous cyst resting on the nail matrix may cause longitudinal grooving of the nail in some cases.

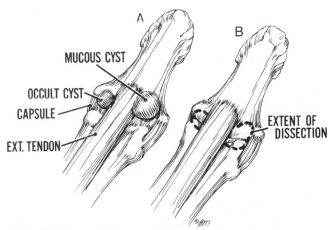

FIGURE 63-31. **A,** The ganglion in situ with its connection to the dorsal joint capsule. A second occult cyst is also illustrated. **B,** The exposed DIP joint after excision.

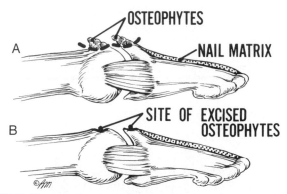

FIGURE 63-32. **A,** The usual osteophytes seen with mucous cysts. **B,** The extent of dissection while avoiding injury to the nail matrix, insertion of the extensor tendon, and articular surface.

extensor tendon to the opposite side. The underlying arthritic process persists and may result in new ganglion formation. Relief of pressure on the nail matrix by ganglion decompression or excision usually restores the nail to its normal appearance. Stiffness is rarely a functional problem.

Other Ganglions of the Hand

Dorsal, volar retinacular, and DIP ganglions constitute over 90% of the ganglions of the hand. Ganglions do occur at other locations, however, and must be approached with the same care and thoroughness.

Carpometacarpal Boss

Clinical Characteristics. Dorsal wrist ganglions may be confused with carpal bosses.[125] A carpal boss is an osteoarthritic spur or prominence that develops at the base of the second and/or third carpometacarpal joints (Fig. 63-33). A firm, bony, nonmobile, tender mass is visible and palpable at the base of the carpometacarpal joints, especially when the wrist is flexed.

Radiologically, the mass is best visualized with the hand in 30 to 40 degrees of supination and 20 to 30 degrees of ulnar deviation ("carpal boss view").[209]

Bosses are more common in women, in the right hand, and between the third and fourth decades.[17] The mass may be asymptomatic, or the patient may complain of considerable pain and aching. A small ganglion is associated with a carpal boss in 30% of cases, thus adding to confusion of it with the more common dorsal wrist ganglion. As with

mucous cysts, successful treatment requires excision of the ganglion as well as the osteoarthritic spurring.

The dorsal osteophytes must be adequately excised so that only cartilage surfaces and not bone are abutting each other (see Fig. 63-35C). Osteoarthritic changes within the joint itself must be ruled out, because, if present, a fusion at the joint might be necessary. A discussion of this possibility must be reviewed with the patient preoperatively, especially when more severe symptoms exist. The potential for persistent symptoms must be emphasized.

Operative Technique. The mass is approached through a transverse or oblique incision over the bony prominence (Fig. 63-34). The extensor digitorum communis and extensor indicis proprius tendons are retracted ulnarward. A ganglion, if present, can be mobilized and excised with its capsular attachments. The osteophytes and carpometacarpal joints are approached through a separate longitudinal incision over each involved joint. Subperiosteal dissection exposes the involved joint with the adjacent osteophytes. The osteophytes are then excised with small osteotomes down to normal cartilage. The dissection may involve the second and third carpometacarpal joints individually or all four opposing surfaces together (Fig. 63-35). The surgical area is palpated through the skin to ensure excision of all palpable prominences.

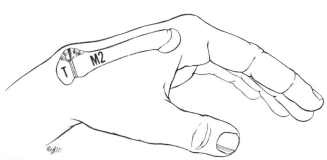

FIGURE 63-33. Carpal boss involving the second carpometacarpal joint. T, trapezoid.

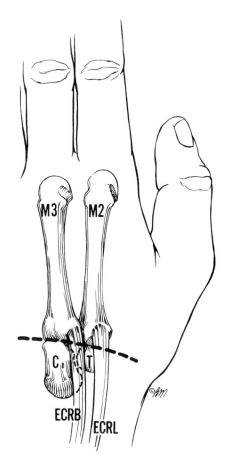

FIGURE 63-34. Incision for carpal boss excision, centered over the second and third carpometacarpal joints. C, capitate; T, trapezoid; ECRB, extensor carpi radialis brevis; ECRL, extensor carpi radialis longus.

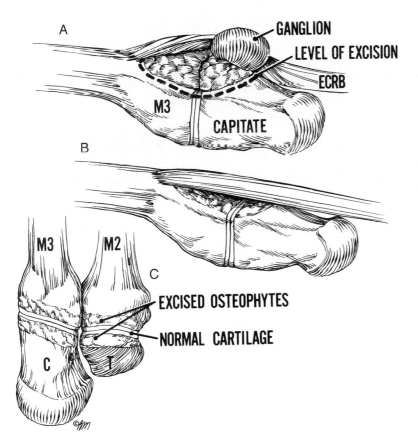

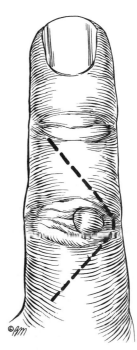

FIGURE 63-35. A, Typical carpal boss and associated ganglion. The extent of bony excision is illustrated. **B,** Excised osteophytes with periosteum and extensor carpi radialis tendon reapproximated. **C,** Exposure after excision of osteophytes involving both carpometacarpal joints (attached extensor carpi radialis longus and extensor carpi radialis brevis not illustrated). C, capitate; T, trapezoid; ECRB, extensor carpi radialis brevis.

The capsule, periosteum, and any adjacent overlying tendon fibers (extensor carpi radialis longus, extensor carpi radialis brevis) are reapproximated over the joint with a few fine inverting sutures, which should not be palpable through the skin.

Postoperative Care. A cast or splint is worn for 4 to 6 weeks to allow adequate ligamentous healing and pain relief.

Complications. The most common complication is the persistence of a mass because of excision of the ganglion alone or inadequate excision of the osteophytes. Pain may persist unless all abnormal abutting surfaces have been excised. Dorsal wrist ganglions can occur over the carpometacarpal joints and must be distinguished from carpal bosses with an associated ganglion. Avoidance of injury to branches of the radial and ulnar sensory nerves is again stressed.

Ganglions of the Proximal Interphalangeal Joint

Clinical Characteristics. Similar to a mucous cyst of the DIP joint, ganglions also occur dorsally over the PIP joint on either side of the extensor tendon. They arise from the joint capsule and usually pierce the oblique fibers between the central slip and lateral band. These cysts are small (3 to 5 mm) and tender and may interfere with joint motion.

Operative Technique. A curved incision over the PIP joint exposes the ganglion (Fig. 63-36). The lateral margin of the lateral band is released from the transverse retaining ligament and retracted dorsally to expose the PIP joint

FIGURE 63-36. Dorsal proximal interphalangeal ganglion with curved skin incision.

(Fig. 63-37). The pedicle from the main cyst can usually be followed through the extensor system into the joint capsule. A small, elliptical incision through the oblique extensor fibers mobilizes the cyst and pedicle. The entire joint capsule and synovial lining are excised between the collateral ligament and extensor insertion on the middle phalanx.

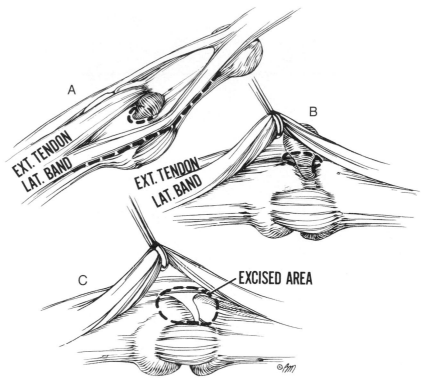

FIGURE 63-37. **A,** Proximal interphalangeal (PIP) ganglion in situ between the extensor tendon and lateral band. An incision along the lateral border of the lateral band and the base of the pedicle is illustrated with a dotted line. **B,** The lateral band has been released and elevated to expose the joint capsule and infratendinous portion of the cyst. **C,** Excision of the cyst and joint capsule reveal the exposed PIP joint.

Postoperative Care. A simple skin closure and dressing followed by early motion are all that is required.

Ganglions of Extensor Tendons

Clinical Characteristics. Ganglions do arise on or within extensor tendons.[579] They usually occur over the metacarpals and are distinguished by their proximal motion with the fingers in extension. They can, however, be confused with dorsal wrist ganglions, carpal bossing, or extensor tenosynovitis. The patient may complain of tenderness, aching, or snapping of the tendon with motion.

Operative Technique. The ganglion is approached through a transverse incision (Fig. 63-38), and the intimate broad attachment to the extensor tendon is readily appreciated. The ganglion is dissected off the extensor tendon with all the synovial tissue surrounding the involved tendon. Rupture of the ganglion is difficult to avoid, but recurrences are rare.

Miscellaneous Locations

Ganglions have been reported from numerous other locations of the hand and wrist and are often associated with other conditions, including the following sites.

First Extensor Compartment (Dorsal Retinacular) Ganglion. Ganglions attached to the first extensor compartment, similar to volar retinacular ganglions, are seen in patients with acute stenosing tenosynovitis (de Quervain's disease) (Fig. 67-39). Therefore, in addition to releasing the tendons (see Chapter 60), the involved tendon sheath and the ganglion can be excised. Injury to the radial sensory nerve should be avoided, and a separate compartment of the extensor pollicis brevis may be present and require release.

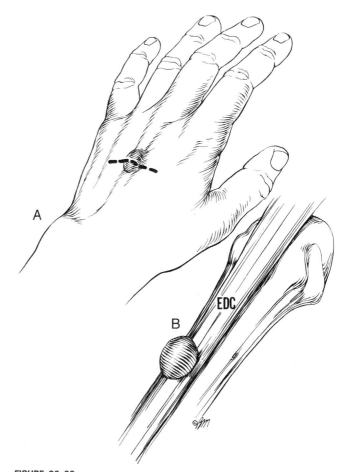

FIGURE 63-38. Extensor tendon ganglion. **A,** The ganglion, tendon, and overlying skin incision. **B,** The ganglion in situ on the extensor tendon. EDC, extensor digitorum communis.

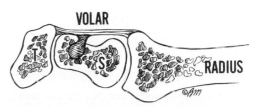

FIGURE 63-40. Intraosseous ganglion of the scaphoid with articular communication. The lesion was successfully treated with curettage and bone grafting. T, trapezoid; S, scaphoid.

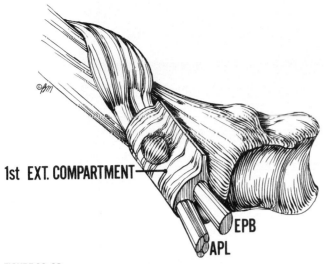

FIGURE 63-39. Dorsal retinacular ganglion. The first extensor compartment with attached ganglion. A separate compartment for the extensor pollicis brevis (EPB) is illustrated. APL, abductor pollicis longus.

Carpal Tunnel. Symptoms consistent with compression of the median nerve have been ascribed to ganglions arising from the volar carpus within the carpal canal.[230,290] A volar wrist ganglion can also extend distally and ulnarward to compress the median nerve. All carpal tunnel releases should be accompanied by exploration of the canal to rule out extrinsic masses, including ganglions.

Guyon's Canal/Distal Ulnar Nerve. Ganglions within the ulnar canal (loge de Guyon) can compress the ulnar nerve and cause motor and/or sensory loss.[68,229,337,485] These ganglions usually arise from joints around the hamate and dissect through the hypothenar muscles or along the motor branch. Ganglions in the palm may lead to isolated atrophy of the first dorsal interosseous muscle.[367] Early excision is imperative and avoids permanent injury to the ulnar nerve.

Intraosseous Ganglions

Although rare and usually an incidental radiographic finding, intraosseous ganglions are being increasingly recognized as a source of wrist pain.[58,117,178,237,286,428,493] Surgical treatment is best delayed, however, until all other possible causes of the patient's discomfort have been excluded. When indicated, curettage and bone grafting will adequately treat the condition. Careful exploration of the joint at the time of surgery helps rule out other undiagnosed causes of the patient's symptoms. Communication between the joint cavity and the intraosseous cyst has not been consistently demonstrated (Fig. 63-40). The histologic features of intraosseous ganglions are identical to those of their soft tissue counterparts.

Epidermal Inclusion Cysts

Epidermal inclusion cysts are thought to result from traumatic implantation of epithelial cells into the underlying soft tissue or bone.* The cells grow over an interval of months to years to produce a painless swelling, most commonly in the fingertip. Erythematous and painful lesions have been described.[523,540] These lesions most commonly

occur in the distal phalanx of the left long finger and thumb in men in the third and fourth decades of life.[239,480] Epidermal inclusion cysts may be seen after traumatic or surgical amputation of the fingertip.[480] Metacarpal involvement is rare, and there are no reported cases occurring in the carpus.[406]

Patients typically note a slowly growing mass involving a finger or thumb tip, although a history of trauma (penetrating injury) may not be recalled. When confined to the soft tissue, the cyst is usually well circumscribed, firm, and slightly movable. Differential diagnosis may be more difficult when the cyst involves bone, in which case radiographs generally show a well-demarcated lytic lesion (Fig. 63-41). Occasionally, cortical penetration can be seen, and the lesion may mimic a malignant or infectious process. More than one fourth of reported lesions have been treated with primary amputation, prior to pathologic diagnosis, out of concern of an aggressive neoplasm or advanced bone destruction.[239]

Patients presenting with a lytic lesion of the distal phalanx should undergo biopsy before consideration of an ablative procedure. Epidermal inclusion cysts are readily treated with marginal excision or with curettage and bone grafting for those lesions involving bone. In those rare cases with advanced bone destruction, amputation may be an alternative. Recurrence is uncommon, and malignant transformation has not been reported.

Foreign Body Lesions

Foreign body lesions are traumatic reactive masses rather than true neoplasms. These lesions are a response to implanted foreign material.† The tissue reaction to foreign material varies with the nature of the foreign substance deposited, the anatomic site involved, the duration of the implant, and the presence or absence of tissue hypersensitivity to the foreign material.[244] This response is the host's method of isolating recognized extraneous material. Glass, wood, and metal are the most common types of particulate matter associated with a foreign body reaction. These lesions are usually relatively superficial in location.

It is important to establish the etiology of these lesions, because the differential diagnosis includes malignant soft tissue neoplasms. A history of penetrating trauma or

---

*See references 48, 88, 126, 181, 228, 239, 310, 380, 406, 467, 480, 523, and 540.

†See references 14, 60, 144, 221, 244, 305, 312, 357, 363, 397, 450, 470, and 529.

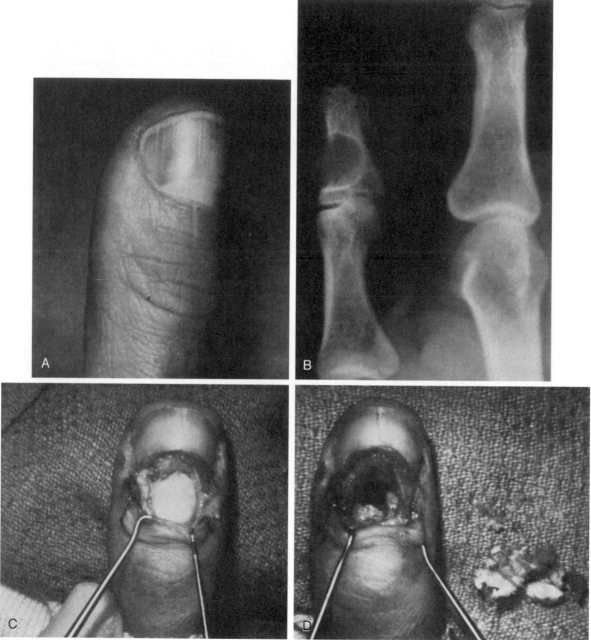

FIGURE 63-41. Epidermal inclusion cyst. A 53-year-old salesman reported that an enlarging deformity of the thumb (**A**) had progressed slowly for some time after a crush injury that occurred at least 18 months earlier. Radiographs showed a well-circumscribed distal phalangeal lesion with a reactive endosteal cortical rim (**B**), typical of bone reaction to a slowly growing soft tissue tumor (**C** and **D**). Marginal excision revealed an epidermal inclusion cyst that was successfully treated by removal and phalangeal curettage.

identification of the foreign body with radiographs or ultrasonography may provide this information.[14,305,470] It may be impossible to distinguish preoperatively between an inclusion cyst, a foreign body reaction, or a soft tissue neoplasm. Excisional biopsy of these relatively small lesions allows pathologic analysis and confirmation of diagnosis and results in a cure of the problem.

Lipomas

Lipomas are common benign fat tumors that occur typically in several locations in the hand,* most commonly subcu-

taneously or intramuscularly. Lipomas have been reported to arise in association with tendon sheaths, in the carpal tunnel, in Guyon's canal, and in the deep palmar space. They present as soft nontender masses that do not transilluminate. Symptoms of nerve compression may be noted if the tumor is in the deep palmar space or in proximity to a major nerve. These lesions are frequently present for several years and may grow slowly. When the lesion is subcutaneous, it is readily recognized by its well-demarcated appearance and

---

*See references 24, 50, 271, 298, 309, 369, 383, 411, 552, 557, and 580.

rubbery consistency. Plain radiographs may reveal a soft tissue shadow, and MRI may be particularly useful by demonstrating signal characteristics that are strongly suggestive of fat, which is often similar to surrounding subcutaneous fat.

Lipomas are usually well demarcated and are readily dissected from surrounding soft tissues, but occasionally the tumor may be immediately adjacent to nerves, making dissection difficult. When the patient's physical examination and radiographs are very strongly suggestive of lipoma, a small lesion may be treated with excisional biopsy. Deep lesions such as those occurring in the carpal tunnel should be studied preoperatively with MRI. If the signal characteristics are not strongly suggestive of lipoma, a small incisional biopsy should be done to establish the diagnosis and prevent operative contamination of the major nerves. Marginal excision of lipomas is generally curative, although recurrence may be seen.

Lipofibromatous Hamartomas

Lipofibromas or lipofibromatous hamartomas are unusual tumors of the peripheral nerves most commonly involving the median nerve when seen in the upper extremity.[195,252, 289,335,376,441,468,469,578] Rare instances of ulnar or radial nerve involvement have been reported.[260] Patients usually present with slowly progressive swelling in the distal forearm or palm, and symptoms of nerve compression may be present. The mass is most commonly noted in childhood or adolescence and is thought to be congenital or developmental in origin. Only rarely is the correct diagnosis made preoperatively. Surgical exploration reveals either diffuse fusiform swelling of the nerve without extension into perineural tissues or a more circumscribed area of involvement. The mass is intimately associated with the nerve fibers and is not readily dissected free. Attempts at partial excision or interfascicular dissection frequently result in permanent loss of motor or sensory nerve function.[252,425] For this reason, biopsy of a cutaneous branch of the nerve has been advocated simply to confirm the diagnosis.[425] Additional surgical treatment is directed only at decompressing the nerve. Spontaneous decrease in tumor size and improved nerve function have been reported after nerve decompression only. If the size of the lesion requires that it be excised, Houpt and associates have advocated complete excision and nerve grafting in children and immediate tendon transfers in adults.[252] Histologic examination of the lesion reveals nerve tissue with surrounding fat cells and a smaller component of fibrous tissue. Long-term follow-up of patients with these lesions has demonstrated slow but progressive loss of nerve function.[335]

Giant Cell Tumors of the Tendon Sheath (Pigmented Villonodular Tenosynovitis)

Giant cell tumor (GCT) of tendon sheath is a benign soft tissue tumor that is the second most common tumor seen in the hand (after ganglions).* Several terms have been used to

---

*See references 2, 7, 45, 214, 226, 247, 264, 267, 270, 275, 292, 362, 382, 404, 413, 445, 472, 475, 476, 484, 512, and 546.

CRITICAL POINTS: EXCISION OF GIANT CELL TUMOR OF TENDON SHEATH

INDICATIONS

- Same as for open incision biopsy
- Suspected giant cell tumor of tendon sheath

TECHNICAL POINTS

- Same as for biopsy.
- When diagnosis is confirmed by biopsy or visual inspection, perform marginal excision.
- Have low threshold for intra-articular exploration or exploration deep to volar plate.

POSTOPERATIVE CARE

- Advise patient of diagnosis and approximate 30% risk of local recurrence.
- Initiate range-of-motion exercises and remove sutures at 7 to 10 days.

---

describe this lesion, including *localized nodular synovitis, fibrous xanthoma,* and *pigmented villonodular tenosynovitis. Giant cell tumor* is not a particularly good term, because the lesion does not uniformly contain giant cells and is not necessarily associated with a tendon sheath. The tumor usually occurs on the volar surface of the fingers or hand, although dorsal involvement is not uncommon. There is a propensity for involvement of the radial three digits and the DIP joint region.[382,475,546] Clinically, the tumor is most often firm, nodular, and nontender. Because it grows slowly, it may be present for a long time before the patient is seen. A sensory deficit may be present when the lesion occurs in proximity to the digital nerves. The lesion does not transilluminate, which helps distinguish it from a ganglion.[475] Plain radiographs may demonstrate a soft tissue mass or pressure erosion of underlying bone.[275] Bone invasion, as may be seen with diffuse pigmented villonodular tenosynovitis, is not typical and suggests a more aggressive neoplasm. Actual bone invasion is rare but has been described.[544] Marginal excision is the recommended treatment, although the reported risk of recurrence is from 5% to 50%.[214,382] The high risk of recurrence is thought to be caused by the presence of satellite lesions or incomplete excision. Statistically significant risk factors for local recurrence include degenerative joint disease, location at the DIP joint, and the presence of radiographic pressure erosion.[440] If extensive joint involvement or degenerative changes are seen, arthrodesis may be necessary after excision. Malignant transformation of GCT of tendon sheath in the hand has not been reported, although a malignant form of GCT of tendon sheath has been well described.[45,270]

Schwannomas (Neurilemomas)

Neurilemoma, or schwannoma, is the most common benign nerve tumor occurring in the upper extremity.[133,145,249,421,]

[433,454,517,518] This lesion arises from the Schwann cell and produces a slowly growing, well-circumscribed, eccentric lesion in the peripheral nerve. Neurilemomas are most commonly seen on the flexor surface of the forearm or hand in the fourth, fifth, or sixth decades. Patients most frequently notice a painless mass, but less commonly there may be a neurologic deficit. Palpation or compression of the lesion may produce radiating pain in a specific nerve distribution. The lesion is often mobile in a transverse direction but not longitudinally. It is frequently misdiagnosed as a ganglion and may have a similar consistency.[249,433,454] MRI may be useful in delineating the lesion, but it may not be possible to distinguish neurilemoma from neurofibroma or malignant peripheral nerve sheath tumor (Fig. 63-42).[518]

Neurilemoma is readily distinguished from other nerve tumors at surgery because typically it is easily dissected free or "shelled out" from the surrounding nerve. Optical magnification and microsurgical technique have been advocated to reduce the risk of postoperative neurologic deficit. The risk of postoperative neurologic deficit in a recent large study was 4%, with a significantly greater risk of deficit for procedures done after incisional biopsy or recurrence.[145] In the overwhelming majority of cases, the lesion can be completely removed and neurologic symptoms, if present preoperatively, are improved. Recurrence is uncommon. Multiple lesions in a single peripheral nerve have been described.[421] There are rare reports of malignant transformation.[95,131]

Neurofibromas

Neurofibromas are benign nerve tumors that arise within nerve fasciculi and are typically more difficult to excise than neurilemomas.[145,249,505,517] Solitary lesions may be seen, but multiple neurofibromas are more common in the setting of neurofibromatosis (von Recklinghausen's disease). Symptoms and clinical findings may be similar to those seen with neurilemomas. At surgery, a more prominent nerve fascicle or group of fascicles may be seen entering and exiting the lesion if both proximal and distal dissection are done under magnification.[145] Excision of the lesion requires transection of the entering and exiting fascicles. Postoperative neurologic deficit is more common than it is after excision of neurilemomas. Progression of motor and sensory nerve deficits has been noted after surgical treatment of plexiform neurofibromas in patients with neurofibromatosis.[145] Surgical treatment of neurofibromas in patients with neurofibromatosis should be reserved for those lesions that are growing or producing progressive symptoms. There is a known risk of malignant degeneration of neurofibromas in patients with neurofibromatosis.[151,505]

Granular Cell Tumors (Granular Cell Myoblastomas)

Granular cell tumor is a neoplasm rarely seen in the forearm and hand.[41,169,182,342,400,548] This lesion appears to arise from neural elements rather than from myoblasts, as originally believed, and it has been noted to occur in close association with nerves (Fig. 63-43).[182,548] Patients usually note a painless mass. Multicentricity has been reported in 10% to 15% of cases.[169] Excision of the tumor has been curative,

although there has been no critical analysis of the need for wide margins at excision.[161] A malignant variant of granular cell tumor has been reported that is rare and difficult to distinguish from the benign lesion.[169] Malignant lesions are highly aggressive and require wide excision and consideration of systemic treatment.

Fibromatoses

Digital Fibroma of Infancy

Digital fibroma of infancy is a benign but very aggressive fibrous lesion seen virtually exclusively in the fingers or toes (Fig. 63-44), with over 80% of cases arising before the age of 1 year.[30,31,47,176,259,281,384,442,535] Digital fibroma of infancy usually occurs in the region of the interphalangeal joints of the fingers. The lesions are usually small, dome shaped, skin colored, and painless. The true natural history of this condition is not known. Observation has generally documented progression with interphalangeal contracture, angular deviation, and bone deformity in severely affected children.[47,176] There are reports of spontaneous resolution of the skin lesions, with some patients having residual deformity.[31,47] Microscopic evaluation has demonstrated intracytoplasmic inclusion bodies, which has resulted in speculation of a viral or myofibroblast etiology for the lesions.

Treatment has included observation, marginal excision, wide excision with coverage, and amputation. No documented cases of metastasis have been reported, but the risk of local recurrence after excision is approximately 60%. Although no firm treatment guidelines exist, it seems prudent to observe these lesions until spontaneous resolution occurs or until early signs of deformity or contracture are seen. Wide excision and skin grafting appear to give the best local control and functional results, but there is a significant risk of local recurrence and even subsequent involvement of adjacent digits.[176]

Juvenile Aponeurotic Fibroma

Fibrous lesions in the hand are commonly seen in childhood and adolescence and are often difficult to classify and treat.[30,513,535] Juvenile aponeurotic fibroma, or calcifying aponeurotic fibroma, is a benign, aggressive fibrous lesion seen in childhood or adolescence that most commonly affects the palm.* This lesion presents as a small painless mass, often intimately associated with tendons or neurovascular structures. The histologic appearance may be difficult to distinguish from fibrosarcoma.

Wide excision allowing for sparing of functional or vital structures is the recommended treatment, but the recurrence rate has been reported to be more than 50%.[91] On rare occasions, amputation has been necessary to control disease.[360] There is one reported case of metastasis after recurrence of juvenile aponeurotic fibroma in the hand, although the metastasis was classified as fibrosarcoma.[302] Local and systemic surveillance should be considered for patients with this lesion. Recurrent lesions may be observed if they do not produce functional impairment and the diagnosis is not in question.[91]

---

*See references 5, 30, 91, 159, 282, 284, 302, 360, 373, 535, and 551.

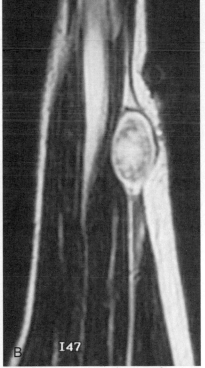

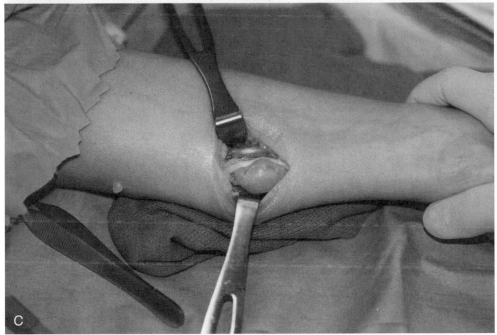

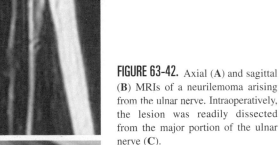

FIGURE 63-42. Axial (**A**) and sagittal (**B**) MRIs of a neurilemoma arising from the ulnar nerve. Intraoperatively, the lesion was readily dissected from the major portion of the ulnar nerve (**C**).

Nodular Fasciitis

Pseudosarcomatous fasciitis, subcutaneous pseudosarcomatous fibromatosis, and *infiltrative fasciitis* are terms that have been used to describe the entity currently called nodular fasciitis. Nodular fasciitis is an uncommon but well-described reactive lesion that is poorly understood and may simulate a sarcoma.[35,67,123,444,514] This lesion most commonly occurs on the volar surface of the forearm and rarely may occur in the hand.[280] Patients most commonly note a rapidly growing small nodule that has been present for a very short time, frequently less than 1 month.[67] There may be a history of local trauma and tenderness on palpation. The histologic appearance has been confused with fibrosarcoma and myxoid liposarcoma, which has led to overtreatment.[514] This diagnosis is rarely anticipated preoperatively. The natural history of nodular fasciitis appears to be self-limited. Recurrence after marginal excision should raise the question of an alternative diagnosis, because even incompletely excised lesions are noted not to recur.[35] The most important issue in treating patients with nodular fasciitis is to

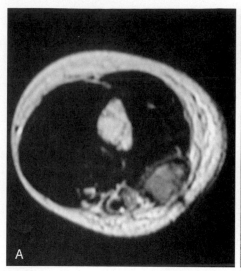
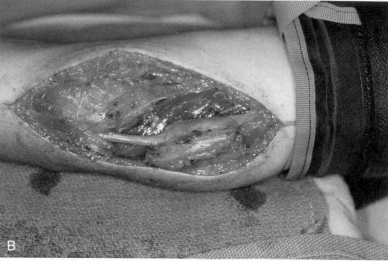

FIGURE 63-43. Axial MRI (**A**) demonstrating a lobulated granular cell tumor arising from the ulnar nerve. At operation (**B**), the tumor was inseparable from the ulnar nerve just proximal to the medial epicondyle.

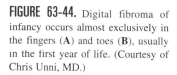

FIGURE 63-44. Digital fibroma of infancy occurs almost exclusively in the fingers (**A**) and toes (**B**), usually in the first year of life. (Courtesy of Chris Unni, MD.)

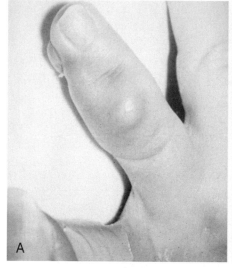
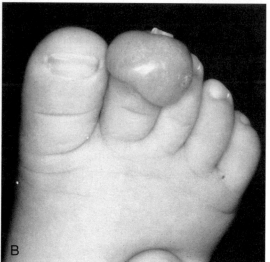

differentiate this lesion from a soft tissue sarcoma and avoid unnecessary aggressive surgical treatment.

MALIGNANT SOFT TISSUE LESIONS

Soft Tissue Sarcomas

Soft tissue sarcomas are relatively rare in the hand and forearm.[66,528] Approximately 6000 new cases of soft tissue sarcoma are diagnosed each year in the United States, and only 15% of these are in the upper extremity.[313] *The majority of these lesions share a common mesodermal origin.* The exception is malignant peripheral nerve sheath tumor, which arises from neuroectoderm. In the majority of patients, no predisposing risk factor can be identified. Certain environmental and genetic risk factors have been implicated as potential causes of soft tissue sarcoma. Patients exposed to radiation[59] and forestry workers exposed to herbicides may have a higher incidence of soft tissue sarcoma.[227] Genetic factors have been implicated in neurofibromatosis and the Li-Fraumeni syndrome.[318,506]

In previous editions of this chapter, individual types of soft tissue tumors were described, based on their presumed cell of origin. It is important to realize that specific cell origin or tumor differentiation of soft tissue sarcoma has limited value in predicting the behavior of the tumor. Biologic behavior of soft tissue sarcomas may be more accurately predicted by the histologic grade of the lesion, which takes into account cell mitotic index, cellularity, tumor necrosis, and anaplasia.[224] The most common histologic subtypes of soft tissue sarcoma seen in the hand are epithelioid sarcoma, synovial sarcoma, and malignant fibrous histiocytoma.[66] Histologic diagnosis may be useful in assessing propensity for regional lymphatic spread.[187,438,510]

Clinical Picture

The clinical presentation of the various types of soft tissue sarcomas in the upper extremity and hand may be similar. Most frequently, patients note a painless mass that may have been present for a long time with recent growth.[66,534] Less commonly, a painful mass may be noted. Epithelioid sarcoma is notable for presentation as an ulcerating nodule that may be mistakenly treated for infection.[510] Soft tissue sarcomas in the hand are frequently misdiagnosed as infection, ganglion, and lipoma. This may lead to inappropriate treatment or delay in treatment.

Physical examination of a patient with a suspicious lesion includes careful assessment of size, location, depth, mobility, and relation to major nerves, vessels, tendon, and bone.

Regional lymph nodes are assessed. Plain radiographs are obtained and may demonstrate soft tissue calcification, fat density, or unexpected bone involvement, which may assist in making a diagnosis (Fig. 63-45). MRI has become increasingly valuable in defining the pathologic anatomy, determining the local extent of disease, and aiding preoperative planning.[137]

Biopsy

Soft tissue masses that are symptomatic, enlarging, or not readily diagnosed by physical examination should be considered for biopsy. Very small lesions that can be excised with a surrounding cuff of normal tissue can be treated with excisional biopsy before a known diagnosis. Large lesions

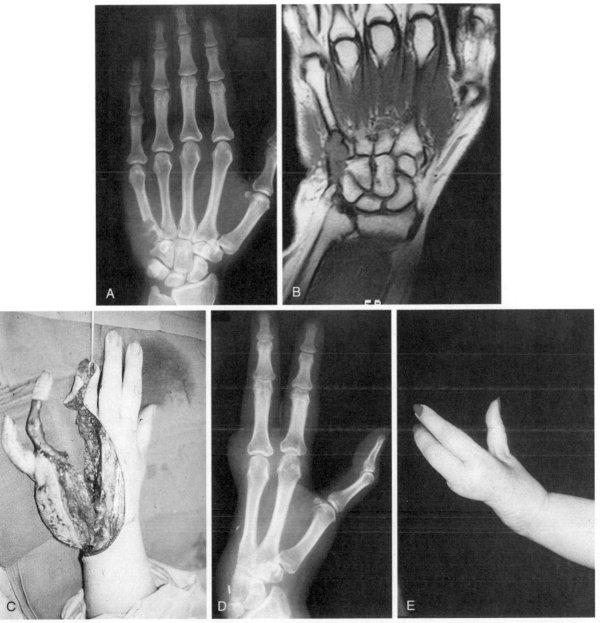

FIGURE 63-45. A 40-year-old woman was diagnosed clinically as having a ganglion and underwent operative exploration. Histologic examination revealed a high-grade pleomorphic soft tissue sarcoma. Postoperative plain radiographs demonstrated extensive fifth metacarpal involvement (**A**). Bone destruction and soft tissue extension were confirmed on coronal MRI (**B**). Re-excision was complicated by positive soft tissue margins. Extended double ray resection (hemiresection of the carpus) (**C-E**) with long finger fillet flap was required to achieve a wide margin.

or those lesions in proximity to major nerves, vessels, or tendons are best treated with incisional biopsy. The decision of how to perform the biopsy is particularly important in the hand, owing to the compact nature of important soft tissues in the wrist and hand. Incisional biopsies or those biopsies in which the tumor is inadvertently violated result in contamination of all tissues included in the exposure. Poorly planned biopsies may compromise the ability to perform limb-sparing surgery. It is best to plan the biopsy to be in line with, or incorporated into, the definitive limb salvage or amputation procedure that may be required in the event of a high-grade malignant diagnosis. Transverse, oblique, and zigzag (Bruner) incisions should specifically be avoided.

Staging

After the diagnosis of a soft tissue sarcoma, systemic staging should be done with CT of the chest and axilla. Soft tissue sarcomas of the upper extremity most commonly metastasize to the lungs or regional lymph nodes.[187,202] Lymph node metastasis occurs in less than 5% of soft tissue sarcomas of the extremities.[187] Epithelioid sarcoma is a notable exception, with a risk of regional lymph node metastasis as high as 42%.[53,70,427,438,510] Soft tissue sarcomas are generally staged based on grade, size, and the presence of metastasis.[158,377] Prognostic factors that have been incorporated into the staging system used at Memorial Sloan-Kettering Cancer Center and by the AJCC include grade, size, depth, and presence of metastasis.[207] Histologic grade is particularly important in predicting the biologic behavior of the lesion and the risk of metastasis.[313] The tumor should also be staged using the Musculoskeletal Tumor Society staging system.[165]

Operative Treatment

Surgery is the primary form of local treatment for patients with soft tissue sarcoma. Treatment of either bone or soft tissue sarcoma requires the surgeon to think and plan for two parts of the operation: resection and reconstruction. At times, a two-team approach may be best. Resection of the lesion is of primary importance. Concerns regarding reconstruction must be given secondary consideration within the context of the particular patient or aggressiveness of the lesion. Compromise of resection margins out of concern for reconstruction will increase the risk of local recurrence and may increase the risk of metastasis and death.[66,321,370,534] Positive margins in the treatment of soft tissue sarcomas in the hand are not readily salvaged or compensated for by the use of external-beam radiation and have been found to be predictive of recurrence.[66,534] *The goal of surgery is complete removal of the tumor through a surrounding cuff of normal tissue.* Wide excision with 2 to 3 cm of normal tissue surrounding the tumor has been advocated.[313,510] Deliberate sacrifice of major neurovascular structures can often be avoided, provided there is meticulous attention to dissection, a margin of normal tissue can be obtained, and neurovascular structures are not surrounded by tumor.[313,465,565] If negative margins cannot be achieved with wide excision, amputation should be very strongly considered.

After wide excision of a large (greater than 5 cm) high-grade lesion, patients require either brachytherapy* or external-beam irradiation in an effort to reduce the risk of local recurrence.[62,63,66,519,528,534] Excision of large low-grade

lesions should be followed with external-beam irradiation. Small (less than 5 cm) high- or low-grade extremity lesions that can be widely excised may not require adjuvant radiation, although this question has not been conclusively answered in the hand.[6,66,313,534] Digit, single-ray, or multiple-ray amputation may often be the best solution for patients with soft tissue sarcoma involving the fingers, thumb, or palm. Wide margins are not readily obtained in the digit or thumb, and the functional result of amputation may be superior to that of digit salvage and reconstruction. Large lesions or those lesions involving the contents of the carpal tunnel may not be amenable to a hand-sparing operation and are often best treated with below-elbow amputation.

The role of chemotherapy in the treatment of soft tissue sarcomas in the extremities is still under investigation.[134,160,432] Chemotherapy may have a small but real overall survival benefit and may increase the disease-free interval in well-selected patients with extremity lesions.[199]

Certain patients with large high-grade lesions may benefit from preoperative chemotherapy in an effort to reduce the size of a lesion to make an unresectable lesion resectable. Patients with large high-grade lesions may be at high risk for metastasis and should be considered for investigational protocols in conjunction with a medical oncologist. Patients presenting with metastasis may also be candidates for chemotherapy and resection of lung nodules.[202]

Patients referred after a primary excision with positive margins should be strongly considered for re-excision or amputation, because the risk for local recurrence in this situation is high.[66,314,534] Patients presenting with metastasis should be treated aggressively locally in the extremity and in the chest, as well as systemically, because survival is possible.[202]

Epithelioid Sarcoma

Epithelioid sarcoma has been reported to be the most common soft tissue sarcoma occurring in the forearm and hand.[†] This tumor is notorious for its innocuous appearance, frequent misdiagnosis, propensity for local recurrence, and regional lymph node metastasis. Epithelioid sarcoma commonly presents as a painless nodule on the volar surface of the digits or palm, which may ulcerate. Misdiagnosis has included infection, Dupuytren's nodules, and other types of sarcoma. The extent of local disease is often not evident by clinical or radiographic examination. This tumor is characterized by a tendency to spread proximally along the course of tendons, lymphatics, and fascial planes without respecting fascial boundaries.[427] A high risk of lymph node involvement has been reported, with several authors recommending lymph node dissection.[427,438,510]

---

*Brachytherapy refers to the use of radioactive implants to deliver radiation over short periods of time. Small flexible catheters are implanted at the time of operation, and, beginning about 5 days after surgery, radioactive implants are loaded into the catheters. These are left in place for 3 to 4 days, during which time high doses of radiation can be given directly to the tissue at risk, with predictable minimal scatter. Another advantage is that this method dramatically shortens the duration of radiation treatment compared with external-beam (5 weeks) therapy. Brachytherapy is more effective for high-grade tumors than for low-grade tumors and should not be considered for the latter.

†See references 53, 70, 74, 167, 170, 427, 438, 486, 491, and 510.

CRITICAL POINTS: TREATMENT OF SOFT TISSUE SARCOMAS OF THE FOREARM AND HAND

INDICATIONS

- Attempted curative treatment of patient with soft tissue sarcoma
- Patient able to tolerate limb salvage and reconstruction

PREOPERATIVE EVALUATION

- Have pathologic diagnosis confirmed by experienced pathologist before surgery.
- Complete staging workup and appropriate consultation before surgery.
- Make preoperative plan detailing positioning, resection steps, and reconstruction options.

TECHNICAL POINTS

- Mark limb salvage incision incorporating prior biopsy tract and any previously contaminated tissue.
- Prioritize tourniquet time to critical portions of the case—usually dissection of neurovascular structures.
- Create flaps while leaving biopsy tract en bloc with the major tumor mass.
- Dissect or sacrifice major nerves and vessels first.
- Leave cuff of normal, uninvolved, nonreactive tissue covering major tumor mass.
- Use nondominant hand to palpate tumor mass and ensure dissection at least one fingerbreadth from tumor when possible.
- Avoid any contamination from tumor.
- Take advantage of fascial or compartment boundaries by dissecting on opposite side of fascia from tumor.
- Sacrifice functional tissues, nerves, tendons, vessels, and bone as needed to achieve negative margins.
- Confirm negative margins of resection with frozen section assessment.
- Consider separate reconstruction team, especially with free tissue transfer.
- Use separate isolated fields and clean instruments and clothing for remote tissue harvest for reconstruction.
- Achieve excellent hemostasis before closure.

POSTOPERATIVE CARE

- Confirm pathologic diagnosis on permanent analysis.

Epithelioid sarcoma must be treated aggressively with a true wide excision, radical resection, or amputation. Epitrochlear and axillary lymph node sampling should be strongly considered, even in the absence of clinically or radiographically detectable disease, because excision of involved nodes has the potential to be lifesaving. The role for sentinel lymph node biopsy, as opposed to prophylactic lymphadenectomy, is under investigation. Forequarter amputation has resulted in cure of patients with proximally recurrent disease or axillary lymph node involvement.[66] Marginal excision, even when combined with external-beam irradiation, has resulted in unacceptably high rates of local recurrence and regional spread and is not a reasonable option in the treatment of epithelioid sarcoma.[510] External-beam irradiation or brachytherapy should be done after wide excision of larger lesions. Chemotherapy should be considered for those patients with lymph node involvement, metastasis, or recurrence.

Synovial Sarcoma

Synovial sarcoma is a high-grade malignant soft tissue sarcoma that commonly arises in proximity to joints, tendons, or bursae.* Although epithelioid sarcoma is generally thought to be the most common soft tissue sarcoma arising in the forearm and hand, synovial sarcoma has been the most common soft tissue sarcoma seen in the hand at Memorial Sloan-Kettering Cancer Center since 1982.[66,534] This tumor most commonly occurs in the region of the carpus and is rarely seen in the fingers. A painless mass over the dorsum of the hand or in the palm, often present for many years, is the most frequent presentation and can lead to the false impression that the lesion is benign. Rare intraneural lesions may be heralded by intense radiating pain not usually seen with schwannoma or neurofibroma. Synovial sarcoma may grow very slowly initially, and the patient may give a history of no apparent growth. Any soft tissue mass that is unexplained and not readily diagnosed based on physical examination or imaging should be sampled to establish an accurate diagnosis.

Soft tissue calcifications may be seen in 20% to 30% of cases on plain radiographs.[139,386] This lesion metastasizes to regional lymph nodes in as many as 25% of patients who develop metastasis.[386] Although the size of synovial sarcoma has been thought to be an important prognostic factor in general case series,[407] small size may not necessarily be associated with a better prognosis for those lesions arising in the hand.[66,139] Recent investigational studies suggest a benefit from the use of intensive or high-dose chemotherapy, particularly in those patients with resectable metastatic disease.[272,461] This tumor is treated as previously discussed for soft tissue sarcomas.

Liposarcoma

Liposarcoma is one of the most common types of soft tissue sarcoma, but it is only rarely seen in the hand.[66,528,534] Histologic subtypes of liposarcoma include well-differentiated, myxoid, round cell, dedifferentiated, and pleomorphic liposarcomas. The differentiation of liposarcoma into its

---

*See references 78, 139, 148, 217, 272, 334, 336, 386, 407, 455, 461, 562, and 573.

various subtypes is useful, because histologic appearance and tumor grade correlate with clinical behavior, risk of metastasis, and prognosis.[169] Clinically, these lesions may resemble lipomas, but more often they are painful and grow more rapidly. The image on MRI may also be similar to that of lipoma (Fig. 63-46). Any lesion diagnosed preoperatively as lipoma based on history, examination, and radiographic studies should be approached as if it were potentially malignant. Any biopsy or excision should not compromise a subsequent limb salvage operation or amputation. Frozen section diagnosis of fat-containing tumors is difficult, and suspicious lesions are best treated after a malignant diagnosis can be confirmed on permanent sections.

Appropriate treatment for liposarcoma is wide excision and adjuvant radiation for large lesions. Amputation may be necessary if wide margins cannot be achieved, particularly for high-grade lesions. Chemotherapy may be considered for very large high-grade lesions or for those patients presenting with or developing metastasis.

Fibrosarcoma

Approximately 30% of soft tissue fibrosarcomas occur in the upper extremity, although hand involvement is extremely rare.[192,302,358,429,439] There may be considerable difficulty in making the diagnosis of fibrosarcoma, particularly in children younger than the age of 5 years, in whom the aggressive histologic appearance of benign fibrous lesions is similar to that of fibrosarcoma. The clinical course of these lesions is different from that of fibrosarcoma, in that they are not known to metastasize.[439] Treatment of high-grade lesions in adults includes systemic staging, wide excision, and

consideration of irradiation and chemotherapy, as previously outlined for soft tissue sarcomas.

Dermatofibrosarcoma Protuberans

Dermatofibrosarcoma protuberans (DFSP) is an uncommon low-grade malignant soft tissue tumor that may be encountered in the forearm and rarely in the hand (Fig. 63-47).[109,158,296,419,443,473,482,522,567] This lesion arises in the dermis and most often presents as a painless violet-red plaque or nodule that may be present for several years. Long-standing lesions may ulcerate or extend deep to the subcutaneous tissues to involve muscle, tendon, and fascia. DFSP has a striking propensity for horizontal spread in the dermis and subcutaneous tissues, and there is a notoriously high risk of local recurrence after even wide excision.

Patients with DFSP must have their disease carefully staged locally before planned excision. MRI is extremely useful in assessing the local extent of disease (see Fig. 63-47). Several reports have suggested a 3-cm margin of resection and inclusion of the deep fascia to minimize the risk of local recurrence.[296,419,473] Retrospective microscopic analysis of resection margins has shown that 75% of lesions can be effectively excised with a 1-cm margin, 80% with a 1.5-cm margin, 85% with a 2-cm margin, and 100% with a 2.5-cm margin.[419] Historically, the risk of local recurrence with DFSP has been 50%. If appropriate wide excision is performed for either primary or recurrent lesions, the risk of local recurrence is reduced to approximately 12%.[473] The risk of metastasis for this low-grade lesion is less than 5%.[473] External-beam irradiation has been of benefit in improving local control in those patients with positive margins,

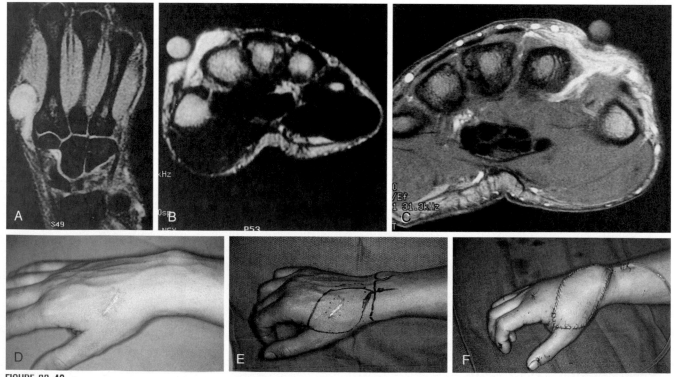

FIGURE 63-46. Preoperative MRI demonstrating a soft tissue mass with signal characteristics similar to subcutaneous fat: coronal (**A**), axial (**B**). After marginal excision for a presumed benign lesion, it is not possible to differentiate residual myxoid liposarcoma, postoperative change, and normal fat on an axial MRI image (**C**). The initial marginal excision biopsy was done through an oblique incision (**D**). Margins were positive. Wide excision (**E**) was done, using a lateral arm free flap for closure (**F**). Re-excision that included a portion of the index metacarpal achieved negative margins.

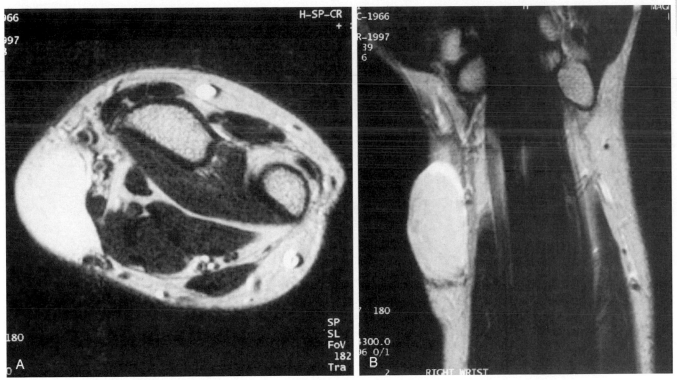

FIGURE 63-47. Axial (**A**) and coronal (**B**) MRI of dermatofibrosarcoma protuberans abutting the radial artery.

although re-excision is generally recommended for patients with positive margins.[522] Soft tissue coverage is frequently required after the generous excision of skin necessary to achieve appropriate margins. Recent reports of Mohs' micrographic surgery have noted excellent short-term local control, although further follow-up is necessary to document the effectiveness of this approach, which is typically intralesional surgery and not commonly used in the treatment of soft tissue sarcoma.[419,443]

Malignant Fibrous Histiocytoma

There are very few reports of malignant fibrous histiocytoma (MFH) occurring in the hand, although 19% of lesions arise in the upper extremity, many of which are in the forearm.* MFH may arise in the soft tissues or as a primary bone tumor. Bone lesions are lytic on plain radiographs and may arise from a preexisting lesion such as Paget's disease or a bone infarct. Multifocal soft tissue lesions in the hand have been reported.[225] These lesions are best treated with wide excision or amputation (Fig. 63-48). Adjuvant radiation is necessary to maximize local control after wide excision of large lesions. There may be a role for chemotherapy in treating very large soft tissue lesions and those lesions arising in bone.[25,543,560]

Malignant Peripheral Nerve Sheath Tumor (Neurofibrosarcoma/Malignant Schwannoma)

Malignant peripheral nerve sheath tumor (MPNST) is the accepted term for malignant soft tissue tumors of neural origin, including neurofibrosarcoma, neurosarcoma, and malignant schwannoma.[†] Approximately 30% of MPNSTs occur in the upper extremity, with 50% of cases arising in the setting of neurofibromatosis (von Recklinghausen's disease). This lesion may be seen as a secondary sarcoma following primary radiation for a different sarcoma or lymphoma.[59,186] MPNST is known for its propensity to grow along peripheral nerves and has an exceptionally high rate of local recurrence, even after amputation. This tumor does not appear to be radiosensitive, nor has chemotherapy been shown to be of benefit.[132,151,553] Wide excision or amputation has been the recommended treatment. Forequarter amputation may be necessary to obtain local control for brachial plexus lesions. Poor prognostic factors include proximal location of the primary lesion, tumor size, and neurofibromatosis. The 5-year survival for patients with MPNST is approximately 40%, with the poorest prognosis in those patients with neurofibromatosis.[151,186,553]

Rhabdomyosarcoma

Rhabdomyosarcoma is a malignant round cell tumor most frequently seen in childhood, but it is uncommon in the hand.[‡] Extremity rhabdomyosarcoma has been associated with a poor prognosis, although upper extremity lesions and distal lesions fare better than lower extremity or more proximal lesions. Alveolar rhabdomyosarcoma is the most common histologic variant seen in the hand and in the past has been thought to confer a poorer prognosis. More intensive chemotherapy regimens appear to have improved the prognosis for patients with this histologic subtype of rhabdomyosarcoma.[120,121]

---

*See references 71, 138, 143, 169, 200, 225, 256, 276, 285, 368, 388, 403, 412, 422, 506, 530, 564, and 568.

†See references 95, 107, 127, 128, 132, 151, 186, 255, 460, and 558.

‡See references 4, 108, 120, 121, 233, 234, 326, 330, 345, 364, 366, 389, 437, 459, 463, and 483.

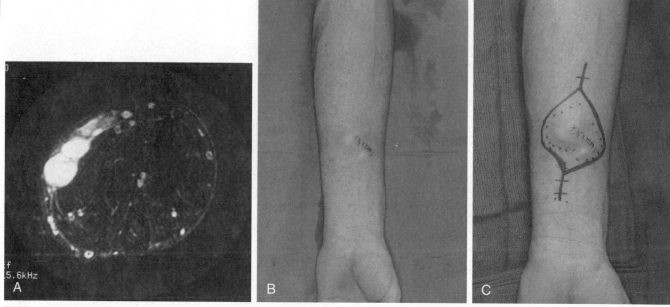

FIGURE 63-48. An MRI of malignant fibrous histiocytoma of the forearm (**A**). An oblique incision was used for incisional biopsy (**B**). (A straight longitudinal incision would have been better, because it is more easily incorporated into a limb-sparing incision at the time of definitive resection.) The planned wide excision included generous skin margins (**C**).

Patient survival in the past 25 years has dramatically improved with the use of effective multiagent chemotherapy and radiation. The extent of disease at presentation and the surgeon's ability to completely remove the lesion with negative margins affect prognosis.[120,121,133,234,364] Limb-sparing surgery through a wide margin has been recommended for obtaining local control in the setting of multiagent chemotherapy. Marginal surgery or gross total excision has been advocated rather than amputation, owing to the ability to improve local control with radiation in those patients who do not have wide margins. Extremity rhabdomyosarcoma appears to have a high risk of regional lymph node metastasis, and pathologic evaluation of lymph nodes has been advocated to improve staging and to direct systemic treatment.[187,345]

Leiomyosarcoma

Leiomyosarcoma is most commonly seen in the viscera and only rarely in the hand.[64,66,76,135,291,311,395,396,434] This lesion appears to arise in areas of smooth muscle and has been seen in the veins in the hand. There is a single case of an apparent benign angiomyoma in the hand recurring as leiomyosarcoma.[396] Some reports have noted a particularly high rate of local recurrence when surgery is not followed with radiation in extremity lesions.[395,434] Leiomyosarcoma is best treated with wide excision and consideration of adjuvant treatment, as previously outlined for the treatment of soft tissue sarcomas in general.

Clear Cell Sarcoma

Clear cell sarcoma, or malignant melanoma of soft parts, is an uncommon soft tissue sarcoma with a propensity to occur in close association with tendons and aponeuroses.* Clear cell sarcoma has been confused with metastatic acral lentiginous melanoma.[555] This lesion has been noted to have both a high risk of local recurrence and a potential for regional

lymph node metastasis as high as 53%.[101] Regional lymph nodes should be carefully assessed both clinically and radiographically during staging. Strong consideration should be given to regional lymph node biopsy in patients with clear cell sarcoma. These lesions are best treated as previously outlined for soft tissue sarcomas.

BENIGN BONE TUMORS

Enchondroma

Enchondromas are benign cartilaginous lesions that are the most common primary bone tumors arising from the bones in the hand.[†] Approximately 35% of all enchondromas arise in the hand, and enchondromas account for as many as 90% of bone tumors seen in the hand.[28,257] Monostotic lesions most commonly occur in the fourth decade, with the majority of lesions occurring between the ages of 10 and 40.[257,527] The proximal phalanx is the most common site of involvement, followed by the metacarpal and middle phalanx. The carpus is rarely involved, although enchondromas have been reported in the scaphoid, lunate, and capitate.[361,399,526]

Patients with monostotic lesions present most commonly with either localized swelling, which may be painless, or after pathologic fracture associated with minor trauma. Enchondroma may also be diagnosed as an incidental finding on plain radiographs. Radiographs typically demonstrate a well-defined lytic lesion, which may be lobulated (Fig. 63-49). Matrix calcification may be seen. Soft tissue extension is not typical and is suggestive of a more aggressive neoplasm.

---

*See references 8, 17, 66, 101, 153, 166, 248, 463, 541, and 555.

†See references 28, 124, 177, 197, 231, 257, 265, 273, 300, 329, 361, 377, 393, 399, 526, 527, 537, 545, and 550.

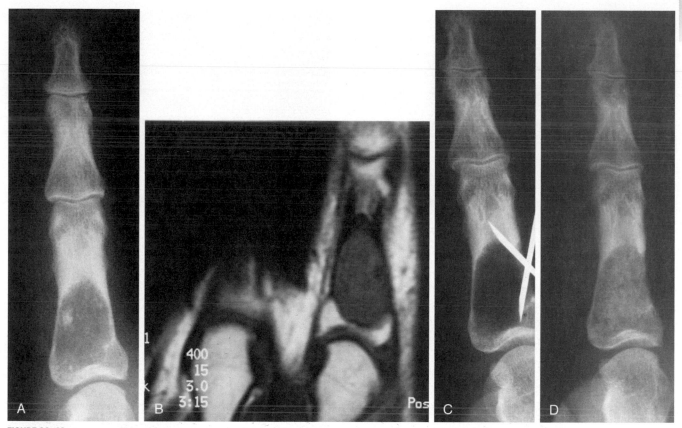

FIGURE 63-49. Enchondroma. A well-demarcated lytic lesion with stippled calcification was seen on radiographs of the proximal phalanx of the index finger (**A**). MRI confirms the intraosseous nature of the lesion (**B**). An open biopsy from ulnar lateral approach confirmed the clinical impression of enchondroma. Intraoperative radiographs after curettage documented complete removal of the lesion (**C**) and complete filling of the cavity with bone graft (**D**).

The diagnosis of enchondroma in the overwhelming majority of cases can be made with plain radiographs without the need for axial images obtained with CT or MRI.

Small asymptomatic lesions with a typical radiographic appearance may simply be observed. Large or symptomatic enchondromas, or those lesions that do not demonstrate a characteristic radiographic appearance, should be treated with biopsy and curettage. Pathologic fractures may be treated acutely, but the evaluating pathologist should be given the clinical history, because the presence of osteoid seen during fracture healing may add confusion to the pathologic diagnosis. Alternatively, the lesion may be treated after the pathologic fracture has healed. There are data to suggest that clinical outcome may be improved if treatment is done after healing of the pathologic fracture.[3]

Enchondromas may be approached dorsally or laterally. The initial biopsy should be done through a limited exposure and the diagnosis confirmed on frozen section before proceeding with wider exposure. Several reports have emphasized the need for thorough curettage, with recurrence being attributed to inadequate curettage.[526] Intraoperative radiographs are useful to be certain of complete removal of all tumor (see Fig. 63-49C). Iliac crest bone graft has been most commonly used to fill the defect left after curettage,[28,300,399,526] although fresh-frozen or freeze-dried irradiated allograft has been used with similar excellent results reported.[28,265] More recently, several authors have reported excellent results with simple curettage without filling the defect with any

material.[219,231,537,550] Although data are limited, whether or not the cavity is filled with any material does not appear to affect the risk of local recurrence. The latter methods eliminate the morbidity of graft harvest and are an alternative to iliac crest bone graft. There is a small but real risk of disease transmission with allograft. It is not clear whether there is an increased risk of fracture if the cavity is not grafted or whether certain lesions are best excluded from this form of treatment. The risk of local recurrence after curettage was 4.5% in the largest published series.[526] Early mobilization may be encouraged in an effort to minimize joint stiffness, provided there is sufficient residual bone stock and stability. Filling the curetted cavity with methylmethacrylate cement has been advocated to ensure immediate stability and facilitate early motion. Malignant degeneration of monostotic enchondromas to chondrosarcoma, although rare, has been well described.[124,393,575]

Author's Preferred Method of Treatment

I prefer to expose phalangeal lesions from a lateral approach rather than dorsally to minimize extensor mechanism scarring and contamination. My current preference is to fill the

CRITICAL POINTS: TREATMENT OF ENCHONDROMA OF THE BONES OF THE HAND

INDICATIONS

- Same as for biopsy
- Lesions at risk for pathologic fracture
- Lesions in which pathologic fracture has previously occurred

TECHNICAL POINTS

- Review case with pathologist in advance and confirm availability of pathologist at surgery.
- Draw limb salvage incision or amputation flaps in case of a final diagnosis of chondrosarcoma.
- Place biopsy incision in line with limb salvage incision or within amputation field.
- Use radial or ulnar lateral incisions when possible.
- Minimize dissection or retraction of the extensor mechanism to minimize postoperative adhesions.
- Consider using Kerrison rongeurs to allow precise bone window creation.
- Confirm diagnosis of enchondroma on frozen section analysis.
- Place needle markers in bone cavity and obtain radiograph to confirm adequate curettage.
- Fill cavity with autograft, allograft, as indicated.

POSTOPERATIVE CARE

- Confirm diagnosis on permanent analysis.
- Initiate early active, active-assisted range-of-motion exercises under supervision.
- Apply splint for 6 weeks or as indicated.
- Monitor for local recurrence (4% to 5% risk).

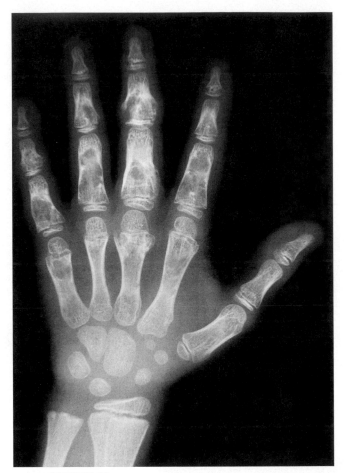

FIGURE 63-50. Multiple enchondromas (Ollier's disease).

curetted cavity with freeze-dried irradiated allograft mixed with the patient's bone marrow. I never use local bone graft from the radius or ulna in treating any bone tumor in the hand, owing to the risk of contamination of the donor field with tumor cells.

Multiple Enchondromatosis (Ollier's Disease)

Multiple enchondromatosis, or Ollier's disease, is an uncommon, nonhereditary skeletal disorder characterized by the presence of multiple enchondromas or cartilaginous masses in the metaphysis and diaphysis of long bones or short tubular bones of the hands and feet.[257] The disease is usually unilateral or predominant on one side. Enchondromas in Ollier's disease can be large and produce significant cosmetic and functional deformity in the hand, as well as brachydactyly (Fig. 63-50). Benign lesions are typically not painful. Growth of the lesion after skeletal maturity, radiographic progression, or the onset of pain should raise the question of malignant transformation. The risk of malignant transformation to chondrosarcoma or osteosarcoma in patients with Ollier's disease is approximately 30%.[177,257,329] Histologic confirmation of chondrosarcoma in these patients is difficult and requires correlation with the clinical findings and radiographs.[329] Patients with Ollier's disease require periodic surveillance with physical and radiographic examination, owing to the risk of malignancy. Progressive nonmalignant deformity has been treated with diaphysectomy and fibula strut grafting.[177]

Maffucci's Syndrome

Maffucci's syndrome is an extremely rare disease that affects the hands in the majority of cases.[257,273,316] The radiographic findings in bone are identical to those seen in Ollier's disease (see Fig. 63-50), but these patients also have multiple hemangiomas, which may be apparent radiographically owing to the presence of phleboliths. Patients with this syndrome are also at high risk for developing both bone and soft tissue sarcomas.[257,273,316]

Periosteal Chondroma

Periosteal chondroma is an uncommon benign cartilaginous lesion that may occur in the phalanges and be confused radiographically with enchondroma and histologically with chondrosarcoma.[51,188,315,356,402,458] Periosteal chondroma is most commonly seen in males in the second or third decade. The second most common location for this lesion is the metaphyseal-diaphyseal junction of the phalanges of the hand.[315] Radiographs typically reveal a subperiosteal lytic lesion with erosion of the underlying cortex, buttressing at the proximal and distal extent, and occasionally an overlying rim of sclerosis (Fig. 63-51). Histologic examination demonstrates an aggressive-appearing cartilaginous lesion that may be confused with chondrosarcoma. This lesion has a benign clinical course but may recur locally if the overlying periosteum is not excised en bloc with the tumor.[402] Marginal excision is usually curative, with local recurrence rates of less than 4%.[315] It is important to attempt to make the diagnosis of periosteal chondroma preoperatively based on plain radiographs to treat the lesion appropriately and to avoid unnecessary amputation that has been reported.[402] Periosteal chondroma most often has a characteristic radiographic appearance: external cortical erosion by a lytic unilobular lesion with a faint overlying calcified rim. The differential diagnosis for this lesion includes enchondroma, juxtacortical chondrosarcoma, periosteal osteogenic sarcoma, and subperiosteal aneurysmal bone cyst.

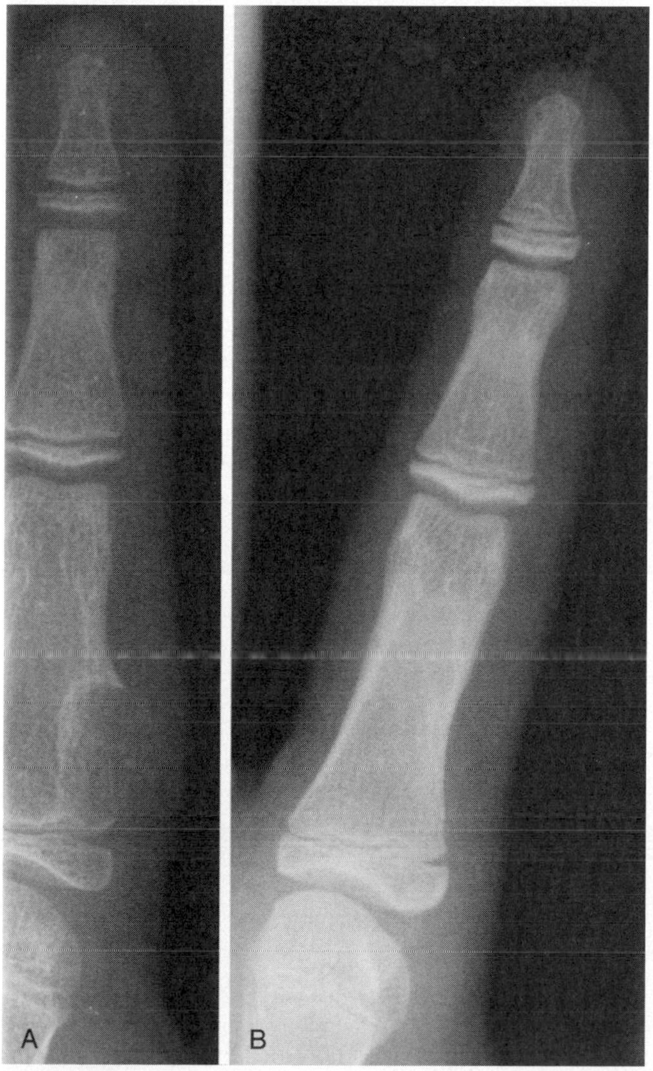

Osteochondroma

Osteochondroma is one of the most common bone lesions seen in the general skeleton, but it is not frequently seen in the hand, except in patients with multiple hereditary exostoses.[93,204,277,372,381] These lesions are osseous growths with a hyaline cartilage cap thought to originate from the physis or regions of tendon insertion.[257] Osteochondromas in the hand are most commonly seen at the distal aspect of the proximal phalanx in the second or third decade of life.[381] The prominence caused by an osteochondroma may result in cosmetic deformity and impaired function by producing a mechanical block to motion. Angular growth disturbance or rotational abnormalities may be seen, particularly with those lesions arising distally in the phalanges.[277] Osteochondromas with a characteristic radiographic appearance that are asymptomatic and do not impair function may be observed. Lesions that produce progressive deformity, pain, or impairment of function should be excised. There is a known risk of malignant transformation of osteochondroma to chondrosarcoma in the general skeleton, but malignant transformation of an osteochondroma in the hand has not been reported.

Bizarre Parosteal Osteochondromatous Proliferation

Osteochondromas are distinct entities and are not related to so-called bizarre parosteal osteochondromatous proliferations.[390,401,542] The latter is a benign, large proliferation of bone and cartilage that appears to arise from the cortical surface and lacks continuity with the medullary cavity. It has an aggressive radiographic and histologic appearance and may be confused with parosteal osteogenic sarcoma.[401] Although there is a high risk of local recurrence after marginal excision, wide or radical excision is not necessary, owing to its benign clinical course.

Subungual Exostosis (Subungual Osteochondroma)

Subungual exostoses are frequently misdiagnosed and may be confused with osteochondromas. This lesion has a cap of fibrocartilage, as opposed to the hyaline cartilage seen with an osteochondroma. Nail removal and excision of the exostosis have been successful in correcting nail deformity, without reported recurrence.[93]

Chondromyxoid Fibroma

Chondromyxoid fibroma is a benign cartilaginous lesion. Fewer than 20 cases have been reported in the hand.[15,44,208,346,481,515] Patients may give a long history of mild pain or swelling. Plain radiographs most often reveal a lytic lesion in the metaphyseal region of the bone. In large bones, the lesion is usually eccentric, but in the hand, it is more commonly central. Cortical expansion and the presence of a sclerotic rim are frequent. Pseudotrabeculation may be seen, and matrix calcification is rare in comparison with enchondroma. The lesion is most common before the age of 30, with a male-to-female ratio of 2:1. Curettage and bone

FIGURE 63-51. **A,** Periosteal chondroma of the proximal phalanx. **B,** Two years after marginal en bloc excision without grafting, normal bone contour has been restored.

grafting have been successful in controlling hand lesions. Recurrence rates of 7% to 25% have been reported with this method of treatment in large case series.[208,481] Local recurrence after curettage and bone grafting for lesions in the hand has not been reported. The most important issue in treating this lesion is making an accurate diagnosis. This lesion has been confused with chondrosarcoma in the past, owing to its aggressive histologic appearance, and amputation has been done unnecessarily.

Osteoid Osteoma

Osteoid osteoma is a benign bone lesion that has been well described in the hand and distal radius.* Five to 15 percent of osteoid osteomas occur in the hand and wrist,[24,161] most commonly in the proximal phalanx and carpus; involvement of the middle phalanx is rare. Those lesions arising in the distal phalanx may be atypical in presentation, with frequent pulp swelling and nail deformity. Radiographs most commonly demonstrate a lytic lesion rather than the classic appearance of reactive sclerosis surrounding a central lucent nidus.[57,122,365,392]

Patients typically present in the late second or early third decade of life with a deep, dull ache that is constant and frequently relieved with nonsteroidal anti-inflammatory drugs. Painless osteoid osteomas in the hand do occur, and in these instances the primary complaint is swelling.[569] Osteoid osteoma of the capitate has been reported to cause symptoms of carpal tunnel syndrome, and lesions of the radial styloid have presented as de Quervain's tenosynovitis.[198,241] Physical examination usually demonstrates well-delineated tenderness and swelling. The classic radiographic appearance is one of reactive sclerosis surrounding a central lucency less than 1 cm in diameter (Fig. 63-52), although lesions that present early may lack these findings. The diagnosis of lesions in the hand is frequently delayed, with a mean time to diagnosis of over 15 months in two large case series.[12,32] Radionuclide bone scan, tomography, and CT may improve diagnostic accuracy and assist in better defining and localizing the lesion before planned surgical treatment.[32,49]

The treatment of osteoid osteoma in the hand or carpus has been surgical excision with either curettage of the nidus or en bloc excision. Persistence of the lesion has been reported if the nidus is not completely excised.[12,32] Successful treatment with prolonged use of nonsteroidal anti-inflammatory drugs (NSAIDs) has been reported for lesions occurring in long bones with a mean symptom duration of 33 months.[295] There is no large report of this type of treatment for lesions occurring in the hand. Prolonged use of NSAIDs may be an alternative to surgical treatment if the clinical and radiographic findings are strongly supportive of a diagnosis of osteoid osteoma and excision or biopsy of the lesion might produce excessive morbidity. This may also offer an alternative for the treatment of recurrent or residual lesions in which the diagnosis of osteoid osteoma had been clearly established previously.

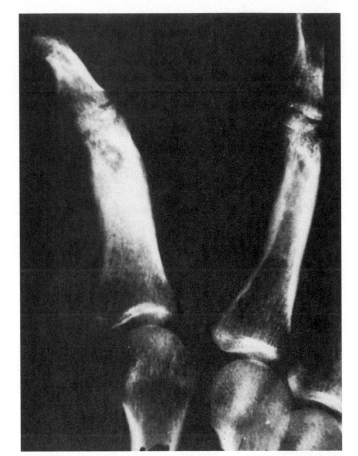

FIGURE 63-52. Osteoid osteoma. A 19-year-old woman presented with a painful proximal phalanx, dramatically relieved with aspirin. Note the classic sclerotic cortical area with a radiolucent nidus. Complete relief of pain followed local resection of the tumor nidus.

Osteoblastoma

Osteoblastoma is a rare benign tumor that is usually larger than 2 cm in diameter and is characterized by osteoid and woven bone production.[212,385] The tumor is most frequently found in the posterior elements of the spine. The histology is similar to that described for osteoid osteoma, but it is important that the tumor be distinguished from osteosarcoma. The differentiation between osteoblastoma and osteoid osteoma is usually based on location and size. Osteoblastoma is more commonly centered in the medullary portion of bones, whereas osteoid osteomas tend to be cortical, medullary, or subperiosteal in location. Local recurrence may be seen in 20% to 30% of cases after curettage and bone grafting in general case series.[252] In circumstances in which the lesion has recurred or has become locally destructive, cure may require marginal or wide excision with subsequent reconstruction.

Unicameral Bone Cyst

Unicameral bone cysts are benign, cystic lesions of uncertain etiology that are extremely rare in the bones of the hand and forearm.* Most information regarding natural

---

*See references 9, 12, 32, 33, 49, 57, 89, 99, 122, 146, 198, 241, 303, 349, 365, 392, 524, 569, and 572.

*See references 55, 80, 83, 84, 174, 262, 269, 343, 430, and 478.

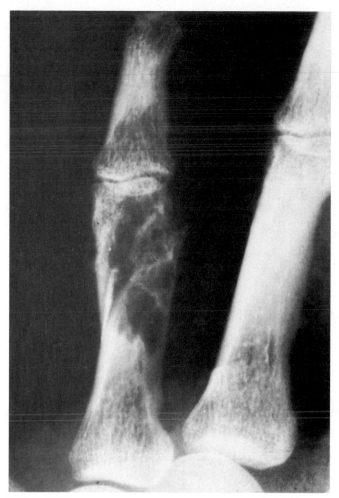

FIGURE 63-53. Solitary (unicameral) bone cyst. An 18-year-old man presented with a pathologic fracture through a bone cyst. Biopsy revealed a cavity with fluid present. Treatment was curettage and bone grafting, and prognosis was excellent.

history and treatment has been gained from the care of proximal humeral and femoral lesions. Unicameral bone cysts are usually asymptomatic until there has been a pathologic fracture. Radiographs demonstrate a lytic metaphyseal lesion with well-defined borders and septa or minor trabeculations (Fig. 63-53). The radiographic differential diagnosis for lesions occurring in the forearm and hand may include enchondroma, aneurysmal bone cyst, and telangiectatic osteogenic sarcoma.

Treatment of unicameral bone cysts has included observation, curettage and bone grafting, drilling, corticosteroid injection, and en bloc excision. Cyst aspiration and corticosteroid injection have become more popular for the treatment of these lesions, owing to the lower risk of complications and similar healing rates achieved when compared with curettage and bone grafting.[80,478] Intraosseous injection may need to be repeated several times to achieve partial or complete healing.[55,269,478] There is no known risk of malignant degeneration of unicameral bone cysts. Indications for treatment, when a diagnosis has been established, are based on the potential for mechanical failure (fracture) and deformity.

 ## Author's Preferred Method of Treatment

Unicameral bone cysts are sufficiently rare in the hand to warrant biopsy in all suspected cases, because the accurate radiographic diagnosis of this entity in the hand or forearm may not be predictable. Although "classic" lesions in the distal radius may be treated by corticosteroid injection, my preference is to treat these with open biopsy, curettage, and bone grafting with allograft after frozen section diagnosis. This technique offers the advantage of an accurate pathologic diagnosis and potentially fewer anesthetics for the patient than may be required with repeated corticosteroid injection.

Aneurysmal Bone Cyst

Aneurysmal bone cyst accounts for approximately 5% of benign bone tumors but only 3% to 5% of all aneurysmal bone cysts occur in the hand.* Hand lesions most commonly occur in the second decade of life, with males and females being equally affected. Metacarpal involvement is more common than phalangeal involvement, and carpal lesions are rare. Radiographic appearance may be similar to giant cell tumor of bone, although more frequently there is an expansile deformity and a thin rim of bone that surrounds the entire lytic lesion (see Fig. 63-54).[191] Soft tissue exten-

---

*See references 27, 42, 52, 73, 97, 106, 191, 201, 229, 319, 320, and 353.

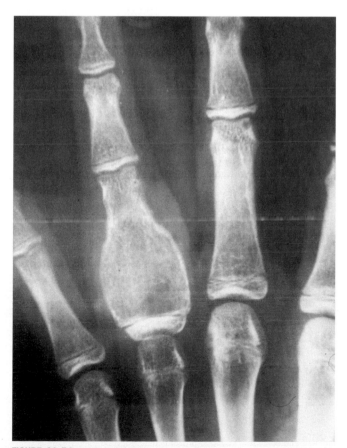

FIGURE 63-54. Lytic expansile lesion with surrounding rim of sclerosis typical of aneurysmal bone cyst.

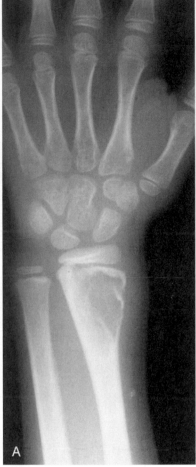
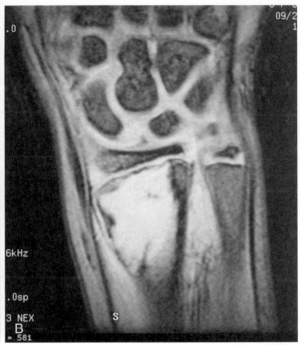

FIGURE 63-55. Aneurysmal bone cyst. **A,** A lytic lesion of the distal radius on plain radiograph. **B,** MRI suggested a fluid-filled lesion. Radiographic interpretation was unicameral bone cyst, but biopsy revealed aneurysmal bone cyst. The lesion recurred 2 months after curettage and bone grafting.

sion is uncommon. Although this lesion may be aggressive locally, it is not known to metastasize. The risk of local recurrence may be as high as 60% after curettage and bone grafting of lesions in long bones.[353,421] The risk of local recurrence in the hand appears to be similar to that seen in long bones (Fig. 63-55).[191] Frassica and coworkers reported the successful use of curettage in six of seven patients, but only three patients were successfully treated at the first operation.[191] Marcove and colleagues reported successful local control in 86% of lesions treated with curettage, cryosurgery, and cementation or bone grafting.[353] Cryosurgery[†] has been used successfully to treat recurrent aneurysmal

bone cyst in the proximal phalanx. Wide excision has been successful in treating metacarpal lesions, and large distal phalangeal lesions have been successfully treated with amputation.[52,73,191,201]

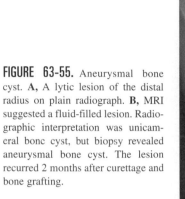

Author's Preferred Method of Treatment

When performing all incisional biopsies on lytic lesions of the bones of the hand, I am equipped and prepared to perform cryosurgery immediately after frozen section diagnosis. Cryosurgery, when used as an adjuvant to curettage, has significantly reduced the risk of local recurrence in long bones and has been used successfully in the hand. I prefer to treat small lesions that have sufficient remaining native bone stock with immediate curettage, cryosurgery, and bone grafting or cementation. Recurrent lesions may be treated with a second curettage and cryosurgery, provided there is sufficient bone stock remaining in the affected bone. Wide excision followed by reconstruction is an alternative for

---

[†]The principle of cryosurgery is to cyclically rapidly freeze the neoplasm or any remaining microscopic disease after curettage, followed by slow warming to room temperature. This produces intracellular crystal formation and cell lysis on rewarming and effectively extends the zone of curettage in a controlled but not precise manner. The technique causes nonselective tissue necrosis based on the temperature produced in the tissues. Rapid freezing is typically accomplished by a direct pour or spray of liquid nitrogen into the tumor cavity after the soft tissues have been isolated and protected. A metal or synthetic cryoprobe that circulates liquid nitrogen is an alternative to the direct pour or spray technique.

large recurrent proximal phalanx or metacarpal lesions. Metacarpal lesions are readily reconstructed with diaphyseal fibula bone graft.

Giant Cell Tumor of Bone

Although giant cell tumor of bone accounts for approximately 5% of benign bone tumors, only 2% of giant cell tumors occur in the hand.[21,23,257] These tumors are considered benign lesions, based on their histology, but they may behave in a locally aggressive fashion, metastasize, and ultimately result in death.[21,23,36,129,189,332,344,457] Lesions that arise in the bones of the hands have a higher risk of local recurrence after intralesional treatment, have a greater propensity to metastasize than those lesions seen elsewhere in the body, and must be approached with great caution.* Local recurrence rates of greater than 80% may be seen after intralesional treatment with curettage, even with the use of phenol as an adjuvant.[21,23] There are several well-documented cases of pulmonary metastases from benign giant cell tumors of bone arising in the hand.[21,23,332,344]

Giant cell tumor of bone most commonly arises early in the fourth decade of life. The most common locations in the hand are the metacarpals and phalanges, although they have been reported in all carpal bones, with the exception of the trapezoid.[1,21,23,183,254,306,333,571] A propensity for multicentricity has been reported.[23,426,571] Patients present with pain and swelling in the affected region or after a pathologic fracture. Radiographs typically demonstrate a lytic lesion with no matrix and indistinct borders, which helps to differentiate this lesion from aneurysmal bone cyst (Fig. 63-56). Cortical expansion, destruction, and soft tissue extension are common. Epiphyseal and eccentric locations typically seen elsewhere in the body are less common in hand lesions, because they frequently involve a major portion of the bone at presentation.

Incisional biopsy should be done through a well-planned approach that can later be incorporated into a salvage operation or amputation. Soft tissues must be protected during the biopsy, because giant cell tumor has a propensity to seed soft tissues, which could result in subsequent soft tissue local recurrence.[21,525] Proximal carpal lesions have been treated with either curettage or proximal row carpectomy.[1,21,183,306,333] Wide excision has been recommended for distal carpal row lesions.[254,306] Isolated curettage and bone grafting in metacarpal and phalangeal lesions is associated with an unacceptably high risk of local recurrence.[21,23,420] There are reports of success with the use of curettage, cryosurgery, and bone grafting or cementation for both metacarpal and phalangeal lesions.[351,354,371] Metacarpal lesions have been successfully treated with ray amputation or wide excision and reconstruction.[20,23,86,238,323,378,487,507] Phalangeal lesions have been successfully treated with amputation or wide excision and reconstruction using toe phalanx transfers.[21,498,538] External-beam irradiation has been effective in the treatment of benign giant cell tumor of bone, but radiotherapy is associated with a risk of malignant

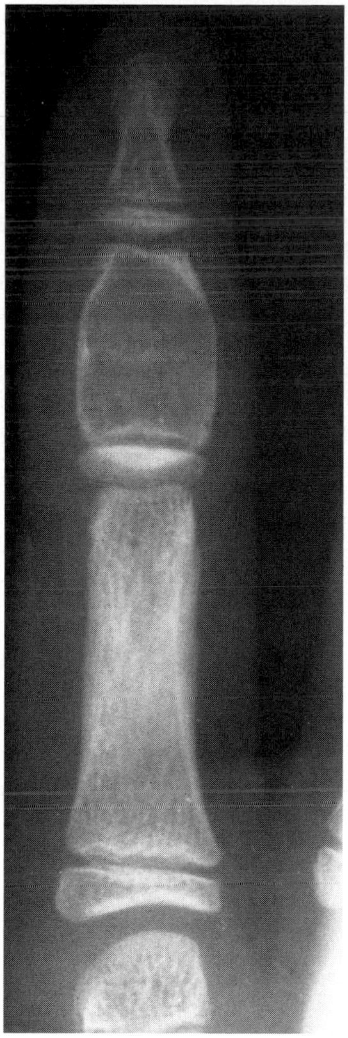

FIGURE 63-56. Giant cell tumor of bone, showing the typical cortical expansion.

transformation as high as 8.7%.[129,453] Malignant giant cell tumor of bone that occurs after external-beam irradiation is fatal in most cases. Chemotherapy has not been shown to be effective for benign giant cell tumor of bone.[36,344,457]

The third most common site of occurrence of giant cell tumor in the body is the distal radius.[257] A review of 225 patients with long bone lesions treated with curettage, burring, application of phenol, and packing of the cavity with methylmethacrylate noted a 25% risk of local recurrence.[405] However, when those cases arising in the distal radius are selectively reviewed, the risk of recurrence is 50%. In the Sloan-Kettering Memorial series, which included radiographically advanced lesions, the risk of local recurrence was reduced to 22% when curettage was combined with cryosurgery.[489] The most predictable method of local control has been wide excision of the distal radius.[387,489,550] Patients with distal radius lesions appear to be at an increased risk for metastasis.[344] Reconstruction after wide excision has been done with intercalary bone grafting for arthrodesis, articular fibula autograft, articular distal radius allograft, and creation of a one-bone forearm.[387,489,550]

---

*See references 21, 23, 79, 81, 85, 155, 211, 215, 405, 420, and 479.

Author's Preferred Method of Treatment

Giant cell tumor of bone should be approached as a low-grade malignancy when it occurs in the hand and wrist. The disease should be staged after the diagnosis with chest radiographs and a bone scan to rule out pulmonary metastasis and multicentric lesions. Phalangeal or metacarpal lesions that perforate the cortex or extend into soft tissues are best treated with amputation or wide en bloc excision and reconstruction. Distal carpal row lesions are best treated with wide excision and limited carpal fusion for reconstruction. Proximal carpal row lesions may be treated with proximal carpal row carpectomy. I consider performing curettage and cryosurgery for those lesions that do not perforate the involved bone and have sufficient remaining bone stock to allow bone grafting. Cryosurgery is associated with significant risks of soft tissue necrosis, wound infection, pathologic fracture, and neurapraxia and should be used only by those experienced with it.[351,354,371] Isolated curettage and bone grafting or curettage, application of phenol, and bone grafting cannot be advocated for the treatment of giant cell tumor of the bones of the hand.

I prefer to treat distal radius lesions that have not perforated the cortex (Campanacci grade I or II lesions) with curettage, burring, cryosurgery, and cementation, as long as there is sufficient remaining native bone stock (Fig. 63-57). Patients with pathologic fracture or large cortical perforation (Campanacci grade IIF or III lesions) are most predictably treated with wide excision of the distal radius. Reconstruction with an intercalary fibula graft and rigid internal fixation gives the most predictable result.

CRITICAL POINTS: GIANT CELL TUMOR OF BONE

PREOPERATIVE EVALUATION

- Lesion should be considered a low-grade malignancy.
- Patients should be staged with CT of chest and total body bone scan.
- Use MRI to determine extent of soft tissue contamination.

INDICATIONS FOR WIDE EXCISION OR AMPUTATION

- Soft tissue contamination precluding the use of curettage with adjuvants
- Amputation for majority of non–distal radius lesions
- Wide excision for distal radius lesions with perforation of more than one cortex

TECHNICAL POINTS

- As for biopsy or wide excision

POSTOPERATIVE CARE

- Surveillance for local recurrence or metastasis for 10 years

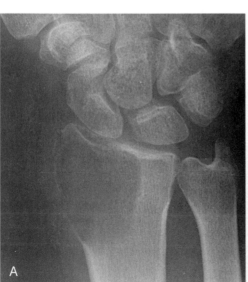
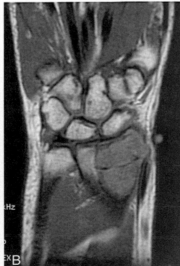
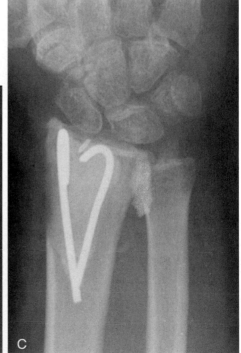

FIGURE 63-57. **A,** An expansile lytic lesion of the distal radius without a reactive sclerotic rim. **B,** MRI further delineates the lesion. Open biopsy revealed giant cell tumor of bone. **C,** A radiograph was taken after curettage, burring, cryosurgery, and cementation with internal Steinmann pin struts.

MALIGNANT BONE TUMORS

Chondrosarcoma

Chondrosarcoma is the most common primary malignant bone tumor that occurs in the hand.* This tumor may arise primarily or may develop in a preexistent benign lesion such as an enchondroma or osteochondroma. The lesion most commonly occurs in patients older than the age of 60. The proximal phalanges and metacarpals are most commonly affected. Only rarely has chondrosarcoma been reported in the distal phalanges or carpus.[192,497] This lesion often presents as a slowly growing, firm, and often painful mass. Radiographs typically reveal a tumor matrix with stippled calcifications, areas of lysis, and poorly defined borders. Extreme cortical expansion, perforation, or extension into the surrounding soft tissues helps to differentiate this lesion from enchondroma (Fig. 63-58). Although there are well-documented instances of metastasis and mortality, the majority of chondrosarcomas are slow-growing lesions that do not metastasize. The prognosis for patients with chondrosarcoma in general is related to the histologic grade of the lesion, although it is not clear that this principle applies to those lesions arising in the hand.[257] The risk of metastasis for lesions occurring in the hand is approximately 10% and usually occurs after local recurrence following intralesional treatment.[268]

A well-planned incisional biopsy should be done for suspicious lesions. It is imperative that the surgeon consult with the pathologist before the biopsy and that the biopsy specimen be reviewed in the presence of the plain radiographs. Interpretation and diagnosis of cartilaginous lesions in the hand, in particular low-grade chondrosarcoma, are extremely difficult.[130] In general, peripheral cartilaginous lesions (i.e., those in the hand) tend to show greater degrees of cellularity and atypia on histologic examination, although the clinical course is that of a benign lesion. Radiographic findings of an inactive or, alternatively, an aggressive lesion may influence the pathologic diagnosis of cartilaginous lesions, and this has great implications for appropriate treatment.

Patients suspected of having chondrosarcoma must have their disease locally and systemically staged. Chondrosarcoma most commonly metastasizes to the lungs, and patients should be evaluated with CT of the chest. Currently, chondrosarcoma of the bones of the hand is best treated surgically with wide en bloc excision or digit or ray amputation. There is investigational interest in intralesional procedures owing to the limited metastatic potential of hand lesions.[54] The potential indications for this less aggressive approach remain to be defined. Chemotherapy is not known to be effective for the vast majority of chondrosarcomas. There may be a role for chemotherapy in the treatment of dedifferentiated chondrosarcoma or mesenchymal chondrosarcoma, but neither of these entities has been reported to occur in the hand.[193,391] There is no role for radiation in the treatment of chondrosarcoma arising in the bones of the hand. Patients must be followed for both local and systemic recurrence, because metastasis may become apparent several years after treatment of the primary lesion.

Osteogenic Sarcoma

Osteogenic sarcoma is the most common primary bone tumor seen in children and adolescents, but it is only rarely seen as a primary lesion in the hand.† When it does occur in the hand, it may be in older patients in the fourth, fifth, and sixth decades, often arising from a preexistent lesion.[22,90,94, 149,410] Survival in patients with osteogenic sarcoma has improved dramatically with the use of systemic chemotherapy, and all patients with high-grade malignant lesions should receive adjuvant chemotherapy.[213,235,324,352,374,375,435]

Patients present with a rapidly enlarging mass that is firm and painful. Plain radiographs may reveal an expansile,

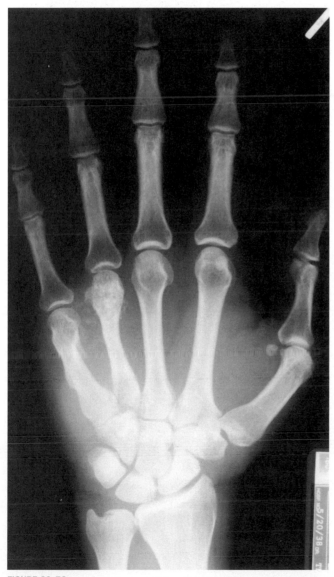

FIGURE 63-58. Chondrosarcoma of the fourth metacarpal. Note the poorly defined borders and extension into the soft tissues.

---

*See references 46, 77, 96, 124, 130, 131, 192, 196, 205, 218, 220, 223, 240, 268, 274, 279, 304, 307, 393, 416, 423, 446, 456, 477, 488, 497, 508, 539, and 575.

†See references 22, 37, 40, 90, 94, 102, 105, 110, 140, 149, 184, 192, 374, 375, 379, 410, 436, 509, and 549.

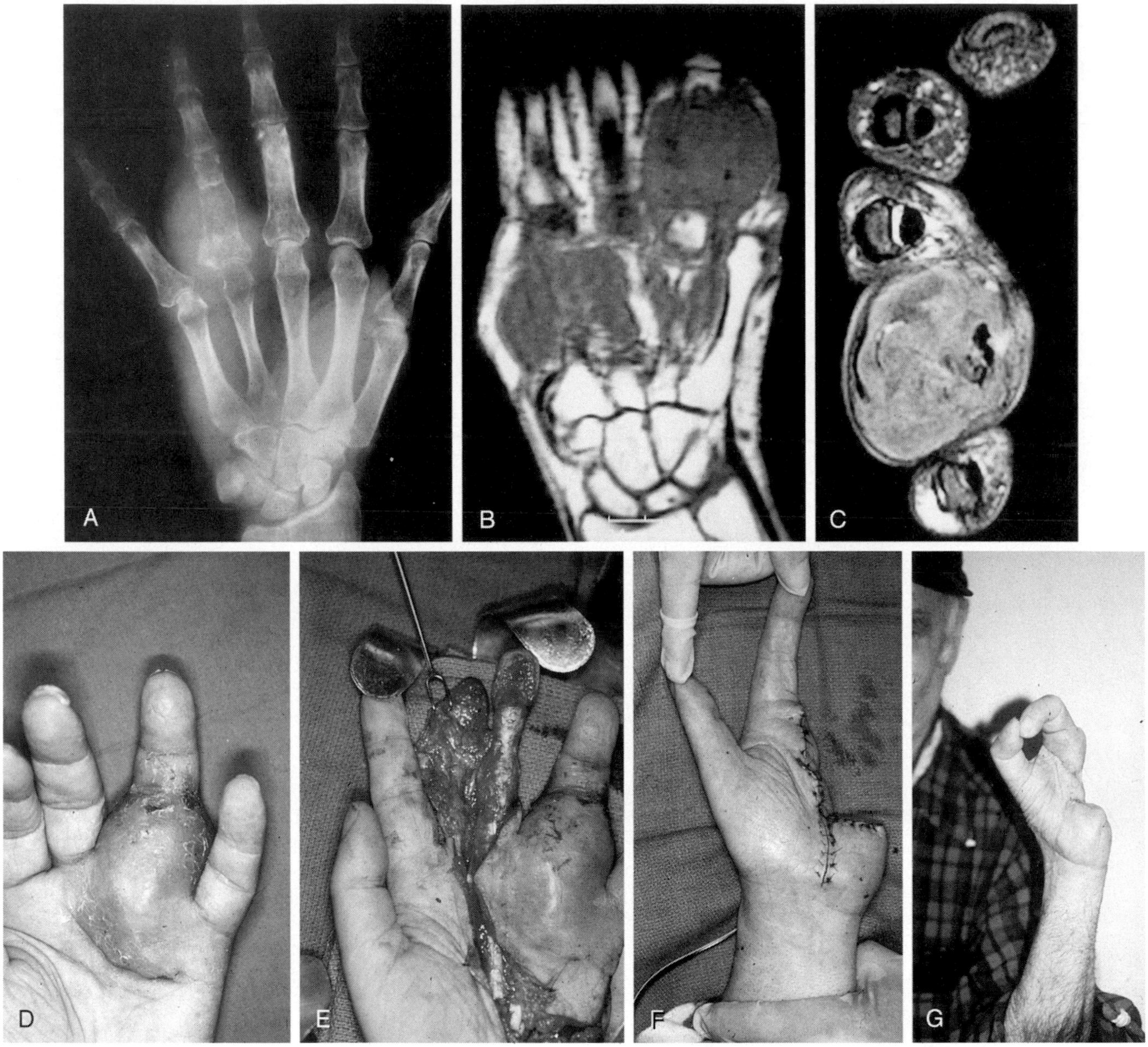

FIGURE 63-59. Osteogenic sarcoma. **A,** A lytic destructive lesion with soft tissue extension in the proximal phalanx of the ring finger. **B** and **C,** MRI demonstrates extensive soft tissue involvement, including the metacarpal head region. This elderly man was unable to tolerate chemotherapy and was treated with triple ray amputation (long, ring, and small fingers). This very large tumor (**D**) was approached palmarly and dorsally, and closure was facilitated with a fillet flap of the long finger (**E**). The appearance after closure (**F**), and useful function (**G**).

sclerotic lesion with malignant new bone formation or with a more lytic or mixed pattern with destruction and soft tissue mass (Fig. 63-59). Parosteal osteogenic sarcoma may present with a surface lesion and soft tissue involvement.[509,549] This lesion most commonly occurs in the proximal phalanges and metacarpals, with only one reported case occurring in the carpus.[40]

A well-planned incisional biopsy should be performed while considering the need for subsequent amputation or a limb salvage procedure. After confirmation of the diagnosis, the lesion should be treated with wide en bloc excision or finger or ray amputation. Before modern chemotherapy, hand lesions were thought to have a better prognosis than those lesions occurring elsewhere in the body.[90,94,110] It is not

clear to what extent adjuvant chemotherapy affects the prognosis of patients with hand lesions,[410] but currently adjuvant chemotherapy is considered to be part of a comprehensive treatment plan.[213,235,324,352,374,375,435] There is no significant difference in survival between the use of chemotherapy before excision (neoadjuvant) and after excision (adjuvant), although neoadjuvant therapy may improve the quality of resection margins and reduce the risk of local recurrence.[375,435] There is no role for external-beam irradiation in the attempted curative treatment of these lesions.[75] Long-term survival after aggressive treatment of local recurrence may be better for those lesions occurring in the hand as compared with general case series, in which the prognosis is extremely poor.[435]

Author's Preferred Method of Treatment

After confirmation of the diagnosis and local and systemic staging, I prefer the immediate initiation of neoadjuvant chemotherapy. Although there may be no significant survival benefit with the use of neoadjuvant as opposed to adjuvant chemotherapy, an effective adjuvant in most cases decreases the size of the tumor and reduces surrounding soft tissue edema. This may facilitate wide en bloc excision or improve the quality of margins at amputation. A good response to chemotherapy appears to reduce the risk of local recurrence after wide excision.[435] Analysis of the resection or amputation specimen allows quantitation of response to chemotherapy, which has prognostic significance and may affect postoperative adjuvant treatment plans.[375] After local treatment, chemotherapy should be promptly resumed, because a delay in the resumption of chemotherapy beyond 23 days adversely affects survival.[375] Prolonged local and systemic surveillance for recurrence or metastasis is mandatory.

Ewing's Sarcoma

Ewing's sarcoma is one of the common primary childhood sarcomas of bone but only rarely arises in the bones of the hand.* This tumor most commonly occurs in the first or second decade of life, with the youngest recorded case occurring in the distal phalanx of a 5-month-old infant.[516] Survival has improved considerably with the use of adjuvant chemotherapy. Local treatment of the tumor in the hand must be done in the context of well-planned and coordinated systemic treatment.[†]

The clinical presentation of Ewing's sarcoma in the hand is very similar to that seen in infection. Pain, swelling, and erythema are common. A significant soft tissue mass is frequently seen. Signs of systemic illness may be present and include fever and elevated white blood cell count and sedimentation rate. There are several reports of misdiagnosis and prolonged treatment for presumed infection.[297,350,359] The tumor most commonly arises in the metacarpals or phalanges, with extensive soft tissue involvement. There is no well-documented case of this tumor arising in the carpus, and middle phalangeal involvement is rare. Radiographs typically reveal a large lytic, destructive, expansile lesion with associated soft tissue involvement. A mixed lytic and sclerotic appearance may be seen.[449,492] MRI is particularly useful in delineating the extent of bone and soft tissue involvement that may not be apparent on plain radiographs (Fig. 63-60).

Incisional biopsy is indicated in those patients presenting with lytic destructive lesions of the bones of the hand. In addition, strong consideration for biopsy must always be given before the initiation of treatment for presumed deep infection, because this is the most common error in diagnosis. The biopsy must be carefully planned and executed in

an effort to avoid additional soft tissue contamination, which may compromise subsequent ablative or limb salvage procedures. The pathologist who will be evaluating the specimen should be consulted in advance, and arrangements should be made to perform cytogenetic analysis, because this will improve the accuracy of diagnosis and assist in the diagnosis of particularly difficult cases.

There is considerable controversy regarding the timing and method used for obtaining local control of tumors in the hand. The radiation oncology literature supports the use of external-beam irradiation to obtain local control in the context of systemic treatment with chemotherapy.[266,293] The hand surgery literature supports the use of ablative surgery with or without the use of external-beam irradiation, as well as in the setting of systemic treatment with chemotherapy.[141,150,173,414] Similar rates of local control with the use of either curative external-beam irradiation or surgery have been reported. It is imperative to obtain local control at the time of primary treatment, because local recurrence has been found to be uniformly fatal in some series.[206] Although survival for those patients with Ewing's sarcoma occurring in the hand or foot appears to be better than for those with more central primary lesions, when those cases occurring specifically in the hand are selectively assessed, the rate of survival is similar to that for lesions elsewhere in the body, with the exception of those tumors arising in the pelvis.

Author's Preferred Method of Treatment

I prefer the immediate initiation of systemic chemotherapy before definitive local treatment. Ewing's sarcoma is a highly lethal malignancy, and there may be a survival benefit in the immediate initiation of systemic treatment without the delay that may occur after normal postoperative healing or a postoperative complication. In addition, the use of an effective preoperative adjuvant in most cases decreases the size of the tumor and facilitates subsequent surgery. The analysis of the resected specimen provides information regarding the effect of chemotherapy and has implications for additional adjuvant treatment, the possible need for postoperative external-beam irradiation, and prognosis. I favor the use of wide en bloc excision or amputation through a wide margin to obtain local control for lesions that occur in the hand. If a wide margin of normal tissue has not been obtained after analysis of the excised specimen, external-beam irradiation should be added to the treatment protocol after the completion of chemotherapy.[415] Although external-beam radiation may be effective in obtaining local control, it may be associated with soft tissue contracture, neuropathy, pathologic fracture, growth inhibition, and radiation-induced malignancy.[317] Wide excision with adequate margins eliminates the need for radiation and avoids the associated morbidity.

Although rates of local control appear to be similar when external-beam irradiation is used as primary treatment for Ewing's sarcoma in the hand, the available data are limited. Autopsy studies have documented residual disease at the

---

*See references 26, 38, 48, 72, 105, 115, 140, 141, 147, 150, 171, 173, 192, 246, 253, 266, 283, 293, 297, 301, 308, 359, 414, 417, 449, 452, 492, 516, and 566.

[†]See references 73, 175, 206, 251, 266, 293, 394, 414, 462, and 533.

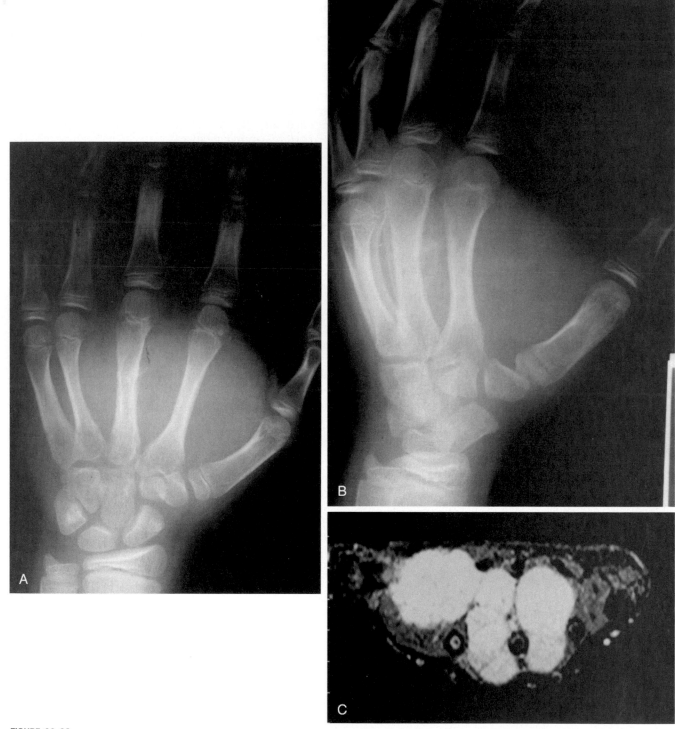

FIGURE 63-60. Ewing's sarcoma. **A** and **B,** Diaphyseal sclerosis and periosteal new bone formation of the third metacarpal on radiography. **C,** MRI demonstrates a large soft tissue mass surrounding the third metacarpal with extensive palmar and radial involvement.

primary site of malignancy in up to 20% of patients who subsequently died of pulmonary metastases when the primary tumor was treated with external-beam irradiation, even in the absence of clinical local recurrence.[532] Local control must be obtained at the time of initial treatment, because local recurrence unquestionably adversely affects patient survival.

Metastatic Tumors

Metastasis to the bones of the hand is uncommon.* Fewer than 0.3% of patients with cancer develop acrometastases.[180]

---

*See references 11, 61, 65, 111, 116, 194, 236, 242, 243, 258, 278, 288, 418, 424, 503, and 574.

Metastasis to the hand usually occurs as a rare, preterminal event and is often part of a widespread dissemination of the primary malignancy. In as many as 50% of patients with acrometastasis, the lesion can mimic a benign condition or can be the first presentation of malignancy or metastatic disease.[236,242,258,424]

Although the distal phalanx previously has been noted to be the most common site of metastasis to the hand, the other phalanges and metacarpals can be equally affected. Involvement of the carpal bones is rare.[258] A predilection for involvement of the dominant hand has been noted.[236] Bronchogenic carcinoma of the lung has been reported as

the primary malignancy in as many as 50% of cases and is the most common metastatic lesion occurring in men (see Fig. 63-61).[236,424] Other reported primary malignancies include renal, esophageal, breast, colon, prostate, thyroid, and bone cancer. In one study the mean time to the development of hand metastases was 16 months after the diagnosis of the primary malignancy.[236]

Clinical findings include the typical signs of inflammation—pain, swelling, and erythema—which may lead to an initial clinical diagnosis of infection. Misdiagnosis is common and has included osteomyelitis, felon, gout, rheumatoid arthritis, reflex sympathetic dystrophy, and trau-

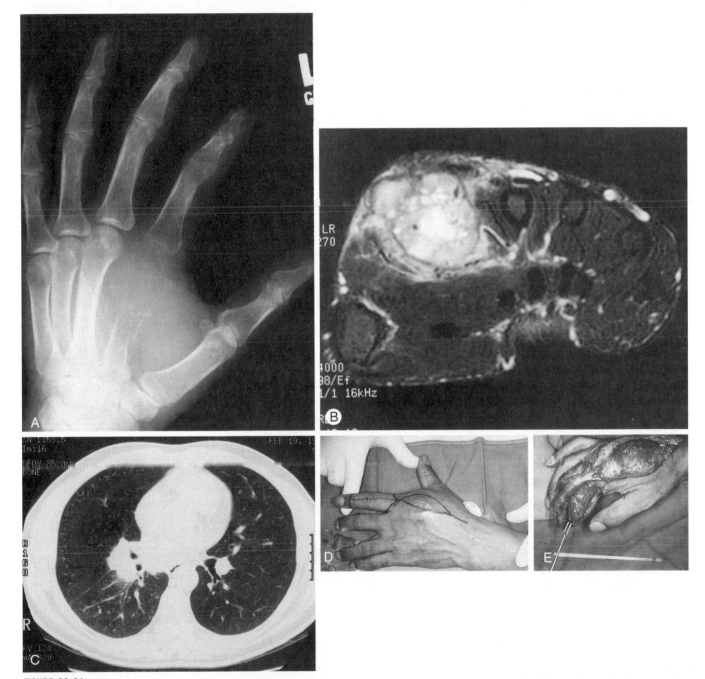

FIGURE 63-61. Metastatic tumor. **A,** In this 46-year-old man with a history of noninvasive bladder cancer and smoking, radiographs demonstrated a destructive lytic permeative lesion of the index metacarpal. **B,** MRI documented the extent of soft tissue involvement. **C,** CT of the chest revealed bilateral masses. An index ray amputation with fillet flap closure was done (**D** and **E**) after confirmation of the diagnosis of metastatic lung cancer.

matic fracture.[65,236,424] Radiographs usually reveal a lytic destructive lesion, although metastatic prostate carcinoma can produce a sclerotic lesion. Extension into adjacent joints is uncommon. Lytic destructive lesions in the bones of the hand should be sampled and cultured without delay in the absence of a known primary malignancy.

Treatment of documented metastases should be directed at relief of pain and preservation of function. Amputation and ray resection are effective in providing palliation and local control of disease. Although amputation has been done for lesions occurring in the carpus, curettage and packing with methylmethacrylate may offer an alternative method of providing local control of small lesions without the associated morbidity of an amputation in a patient who is terminally ill. External-beam irradiation may be used in patients with multiple or inoperable lesions, although pain relief is less predictable.[65] Systemic staging should be done after the diagnosis of the metastasis and consideration given to systemic treatment in consultation with an oncologist. The median survival for patients with metastases to the hand is approximately 6 months and is related to the primary malignancy. Early diagnosis may improve morbidity, particularly when the metastasis is the primary symptom of an undiagnosed malignancy.

The treatment of isolated renal cell carcinoma to the hand deserves special consideration. Long-term survival and prolonged disease-free interval have been reported after the resection of isolated metastatic renal cell carcinoma to the extremities.[10,536] A long interval between presentation of the primary lesion and the detection of isolated metastasis as well as distal extremity metastasis have been correlated with longer survival. Isolated renal cell carcinoma metastasis to the hand should be approached similar to that of a primary bone sarcoma.

ANNOTATED REFERENCES

3. Ablove RH, Moy OJ, Peimer CA, Wheeler DR: Early versus delayed treatment of enchondroma. Am J Orthop 29:771-772, 2000.

This article compares the results of early and delayed treatment of patients presenting with pathologic fracture through enchondroma in the hand. The results suggest improved outcome with delayed treatment after healing and early recovery of range of motion.

18. Angelides AC, Wallace PF: The dorsal ganglion of the wrist: Its pathogenesis, gross and microscopic anatomy, and surgical treatment. J Hand Surg [Am] 1:228-235, 1976.

This classic article reviews the pathogenesis, anatomy, and treatment of dorsal carpal ganglion cysts.

21. Athanasian EA, Wold LE, Amadio PC: Giant cell tumors of the bones of the hand. J Hand Surg [Am] 22:91-98, 1997.

A 50-year retrospective review is presented of treatment of giant cell tumor of bone of the hand at a single institution. Local recurrence was seen in approximately 80% of patients treated with curettage, and metastasis was seen concurrent with local recurrence in two patients. Wide excision or amputation is advocated as definitive treatment for giant cell tumor of bone when it occurs in the hand.

33. Bednar MS, Maywood IL, McCormack RR Jr, et al: Osteoid osteoma of the upper extremity. J Hand Surg [Am] 18:1019-1028, 1993.

A retrospective review of a large group of patients with osteoid osteoma is presented. The study documents the difficulty and delay in diagnosis and response to curettage.

66. Brien EW, Terek RM, Geer RJ, et al: Treatment of soft-tissue sarcomas of the hand. J Bone Joint Surg Am 77:564-571, 1995.

A retrospective review of 24 cases of soft tissue sarcoma occurring in the hand during a 10-year period at Memorial Sloan-Kettering Cancer Center is discussed. Synovial sarcoma was the most frequent diagnosis. Local recurrence was frequent when positive margins were identified after resection. Adjuvant radiation could not compensate for inadequate margins. Several of the patients with positive margins ultimately died. The authors advocated achieving negative margins with amputation if needed and re-excision in the event of positive margins.

145. Donner TR, Voorhies RM, Kline DG: Neural sheath tumors of major nerves. J Neurosurg 81:362-373, 1994.

A large retrospective review of schwannoma and neurofibroma documented risks of permanent neurologic deficit after excision and factors that increase risks, including reoperation and prior biopsy.

191. Frassica FJ, Amadio PC, Wold LE, Beabout JW: Aneurysmal bone cyst: Clinicopathologic features and treatment of ten cases involving the hand. J Hand Surg [Am] 13:676-683, 1988.

This is one of the largest retrospective studies of aneurysmal bone cyst in the hand with results similar to general case series for lesions treated with curettage alone.

199. Frustaci S, Gherlinzoni F, De Paoli A, et al: Adjuvant chemotherapy for adult soft tissue sarcomas of the extremities and girdles: Results of the Italian randomized cooperative trial. J Clin Oncol 19:1238-1247, 2001.

These researchers report a prospective randomized trial of the use of chemotherapy for the treatment of extremity soft tissue sarcoma. Increased disease-free survival was seen at 2- and 5-year follow-up. The study supports the use of chemotherapy in selected patients with extremity soft tissue sarcoma.

210. Gingrass MK, Brown RE, Zook EG: Treatment of fingernail deformities secondary to ganglions of the distal interphalangeal joint. J Hand Surg [Am] 20:502-505, 1995.

This report outlines a useful technique for approaching mucous cysts while minimizing skin complication risk. The base of the lesion is excised without excising the entire lesion. Excellent results were seen with low complication.

214. Glowacki KA, Weiss APC: Giant cell tumors of tendon sheath. Hand Clin 11:245-253, 1995.

This is a comprehensive review of the history, pathogenesis, and treatment of giant cell tumor of tendon sheath when it occurs in the hand. The study demonstrates a local recurrence risk range between 5% and 50%.

236. Healey JH, Turnbull ADM, Miedema B, Lane JM: Acrometastases: A study of twenty-nine patients with osseous involvement of the hands and feet. J Bone Joint Surg Am 68:743-746, 1986.

This is a large retrospective review of acrometastasis at a major cancer center. Limited survival was seen after diagnosis with duration correlating with the primary site of disease. Palliative treatment was advocated.

314. Lewis JJ, Leung D, Heslin M, et al: Association of local recurrence with subsequent survival in extremity soft tissue sarcoma. J Clin Oncol 15:646-652, 1997.

This identifies local recurrence as a poor prognostic factor for patients with extremity soft tissue sarcoma, particularly if the primary tumor was high grade and large (>5 cm). Aggressive local treatment and consideration of chemotherapy were advocated for these high-risk patients. The authors noted that although local recurrence was associated with a worse prognosis, statistical analysis did not identify local recurrence to be causative of subsequent metastasis. It was speculated that biologic primary tumor factors increase the risk of both local recurrence and metastasis.

335. Louis DS, Hankin FM, Greene TL, Dick HM: Lipofibromas of the median nerve: Long-term follow-up of four cases. J Hand Surg [Am] 10:403-408, 1985.

This report documents the long-term progressive deterioration of function in patients with lipofibromatous hamartoma.

348. Mankin HJ, Lange TA, Spanier SS: The hazards of biopsy in patients with malignant primary bone and soft-tissue tumors. J Bone Joint Surg Am 64:1121-1127, 1982.

This classic article documents the increased risk of local recurrence, amputation, and death associated with poorly performed biopsy of malignant bone and soft tissue sarcomas of the extremities. A recommendation was made to refer all patients suspected of having malignant bone or soft tissue lesions to a tumor center for biopsy.

375. Meyers PA, Heller G, Healey JH, et al: Chemotherapy for nonmetastatic osteogenic sarcoma: The Memorial Sloan-Kettering Experience. J Clin Oncol 10:5-15, 1992.

This study identifies primary site, alkaline phosphatase, lactase dehydrogenase, histologic response to chemotherapy, and race as independent predictors of prognosis for young patients with high-grade, nonmetastatic osteogenic sarcoma of bone. No survival benefit was identified whether chemotherapy was initiated before definitive surgical treatment or after induction. A survival benefit was noted in patients who resumed chemotherapy within 23 days of definitive surgical treatment.

405. O'Donnell RJ, Springfield DS, Motwani HK, et al: Recurrence of giant-cell tumors of the long bones after curettage and packing with cement. J Bone Joint Surg Am 76:1827-1833, 1994.

This multicenter retrospective study found a general local recurrence risk of 25% for patients with extremity giant cell tumor of bone treated with curettage, phenol, and cement. When distal radius tumors in the study are selectively reviewed, the local recurrence risk was 50%.

410. Okada K, Wold LE, Beabout JW, Shives TC: Osteosarcoma of the hand: A clinicopathologic study of 12 cases. Cancer 72:719-725, 1993.

This study reviews a small number of patients treated at the Mayo Clinic as well as patients in consultation files. Overall survival was very good even in the absence of chemotherapy. The authors question the need for chemotherapy for osteogenic sarcoma when it occurs in the hand. They make no differentiation of importance of tumor grade or volume in determining prognosis or implication for chemotherapy.

415. Ozaki T, Hillmann A, Hoffmann C, et al: Significance of surgical margin on the prognosis of patients with Ewing's sarcoma. A report from the Cooperative Ewing's Sarcoma Study. Cancer 78:892-900, 1996.

This retrospective analysis reviews the impact of the quality of surgical margins and adjuvant radiation on the prognosis of patients with Ewing's sarcoma. The lowest risk of local recurrence was seen when wide margins were achieved at definitive surgical treatment. External-beam irradiation had only a small beneficial impact on local recurrence

risk in patients with positive margins. The benefit did not approximate the results seen with widely negative margins only. This study highlights the importance of achieving widely negative margins in minimizing local recurrence risk in patients with Ewing's sarcoma treated with limb-sparing surgery.

427. Peimer CA, Smith RJ, Sirota RL, Cohen BE: Epithelioid sarcoma of the hand and wrist: Patterns of extension. J Hand Surg [Am] 2:275-282, 1977.

This study demonstrates the dramatic and unique propensity for epithelioid sarcoma to spread proximally in an extremity. The findings have implications for the need for widely negative margins when treating patients with this disease and support the practice of MRI evaluation of the forearm in patients with epithelioid sarcoma of the hand.

465. Rosenberg SA, Tepper J, Glatstein E, et al: The treatment of soft-tissue sarcomas of the extremities: Prospective randomized evaluations of (1) limb-sparing surgery plus radiation therapy compared with amputation and (2) the role of adjuvant chemotherapy. Ann Surg 196:305-315, 1982.

A landmark study prospectively compared limb salvage versus amputation for soft tissue sarcoma of the extremities. The study demonstrated higher risk of local recurrence for the limb salvage patients but equal survival. The findings were used to support the concept of wide excision of tumors and limb-sparing surgery. The study has subsequently been criticized for being underpowered.

478. Scaglietti O, Marchetti PG, Bartolozzi P: Final results obtained in the treatment of bone cysts with methylprednisolone acetate (Depo-Medrol) and a discussion of results achieved in other bone lesions. Clin Orthop 165:33-42, 1982.

This classic retrospective study demonstrated the efficacy of intraosseous steroid injection for unicameral bone cysts of the extremities. On average, 3.8 injections were administered. Roughly 50% of patients had no recurrence, 25% had partial recurrence, and 25% needed additional treatment.

489. Sheth DS, Healey JH, Sobel M, et al: Giant cell tumor of the distal radius. J Hand Surg [Am] 20:432-440, 1995.

This retrospective study demonstrated the results of curettage and cryosurgery for distal radius giant cell tumor of bone. Many of the patients had advanced disease (Campanacci stage 3). Local recurrence was seen in approximately 17% of patients.

527. Takigawa K: Chondroma of the bones of the hand: A review of 110 cases. J Bone Joint Surg Am 53:1591-1600, 1971.

This is the largest report of enchondroma occurring in the hand. This study demonstrated a 4.5% local recurrence risk after curettage. Recurrences were attributed to inadequate primary curettage.

550. Vander Griend RA, Funderburk CH: The treatment of giant-cell tumors of the distal part of the radius. J Bone Joint Surg Am 75:899-908, 1993.

All stage III patients were treated with wide excision and nonvascularized fibula grafting with internal fixation using a long 3.5-mm dynamic compression plate. No local recurrences were seen and all patients achieved bony union. This paper highlights the importance of rigid fixation rather than the vascularity of the fibula bone graft in achieving union.

570. Wittig JC, Simpson BM, Bickels J, et al: Giant cell tumor of the hand: Superior results with curettage, cryosurgery, and cementation. J Hand Surg [Am] 26:546-555, 2001.

This small case series demonstrated the successful use of curettage, cryosurgery, and cementation for giant cell tumor of bone in the hand as opposed to wide excision or amputation.

CHAPTER 64

Vascular Disorders

L. Andrew Koman, David S. Ruch, Beth Paterson Smith, and Thomas L. Smith

GENERAL CONSIDERATIONS

Although uncommon, disorders of the upper extremity vascular system may cause significant morbidity. In this chapter we discuss the evaluation, pathoanatomy, and treatment of post-traumatic, occlusive, vasospastic, and arteriovenous processes affecting the upper extremity vasculature.

Preoperative Evaluation

Symptomatic vascular disorders of the upper extremity interfere with health-related quality of life, compromise function, and negatively impact patients and society. Although significant upper extremity peripheral vascular disease is less prevalent than comparable lesions in the lower extremity, heart, or brain,[102] upper extremity vascular morbidity is a significant societal burden.[157,208,339] Aberrant microvascular flow secondary to acute or chronic trauma, congenital deformity, systemic processes, or genetic influences affects over 10% of the general population and 20% to 30% of premenopausal women.[157,208,339] Vascular insufficiency or *incompetency* may produce pain, cold intolerance, numbness, digital ulceration, and/or gangrene. Symptoms associated with abnormal perfusion may occur secondary to congenital or acquired events that affect vascular structures (e.g., thrombosis or occlusion), vascular function (e.g., abnormal autonomic/vasomotor control), or both.[103] Vascular insufficiency occurs when blood flow fails to meet cellular metabolic demand, with resultant cellular ischemia, cellular injury, and pain.

Vascular insufficiency may occur after structural arterial damage or in the presence of injury to the structures innervating the vasculature. It may also be secondary to acquired vasomotor dysfunction after trauma.[169,176] In the majority of cases, vascular damage—transection, thrombosis, embolism—occurs in the presence of adequate collateral circulation and symptoms are minimal. However, in the presence of increased sympathetic tone from reflex vasospasm, a concomitant nerve injury, bone or soft tissue injury, or premorbid vasomotor control abnormalities, otherwise adequate collateral vessels may be compromised by spasm and subject to functional vascular compromise and to further decreases in tissue perfusion, with resultant ischemic symptoms and signs (Fig. 64-1). An arterial injury that occurs at a crucial location or in the absence of adequate collateral circulation may result in ischemia, reflex increase in sympathetic tone, further arterial spasm, and eventual tissue death unless intervention occurs (see Fig. 64-1). *Critical vascular injury results in distal cell death and gangrene* (Table 64-1).

Preoperative evaluation requires an assessment of the integrity of arterial and venous channels, the adequacy of compensatory or collateral capability, and the appropriateness of both macrovascular and microvascular control systems. Symptoms and signs of vascular insufficiency may be secondary to structural vascular damage (e.g., thrombosis, embolism), to congenital malformation(s) (e.g., arteriovenous shunting), to iatrogenic interventions (e.g., vascular access procedures), or to a combination of these conditions. Therefore, a detailed history, physical examination, and appropriate testing are required to delineate the pathoanatomy responsible for morbidity and to identify optimal interventional strategies.

The causes of vascular disorders include trauma, iatrogenic events, chronic processes, metabolic abnormalities, genetic factors, congenital processes, and systemic disease (Table 64-2). However, failure to provide adequate nutritional blood flow to the extremity is the common final pathway. Therefore, operative and nonoperative interventions must be designed to correct perfusion inadequacies.

History

The patient's clinical history is vital in establishing the correct diagnosis. Important details obtained from the patient include a description of penetrating and/or nonpenetrating trauma, the presence of repetitive insults, documentation of the existence of familial or sporadic blood dyscrasias or abnormalities, the presence or absence of swelling, a history of drug exposure or tobacco use, the occurrence and frequency of Raynaud's events, and the extent of cold sensitivity, numbness, weakness, and/or pain. *Unilateral Raynaud's phenomenon suggests occlusive disease and, when combined with nonhealing ulcerations, necrosis, and/or impending gangrene, should be considered pathognomonic of vascular compromise from thrombosis or embolism.*

Quantifying symptomatic complaints and defining functional impairment may be facilitated by using validated questionnaires (instruments); these questionnaires facilitate

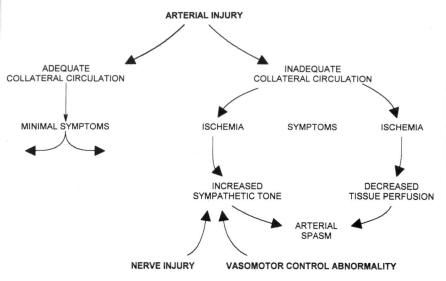

FIGURE 64-1. Vascular injury precipitates a vicious cycle of symptoms if insults occur at a crucial location, are associated with concomitant or preexisting abnormalities of vasomotor control, and/or accompany nerve injury. (From Koman LA [ed]: Bowman Gray School of Medicine Orthopaedic Manual. Wake Forest University Orthopaedic Press, Winston-Salem, NC, 1997, with permission.)

Table 64-1
DEFINITIONS

"Critical" vascular events result in tissue death and necrosis without intervention.

"Noncritical" vascular events occur when a vascular structure is damaged or destroyed (e.g., laceration of an artery) and collateral circulation is sufficient to prevent cell death or damage.

Vascular competency is the ability to appropriately modulate thermoregulatory and nutritional blood flow to fulfill metabolic requirements and maintain core temperature.

Vascular/arterial insufficiency occurs when nutritional blood flow is inadequate to maintain cellular viability.

Thermoregulatory flow is the portion of total digital flow that does not support cellular metabolism.

Nutritional flow is the portion of total digital flow that provides material for cellular metabolism.

Table 64-2
VASCULAR DISORDERS

Acute Injury
Arteries
Veins

Iatrogenic Events
Cannulation injury
Vascular access

Chronic Processes
Occlusive disease
  Thrombosis
  Aneurysm
  Embolism
Vasospastic disease
Combined (vaso-occlusive)

Congenital/Genetic
Arteriovenous malformations
Connective tissue diseases
  Ehlers-Danlos (aneurysms)
Abnormalities of coagulation

initial examinations, improve follow-up determinations of progress, and aid in the evaluation of interventional modalities.[5] Available instruments include the Rand Short Form 36,[317,318,346] the American Academy of Orthopaedic Surgeons Disabilities of the Arm, Shoulder, and Hand Outcomes Data Collection Instrument,[6] the McGill Pain Questionnaire,[228] the Carpal Tunnel Instrument,[192] and the McCabe Cold Sensitivity Severity Scale.[218] These instruments provide objective and reproducible quantitative assessments of the magnitude, duration, and frequency of symptoms and define the effects of vascular compromise on health-related quality of life.

Physical Examination

A complete physical examination of the hand includes an evaluation of the entire upper extremity and neck. An assessment should include the following evaluations: capillary refill; turgor; skin integrity, including the presence or absence of ulceration or gangrene; documentation of the presence of fungal infestation of the nails; and quality of the peripheral

pulse. Nail folds may be examined for evidence of collagen vascular disease or embolism with an ophthalmoscope[210] or epi-illumination microscope.[176] The presence of masses and/or bruits is determined by palpation or auscultation. An Allen test at the wrist and/or proximal phalanges provides information regarding arterial perfusion patterns and may identify occlusive disease (Fig. 64-2).[3] An objective assessment of collateral circulation can be obtained by capillary refill time, plethysmographic tracings, or pulse volume measurement after release of the patent vessel[110] (see Fig. 64-2; Table 64-3).

If occlusion or embolism is suspected, the physical examination is augmented by an evaluation of vascular perfusion using a hand-held ultrasound Doppler instrument. Careful ultrasound Doppler mapping can identify area(s) of occlusion or compromise and may provide an assessment of collateral flow (Fig. 64-3). Sequential occlusion of the radial

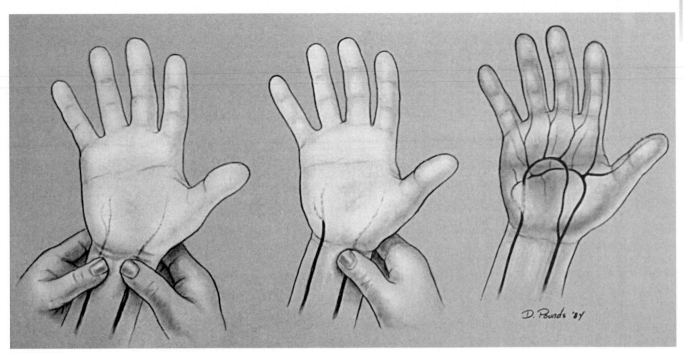

FIGURE 64-2. The Allen test is represented schematically. Blood is exsanguinated from the hand, and both the radial and ulnar arteries are compressed (**left**). After release of the ulnar artery (**middle**), no blood flow passes through the occluded artery, and the palm remains pale. With release of the radial artery (**right**), the entire hand will fill rapidly through the radial artery if the arch is complete. The order of the testing maneuvers can be reversed to test the radial artery in a similar fashion. The test is best described as demonstrating flow or no flow through a specific artery. (From Koman LA: Diagnostic study of vascular lesions. Hand Clin 1:217-231, 1985, with permission.)

Table 64-3
DIRECT VASCULAR EVALUATION

Test Measured	Anatomic Structure	Functional Performance	Primary Component of Flow
Digital plethysmography	0	+ + ½	Total flow
Segmental arterial pressure	+	+ +	Total flow
Real-time ultrasonography	+ + ½	+	Total flow
Doppler perfusion imaging	+	+ +	Thermoregulatory (total flow)
Laser Doppler fluxmetry	0	+ +	Nutritional and thermoregulatory
Duplex Doppler	+ +	+ +	Total flow
Skin surface temperature	0	+ +	Total flow
Vital capillaroscopy	+ + +	0	Nutritional flow
Technetium 99m	+	+ +	Total flow
Magnetic resonance angiography	+ +	+	Total flow
Arteriography	+ + +	+	Total flow

+ = fair; + + = good; + + + = excellent; 0 = not applicable.

and ulnar artery while monitoring distal flow with a Doppler ultrasound probe delineates the source of arterial inflow or the presence of collateral channels.

Diagnostic Testing and Evaluation
A noninvasive, or nonsurgical, minimally invasive vascular evaluation includes (1) Doppler ultrasound or pulse echo ultrasonography, (2) digital plethysmography (pulse volume recording [PVR]), (3) segmental arterial pressures, (4) color duplex imaging (CDI), (5) laser Doppler perfusion imaging (LDPI), (6) laser Doppler fluxmetry (LDF) measurements, (7) skin surface temperature measurements, (8) vital capil-

laroscopy, (9) technetium-99m three-phase bone scanning, (10) magnetic resonance angiography (MRA), and (11) contrast angiography. *An evaluation of vascular competency should define vascular structure and function under stressed and nonstressed conditions.* Therefore, a combination of vascular studies may be necessary to perform a comprehensive evaluation[161,176,295,335] (Table 64-3).

Ultrasound
Doppler ultrasound and pulse echo ultrasound use sound waves to evaluate vascular perfusion and/or anatomy. Doppler ultrasound analyzes variations in the ultrasound

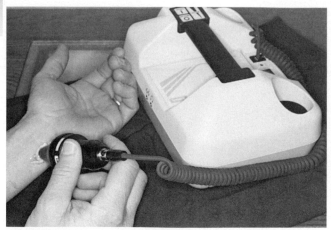

FIGURE 64-3. A hand-held Doppler probe provides an audible evaluation of vascular perfusion. (From Koman LA [ed]: Bowman Gray School of Medicine Orthopaedic Manual. Wake Forest University Orthopaedic Press, Winston-Salem, NC, 1997, with permission.)

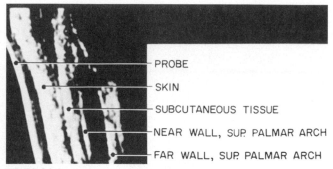

FIGURE 64-4. Ultrasonic B-mode imaging of the distal ulnar artery and superficial arch. During dynamic imaging, movement of the near and far wall may be observed from diastole to systole. (From Koman LA, Urbaniak JR: Ulnar artery thrombosis. Hand Clin 1:311-325, 1985, with permission.)

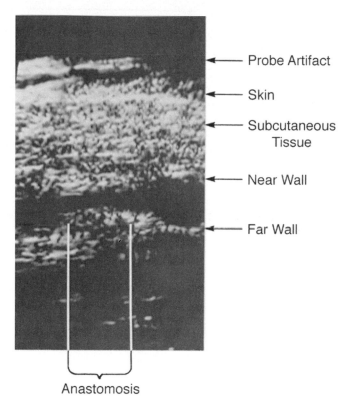

FIGURE 64-5. Longitudinal static image obtained during B-mode ultrasonography demonstrating the anastomotic site after end-to-end repair of an ulnar artery. The narrowing at the anastomotic site is visible. (From Koman LA, Bond MG, Carter RE, et al: Evaluation of the upper extremity vasculature with high-resolution ultrasound. J Hand Surg 10A:249-255, 1985, with permission.)

frequency (wavelength) produced when sound generated from a piezoelectric crystal is reflected by moving red blood cells.[322,323] The strength or loudness of the audible signal depends on beam placement in relationship to midstream flow. The pitch of the signal depends on the velocity of the moving red blood cells, as well as beam placement. However, with this technique velocity does not equal flow, because the cross-sectional area of the vessel must also be known in addition to blood flow velocity.[322,323]

Continuous-wave Doppler units contain a sending and receiving crystal, and pulsed Doppler units contain one crystal for both functions. Both types of units allow the differentiation of arterial from venous signals, permit an assessment of normal pulsatile or triphasic flow from monophasic flow, and facilitate the mapping of vascular channels.[37] Doppler ultrasound provides dynamic flow information and permits the identification of areas of abnormal flow characteristics.

Pulse echo ultrasonography uses sound "echo" to generate a two-dimensional image of deep structures. "B-mode," or "brightness mode," is the most common technique used clinically. Rapid pulse sequences allow real-time visualization of moving vessels, provide estimates of wall thickness and lumen diameter during diastole and systole, document postoperative intraluminal changes, and aid in arterial cannulation[171,181,237] (Figs. 64-4 and 64-5).

Digital Plethysmography (Pulse Volume Recordings)

Plethysmography, from the Greek *plethys* or "full," is a technique that quantitates flow by the analysis of limb or digit volume change.[276,290,342] Volume changes may be assessed by strain gauges (e.g., mercury in rubber), impedance sensors, air-filled cuffs, or photosensors.[37,321] Air-filled cuffs connected to pressure transducers and photoplethysmographs are used most commonly in clinical practice. PVRs demonstrate arterial compliance and vascular perfusion through analogue tracings. Plethysmography of normal arteries produces triphasic patterns, whereas vessels compromised by occlusive disease or stenosis demonstrate characteristic flow dynamics documented by plethysmographic tracings (Fig. 64-6).[37,166]

PVRs have been used (1) to detect vaso-occlusive disease, (2) to differentiate vasospastic from vaso-occlusive disease,[327] (3) to diagnose radial or ulnar artery occlusion,[165,181] (4) to predict the results of surgical sympathectomy,[350,351] (5) to study the effects of drug interventions or medical management,[166,327] and (6) as a research tool.[165,166]

PVRs are noninvasive, reproducible, and inexpensive. Valuable vascular information is available when PVRs are used in conjunction with clinical data and data from other studies. Although limited in the localization of subclavian

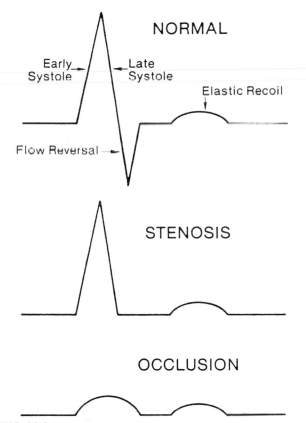

NORMAL

Early Systole ⟶   ⟵ Late Systole

Elastic Recoil ↓

Flow Reversal ⟶

STENOSIS

OCCLUSION

FIGURE 64-6. **Top,** The normal triphasic arterial wave pattern is schematically depicted. **Bottom,** The changes that occur with stenosis and occlusion are demonstrated. (From Koman LA: Diagnostic study of vascular lesion. Hand Clin 1:217-231, 1985, with permission.)

lesions, the dynamic information generated by PVRs complements static structural data from contrast arteriography. The differentiation of occlusive from vasospastic disease and the ability to define partial occlusions of hemodynamic significance that do not affect blood pressure support the diagnostic capability of this technique.[166]

Segmental Arterial Pressure

Segmental pressures are obtained by combining occlusive cuffs and Doppler units to obtain systolic blood pressure measurements.[37] Pressure patterns and ratios can be obtained and compared between levels. Thus, a radial-brachial index (RBI) and a digital-brachial index (DBI) can be calculated. A DBI or RBI of 0.7 or less indicates that arterial flow to the hand or digit is inadequate and supports medical and/or surgical intervention.[360] A DBI greater than 0.7 suggests adequate vascular flow. Heavily calcified vessels such as those seen in patients with diabetes may produce falsely high pressures.[351,360]

Color Duplex Imaging

Color duplex imaging (CDI) accurately demonstrates thrombosis in large vessels and is routinely used to examine carotid arteries and evaluate veins for thrombosis.[100,143] The technique combines ultrasound imaging techniques and color-coded Doppler evaluation. In the upper extremity, indications for this imaging technique include evaluation of

masses, identification of perfusion abnormalities, determination of anomalous vasculature, and postoperative evaluation and/or monitoring.[292,301,332] CDI is advocated for the discrimination of ganglia from aneurysms or pseudoaneurysms.[143] Although it provides less anatomic information than the "gold standard" of arteriography and venography, the advantages of this technique include lower cost, no radiation exposure, complete noninvasiveness, repeatability, and dynamic acquisition of flow data and characteristics.[75,100,320]

Skin Surface Temperature

Digital skin temperature measurements provide estimates of total digital blood flow.[58,59] Because the hands have minimal muscle mass, heat produced from metabolic activity is negligible. Digital skin blood flow is proportional to the skin surface temperature at temperatures below 30° C. At higher temperatures, skin blood flow rises disproportionately to temperature, with large volumes of flow shunted through arteriovenous anastomoses. At temperatures between 20° C and 30° C there is a direct, nearly linear correlation between blood flow and skin temperature, and therefore digital cutaneous temperature is indicative of and proportional to total flow. *Care must be taken to avoid overinterpreting isolated temperature data.* Digital temperature measurements cannot evaluate rapid fluctuations in digital perfusion or differentiate between the thermoregulatory and nutritional components of blood flow. The evaluation of digital temperatures, especially when monitored in response to stress, provides objective evidence of autonomic performance.[253]

Thermography

Thermography techniques accurately measure skin surface temperatures over large areas (accurate to 0.1° C). Thermographic images provide large quantities of data, permit the simultaneous comparison of both extremities, and are capable of capturing sequential and timed responses to interventions. However, isolated temperature data generated by thermographic techniques are subject to the same limitations as small surface temperature probes and, without the use of a physiologic stressor, are not reproducible. Interpretation of thermographic data must be tempered by the knowledge that (1) there is normally heterogeneity of vascular perfusion through hand skin surfaces, (2) microvascular perfusion on the palmar and dorsal surfaces is not normally symmetrical, (3) temperature readings greater than 30° C are not directly related to perfusion, (4) repeated measures over time of the same areas or contralateral areas require the use of a stress maneuver to ensure reproducible results, and (5) large volumes of data do not increase the significance or validity of an observation.[176,345]

Laser Doppler Fluxmetry

Laser Doppler fluxmetry evaluates cutaneous microvascular perfusion with good temporal resolution. LDF measurements are restricted to evaluating the motion of blood cells in the area directly beneath the probe. The depth that laser light penetrates is dependent on the wavelength of coherent light and the configuration of the fiberoptic fibers, the ability of the laser light to penetrate the tissue, and the thickness of the stratum corneum. The thickness of the stratum corneum affects what vessels are evaluated (i.e., thin-skinned areas are evaluated at a greater depth than vessels beneath thicker skin). Red blood cell motion within vascular beds is detected by the probe; the signal produced by the probe is analyzed by means of the Doppler shift in the wavelength, which is proportional to the average velocity and number of the red blood cells moving beneath the probe. This technique provides real-time, noninvasive measurement of cutaneous perfusion.[254]

Isolated Cold Stress Testing

Isolated cold stress testing (ICST) was developed to provide an evaluation of the response of the digital blood vessels to physiologic stress.[172,176,274] The stressor is provided by exposing the hands to moderately cool air (5° C to 8° C) by inserting the hands into a modified refrigeration unit. Digital temperatures and cutaneous perfusion are monitored before, during, and after application of the stress. To perform the test, thermistors are applied to the pulp of each digit. The thermistors are linked to a computer so that temperatures are sampled frequently (every 10 seconds) to monitor total flow.[172,176] An estimate of cutaneous perfusion and a direct observation of rapid fluctuations in flow are monitored by an LDF probe. The LDF probe is attached to one finger of each hand. The temperature and LDF data may then be analyzed by statistical methods or graphic analysis.[176,257,310]

With the use of moderately cold stress, ICST provides an evaluation of vasomotor and autonomic responses before, during, and after a controlled stress. In view of the limitations of the information about blood flow obtained from temperature measurements alone, simultaneous LDF adds important information and allows an assessment of microvascular function, vascular responsiveness and tone, and microvascular recovery.[176] Patients without morbid pathology may demonstrate *two normal* patterns of response[274] characterized by parallel temperature and laser Doppler responses.[274] Normal responses include cold and warm response patterns. Women are five times more likely than men to exhibit a cold response pattern characterized by a decrease in digit temperature and microvascular perfusion with cooling. The warm pattern shows little sympathetic modulation of vascular tone before, during, or after the hands are exposed to cold. The warm pattern is observed twice as often in men as in women[176,274] (Fig. 64-7).

Laser Doppler Perfusion Imaging

Laser Doppler perfusion imaging uses the Doppler principle to provide a microvascular perfusion profile of a defined area.[345] In contrast to standard LDF, the laser perfusion imager measures cutaneous perfusion over a 12 × 12-cm surface and produces a color-coded image or a gray-scale measure without requiring direct contact with the skin or tissue surface. An optical scanner controlled by stepping motors is positioned 15 cm over the measurement site, allowing up to 4096 discrete laser scans in a 12 × 12-cm area. Perfusion is measured at each site, and a final composite scan is produced by a computer and customized software. This technique assesses both thermoregulatory and nutritional components of flow, does not require direct contact of a probe with the patient to obtain a measurement, and provides a spatial distribution of cutaneous microvascular perfusion over a significant surface area. Studies using LDPI have demonstrated significant heterogeneity of perfusion in the palmar and dorsal surfaces of the hands and feet and significant variation between the right and left sides of the body[295,345] (Fig. 64-8). This technique permits an assessment of perfusion after surgical intervention.[30]

Vital Capillaroscopy

Vital capillaroscopy provides a noninvasive analysis of blood flow in nutritional papillary capillaries. The orientation of nail fold capillaries parallel to the skin surface provides the most direct approach to analysis; however, specialized systems allow an evaluation of the nutritional capillaries of other areas of the body.[27,90,91] Epi-illumination microscopy is used to evaluate the arterial and venous loops of the papillary capillaries with regard to static morphometry and dynamic flow characteristics (Fig. 64-9). The flow and morphology of nutritional vessels are analyzed by direct dynamic videophotometric capillaroscopy.[176,209] Specialized computer techniques provide measurements of capillary diameter, red blood cell velocity, and total flow.[90,176,264,265] The use of sodium fluorescein can provide additional information.[28] Because resting capillary blood flow varies widely among individuals, a dynamic intervention (stress) is required to assess blood flow response patterns and permit quantitative comparison. Stress may be induced by occlusion and reactive hyperemia[91,92] and by direct or indirect exposure to thermal (hot or cold) or psychological challenge.[176] Quantitative capillary analysis is difficult in 10% to 12% of subjects because individual capillary visibility is hampered by vessel orientation, length of the capillary loop, hyperkeratotic skin, or dense pigmentation.[209]

Currently, *dynamic capillary videomicroscopy is the only technique that permits direct assessment of nutritional perfusion.* No other technique allows direct assessment of nutritional flow, permits direct evaluation of the external arteriovenous shunting, or provides direct feedback on the microvascular effects of disease or medical interventions.[176] The technique is noninvasive, repeatable, and specific; repeated measures of a specific capillary loop(s) or capillary bed(s) provide a powerful analytic tool. Because the morphometry of individual capillaries of the skin normally does not change over many months, the same capillary can be studied over time.

Bone Scintigraphy

Radionuclide imaging (RI) or bone scintigraphy can be used to (1) provide a two-dimensional assessment of upper extremity vascular anatomy, (2) document spatial and temporal patterns of vascular distribution, and (3) quantify perfusion characteristics. The technique uses large field-of-view gamma scintillation cameras available in standard nuclear medicine facilities. The intravascular distribution of technetium-99m pertechnetate or diphosphonate after intravenous injection produces the radionuclide angiogram, the first phase of a "three-phase nuclear bone scan" (Fig. 64-10). In the second phase, or "blood pool image," sequential 3- to 5-second imaging periods over a 60- to 90-second period provide objective data outlining perfusion pathways and relative flow dynamics. The third phase is a standard delayed bone scan. Many vascular lesions have a "typical" radionuclide scan appearance.[138] Radionuclide imaging may be diagnostic in occlusive disease, aneurysms, and arteriovenous malformations (AVMs) (Fig. 64-11)[232]; may provide significant prognostic information after frostbite[227,297]

Subject: MA Left Hand 9/01/93

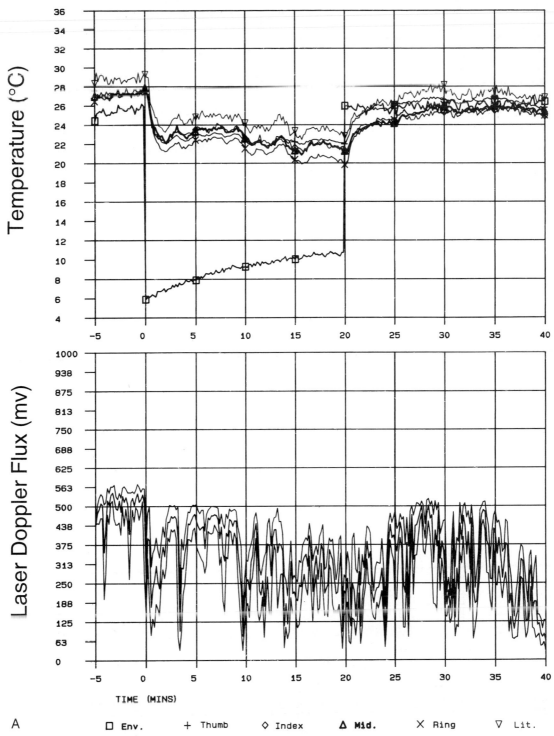

A □ Env. + Thumb ◇ Index △ **Mid.** ✕ Ring ▽ Lit.

FIGURE 64-7. Normal pattern of temperature *(top)* and laser Doppler *(bottom)* observed during isolated cold stress testing. Normal patterns include a warm response (**A**) and a cold response (**B**). (From Koman LA [ed]: Bowman Gray School of Medicine Orthopaedic Manual. Wake Forest University Orthopaedic Press, Winston-Salem, NC, 1997, with permission.)

Continued

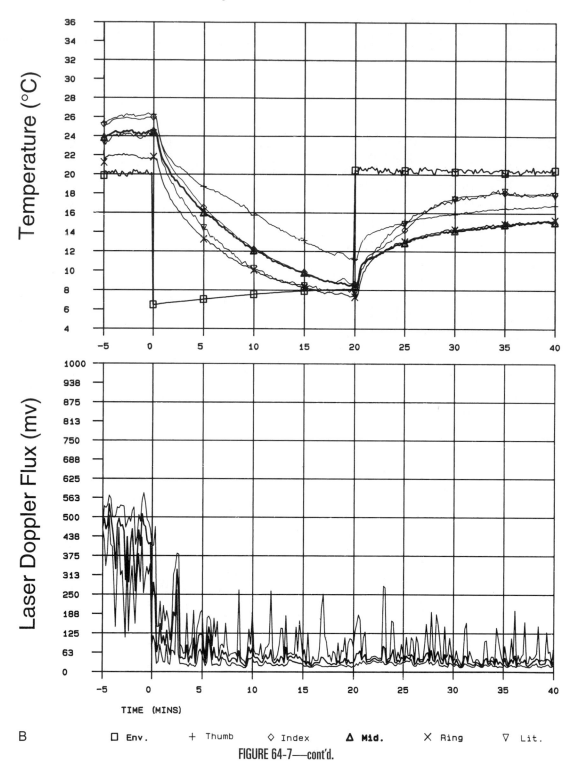

Subject LS: Left Hand 4/11/96

B   □ Env.   + Thumb   ◇ Index   ▲ **Mid.**   ✕ Ring   ▽ Lit.

FIGURE 64-7—cont'd.

or electrical injury; and may identify significant abnor-malitics in vasospastic conditions before the escalation of symptoms.[213,214] Radionuclide images provide specific diag-nostic information. Occlusive disease produces a sharp interruption of tracer flow with a delay in perfusion of distal sites, as judged by the appearance of radiotracer in sequen-tial frames. Collateral vessels may or may not be visualized, but the extent of radiotracer and the time delay of appear-ance provide a visual or quantitative estimate of perfusion. Quantitative information is available by using time-activity data. Absence of radiotracer activity distal to occlusive disease is a poor prognostic sign and portends ischemic

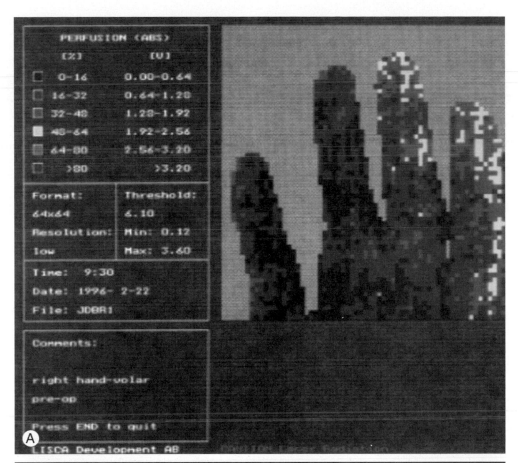

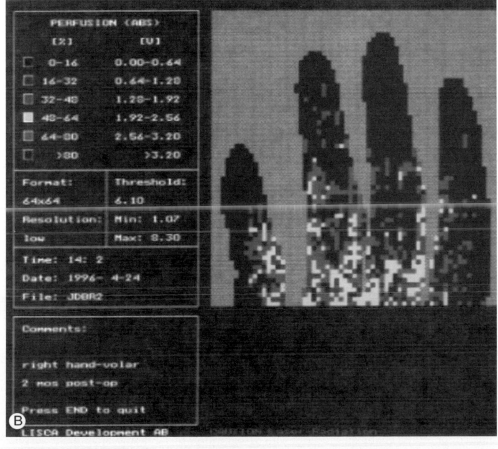

FIGURE 64-8. A, Laser Doppler perfusion image of a patient with a thrombosed ulnar artery and ischemia. Decreased flow is observed in the index, long, ring, and little fingers; the little and ring fingers demonstrate significantly less flow than the other digits. B, Postoperative laser Doppler perfusion image demonstrating increased perfusion throughout the hand. (From Koman LA [ed]: Bowman Gray School of Medicine Orthopaedic Manual. Wake Forest University Orthopaedic Press, Winston-Salem, NC, 1996, with permission.)

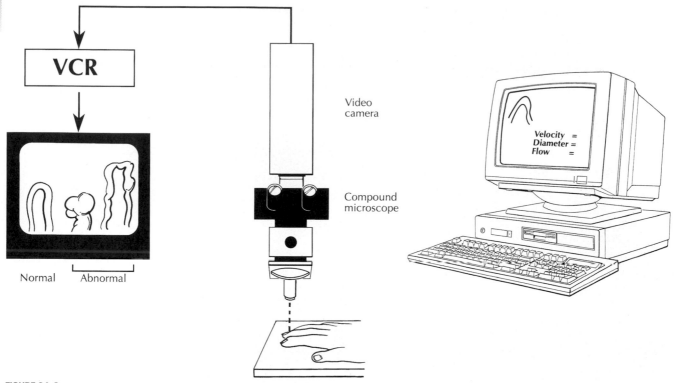

FIGURE 64-9. Vital capillaroscopy allows direct evaluation of cutaneous nutritional papillary capillaries and permits direct measurement of nutritional blood flow—a component of total digital blood flow. Abnormal capillary morphology may permit the diagnosis of systemic diseases. (From Koman LA [ed]: Bowman Gray School of Medicine Orthopaedic Manual. Wake Forest University Orthopaedic Press, Winston-Salem, NC, 1996, with permission.)

symptoms and possible necrosis. Conversely, rapid detection of radiotracer activity distal to vascular injury or occlusion confirms the presence of collateral flow. AVMs will often exhibit characteristic patterns that correlate with the extent of arterial, venous, arteriovenous, and/or capillary involvement.

Magnetic Resonance Angiography

Techniques of high-resolution magnetic resonance angiography (MRA) allow the visualization of upper extremity arterial and venous vascular structures.[67] Adequate image resolution requires surface coils and a mid- to high-field scanner with a large signal-to-noise ratio. Visualization is achieved by the use of "bright blood" spin-echo or "dark blood" gradient-echo techniques; intravenous gadolinium diethylenetriamine penta-acetic acid (DTPA) contrast enhancement is necessary for small vessels and/or low-flow states.[138] Fine detail requires specialized computer software with specific signal processing and the use of thin-slice data obtained by the suppression of nonvascular tissue signals.[138] Useful image production demands the conversion of 1.5- to 2.5-mm axis signals to produce a projection angiogram of arterial (Fig. 64-12) or venous structures. Two-dimensional and three-dimensional phase-contrast techniques permit imaging in low-flow states and the acquisition of velocity and volume (flow) data and directional information.[46,71] When compared with cut film arteriography or digital subtraction techniques, MRA produces no ionizing radiation, cannot initiate allergic reactions because the technique does not require the injection of iodinated or other contrast agents, eliminates remote side effects, diminishes study-

induced vasospasm, provides imaging through radiodense casts or splints, and does not require arterial catheters or injections.[74] Conventional radiographic techniques currently provide more detailed data, produce higher resolution, are available in more locations, do not require sophisticated computer and personnel support, and are less likely to produce claustrophobia. The use of MRA continues to evolve and the use of gadolinium-enhanced elliptically recorded three-dimensional pulse sequence MRA demonstrates good correlation with ulnar and radial occlusion and can identify embolic events.[354]

Contrast Angiography

Arteriography. Contrast arteriography provides the best anatomic detail and structural information on upper extremity vasculature and remains the "gold standard" in the static evaluation of extremity vasculature. Since the technique was introduced by Seldinger in 1953, there have been significant refinements in contrast material, equipment, and imaging devices.[304] Computed digital imaging combined with subtraction techniques enhances images and requires the use of less contrast material (Figs. 64-11 and 64-13). Rapid image sequences provide dynamic information with respect to flow direction, source of collateral flow, the degree and presence of retrograde vessel filling, and venous outflow. Information is optimized by the use of (1) new isosmolar contrast agents; (2) intra-arterial vasodilators (e.g., tolazoline [Priscolene]); (3) femoral access with visualization of the aortic arch, great vessels, and brachial artery; (4) subtraction techniques that minimize

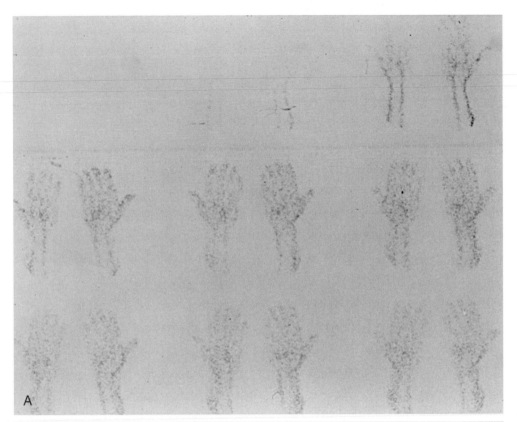

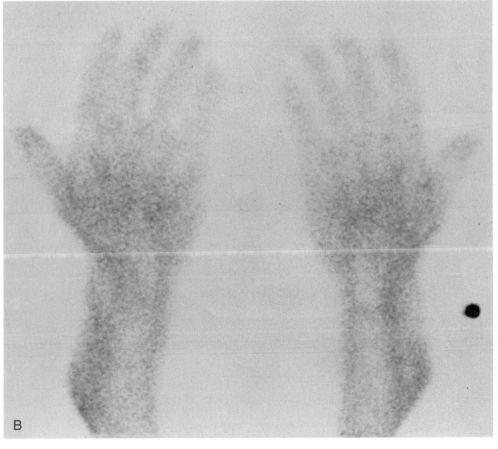

FIGURE 64-10. The first two phases of a three-phase bone scan reflect vascular perfusion. During the dynamic phase (**A**), images represent radio tracer accumulated over 3- to 5-second intervals. Visual representation of arterial flow is possible. The "blood pool" image (**B**) demonstrates and quantifies the accumulation of radiotracer during a fixed period of time (usually 60 to 180 seconds). Soft tissue perfusion of the entire hand or specific areas may be evaluated. (From Koman LA [ed]: Bowman Gray School of Medicine Orthopaedic Manual. Wake Forest University Orthopaedic Press, Winston-Salem, NC, 1996, with permission.)

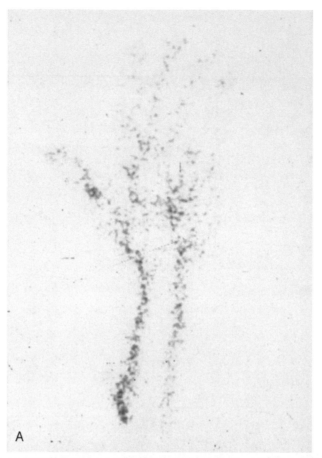

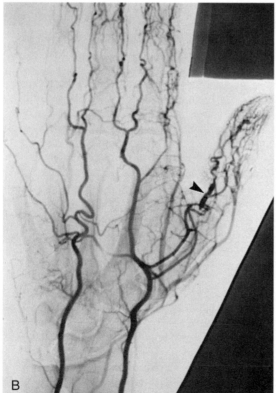

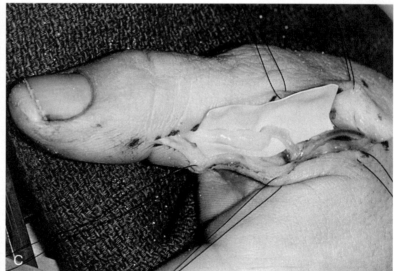

FIGURE 64-11. Radionuclide scan (**A**) demonstrating increased uptake by an aneurysm in the princeps pollicis artery of the right thumb. Arteriogram (**B**) and clinical photograph (**C**) showing the lesion *(arrowhead in **B**)* producing an abnormal bone scan. (From Koman LA [ed]: Bowman Gray School of Medicine Orthopaedic Manual. Wake Forest University Orthopaedic Press, Winston-Salem, NC, 1997, with permission.)

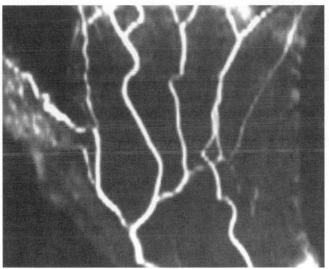

FIGURE 64-12. Magnetic resonance angiography demonstrating arterial structures. (From Holder LE, et al: Nuclear medicine, contrast angiography, and magnetic resonance imaging for evaluating vascular problems in the hand. Hand Clin 9:85-113, 1993, with permission.)

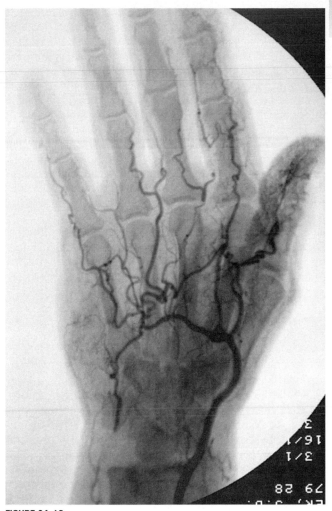

FIGURE 64-13. Arteriogram demonstrating occlusive disease involving the superficial common arch and the origins of the common digital vessels. Multiple occlusive (thrombosed) areas throughout the digits are visible. (From Koman LA [ed]: Bowman Gray School of Medicine Orthopaedic Manual. Wake Forest University Orthopaedic Press, Winston-Salem, NC, 1997, with permission.)

background and bone shadow interference; and (5) close communication with the radiologist before and, if necessary, during the procedure.[277] *The value of communication cannot be overstated*; maximum information requires clinical input and studies designed to answer specific questions. Potential problems, concerns, and complications associated with arteriography include (1) injury to the artery at the injection site, (2) dislodgement of emboli, (3) catheter-induced vasospasm, (4) failure to visualize distal arterial reconstruction because of vasospasm, (5) allergic reaction to contrast agents, and (6) inadequate visualization of "superficial" radial and/or ulnar vessels. *Although there are multiple normal variations of palmar circulation, all normal patients have three common volar digital arteries at the level of the metacarpophalangeal joint.*

Closed-System Venography

The evaluation of AVMs may be enhanced by the use of closed-system venography, in which venous injection of contrast agents is performed distal to a proximal tourniquet. Although venous data are available in later phases of contrast cut film arteriography, direct venous injection may be necessary to delineate the full extent of predominantly venous and/or capillary AVMs.[108]

Importance of Stress. The use of stress in the evaluation of upper extremity vascular perfusion is necessary to determine functional performance capacity and capability. Stress may be necessary to define the adequacy of collateral flow after occlusive disease and is often diagnostic in elucidating functional microcirculatory dynamics and flow characteristics in vasospastic conditions. A complete evaluation of vascular function requires analysis of flow before, during, and after a controlled and repeatable stress. The type of stress used can vary and can include thermal (heat or cold), anoxic (tourniquet), or emotional. Analysis of flow should include an assessment of total flow as well as its thermoregulatory and nutritional components.[91,92,176]

Authors' Preferred Approach

The goal of diagnostic testing is to determine the *structural* configuration of upper extremity vasculature and the *functional* capability of the system to respond to stress. Patient-oriented management requires an understanding of both the anatomy and function of the vascular system. Physical examination, wrist and digital Allen testing, and hand-held Doppler mapping are used to guide additional testing. Digital blood pressure is measured, and a DBI or radial/ulnar brachial index is calculated. Appropriate tests then are chosen to delineate structural abnormalities, determine the quality of the collateral circulation, and define the functional integrity of the extremity. Structural and anatomic details are defined by using B-mode ultrasonography and contrast arteriography. For complex vascular disorders, the definitive structural detail provided by arteriography remains the gold standard in the majority of instances.

However, surgical exploration after noninvasive testing is appropriate.[166,350] Evaluation of functional control requires exposure of the patient to a stressor. We prefer ICST and the use of digital temperature and LDF measurements to assess functional control. Because these modalities are not available universally, any technique that provides rapid responses to stress (verbal, thermal, hypoxic) will provide valuable information and facilitate decision making (Table 64-3).

The goal of our diagnostic testing is to (1) determine the appropriateness of vascular control; (2) assess the extent and type of vessel abnormality in terms of thrombosis, embolism, and/or aneurysm; (3) define the quality and quantity of collateral vessels; and (4) evaluate distal vessel reconstitution or patency. *The DBI is important. If the DBI is less than or equal to 0.7, vascular reconstruction should be performed if possible and the risk-benefit is justified. Optimal preoperative evaluation of structural damage and the adequacy of distal patency (run-off) may be assessed by arteriography, MRA, or ultrasound techniques.*

Anatomy and Physiology

Vascular networks in the upper extremity (1) deliver metabolic and nutritional requirements to cellular structures, (2) clear metabolic waste, and (3) contribute to the maintenance of core body temperature. Upper extremity symptoms occur secondary to the failure of vascular structural integrity or because of functional inadequacies. Critical arterial insufficiency produces cell death and tissue necrosis. However, the majority of pathologic vascular events are subcritical and produce symptoms and functional compromise without gangrene. Vascular compromise may result from insult(s) to anatomic structure(s) or physiologic control mechanism(s). The ability of the vascular supply to respond appropriately to stress is defined as *vascular competency* (see Table 64-1) and depends on vascular anatomy, vasomotor tone, systemic factors, and end-organ metabolic requirements.

Vascular insufficiency, synonymous with vascular incompetency, is defined as arterial inflow inadequate to maintain cellular metabolism and occurs (1) if perfusion is inadequate because of structural abnormality (e.g., critical brachial artery injury) and/or (2) if the vascular system is controlled inappropriately (e.g., vasospasm secondary to collagen vascular disease). *Vascular competency* requires appropriate volume and distribution of blood flow during stressed and nonstressed conditions and adequate nutritional perfusion for normal cellular function.

Arterial Anatomy

In the majority of extremities, parallel and interconnected arteries provide a collateral blood supply to the hand via the radial and ulnar arteries.[13] "Superficial" radial or ulnar arteries originate in the brachium (arm) rather than arising from the classic origin within the proximal forearm.[139] Failure to recognize this anatomic variation during testing (e.g., arteriography) or surgical exploration may confound the diagnosis. In most patients, the major blood supply to the hand is provided via the *superficial palmar arch* (i.e., the

continuation of the ulnar artery) and the *deep palmar arch* (i.e., the continuation of the radial artery). However, a large median or interosseous artery may also be present (Fig. 64-14). In a study of 120 normal subjects, 57% of radial arteries provided dominant flow to three or more digits. The ulnar artery and superficial arch supplied three or more digits in 21.5% of hands; flow from radial and ulnar vessels was equal in 21.5% of extremities.[165] The deep palmar arch or superficial palmar arch is defined as *complete* if there is a significant connection to a branch from another independent arterial limb. The superficial palmar arch is *"completed"* by branches from the deep palmar arch, the radial artery, or the median artery in 78.5% of extremities and is *incomplete* in 21.5% of hands.[54] The deep palmar arch is less variable and is completed by the superior deep branch of the ulnar artery, the inferior deep branch of the ulnar artery, or both in 98.5% of extremities (see Fig. 64-14).[54] In the majority of extremities (86% to 98.5%), all five digits receive arterial inflow at the level of the proper digital artery or the common digital artery from both the deep and superficial arches.[54,80,81] Collateral flow between the radial and ulnar systems exists in a myriad of anatomic configurations.[54,80,81,186] However, *all reported variations of arterial anatomy include the presence of three palmar common digital arteries at the level of the metacarpophalangeal joint*[54,80,179,268] (see Fig. 64-14). This observation simplifies the differentiation of pathologic events from normal anatomic variants, which should include a minimum of three palmar common digital vessels.[181]

In general, digital perfusion occurs through a dual blood supply via the radial and ulnar proper digital vessels. In most hands, the proper digital vessels of the radial aspect of the thumb and index finger and the ulnar aspect of the little finger are smaller than the parallel proper digital artery.[13] The diameter of the ulnar digital vessels in the thumb, index, and long fingers is greater than that of the parallel radial vessels; in the ring and small finger, the radial digital vessels are slightly larger.[332] The majority of the multiple branches and interconnections that occur throughout the digit are located in superficial areas close to the skin surfaces.[57,59] Large numbers of vessels are clustered within the digital pulp.[118]

The vascular anatomy of the thumb is variable from the radial artery, deep arch, and/or superficial arch. In the classic pattern, the palmar blood supply to the thumb arises from the first of the four palmar metacarpal arteries, which is commonly designated the "princeps pollicis" artery.[49,54,241] The "radialis indicis," a vessel that supplies the radial aspect of the index, originates from either the princeps pollicis or the deep arch. Before passing through an arcade formed within the first dorsal interosseous muscle, the radial artery gives rise to the large dorsal artery of the thumb, which passes distally to supply the digit. The princeps pollicis may arise from the first dorsal metacarpal artery, the deep arch, the first palmar metacarpal artery, or the terminal branch of the superficial palmar arch.[145,241] There are consistently four vessels that supply the thumb: the palmar ulnar, palmar radial, dorsal ulnar, and dorsal radial arteries.[145]

Microvascular Beds

The microvascular components of distal extremity circulation are defined as vessels less than 100 μm in diameter.

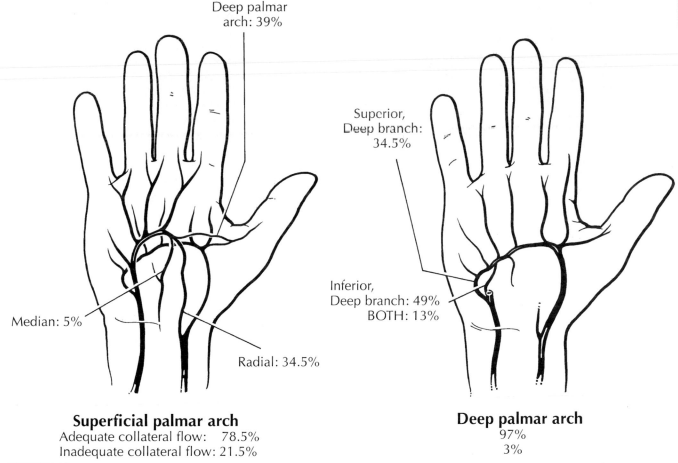

FIGURE 64-14. The superficial palmar arch is completed by branches from the deep palmar arch, radial artery, or median artery in 78.5% of patients; the remaining 21.5% are "incomplete." The deep palmar arch is completed by the superior branch of the ulnar artery, the inferior branch of the ulnar artery, or both in 98.5% of patients. (Modified from Koman LA, Urbaniak JR: Ulnar artery thrombosis, pp 75-83. *In* Brunelli G (ed): Textbook of Microsurgery. Milan, Masson, 1988, with permission.)

Microvascular functions are to (1) deliver nutrients to microvascular beds, (2) provide adequate capacity for arteriovenous thermoregulatory flow, and (3) drain nutritional and thermoregulatory beds. The capacity of the collective microcirculation is considerable, and large fluctuations in its volume are common (Fig. 64-15).

The 100-μm and smaller vessels that constitute the microcirculation deliver oxygen, provide nutrients, and clear metabolic waste at a cellular level. Under normal circumstances, nutritional flow is relatively constant; however, significant fluctuations in total flow can occur and are accomplished by the regulation of blood flow through thermoregulatory arteriovenous anastomoses. Human digit skin microcirculation is composed of *nutritional* papillary capillary beds and non-nutritional *thermoregulatory* vessels.[80] Distribution of flow between and within these beds varies by anatomic region. However, under normal conditions in the digits, 80% to 90% of the total flow passes through thermoregulatory beds and the remainder flows through nutritional capillaries (see Fig. 64-15).[57,59,92] Under normal conditions, the majority of total flow is involved in thermoregulation. In pathologic states, the cellular hypoperfusion that produces symptoms and/or permanent injury may be secondary to decreased total flow, abnormal distri-

bution of the nutritional and thermoregulatory components of flow, or both. After arterial occlusion, total flow may be reduced to critical levels and flow redistribution into nutritional beds may be necessary to avoid cell injury or death. In the presence of severely diminished total flow and excessive microvascular distribution into non-nutritional thermoregulatory beds, cell death or damage may occur despite the presence of "potential flow" adequate to sustain cellular viability. Therefore, in many vascular disorders, distribution of the components of total flow may vary from expected norms and may cause and/or contribute to the clinical problem.

Venous Anatomy

There is a rich venous network that includes superficial dorsal and volar arteries and deeper veins paralleling arteries and arterioles. The basilic and cephalic vessels are the largest named vessels. In addition, a rich subdermal plexus is capable of sustaining venous return and is involved in thermoregulation.

Control Mechanisms

In normal extremities, blood flow in the hands and digits depends on sympathetic tone, metabolic demand(s), environmental event(s), local factors, and circulating humoral

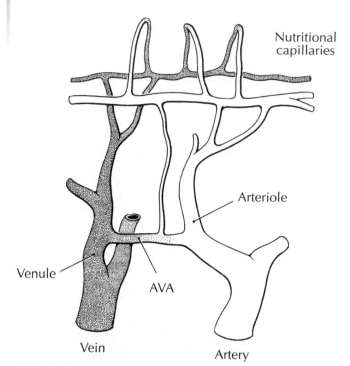

FIGURE 64-15. Schematic diagram of a microvascular bed from the skin surface. Nutritional perfusion occurs in papillary capillaries and is dependent on appropriate arteriovenous shunting. Excessive shunting through arteriovenous anastomosis (AVA) prevents or limits nutritional flow. (From Koman LA [ed]: Bowman Gray School of Medicine Orthopaedic Manual. Wake Forest University Orthopaedic Press, Winston-Salem, NC, 1997, with permission.)

mediators.[128,129] Digital circulation is controlled by locally released or circulating metabolites and mediators that induce vasoconstriction or vasodilatation. Vasoconstriction is controlled predominantly by α-adrenergic neurotransmitters,[1,58,59,128,129,252,289,338] and vasodilatation, which until recently was considered a passive phenomenon, is initiated by a variety of compounds (e.g., nitric oxide).[73,86,97,104,125,182,242] Active vasoconstriction and vasodilatation may be initiated by *central control processes* mediated through peripheral neural structures (e.g., autonomic nervous system) or circulatory factors (e.g., hormones) or by *local autoregulation*, which may be *metabolic* and/or *myogenic*.

Adrenergic neurotransmitters (agonists) and/or vasoactive compounds stimulate the constriction or dilation of vascular smooth muscle. Adrenergic receptors include subtypes that act presynaptically and postsynaptically (Fig. 64-16). Receptor subtypes (α_1 and α_2) are distributed along vascular channels based on vessel size and function. In general, the ratio of α_1 to α_2 receptors decreases as vessels become smaller. Postsynaptic α_1 and α_2 receptors cause vasoconstriction when stimulated. Presynaptic α_2-receptor stimulation decreases or moderates vasoconstriction by inhibiting norepinephrine release from the nerve terminal. Circulating factors contribute to both vasoconstriction and vasodilatation, and there is evidence that non-neural β-adrenergic vasodilators exist.[99] Active vasodilatation is mediated through mechanisms that include nitric oxide.

On a local level, *metabolic* and *myogenic autoregulation* affects vascular tone and microvascular perfusion. Under normal circumstances, microvascular nutritional perfusion matches metabolic needs. Local metabolites and factors

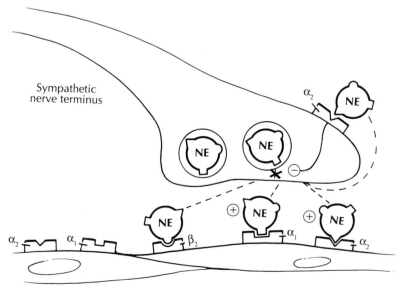

FIGURE 64-16. Sympathetic nerve terminals release norepinephrine (NE) and produce vasoconstriction via postsynaptic α_1 and α_2 receptors or inhibit NE release via presynaptic α_2 receptors. Stimulation of postsynaptic β_2 receptors relaxes vascular smooth muscles. (From Koman LA, Smith BP, Smith TL: Stress testing in the evaluation of upper extremity perfusion. Hand Clin 9:59-83, 1993, with permission.)

produce specific effects on different microvascular beds.[282] Metabolic autoregulation occurs in response to local metabolic needs and is mediated by decreased oxygen levels and the buildup of adenosine and potassium.[282] When nutrients are required to prevent cell death or provide energy, metabolic autoregulation responds by opening flow into nutritional channels. In the presence of diminished metabolic demands, constriction of microvascular beds redistributes flow away from nutritional microvessels. Simultaneously, myogenic autoregulation adjusts arterial caliber to maintain appropriate microvascular pressure during transient changes in systemic arterial pressure. Myogenic autoregulation is mediated via transmural pressure and stretch-operated calcium channels.[89,134,263]

Normal microcirculatory flow in the digits is cyclic, with increasing and decreasing perfusion determined, in part, by environmental temperature.[21,39,52,129,248,249,353] Blood flow characteristics are affected by basal autonomic tone, systemic blood pressure, and autoregulation.[89] For example, arterioles constrict reflexively and wall tension is returned to its predilation state if arteriolar wall tension increases secondary to an increase in transmural pressure. Myogenic autoregulation of the skin microcirculation limits the cutaneous perfusion changes accompanying postural change and minimizes edema secondary to limb dependency.[282]

The microcirculation is also affected by endothelial factors within the blood vessels. Once, the endothelium was thought to be a passive layer of cells lining the blood vessels that facilitated smooth, nonturbulent flow. Now the endothelium is recognized as an active tissue responsible for elaborating both vasodilatory and vasoconstrictor substances. *Nitric oxide,* an endothelium-derived relaxing factor, produces active vasodilatation, and *endothelin,* also produced by the vascular endothelium, is a potent vasoconstrictor. Both compounds are released from vascular endothelial cells to regulate vascular flow, and inappropriate balance of these compounds may induce pathologic conditions.

Peripheral nerve function is important for microvascular control, and normal perfusion requires intact and functioning peripheral nerves. Sympathetic nerve fibers accompanying vascular channels innervate the vessels in the forearm and hand and penetrate the arterial and venous walls after traveling in perivascular tissue.[236] Peripheral sympathetic fibers are predominantly unmyelinated (group C fibers) and travel variable distances within peripheral nerves before pursuing a perivascular route.[273] In the hand and digits, common and proper digital nerves have sympathetic fibers that connect to correspondingly sized vessels. Neural tissue, which is composed predominantly of sympathetic fibers, accompanies most arteries. The nerve of Henle, the sympathetic arterial branch accompanying the ulnar artery, supplies several large segments to the ulnar artery during its course from the forearm to the hand.[273] Resection of sympathetic nerve branches to vessels combined with periadventitial dissection of ascending and descending nerve branches within perivascular tissue reduces vasoconstrictor tone. This nerve disruption is the basis for peripheral sympathectomy for managing vasospastic disease.[82,95,175,236,351]

In vasospastic disorders, abnormal vascular control may be secondary to (1) abnormal vascular (receptor) responsiveness to agonists and/or antagonists, (2) receptor upregulation, (3) abnormal receptor subtype distribution throughout the microcirculation, (4) inappropriate vasodilator/vasoconstrictor mechanisms mediated through nitric oxide, (5) aberrant myogenic and metabolic control mechanisms, and/or (6) the presence of increased local vasoactive metabolites.[51,236]

Historical Review

- William Hunter (1704): ligation of artery proximal to aneurysm (popliteal); described traumatic aneurysm
- Von Winiwarber (1879): description of thromboangiitis obliterans
- Mata (1888): endoaneurysmorrhaphy
- Murphy (1905): resection of cervical ribs for brachial artery impingement
- Leriche (1937): sympathectomy as an effect of excision and ligation of an artery
- Korean conflict (1952): demonstration of successful arterial repairs
- Allen (1962): description of Allen test
- Kleinert (1965): revascularization of superficial palmar arch
- Flatt (1980): digital artery sympathectomy
- Koman (1995): palmar and wrist sympathectomy for secondary Raynaud's phenomenon

Types of Operations and Treatment

Operative options for vascular disorders depend on the underlying pathology and include ligation and resection, primary repair, reversal interposition vein grafting, nonreversed or in-situ vein grafting and valve incision, arterial grafting, bypass grafting, arteriovenous reversal, and sympathectomy. These techniques are discussed in detail in the following sections.

ACUTE VASCULAR INJURY: ARTERIAL

Acute vascular injury may occur during blunt (closed) or penetrating (open) extremity trauma or from iatrogenic injury. Crush injuries after blunt trauma and/or secondary to fracture-dislocation are less common causes of vascular injury but may affect the arterial and venous system. Upper extremity arterial trauma represents 30% to 50% of all peripheral vascular injuries. The majority of these injuries involve the brachial artery, with 90% penetrating injuries.[142] The onset of symptoms and signs of acute vascular injury may be delayed as the combination of swelling, hypotension, and intimal injury combine to cause late thrombosis and vascular insufficiency. Traumatic insults associated with severe crushing may cause thrombosis, hemorrhage, and/or incomplete vessel injury with the development of aneurysm(s), compartment syndrome(s), progressive thrombosis, and distal embolization.[19] Whereas the diagnosis of significant arterial and/or venous injuries secondary to traumatic lacerations is often obvious, vascular injuries after penetrating trauma may be insidious and, therefore, present management dilemmas.[288] Innocuous entry wounds can mask significant arterial injuries and thus make distal assessment of perfusion a critical aspect of patient evaluation. Management of acute vascular injuries requires (1) an understanding of the physiology of symptoms associated with vascular trauma; (2) a thorough knowledge of the pertinent vascular anatomy; (3) an assessment of associated soft tissue, osseous, and neural injury; and (4) an appreciation of the natural history of the treated and untreated injury.[22]

Preoperative Evaluation

History

Evaluation of acute trauma in the upper extremity requires a high index of suspicion. Vascular compromise may occur after fractures or in the presence of innocuous wounds. After penetrating trauma, there is usually a history of external bleeding, which may result in hypotension.[189] In a series of 66 patients with upper extremity arterial injuries, 62% had a history of profuse external bleeding and 18% were hypotensive.[189] Physical findings include expanding or pulsatile hematomas, thrills, bruits, and decreased peripheral pulse.[189] The presence of a bruit or thrill, absent arterial pulses, hypotension, and associated neurologic deficits correlate highly with arterial injury.[230]

Examination

The presence of a distal pulse is not a reliable assessment in the evaluation of vascular integrity. Peripheral pulses are palpable in approximately one fourth of patients with brachial artery disruption and in 50% of patients with an isolated radial or ulnar artery injury.[189,262] After arterial damage, palpable pulses are secondary to retrograde flow through preexisting collateral circulation or wave transmission through the injured segment.[115] The Allen test is extremely accurate in documenting arterial patency[115] and therefore is a more reliable indicator of vascular integrity than the presence of a pulse.[115] The Allen test may be conducted in conjunction with Doppler ultrasound evaluations to document the direction of flow and the quality of the collateral circulation.[176] An arterial injury is of concern; and if a pulse is palpable, the parallel artery should be occluded and the persistence of the pulse ascertained. Loss of the pulse suggests an injury proximal to the area palpated, and maintenance of a pulse is secondary to retrograde flow.

Diagnostic Testing

Noninvasive Diagnostic Techniques

Doppler ultrasound, pulse echo ultrasonography, and duplex Doppler provide rapid and accurate diagnostic information in the acute care situation. Hand-held Doppler evaluation, performed with and without parallel vessel compression, permits an assessment of arterial flow and allows the determination of whether blood flow is antegrade or retrograde. Pulse echo real-time ultrasonography and CDI can be used rapidly at the bedside. The measurement of digital blood pressure during an initial evaluation, during a surgical exploration, or in the postoperative period provides an objective measure of the net arterial pressure in different parts of the hand.

Invasive

The role of *arteriography* in the assessment of acute extremity trauma has been studied extensively and remains controversial.[8,101,123,303,348] Arteriography is *not* a cost-effective screening modality and should *not* be used routinely to rule out or delineate arterial injury after penetrating trauma or closed injury without clinical suspicion of arterial injury or compromise. In a review of 99 arterial injuries during combat, preoperative arteriography was "usually not necessary" and there were no primary amputations.[246] Indications for arteriography must be based on the clinical situation. After the recognition of clinically significant penetrating arterial damage, surgical exploration is indicated unless (1) direct vascular evaluation compromises the patient and/or extremity, (2) multilevel arterial damage is possible or probable (e.g., shotgun wound), and/or (3) extensive thrombosis or embolism is a clinical concern (e.g., injection or cannulation injuries). Relative indications for arteriography after blunt trauma include (1) suspicion of a proximal traction injury or distal occlusion (thrombosis or embolism), (2) correction of a partial arterial injury (e.g., intimal flap), and/or (3) suspicion of a false aneurysm.

Intraoperative Assessment

Exploration of penetrating and nonpenetrating arterial trauma often is required to determine the extent of the damage and directly assess the quality of the collateral circulation. "Backflow" provides an indication of collateral flow by clinical grading of the quality of pulsatile flow or quantitative measurement of retrograde blood pressure.[109,114,181,255] Whereas excellent retrograde flow (DBI > 0.7) confirms adequate collateral circulation, poor retrograde flow may be transient secondary to vasospasm and/or hypotension and is not predictive of potential collateral flow after recovery from anesthesia. Intraoperative assessment may be accomplished by estimating capillary refill or pulp turgor or by a quantitative technique such as digital plethysmography, laser Doppler fluxmetry, or digital blood pressure measurements.

Anatomy and Physiology

After acute arterial injury, patient symptoms depend on the adequacy of the collateral circulation, post-traumatic sympathetic tone, and the status of vasomotor control mechanisms (see Fig. 64-1). In general, patients with an arterial injury, adequate collateral circulation, and normal vasomotor control may experience minimal symptoms, meaning that vascular reconstruction is not mandatory. However, an underlying neurologic, soft tissue, or osseous injury may alter sympathetic control and result in ischemic symptoms from an otherwise insignificant injury. Furthermore, vasospasm of the remaining intact vessel(s) may decrease tissue perfusion, resulting in symptoms and signs of vascular insufficiency. Thus, *adequate anatomic vasculature* may be compromised by *inappropriate functional control*, with consequent vasospasm and arteriovenous shunting resulting in hypoperfusion. In patients with arterial injury and inadequate collateral circulation, distal ischemia increases sympathetic tone, produces additional arterial spasm, decreases tissue perfusion, induces ischemia, and potentiates symptoms. In addition, the effects of the arterial injury may be magnified in the presence of a concomitant nerve injury or underlying vasomotor control abnormality (see Fig. 64-1).

Natural History After Acute Arterial Injury

Upper extremity arterial damage is common, may occur after penetrating or blunt trauma, and is frequently associated with other significant soft tissue or osseous injuries.[116,272] Complex injuries that involve disruption of the brachial artery or extensive damage to both the radial and ulnar arteries are often classified as *critical*.[11] Critical injuries include injuries that, in the absence of arterial reconstruction, will produce tissue necrosis requiring amputation.[9,31,70] Although isolated brachial artery injuries in the supracondylar area may have adequate collateral circulation, most authorities recommend revascularization in the presence of significant associated trauma and/or signs of arterial insufficiency.[146,223,284,355] Vascular injuries associated with a significant amputation rate, if they are not reconstructed, include brachial artery injury above the origin of the profunda brachii and forearm injuries involving both the radial and ulnar arteries.[70] Axillary injuries sustained during war usually require reconstruction.[246]

Although a closed brachial artery injury associated with a supracondylar fracture in children is reported to do well without arterial reconstruction, arterial reconstruction is recommended if signs or symptoms of arterial insufficiency exist after fracture reduction.[45,60,107,195,293,305,333] In children with a pulseless, but perfused and asymptomatic hand, observation of the injury is appropriate after reduction and rigid fixation of the fracture. Indications for exploration and reconstruction include (1) clinical evidence of hypoperfusion, (2) impending or occurring compartment syndrome, or (3) a persistent DBI of less than 0.7.[361]

The majority of acute isolated upper extremity vascular injuries do not require surgical reconstruction to maintain tissue viability and normal function. A rich collateral network at the elbow, in combination with paired major vessels distal to the elbow, provides protection from catastrophic vascular damage in the majority of instances; however, injury to an isolated radial or ulnar artery may still result in *critical* ischemia with subsequent gangrene of all or a portion of the hand.[109,224]

Penetrating trauma accounts for over 80% of acute vascular injuries in the upper extremity.[29,142,262,315] Careful evaluation of these injuries is important because high-energy fractures or dislocations often are associated with acute arterial trauma. The entry wound produced by a high-energy gunshot may appear innocuous yet produce arterial contusion with delayed thrombosis and progressive ischemia. Supracondylar humerus fractures, fracture-dislocations of the elbow, and dislocation of the elbow can injure the intima and media of the brachial artery with subsequent thrombosis.[56,105,120]

Historical Review

- Boswick (1967): 100% thrombosis of repair of forearm arteries
- Gelberman (1979): natural history after radial and ulnar artery injury
- Gelberman (1982): results of radial, ulnar, and combined radial and ulnar artery repair(s)

Treatment of Acute Arterial Injury

Critical Arterial Injury

A critical arterial injury produces cell death and may require amputation. The extent of tissue damage is affected by vasomotor tone, systemic factors, and postinjury management. Preexisting abnormal sympathetic sensitivity (vasospasm) may expand the zone of injury and systemic insults (e.g., shock), or remote damage may decrease perfusion pressure and potentiate the vascular insult. During World War II, amputation after arterial injury occurred in 26% of brachial artery injuries below the origin of the profunda brachii and in 55% of injuries above this level. If both the radial and ulnar arteries were injured in the forearm, the amputation rate was 39%, whereas for isolated single vessel injuries the amputation rate dropped to 5%.[9]

Successful reconstruction of critical injuries prevents distal gangrene and is indicated if limb salvage is an appropriate clinical goal. If both vessels (radial and ulnar) in the forearm are injured and both are repaired, the probability of one vessel in the forearm remaining patent is high.[116,195] The use of vein grafts does not lower patency rates in critical vessel injury in either the upper or lower extremities.[159,222] Factors that influence limb salvage include soft tissue coverage, bony stability, the extent of myonecrosis, and the presence or absence of infection. Low-grade infection affecting an anastomotic suture line produces a hypercoagulable state and exponentially increases the likelihood of thrombosis. Poor soft tissue coverage, unstable fractures, and myonecrosis decrease the probability of maintaining patency and achieving limb salvage after revascularization.[246]

Isolated Noncritical (Radial/Ulnar) Artery Laceration

In general, acute isolated lacerations of the radial or ulnar artery in the forearm do not produce critical events.[109] In the absence of associated neural or osseous injury, unrepaired single vessels with adequate collateral circulation do not produce significant symptoms, impaired function, or cold intolerance. Over time, flow will increase in the intact parallel vessel, digital blood pressure will remain diminished in the digits directly served by the damaged vessel, and digits perfused by direct flow from the undamaged artery will demonstrate a normal DBI.[111,166] Evaluation of the effects of radial artery harvest on collateral forearm flow confirms these findings with diminished thumb index perfusion from 1.25% to 0.84% and an increase in ulnar artery flow.[34] The effect of an unrepaired single vessel laceration on nerve recovery after neurorrhaphy is unclear; reports relating the effect of a patent repaired ulnar artery on ulnar nerve recovery are contradictory.[111,188,245] Significant arterial compromise exists when injuries (1) occur distal to collateral inflow, (2) propagate extensive thrombi that block the origins of collateral vessels, (3) dislodge or produce distant emboli, and/or (4) compromise distal inflow because of their anatomic location. In the presence of congenital or preexisting vascular damage or because of anatomic location, otherwise insignificant arterial disruption may cause cell death and require arterial reconstruction to maximize health-related quality of life.[176]

Reconstruction of noncritical arterial injuries is advocated to (1) restore parallel flow in case of future injury, (2) prevent cold intolerance, (3) enhance nerve recovery,[42,164,188,305a] and/or (4) facilitate healing. Unfortunately, patency rates with microvascular technique are less than perfect, and data justifying prolongation of operating time and/or transfer to specialized facilities are incomplete. Although patency rates have improved since 1967, when a 100% postoperative thrombosis rate was reported,[31] the published patency rates of single vessel repairs vary from 47% to 82%.[116,324]

The etiology of post-repair thrombosis after repair performed by experienced personnel under favorable conditions has been attributed to a variety of factors, including surgical technique, tension on the repair site, unrecognized vascular injury, mechanism of injury, timing of repair, distal stump pressure, gender, and vessel injured.[114,255] The causes of vascular thrombosis are multifactorial; experienced surgeons should anticipate a 10% to 20% thrombosis rate even under "nearly ideal" conditions.

Indications for Arterial Reconstruction

Arterial reconstruction is indicated after *critical* injury and noncritical injury to maintain pulsatile digital flow capable of responding to stress. In general, the following injuries are optimally managed by vascular repair/reconstruction: (1) axillary or brachial artery injury, (2) combined radial *and* ulnar artery injury, and (3) radial *or* ulnar artery injury associated with "poor" collateral circulation. Relative indications for repair/reconstruction include (1) combined vascular and neural injury, (2) extensive distal soft tissue injury, and (3) the technical ability to achieve repair without compromising the patient's general well-being or unduly prolonging the operative time. Penetrating "war" injuries involve fragmentation damage, high-velocity projectile injury, and shotgun pellets. Presentation of patients with these injuries in shock is common, as reported by 39% of 99 patients treated between 1991 and 1994.[246] In this series, arterial reconstruction of axillary injury was always necessary; some brachial injuries were not critical. In the 39% of the patients who presented in shock, end-to-end repair was possible in 38%, vein grafts were required in 56%, and severe wound infection complicated 22%, with an overall amputation rate of 10%.[246]

CRITICAL POINTS: DECISION TO REPAIR ACUTE ARTERIAL INJURY

INDICATION

- Evidence of ischemia
  - Decreased capillary refill, turgor
  - Allen test > 6 seconds after release
  - Digital brachial index ≤ 0.7

PITFALLS

- Fasciotomy if reperfusion injury likely or probable
- Repair of damaged vessel

Authors' Perspective and Preferred Method of Treatment

The need for arterial reconstruction requires an assessment of the adequacy of the collateral circulation and is based primarily on clinical judgment. Preoperative and/or intraoperative assessment of the injured area regarding color, capillary refill, turgor, and backbleeding combined with quantitative measures of perfusion provides an estimate of adequacy of the collateral circulation. Arterial reconstruction should be considered part of a patient-oriented plan and, assuming that limb salvage is appropriate, should be undertaken to restore circulation in critical injuries or in the presence of "poor" collateral circulation.[170] The final decision regarding arterial reconstruction is made in the operating room, often after exploration of the injury. Once the injured structures have been identified and isolated and potential bleeding sites controlled, the extremity may be assessed. Bleeding from lacerated vessel ends is controlled by atraumatic vascular clamps; then the tourniquet is released. Capillary refill and turgor of the distal extremity and digits are assessed and "backflow" evaluated after clamp and/or tourniquet release. The distal stump may be cannulated and "backflow" measured, digital blood pressure may be quantified with a sterile Doppler probe and cuff, and/or digital plethysmography may be performed.[170] A DBI of 0.7 or greater suggests adequate perfusion.[270,327,360] If collateral flow is judged to be "poor," arterial reconstruction is performed. If collateral flow is "good," reconstruction is optional and ligation(s) is an appropriate option at the discretion of the operating surgeon. If symptoms secondary to decreased arterial perfusion occur in the perioperative period, elective arterial reconstruction may be performed without compromising long-term symptoms or function. *At this time, the standard of care does not require arterial repair of isolated and noncritical vessels. Subsequent symptoms requiring postoperative transfer to a facility for revascularization are appropriate assuming that adequate preoperative, intraoperative, and postoperative evaluation and assessment are performed.*

Brachial artery lacerations, particularly those injuries occurring above the origin of the profunda brachii, are reconstructed unless there is a specific clinical contraindication. In combined radial and ulnar artery injury, one or two vessels are reconstructed. If possible, both vessels are reconstructed. If only one vessel is to be repaired, selection of the most appropriate vessel for reconstruction is controversial. Although the ulnar artery is larger anatomically, the radial artery often provides more flow or is equal in flow to the ulnar artery in 88% of patients.[165] The authors routinely reconstruct both vessels. If only one can be repaired without significant additional intervention, distal perfusion is assessed after repair and the decision regarding the second vessel is based on clinical judgment.

Surgical Reconstruction of Acute Vascular Injury

Exposure

Acute injuries are explored under magnification, and a tourniquet may be used to control bleeding. Extensile incisions are made to incorporate traumatic wounds. Extensive transverse wounds are often extended by perpendicular longitudinal extensions (Fig. 64-17). Transected and injured structures, if not easily recognizable, are identified proximally and distally in normal tissue, mobilized, and tagged with vascular tapes or loops. Dead and necrotic tissue is excised, and wound margins are trimmed. If clinically indicated, a fasciotomy is performed. Rigid skeletal fixation is performed before vascular repair in cases involving skeletal trauma. In critical injuries, arterial and/or venous shunting may be used to prevent excessive warm ischemia.[256]

Vessels are dissected away from surrounding tissue, and atraumatic vascular clamps are placed on either side of the repair site. Vessel ends are evaluated under magnification and trimmed to include only normal tissue. Evidence of diffuse crush injury, damaged endothelium, exposed media, or extensive thrombosis suggests vessel compromise and requires resection back to levels of "normal vessel." Clinical concern with regard to vessel integrity may be managed by resection (resection of the damaged vessel to include an undamaged branch both proximally and distally). This is the most reliable guarantee that undamaged vasculature remains. The vessel may then be placed in an approximating clamp and repaired in end-to-end fashion. Undue tension may be managed by the use of reversed interposition vein

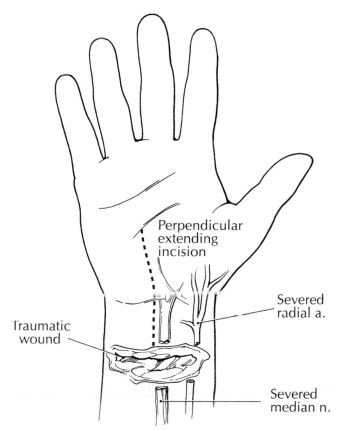

FIGURE 64-17. Schematic representation of treatment of a traumatic wound involving transaction of the radial artery and the median nerve. During arterial reconstruction, transverse wounds may be extended by perpendicular longitudinal incisions to facilitate exposure and to protect repaired structures when wound closure is not possible. (From Koman LA [ed]: Bowman Gray School of Medicine Orthopaedic Manual. Wake Forest University Orthopaedic Press, Winston-Salem, NC, 1997, with permission.)

grafting, in-situ vein grafting with valvulotomy, antegrade grafting with valvulotomy, proximal and distal arterial mobilization, acute arterial lengthening, bone shortening,[270] or joint flexion (with external fixation or casting, where appropriate).

Types of Operations

End-to-End Vascular Repair. The decision to perform an end-to-end repair is based primarily on tension at the anastomotic site. In sharp nonsegmental injuries, a tension-free anastomosis is usually possible after resection of damaged vessel ends, moderate mobilization of the artery, and ligation of nonessential branches. Although acute intraoperative arterial lengthening has been reported,[296] difficulty in approximating vessel ends is managed most frequently by vascular grafts.[170] The vessel ends are trimmed, the adventitia is excised, and the intima is inspected. Repair is performed with the aid of an operating microscope. The vessel is held in place by an appropriately tensioned vascular double-armed clamp. After irrigation with heparinized physiologic saline, interrupted sutures are placed circumferentially using a triangulation technique. Forearm-level injuries are repaired with nonabsorbable 7-0, 8-0, or 9-0 nylon sutures on an appropriately sized needle. Systemic heparin (1000 to 3000 U) is given before clamp release and intermittently during the operative period. Postoperative heparin is not used routinely. Our postoperative pharmacologic routine includes dextran 40 at 20 mL/hr and/or salicylates (81 mg/day). Before wound closure, the tourniquet is deflated and anastomotic patency is assessed. Wounds are closed, and closed-suction Silastic drains are used at the surgeon's discretion.

Grafting for Vascular Reconstruction

Reversed Interposition Grafting
Vascular grafts frequently are necessary to overcome gaps after resection of damaged blood vessel.[127] Reversed interposition vein grafts are the most frequent choice in compensating for inadequate arterial length. Either the cephalic vein from the forearm or the distal saphenous vein from the leg is harvested for grafting. Although veins may be stripped through small transverse incisions, longitudinal exposure and meticulous dissection of the vein under direct vision minimizes damage to the vein or accompanying sensory nerves (e.g., superficial radial nerve in the forearm and saphenous nerve in the leg). Endoscopic vein harvest has been advocated in the lower extremity. Branches are ligated with 4-0 or 5-0 absorbable or nonabsorbable suture or coagulated with a bipolar cautery unit. A segment of vein 15% to 20% longer than the measured defect is harvested. In general, veins are harvested from outside the zone of injury. However, in low-velocity supracondylar pediatric practices, reconstruction of the brachial artery has been successful using the basilica vein from the zone of injury.[195] The vein is then dilated so that it can be inspected for injury and the valves are compressed. Any vein deficits are repaired or a new vein is harvested. The vein is then reversed and positioned in the forearm. After placing the reversed vein graft and one end of the artery in a double-armed vascular clamp, the vessels are prepared under the operating microscope by

CRITICAL POINTS: END-TO-END ARTERIAL REPAIR

INDICATION

- Acute arterial injury, thrombosis, or embolism in which normal vessel can be approximated without tension

PREOPERATIVE EVALUATION

- Clinical assessment
  - Capillary refill
  - Turgor
  - Pulses
- Doppler ultrasound
- Digital blood pressure
- Arteriography, if remote trauma or insult considered

PEARLS

- Normal intima and media are crucial for success.
- Graft if in doubt about too much tension.
- If vessel is suspect, resect it proximally and distally to patent branches.

TECHNICAL POINTS

- Use extensile exposure.
- Mobilize vessel completely.
- Ligate, clip, or bipolar branches.
- Resect damaged vessel; cut ends sharply.
- Inspect using microscope.
- Repair with appropriate magnifications.

- Avoid tension; graft as needed.
- Utilize vascular approximation double bay clamps, if possible.
- Use interrupted suture technique (triangulation helpful).
- Avoid excessive suture and do not tie too tightly.
- Use smallest suture appropriate.
  - 7-0 to 8-0 for radial/ulnar arteries
  - 8-0 to 10-0 for palmar and digital vessels
- Close wound over Silastic drain if required.
- Administer intraoperative heparin, if appropriate.

PITFALLS

- Repair of damaged vessel
- Excessive tension

POSTOPERATIVE CARE

- Anticoagulation with dextran 40 or unfractionated heparin for 3 to 5 days; factor Xa inhibitors or fractionated heparin for 2 to 12 weeks
- Antiplatelet agents (aspirin, ibuprofen, for 2 to 12 weeks)
- Smoking cessation (e.g., nicotine patch)

RETURN TO WORK

- Depends on associated injury
- Light duty for 7 to 14 days
- At 4 to 6 weeks, normal duty

---

dissecting adventitial tissue and trimming the graft to the appropriate length. Size discrepancies between the lumens are managed by angling the cut in the smaller vessel up to 30 degrees, by excising a "V" from the larger vessel and closing it in linear fashion, by a linear cut in the smaller vessel to create a "V," or by a sleeve anastomosis (Fig. 64-18). Vascular repair is done with nonabsorbable 7-0, 8-0, or 9-0 suture in an interrupted or a "sleeve" anastomosis technique. The latter may be chosen to overcome an anastomosis between a small proximal artery and a large vein.[359] For this technique, two or three 8-0 sutures are placed through the larger vessel (e.g., vein graft) from the adventitia into the intima, then through the adventitia of the smaller artery, and back through the intima and adventitia of the first vessel (see Fig. 64-18). The larger vessel wall is entered at a point three to five times the arterial wall thickness from the vein edge. The smaller vessel is then pulled into the larger. Clamps are removed and leaks are stopped with circumferential partial-thickness sutures.[359]

In-Situ and Nonreversed Vein Grafting

The advantage of in-situ and nonreversed interposition grafting is marginal in brachial or forearm injury in which short segments (<5 cm) and minimal size discrepancy exist between the proximal and distal arterial stumps. However, in situations that involve a significant size discrepancy between the proximal and distal vessels (e.g., a brachial artery graft to a radial or ulnar artery in the distal forearm or hand) and larger segments (>7 cm), the proximal reversed interposition segment that is anastomosed to the smaller vessel may be much larger than the distal artery, thereby complicating the procedure. Nonreversed grafts in which the valves are incised or excised reduce this problem and may provide branching segments for multiple distal grafts. *If vein grafts are not reversed, all valves must be incised before revascularization* (Fig. 64-19). The risk of inadvertent vein damage is the limiting factor in vein valvulotomy. For this reason, a majority of surgeons prefer reversed interposition vein grafting.

Bypass Grafting

Vein grafts are frequently used to bypass damaged areas in the lower extremity and also can be used in the upper extremity. Grafts include reversed interposition veins, in-situ vein segments, nonreversed valve-incised veins, arterial segments, and synthetic or allograft material. After controlling bleeding, arteries proximal and distal to the zone of injury are dissected and vascular loops are placed to identify

CRITICAL POINTS: VENOUS INTERPOSITION GRAFTS FOR REPAIR OF ARTERIES

INDICATIONS

- Extensive arterial damage that does not permit end-to-end repair without tension
- Segmental injuries
- Extensive soft tissue damage requiring rerouting of the vessel

PREOPERATIVE EVALUATION

- Clinical need for vessel repair
- Extensive damage

PEARLS

- Graft if in doubt about too much tension.
- Orientation of the graft and size match are crucial.
- Resect damaged vessel, proximally and distally, to normal-appearing structure; presence of a patent branch supports undamaged vessel.

TECHNICAL POINTS

- Use extensile exposure.
- Harvest graft 15% to 20% longer than defect and trim after initial anastomosis.

- Excision of native thrombosed and damaged vessel is usually appropriate in the distal upper extremity. Bypass grafting at forearm, elbow, and brachial levels may be indicated.
- Reverse vein graft or excise valves.
- Dilate to open valves and decrease spasm. If there is concern over valves, valvulotomy may be performed.
- Set tension to prevent kinking.
- Administer intraoperative heparin.

PITFALLS

- Not reversing graft with intact valves
- Redundant: graft that twists causing turbulence
- Not dilating graft to open valves
- Not confirming patency

POSTOPERATIVE CARE

- Anticoagulation during hospitalization
- Aspirin, 81 mg daily × 3 months
- Avoid repeated trauma
- Light duty for 7 to 14 days
- Reduced hand trauma for 4 to 6 weeks

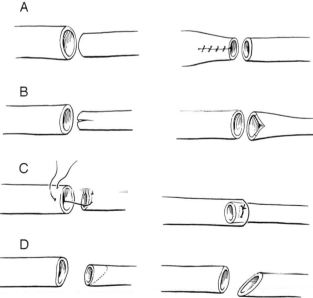

FIGURE 64-18. Mechanisms to overcome size discrepancies during arterial repair. **A,** The larger vessel may have a "V"-shaped portion excised and then closed. **B,** Conversely, the smaller vessel may be split longitudinally and then expanded to fit the larger vessel. **C,** If the smaller vessel provides proximal inflow, it may be intussuscepted into the larger vessel via a sleeve-type technique. **D,** Small discrepancies may be diminished by a 30-degree angled or beveled cut of the smaller vessel followed by a gentle dilation. (From Koman LA [ed]: Bowman Gray School of Medicine Orthopaedic Manual. Wake Forest University Orthopaedic Press, Winston-Salem, NC, 1997, with permission.)

them. A suitable length of graft is dissected, usually from the lower extremity. The distal saphenous vein is exposed through one or more longitudinal incisions, venous branches are ligated, the saphenous nerve is protected, and the vessel is harvested. Valves are incised with a valvulotome, or the vessel is reversed. End-to-side anastomoses are performed proximally and distally with interrupted 7-0, 8-0, or 9-0 sutures (see Fig. 64-19B).

Temporary Shunting

In critical injuries, prolonged warm ischemia can be prevented or minimized by temporary shunting using commercially available shunts or heparinized Silastic catheters. Shunts are placed under direct vision proximally and distally. The minimal dissection necessary to avoid iatrogenic damage is performed, shunts are placed, and the distal extremity is perfused. Fasciotomy may be necessary for overt or impending compartment syndrome.[112,117,256] Early restoration of arterial perfusion using a temporary shunt "can eliminate the adverse effects of prolonged ischemia and enables the surgeons to manage other associated injuries in an unhurried manner."[312]

Arterial Grafts

Arterial autografts are used infrequently in extremity revascularization. Advantages of arterial autografts over venous autografts include better size match, absence of concern over orientation, longer theoretic patency, and ease of dissection. However, few adequately sized donor arterial grafts are available. If reconstruction of one artery is

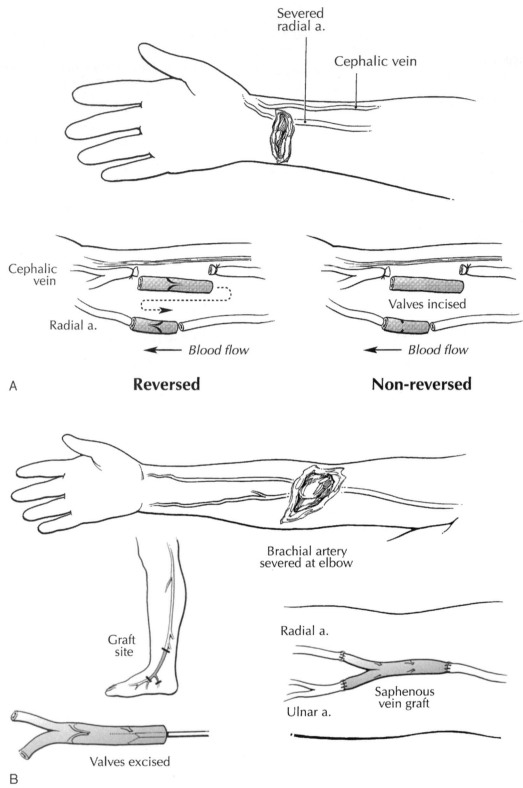

FIGURE 64-19. **A,** Interposition vein grafting may be used to repair damaged arterial segments that would be under tension with an end-to-end repair. Reversed interposition grafts may be obtained from local veins (e.g., cephalic) after reversal. Alternatively, nonreversed veins may be used if the valves are incised *(lower right)*. **B,** Severe injuries that involve the brachial artery or the radial and ulnar artery may be managed by branched vein grafts. Either reversed interposition or nonreversed (with valves incised) interposition vein grafts may be used. (From Koman LA [ed]: Bowman Gray School of Medicine Orthopaedic Manual. Wake Forest University Orthopaedic Press, Winston-Salem, NC, 1997, with permission.)

contraindicated and sufficient undamaged vessel is available, its use as an interposition graft is appropriate.

Postoperative Management and Expectations

Post-repair protocols depend on the mechanism of vascular damage and associated soft tissue and bony injury. Patients with uncomplicated venous grafts are anticoagulated for 3 to 5 days with dextran 40 and aspirin. If there is concern over repair in the presence of proximal or distal vessel damage, anticoagulation with unfractionated heparin, low molecular weight heparin, factor Xa inhibitor, or hirudin is indicated. Rarely is chronic anticoagulation with warfarin (Coumadin) necessary.

Postoperative management depends on the associated soft tissue and/or bony injuries, the mechanism of arterial injury, and the critical importance of the revascularization. Recommendations for anticoagulation are based on empirical observations and experience. Clean lacerations without extensive muscle damage or significant bony or neurologic injury require minimal anticoagulation (e.g., short-term dextran 40 and aspirin for 3 to 5 days followed by aspirin alone (81 mg/day) for 3 months. However, critical injury resulting from a crush or avulsion mechanism may require heparin (either unfractionated, low molecular weight) or a factor Xa inhibitor or hirudin for 5 to 10 days followed by aspirin (81 mg/day).

Immediate postoperative joint range of motion is encouraged with the patient in a bulky dressing that may be removed at 3 to 5 days. Patients can resume light duty 5 to 14 days after surgery but should avoid trauma to the repair site.

ACUTE VASCULAR INJURY: VENOUS

Little has been written about acute isolated venous injury. The extensive redundancy of the forearm and arm superficial venous system combined with the large capacity of the subdermal plexus permits the ligation of most injured veins without morbidity.[221] However, venous injury associated with degloving of the skin and loss of the cephalic and basilic veins may produce outflow obstruction, associated compartment syndrome, and ischemic necrosis. Venous insufficiency after upper extremity trauma is managed by reconstruction of the cephalic and basilic veins or two or more superficial veins. Vein grafts may be necessary for the reconstruction. Such reconstruction does not reduce patency rates and, in fact, may allow placement of the anastomoses outside the zone of injury.[183]

Authors' Perspective

The decision to repair/reconstruct acute venous injury is dependent on the condition of the extremity after exploration/débridement and the appearance of the hand. If physical examination of the hand demonstrates a distended, somewhat bluish appearance with increased turgor, venous outflow must be critically assessed. If pulsations ("throbbing") are palpable in the pulp and if the wound edges distal to the injured segment reveal pulsatile flow from venous struc-

tures, the available compromised venous outflow may be inadequate.

An extensile incision and careful mobilization of the venous structures from surrounding soft tissue are important. Branches preventing vein mobilization are ligated. Repair of the cephalic and/or basilic vein is the first priority within the forearm or arm; the brachial and axillary veins may be repaired in the upper brachium or axillae. If these vessels cannot be reconstructed, the largest accessible veins are dissected. We do not hesitate to perform a vein graft to obtain adequate flow. The number of large superficial veins that are necessary to provide adequate outflow is unknown; however, we routinely attempt to reconstruct two veins for each artery at the forearm level during replantation of a complete amputation. Under magnification (usually an operating microscope), each vein is repaired with 7-0, 8-0, 9-0, or 10-0 nonabsorbable suture attached to an appropriately sized needle.

CANNULATION INJURIES

Preoperative Evaluation

The frequent need for arterial blood studies, indwelling arterial catheters, and cardiac catheterization has led to an increased incidence of cannulation injuries, most frequently involving the brachial and radial arteries.[17,286] In patients undergoing brachial artery cannulation for cardiac catheterization, surgical repair/reconstruction of the brachial artery is necessary in 0.5% to 0.7% of patients after cardiac catheterization.[230] Repeated injuries to the arterial lumen after attempts at obtaining blood from the artery cause an increased likelihood of (1) pseudoaneurysm formation, (2) creation of an arteriovenous fistula (AVF), and (3) acute thrombosis with possible distal embolization. The incidence of occlusion of the radial artery after cannulation has been estimated at approximately 23%; however, recanalization of the occluded vessel generally occurs.[352] Despite the probability of recanalization of the vessel, acute ischemia and distal embolization have been reported.[12,207]

Vascular insufficiency is suggested by pallor, decreased refill, and/or petechiae and may be confirmed by the Allen test and/or Doppler evaluation. Arteriography should be used only to answer specific clinical questions and may be contraindicated after cannulation events because associated compromising medical conditions are frequent. Brachial artery thrombi have the highest probability of distal embolization and ischemia. Management of ischemia after cannulation injuries depends on the patient's medical status. Therefore, exploration of the involved vessel in the intensive care unit or operating room under local anesthesia may be necessary and prudent.

Management and Surgical Treatment

Management options include one or more of the following: thrombolytic therapy, surgical reconstruction, thrombectomy, and embolectomy. In an acute situation, the involved vessel is exposed and the extent of injury assessed. Vessel lacerations and intimal flaps are common injuries complicated by hematoma, pseudoaneurysm formation, thrombosis, and/or embolism. Results after exploration, primary repair, patch grafting, and vein grafting are excellent. Wound complications are infrequent and manageable.[220] Thrombolytic therapy may be considered for patients without complicating medical conditions but should be avoided in the immediate postoperative period after extensive nonvascular surgery.

Authors' Perspective

The loss of a radial pulse without ischemic symptoms distally is *not* an indication for emergency surgery. The extremity may be observed clinically in an awake and alert patient; surgical intervention is dictated by the patient's clinical condition. In an anesthetized or unconscious (e.g., head injury) patient, objective monitoring is recommended and is achieved by the placement of temperature or laser Doppler probes or by distal pressure measurements of the affected extremity.

Brachial and radial arterial injuries after cannulation or indwelling catheter placement are evaluated for the presence of pseudoaneurysm, arteriovenous fistula, and distal embolization by using the Allen test, hand-held Doppler, color duplex Doppler, and/or the digital brachial index. If symptoms and signs suggest vascular compromise (e.g., DBI ≤ 0.7), heparin is used unless contraindicated. Alternative pharmacologic options to unfractionated heparin include low-molecular-weight heparin, factor Xa inhibitors, and hirudin. Arteriography is indicated to answer specific clinical questions or to explain contradictory findings. Suspicion of a proximal event unrelated to the cannulation injury is an indication for arteriography. If symptoms and signs of arterial compromise persist, surgical exploration is indicated to determine the extent of arterial damage. The use of thrombolytic agents is contraindicated in the presence of pseudoaneurysm or vascular laceration or in most postoperative conditions (e.g., after heart surgery). Surgical management of arterial injuries is indicated in the presence of distal ischemia, active bleeding, or aneurysmal expansion. Appropriate surgical techniques include resection and ligation, arterial reconstruction, and/or thrombectomy/embolectomy.

ARTERIAL INJECTION INJURY

Preoperative Evaluation

Mechanism of Injury

Arterial injection injuries occur inadvertently with workplace exposure, are initiated during medical procedures, or may be self-inflicted during drug abuse. Distal ischemia is reported after inadvertent or inappropriate injection of a variety of pharmaceutical agents (e.g., barbiturates, propoxyphene, and nonparenteral narcotics). Severe vascular events occur after workplace injury involving solvents, paint products, and lubrications injected through high-pressure devices. Fortunately, intra-arterial injection is infrequent in workplace injuries.[2,119,269] Injection injuries can result in acute, severe extremity ischemia on the basis of secondary vasospasm, chemical endarteritis, arterial blockage by acid crystals, and activation of the clotting cascade.[2,307]

The diagnosis of injection injuries is based on a clinical history of exposure to a high-pressure source, a high-risk medical procedure, or drug abuse. Acute symptoms of arterial insufficiency are often accompanied by swelling, numbness, and discoloration. Injection wounds often appear innocuous, but the combination of the mass of injected material and chemically induced inflammation produces secondary vasospasm and/or thrombosis and skin and soft tissue necrosis. Diagnostic modalities to determine segmental and reconstructable occlusive disease are appropriate and include Doppler evaluation, CDI, and arteriography. Unfortunately, end-artery occlusion within microvascular beds is common, and systemic anticoagulation with systemic support is the only option (Fig. 64-20).

Management and Surgical Options

Treatment options include vasodilators, thrombolytic agents (e.g., urokinase), steroids, unfractionated heparin, low-molecular-weight heparin, factor Xa inhibitors, and low-molecular-weight dextran.[36] Surgical management includes revascularization of injured and repairable segments, fasciotomy, and, in some cases, amputation(s). Revascularization procedures after arterial injection injuries are difficult because of the frequent involvement of small and distal vessels and/or the presence of diffuse distal vascular injury. However, if surgical exploration and/or arteriography demonstrates discrete and reconstructable obstruction(s), early exploration and embolectomy/thrombectomy and/or arterial repair are possible.[53] Associated compartment syndromes are common; therefore, a high index of suspicion is warranted when observing these patients. A compartment syndrome can occur in the digits, hands, or forearm and is an indication to perform a fasciotomy.[119]

Authors' Preferred Methods of Treatment

Treatment involves one or more techniques, which may be used sequentially or simultaneously. Management depends on the etiologic agent, the extent of damage, the type of agent, and the location of arterial compromise. After clinical examination, including Doppler ultrasonography, contrast arteriography is performed to determine whether reconstructable segmental occlusion is present and to evaluate the extent of distal microvascular compromise. Diffuse thrombosis and/or embolism involving vessels of any size is managed with thrombolytic therapy (e.g., urokinase), oral vasodilators, and close observation of the patient. Discrete, distal small vessel occlusion is less amenable to urokinase, so in these cases, heparin is used. Evidence of elevated interstitial pressure is monitored or addressed with fasciotomy, as needed. Revascularization and/or thrombectomy is performed if technically possible and clinically indicated. Repeat arteriography is often necessary to document the extent of large versus small vessel involvement and to evaluate the effects of medical thrombolytic management.

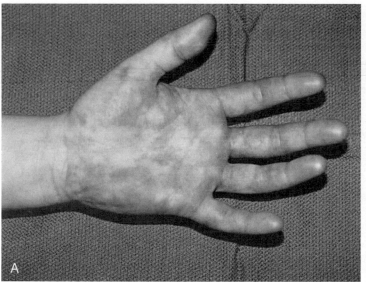
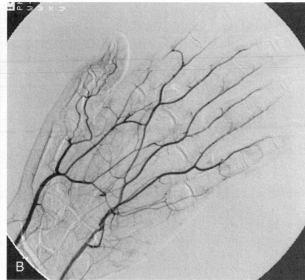

FIGURE 64-20. **A,** Clinical picture of a patient after an inadvertent arterial injection of oral prescription medication. **B,** The arteriogram of the same patient demonstrates multiple distal embolic events to the digital arteries. (From Koman LA [ed]: Bowman Gray School of Medicine Orthopaedic Manual. Wake Forest University Orthopaedic Press, Winston-Salem, NC, 1997, with permission.)

CHRONIC VASCULAR EVENTS: THROMBOSIS, ANEURYSM, EMBOLUS, AND ARTERIOVENOUS FISTULA

Chronic symptoms secondary to occlusive disease in the upper extremity may be the result of trauma, atherosclerosis, proximal embolic events, systemic disease, and/or hypercoagulable states. Significant arterial occlusion produces ischemia, vasospasm, and stress-induced symptoms; venous involvement may produce cyanosis and/or edema. Nonembolic occlusive disease occurs after damage to the intima and media and in the presence of a hypercoagulable environment and stasis. Symptoms and signs depend on the existing collateral vessels and the appropriateness of mechanisms that control vasomotor/autonomic function (see Fig. 64-1). Although the etiologic mechanisms involved in atherosclerosis and chronic trauma vary, the histologic picture, pathodynamics, and clinical consequences are similar. However, the prognosis is related to the etiology. For example, post-traumatic ulnar artery thrombosis has a much better prognosis than Buerger's disease. Symptomatic chronic vascular events produce pain, cold intolerance, and numbness and may cause ulceration, segmental cell death, and/or gangrene. The relationship of trauma to occlusive disease is well documented among laborers who use their palms as a hammer[55,88,179,181,199,200,343,362] or in individuals who participate in activities with repetitive palmar stress (e.g., baseball catchers).[202]

Repetitive trauma may produce localized thrombosis on the basis of periadventitial scarring and compression.[50,181] Alternatively, trauma may cause damage to the intima and media, disruption of the internal elastic lamina, exposure of endothelial collagen, and aneurysmal dilatation and/or thrombosis (Fig. 64-21). In the presence of atherosclerosis or systemic disease, vessels appear to be more susceptible to trauma, and occlusion/aneurysm is more frequent.[152,173] Regardless of the etiology, arterial thrombosis and/or embolism may be categorized by the level and extent of occlusion, the adequacy of collateral flow, and sympathetic tone (Table 64-4).[177] Group I patients, with good collateral circulation and normal autonomic responses, have minimal symptoms and rarely require surgery. Group II patients often respond to oral medications, resection, and ligation (Leriche sympathectomy), and arterial reconstruction is optional. Group III patients require arterial reconstruction.[68,173,361]

POST-TRAUMATIC OCCLUSIVE DISEASE

Preoperative Evaluation (Ulnar/Radial Artery Thrombosis)

History and Physical Examination

Thrombosis of any artery in the upper extremity may be encountered after trauma. Compromise of the ulnar artery and proximal superficial palmar arch is the most common type of upper extremity occlusion and is well described as ulnar artery thrombosis or "hypothenar hammer syndrome."[55,68,142,164,175,179,247,335,340] Symptoms of pain, cold sensitivity, numbness, and weakness occur after thrombosis or occlusion of the ulnar artery within the confines of Guyon's canal[181,306] (Fig. 64-22). Repetitive trauma with disruption of the internal elastic lamina may produce aneurysmal dilatation with mural thrombi, complete occlusion, and/or distal embolic events (see Fig. 64-21).[181] Signs include the presence of a pulsatile or pulseless mass, absent flow through the ulnar artery by the Allen test, decreased ulnar sensibility, nail bed changes, decreased refill, diminished turgor, ulceration, and/or gangrene. Fortunately, ulceration and gangrene rarely occur. Ulnar artery thrombosis occurs most frequently in male laborers in the fifth decade of life. Patients often report a history of using the palm of the hand as a hammer and using tobacco products. Thrombosis and aneurysms are reported in individuals

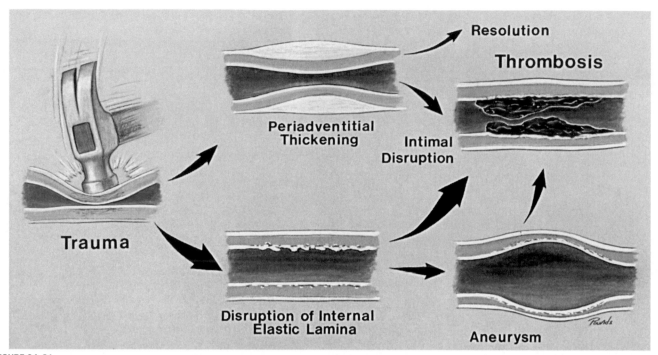

FIGURE 64-21. Mechanisms of occlusion and aneurysm formation in the ulnar artery may include acute or repeated trauma, which may cause direct intimal damage or periadventitial scarring. Periadventitial thickening may constrict the vessel and obstruct flow. Flow may be restored by surgical intervention. Without intervention, additional injury with intimal damage and exposed media may result in thrombosis and/or aneurysmal dilatation. (From Koman LA [ed]: Bowman Gray School of Medicine Orthopaedic Manual. Wake Forest University Orthopaedic Press, Winston-Salem, NC, 1997, with permission.)

Table 64-4

WAKE FOREST CLASSIFICATION OF OCCLUSIVE/VASOSPASTIC/VASO-OCCLUSIVE DISEASE

Group		Etiology
I	Raynaud's disease	Idiopathic
II	Raynaud's phenomenon	Collagen vascular disease
	A Adequate circulation	
	B Inadequate circulation	
III	Secondary vasospasm/occlusive disease	Vascular injury
	A Adequate collateral circulation	Occlusion/embolus
	B Inadequate collateral circulation	
IV	Secondary vasospasm	Nonvascular injury Nerve/bone/soft tissue damage

participating in sports,[26] including baseball,[202] golf,[238] body building,[40] and wrestling[331] and in hand clapping in over-enthusiastic fans.[259] Thrombosis of the radial artery, deep arch, and/or common digital vessels may also occur. Radial artery thrombosis often involves the deep branch of the radial artery within the anatomical snuff-box.[294] Physical examination reveals a pulsatile mass in fewer than 10% of patients. The absence of flow through the suspected artery during an Allen test confirms the clinical diagnosis. However, recanalized thrombosed vessels and/or aneurysms may demonstrate flow in spite of abnormal hemodynamics and the presence of distal emboli.

Diagnostic Testing

Doppler ultrasound, duplex scanning, plethysmography, DBIs, stress testing, magnetic resonance imaging (MRI), and arteriography help delineate structural and functional flow characteristics of vessels and provide insight into the optional management necessary *to restore pulsatile flow capable of responding to stress.*[35,69,176,354]

Types of Operations and Treatment

Management options include (1) smoking cessation, (2) environmental and behavioral modifications, (3) oral pharmacologic intervention, (4) biofeedback, (5) resection and ligation of involved segment(s) (Leriche-type sympathectomy), (6) cervicothoracic sympathectomy, (7) thrombolytic therapy, and (8) surgical reconstruction. The choice of treatment depends on sympathetic tone, adequacy of the collateral circulation, and functional capability. Symptoms secondary to anatomic damage (e.g., arterial thrombosis) are managed by either *increasing collateral flow* or *restoring primary arterial flow* (Table 64-5). Symptoms secondary to abnormal functional (physiologic) control require alteration in vasoconstrictive/vasodilatory tone.

Increasing collateral flow by altering vasoconstrictor tone may be accomplished by a variety of behavioral and environmental methods.[208,231] Cessation of the use of tobacco products (cigarettes and smokeless tobacco) is crucial. Nicotine patches may be used for smoking cessation and do not affect nutritional microcirculatory perfusion adversely.[103]

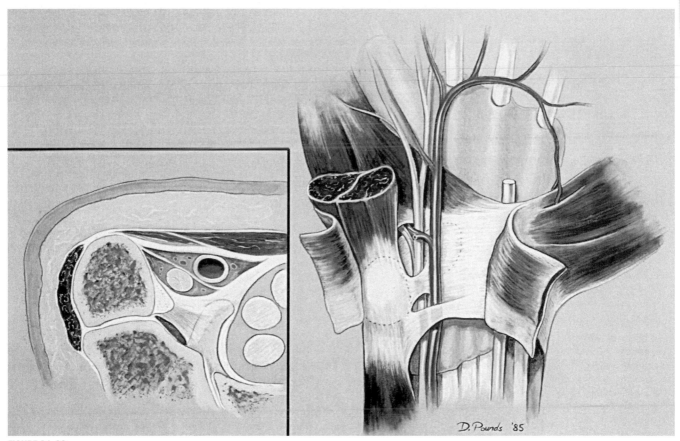

FIGURE 64-22. Schematic drawing of the ulnar artery within Guyon's canal. (From Koman LA [ed]: Bowman Gray School of Medicine Orthopaedic Manual. Wake Forest University Orthopaedic Press, Winston-Salem, NC, 1997, with permission.)

Total flow may be maximized by the use of vasodilators such as tolazoline and chlorpromazine (Thorazine); nutritional flow may be enhanced by calcium channel antagonists or adrenergic antagonists/agonists. Partial sympathectomy may be affected by intra-arterial medications (e.g., guanethidine) or epidural or brachial plexus sustained blocks, implanted dorsal column stimulators,[94,131,147,198] or surgical procedures. Surgical options to decrease abnormal sympathetic tone include resection/ligation of the thrombosed segment (Leriche sympathectomy), adventitial dissection (peripheral or periarterial sympathectomy), and cervicothoracic sympathectomy.

Classification based on anatomic and physiologic pathology aids in the selection of appropriate treatment options (see Tables 64-4 and 64-5). Patients with "secondary vasospasm" and occlusive disease (group III) will have either *adequate* collateral circulation or *inadequate* collateral circulation. The majority of patients will have adequate collateral circulation (group IIIA) and will exhibit secondary vasospasm that compromises otherwise adequate collateral circulation. These patients require minimal intervention and, in general, will respond to sympatholytic medications or sympathectomy techniques, including resection of the thrombosed segment and ligation.

Medical management of group IIIA patients includes the use of biofeedback and oral pharmacologic interventions combined with environmental modifications including, but not limited to, cessation of tobacco use, avoidance of caffeine, and minimization of cold exposure by the use of

gloves, hats, and/or scarfs. Initial pharmacotherapy options include calcium channel blockers and mild sympatholytics (see Complex Regional Pain Syndrome, Chapter 57). Surgical options either decrease vasoconstrictor tone or restore blood flow. Options to decrease vasoconstrictor tone include cervicothoracic sympathectomy (not discussed in this chapter), resection and ligation of thrombosed vessels (Leriche-type sympathectomy), and periarterial/peripheral sympathectomy. The last option, considered a salvage procedure, is reserved for otherwise unreconstructable disease with *adequate* collateral flow. Techniques to restore arterial flow are indicated if collateral flow is judged to be inadequate. *Group IIIB patients, who have secondary vasospasm and inadequate circulation, require arterial reconstruction for maximal recovery.* Methods to restore arterial flow include thrombolytic agents and a variety of reconstructive arterial surgery techniques.

Thrombolytic Therapy

A reported alternative to surgery is the use of anticoagulants for upper extremity occlusive disease. Indications include embolic events,[15,270] nonembolic thrombosis,[61,326,358] or intra-articular injection injury with medium-vessel occlusion.[32,270,326,358] Arteriographic diagnosis is achieved by using a modified Seldinger technique through femoral access. If thrombolytic therapy is selected, a small catheter is introduced percutaneously into the brachial artery and the catheter is advanced into the thrombus or as close as possible to the thrombosis. Urokinase, a tissue plasminogen activator, was

Table 64-5
TREATMENT OPTIONS FOR SYMPTOMATIC THROMBOSIS

Increase Collateral Flow
Reduce vasoconstrictor tone
  Eliminate tobacco
  Biofeedback

Increase Nutritional Flow
Calcium channel blockers (e.g., nifedipine)

Sympathectomy
Chemical
  Intra-arterial (e.g., bretylium tosylate)
  α and β Blockers
Continuous autonomic blockage (e.g., sustained brachial plexus blockade)
Dorsal column stimulator
Surgical
  Resection of thrombosed segment and ligation (Leriche)
  Adventitial dissection (peripheral/periarterial)
  Cervicothoracic

Restore Circulation
Resection and end-to-end repair
Thrombectomy
Resection and vein graft
Arterial bypass
Thrombolytic therapy
Arteriovenous reversal
Omental resurfacing

frequently used as a thrombolytic agent.[61,79,349] It was infused intra-arterially at 50,000 to 100,000 U/hr. In the United States, newer thrombolytic agents (e.g., Retevase) are utilized and urokinase is no longer available.

Frequent arteriographic imaging (6- to 12-hour intervals) is necessary to document the status of the thrombolytic therapy. During the process, which may last from 1 to 4 days, monitoring in an intensive care unit is necessary because complications from local or distant spontaneous hemorrhage are common.[136] Thrombolytic therapy is effective in the treatment of symptoms secondary to subclavian artery thrombosis,[225,326] ulnar artery thrombosis,[358] and embolic disease.[270] Evaluation of short-term results of thrombolytic therapy defines success as the restoration of patency. In a series of 12 acute and subacute events in patients with ischemic digits, intravenous urokinase altered amputation levels, "optimize(d) distal runoff," improved surgical options, and limited tissue loss.[150] However, the conversion of a thrombosed ulnar artery aneurysm to a patent aneurysm requires follow-up to determine whether this is a "success" or failure of new technology with regard to patient outcomes. Post thrombolysis, 3 to 6 months of anticoagulation with warfarin is recommended. Long-term patency rates after this procedure are unknown.

Resection and Ligation (Leriche-type Sympathectomy)—Technique

Ulnar Artery Thrombosis
The ulnar artery is approached through a longitudinal incision that crosses the wrist crease in either an oblique or perpendicular fashion. The ulnar artery and nerve are identified 3 to 5 cm proximal to the wrist crease, and a vascular loop is placed around each structure. By dissecting in a proximal-to-distal direction, the distal ulnar artery and superficial arch are mobilized by freeing the artery from all surrounding tissue and accompanying venae comitantes. Venae comitantes are cauterized with a bipolar technique or ligated by using small absorbable or nonabsorbable suture. The following structures are visualized: (1) a patent arterial branch proximal to the wrist crease, (2) the arterial branch(es) accompanying the deep motor branch of the ulnar nerve, (3) the origin of the proper digital artery to the little finger, and (4) the origins of the common digital arteries from the superficial arch. Thrombosis extending beyond the common digital arteries is an indication for arterial reconstruction. If the thrombus is well contained and the collateral vasculature is adequate (group IIIA) as determined by preoperative testing, direct observation, and/or intraoperative testing, the thrombosed artery is resected and ligated. Then the wound is closed; a small suction drain may be used if judged necessary by the operating surgeon.

Radial Artery Thrombosis
Although less frequently involved than the ulnar artery, the radial artery may also become occluded. The deep branch within the anatomical snuff-box is often involved. During radial artery dissection, the branches of the superficial radial nerve are protected. As the vessel enters the thumb/index web space, often it is necessary to mobilize the artery by ligating several small, deep branches. If a short segment is involved and there is adequate collateral flow, the artery may be resected and ligated.[287]

Arterial Reconstruction

End-to-End Repair
End-to-end repair is rarely possible. After resection of chronically occluded vessels, end-to-end repair is difficult because of tension at the repair site. It is important to maximize patency by removing sufficient damaged artery. After resection of moderate-length sections in patients with tortuous vessels, end-to-end repair has been reported. Exposure for end-to-end repair must be available. Critical evaluation of anastomotic sites is crucial or compromised vessel(s) will be included in the reconstruction and the likelihood of rethrombosis will be high[164] (see Critical Points, page 2286).

Embolectomy
Embolectomy is used less frequently in the upper extremity than in the lower extremity. However, this procedure provides valuable treatment for selected patients. Embolectomy often is used in conjunction with thrombolytic agents (e.g., Retevase) and may be used after proximal resection of thrombosed areas and arterial reconstruction. The use of embolectomy catheters within the hand and digits is difficult and may produce vascular damage.[270]

After obtaining appropriate imaging studies to verify the extent and location of embolic events, an arteriotomy is performed at either the wrist or elbow. The artery (either radial, ulnar, or brachial) is exposed with an extensile/longitudinal incision. A linear arteriotomy is performed after obtaining proximal and distal arterial control with vascular loops, vascular clamps, and/or a tourniquet. Alternatively, the arteriotomy may be performed through a side branch or directly into the lumen after resection of an aneurysm (Fig. 64-23). A bolus of 2000 to 5000 U of heparin is given systemically before arteriotomy or inflation of the tourniquet. Irrigation is accomplished with heparinized balanced salt solution. The size of Fogarty catheter chosen is based on the size of the arteries involved. In general, 1- to 1.5-mm catheters are used within the distal palm whereas 2- to 3-mm catheters are appropriate for use at the wrist and forearm level. The use of embolectomy/thrombectomy catheterization distal to the mid palm or distal palm is difficult to perform without producing iatrogenic injury. The integrity and size of the catheters are checked before insertion. A catheter that is too large will damage the artery and induce additional thrombosis; use of a catheter that is too small will be ineffective in removing the obstruction. The catheter is inserted proximally and advanced distally while maintaining a negative force on the syringe to reduce balloon expansion. Catheters are marked to aid the surgeon in judging the insertion distance.

Embolectomy in the palm and digits is rarely indicated and, if performed, should be done with distal arteriotomies under direct vision of the involved vessels. For example, if at exploration a small and newly formed embolus is visualized within the common digital artery distal to an ulnar artery aneurysm, embolectomy may be performed. After resecting the aneurysm, a 1.5-mm Fogarty catheter is advanced under direct vision distal to the embolus, the balloon is inflated, and the lesion is removed (see Fig. 64-23).

The use of Fogarty catheters within the hand is "fraught with hazard because of the potential for damaging vessels"[270] and requires a careful risk-benefit assessment. The arteriotomy is repaired with interrupted suture under appropriate magnification (e.g., operating microscope or loupes). After successful embolectomy, systemic anticoagulation therapy is administered for 5 to 7 days. This systemic therapy should be followed by an oral anticoagulant based on clinical considerations.

Reversed Interposition Vein Grafting

Graft material is often required to manage the arterial defect after resection of an occluded and damaged artery. The most common graft material is autologous vein, which is reversed because of the presence of valves in the venous system. Veins may be used from the upper and lower extremity. The cephalic, basilic, distal saphenous, and distal lesser saphenous veins are used most frequently. Veins may be harvested through a simple longitudinal incision, multiple short longitudinal incisions or transverse incisions with the aid of a vein stripper, or under endoscopic visualization. Proper vein preparation requires atraumatic technique, hemostatic control of

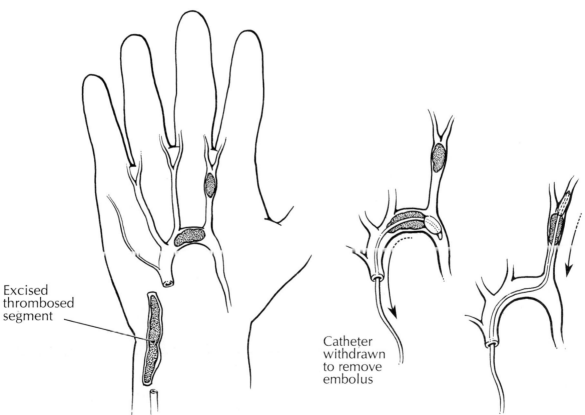

Excised thrombosed segment

Catheter withdrawn to remove embolus

FIGURE 64-23. After resection of the thrombosed segment of the ulnar artery, the superficial arch is visualized, and under direct vision, the embolectomy catheter is then passed through the clot. Once the catheter has passed the clot, the balloon is inflated and the catheter is withdrawn to remove the embolus. An embolectomy catheter should be used with caution in the small vessels in the hand. In general, if there is concern with regard to dislodging clot and producing a more distal embolus or concern that removal of the clot will be incomplete, excision followed by grafting or bypass should be considered. (From Koman LA [ed]: Bowman Gray School of Medicine Orthopaedic Manual. Wake Forest University Orthopaedic Press, Winston-Salem, NC, 1997, with permission.)

all branches, and maintenance of appropriate vessel length and rotation at the repair site (Figs. 64-24 and 64-25).

For ulnar lesions, the incision parallels the thenar crease, zigzags in the palm, and extends proximally parallel to the flexor carpi ulnaris tendon midway between that tendon and the palmaris longus. A radial lesion is approached by a longitudinal incision proximal to the wrist that crosses obliquely to the dorsum of the hand over the anatomical snuff-box (navicular). Tourniquet control is helpful, and dissection under magnification is suggested.

The involved artery and/or nerve is identified proximally to the wrist crease and tagged with rubberized loops. The artery is dissected and mobilized, and the major branches are identified but not divided. Proper dissection will allow direct visualization of the distal ulnar artery, the entire superficial arch, and the origins of the common digital vessels or radial artery, superficial radial, princeps pollicis, and deep arch. The artery and its branches are inspected and evaluated in terms of shape, color, and resilience; in addition, obviously thrombosed or aneurysmal areas are identified for later resection.

All abnormal vessels should be resected. The length of excised vessel is determined by removing the obviously thrombosed portion with serial inspection and resection of all abnormal vessel, aided by the operating microscope. Partial reconstitution of the lumen (recanalization) may be encountered and should not be confused with undamaged vessel. An asymmetrical lumen with loose-appearing intima

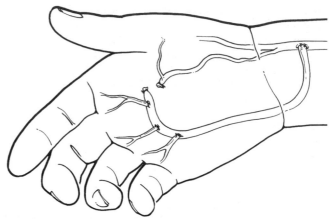

FIGURE 64-24. Schematic of arterial reconstruction using a 14-cm reversed interposition vein graft. The ulnar artery was not suitable at the level of the mid forearm; therefore, end-to-side anastomosis to the radial artery was performed. Because of the size discrepancy, the distal vein was ligated and three end-to-side repairs were performed. (From Koman LA [ed]: Bowman Gray School of Medicine Orthopaedic Manual. Wake Forest University Orthopaedic Press, Winston-Salem, NC, 1996, with permission.)

and thickened media still within the zone of damage represents recanalization of a thrombotic area. The intima should be inspected carefully for asymmetry, tears, redundancy, or exposed media. Damaged or exposed media proximal or distal to the arterial reconstruction will compromise patency.

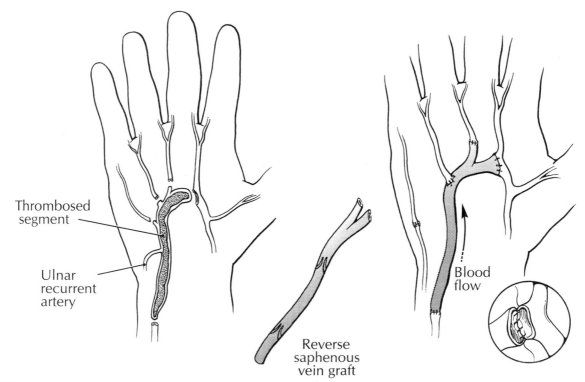

Thrombosed segment

Ulnar recurrent artery

Reverse saphenous vein graft

Blood flow

FIGURE 64-25. Complex reversed interposition grafts may be necessary to reconstruct extensive occlusive disease. This patient (see scanning laser Doppler imager, Fig. 64-8) had severe symptoms and pregangrenous digits. Exploration confirmed the arteriographic findings: thrombosis extending from the wrist crease to the origin of the common digital artery to the long-index finger and abnormal radial and ulnar vessels at the wrist. Reconstruction required a 13.5-cm graft from the saphenous system. During harvest, a "Y" branch was suitable for repair. Distal anastomosis included end-to-side anastomosis of the common digital to the ring-little finger into the vein graft, end-to-end repair of the vein branch to the common digital artery to the long-ring finger, and a complex end-to-end repair of the proximal vein to the junction of the common digital index-long finger and superficial radial artery. The inferior ulnar recurrent is anastomosed to the proper digital artery to the ulnar side of the little finger. (From Koman LA [ed]: Bowman Gray School of Medicine Orthopaedic Manual. Wake Forest University Orthopaedic Press, Winston-Salem, NC, 1997, with permission.)

Resection of patent but compromised vessels involving proximal or distal collateral inflow or the origin of a common digital artery commits the surgeon to arterial reconstruction. "Resection to normal vessel" under the operating microscope is important and must be performed if patency rates are to be maximized. If possible, it is preferable to resect proximally and distally until there is a patent branch within the specimen. Once all damaged vessels are resected, distal outflow may be assessed by observing "backflow," measuring digital-brachial pressure, and/or measuring backpressure with a catheter or digital plethysmography after deflating the tourniquet. The size of the defect and the number of anastomoses necessary for its repair then are determined (see Fig. 64-24).[170]

A vein graft of appropriate length may be obtained from either the upper or the lower extremity. The distal cephalic or basilic vein within the forearm or the greater or lesser saphenous veins within the foot and lower leg provide excellent graft material. Satisfactory results have been reported with grafts from both the upper and lower extremities.[170,179,181] Vessels are harvested through multiple transverse incisions, through two transverse incisions aided by a vein stripper, or through an extensile longitudinal exposure. Bleeding from venous branches is prevented by ligation, vascular clips, and/or bipolar cauterization. During harvest and transport of the graft it is important to maintain the graft's proper orientation and length.[235] We prefer to harvest the saphenous vein at the ankle to midcalf level. Veins are harvested through longitudinal incisions under tourniquet control. The skin over prominent veins is marked, the leg is exsanguinated with an Esmarch bandage, and the tourniquet is inflated. Under magnification, the saphenous vein is identified at the medial malleolar level and a vessel loop is placed. The saphenous nerve is identified and protected, if possible. If the vein is suitable in size and consistency, the incision is extended proximally and distally, the vessel is dissected free, and all branches are identified. On occasion, proximal branching is appropriate for a distal "Y" anastomosis (see Fig. 64-25). These valve-free proximal branches, when available, simplify reconstruction of multiple common branches of the superficial arch. Large and medium branches are ligated with 4-0 polyglycolic acid suture, and small branches are coagulated with a bipolar cautery. Silver clips may be used for obtaining hemostasis, although they may dislodge from short branches. Often a 5- to 7-cm length of vein with few branches is found immediately above the medial malleolus.

The entire donor vessel for grafting is mobilized in situ, the adventitia is exposed by removal of loose areolar tissue, and the vessel is measured with a ruler. After adequate vessel length is ensured (10% to 30% more than is estimated to perform the graft is harvested), the proximal vessel is ligated with 4-0 suture, clamped with a small hemostat, and transected between the ligature and the hemostat. To maintain proper orientation of the vessel, the hemostat is left in place and not removed until the vascular repair is initiated. The distal vessel is then ligated and transected, and the graft is harvested. The distal vein, which will become the proximal artery, is not clamped for orientation purposes. A consistent pattern of clamping decreases the likelihood that the proximal-distal orientation will become confused.

A blunt cannula is inserted into the open distal vein, the vein is distended with heparinized saline, valves are dilated forcibly, and leaks or injuries are exposed. Any injuries must be repaired. Leaks from branches may be tied with either 8-0 nylon circular suture or suture ligature. The latter is achieved by passing the needle through the stump of the branch and then tying the suture circumferentially. Silver clips and bipolar cautery are used to obtain hemostasis. Small lacerations in the vessel may be repaired; however, a significantly compromised vessel should be discarded and replaced.

The length of vein required and the number of distal anastomoses are determined before the vein is harvested. The size of the vein graft is based on the in-situ measurement, and final length adjustment is made after inflow has been established. *The vein graft must be reversed or the valves incised.* In general, the proximal end-to-end anastomosis is performed first, the patency of that repair is determined, and then the distal repair is performed. If the distal configuration of the graft is complex or if satisfactory exposure is difficult to achieve, the distal segment may be anastomosed first. Size discrepancies are managed by a 30-degree oblique cut in the artery, an "open V" in the artery, or a "closing V" in the vein graft (see Fig. 64-18). The suture most frequently used is 8-0 or 9-0 nylon on a 100- to 135-μm needle. Stay sutures are placed at 120 degrees, the front wall is repaired with interrupted sutures, the vessel is turned, and the "back" wall is repaired. Approximating vascular clamps are useful for vessel alignment and hemostasis. It is crucial to place all sutures through the intima to avoid back-wall or side-wall tethering, maintain vessel alignment, and correct any technical errors.[170,235]

In short grafts involving the ulnar artery and superficial arch, both end-to-end repairs may be completed before the tourniquet is deflated. When reconstructing the radial artery within the anatomical snuff-box, the distal anastomosis to the deep arch and princeps pollicis is performed before the proximal repair, to facilitate exposure of the back wall. In larger or more complex grafts, deflating the tourniquet briefly to confirm flow through the vein graft is beneficial. All repairs are performed with an operating microscope. After the proximal repair is achieved, the distal anastomosis(es) is performed. The graft is trimmed to size (10% longer than the defect), distended with heparinized physiologic saline, and placed in its new bed in the wrist or palm. The graft should not be twisted. Distal repairs are performed with 8-0 or 9-0 nylon suture on 100- to 135-μm needles. Vessel size discrepancies are managed in a manner similar to that used in the proximal repair. Significant differences in vessel size may be best handled by creating a blind pouch (ligation of the end on the vessel) and an end-to-side repair (see Fig. 64-24). If two or more distal anastomoses are necessary, variables involving end-to-end and end-to-side repairs can be achieved in series. Complex reconstructions are necessary on occasion and may include end-to-side anastomoses proximally and distally (see Fig. 64-24), "Y" grafts (see Fig. 64-25), and bypass grafting (Fig. 64-26).

Systemic intraoperative heparin is given as one or two 2000- to 5000-U boluses immediately before the tourniquet is released. All vessels used in grafts are irrigated with heparinized balanced solution(s). Dextran 40 infusion

20 mL/hr is initiated in the operating room. In general, heparin is not necessary postoperatively; however, if the anastomosis is compromised by abnormal distal vessels and/or marginal runoff, systemic anticoagulation should be considered.[170]

After all the anastomoses have been completed, the tourniquet is deflated, the clamps removed, and the repair(s) checked for patency or leaks. After obtaining hemostasis, the wound is closed in a single layer from the wrist to the digit(s). Simple and/or vertical mattress and/or horizontal mattress sutures of 4-0 nylon are used in the hand. Subcutaneous sutures may be used proximal to the wrist, but the fascia is not repaired. A single Silastic 7-French drain is placed adjacent to but not touching the vein graft at the surgeon's discretion.

A large bulky hand and forearm dressing with dorsal plaster is applied from the fingertips to the elbow with the hand in a functional position. The drain is left in place 12 to 36 hours. The circulation in the hand is assessed every hour for 6 hours and then every other hour for 24 hours. Smoking, smokeless tobacco, and caffeine consumption are avoided. The patient is placed in a warm, quiet environment. Dextran 40 infusion is continued at 20 mL/hr for 2 to 5 days, and salicylates (81 mg/day) are administered. If sedation is necessary, chlorpromazine (25 mg orally three times daily) is used. Narcotic analgesia may be used as necessary.

In-Situ and Nonreversed Vein Grafts

The use of in-situ and nonreversed interposition grafts requires incising the valves. The exposure and technique are similar to that for reversed interposition grafting with the exception of vein placement and valvulotomy[270] (see Fig. 64-19).

Arterial Grafting

The use of "expendable" donor arteries has not been described for upper extremity reconstructions. However, current data in the thoracic literature support the use of arteries in preference to veins for coronary artery bypass and document the "expendability" of the internal mammary and radial arteries. Therefore, the use of a contralateral radial artery graft for a "critical" upper extremity vascular event provides an alternative to vein grafting.

Bypass Grafting

Although infrequently used, bypass grafts are occasionally necessary in the upper extremity. Reversed in-situ, interposition, or nonreversed vein grafts may be used from the parallel forearm vessel or from the brachial artery to a distal artery (see Fig. 64-26).

Arterialization of Venous Flow

Patients with inadequate distal arterial reconstitution or poor outflow secondary to arteriosclerosis or end-stage vaso-occlusive or embolic disease may be treated with arteriovenous reversal.[14,124,144,160,244,251,270] This procedure attempts to bypass the valves in the venous system and reverse flow through arteriovenous anastomoses to nutritional vascular beds.[14,124,160,270] The proximal artery is identified, branches of the in-situ venous system are ligated, valves are incised, and

arterial flow is established through the venous system to the metacarpophalangeal level. If adequate arterial flow is delivered to vessels 150 μm or smaller, there is a minimum of valves distal to this point, arterial pressure flow renders distal valves incompetent, and flow reversal within the microcirculation is possible.[270]

Salvage Procedures (Omental Transfer)

Resurfacing and revascularization with free tissue transfers are occasionally appropriate. Omental transfer has been proposed for resurfacing ischemic extremities. Ischemic distal areas may be resurfaced by omental free tissue transfers nourished by proximal arterial and venous anastomoses.[270]

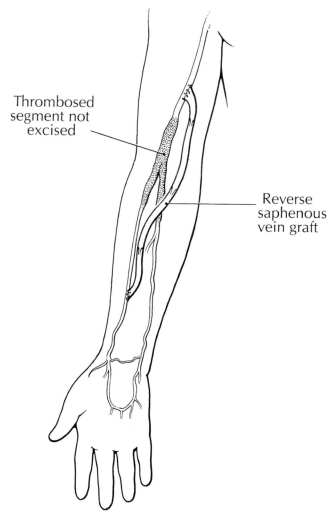

FIGURE 64-26. Bypass grafting in the upper extremity is often advisable. For example, in this patient with severe occlusive disease associated with diabetic vasculitis and nephropathy and chronic dialysis, the brachial artery and the origins of both the radial and ulnar artery are thrombosed (*solid lines*). Rather than dissecting the entire brachium and forearm, bypass grafting was performed with end-to-side repair into the brachial artery proximally and an end-to-side repair into the radial artery distally. A reversed interposition graft of 34 cm was used. (From Koman LA [ed]: Bowman Gray School of Medicine Orthopaedic Manual. Wake Forest University Orthopaedic Press, Winston-Salem, NC, 1997, with permission.)

Authors' Preferred Method

If the DBI is less than 0.7 through the collateral circulation after resection and ligation, arterial reconstruction is appropriate. Resection of all damaged vessels is critical, and grafts of 5 to 12 cm are common. End-to-end repair is appropriate in well-defined aneurysm if after resection there is no tension at the anastomotic site. We prefer resection of the involved segment and a reversed saphenous vein in most cases. Nonreversed valvulotomized grafts facilitate surgery but are infrequently required.

Indications for Arterial Reconstruction

Arterial reconstruction is appropriate in selected patients with adequate circulation (groups IIA and IIIA), assuming that the risk-benefit relationship is appropriate. In patients with inadequate collateral circulation (groups IIB and IIIB), revascularization is indicated if technically possible, and the risk-reward ratio is positive. Physical findings after surgical exploration that support arterial reconstruction include (1) absence of a parallel arterial limb, (2) two or more levels of occlusion that compromise potential collateral flow, (3) thrombosis extending beyond the origin(s) of the common digital vessels, and (4) incomplete deep and superficial arches. The major indication for arterial reconstruction is inadequate perfusion with a DBI of less than 0.7; and if an appropriate risk-benefit exists, arterial reconstruction should be performed.

Treatment

Reconstruction

After exploration of the involved arterial tree, damaged and/or compromised arterial segments are excised and reconstruction is achieved by end-to-end repair or reversed interposition grafting. End-to-end repair is difficult to achieve except in short segment involvement or in association with tortuous vessels.[164] Repair should not be performed with the vessel under tension. Interrupted 7-0 to 9-0 sutures on appropriately sized needles are used. Although grafting can be achieved by the use of reversed interposition vein grafts, antegrade veins with incised valves, arterial grafts, or prosthetic grafts, we prefer reversed interposition vein grafts. Vessels are exposed, the vasculature is evaluated, and resection and ligation or repair are initiated. Identification of damaged areas is important so that these areas can be excised. Often, areas of the vessel that remain patent have damaged internal elastic lamina and are at great risk for future thrombosis. If possible, it is best to resect a central vessel segment that includes patent branches proximally and distally. This technique maximizes the probability that the remaining vessel will be undamaged. An appropriately sized graft is then harvested either from the upper or lower extremity. Although we will use the cephalic and basilic veins, the distal saphenous vein is our donor graft of choice. Use of the contralateral radial artery is a potential option in selected patients who do not have appropriate donor veins.

Grafts may be left in situ while the valves are incised or they may be reversed; we prefer the latter. In-situ grafts overcome the size discrepancy created by reversed grafts in which the larger proximal end must be anastomosed to the smaller distal artery. Multiple terminal branches are common in antegrade grafts with incised valves and are more difficult to find in reversed vein grafts. In-situ placement, valvulotomy, and end-to-side repair are accomplished with an operating microscope. The grafts must be tensioned appropriately so that they are not tortuous, will not kink, and are straight.[235]

Excision and Ligation

If DBI is 0.7 or greater, excision and ligation is an appropriate option in a high-risk patient, defined as someone who will, or is likely to, continue to use the hand as a hammer, has an abnormal coagulation profile (e.g., abnormal protein S or C), refuses to stop smoking, or has other comorbidities that will compromise patency. The artery is exposed and ligated, and the thrombotic segment is excised.

Postoperative Management and Expectations

Excision and Ligation

Postoperative care for resection and ligation requires an overnight or short hospital stay. If there is no drainage, the drain is removed and the patient is discharged. No anticoagulation is necessary. Sutures are removed at 10 to 14 days after surgery. Return to work is based on job type; the hand is protected for 2 to 6 weeks. No restrictions are necessary after 6 weeks. Some residual cold sensitivity, soreness, pillar-type palm pain, and ulnar nerve irritability are expected. At 6 to 12 weeks, no athletic or work restriction is necessary if the patient is asymptomatic.

Reconstruction

Intraoperative and postoperative anticoagulation depends on the pathology. In general, we utilize a single bolus of unfractionated heparin (1,000 to 2,500 IU, IV push) immediately before clamps are removed or the tourniquet is deflated. Eighty-one milligrams of aspirin is given in the recovery room. Dextran 40 is administered intravenously at 10 to 20 mL/hr for 3 to 5 days. Aspirin (81 mg) is continued for 3 months.

If there is extensive vascular damage or compromise, full heparinization with unfractionated heparin and conversion to warfarin is advisable. Alternatives include therapeutic unfractionated heparin for 18 to 24 hours and conversion to low-molecular-weight heparins or fondaparinux.[206] The patient is instructed to avoid direct trauma to the graft, to check the graft for a pulse and to call if it changes, and to discontinue smoking.

Conversely, reconstruction is ideally managed with 3 to 5 days of anticoagulation therapy. If a "good" vessel is able to be repaired, dextran 40 at 20 mL/hr is used for 3 to 5 days, and the patient is discharged on aspirin. Sutures are removed at 10 to 14 days. Protection of the graft is important forever. Using the hand as a hammer is forbidden. We instruct patients to check their graft pulse and call if it diminishes or disappears. Cold sensitivity and palm tenderness are expected. Patency of upper extremity grafts are satisfactory.[76] Re-thrombosis may occur and has been observed at 10 years.

Impact of Arterial Reconstruction on Symptoms, Function, and Microcirculatory Flow

In the absence of good collateral circulation, arterial reconstruction reduces symptoms of pain, improves function, increases distal arterial perfusion, promotes healing of ulcerations, and prevents gangrene in extremities characterized by inadequate collateral circulation.[176,177,226,291,295] Successful reconstruction of occlusive lesions proximal to unreconstructable lesions increases total digital flow and nutritional flow distal to nonoperable digital occlusions while simultaneously decreasing symptoms, increasing function, and positively impacting health-related quality of life[173,177] (Fig. 64-27). In contradistinction, symptomatic improvement from Leriche or peripheral sympathectomy in patients whose digits have vaso-occlusive disease occurs via an increase in the ratio of nutritional to total flow without increasing total microvascular perfusion.[177]

Expectations

Patency rates of 80% to 90% can be expected; however, at 5 to 10 years, re-thrombosis can occur and symptoms often return if the original injury was significant (DBI ≤ 0.7). In 106 reported reconstructions of the ulnar artery for chronic occlusive disease, patency was reported in 87 (82%).[68,93,179,181,226,361]

EMBOLISM

Preoperative Evaluation

Presentation and Natural History

In contradistinction to occlusive disease, which may be insidious in onset, embolization often produces acute pain, pallor, and pulselessness. Ischemia will produce muscle paralysis after embolus/thrombosis proximal to muscle units, but it is not present in distal events. Secondary vasospasm may compromise undamaged collateral flow, and necrosis is common in untreated digits. The classic "blue finger" progresses to white and then black. The degree of damage depends on the quantity of emboli, the extent of undamaged collateral vessels, the presence or absence of continued embolic events, and the source of the emboli.

Common sources of upper extremity emboli are the heart, subclavian artery, and the superficial palmar arch. Upper extremity embolic events account for fewer than 20% of arterial emboli.[16,20,152] Seventy percent of upper extremity emboli are of cardiac origin. Emboli from the subclavian artery are the most frequent arterial source and are commonly produced by mural thrombi secondary to thoracic outlet compression and post-stenotic dilatation.[16,156,308] Cardiac emboli are created by mural thrombi that form after myocardial infarction or in association with atrial fibrillation. In general, cardiac emboli are large and affect the brachial artery, and emboli of arterial origin are smaller and affect wrist-level and digital-level vessels. Emboli from aneurysms or thrombotic events in the wrist and palm occur and primarily affect the common and proper digital arteries. Arterial emboli are frequently observed after surgical thrombectomy or revision of hemodialysis graft thrombosis.[334]

Diagnosis

Acute changes in upper extremity flow affecting multiple terminal vessels suggest embolic events. Symptoms of pain, pallor, pulselessness, and/or paralysis are not specific, but acute onset suggests an arterial origin. Petechiae and varying degrees of cyanosis are common. The extent and location of symptoms are rapidly determined by obtaining segmental pressures. Evaluation should include a complete history and physical examination, including referral evaluations for embolic events and echocardiography. Arteriography, MRA, and duplex Doppler may help localize the source of the emboli.

Treatment and Types of Operations

Anticoagulation using heparin sulfate and embolectomy are the treatment of choice for large emboli.[96] After embolectomy, heparin therapy is followed by warfarin therapy for approximately 3 months. Reperfusion may result in a compartment syndrome that must be released. Embolic events in the hand and the excision of embolic sources may require surgical exploration. Thrombolytic agents may be used in acute situations that do not respond to heparinization. There is laboratory and clinical support for the use of low-molecular-weight heparins[77,206] and pentasaccharides.[87]

ANEURYSM

Preoperative Evaluation

Presentation and Natural History

Aneurysms of the upper extremity may be divided into two types: false and true (Table 64-6). False aneurysms, or "pseudoaneurysms," occur after penetration of the vessel wall and subsequent hemorrhage and extravasation. The resultant hematoma in the soft tissues organizes, fibroses, and recanalizes. The lumen of this false vessel is in continuity with a true vessel and is distinguished from it by the absence of an endothelial layer lining the vessel. False aneurysms are seen most commonly after traumatic and iatrogenic incidents; however, they may be initiated in the absence of penetrating trauma.[298,360] True arterial aneurysms result from injury to the vessel that permits gradual dilatation of the vessel. A true aneurysm is usually more uniform in shape, as opposed to the saclike appearance of a pseudoaneurysm. Whereas false aneurysms commonly result from penetrating trauma, true aneurysms occur most frequently in areas of the arterial circulation that are exposed to repetitive trauma (e.g., the distal ulnar artery and superficial arch).[106,137,152,187,219]

The incidence of false aneurysms after penetrating trauma is unknown. Upper extremity false aneurysms accounted for 27% of all false aneurysms recorded in the Vietnam vascular registry.[284,285] False aneurysms are encountered most frequently in the area of the volar wrist and antecubital fossa and may involve the radial artery within the anatomical snuff-box, the palmar arch, and the digits.[164,187,217,234,258,309,316] In general, false aneurysms are more likely to involve the axillary, brachial, anterior interosseous, and radial arteries. Aneurysms of the ulnar and digital vessels are evenly

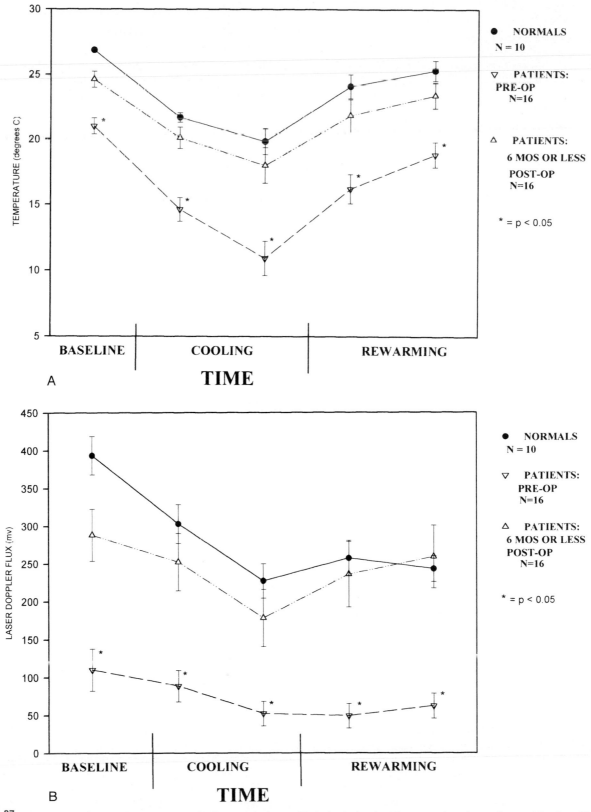

FIGURE 64-27. Digital temperatures (**A**) and laser Doppler flux measurements (**B**) during isolated cold stress testing of normal control hands and hands of patients with vaso-occlusive disease preoperatively and postoperatively. After successful arterial reconstruction, digital temperatures and laser Doppler measurements improved, thus confirming statistically significant increases in both total and nutritional flow. (From Koman LA [ed]: Bowman Gray School of Medicine Orthopaedic Manual. Wake Forest University Orthopaedic Press, Winston-Salem, NC, 1997, with permission).

Table 64-6
ETIOLOGY OF ANEURYSMS

False	True
Penetrating	Arteriosclerotic
Stab wounds	Congenital
Gunshot wounds	Metabolic
Arterial punctures	Disease-related
Arterial catheterization	Osteogenesis imperfecta
Surgical	Kawasaki's syndrome
Vascular repair/reconstruction	Buerger's disease
Regional blockade with local	Cystic adventitial
anesthetics	Hemophilic
Nonpenetrating	
Fractures	
Crush	
Hemophilic recurrent bleeding	
Mycotic infection	

distributed between the true and false type.[137] True aneurysms can occur after iatrogenic injury.

Diagnosis

The presence of an expanding mass and/or distal ischemic events are the usual manifestations of an upper extremity aneurysm. The time interval between the trauma and clinical appreciation of an aneurysm can vary considerably, ranging between 2 weeks and 12 years.[85] Signs and symptoms of vascular insufficiency are uncommon. Aneurysms are commonly observed as a painless, palpable mass.[163] Symptoms of localized pain from soft tissue and/or neural compression occur secondary to a mass effect; distal signs and symptoms occur most frequently from embolization.[163] The natural history of both true and false aneurysms is characterized by a slow progression leading to thrombosis and/or the production of emboli.[219]

Aneurysms are readily identified by Doppler ultrasonography and color duplex scanning. "B"-mode imaging is very effective in identifying aneurysms.[181] Arteriography will delineate distal embolic events, identify reconstructable distal vessels, and differentiate the aneurysmal mass from an arteriovenous malformation, neural tumor, or malignancy. Arteriographic evaluation is the gold standard for identification of aneurysms and allows an assessment of collateral flow, aids in preoperative planning, and defines the extent of damage.[10]

Management and Types of Operations

Treatment options for aneurysms include (1) resection and ligation, (2) excision of the damaged wall and "patch" grafting, (3) resection with end-to-end repair, and (4) resection with an interpositioned graft. Resection of the aneurysm and proximal and distal ligation of a noncritical radial or ulnar artery aneurysm are suggested as efficacious.[85,201] However, brachial vessels or critical vessels require arterial reconstruction.[201] Ulnar artery aneurysms comprise the largest group of both true and false aneurysms.[219] Management options include resection with ligation, end-to-end repair, or grafting; the option used depends on collateral flow and vasomotor tone.[126,137,163,180]

Authors' Preferred Method of Treatment

Aneurysmal dilatation produces blood flow turbulence, thrombosis, recanalization, and/or embolism. Because of this association between aneurysms and thrombosis with distal emboli, surgical treatment of both true and false aneurysms is recommended. Selection of the appropriate intervention is based on physiologic considerations (see Table 64-5). Aneurysms can occur in the presence of adequate or inadequate circulation and are seen with or without distal occlusive and/or embolic disease. Arterial reconstruction using end-to-end repair, reversed interposition vein grafting, or other techniques is indicated if collateral flow is inadequate to provide pulsatile digital perfusion and/or if occlusive or embolic events are distal to the aneurysm. In the presence of adequate collateral flow providing uniform digital pulp microcirculatory perfusion, resection and ligation are appropriate. Preoperative and intraoperative assessment techniques are discussed in the sections on acute injury and occlusive disease. Until further data are available, thrombolytic therapy is relatively contraindicated as the final treatment of upper extremity aneurysms.

ACQUIRED ARTERIOVENOUS FISTULA

Preoperative Evaluation

Arteriovenous fistulas (AVFs) occur after trauma or infection or are created surgically to provide circulatory access for patients undergoing hemodialysis.[285] An AVF secondary to trauma or infection may produce distal ischemic symptoms by the creation of a "steal" phenomenon. Frequently, a thrill or bruit is present. The creation of an AVF for hemodialysis may produce distal ischemic and/or neurologic sequelae. Although most patients tolerate an AVF, complications are not uncommon.[41,229,319] Following end-to-end radial artery-to-cephalic vein anastomosis, ischemic and neural complications are related to a steal phenomenon and/or distal emboli.[219,279] Side-to-side anastomoses between the radial artery and cephalic vein (radiocephalic AVF) reduce thumb digital blood flow by 40% because of proximal shunting (steal phenomenon) and may produce arterial insufficiency.[41,78] Occlusion of the radial artery distal to the fistula eliminates the retrograde steal phenomenon and increases thumb blood pressure significantly.[41,78] Dialysis-associated steal syndrome (DASS) occurs in 1% of side-to-side radiocephalic fistulas and in 6.4% of patients who have undergone forearm loop grafts.[260] Shunts may cause high-output cardiac failure characterized by progressive cardiomyopathy, fatigue, and dyspnea on exertion[7] and may produce a higher than expected incidence of median and ulnar neuropathy.[132,148,278] The incidence of median mononeuropathy after radiocephalic anastomosis approaches 70% and is significantly higher than the 2% incidence in contralateral hands.[167] Neurologic symptoms are produced by neural ischemia, elevated interstitial pressure, diminished systolic pressure in the presence of preexisting elevated carpal canal pressure, and/or venous distention compressing neural structures. Shunt reversal may alleviate symptoms of arterial insufficiency secondary to inappropriate shunting;

however, neurolysis of the involved nerves may be required.[278] After revision or thrombectomy for thrombosed AVF, distal embolic events are common.[334]

Treatment and Types of Operations

Management options for symptoms secondary to an AVF include ligation, banding, and observation. Surgical ligation may be necessary if recurrent thrombus formation results in distal embolization. Banding or narrowing of the shunt increases resistance through the shunt, increases blood flow distally in the digits, and may reverse symptoms. Banding is indicated if occlusion of the radial artery distal to the fistula causes a documented increase in distal perfusion.[267] Persistence of excessive arteriovenous shunting may produce severe neurologic and/or ischemic sequelae, which will respond to shunt revision and banding or "takedown" of the shunt. Documentation of digital blood pressure before and after occlusion of the radial artery below the fistula provides valuable information in symptomatic patients with a digital-brachial pressure index of less than 0.64.[260] Treatment must be patient oriented and must recognize the importance of vascular access in dialysis-dependent patients. In general, severe symptoms following an AVF require surgical intervention. In the presence of preexisting or acquired occlusive disease distal to the AVF, severe symptoms are frequent and are alleviated most effectively through elimination of the vascular steal and/or by arterial reconstruction of occlusive disease. However, periarterial sympathectomy is not generally helpful.

Authors' Preferred Method of Treatment

Treatment of ischemia in patients with AVFs is difficult and requires involvement of the patient, the nephrologist, and the vascular surgeon. Patients often have (1) necrotic digital tips requiring amputation, (2) cyanotic digits, and/or (3) neurologic impairment. An evaluation in conjunction with the renal transplant/vascular surgery team is important. Digital blood pressure and peripheral nerve conduction velocity (PNCV) measurements are used to guide the decision process. If temporary occlusion of the radial artery distal to the shunt improves symptoms and capillary refill and the DBI is less than 0.5, banding or ligation of the shunt should be considered. If PNCVs are abnormal and the DBI is greater than 0.7, associated neurologic complaints may be reduced by neurolysis with ligation or excision of any venous engorgement causing nerve compression. If PNCVs are normal, distal perfusion is poor, the DBI is less than or equal to 0.5, and graft reversal represents an unacceptable burden, bypass grafting from the brachial artery to a vessel distal to the fistula is considered.

ATHEROSCLEROSIS

Although atherosclerosis occurs in the upper extremity, lower extremity atherosclerotic involvement is more frequent. Symptomatic upper extremity atherosclerosis most commonly affects the innominate and subclavian arteries. Pathologic findings include the formation of characteristic plaque in the intima and subintimal media.[102] Symptomatic left subclavian disease occurs three times more frequently than right-sided symptoms.[133,360] Diagnosis is supported by noninvasive vascular studies and Allen testing and is confirmed by duplex Doppler or arteriography. Treatment depends on functional and anatomic factors and is similar to the treatment of occlusive disease associated with trauma.

ARTERITIS

Thromboangiitis obliterans (TAO) or Buerger's disease is an inflammatory occlusive disease of small and medium-sized vessels.[38,266] Classic clinical characteristics of TAO include lower extremity involvement in young and predominantly male smokers.[155,261] In a study from Japan, 5.1% of 749 men and 76 women had upper extremity involvement only; 167, or 20.2%, had both upper and lower extremity involvement.[300] However, the male-to-female ratio of patients with TAO is declining, with older patients seen more frequently and upper extremity involvement more common.[261] Arteriographic findings typical of TAO include (1) small- and medium-vessel involvement, (2) segmental occlusive disease, (3) distal disease greater than proximal, (4) collateralization bypassing occlusive segments, and (5) normal proximal (e.g., brachial) vessels. Although arteriographic differentiation from atherosclerosis is relatively obvious, TAO is difficult to differentiate from scleroderma and collagen vascular disease. Histologically, arterial and/or venous thrombosis with lymphocytic and polymorphonuclear leukocyte infiltration into the thrombus and vessel wall is observed with TAO.[185] Cessation of smoking decreases disease progression and the incidence of amputation. Treatment is directed toward the relief of vasospasm and restoration of anatomic channels by vascular reconstruction, if necessary.[155,197,360] Upper extremity arteritis is encountered in giant cell arteritis,[203] Wegener's granulomatosis, Takayasu's arteritis,[203] polyarteritis nodosa,[18] collagen vascular disease, and in association with neoplastic disease.[203,360]

VASOSPASTIC DISEASE

Preoperative Evaluation

Under normal conditions, arterial vasoconstriction maintains blood pressure by the peripheral modulation of vascular resistance, directs blood to nutritional capillary beds, allows appropriate thermoregulatory control, and prevents excessive blood loss after trauma. However, inappropriate *vasospasm* produces symptoms of pain and cold intolerance, interferes with health-related quality of life, and may contribute to digital ulceration and/or gangrene in the presence of occlusive disease. Vasospastic conditions are pathologic and cause inappropriate arterial and/or venous tone that persists in the presence of physiologic demands for increased flow. Inappropriate cold sensitivity, the most common symptomatic manifestation of vasospastic states, is frequent and affects 5% to 10% of the general population and 20% to 30% of premenopausal women.[157,208,339] Vasospastic states are defined as *primary* in the absence of an identifiable etiology or *secondary* in the presence of a causal condition. Using this terminology, Raynaud's disease is *primary* and all other conditions are *secondary* (Tables 64-7 and 64-8).

An examination to diagnose vasospastic disease includes a complete history, physical examination, and laboratory testing. Historical data should delineate vaso-occlusive from vasospastic conditions and should document the frequency and durations of episodes of pain, cold intolerance, and/or Raynaud's phenomenon. In addition, detailed information regarding smoking, exposure to trauma at work or play, episodes of frostbite, and symptoms of systemic collagen vascular disease are recorded. The use of standardized patient questionnaires and validated instruments facilitates the collection of this information. *The existence of non-healing ulcerations and/or impending gangrene associated with unilateral Raynaud's symptoms is presumptive evidence of thrombosis or embolism.*

The physical examination includes an evaluation of pulses, trophic change, ulcerations, and infections. Allen testing at the wrist and the digit should be performed, and Doppler mapping of palmar and dorsal vessels aids in making the diagnosis.[168] Classically, Raynaud's phenomenon occurs in three stages associated with three colors. The involved digit(s) progresses from *normal* to *blanched* (white) to *cyanotic* (blue) to *ruborous* (red). Sympathetic hyperactivity stimulated by exposure to cold or other stresses initiates intense vasospasm with cessation of arterial inflow and the production of a white, blanched, and cool digit. Stasis within the digit produces deoxygenated, pooled blood that appears cyanotic or bluish and produces the characteristic blue hue seen in the second stage of the phenomenon. The rubor (redness) in the third phase is secondary to reactive hyperemia from a rebound vasodilatation initiated by ischemia; reperfusion is associated with burning pain and/or dysesthesias. In addition, capillary refill, turgor,

Table 64-7
CRITERIA DEFINING RAYNAUD'S DISEASE

Characteristic triphasic digital color changes

Bilateral hand involvement

Absence of occlusive disease

Absence of gangrene or trophic changes (fingertip trophic findings permissible)

Absence of identifiable systemic disease (e.g., collagen vascular disorder)

Symptoms of at least 2 years' duration

Female predominance

skin integrity, and sensibility are evaluated. Suspicion of neurologic dysfunction and neurologic symptoms should be confirmed by appropriate nerve conduction studies. Routine laboratory blood work for hematologic or collagen vascular abnormalities is appropriate.

The noninvasive vascular evaluations outlined previously may be used to delineate the structural and functional influences on perfusion characteristics of the upper extremity. Digital plethysmography and temperature measurements with and without the application of a stressor are most commonly performed. Arteriography continues to be the gold standard for delineating upper extremity structural abnormalities; however, response to stress is necessary to fully define functional control properties.

A diagnostic strategy should be designed to delineate physiologic events (i.e., vessel structure, vascular function/control, and intravascular "blood" components) *and* to determine precipitating local or systemic processes or disease (e.g., collagen vascular disease, arterial occlusion, neurovascular compression, hematologic abnormality, trauma, drugs or toxins, central nervous system disease, or *primary* vasospasm). Specifically, diagnostic goals should (1) differentiate vasospastic from vaso-occlusive states, (2) separate

Table 64-8
RAYNAUD'S DISEASE VERSUS RAYNAUD'S PHENOMENON

Characteristic	Disease	Phenomenon
History		
Triphasic color change	Yes	Yes
Age > 40	No	Yes
Progression rapid	No	Yes
Underlying disease	No	Yes
Female predominance	Frequent	Occasional
Physical examination		
Trophic findings (ulcer, gangrene)	Infrequent	Frequent
Abnormal Allen test	No	Common
Asymmetrical findings	Infrequent	Frequent
Laboratory testing		
Blood chemistry	Normal	Frequently abnormal
Microangiology	Normal	Frequently abnormal
Angiography	Normal	Frequently abnormal

Raynaud's disease from secondary Raynaud's phenomenon, and (3) evaluate the effects of structural compromise versus functional impairment. Wrist-level and digital Allen testing is a valuable screening test for distal occlusive disease and may be enhanced by digital plethysmography and segmental arterial pressures. Pressure gradients greater than 20 mm Hg between two levels in the same extremity or between the affected and contralateral extremity or a DBI of less than or equal to 0.7 suggests stenosis or occlusion.[37,166,233]

Collagen vascular disease can be diagnosed by using vital capillaroscopy to document characteristic nutritional nail fold capillary morphologic findings, including telangiectasia, abnormal capillary budding, and/or blunted, dilated, or deformed papillary capillaries. These findings are pathognomonic for collagen vascular disease.[210] Vital capillaroscopy is currently the only clinical method that directly assesses the nutritional components of digital blood flow.[176] Quantitative and qualitative assessments of digital perfusion are necessary to make an appropriate diagnosis and plan medical care. Detailed assessments of digital temperature, LDF measurements of cutaneous perfusion, and vital capillaroscopy before and after the application of a stressor allow a determination of the extent of arteriovenous shunting, the adequacy of nutritional flow, and an estimate of total available flow. LDF measures nutritional perfusion and provides data regarding thermoregulatory flow components. Temperature and plethysmographic data reflect total perfusion.[175,176] Allen testing and pulse volume recordings provide data regarding vascular structure, which may be maximally delineated by contrast arteriography or MRA if available. These structural data are complemented by stress testing, which provides a functional assessment of extremity flow. *A combination of both structural data and functional information is mandatory for an optimal evaluation.* Our indications for arteriography include potential surgical intervention, unilateral Raynaud's phenomenon, progressive digital gangrene or ulceration, suspected occlusive or embolic disease, and/or clinical concerns regarding vascular structural integrity.

The use of contrast arteriography provides the best overall assessment of upper extremity pathology, as well as the optimal evaluation of structural vascular integrity. For patients with decreased perfusion and/or vasospasm, diagnostic capability is enhanced by iso-osmolar contrast agents, the use of intraarterial vasodilators (e.g., tolazoline or nitroglycerin), and the consideration of regional anesthetic block (e.g., axillary block). Vasospasm can prevent visualization of vasculature that is adequate structurally and should be addressed during arteriography.

The use of clinical examination, Allen testing, PVR, ICST with digital temperature and LDF measurements, and vital capillaroscopy allows the physiologic staging of patients to determine their vascular structural anatomy and functional control (see Tables 64-3 and 64-4). Staging is performed to determine the presence or absence of (1) adequate circulation, (2) occlusive disease, and (3) abnormal control mechanisms.

Patients with vasospastic symptoms and abnormal anatomic control without occlusive disease (i.e., group I [Raynaud's disease]) will frequently respond to nonoperative modalities. In group II (Raynaud's phenomenon

secondary to collagen vascular disease) and group III (vasospasm secondary to occlusive disease) patients, structural and functional information guides treatment decisions. The presence or absence of adequate collateral circulation is of paramount importance. In patients with inadequate collateral circulation, vascular reconstruction is indicated, if possible. Although patient symptoms may be reduced by nonoperative methods or peripheral sympathectomy, the prognosis is guarded. Patients in group IV (secondary vasospasm and normal vasculature) will improve with correction of the initiating traumatic event or with appropriate pharmacologic intervention.

 # Anatomy

Pathophysiology

Symptoms in vasospastic conditions result from inadequate *vascular structure,* inappropriate *vascular control* mechanisms, or a combination of both.[176] Adequate tissue perfusion requires (1) delivery of blood to nutritional capillary beds in sufficient quantity to fulfill metabolic needs, (2) appropriate oxygen-carrying capacity, and (3) diffusion of oxygen through intravascular spaces to functioning cellular structures. In the majority of patients, the metabolic and oxygen-carrying capacity within the vascular system is adequate. In the absence of intravascular fibrosis and/or cell death, symptoms are secondary to inadequate delivery of blood products at a cellular level (ischemia). Vasospasm decreases total flow, shunts blood through non-nutritional thermoregulatory pathways, or both. For example, after vascular injury, local and systemic factors may produce inappropriate vasospasm that decreases large vessel collateral flow and shunts existing flow in small vessels into non-nutritional channels. Occlusion of the ulnar artery has been reported before the diagnosis of systemic sclerosis.[184,325,330] Physiologic staging allows vasospastic conditions to be categorized (see Table 64-4). Group I patients have idiopathic Raynaud's disease characterized by normal vascular architecture, no identifiable underlying etiology, and the presence of vasospasm. Group II patients exhibit Raynaud's phenomenon secondary to collagen vascular disease and may be divided into those with normal circulation (A) and those with compromised circulation (B). Group III patients have secondary vasospasm as a result of vascular injury and may be classified into those with uncompromised collateral flow (A) and those with abnormal collateral flow (B). Group IV patients without preexisting or acquired structural/vascular abnormality have secondary vasospasm after sustaining an injury to nerves, soft tissue, bone, or a combination of two or more. These categories provide criteria to base treatment on anatomic and physiologic considerations.

The clinical manifestations of vasospastic states are secondary to inadequate nutritional perfusion, insufficient delivery of oxygen and metabolites to cellular structures, and the development of an anaerobic and acidotic tissue environment. Therefore, therapeutic approaches should be designed to increase microvascular flow and maximize capillary perfusion. Vasospastic disease, occlusive disease, and vaso-occlusive disease are interrelated. Occlusive disease occurs via Virchow's triad (i.e., stasis and intimal and medial trauma in the presence of a hypercoagulable state). After extremity trauma, vasospasm decreases flow with subsequent relative stasis. The presence of local hypercoagulable states is common. When hypercoagulability is coupled with trauma, exposed media, and stasis, occlusive disease occurs.

Definitions

Raynaud's phenomenon, a clinical sign, describes the characteristic and intermittent color changes that occur in acral skin after exposure to cold or to stress; however, the term does not identify etiologic factors or define pathologic events. *Raynaud's disease* is a distinct clinical entity defined by established criteria that include Raynaud's phenomenon (see Table 64-7).[4] Raynaud's disease is the only *primary* vasospastic disorder; all others are *secondary*. Vasospastic disorders may be multifactorial, with the only requirement for the use of this nomenclature being evidence of the classic triphasic color change associated with arterial vasospasm, autonomic dysfunction, or vasomotor disturbance (see Table 64-8).

Treatment

Although the majority of patients can be managed with nonoperative modalities, treatment of vasospastic disorders must be individualized. Management options include medical therapy, biofeedback, microvascular reconstruction, and digital sympathectomy.

Nonoperative Treatment

Environmental Modification

Environmental modification includes cessation of smoking, avoidance of cold environments, alteration of activities to eliminate those that precipitate symptoms, use of protective garments, use of biofeedback techniques, and drug therapy. Cessation of smoking is the most important of these modifications. Patients who live in cold climates experience more significant pathology than those who live in warm climates. Patients must understand the importance of wearing hats, scarves, and mittens. They should be aware of the relationship between cold exposure to the occipital/cervical area and the reflex vasospasm of hands and feet.[172] Hands can be protected by mittens or hand-held heating devices, which are available from a variety of nonmedical and medical supply houses.

Biofeedback

Biofeedback, training to develop central nervous system control over peripheral autonomic functions, involves instruction in methods that allow the conscious regulation of autonomic body processes. External monitors are used initially so that the patients can observe the elevation in their digital temperatures by changing their rate of breathing or thought processes. Controlled investigations have demonstrated that normal patients and patients with vasospastic conditions can increase finger temperature and finger blood flow significantly by using temperature biofeedback.[98] Biofeedback alleviates symptoms most effectively in patients with Raynaud's disease, vasospasm from nonneural or nonvascular etiology, and Raynaud's phenomenon with adequate collateral circulation. The results of biofeedback are much less favorable in patients with inadequate collateral circulation (groups IIB and IIIB).

Pharmacologic Management

The goal of pharmacologic intervention is to interrupt or mitigate the sympathetic hyperactivity associated with vasospastic and vaso-occlusive disease. Pharmacologic intervention works best in patients with adequate collateral circulation. In patients with adequate collateral circulation but significant vasospasm, the use of pharmacologic agents may redistribute flow to nutritional capillary beds and prevent inappropriate shunting.[176] Currently, calcium channel antagonists are the drugs of choice for vasospastic symptoms, provide the most reliable palliation of symptoms, have an acceptable level of side effects, and present an excellent risk-benefit ratio.[65] Calcium channel antagonists affect receptor control of the vasculature by preventing calcium influx in vascular smooth muscle and diminish sympathetically driven vasoconstriction. Nifedipine (10 to 30 mg orally three times daily or in long-acting form [30 to 60 mg/day]) is the drug most frequently used. Both tricyclic antidepressants (TCAs) and selective serotonin reuptake inhibitors (SSRIs) have proved efficacious in the management of vasospastic symptoms. TCAs have both an analgesic and sedative effect that relieves pain and helps insomnia. Postganglionic presynaptic reuptake of amine neurotransmitters is diminished by TCAs, thereby decreasing sympathetic tone. The most common TCA used is amitriptyline (Elavil, 25 to 75 mg orally every night). The dose can be titrated to effect, and the effective dose is usually much lower than necessary to treat organic depression. TCAs should be prescribed cautiously because of their side effects: orthostatic hypotension, anticholinergic effects, and seizures. Such SSRIs as fluoxetine (Prozac), sertraline (Zoloft), and paroxetine (Paxil) theoretically reestablish autonomic balance by interfering with serotonin reuptake. By stimulating serotonin-mediated neural pathways, sympathetic tone is partially ameliorated. The antidepressant effect helps patients cope with the pain and frustration of Raynaud's phenomenon. In general, SSRIs are taken once a day with the dose titrated to effect. Side effects include nausea, headaches, insomnia, and anorexia; however, these side effects generally resolve after tolerance to the drug develops.

Unfortunately, drugs that directly affect sympathetic tone are often difficult for patients to tolerate.[47,65,356] Prazosin and terazosin (postsynaptic adrenergic α_1 antagonists) may be given orally to induce vasodilatation, but side effects such as orthostatic hypotension are commonly associated with their use. Clonidine (a presynaptic α_2 agonist that is sympatholytic) can be administered orally or topically as a patch but may be poorly tolerated because of the frequent side effects of dry mouth and drowsiness.[65]

Operative Treatment

Surgical options may restore nearly normal physiologic function or provide short to intermediate-term palliation for patients with vasospastic disease or occlusive disease. Group IV patients with nonvascular injury seldom require operative procedures to modify vascular or sympathetic tone and are not discussed in this section. Successful surgical intervention depends on the underlying etiology, the extent and location of the vascular insults, and the extent of irreversible end-organ damage. For example, patients with vaso-occlusive disease secondary to atherosclerosis have an ongoing disease process that is not directly affected by surgery. Surgical options include reconstruction of occluded vessels and/or modification of sympathetic tone. The former may be achieved by (1) resection of occluded vessel(s) and end-to-end repair, (2) resection of occluded vessel(s) and reconstruction with graft material, and (3) bypass grafting of the occluded vascular areas. Sympathetic tone may be altered by (1) proximal cervicothoracic sympathectomy, (2) Leriche sympathectomy (resection of thrombosed or occluded vessels and ligation), or (3) peripheral periarterial sympathectomy, and (4) arterial reconstruction.[84,95,335,351]

Alteration of Sympathetic Tone

Proximal Sympathectomy (Cervicothoracic). Cervicothoracic sympathectomy may be used to decrease sympathetic tone and improve peripheral blood flow by ablating the cervical sympathetic trunk.[311] The procedure may be performed through an axillary or cervical incision. Short-term efficacy of this procedure is well documented; however, after 6 to 12 weeks, sympathetic tone may return or actually increase. Posterior cervicothoracic sympathectomy by phenol injection under computed tomographic control is reversible and may be of benefit during collateral vessel maturation. The authors do not recommend ablative cervicothoracic sympathectomy.

Peripheral (Periarterial) Sympathectomy. Peripheral sympathectomy may be achieved by ligation and excision of the involved vascular segment (Leriche sympathectomy) or by adventitial dissection of arterial trunks and transection of neural connections between arteries and paired peripheral nerves (periarterial sympathectomy).[95,175,236,351] Symptoms either in single digits or the entire hand may be addressed with periarterial sympathectomy.[175,313,351]

Leriche Sympathectomy Technique. The excision of a thrombosed segment of artery and proximal and distal ligation promotes collateral circulation, interrupts local nociceptive input, provides distal sympathectomy, and produces amelioration of symptoms in patients with adequate collateral flow compromised by increased sympathetic tone.[175,191,335] However, if collateral circulation is inadequate or multiple levels of occlusion are present, a Leriche-type sympathectomy may not provide palliation. The area of occlusion is determined by clinical examination and appropriately selected imaging modalities. Through an extensile incision the artery is identified and dissected proximally and distally. It is preferable to begin in an area of "nearly" normal tissue and continue the dissection into the area of occlusion. In the case of the ulnar artery, the nerve of Henle as well as other connections with the ulnar nerve are transected while the ulnar nerve is protected. The proximal

and distal arterial stumps are then ligated, and the wound is closed in layers.

Peripheral/Periarterial Sympathectomy Technique. Modifications of Flatt's technique[95] have been described by Wilgis and Koman.[66,175,350,351] Peripheral sympathectomy interrupts the sympathetic connections from the peripheral nerves to the peripheral arteries, as well as the sympathetic fibers that travel within the adventitia of peripheral arteries.

Digital Sympathectomy Technique (Flatt and Wilgis). The digital arteries and nerves are identified through Bruner zigzag incisions extending from the distal palmar crease to the midportion of the proximal phalanx. All connections

---

CRITICAL POINTS: PALMAR/WRIST SYMPATHECTOMY

INDICATIONS

- Refractory to medications
- Nonhealing ulcer
- Gangrene requiring amputation

PREOPERATIVE EVALUATION

- Evaluation of arterial structure (e.g., arteriogram)
- Assessment of functional control

PEARLS

- Strip adventitia for 0.5 to 2.0 cm for each vessel.
- Include radial, ulnar, deep arch, superficial arch, and common digitals × 3; proper digital is optional.
- Insert drain for 4 to 18 hours.
- Reconstruct, if possible.

TECHNICAL POINTS

- Hemostasis
- Extensile exposure and thus release of vertical fascial structures
- Vessel loops
- Macrodissections followed by microscopic-assisted adventitial dissections

POSTOPERATIVE CARE

- Bulky dressing
- Drain
- Sutures at 10 to 14 days

ATHLETIC PARTICIPATION

- Not usually applicable

between the digital nerve and artery are transected, and the adventitia of the digital artery is stripped from the artery under visualization with the operating microscope[95,236,351] (Fig. 64-28).

Palmar/Hand Sympathectomy Technique (Koman). To achieve a sympathectomy of all four digits and the thumb,

the radial artery and ulnar artery, the superficial arch, the three common volar digital arteries, and the deep arch are visualized. Three palmar incisions are required: two parallel 3-cm longitudinal incisions at the wrist and an oblique incision in the palm (Fig. 64-29). The radial and ulnar arteries are identified, and connections between the arteries and nerves over the 3-cm area are transected. The adventitia

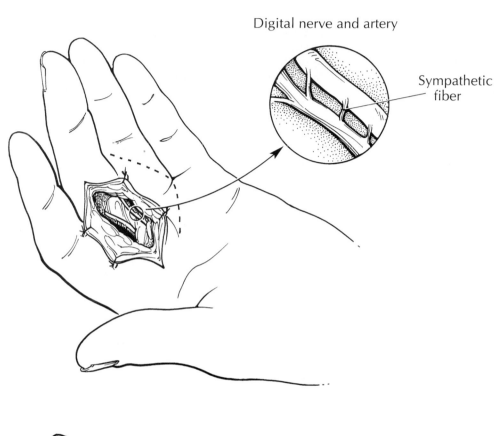

Digital nerve and artery

Sympathetic fiber

FIGURE 64-28. Digital periarterial sympathectomy (Flatt/Wilgis technique) is accomplished through a zigzag volar (Bruner) incision. The adventitia is cleaned of sympathetic fibers, and all connections with the accompanying peripheral nerve are transected. The initial dissection is performed under loupe magnification with subsequent dissection using an operating microscope. (From Koman LA [ed]: Bowman Gray School of Medicine Orthopaedic Manual. Wake Forest University Orthopaedic Press, Winston-Salem, NC, 1997, with permission).

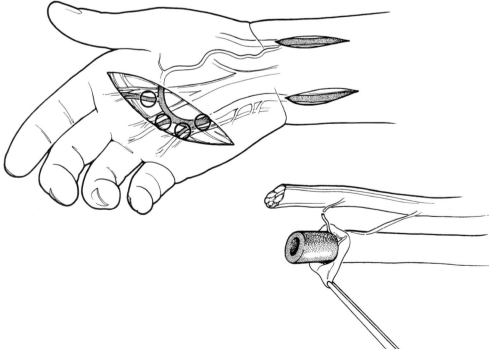

FIGURE 64-29. Schematic representation of periarterial sympathectomy of the hand. Longitudinal incisions are used to expose the radial and ulnar artery, and an oblique incision is used in the palm to expose the superficial arch and the origins of the common volar digital arteries (Koman technique). A separate incision (not shown) may be used over the anatomic snuffbox to expose the radial artery. After initial dissection under loupe magnification, the operating microscope is used to strip the adventitial fibers from the vessels and sever connections with parallel peripheral nerves. (From Koman LA [ed]: Bowman Gray School of Medicine Orthopaedic Manual. Wake Forest University Orthopaedic Press, Winston-Salem, NC, 1997, with permission).

of the radial and ulnar arteries is dissected under the operating microscope for a length of 2 cm. Through a transverse incision in the palm, the distal portion of the ulnar artery, the proximal portion of the superficial arch, and the origins of the three common volar digital arteries are identified. With the aid of an operating microscope, all connections from the peripheral nerves to the arteries are severed, and the adventitia containing neural tissues is dissected from the arteries. Through a fourth dorsal incision in the anatomic snuff box, the deep branch of the radial artery and origin of the deep arch are exposed and mobilized to remove the adventitia; a fourth incision is used if significant symptoms are present in the thumb[175] (see Fig. 64-29).

Arterial Reconstruction. Arterial reconstruction is performed for patients with vaso-occlusive disease to restore arterial inflow. The presence of reconstructable distal arterial channels is necessary and does not exist in many diseased extremities.[335]

Vascular reconstruction is indicated, if possible, in patients with refractory symptoms and inadequate collateral circulation (groups IIB and IIIB).[175,335] Vascular reconstruction in group IIA and IIIA patients should be individualized (see Occlusive Disease). The goal of surgical reconstruction is to increase digital perfusion pressure and nutritional flow in ischemic digits.[176,233] This is accomplished by structural restoration of arterial inflow via end-to-end or graft repair and functional modification of sympathetic tone resulting from the peripheral sympathectomy associated with the vascular resection. Successful arterial reconstruction in patients with underlying collagen vascular disease increases total digital flow and nutritional flow, diminishes symptoms, and promotes healing of ulcers.[151,153,173-175]

In patients with inadequate collateral circulation, reconstructable proximal occlusive disease (e.g., thrombosis of the ulnar artery and superficial palmar arch), *and* unreconstructable distal occlusion (e.g., both proper digital arteries at the proximal interphalangeal joint level), successful reconstruction of the former will increase total digital flow and nutritional flow, decrease symptoms, and allow ulcers to heal.[151,153,154,174,175,177] In contradistinction, Leriche resection of the proximal occluded segment combined with peripheral digital/palmar sympathectomy improves nutritional flow but does not increase total flow.[178]

Surgical Technique

Arterial reconstruction is performed through extensile incisions that expose (1) the ulnar, superficial palmar, and common digital arteries or (2) the radial artery at the wrist and the radial artery and deep arch within the anatomical snuff-box. With the use of 2.5× to 4.5× loupe magnification, the vessels are identified proximal and distal to the occluded areas as determined by preoperative evaluation. The vessels are dissected from the accompanying venous connections, and connections with peripheral nerves are transected. The artery is inspected for abnormal shape, color, or resilience, and all thrombosed or aneurysmal areas are resected. The vessel then is inspected under the operating microscope for evidence of damage to the intima or media. If possible, the involved vessel is resected distally and proximally to patent branches within the specimen. The technique for arterial reconstruction is similar to that used in occlusive disease.

Authors' Preferred Method of Treatment

The selection of treatment modalities is determined by each patient's individual pathophysiology and is goal specific. Treatment decisions are aided by knowledge of vascular structural and functional characteristics and the classification of the vasospastic state (see Table 64-4). For example, patients in group IIB (Raynaud's phenomenon with inadequate circulation) are the most refractory to treatment and have the highest incidence of ulceration. Conversely, patients in group IV (secondary vasospasm from a nonvascular injury) have the best prognosis, rarely have ulceration(s), progress infrequently to gangrene, and often respond to oral medications or biofeedback. Physiologic staging (i.e., an analysis of both structure and function) is crucial in selecting the most appropriate treatment modality. *Regardless of the etiology or classification, the treatment goal should be directed at appropriate distribution of digital flow to provide nutritional capillary flow sufficient to meet metabolic demands under both stressed and nonstressed conditions.* Environmental modifications, pharmacologic agents, and biofeedback are often effective in group I (Raynaud's disease), group IIA (Raynaud's phenomenon with adequate circulation), and group IV (secondary vasospasm without arterial compromise). These patients have "normal vasculature" but abnormal vascular reactivity secondary to abnormal sympathetic control. In patients with inadequate collateral circulation or inadequate circulation (groups IIB and IIIB), the prognosis is guarded unless arterial reconstruction can be successfully achieved. The use of periarterial sympathectomy in patients with inadequate circulation is a salvage procedure.

The selection criteria for candidates appropriate for periarterial sympathectomy are controversial. Increased digital temperatures or PVR and decreased symptoms after wrist or digital block with lidocaine or bupivacaine confirm abnormal sympathetic tone and indicates that sympathectomy will provide palliation. However, patients with vaso-occlusive disease and adequate collateral circulation are unlikely to experience increased digital temperature(s), a reflection of total flow, although nutritional flow will be maximized, inappropriate arteriovenous shunting will be decreased, ulcers will heal, and symptoms will decrease. It is this group of patients who will benefit the most from periarterial sympathectomy.[175]

Postoperative Management and Expectation

Raynaud's phenomenon associated with collagen vascular disease is incurable. Therefore, surgery is designed to provide palliation. Postoperative care after sympathectomy requires only wound care. If arterial reconstruction has been performed, short-term heparin, low-molecular-weight dextran, and aspirin (81 mg/day) are indicated. If anastomoses are performed through marginal vessels, long-term (3 to 6 months) anticoagulation with warfarin after heparin therapy is appropriate. Theoretically, 7 to 21 days of low-molecular-weight heparin or fondaparinux are beneficial although this has not been reported in the peer-reviewed literature.

Peripheral sympathectomy is palliative. Acute ulcer healing is common; however, the recurrence of problems depends on the underlying disease. Patency after arterial reconstruction depends on the activity of the underlying disease.

CONGENITAL ARTERIOVENOUS MALFORMATIONS

Preoperative Evaluation

Congenital vascular anomalies have been divided into numerous categories.[72,196,204,205,280,281,329] The groupings of Malan and Puglionisi[205] are most commonly referenced. These groupings divide congenital vascular problems into *dysplasia* (normal formations with structural deviations) or *hamartias* (anomalous formations of normally present tissues).[204,205] The management of congenital vascular malformations is hindered by the myriad of descriptors and groupings without pathophysiologic significance. *Lesions are primarily arterial, venous, capillary, or a combination.* They should be designated with regard to the presence or absence of (1) clinical significance, (2) pain, (3) hemodynamic significance, and/or (4) structural damage. Lesions are invariably more extensive than they appear on first examination.

Signs and Symptoms

Congenital anomalies are rare and may involve all areas of the body with the upper extremity involved in 30% to 60% of patients.* Approximately 50% of lesions are clinically recognized before the age of 2, whereas 60% are of concern to the family or physician by age 10.[140,204]

Although present since birth, lesions frequently are noted after trauma, an event that may stimulate vascular proliferation or produce hemorrhage.[64,275] Common initial symptoms include pain (40%), swelling (50%), or a noticeable mass (30%).[33,62,130,357] Less frequently, patients complain of ischemic ulcers,[64] asymmetrical warmth,[140] paresthesias, and hyperhidrosis.[62] Signs of congenital venous malformations include asymmetrical enlargement, varices, thrills, bruits, trophic changes, skin discoloration, edema, decreased distal pulses, and joint stiffness[62,204,344] (Fig. 64-30).

Diagnostic Testing

Plain radiographs demonstrate pathognomonic phleboliths in 50% of extremities, and soft tissue masses are observed frequently (65%).[24,43,314] Arteriography is indicated if surgical intervention is being considered and may be augmented by closed-system venography or MRA.[108,141,162,243] Four radiographic patterns of congenital AVFs have been described[25]; however, these patterns do not provide clinically significant prognostic information. Computed tomography may better define the extent of bone or soft tissue involvement. In patients with ischemic pain and/or

*See references 44, 122, 140, 158, 190, 193, 194, 280, 281, and 329.

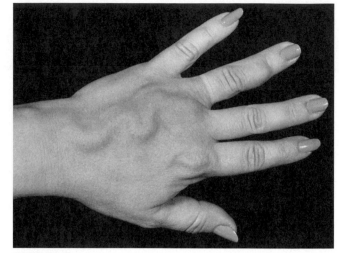

FIGURE 64-30. Clinical photograph of a hand with predominantly venous congenital malformations. Upper extremity dilated venous structures are pathognomonic for congenital vascular malformations. (From Koman LA [ed]: Bowman Gray School of Medicine Orthopaedic Manual. Wake Forest University Orthopaedic Press, Winston-Salem, NC, 1997, with permission).

ulcerations, nutritional deprivation in the presence of increased total flow may be demonstrated.[176]

Treatment and Types of Operations

Congenital vascular malformations are difficult to treat, and surgical intervention should be used as a last resort. Recurrence is common, and a definitive "cure" is unlikely. Malformations are frequently more extensive than the clinical appearance suggests. Intervention is dependent on the symptoms, the location of the malformation, and the predominant vessels involved. Low-flow venous malformations often can be managed by compression garments, and nonoperative methods should be used if possible. "The futility of any attempt to cure by surgical means any but the simplest and most sharply localized of these lesions"[328] is universally accepted with regard to the management of AVMs.

Nonoperative Management

Intra-arterial embolization is possible but difficult to use in lesions within the upper extremity because of the frequent complications of ischemic neuritis and ischemic pain.[121,218] Therefore, selective embolization is used primarily to decrease flow in high-flow AVMs before surgical excision and/or amputation. Symptoms are related to distal ischemia and may be diminished by vasoactive drugs that decrease shunting and/or increase nutritional flow. In addition, calcium channel antagonists and α-adrenergic agonists/antagonists may reduce symptoms.

Operative Management

Options for surgical management include (1) excision of the malformation, including ligation of the feeding artery and draining vein; (2) ligation of the feeding artery and draining vein; (3) excision of the fistula with arterial repair; or (4) "quadruple ligation with distal and proximal artery and vein ligation."[271] Successful surgical excision is compromised by the activation of quiescent arteriovenous channels, creation of distal ischemia, involvement of muscle and bone, and stimulation of angiogenesis.[113,196,211,216] Moreover, significant AVMs generally have exceedingly complex structures and are composed of multiple feeding and draining vessels. Operative approaches are performed for palliative or curative reasons. However, the latter is exceedingly difficult to achieve short of terminal amputation whereas the former is complicated by a high rate of recurrence.

Palliative Options

Ligation of feeding vessels and/or subtotal arteriovenous malformation excision in stages with ligation of inflow/outflow is advocated[63,72,113,302,341] with and without arterial reconstruction. Ligation of feeding arteries and communicating vessels provides significant symptomatic relief; however, recurrence is common and amputation may be necessary.

En Bloc Resection

Intercalary and localized AVMs may be excised en bloc, although this may require arterial reconstruction. Preoperative staging, including MRI to evaluate bone and soft tissue involvement and arteriography with venous imaging, is used to delineate the malformation. The identified malformation is isolated and excised so that only neural structures and/or a skeletonized artery remains. If an artery is left, all branches are ligated. Terminal AVMs may be deleted by transverse amputation or ray resection.

 Authors' Perspective

Pain associated with AVMs is often secondary to nutritional deprivation in spite of a significant volume of total flow. Calcium channel blockers and α_2 agonists may alleviate the pain in some patients. Operative intervention should be used as a salvage procedure. Lesions are invariably larger than they appear clinically, and recurrence or proximal angiogenesis even with en bloc resection and amputation is common.

HEMANGIOMAS

Preoperative Evaluation

Hemangiomas, as defined by Mulliken and coworkers, are true tumors that are generally seen within the first 4 weeks of life and have a characteristic growth cycle.[239] Only 30% of these lesions appear at birth; however, 70% to 90% are visible by 4 weeks of age.[347] The first phase of growth is very rapid and corresponds to endothelial cell proliferation and multilaminate basement membranes.[239] This rapid growth phase lasts 10 to 12 months, and during this time the tumor may change from a red-purple lesion to a large, bright red or bright blue color. Growth of the mass may even outstrip skeletal growth during this first year, thus raising the concern of malignancy.[337] The second phase, during which the mass appears to grow at a rate proportional to the

rest of the child, is marked by the color fading from bright red to a dull red or purple. The deeper the lesion, the more bluish it appears.[240] Finally, the third phase is involutional, during which the lesions become softer and shrink with gradual fading of the discoloration. By age 5, 50% of the lesions have regressed; and by age 7, 70% of the lesions have involuted.[240] Often a skin wrinkle consisting of a fibrolipomatous mass with an associated telangiectasia may remain.

Hemangiomas are three times more common in females, which has led some investigators to question a hormonal basis for the lesion.[299] Others have questioned an excess of angiogenic factors; however, no single factor appears responsible.[219] Although the majority of rapidly growing lesions that appear early (before 5 months) undergo involution, some lesions fail to disappear by age 7.[23] Noninvoluting lesions are usually capillary or cavernous hemangiomas by histologic criteria. Noninvoluting capillary hemangiomas are usually a "port-wine stain" or nevus flammeus, whereas noninvoluting cavernous hemangiomas usually have an arteriovenous flow that perpetuates the lesion and may be either a high-flow or low-flow lesion.[250]

Diagnosis

Hemangiomas may be difficult to distinguish from vascular malformations or even sarcomas during the initial phase of rapid growth. Radiographs typically demonstrate a soft tissue shadow, and calcifications may be present. Ultrasonography, including color duplex, is a simple, inexpensive, and noninvasive means of evaluating the size and flow characteristics of the lesion and is ideal for evaluating hand and wrist lesions. Computed tomography with contrast medium enhancement will demonstrate hemangiomas to be homogeneous lesions with well-defined borders.[239] AVMs lack this homogeneous pattern and show diffuse vessels with no parenchyma, with eccentric vessels being present in low-flow lesions and tortuous arteries in high-flow lesions.[239] MRI has been demonstrated to accurately define proximity to deep structures, as well as distinguish these lesions from sarcomas. MRI with gadolinium also assists in distinguishing capillary malformations from sympathetic malformations.[336]

The need for arteriography has diminished with the increasing availability of MRI. Upton and Coombs indicated the relative advantages of MRI, including its noninvasiveness and appreciation of the proximity of neural structures.[336] We currently use MRI to confirm the clinical diagnosis and to visualize skeletal muscle hemangiomas.

Management

Management of hemangiomas is usually conservative because the majority will involute by the age of 7 years. Treatment is therefore directed at associated complications, including bleeding, ulceration, and infection. Hemorrhage, particularly in the neonatal period, may require compression dressing, elevation, and blood products. One rare complication associated with hemangiomas is the Kasabach-Merritt syndrome. This syndrome is manifested as a diffuse coagulopathy secondary to platelet trapping within the hemangioma. Treatment is directed toward managing the underlying coagulopathy and includes the administration of platelets, fresh frozen plasma, and pressure support.[83]

Ulcerations and superficial infections secondary to hemangiomas usually respond well to dressing changes and antibiotics.[239] Surgical management may be indicated in noninvoluting lesions in which the diagnosis is in question or symptoms (ulceration, bleeding, or recurrent infection) are encountered.

The surgical technique involves meticulous attention to isolation and ligation of feeder vessels with complete excision of the lesion. Adjunctive therapy with either cryosurgical or yttrium-aluminum-garnet laser ablation has been advocated; however, it is difficult to assess the success of these treatments because of the natural history of involution of these lesions.[250]

The prognosis after excision is dependent on the degree of soft tissue infiltration. Johnson and coworkers noted that diffuse lesions had a much higher recurrence rate.[149] Three of the 20 patients in their series with diffuse lesions required amputation after multiple recurrences.[149] Recurrence of small lesions may still be curable with repeated ligation; however, large recurrences may require amputation.[250]

GLOMUS TUMORS

Glomus tumors are benign vascular hematomas containing all of the cells of a normal glomus apparatus. The normal glomus lies in the reticular layer as an arteriovenous anastomosis in the dermis and functions as a thermoregulatory control mechanism. The apparatus itself consists of (1) an afferent vessel, (2) a Sucquet-Hoyer canal consisting of a channel surrounded by large polygonal cells, and (3) multiple shunts in the glabrous skin of the hand and beneath nail beds. Histologic findings include endothelial pericytes and numerous nonmyelinated nerve fibers. These findings explain the classic triad of symptoms seen: (1) cold hypersensitivity, (2) paroxysmal pain, and (3) pinpoint pain.

Glomus tumors are typically characterized by painful, subcutaneous nodules usually located in the subungual region of the digits.[48] Up to 75% of these lesions are found in the hand, and 65% are located in the fingertip.[48] Symptoms are remarkable in the severity of the sharp lancinating pain brought on by either cold exposure or even light touch. Physical examination is unremarkable in 50% of lesions; however, localized bluish discoloration in the nail bed, with or without nail plate ridges, strongly suggests the diagnosis.[283] Cold sensitivity may be provoked by ice bath immersion or by spraying the lesion with ethyl chloride, which causes well-localized pain.

These lesions appear as a dark, well-delineated lesion on T1-weighted and bright on T2-weighted MRI. MRI has been successful at pinpointing lesions as small as 5 mm in the fingertip.[212]

Classification

Glomus tumors have been classified into three groups: (1) solitary lesions, (2) multiple painful lesions, and (3) multiple painless lesions.[135] Such a classification is useful in that the surgeon must consider residual lesions should surgical excision result in continued symptoms.

Treatment

The treatment for symptomatic lesions is surgical excision. Lesions in the nail bed are exposed after removal of the nail. A longitudinal incision is made in the sterile matrix. The matrix is elevated on either side to expose the lesion. Care must be taken to avoid leaving either residual tumor or other lesions in the same fingertip. Maxwell and associates reported that 25% of patients have multiple lesions and stressed the need for thorough surgical exploration.[215] More proximal lesions, particularly at the level of the germinal matrix, may be exposed through a dorsolateral incision at the junction of the glabrous skin. This permits exposure of the lesion without damage to the germinal matrix. Recurrence may be as high as 20%.[215] If symptoms continue longer than 3 months after excision, the surgeon should strongly consider re-exploration because the incidence of multiple lesions is so high.[215]

ANNOTATED REFERENCES

109. Gelberman RH, Blasingame JP, Fronek A, Dimick MP: Forearm arterial injuries. J Hand Surg [Am] 4:401-408, 1979.

This article details the natural history of arterial injuries in the forearm. After isolated injury to the radial or ulnar artery, flow in the remaining vessel will increase, digital blood pressure in the distribution of the damaged vessels will decrease, and cold sensitivity will occur.

116. Gelberman RH, Nunley JA, Koman LA, et al: The results of radial and ulnar arterial repair in the forearm. J Bone Joint Surg Am 3:383-387, 1982.

Repair of noncritical arterial injuries—even when repaired by experienced surgeons using microvascular techniques—has a high rate of failure. Conversely, in critical injuries, patency of one vessel is common.

164. Kleinert HE, Volianitis GJ: Thrombosis of the palmar arterial arch and its tributaries: Etiology and newer concepts in treatment. J Trauma 4:447-457, 1965.

Classic description of repairs of the ulnar artery and superficial palmar arch.

173. Koman LA, Ruch DS, Aldridge M, et al: Arterial reconstruction in the ischemic hand and wrist: Effects on microvascular physiology and health-related quality of life. J Hand Surg [Am] 23:773-782, 1998.

Documentation of the microvascular circulatory effects of peripheral sympathectomy (PAS). This article demonstrates that PAS in patients with scleroderma is effective and provides the first description of sympathectomy in the palm and at the wrist.

175. Koman LA, Smith BP, Pollock F, et al: The microcirculatory effects of peripheral sympathectomy. J Hand Surg 5:709-717, 1995.

This article documents that successful arterial reconstruction in patients with inadequate collateral circulation improves digital perfusion, which correlates with symptoms, function, and health-related quality of life.

179. Koman LA, Urbaniak J: Ulnar artery insufficiency: A guide to treatment. J Hand Surg 1:16-24, 1981.

This manuscript outlines reconstructive options for ulnar artery thrombosis and provides a treatment algorithm that includes operative and nonoperative techniques.

218. McCabe SJ, Mizgala C, Glickman L: The measurement of cold sensitivity of the hand. J Hand Surg [Am] 16:1037-1040, 1991.

The development and validity of an instrument that evaluates cold intolerance is presented.

294. Ruch DS, Aldridge M, Holden M, et al: Arterial reconstruction for radial artery occlusion. J Hand Surg [Am] 25:282-290, 2000.

Indication, technique, and result of radial artery reconstruction for symptomatic occlusion.

351. Wilgis EF: Digital sympathectomy for vascular insufficiency. Hand Clin 1:361-367, 1985.

Description of digital artery sympathectomy and summary of results.

361. Zimmerman NB, Zimmerman SI, McClinton MA, et al: Long-term recovery following surgical treatment for ulnar artery occlusion. J Hand Surg [Am] 19:17-21, 1994.

Expected outcome following arterial reconstruction for ulnar artery thrombosis in patients with a digital brachial index of less than 0.7. It also demonstrates good results of resection and ligation of occluded vessels if index is 0.7 or more.

INDEX

Note: Page numbers followed by the letter f refer to figures; those followed by the letter t refer to tables.

Guancthidine blockade, for neuroma, 1104
Gumma, syphilitic, 104
Gutters, lateral and medial, arthroscopic
    visualization of, in thrower's elbow, 968,
    969f
Guyon's canal
    anatomy of, 1023, 1023f
    ganglion in, 2237
Guyon's canal compression, 1022–1024
    postoperative care in, 1024
    recommended treatment of, 1023–1024
Guyon's canal release, recurrent, 1044

H

H incision, distal interphalangeal joint opening
    through, 79, 79f
Haddad-Riordan technique, of total wrist
    arthrodesis, 524–525, 525f
Hahn-Steinthal injury, in capitellum fracture,
    816, 817f
Hair, preoperative removal of, 11
Halstead maneuver, for thoracic outlet
    syndrome, 1057, 1058f
Hamartoma, lipofibromatous, 2239
Hamate, fracture of, 764–765, 764f–765f
    incidence of, 711t
    recommended treatment of, 765
Hamulus, fracture of, 764, 765f
    nonunion of, bone grafting for, 765
Hand deformity(ies). *See also specific deformity.*
    after brain injury or stroke, 1262–1267
        fractures as, 1262
        impaired active function as, 1263, 1264f
        impaired passive function as, 1263, 1265f
        intrinsic, 1266–1267, 1266f–1267f
        intrinsic-minus, 1267
        spasticity as, 1262–1263, 1262t
        thumb-in-palm deformity as, 1263–1266,
            1265f
    in Apert's syndrome, 1388–1391. *See also*
        Apert's sundrome.
Hand function, in cerebral palsy, grading of,
    1200–1201, 1201t
Hand postures, dysfunctional, 2046,
    2046f–2047f
Hand preparation
    in finger reconstruction, 1421–1422, 1421f
    in microvascular toe transfer, for hypoplastic
        digits, 1426
Hand support, elevated, in postoperative period,
    22, 23f
Hand surgery instruments, 17, 18t, 19, 19f–21f
Hand therapy, for complex regional pain
    syndrome, 2030
Hangnail, 408
Hansen's disease, 116–129
    classification of, 117, 118t, 119
    claw hand in, 128, 1183
    clinical, bacteriologic, histologic, and
        immunologic features of, 118t
    clinical pathology of, 116–117
    diagnosis of, 119–123
        cardinal signs in, 119–121, 119f–121f
        tests in, 12t, 121–123
    epidemiology of, 116
    microbiology of, 116
    nerve involvement in, common sites of,
        119–120, 119f
    reactions in, 123–125
        classification of, 125t
        treatment of, 125, 126t
    rehabilitation for, 129

Hansen's disease *(Continued)*
    resource materials for, 129
    treatment of, 123–128
        for compression neuropathy, 125–126, 126f
        for deformities, 128
        for nerve abscess, 126–127, 127f–128f
        for reactions, 125, 126t
        multidrug therapy in, 123
        pain relief in, 123–127, 124f
        preservation of sensation in, 127–128
        restoration of sensibility in, 128
    ulnar nerve palsy due to, 1161, 1162, 1166.
        See also Ulnar nerve palsy.
Harashina procedure, modified, of suture
    placement, 1544–1545, 1546f
Harmon's procedure, for multiple muscle
    transfer, in brachial plexus injury, 1358
Healing time, for phalangeal shaft fracture,
    313–314
Heat therapy, for sporotrichosis, 110
Hemangioma, 2311–2312
Hemarthrosis, of elbow, aspiration of, 848, 848f
Hematoma
    after dorsal tenosynovectomy, 2063
    formation of
        after free flap transfer, 1726
        after skin grafting, 1646
        in Dupuytren's contracture surgery, 182
            avoidance of, 178–179
    subungual, management of, 389–391, 391f
Hemiarthroplasty. *See also* Arthroplasty.
    silicone, of carpometacarpal joint, of thumb,
        475
Hemipulp flaps, transfer of, from toes to fingers,
    1850, 1851f
Hemiresection-interposition arthroplasty, for
    radioulnar joint arthritis, 631–633, 632f
Hemophilic arthropathy, joint destruction
    associated with, 977
Hemorrhage. *See* Bleeding.
Hemostatic mechanism(s), in microvascular
    repair, 1561–1564
    cascade pathway and, 1561–1562, 1564f
    fibrinolysis and, 1564
    hypercoagulability and, 1562–1563
    platelets and, 1561, 1562f–1563f
Henry approach, to radial tunnel syndrome,
    1038, 1038f–1039f
Heparin
    after free flap transfer, 1727
    after microvascular surgery, 1564
    after replantation procedures, 1583
    postoperative, for thrombosis, 2299
    preoperative use of, discontinuation of, 48
Herbert classification, of scaphoid fractures,
    717, 718f
Herbert screws. *See also* Screw fixation.
    comparision of screw types with, 723
    for acute scaphoid fracture, technique of, 723,
        724f, 725
    for distal humeral fracture, 831
    for metacarpal head fracture repair, 279f
Hereditary multiple exostosis, of forearm,
    1502–1505
    classification of, 1502, 1503f
    clinical features of, 1502
    epidemiology of, 1502
    imaging of, 1502
    surgical treatment of
        contraindications to, 1504
        indications for, 1502–1504
        outcome of, 1505
        techniques in, 1504–1505, 1504f
Herpes simplex virus (HSV) infection, of
    fingers, in AIDS patients, 152–153

Herpetic whitlow, 87–88
Heterodigital flaps, for soft tissue defects of
    thumb, 1871–1882
    cross-finger, 1871–1872, 1872f–1873f
        dual-innervated, 1876, 1878f–1880f
        innervated, 1873
        radial-innervated, 1873–1876, 1875f, 1877f
    neurovascular island pedicle, 1876,
        1880–1882, 1881f
Heterodigital island transfer, of joints,
    1817–1818, 1818f
Heterotopic ossification
    after brain injury, 1241–1242, 1243f
        about shoulder, 1251
    after elbow contracture release, 956
    after humeral fracture, 841–842, 841f
    after radial head fracture, 879
    after ulnar fracture, 905
    postburn, 2177
Hexachlorophene, as preoperative antiseptic, 10t
H-flap, thenar, Smith and Albin, for
    reconstruction of amputated fingertip,
    1946–1947
High-pressure injection injury, 91
High-velocity injuries, to radius, 650, 654f
High-voltage injury. *See* Electrical injury.
Hinged fixation
    after elbow contracture release, 951,
        952f–953f
        Morrey column procedure of, 952
    in complex elbow dislocation repair, 917–918
Hirudin, in microvascular surgery, 1564–1565
Hirudo medicinalis, 84. *See also* Leeches.
Histiocytoma (dermatofibroma), 2197
    malignant fibrous, 2247, 2248f
Histoplasmosis, 113
Hockey stick incision, for felon drainage, 62,
    63f
Holstein-Lewis fracture, radial nerve palsy
    associated with, 1127
Homodigital transfer, interphalangeal joint,
    distal-to-proximal, 1818–1819, 1819f
Hook of hamate, fracture of, 764–765, 765f
    recommended treatment of, 765
Hooked nail deformity, 404–405, 406f
Horner's sign, in brachial plexus injury, 1320,
    1320f
Hospital treatment, of snake bites, 2008–2012
Hotchkiss classification, of radial fractures, 849,
    851t
Hotchkiss fracture
    type I, 855f
    type II, 863f–864f, 867f
    type III, 868f, 871f
House reconstruction, in tetraplegic patient
    one-stage, 1284–1285, 1285f
    two-stage, 1286–1287, 1288f–1289f
HOX gene mutation, in limb deformation,
    1376–1377, 1378f, 1393
Huber opponensplasty, in median nerve palsy,
    1140–1141, 1140f, 1142f
Hui-Linscheid procedure, in triangular
    fibrocartilage complex reconstruction, 622,
    622f
Human bites
    extensor tendon injuries caused by, 207–209
        recommended treatment of, 209, 209f
    infections caused by, 84–86, 85f, 207
Human immunodeficiency virus (HIV) infection
    CD4+ T cell count in, 151, 152, 153t
    clinical manifestations of, 152–153, 152t
    etiology and epidemiology of, 151–152
    prevention of, 155
    prognosis of, 154–155
    resources for, 157

Midcarpal joint (*Continued*)
portals of, for arthroscopy of wrist, 772–773, 773f–774f
diagnostic, 775
stabilizing mechanism of, 540, 541f
Midcarpal ligaments, 538
Midhumeral axillary block, 40
Midlateral incisions, of amputated digit and stump, 1576–1577, 1577f
Midpalmar space
anatomy of, 71
infections of, 70–71, 71f
complications of, 77
treatment of, 73–74, 73f, 76
Milker's interdigital granuloma, 146
Milker's nodule, 156–157
Millard "crane principle," of abdominal burying of digits, 1612–1613, 1613f
Millender-Nalebuff fusion, of rheumatoid wrist, 525–526, 526f
modified, 526, 526f
Miller's criteria, of extensor tendon function, 192t
Minocycline, for Hansen's disease, 123
Mirror hand, 1395–1398, 1395f
classification of, 1395t
etiology of, 1396, 1396f
management of, 1396, 1396f–1397f
Mitsuda reaction, in Hansen's disease, 121
Miura and Komada technique, of cleft hand surgery, 1408, 1410, 1411f
Moberg advancement flap, 1663–1664, 1664f 1666f. See also Skin flaps.
Moberg's techniques, in tetraplegia
of deltoid-to-triceps transfer, 1276–1277, 1277f
of passive key pinch reconstruction, 1282, 1283f
Moermans' small curved incision, for Dupuytren's contracture, 170, 170f
Mohs' procedure, for excision of skin tumor, 2193
Mole (melanocytic nevus), 2197–2199, 2198f. See also Nevus(i).
atypical, 2200
Monitoring techniques, of reperfusion failure, in microvascular surgery, 1559
Mononeuritis, 1019, 1035
Monteggia fracture
classification of, 892–893, 893f
plate fixation of, 899f, 900, 901f
posterior, 894, 895f
Morphine
for sedation, in pregnancy, 48
preanesthetic sedation with, 26
Morrey column procedure, for stiff elbow, 948–955
access to anterior capsule in, 949
after head trauma and brain injury, 950–951, 950f
after humeral fracture nonunion, 950
after humeral fracture reduction and fixation, 950
distraction arthroplasty in, 952
exposure of posterior capsule in, 949
hinged fixation after release in, 952, 952f–953f
patient position and skin incision in, 948–949
postoperative care in
adjuvant therapy for heterotopic ossification in, 951, 953–954
immediate, 949
physical therapy and splinting in, 954–955, 954f–955f
Mortality, in necrotizing fasciitis, 89–90

Motion, complete failure to achieve, after elbow contracture release, 956–957
Motor control
clinical scale of, 1238t
impaired, in stroke patient, 1238
in limb deformity
clinical evaluation of, 1248–1249, 1249f
laboratory evaluation of, 1249–1250, 1250t
Motor nerve, repair of, in free muscle transfer for finger flexion, 1765–1766
Motor paralysis, in ulnar nerve palsy, patterns of, 1161
Motor rehabilitation, after toe-to-finger transfer, 1861–1862
Moxifloxacin, for tuberculosis, 141t
MRA (magnetic resonance angiography), of vascular disorders, 2274, 2277f
MRI. See Magnetic resonance imaging (MRI).
Mucormycosis, 113–114
Mucous cyst, 2233–2234, 2233f–2234f
Multidrug therapy
for Hansen's disease, 123
for mycobacterial tenosynovitis, 135
for tuberculosis, 140, 141t
Multiple enchondromatosis, 2250, 2250f
Multiple exostosis, hereditary, of forearm, 1502–1505, 1503f–1504f
Multiple warts, 149
Multiple-digit injury(ies)
ray amputation in, 1961, 1963–1964, 1964f–1965f
replantation after, 1570, 1571f
Muriatic acid, tissue damage characteristics of, 2184t
Muscle(s). See also named muscle.
applied physiology of, 1758–1759, 1759f–1761f
contraction of, 1758, 1759f–1760f
dysfunction of, after metacarpal fracture, 301
evaluation of, in mangling injuries, 1593
fibula with, in vascularized grafting, 1787
forearm, work capacity of, 1116, 1116t
free transfer of, 1757–1775, 1757f
applied physiology in, 1758–1759, 1759f–1761f
cortical plasticity and motor relearning in, 1774–1775
for biceps reconstruction, 1770–1772, 1771f, 1773f
for brachial plexus injury, 1349–1356
complete, 1351–1356
complications of, 1355
donor muscle selection in, 1352
outcome in, 1355–1356, 1356f–1357f
postoperative protocol in, 1355
technique of, 1352–1354, 1353f–1354f
donor muscle selection in, 1350
stability of proximal joints in, 1349–1350
for deltoid reconstruction, 1772–1774, 1774f
for elbow flexion, 1350–1351, 1351f
for finger extension, 1767–1770, 1769f, 1770t, 1771f
for finger flexion, 1765–1767, 1766f
for triceps reconstruction, 1772
gracilis preparation for, 1760–1761, 1762f–1764f
latissimus dorsi preparation for, 1761–1762
patient selection for, 1758t
preoperative planning in, 1762–1765, 1764f
principles of, 1757–1758, 1758f, 1758t
in thumb extension, 187
in wrist extension, 187, 189
incomplete relaxation of, intravenous regional anesthesia and, 45

Muscle(s) (*Continued*)
multiple transfer of, for brachial plexus injury, 1357–1360, 1359f, 1361f–1362f
of elbow, lengthening of, in cerebral palsy, 1207–1208
of thumb, innervation of, 1131
recovery of, in brachial plexus palsy, defining and grading, 1300, 1300f, 1300t
selection of, for opponensplasty, 1133–1134, 1134t
synergistic transfer of, in tendon transfers, 1117
Muscle grading system
in brachial plexus palsy, 1300, 1300t
in tetraplegia, currently accepted, 1271, 1272t
Muscle graft(s)
damaged nerve replacement with
in Hansen's disease, 128
in neuromas, 1110, 1110f
freeze-thawed, 1094
Muscle slide operation, for compartment syndrome, in Holden I (moderate), 1998–2001, 1999f–2002f
Muscle tightness, in cerebral palsy
evaluation of, 1198–1199
surgical treatment of, 1230–1233, 1230f–1231f, 1233f
Muscular neurotization, in nerve injury repair, 1094. See also Neurotization.
Musculocutaneous flaps. See also Skin flaps; *specific muscle, e.g.,* Latissimus dorsi flap.
axial-pattern, 1650, 1650f
free, 1716, 1719. See also Free flaps.
donor sites for, 1718t–1719t
regional, 1685–1686, 1689f
Musculocutaneous nerve neurotization, for brachial plexus injury, 1341–1342
partial ulnar nerve transfer with, 1345–1347, 1346f
recommended method of, 1343–1345, 1344f
Musculocutaneous neurectomy, for cerebral palsy, 1205
Musculoskeletal tumor(s), 2211–2221. See also Bone tumor(s); Soft tissue tumor(s).
benign, treatment of, 2216
biopsy of, 2215–2216, 2215f
classification and staging of, 2212–2213, 2212t, 2213t
diagnosis of, 2211–2212
evaluation protocol for, 2213–2216, 2214f
excision of, 2216–2221
from distal forearm, 2221, 2225f–2227f
from finger metacarpals, 2219–2220, 2220f–2224f
from first metacarpal, 2217, 2219, 2220f
from phalanx
distal, 2217, 2217f
middle, 2217, 2218f–2219f
from wrist, 2221, 2224f
principles of, 2217–2221
imaging of, 2213–2214
laboratory studies of, 2213
location of, 2212–2213
malignant, treatment of, 2216–2217
metastatic, 2213
Musculotendinous junction, extensor tendon rupture at, 216
Mycetoma, 101–103, 102f
Mycobacterium(a), atypical
growth rates of, 132t
infections with, 131–140. See also *specific infection.*
chronic, 95t
diagnosis of, 142–143
"eight-pack" tissue culture for, 96–97, 96t